Fourteenth Edition

TEXTBOOK OF MEDICINE VOLUME I

Edited by

PAUL B. BEESON, M.D.

Distinguished Physician, United States Veterans Administration,
University of Washington School of Medicine;
Formerly Nuffield Professor of Clinical Medicine, University of Oxford

WALSH McDERMOTT, M.D.

Professor of Public Affairs in Medicine, Cornell University Medical College;
Attending Physician, The New York Hospital; Special Advisor to the
President, Robert Wood Johnson Foundation

W. B. SAUNDERS COMPANY · Philadelphia · London · Toronto 1975

W. B. Saunders Company: West Washington Square
Philadelphia, PA 19105

12 Dyott Street
London WC1A 1DB

833 Oxford Street
Toronto, Ontario M8Z 5T9, Canada

Listed here are the latest translated editions of this book, together with the language of the translation and the publisher:

Portuguese (13th Edition) – Editoria Guanabara Koogan, Rio de Janeiro, Brazil
Serbo-Croat (11th Edition) – Medicinska Knjiga, Belgrade, Yugoslavia
Spanish (13th Edition) – Nueva Editorial Interamericana S.A., de C.V., Mexico

Textbook of Medicine

Single Vol: ISBN 0-7216-1660-7
Vol I: ISBN 0-7216-1661-5
Vol II: ISBN 0-7216-1662-3

Last digit is the print number: 9 8 7 6 5 4 3 2 1

DEDICATED TO THE MEMORY OF

RUSSELL L. CECIL, 1881–1965

and

ROBERT F. LOEB, 1895–1973

Great teachers of medicine
who in their editorial partnership were able
to better the lives of thousands more patients
and students than they ever got to see.

Preface

This fourteenth edition of the Textbook of Medicine is dedicated in warm and respectful affection to the memory of Russell L. Cecil and Robert F. Loeb. Their influence goes on in the essential character created and maintained by them for the book and in the long-range effects they have had as teachers and editors. Although their names no longer appear on the title page, the book still carries their imprint throughout.

Each played a different yet essential part in the development of this textbook. In the mid-1920's, Dr. Cecil had the wisdom to perceive that a single-authored text in medicine would no longer suffice and created the first multiauthored textbook of medicine. Twenty years later he had the further wisdom to perceive that the scientific base of medicine had so enlarged that his own background in science was no longer sufficiently contemporary. Hence he invited Dr. Loeb to join him as coeditor. This marriage of the private physician–professor and the full-time academic professor was a very happy one; each complemented the other perfectly. Both were dedicated to the idea of getting the key concepts and useful practices of the specialist and the scientist into a form that could be employed by physicians and medical students. Under the coeditorship of Dr. Loeb the textbook changed subtly. It became less the repository of established doctrine and more the expression of advanced, ongoing ideas in medicine.

Dr. Cecil tended to worry more about the physician and Dr. Loeb about the medical student; yet each was deeply interested in both. Each had ample claims to distinction quite aside from the book, and in the course of their long careers, each benefited many people. It was their joint editorial venture, however, that allowed them to exert a healing influence on the many thousands of patients they never got to see and a learning influence on the many thousands of students who could not know personally their extraordinary dedication to teaching. This lengthened shadow is a very real part of their memorial and our legacy.

It is appropriate at this time to mention others who have shared editorial responsibilities of the textbook throughout its 14 editions. There has always been an Associate Editor responsible for the section on Diseases of the Nervous System. In the first seven editions Foster Kennedy served in that capacity. Harold Wolff took over for the eighth through eleventh editions and has been followed by Fred Plum. Walsh McDermott served as Associate Editor from the sixth edition, and in the eighth edition Alexander Gutman also joined in that role.

By its tenth edition (1959) when this textbook had attained world recognition and probably the widest use of any English language textbook of medicine, Cecil and Loeb retired from academic medicine and from their joint editorship. The W. B. Saunders Company invited us to succeed them as coeditors, and we gladly accepted with the goal of striving to maintain the high standards set by our predecessors. We invited four others to serve with Dr. Plum as Associate Editors. They were Alexander Bearn, Hereditary Diseases; Philip Bondy, Endocrine and Metabolic Diseases; Carl Moore, Hematologic and Hematopoietic Diseases; and Marvin Sleisenger, Gastrointestinal Diseases. At the time of preparing the twelfth edition, Dr. Bondy had to withdraw because of other responsibilities and was succeeded by Nicholas Christy.

When the planning for the present edition was just getting under way, Carl Moore died suddenly, to be mourned by friends and students everywhere. He had contributed powerfully to the development of his section on Hematologic and Hematopoietic Diseases, and because of his great experience and breadth of understanding had been able to write about one quarter of that section himself. We believe that his Introduction to Hematologic Diseases in the eleventh to thirteenth editions deserves to rank with another Cecil "classic," Fuller Albright's Introduction to the Endocrine section, which appeared in the seventh to tenth editions. We prized Moore's association with the book not only for the standard of his own section but also for his advice about organization of the entire work.

We welcome to the present edition a new colleague, Ralph Nachman, as Associate Editor for Hematologic and Hematopoietic Diseases. Thus the Cornell Medical Center tradition in editorship of this book and the Moore tradition of excellence in editorship of Hematology remains strong.

There are 200 contributors to the present edition, of whom 72 are making contributions for the first time. In addition, a considerable number of contributors to previous editions have elected to rewrite rather than simply revise, so that fully half the present edition is assembled from new manuscripts. As Editors, we have accepted responsibility for maintaining reasonable balance in the length and style of contributions. In consultation with the expert editorial staff of the Saunders Company, we have again given special attention to the headings of sections, chapters, and paragraphs in order to make the book as easy to use as possible. In the Table of Contents we have reverted to a style employed in some of the earlier editions, which we think makes for easier use than that in some more recent editions. We have also introduced a system of cross-reference by chapter, which is made easier by printing the chapter number in the running head of each right-hand page.

A major goal in this edition has been to give as much information as practical about therapy. Each contributor has been specially requested to pay attention to this point. Furthermore, we have introduced five new chapters solely about treatment: Antimicrobial Therapy, Cytotoxic and Immunosuppressive Agents, Medical Treatment of Hormone-Dependent Cancers, Respiratory Failure and Its Management, and Diet Therapy in Acute and Chronic Disease. A new essay appears in Part I, dealing with Care of the Patient with Terminal Illness. Various other areas in which treatment is complex have been given additional space, e.g., management of renal insufficiency, management of shock and heart failure, use of anticonvulsant drugs, treatment of pain, and the problems of drug intoxications and addictions.

We view seriously our responsibility as custodians of what has become a classic medical text during the past half century; yet we realize full well that for the expert quality of the substance, it is the contributors who must be thanked. We do this with gratitude.

But contributors and editors acting alone would not make a book; there are others we must thank. We should like to acknowledge the help and dedication of our secretaries, Miss Phyl Woolford and Mrs. Irma Sway. We are deeply indebted to our editorial assistant, Mrs. Helen Miller of New York, who for four editions has served as the major link between contributors, the publisher, and ourselves and has carried out the task faultlessly. We continue to find it a pleasure to work with all the people of the Saunders Company and especially wish to thank David Kilmer for his careful editing.

As this is the last edition that will have the benefit of his experience and wisdom, we insist, despite his protest, on paying homage to John Dusseau, Editor and Vice-President. In the finest tradition of the book publisher's role, he has continuously served as confidant, friend, sensitive critic, and counselor. To work with him has been our great good fortune.

PAUL B. BEESON
WALSH MCDERMOTT

Contributors

ALBERT J. AGUAYO, M.D.

Mechanical Lesions of the Nerve Roots and Spinal Cord

Associate Professor of Neurology and Neurosurgery, McGill University. Associate Physician, The Montreal General Hospital, Montreal, Quebec, Canada.

MARGARET J. ALBRINK, M.D.

Obesity

Professor of Medicine, West Virginia University School of Medicine. Member of Medical Staff, West Virginia University Hospital, Morgantown, West Virginia.

THOMAS P. ALMY, M.D.

Disorders of Motility

Third Century Professor of Medicine, Dartmouth Medical School. Staff Member, Mary Hitchcock Memorial Hospital, Hanover, New Hampshire; Consultant in Medicine, Veterans Administration Center, White River Junction, Vermont.

GERALD D. AURBACH, M.D.

Parathyroid

Chief, Metabolic Diseases Branch, National Institute of Arthritis, Metabolism, and Digestive Diseases, National Institutes of Health, Bethesda, Maryland.

K. FRANK AUSTEN, M.D.

Connective Tissue Diseases ("Collagen Diseases") Other Than Rheumatoid Arthritis: Introduction; Periarteritis Nodosa

Theorore B. Bayles Professor of Medicine, Harvard Medical School. Physician-in-Chief, Robert B. Brigham Hospital, Boston, Massachusetts.

J. RICHARD BARINGER, M.D.

Herpes Simplex Encephalitis

Associate Professor (in Residence) and Vice-Chairman, Department of Neurology, University of California, San Francisco. Chief, Neurology Service, Veterans Administration Hospital, San Francisco, California.

ALEXANDER G. BEARN, M.D.

Genetic Principles: Introduction; Pedigree Analysis in Inherited Disease; Inborn Errors of Metabolism and Molecular Disease; Polygenic and Multifactorial Inheritance; Pharmacogenetics; Population Genetics; Heredity and Environment; Congenital Malformations; Prevention and Management of Genetic Disease; Acalasia; Albinism; Dysautonomia; Laurence-Moon Syndrome; Lipoatrophic Diabetes; Lipoid Proteinosis; Marfan's Syndrome; The Mucopolysaccharidoses; Wilson's Disease; Werner's Syndrome

Professor and Chairman, Department of Medicine, Cornell University Medical College. Physician-in-Chief, The New York Hospital, New York, New York.

MARGARET R. BECKLAKE, M.D., F.R.C.P.

Physical and Chemical Irritants

Professor, Departments of Experimental Medicine and of Epidemiology and Health, McGill University. Associate Physician, Royal Victoria Hospital, Montreal, Quebec, Canada.

PAUL B. BEESON, M.D.

On Becoming a Clinician; Granulomatous Diseases of Unproved Etiology; Introduction; Polymyalgia Rheumatica and Cranial Arteritis; Lethal Midline Granuloma; Wegener's Granulomatosis; Weber-Christian Disease; Fibrosing Syndromes; Eosinophilic Syndromes; Viral Diseases (Presumptive); Infective Endocarditis; Familial Mediterranean Fever

Distinguished Physician, United States Veterans Administration, University of Washington School of Medicine, Seattle, Washington. Formerly Nuffield Professor of Clinical Medicine, University of Oxford, England.

ABRAM S. BENENSON, M.D.

Typhoid Fever

Professor and Chairman, Department of Community Medicine, University of Kentucky College of Medicine, Lexington, Kentucky.

JOHN E. BENNETT, M.D.

Nocardiosis; Cryptococcosis, Mucormycosis; Aspergillosis; Candidiasis

Head, Clinical Mycology Section, Laboratory of Clinical Investigation, National Institute of Allergy and Infectious Diseases, Bethesda, Maryland.

ERNEST BEUTLER, M.D.

Galactosemia

Clinical Professor of Medicine, University of Southern California. Chairman, Division of Medicine, City of Hope Medical Center, Duarte, California.

CHARLES E. BILLINGS, M.D.

Electric Shock

Professor of Preventive Medicine, The Ohio State University College of Medicine. Attending Physician, University Hospitals, Columbus, Ohio.

PHILIP K. BONDY, M.D.

Medical Treatment of Hormone-Dependent Cancers

Cancer Research Campaign Professor of Medicine and Consultant in Medicine, Ludwig Institute of Cancer Research, Sutton. Honorary Consultant, Royal Marsden Hospital, Sutton, Surrey, England.

THOMAS H. BOTHWELL, M.D., D.Sc., F.R.C.P.

Hemochromatosis

Professor of Internal Medicine, University of the Witwatersrand Medical School. Chief Physician, Johannesburg Hospital, Johannesburg, South Africa.

MICHAEL C. BRAIN, D.M.

The Anemias: Introduction; Aplastic Anemia; Sideroblastic Anemia; Myelophthisic Anemia

Professor of Medicine, McMaster University. Physician, McMaster University Medical Centre and Civic Hospitals, Hamilton, Ontario, Canada.

LLOYD L. BRANDBORG, M.D.

Neoplastic Diseases of the Alimentary Tract: Introduction; Neoplasms of the Esophagus; Malignant Neoplasms of the Stomach; Benign Neoplasms of the Stomach

Clinical Professor of Medicine, University of California, San Francisco. Chief, Gastroenterology Section, Veterans Administration Hospital, San Francisco; Consultant, Letterman General Hospital, Oakland Naval Hospital, U.S. Public Health Service Hospital, San Francisco, David Grant Air Force Base, California, and William Beaumont General Hospital, El Paso, Texas.

NEAL S. BRICKER, M.D.

Acute Renal Failure

Professor and Chairman, Department of Medicine, Albert Einstein College of Medicine, Bronx, New York.

WALLACE BRIGDEN, M.D., F.R.C.P.

Disease of the Myocardium

Lecturer in the London Hospital Medical School and the Institute of Cardiology. Consultant Physician to the London Hospital and Physician to the Cardiac Department; Physician to the National Heart Hospital, London, England.

ELMER B. BROWN, M.D.

Acute Hemorrhagic Anemia; Anemia Associated with Infection and Chronic Systemic Diseases; Hypochromic Anemias

Professor of Medicine, Washington University School of Medicine. Associate Physician, Barnes Hospital, St. Louis, Missouri.

ANTHONY D. M. BRYCESON, M.D., F.R.C.P.E., D.T.M.&H.

Leishmaniasis

Senior Lecturer, London School of Hygiene and Tropical Medicine. Consultant Physician, Hospital for Tropical Diseases, London, England.

GEORGE F. CAHILL, Jr., M.D.

Diabetes Mellitus

Professor of Medicine, Harvard Medical School. Director, Joslin Research Laboratories; Harvard Physician, Peter Bent Brigham Hospital, Boston, Massachusetts.

PAUL CALABRESI, M.D.

Cytotoxic and Immunosuppressive Agents

Professor and Chairman, Department of Medicine, Brown University. Physician-in-Chief, Roger Williams General Hospital and Women's and Infants' Hospital of Rhode Island, Providence; Consultant, Rhode Island Hospital, Providence Veterans Administration Hospital, and The Miriam Hospital, Providence, and The Memorial Hospital, Pawtucket, Rhode Island.

PAUL P. CARBONE, M.D.

Lymphoreticular Neoplasms: Introduction; Lymphocytic and Histiocytic Lymphomas; Burkitt's Lymphoma

Associate Director for Medical Oncology, National Cancer Institute, Bethesda, Maryland.

HUGH CHAPLIN, Jr., M.D.

Hemoglobinuria; Transfusion Reactions

Professor of Medicine and Preventive Medicine, Washington University School of Medicine. Associate Physician, Barnes Hospital, St. Louis, Missouri.

CHARLES L. CHRISTIAN, M.D.

Diseases of the Joints

Professor of Medicine, Cornell University Medical College. Physician-in-Chief, Hospital for Special Surgery, New York, New York.

NICHOLAS P. CHRISTY, M.D.

Diseases of Metabolism: Introduction; Diseases of the Endocrine System: Introduction; The Anterior Pituitary; Endocrine Syndromes Associated with Cancer

Professor of Medicine, Columbia University College of Physicians and Surgeons. Director, Medical Service, The Roosevelt Hospital; Visiting Physician, Francis Delafield Hospital; Associate Attending Physician, The Presbyterian Hospital, New York, New York.

LEIGHTON E. CLUFF, M.D.

Shigellosis; Cholera; Diseases Caused by Malleomyces; Anthrax; Listeriosis; Erysipeloid of Rosenbach

Professor of Internal Medicine, University of Florida. Chairman, Department of Medicine, University of Florida Teaching Hospitals, Gainesville, Florida.

JAY D. COFFMAN, M.D.

Diseases of the Peripheral Vessels

Professor of Medicine, Boston University School of Medicine. Section Head, Peripheral Vascular Department, University Hospital, Boston, Massachusetts.

C. LOCKARD CONLEY, M.D.

Hemoglobin, the Hemoglobinopathies, and the Thalassemias

Professor of Medicine, The Johns Hopkins University School of Medicine. Head, Hematology Division, The Johns Hopkins University and Hospital, Baltimore, Maryland.

REX B. CONN, M.D.

Normal Laboratory Values of Clinical Importance

Professor of Laboratory Medicine, The Johns Hopkins University. Director, Department of Laboratory Medicine, The Johns Hopkins Hospital, Baltimore, Maryland.

ROBERT B. COUCH, M.D.

Mycoplasmal Diseases

Professor of Microbiology and Immunology and Medicine, Baylor College of Medicine. Attending Physician, The Methodist Hospital, Houston; Attending Physician in Medicine, Ben Taub Hospital, Houston, Texas.

ALEXANDER CRAMPTON SMITH, M.A., M.B., Ch.B., F.F.A.R.C.S.

Tetanus

Nuffield Professor of Anaesthetics, University of Oxford, England. Consultant Anaesthetist (Honorary), Oxfordshire Area Health Authority (Teaching).

ANTHONY N. DAMATO, M.D.

Cardiac Arrhythmia

U.S. Public Health Service Hospital, Staten Island, New York.

LESLIE J. DeGROOT, M.D.

The Thyroid

Professor of Medicine, University of Chicago School of Medicine, Chicago, Illinois.

ROGER M. DES PREZ, M.D.

Tuberculosis; Extrapulmonary Tuberculosis

Professor of Medicine, Vanderbilt University School of Medicine. Chief, Medical Service, Veterans Administration Hospital, Nashville. Visiting Staff, Vanderbilt University Hospital, Nashville, Tennessee.

BERTRAM D. DINMAN, M.D., Sc.D.

Carbon Monoxide Poisoning

Non-resident lecturer, University of Michigan School of Public Health. Medical Director, Aluminum Company of America, Pittsburgh, Pennsylvania.

PHILIP R. DODGE, M.D.

Infections and Inflammatory Diseases of the Central Nervous System and Its Coverings: Introduction; Aids to Diagnosis in Intracranial and Intraspinal Inflammatory Disease; Spinal Epidural Infections; Transverse Myelitis or Myelopathy; Syphilitic Infections of the Central Nervous System

Professor of Pediatrics and Neurology and Head, Edward Mallinkrodt Department of Pediatrics, Washington University School of Medicine. Medical Director, St. Louis Children's Hospital; Pediatrician-in-Chief, Barnes Hospital, St. Louis, Missouri.

WILBUR G. DOWNS, M.D.

Yellow Fever

Clinical Professor of Epidemiology, Yale University School of Medicine, New Haven, Connecticut.

DAVID A. DRACHMAN, M.D.

Dizziness and Vertigo

Professor of Neurology, Northwestern University School of Medicine. Attending Physician and Chief of Neurology, Passavant Pavilion, Northwestern Memorial Hospital, Chicago, Illinois.

PIERRE M. DREYFUS, M.D.

Nutritional Disorders of the Nervous System

Professor of Neurology, University of California, Davis. Chief of Neurology, Sacramento Medical Center, Sacramento, California.

PETER JAMES DYCK, M.D.

Diseases of the Peripheral Nervous System

Professor of Neurology, Mayo Medical School, Rochester, Minnesota.

DAVID L. EARNEST, M.D.

Other Diseases of the Colon, Rectum, and Anus

Assistant Professor of Medicine, University of California School of Medicine, San Francisco. Staff Gastroenterologist, San Francisco General Hospital, San Francisco, California.

RICHARD V. EBERT, M.D.

Abnormal Air Spaces; Diffuse Lung Disease

Professor of Internal Medicine, University of Minnesota Medical School, Minneapolis, Minnesota.

HAROLD V. ELLINGSON, M.D., Ph.D., M.P.H.

Motion Sickness and Problems of Air Travel

Professor and Chairman, Department of Preventive Medicine, Ohio State University College of Medicine, Columbus, Ohio.

KARL ENGELMAN, M.D.

The Adrenal Medulla and Sympathetic Nervous System; The Carcinoid Syndrome

Associate Professor of Medicine and Pharmacology, University of Pennsylvania School of Medicine. Chief, Hypertension and Clinical Pharmacology Section, and Director, Clinical Research Center, Hospital of the University of Pennsylvania, Philadelphia; Attending Physician, Veterans Administration Hospital, Philadelphia General Hospital, and Children's Hospital of Philadelphia, Pennsylvania.

ALVAN R. FEINSTEIN, M.D.

Science, Clinical Medicine, and the Spectrum of Disease; Neoplasms of the Lung

Professor of Medicine and Epidemiology and Director, Johnson Clinical Scholar Program, Yale University School of Medicine. Attending Physician, Yale–New Haven Hospital, New Haven; Chief, Clinical Biostatistics, West Haven Veterans Administration Hospital, West Haven, Connecticut.

F. ROBERT FEKETY, Jr., M.D.

Staphylococcal Infections

Professor of Internal Medicine, University of Michigan Medical School. Attending Physician, University Hospital, Ann Arbor, Michigan.

HARRY A. FELDMAN, M.D.

Meningococcal Disease

Professor and Chairman, Department of Preventive Medicine, State University of New York, Upstate Medical Center. Attending Physician, State University and Silverman Hospitals; Consultant, Syracuse Psychiatric Hospital, Syracuse, New York.

PHILIP FELIG, M.D.

Nutritional Maintenance and Diet Therapy in Acute and Chronic Disease

Associate Professor of Medicine and Director, General Clinical Research Center, Yale University School of Medicine. Attending Physician, Yale–New Haven Hospital, New Haven; Consultant in Metabolism and Endocrinology, Veterans Administration Hospital, West Haven, Connecticut.

THOMAS F. FERRIS, M.D.

Renal Disease in Pregnancy

Professor of Medicine, Ohio State University. Director, Division of Renal Diseases, Ohio State University Hospitals, Columbus, Ohio.

SYDNEY M. FINEGOLD, M.D.

Disease Due to Nonsporeforming Anaerobic Bacteria

Professor of Medicine, Department of Medicine, UCLA School of Medicine. Chief, Infectious Disease Section, Veterans Administration Wadsworth Hospital Center, Los Angeles, California.

ALFRED P. FISHMAN, M.D.

Heart Failure; Shock

William Maul Measey Professor of Medicine, University of Pennsylvania School of Medicine. Director of Cardiovascular-Pulmonary Division, Hospital of the University of Pennsylvania; Attending Physician, Philadelphia General Hospital, Philadelphia, Pennsylvania.

ROBERT A. FISHMAN, M.D.

Intracranial Tumors and States Causing Increased Intracranial Pressure

Professor and Chairman, Department of Neurology, School of Medicine, University of California, San Francisco. Attending Neurologist, Veterans Administration Hospital, Fort Miley, San Francisco General Hospital, and Letterman General Hospital, Presidio, San Francisco, California.

EDMUND B. FLINK, M.D., Ph.D.

Heavy Metal Poisoning

Professor and Chairman, Department of Medicine, West Virginia University School of Medicine. Chief, Medical Service, West Virginia University Hospital, Morgantown, West Virginia.

DONALD S. FREDRICKSON, M.D.

Lipid Storage Disorders

President, Institute of Medicine, National Academy of Sciences, Washington, D.C.

NORBERT FREINKEL, M.D.

Hypoglycemic Disorders

Kettering Professor of Medicine, Professor of Biochemistry, and Director, Center for Endocrinology, Metabolism and Nutrition, Northwestern University Medical School. Director, Endocrine-Metabolic Clinics, Northwestern University Medical School; Attending Physician, Northwestern Memorial Hospital, Chicago; Consultant in Endocrinology, Veterans Administration Research Hospital, Chicago, Illinois.

PARK S. GERALD, M.D.

Chromosomes and Their Disorders

Professor of Pediatrics, Harvard Medical School. Chief, Clinical Genetics Division, Children's Hospital Medical Center, Boston, Massachusetts.

NORMAN GESCHWIND, M.D.

Focal Disturbances of Higher Nervous Function

James Jackson Putnam Professor of Neurology, Harvard Medical School. Director, Neurological Unit, Boston City Hospital, Boston, Massachusetts.

GILBERT H. GLASER, M.D., Med.Sc.D.

The Epilepsies

Professor of Neurology and Chairman, Department of Neurology, Yale University School of Medicine. Neurologist-in-Chief, Yale–New Haven Hospital, New Haven; Consultant Neurologist, Veterans Administration Hospital, West Haven, Connecticut.

ROBERT A. GOOD, Ph.D., M.D.

The Primary Immunodeficiency Diseases

Professor of Medicine and Pediatrics, Cornell University Medical College. President and Director, Sloan-Kettering Institute for Cancer Research. Attending Physician and Director of Research, Memorial Hospital for Cancer and Allied Diseases, New York, New York.

ROBERT A. GOODWIN, Jr., M.D.

Pulmonary Tuberculosis; Diseases Due to Mycobacteria Other Than M. tuberculosis and M. leprae

Professor of Medicine, Vanderbilt University School of Medicine. Chief, Pulmonary Disease Section, Veterans Administration Hospital, Nashville; Visiting Staff, Vanderbilt University Hospital, Nashville, Tennessee.

MORTON I. GROSSMAN, M.D., Ph.D.

Peptic Ulcer: Pathogenesis and Pathology

Professor of Medicine and Physiology, UCLA School of Medicine. Senior Medical Investigator, Wadsworth Veterans Administration Hospital, Los Angeles, California.

THORSTEIN GUTHE, M.D., M.P.H.

Treponemal Diseases; Relapsing Fevers; Phagedenic Tropical Ulcer; The Rat-Bite Fevers

Head, Medical Department, Elkem-Spigerverket, Oslo, Norway. Former Chief Medical Officer, Venereal Diseases and Treponematoses, World Health Organization, Geneva, Switzerland.

ROBERT J. HAGGERTY, M.D.

Common Accidental Poisoning

Professor and Chairman, Department of Pediatrics, University of Rochester School of Medicine and Dentistry. Pediatrician-in-Chief, Strong Memorial Hospital; Consulting Pediatrician, Genesee Hospital and Rochester General Hospital, Rochester, New York.

CONSTANTINE L. HAMPERS, M.D.

Dialysis

Assistant Clinical Professor of Medicine, Harvard Medical School. Senior Associate in Medicine, Peter Bent Brigham Hospital, Boston, Massachusetts.

JAMES B. HANSHAW, M.D.

Cytomegalovirus Infections

Professor of Pediatrics and Microbiology, University of Rochester School of Medicine. Pediatrician-in-Chief, The Genesee Hospital, Rochester, New York.

EDWARD D. HARRIS, Jr., M.D.

Systemic Sclerosis

Associate Professor of Medicine, Dartmouth Medical School. Staff Physician, Mary Hitchcock Memorial Hospital, Hanover; Chief, Connective Tissue Disease Section, Dartmouth/Hitchcock Medical Center, Hanover, New Hampshire.

RICHARD J. HAVEL, M.D.

Disorders of Lipid Metabolism

Professor of Medicine and Director, Cardiovascular Research Institute, University of California School of Medicine. Attending Physician, University of California Hospitals, San Francisco, California.

ROBERT P. HEANEY, M.D.

Bone Physiology and Calcium Homeostasis; The Osteoporoses; The Osteomalacias; Osteitis Fibrosa; Bone Intoxications

Professor of Medicine, Creighton University School of Medicine. Vice President for Health Sciences, Creighton University, Omaha, Nebraska.

VICTOR HERBERT, M.D., J.D.

Megaloblastic Anemias

Clinical Professor of Pathology and Clinical Professor of Medicine, Columbia University College of Physicians and Surgeons. Medical Investigator and Director of the Hematology and Nutrition Laboratory, Veterans Administration Hospital, Bronx, New York.

ALBERT HEYMAN, M.D.

Syncope; Hyperventilation

Professor of Neurology, Duke University Medical Center. Attending Neurologist, Duke University Medical School and Durham Veterans Administration Hospital, Durham, North Carolina.

HOWARD H. HIATT, M.D.

Man and His Environment

Dean, Harvard School of Public Health, and Professor of Medicine, Harvard Medical School. Board of Consultation in Medicine, Beth Israel Hospital; Consultant, Peter Bent Brigham Hospital and Children's Hospital, Boston, Massachusetts.

PATRICK J. HOGAN, M.D.

Pericarditis

Instructor of Internal Medicine, Baylor College of Medicine. Staff, Methodist Hospital, Houston, Texas.

JAMES F. HOLLAND, M.D.

The Acute Leukemias

Professor and Chairman, Department of Neoplastic Diseases, and Professor of Medicine, Mt. Sinai School of Medicine of the City University of New York. Director, The Cancer Center, and Attending Physician, Mt. Sinai Hospital, New York, New York.

EDWARD W. HOOK, M.D.

Pneumococcal Pneumonia; Salmonella Infections Other Than Typhoid Fever

Henry B. Mulholland Professor and Chairman, Department of Medicine, University of Virginia School of Medicine. Physician-in-Chief, University of Virginia Hospital, Charlottesville, Virginia.

DOROTHY M. HORSTMANN, M.D.

Mumps; Viral Meningitis and Encephalitis

Professor of Epidemiology and Pediatrics, Yale University School of Medicine. Attending Pediatrician, Yale–New Haven Hospital, New Haven, Connecticut.

JOHN BERNARD LLOYD HOWELL, M.D., Ph.D.

The Diaphragm; The Chest Wall; Chronic Obstructive Lung Disease: Introduction; Chronic Bronchitis; Bronchiectasis; Asthma: Acute Reversible Airway Obstruction; Chronic Airway Obstruction; Localized Airway Obstruction

Professor of Medicine, University of Southampton Medical School. Consultant Physician, Southampton University Hospitals Group, Southampton, England.

CHARLES M. HUGULEY, Jr., M.D.

The Chronic Leukemias

Professor of Medicine, Emory University School of Medicine. Attending Hematologist and Oncologist, Emory University Hospital and Grady Memorial Hospital, Atlanta, Georgia.

J. WILLIS HURST, M.D.

Diseases of the Aorta

Professor and Chairman, Department of Medicine, Emory University School of Medicine, Atlanta, Georgia.

JON I. ISENBERG, M.D.

Peptic Ulcer: Diagnostic Studies and Medical Treatment

Associate Professor of Medicine, University of California at Los Angeles. Chief, Gastroenterology Section, Wadsworth Veterans Administration Hospital, Los Angeles, California.

GEORGE GEE JACKSON, M.D.

The Common Cold; Rhinoviral Respiratory Disease; Viral Pharyngitis, Laryngitis, Croup, and Bronchitis; Adenoviral Infections; Respiratory Syncytial Viral Disease; Parainfluenza Viral Diseases

Professor of Medicine and Chief, Section of Infectious Diseases, Abraham Lincoln School of Medicine, University of Illinois College of Medicine. Attending Physician, University of Illinois Hospital, Chicago; Consultant in Infectious Diseases, Westside Veterans Administration Hospital, Chicago, Illinois.

ERNST R. JAFFÉ, M.D.

Methemoglobinemia and Sulfhemoglobinemia

Professor of Medicine and Head, Division of Hematology, Albert Einstein College of Medicine. Attending Physician (Medicine), Bronx Municipal Hospital Center, Hospital of the Albert Einstein College of Medicine, and Lincoln Hospital, Bronx, New York.

DAVID GERAINT JAMES, M.A., M.D. (Cambridge), F.R.C.P.

Sarcoidosis

Dean, Royal Northern Hospital, London, England; Consultant Ophthalmic Physician, St. Thomas' Hospital, London. Clinical Professor of Medicine, University of Miami, Florida. Consulting Physician, Sydney Hospital, Sydney, Australia.

HENRY D. JANOWITZ, M.D.

Chronic Inflammatory Diseases of the Intestine

Clinical Professor of Medicine, Mount Sinai School of Medicine. Head, Division of Gastroenterology, Mount Sinai Hospital, New York, New York.

ERNEST JAWETZ, M.D., Ph.D.

Trachoma and Inclusion Conjunctivitis; Lymphogranuloma Venereum

Professor of Microbiology and Medicine, University of California Medical Center, San Francisco, California.

GRAHAM H. JEFFRIES, M.B., Ch.B. (N.Z.), D.Phil. (Oxon.)

Diseases of the Liver

Professor and Chairman, Department of Medicine, The Milton S. Hershey Medical Center, Pennsylvania State University College of Medicine. Chief, Medical Service, The Milton S. Hershey Medical Center Hospital, Hershey, Pennsylvania.

KARL M. JOHNSON, M.D.

Arthropod-Borne Viral Fevers, Viral Encephalitides, and Viral Hemorrhagic Fevers: Introduction; Dengue; West Nile Fever; Fevers Caused by Group A Arboviruses: Chikungunya, O'nyong-nyong, Mayaro, and Ross River; Rift Valley Fever; Sandfly Fever; Arthropod-Borne Viral Encephalitides; Viral Hemorrhagic Fevers: Introduction; Hemorrhagic Fever Caused by Dengue Viruses; Crimean Hemorrhagic Fever; Hemorrhagic Diseases Caused by Arenaviruses: Argentine and Bolivian Hemorrhagic Fevers and Lassa Fever; Epidemic Hemorrhagic Fever: Hemorrhagic Nephrosonephritis

Director, Middle America Research Unit, National Institute of Allergy and Infectious Diseases, National Institutes of Health, U.S. Public Health Service, Balboa Heights, Canal Zone.

RICHARD T. JOHNSON, M.D.

Viral Infections of the Nervous System: Introduction; Herpes Zoster; Slow Infections of the Nervous System

Professor of Neurology and Associate Professor of Microbiology, The Johns Hopkins University School of Medicine. Neurologist, The Johns Hopkins Hospital, Baltimore, Maryland.

ROBERT L. JOHNSON, M.D.

Alterations in Atmospheric Pressure

Deputy Chief, Biomedical Research Division, Life Sciences Directorate, Lyndon B. Johnson Space Center, Houston, Texas.

THOMAS C. JONES, M.D.

Malaria; Pneumocystosis; Trichomoniasis; Toxoplasmosis

Assistant Professor of Medicine and Public Health, Cornell University Medical College. Assistant Attending Physician, The New York Hospital, New York, New York.

FRED S. KANTOR, M.D.

Serum Sickness; Drug Allergy; Allergic Rhinitis; Vasomotor Rhinitis; Urticaria; Angioneurotic Edema; Insect Stings

Professor of Medicine, Yale University School of Medicine. Attending Physician, Yale–New Haven Hospital, New Haven, Connecticut.

ALBERT Z. KAPIKIAN, M.D.

Enteroviral Diseases

Head, Epidemiology Section, Laboratory of Infectious Diseases, National Institute of Allergy and Infectious Diseases, National Institutes of Health, Bethesda, Maryland.

NATHAN G. KASE, M.D.

The Ovaries

Professor and Chairman, Obstetrics and Gynecology, Yale University School of Medicine. Chief of Service, Yale–New Haven Hospital, New Haven, Connecticut.

DONALD KAYE, M.D.

Gonococcal Disease

Professor and Chairman, Department of Medicine, The Medical College of Pennsylvania. Chief of Medicine, Hospital of the Medical College of Pennsylvania, Philadelphia; Consultant in Medicine, Veterans Administration Hospital, Philadelphia, Pennsylvania.

C. HENRY KEMPE, M.D.

Variola and Vaccinia

Professor of Pediatrics, University of Colorado Medical Center. Consultant, Colorado General Hospital, Children's Hospital, Fitzsimons Army Hospital, and Veterans Administration Hospital, Denver, Colorado.

DAVID N. S. KERR, M.S., F.R.C.P.

Role of the Kidney in Health and Disease; Investigation of Renal Function; Chronic Renal Failure

Professor of Medicine, University of Newcastle upon Tyne. Consultant Physician, Royal Victoria Infirmary, Newcastle upon Tyne, England.

EDWIN D. KILBOURNE, M.D.

Introduction to Viral Diseases; Influenza; Measles; Rubella; Exanthemata Associated with Enteroviral Infections

Professor and Chairman, Department of Microbiology, Mount Sinai School of Medicine of the City University of New York, New York.

THOMAS KILLIP, M.D.

Coronary Artery Disease

Professor of Medicine, Northwestern University Medical School. Chairman, Department of Medicine, Evanston Hospital, Evanston, Illinois.

PRISCILLA KINCAID-SMITH, M.D., F.R.A.C.P., F.R.C.P., D.C.P.

Treatment of Irreversible Renal Failure by Transplantation and Dialysis: Introduction; Renal Transplantation

Reader in Medicine, University of Melbourne. Physician-in-Charge, Department of Nephrology, Royal Melbourne Hospital, Melbourne, Australia.

SEYMOUR J. KLEBANOFF, M.D., Ph.D.

Neutrophil Function; Neutrophil Dysfunction Syndromes

Professor of Medicine, University of Washington School of Medicine, Seattle, Washington.

RICHARD KNIGHT, M.B., B.Chir., M.R.C.P., D.T.M.&H.

Amebiasis

Lecturer, Liverpool School of Tropical Medicine, Liverpool, England. Clinical Assistant to Tropical Unit, United Liverpool Visiting Fellow, and Physician, Department of Clinical Sciences, University of Papua, New Guinea.

VERNON KNIGHT, M.D.

Brucellosis

Professor of Medicine and Professor and Chairman, Microbiology and Immunology, Baylor College of Medicine. Senior Attending Physician, The Methodist Hospital, Houston; Attending Physician, Ben Taub General Hospital, Houston, Texas.

HILARY KOPROWSKI, M.D.

Rabies

Director, The Wistar Institute, Philadelphia, Pennsylvania.

O. DHODANAND KOWLESSAR, M.D.

Diseases of the Pancreas

Professor of Medicine, Thomas Jefferson University, Jefferson Medical College. Director, Division of Gastroenterology, and Director, Clinical Research Center, Jefferson Medical College and Thomas Jefferson University Hospital, Philadelphia, Pennsylvania.

RICHARD M. KRAUSE, M.D.

Rheumatic Fever

Professor and Senior Physician, Rockefeller University, New York, New York.

CALVIN M. KUNIN, M.D.

Enteric Bacterial Infections; Urinary Tract Infections and Pyelonephritis

Professor of Internal Medicine, University of Wisconsin School of Medicine. Chief, Medical Service, Veterans Administration Hospital, Madison, Wisconsin.

HENRY G. KUNKEL, M.D.

Immune Disease: Introduction

Professor, Rockefeller University. Adjunct Professor of Medicine, Cornell University Medical School, New York, New York.

HAROLD P. LAMBERT, M.D., F.R.C.P.

Food Poisoning

Professor of Microbial Diseases, St. George's Hospital Medical School, University of London. Consultant Physician, St. George's Hospital, London, England.

DAVID H. LAW, M.D.

Gastrointestinal Bleeding

Professor of Medicine (Vice-Chairman), University of New Mexico School of Medicine. Chief, Medical Service, Albuquerque Veterans Administration Hospital, Albuquerque, New Mexico.

ALEXANDER LEAF, M.D.

Posterior Pituitary

Jackson Professor of Clinical Medicine, Harvard Medical School. Chief, Medical Services, Massachusetts General Hospital, Boston, Massachusetts.

AARON B. LERNER, M.D.

Disorders of Melanin Pigmentation

Professor of Dermatology, Yale University School of Medicine. Professor and Chairman, Department of Dermatology, Yale–New Haven Hospital, New Haven, Connecticut.

HERBERT L. LEY, Jr., M.D., M.P.H.

Rocky Mountain Spotted Fever; Tick-Borne Rickettsioses of the Eastern Hemisphere; Rickettsialpox; Scrub Typhus; Trench Fever; Q Fever; Bartonellosis

Medical consultant in foods and drugs, Bethesda, Maryland.

GRANT W. LIDDLE, M.D.

Adrenal Cortex

Professor and Chairman, Department of Medicine, Vanderbilt University. Physician-in-Chief, Vanderbilt University Hospital, Nashville, Tennessee.

PHILIP H. LIEBERMAN, M.D.

Eosinophilic Granuloma and Related Syndromes

Associate Professor of Pathology, Cornell University Medical School. Chief, Surgical Pathology Service, Memorial Hospital for Cancer and Allied Diseases, New York, New York.

HAROLD I. LIEF, M.D.

Medical Aspects of Sexuality

Professor of Psychiatry, School of Medicine, University of Pennsylvania. Director, Division of Family Study, Marriage Council of Philadelphia, and Center for the Study of Sex Education in Medicine, all affiliates of the School of Medicine of the University of Pennsylvania, Philadelphia, Pennsylvania.

MORTIMER B. LIPSETT, M.D.

The Testis

Professor of Medicine, Case Western Reserve School of Medicine. Director, The Cancer Center, Cleveland, Ohio.

JOHN N. LOEB, M.D.

Mode of Action of Hormones

Associate Professor of Medicine, College of Physicians and Surgeons, Columbia University; Adjunct Assistant Professor, Rockefeller University. Associate Attending Physician, Presbyterian Hospital, New York, New York.

DANIEL S. LUKAS, M.D.

Pulmonary Hypertension

Associate Professor of Medicine, Cornell University Medical College. Chief, Cardiopulmonary Service, and Attending Physician, Memorial Hospital for Cancer and Allied Diseases; Associate Attending Physician, The New York Hospital, New York, New York.

PHILIP D. MARSDEN, M.D.

Leeches as Agents of Disease; Arthropoda of Medical Importance; Venomous Arthropods; Protozoan and Helminthic Diseases: Introduction; Protozoan Diseases: Introduction; Other Protozoan Diseases: Introduction; Giardiasis; Balantidiasis; Coccidiosis; Primary Amebic Meningoencephalitis; Helminthic Diseases: Introduction; The Cestodes; Hermaphroditic Flukes; The Nematodes; Tropical Pyomyositis; Eosinophilia in Relation to Helminthic Infections

Visiting Professor of Tropical Medicine, University of Brasilia. Physician, General Medical Service, Sobradinmo Hospital. Visiting Professor of Public Health, Cornell University Medical College. Senior Lecturer, Department of Clinical Tropical Medicine, London School of Hygiene and Tropical Medicine. Physician, Hospital for Tropical Diseases, London, England.

JOHN H. McCLEMENT, M.D.

Diseases of the Pleura

Professor of Medicine, New York University School of Medicine. Director, Chest Service, Bellevue Hospital, New York; Attending Physician, University Hospital, New York, New York.

FRED R. McCRUMB, Jr., M.D.

Plague

Special Assistant to the Director, Fogarty International Center, National Institutes of Health, Bethesda, Maryland.

WALSH McDERMOTT, M.D.

Medicine in Modern Society; Chemical Contamination of Water and Air; Introduction to Microbial Diseases; Foot-and-

Mouth Disease; Bacterial Diseases: Introduction; Pneumonia: Introduction; Hemophilus influenzae Infections; Granuloma Inguinale; Drugs and Microbes

Professor of Public Affairs in Medicine, Cornell University Medical College. Attending Physician, The New York Hospital, New York, New York. Special Advisor to the President, Robert Wood Johnson Foundation, Princeton, New Jersey.

FLETCHER H. McDOWELL, M.D.

Cerebrovascular Diseases

Professor of Neurology, Cornell University Medical College. Attending Neurologist, The New York Hospital; Medical Director, Burke Rehabilitation Hospital, New York, New York.

PAUL R. McHUGH, M.D.

Dementia; Psychologic Illness in Medical Practice; Psychologic Testing in Clinical Medicine

Professor of Psychiatry and Chairman, Department of Psychiatry, University of Oregon Medical School, Portland, Oregon.

GORDON MEIKLEJOHN, M.D.

Colorado Tick Fever

Professor and Chairman, Department of Medicine, University of Colorado Medical School. Staff, Colorado General Hospital, Denver General Hospital, Veterans Administration Hospital, and Fitzsimons Army General Hospital, Denver, Colorado.

JACK H. MENDELSON, M.D.

Alcohol Abuse and Alcohol-Related Illness

Professor of Psychiatry, Harvard Medical School. Director, Alcohol and Drug Abuse Research Center, McLean Hospital, Belmont, Massachusetts.

JAMES H. MEYER, M.D.

Peptic Ulcer: Complications and Surgical Treatment

Assistant Professor of Medicine, University of California, San Francisco. Staff, Veterans Administration Hospital, San Francisco, California.

ROBERT B. MILLMAN, M.D.

Drug Abuse, Addiction, and Intoxication: Introduction; The Opiates; Central Nervous System Depressants; Central Nervous System Stimulants; Cannabis; Psychedelics; Miscellaneous Inhalants

Assistant Professor of Public Health, Cornell University Medical College; Adjunct Assistant Professor, Rockefeller University. Director, Adolescent Development Program, The New York Hospital–Cornell Medical Center and Rockefeller University, New York, New York.

SHERMAN A. MINTON, Jr., M.D.

Snakebite; Marine Venoms

Professor of Microbiology, Indiana University School of Medicine, Indianapolis, Indiana.

STEPHEN I. MORSE, M.D.

Whooping Cough

Professor and Chairman, Microbiology and Immunology, State University of New York, Downstate Medical Center, Brooklyn, New York.

ARNO G. MOTULSKY, M.D.

Genetic Counseling

Professor of Medicine and Genetics, University of Washington. Attending Physician, University Hospital, Seattle, Washington.

FRANCIS P. MULDOWNEY, M.D., F.R.C.P.

Obstructive Nephropathy

Research Professor of Medicine, University College, Dublin. Physician in Charge, Metabolic and Renal Unit, St. Vincent's Hospital and National Maternity Hospital, Dublin, Ireland.

EDWARD S. MURRAY, M.D., M.P.H.

Rickettsial Diseases: Introduction; The Typhus Group

Professor of Microbiology, Harvard School of Public Health, Cambridge, Massachusetts.

W. P. LAIRD MYERS, M.D.

The Care of the Patient with Terminal Illness

Professor of Internal Medicine, Cornell University Medical College. Chairman, Department of Medicine, and Attending Physician, Memorial Sloan-Kettering Cancer Center; Member, Sloan-Kettering Institute for Cancer Research; Attending Physician, The New York Hospital, New York, New York.

RALPH L. NACHMAN, M.D.

Hematologic and Hematopoietic Diseases: Introduction; Hemorrhagic Disorders: Disorders of Primary Hemostasis

Professor of Medicine, Cornell University Medical College. Attending Physician, The New York Hospital, New York, New York.

JAMES R. NELSON, M.D.

Hearing Loss

Adjunct Associate Professor of Neurosciences, University of California School of Medicine, La Jolla. Attending Neurologist, University Hospital of San Diego County, San Diego, and Veterans Administration Hospital, La Jolla, California.

THOMAS F. O'BRIEN, Jr., M.D.

Neoplasms of the Small Intestine; Neoplasms of the Large Intestine

Associate Professor of Medicine, Bowman Gray School of Medicine. Chief, Gastroenterology Section, North Carolina Baptist Hospital, Winston-Salem; Member, Courtesy Staff, Forsyth Memorial Hospital, Winston-Salem, North Carolina.

ROBERT K. OCKNER, M.D.

Vascular Diseases of the Intestine; Diseases of the Peritoneum

Associate Professor of Medicine, University of California School of Medicine, San Francisco. Attending Physician, University of California–Moffitt Hospitals, Ft. Miley Veterans Administration Hospital, and San Francisco General Hospital, San Francisco, California.

W. E. ORMEROD, M.A., D.Sc., D.M.

African Trypanosomiases

Reader in Medical Protozoology, London School of Hygiene and Tropical Medicine, London, England.

ELLIOTT F. OSSERMAN, M.D.

Plasma Cell Dyscrasias

American Cancer Society Professor of Medicine and Associate Director, Institute of Cancer Research, Columbia University College of Physicians and Surgeons. Visiting Physician, Francis Delafield Hospital, New York; Attending Physician, Presbyterian Hospital, New York, New York.

DEMOSTHENES PAPPAGIANIS, M.D., Ph.D.

Coccidioidomycosis

Professor and Chairman, Department of Medical Microbiology, School of Medicine, University of California, Davis, California.

SOLOMON PAPPER, M.D.

Chronic Pyelonephritis

Distinguished Professor of Medicine, University of Oklahoma College of Medicine. Distinguished Physician, Oklahoma City Veterans Administration Hospital, Oklahoma City, Oklahoma.

RUSSEL H. PATTERSON, Jr., M.D.

Injuries of the Head and Spine

Professor of Surgery (Neurosurgery), Cornell University Medical College. Attending Surgeon-in-Charge, The New York Hospital, New York, New York.

WILLIAM STANLEY PEART, M.D., F.R.C.P., F.R.S.

Arterial Hypertension

Professor of Medicine, St. Mary's Hospital Medical School (University of London), London, England.

JOSEPH K. PERLOFF, M.D.

Congenital Heart Disease

Professor of Medicine and Pediatrics, University of Pennsylvania. Chief, Cardiovascular Section, University of Pennsylvania School of Medicine, Philadelphia, Pennsylvania.

ROBERT G. PETERSDORF, M.D.

Bacterial Meningitis

Professor and Chairman, Department of Medicine, University of Washington School of Medicine. Physician-in-Chief, University of Washington Hospital, Seattle, Washington.

FRED PLUM, M.D.

Disorders of the Nervous System and Behavior: Introduction; Consciousness and Its Disturbances: Introduction; The Pathogenesis of Stupor and Coma; Sleep and Its Disorders; Acute Drug Poisoning; Headache; Idiopathic Autonomic Insufficiency; Acute Anterior Poliomyelitis; Abnormalities in Respiratory Control

Ann Parrish Titzell Professor of Neurology, Cornell University Medical College. Neurologist-in-Chief, The New York Hospital, New York, New York.

JEROME B. POSNER, M.D.

Delirium and Exogenous Metabolic Brain Disease; Pain; Nonmetastatic Effects of Cancer on the Nervous System

Professor of Neurology, Cornell University Medical College. Chief, Neuropsychiatric Service, Memorial Sloan-Kettering Cancer Center; Attending Neurologist, The New York Hospital, New York, New York.

OSCAR D. RATNOFF, M.D.

Hemorrhagic Disorders: Coagulation Defects

Professor of Medicine, Case Western Reserve University School of Medicine. Career Investigator of the American Heart Association; Visiting Physician, University Hospitals of Cleveland, Cleveland, Ohio.

SEYMOUR REICHLIN, M.D., Ph.D.

The Control of Anterior Pituitary Secretion; The Pineal

Professor of Medicine, Tufts University School of Medicine. Senior Physician and Chief, Division of Endocrinology, Tufts–New England Medical Center, Boston, Massachusetts.

EDWARD H. REINHARD, M.D.

Polycythemia

Professor of Medicine, Washington University School of Medicine. Associate Physician and Director of the Blue Medical Service, Barnes Hospital, St. Louis; Member of Consulting Staff, Jewish Hospital and Veterans Administration Hospital, St. Louis, Missouri.

DONALD J. REIS, M.D.

Degenerative and Heredofamilial Diseases of the Central Nervous System

Professor of Neurology, Cornell University Medical College. Attending in Neurology, The New York Hospital, New York, New York.

RICHARD B. ROBERTS, M.D.

Antimicrobial Therapy

Associated Professor of Medicine and Head, Division of Infectious Diseases, Cornell University Medical College. Associate Attending Physician, The New York Hospital and Memorial Sloan-Kettering Cancer Center, New York, New York.

HEONIR ROCHA, M.D.

Diphtheria; Chagas' Disease

Professor and Chairman, Department of Medicine, University of Bahia School of Medicine, Bahia, Brazil.

DAVID E. ROGERS, M.D.

Psittacosis

President, The Robert Wood Johnson Foundation, Princeton, New Jersey.

SAUL A. ROSENBERG, M.D.

Hodgkin's Disease

Professor of Medicine and Radiology, Stanford University School of Medicine. Chief, Division of Oncology, Stanford University Hospital, Stanford, California.

JOHN ROSS, Jr., M.D.

Acquired Valvular Heart Disease

Professor of Medicine and Head, Cardiology Division, Department of Medicine, University of California, San Diego, School of Medicine. Attending Physician, University Hospital, San Diego County, La Jolla, California.

WENDELL F. ROSSE, M.D.

Hemolytic Disorders: Extracorpuscular Mechanisms

Professor of Medicine, Duke University Medical Center.

Chief of Medical Service, Veterans Administration Hospital, Durham, North Carolina.

LEWIS P. ROWLAND, M.D.

Diseases of Muscle and Neuromuscular Junction

Henry L. and Lucy Moses Professor of Neurology, College of Physicians and Surgeons, Columbia University. Director, Department of Neurology, Neurological Institute, Presbyterian Hospital, New York, New York.

GERALD F. M. RUSSELL, M.D., F.R.C.P., F.R.C.P.Ed., F.R.C.Psych.

Anorexia Nervosa

Professor of Psychiatry, Royal Free Hospital School of Medicine, University of London. Consultant Psychiatrist, Royal Free Hospital, London, England.

JAY P. SANFORD, M.D.

Hospital-Associated Infections: Endogenous Microbial Disease; Klebsiella and Other Gram-Negative Bacterial Pneumonias; Leptospirosis

Professor of Internal Medicine, University of Texas Southwestern Medical School. Chief, Infectious Disease Service and Microbiology Laboratory, Parkland Memorial Hospital, Dallas; Consultant in Internal Medicine, Dallas and Temple, Texas, Veterans Administration Hospitals, Brooke General Hospital, and Wilford Hall USAF Hospital, San Antonio; Attending Physician, Parkland Memorial, Presbyterian, and St. Paul Hospitals, Dallas, Texas.

PAUL D. SAVILLE, M.D., F.R.C.P.

Osteomyelitis; Osteonecrosis; Congenital and/or Hereditary Disorders Involving Bone; Paget's Disease of Bone: Osteitis Deformans; Fibrous Dysplasia; Hypertrophic Osteoarthropathy; Tumors of Bone

Professor of Medicine, Creighton University and University of Nebraska. Director, Metabolic Research Laboratory, and Chief, Rheumatology Service, Creighton University; Chief of Rheumatology, University of Nebraska, Omaha, Nebraska.

LABE C. SCHEINBERG, M.D.

The Demyelinating Diseases

Professor of Neurology, Albert Einstein College of Medicine. Director of Neurology, St. Barnabas Hospital, Bronx, New York.

RUDI SCHMID, M.D., Ph.D.

Porphyria

Professor of Internal Medicine, University of California, San Francisco, School of Medicine. Attending Physician, Moffitt-University Hospital, San Francisco, California.

RICHARD P. SCHMIDT, M.D.

Neurologic Diagnostic Procedures

Dean, College of Medicine, and Professor of Neurology, State University of New York, Upstate Medical Center. Attending Neurologist, University Hospital, Syracuse; Consultant, Veterans Administration Hospital, Syracuse, New York.

GEORGE E. SCHREINER, M.D.

Toxic Nephropathy; Cysts of the Kidney; Tumors of the Kidney; Miscellaneous Renal Disorders

Professor of Medicine, Georgetown University School of Medicine. Director, Nephrology Division, Georgetown University Hospital, Washington, D. C.

PETER H. SCHUR, M.D.

Systemic Lupus Erythematosus

Associate Professor of Medicine, Harvard Medical School. Physician, Robert B. Brigham Hospital, Boston; Senior Associate in Medicine, Peter Bent Brigham Hospital, Boston, Massachusetts.

WILLIAM B. SCHWARTZ, M.D.

The Nephropathy of Potassium Depletion; The Nephropathy of Hypercalcemia; Renal Tubular Acidosis; The Nephropathy of Acute Hyperuricemia; Balkan Nephritis; Analgesic Nephropathy; Disorders of Fluid, Electrolyte, and Acid-Base Balance

Endicott Professor of Internal Medicine, Tufts University School of Medicine. Physician-in-Chief, Tufts–New England Medical Center Hospital, Boston, Massachusetts.

NEVIN S. SCRIMSHAW, Ph.D., M.D.

Nutrient Requirements; Assessment of Nutritional Status; Nutrition and Infection; Kwashiorkor, Marasmus, and Intermediate Forms of Protein-Calorie Malnutrition; Undernutrition, Starvation, and Hunger Edema; Deficiencies of Individual Nutrients: Vitamin Diseases

Professor of Human Nutrition and Head, Department of Nutrition and Food Science, Massachusetts Institute of Technology, Cambridge, Massachusetts.

CHARLES R. SCRIVER, M.D., C.M., F.R.S.C.

Inborn Errors of Amino Acid Metabolism

Professor of Pediatrics and Associate Professor of Biology, McGill University. Physician, Montreal Children's Hospital; Director, DeBelle Laboratory for Biochemical Genetics, McGill University–Montreal Children's Hospital Research Institute, Montreal, Quebec, Canada; Co-Director, MRC Genetics Group.

SOL SHERRY, M.D.

Thromboembolic Diseases

Professor and Chairman, Department of Medicine, Temple University School of Medicine. Physician-in-Chief, Temple University Hospital, Philadelphia, Pennsylvania.

JAMES B. SIDBURY, Jr., M.D.

Glycogen Storage Disease; Pentosuria; Fructosuria and Hereditary Fructose Intolerance

Professor of Pediatrics, Duke University School of Medicine, Durham, North Carolina.

DONALD H. SILBERBERG, M.D.

Encephalitic Complications of Viral Infections and Vaccines

Professor of Neurology, School of Medicine, University of Pennsylvania. Neurologist, Hospital of the University of Pennsylvania; Consultant in Neurology, Veterans Administration Hospital, Philadelphia, Pennsylvania.

RICHARD T. SILVER, M.D.

Leukemoid Reactions; Myeloproliferative Disorders

Professor of Clinical Medicine, Cornell University Medical College. Attending Physician, The New York Hospital, New York, New York.

MARVIN H. SLEISENGER, M.D.

Diseases of the Digestive System: Introduction; Diseases of Malabsorption; Other Inflammatory Diseases of the Intestine

Professor and Vice Chairman, Department of Medicine, University of California, San Francisco. Chief, Medical Service, Ft. Miley Veterans Administration Hospital, San Francisco, California.

JAMES P. SMITH, M.D.

Respiratory Failure and Its Management

Clinical Associate Professor of Medicine, Cornell University Medical College. Associate Attending Physician and Head, Respiratory Care Unit, The New York Hospital, New York, New York.

LLOYD H. SMITH, Jr., M.D.

Primary Hyperoxaluria; Disorders of Purine Metabolism; Disorders of Pyrimidine Metabolism

Professor and Chairman, Department of Medicine, School of Medicine, University of California, San Francisco, California.

CHARLES J. STAHL, M.D.

Drowning

Professorial Lecturer in Forensic Science, Graduate School of Arts and Sciences, The George Washington University. Captain, Medical Corps, United States Navy. Chief, Forensic Sciences Division, and Registrar, Registry of Forensic Pathology, Armed Forces Institute of Pathology, Washington, D.C.; Consultant in Forensic Pathology, Professional Division, Bureau of Medicine and Surgery, Department of the Navy, Washington, D.C.

GENE H. STOLLERMAN, M.D.

Streptococcal Diseases: Introduction; Group A Streptococcal Infection; Clinical Syndromes of Group A Streptococcal Infection; Treatment of Group A Streptococcal Infection and Chemoprophylaxis of Nonsuppurative Complications; Prophylaxis of Streptococcal Infection

Professor and Chairman, Department of Medicine, University of Tennessee College of Medicine. Physician in Chief, City of Memphis Hospital, Memphis, Tennessee.

MORTON N. SWARTZ, M.D.

Parameningeal Infections

Professor of Medicine, Harvard Medical School. Chief, Infectious Disease Unit, Massachusetts General Hospital, Boston, Massachusetts.

WILLIAM C. THOMAS, Jr., M.D.

Renal Calculi

Professor of Medicine, University of Florida College of Medicine. Associate Chief of Staff for Research, Veterans Administration Hospital, Gainesville, Florida.

H. RICHARD TYLER, M.D.

Polymyositis and Dermatomyositis

Associate Professor of Neurology, Harvard University. Physician and Head, Section of Neurology, Peter Bent Brigham Hospital, Boston; Consultant in Neurology, Children's Hospital Medical Center, Beth Israel, Hospital for Women, Robert B. Brigham Hospital and West Roxbury Veterans Administration Hospital, Boston, Massachusetts.

JOHN P. UTZ, M.D.

Actinomycosis; The Mycoses: Introduction; Histoplasmosis; Blastomycosis; Paracoccidioidomycosis; Maduromycosis; Chromomycosis; Sporotrichosis

Professor of Medicine, School of Medicine, Georgetown University, Washington, D.C.

WILLIAM N. VALENTINE, M.D.

The Leukopenic State and Agranulocytosis; Infectious Mononucleosis

Professor of Medicine, University of California at Los Angeles. Senior Attending Physician, Veterans Administration Center, Los Angeles, California.

NIEL WALD, M.D.

Radiation Injury

Professor and Chairman, Department of Radiation Health, and Professor of Radiology, Graduate School of Public Health and School of Medicine, University of Pittsburgh. Active Medical Staff (Radiology) and Director, Radiation Medicine Department, Presbyterian-University Hospital, Pittsburgh; Consultant Staff, Children's Hospital of Pittsburgh, Pittsburgh, and Aliquippa Hospital, Aliquippa, Pennsylvania.

JOHN H. WALSH, M.D.

Peptic Ulcer: Clinical and Endocrine Aspects

Associate Professor of Medicine, University of California, Los Angeles, California.

KENNETH S. WARREN, M.D.

Schistosomiasis

Associate Professor of Medicine, Case Western Reserve University School of Medicine. Assistant Physician, University Hospitals, Cleveland, Ohio.

M. F. R. WATERS, M.A., M.B., M.R.C.Path., F.R.C.P.

Leprosy

Member of the Senior Scientific Staff, British Medical Research Council. Director, Leprosy Research Unit, National Leprosy Control Centre, Sungei Buloh, Selangor, Malaysia.

LAWRENCE W. WAY, M.D.

Diseases of the Gallbladder and Bile Ducts

Associate Professor of Surgery, University of California School of Medicine, San Francisco. Chief of Surgery, Ft. Miley Veterans Administration Hospital, San Francisco, California.

PAUL WEBB, M.D.

Disorders Due to Heat and Cold

Principal Associate, Webb Associates, Yellow Springs, Ohio. Associate Professor of Preventive Medicine, The Ohio State University.

ROBERT I. WEED, M.D.

Diseases of the Spleen

Professor of Medicine and of Radiation Biology and Biophysics, University of Rochester School of Medicine and Dentistry. Staff, Strong Memorial Hospital, Rochester, New York.

CLAYTON E. WHEELER, Jr., M.D.

Orf; Molluscum Contagiosum; Certain Cutaneous Diseases with Significant Systemic Manifestations: Introduction;

Cutaneous Manifestations of Internal Malignancy; Erythemas; Contact Dermatitis; Behçet's Disease; Pemphigus; Acanthosis Nigricans; Mast Cell Disease; Lethal Cutaneous and Gastrointestinal Arteriolar Thrombosis; Angiokeratoma Corporis Diffusum; Incontinentia Pigmenti; Hereditary Anhidrotic Ectodermal Defect; Neurofibromatosis of von Recklinghausen; Ainhum; Toxic Epidermal Necrolysis; Ehlers-Danlos Syndrome; Pseudoxanthoma Elasticum

Professor of Dermatology, University of North Carolina School of Medicine. Chairman, Department of Dermatology, North Carolina Memorial Hospital, Chapel Hill, North Carolina.

M. HENRY WILLIAMS, Jr., M.D.

Respiratory Disease: Introduction; Pulmonary Structure and Function: Introduction; Ventilatory Function; Conducting Airways; Alveolar Structure and Function; Pulmonary Circulation; Disability Evaluation; Hypoxemia

Professor of Medicine, Albert Einstein College of Medicine. Director, Chest Service, Bronx Municipal Hospital Center, Bronx, New York.

EMANUEL WOLINSKY, M.D.

Clostridial Diseases: Introduction; Clostridial Myonecrosis; Other Clostridial Diseases; Clostridial Gastroenteritis

Professor of Medicine, Case Western Reserve University School of Medicine. Chief, Division of Infectious Diseases, and Director of Microbiology, Cleveland Metropolitan General Hospital, Cleveland, Ohio.

THEODORE E. WOODWARD, M.D.

Tularemia

Professor of Medicine, University of Maryland School of Medicine. Physician-in-Chief, University of Maryland Hospital, Baltimore, Maryland.

OLIVER M. WRONG, D.M., F.R.C.P.

Glomerular Disease

Professor of Medicine, University College Hospital Medical School, London. Consultant Physician, University College Hospital, London, England.

JAMES B. WYNGAARDEN, M.D.

The Use and Interpretation of Laboratory-Derived Data

Professor and Chairman, Department of Medicine, Duke University Medical School, Durham, North Carolina.

MELVIN D. YAHR, M.D.

The Extrapyramidal Disorders: Introduction; The Parkinsonian Syndrome; Essential Tremor; Senile Tremor; The Choreas; Tics; Athetosis; Dystonia Musculorum Deformans; Spasmodic Torticollis; Hemiballism

Henry P. and Georgette Goldschmidt Professor of Neurology and Chairman, Department of Neurology, Mt. Sinai Hospital. Neurologist-in-Chief, Department of Neurology, Mt. Sinai Medical Center, New York, New York.

LAWRENCE E. YOUNG, M.D.

Hemolytic Disorders: Introduction; Intracorpuscular Abnormalities

Alumni Distinguished Service Professor of Medicine, University of Rochester School of Medicine and Dentistry. Director, University of Rochester Associated Hospitals Program in Internal Medicine, Rochester, New York.

Contents

VOLUME I

PART I. THE NATURE OF MEDICINE

PART II. GENETIC PRINCIPLES

PART III. ENVIRONMENTAL FACTORS IN DISEASE

PART IV. IMMUNE DISEASE

PART V. CONNECTIVE TISSUE DISEASES ("COLLAGEN DISEASES") OTHER THAN RHEUMATOID ARTHRITIS

PART VI. DISEASES OF THE JOINTS, *Charles L. Christian*

PART X. DISORDERS OF THE NERVOUS SYSTEM AND BEHAVIOR

PART XIII. RENAL DISEASES

PART XIV. DISEASES OF THE DIGESTIVE SYSTEM

PART XV. DISEASES OF NUTRITION

SECTION FIFTEEN. HEMORRHAGIC DISORDERS: COAGULATION DEFECTS, *Oscar D. Ratnoff,* 1564

PART XVII. DISEASES OF METABOLISM

PART XVIII. DISEASES OF THE ENDOCRINE SYSTEM

PART XIX. DISEASES OF BONE

PART XXII. NORMAL LABORATORY VALUES OF CLINICAL IMPORTANCE

Part I
THE NATURE OF MEDICINE

1. ON BECOMING A CLINICIAN

Paul B. Beeson

This essay is addressed to the student entering upon the study of clinical medicine. To leaf through a modern medical textbook for the first time must be a daunting experience for you. How can anyone hope to master so much scientific and technical information? The task *is* difficult, indeed impossible. Nevertheless, some encouragement should come from observing that senior medical students and young doctors on the hospital staff appear to have made a satisfactory adjustment to the challenge. Furthermore, as your acquaintance with clinical teachers grows, you will observe that although each of them has special knowledge and experience in some area of clinical medicine, he makes no pretense of knowing it all. You will also find that clinicians frequently disagree, and that each of them comes to wrong conclusions from time to time. Clinical teachers must in fact appear to be very different from those under whom your preclinical work was done. Biochemists and pharmacologists have "hard" facts to propound. We, on the other hand, deal with such commodities as pain and nausea. We must accept any kind of problem. We cannot insist on working with inbred strains of people, we cannot control the environment from which they come, we know that their recollection of past events is faulty, and we cannot reduce them to subcellular fractions in order to determine what is going on. We must even question the opinions of our colleagues. We live, therefore, in an atmosphere of doubt and uncertainty, and make our decisions and take our actions on the basis of probabilities. You will have the same handicaps, and you too will make mistakes. Simply try to ensure that each mistake constitutes a learning experience which leaves you a better doctor.

A word of encouragement can be inserted here. Students as a rule accommodate to clinical medicine with astonishing speed. I never cease to be surprised at the progress they make during the first few years. They learn by their own study and practice, by attending lectures and conferences, by observing senior people at work, and by informal discussions with fellow students and housemen in ward offices, corridors, and dining rooms. Good-natured arguments facilitate the process, because debate tends to fix the information that emerges. In that connection you will find it helpful to adopt a habit of offering your point of view tentatively rather than in the form of a positive assertion.

But how should you *begin* the study of clinical medicine? I have not found it helpful (except as an editor!) to read a book like this in systematic cover-to-cover fashion. In my judgment, you should use it the way the mature clinician does, as a place in which information can be obtained about problems being dealt with at the time. Inasmuch as common disorders occur commonly, this practice will in good time ensure that you will have read and thought about such frequently encountered disorders as peptic ulcer, angina pectoris, and urinary tract infection. Furthermore, although at first glance a medical text seems to be a sort of dictionary describing hundreds of unrelated entities, you will find that knowledge of one helps the study of another, because there often are dovetailing aspects or useful contrasts. You should make it a rule to examine the references which accompany the discussions, and to consult some of them. That is the kind of study doctors must carry on for themselves throughout life. Reading in connection with specific clinical problems is likely to provide knowledge that sticks.

What about the many uncommon maladies described in textbooks? The student of any age really needs only to know how to find out about them. One test of a good doctor is whether he can come to a correct diagnosis even though he has never met the disease before.

Medical knowledge and practice are continually changing. In order to incorporate the steady flow of new information, a textbook must be extensively rewritten every few years. Let me illustrate this by citing an example of changes that have taken place during my own clinical career. The third edition of this book, which appeared in 1933, the year I graduated from medical school, contained a chapter on nephritis by H. A. Christian, Professor of Medicine at Harvard and Physician-in-Chief to the Peter Bent Brigham Hospital. Christian had been a leader in American medicine since early in the century and had made important contributions to a wide range of subjects. His name is still attached to the Hand-Schüller-Christian and Weber-Christian syndromes. His chapter on nephritis employed this classification:

1. Acute and subacute nephritis
    (a) With renal edema (nephrosis syndrome)
    (b) Hemorrhagic nephritis
2. Chronic nephritis
    (a) With renal edema
    (b) Without renal edema
3. Essential hypertension progressing into chronic nephritis
4. Renal arteriosclerosis progressing into chronic nephritis

His approach to renal disease was based on history, physical examination, blood pressure, urinalysis, and observation of the clinical course. Most of today's "routine" biochemical determinations were not available to him, though he knew of course that elevated blood urea and acidosis are characteristic of renal failure. His treatment of all forms of nephritis was mainly rest and diet. Now compare that perspective of kidney disease with the discussions in the current edition, in chapters on Investigation of Renal Function, Glomerular Disease, Acute Tubular Necrosis, Nephrotic Syndrome, Arterial Hypertension, Chronic Pyelonephritis, Renal Disease in Pregnancy, the Nephropathy of Potassium Depletion, Hypercalcemia and Hyperuricemia, and Disorders of Fluid and Electrolyte Balance. You will note that the trend in terminology has shifted from purely descriptive to pathogenetic. Our current concepts and management have resulted from intensive study of renal diseases by clinicians who have specialized in the field and have been able to apply new biochemical, physiologic, and immunologic approaches, using sophisticated clinical chemistry, renal biopsy, electron microscopy, immunofluorescence, and similar procedures. Today's management makes use of a variety of effective pharmacologic preparations: diuretics, antimicrobials, corticosteroids, antihypertensives, and cytotoxic agents. Our understanding of fluid and electrolyte dynamics is based upon ready availability of good clinical biochemical methods. Our ultimate forms of treatment—hemodialysis and renal transplantation—involve scientific and technical developments scarcely imaginable in Christian's day.

The example cited is in no way unusual. Similar advances characterize every branch of general medicine. This kind of progress has been achieved largely by full-time clinical scientists working in medical schools and research institutes all over the world. They have concentrated on specific problems and have been greatly aided by new knowledge and techniques developed by other workers in biologic and physical sciences. Such investigation-in-depth is essential to the advancement of clinical medicine. We have for all time departed from the era of clinical "giants" like Christian who could be looked upon as authorities in many aspects of internal medicine. That is why a modern textbook must be compiled from the writings of scores of contributors.

The medical student should be aware that our exciting advances in medicine have *created* some serious new problems. Our therapy now makes use of powerful drugs, all of which can do harm. Few hospital patients receive less than half a dozen different medications. In addition to intrinsic toxicity these can interact with each other to produce unwanted effects. A substantial part of hospital medicine today is in fact devoted to overcoming untoward effects of therapy. Knowing when to stop a certain treatment is as important as knowing when to bring it into use. There are risks too in many of our present diagnostic procedures, e.g., a 1 per cent incidence of death or serious complication from coronary or cerebral angiography. We must acknowledge that the recent scientific and technologic explosion in clinical medicine has created its own kind of "pollution."

Having recognized the essential role of the specialist investigator in bringing about what are really immense advances in clinical medicine, we should give some consideration to the impact of this on trends in the practice of medicine as well as the training of future doctors. Does it follow, because we owe our advances in medical sciences to specialists, that the best medical care must be given by specialists? Shall we say to young people now entering the profession that the age of specialization is here, and advise each of them to select a narrow field for his or her medical practice?

I believe that in the actual provision of medical care there is still need for the generalist. Diseases do not always present themselves in pure culture, and in fact the perspective of the clinical scientist can sometimes be skewed. It seems fair to say, for example, that a good family doctor (now, alas, in short supply in America) can deal effectively with the great majority of episodes for which patients seek a doctor's help. When we focus on internal medicine, the field with which this book is concerned, it can be said with assurance that the well-trained internist, e.g., one who has been certified by the American Board of Internal Medicine or has attained Membership of the Royal College of Physicians, is capable of dealing with most medical illnesses, including those for which hospital care is required. To do that in exemplary fashion is, however, a full-time job, which does not permit substantial parts of the doctor's time and effort to be devoted to research. Inasmuch as a major responsibility of a university is acquisition of new knowledge, the funds available for salaries in medical school departments go mainly to doctors who are active investigators. Consequently, the medical student and the house officer in a teaching hospital may need to be reminded that outside the medical school orbit much excellent medical care is provided by generalist physicians. In the setting of a teaching hospital the clinical investigator can be a superb teacher of undergraduate and graduate medical students, and can, by combining forces with many other specialists in the institution, provide sophisticated medical service for the patients. This, however, is an expensive and somewhat inefficient way of offering medical care which, though well suited to the diverse functions of a teaching institution, does not make a realistic pattern for professional care in the larger community. Specialized skill, although essential to any good system of medical care, is not needed in the proportion found among the members of medical school faculties.

Can we have it both ways, even in our teaching centers? I think this is possible and desirable. Pressure from within and without will probably dictate some revising of present medical school priorities, though the schools must always support a high proportion of specialist investigators. But even today one finds occasional excellent generalists in medical schools, people who like the environment but do not wish to engage personally in research. They are likely to be the doctors who take care of their colleagues and their colleagues' families. They find satisfaction in dealing with a broad range of clinical problems and are willing to devote all their energies to clinical practice. They are confident of their ability to deal with most of the problems that come to them, yet have no hesitation about calling for specialist advice when they need it. They exercise some discrimination in their diagnostic approach and know when to cut corners.

One of the most important qualities needed by today's physician is ability to restrain his curiosity. He must constantly remind himself that a potentially injurious diagnostic procedure should only be carried out when possible benefit to the patient justifies the risk. A diagnostic test should never be done just for the sake of "thoroughness," that is to say, before someone else suggests that it be done, or because a specialist feels he must do it to protect his own reputation, "just in case. . . ." Let us speculate on how a good doctor would go about the care of an elderly patient who has recently developed obstructive jaundice. The *probability* is that this patient has neoplastic disease not amenable to surgery or chemotherapy. There is, however, the possibility that the biliary obstruction is caused by some other lesion such as stone or nonmalignant tumor. The doctor has many options. He can make use of a variety of remarkably accurate diagnostic procedures: barium x-ray studies, isotopic scan of the liver or pancreas, laparoscopy, needle biopsy of the liver, celiac angiography, or endoscopic probing of the duodenum (for cytology, or for cannulation and retrograde visualization of the biliary or pancreatic ducts). It is tempting to proceed with some or all of these procedures, because a precise diagnosis may well be achieved. But that may not be in the patient's interest in view of high probability of incurable disease. The doctor in charge can discuss with colleagues the chances of curative surgery or chemotherapy. Or he can do nothing further, feeling that the sensible option is to allow the disease to run its course, and spare the patient the discomfort, dangers, and expense of elaborate study. He may, however, choose a compromise: calling on a surgeon to operate without further delay, while the patient's general condition is still good, in order to treat definitively a nonmalignant lesion if there be one; or, if the obstruction is due to cancer, to divert the flow of bile into the intestine. This course would be likely at least to give the patient some months of comfortable life, even though the cancer is not treated. The good doctor will then "stay with" the patient, meeting problems as they come, as described so well by Dr. Myers in Ch. 3.

I close by offering a few precepts: (1) Each patient must be given *enough of your time.* Sit down; listen to him; ask thoughtful questions; examine him carefully; go back and do it again. So many medical mistakes are simply due to failure of the doctor to give enough time. (2) Work to develop your *ability to study* about your patient's clinical problems. (3) Train yourself to *concentrate on each problem to the exclusion of all else.* Here is the way Trotter, a great English neurosurgeon, put it:

> . . . As long as medicine is an art, its chief and characteristic instrument must be human faculty. We come therefore to the very practical question of what aspects of human faculty it is necessary for the good doctor to cultivate. . . . The first to be named must always be the power of attention, of giving one's whole mind to the patient without the interposition of oneself. It sounds simple but only the very greatest doctors ever fully attain it. It is an active process and not either mere resigned listening or even politely waiting until you can interrupt. Disease often tells its secrets in a casual parenthesis. . . .

If you will give each patient the time he deserves, if you will learn to concentrate, and if you can then study appropriately, you will have much of what it takes to care for people, even in today's world.

2. SCIENCE, CLINICAL MEDICINE, AND THE SPECTRUM OF DISEASE

Alvan R. Feinstein

A textbook of medicine contains concepts and data for at least two distinctly different types of clinical decisions. With *explicatory** decisions, doctors choose names, causes, and mechanisms that provide intellectual explanations for the ailments observed in patients. With *interventional* decisions, doctors choose therapeutic strategies intended to prevent or to remedy the ailments.

The explicatory decisions are often regarded as the main scientific activity of clinical medicine. For diagnostic selections, modern technology has allowed diseases to be identified more precisely than ever before. The morphologic abnormalities that formerly could be demonstrated only at necropsy are now often revealed during life with the aid of roentgenography, biopsy, cytology, or surgical exploration; and many other ailments that cannot be depicted morphologically are identified with the aid of chemical, microbial, electrophysiologic, or other laboratory procedures. For ideas about causes and mechanisms of disease, doctors have received scientific confirmation both from the diagnostic tests performed in individual patients and from the many experimental models that have been tested during clinical investigation. The explicatory decisions thus enable doctors to apply at the bedside the major advances that laboratory research has brought to diagnostic medical science.

A doctor's interventional decisions, on the other hand, are often regarded mainly as art. The pharmaceutical, surgical, and other agents used for therapeutic intervention are highly developed scientifically, but the decisions themselves are still often made as acts of judgment, generally unsupported by the type of scientific evidence that sustains the explicatory activities. The available evidence to prove the value of a treatment may be quantitatively defective, consisting mainly of anecdotal reports of clinical experiences that have not been thoroughly enumerated; or the evidence may seem qualitatively unappealing, depending on such "soft" data as a patient's pain, a family's anxiety, or an employer's forbearance.

With medical activities demarcated into explicatory science and interventional art, a medical student (or a practicing clinician) often develops the belief that the purely clinical work of patient care does not present any scientific challenges. According to this belief, a clinician's principal science is contained in the "workup" that reveals diagnostic names and pathogenetic mechanisms. Once this challenge is completed, no further scientific thinking may seem necessary. After choosing a therapeutic agent according to the established diagnosis, the clinician would need only the arts of human perception and communication for telling the patient what is wrong and what is planned.

Despite popular acceptance, this demarcation of art and science in clinical work has at least three major inaccuracies. The demarcation is based on the idea that science consists only of explication, but science contains another major component: prediction. In dealing with a sick patient, a clinician is scientifically challenged not merely to explain what is wrong and how it went wrong, but also to predict what may happen and how its occurrence can be altered. To perform these predictions, a clinician must make the type of interventional decisions with which prognosis is estimated, therapy chosen, and results evaluated. A second conceptual error arises from the belief that the choice of treatment depends almost entirely on a diagnostic citation. Although diagnosis is usually an important first step, the scientific selection and appraisal of therapy require analysis of data much more intricate than the mere identification of a disease. The most cogent information often includes symptoms, signs, and other clinical phenomena rather than a diagnostic title alone. A third misconception is the idea that important clinical phenomena cannot be expressed in "hard" scientific terms because the descriptions usually contain verbal categories rather than measured dimensions. The fallacy here is that "hard" information must be precise and reproducible, but it need not be dimensional. Some of the outstanding accomplishments of biologic science—including the work of Darwin, Virchow, and modern geneticists and electron microscopists—have been based on precise, reproducible, but nondimensional descriptions. With better standards of observation and classification, the verbal categories of "soft" clinical data could readily be improved into "hard" scientific quality.

Even when these attributes of clinical work are recognized, they may be regarded as scientifically unimportant because ordinary medical practice does not provide the experimental challenges offered by laboratory re-

*The word *explicatory* is used here to refer to diagnostic citations or pathogenetic explanations or both.

search. This belief is also inappropriate, however, because every act of clinical therapy is constructed in the same architectural sequence used for an experiment: a prepared entity is exposed to a planned maneuver and undergoes an observed response. This basic construction of an experiment can be used to outline all of a doctor's interventional decisions in clinical practice.

Despite similar challenges in the applicability of scientific methods, the "experiments" of the laboratory and bedside contain major differences in goals, reasoning, and procedures. In motive, the laboratory investigator seeks to understand how nature works and what it does; the clinician wants to change what nature has done or to thwart what it might do. In hypothesis, the laboratory investigator is innovative, wanting to test a new idea; the clinician is repetitive, wanting to reproduce the successful result achieved with the therapy used in a similar situation of the past. In cause-effect comparisons, the laboratory investigator can contrast the results of a concurrent "control group"; the clinician often relies on the "historical controls" of previous experience. In choice of data, the laboratory investigator can confine his observations only to the immediate events that seem most pertinent; the clinician must note all phenomena that can indicate a change in the patient's medical condition and way of life. These major differences in orientation require different strategies for the scientific methods used in the experiments of laboratory explication or clinical intervention, but both sets of activities offer the intellectual challenges of planning and evaluating an experiment.

In contemporary medicine, however, the methods used for acquiring and analyzing clinical data are not yet as scientifically well developed as the techniques that have been employed in laboratory research. Consequently, a doctor's explicatory decisions are often supported by excellent scientific evidence, but the interventional decisions are not. The purely clinical activities of contemporary medicine may thus seem more like art than science. The scientific improvement of this clinical art offers a prime target for future research, but in the meantime the reader of any compendium of clinical knowledge must deal with the state of the art in its existing form. The rest of this chapter will be concerned with certain caveats to help warn about some of the imperfections, and with a few suggestions to help resolve some of the difficulties.

One of the principal problems arises from the complex clinical spectrum associated with a disease. With increasing frequency in modern medicine, diseases are diagnostically identified as abnormalities not in a patient's clinical state (such as fever, jaundice, or chest pain), but in a paraclinical entity. The paraclinical abnormalities of disease can be diagnostically cited in such terms as morphologic structure *(coronary artery disease, carcinoma)*, biochemical function *(diabetes mellitus, hyperthyroidism)*, physiologic function *(atrial fibrillation, malabsorption)* or microbial invasion *(viral infection, meningococcemia)*. Although the aid of modern diagnostic technology allows these paraclinical abnormalities to be diagnosed with unprecedented specificity and consistency, the principal "lesion" of each such paraclinical disease has an associated spectrum of diverse clinical manifestations that may not always occur specifically or consistently.

Some of the clinical manifestations represent the primary effects of the disease's principal abnormality, whereas other manifestations can be regarded as secondary effects or complications. In coronary artery disease, for example, angina pectoris is a primary effect and congestive heart failure is secondary. In peptic ulcer, pain is a primary effect and pyloric obstruction is secondary. Since different primary and secondary manifestations can appear alone or in various overlapping combinations, the disease in a particular patient may occur with some, all, or none of the possible clinical manifestations. An illustration of the diverse clinical spectrum that can be associated with a single disease is shown in the Venn diagram for lung cancer in Ch. 540. Certain patients with lung cancer may be wholly asymptomatic; others can have primary features, such as hemoptysis; others can have the secondary features of systemic or metastatic manifestations; and yet others may have various combinations of these primary and secondary elements. The complexity of a disease's spectrum will thus produce subsets of patients who have the same diagnosis but different clinical manifestations, and who may also differ in prognosis and therapy.

The existence of these different subsets creates important defects in any "textbook picture of disease." Since the author can seldom describe all the diverse possibilities, the "classic" textbook description is usually based on the most common or pathognomonic manifestations. The reader who expects that the disease will always occur in this classic manner may then be surprised, perplexed, or dismayed by the many occasions in which a patient appears from a less common subset. A quantitative example of subset distributions is shown in the disease spectrum shown in Ch. 540. The most common single subset in the 1032 instances of lung cancer consisted of 340 patients with the concurrence of pulmonic and systemic manifestations; but 70 patients were wholly asymptomatic, and 34 had metastatic features only. Similarly, coronary artery disease can occur without angina pectoris in certain patients who have no symptoms or in others with manifestations only of congestive heart failure; hepatitis may first be found as advanced cirrhosis in a patient who never had jaundice.

The occurrence of an asymptomatic subset in a disease's spectrum is responsible for the frequent practice of "screening" in modern medicine. The purpose of the screening tests is to find the disease in circumstances in which it has produced no overt manifestations to arouse diagnostic suspicion. The occurrence of the many diverse subsets in a disease's spectrum is also responsible for some of the major current difficulties in evaluating prognosis and therapy. Despite similarity in diagnosis, the patients in the different subsets may have striking differences in prognosis. For example, Table 1 in Ch. 540 shows that the six-month survival rate for patients with lung cancer was 44 per cent, but the rate ranged from 84 per cent in the localized asymptomatic subset to 14 per cent in the worst of the metastatic subsets. In acute myocardial infarction, a patient with only chest pain has a much better prognosis than a patient with shock and pulmonary edema.

These natural prognostic distinctions will substantially affect the selection and appraisal of therapy. Since the "experiments" of routine clinical treatment are based on a repetitive hypothesis, a doctor chooses treatment for an individual patient by reviewing previous clinical experience, recalling the patients with similar manifestations, noting the outcomes of the therapy given to the "resemblance group," ascertaining which treatment gave the best result, and trying to reproduce that success in the current patient. To select the appropriate resemblance group, the doctor must have data for suitably demarcated subsets of patients.

Such data may not always be available. The results of previous treatment are often reported for all patients with the same disease, regardless of subsets; or the subsets distinguished in the reported results may be different from the particular one in which a subsequent patient is encountered. The absence of these details often creates difficulty in choice of treatment for an individual patient and arouses controversy in comparative evaluations of treated groups. One physician, treating diabetes mellitus with Regimen X, may have had a group of patients whose prognostic expectations were substantially different from those of another physician's patients treated with Regimen Y. One surgeon's Stage I cancer patients may be predominantly asymptomatic, whereas another surgeon's Stage I patients may have a high proportion of weight loss and fatigue. During arguments about the merits of the compared therapy, the clinicians may not realize that some of the crucial post-therapeutic differences arose not from different methods of treatment, but from prognostic differences in the subsets who constituted the treated groups.

To this complexity of clinical subsets for a single disease is added the further complexity introduced by comorbidity and demography. Since an individual patient may have more than one disease, the presence of associated ailments will create extra subsets in the spectrum of the "principal" disease, and may produce pathologic effects that alter prognosis and treatment in those subsets. The number of potential subsets for a disease becomes even larger when the cited clinical and co-morbid demarcations are augmented by such demographic features as age, race, sex, and occupation.

This enormous variability of individual patients and diseases would pose insurmountable problems in clinical decisions if each decision depended on determining a unique subset for that patient and on having adequate background information for previous experience with that subset. Fortunately, many small subsets can be combined into larger "determinant" groups for which therapeutic decisions can be based on satisfactory amounts of previous data or experience. For example, a patient with acute rheumatic fever is usually treated with salicylate if there is no clinical evidence of carditis, and with steroids if severe carditis is present. In this decision, the *no carditis* and *severe carditis* groups act as therapeutically determinant subsets, regardless of the many smaller subgroups into which the patients could be classified by virtue of demography or other clinical phenomena. The selection of therapeutically determinant "super" subsets has traditionally been a fundamental decision in clinical judgment. With the availability of electronic data processing and computers to help in the analysis of previous experience, future judgments can be supported with an improved quantification in both subsets and data.

A different type of therapeutic intervention is aimed not at a disease or a determinant subset, but at a specific clinical manifestation, such as pain, constipation, or insomnia. Thus a patient may receive an antimicrobial drug for the disease pneumococcal pneumonia, but codeine for the associated symptom of pleuritic pain; radiation or chemotherapy may be given for Hodgkin's disease and blood transfusions for the associated weakness and anemia. For patients with acute myocardial infarction, the only treatment directed at the disease itself is bed rest. All other treatments are chosen according to the associated clinical manifestations: e.g., narcotics or analgesics for pain, diuretics or digitalis for congestive heart failure, and appropriate agents for arrhythmia.

For the many minor ailments encountered in primary medical care or family practice, a specific disease may not be diagnosed and treatment may be intended only to relieve symptoms. Encountering such ailments as an upper respiratory infection, a sprained muscle, or a gastrointestinal upset, the practitioner may decide prognostically that the ailment is self-limited and does not require more extensive diagnostic or therapeutic efforts. Another common event in general medical practice is a temporary, acute exacerbation of a chronic major ailment that has been relatively stable. In these events, which may occur in such conditions as chronic alcoholism, irritable colon syndrome, or neurotic anxiety, patients are also often treated for symptoms only.

In all the circumstances just described, the clinician's scientific challenges in interventional decisions were to determine the target(s) to be treated and to choose the best mode(s) of therapy. A different set of challenges consists of evaluating the patient's condition afterward to decide what the treatment accomplished and whether it has been successful. For this purpose, the clinician again often uses individual manifestations, rather than a disease diagnosis, as an index of accomplishment. Furthermore, the evaluation of a particular response may depend on graded subsets composed of changes in clinical manifestations. Thus the effect of treatment on congestive heart failure may be called *excellent* if both dyspnea and edema disappear; *fair* if one disappears while the other remains; and *poor* if both remain.

The data used to identify transitions in clinical state often require additional details that may not have been necessary for decisions about diagnosis, prognosis, and therapy. For example, a description of substernal chest pain provoked by exertion and relieved by rest will often suffice for a clinical diagnosis of coronary artery disease, but the evaluation of response of the angina to treatment will usually depend on further information about its frequency and the associated amounts of exertion or rest. Similarly, the amount of jaundice may not be crucial for a diagnosis of hepatitis, but may be a valuable index of therapeutic response. Other examples of clinical details that are sometimes diagnostically unimportant but therapeutically valuable are the patient's weight (in treatment of edematous congestive heart failure), the size of a massive spleen (in treatment of chronic monocytic leukemia), the frequency of bowel movements (in treatment of various gastrointestinal disorders), and the frequency of urination (in treatment of cystitis or prostatitis).

The challenges of directly communicating with patients are often regarded as a nonscientific form of clinical art, mainly because the contents of the communications, which are much more complex than any of the complexities already cited, create diverse data and subsets that are even more difficult to specify. Nevertheless, many of the decisions made during these communications require the intellectual discipline used by a scientist to select suitable information, organize data, recapitulate previous experience, and evaluate responses. The discipline of scientific reasoning may not contribute to a clinician's creative insight and artful perception in dealing with the personal attributes of people, but without such reasoning the insight and perception will often be used ineffectually.

Whether a practicing doctor is involved in decisions of communication, explication, or intervention, clinical medicine will always contain and unite elements of both art and science. The complexity of people and human ailments will demand many artful judgments that cannot be expressed in scientific terms, but a scientific discipline is required for the optimal use of modern technology in identifying, explaining, preventing, or treating the ailments. To be properly adapted to its human recipients, this scientific discipline must contain suitable provision for the important personal and clinical information that is not perceived with "scientific" equipment or expressed in "scientific" dimensions. The art and science of clinical medicine are intermingled, symbiotic, and inseparable. Without the art, there can be no data for the science. Without the science, there can be no reason for the art.

3. THE CARE OF THE PATIENT WITH TERMINAL ILLNESS

W. P. L. Myers

There is perhaps no more controversial medical issue of our time than that dealing with the care of the patient with terminal illness. Endless articles in the lay press dealing with death and dying, death with dignity, a patient's right to die, euthanasia, and so forth are testimony to the enormous interest and concern of the public and to the confusion that abounds. It is not the intent of this chapter to sort out these conflicting attitudes and beliefs, but rather to provide an approach to the problem for the student of medicine. Final answers cannot be written, but the reader will find an approach that is based on long personal experience with terminal illness and on the premise that it is the individual that matters. It is necessary to understand this at the outset, because an entirely different approach could be adopted if one proceeded on the premise that it is the greatest good for the greatest number of people that matters.

The Hippocratic oath demands of each of us that we practice our art for the benefit of our patients. Implicit in this charge is the preservation of life. Nowhere in the original or in its modern version does the word "prolong" appear, with respect to a patient's life. "Prolong" is a word that has come to mean the unnecessary continuation of life in a setting in which, usually in the eyes of a patient's family, recovery is impossible. It is a word most used by the laity because, in general, physicians do not view their efforts in these terms. They are more likely to take the long view and consider that their efforts should be to preserve life, since such efforts are in the main to be equated with what is beneficial for the patient. Therapeutic efforts in a seemingly hopeless situation can be viewed by the patient's family as needless efforts to prolong life, whereas the physician, from his vantage point of seeing a disease in perspective, may regard the same efforts as fully justifiable in terms of his obligation to the patient. The dilemma that arises, however, is that there are those who reasonably question preservation of life as the sole objective of treatment. The physician must always act in his patient's interests, but undoubtedly there are situations in which these are not best served by endless efforts to preserve life. Where does the physician draw the line? How is he to tell when to pursue treatment aggressively and when not to? Are there any guideposts?

MEDICAL ANALYSIS OF TERMINAL ILLNESS

It is important at the outset to define "terminal illness," because an accurate medical analysis of a given situation is the keystone for all future considerations, both medical and humanitarian. How can we tell if a patient is terminally ill? This determination may tax all the skills a physician can muster, and yet he may end up defining a patient as terminally ill who would not be so regarded by another doctor. We must begin somewhere, however, and there is no better place to begin than to be sure that the medical details have been set forth and have been analyzed in the fullest. It has been said that all problems could be solved if one only knew the right questions to ask. One approach to the matter of determining whether a patient is, in fact, terminally ill is for the physician to ask himself a few brief questions. The seven questions listed below are presented with a cancer patient in mind, but they can serve as a model for this approach to other diseases as well:

1. Has the patient had a complete history and physical examination?
2. Is there histologic evidence of cancer, and where is the primary site?
3. Is the presenting problem caused by a second primary cancer?
4. What is the extent of the disease?
5. What medical complications, both those caused by the tumor and those unrelated to the tumor, exist?
6. What was the previous treatment, and was it adequate?
7. Is the disease process active and progressive or chronic and stable?

The answers to these questions are fundamental to the proper assessment of a patient's illness, all the more so if he has been categorized as terminally ill. The questions are considered in greater detail as follows:

Question 1: Has the patient had a complete history and physical examination? It is almost embarrassing to include such a question in a list of this sort, but many patients have been improperly designated as being terminally ill because of what *appears* to be, without the benefit of a complete history and physical examination. Unfortunately the reason for this is that such patients frequently are seen initially by those who lack interest or who are guided by an attitude of hopelessness, especially when it comes to cancer. The following case will serve to emphasize the importance of a complete history and physical examination:

The patient was a 62-year-old white man from Central America who had had mild intermittent diarrhea for several years. Six months before admission he had been treated for malignant lymphoma, histiocytic type, of the stomach. He did well subsequently, but in the week prior to admission he developed anorexia followed by watery diarrhea and rectal bleeding. He had been treated with prednisone, 30 mg daily, for five days before admission. On admission he was found to be febrile and his abdomen was distended and tender, but there was no rebound tenderness. His stool was positive for blood. There was no peripheral lymphadenopathy. It was assumed that he had recurrent intra-abdominal malignant lymphoma, and when he went into shock the day after admission, he was considered to be terminally ill. He responded briefly to medical measures, but shock recurred and he died on the third day after admission. Autopsy disclosed diffuse colonic amebiasis with perforation and peritonitis. There was no evidence of recurrent malignant lymphoma.

In retrospect, further inquiry into the patient's history of intermittent diarrhea should have been made, especially in view of the fact that he came from Central America. The presence of fever, abdominal distention, and rectal bleeding, even without overt signs of perforation at the time of admission, should have led to a more careful examination, in particular a proctoscopic examination, to establish the correct diagnosis. Even so, the patient might not have recovered, but at least he would have had treatment directed against the correct disease, which in this instance was non-neoplastic.

Question 2: Is there histologic evidence of cancer, and where is the primary site? Consignment of patients to the ranks of the "terminally ill" has occurred all too often without histologic evidence of cancer and especially without attempts to define a primary site, if a histologic diagnosis of cancer has been made. The latter does not always have a therapeutic implication, but often it does, notably in those instances in which tumors originate in the breast, prostate, and thyroid. The following is a case in point:

The patient was a 50-year-old man seen in the clinic because of abdominal complaints and back pain. Evidences of tumor were noted intra-abdominally as well as in the lungs and left supraclavicular area. The impression was that he had metastatic carcinoma probably of gastrointestinal tract origin, despite negative gastrointestinal x-rays. A subsequent biopsy of the left supraclavicular lymph node was interpreted as "metastatic carcinoma." The hopeless attitude expressed by one of the patient's attending physicians was brought out by the following note he entered in the patient's record:

"This unfortunate patient has hopeless cancer as evidenced by left supraclavicular nodes. Biopsy shows metastatic adenocarcinoma. The exact site of primary is not apparent. This is now a purely academic question. He has hopeless cancer originating in the upper abdomen and is suitable only for terminal care."

Fortunately, other physicians did not share this opinion, and, in the attempt to discover a primary site, an acid phosphatase was obtained. This proved to be markedly elevated, indicating a diagnosis of metastatic carcinoma of the prostate. After orchiectomy and estrogen therapy, a chest film showed regression of mediastinal disease, and the patient remained alive with his disease in remission for many months. He finally died about three and a half years after having been regarded by one physician as being suitable only for terminal care.

Question 3: Is the presenting problem caused by a second primary cancer? It is difficult for a patient, once treated for cancer, not to have all subsequent clinical disease interpreted as manifestations of the original cancer. A patient previously treated for cancer of the pancreas may now have advanced metastatic disease and correctly be considered terminally ill. But if the metastatic disease is, in fact, caused by a second primary cancer such as carcinoma of the breast, the patient may respond dramatically to hormonal treatment and be anything but terminally ill. This possibility must always be kept in mind, particularly when there has been an appreciable time interval between the diagnosis of the original tumor and the appearance of metastatic disease.

Question 4: What is the extent of the disease? The accurate assessment of the extent of a cancer is the major determinant of treatment. In general, surgery and radiotherapy are utilized for localized and regional disease, whereas systemic treatment is applied to disseminated disease. Patients whose extent of disease is incorrectly evaluated may receive the wrong treatment or may inappropriately be considered to be terminally ill. Obviously, jaundice in a patient with known cancer may or may not represent metastatic disease. Only by judging each manifestation on its own merits can a correct assessment of the extent of disease be made. Again, a case report will serve to emphasize this point:

A 41-year-old man was admitted to the hospital because of suspected recurrent islet cell cancer of the pancreas. He had undergone a subtotal pancreatectomy and splenectomy elsewhere, and although the operation was thought to have been curative, the patient subsequently developed recurrent hypoglycemia. He was referred for chemotherapy. Examination revealed slight hepatomegaly but no intra-abdominal masses. Although a celiac arteriogram and a liver scan suggested that a large metastasis was present in the right lobe of the liver, it was *not assumed* that the patient had nonresectable cancer. At operation, it was established that, contrary to the preoperative laboratory data, no metastasis existed in the liver and it was possible to resect a residual tumor in the head of the pancreas by means of a Whipple procedure. The patient is alive some three years later and is without evidence of recurrent disease.

In this case, an accurate appraisal of the extent of disease, as determined at surgery, led to definitive and hopefully curative treatment. Had the extent of disease been *assumed* to be nonresectable, the patient would have been subjected to noncurative forms of treatment.

Question 5: What medical complications, both those caused by the tumor and those unrelated to the tumor, exist? This question is really a corollary to the last one but deserves special emphasis because a metabolic or infectious complication may be more life-threatening than the underlying cancer, and often if properly identified and treated, the patient may not needlessly lose his life. The following case is illustrative:

A 64-year-old woman was admitted to the hospital with a diagnosis of mammary carcinoma metastatic to the brain. Two years previously she had undergone a left radical mastectomy for infiltrating duct carcinoma of the breast. She had had positive axillary nodes and received postoperative radiation therapy. She remained well until seven weeks before admission when she developed double vision and dysphagia. On examination she had bilateral ptosis and motor weakness of cranial nerve V bilaterally without sensory impairment. Shortly after admission she underwent emergency tracheostomy for severe stridor, and radiation therapy to the brain was begun. At this point a resident physician, unwilling to assume that everything was caused by metastatic cancer, observed: "This lady really has little evidence for spread of her breast carcinoma. . . . I am hard put to assign her neurologic signs to an anatomic lesion, especially bilateral jaw weakness without any impairment of the sensory component of cranial nerve V. Right now she has marked ptosis bilaterally and paresis of gaze in all directions – without any pupillary abnormalities! The quick fatigue in the jaw muscles brings up myasthenia gravis which could explain all her signs."

A test with edrophonium chloride confirmed the resident's suspicions and a diagnosis of myasthenia gravis was made. The radiation therapy to the brain was stopped and the patient has done very well on medical management of her myasthenia and has had no demonstrable recurrence of breast cancer during these past four years.

Question 6: What was the previous treatment, and was it adequate? Corollary: Was previous treatment in any way responsible for the patient's present problems? At times "terminal" situations arise because patients have not received adequate treatment. No patient should be so regarded without a careful review of the type and adequacy of prior treatment, including treatment of coexistent diseases unrelated to the primary one. Of course previous treatment may also cause problems which can be misinterpreted as manifestations of the underlying malignancy. For example, a rare but remarkable complication of radiotherapy, that of radiation nephritis, is illustrated by the following case:

The patient, a 63-year-old man, was admitted to the hospital for what ultimately proved to be a spindle and giant cell sarcoma of the duodenum which was treated by radiotherapy to the upper abdomen. Two months later, the patient was re-explored and radon seeds were inserted throughout the residual tumor mass. Six months later and during the ensuing 18 months the patient's course was marked by the gradual appearance of recurrent fluid accumulation (peripheral, peritoneal, pleural), hypertension, anemia, thrombopenia, albuminuria, and azotemia. He eventually succumbed to renal failure some 26 months after the initial radiotherapy had been given.

From a clinical viewpoint, the patient had been regarded as having had recurrent intra-abdominal cancer on the basis of a cytologic examination of the peritoneal fluid which was reported to have revealed malignant cells. However, at autopsy none of the organs or tissues showed evidence of residual tumor or metastases. The kidneys presented the classic picture of radiation nephritis, and in retrospect it was apparent that this lesion was responsible for the clinical findings. Had it been recognized that the patient did not have recurrent cancer but rather the renal complications of radiation therapy, it is possible that more aggressive measures directed at his renal failure might have altered the outcome.

Question 7: Is the disease process active and progressive or chronic and stable? There are many so-called terminal diseases, metastatic cancer among them, that pursue a chronic course. A patient may have metastases from a cancer for which we have no specific therapy and he may therefore be "written off" as terminally ill. However, the natural history of the cancer in that patient may not be progressive, and the physician should take this into account when forming his own appraisal of a patient with an incurable illness. In addition, rare but clearly documented, inexplicable remissions of advanced cancer have occurred, and these serve to remind us of the incompleteness of our knowledge and the fallibility of our judgments.

THE TRULY "TERMINAL" PATIENT

If the physician has asked the aforementioned questions and has satisfied himself that, in fact, his patient is nearing death from an illness which is progressive, unrelenting, and disseminated and which cannot be arrested or reversed in our present state of knowledge (or perhaps more accurately, ignorance), how then should he manage the problem? Here again, he should have an approach or way of thinking about the over-all problem and should use the technique of asking himself some further critical questions. The principal questions are these:

1. What does the patient know about his situation?
2. What is the patient's attitude regarding the prospect of death?
3. Does he have pain and, if so, is it being relieved?
4. Is the patient being comforted physically, mentally, and spiritually?
5. Is the physician prepared to give of himself to the patient and "go down to the wire" with him? As a corollary, is the physician willing to continue to think about the problems his patient presents until the end?
6. What is the attitude of the patient's family, and how is it being dealt with?
7. Is the patient undergoing experimental study, and, if so, are humanitarian principles being observed or compromised?

There may be other questions one could ask, but these will serve most situations, and they should be considered in some depth.

Question 1: What does the patient know about his situation? Too often the physician fails to ask this question and, if he does, he does not record it on the patient's chart, so there is no general knowledge of this among the various personnel caring for the patient. This, in turn, leads to a lack of coordination in treatment efforts. The care of a patient can be improved substantially if his understanding of his illness is brought to light and recorded in a manner that will permit all medical and nursing personnel involved to know and act accordingly.

By asking a patient what he understands about his illness, the physician provides an opportunity for the patient to tell the physician, directly or indirectly, how much he wants to know. Some patients are quite content to leave it all to the doctor, but usually, if given the opportunity, they will ask questions. There is no standard answer to a patient's question, but the physician should be truthful insofar as his answer goes. *Truth can always be supported by hope;* an outlook with a grave prognosis can be coupled, in a compassionate manner, with a positive statement regarding what the physician plans to do and how other patients have responded under similar circumstances. Although this approach is not uniformly followed by the medical profession, it is increasingly so, because doctors have come to know that the erosion of trust between themselves and their patients, created by a failure to tell a patient as much truth as the doctor believes the patient seeks to know, is a more severe blow to the patient than dealing with the truth. There is no need, however, to tell the patient all the details, particularly in view of the fact that our fallibility could lead us to tell a patient more than we know. In addition, by seeking to know what the patient understands, the physician can correct misconceptions which are often the basis of fear and anxiety. Relief of these major burdens of a terminally ill patient should be of primary concern to the physician.

Attempts by a patient's family to persuade the physician to go along with an outright lie regarding the patient's illness should never be acceded to. Good intentions were never more misplaced; the lie creates further problems and is an insult to the patient. In addition, seriously ill patients usually know they are seriously ill, and explanations that do not seem likely create fear that the patient's doctor does not know the real diagnosis. This torment can be worse than the knowledge of the primary illness.

Question 2: What is the patient's attitude regarding the prospect of death? Attitudes toward death and dying are being more openly discussed and analyzed than ever before. The patient stricken with a fatal illness has been noted as going through various stages which have been categorized, progressively, as denial, anger, bargaining, depression, and, ultimately, acceptance (Kübler-Ross). This dissection is useful because it can form a basis for a physician's approach to his patient. For example, understanding that a patient's anger (which may be directed at the physician) is part of the unfolding reaction to his illness permits the physician to deal with this in a helpful rather than defensive manner. Learning about a patient's attitude takes time which a physician may be unwilling or unable to spend. In addition, a physician may be at a loss as to how to broach the subject, although usually this only requires that one give a patient the realization that he will be listened to. This obviously entails choosing a proper time, such as returning to see the patient after regular rounds. The press of time may not always permit this, and under these and other circumstances, the physician would do well to enlist the help of a clergyman or rabbi, preferably the patient's, or if he doesn't have one, the hospital chaplain or rabbi.

There are times when a patient will feel freer to discuss his or her attitude about death with the spiritual adviser than with the physician, and the adviser can be of enormous help in these situations. The fear of death is a human emotion widely considered in any discussion of death and dying, but the fear of *not* dying has received little attention. Patients may seek assurances from a clergyman that death is imminent, believing that the physician will not provide such assurances because doing so would be a denial of his role in preserving life.

Those who have had experience in the care of dying patients will not have failed to be impressed with the peace that patients experience when they have become convinced of the inevitability of their own death. Rhoads has written of this penultimate moment: "It was as if tearing away the veil of uncertainty at the same time released him from fear. He became calm, gentle, considerate of those about him, assuming a new dignity, as if he had already partly crossed the threshold."

Question 3: Does the patient have pain, and, if so, is it being relieved? The specter of death being painful is firmly rooted in the lay mind, and there is no doubt that osseous metastases, nerve root compression or infiltration, ischemic neuritis, and so forth can cause great pain. Yet pain as a major feature of terminal illness is uncommon. When it occurs it is essential that it be relieved; there is no excuse for a terminal illness being marked by uncontrolled pain except that the physician has not fully analyzed the cause of the patient's pain and utilized those measures available to him for control.

The skillful use of narcotics, radiotherapy, nerve blocks, and, rarely, cordotomy can all be applied individually and together to achieve control. Clearly, however, relief of pain will best be achieved by a careful analysis of its cause and by measures directed against the cause. Thus pain in the thigh in a patient with metastatic cancer may be referred pain or it may represent metastases in the femur. Radiotherapy directed to the wrong area will not relieve pain, and it is the primary physician's responsibility to see to it that treatment is directed against the cause.

In a terminal illness narcotics should not be withheld for fear of addiction, assuming the physician has made an accurate determination that the illness is in its terminal stages. Often doctors achieve less than satisfactory results because they fail to adjust the dose of the narcotic to fit the situation. There are no rigid rules of dose and time intervals, but rather these must be adapted to each patient's need. Oral administration of narcotics will usually suffice in all but the most serious pain problems if the dose and time intervals have been carefully adjusted. At times, physicians worry too much about the development of tolerance. Of course, the risk of tolerance will increase with increasing doses of a narcotic, but cross-tolerance between narcotics is incomplete and substitution of one narcotic for another may often be helpful if tolerance does become a problem. Also the combination of non-narcotic analgesics with narcotics may permit adequate pain relief with lower doses of narcotics and hence a lower risk of developing tolerance. The guiding principle, then, is to be flexible in adopting a program that is suitable for each individual patient and not to be too concerned with standardized regimens.

The subject of pain and its management is considered in Ch. 349.

Question 4: Is the patient being comforted physically, mentally, and spiritually? It is important to draw a distinction between measures undertaken as primary treatment for a disease and those undertaken for the patient's comfort. The latter are often misinterpreted by the laity as needless efforts to prolong life, whereas in the terminally ill patient they are only intended for the relief of discomfort. These measures might include antimicrobial drugs to relieve high fever and drenching sweats caused by infection, oxygen to relieve air hunger, an indwelling catheter to prevent decubitus ulcers secondary to incontinence, and intravenous fluids to relieve thirst and dehydration. These measures do not prolong the life of a dying patient; they, like the relief of pain, merely make more tolerable the period of dying. Yet they have become the targets of those who do not understand and who therefore accuse the medical profession of preventing patients from "dying with dignity." Departing this life in a dignified manner is a noble objective and is often achieved, but in many instances it is not. Dignity is defined in one dictionary as "the presence of poise and self-respect in one's deportment to a degree that inspires respect." This is a reasonable definition; but in those instances in which dignity is lost, it is the illness that is responsible, not the physician, unless through the *injudicious* ordering of drugs, he renders his patient incompetent and robs him of his chance to meet his final hour with courage and character.

Dignity is a quality of human character that is a consequence of what lies within the soul. It is not something that can be taken away by another person. It may lie dormant only to appear under adverse circumstances, such as the prospect of death, or it may be in evidence in all that a person does. Those who have had experience in the treatment of dying patients have often been struck by their fortitude of character and spirit. The medical profession is privileged to go through life with this particular view of humanity, which may only rarely be revealed to people in other walks of life.

Having attended to the patient's physical comfort, the concerned physician will see to it that, to the best of his ability, he brings about mental comfort to the patient. Fear and anxiety are too often left unattended. Narcotics may be useful in allaying both, but even more important is the understanding that physicians can bring to their patients by listening and by giving a patient the realization that his burden is shared by the physician: these, plus a careful interpretation to the patient concerning what is happening to him. Fear can often be counteracted with knowledge and understanding better than with any drug in the pharmacopeia. Lewis Thomas has alluded to the observations of Osler and his own experience that there appears to be no such thing as the agony of death. Regarding the ultimate moment of death he has cited observations that there may be a physiologic mechanism which somehow relieves the patient of all fear and anguish. As we learn more about the pathophysiology of dying, we will undoubtedly come to understand more about such a possible mechanism.

Finally, is the patient being comforted spiritually? A visit by a clergyman is not necessarily synonymous with spiritual comfort, because some patients do not experience comfort under these circumstances, despite the best efforts of the clergyman. It all depends on the patient's background, and this must be known to his physician. Spiritual comfort can come in many forms, and the doctor who really cares about his patient will see to this aspect of his needs. Usually, however, the clergyman is indispensable in providing spiritual comfort. The physician and clergyman need each other, and the patient needs them both. It has been observed that what a physician can provide a patient in these circumstances will depend upon his own beliefs and his coming to terms with his own mortality. If he views life as simply a biologic accident, one in which consciousness dies with the flesh, and one in which there is no divinity in each person, he will be in no position to help his patient in a spiritual sense. If, on the other hand, he views life as a continuum and divine guidance as something operative in all lives, his manner, compassion, gentleness, and understanding will not be lost on the patient seeking spiritual solace. In considering the question of consciousness and what happens to it, Thomas has written: ". . . there is still that permanent vanishing of consciousness to be accounted for. Are we to be stuck forever with this problem? Where on earth does it go? Is it simply stopped dead in its tracks, lost in humus, wasted? Considering the tendency of nature to find uses for complex and intricate mechanisms, this seems to me unnatural. I prefer to think of it as somehow separated off at the filaments of its attachment and then drawn like an easy breath back into the membrane of its origin, a fresh memory for a biospherical nervous system, but I have no data on the matter."

Question 5: Is the physician prepared to give of himself to the patient and "go down to the wire" with him? As a corollary, is the physician willing to continue to think about the problems his patient presents until the end? The phrase "dying a little with each patient" perhaps sounds trite, but it is a useful way of indicating the eventuality of real commitment to a patient. There is no substitute for making sure that your patient never once worries about being abandoned. Of course, no true physician would ever really abandon his patient, but I am speaking of a greater commitment: one that makes the patient know that you are there at all times, at the very least in spirit. Most people face illness with courage, hope, a willingness to place their trust in others, and a capacity to endure. They do this quietly, not seeking praise but simply because this is the way they are made. For a doctor to abandon a fellow human being at such times, through some well-meant but misguided effort to hurry him out of the world, is breaking the faith that he has pledged to all patients.

Now, any position that one takes can be pushed to absurdity, and clearly certain judgments must be taken every day as part of a doctor's life in determining what should or should not be done for a patient. If a patient with far-advanced cancer, whose disease has been resistant to treatment, has a cardiac arrest, he obviously should not be resuscitated. Likewise, one does not transfuse such a patient to maintain a normal hemoglobin, and so on. Therapeutic intervention need *not* be undertaken just because it *can* be undertaken. Nevertheless, these judgments are thinking judgments, and are made in the context of the earlier remarks. There is often a lot of living that has still to be "lived through" between the diagnosis of a terminal illness and death, and it is the quality of that living which should concern a physician. Helping a patient out of this world usually demands more skill, and certainly more understanding, than helping him into the world. Nevertheless, this can be done without abandoning the principles that guide physicians throughout their lives; if they will but continue to think, they will make decisions as nearly right as they can be.

A. E. Clark-Kennedy has written the following about the moral problem of preserving life: "According to Christian teaching, life is a gift, and the doctor is under a moral obligation to keep his patient alive as long as he can by means put into his hands. . . . A man has been given his life and it is not for him to opt out of it. But even Roman Catholic moralists hold that a doctor is only under an obligation to keep his patient alive as long as life can be reasonably maintained. Further, he need only use ordinary methods. These are those easily available." The key words are "reasonably," "ordinary," and "easily available." Obviously what is reasonable, ordinary, and easily available in a big university hospital will differ from what those terms would mean in a remote hospital in Africa. Further, these terms are also subject to the individual physician's interpretation. In this connection, this same author goes on to identify as "extraordinary" methods of treatment: "palliative surgery such as . . . oophorectomy, adrenalectomy, and even hypophysectomy in carcinoma of the breast." These surgical procedures are certainly available in many countries, but he has chosen to identify them as "extraordinary"; in the United States they would not generally be so regarded. Remissions of metastatic breast cancer have at times been so striking after endocrine surgery (in one recent case report, as long as 25 years after oophorectomy) that there is little doubt as to the value of these procedures in some patients.

One must also consider the thought that physicians may persist in their efforts to preserve life in the realization that they see and know only in part and that some unforeseen event may occur to alter an outcome which the physician, in his fallibility, has come to expect. Further, a patient is less apt to be fearful that his doctor will try to sustain his life than he is that the doctor will give up, notwithstanding the popular idea that healthy persons, contemplating terminal illness, usually express the wish to be allowed to die quickly. Recently, formalized documents have been executed as "living wills," and, although they are not legally binding, they are supposed to give some indication as to what a person wants in a terminal illness. These wills state, in part, that the signer "be allowed to die and not be kept alive by artificial means or heroic measures." As noted, these pronouncements are generally made by people who are healthy. Sick people do not usually express these sentiments, perhaps because of denial or because, facing death, they want to live. There is, of course, a middle ground which responsible physicians should take. They should not, on the one hand, aggressively resuscitate a patient who has had prolonged cerebral anoxia after cardiac arrest, or, on the other hand, consign a terminally ill patient to a state of stupor with morphine just to be relieved of the awesome burden of caring for him.

One attempt to articulate the middle ground has been as follows: "When, in the opinion of the attending physicians, measures to prolong life which have no realistic hope of effecting significant improvement will cause further pain and suffering to the patient and the family, we support conservative, passive medical care in place of heroic measures in the management of a patient afflicted with a terminal illness" (New York Academy of Medicine, 1973). Although the word "prolong" appears in this statement, it is qualified by referring to measures which have "no realistic hope of effecting significant improvement," and in this sense it does not conflict with earlier statements about the use, or misuse, of the word "prolong." This statement puts the burden of these decisions squarely on the attending physicians, where it belongs. This burden implies that a doctor will continue to try to analyze what is happening to his patient, but that what action he takes will be dictated by the over-all circumstances. Note also the reference to "physicians," to indicate that decisions to stop active medical care are usually best taken in consultation with one's colleagues.

Question 6: What is the attitude of the patient's family, and how is it being dealt with? Failure of the medical profession to explain to families what is happening to their terminally ill relatives is the cause of many of the articles published in newspapers and magazines about the increasing insensitivity of doctors. One hears repeatedly from families that "no one tells them anything." It is imperative that at least one member of the family, usually the next of kin, be fully informed of the patient's illness by the responsible physician. This should not be a single session but should be reviewed several times during the course of the patient's illness so that members of the family may have as complete an understanding as is possible for laymen to have. This does not mean that the physician has to have individual sessions with every member of the family; his time obligations must be respected. If a number of relatives are involved, it may be useful to meet with them together, because the physician's explanations, relayed by one member to others in the family, are subject to wide distortions.

It is wise to tell the family what you are doing and why, so that they will not harbor misconceptions. If you are giving fluids, antimicrobials, or oxygen, explain that these are designed for the patient's comfort. If members of a family understand, they will be more helpful and supportive to the patient; but if they are kept in the dark, they may sublimate their anxiety into hostility toward everyone and everything connected with their dying relative.

Further, physicians should give families an opportunity to express their own feelings. Guilt, frustration, and fear are all intermingled with grief, and someone must let the family know that their feelings are normal, that such feelings happen to everyone, and that those caring for the patient understand. No one can do this better than the responsible physician, and he should not delegate this to someone else.

The family also needs to have some reasonable projection as to the patient's life expectancy, but it is unwise to be too specific. Only the inexperienced claim such clairvoyance. Also they should know what to expect in terms of new developments in the patient's course. If the natural history of the disease permits some projections, this information should be shared. Finally, it is important not to engage in speculations as to what might have been had this or that been done or not done earlier in the patient's illness. The family likewise should be discouraged from making such speculations themselves, because they serve no useful purpose and may needlessly promote anxiety and bitterness.

Question 7: Is the patient undergoing experimental study, and, if so, are humanitarian principles being observed or compromised? Although this chapter is not concerned primarily with human experimentation, it is necessary to give this important subject some consideration in the context of the care of the terminally ill, because often new procedures or treatments are undertaken for the first time in humans with a limited life expectancy. Under these circumstances the approach of the physician to the terminally ill patient must, of necessity, be modified. In his quest for new knowledge, however, he must be prepared to see to it that the rules under which human experimentation is carried out are strictly observed.

Some have proposed that experiments done not for the immediate good of the patient but for the general welfare of mankind should be carried out by those who do not simultaneously have responsibility for the clinical care of the subject. Thus patients who are the subjects of such experiments would have two physicians: a physician-friend and a physician-investigator. Such a system would avoid the subtle alterations of reasoning that may take place when one physician tries to be both. However, if an investigator is true to himself, to his patient, and to the ethical principles which should guide his professional life, it is quite feasible for the same physician to be both friend and investigator. This relationship between investigator and investigatee has been defined by Guttentag as ". . . a partnership between the two, resulting from the fact of their being fellow human beings. . . ." He characterizes this relationship as one of "mutual trust and confidence, of openness between experimenter and subject." In the last analysis, then, the ethics of human experimentation arise from those of the individual investigator and from his perceptions and integrity in dealing with another human being. The essence of experimentation by one human being on another has been captured in this quotation from Paul Tillich:

> Man becomes man in personal encounters. Only by meeting a "thou" does man realize he is an "ego." No natural object within the whole universe can do this to him. Man can transcend himself in all directions in knowledge and control. He can use everything for his purposes. Nobody can say where the final limits of human power lie. In his encounter with the universe, man is able to transcend any imaginable limit. But there is a limit for man which is definite and which he always encounters, the other man. The other one, the "thou," is like a wall which cannot be removed or penetrated or used. He who tries to do so, destroys himself.

All human experimentation is based upon the integrity of the individual investigator and the obtaining of informed consent, freely given. Various codes have been developed, beginning with the Nuremberg Code in 1947, and in one form or another they contain the following provisions:

1. Prior voluntary consent must be obtained from all subjects.
2. The study must hold promise of results for the good of society unprocurable by other means.
3. The study must be based on animal experimentation.
4. It must avoid all unnecessary physical and mental suffering.
5. The degree of risk must never exceed that determined by the humanitarian importance of the problem.
6. It must be conducted only by scientifically qualified persons.
7. The human subject must always be at liberty to withdraw.
8. The scientist must be prepared to terminate the study if the subject is endangered to the point of disability or death.

Informed consent is still the most difficult thing to achieve, and the physician, in obtaining this, must keep in mind the following additional principles as outlined by the Board of Regents of the University of the State of New York:

(1) . . . it is the patient, and not the physician, who has the right to decide what factors are or are not relevant to his consent, regardless of the rationality of his assessment. . . . A physician has no right to withhold from a prospective volunteer any fact which he knows may influence the decision.

(2) . . . the physician, when he is acting as experimenter, has no claim to the doctor-patient relationship, that, in a therapeutic situation, would give him the generally acknowledged right to withhold information if he judged it in the best interest of the patient.

(3) No person can be said to have volunteered for an experiment unless he had first understood what he was volunteering for. Any matter which might influence him in giving or withholding consent is material. Deliberate nondisclosure of the material fact is no different from deliberate misrepresentation of such a fact.

Physicians dealing with terminal patients who are the subjects of experimentation must assure themselves that all these principles are being observed.

In conclusion, there is no greater test of the qualities of a physician than that imposed by the care of the terminally ill. It calls upon the doctor to exercise medical skill and at the same time to become involved with a fellow human being in the most trying and yet most ennobling of human relationships. How his patient fares will be determined in large part by how the physician meets this test.

Clark-Kennedy, A. E.: Man, Medicine and Morality. Hamden, Conn., Shoe String Press, 1970, pp. 196, 200.
Kübler-Ross, E.: On Death and Dying. New York, The Macmillan Company, 1969.
New York Academy of Medicine: Statement on Measures Employed to Prolong Life in Terminal Illness. Bull. N.Y. Acad. Med., 49 (2nd ser.):349, 1973.
Rhoads, P. S.: Management of the patient with terminal illness. J.A.M.A., 192:661, 1965.
Thomas, L.: The long habit. N. Engl. J. Med., 286:825, 1972.
Tillich, P.: Love, Power and Justice: Ontological Analyses and Ethical Applications. New York, Oxford University Press, 1960, p. 78.

4. MEDICINE IN MODERN SOCIETY

Walsh McDermott

Medicine is not a science but a learned profession deeply rooted in a number of sciences and charged with the obligation to apply them for man's benefit. So complex a process could hardly be reduced to a neat symmetrical design and fitted within the covers of a book. Yet this subject, the beneficial uses of medical science, is not without any design at all—it has a conceptual base on which all medical teaching and all medical books should rest. To consider this base, or certain aspects of it, seems proper at the start of a textbook of medicine. Although the book itself is addressed to medical students and graduate physicians of all ages, this essay is presented mainly for those now entering the profession.

One part of the conceptual base is set forth above in the opening sentence that ends ". . . to apply them for man's benefit." Traditionally this applying is made with compassion and in accord with a widely recognized moral and ethical code. The responsibilities of medicine are thus threefold: to generate scientific knowledge and to teach it to others; to use the knowledge for the health of an individual or a whole community; and to judge the moral and ethical propriety of each medical act that directly affects another human being. These three areas of responsibility command the efforts of individuals from a wide range of scientific disciplines and professions. The physicians who actually apply the knowledge, however, are of two sorts: those who deal through a personal encounter with one patient at a time and those who deal with people as groups.

The activities of both sorts of physicians are based on the concept that each disease entity has its own pathogenic chain—the whole series of events that determine its causation and maintenance—and that understanding this chain for a particular disease not only permits clearer recognition of its clinical manifestations, but reveals any weak links that might be exploited for prevention or therapy.

Approach to the body of knowledge organized in this way (both in books and elsewhere) is made from one of two viewpoints. The physician in public health or community medicine is constantly reaching for ways in which pathogenic chains can be broken by some continuing intervention that affects a number of people at once, e.g., to reduce the incidence of goiter by putting iodine in table salt. By contrast, physicians acting through the personal encounter system will search the same knowledge sectors and with educated discrimination will extract those elements appropriate for the solution of a problem in an individual. The viewpoints from which the knowledge is scrutinized are different, but the body of knowledge about each disease is the same. Textbooks about diseases and their pathogenic chains serve both these viewpoints and form important instruments for this process of the beneficial uses of science.

The physician who treats one patient at a time and the physician who deals with a community as a whole both exert compassion, but it is of two quite different sorts. The compassion exercised by the physician who treats individuals takes the form of a cultivated instinct to lend support and comfort to a particular fellow human being. By contrast, the "group" compassion of the public health or community physician necessarily takes the form of what the writer has previously termed "statistical compassion." By this is meant an imaginative compassion for people whom one never gets to see as individuals and, indeed, can know only as data on a graph. This compassion—the deep-seated instinct to try to help those whom one never gets to see—is a characteristic form of motivation for political leaders and other social activists, and "statistical" successes bring them major satisfactions. Such is really not the case with most physicians, who usually do not derive as much satisfaction from seeing improvement on a graph as they do from seeing improvement in an individual. *Indeed, part of the self-selection in choosing medicine as a career seems to be a self-image of a person whose professional activities are to relate directly with individuals rather than with groups.* Thus the system of public health or community medicine—based on physicians *not* seeing patients as individuals—runs contrary to most medical instincts. Yet until we have significant numbers of physicians for whom "statistical compassion" is as rewarding as it is to the leaders in certain other walks of life, we will fail as a society to derive the full measure of the benefits of our medical science.

The scientific basis of medicine had been building up throughout the whole nineteenth century, but the *uses* of that science in the sense of decisively altering or preventing disease were largely accomplished through the public health or "community" physicians who dealt with people as groups. Chlorination of water supplies and the pasteurization of milk are cases in point. It was not until the discovery of insulin in 1921, and not really until the advent of the modern antimicrobial era 40 years ago, that the clinical physicians had much in the way of decisive therapies or preventives derived from science. Since that time most of the practical uses of biomedical science and technology have been of a nature fitted to the clinical or personal system, and, despite recent efforts, the other system has been allowed to languish. Indeed, the evolution of the highly complex and extraordinarily effective instrument that is today's university-based medical center has been almost exclusively devoted to the one system – the personal encounter system of one patient at a time.

We could tolerate this so long as what medicine had to offer was technologically simple and physicians were spread out across the whole of society much more evenly than they are now. But the coincidence of massive scientific innovation and wide social change has created a situation in which the application of medical science for man's benefit can no longer be managed by just one of the two systems – we desperately need both.

For there are two critically different populations involved, each of which is the primary responsibility of one of the systems. These two populations are the *constituency* and the *community.* The members of the constituency represent a progressively selected group, in part self-selected, and the selection is based on the presence of a medical problem, frequently one that is quite complex. Each member, in effect, has *voted* to obtain the services of a physician (or center or medical group) and has cast this vote as an individual without reference to others. The constituency is thus a collection of individuals who share in common only the fact that each has perceived a self-problem of illness or disease. It is the group known familiarly as the physician's "practice." The community, by contrast, is made up of people distinguished by the possession in common of some factor not directly related to disease. Usually, but not invariably, this common factor is a domicile located within some geographically defined boundary. In health terms, therefore, the community is a wholly unselected group, and at any one point in time many more of its members are well than are sick. *The community and the constituency thus differ strikingly in the prevalence of significant illness and disease. Because of this difference, an institutional form appropriate to meet the needs of one group would be markedly different from the form appropriate for the other.* Our challenge today is to develop such a two-type institutional form so that the needs of both groups may be equally served.

What the community needs is recognition of weakness in pathogenic chains that may be exploited in the prevention of disease. For nonpreventable disease the community needs straightforward medical care close to home, safeguarded by continuous mechanisms for identifying those who need care in the first place and mechanisms for sifting the few who need complex care from the many who do not. These few join the constituency – that self-selected group of people derived from a much larger population base than could be satisfactorily served by a single personal encounter physician. What the properly sifted members of the constituency need is an institution that can offer a complete array of talents appropriate for the solution of any currently solvable medical problem, no matter how rarely occurring or complicated it might be. Whether for the community or for the constituency, the actual provision of the care is the responsibility of the personal encounter physician. Community medicine (or the larger public health system of which it is a part) is thus responsible *not* for the delivery of personal health services to the members of a community, but for ensuring that the community receives the proper health services of all sorts. And prominent among these are the invention of better mechanisms than we have now for both the continuous community scan of who needs care at any moment and appropriate entry points for the care of those identified. Neither of these two systems is inherently of greater social value than the other, but in the course of developing the personal encounter system to its present high point of technologic effectiveness for the individual, we have failed to mount a comparable effort for the nourishment of the other system responsible for the medical welfare of every member of the group. Without such a healthy watchdog we have allowed the personal encounter system to become unevenly distributed throughout our population. The speedy correction of this imbalance is the critical challenge facing medicine today, and how well we meet it will determine the role of the physician in society. For the imbalance of the two systems affects our efforts for the beneficial uses of science not only at the level of medical care for the community and the constituency, but in those even larger matters that have to do with how the developing individual can be aided in his or her continuous interaction with the environment.

It is not possible to do justice to all these issues in this book, although some are indeed considered. For others, certain key references to the valuable literature that has been developing in recent years are set forth below. There remain a few, however, that are so vital to the conceptual base forming the theme of this chapter that they deserve special mention.

Moral judgments must be made by the physician engaged in individual patient care, but they are to be made on his own professional acts and those of his colleagues, not on the actions of those who sought his care. Any moral judgments he might make on his patients' behavior are private matters to be kept within himself; he must not permit them to influence his own professional acts. This has long been the medical tradition, and it is important that it not be forgotten in the tumult of today's world of clashing value systems. The prospect of moral and ethical problems of an essentially new type is also now emerging before us. There is general awareness that advances in medical science are leading to various ethical conflicts that have to be faced by the personal encounter physician. What is less well recognized, however, is that this situation will also become socially serious for the nonclinical system, whether it be called public health or community medicine. Critical phenomena in human development formerly thought to represent the hand of fate are now found to be, at least in part, environmentally determined, and hence manipulable – such matters as the full expansion of an individual's intelligence or perhaps his or her degree of educability. If we develop the power to significantly influence such critical matters – and scientifically we are getting closer to it every day – we may find ourselves faced with seeking to protect the "interests" of an unborn or newborn child in the receipt of a particular intervention against the "rights" of its parents to be free from outside interference. And this question of how to ensure the best opportunity for the individual without destroying family structure in the process will not be an ethical problem to be faced by medicine in rare instances, but one that will involve whole societies. Yet we cannot run away from such questions, for it is the wise application of our science and technology, made with either form of compassion, that allows us to approach one of our major goals—that of ensuring that every child born into the world has the maximal chance to make his run through life's most productive years.

Finally, we must heed a concept of medicine that is ageless. In the life of an individual there ultimately may come a time when all the knowledge so carefully presented by the contributors to this book no longer has usefulness, yet life must go on, at least for a time. Whenever this happens, and it happens every day, it is up to each of us to follow to the fullest measure the charge laid down long ago for "the physician to become himself the treatment."

Beeson, P. B.: Some good features of the British National Health Service. Arch. Intern. Med., 133:708, 1974.

Dubos, R.: So Human an Animal. New York, Charles Scribner's Sons, 1969.

McDermott, W.: Demography, culture, and economics and the evolutionary stages of medicine. *In* Kilbourne, E. D., and Smillie, W. G. (eds.): Human Ecology and Public Health. 4th ed. New York, The Macmillan Company, 1969.

Morison, R. S.: Where is biology taking us? Science, 155:429, 1967.

Rogers, D. E.: The doctor must himself become the treatment. Lecture given at the University of North Carolina. February 20, 1974. The Pharos (to be published).

Part II
GENETIC PRINCIPLES

5. INTRODUCTION

Alexander G. Bearn

It is a convenient if misleading abstraction to consider that all diseases of man are due either to the action of environmental agents or to hereditary influences. This simplistic view has been nurtured by innumerable studies that relegate a disease into one or the other category. It is more correct, however, as well as more rewarding, to consider that both environmental and hereditary influences play a role in the etiology of disease. In some conditions genetic influences are clearly decisive, whereas in others the disease appears to be independent of the genetic constitution of the patient. In most diseases, both genetic and environmental factors play a detectably influential role. The science of human genetics is concerned primarily with the recognition of hereditary variations in man. Most of these variations are not harmful; indeed they are beneficial, for they confer on the species the capacity to adapt to an ever-changing environment. But when these variations are extreme and are associated with clinical disease, they come within the realm of the physician. Since medical genetics is an applied science, certain general genetic principles will be discussed before considering in detail the direct application of genetics to clinical medicine.

After the establishment of the principle of genetic transmission by Gregor Mendel, Johannsen, in 1909, introduced the word *gene* to denote a unit of heredity. A structural gene is now defined, operationally, as a functional unit of inheritance situated on a chromosome and responsible for the synthesis of a specific polypeptide. It has been estimated that there are probably no less than 100,000 genes in man. Since the number of well documented examples of genetic variability is of the order of 1000, it is apparent that despite the acceleration in discovery of new genetic entities 99 per cent of the human genome remains to be discovered.

The chemical nature of a gene was unrecognized until 1944, when a soluble extract derived from pneumococci of one genotype was found to effect a stable heritable change when added to a growing culture of pneumococci of another genotype. The prompt identification of the transforming substance present in the extract as deoxyribonucleic acid (DNA) launched the present era of molecular biology. The genetic information encoded in the DNA that determines polypeptide structure is transcribed through the synthesis of another macromolecule, ribonucleic acid (RNA). Part of this RNA is termed *messenger RNA* (mRNA), and the linear amino acid sequences in the polypeptide chain are precisely determined by the linear sequences of the coding units (*"codons"*—see below) in the mRNA. These relationships are often referred to as the central dogma of molecular biology, and can be depicted schematically:

$$\text{DNA} \xrightarrow{\text{transcription}} \text{RNA} \xrightarrow{\text{translation}} \text{polypeptide}$$

The universality of this biologic truth was momentarily shaken by the discovery in 1970 that several RNA animal tumor viruses contain polymerase activity (reverse transcriptase) which uses RNA as a template for the synthesis of double-stranded DNA and thus reverses the familiar direction of genetic transcription. This discovery raised the possibility that an RNA-dependent DNA polymerase might indicate the presence of an oncogenic virus. Although this enzyme has now been detected in certain nononcogenic viruses as well, the function of viral reverse transcriptase remains a question of central biologic importance in the problem of neoplasia.

Deoxyribonucleic Acid (DNA). Deoxyribonucleic acid is constructed from three essential components: the five-carbon sugar 2-deoxy-D-ribose; phosphoric acid, which confers on DNA its acidic properties; and nitrogenous bases. Two of the bases are purines, adenine (A) and guanine (G), and two are pyrimidines, thymine (T) and cytosine (C). In 1953 Watson and Crick assembled the available physical and chemical data on DNA into the present model for the structure of DNA. Two polynucleotide chains are twisted together to form a double helix. The two chains are held together by hydrogen bonds between the bases which face inward forming the core, and the phosphate-sugar groups form an external helical backbone. Adenine must always pair with thymine (A-T), and guanine with cytosine (G-C). The result of this pairing leads to a precise complementary relationship between the bases on the two chains. Thus, if part of the base sequence were TTGCC, the corresponding portion of the complementary strand would read AACGG.

Replication of DNA. One of the chief attractions of the Watson-Crick model for DNA is that it contains a built in system for self-replication. As the double helix of a parent molecule unwinds, the sequence of bases in each strand acts as a template for the synthesis of a new strand of DNA in two daughter molecules. The replication is catalyzed by the enzyme DNA polymerase and has been termed *semiconservative,* because both parental strands are conserved in the next generation, each now paired with a newly synthesized complementary partner.

Ribonucleic Acid (RNA). Ribonucleic acid differs from deoxyribonucleic acid in three important ways. (1) The sugar D-ribose replaces the 2-deoxy-D-ribose of DNA. (2) The pyrimidine base uracil (U) replaces the thymine of DNA. (3) RNA is a single-stranded polymer in contrast to double-stranded DNA.

Messenger Ribonucleic Acid (mRNA). Messenger RNA is formed by the transcription of one of the strands of DNA and is catalyzed by the specific enzyme RNA polymerase (transcriptase). The sequence of bases in mRNA is identical to that in the corresponding uncopied strand of DNA except that uracil replaces thymine. In this way single-stranded RNA carries into the cytoplasm the genetic information originally encoded in nuclear DNA. In bacteria, mRNA has a half-life of about two minutes, and it has been calculated that during this time 10 to 20 molecules of protein can be synthesized. In cells of higher organisms the bulk of mRNA appears to be much more stable, and may remain functional for two to three days and direct the synthesis of several thousand molecules of protein.

Transfer RNA (tRNA). Before amino acids are assembled into polypeptide chains they must first be "activated." This activation is accomplished by the enzyme amino-acyl-tRNA synthetase which attaches the phosphate group of adenine to the carboxyl group of an amino acid to form amino-acyl-adenylate. The activated amino acid is now joined to another type of RNA called transfer RNA. Mammalian cells contain more than 20 different transfer RNA's, and at least one transfer RNA is specific for each of the amino acids. Each transfer RNA molecule is folded into a cloverleaf pattern and has two recognition sites. One site binds the "activated" amino acid, whereas the second, often called the anticodon, recognizes the codon in the mRNA. Thus the fidelity of translation is assured by the specific binding of the amino acid, with the tRNA catalyzed by the specific activating enzyme and by complementary pairing of the anticodon of tRNA with the codon of the mRNA.

Ribosomal RNA (rRNA). More than 80 per cent of the RNA of most cells is found in small cytoplasmic particles, closely associated with the endoplasmic reticulum, called ribosomes. These ribosomal particles represent the protein synthetic machinery of the cell and consist of about half protein and half RNA. There are some 50 different proteins in a single ribosome; the RNA does not contain any genetic information, and its function is unknown. Mammalian ribosomes have a diameter of approximately 200 Å and a sedimentation coefficient of 80 S, and dissociate into 60 S and 40 S subunits in low concentrations of magnesium ion. Messenger RNA, bearing the instructions for protein synthesis, must become attached to the ribosomes on which the polypeptide is synthesized. In bacteria, mRNA contains several "sticky points" which enable it to adhere to the smaller ribosomal subunit. When this has occurred, the larger ribosomal subunit becomes attached to form the final functional ribosome, and the sequential assembly of amino acids into protein begins.

Protein Synthesis. Translation is initiated as soon as mRNA becomes bound to the ribosomes. In bacteria the initiation of translation is effected by the codon, AUG, which binds a specific tRNA, n-formylmethionyl-tRNA, to the ribosome complex. The second codon then recognizes its specific tRNA, and the second amino acid in sequence is brought into alignment. A peptide bond is formed between the two amino acids, and the ribosome moves along the mRNA so that the third codon, recognizing its tRNA, brings the third amino acid into position with further elongation of the peptide chain (Fig. 1). The information that a polypeptide chain is completed and that its synthesis must be terminated is specified by a special chain-terminating codon. A ribosome takes about ten seconds to read an entire mRNA molecule of average length, and a single mRNA molecule may move over the surfaces of several ribosomes simultaneously. This explains why a cell needs relatively little mRNA to synthesize a great deal of protein. A molecule of mRNA attached to several ribosomes simultaneously is called a polyribosome; polyribosomes synthesizing hemoglobin (a protein of molecular weight 64,500), on the average, contain four to six ribosomes.

Codons. Because most proteins normally contain 20 different amino acids and because DNA has only four different nucleotide bases, it is evident that more than one base is required to prescribe for a particular amino acid. It is now known that a sequence of three bases (a codon) is needed to code for each amino acid, and that the code is nonoverlapping. Thus a gene with 1500 nucleotide pairs would determine the sequence of a polypeptide chain consisting of 500 amino acids. Since the four-letter code is triplet in nature, there are 64 ($4 \times 4 \times 4$) possible codons, of which 61 have been shown to code for one of the 20 amino acids. The three remaining codons represent signals that the polypeptide chain is completed and are called chain-terminating codons. Two codons serve to initiate polypeptide synthesis as well as to insert amino acids and are sometimes designated chain-initiating codons. One of the unresolved problems of eukaryotic organisms such as man is that they possess more DNA in their genome than is needed for genetic information. Multiple copies of structural genes almost certainly occur and may account for much of the redundancy. The genetic code is said to be *universal* in the sense that all plant and animal species have thus far been found to use the same genetic code, and *degenerate* because certain amino acids can be specified by more than one triplet.

Certain acridine dyes induce mutations in bacteriophage by inserting an extra nucleotide into the pre-existing (normal) sequence. Because of this extra nucleotide, the reading frame becomes altered distal to the point of insertion and results in a disruption of normal protein synthesis. The correct reading frame of the code can be restored by a deletion of another nucleotide (or by the insertion of an additional two extra nucleotides) distal to the insertion. This model makes the prediction that a double mutant, consisting of an insertion followed by a deletion, will result in a polypeptide chain with an altered amino acid sequence between the two mutations. If the segment of DNA between the two mutations is short, and does not code for amino acids vital for functional specificity, a protein with a normal function may still be produced. A mutation in the codon which terminates the reading of the code is referred to as a terminator mutation. Three variant hemoglobins (Hb Constant Spring, Hb Tak, and Hb Wayne) have been reported in which either the α or β chain has been elongated. In Hb Constant Spring and Hb Tak the increased length of the molecule is due to a terminator mutation, whereas in Hb Wayne the increased chain length is caused by a frame-shift mutation.

Structural Genes, Control Genes, and the Structure-Rate Hypothesis. The most extensive understanding of genetic regulatory mechanisms has stemmed from the investigations of the β-galactosidase enzyme system in *Escherichia coli.* These studies have led to the formulation of new concepts of regulation in bacteria, according to which a hierarchy of control genes and structural genes has been established. Thus, whereas certain genes (structural genes) are responsible for the actual synthesis of specific protein and enzymes, and contain the DNA code which specifies their amino acid sequences, other genes (control genes) are responsible for the regulation of the production of these proteins. Although the distinction between a control gene mutation and a structural gene mutation can be resolved in microorganisms by tracing the mutation to a locus within or outside the structural gene, techniques for a similar analysis in man are not yet available. It is increasingly clear, however, that the regulation of gene function in man is far more complex than in bacteria, and the application of the Jacob-Monod model is undoubtedly a misleading oversimplification.

A dramatic example of a structural gene mutation in man was most clearly demonstrated when Ingram re-

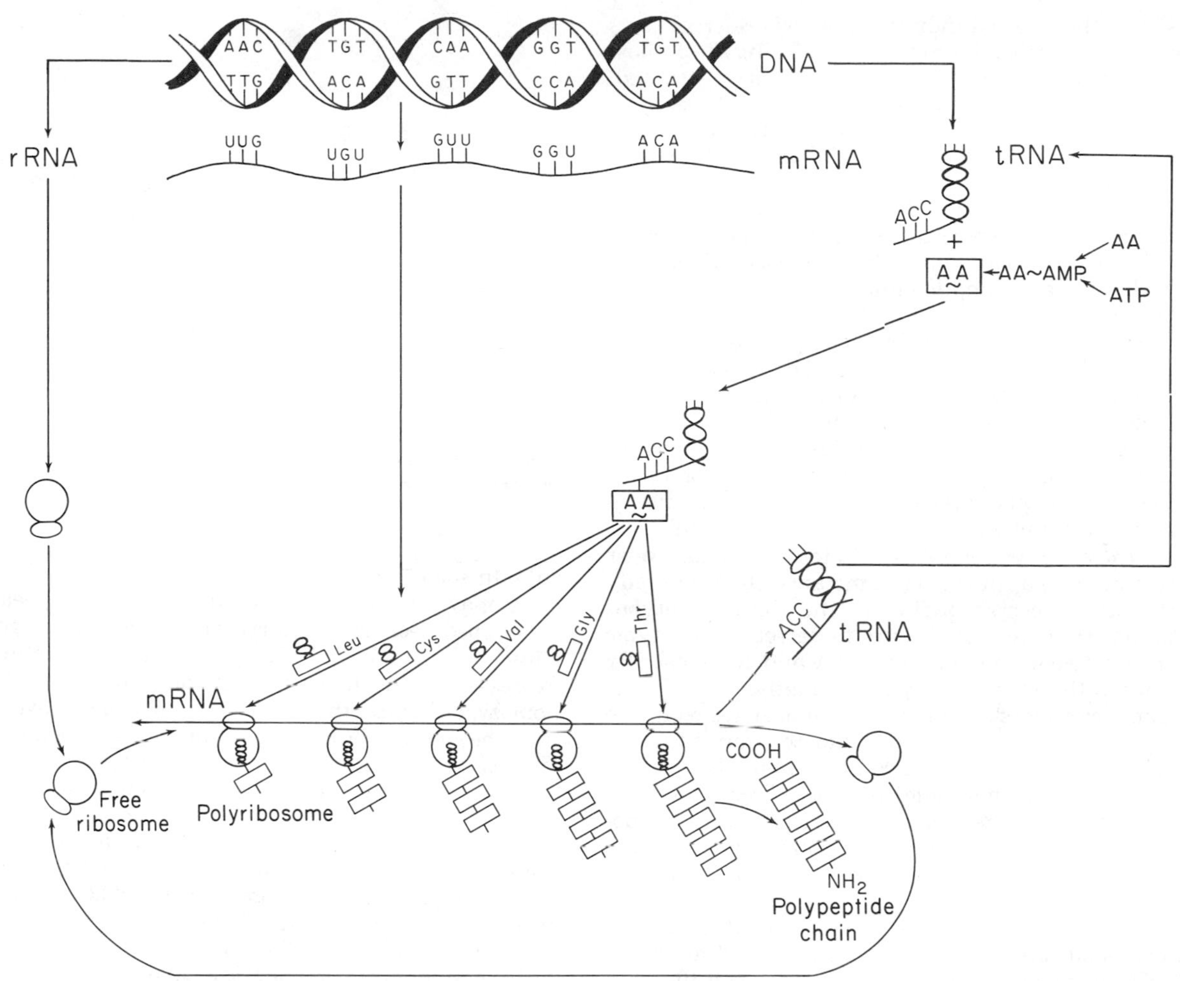

Figure 1. A schematic diagram of the genetic control of protein synthesis. A=adenine, T=thymine, G=guanine, C=cytosine, U=uracil. The codons indicated represent code words for the amino acids indicated. The messenger RNA (mRNA) moves across the ribosomes in the direction of the arrow. tRNA=transfer RNA; rRNA=ribosomal RNA. (For details see text.)

ported in 1956 that sickle cell hemoglobin differed from normal hemoglobin in a single amino acid substitution. Since that time a very large number of structural mutants have been identified in man, and in many instances the precise amino acid substitution has been identified. The question of whether, in man, there are also control gene mutations which so drastically affect synthesis that only very small quantities of a structurally normal protein are formed has been less easy to document.

Although many of the hereditary diseases studied by Garrod are characterized by the synthesis of a decreased quantity of an enzyme of apparently normal structure, rigorous structural studies have seldom been performed. The apparent absence of a specific protein in certain genetic disorders may be due to a structural gene mutation that has resulted in the synthesis of a modified protein which has become immunologically, enzymatically, and chemically unrecognizable. The growing concept that the gene controlling the structure of a protein also influences the amount of protein synthesized has been termed the structure-rate hypothesis. In most instances the mutational event leads to decreased synthesis; rarely, however, an increased synthesis of the mutant protein may occur. An increased enzymatic activity has been observed in G6PD Hektoen, a structural mutant in the glucose-6-phosphate dehydrogenase system, and in a pseudocholinesterase mutant designated Cynthiana (see Ch. 740). In certain inherited diseases the primary biochemical abnormality probably resides in a decreased or defective synthesis of messenger RNA. In thalassemia a decreased synthesis of the β globulin chain of normal hemoglobin is associated with a deficiency of functional mRNA for globin chains. In those rare forms of thalassemia in which β chain synthesis is totally absent, a deletion of the DNA sequences coding for the β chain mRNA is responsible for the lack of globin synthesis.

Watson, J. D.: Molecular Biology of the Gene. 2nd ed. New York, Benjamin, 1970.

6. PEDIGREE ANALYSIS IN INHERITED DISEASE

Alexander G. Bearn

Inspection and analysis of human pedigrees form the basis for an understanding of the application of the laws of Mendel to human disease. Analysis of a pedigree begins with the affected individual, who is referred to as the propositus, proband, or index case. Using the propositus as the point of departure, a pedigree is constructed, and the pattern of the pedigree is analyzed. It is worth emphasizing, however, that the construction of human pedigrees beyond first- and second-degree relatives is an occupation more likely to please the physician than to provide a deeper genetic understanding of the patient's disease. Human memories are notoriously untrustworthy, and great care must be exercised when very large pedigrees are compiled and recorded.

Autosomal Inheritance. When there are two alleles, A and a, at a locus, three possible genotypes exist, which can be represented AA, Aa, and aa. The genotypes AA and aa are called *homozygotes*; Aa is a *heterozygote*. A gene can be recognized only by the effect it produces; thus in the strictest sense it is incorrect to speak of dominant or recessive genes, but only of dominant or recessive effects. If the phenotype Aa cannot be easily distinguished from the phenotype AA, but is clearly different from aa, the effect of gene A is said to be dominant over the effect of gene a. In this circumstance there are only two phenotypes corresponding to the three genotypes AA, Aa, aa. However, the failure to detect a phenotypic difference between the genotypes AA and Aa is usually testimony to the insensitivity of the methods employed. If the gene product of A and a can both be detected in the heterozygote Aa, the genes are said to exert an effect which is *co-dominant*. In many ways it would be preferable to discard the terms "dominant" and "recessive" and instead to state whether the genes concerned are phenotypically expressed in a single or double dose; for the sake of convenience, however, the terms are often retained.

Autosomal Dominant Traits. Autosomal genes are those genes situated on chromosomes other than the X and Y. Dominant traits are defined as those traits that are fully manifested by the presence of a gene in the heterozygous state. Thus far, approximately 1000 well established autosomal dominant traits have been identified in man. Satisfactory examples of dominant traits are those responsible for the formation of certain blood group antigens. In the ABO system, the genes controlling the formation of A and B substances are dominant over O. Thus it is not ordinarily possible to distinguish serologically AA from AO individuals, or BB from BO individuals. However, heterozygous individuals of type AB can be recognized because the product of genes A and B can be detected.

An autosomal dominant trait can be recognized in human pedigrees by its transmission from one generation to the next. Except for sporadic cases in which a fresh mutation in the germ cell has arisen in either the father or the mother, and provided illegitimacy can be excluded, every affected individual has at least one affected parent and may have affected offspring and sibs (Fig. 2). The more severe the condition, the larger is the proportion of sporadic cases caused by fresh mutation. According to mendelian laws, a heterozygous affected individual married to a normal homozygote will, on the average, transmit the trait to half his offspring, both sexes being equally affected. Neurofibromatosis, Huntington's chorea, and achondroplastic dwarfism are examples of dominant traits of clinical significance.

In contrast to recessive disorders, most dominant traits in man frequently exert only mild effects, and marked variation in the expression of the trait is the rule. In some instances the expression of the abnormal gene may be so weak that a generation appears to be skipped because the carrier of the abnormal gene is clinically normal. When a gene that can be clinically expressed in the heterozygous condition occurs in the homozygous state, the effect is usually more severe and may be lethal. Although examples are common in species in which experimental matings can be constructed, such examples are exceptional in man, because marriage of two clinically affected heterozygotes is rare. An increased paternal age effect has been demonstrated among parents of sporadic cases of achondroplastic dwarfism, Marfan's syndrome (see Ch. 933), and certain other dominantly inherited disorders.

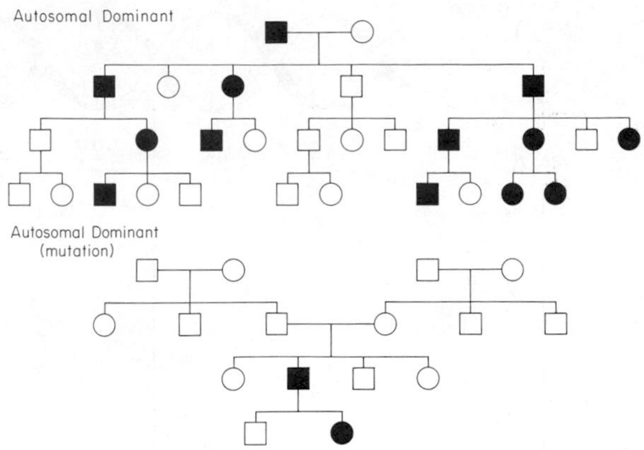

Figure 2. Pedigrees of autosomal dominant traits. In the lower pedigree the normal parents of the affected individual suggest the possibility of a new mutation. (For details see text.)

The molecular basis for the more than 1000 genetically dominant diseases now known is quite obscure. It is of interest that in contrast to recessively inherited diseases in which an impairment of enzyme function is the rule, defective enzymes are only rarely found in dominant diseases. A deficiency of the inhibitor of the first component of complement, *C1-esterase inhibitor*, in hereditary angioneurotic edema and a deficiency of *uroporphyrinogen-1-synthetase* in porphyria are exceptions to this general rule (see Ch. 76 and 942). It appears that in most dominantly inherited disorders the abnormal gene determines a protein with a structural rather than an enzymatic function. Several hemolytic disorders are due to the presence of a single unstable mutant hemoglobin (see Ch. 746 to 751). The presence of one of these abnormal hemoglobin genes is sufficient to shorten the life of the red cells.

Autosomal Recessive Traits. In an autosomal recessive trait, the father and the mother of the affected individual are usually normal, as are more distant ancestors. On the average, one fourth of the brothers and sisters of the index case will be affected. If the trait is rare, an increased consanguinity will be observed among the parents of those affected. According to mendelian laws, two normal parents, both heterozygous for a recessive trait, will produce offspring of whom, on the average, one quarter will be homozygous for the normal allele, one quarter homozygous for the abnormal allele and thus affected, and one half heterozygous for the abnormal allele, like the parents. Affected individuals usually have phenotypically normal offspring who are all carriers of the abnormal gene. If an affected individual marries an individual heterozygous for the same gene, one half of the offspring will be affected and one half will be heterozygous carriers (Fig. 3). Approximately 800 well established recessive traits have been identified in man.

Certain aspects of the segregation ratio in autosomal recessive conditions must be emphasized. Because of the small size of families and because ascertainment of the family is usually through an affected member, the mean observed proportion of affected individuals will be greater than expected. Only when the size of the sibships is large will the expected ratio of one affected to three unaffected be realized in pooled data. Thus the analysis of the expected ratio in families of various sizes requires a correction factor whose magnitude depends on the number of children in the sibship. The simplest correction is to subtract in each family the index case from the total number of affected individuals and then determine the proportion of affected children among the remaining sibs.

The disadvantage of the term "recessive" is emphasized by the increasing number of instances in which refined biochemical observations enable the recognition of the trait in the clinically normal heterozygote. Indeed, because of its importance in genetic counseling, the detection of healthy heterozygous carriers of genes that in the homozygous condition cause overt disease is becoming one of the most significant aspects of medical genetics. In recent years, the biochemical detection of heterozygotes for autosomal recessive diseases has been greatly facilitated by the development of techniques to culture skin fibroblasts. Although the culturing of human fibroblasts has been relatively uninformative in dominant disorders, in approximately 25 per cent of all autosomal recessive diseases the precise biochemical defect can be detected in cultured fibroblasts derived from a simple skin biopsy.

X-Linked Inheritance. *Dominant X-Linked Traits.* This mode of inheritance is uncommon. Heterozygous affected females will transmit the trait to both sexes with a frequency of 50 per cent. Affected males will transmit the trait to all their daughters, but to none of their sons (Fig. 4). This rule of X-linked dominant inheritance enables critical distinction from traits inherited in an autosomal dominant fashion, in which an affected male transmits the trait to both sons and daughters. The variability of expression of an X-linked dominant trait is less in males than in females. If the trait is uncommon, the incidence in females is roughly twice that in males. The erythrocyte antigen Xg^a and vitamin D resistant rickets (hypophosphatemic rickets) are inherited as X-linked dominant traits. Approximately 100 loci have been identified on the human X chromosome.

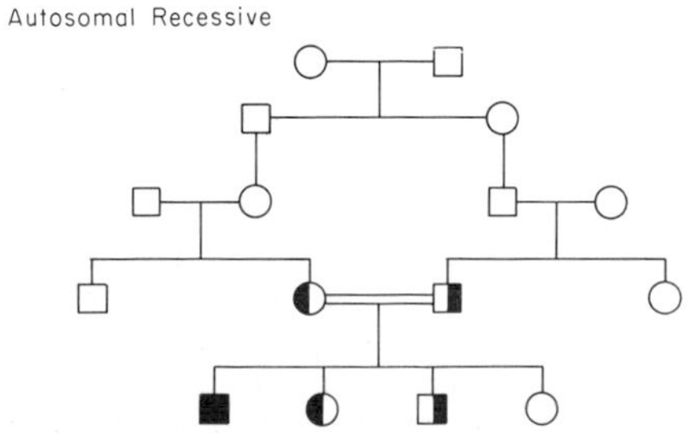

Figure 3. Pedigree of autosomal recessive trait. Note: both parents are heterozygous. One sib is affected, two are carriers, and one is normal. Double line (═) indicates that parents are related by descent (first cousins).

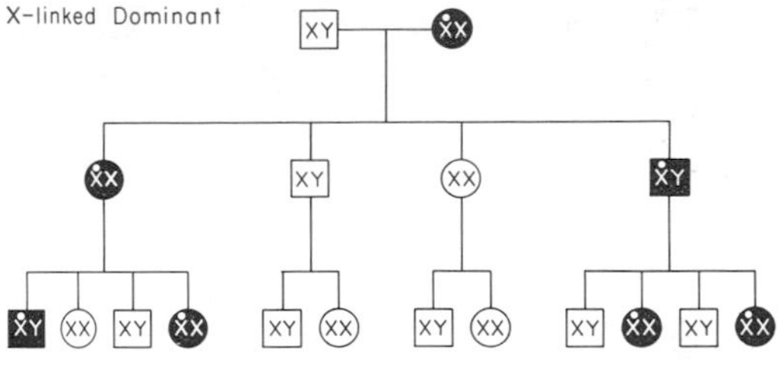

Figure 4. Pedigree of dominant X-linked trait. The X chromosome bearing the abnormal gene is designated by a small white dot.

Recessive X-Linked Traits. Recessive X-linked traits are relatively common. On the average, half the sons of normal heterozygous females will be normal, and half will be affected. If the trait is rare, parents and relatives will be normal except for male relatives in the female line; for instance, on the average, one half of the maternal uncles will be affected. An affected male married to a normal female will have normal offspring. All their daughters will be carriers, and they, in turn, can transmit the trait to the next generation. The rare event of an affected male married to a carrier female will result in equal proportions of affected male and female offspring. The unaffected males will be genotypically normal; the unaffected females, however, will be heterozygous carriers (Fig. 5). The common red-green color blindness is inherited as an X-linked recessive trait; other, less common traits include hemophilia (see Ch. 797), pseudohypertrophic muscular dystrophy (see Ch. 476), congenital agammaglobulinemia (Bruton) (see Ch. 62), and the Wiskott-Aldrich syndrome (see Ch. 69). In the general population the frequency of affected females will be roughly the square of the frequency of affected males.

The Lyon Hypothesis. Since the human female bears two X chromosomes, it might have been expected that the concentration of proteins determined by genes on the X chromosome would be twice that observed in males who have only one chromosome. Thus it might have been expected that the concentration of factor VIII (antihemophilic factor) in females would be twice that found in males. This is not the case, and the explanation is provided by a hypothesis first advanced by Mary Lyon.

In all adult females only one of the two X chromosomes is genetically active. Early in differentiation one of the X chromosomes becomes inactive and forms the Barr body. Inactivation is random; but once one of the two X chromosomes in any cell is inactivated, the same X chromosome remains inactive during all its subsequent cell divisions. For example, in X-linked hemophilia, on the average, only half the X chromosomes are genetically active and synthesizing antihemophilic globulin, and thus the amount of antihemophilic globulin synthesis is approximately the same in males and females. Greater variability in expression of an X-linked trait is a natural consequence of the Lyon hypothesis. The number of cells determining a specific function at the time of inactivation is small, and thus chance alone could influence the number of such cells inactivated.

Y-Linked Inheritance. If a trait is determined by a gene in the Y chromosome, it will be transmitted through the father to all his sons and none of his daughters. Thus far, the only genes that have been shown to be located in the Y chromosome are those that determine "maleness." (See also XYY Syndrome in Ch. 859.)

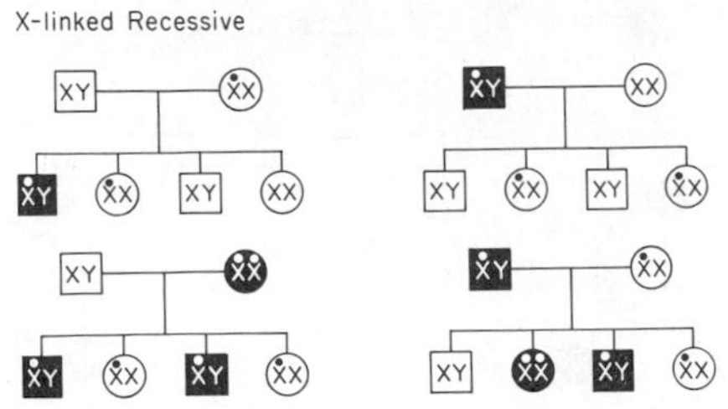

Figure 5. Pedigrees of recessive X-linked trait. The X chromosome bearing the abnormal gene is designated by a small white dot.

Sex Limitation. Autosomal genes that are expressed only in males may mimic sex-linkage but can be formally distinguished if affected individuals reproduce. If a gene is on an autosome, affected males can transmit the trait to their sons; if the gene is on the X chromosome, they cannot.

Modification of Gene Expression. The manifestation of an abnormal gene is influenced not only by its normal allele, but also by alleles at other loci, and by environment. The terms expressivity and penetrance have been employed to describe the variable manifestation of a gene. These vague words are usually best avoided unless they can be used with precision, e.g., it would be precise but cumbersome to say that the gene for Huntington's chorea is 0 per cent penetrant at the age of 10 and 95 per cent penetrant at 65. Some genetically determined traits such as those determining the blood antigens are present at birth, whereas others such as Huntington's chorea appear only in adult life. A negative correlation between the age of onset of a trait in parents and sibs suggests that the expression of a gene may be influenced by the type of normal allele present. The effect can be seen in certain dominant diseases such as the nail-patella syndrome and in the dominant form of muscular dystrophy. The concept of anticipation, which asserts that hereditary diseases tend to have a progressively earlier age of onset with successive generations, is a statistical artifact which is based on a bias of ascertainment.

Consanguinity. It is mandatory in taking a family history to inquire whether there is parental consanguinity. When confronted with a patient, particularly a child, whose disorder does not fit any clear-cut diagnosis, the history of consanguinity in the parents is often the first clue that the patient is suffering from a rare, recessively inherited disorder. In all autosomal recessive disorders the affected individual has inherited one abnormal gene from each parent. It is thus evident that an individual will be more likely to inherit the same allele from each parent if the two parents have genes inherited from a common ancestor. First cousins have, on the average, one eighth of their genes derived from a common ancestor. When the two first cousins marry, their offspring will have, on the average, one sixteenth of their genes derived from the common ancestor. It is frequently of interest to calculate the expected frequency of first-cousin marriages among parents of those with rare autosomal recessive disorders. Providing that the frequency of the disease in the population can be estimated and the frequency of first-cousin marriages in the general population is known, the calculation can be made according to the following formula. If k is the frequency of first-cousin marriages in a rare recessive disease, then as a first approximation $k = c/16q$, where c is the frequency of first-cousin marriages in the general population and q is the frequency of the abnormal gene. The frequency of cousin marriages is variable. In some isolated populations a frequency of as high as 30 per cent has been recorded, whereas in the United States in an urban population the frequency may be as low as 0.05 per cent. Let us suppose a recessively inherited disease has a frequency in the population of 1 in 10,000 (q^2); then the frequency of the gene, which in double dose causes the disease, is 1 in 100 (q). If the frequency of consanguinity in the general population is 0.5 per cent, then k, the parental consanguinity, is 3 per cent, a six-fold increase over normal. If the disease is much rarer, 1 in 100,000, then 10 per cent of the individuals affected by the disease will have parents who are first cousins. As the frequency of c increases, the expected frequency of parents who are first cousins will also increase. In some geographically isolated populations c may reach as high as 2 per cent. If a recessively inherited disease in such an isolate has a frequency of 1 in 100,000, 40 per cent of the parents of the affected individuals will be first cousins.

It is important to realize that an increased frequency of consanguinity will not be observed if the recessive disease is common. Thus in cystic fibrosis of the pancreas, which has a frequency of approximately 1 in 2500, no increase in parental consanguinity can be detected. Although the frequency of albinism in the general population is approximately 1 per 20,000, the unexpectedly high consanguinity in the parents ($k = 20$ per cent) of some patients is due to the existence of more than one gene for this condition. No increase in consanguinity would be expected in dominant or X-linked traits.

Although in most populations the consanguinity rate is approximately 1 per cent or less, and in general is decreasing, certain geographic and cultural isolates remain in which there is a high coefficient of inbreeding. These isolates may shelter rare genes which because of the high consanguinity rate are likely to become manifest. More than 90 per cent of patients described with the Ellis–van Creveld syndrome have been found in the Old Order Amish living in Pennsylvania, Ohio, Indiana, and Ontario. Other rare recessive diseases found within this genetic isolate include pyruvate kinase deficiency, a form of dwarfism associated with hypoplasia of the cartilage and hair, and a form of limb-girdle muscular dystrophy. It is worth remembering that, in general, the offspring of first-cousin marriages are slightly more likely to have congenital malformations, as well as mental and physical defects, than are children from unrelated parents.

Association. The occurrence of two traits in the same person more often than would be expected by chance is called association. A consistent positive association between blood group A and carcinoma of the stomach, and between duodenal ulceration and blood group O, has long been recognized. Such an association may be due to many causes, and does not indicate that the genes controlling blood group antigens are on the same chromosome as those associated with the development of duodenal ulceration. If an association is found between two characters in the general population, it is important to determine whether the association persists when the two characters are examined in sibships. If geographic or social stratification is the cause of the association, the correlation will disappear. If, for example, a mixed population of Africans and Europeans is examined, a positive association between cDe Rhesus blood group (common in African populations) and dark skin color would be found. This association would disappear if individual sibships were examined.

Sometimes two characters are associated because they are due to the action of a single gene. Thus clouding of the cornea and mental retardation are two traits that are associated in Hurler's syndrome. The two traits are not caused by two genes, but are due to a single gene with a so-called pleiotropic effect. When a gene causes a pleiotropic effect, the association found in the general population persists when sibships are examined. Pleiotropic effects of genes are common, and may be of clinical importance. Familial intestinal polyposis (see Ch. 669) is an early consequence of the effect of a gene that later commonly leads to carcinoma of the colon.

Autosomal Linkage. The site of a gene on a chromosome is termed a *locus*. Alternative forms of genes which occupy corresponding sites on homologous chromosomes are called alleles. Applied to human genetics, Mendel's law of independent assortment states that traits controlled by two or more pairs of allelic genes will be transmitted to the children of the next generation, either together or separately, by chance alone. The law holds only for genes situated on different chromosomes or at widely separated loci on the same chromosome. However, if two genes occupy closely adjacent sites on the same chromosome, they tend to segregate together and are said to be linked. The occasional segregation of linked genes is due to crossing over at meiosis. The frequency of crossing over gives an estimate of closeness of the linkage. It is important to remember that even if two genes are present on the same chromosomes, they will appear unlinked if they are so far apart that free (50 per cent) recombination between two loci can take place.

The application of somatic cell genetics as well as the development of more discriminating methods for chromosome identification has enabled the assigment of specific loci to individual autosomes. Structural loci can already be assigned to 19 of the 22 autosomes. In many instances more than one genetic locus can be assigned to a particular chromosome. Chromosome 1 has 15 loci assigned, including the Rh locus. Chromosomes 3, 8, and 9 still await the assignment of specific loci.

Linkage of two genes, that is, close enough proximity of their loci on the chromosome that crossing over between the two loci is insufficient to lead to independent segregation, does not cause association of the two characters in the general population. In any one sibship the two characters may be associated, in which case the genes are on the same chromosome and are said to be linked in coupling (cis configuration). If the characters are dissociated, the genes responsible are distributed on each of the two homologous chromosomes and are described as being linked in repulsion (trans configuration). A common error is to suppose that the association of two characters in the single sibship implies genetic linkage. If true linkage exists and sufficient pedigrees are collected, an equal number of sibships will be found in which the two characters are not in repulsion. There are several known instances of autosomal linkage in man, including the ABO blood group locus and the locus for the nail-patella syndrome; the Rh blood groups and one form of elliptocytosis; and Lutheran blood group and the secretor locus (which determines whether soluble ABO blood substances are present in saliva and other body fluids). The loci determining the β and δ chains of hemoglobin are also very closely linked (see Ch. 746). The mathematical procedures devised to detect linkage have been greatly aided by the development of computer techniques.

Linkage has one important practical consequence for clinical medicine. If a mutant causing a serious inherited disease is closely linked to one causing a common trait, healthy carriers of the disease may be detected in unaffected members of the family by the presence or absence of the common trait. It would, of course, be important to know whether the two linked genes in the family under investigation were in the coupling or repulsion phase. Accurate information regarding the phase can be obtained by studying the distribution of the two traits in three generations.

The Histocompatibility Locus and Susceptibility to Disease. It is increasingly evident that much of clinical medicine in the coming decades will be concerned with the identification of those individuals who have an enhanced susceptibility to a particular disease. Smoking and lung cancer is the classic example of an environmental determinant of a human disease, whereas a deficiency of serum alpha-1-antitrypsin is an example of a genetic determinant in pulmonary emphysema.

In recent years the major histocompatibility locus (HL-A) has emerged as an important locus which can determine increased susceptibility to disease. There is a high degree of polymorphism at this locus, and a particular allele may determine a particular disease susceptibility.

Acute anterior uveitis, Reiter's syndrome, and ankylosing spondylitis occur in an increased frequency among patients carrying HL-A27. The data on classic ankylosing spondylitis are particularly impressive. In some series, 95 per cent of patients with the disease and 50 per cent of their first-degree relatives possess the antigen. Since the HL-A27 antigen is present in approximately 5 per cent of the normal white population, it can be calculated that ankylosing spondylitis is 20 times more likely to occur in individuals who possess this antigen. Gluten-sensitive enteropathy occurs in a high frequency among patients expressing the histocompatibility antigen HL-A8, and psoriasis among those expressing HL-A13.

The reasons for these associations are not clear; in some instances the HL-A antigen may be related to an antigen of the infecting organism. It is also possible that because of linkage disequilibrium certain alleles at adjacent loci are maintained in coupling. In this way the genes influencing the manifestations of ankylosing spondylitis could remain closely associated with a particular allele at the HL-A locus. The possibility that specific immunoresponse genes may play a decisive role in the etiology of certain diseases has been raised by these observations.

McKusick, V. A.: Human Genetics. 2nd ed. Englewood Cliffs, N. J., Prentice-Hall, 1969.
McKusick, V. A., and Claiborne, R. (eds.): Medical Genetics. New York, HP Publishing Company, 1973.
Nora, J. J., and Fraser, F. C.: Medical Genetics: Principles and Practice. Philadelphia, Lea & Febiger, 1974.
Stern, C.: Principles of Human Genetics. 3rd ed. San Francisco, W. H. Freeman, 1973.

7. INBORN ERRORS OF METABOLISM AND MOLECULAR DISEASE

Alexander G. Bearn

Development of the concept of an inborn error of metabolism by Archibald Garrod in the first decade of this century was one of the most brilliant insights in the history of genetics, for it introduced the seminal hypothesis that the primary action of a gene is to control the synthesis of a specific enzyme. Subsequent work has fully substantiated Garrod's belief that the block in a metabolic pathway arises from an inherited deficiency of a specific enzyme. More recently the term inborn error of metabolism has been extended to include hereditary alterations in proteins that have no enzymatic functions.

The development of precise chemical methods that enable a comparison to be made between normal and genetically altered proteins led to the introduction of the term *molecular disease,* to emphasize that the difference between a normal and an affected individual might reside in the substitution of a single amino acid residue in the primary sequence of a protein molecule. Although the metabolic block may affect protein, carbohydrate, lipid, nucleic acid, porphyrin, or pigment metabolism, the *primary* abnormality invariably lies in the genetic specification of the synthesis of a protein.

In some inborn errors of metabolism the mutational event simply affects the active site of the enzyme. In these instances, although the enzyme will be functionally altered, the presence of cross-reacting material can be detected by immunologic methods. In other instances the mutation results in a protein which is functionally inert, and no cross-reacting material can be detected immunologically. Using the terminology of microbial genetics, the former class of mutants is frequently termed CRM (cross-reacting material) (+) and the latter CRM (−). At the pseudocholinesterase locus, for instance, 17 CRM (+) mutants and 18 CRM (−) mutants have been recognized. In the Lesch-Nyhan syndrome there are 21 CRM (+) mutants, and no CRM (−) have been described. Even when there is no apparent cross-reacting material detectable by immunologic methods, the protein, although no longer recognizable by antisera developed against the normal protein, may be present.

Some of the clinical conditions for which a demonstrated abnormality in a specific protein has been observed are listed in Table 1. In most of these a deficiency in a specific enzymatic activity is demonstrable, whereas in others a normal quantity of a structurally abnormal nonenzymic protein is synthesized. The classic example of a "molecular disease" affecting a nonenzyme is sickle cell anemia, in which the only difference between normal and sickle cell hemoglobin is the substitution of a valine for a glutamic acid in the β chain of hemoglobin.

It is increasingly being recognized that many of the inborn variations in metabolism are unassociated with clinical disease (Table 2). These biochemical variations represent the more conspicuous examples of the importance of human biochemical diversity. In some instances they provide a critical genetic background for the expression of an environmentally controlled disorder; in others the physiologic effect of the genetic variation is not apparent.

Genetic Heterogeneity. It is becoming increasingly axiomatic that identical or closely similar clinical syndromes may be determined by different mutant genes. In some instances, the mutations may be at different loci (nonallelic genes) (Table 3), whereas in others they occur at the same locus (allelic genes). In an individual cistron, genes may be allelic at the same codon (eualleles) or at a different codon (heteroalleles). In hemoglobins S and C the mutations occur at the same codon and are thus examples of eualleles. Hurler's and Scheie's syndromes are examples of heteroalleles, for in these instances the mutations occur at different codons but in the same cistron (see Ch. 934 and 935).

Even before the syndromes of recessive albinism yielded to biochemical probes, it was evident that the two clinical syndromes must be caused by genes at different loci, because it was well known that two albinos may marry and produce normally pigmented offspring. Indeed, it is a safe generalization to assume that the majority of inherited diseases presently regarded as homogeneous entities represent the clinical effects of different mutant genes.

Genetic heterogeneity can be detected at several different levels of biologic organization. Although Hurler's and Hunter's syndromes appear clinically similar, genetic heterogeneity is evident, because family studies indicate that Hurler's syndrome is controlled by a gene on an autosome, whereas in Hunter's syndrome the disease is X-linked. Similar variations exist among the spastic paraplegias: some pedigrees indicate autosomal inheritance, whereas others are clearly X-linked. Genetic heterogeneity can be demonstrated in recessive deaf mutism, and nonallelism can be definitely inferred, because marriage between deaf mutes, as with marriage between albinos, can result in normal offspring. Sometimes genetic heterogeneity can be strongly suspected from examining the clinical spectrum of a disease, as is the case in the various inherited mucopolysaccharidoses. When the syndromes associated with nonspherocytic anemias are examined biochemically, it is evident that they are due to a number of different genes. Heterogeneity among the X-linked hemophilias is strongly suggested as a result of functional and immunologic studies of factor VIII in different families. Heterogeneity is also evident in families exhibiting C′3 esterase deficiency. In some instances "genetic compounds" result in additional phenotypic variation. These genetic compounds arise when the individual carries two different mutant alleles. Hemoglobins S and C are controlled by euallelic genes, and individuals who have hemoglobin SC disease can thus be said to illustrate the phenotypic consequences of a genetic compound (euallelic homozygotes).

Now that it is firmly established that genes control the specificity of particular proteins, genetic heterogeneity can also be detected by techniques that discriminate between closely similar protein molecules. The application of electrophoretic techniques to serum protein and red cell enzymes has disclosed a surprising degree of heterogeneity in normal persons. However, any estimate of genetic heterogeneity based on the application of electrophoretic techniques will be too low, because it seems that less than half the mutational events leading to a specific amino acid substitution will result in an altered net charge of the protein.

Screening for Inborn Errors of Metabolism. The central purpose of any screening program is the detection of in-

TABLE 1. Inborn Errors of Metabolism

Disorder	Primary Defect	Carrier Detection	Prenatal Diagnosis
Amino acid metabolism:			
Phenylketonuria	Phenylalanine hydroxylase	+	
Albinism I	Tyrosinase		
II	?		
Tyrosinemia	p-Hydroxyphenylpyruvate oxidase		
Tyrosinosis	Tyrosine transaminase		
Homocystinuria	Cystathionine synthetase	+	(+)
(a) Pyridoxine responsive			
(b) Pyridoxine unresponsive			
Cystathioninuria	Cystathionase	+	(+)
Alcaptonuria	Homogentisic acid oxidase		
Maple syrup urine disease	Oxidative decarboxylase of branched chain ketoacids	+	+
Intermittent branched-chain ketoaciduria	Oxidative decarboxylase of branched chain ketoacids		(+)
Hypervalinemia	Valine transaminase	+	(+)
Isovaleric acidemia	Isovaleryl-CoA-oxidase		
Beta-hydroxyisovaleric aciduria	Beta-methylcrotonyl-CoA-carboxylase	+	
Methylmalonic aciduria			+
(a) Vitamin B_{12} responsive	Deoxyadenosyl transferase		
(b) Vitamin B_{12} unresponsive	Methylmalonyl-CoA-mutase		
Hyperammonemia I	Carbamyl phosphate synthetase		(+)
II	Ornithine transcarbamylase	+	(+)
Citrullinemia	Argininosuccinic acid synthetase	+	(+)
Argininosuccinicaciduria	Argininosuccinase	+	(+)
Hyperargininemia	Arginase	+	(+)
Hyperlysinemia	Lysine-ketoglutarate reductase		
Saccharopinuria	Aminoadipic semialdehyde-glutamate reductase		
Histidinemia	Histidase	+	
Hyperprolinemia I	Proline oxidase	+	
II	Δ'-pyrroline-5-carboxylate dehydrogenase	+	
Hydroxyprolinemia	Hydroxyproline oxidase (?)		
Glycylprolinuria	?		
Ketotic hyperglycinemia	Propionyl-CoA-carboxylase	+	(+)
Nonketotic hyperglycinemia	Glycine decarboxylase (?)		
Hyper-beta-alaninemia	Beta-alanine-alpha ketoglutarate amino transferase		
Carnosinemia	Carnosinase		
Hypersarcosinemia	Sarcosine dehydrogenase	+	
Cystinosis	?	+	(+)
Hartnup disease	Tubular reabsorption of monoamino-monocarboxylic acids	+	
Cystinuria (three types)	Transepithelial transport of cystine and dibasic amino acids	+	
Iminoglycinuria	Transport of imino acids and glycine	+	
Carbohydrate metabolism:			
Pentosuria	Xylitol dehydrogenase	+	
Fructosuria	Liver fructokinase		
Fructose intolerance	Fructose-1-phosphate aldolase		
Fructose-1,6-diphosphatase deficiency	Fructose-1,6-diphosphatase	+	
Glycogenosis I	Glucose-6 phosphatase	+	
II	Alpha-1,4-glucosidase	+	+
III	Amylo-1,6-glucosidase	+	(+)
IV	Amylo(1-4 to 1-6)-transglucosidase	+	(+)
V	Muscle phosphorylase		
VI	Liver phosphorylase	+	
VII	Muscle phosphofructokinase	+	
VIII	Liver phosphorylasekinase	+	
Galactosemia	Galactose-1-phosphate uridyl transferase	+	+
Galactokinase deficiency	Galactokinase	+	
Hyperoxaluria I	Alpha-ketoglutarate:glyoxalate carboligase		
II	D-Glyceric dehydrogenase		
Renal glycosuria	?		
Pyruvate decarboxylase deficiency	Pyruvate decarboxylase	+	(+)
Lactase deficiency	Lactase		
Sucrase-isomaltase deficiency	Sucrase, isomaltase		
Glucose-galactose malabsorption	?	+	
Hurler's syndrome	Alpha-L-iduronidase	+	(+)
Hunter's syndrome	Sulfoiduronate sulfatase	+	(+)
Sanfilippo's syndrome A	Heparan sulfate sulfatase		
B	N-acetyl-alpha-glucosaminidase		
Morquio's syndrome	?		
Scheie's syndrome	Alpha-L-iduronidase		
Maroteaux-Lamy syndrome	?		
I-cell disease	?		
Mannosidosis	Alpha-mannosidase		(+)
Fucosidosis	Alpha-1-fucosidase		(+)
Gaucher's disease (three types)	Glucocerebrosidase	+	+
Globoid cell leukodystrophy	Galactocerebroside Beta-galactosidase	+	+

(Table continues on following page.)

TABLE 1. Inborn Errors of Metabolism (*Continued*)

Disorder	Primary Defect	Carrier Detection	Prenatal Diagnosis
Lipid metabolism:			
Hyperlipoproteinemia	Lipoprotein lipase	+	
Hypercholesterolemia	?		
Hypertriglyceridemia	?		
Combined hyperlipidemia	?		
Abetalipoproteinemia	Betalipoproteins		
Hypobetalipoproteinemia	Low density lipoproteins		
Tangier disease	Alpha lipoproteins	+	
Norum disease	Lecithin:cholesterol acetyl transferase		
Gangliosidosis GM_1 (types I and II)	Beta galactosidase	+	+
Gangliosidosis GM_2 (Tay-Sachs)	Hexosaminidase A	+	+
Gangliosidosis GM_2 (Sandhoff)	Hexosaminidase A and B	+	+
Fabry's disease	Ceramide trihexosidase	+	+
Metachromatic leukodystrophy I	Arylsulfatase A	+	+
II	Arylsulfatase A, B, C, and steroid sulfatase	+	
Lactosylceramidosis	Lactosylceramidase		
Niemann-Pick disease	Sphingomyelinase		+
Wolman's disease	Acid lipase		
Cholesterylester storage disease	?		
Cerebrotendinous xanthomatosis	?		
Refsum's disease	Phytanic acid alpha hydroxylase	+	(+)
Nucleic acid metabolism:			
Gout	?		
Lesch-Nyhan syndrome	Hypoxanthine-guanine phosphoribosyl transferase		+
Hyperuricemia	Adenine phosphoribosyl transferase	+	
Xanthinuria	Xanthine oxidase		
Xanthurenic aciduria	Kynureninase		
Orotic aciduria I	Orotidylic pyrophosphorylase and decarboxylase	+	(+)
II	Orotidylic decarboxylase		
Xeroderma pigmentosum	UV-specific endonuclease		
Porphyrin and heme metabolism:			
Erythropoietic porphyria	Uroporphyrinogen-III cosynthetase	+	(+)
Acute intermittent porphyria	Uroporphyrinogen-I synthetase	+	
Porphyria variegata	?		
Coproporphyria	?		
Porphyria cutanea tarda	?		
Protoporphyria	?		
Crigler-Najjar syndrome (two types)	Glucuronyltransferase		
Gilbert's syndrome	Bilirubin uptake		
Dubin-Johnson syndrome	Bilirubin excretion		
Erythrocyte metabolism:			
Hemolytic anemia	Pyruvate kinase	+	
	Hexokinase	+	
	Glucosephosphate isomerase	+	
	Triosephosphate isomerase	+	
	2,3-Diphosphoglyceromutase	+	
	Phosphoglycerate kinase	+	
	Glucose-6-phosphate dehydrogenase	+	(+)
	6-Phosphogluconate dehydrogenase		
	Glutathione reductase		
	Glutathione peroxidase		
	Glutathione synthetase		
Methemoglobinemia	NADH-methemoglobin reductase	+	
Leukocyte metabolism:			
Myeloperoxidase deficiency	Myeloperoxidase	+	
Chronic granulomatous disease	?	+	
Chédiak-Higashi syndrome	?	+	

(*Table continues on opposite page.*)

dividuals in whom it is likely that a specific hereditary disease will develop and against which preventive or therapeutic measures are potentially available. Screening for genetic diseases can be performed at three principal phenotypic levels. In many instances the recognition of overt clinical disease represents the only phenotypic level at which the inborn error can be recognized. Thus in Huntington's chorea no biochemical abnormality has been found to be characteristic of the disease, and early recognition of signs and symptoms represents the only means to arrive at a diagnosis. Early diagnosis of polyposis of the colon is important because of the frequency of malignant transformation. The recognition of genital abnormalities at birth in females may aid in early detection of the adrenogenital syndrome. Inborn errors can also be recognized by the presence of an abnormal metabolite in physiologic fluids. The enzymatic deficiency may lead to an accumulation of the substrate

TABLE 1. Inborn Errors of Metabolism (*Continued*)

Disorder	Primary Defect	Carrier Detection	Prenatal Diagnosis
Abnormalities of plasma proteins:			
Analbuminemia	Albumin		
Atransferrinemia	Transferrin		
Afibrinogenemia	Fibrinogen		
Alpha$_1$-antitrypsin deficiency	Alpha$_1$-antitrypsin	+	
Acatalasia	Catalase	+	(+)
Suxamethonium sensitivity	Pseudocholinesterase		
Hereditary angioedema	C$\overline{1}$-inhibitor		
C1q deficiency	C1q		
C1r deficiency	C1r		
C2 deficiency	C2		
C3 deficiency	C3		
X-linked agammaglobulinemia	?		
Severe combined immunodeficiency	Adenosine deaminase (?)		
Selective IgA deficiency	?		
X-linked immunodeficiency with increased IgM	?		
Hemophilia A	Factor VIII	+	
Hemophilia B	Factor IX	+	
von Willebrand's disease	?		
Hageman trait	Factor XII	+	
PTA deficiency	Factor XI	+	
Parahemophilia	Factor V	+	
Hypoprothrombinemia	Factor II	+	
Factor VII deficiency	Factor VII	+	
Factor X deficiency	Factor X	+	
Fibrin-stabilizing factor deficiency	Factor XIII	+	
Hormone and vitamin metabolism:			
Adrenogenital syndrome	21-Hydroxylase		+
	11-Hydroxylase		
	3-Beta-hydroxysteroiddehydrogenase		
	17-Hydroxylase		
	Desmolase		
Aldosterone deficiency	18-Hydroxylase		
Familial goiter	Iodide transport		
	Peroxidase		
	Iodotyrosine coupling		
	Iodotyrosine deiodinase		
	Thyroglobulin synthesis		
Renal diabetes insipidus	?	+	
Vitamin D dependent rickets	25-Hydroxycholecalciferol-1-hydroxylase		
Formiminotransferase deficiency	Formiminotransferase		
Miscellaneous:			
Cystic fibrosis	?		
Wilson's disease	?	+	
Hemochromatosis	?		
Menkes' kinky hair syndrome	Intestinal copper absorption		
Sulfite oxidase deficiency	Sulfite oxidase deficiency		
Hypophosphatasia	Alkaline phosphatase (?)		
Lysosomal acid phosphatase deficiency	Acid phosphatase	+	+
Renal tubular acidosis I	Gradient defect		
II	Bicarbonate wastage		

(+) = Prenatal diagnosis may prove to be possible, because the defect is expressed in cell culture.

for the reaction catalyzed by the normal enzyme and to a deficiency of the product. An increased level of blood galactose in galactosemia and of phenylalanine in phenylketonuria are examples in which the disturbance of the normal metabolic relationships leads to detection of disease.

Since genes control the synthesis of proteins, the most direct way of identifying an inborn error is to utilize a screening program which detects a qualitative change in the structure of the protein, e.g., electrophoretically, or by its altered enzymatic or immunologic activity. Mass screening for inborn errors of metabolism in the general population is expensive and time consuming, and a careful estimate of the cost of such a program must be balanced against the potential gains. When this is done, the cost for most countries would seem to be prohibitive. For the moment it seems wiser to focus on those families and populations who are particularly at risk and for whom effective therapy for the inborn errors of metabolism is available. Screening for Tay-Sachs disease among Ashkenazic Jews and sickle cell hemoglobin among black populations are examples of screening programs which, when carefully carried out, can be of undoubted benefit. Amniocentesis and expanding usefulness of cultured fibroblasts to identify certain inborn errors of metabolism before birth can be expected to increase sharply in the years ahead and will increase the usefulness of screening programs.

TABLE 2. A Selection of Common Inherited Polymorphisms

Blood groups, e.g., ABO, MNS, Rh
Leukocyte groups
Platelet groups
Histocompatibility antigens (HL-A system)
Hemoglobin (α, β, γ, δ-chains)
Myoglobin
Serum proteins:
Albumin
Alpha$_1$-antitrypsin
Group-specific component (Gc)
Haptoglobin (α, β-chains)
Ceruloplasmin
Alpha$_2$-macroglobulin (Xm)
Complement (C3, C4)
Beta-lipoprotein (Ag-, Ld-, Lp- types)
Transferrin
Fibrinogen
Immunoglobulins (Am, Gm, InV)
Enzymes:
Glucose-6-phosphate dehydrogenase
Phosphoglucomutase (PGM 1, 2, 3)
Phosphohexoseisomerase
Lactate dehydrogenase
Adenine phosphoribosyl transferase
Hypoxanthine-guanine phosphoribosyl transferase
Peptidases (A, B, C, D, E)
Pseudocholinesterase (E1, E2)
Amylase
Phenylthiocarbamide testing
Beta-aminoisobutyric aciduria
Color blindness

TABLE 3. Some Illustrative Examples of Genetic Diseases Showing Nonallelic Heterogeneity

Albinism
Cystic fibrosis
Deafness
Diabetes insipidus, neurohypophyseal type
Osteogenesis imperfecta
Pituitary dwarfism
Retinitis pigmentosa
Sanfilippo's syndrome A and B

Harris, H.: The Principles of Human Biochemical Genetics. *In* Neuberger, A., and Tatum, E. L. (eds.): Frontiers of Biology. Vol. 19. New York, American Elsevier Publishing Company, 1970.

McKusick, V. A.: Mendelian Inheritance in Man: Catalogs of Autosomal Dominant, Autosomal Recessive, and X-linked Phenotypes. 4th ed. Baltimore. The Johns Hopkins Press, 1975.

8. POLYGENIC AND MULTIFACTORIAL INHERITANCE

Alexander G. Bearn

Traits determined by the collaboration of many genes at different loci are called polygenic, in contrast to those traits which are determined by a single gene (monogenic). Most of the differences among normal people are determined by the interaction of many genetic and environmental factors (multifactorial inheritance).

Polygenic inheritance, in which many genes each contribute a minor effect, is best established for those traits which show continuous variation in the form of a "normal" distribution curve. Height is an example of a polygenic (and multifactorial) trait in which the extremes of the normal distribution are not considered abnormal. The degree of resemblance among relatives can be deduced from the number of genes they share in common. Dizygotic twins, however, will have 50 per cent of their genes in common, as will all sibs. Parents and children also have 50 per cent of their genes in common. Thus it would be expected that if one parent is 6′0″ and the other 5′6″, all the children, on the average, would be 5′9″. Polygenic models have been advanced for inheritance of high blood pressure, diabetes mellitus, and rheumatoid arthritis, as well as a variety of congenital defects.

In clinical medicine polygenic and multifactorial inheritance should be suspected when the disease under consideration is "known to run in families," and when, in addition, examination of the affected and unaffected sibs in any sibship does not support inheritance in a simple dominant or recessive fashion. When this occurs, it is reasonable to suspect that within such families a large number of "risk genes" are present. "Risk genes" are of course present in the normal population, but in low frequency. If in any one individual there is a particularly large number of high "risk genes," the latent disorder becomes overt. This phenomenon is known as the "threshold effect" (Fig. 6). When examining a pedigree for a possible polygenic inheritance pattern, it is worth remembering that polygenic inheritance becomes more likely if in the empiric risk figure for the disease the frequency of affected sibs increases with the number of affected sibs already born. This latter fact is particularly important in genetic counseling. The elegance and complexity of the mathematical models advanced for polygenic-multifactorial disease should not obscure the fact that each of the "risk genes" has, like any other gene, a specific biochemical consequence. Eventually,

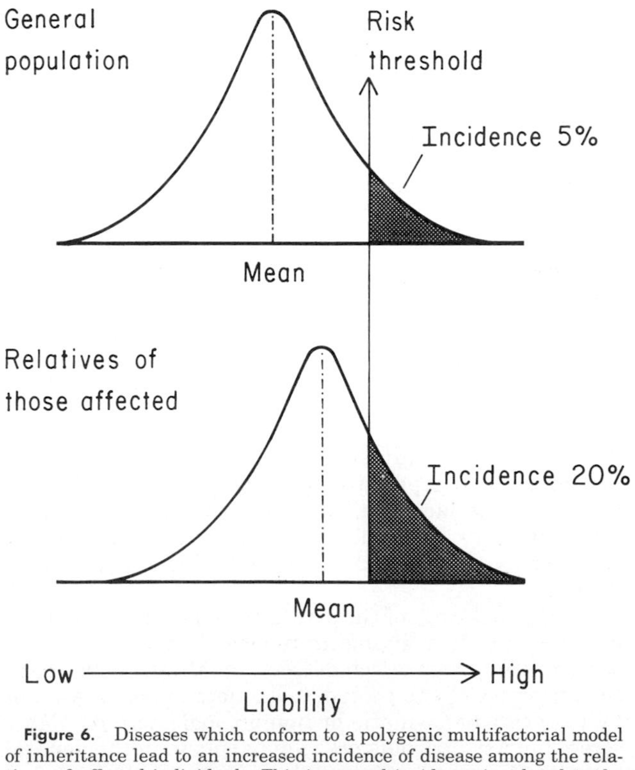

Figure 6. Diseases which conform to a polygenic multifactorial model of inheritance lead to an increased incidence of disease among the relatives of affected individuals. This increased incidence is related to the lowering of the "risk threshold" and is most evident among close relatives (sibs, uncle-niece, first cousins).

the vague concept of genetic susceptibility of polygenic inheritance must yield to the central dogma that genes control the synthesis of specific proteins each of which has specific enzymatic functions.

Carter, C. O.: Genetics of common disorders. Br. Med. Bull., 25:52, 1969.

9. PHARMACOGENETICS

Alexander G. Bearn

It has long been recognized that certain people respond unusually to the administration of specific drugs. In some instances the altered reaction has an immunologic basis, in others it appears to be idiosyncratic without obvious cause; and in some the difference appears to be contingent on the genetic constitution of the host. Pharmacogenetics is concerned with those deviant responses to specific drugs that are genetically determined. The breakdown and disposal of drugs in the body are usually dependent on a series of specific gene-controlled enzymatic reactions. Mutant genes in the population that alter these reactions can result in serious clinical consequences.

Inherited Diseases Discovered or Precipitated by the Use of Drugs. Several diseases have been disclosed or precipitated as a direct result of the administration of drugs which for their proper metabolic disposal require an intact enzyme system. In the absence of pharmacologic overload, the defective enzyme system does not cause disease.

Glucose-6-Phosphate Dehydrogenase Deficiency. A severe hemolytic anemia (favism) may be produced by the ingestion of the broad bean *Vicia fava.* The anemia is due to deficiency of the X-linked enzyme glucose-6-phosphate dehydrogenase in the erythrocytes of susceptible subjects (see Glucose-6-Phosphate Dehydrogenase in Ch. 740). It is of interest that a deficiency of the enzyme is a necessary but not sufficient cause for the anemia that follows ingestion of fava beans. Additional genetic factors, presently poorly identified, are also required if the disease is to be manifest. Severe neonatal jaundice in the Mediterranean basin and Far East may occasionally be associated with glucose-6-phosphate dehydrogenase deficiency.

Persons with glucose-6-phosphate dehydrogenase deficiency are particularly susceptible to hemolytic reactions after administration of the antimalarial drug primaquine and certain other drugs, including aspirin and phenacetin. The mutation in the black population is characterized by a mean enzyme activity of 10 to 20 per cent of normal, and the increased susceptibility to hemolysis is restricted to the older red cells. The risk of hemolysis is significantly less than in the Mediterranean type of glucose-6-phosphate dehydrogenase deficiency in which the residual enzymatic activity is less than 5 per cent of normal and increased susceptibility to hemolysis occurs in young as well as old cells. Interestingly, a severe hemolytic anemia may occur during the course of acute viral hepatitis and infectious mononucleosis in individuals with deficiency of glucose-6-phosphate dehydrogenase. The trait is present in about 10 per cent of blacks in the United States and may reach as high as 35 per cent in certain African and Mediterranean populations. The deficiency provides some protection against falciparum malaria and accounts for the persistence of the gene at a very high level in these populations. The relationship of glucose-6-phosphate dehydrogenase deficiency and resistance to falciparum malaria affords one of the better examples of a balanced polymorphism in which a heterozygous advantage can be clearly demonstrated.

Isoniazid. When a group of individuals is given a standard dose of the antituberculosis drug isoniazid (INH), two subpopulations can be identified. In one group the blood level of isoniazid is high and very little acetylated INH is excreted in the urine (slow inactivators), whereas in the second group the blood isoniazid is considerably lower and acetylated INH appears in the urine in large quantities (rapid inactivators). Twin studies show a similar metabolic response in monozygotic twins, whereas notable differences are apparent in dizygotic twins. Pedigree analysis indicates that the capacity to acetylate isoniazid is inherited as a simple recessive trait. The "slow inactivators" lack the liver enzyme N-acetyltransferase present in "rapid inactivators." Although it is clinically reassuring that rapid acetylators show an impairment of the antituberculosis effect of the drug, slow acetylators are more likely to encounter undesirable side effects such as peripheral neuropathy, a mischance which can be avoided if pyridoxine is administered concomitantly. It is of some clinical importance that the absence of the acetylating enzyme also makes more likely the toxic effects of the antiepileptic drug phenelzine and the antihypertensive agent hydralazine, because both these agents are acetylated by N-acetyltransferase.

The gene determining N-acetyltransferase deficiency occurs in 60 per cent of the black and white populations, but in only 10 per cent of Eskimo and Japanese populations. This polymorphism is of particular interest, because the aberrant gene has no clinical effect unless drugs which require acetylation for their metabolism are administered.

Suxamethonium (Succinylcholine). Suxamethonium is a commonly employed short acting muscle relaxant. Its short action is due to the rapidly inactivating influence of the serum enzyme cholinesterase. Genetic variants of the enzyme are known which fail to hydrolyze suxamethonium and as a consequence cause a prolonged, but fortunately rarely fatal, apnea. This increased sensitivity to suxamethonium occurs in about 1 in 3000 patients and can be caused by a large number of different alleles at the pseudocholinesterase locus.

Hemoglobin Zürich and Other Drug-Sensitive Hemoglobins. The red cells from patients with the unstable hemoglobins (Zürich, Shepherd's Bush, and Torino) exhibit an unusual tendency to hemolysis when exposed to certain drugs. The sulfonamides are particular offenders, but all drugs which cause hemolysis in patients with glucose-6-phosphate deficiency may be potentially harmful.

Anticoagulant Resistance. Two families have been reported in which some members are extremely resistant to warfarin and other coumarin congeners. Approximately ten times the usual dose of warfarin was needed to increase the prothrombin time to an expected level. This provides an example in which resistance to a drug is genetically determined. The frequency of the trait is undoubtedly rare.

Glaucoma. Repeated instillation of glucocorticoids

into the eye is followed by an increase in intraocular pressure. The ocular response is controlled by a pair of allelic genes. Those individuals, perhaps 5 per cent of the population, who have an unusually brisk response to the instillation of glucocorticoids are particularly liable to develop glaucoma.

Porphyria. The well known sensitivity of individuals with porphyria to barbiturates, particularly the short-acting compound thiopental (thiopentone), is a classic example of a genetically determined altered response to a drug.

Malignant Hyperthermia. This is an autosomal dominantly inherited condition causing a frequently fatal hyperthermia associated with muscle rigidity that may follow the administration of anesthetic agents such as halothane, succinylcholine, or methoxyflurane. It is particularly important to inform affected individuals that half of their first-degree relatives are at a similar risk. This condition occurs in 1 out of 20,000 anesthetized patients.

Vesell, E. S.: Advances in pharmacogenetics. *In* Steinberg, A. G., and Bearn, A. G. (eds.): Progress in Medical Genetics. Vol. 9. New York, Grune & Stratton, 1973, p. 291.

10. POPULATION GENETICS

Alexander G. Bearn

Gene Frequency. Although genes are expressed in individuals, it is often of interest to consider the distribution of mutant genes in the general population. The basis of population genetics is the Hardy-Weinberg law, which was formulated in a context of concern that a dominant trait would eventually displace a normal trait in the population. In particular, it arose in response to the fallacious assertion that if brachydactyly is a dominant trait, then "in the course of time, one would expect in the absence of counteracting factors to get three brachydactylous persons to one normal."

If the frequency of a particular gene A is p, then its alternate allele a is $(1-p)=q$; the population will consist of individuals of three genotypes: those who are homozygous AA, those who are heterozygous Aa, and those who are homozygous aa. The frequency of these genotypes in a randomly mating population will be in the proportion p^2 (AA), 2pq (Aa), and q^2 (aa). One important consequence of this formulation is that whatever the initial frequency of the genes A and a in the population, the proportion of the three genotypes will tend to remain constant during succeeding generations, providing that the three genotypes are equally fertile. If the mating in the population is not random or if there is not equal viability of the three genotypes, the frequency calculations require considerable adjustment, and in small populations substantial changes in gene frequency may occur simply as a matter of chance.

The Hardy-Weinberg law has a very useful practical consequence. If the frequency of a recessive disease in a particular population is known, the frequency of heterozygous carriers as well as the frequency of the abnormal gene can be calculated. Thus for a recessively inherited disease aa (q^2) with a frequency of 1 per 10,000, the frequency of the gene a (q) will be the square root of 1/10,000 or 1/100. The frequency of heterozygous carriers will be $2 \times p \times q = 2 \times 99/100 \times 1/100$ or approximately 1/50. Thus for this particular inherited disease there will be 200 clinically unaffected carriers of the abnormal gene in the population for every affected individual. Cystic fibrosis of the pancreas, the most frequent recessively inherited disease in the white population, has a frequency of approximately 1 in 2500 (q^2); thus the frequency of heterozygous carriers is approximately 1 in 25 (2pq).

Mutation and Selection. A mutation is a stable heritable change in the genetic material. This change may affect a single locus, or it may consist of chromosome breakage with loss or rearrangement of the fragments. In molecular terms a point mutation can be regarded as an alteration, addition, or deletion of one of the bases of the DNA molecule. The simplest mutational event is the substitution of one nucleotide for another in the DNA sequence. Although this usually results in the substitution of one amino acid for another in the polypeptide chain (e.g., glutamic acid at position 6 of the beta polypeptide chain is replaced by valine in hemoglobin S), it is not invariable, because several different triplets can code for the same amino acid. Mutations which either insert or delete nucleotide into the genetic code usually cause more extensive substitutions in the polypeptide synthesis than single nucleotide substitutions. It will be recalled that the genetic code is read as successive triplets; an insertion or deletion will upset the regularity of the triplets, and the translation of the code into amino acids distal to the point of insertion or deletion will be altered. From what is known about the genetic code, about 75 per cent of mutations will result in a single base change, resulting in the substitution of one amino acid for another; about 20 per cent of the mutations will be synonymous, in which the base change in the codon does not change the amino acid specified; and in about 5 per cent the base triplet change will result in a nonsense triplet, leading to a chain termination and the synthesis of a polypeptide lacking a variable portion of its carboxyl terminal amino acid sequence. The effect of a mutation in a somatic cell is restricted to the life of an individual, whereas mutation in the germ line can be transmitted to future generations. The natural mutation rate can be greatly increased by x-rays, ultraviolet rays, increased temperature, and various chemical mutagens such as nitrogen mustard, ethylene sulfonate, and 5-bromouracil. Chemical mutagens are thought to achieve their effects by direct structural modification of a purine or pyrimidine base, or by substitution of a base analogue for one of the normal bases.

The germinal mutation rate is usually expressed as the number of mutations per locus per generation. The average spontaneous mutation rate is usually expressed as the number of mutations per locus per generation. The average spontaneous mutation rate for a number of autosomal, recessive, and X-linked traits is 3×10^{-5}. One common, often unavoidable, error in estimating mutation rates in man is the failure to recognize that indistinguishable clinical syndromes can be caused by different genes (see Genetic Heterogeneity in Ch. 7). Thus the frequencies deduced by the elegant studies of Haldane on mutation rate for hemophilia must be revised downward, because Christmas disease, another bleeding disorder determined by a gene on the X chromosome, had not been discovered when the original calculations were made. Since heterogeneity appears to be the rule in inherited disease, all estimates of mutation rate are likely to be high. Nonhereditary conditions which mimic mutations are termed phenocopies and will also lead to overestimation of mutation rates. Spontaneous mutation rates tend to increase with advancing age. The occurrence of new mutations for chondrodystrophy is almost linearly related to paternal age. It is approximately three times more likely for a chondrodystrophic child to be born of unaffected parents if the father is 45 years of age or older than if he is 25 years old.

The frequency of most genes in the population is relatively stable. When a gene is rare and severely disadvantageous, the mutation rate is balanced by the elimination of the disadvantageous gene by natural selection. The frequency of the disadvantageous gene, however, can be stabilized at a high level if the heterozygotes are slightly favored and leave a greater number of progeny than either homozygote. The concept of *balanced polymorphism* has been defined as the existence of two or more discontinuous forms of a species in such proportion that the rarest of them cannot be maintained at its frequency in the population by recurrent mutation. As a general proposition, if the rarer of the two allelic forms occurs in a frequency that is greater than 1 per cent, the existence of balanced polymorphism should be entertained. An example of such a balanced polymorphism is the increased resistance of individuals heterozygous for sickle cell trait to falciparum malaria. Although patients with sickle cell disease (homozygotes) usually die before they can reproduce and thus cannot transmit the gene to the next generation, the incidence of the sickle cell trait may reach 40 per cent in certain West African populations. Theoretically, the high frequency of the sickle cell gene could be maintained if the heterozygote were 25 per cent more fit than the so-called normal homozygote. It has now been shown unequivocally that death from falciparum malaria is much less frequent in carriers of the sickle cell trait than in noncarriers, and thus the heterozygote does have an advantage. How much of the advantage is due to differential mortality and how much to differential fertility is uncertain, but this example serves to emphasize that the effect of genes can be assessed only in relation to a particular environment. It is, however, being slowly appreciated that the example of balanced polymorphism provided by the advantage to individuals heterozygous for the sickle cell trait may be atypical. In most instances a distinct advantage for the heterozygote cannot be demonstrated, and the possibility that certain polymorphic traits are genetically neutral is becoming increasingly discussed.

Muller introduced the term *genetic load* to describe the total genetic disability of a population. It is composed of the *mutational load,* the load caused by recurrent mutations from a normal to a lethal or sublethal gene, and the *segregational load,* which is due to the segregation of harmful genes from favorable heterozygotes. The sickle cell gene is maintained in the population because of its heterozygous advantage, and thus contributes to the segregational load. It has been estimated that, on the average, each person has three to six genes which, if homozygous instead of heterozygous, would be lethal. The relative contribution of the segregational and mutational loads to the total load is unsettled.

Stern, C.: Principles of Human Genetics. 3rd ed. San Francisco, W. H. Freeman and Company, 1973.

11. HEREDITY AND ENVIRONMENT

Alexander G. Bearn

To disentangle the relative importance of genetic and environmental influences in the causation of disease is an important but frequently difficult undertaking. In many diseases, the genetic influences are major and environmental influences are trivial, whereas in others the environment plays a major role and the genetic constitution is unimportant. For example, the genetic constitution is solely responsible for the appearance of erythrocyte antigens, the environment being without detectable influence. Many of the inborn errors of metabolism are determined by a single gene that is necessary for their expression. However, the phenotypic expression of genetic diseases such as phenylketonuria and galactosemia can be impressively influenced by alteration of the diet.

Paradoxically, the greatest difficulty in assessing relative roles of genetic and environmental influences is encountered with the common diseases of man. In disorders such as essential hypertension, coronary artery disease, and schizophrenia several genes influence the disease, but environmental factors are also highly relevant. It is important to recognize that a familial concentration of cases will be expected even when the trait is multifactorially inherited. If the frequency of a multifactorially determined trait is n, it can be shown that the frequency of the trait in first-degree relatives (parents and sibs) will be approximately $\sqrt{n}$. Although in many infections the environmental agent is crucial, the importance of the genotype of the host should not be discounted. It seems likely that, in the past, infectious diseases were powerful selective agents, and the ability to survive epidemic disasters was probably dependent, at least in part, on the individual's genotype.

Comparative studies of identical and nonidentical twins, although traditionally regarded as being of great pertinence, have not enabled sharp distinctions between hereditary and environmental influences to be drawn. Even when identical twins are reared apart, they have shared a similar environment before birth, and dogmatic conclusions are treacherous. Nevertheless, with proper regard for their limitations, studies on twins are frequently informative.

More recently, the traditional if somewhat specious nature-nurture polemic has been illuminated by fundamental studies on gene regulation. Evidence has now accumulated which suggests that, at any given time, as much as 80 per cent of the genetic material in the cells of higher organisms is inactive. This inactivation can be reversed by certain environmental influences, and the previously inactive genes can be restored to activity. Certain steroid hormones possess the capacity to influence gene activity, and a number of these have now been shown to influence directly the synthesis of mRNA and tRNA. Indeed, the administration of estrogen to a rooster can activate genes in the rooster's liver cells so that they synthesize egg yolk proteins—proteins more useful to the molecular biologist than to the rooster.

McKusick, V. A.: Human Genetics, 2nd ed. Englewood Cliffs, N. J., Prentice-Hall, 1969.
Stern, C.: Principles of Human Genetics. 3rd ed. San Francisco, W. H. Freeman and Company, 1973.

12. CONGENITAL MALFORMATIONS

Alexander G. Bearn

The term congenital malformation is usually applied to important structural defects present at birth that are not caused by a birth injury. The relative importance of congenital malformation has increased as more effective control has been exercised over the environmental agents of disease. In 1900, in the United States, approximately 3.3 per cent of the total infant mortality could be ascribed to congenital malformations, whereas in 1964 congenital malformations accounted for 25 per cent of the total infant mortality. During the first 15 years of life congenital malformations are responsible for approximately 15 per cent of the annual death rate. It has also been estimated that 7 per cent of children have a congenital malformation of consequence recognizable by the age of one year, yet only 43 per cent of such malformations are detectable at birth. In most malformations no major etiologic factor can be identified, and it must be presumed that their existence depends on complicated interactions of genetic and environmental influences or on particular genetic combinations. The frequency of many congenital malformations is compatible with a polygenic model with a threshold beyond which there is a risk of malformation. First-degree relatives (sibs and children) of an individual with a congenital malformation are at greater risk than members of the general population. This is because first-degree relatives will have a curve of distribution of high risk genes approximately halfway between the general population and those affected. The first-degree relatives of a patient with cleft lip and cleft palate are approximately 40 times more likely to develop the malformation than the population at large. The approximate frequency and sex ratio of the major malformations per 1000 births are illustrated in Table 4.

Genetic Factors. With the exception of mongolism (trisomy 21), relatively few congenital malformations can be ascribed to specific genes or autosomal chromosomal abnormalities. Congenital hydrocephalus is occasionally inherited in an X-linked fashion. Congenital pyloric stenosis is five times more frequent in males, and hare lip and cleft palate twice as common. Congenital dislocation of the hip and spina bifida are more frequent in females. Twin studies and pedigree patterns seldom provide any useful genetic information in the common malformations. The offspring of consanguineous marriages show a slight increase in the frequency of congenital malformations.

TABLE 4. Approximate Frequency and Sex Ratio of Common Congenital Malformations

Malformation	Frequency/1000 Births (Range)*	M:F
Congenital heart disease	4.5 (1.0–10.0)	1:1
Pyloric stenosis	4.0 (0.5–4.0)	4:1
Talipes equinovarus	1.8 (0.6–6.8)	2:1
Myelomeningocele	1.5 (0.5–4.4)	1:1
Down's syndrome (mongolism)	1.6	1:1
Hydrocephalus†	1.2 (0.3–4.2)	1:1‡
Anencephaly	1.0 (0.1–7.0)	1:2
Congenital dislocated hip	1.0 (0.5–60.0)	1:6
Cleft lip ± cleft palate	1.0 (0.5–4.0)	2:1
Klinefelter's syndrome	1.0	1:0

*Reported range in various studies and populations.
†Without spina bifida.
‡Excluding X-linked recessive hydrocephalus.

Environmental Factors. Contrary to popular belief, there is little direct evidence that environmental factors such as viral diseases, maternal ingestion of drugs, or maternal irradiation makes a significant contribution to the *common* malformations, although each of these factors materially increases the frequency of certain *specific* malformations. Recent evidence suggests that approximately 70 per cent of mothers exposed to rubella during the first trimester give birth to children with severe congenital defects, including cataracts, deafness, heart disease, and neonatal thrombocytopenic purpura.

Some evidence indicates that first-born children are more likely to have a congenital defect than later children. This is particularly true of anencephaly, congenital dislocation of the hip, talipes equinovarus, and pyloric stenosis. Striking regional differences in the incidence of congenital defects have been recognized, and have been well documented for anencephaly and spina bifida. An increased frequency of congenital dislocation of the hip in Lapps and certain American Indians is well recognized. An inexplicable but marked seasonal variation in the incidence of certain malformations has also been reported. It has been estimated that nearly one third of the pregnancies complicated by hydramnios result in congenital malformations.

The risk that a congenital malformation will recur with subsequent pregnancies depends on the specific abnormality and its cause. For the three most common neurologic malformations, anencephaly, hydrocephalus, and spina bifida, the recurrence rate in subsequent children is approximately 4 per cent after the first malformation, but much higher after two malformations. If it is recalled that the recurrence rate for a simple recessively inherited disease is 25 per cent, the role of genetic factors in congenital malformation can be put in perspective.

Drug-Induced Embryopathy. Fetal malformations can be regarded as the consequence of developmental unpunctuality, and are liable to follow environmental insults during the first three months of fetal life. There is growing evidence that errors in embryonic development are particularly likely to arise between the sixth and eighth weeks. It is therefore clearly prudent to minimize frivolous medication during the first three months of pregnancy. The importance of drugs as possible etiologic agents in congenital malformations has been emphasized, and perhaps overemphasized, by the thalidomide tragedy. Indeed, it is virtually impossible to specify a drug that will *not* result in an increased frequency of congenital malformations when administered to a sufficiently large panel of different laboratory animals. To assume that a drug that causes a congenital malformation in one species will necessarily cause one in man is as misguided as to assume that if a drug is harmless in animals, it will be harmless in man. It is certainly worth emphasizing that had thalidomide merely increased the frequency of a common malformation, such as cleft lip or cleft palate, rather than the strikingly tragic malformation of phocomelia ("seal extremities"), the causal association might still be unrecognized. During the two- to three-year period during which thalidomide (alpha-phthalimidoglutarimide) was freely available, approximately 7000 infants throughout the world were born with thalidomide-induced deformities. Only thalidomide, the antitumor drug aminopterin (4-aminopteroyl glutamate), and progesterone, administered during pregnancy, have been reported to be definitely teratogenic to man.

Warkany, J.: Congenital Malformations. Chicago, Year Book Medical Publishers, 1971.

CHROMOSOMES AND THEIR DISORDERS

Park Gerald

13. INTRODUCTION

Modern human cytogenetics began in 1956, when Tjio and Levan employed techniques that had been created for use with other organisms to demonstrate the presence of 46 chromosomes (23 pairs) in cultured human fibroblasts. The field became of major medical importance with the observation in 1959 that an additional chromosome was present in patients with Down's syndrome (mongolism). It was soon thereafter brought to clinical maturity when simple means were discovered for obtaining chromosome preparations with cultured leukocytes from peripheral blood.

Modern cytogenetics entered its second and present period of growth with the introduction of a fluorescent stain which permitted identification of each of the 22 pairs of non-sex chromosomes (autosomes) as well as the 2 sex chromosomes (XX in the female and XY in the male). Additional staining procedures have since been developed which provide further evidence for the uniqueness of each chromosome pair and even of individual regions within chromosomes.

Frequency of Chromosomal Abnormalities. Chromosomal abnormalities occur with greatly different frequencies at various times in life. The highest frequency and the greatest variety are found among spontaneous abortuses, 30 to 40 per cent of whom have a major chromosomal defect. Among liveborn infants, about 6 per 1000 have a chromosomal defect sufficiently severe to cause disability at some time in their lives. About half of these abnormalities involve the autosomes, whereas the remainder are sex chromosomal disorders. Among adults in the general population, the abnormalities are largely confined to the sex chromosomal disorders.

There are clinically definable subgroups within these population segments that have an increased risk for a chromosomal disorder. Infants with multiple congenital defects, for example, have a 5 to 10 per cent probability of possessing a major autosomal abnormality. The occurrence in a family of individuals with a similar group of congenital malformations is often the result of an inheritable chromosomal disorder. Such families may also have an increased number of spontaneous abortions. Sex chromosomal disorders occur with increased frequency among infertile males and among women with primary amenorrhea. They are also found to be unusually frequent among males incarcerated in penal institutions.

Preparation of Cells for Chromosomal Analysis. The chromosomes in the nondividing (interphase) cell are so extended and intertwined that they cannot be individually distinguished. During cell division (mitosis), however, they become greatly condensed and are then visible as separate entities. Dividing cells can be arrested in that phase of mitosis (metaphase) at which the chromosomes are most contracted by treatment with colchicine. By the use of colchicine and by swelling the cells in hypotonic solution to increase the separation of the chromosomes, preparations can be produced in which each chromosome is clearly visible.

Dividing cells can be obtained directly from bone marrow or by culturing a small piece of skin. The procedure required for obtaining either of these specimens, however, is unpleasant for the patient. In addition, skin cells must be cultured for several weeks before a sufficient number of dividing cells is present. Fortunately, the normally nondividing leukocyte from peripheral blood can be stimulated to divide when exposed to phytohemagglutinin (PHA). PHA appears to act only on lymphocytes (specifically, thymus-dependent lymphocytes). Stimulated lymphocytes undergo a transient wave of mitosis that reaches a peak in three to four days. By a combination of PHA, colchicine, and hypotonic treatments, suitable chromosome preparations can be obtained from a few drops of capillary blood.

In view of the simplicity of the procedure, most chromosomal analyses are now carried out with peripheral blood specimens. Bone marrow cells may nonetheless be used in the study of diseases, such as myelogenous leukemia, which are confined to these cells. Skin cells may be examined when a difference between the skin cell and lymphocyte chromosome complement is suspected, or when blood samples cannot be obtained, as in abortuses.

Amniocentesis. The amniotic fluid comprises a special source of fetal cells which has attained great practical importance in recent years. Ten to 20 ml of fluid can be withdrawn with apparent safety as early as the fourteenth to fifteenth week of gestation. The amniotic cells may be examined directly for sex determination by staining for the Barr body (sex chromatin mass) or for the Y body, as will be described later. More commonly, they are cultured and the dividing cells are treated to obtain metaphase preparations by the methods previously mentioned. Amniotic cells are unusual in that tetraploid cells (cells with two complete chromosomal complements) occur with significant frequency even when the fetus is cytologically normal. This may indicate that amniotic cells may arise in part from the fetal membranes and may not be totally representative of the fetus proper. Chromosomal examination of the fetus may alter in the future if attempts to obtain fetal blood or skin biopsies through an amnioscope are successful.

Amniocentesis for chromosomal analysis can be considered for those pregnancies in which the risk of a chromosomally abnormal fetus is thought to be significantly greater than the risk of damage to the fetus from the amniocentesis procedure itself (see Ch. 18).

Methods of Chromosome Identification. The chromosomes present in metaphase have replicated but have not yet longitudinally divided, as would have occurred if mitosis had proceeded further. The unseparated parts are known as *sister chromatids,* or *chromatids,* and remain attached together at the centromere (Fig. 1). This leads to an X-like or inverted V configuration. The portions of a chromatid extending above and below the centromere are the chromosome arms. Chromosomes are

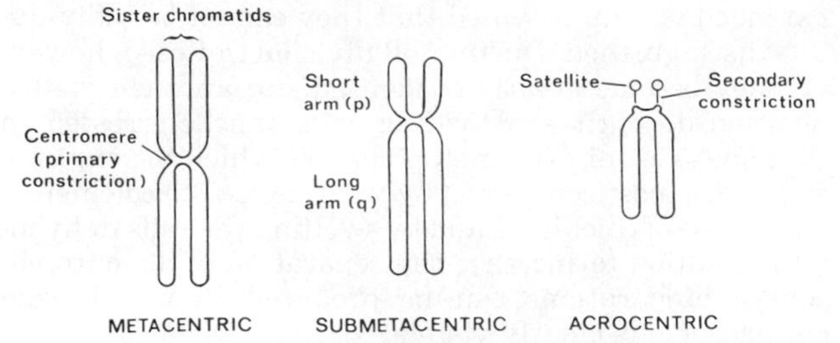

Figure 1. Schematic representation of human metaphase chromosomes and the terms commonly used to describe their gross morphologic features.

described as metacentric, submetacentric, or acrocentric, according to the position of the centromere (Fig. 1). The acrocentric chromosomes frequently possess a small amount of chromosomal material, called a satellite, connected to the short arm by a constricted region (the secondary constriction). Secondary constrictions are also found near the centromere on the long arms of chromosomes 1, 9, and 16.

When conventional stains are used, the chromosomes display no longitudinal features other than the centromere and secondary constrictions (Fig. 1). When certain fluorescent stains, such as quinacrine mustard, are applied directly or when Giemsa stain is used after various pretreatments (e.g., trypsin, urea, heat), the chromosomes display a characteristic banded appearance (Fig. 2). The location and morphology of the individual bands in each chromosome are sufficiently constant that a system of nomenclature for each band has been devised (Fig. 3). This is becoming of great importance, because it is now possible to associate a particular gene with a par-

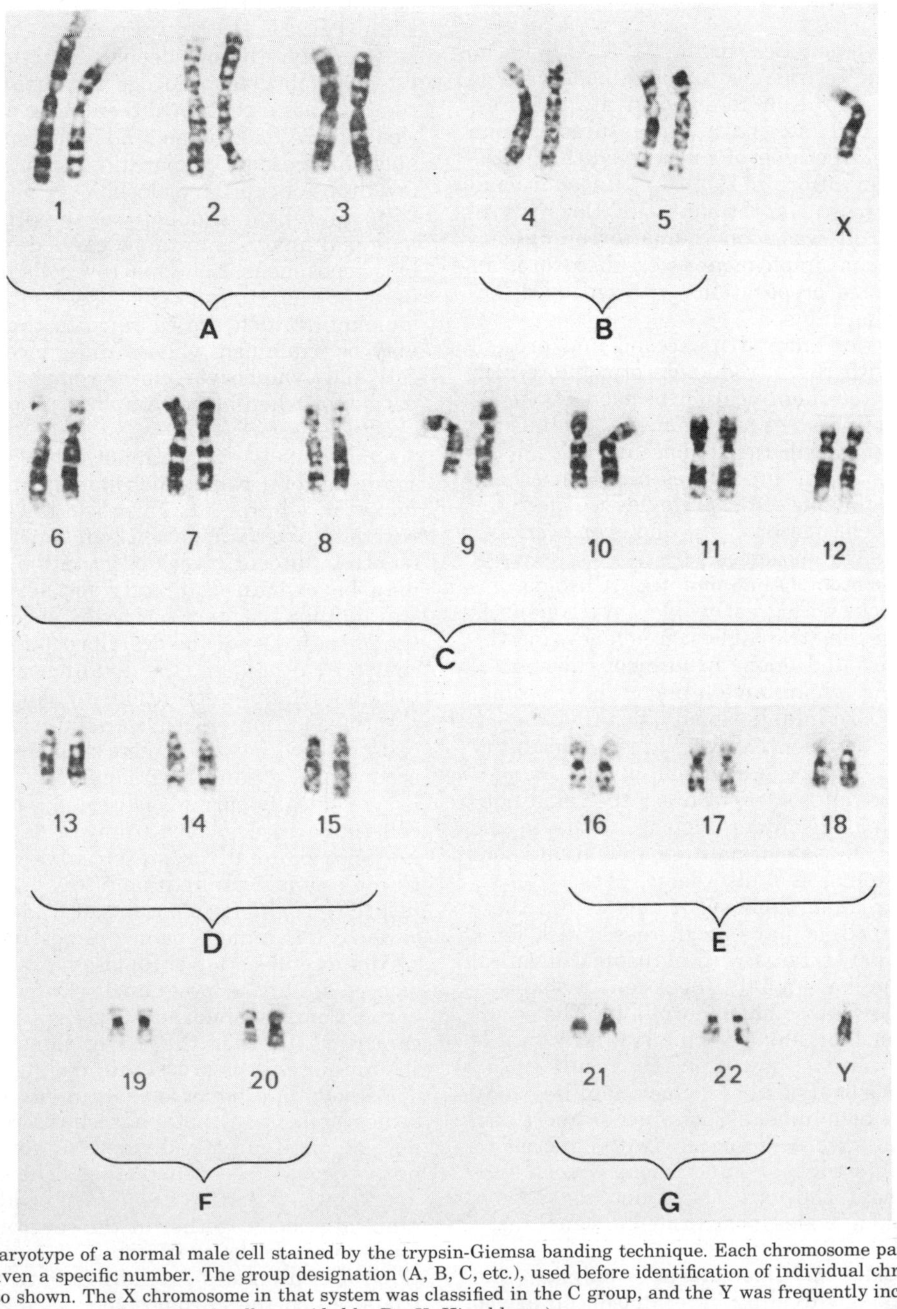

Figure 2. Karyotype of a normal male cell stained by the trypsin-Giemsa banding technique. Each chromosome pair can be identified and is given a specific number. The group designation (A, B, C, etc.), used before identification of individual chromosomes was possible, is also shown. The X chromosome in that system was classified in the C group, and the Y was frequently included in the G group. (Constructed from a karyotype kindly provided by Dr. K. Hirschhorn.)

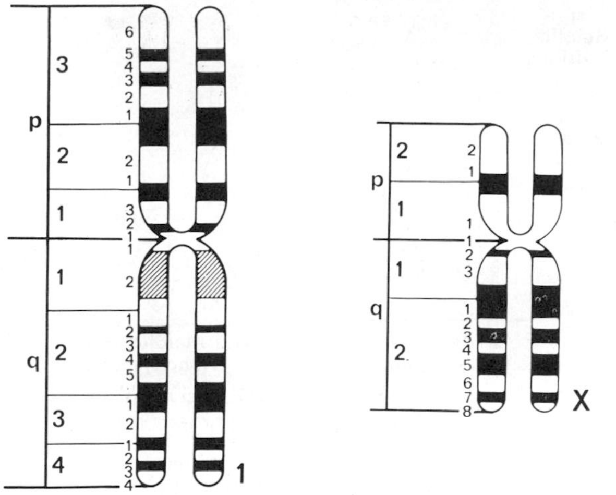

Figure 3. Schematic representation of human chromosomes 1 and X, showing their standardized banding patterns. A numbering system for the individual bands was adopted at the Paris conference (1971) on Standardization in Human Cytogenetics (Birth Defects Original Article Series, 8:1, 1972). The Rh blood group locus is in chromosome 1 near band 34 on the short arm. The loci for the following enzymes have been tentatively localized to regions in the long arm of the X: phosphoglycerate kinase (near band 13), hypoxanthine-guanine phosphoribosyl transferase (near band 26), and glucose-6-phosphate dehydrogenase (near band 28).

ticular band by such techniques as somatic cell hybridization.

The chromosomes from a single metaphase are customarily arranged in a standardized format, known as a *karyotype* (Fig. 2). Conventionally, the chromosomes are arranged in pairs and are ordered on the basis of decreasing length. Since the chromosome pairs could not be individually identified when the first karyotypes were prepared, chromosomes with similar morphology were originally classified into groups (A to G). Now that each pair can be recognized, the autosomes are numbered from 1 to 22, and the sex chromosomes are identified as X and Y (Fig. 2).

Nomenclature for Chromosomal Abnormalities. In the shorthand notation now generally used to describe the chromosome complement of an individual, the number of chromosomes is specified first, followed by the listing of the sex chromosomes. In this notation the normal female karyotype is 46,XX and the normal male is 46,XY. Any deviations from the normal karyotype are written after the sex chromosome listing. An individual autosome is referred to by number, its upper (shorter) arm by p and its lower arm by q. A plus or a minus sign written *after* the p or q indicates an increase (+) or decrease (−) in length of the arm. When written before a designated chromosome, the sign indicates that the chromosome is extra (+) or missing (−). (Examples: 46,XY,18q− describes a male with 46 chromosomes, including one chromosome 18 whose long arm is diminished in length; 47,XX,+21 describes a female with 47 chromosomes, including an extra chromosome 21 in addition to the 46 chromosomes of the normal karyotype.)

The Barr Body and the Y Body. Despite the detail revealed by the various banding techniques, none is able to distinguish between the two X chromosomes of the normal female. It is known that only one X chromosome is active in any cell; each X chromosome in excess of one condenses to form a sex chromatin mass (Barr body) visible at the periphery of the nucleus. The number of X chromosomes may be indirectly determined by examination of buccal mucosal cells for the number of Barr bodies.

Condensed, inactive X chromosomes are also delayed in the timing of their DNA synthesis, relative to the active X chromosome. The late-replicating X chromosome can be identified by autoradiography using tritiated thymidine.

In over 99 per cent of males, the distal part of the long arm of the Y chromosome fluoresces brilliantly after staining with quinacrine. The intensity is sufficiently great that this region can be seen as a spot of fluorescence, the Y body, in the interphase nucleus. Y-bearing cells can thereby be recognized in cells from blood, hair follicles, and tissue sections, and even in sperm.

Polymorphic Variations in the Human Karyotype. In addition to those alterations in the karyotype which are directly or potentially associated with disease, some variations are known which are apparently without consequence to the individual who possesses them or to his progeny. These polymorphic variations, as they are called, may represent changes in the DNA sequence of the chromosomal region concerned. They are transmitted to progeny as part of the chromosome which contains them. The more commonly recognized variations of this type occur in the length of the short arms of the acrocentric chromosomes, the size of their satellites, the length of the fluorescent segment in the long arm of the Y, and the length of the secondary constrictions of 1, 9, and 16.

14. MEIOTIC AND MITOTIC NONDISJUNCTION

Meiotic Nondisjunction. Since gametes (sperm or ova) contain only half as much genetic material as a somatic cell, the behavior of the chromosomes during their formation is obviously a unique process, to which the term meiosis is applied. Of the many steps involved in meiosis, those of concern here are only the steps that lead to a reduction in the chromosome number from 46 in the precursor cell to 23 in the gamete. Meiosis consists of two successive stages or divisions (Fig. 4). During first meiotic division, each replicated chromosome pairs with its identical partner. Next, each member of a pair enters one of the two new daughter cells formed. During second meiotic division, sister chromatids separate at the cen-

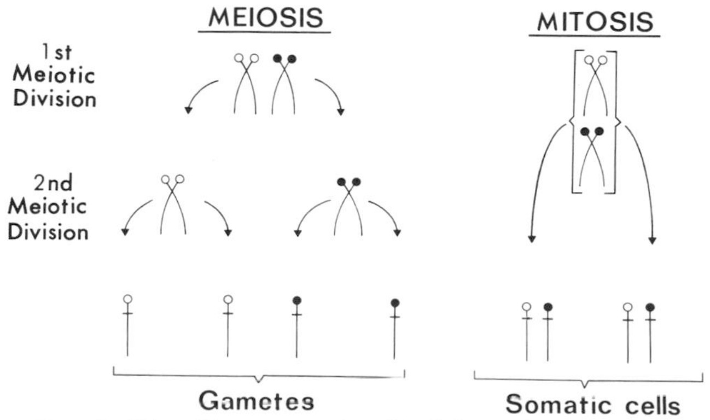

Figure 4. Schematic representation of the behavior during meiosis of a single pair of acrocentric chromosomes, contrasted with their behavior during mitosis. The round bodies on the short arms represent the satellites which are characteristically present on acrocentric chromosomes.

tromere, analogous to their behavior in mitosis, and the two new chromosomes enter the two daughter cells produced at this state (Fig. 4). Of the four cells formed from a gonadal precursor cell, each contains one chromosome from every autosomal pair and one sex chromosome (either an X or Y). (In the formation of the female sex cell, only one of the four cells becomes a functional ovum. In the male, all four cells become spermatozoa.)

Maintenance of the normal chromosome number in the gametes requires the separation of the paired chromosomes at first meiotic division and the separation of sister chromatids at second meiotic division. The failure to disjoin properly (nondisjunction) at either first or second meiotic division will produce gametes with abnormal numbers of chromosomes (Fig. 5). This will result in formation of an individual with an abnormal number of chromosomes in each cell. By using marker genes or polymorphic variations (Fig. 5), it is sometimes possible to identify the parent in whom the nondisjunction occurred and even to distinguish between first and second meiotic division nondisjunction. It is now known that nondisjunction can occur during gametogenesis in either the male or the female and during either first or second meiotic division. Some types of meiotic errors, however, are more likely to be associated with certain kinds of chromosomal abnormalities than with others (see below).

Mitotic Nondisjunction. Mitosis resembles second meiotic division in that sister chromatids become separated, with one of the two newly formed chromosomes going to each of the daughter cells. Failure of separation (mitotic nondisjunction) of the chromatids may occur and lead to creation of two cell lines, one with 47 chromosomes and one with 45 chromosomes. If mitotic nondisjunction occurs at the first cleavage division of the zygote (the cell formed by union of ovum and sperm), an individual with two cell lines (if both cell lines are viable), neither of which is normal in karyotype, will result. If mitotic nondisjunction occurs subsequent to the first cleavage division, a third and normal cell line will be present.

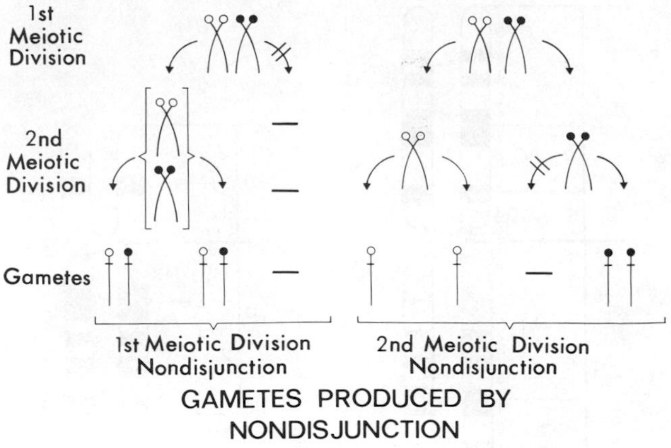

Figure 5. Production of gametes with an altered number of chromosomes by the two types of meiotic nondisjunction. When polymorphic variation in the satellites of acrocentric chromosomes occurs, a distinction may be made between first and second meiotic nondisjunction of these chromosomes.

Individuals with two or more chromosomally distinct cell types are referred to as mosaics. Mosaicism usually results from mitotic nondisjunction or anaphase lag loss. In the latter, sister chromatids separate properly at mitosis, but one of the newly formed chromosomes fails to be incorporated in a daughter cell. This leads to creation of a new cell line with one chromosome less than the main cell line.

15. CHANGES IN CHROMOSOME NUMBER

Chromosomal abnormalities limited to a change in chromosome number are usually the consequence of nondisjunctional errors. This abnormality is much more common than the group of disorders which result from change in chromosomal structure. The presence of an ad-

Clinical and Cytogenetic Characteristics of Common Syndromes Associated with Change in Chromosome Number

Autosomal Abnormalities	Common Name	Approximate Frequency among Liveborn Infants	Mechanism of Origin	Major Clinical Findings
47, +21	Trisomy 21 or Down's syndrome	1:1000	Material first meiotic division nondisjunction	Mental retardation, abnormal brain development (microgyria), characteristic facies, marked hypotonia
47, +18	Trisomy 18 or Edwards' syndrome	1:11,000	Probably maternal meiotic nondisjunction	Mental retardation, severe failure to thrive, periarticular limitation of motion of distal interphalangeal joints
47, +13	Trisomy 13 or Patau's syndrome	1:15,000	Probably maternal meiotic nondisjunction	Mental retardation, abnormal brain development (arrhinencephaly), cleft palate (and cleft lip), ocular colobomata, postaxial polydactyly
Sex Chromosomal Abnormalities				
45, X (45, XO)	Turner's syndrome	1:6000	Maternal (22%) or paternal (78%) meiotic nondisjunction	Short stature, failure of secondary sexual development, pterygium colli, neonatal edema of hands and feet
47, XXX	Triple X syndrome	1:2000	Possibly maternal meiotic nondisjunction	Usually clinically normal; may be mentally retarded and deficient in secondary sexual development
47, XXY	Klinefelter's syndrome	1:2000	Maternal (61%) or paternal (39%) meiotic nondisjunction	Mild increase in stature, micro-orchidism, infertility, gynecomastia, behavioral changes
47, XYY	XYY syndrome	1:2000	Paternal second meiotic division nondisjunction	Significantly increased stature, behavioral changes

ditional autosome (trisomy) occurs with reasonable frequency, whereas the absence of an autosome is almost never found among liveborn individuals.

A change in the number of sex chromosomes is less deleterious than a change in the number of autosomes. Individuals with as many as three extra sex chromosomes are able to survive, although they are usually mentally defective and congenitally malformed. Individuals with a single sex chromosome (one X chromosome) are, surprisingly, only moderately affected. Individuals with only Y chromosomes, that is, without any X chromosome, have never been found.

The clinical features associated with the more frequently encountered changes in chromosome number are given in the accompanying table. Each type of chromosomal aberration is associated with a relatively characteristic group of clinical findings. It is therefore highly probable that the clinical findings associated with each chromosomal aberration are at least in part determined by the specific genes present on the chromosome involved.

16. CHANGES IN CHROMOSOMAL STRUCTURE

Chromosomal Breakage. Changes in chromosomal structure are largely the consequence of chromosomal breakage. The constancy of the human karyotype from cell to cell and from individual to individual conceals the true frequency with which the continuity of the genetic material is interrupted. In most instances, a break in a chromosome is quickly repaired, with restoration of the normal chromosome structure and without harmful consequences. The exceptions to this are of two kinds and include, on the one hand, the production of chromosomal rearrangements and, on the other hand, diseases characterized by the presence of unrepaired chromosomal breaks.

Chromosomal Rearrangements; Reciprocal Translocations. If two or more chromosomal breaks occur simultaneously in the same cell, the repair process occasionally may unite the chromosomal fragments incorrectly, with production of a chromosomal rearrangement (Fig. 6). One of the most common rearrangements encountered is that which is produced by an exchange of terminal chromosomal segments between two different chromosomes, with formation of a reciprocal translocation (Fig. 6*A*). A reciprocal translocation occurring between two acrocentrics, with the chromosomal breakpoints in each being located very near to the centromere, is given the special name of *centric fusion translocation* (Fig. 6*B*). The two most common rearrangements observed in man are centric fusions between chromosomes 14 and 21 and between chromosomes 13 and 14. The minute chromosome produced during a centric fusion translocation (Fig. 6*B*) is usually lost so that a cell with only 45 chromosomes results. The minute chromosome appears to have little essential genetic material, because its loss has no effect on the cell or the individual.

The types of rearrangement illustrated in Figure 6 apparently produce no change in the amount of genetic material in the cells in which they occur. Such rearrangements are described as *balanced rearrangements,* and the individuals who possess them are carriers of the balanced rearrangement.

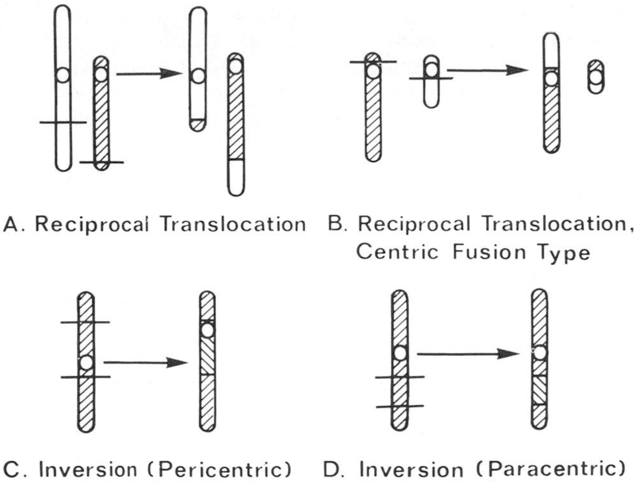

Figure 6. Schematic representation of the mechanisms underlying some type of chromosomal rearrangements. The horizontal lines represent the points of chromosomal breakage and reunion. The chromosomes are depicted as having single chromatids (i.e., they are unreplicated). It is not known, however, whether rearrangements usually occur before or after replication.

Transmission of a Reciprocal Translocation. When meiosis occurs in a reciprocal translocation carrier, the translocated chromosomes will pair with each other, as well as with their untranslocated partners. Separation of the individual members of this pairing group is often quite abnormal, with any one, two, three, or four chromosomes being incorporated in a single gamete. Since gross amounts of genetic imbalance are poorly tolerated, only a few of the possible abnormal types of progeny will be liveborn. The remaining abnormal types may appear as abortuses or may not be detected at all (because the embryo expires before implantation).

The variety of liveborn progeny expected depends dramatically upon the specific reciprocal translocation. A carrier of a centric fusion translocation between chromosomes 14 and 21, for example, will produce equal numbers of children with the balanced rearrangement and children who are chromosomally normal. A smaller number will have the genetic equivalent of an extra chromosome 21 (and have Down's syndrome), the only type of abnormal progeny produced by this rearrangement able to survive until birth.

Individuals with balanced or unbalanced reciprocal translocation may also be born of chromosomally normal parents. In this case the reciprocal translocation is assumed to have originated during gametogenesis.

Occasionally, a somatic cell may develop a chromosomal rearrangement which may then be passed on to its cellular descendants. This has been observed particularly in some forms of leukemia and in some solid tumors. Chronic myelogenous leukemia, for example, is characterized by a rearrangement (probably a reciprocal translocation) occurring in the leukemic cells which involves chromosome 22 and another autosome, usually chromosome 9. One chromosome 22 in this case has the appearance of a 22q− and is referred to as the Philadelphia chromosome (Ph^1) (see Ch. 764).

Chromosomal Rearrangements; Deletions. A chromosome may undergo breakage so that an interstitial or a terminal segment of one arm is lost. These abnormalities are known as *chromosomal deletions.* In general they are sporadic, because the abnormality is not present in the ancestors of the affected individual. The loss of genetic material leads to production of multiple congenital malformations if an autosome is involved or to abnormal sexual development if a sex chromosome is affected. The most commonly encountered autosomal chromosomal deletion syndromes have the karyotypes 46,XX or XY,5p− (the cri du chat syndrome) and 46,XX or XY, 18q−.

Diseases Associated with Unrepaired Chromosomal Breaks. There are three diseases (Bloom's syndrome, Fanconi's anemia, and ataxia telangiectasia) now known in which unrepaired chromosomal breakage commonly occurs with several times the frequency observed in normal individuals. Each of these diseases is inherited as an autosomal recessive condition. In addition to the unrepaired breaks, other cytogenetic abnormalities are present with an abnormally high frequency. These include chromosomal rearrangements, deletions, *"fusion figures,"* and *endoreduplication* (in Fanconi's anemia). The fusion figures appear to result from a break in a single chromatid in each of two chromosomes, followed by union of the ends from nonsister chromatids. Endoreduplication is a different type of cytogenetic abnormality and results when two cycles of chromosomal replication occur without an intervening cell division—each metaphase chromosome possesses four juxtaposed sister chromatids instead of the normal two. Although chromosomal breaks and rearrangements as well as fusion figures are perhaps likely consequences of an abnormality in the DNA repair process, it is not yet possible to visualize a rational connection of this with endoreduplication.

Clinically, these three syndromes are also associated with congenital malformations and a predisposition to malignancy. Cultured fibroblasts from patients with Fanconi's anemia are unusually likely to undergo transformation (a change which superficially at least resembles the development of malignancy) when exposed to the SV-40 virus. This increase in frequency of transformation is also observed with fibroblasts from Fanconi's heterozygotes.

Ford, E. H. R.: Human Chromosomes. New York, Academic Press, 1973.
Levine, H.: Clinical Cytogenetics. Boston, Little, Brown & Company, 1971.
Miller, O. J., Miller, D. A., and Warburton, D.: Application of new staining techniques to the study of human chromosomes. Prog. Med. Genet., 9:1, 1973.

17. PREVENTION AND MANAGEMENT OF GENETIC DISEASE

Alexander G. Bearn

The cardinal principles underlying the prevention and management of disease are similar, whether the disease is determined primarily by environmental agents or by genetic influences, and in both instances accurate diagnosis is a prerequisite. Treatment of the patient with inherited disease must not depend exclusively on alleviation of the metabolic defect; symptomatic treatment is often of great value, and the need for sympathetic handling of a patient with a disease that is inherited, and which may be transmitted to subsequent generations, is paramount.

Although in this chapter considerable emphasis is placed on specific, individually rare, genetic syndromes, it must be realized that the magnitude of the genetic component in the causation of all disease must be assessed if control and treatment of the disease are to be optimal. Indeed, it has been a tragic misconception, too long held, that in contrast to disease caused by environmental agents, there is no effective prevention or treatment for inherited diseases. This misguided view is quickly drained of validity when it is remembered that the expression of a disease process requires the interaction of environmental and genetic influences. Realization that 20 per cent of the hyperlipidemic survivors of a myocardial infarct occurring under the age of 60 suffer from a monogenic inherited hyperlipidemic disorder suggests that it is prudent to investigate the first-degree relatives of such individuals to ascertain those particularly at risk. Moreover, an understanding of the genetic aspects of such common diseases as obesity, hypertension, and emphysema is necessary for a comprehensive approach to prevention and management. Furthermore, an awareness of genetic influences in the metabolism of many drugs will increase the effectiveness of a physician confronted with a variety of puzzling clinical syndromes.

In the balance of this chapter attention is drawn, in particular, to those specific modalities of treatment which can be applied to inherited disease, and which stem from an understanding of the nature of the primary molecular defect. Therapeutic manipulation of the cellular environment in which the gene must act and display its nature is an approach more tractable and less perilous than direct interference with the genetic material itself.

Restriction of Substrate. General dietary restriction is often an effective way to reduce the excessive substrate that accumulates behind an inherited metabolic block. A general reduction in protein intake will improve the clinical manifestations of a number of rare inherited diseases affecting the urea cycle, including arginosuccinicaciduria, citrullinemia, and hyperammonemia. In some rather more common diseases, such as phenylketonuria and galactosemia, specific dietary restrictions are needed. The elimination of phenylalanine from the diet of phenylketonuric infants, if instituted before two years of age, is increasingly recognized as effective therapy. Similarly, elimination of galactose in the neonatal period for patients with galactosemia has resulted in an increased mental alertness, as well as the prevention of cataracts in those individuals who have a recessively inherited galactokinase deficiency. Defective oxidation of phytanic acid is the specific inherited defect in Refsum's disease; dietary restriction of this lipid will significantly ameliorate the symptoms of this disorder.

Provision of the Biologically Active End-Product. An inherited enzymatic defect will lead not only to an accumulation of the substrate on which the enzyme normally acts but also to a decrease in the end-product. When the end-product is of key biological importance, simple replacement will overcome the consequences of the metabolic block. Many instances of familial goiter associated with a deficiency of a specific enzyme can be effectively prevented by the administration of thyroid hormone. Human growth hormone is effective treatment of the recessively inherited form of pituitary dwarfism, and the ill effects of X-linked diabetes insipidus can be prevented by supplying antidiuretic hormone. Oroticaciduria, in which there is an inherited deficiency of enzymes that transform orotic acid to uridine, can be effectively circumvented by providing the uridine-starved cells with exogenous dietary uridine. Dietary phosphorus will overcome the excessive urinary loss of phosphate in X-linked hypophosphatemic rickets, and administration of dietary copper will effectively combat the inherited copper deficiency of Menkes' syndrome.

Removal of a "Toxic Product." In some hereditary diseases the accumulation of a "toxic product" may be responsible for the manifestations of the disease, and removal of the excess material may reverse the phenotypic consequences of the abnormal gene. Removal of the increased tissue copper in Wilson's disease by penicillamine is a particularly striking example of the effectiveness of this form of treatment. Similarly, removal of iron in hemochromatosis by phlebotomy is another example of therapy designed to remove accumulated toxic material.

Augmentation of Enzymatic Activity. Active efforts are being directed toward increasing the residual enzymatic activity that is usually present in patients with autosomal recessively inherited diseases. The administration of barbiturates, for example, to patients with the Crigler-Najjar syndrome has been found to increase the activity of the enzyme glucuronyl transferase, and simultaneously to decrease the serum bilirubin level.

Many biologically important enzymes require essential cofactors for their activity. In some inborn errors of metabolism the mutational event affects the ability of the enzyme to combine with cofactor. Pyridoxine (vitamin B_6) is a cofactor for the enzyme cystathionine synthetase. In more than half the patients with cystathioninuria, in whom there is a decrease in activity of this enzyme, the defect can be overcome by administration of large doses of pyridoxine. Similarly, the metabolic ketoacidosis of some patients with methylmalonic aciduria can be overcome by the administration of pharmacologic doses of the cofactor vitamin B_{12}.

Enzyme Replacement. Direct replacement of the missing enzyme is an attractive and direct approach to the treatment of recessively inherited disease, and although there are a number of substantial obstacles to this simple concept, progress is being made. It should be emphasized, however, that to be effective the enzyme must not only retain its biologic activity when administered to the patient, but must also gain access to the organs and cellular organelles in which excessive substrate has accumulated. Moreover, since the infused enzyme will have a finite half-life, continuous administration or gradual release from an implanted "depot store" must be achieved. Enzyme infusions have been attempted in the mucopolysaccharidoses, in which their therapeutic effect is still unproved, and in metachromatic leukodystrophy, in which the effect is rather more promising.

Surgical Treatment. Numerous examples of the application of surgery to the treatment of inherited disease could be cited. This is particularly likely to be effective in diseases transmitted in a mendelian dominant fashion. The prevention of neoplastic transformation in polyposis of the colon and the removal of the spleen in hereditary spherocytosis are examples of inherited diseases in which surgery can play an important therapeutic role. It should not be overlooked that surgery is a quick and permanent cure for polydactyly as well as for certain other dominantly inherited defects.

Allotransplantation of the organ in which the deficient enzyme is normally synthesized has been attempted in a variety of inherited diseases. Renal transplantation has been performed in patients with Fabry's disease and in cystinosis. In Fabry's disease renal transplantation appears to ameliorate the manifestations; in cystinosis allotransplantation is effective in overcoming uremic nephropathy but does not affect the disease itself. Although in general the results are encouraging, considerably more work will be needed before organ transplantation can be recommended as a routine therapeutic measure in any inborn error of metabolism. Bone marrow transplantation is presently the only effective therapy in patients with severe combined immunodeficiency disease.

18. GENETIC COUNSELING

Arno G. Motulsky

Genetic counseling provides information concerning the risks of occurrence of genetic disorders and the reproductive options available to prospective parents. Since genetic factors play an etiologic role in many different diseases, genetic counseling has become an important component of patient management. If there is a significant risk that a given disease will recur in future children, physicians should provide or arrange for genetic counseling even if the patient or parents do not specifically request such advice. Genetic counseling not only gives factual information but also adapts the communication process to the needs of the individual patient and his family. Alleviation of guilt and explanations regarding the nature and severity of the disease under study are always required. The natural history of the disease, including its variability from patient to patient as well as the potential personal, medical, and social burden, must be conveyed.

Diagnosis. Accurate diagnosis is a prerequisite for genetic counseling. Similar-appearing diseases may be inherited by different modes of transmission (heterogeneity) or may not be genetic at all. Accurate diagnosis requires a carefully obtained family history which is best denoted by conventional pedigree symbols. Information about relatives regarding age, onset of a given disease, health status, and cause of death is obtained. Knowledge of the ethnic origin of the family may be helpful in considering certain genetic diseases; Tay-Sachs disease is common in Jews of European origin, and cystic fibrosis is rare in blacks. Advanced maternal age is a predisposing factor to chromosomal errors such as Down's and Klinefelter's syndromes. Advanced paternal age may be found when new mutations for autosomal dominant diseases such as Marfan's disease or achondroplasia are suspected. Historic data on the immediate family are more accurate than information regarding more remote relatives. Occasionally, physicians' and hospital records have to be obtained for documentation of suspected diseases. Genetic diseases manifesting anomalies of stature or a characteristic physiognomy can sometimes be recognized in photographs of family members. If the parents are related, or if both the father's and mother's ancestors originated from a restricted rural area, autosomal recessive inheritance should be considered as the possible cause for an obscure disease. The mode of inheritance together with the clinical and laboratory findings of a given patient may be helpful in defining various subtypes of clinically similar-appearing genetic disorders such as Hurler's (autosomal recessive) and Hunter's (X-linked recessive) disease, or Marfan's disease (autosomal dominant) and homocystinuria (autosomal recessive). Diagnosis and appropriate counseling for the majority of genetic diseases require knowledge of the clinical and genetic features of the disease rather than special "genetic tests." Suitable cytogenetic and enzymatic tests should be available in the investigation of some conditions. However, because chromosomal aberrations usually are sporadic events and do not run in families, chromosomal analyses are not helpful for counseling in most genetic diseases.

Recurrence Risks. If a disease is transmitted by a mendelian or monogenic pattern, recurrence risks can be well defined. Lack of clinical manifestation (diminished penetrance) or variable expression is particularly frequent in autosomal dominant disorders. In addition to the information that a given gene will be transmitted with a certain probability, the actual recurrence risk of the clinical symptomatology and the risk for severe manifestations associated with that gene must be communicated to the patient. As an example, only 10 to 20 per cent of the gene carriers for Waardenberg's syndrome (autosomal dominant) are deaf. Deafness, rather than the pigmentary and eye anomalies associated with that condition, is disabling, and the problems and recurrence risks of deafness must be stressed during genetic counseling. Some genetic diseases transmitted by an autosomal dominant mechanism, such as polycystic kidneys and Huntington's chorea, only express themselves clinically in the middle-aged. The risk for unaffected offspring of patients, which is 50 per cent at birth, becomes progressively less as a person remains unaffected beyond the age at which these diseases first manifest. Curves plotting the age of onset can be used to quantitate these risks. McKusick's catalogue of mendelian disorders gives helpful short descriptions and literature citations for the known mendelian genetic diseases.

Since in polygenic conditions the number of genes and their relative contributions are unknown, genetic theory does not allow prediction of genetic risks, and so-called empiric risk figures must be relied on for counseling. Similarly, the transmission of viable chromosomal aberrations, such as translocations, does not usually follow mendelian principles, and counseling must also be based on empirically derived risk figures. Empiric risk figures are obtained from observing the frequency of recurrence of the disease in many affected families. Fortunately, recurrence risks for polygenic diseases are rarely higher than 5 per cent. Because empiric risks are derived from genetically heterogeneous families, they do not have the scientific precision of recurrence risks for mendelian disease. Risk assessment requires recognition of the occasional monogenic variant among the broad category of a common disease by careful consideration of the family history and possible differentiating clinical and laboratory features. For instance, autosomal dominant familial hypercholesterolemia is found in 5 per cent of patients who have a myocardial infarction at or below age 60.

Absolute recurrence risks are more meaningful to a family than relative risks. A 1000-fold increase in recurrence risk for a certain disease in a family appears frightening. However, for a condition which occurs in 1 of 100,000 births, a 1000-fold increase means that the absolute or actual risk of recurrence is only 1 per cent – a rather low risk. In mendelian diseases the recurrence risk is fixed (e.g., 25 per cent for autosomal recessive disease), whether several or no affected children preceded. In polygenic diseases, if several sibs are affected in a given family, more disease-producing genes are operative in that sibship, and the risk for future offspring becomes higher.

The meaning of genetic risks must be conveyed in terms understandable to patients. Qualitative terms such as "high" for 50 per cent risks, "substantial" for 25 per cent risks, and "low" for risks of 5 per cent or less may be helpful for optimal communication. The probability that approximately 3 per cent of all children of normal couples will develop serious birth defects, genetic disease, or mental retardation should be communicated as a measure against which the additional risks can be gauged.

Once the significance of the recurrence risk and the contribution of heredity to the disorder have been considered, reproductive alternatives which are meaningful within the social, emotional, and religious framework of the particular family must be discussed. Occasionally, it may be appropriate to give firm and directive advice. More generally, genetic counseling should be nondirective and should provide the necessary information to allow a couple to make their own decisions regarding future reproduction. A genetic counselor should not force his values on those who seek his advice. On the other hand, a scientifically cool and aloof stance is not sufficient, and a sympathetic discussion of the many problems faced by the family is required.

Heterozygote Detection. Heterozygote detection is particularly important in sisters of males affected with X-linked recessive diseases such as hemophilia and Duchenne type muscular dystrophy, because regardless of their husband's genetic constitution, there is a 50 per cent risk that the sons of female carriers will be affected. In contrast, autosomal recessive disease becomes evident only when *both* parents are carriers, and a heterozygote sib of an affected patient must mate with another heterozygote for the disease to occur. The chance that an unrelated mate will be a carrier is usually quite low. Specialized laboratory tests for carrier detection (such as creatine phosphokinase enzyme assays in Duchenne muscular dystrophy) may be helpful but must be carefully standardized on normal subjects and known heterozygotes before applying them for individual carrier identification. Detection of carriers is relatively simple in the hemoglobinopathies, and an increasing number of heterozygote states for various enzyme deficiencies such as Tay-Sachs disease can be recognized.

Reproductive Options. Fragmentary data suggest that couples who sought genetic counseling have had fewer children if the genetic risk was more than 10 per cent. If a couple decides that the risks for further reproduction are too high, several options besides contraception sometimes must be discussed. Adoption is becoming less practicable because fewer babies are available. Sterilization of either husband or wife may be considered, but it must be emphasized that this is an irreversible procedure. Thus sterilization is undesirable for prevention of autosomal recessive conditions, because remarriage after possible divorce or death could eliminate the genetic risks almost entirely. Artificial insemination by a donor other than the husband may be acceptable to occasional couples to prevent autosomal recessive disease or autosomal dominant disease contributed by the husband.

Intrauterine Diagnosis. Amniocentesis performed during the fourteenth to sixteenth week of pregnancy allows the diagnosis of genetic disease in fetuses. When performed by a trained gynecologist, the procedure has proved safe to mother and fetus. During amniocentesis amniotic fluid containing cells of fetal origin is aspirated transabdominally. After a 10- to 20-day period of cell culture, chromosomes can be visualized to ascertain fetal sex and to detect various chromosomal aberrations. Many enzyme deficiencies can be detected by suitable assays. An increased level of α-fetoprotein is frequently observed in spina bifida and other neural tube malformations. Amniocentesis is therefore indicated in the following conditions: (1) chromosomal aberrations, (2) detection of male fetuses who have a 50 per cent risk of being affected with serious X-linked diseases, (3) inborn errors of metabolism which can be detected by amniotic cell assay, and (4) spina bifida and anencephaly. Most amniocenteses are performed in pregnant women over 38 to 40 years of age who have a significant chance of carrying babies with Down's syndrome or in women who had a previous child with that disorder. In both situations the recurrence risk is 1 to 2 per cent; this risk becomes significantly higher if either parent is a translocation carrier for Down's syndrome (5 per cent for male carriers and 20 per cent for female carriers).

Intrauterine diagnosis provides a definite diagnosis and replaces statistical likelihood with certainty. Parents may select abortion if the fetus is affected and, with monitoring of future pregnancies by amniocentesis, may be assured unaffected children.

Detection of Genetic Disease in Relatives. Optimal genetic counseling in some diseases includes the testing of relatives at risk. In some conditions the detection of latent disease in sibs and other relatives, if followed by suitable therapy, may be lifesaving. A sib of a patient with Wilson's disease (autosomal recessive) has a 25 per cent chance of being affected but may be too young to exhibit overt symptoms. Sibs of patients with hereditary polyposis of the colon (autosomal dominant) have a 50 per cent chance of being affected and therefore carry the certain risk of developing malignant transformation of one of the many polyps. In general, vigorous attempts should be made to examine relatives, using appropriate tests, when a genetic condition causes serious preventable or treatable disease. Possible carriers for serious X-linked diseases (such as hemophilia) and for chromosomal carrier status (such as Down's syndrome associated with translocation) should be sought in families for prevention by intrauterine diagnosis and possible abortion.

Genetic Screening. Genetic counseling has usually been retrospective and has followed the advent of a sick child or relative. In prospective counseling, advice is given before a sick person is born. Such an approach is possible for common autosomal recessive diseases such as sickle cell anemia, thalassemia major, and Tay-Sachs disease in populations with high frequencies of these genes. Eight per cent of the American black population are carriers of the sickling gene, and 4 per cent of the American Jewish population of European extraction are carriers of the Tay-Sachs gene. Mass screening for heterozygote detection followed by suitable genetic counseling has been proposed.

Identification of the sickle cell trait before reproduction permits the prevention of sickle cell anemia if carriers refrain from mating with each other or if those already married have no children. Such programs raise many ethical and social problems, and it is doubtful whether mating and reproductive choices which are logical from the points of view of medicine, genetics, and public health would actually be made. Unfortunately, many sickling screening programs have been established without adequate counseling. Often the mistaken notion has been promoted that the sickle cell trait represents a mild form of sickle cell disease. Needless anxiety and occupational discrimination against sickle cell trait carriers have resulted. Screening programs for Tay-Sachs disease have been more successful because intrauterine detection of this condition is possible.

With the present tendency for couples to have smaller families, there is greater concern that children should be healthy, and thus genetic counseling will become more important. The principles of genetic counseling are simple and should be mastered by every physician. Although for complex genetic problems referral to a genetics clinic in a medical center is necessary, increased education in the principles of human genetics will enable genetic counseling to be undertaken by primary care physicians in many instances.

Clow, C. L., Fraser, F. C., Laberge, C., and Scriver, C. R.: On the application of knowledge to the patient with genetic disease. *In* Steinberg, A. G., and Bearn, A. G. (eds.): Progress in Medical Genetics. Vol. IX. New York, Grune & Stratton, 1973.

McKusick, V. A.: Mendelian Inheritance in Man. Baltimore, The Johns Hopkins Press, 1971.

Nora, J. J., and Fraser, F. C.: Medical Genetics: Principles and Practice. Philadelphia, Lea & Febiger, 1974.

Part III
ENVIRONMENTAL FACTORS IN DISEASE

19. MAN AND HIS ENVIRONMENT

Howard H. Hiatt

All disturbances in health reflect the interplay of environmental and genetically determined host factors. In that sense a textbook of medicine is concerned in its entirety with a consideration of man and his environment. However, the complexity of environmental factors affecting health makes it appropriate to offer a few introductory generalizations about them. Further, attention to how alteration of environmental factors can prevent or ameliorate disease is particularly urgent at this time of justifiable concern with the limitations and economic costs of therapeutic medicine.

The dimensions of man's environment are suggested when we consider that it encompasses everything that impinges on man other than the genes of the germ cell. Indeed, studies in other forms indicate that the genetic apparatus itself often includes material that was once "environment." For example, a bacterial cell may become resistant to an antimicrobial drug as a result of infection with a virus containing the information necessary for the synthesis of enzymes that inactivate the drug. Not only is the bacterium thus able to make the enzymes in question, but because viral nucleic acid may become a part of the genetic apparatus of the cell, the cell can pass on to its progeny the capacity to inactivate the drug. A related phenomenon may explain the presence of tumor viral nucleic acid in certain animal cells. The expression of the nucleic acid in terms of tumor production may require one or more further environmental exposures—for example, to x-rays or to a chemical. This multifactorial etiology is characteristic of all diseases, and the complex interaction of causes has been likened by MacMahon and Pugh to a "web" of causation. Fortunately, effective action does not require complete unraveling of such webs—the disruption of any one thread may be sufficient to induce a favorable change in health status.

DETERMINANTS OF RESPONSE TO ENVIRONMENTAL FACTORS

It has long been recognized that many environmental substances are harmful only to individuals of a specific genetic constitution. Individuals with genetic defects in metabolic pathways may be poisoned by substances that are readily tolerated by most people. An example is the damage done by the muscle relaxant drug suxamethonium to people with abnormal forms of the enzyme pseudocholinesterase. A diet containing "normal" amounts of phenylalanine will be profoundly damaging to persons homozygous for a particular gene. People unable to convert certain dietary constituents to biologically active forms, such as those with vitamin D resistant rickets, will manifest deficiency states even when receiving the substance in amounts adequate for "normal" individuals. Such conditions are worthy of special emphasis, for although they are infrequent, they are but recognized manifestations of individual variations that are ubiquitous. Responses to drugs, chemicals, microorganisms, stress, and other environmental factors, particularly at low doses, reflect in part the genetically determined constitution of the person exposed. Differences from the "normal" in lipoprotein profiles have already been well documented in the families of patients with complications of atherosclerosis; thus genetic predisposition probably makes the cardiovascular system of certain people more susceptible to the ravages of such known potentially harmful factors as hypertension, obesity, and too little exercise. Similarly, individual susceptibility likely explains in part why many but not all cigarette smokers develop lung cancer. Critical to preventive medicine is the development of methods for identifying people for whom specific environmental factors are hazardous, so that appropriate measures can be directed at those at risk.

Response to environmental factors is greatly affected by other environmental conditions prevailing at the time of exposure. One example is a drug the administration of which leads to altered metabolism of, and thereby to altered action of, a second drug. Another is the effect of nutritional status on the response to infectious agents; malnutrition may explain at least in large part why the fatality rate from measles is so much greater in rural Guatemala than in the United States. An individual with compromised function as a result of earlier exposure to one environmental factor may be particularly prone to the effects of another; for example, people with pneumoconiosis are sensitive to carbon monoxide and those with coronary artery disease to carbon disulfide.

Timing of exposure may also be important, particularly during prenatal life. A few of the known congenital malformations and spontaneous abortions have thus far been traced to identified environmental insults, but over 80 per cent are of unknown cause. Drugs, other chemicals, viruses, bacteria, carbon monoxide, and ionizing radiation are among factors known to cause congenital malformations, but only if exposure occurs during the first trimester of pregnancy. Thalidomide, for example, given to a pregnant woman can cause serious anomalies in the offspring. Exposure early in the sensitive period leads to ear anomaly, later to arm deformity, and later yet to leg deformity. Exposures after the first trimester produce no anomalies.

Environmental factors may affect the incidence or the course of a disease, or both; the condition of the host at the time of exposure helps determine which. For example, in mice, x-rays may activate a pre-existing tumor virus, thereby producing cancer. However, even in the absence of latent oncogenic viral DNA, x-rays may themselves lead to cancer by inducing a mutation of cellular DNA. Finally, by their lethal effects on cells, x-rays may be used to destroy cancer, and thus are used therapeutically. Similarly, diethylstilbestrol will produce temporary remissions of breast cancer in some patients; however, it is also known to lead to the appearance of cancer, and some young women have developed cancer of the vagina after exposure to diethylstilbestrol during intrauterine life 20 years earlier. Since many environmental factors cause disease only after latent periods measured in decades, alertness and continued monitoring of potential hazards are required.

CLASSIFICATION OF ENVIRONMENTAL FACTORS

In considering the variety of environmental factors known to be harmful to health, it must be emphasized that the field is in a state of flux, and there are few broadly accepted organizing principles. In developing countries the environmental influences of principal importance are naturally occurring, whereas in Europe and North America, where many of these have been controlled, attention is now focused increasingly on the health hazards of environmental conditions created by man. Some factors are detrimental to health when present in excess, and others when deficient; many lead to problems under either circumstance. Many and probably most environmental factors injurious to health have yet to be identified, and new ones are constantly appearing as a result of increased population, increased affluence, and technologic advances.

A prevailing classification breaks down the principal environmental factors into chemical, physical, biologic, and social. A few examples of each follow.

Chemical Factors. The role of chemicals in inducing human disease is variable and complicated. No chemical can be considered completely nontoxic, even though many are required in small amounts for physiologic processes. For example, the benefits of small amounts of fluoride on tooth development are now accepted. Studies of disease patterns in areas of hard and soft water supply suggest that one or more trace metals may offer some protection against atherosclerosis. Lead, arsenic, mercury, cadmium, cobalt, selenium, tin, manganese, and other metals can produce acute poisoning and may be introduced by contaminated food or water. Polychlorinated biphenyls, organochlorine, and organophosphorus insecticides may gain access via the same route. A variety of chemicals, including silica, asbestos, lead, and many solvents, may be present in toxic amounts in the air, particularly in and near industrial plants.

Over 10,000 synthetic compounds are now in commercial production in amounts between 500 and 1 million kilograms per year. Some are carcinogenic, some mutagenic, and some teratogenic. Because the long-term effects of a substance cannot be known with certainty for decades, testing for chronic as well as acute effects should be carried out before widespread human exposure is permitted. However, since it is impossible to test comprehensively all new compounds, it is particularly important to pay attention to those structurally related to other substances known to be toxic. In many instances in which relation between cancer and environmental exposure is well established, the specific chemicals responsible remain to be identified, as for example the carcinogenic constituents of cigarette smoke.

Physical Factors. Home accidents account for 1 to 2 per cent of all deaths in the United States and Europe, and automobile accidents cause 150,000 deaths and 6 million injured per year in those two areas. Modern transportation has had detrimental effects on health in addition to the loss of life and limb caused by automobile accidents; there is evidence that one factor contributing to coronary artery disease is lack of exercise.

Excessive heat, cold, and noise are harmful, as are both nonionizing and ionizing radiation. Less than 2 per cent of our total exposure to ionizing radiation comes from occupational sources and fallout consequent to nuclear weapons testing and nuclear power development. Almost one third of our exposure is from medical diagnostic procedures, and two thirds from natural sources. However, with increasing dependence on nuclear power certain in the years ahead, this could change significantly. The effect of ionizing radiation on the gene pool is cumulative. The most important somatic effect is carcinogenesis. Whether radiation effects contribute to mortality from causes other than cancer is uncertain.

Biological Factors. Man may be exposed to pathogenic bacteria, viruses, and parasites through inspired air, ingested food and water, and skin contact. The soil is a common source of pathogenic microorganisms and parasites, and many occupations have special biologic hazards, such as anthrax and brucellosis. Many infectious agents produce both acute and chronic disease. Some virus-induced conditions, such as kuru, become manifest only after a latent period of years. Although there have been many claims and much speculation, no unequivocal evidence yet exists for a microbiologic agent as a cause of cancer in man. However, it is likely that at least some forms of human cancer are viral in origin.

Social Factors. Social factors, including economic, psychologic, and cultural factors, all affect health. There is evidence that schizophrenia, crime, suicide, alcoholism, and drug abuse have higher rates in impoverished and crowded areas. Infant mortality is as much as three times higher in the poverty sectors than in more affluent parts of the same cities. Pasamanick and Knobloch (1962) have shown that although black and white infants manifest no differences in developmental tests at 40 weeks of age, by three years the performance of black children is significantly behind that of the white. Whether poverty itself, poor housing, inadequate diet, less education, a combination of these, or other factors are responsible is yet to be established. However urgent the need for more knowledge in this area, existing information is sufficient to provide strong incentive for improving conditions.

Examination of mortality data reveals that major improvements in health have resulted to a much greater extent from changes in a variety of environmental factors than from medical measures. This is particularly apparent in studies of deaths from infectious diseases in the preantimicrobial era (see accompanying figure). Although precise explanations for the dramatic health improvements in the eighteenth, nineteenth, and early twentieth centuries are not available, there is reason to believe that they resulted from better nutrition, removal of hazards from the physical environment by improved water supply and sewage disposal, and a decrease in the birth rate. Other factors may also have contributed, including changes in the virulence of some of the microorganisms, notably the streptococci.

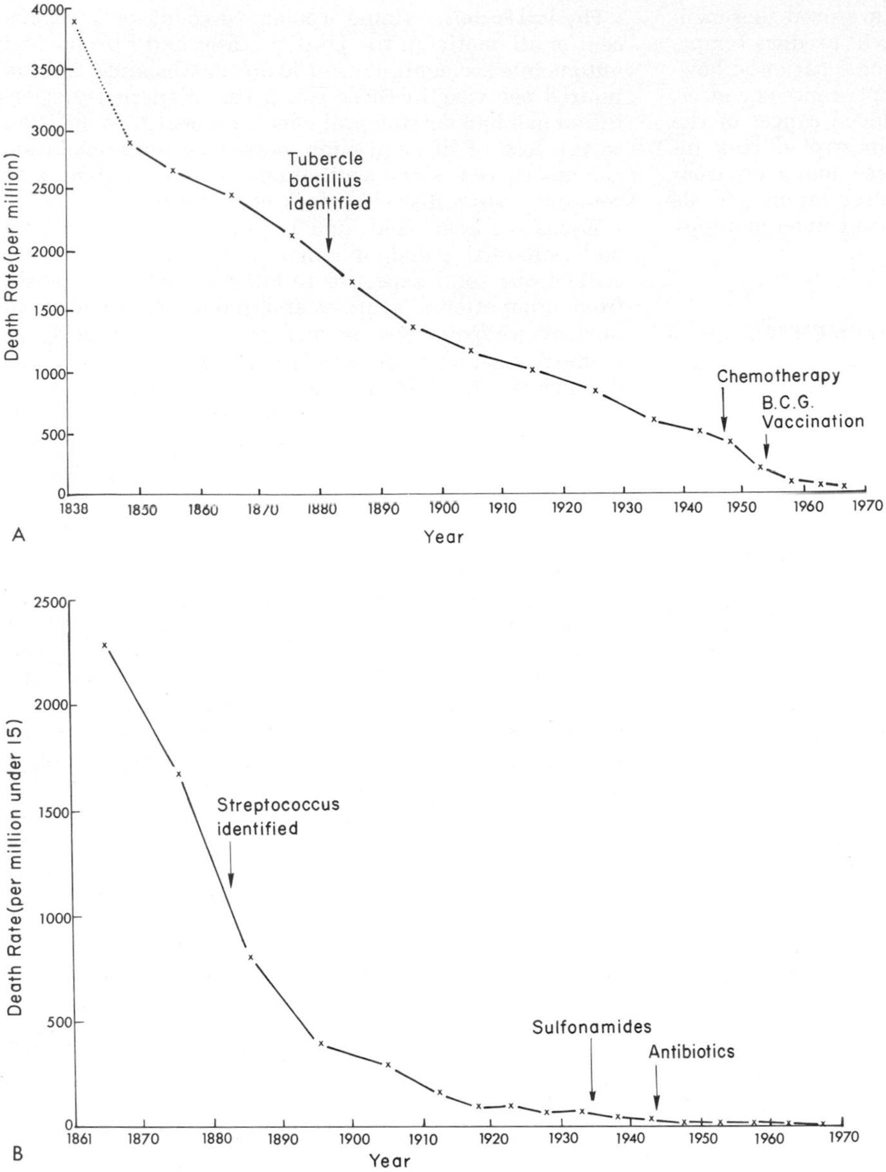

A, Respiratory tuberculosis: mean annual death rate, England and Wales. *B*, Scarlet fever: mean annual death rate of children under 15, England and Wales. (From McKeown, T., and Lowe, C. R.: An Introduction to Social Medicine. Oxford, Blackwell, 1974.)

BEHAVIORAL CHANGE

It was earlier pointed out that in order to prevent or alter an illness we do not always require an understanding of the mechanism whereby an environmental factor contributes to it, and often not even a precise identification of the specific offending factor. On the other hand, however difficult it may be to establish a cause-and-effect relationship between environmental factor and disease, it may be far more difficult to exploit such knowledge. Consider, for example, our failures to achieve the attitudinal and behavioral changes required to take advantage of the knowledge that gonorrhea is transmitted sexually and that a variety of pulmonary and cardiac diseases are aggravated by cigarette smoking. One important step is, of course, behavioral change in the physician. It is unlikely that even the most enlightened patient will be appropriately moved by statistics relating cigarettes, obesity, or lack of exercise to disease if those statistics are offered by his physician who himself pays them no heed. Further, just as the physician who has diagnosed a condition that requires penicillin must ensure that the drug is received, so he must do everything possible to achieve the environmental changes that he feels are dictated by his patient's health.

Much of the health benefit resulting from a recognition of responsible environmental factors and their alteration can be achieved only through action directed at population groups. Here the responsibilities of the physician include participation with other members of society in those actions necessary to achieve the desired ends.

CONCLUSIONS

An examination of the present state of knowledge of the relationships of environmental factors and health leads to certain conclusions. First, there is great need for careful and extensive data collection and analysis. The paucity and unreliability of available data and the complexity of the problems that confront us have led too often in this chapter and in this book to the use of such expressions as "is believed to," "may," "conflicting reports exist," and so on, and undoubtedly even more often to our overlooking associations. Better patient records and information systems are required to help correlate data concerning illness, drugs, chemicals, and physical, nutritional, social, and other environmental factors that affect health in order to alert society to dangers as early as possible. However, even these will never replace the contribution of the astute physician who regards every patient not only as a human being in need of attention and devotion, but also as one presenting a problem in need of a solution. It is relevant to recall that rubella and thalidomide were recognized as teratogens not in a research laboratory or by a computerized medical record system, but by astute clinicians in the course of their practice.

The most sophisticated techniques of modern science will help demonstrate mutagenic, carcinogenic, teratogenic, and other effects of environmental factors on human cells and test organisms. Modern technology can contribute greatly needed quantification to environmental health studies. We require methods for assessing the effects of a variety of factors on human behavior and emotions and on other mental functions, although precise methodology in this area is likely to be a long way in the future. Cost-benefit studies, both medical and economic, are necessary for the physician to make enlightened decisions concerning the risks to which diagnosis and treatment inevitably expose his patient. The risk of anaphylaxis to penicillin is surely worth taking in the individual with pneumococcal pneumonia who has never had the drug previously. The risk of thromboembolic disease from oral contraceptives now seems reasonable in the young woman seeking birth control. (Whether this will continue to be the case when all their health effects are uncovered remains uncertain.) Many other more difficult choices exist, and with the growing medical armamentarium and increasing information concerning the effects of drugs, chemicals, and procedures, many more difficult decisions are placed daily before the physician in his practice.

In recent decades there have been no major improvements in over-all mortality rates from the principal killers, cardiovascular disease and cancer.* More than 80 per cent of cases of cancer in the United States are thought to be the result of potentially controllable environmental factors. Similarly, a variety of environmental factors are known to aggravate cardiovascular disease. These and related facts make mandatory increased attention to preventive measures. The exciting implications of the application of our rapidly growing understanding of biology and chemistry to medical problems are widely recognized, and fundamental and clinical research has been and must continue to be encouraged. However, it is at least equally important that we address the present neglect of the benefits that can be achieved from available knowledge. Social and individual action could surely lead to the prevention or amelioration of many diseases, including several that are occupationally related. In this area the physician is often in a unique position to help identify problems and contribute to campaigns to alter responsible conditions.

Gregg, N. M.: Congenital cataract following German measles in mother. Trans. Ophthalmol. Soc. Australia, 3:35, 1942.

*However, some changes, including a marked increase in survival of children with acute leukemia and a decline in age-adjusted death rates from coronary heart disease, are not reflected in the over-all data.

Health Hazards of the Human Environment. Geneva, World Health Organization, 1972.
MacMahon, B., and Pugh, T. P.: Epidemiology: Principles and Methods. Boston, Little, Brown & Company, 1970.
McBride, W. G.: Thalidomide and congenital abnormalities. Lancet, 2:1358, 1961.
McKeown, T., and Lowe, C. R.: An Introduction to Social Medicine. 2nd ed. Oxford, Blackwell, 1974.

20. CHEMICAL CONTAMINATION OF WATER AND AIR

Walsh McDermott

Chemical contamination may occur in one's own special environment, notably in one's work-place, such as factory or kitchen, or it may occur in the environment we share with the community at large. Both types of contamination stem in large measure from our skill in manipulating chemicals. As the use of this skill continues, new chemical threats are constantly being introduced. This occurs at a considerably faster rate in the special environments of small clusters of people than it does in the environment at large. Within these small groups the effects of a particular chemical contamination can be quite serious and may even be fatal. Once the presence of a particular chemical is identified as a threat to health, however, its dangers can be neutralized in some way, or its use in the process or the product can be abandoned. It is the *initial* identification that may be quite difficult. For the health damage produced by a particular chemical may take the form of a well known disease entity—asthma or primary carcinoma of the liver, to mention two actual examples. To detect a correlation between one or only a few instances of a well known disease and some one of the many chemicals in a particular "occupational" environment is obviously difficult. Yet the feat must be accomplished early; otherwise conceivably large numbers of people might be seriously harmed. A constant vigilance and a keen epidemiologic sensitivity must be a prominent part of the skill of clinicians engaged in occupational medicine. In a sense these are the pioneers at the outermost frontier of the subject of environmental contamination. Likewise, the physician not engaged in occupational medicine should be quick to consult the medical staff of his patient's work-place when some disease arises in a setting that might be viewed as representing something of a surprise.

Some of the more common chemical offenders are discussed in the chapters that follow and in Ch. 535 to 537. Because the chemical nature of occupational environments is ever changing, however, for comprehensive coverage the practitioner or student must consult the periodical literature or textbooks in occupational medicine. Of necessity, therefore, the present discussion is limited to chemicals in our larger environment, particularly chemicals in the water or air.

Like so many problems in medicine today, the one presented by chemical contamination of our air and water is only partly medical. The effects of contaminants on an individual would be medical; yet the forces that expose the individual to the contaminants would be technologic, economic, or cultural. As modulation of these forces requires social action on a broad scale, the physician's role has to be chiefly one of educator and counselor for those of his patients who are concerned citizen activists and for the public authorities. But the physician is frequently "a concerned citizen" too. It is imperative, therefore, that while serving as counselor or educator he be able to distinguish between his advice given as a physician based on scientific and professional evidence relating to *human health,* and his advice given as a concerned citizen—albeit one with a fairly broad background in biology.

The crux of the matter is that with a very few exceptions (see below) the risks to health posed by chemical contamination of our air or water are not tangible disease realities of the sort with which the physician is accustomed to deal. Instead the fact that there are health risks at all is an intellectual judgment based mainly on biologic analogies rather than on evidence established by direct medical observations. To be sure, the physician is well schooled in making judgments among offsetting risks, but he is usually dealing with risks all of which loom for the immediate future of his patient. In weighing chemical threats from the environment, however, he must frequently offset health gains that are clear and immediate against health risks that are far off and theoretical, and indeed might become a problem only for some future generation.

A splendid example of such offsetting threats may be seen in the chemical contamination of our streams and lakes, some of which serve as community water supplies. The availability of this water made it possible to build the United States as an urbanized society, but to do so required the development of a technology whereby the water could be decontaminated of its threats to health. These threats were all actual disease-producing agents. Because they were living organisms they had the property of death and dissolution, and a highly effective technology was based on these biologic properties. For the past 50 years or so, however, on an increasing scale, we have been contaminating the water not only with our microbes but with the direct or indirect products of our chemical industry. Whereas our microbes are biodegradable, many of these chemicals are not; indeed some are not simplified at all, either by biologic degradation or by any other process of decay. Technologic solutions for this part of the problem are to be expected in the form of substituting more readily degradable pesticides and detergents. The over-all problem, however, cannot be solved purely through technologic means. For the chemical contamination, like that by man's microbes, is part of his aura and is derived from his presence and way of life. To change the aura significantly would require major changes in the way of life; yet it is only the microbial part of his aura that can be clearly incriminated as producers of disease.

Microbes, however, can contribute to the process by more ways than one. The methylation of inorganic mercury in large bodies of water appears to take place through microbial action. This microbial process is of the greatest importance; it converts a form of mercury of rather low toxicity for man into one that is quite dangerous, because, unlike inorganic mercury, methyl mercury is readily absorbed and distributed throughout the tissues of man. Strictly speaking, the *demonstrable* dangerous contamination is in the food chain, i.e., the fish; but as fish cannot methylate inorganic mercury, it is clearly a contaminant of the water. Indeed two outbreaks in Japan (the Minamata Bay and River and the Agono River) of serious disease from methyl mercury acquired through this *microbe to water to fish to man* route represent one of the few solid examples of human disease from chemical contamination of a large body of water.*

The many offsetting factors that must be weighed in a judgment on the health risks of chemical contamination of water in general are well illustrated by the story of chlorophenothane (DDT). Indeed the DDT situation may be regarded as a fine prototype of the whole problem. As a pesticide this chlorinated hydrocarbon has been marvelously effective in enhancing agricultural productivity; unfortunately it is relatively stable chemically over a wide range of conditions and thus persists for long periods in the environment. Here it produces a number of unsought ecologic effects. These include critically harmful disturbances of the calcium metabolism of predatory birds; interference with various forms of marine life; and persistence in the food chain whereby it can accumulate in the tissues of a number of organisms, including man. All these effects are reason enough for insisting on strict controls on the use of DDT and on an intensive effort to develop less stable but comparably effective substitutes. Moreover, the property of accumulation in human tissue is obviously disquieting from the standpoint of human health. Thus far, however, there is no evidence that this accumulation has led to recognizable disease in humans. The World Health Organization in a 20-year experiment involving more than 200,000 DDT spraymen has received no reports of toxic effect except from accidental swallowing, and even that caused no deaths. No adverse effects were observed in a clinical study of chronic low-grade exposure in which a group of volunteers received daily for 18 months a dosage 200 times the estimated usual exposure from food (Hayes, W. S., et al., 1956).

The physician must offset the theoretic risk that these accumulations might ultimately lead to human disease against the demonstrable health gains from controlling some of the world's major diseases such as malaria (or filariasis) and those caused by arboviruses and rickettsia. And at the present time, there is no wholly satisfactory substitute for DDT in disease control. Faced with this choice between the clear and present danger of vector-borne diseases and the theoretic risk that tissue accumulation of low concentrations of DDT might lead to disease a few decades hence, the physician has no choice but to opt for continued use of DDT under proper control. Yet in making this choice—and the DDT situation can be viewed as the prototype of many more—he must be keenly aware of the critical nature of the factors it was *not* possible to include in the decision.

For to say that low-grade continued exposure to DDT has produced no recognizable disease in man is not to say that it exerts no *physiologic effects.* On the contrary, it is a potent inducer of the microsomal enzyme system of the liver. As this system plays a critical role in the metabolism of drugs and other chemicals introduced to the body from the outside, it serves as a major protective mechanism against chemical threats from the environment, and hence consideration of its workings is appropriate.

The activity of the microsomal enzyme system is minimal at birth and in early life but increases steadily

*The current problem concerning contamination of the environment by mercury is not limited to, or even principally, one of contamination of water, but has to do with the presence of methyl mercury in foodstuffs (see references at end of chapter).

throughout adulthood. It is inducible; and the buildup of enzymatic capability as the individual grows older is thought to be a reflection of increasing experience with chemicals from the environment acting as inducers. Activity of the system induced by one chemical may also be effective on another. Consequently when more than one drug (or adventitious chemical) are being taken into the body simultaneously, the metabolic disposition of one of the drugs can be significantly altered by the presence and inducing capabilities of the other drug or adventitious chemical. Such "cross-over" effects have obvious implications for multiple drug therapies and conceivably might also attain significance when one of the chemical compounds was an environmental contaminant. The only endogenous materials metabolized via the hepatic microsomal system are the steroid hormones, and their hydroxylation can be considerably enhanced when the system is induced. In theory, therefore, it could be imagined that the presence of DDT with its known potency as an inducer of the hepatic microsomal system could lead to an increased demand for the synthesis of some hormone. There is no evidence that such a DDT phenomenon with steroid hormones actually occurs. But the postulated phenomenon can serve as an imaginary example of how an adventitious chemical in the environment could alter the course of bodily metabolic activities *through an adaptive hepatic system that is known to exist.*

The question arises whether the decades-long stimulation of such an adaptive mechanism in an individual carries with it a risk to the total organism or whether, on balance, such continued stimulation is a good thing. In general, the many bodily systems that work toward homeostasis are regarded as normal processes whose continued operation is not harmful in itself. But some of these systems require the synthesis of protein, and this requires an allocative process involving protein precursors. In effect, therefore, as emphasized by V. R. Potter, there is a "physiologic cost" involved in each of these adaptive enzymatic processes in the sense that one is accomplished at some cost to all possible others. When the "triggering" of the system comes chiefly from the external environment, as in the hepatic microsomal system, the long-continued engagement with a wealth of chemical stimuli conceivably might result in "physiologic costs" that would be harmful to the organism. This could be so; conversely, as our knowledge advances, the notion may prove to have been ridiculously naïve. Our current state of knowledge simply does not permit judgment of the question at this time. It is really the fact that we are dealing with so many "unknowns" that serves to temper any tendency to complacency based on the present absence of detectable disease resulting from chemical contamination of water. For any situation in which a variety of chemicals pass through a series of living systems that at some stage may include the human body is bound to be not only complex but a situation that is continuously subject to change. It is this fact—that the door is wide open for trouble rather than that trouble has already occurred—that characterizes our present situation with respect to possible adverse effects on health from chemical contaminants of our water.

One expressed fear about pesticides in the water also concerns contamination of the air, specifically that the world's newly released oxygen content might be undergoing subtle reduction. Approximately 60 per cent of the world's newly released oxygen each year comes from the activity of oceanic plant life which it was feared might be harmed by the pesticide pollution of the oceans. However, careful studies of Machta and Hughes (1970) have revealed that there has been no change in the world atmosphere's content of oxygen in the 60-year period from 1910 to 1970. Their "negative" data can now serve as a baseline for monitoring this question throughout the future. Fears of reduction in the global oxygen supply from combustion on land can be set completely to rest by examining the quantitative aspects of the question.

With respect to chemical contamination of the air, the challenge to the physician is the same as with water, namely, he must learn to distinguish at any one point in time between what are presently demonstrable health hazards and what are *current stimuli* that conceivably might be generating health effects to be recognized only several decades later. In broad terms two distinct types of widespread chemical contamination exist: a "London type," composed principally of sulfur compounds from burning coal or certain grades of oil, and a "Los Angeles" type, composed mainly of petroleum products introduced into the atmosphere principally from automobiles, and consisting chiefly of carbon monoxide, carbon dioxide, oxides of nitrogen, lead, and unburned or partially oxidized hydrocarbons. None of these chemicals are present in concentrations sufficiently high in themselves to produce acute toxicity in man. In the Los Angeles type of contamination the visible and palpable "smog" is a result of *sunlight* acting on certain of these discharged chemicals to produce more reactive chemicals, whereas in London it frequently results from *fog* physically trapping the sulfur compounds from the coal. Both types exist in both countries, but in the United States it is the hydrocarbon type that is our basic problem. It is overlaid in certain localities by the sulfur type, for the use of coal varies considerably from region to region. It is highly probable that with both types, one of the important end-results—irritation of certain body and plant cells—is much the same.

In terms of presently demonstrable effects on health the evidence is convincing that the irritation from chemicals in the air is definitely harmful to persons who have sustained damage to their cardiovascular or bronchopulmonary systems, notably that apparently enlarging number of patients with chronic obstructive pulmonary disease (see Ch. 502 to 507). The physician is on quite solid ground in attempting to protect his patients with damaged lungs or bronchi from the aggravating effects of chemically polluted urban air. Sometimes this can be accomplished by emigration, sometimes by window fans with filters. Often, however, particularly among urban poverty groups, it cannot be accomplished at all. For these unfortunates, and indeed for the majority of those with chronic pulmonary disease in all socioeconomic groups, protection, if it is to come, will have to come from the community efforts now in progress in many localities to reduce chemical contamination of the air.

In terms of presently demonstrable effects it must be appreciated that virtually the entire "health case" for reducing the chemical contamination of the air rests on the protection of this population with damaged cardiopulmonary systems. For no convincing case has yet been assembled to the effect that bronchopulmonary disease with its frequent cardiac sequels can be *initiated* by continued exposure to the chemical contamination of urban air. This is not to say there is no medical case at all for continued efforts to minimize contamination of the air for the sake of the far larger population with undamaged bronchopulmonary structures. On the contrary, such a case does exist. The physician must recognize clearly, however, that the case for action to protect the population at large is of quite a different nature from that for action to protect those already damaged. For those damaged the evidence is of a conventional medical sort, i.e., it is based on systematic clinical, laboratory, and epidemiologic observations. For the population at large, however, the case is not derived from actual scientific observations. On the contrary, *as in the case of chemical contamination of the water,* the argument for decontaminating the air can be no more than an intellectual judgment based mainly on biologic analogies.

There is one difference between the problems with air and with water. As mentioned previously, at present there is no recognized disease of unknown pathogenesis that seems to have any relationship to widespread chemical contamination of water. By contrast, in the disease complex of bronchitis and emphysema (chronic obstructive pulmonary disease), there *is* a commonly occurring disease grouping of unknown pathogenesis that starts in early middle age, is clearly aggravated by chemicals in the air, and hence might also be *initiated* by them. But to demonstrate convincingly that such a causative relationship exists is a difficult task that has not yet been accomplished despite careful and intensive studies of laboratory animals and man. The epidemiologic problems involved have to do with the great difficulties in separating for analysis the various factors of conceivable relevance such as cigarette smoking and degree of expsoure to particular chemicals in the air. After the first five years of planned long-term studies in The Netherlands (Vlagtwedde/Vlaardingen), it was not possible to demonstrate that residence in areas of high air pollution was associated with an unusual incidence of bronchopulmonary abnormalities. The factor of age seemed to produce a far greater decrease of pulmonary function than smoking or living in a polluted area. Conceivably the *impact* of the chemicals that led ultimately to disease might be something that occurs relatively early in life. Studies in young children in the United Kingdom suggest that continued exposure to high levels of pollution increases the risk of serious respiratory disease in children (Colley and Reid, 1970).

But the major problem is how to study what are in effect "water dripping on stone" effects. The chemicals now contaminating the air, taken singly or collectively, are not present in quantities that produce detectable bronchopulmonary damage in the short run. Thus if the "current stimuli" represented by these chemicals play a significant role in the pathogenesis of such a major disease grouping as chronic bronchopulmonary disease, the effects presumably would take the form of steady but individually minute episodes of damage that ultimately fail to heal completely and emerge to significance only when accumulated over decades. Questions of this type, i.e., 30- to 40-year effects in humans, are far more difficult to answer than questions of the role of environmental contaminants on plant life or other elements of the nonhuman ecology.

To be sure, the physician in his role of public educator and counselor should support well organized efforts to develop the new methods and new research institutional arrangements necessary for the productive study of these medical questions of this essentially new type. But he should also not fail to stress that because of the very nature of these questions as they apply to *human health,* it seems highly unlikely that answers concerning air pollution as an initiator of disease will be forthcoming in the near future. Whatever action is to be taken, therefore, must be based on the medical information that is available now. From the standpoint of health, therefore, we are left with the following dilemma. On the one hand, most of the actions necessary to abolish air pollution as a potential danger to health are costly and likely to prove quite disruptive to the economy and the whole style of life. To campaign for these actions in the name of health without a convincing scientific case that the evils to be corrected represent a widespread danger to health might be unwise. On the other hand, if, a few decades hence, it were shown convincingly that long-continued chemical contamination of the air *of the present sort* did have the property of initiating chronic bronchopulmonary disease, the proportion of the population of any industrialized country that would by then have been irreversibly affected would be large indeed.

There seems to be no obvious solution for this dilemma so long as the major case for minimizing air pollution is viewed as being primarily a "health matter" and health is considered principally in terms of detectable disease. But there are more subtle aspects to health than definable disease, including even definable mental disease. There is the whole affect involved in one's response to one's environment. The intense love of their city shown by so many Leningraders when it was under siege in World War II is a case in point. These are not the kinds of phenomena that lend themselves readily to comparative weighing in the scale against the major economic factors that might be disrupted in "air reform." Nevertheless, they deserve attention too.

What it comes down to is that, except for those already afflicted with cardiopulmonary disease, the present chemical pollution of urban air is not really a health problem in the orthodox sense; it is a widespread *social* evil that is quite unacceptable on a number of counts, of which the possible health effects are only one (Dubos, 1970). Viewed in this way it becomes the physician's role to characterize continuously what is known or seems highly probable about the health aspects of the matter. Included should be encouragement of attempts to develop more sensitive methods for the essentially permanent monitoring of the possible effects of long-continued chemical stimuli. The physician presents this knowledge not as a determining reason in itself for air control, but as only one portion of a total argument for cleansing this part of our external environment. Once the medical contribution can be regarded as but one contribution to a much larger total effort, the physician can escape from the trap of seeming to be minimizing the significances of a particular form of contamination of the air on the grounds that it is not a *known* danger to health. For the physician to operate in such a cooperative professional-social role is not new; most of the impressive twentieth century accomplishments of medicine in extending life expectancy from birth were made in exactly this way.

Burns, J. J.: Interaction of environmental agents and drugs. Environ. Res., 2:352, 1969.

Conney, A. H., et al.: Effects of pesticides on drugs and steroid metabolism. Clin. Pharmacol. Ther., 8:2, 1967.

Dubos, R.: Reason Awake! Science for Man. New York, Columbia University Press, 1970.

Goodman, L. S., and Gilman, A.: The Pharmacological Basis of Therapeutics. New York, The Macmillan Company, 1965.

Keil, J. E., Sandifer, S. H., Finklea, J. H., and Priester, L. E.: Serum vitamin A elevation in DDT-exposed volunteers. Bull. Environ. Contam. Toxicol., 9:317, 1972.
Lu, F. C., Berteau, P. E., and Clegg, D. J.: *In* FAO/IAEA/ILO/WHO: Mercury contamination in man and his environment. IAEA Techn. Rep. Ser. No. 137, 1972, p. 67.
Machta, L., and Hughes, E.: Atmospheric oxygen in 1967 to 1970. Science, 168:1582, 1970.
Royal College of Physicians: Air Pollution and Health. London, Pitman Medical and Scientific Publishing Company, Ltd., 1970.
Sweden, National Institute of Public Health. Nord. Hyg. T. Suppl. 4, 1971.

FOOD POISONING

Harold P. Lambert

21. INTRODUCTION

Food may cause illness in three ways. The most common varieties are produced by *contamination with microorganisms or their products.* Although the gastrointestinal tract is an important mode of entry for many viral, bacterial, and parasitic agents of disease, the term "food poisoning" is conventionally restricted to two main types of syndromes: various forms of acute gastroenteritis caused by bacteria or their products in food; and neurologic syndromes such as botulism or paralytic shellfish poisoning caused by the toxic products of microorganisms. Second, food may be *contaminated by poisonous chemicals.* Examples include heavy metal poisoning by mercury, antimony, cadmium, arsenic, or zinc; poisoning by simple salts such as sodium fluoride or potassium chlorate; and poisoning by organic compounds such as insecticides and orthotricresyl phosphate. Third, *poisonous plants or animals may be eaten in error.* The material may be inherently poisonous, as are some species of mushroom and many other plants; or it may have become secondarily poisonous by incorporating a substance toxic to man during its own food cycle, as in certain forms of shellfish and fish poisoning.

22. BACTERIAL FOOD POISONING

The infectious type of bacterial food poisoning requires the ingestion of living organisms, albeit often in very large numbers, and their subsequent multiplication in the gastrointestinal tract. The most important example of this type of illness is Salmonella gastroenteritis, which is dealt with in Ch. 213. Shigella species may give rise to very similar syndromes, but these are not conventionally classified as episodes of food poisoning, although water- or food-borne outbreaks of Shigella infection do sometimes occur. In the toxin type of bacterial food poisoning, such as that associated with staphylococci, the illness is caused by toxin formed in food before its ingestion, and does not depend on the ingestion of living organisms. Although a generally useful concept, the distinction between the "infection" and "toxin" types of food poisoning has become less rigid than formerly with the demonstration and partial identification of a number of enterotoxins produced by bacterial gut pathogens, including those which produce disease only when ingested as living organisms.

STAPHYLOCOCCAL FOOD POISONING

Etiology and Epidemiology. This common form of food poisoning is caused by the multiplication of an enterotoxin-forming strain of Staphylococcus in the food before ingestion. Contamination of food with staphylococci is extremely common, because the organism can be grown from the hands of about 50 per cent of people. Heavy growth may often be obtained from apparently noninfected minor cracks and cuts on the skin. Staphylococci of human origin contaminating meat or confectionery constitute the source of most outbreaks, but about 10 per cent of them are milk borne, and the organism is then usually of bovine origin. The conditions needed to cause food poisoning of this type are contamination of a suitable food—most foods will support the growth of staphylococci—and a period of some hours after preparation during which the organisms are able to multiply. This may occur during a period of slow cooling after cooking or if food is held at ambient temperature in a warm climate after preparation. Later reheating or even boiling will not then prevent illness, because this is caused by preformed, heat-stable toxin and not by the ingestion of living staphylococci.

Pathogenesis. Detailed study of staphylococcal enterotoxin has been hindered by many technical difficulties. Strains which form enterotoxin are almost always coagulase positive, but enterotoxin production is otherwise not related to any easily measurable metabolic activities. Moreover, study of the toxin has hitherto been limited by lack of a satisfactory animal model; most workers use intraperitoneal injection of toxin in kittens as the test system. Some progress has been made in recent years, notably the differentiation of four antigenic types: enterotoxins A, B, C, and D. Enterotoxin B has been isolated in relatively pure form by Bergdoll and his colleagues. The types are antigenically specific and do not cross-react, but one staphylococcal strain may produce more than one type. The toxin, like the crude extracts, is relatively heat resistant and resistant to trypsin. Its precise mode of action is still in dispute, but experiments in monkeys suggest that this so-called enterotoxin probably has its primary site of action in the central nervous system, and that vomiting is a centrally induced response.

Clinical Manifestations and Treatment. The period between ingestion and illness is short, one to six hours, occasionally a little longer, and the illness is characterized by abdominal cramping pain with violent and often repeated retching and vomiting. Diarrhea is variable; it may be profuse, mild, or absent entirely. Although often violent, staphylococcal food poisoning is short lived, usually subsiding in six or eight hours and rarely lasting as long as 24 hours. It may occasionally threaten life in patients who are old or suffering from other serious disease. The patient is often recovering when first seen by a doctor, but may require an intramuscular injection of prochlorperazine, 12.5 mg or metaclopramide, 10 mg, to control vomiting. Patients with evidence of serious depletion of extracellular fluid may require intravenous treatment using isotonic sodium chloride with added potassium.

Prevention. Careful training of food handlers in personal hygiene and immediate refrigeration of foods not due for immediate consumption are the most important preventive measures. Enterotoxin is not produced at ordinary domestic refrigerator temperatures. Foods should not be left to cool slowly, especially in large containers, and should be taken from the refrigerator and reheated, if this is required, immediately before serving.

Epidemiologic work on outbreaks of staphylococcal food poisoning involves standard methods of bacteriophage typing in identifying the source of the responsible strain. Since, however, terminal heating may kill the organisms in food without inactivating enterotoxin, staphylococci may not be grown from food under suspicion. Animal assays for the detection of enterotoxin are now being replaced by serologic methods based on gel diffusion after preliminary extraction and concentration.

CLOSTRIDIAL FOOD POISONING

Etiology. *Clostridium perfringens* type A is responsible for about one third of the reported cases of food poisoning both in the United States and in Great Britain. It occurs in fairly large outbreaks, with an average of 35 affected people in each episode. The organism is ubiquitous. Strains can be isolated from the feces of man and of most domestic and farm animals, and samples of raw meat may often be contaminated with this organism. It has also been found in flies, soil, and dirt from kitchens. The conditions necessary for an outbreak are well defined. A meat or poultry dish, in the form of either a stew or a solid preparation such as a joint, pie, or mince, is cooked at a temperature not higher than 100° C, allowing the spores to survive. During a period of slow cooling the spores germinate, this process being provoked by "heat shock"; rapid multiplication of vegetative forms is encouraged by the rich medium and the low oxidation-reduction potential after cooking. These conditions are especially likely to apply with a large bulk of food, in which slow cooling and anaerobic conditions are likely to occur. Food eaten cold or merely warmed before serving may then cause an outbreak of food poisoning.

Pathogenesis. Human volunteer experiments indicate that ingestion of living organisms is necessary for the production of this form of food poisoning, and the responsible strain may often be found in large numbers in the feces of affected patients. Strains of *Cl. perfringens* type A which cause food poisoning do not differ from other strains in any way easily identifiable by routine methods, although outbreaks in Britain have most commonly been caused by strains with heat-resistant spores. The pathogenesis of the disease has yet to be defined in detail. It was believed for some time that phosphoryl choline, an end product of the action of alpha toxin (= lecithinase-phospholipase-C) was responsible for the outpouring of fluid into the bowel, but this substance has no effect in experimental systems and is probably inactive in the bowel. Recently, however, partial purification has been achieved of a toxin from strains which cause diarrhea in human volunteers as well as accumulation of fluid in isolated loops of rabbit ileum. The toxin is a heat-labile, nondiffusible protein, antigenic and different from other known toxins produced by *Cl. perfringens*.

Clinical Manifestations. The incubation period is 8 to 12 hours after ingestion of the infected food, occasionally as little as 6 or as long as 24 hours. The main features are diarrhea and griping abdominal pain. The feces are liquid but do not contain blood or mucus. A small proportion of patients suffer from nausea and vomiting. The illness is usually not severe, lasts less than 24 hours, and is unaccompanied by systemic disturbance or fever. A few deaths have been recorded in old or infirm patients.

Drug treatment is rarely necessary, but in longer attacks a kaolin mixture may be given, and patients with severe abdominal pain may need an analgesic.

Prevention. Preferably food should be served immediately after cooking. If it has to be kept, it should be rapidly cooled and held at a safe temperature. Cooked meat should always be kept either cold, below 5° C, or hot, over 60° C. Careful techniques of food hygiene are especially important in institutions in which large amounts of meat or poultry are cooked.

ENTERITIS NECROTICANS
(Pig-Bel)

Outbreaks of severe intestinal disease have been associated with ingestion of *Cl. perfringens* type C. A large outbreak was reported from Germany in 1948, and a similar syndrome known as pig-bel has more recently been described from parts of New Guinea in which pig feasts have an important economic and social function. The syndrome is characterized by severe abdominal pain, bloody diarrhea, and vomiting. Operation or autopsy reveals a severe hemorrhagic jejunitis and ileitis. Some patients die and some recover after resection of strangulated, perforated, and necrotic bowel. Others may pass through the acute phase to develop chronic small bowel obstruction and malabsorption, and some recover completely.

VIBRIO PARAHAEMOLYTICUS FOOD POISONING

V. parahaemolyticus is a halophilic marine vibrio long recognized as an inhabitant of coastal waters of Japan and as a cause of gastroenteritis associated with sea foods. More recently it has been found in American and British coastal sea waters. Techniques for its isolation and differentiation from nonpathogenic marine vibrios are now well established.

In Japan gastroenteritis of this type is confined to the summer months. It is the most common cause of infective food poisoning in Japan, accounting for 59 per cent of 22,000 cases of identifiable cause in 1963. *V. parahaemolyticus* causes an infectious type of gastroenteritis and is associated with ingestion of raw fish or shellfish. Outbreaks in Japan have been associated with semidried young sardines, and especially with sushi, a food composed of cooked rice, raw fish, and shellfish. In 1971 three outbreaks of *V. parahaemolyticus* were identified in the United States, associated with ingestion of indigenous crabs and shrimps.

Incubation periods varying from 2 to 66 hours have been recorded, but the most frequent interval between ingestion and infection is 12 to 24 hours. The chief clinical features are severe diarrhea accompanied by cramping abdominal pain, nausea, and vomiting. Most patients also exhibit systemic symptoms of fever, chills, and headache. Less commonly the organism causes a dysenteric form of illness with fever and bloody diarrhea. The illness lasts for one to five days, and recovery appears to be complete. As with staphylococcal and clostridial food poisoning, the disease is rarely fatal, but old and debilitated patients may be at special risk.

BACILLUS CEREUS FOOD POISONING

Bacillus cereus is an aerobic, spore-bearing, gram-positive bacillus of wide natural distribution, and several outbreaks of food poisoning have been associated with high counts of the organism in the responsible food. Contamination has been traced to corn flour, rice, and other dried foods. In large outbreaks in Norway affecting as many as 600 people, the incubation period was 12 hours, and the main features were watery diarrhea, abdominal pain, and nausea lasting about 12 hours. More recently, fried rice in restaurants has been incriminated. Large quantities of rice are prepared and kept at warm kitchen temperatures for many hours, small portions being refried for a few minutes as orders are placed. In one such episode the rice contained 450×10^6 organisms per gram. The incubation period has been as short as 15 minutes to 3 hours when large inocula such as these are ingested.

OTHER FORMS OF BACTERIAL FOOD POISONING

Many outbreaks cannot be assigned to one of the specific pathogens generally accepted as a cause of food poisoning, but many other bacteria have been implicated at one time or another as possible causes of acute gastrointestinal illness. The evidence is often inconclusive and is frequently based on high counts of the presumptive pathogen in samples of food which may have been kept at room temperature for long periods before reaching the laboratory, or on the isolation from patients' stools of organisms which form part of the normal fecal flora. Volunteer studies have often proved equivocal. With these reservations, it seems likely that diarrhea and vomiting may occasionally be caused by a considerable variety of bacteria, if circumstances have allowed their multiplication to high enough concentrations before ingestion. The genera most often implicated have been the enterococci (group D streptococci) and various members of the Enterobacteriaceae, notably *E. coli*, Proteus, Providencia, Pseudomonas, and Citrobacter.

23. BOTULISM

Etiology. Botulism is a life-threatening illness characterized by muscle paralysis and variable gastrointestinal symptoms. It is caused by absorption from the gastrointestinal tract of ingested toxin produced by *Clostridium botulinum*. Botulism resulting from wound infection by this organism has also been recorded several times.

Incidence. The unexpectedness of outbreaks of botulism, the dramatic and frightening nature of the illness, and its high mortality have attracted much attention from both laymen and doctors, but botulism is in fact an uncommon disease. From 1899 to 1969 there were 659 outbreaks in the United States, with 1696 cases and 959 deaths. Outbreaks have also been recorded in many other countries, especially in Canada, Japan, Western Europe, Scandinavia, and the U.S.S.R.

Epidemiology. The six strains of *Cl. botulinum* cause disease in man and in a variety of animals. Human disease is caused by types A, B, and E and occasionally by type F. Toxins produced by the different types are antigenically distinct. *Cl. botulinum,* a spore-bearing anaerobic bacillus, is widely distributed in nature. The organism has been identified in many parts of the world, in cultivated and virgin soils, in a variety of marine environments, and in many animals and animal products. The distribution of types varies in different areas, so that type A botulism is more common than type B in the United States, especially in the Western states, whereas in Europe this order is reversed. In recent years type E has superseded both types A and B in frequency. Type E organisms are especially but not exclusively associated with the aquatic environment in northern latitudes, being found in the sea bed of coastal and lake waters and in the intestinal tract of fish. However, types A and B may also be associated with a marine source.

Pathogenesis. Contamination of fresh food by spores of *Cl. botulinum* does not cause botulism. The spores must have germinated and toxin must have been produced by the vegetative organisms. Spores are destroyed at a temperature of 121° C or greater, as used in commercial canning processes, but can usually survive a temperature of 100° C. Type E spores are relatively heat sensitive, but smoking and light cooking may not kill them, so that food processed in these ways or preserved in the raw state may act as a vehicle of the disease. Another factor predisposing to type E botulism is the production of toxin by this organism at temperatures as low as 5° C. The cooking or preserving process is conducive to the germination of spores and, by reason of the lowered redox potential, to multiplication of the vegetative forms. Multiplication is inhibited in acid media, and botulism is rarely associated with food of pH below 4.5. All types of botulinum toxin are heat labile, and botulism could be entirely prevented by terminal heating for 20 minutes at 80° C or for 10 minutes at 90° C.

The types of food associated with botulism as a result of these contributory factors vary, with local food customs, from country to country. In the United States home-preserved vegetables constitute the most frequent source, followed by preserved fruit and fish products. Meat and meat products are more commonly responsible in Europe. Preserved fish is the chief source of botulism in Japan, Scandinavia, and the U.S.S.R. Although most outbreaks are associated with domestic methods of preparing and preserving foods, outbreaks from commercially prepared foods also occur. Recent sources have included canned tuna fish, canned vichyssoise, and vacuum-packed smoked fish.

Ingested toxin is rapidly absorbed from the gastrointestinal tract. Toxemia may be demonstrated for periods of up to ten days or even three weeks, and it is possible that toxin continues to be absorbed from the bowel for some days after ingestion. Type E toxin is potentiated by proteolytic enzymes, including trypsin, and this phenomenon has been invoked as a mechanism which contributes to the pathogenicity of this type. Botulinum toxin is active in extremely low doses, nanogram quantities of pure toxin being lethal to mice. It prevents conduction in peripheral nerves by a presynaptic block, thus preventing release of acetylcholine without direct action on the acetylcholine release mechanism. Anticholinesterase drugs do not affect its action.

Clinical Manifestations. Illness usually begins between 12 and 36 hours after ingesting the toxin-containing food. The first manifestations are often gastrointestinal, especially in type E disease, with nausea, vomiting, abdominal pain, and distention. Other common early symptoms are weakness, unsteadiness, and dryness of the mouth and throat. Neurologic symptoms may accompany the early gastrointestinal illness or may follow at an interval of 12 to 72 hours. Early features are blurring of vision, dysphagia, dysarthria, and weakness of a variety of muscles. Weakness spreads as the disease advances, affecting especially the respiratory system, the external ocular muscles, and muscles of the neck and proximal limb groups. The pupils are usually dilated and fixed, and retention of urine is common. Deep tendon reflexes are preserved. The patient remains mentally clear, and fever is not observed except as a terminal event. Paralysis may continue for many days or weeks.

One recent outbreak of type A botulism showed atypical features; the pupillary reactions remained normal, and two of the six patients showed myasthenic features not usually observed in botulism. Defects of cardiac conduction have occasionally been noted.

The chief causes of death are respiratory or bulbar paralysis or both, along with the infective complications resulting from these paralyses.

Diagnosis. The illness is easily recognized if a group of patients, known to have eaten food of a type associated with botulism, present with characteristic symptoms. By contrast, diagnosis of the individual patient, in whom there may be no suspicion that the illness is a form of food poisoning, has often proved extremely difficult. The gastrointestinal features may be so severe as to simulate intestinal obstruction, and the epigastric pain may be mistaken for that of myocardial infarction. The dry and sometimes painful throat may suggest various forms of acute pharyngitis, and the combination of sore throat and neurologic disease can cause confusion with diphtheria. The neurologic illness has been mistaken for acute polyneuritis (Guillain-Barré syndrome), encephalitis, a stroke, or myasthenia gravis. The dry mouth and fixed dilated pupils suggest atropine poisoning, as is produced by *Datura stramonium* (jimson weed). Paralytic poisoning caused by shellfish or by puffer fish (see below) is accompanied by prominent sensory symptoms not found in botulism.

Circulating toxin may sometimes be detected in the patient's blood, even long after onset of the disease. It is detected by intraperitoneal injection in mice, controls simultaneously receiving antiserum of the different types. Suspected food is also tested for toxin in the same way, and the organism is sought by anaerobic culture.

Treatment. Since the greatest risk of botulism is respiratory failure, treatment is dominated by the prevention and management of this complication. Bulbar paralysis is treated by early tracheostomy, employing a cuffed endotracheal tube. Coincident or supervening respiratory muscle paralysis indicates the need for artificial ventilation applied through the tracheostomy. Specific antitoxin is probably effective in reducing the mortality of type E botulism. Although there is no such evidence in other forms of botulism, the high mortality of the disease and the difficulty of obtaining statistically valid data justify the use of antitoxin in all forms of the disease. Antitoxin should be given irrespective of the duration of illness when the diagnosis is made, because toxin may be present in the blood for many days. Unless the type of botulism is definitely known, multivalent antitoxin should be administered, because the type cannot be reliably inferred from the food source. After a preliminary test for hypersensitivity to horse serum, two vials of trivalent antitoxin (each containing 7500 IU type A, 5500 IU type B, and 8500 IU type E antitoxin) are administered by intravenous injection, and this is repeated in two to four hours. For botulism of known type, preparations containing A and B antitoxin or E antitoxin alone are available, as is a small stock of monovalent F antitoxin.

Until 1968 no method had been proposed by which the effects of botulinum toxin could be counteracted, but recently guanidine has been claimed as a useful adjunct in treatment. Both clinical and electromyographic improvement were observed in a number of patients who received guanidine by nasogastric tube in a dose of 15 to 50 mg per kilogram per day.

Since it is uncertain whether the long duration of toxemia in botulism is attributable to continued absorption from the bowel, gastric aspiration and colonic washouts are also used in treatment. A solution of sodium bicarbonate may be left in the stomach to promote breakdown of toxin.

Prognosis. The over-all mortality of botulism is high, 60 to 70 per cent for type A, 10 to 30 per cent for type B, and 30 to 50 per cent for type E. Patients with type E botulism tend to die more quickly than those affected by other types, usually within three days of onset. Improved management of respiratory failure should lower the death rate, especially because patients who survive the stage of severe paralysis can recover completely.

24. POISONOUS PLANTS AND ANIMALS

PARALYTIC SHELLFISH POISONING

Shellfish may act as the vehicle of transmission of many pathogens, for example, infective hepatitis, *Vibrio parahaemolyticus* gastroenteritis, and diarrhea and vomiting of unknown cause. Ingestion may also give rise to an acute neurologic syndrome caused by the transmission to man of a neurotoxin acquired by shellfish from plankton on which they feed. Outbreaks are especially likely to follow a sudden increase in the population of dinoflagellate protozoa, the "red tide." The main responsible species in the Pacific Ocean is *Gonyaulax catanella,* which produces the paralytic poison *saxitoxin,* first isolated from the Alaskan butterclam *Saxidomus giganteus.* The toxin of *G. tamarensis,* responsible for outbreaks on Atlantic coasts, produces the same pharmacologic effects, although it may not be identical with saxitoxin. The toxins are water-soluble, heat-stable compounds, rapidly absorbed from the gastrointestinal tract and active in vitro at concentrations of 1 to 10 μg per milliliter. They act on vertebrate nerve fibers and on skeletal muscle fibers, abolishing action potentials by preventing depolarization.

Clinical Manifestations. Symptoms may begin as soon as 20 minutes after ingestion, with paresthesias of the hands and mouth, weakness of the limbs, and a floating feeling. Other common features are ataxia, headache, and vomiting, whereas in severe cases bulbar and respiratory paralysis supervene and may cause death. Mortality rates between 5 and 18 per cent have been reported in various outbreaks, but the illness is less likely to be severe if water used in cooking the shellfish has been discarded. Treatment is that of respiratory paralysis. No specific treatment is available, but patients are likely to recover if they survive the first 12 hours of the illness.

A different form of paralytic shellfish poisoning is associated with ingestion of red whelk, *Neptunea antiqua.* This is caused by tetramine (tetramethylammonium hydroxide) which is produced in the salivary glands of this mollusk and causes curare-like effects on muscle.

FISH POISONING

A number of different mechanisms are involved in fish poisoning. Some species are inherently poisonous; the toxins of other species are acquired from organisms on which they feed; yet another form of fish poisoning is caused by breakdown products of bacterial action.

Ciguatera Poisoning. This can be acquired from a large number of species, about 300 in all, whose common characteristic is the narrow range of reef or coastal tropical waters which they inhabit. The toxin is thought to originate in blue-green algae consumed by herbivorous fish which are in turn the prey of carnivorous species. The toxin accumulates in the tissues and is excreted very slowly. Poisoning of this type is difficult to prevent, because the toxin is stable to heat, cold, and drying, and the taste and smell of the fish are unaffected. Symptoms commonly begin several hours after ingestion, but may be almost immediate. Nausea and vomiting are followed by paresthesias of the face, mouth, and limbs, dizziness, ataxia, muscular weakness, and severe muscle pain. The patient may die from respiratory paralysis during the first day, and in nonfatal cases the neuritic symptoms may persist for many weeks. No immunity is gained by an attack; indeed, a second episode of poisoning may be more severe.

Tetraodon Poisoning. Many puffer fish found in the Pacific, Atlantic, and Indian Oceans are inherently toxic. The neurotoxin contained in their viscera *(tetraodontoxin)* is identical with that formerly known as tarichatoxin, found in the Californian newt *Taricha torosa.* Its mode of action is similar to that of saxitoxin, and this is reflected in the syndrome of tetraodon poisoning which bears clear resemblances to paralytic shellfish poisoning (see above). Symptoms begin soon after ingestion and include paresthesias, dizziness, ataxia, and paralysis, often together with diarrhea, vomiting, and abdominal pain. The patient may die of respiratory paralysis.

Scombroid Poisoning. Some species of the mackerel family, such as tuna and bonito, are susceptible to decomposition by *Proteus morganii.* Toxic products result from the breakdown of histidine normally contained in fish flesh. Within a few minutes of ingesting contaminated fish, the patient develops nausea, vomiting, headache, epigastric pain, dysphagia, dryness of the mouth, and severe urticaria. The illness usually lasts less than 24 hours.

Other Fish Poisons. Neurologic symptoms may follow ingestion of several other types of fish. Some of the toxins responsible are probably acquired from dinoflagellates, as in paralytic shellfish poisoning, but the source of other neurotoxins is still uncertain. In addition to these forms of fish poisoning, some species of the Gempylid group such as castor oil fish and snake mackerel contain a purgative oil, whereas the roe of some freshwater fish is toxic during the reproductive period, causing acute gastrointestinal symptoms with headache and fever.

MUSHROOM POISONING

In poisoning by muscarine-containing species such as *Amanita muscaria* (fly agaric) and *Amanita pantherina,* symptoms begin two or three hours after ingestion and consist of abdominal cramp, sweating, salivation, miosis, and bradycardia. Poisoning by these species is rarely fatal. By contrast, death-cup poisoning, by *Amanita phalloides* and *Amanita verna,* carries a mortality of 30 to 50 per cent or more. Two groups of toxins are contained in these mushrooms. Cyclic heptapeptides known as *phallotoxins* cause the violent symptoms of abdominal pain, vomiting, and diarrhea which begin 6 to 15 hours after ingestion. Symptoms then remit for about 48 hours. During this time tests of liver function become abnormal, and signs of hepatic and renal failure then develop, often accompanied by confusion, coma, and paralysis of the extremities. This phase of the illness is probably caused by cyclic octapeptides known as *amatoxins.*

No specific treatment is available, but the stomach should be emptied by induced vomiting or gastric lavage, and atropine administered if muscarinic effects are observed. Otherwise, the general principles of management in acute hepatic and renal failure should be observed. For example, peritoneal dialysis or hemodialysis may be necessary in renal failure, and modern methods of managing acute hepatic failure may help to reduce the high mortality.

In experimental conditions, the mortality rate in mice poisoned by alpha-amanitin (the principal amatoxin of *A. phalloides*) is much reduced by administration of a number of agents—penicillin and sulfamethoxazole, penicillin and phenylbutazone, and chloramphenicol—which are thought to act by displacing toxin from plasma albumin-binding sites and thus promoting its excretion. Whether this approach to treatment would be useful in human mushroom poisoning is unknown.

POISONING BY FLOWERING PLANTS

An immense number of plant species may contain constituents toxic to man, and only a few of the more common and important forms of plant poisoning can be considered here.

The first examples are all members of the family of *solanaceous plants,* in which toxic species are especially well represented.

Atropa belladonna (deadly nightshade) poisoning is caused by ingestion of the prominent black berries, which contain a number of alkaloids of the belladonna group. The symptoms and signs are those of atropine poisoning: dry mouth, dry skin, blurring of vision, dilated pupils, tachycardia and excitement, hallucinations, and delirium followed by coma—"hot as a hare, blind as a bat, dry as a bone, red as a beet, and mad as a hen."

Datura stramonium (thorn apple, jimson weed) also contains stramonium alkaloids, as do other species of this genus, and they may cause poisoning by ingestion of their seeds, of extracts of leaves, and even of nectar.

Clinical manifestations are generally similar to those of atropine poisoning.

Other familiar members of the Solanaceae are *Solanum americanum* and *S. nigrum* (common nightshade, black nightshade), *S. dulcamara* (woody nightshade, bittersweet), *Hyoscyamus niger* (henbane), and the potato plant, of which the green parts and tuber sprouts may be poisonous. Plants of this group contain a mixture of the stramonium alkaloids and of solanine, itself a mixture of alkaloids.

No specific treatment is available for these forms of poisoning. Peripheral effects caused by atropine can be antagonized by pilocarpine, but this does not affect its cerebral actions. Vomiting should be induced or the stomach emptied by gastric lavage.

The family Umbelliferae also includes many toxic species, in addition to familiar food species such as carrot, parsnip, and celery. *Conium maculatum* (hemlock) is a common weed which contains several toxic alkaloids causing nausea and vomiting, progressive weakness, respiratory paralysis, and convulsions. Various species of Cicuta, the water hemlocks, are also toxic, the root containing cicutoxin, an unsaturated alcohol. Ingestion is followed by vomiting, salivation, delirium, convulsions, and paralysis.

25. CHEMICAL FOOD POISONING

Various forms of metallic poisoning are discussed in Ch. 27 to 33 and Ch. 626. Occasionally patients react idiosyncratically to a normal constituent of food, or to a food additive or preservative. The headache and hypertension induced by certain foods in patients receiving monoamine oxidase inhibitors are attributable to their natural tyramine content. The two examples which follow illustrate peculiar reactions to additives in food.

Chinese Restaurant Syndrome. A few people develop dramatic symptoms 10 to 20 minutes after eating some kind of Chinese food. These include tingling and burning in the back of the neck, radiating to the upper back, arms, and front of the chest. Some of them experience throbbing pain in the temples and infraorbital region. The symptoms fluctuate in severity and usually last for 45 minutes to 2 hours. The cause of this syndrome has been much disputed, but is probably the monosodium glutamate used in seasoning certain Chinese foods.

Hot Dog Headache. A patient experienced several hours of bitemporal headache and facial flushing, starting within 30 minutes of eating certain kinds of cured meat. His symptoms were shown to be caused by sodium nitrite used in the curing process.

Cherington, M. and Ryan, D. W.: Botulism and guanidine. N. Engl. J. Med., 282:195, 1970.

Dadisman, T. A., Nelson, R., Molenda, J. R., and Garber, H. J.: *Vibrio parahaemolyticus* in Maryland. 1. Clinical and epidemiological aspects. Am. J. Epidemiol., 96:414, 1972.

Editorial: Death cap poisoning. Lancet, 1:1320, 1972.

Evans, M. H.: Mechanism of saxitoxin and tetrodotoxin poisoning. Br. Med. Bull., 25:263, 1969.

Gangarosa, E. J., Donadio, J. A., Armstrong, R. W., Meyer, K. F., Brachman, P. S., and Dowell, V. R.: Botulism in the United States, 1899–1969. Am. J. Epidemiol., 93:93, 1971.

Koenig, M. D.: Drutz, D. J., Mushlin, A. I., Schaffner, W., and Rogers, D. E.: Type B botulism in man. Am. J. Med., 42:208, 1967.

Koenig, M. G., Spickard, A., Cardella, M. A., and Rogers, D. E.: Clinical and laboratory observations on type E botulism in man. Medicine, 43:517, 1962.

Loewenstein, M.: Epidemiology of *Cl. perfringens* food poisoning. N. Engl. J. Med., 286:1026, 1972.

Murrell, T. G. C., Roth, L., Egerton, J., Samels, J., and Walker, P. D.: Pig-bel; enteritis necroticans. Lancet, 1:217, 1966.

Nakamura, M., and Schulze, J. A.: *Clostridium perfringens* food poisoning. Ann. Rev. Microbiol., 23:359, 1970.

Riemann, H. (ed.): Food-borne infections and intoxications. New York, Academic Press, 1969.

Ryan, D. W., and Cherington, M.: Human type A botulism. J.A.M.A., 216:513, 1971.

Zen-Yoji, H., Sakai, S., Terayama, T., Kudo, Y., Ito, T., Benoki, M., and Nagasaki, M.: Epidemiology, enteropathogenicity and classification of *Vibrio parahaemolyticus*. J. Infect. Dis., 115:436, 1965.

26. COMMON ACCIDENTAL POISONING

Robert J. Haggerty

Definition. The term "accidental poisoning" is usually limited to clinical illness that results from the introduction of exogenous chemicals into the body. These chemicals may be medications in excessive dose, other chemicals not intended for human metabolism, or biologic products, both plant and animal. The term, however, generally excludes disease produced by toxic products of microorganisms. An accident is (1) an observable tissue or biochemical injury that is (2) unplanned. This definition is too restrictive for accidental poisoning, for in many instances the physician is called upon to treat patients who have only ingested a poison but do not yet have any observable symptoms or signs of tissue or biochemical injury. Also, although most poisonings are unplanned in children, the same tissue or biochemical damage occurs when a chemical is introduced for homicidal or suicidal intent.

Etiology. Accidental poisoning is best understood as a problem of multiple causes – the interaction of an agent (the poison) with a host (the patient) in a particular environment. The major agents and the number of accidental poisoning deaths caused by each are listed in Table 1. In nonfatal accidental poisoning the agents responsible are quite different from those in fatal cases. The most common agents responsible for nonfatal accidental poisoning are listed in Table 2, together with the number of such accidents in different age groups. Strictly speaking, these are the etiologic agents, but to understand why a particular poisoning occurs requires knowledge of the interaction of the agent, environment, and host; this is discussed under Pathogenesis.

The route of entry of the poison (agent) is most often oral for solids and liquids, but may occasionally be by absorption through skin, rectum, or lung, or by parenteral injection.

Incidence. Nearly 3000 accidental poison fatalities occur each year in the United States. Only 10 per cent of these occur in children, but nearly two thirds of all accidental poisonings occur in preschool children. Not so evident from Table 2 is the second peak in the late teens and early twenties owing to suicide attempts. In children there are from 300 to 1000 nonfatal poison ingestions for each poison fatality. Some estimates place the total number of nonfatal poisonings as high as 300,000 to 500,000 per year in children in the United States. It is

TABLE 1. Mortality: Agents Responsible for Accidental Poison Deaths in the United States, 1969

	Less Than 5 Years of Age	Total
Medications		
Salicylates and analgesics	68	554
Sedatives and hypnotics	8	687
Psychotherapeutic drugs	12	103
Others	49	467
Total drugs	137	1811
Household products		
Alcohol	1	189
Petroleum and solvents	29	67
Pesticides	25	56
Heavy metals	18	39
Other	32	725
Total other than medications	105	1076
Grand total	242	2887

the most common medical, i.e., nonsurgical, emergency seen in preschool children. In one study, 12 per cent of all two-year-old children had experienced an accidental poisoning within the previous year. In addition to differences in the agents responsible for fatal as compared with nonfatal poisoning, the agents responsible for accidental poisoning vary considerably in their frequency between children and adults. Salicylates are the most common agent involved in children, whereas barbiturates and carbon monoxide are more common in adults. A multitude of household products (such as cleansers, solvents, and insecticides) are potentially poisonous and are available in the American home. They are more likely to be the cause of childhood than of adult poisonings.

Epidemiology. There are more epidemiologic data available on the role of the agent in causing accidental poisoning than on the host and environmental factors, and very few data on the complex interrelations of these three factors in causing accidental poisoning (Wehrle et al.). Most of the available information is of the retrospective epidemiologic type for accidental poisoning in children. It documents incidence by age (peak childhood age one to four years), sex (males more than females, except for the poison suicides of the late teens and early twenties), socioeconomic class (no difference), season (no overall significant variation, although there are some special variations such as medications that are more frequent in the winter and pesticides in the summer), hour of day (peak in midmorning), geographical area (lye and petroleum distillates more common in the South), and place where poisoning occurred (kitchen, bedroom, and bathroom are most common). Unfortunately, this information has not led to effective prevention, for the death *rate* for all age groups from accidental poisoning has remained steady for the past two decades at about 1 per 100,000 for all age groups. There has been a significant decrease in both the *actual number* of deaths in children under five years of age from accidental poisoning (from 422 in 1958 to 242 in 1969) and in the *rate* (from 2.5 per 100,000 in 1958 to 1.5 in 1969). The most dramatic drop has occurred in aspirin poisoning. Over 20,000 total ingestions were reported to the National Clearinghouse in 1965 and only about 8000 in 1972, whereas the number of all ingestions reported actually increased. The reasons are probably multiple, but are likely to be from public and professional education, better therapy, safety enclosures for dispensing medicines (Schertz et al.), and limitation of the number of tablets in children's aspirin (1 1/4 grains) to 36 per bottle.

Since poisonous agents such as aspirin are available in nearly every home, the very real question is why more children are not poisoned when one considers the ubiquity of potentially poisonous agents.

Some children seem peculiarly susceptible to accidental poisoning (Sobel and Margolis). A child with a history of one poisoning episode is nine times as likely to have a second episode in the following year than is a child from a matched control group. Poisoned as compared to nonpoisoned control children appear to have different personalities. They are more impulsive and overactive and are likely to strike back when disciplined, to have more disturbed relationships with their parents, and to have other behavior problems. Their social environment is also different, for their parents are more likely to have marital problems, to be suffering acute illness at the time of the ingestion, or to show a more distant and tense family relationship. Whether this knowledge can lead to identification of the high-risk group before poisoning occurs and whether one can change the incidence of poisoning in this high-risk group are not known; prevention by alteration of social and environmental therapy has never been documented. Among adults, suicide and homicide by poisoning obviously present a very different

TABLE 2. Most Common Agents Responsible for Accidental Poisoning Reported to the National Clearinghouse for Poison Information Centers, 1972*

	<5 Yrs.	5–14 Yrs.	15+ Yrs.	Unknown	All Ages
Medicines	47,625	4742	27,044	4721	84,132
Aspirin	8146	734	1871	310	11,061
Other internal	30,919	3570	24,294	3674	62,457
External	8560	438	879	737	10,614
Cleaning and polishing agents	17,369	852	1203	1819	21,243
Petroleum products	4571	429	610	472	6082
Cosmetics	8660	194	191	491	9536
Pesticides	5336	530	745	1043	7654
Turpentine, paints, etc.	6282	370	479	620	7751
Plants	5503	772	449	663	7387
Gases and vapors	157	178	564	379	1278
Miscellaneous	8599	1731	1357	1578	13,265
Unknown	916	248	1182	150	2496
	105,018	10,046	33,824	11,936	160,824

*Data from National Clearinghouse for Poison Information Centers, May–June, 1973.

epidemiologic picture. Unlike immunization for infectious diseases, no one method of control can be expected to be effective for all types of poisoning.

Prevention. Prevention of accidental poisoning, in spite of these negative statements about its effectiveness, should be attempted by many groups, including physicians. Better labeling of household products and prescriptions is of importance, but it should be remembered that children of the age most often poisoned cannot read. Parents should store such medications in safe places, but locked medicine cabinets are of little practical use because they are usually left unlocked when in use. Physicians treating adults should especially warn grandparents that the digitalis, quinidine, or other potent drugs they are receiving are toxic to small children and are often taken by the child from the grandmother's pocketbook. When prescribing analgesics, especially aspirin, for an acute illness in adults, the physician should warn that these are poisonous to children and should prescribe only the minimal amounts needed for an illness. All prescriptions should be dispensed in safety cap enclosures. New laws also require household cleansers to be dispensed in safety cap containers and should be effective. A common scenario of an accidental poisoning starts with a mother with an influenzal syndrome who may have aspirin prescribed; she falls asleep, and her two-year-old child ingests a fatal amount of aspirin left on the bedside table. Other acute family crises, social as well as medical, also seem to be factors in the pathogenesis of childhood poisoning (Meyer et al.). The physician who cares for such adult crises may be the most effective person to prevent childhood accidental poisonings by seeing that adequate supervision of children is arranged when parents are sick or upset.

Most poisonings in adults are the result of suicide attempts, and of course prevention is aimed at recognition of the person at risk.

Community aspects of poison prevention include public education concerning the hazards of poisons. The Federal Hazardous Substances Labeling Act requires special labeling of hazardous substances and the listing of toxic ingredients on the label. This important step is but one of many that have been taken by the community in an effort to reduce the frequency of accidental poisoning.

National Poison Prevention Week during the third week in March serves as a focal point for health education programs. But to have any chance of success, such measures should be carried out throughout the year. The rapid development of poison information centers since the first one was formed in Chicago in 1953 to the now more than 500 in the United States is another important community action. The National Clearinghouse for Poison Information Centers of the Public Health Service coordinates activities of the local centers and is a valuable repository of information, both for treatment of poisoned patients and for preventive programs. The Association of Poison Control Centers, a voluntary national group, has produced educational material designed to prevent poisonings, has established standards for operation of poison control centers, including an approved list of antidotes, their indications, and doses, and has promoted scientific study of poisonings. It seems clear that these multiple approaches to prevention of poisoning need to be continued, but there is a need to critically evaluate their effectiveness and to add imaginative new programs aimed at prevention.

Diagnosis. Diagnosis of accidental poisoning is made from (1) the label on the poison container, (2) the characteristic signs and symptoms in the patient, and (3) chemical analyses, in that order of importance. In most cases of acute poisoning, especially in children, there is no problem in determining that ingestion of a poison has occurred. The patient is often observed to ingest the poison or is found with the empty container. Here the problem is only to determine the chemical ingredients of the compound ingested, how much was taken, and what toxicity is to be expected. On the other hand, unlabeled prescriptions or trade-name household products (of which there are estimated to be over 250,000 potentially poisonous ones available in American homes) may present a serious problem in identification of the precise chemical involved. Poison information centers are especially equipped to deal with this aspect of diagnosis, for they keep on file trade names of potentially poisonous products and their ingredients. Most operate 24 hours a day and are listed in the telephone book. Information on management will also be provided by these centers. Of great use to the physician in diagnosis of poisoning, as well as in therapy, is a book (Gleason et al.) which contains a section with over 17,000 trade-name household products, their ingredients, toxicity, symptoms, and treatment.

When the label is missing, identification of the poison may be aided by knowing that certain ingredients are common to household products used for the same specific purpose; e.g., most solvent cleansers contain ketones or hydrocarbons. Federal labeling legislation, which requires most hazardous household chemicals to bear a label that plainly lists ingredients, has helped in diagnosis. *The label on the container is the single most useful diagnostic bit of information in accidental poisoning.*

When the patient has not been observed to ingest a poison, the problem of diagnosis may be great. Although some poisons produce pathognomonic signs or symptoms, most do not. Almost any acute disease may be simulated, and the range of symptoms and signs that may result is so vast that one can only advise that any symptoms or signs of unknown cause must be suspected of being due to poisoning until proved otherwise. Lists of such symptoms and signs with the various poisons that can produce them are available in standard toxicology texts.

Toxicologic analysis of body fluids or of the ingested substance itself plays a numerically small but important role in the diagnosis of accidental poisoning. Its main usefulness is for certain common medications, e.g., the ferric chloride urine screening test for salicylates and phenothiazines, and barbiturate or salicylate determinations of blood specimens; and for some heavy metal determinations (lead, thallium, mercury). It is usually impossible for a chemist to analyze a specimen of a completely unknown poison. Even when analysis is possible, the results will not be available for several hours or days; and except for certain patients with chronic poisoning, treatment must be begun much sooner than that. In those few instances in which analysis is useful, it is usually much easier to analyze the remains in the container from which the poison came than to analyze body fluids in which great dilution of the poison has occurred. Recent developments suggest that chemical analysis may play a more important role in the future. Such techniques as thin-layer and gas chromatography make possible the identification of the minute amounts of poisons present in body fluids.

Once the poison that was ingested has been identified,

TABLE 3. Toxicity Rating*

Rating	Probable Lethal Dose mg/kg	For 70 kg Man
6–Super toxic	< 5	A taste < 7 drops
5–Extremely toxic	5–50	7 drops to 1 tsp
4–Very toxic	50–500	1 tsp to 1 oz
3–Moderately toxic	500 mg–5 gm	1 oz to 1 pint
2–Slightly toxic	5–15 gm	1 pint to 1 quart
1–Practically nontoxic	> 15 gm	> 1 quart

*From Gleason, M., Gosselin, R., Hodge, H., and Smith, R.: Clinical Toxicology of Commercial Products. 4th ed. Baltimore, Williams & Wilkins Company, 1973.

there remains the problem of determining its potential for harm to the patient. This depends on the amount ingested and the toxicity of the agent. The amount can sometimes be estimated by observers who may have seen the patient ingest the poison and by the amount remaining in the container. The toxicity of a particular poison can be assessed by reference to known data on LD_{50} and minimal lethal dose. A table has been prepared that is most useful in then estimating the degree of risk to the patient (Table 3).

Treatment. A common mistake in the therapy of acute poisoning is to search for a specific antidote, of which there are very few, and to delay general therapy, which may be very effective and which is all that is available for the majority of poisonings.

General principles of therapy are (1) elimination of the poison from the body, (2) inactivation of the poison, and (3) supportive measures.

Elimination of the Poison. INDUCED EMESIS. One of the most common poison problems brought to the physician is that of a child or adult who has just ingested a potential poison but is still asymptomatic. The most important part of therapy is removal of the poison from the stomach before significant absorption can occur. It is now clear that gastric lavage, the time-honored method for removal of gastric contents, is much *less* effective than induced vomiting because the stomach normally traps large quantities of material in several pouches inaccessible to the lavage tube. The most effective way to induce vomiting is to administer a large dose of syrup of ipecac (15 ml for a child one to four years old, 30 to 45 ml for adults), followed by a repeat dose if no vomiting occurs within 20 minutes (Robertson). This dose is considerably larger than is recommended in older texts, but it has been found safe and much more rapidly effective than smaller doses. Many physicians now prescribe a 1-ounce bottle of syrup of ipecac when children reach age one in order that parents will have it on hand in case of need. Vomiting is more complete if the patient drinks several ounces of fluid three to five minutes after administration of the syrup of ipecac. Mechanical induction of vomiting by gagging, although having the merit of speed, is so often not effective that it is not the first choice of methods. Parenteral administration of apomorphine (1 mg for a one- to three-year-old, 6 mg for an adult) has received renewed interest as a very effective emetic, especially if Naloxone (adult dose, 0.4 mg) is then used as an antidote for the depressant effects, once vomiting has occurred. Vomiting should be induced even if several hours have elapsed after ingestion, for many poisons remain for long periods in the stomach when ingested in large quantities. Other methods of inducing vomiting such as use of a solution of powdered mustard or soap suds are not very effective.

CAUTIONS REGARDING INDUCED EMESIS. The only contraindications to induced emesis in the treatment of accidental poisoning are in patients who have ingested caustics (lyes, acids, etc.), strychnine, and hydrocarbons, and in the comatose patient. With any cause of altered consciousness, gag reflex may be altered sufficiently to increase the risk of aspiration. Ipecac does not work well if antiemetics or some tranquilizers with antiemetic properties have been ingested. Whether one should remove hydrocarbons by careful gastric lavage is still a disputed point. A collaborative study suggests that it may be of slight advantage. At least lavage does not seem to be dangerous, but emesis should not be used to remove hydrocarbons. Saturated salt and sodium bicarbonate solutions should not be used as emetics.

GASTRIC LAVAGE. Even though less effective than emesis, gastric lavage is indicated for comatose poisoned patients to remove the poison from the stomach with less risk of aspiration than with emesis. A large-bore gastric lavage tube should usually be employed, and the stomach should be irrigated with copious amounts of water or physiologic saline. Aspiration can be prevented by having the patient lie on his side with the head slightly lower than the body. Sodium bicarbonate should not be used because it increases absorption of many poisons (salicylates) and causes large amounts of carbon dioxide to be released in the stomach, increasing the risk of aspiration.

OTHER METHODS OF POISON REMOVAL. No data are available on the *effectiveness of catharsis* or *colonic irrigations.* Most do not use cathartics today, for ipecac will cause catharsis and there is often diarrhea produced by the original poison.

Exchange transfusion has proved useful for removal of some poisons when plasma protein binding makes any form of dialysis less effective, i.e., with boric acid and some barbiturates.

Peritoneal dialysis and hemodialysis are effective means of removing many poisons. For preschool children, and even for many adults, peritoneal dialysis (Etteldorf et al.) is preferred because proper equipment and an experienced team for hemodialysis are less available. Use of commercially prepared solutions that contain properly balanced electrolytes and albumin, together with simple multiple-holed polyethylene tubing for insertion into the peritoneal cavity, provides a relatively convenient and simple technique. In certain adult patients in whom renal failure from the poisoning is the major problem, e.g., ethylene glycol poisoning, or for whom prolonged dialysis is needed, hemodialysis has proved very useful.

The kidney is the most effective organ for removal of many poisons. If renal function was normal prior to the poisoning, this route of excretion should be facilitated by adequate fluids, usually intravenously, and in some situations by the use of *osmotic diuretics,* such as mannitol (Cirksens et al.). In salicylate poisoning renal excretion is enhanced as much as twentyfold by making the pH of the urine alkaline with sodium bicarbonate. For patients who are seriously ill, several of these routes of elimination of the poison should be used simultaneously, i.e., gastric lavage, enhancement of urinary excretion, and peritoneal dialysis.

Inactivation of the Poison. A time-honored agent designed to inactivate many poisons has been the "universal antidote" made of two parts charcoal, one part tannic acid, and one part magnesium oxide. This mixture is of no value, but there are new data to support the use of specially prepared activated charcoal to absorb poisons in the intestinal tract. Five to 6 teaspoonfuls of such charcoal (not burnt toast) mixed in a glass of water should be swallowed or administered by gastric tube and then, after absorption has occurred, within 30 minutes, removed from the stomach (Holt and Holz). Neutralization of ingested acids or alkalis is probably of little value, because the tissue necrosis that results from such poisons occurs almost immediately upon contact. The use of demulcents, such as olive oil or milk, makes the patient who has ingested an irritant poison more comfortable but probably does little else and should be avoided if the poison is fat-soluble.

Supportive Measures. More lives are likely to be saved by careful, early, symptomatic treatment of complications such as peripheral vascular collapse, respiratory obstruction, urinary retention, fluid imbalance, and central nervous system excitement or depression than by frantic and usually unsuccessful search for specific antidotes. All these complications are treated by the standard methods that are used when they are due to other causes.

Poisonings for Which Specific Antidotes Exist. *Cyanide poisoning* produces death within minutes. Specific antidotes are available, but unless poisoning occurs in a laboratory there is rarely time to administer them. The antidotes are sodium nitrite injected intravenously (6 to 8 ml per square meter of body surface of a 3 per cent solution at a rate of 2.5 to 5 ml per minute), which produces methemoglobinemia, followed by sodium thiosulfate intravenously (50 ml of a 25 per cent solution). Amyl nitrite inhalation may be of value immediately while the sodium nitrite is being prepared.

Heavy metal poisoning can often be successfully treated by various chelating agents—BAL, EDTA, or penicillamine (see Ch. 27 to 33 and 626).

Iron salts produce acute gastroenteritis, shock, liver necrosis, and, frequently, death. As few as 10 tablets of the usual size (0.3 gram) may be fatal. The specific antidote, desferrioxamine, is useful intravenously to bind absorbed iron (2.0 grams in 5 per cent of levulose solution intravenously, dose 90 mg per kilogram); 140 mg of desferrioxamine can bind about 1 gram of ferrous sulfate—200 mg of iron. It is contraindicated orally, for it probably enhances absorption. Fluid replacement, including blood plasma, should be used for shock.

Morphine and other opium derivatives can be successfully antagonized by Naloxone HCl (adult dose 0.4 mg), repeated up to three times at three-minute intervals. If no improvement occurs, another cause of symptoms should be suspected. Since the action of the antagonist lasts only one to two hours and that of morphine for six or more hours, repeat doses may be needed after two hours (see Ch. 341).

Phosphate ester insecticides such as parathion are powerful anticholinesterases. In addition to peripheral parasympathetic stimulation they produce voluntary muscle paralysis, the most serious being to the muscles of respiration. Red cell cholinesterase is a valuable laboratory test to make the diagnosis and to follow therapy. Atropine in very large doses of 1 mg subcutaneously for a child, 2 to 3 mg for an adult, every 15 to 60 minutes until symptoms subside will antagonize these peripheral parasympathomimetic toxic effects. 2-Pyridine aldoxime methiodide (PAM), a cholinesterase regenerator, is dramatically effective in relieving skeletal muscle paralysis (1 gram intravenously over a five- to ten-minute period and repeated as a slow intravenous drip as needed for respiratory paralysis). Atropine is used first. PAM is not used alone. Airway obstruction must be treated by aspiration, positioning, and occasionally tracheostomy.

Treatment of Specific Common Poisons. A few words should be said about general management of the most common poisonings, but reference to standard texts is necessary for details of treatment of these as well as for the many poisonings that cannot be discussed here.

Amphetamine poisoning is common from an overdose of reducing pills or pep pills. After removal from the stomach, chlorpromazine should be administered in full dose to counteract mania and delirium. Barbiturates should not be used because the late-stage depression that occurs with amphetamines may be compounded.

Atropine poisoning may be produced by overdose or accidental ingestion of the drug or by accidental ingestion of one of several plants, such as the jimson weed. Symptoms include those of parasympathetic blocking, intense erythema, fever, and delirium. Peripheral parasympathetic blockade can be treated with pilocarpine, but this will not counteract the more serious central nervous system symptoms, which must be treated symptomatically with sedatives such as chloral hydrate or paraldehyde.

DDT and other chlorinated hydrocarbon insecticides are relatively uncommon causes of acute poisoning, for fatal doses in man are in the range of 250 mg per kilogram, and this amount is difficult to ingest. Central nervous system stimulation and convulsions are the most serious symptoms. Treatment is entirely symptomatic.

Hydrocarbon ingestion, especially of gasoline and kerosene, produces a severe pneumonia due mainly to direct aspiration into the lung rather than to bloodstream transport to the lungs. Most of the aspiration probably occurs during the initial swallow, but some may also occur during subsequent vomiting. *Emesis is therefore contraindicated.* If large amounts have been ingested, careful lavage is useful. The head should be lower than the chest to prevent aspiration, and the procedure should be performed with a small Levin tube passed through the nose. This is most effective if done before vomiting and consequent aspiration can occur. Varying degrees of central nervous system depression occur, but this rarely needs therapy except with lighter fluid, a common poisoning today with the use of outdoor charcoal cooking. It should be removed by lavage. Probably the only effective therapy for the patient with severe pneumonia is oxygen. Although adrenocortical steroids and prophylactic antimicrobials have been used, there is little evidence that they are the crucial element in successful therapy of this poisoning. Again lighter fluid is the exception, and adrenal steroids do seem useful for pneumonia caused by this agent.

Carbon tetrachloride produces prompt central nervous system depression and abdominal pain. Early death is due to depression of vasomotor and respiratory centers and convulsions. If the patient survives this, he may develop renal and hepatic necrosis. The management at this stage is the same as for other causes of failure of these organs.

Methyl alcohol can cause severe metabolic acidosis and blindness with a fatal dose from as little as 2 ounces. Treatment includes emesis, ethyl alcohol to inhibit the metabolic oxidation of methanol (whiskey, 30 ml every three to four hours for adults), and sodium bicarbonate intravenously for the metabolic acidosis.

Lye and other caustics produce severe, deep burns of the esophagus that may perforate or may later cause esophageal stenosis. Initial pain, airway obstruction, and shock are treated symptomatically. Early esophagoscopy, to determine whether burns have occurred, is followed by cortisone if burns are found. After several days for healing to progress, careful dilatation of the esophagus can be begun. Management should be a team effort with the esophagoscopist.

Salicylate poisoning is the single most common cause of poisoning in children. Emesis should always be carried out if the patient is awake, even though several hours have elapsed after ingestion. Salicylates produce an initial respiratory alkalosis that is transient in children but less so in adults, followed by severe metabolic acidosis, dehydration, and loss of body potassium. With severe poisoning several routes of elimination may have to be used, i.e., by increasing urinary excretion and by peritoneal dialysis. Initial hydration should be vigorous to initiate brisk diuresis, and the fluids should include sodium bicarbonate, 14 to 20 ml of 7.5 per cent solution per 500 ml of fluid. Once diuresis has begun, potassium salts, approximately 35 mEq per liter of fluid, should be added to the solution. Monitoring of serum pH and electrolytes and adjustment of fluid and electrolyte administration appropriately are important for optimal therapy. Milder degrees of poisoning can usually be treated with alkali and intravenous fluids alone. Other symptoms, such as respiratory depression or convulsions, are treated symptomatically.

Cirksens, W. J., Bastian, R. C., Malloy, J. P., and Barry, K. G.: Use of mannitol in exogenous and endogenous intoxications. N. Engl. J. Med., 270:161, 1964.

Etteldorf, J. N., Dobbins, W. T., Summitt, R. L., Rainwater, W. T., and Fischer, R. L.: Intermittent peritoneal dialysis using 5 per cent albumin in the treatment of salicylate intoxication in children. J. Pediatr., 58:226, 1961.

Gleason, M., Gosselin, R., Hodge, H., and Smith, R.: Clinical Toxicology of Commercial Products. 4th ed. Baltimore, Williams & Wilkins Company, 1973.

Holt, L. E., Jr., and Holz, P. H.: Activated Charcoal as an Antidote for Poisons. Nat. Clearinghouse Poison Control Cent. 1963, Jan.-Feb., pp. 1–3.

Meyer, R. J., Roelofs, H. A., Bluestone, J., and Redmond, S.: Accidental injury to the preschool child. J. Pediatr., 63:95, 1963.

Robertson, W. O.: Syrup of ipecac—a slow or fast emetic? Am. J. Dis. Child., 103:136, 1962.

Schertz, R. G., Latham, G. H., and Stracener, D. E.: Child-resistant containers can prevent poisonings. Pediatrics, 43:84, 1969.

Sobel, R., and Margolis, J. A.: Repetitive poisoning in children: A psychosocial study. Pediatrics, 35:641, 1965.

Wehrle, P. F., DeFreest, L., Penhollow, J., and Harris, V. G.: The epidemiology of accidental poisoning in an urban population. III. Pediatrics, 27:614, 1961.

HEAVY METAL POISONING

Edmund B. Flink

27. INTRODUCTION

Many features of poisoning by the heavy metals are similar. The important metals from the standpoint of toxicology are arsenic, lead, mercury, antimony, cadmium, and thallium. The toxic and lethal doses of each metal are small. Antimony, arsenic, lead, mercury, and thallium all have effects on enzymes of the body. Antimony, arsenic, and mercury poison sulfhydryl groups. Mercuric ions even in fairly dilute solutions denature proteins and cause protein precipitation. Thallium and cadmium have recently assumed importance industrially.

Other metals may be toxic also. *Beryllium* intoxication is discussed in Ch. 526, and *bismuth, copper, gold, iron, silver, and uranium* intoxications are discussed in Ch. 626. *Barium* ions cause epigastric pain, nausea, vomiting, diarrhea, chills, cramps, muscle contractions, convulsions, hypertension, tachyarrhythmia, and cardiac arrest. Sodium sulfate or magnesium sulfate should be given immediately to precipitate the barium as sulfate. *Cobalt* was added to beer from 1957 to 1967. Ingestion of large volumes of this beer caused serious and often fatal myocardiopathy. Cobalt has been eliminated as an additive. *Manganese* poisoning occurs in mining and smelting of manganese ores. Damage to the basal ganglia of the brain occurs with attendant Parkinson-like symptoms. When symptoms begin, removal from exposure is mandatory. Proper ventilation of mines and processing plants will prevent intoxication.

Dubois, K. P., and Geiling, E. M. K.: Textbook of Toxicology. New York, Oxford University Press, 1959.

Gleason, M. N., Gosselin, R. E., Hodge, H. C., and Smith, R.: Clinical Toxicology of Commercial Products. 4th ed. Baltimore, Williams & Wilkins Company, 1973.

Goodman, L. S., and Gilman, A.: Pharmacological Basis of Therapeutics. 4th ed. New York, The Macmillan Company, 1970.

28. ARSENIC POISONING

Exposure. Many household and garden pesticides contain arsenous oxide, copper acetoarsenite (Paris green), or calcium or lead arsenate. Drugs that contain arsenic include sodium cacodylate, Fowler's solution, and the arsphenamines (now obsolete). Fowler's solution continues to be used in treatment of asthma in certain regions. Fruits sprayed with insecticides may contain enough arsenic to be toxic. Bootlegged whiskey has occasionally been contaminated with arsenicals. Arsenic trioxide (As_2O_3) or white arsenic has been a favorite for homicidal purposes. Accidental ingestion of arsenic-containing poison continues to be an important source of exposure especially for children.

Although toxic exposure occurs in a variety of industries, only a few cases are reported. Poisoning does occur among agricultural workers using insecticide sprays or dust. Arsine (AsH_3) is a very serious industrial hazard. It is produced accidentally by the exposure of nascent hydrogen to arsenic trioxide.

Arsenic is stored in liver, nervous system, nails, hair, and other viscera and can be detected in them after excretion in urine has ceased. A single dose requires 10 to 70 days for excretion, so accumulation is possible from small daily doses.

The minimal lethal dose of arsenic trioxide (As_2O_3) is 60 to 180 mg, but there is a great variability in susceptibility. The lethal dose of arsine is smaller than this.

Manifestations. *Acute poisoning* may be overwhelming and may produce shock and death within 20 minutes to 48 hours. Ingestion of smaller doses causes vomiting, diarrhea, abdominal pain, and muscle cramps, but does not cause corrosion of mucous membranes. If the victim survives acute poisoning, he may recover without sequelae, or he may develop symptoms of chronic poisoning.

Intravascular hemolysis and renal damage are characteristic of arsenic poisoning, so hemoglobinuria, nausea, vomiting, and abdominal pain develop within six hours after exposure. This initial illness may be quickly fatal, or recovery may begin in a few days. Instances of chronic arsine poisoning have been reported.

Chronic poisoning results from repeated ingestion of small doses. This is the usual method for homicide. Weight loss, diarrhea or constipation, nausea, anorexia, fatigue, drowsiness, peripheral neuropathy, headache, confusion, pigmentation and scaling of the skin, hyperkeratoses of palms and soles, and transverse white lines of all fingernails (Mee's lines) are the important symptoms and signs. Hyperkeratoses may go on to malignant changes in the form of multiple basal cell cancers (Bowen's disease). Perforation of the nasal septum is common. Myocardiopathy induced by arsenic may be fatal.

Hematologic findings of chronic arsenic poisoning include anemia, leukopenia, thrombocytopenia, basophilic stippling, and disturbed erythropoiesis, and myelopoiesis.

Diagnosis. The diagnosis can be established by determining arsenic in the urine. Normal persons excrete an average of 0.015 mg per day, with a range of 0.005 to 0.04 mg. Most patients with manifestations of arsenic poisoning excrete more than 0.1 mg per day.

As in lead poisoning, urine coproporphyrin III excretion is increased markedly, but delta amino levulinic acid is not increased in experimental arsenic poisoning in rabbits and probably not in human intoxication.

Hair and nails store arsenic, so analysis of arsenic content may be of diagnostic value, particularly after removal of the patient from exposure. Hair and nail samples must be very carefully washed to exclude adhering dust and extraneous material. Normal values have ranged from 0.025 to 0.088 mg per 100 grams of hair. Over 0.1 mg per 100 grams is abnormal.

Treatment. When a poison has been ingested, immediate induction of emesis or gastric lavage is of prime importance. Dimercaprol (BAL) should be given immediately. The initial intramuscular dose of BAL is 2.5 to 3.0 mg per kilogram of body weight, followed by the same dose every four hours for six doses. For very severe poisoning, the initial dose should be 5.0 mg per kilogram, followed by 2.5 mg per kilogram, as indicated above, with additional doses at 6- to 12-hour intervals for six doses, depending on the status of the patient. BAL has not proved to be effective in arsine poisoning or in chronic poisoning, probably because the damage has already occurred. Removal from exposure in chronic poisoning is mandatory and usually suffices.

Severe anemia must be treated by transfusion. Treatment of acute renal insufficiency requires the same considerations as that resulting from a variety of causes.

Prevention. Proper storage and labeling of poisons in general should prevent accidental poisoning of children. Avoiding direct contact with insect sprays and wearing appropriate masks when using dusting powders will control this industrial exposure.

Heyman, A., Pfeiffer, J. B., Jr., Willet, R. W., and Taylor, H. M.: Peripheral neuropathy caused by arsenical intoxication: A study of 41 cases with observation of the effects of BAL. N. Engl. J. Med., 254:401, 1956.

Kyle, R. A., and Pease, G. L.: Hematologic aspects of arsenic intoxication. N. Engl. J. Med., 273:18, 1965.

Vallee, B. L., Ulmer, D. D., and Wacker, W. E. C.: Arsenic toxicology and biochemistry. A.M.A. Arch. Industr. Health, 21:132, 1960.

29. LEAD POISONING

Etiology. Exposure to lead in the home is chiefly by ingestion of white lead paint scales by children (pica), from new water systems in which white lead has been used in joints of pipes, by ingestion of soluble lead salts in foods, wines, and distilled liquors, by use of pewter dishes, and by use of tetraethyl lead gasoline for cleaning purposes. Drinking of "moonshine" whiskey distilled by use of an auto radiator as a condenser has resulted in epidemics of acute lead poisoning and constitutes an important cause of lead poisoning of adults.

Ingestion of lead paint scales by young children in areas of poor and old housing constitutes the greatest problem in the United States today. In New York City 4000 cases of lead poisoning were found in 1970 and 1971 because of increased interest and availability of appropriate tests. The incidence in children is greatest in summer months and reaches a peak at the age of one to three years. Black children are at greatest risk. Siblings of children with lead intoxication should be examined also, because about a third of them have been found to have serious exposure.

Lead is dissolved and absorbed from the gastrointestinal tract, deposited in the liver, and then released into the systemic circulation. The respiratory tract epithelium may absorb lead fumes or may propel particles into the pharynx, where they are swallowed. Tetraethyl lead and related compounds may be absorbed through the skin. Soluble lead salts, such as lead acetate or lead carbonate, are readily absorbed and can cause acute poisoning when ingested.

There are many industrial uses of lead and, therefore, many opportunities for exposure. In recent years the industrial consumption of lead in the United States has averaged about 1,110,000 tons a year. The industries using or producing lead are petroleum, mining and smelting, storage battery manufacture, printing, paint and pigment, ceramic and glass, construction (mainly plumbing and insulation), ammunition, wrecking and salvage (acetylene torch and electric arc volatilizing lead paints and alloys), battery reclaiming, and brass polishing. Any procedure that produces lead vapor, mist, or dust exposes workers to inhalation and absorption of lead from respiratory tract epithelium.

The lead-using trades have set up standards and checking procedures that have controlled industrial hazards well. Smoking and eating are restricted to uncontaminated areas. Washing hands and changing clothes before eating and leaving work are the most important personal preventive measures. The gasoline industry has rigid standards for tetraethyl lead workers, but exposure to dangerous amounts still occurs when there is a break in procedure. Cleaning and repairing large storage tanks pose a particular hazard.

Pathology. In chronic poisoning no gross or microscopic lesions are pathognomonic of lead poisoning. Lead is stored in an inert form in bone and is not harmful except when mobilized. Most of the remaining lead is found in the bone marrow, blood, liver, and kidneys. An increased amount of lead in tissues indicates exposure but not necessarily toxicity. Absence of an increased concentration of lead in tissues practically excludes lead poisoning.

In the encephalopathic type, small perivascular hemorrhages, necrosis of cells, and serous exudate around blood vessels may be found anywhere in the brain. In children with acute poisoning, nuclear inclusions are found in liver cells and renal tubular cells. Occasionally inclusions are found in renal tubule cells of lead workers. In Australia chronic lead exposure from the dust of white lead paint has been incriminated as a common cause of chronic renal failure in young adults.

Clinical Manifestations. Lead poisoning is usually divided into acute and chronic forms. Although "chronic poisoning" correctly describes prolonged exposure, manifestations often are acute. It is convenient for descriptive purposes to divide symptomatology into an alimentary form, a neuromuscular form, and an encephalopathic form.

Anemia and attendant pallor and weakness are present in most patients with chronic exposure. *Insomnia, headache, dizziness,* and *irritability* are common symptoms without evidence of more serious encephalopathic disturbances. In a patient with poor oral hygiene, lead sulfide is deposited along the gingival margin of some or all teeth and produces a blue-black *"lead line." Stippling of the retina* adjacent to the optic disc has been described as an early sign in lead poisoning. Chronic renal failure results from chronic lead intoxication. *Saturnine gout* is particularly common in lead poisoning from "moonshine" whiskey. The renal clearance of uric acid decreases.

Alimentary Form. *Painter's* or *lead colic* is the cardinal feature and is the result of spasm of the bowel. Constipation is a natural consequence, and nausea, vomiting, and weight loss are common. Colic is intermittent and often severe enough to double the patient up. Between attacks there is merely a sense of pressure. Absence of tenderness differentiates the condition from appendicitis or other causes of peritoneal inflammation. Relief actually may be produced by pressure on the abdomen. Colic is not invariably present.

Neuromuscular Form. Extensor muscles of the upper extremities are more often paralyzed than flexors or lower extremity muscles. *Wrist drop* is a common and characteristic example. Muscle soreness and stiffness or hypertonus precede and accompany paralysis. The absence of sensory disturbance is important in differentiating this from other forms of peripheral neuropathy. Paralysis is confined to a functional muscle group and is not determined by the distribution of an entire motor nerve. Atrophy may occur after longstanding paralysis and may result in incomplete recovery of muscle function after termination of exposure (see Ch. 456 to 474).

Encephalopathic Form. At present this occurs primarily in children. The diagnosis is not suspected until a large amount of lead has been ingested. Because of the good safeguards in industry now, it rarely occurs in adults and then only after massive exposure to lead fumes or tetraethyl lead in a salvage operation, in cleaning large gasoline storage tanks, or in accidental breaks in techniques. Tetraethyl lead is lipid-soluble, so that exposure results almost exclusively in the encephalopathic form.

The presenting manifestations include *convulsions, mania, delirium,* or *coma.* There may be a history of antecedent behavioral changes such as irritability, insomnia, restlessness, loss of memory, hallucinations, and confusion.

Children may suddenly become very ill. Increased intracranial pressure may occur and is manifested by projectile vomiting, lethargy, convulsions, and coma. In very young children fontanelles bulge. The optic discs may not reflect increased pressure when the process is very acute in onset. Scattered neurologic findings indicate cerebral and cerebellar abnormalities. Blindness and deafness may occur and persist.

Laboratory Findings. The hematologic findings depend on the action of lead on hemoglobin synthesis. Lead interferes with enzymes ALA synthetase, ALA dehydrase, and heme synthetase. ALA and coproporphyrin III accumulate and are excreted in the urine in excessive amounts, and protoporphyrin accumulates in erythrocytes as a result of the blocks in synthetic process. Normally 2 mg of ALA or less is excreted per 24 hours. Lead poisoning results in a 20- to 200-fold increase in excretion of ALA. ALA excretion is a sensitive indicator of lead intoxication. Normally 60 to 280 μg of coproporphyrin is excreted per 24 hours.

In lead poisoning free erythrocyte protoporphyrin (FEPP) ranges from 300 to 3000 μg per 100 ml (normal 15 to 60) and free erythrocyte coproporphyrin (FECP) ranges from 1 to 20 μg per 100 ml (normal 0 to 2). It is noteworthy that iron deficiency anemia and thalassemia result in FEPP values that overlap those of lead poisoning, but the range is not quite as great. If a fresh wet film of blood of a patient with lead poisoning is examined under ultraviolet light, 75 to 100 per cent of the erythrocytes have a red fluorescence. This fluorescence is the result of increased FEPP.

Lead poisoning and *hereditary acute intermittent porphyria* have manifestations that are similar. Both are characterized by colicky abdominal pain, mental symptoms, and paralysis. Acute intermittent porphyria regularly has a great increase in porphobilinogen excretion and uroporphyrin excretion, but lead poisoning usually does not result in excessive excretion of either substance.

Normochromic microcytic anemia, decreased red cell life span, decreased osmotic fragility, but increased mechanical fragility are found. Acute hemolytic anemia with hemoglobinemia, hemoglobinuria, and renal damage occur occasionally in acute poisoning. Death from shock may occur in two to three days. *Basophilic stippling* is nonspecific, is rarely found in tetraethyl lead intoxication, is seldom found in acute poisoning of children, and cannot be relied on for screening purposes. Nevertheless, it frequently furnishes the initial clue for clinical recognition of chronic lead poisoning.

Aminoaciduria, renal glycosuria, fructosuria, hyperphosphaturia, and citraturia result from changes in the epithelium of the proximal convoluted tubules. Other toxins also cause these manifestations. The changes are usually reversible.

Diagnosis. In children, particularly, the normal blood level is low. If the higher range is used with the upper limit of some 0.06 mg per 100 grams, children with serious acute poisoning will have normal levels (see accompanying table). In adults the upper limits of normal coincide with the mean of "safe" exposure.

A diagnosis of tetraethyl lead intoxication is made on the basis of history of exposure. Urine lead determination is the most valuable test. Blood values usually are normal.

Because of the medicolegal implications, it is important to be certain that there is evidence of increased lead excretion. Detection of an earlier exposure may be accomplished by the use of 1.0 gram intravenously of calcium disodium edetate (CaEDTA). Striking augmentation of lead excretion to over 1.0 mg per day usually

Normal and Abnormal Values in Exposure to Lead

	Adults		
	Normal Industrial Exposure	*"Safe" Industrial Exposure*	*Dangerous Industrial Exposure*
Urine mg per liter	Range: 0.00 to 0.06 Mean: 0.03	0.01 to 0.15 0.08	0.08 to 0.4 0.2
Blood mg per 100 grams	Range: 0.01 to 0.05 Mean: 0.03	0.01 to 0.07 0.06	0.07 to 0.2 0.09
Feces mg per specimen	0.25	0.6 to 1.0	1.1+
		Children	
		Normal Range	*Poisoning*
Blood mg per 100 grams	British series American series	0 to 0.04 0.003 to 0.055	0.04 to 0.4 0.06+

occurs. This proves previous exposure but not intoxication.

Collection of samples for analysis must be done with great care to avoid contamination. Pyrex bottles or polyethylene flasks should be rinsed with nitric acid and distilled water. Urine and stool specimens should be passed directly into acid-cleaned containers. Tissues should be placed directly in acid-cleaned containers.

Blood now can be collected in special vacutainer 20 ml tubes (Becton, Dickinson Company) with pure gum rubber stoppers. These tubes have been chemically cleaned for lead analyses. The needle is a straight stainless steel tube. Duplicate samples are desirable.

Lead determinations on blood and urine can now be performed quickly and accurately, using an atomic absorption spectrophotometer. All state and many large city departments of health have such facilities available.

Treatment. Cessation of exposure is of prime importance. A saline cathartic should be given to rid the gut of any unabsorbed lead before chelation of lead is attempted, especially in the encephalopathic form in children.

Colic may be controlled temporarily by intravenous infusion of 1.0 gram of calcium gluconate. The infusion may be repeated as needed.

Fluid intake should be high unless there is increased intracranial pressure. Electrolyte concentrations should be determined and corrected if abnormal.

Chelation of lead by calcium disodium edetate, U.S.P. (CaEDTA), is now the initial treatment of choice for inorganic lead and tetraethyl lead intoxication and is much more effective than any previous method. The chelated lead is excreted in the urine. CaEDTA in doses of 1 to 2 grams per day for an adult and not more than 75 mg per kilogram for a child is given in six to twelve hours intravenously. This dose is repeated for two to three days with a five- to ten-day rest period between courses. Nephropathy has resulted rarely from therapy, but this usually has occurred with larger doses than those outlined above. If symptoms are severe, treatment should not be delayed to obtain results of lead analyses. Lead excretion should be determined during as well as before treatment.

D-Penicillamine not only chelates lead but also supplies sulfhydryl groups. A dose of 30 mg per kilogram up to a total of 2.0 grams per day in four divided doses given orally is satisfactory. It is particularly useful to follow the initial CaEDTA therapy. It has the additional advantages that it can be given orally continuously, and that it is much less toxic than CaEDTA. For moderate lead intoxication, penicillamine is the agent of choice. Successful treatment with CaEDTA or penicillamine results in a return of ALA and coproporphyrin excretion to normal. Erythrocyte protoporphyrin declines very slowly after successful treatment.

The most serious manifestation is lead encephalopathy, which requires prompt and skillful treatment. Increased intracranial pressure may occur suddenly and must be treated vigorously. Infusion of urea solution in a dose of 100 mg per kilogram to 1000 mg per kilogram as 30 per cent urea in 10 per cent glucose solution or of mannitol solution (20 per cent) in a dose of 7 to 10 ml per kilogram can alleviate increased pressure effectively, but the benefit may last only a day or two, and repetition may be necessary. Dexamethasone sodium phosphate in a dose of 10 mg intravenously initially followed by 4 to 6 mg intramuscularly every four to six hours in adults is an effective alternative. Craniotomy may even be required for relief of pressure. Chelation of lead with CaEDTA must be started immediately for patients who are gravely ill.

Physiotherapy is important for patients with neuropathy. Splinting to support the weak extremity prevents overstretching of muscles; otherwise, permanent disability can follow.

Prognosis. In the gastrointestinal form the outlook is good for complete recovery after adequate treatment and prevention of re-exposure. Recovery from paralysis is usually complete even after many months of paralysis.

Encephalopathy is very serious. It causes a mortality rate of 25 per cent or more, and often leaves mental retardation and various permanent neurologic lesions in those who survive. In adults permanent blindness, extraocular muscle paralysis, or other lesions may result. The acute form caused by tetraethyl lead either is fatal or is followed by complete recovery. There is great urgency in treatment of this form. One cannot wait to get results of lead analysis before starting treatment.

Albahary, C.: Lead and hemopoiesis. Am. J. Med., 52:367, 1972.
Ball, G. V., and Sorensen, L. B.: Pathogenesis of hyperuricemia in saturnine gout. New Eng. J. Med., 280:1199, 1969.
Beattie, A. D., Moore, M. R., and Goldberg, A.: Tetraethyl-lead poisoning. Lancet, 2:12, 1972.
Byers, R. K.: Lead poisoning. Review of literature and report on 45 cases. Pediatrics, 23:585, 1959.
Einarsson, O., and Lindstedt, G.: Nonextraction atomic absorption method for the determination of lead. Scand. J. Clin. Lab. Invest., 23:367, 1969.
Feldman, F., Lichtman, H. C., Oransky, S., Ana, E. S., Reiser, L., and Malemud, C. J.: Serum delta aminolevulinic acid in plumbism. J. Pediatr., 74:917, 1969.
Fleming, A. J.: Industrial hygiene and medical control procedures. Arch. Environ. Health, 8:266, 1964.
Guinee, V. F.: Lead poisoning. Am. J. Med., 52:283, 1972.

30. MERCURY POISONING

Etiology. Acute mercury poisoning results from accidental or intentional ingestion of soluble mercuric salts such as mercuric chloride ($HgCl_2$, corrosive sublimate) and is characterized by very serious corrosive effects on the entire gastrointestinal tract and serious renal tubular cell damage.

Mercury is a liquid and is highly volatile at room temperature. In 1957 over 4 million pounds of mercury were used in the United States. It is used widely in medical research and clinical pathology laboratories, as well as in the manufacture of scientific instruments, electric meters, mercury vapor lamps, amalgams with copper, tin, silver or gold, in solders, and in the production of organic mercurial compounds. Mining cinnabar (HgS), refining mercury from it, and cleaning mercury distilling apparatus involve substantial hazards. Photoengraving, bronzing, and the production of certain paint colors such as vermilion and antifouling agents for hulls of ships all use mercury compounds.

As little as 0.1 gram of $HgCl_2$ may cause poisoning, but fatal doses are usually in excess of 1.0 gram. It is caustic and produces cell destruction by protein precipitation on direct contact. In more dilute solutions, such as concentrations effected by absorption from the intestinal tract after ingestion of a toxic dose, its effect is primarily due to selective affinity for sulfhydryl (-SH) groups of proteins, especially of enzymes. This property is counteracted by dimercaprol.

Chronic mercury poisoning results from inhalation of mercury vapor or ingestion of small amounts of mercuric nitrate or other salts, and is characterized by mental symptoms and stomatitis.

Alkyl mercury compounds (ethyl and methyl mercury) have become an important environmental problem. The compounds are soluble in organic solvents, and the covalent carbon-mercury bond is not degraded by biologic processes. Methyl mercury particularly is found in tuna and swordfish taken from waters heavily contaminated with mercury. Epidemics have occurred in Minamata and Niigata, Japan, and in several countries where seed grain treated with alkyl mercury compounds (as antifungal agents) has been diverted into food. Nearly complete intestinal absorption occurs; the liver excretes most of it into the intestine, resulting in continuous enterohepatic circulation. Methyl mercury passes the placental barrier very well and accumulates in the fetus with resultant cerebral palsy and mental retardation of the child.

ACUTE POISONING

See Ch. 626.

CHRONIC POISONING

Clinical Manifestations. *Stomatitis.* Excessive salivation and a metallic taste are common. A blue line develops along the gingival margin. Gums become hypertrophied, bleed easily, and are sore. The teeth become loose.

Erethism. The term "erethism" is applied to the psychic disturbance characterized by irritability, shyness, and deterioration of family and social activities, suggesting hyperthyroidism. Since felt hat makers formerly used mercury salts in the manufacturing process and often became "mad," these symptoms gave rise to the phrase "mad as a hatter."

Tremors. Tremors of the eyelids, lips, tongue, fingers and extremities are characteristic of chronic poisoning. Coarse jerky movements and gross incoordination interfere with fine movements such as writing and eating. Atrophy of the cerebellar cortex and, to a lesser extent, of the cerebral cortex occurs. Microscopic changes occur in the granular layer of the cerebellum, ganglion cells, and posterior columns.

Nephrotic Syndrome. Contact with ammoniated mercury and other compounds has caused proteinuria and frank nephrotic syndrome. Removal from exposure is mandatory, so a careful history of medicinal or occupational exposure is needed.

Hypersensitivity. Hypersensitivity reactions to mercurial diuretic agents include asthma, urticaria, exfoliative dermatitis, and sudden death. Fatal accidents can be prevented by avoiding intravenous injections. Death is usually due to ventricular fibrillation.

Hypersensitivity to calomel (HgCl) results from long-term ingestion of HgCl. Hypersensitivity to ammoniated mercury or other compounds results from topical application. Fever, morbilliform rash, leukopenia, eosinophilia, and enlargement of the spleen and lymph nodes characterize this condition. Mercury fulminate used in percussion caps and detonators may cause dermatitis of exposed parts, with pruritus, papules, vesicles, and pustules.

Acrodynia or "Pink Disease." This disorder of infants and young children is characterized by irritability, insomnia, stomatitis, loss of teeth, hypertension, erythema of fingers, toes, nose, cheeks, and buttocks, and even acral gangrene. Fever, leukocytosis, and albuminuria occur. In 1948 Warkany and Hubbard suggested that sensitivity to mercury might be the cause, and that hypothesis is now fairly generally accepted. The diagnosis is established by finding excretion of more than 0.1 mg of mercury per day in the urine. An organic mercury compound, phenyl mercuric propionate, has been incorporated into house paint to prevent growth of mold. This paint has been incriminated as a source of toxic exposure.

ORGANIC MERCURY INTOXICATION

Ethyl and methyl mercury compounds have an affinity for the central nervous system and produce fatigue, headache, loss of memory, apathy, emotional instability, paresthesia, generalized ataxia, deafness, dysarthria, progressive visual deterioration, dysphagia, and, occasionally, coma and death. Changes in the central nervous system similar to the lesions of chronic mercury poisoning are found.

Diagnosis. Industrial exposure and characteristic symptoms usually make recognition of chronic mercury poisoning relatively straightforward, but, in the absence of known exposure, the diagnosis may be elusive. Patients with chronic mercury poisoning excrete in excess of 0.3 mg of Hg per liter of urine. Normal values range from 0.0001 to 0.001 mg per liter. An excretion of 0.1 mg per liter is considered evidence of toxic exposure. In instances of exposure to metallic mercury for more than five years, a brown reflex from the anterior lens capsule can be seen by slit lamp. Some observers consider it an early sign of mercury poisoning. Albuminuria and hematuria are common findings in chronic poisoning.

Treatment. Removal of the patient from all possible exposure is of paramount importance. The use of BAL in chronic poisoning has not been established as effective treatment. However, n-acetyl-DO-penicillamine, in a dose of 500 mg four times a day, increases mercury excretion and has been used successfully in therapy of chronic mercury poisoning and acrodynia. This treatment is ineffective in methyl mercury poisoning, but promising results have been obtained here, using ion-absorbing resin to interrupt the enterohepatic circulation of mercury.

Prognosis. Recovery is slow even after removal from exposure. Patients with advanced intoxication fare poorly. Only 15 per cent of the more severely involved patients recovered completely in one series. Signs of cerebellar and cerebral damage persisted and prevented return to normal activities.

Prevention. Removal of $HgCl_2$, calomel, and mercury ointments from the market would eliminate acute poisoning and many instances of chronic poisoning. Good safe substitutes are available for each compound. Elimination of mercuric nitrate from the felt-processing industry has already occurred. Mercury salts for fingerprinting by police departments have been replaced by barium, zinc, or bismuth. Silver has replaced mercury in the manufacture of mirrors.

Mercury-containing paints should have a warning label "For Outside Use Only." Mercury cannot be replaced in many electrical apparatuses and scientific instruments. Proper exhaust ventilation, scrupulous avoidance of any exposed metallic mercury, and good personal hygiene are necessary precautions. The maximal allowable concentration of Hg has been set at 0.1 mg per cubic meter of air. Medical supervision is necessary wherever potential exposure exists. Neurologic signs and especially visual field changes, tremor, ataxia, and dysarthria are serious danger signals.

Battigelli, M. C.: Mercury toxicity from industrial exposure. A critical review of the literature. J. Occup. Med., 2:337, 1960.

Hirschman, S. Z., Feingold, M., and Boylen, G.: Mercury in house paint as a cause of acrodynia. N. Engl. J. Med., 269:889, 1963.

Joselow, M. M., Louria, D. B., and Browder, A.: Mercurialism. Environmental and occupational aspects. Ann. Intern. Med., 76:119, 1972.

31. ANTIMONY POISONING

Antimony and potassium tartrate (tartar emetic) is used for emetic purposes, and other organic antimony compounds are used in treatment of schistosomiasis, filariasis, and certain fungal infections. Antimony is encountered in metallurgic processes, mining and smelting, and in rubber manufacturing, but industrial poisoning is rare. Finely divided antimony is more toxic than compounds of antimony. Trivalent antimony combines with sulfhydryl groups of enzymes. The symptoms of acute poisoning are similar to those of acute arsenic poisoning. Vomiting is a prominent symptom. Dimercaprol (BAL) is an effective agent for treatment of antimony poisoning, and the regimen is like that for arsenic and mercury. Dermatitis and conjunctivitis occur from exposure to dust in the smelting process. Stibine (SbH_3) is more volatile than arsine and is very toxic also. It attacks the central nervous system and causes acute hemolysis. Death occurs when there is a 0.01 per cent concentration in the air. The chemical process of formation and the effects are like those of arsine.

32. CADMIUM POISONING

Cadmium sulfide is associated with zinc minerals and particularly with zinc sulfide. Cadmium exposure can occur in the manufacture of alloys, vapor lamps, and storage batteries, grinding and polishing alloys, cadmium plating, welding, zinc ore smelting, and glass blowing. Inhalation of cadmium fumes results in pulmonary edema, followed in two to three days by proliferative interstitial pneumonia. Various degrees of permanent lung damage and fibrosis occur. Cadmium can be inhaled in fatal concentrations without enough discomfort to warn the worker. The inhalation of fumes with cadmium produces dryness of throat, cough, headache, vomiting, sensation of constriction in the chest, severe dyspnea, and prostration. There is no effective treatment except symptomatic treatment of pulmonary edema. Foods prepared and stored in cadmium-plated containers may be contaminated sufficiently to cause poisoning. Cadmium ingestion usually does not produce fatal poisoning, but causes rather violent gastrointestinal symptoms, with sudden onset 20 to 30 minutes after eating.

33. THALLIUM POISONING

Thallium sulfate (Tl_2SO_4) is an extremely toxic cumulative poison (lethal dose 0.2 to 1.0 gram). It has a mild metallic taste. Thallium is absorbed from the gut and from the intact skin. It has had wide use as a rodent, ant, and cockroach poison. Because of serious and frequent accidental and deliberate (homicidal) toxicity, the U.S. Department of Agriculture banned thallium formulations for household use in 1965. Unfortunately, some of it can still be found on shelves in homes and stores.

Alopecia is a very important and unique sign. *Accumulation in nervous tissue* accounts for critical symptoms which include ataxia, choreiform movements, vomiting, constipation, restlessness, delirium with hallucinations and delusions, and, finally, coma. Blindness, loss of other special senses, facial paralysis, paresthesias, and peripheral neuropathy occur. Central lobular necrosis of the liver and renal damage also occur. Liver radiopacity increases in some patients. Urinary excretion of 10 mg per day or more indicates serious poisoning.

Various therapeutic trials, including dithiocarb, dithizone, BAL, and KCl, have been used but either have failed to bring improvement or may even be dangerous because of mobilization of thallium and redistribution to the brain. Gastric lavage should be done immediately after diagnosis up to four hours after exposure. Prussian blue (potassium ferric hexacryanoferrate II) is an excellent chelator of thallium by exchange of potassium for thallium. Prussian blue is not absorbed from the gut and is nontoxic. It must be introduced into the duodenum by tube because of gastric dilation produced by thallium. The recommended dose of colloidal solution is 250 mg per kilogram per day in two to four divided doses. A vigorous laxative such as castor oil is necessary for the first day or two. After this an osmotic agent such as 50 ml of 15 per cent mannitol solution will suffice. Therapy should continue until thallium excretion is less than 0.5 mg per 24 hours.

Huff, J. E.: Special communication: Thallium poisoning. Clin. Toxicol., 5:89, 1972.

Kamerbeck, H. H., Rauws, A. G., TenHam, M., and VanHeijst, A. N. P.: Prussian blue therapy of thallotoxicosis. Acta Med. Scand., 189:321, 1971.

34. CARBON MONOXIDE POISONING

Bertram D. Dinman

Definition. Carbon monoxide, a product of incomplete combustion of carbonaceous materials, is an odorless, colorless gas; its density is slightly less than air. The gas is commonly produced by the internal combustion engine, poorly vented heating devices, or gas refrigerators. Certain industrial operations such as those associated with blast furnaces and coke ovens, foundry cupolas, petroleum refineries, and underground mines also present risks of serious carbon monoxide intoxication. Less severe but potential exposures may exist in automobile repair shops, among traffic policemen, or in arc welding. Frank intoxication caused by vehicular exhausts is usually due to impaired integrity of exhaust systems and/or the automobile body. Poisoning associated with engine operation for in-car heating purposes occurs only with such defects or when the motor is run in confined spaces, e.g., deep snowdrifts, garages. Natural gas has replaced manufactured gas in the United States; since the former is free of carbon monoxide, illuminating gas per se no longer presents any risk of injury. However, carbon monoxide may be produced by the incomplete combustion of natural gas in faulty heating or other gas-burning apparatus. Chronic cigarette smokers develop 3 to 8 per cent carboxyhemoglobin (COHb) concentrations. Although the foregoing exogenous sources of carbon monoxide have long been recognized, the phenomenon of endogenous carbon monoxide production is now well established; as a result of cleavage of the α-methylene bridge in the heme portion of hemoglobin, 0.3 to 1.0 ml per hour is normally produced. This leads to a normal blood COHb concentration of 0.5 to 0.8 per cent.

Pathogenesis. Since carbon monoxide usually exists in a gaseous form, the only significant portal of entry is via the respiratory tract. The gas diffuses across the alveolar membrane in amounts proportional to the pressure gradient for carbon monoxide between alveolar air and blood. The rate of uptake is directly proportional to the respiratory rate, duration of exposure, and carbon monoxide concentration in air. The high affinity of carbon monoxide for hemoglobin (218 times greater than that of oxygen) is responsible for its primary pathologic effect, i.e., reduction of erythrocytic oxygen-carrying capacity. As a result, all signs, symptoms, and pathologic alterations are those of tissue hypoxia. In addition to reducing blood oxygen tension, carbon monoxide in association with hemoglobin (i.e., carboxyhemoglobin) impedes that pigment's discharge of oxygen at the capillary bed. Thus capillary oxygen tensions must be decreased lower than normal in order to dissociate oxygen from the erythrocyte to the tissues. This impairment of oxygen dissociation is expressed by a shift in the oxyhemoglobin curve to the left. Such effects are further complicated in that respiratory chemoreceptors respond only to decreased blood oxygen tension; since this is not decreased (i.e., there is simply a decrease in blood oxygen content), physiologic compensatory mechanisms are not brought into play.

Aside from the formation of carboxyhemoglobin and the resultant hypoxia, there is little evidence that carbon monoxide has any significant direct effect upon tissue except at extremely high concentrations.

Pathology. Carboxyhemoglobin is characteristically cherry red in color. Accordingly, the tissues and skin of poisoned individuals always grossly present a characteristic pink color when blood levels of carboxyhemoglobin exceed 30 per cent concentration levels. (Rarely, severely poisoned individuals may not manifest this change at autopsy; this results from reduction of COHb below the 30 per cent level owing to therapeutically induced respiratory clearance prior to death.) The skin may present areas of vesiculation and ulceration at pressure points. Ischemic necrosis of the cardiac papillary muscles and renal tubular degeneration may be noted. Although animal experiments suggest that repeated carbon monoxide exposures may accelerate the development of coronary atherosclerosis, the design of these experiments makes extrapolation of the results to humans difficult. Although the brain of patients dying of acute intoxication (i.e., within the first 24 hours) is congested, pink, and edematous, under these conditions this organ does not usually demonstrate specific, localized degenerative lesions. However, those surviving this acute episode can later develop diffuse degenerative changes prominently involving the cerebral cortex, globus pallidus, cerebellum, and basal ganglia. It is frequently stated that carbon monoxide–induced lesions have a predilection for certain locations in the brain, e.g., basal ganglia, hippocampal region, but in fact a consistent pattern of brain localization is not evident.

Clinical Manifestations. This disease is characteristically an acute poisoning. Although chronic forms of carbon monoxide intoxication have been claimed to exist, they are not adequately documented. Repeated episodes of mild acute poisoning can occur without cumulative effects.

The clinical picture of carbon monoxide poisoning is closely correlated with the blood concentration of carboxyhemoglobin. Although levels of less than 10 per cent COHb are said to produce no clinical effects, subtle changes of central nervous system function have been consistently demonstrated at the 5 to 10 per cent COHb level (e.g., increased visual threshold, impaired higher cognate function). In addition, precipitation of anginal episodes has been noted in patients with coronary artery disease during exercise with COHb levels of 3 to 5 per cent.

Although frontal, bandlike headaches may be experienced in the 10 to 20 per cent COHb range, more commonly these occur at the upper reaches of this range. In the 20 to 30 per cent COHb range the headaches become more severe. Dyspnea on exertion may be the only other manifestation. At the 30 to 40 per cent COHb levels, headaches become very severe, and are associated with nausea and vomiting, weakness, dizziness, dimness of vision, and possibly collapse. At the 40 to 50 per cent COHb level, ataxia, syncope, and collapse may be observed, in addition to tachycardia and tachypnea. As blood levels of 50 to 60 per cent COHb supervene, there may be coma associated with intermittent convulsions, and Cheyne-Stokes respiration may develop. In the 60 to 70 per cent COHb range, coma deepens, intermittent convulsions occur, and there is clinical shock. Death may terminate such exposures, although profound shock, respiratory and cardiovascular failure, and death have been reported to be delayed until 70 to 80 per cent COHb concentrations are attained. In severe cases, leukocytosis, proteinurea, glycosuria, hematuria, and cylindruria are usually demonstrated, in addition to temperature elevation of 39° C or more.

Diagnosis. Diagnosis is established by quantitative determination of blood carboxyhemoglobin concentration; analysis of alveolar air for carbon monoxide correlates well with blood COHb. The method of Coburn, utilizing a nondispersive infrared meter, is highly accurate; the helium-ionization detector equipped gas chromatograph also provides high sensitivity. Although spectrophotometry has long been used, its sensitivity and specificity are less than with more modern techniques.

The cherry-red skin and mucous membrane coloration are highly characteristic of carbon monoxide poisoning. However, it is not readily detected until a 30 to 35 per cent COHb concentration is attained.

Treatment. The patient must be immediately removed from the contaminated environment. In mild cases clearance of carbon monoxide from the blood is spontaneously accomplished if respiration is sustained. Fresh air and absolute rest are sufficient in such cases; attempts at exertion of any type within four to six hours can cause a rapid recrudescence of signs and symptoms. In the event of unconsciousness—no matter how transient—hospital management and emergency treatment are indicated. Respiration must be sustained by whatever method is available—i.e., artificial respiration, intermittent positive pressure breathing apparatus. Regardless of the level of COHb initially found, normal air breathing will result in 50 per cent clearance of blood carbon monoxide in about 250 to 300 minutes; 100 per cent oxygen inhalation will achieve a similar reduction of carbon monoxide loading in 35 to 80 minutes, and oxygen at three atmospheres of pressure results in the same clearance in about 25 minutes. The use of a 95 per cent oxygen–5 per cent carbon dioxide mixture hastens oxygenation, largely owing to the Bohr shift.

Persistence of coma and the presence of shock require the usual supportive treatments. Induction of hypothermia may help prevent irreversible brain damage.

Prognosis. Patients who do not become comatose usually recover without permanent sequelae. Persistence of hyperthermia, shock, or acute hypoxia-induced clinical laboratory signs for two days after intoxication holds a grave prognosis. Among those who survive such severe intoxication, a small proportion will demonstrate residual changes—e.g., major seizures, dysphasia, parkinsonism or varying degrees of hyperkinesia, mental impairment. Such severely affected patients usually manifest such signs within one week of the acute episode. However, in approximately half of these severe cases there may be apparent recovery followed by relapse after a latent period of one to three weeks. In either case, if recovery is to supervene, it should be expected within two years of the acute episode.

Coburn, R. F. (ed.): Biological effects of carbon monoxide. Ann. N.Y. Acad. Sci., 174:430, 1970.

Haldane, J.: The action of carbonic oxide in man. J. Physiol. (London), 18:430, 1895.

Meigs, J. W.: Acute carbon monoxide poisoning. An analysis of one hundred five cases. A.M.A. Arch. Indust. Hyg. Occup. Med., 6:344, 1952.

Peterson, J. E., and Stewart, R. D.: The post-exposure relationship of carbon monoxide in blood and expired air. Arch. Environ. Health, 21:165, 1970.

Richardson, J. C., Chambers, R. A., and Heywood, P. M.: Encephalopathy of anoxia and hypoglycemia. Arch. Neurol., 1:178, 1959.

Shillito, F. H., Drinker, C. K., and Shaughnessey, T. J.: The problem of nervous and mental sequelae in carbon monoxide poisoning. J.A.M.A., 106:669, 1936.

DISORDERS DUE TO HEAT AND COLD

Paul Webb

35. INTRODUCTION

When thermoregulation fails or is overwhelmed, life-threatening disorders develop from severe heat stress or cold stress. Profound hypothermia is the result of serious loss of body heat, whereas a major accumulation of body heat produces heat stroke. Both conditions require prompt and vigorous treatment. There are other, less serious disorders from heat exposure, in which heat is not stored in large quantity; these are the more common and more easily managed heat syncope and heat exhaustion. Cold and heat can cause local tissue injury, of course, as in frostbite, immersion foot, and burns, but this chapter deals only with the general disorders.

36. HEAT STROKE

A medical emergency, heat stroke is easily diagnosed when it is expected. Thus when military men begin training in hot climates or when seamen work in the engine rooms and galleys of ships in tropical waters, heat casualties are common, and some of them may be heat stroke. In young, healthy men who have been working hard in heat, unconsciousness, high body temperature, strong rapid pulse, and hot flushed skin are presumptive evidence of heat stroke in the absence of another obvious diagnosis such as head injury or massive infection. But in older people who have not been exerting themselves in hot work places, the diagnosis of heat stroke is not so obvious. Deaths from "excessive heat and insolation" in the United States range from 1 to 12 per 100,000 in people over 65, and many cases are missed or not reported. Heat deaths in the elderly are presumably similar in mechanism to classic heat stroke.

Prodromal symptoms, which may not be notable, include faintness, dizziness, staggering, headache, and nausea. There is a clear history of heat exposure or of heavy exertion in heat. Classically the patient in heat stroke is unconscious, although any degree of impairment of the central nervous system may present initially, from lethargy, confusion, or irrational agitation, to coma and convulsions. The body temperature is high, 40° C (104° F), or higher measured in the rectum; but if the patient is not seen immediately, and if even simple measures have been started to relieve heat stress and to start cooling, the body temperature may be lower. The pulse is strong, and its rate is usually 140 or higher. Blood pressure measurement will show a normal or elevated systolic pressure and a lowered diastolic pressure. However, in the late and severe stage of the disorder, blood pressure is low as the circulation fails. The skin is flushed, and sweating may be present, or—a bad sign—reduced or absent. Heat stroke is easily distinguishable from heat syncope or heat exhaustion, with their mildly elevated body temperatures, transient disturbances of consciousness, and mild circulatory signs. Heat stroke results from excessive heat storage, with high cardiac output, cutaneous vasodilation, and low peripheral resistance. Cessation of sweating and circulatory failure are late signs. There is evidence that the heart failure is right-sided, with low resistance in the systemic circulation and high resistance in the pulmonary circulation.

One should not always expect to see all the signs of heat stroke in an elderly person whose circulatory function is not what it used to be, and in whom there may be some pre-existing infectious disease. The diagnosis should be thought of if body temperature stays high and circulation is failing. Heat deaths during heat waves typically increase one or two days after the heat wave begins, and continue for one or two days after it is over. Predisposing factors are age, obesity, lack of acclimatization, and preceding infection or gastrointestinal upset.

The greater the heat storage and the longer it has been present, the worse the prognosis. Damage is done by general cellular degeneration and widespread hemorrhages, especially those in the central nervous system, kidneys, and liver. Laboratory findings in severe cases include reduced blood coagulation, low prothrombin, and low platelet count; low urine volume, high specific gravity, albumin, and renal casts; elevated blood urea; hemoconcentration; low serum potassium and normal to high serum chloride; changes in liver function; elevation of serum enzymes; and a hyperdynamic circulatory pattern unless circulatory failure has already developed.

Treatment of heat stroke should begin at once. Its aim is to lower body temperature and to support the circulation. Effective cooling methods, in ascending order of effectiveness, are wet towels and a strong fan in a cool dry room; icebags over much of the body; water-cooled sheets such as are used to induce hypothermia; and a tub bath of cold water. The higher the body temperature, the more aggressive the cooling technique should be. Sedation may be needed to control the patient, who may struggle or who may begin to convulse. A tranquilizing cocktail of pethidine, chlorpromazine, and phenergan may be used to prevent both convulsions and shivering, or simpler means of calming a person may suffice. Cooling should be continued until the rectal temperature goes below 38° C. After the initial lowering of body temperature, continued temperature monitoring is vital, for strong cooling may produce an after-drop of temperature, and somewhat later, patients will often start to store heat again despite being in a thermally comfortable environment.

Shock must be treated with fluid replacement and possibly isoproterenol. Fluid therapy should be started judiciously, with the amount and electrolyte content guided by laboratory findings. Other supportive measures are begun when problems are identified, e.g., platelet transfusions or renal dialysis.

37. HEAT SYNCOPE

A person who becomes dizzy or suddenly tired after exercising in the heat may abruptly faint. As soon as he is recumbent, and especially if he is removed from direct exposure to heat, he recovers. In contrast to the patient with heat stroke, the person with heat syncope has a cool, sweaty, pale skin; his pulse is weak and either mildly elevated—100 to 120 beats per minute—or slow, as in vasovagal syncope. His blood pressure falls just before fainting, and recovers quickly when he lies down or sits with head lowered.

Lack of acclimatization and lack of training for the exercise undertaken predispose to heat syncope. Cutaneous vasodilation and blood pooling in the erect position contribute to the hypotension. Treatment is a matter of allowing the person to rest, cool down a little, and drink some extra liquid.

38. HEAT EXHAUSTION

Taking much longer to develop than heat syncope (often several days), heat exhaustion results from loss of fluid or loss of fluid and salt. The symptoms of prolonged water depletion are thirst, fatigue, giddiness, elevated body temperature, oliguria, and finally delirium. The water depletion results from sweating and inadequate replacement by drinking, whether voluntary or involuntary. Voluntary dehydration in heat—the failure to replace water loss even though water is available—is common, but most people catch up at the end of the day when they get out of the heat. In the tropics it is sometimes not possible to cool off at night or keep up with water replenishment. This causes problems for the non-native dweller especially.

When both water and salt become depleted, muscle cramps are added to the picture of fatigue, nausea, and giddiness. The urine chloride will be low to absent, and serum chlorides reduced.

Heat exhaustion is treated by rest in bed away from heat, and restoration of body water, or water and electrolytes. Cool liquids should be given by mouth, up to 6 or 8 liters the first day. If body temperature does not return to normal spontaneously, alcohol sponging or wet towels and a fan may be used. If the patient cannot drink, intravenous therapy should be started. Continuation of fluid and electrolyte replacement should be guided by laboratory analyses.

Prevention of heat exhaustion is a matter of ensuring an adequate fluid intake, which means enough to replace losses from sweating. These losses can be as high as 6 to 8 liters per day in men working hard in hot dry conditions. People who are not yet acclimatized to heat need supplemental salt, because their sweat contains more electrolyte than that of the acclimatized. A daily intake of 15 to 25 grams of NaCl is recommended for newcomers to hot environments; about 10 grams of this can be consumed with a meat-containing diet. The additional 5 to 15 grams is best taken in the form of salted fruit drinks and enteric-coated salt tablets. But if water and fluids are in short supply, salt tablets should not be used. The routine use of salt tablets in hot situations is no longer encouraged except possibly for people who have little experience, and then only during the first days of becoming acclimatized.

39. HYPOTHERMIA

When the rectal temperature is below 35° C (95° F), hypothermia is said to be present. This major loss of body heat occurs in hikers and climbers exposed to cold, in elderly people who live alone in meagerly heated homes, in people who have been drinking heavily and have fallen asleep out of doors, in accident victims, and in people accidentally immersed in cold water. In profound hypothermia people are often assumed to be dead, for their vital signs are so depressed as to be missed even by trained observers. If only a clinical mercury thermometer is available, it will fail to register low enough to point to the diagnosis.

Estimates of the frequency of hypothermia vary widely, but the incidence is possibly higher than anyone suspects. In England it has been shown that elderly people are often forced to tolerate being chronically depleted of body heat, and the same may well be true in the United States for isolated old people. This would seem to be an ideal initial condition from which to develop hypothermia. Added hunger, fatigue, or minor injury could increase the heat depletion by rendering such people helpless. Drugs such as chlorpromazine may also contribute to it.

A person in profound hypothermia is in coma and cold to the touch. The skin is pale, usually grayish in color; the neck and extremities resist bending. No peripheral pulse can be found, breathing appears to be absent, and pupillary reflexes are absent. If a low-reading thermometer can be found, the rectal temperature will show 30° C or lower. Less profound hypothermia differs in degree; there will be some signs of consciousness, reaction to pain, a detectable if slow pulse, and flexible joints.

Additional findings are hypotension; cardiac irregularities on the EKG, typically atrial fibrillation and a J wave associated with the QRS complex; low pH in the blood from metabolic acidosis, especially in patients whose hypothermia was preceded by exhaustion and prolonged shivering; low blood CO_2 content; and high blood glucose.

Rewarming is the first order of business, and a decision must be made about passive or active rewarming and, if active, whether by external or core first means. A person who is still somewhat conscious, who has a reasonable heart rhythm, and whose rectal temperature is between 31 and 35° C is probably best handled by rewarming in a warm room or in a bed with blankets. If a person is acutely hypothermic from cold water immersion, the preferred approach is immersion in a warm tub bath whose temperature is kept at 40 to 42° C. A person with slowly developed hypothermia, in whom fatigue, injury, or old age has produced a poor condition beyond the hypothermia, should probably be warmed actively but less aggressively, e.g., with a heating blanket kept at 37° C. Rewarming the core first may be undertaken for profound hypothermia, for there is grave danger of ventricular fibrillation at heart temperatures from 27 to 30° C. The core-warming method avoids the early return of cold blood from the arms, legs, and skin, which commonly causes an unwanted after-drop in central temperature during external rewarming. But the methods of core-warming first are not simple ones; warm peritoneal dialysis and an extracorporeal blood circuit with a heater are examples.

Other than a determined approach to restoring body heat, the management of hypothermia should be as conservative as circumstances warrant, i.e., trauma or infection must be heeded. Respiratory support, for example, should include intubation or tracheostomy only if absolutely necessary. These procedures affect an already irritable heart. Cardiac irregularities should be watched rather than treated; if arrest occurs, it should be treated by external cardiac massage, and use of a defibrillator for ventricular fibrillation. Fluid therapy should be guided by laboratory findings rather than by some predetermined rule; thus one should combat acidosis or hypokalemia specifically if present.

Anderson, S., Herbring, B. G., and Widman, B.: Accidental profound hypothermia. Br. J. Anaesth., 42:653, 1970.

Ellis, F. P.: Mortality from heat illness and heat-aggravated illness in the United States. Environ. Res., 5:1, 1972.

Fernandez, J. P., O'Rourke, R. A., and Ewy, G. A.: Rapid active external rewarming in accidental hypothermia. J.A.M.A., 212:153, 1970.

Fox, R. H., Woodward, P. M., Exton-Smith, A. N., Green, M. F., Donnison, D. V., and Wicks, M. H.: Body temperatures in the elderly: A national study of physiological, social, and environmental conditions. Br. Med. J., 62:200, 1973.

Leithead, C. S., and Lind, A. R.: Heat Stress and Heat Disorders. Philadelphia, F. A. Davis Company, 1964.

O'Donnell, T. F., Jr., and Clowes, George H. A., Jr.: The circulatory abnormalities of heat stroke. N. Engl. J. Med., 287:734, 1972.

Patton, J. F., and Doolittle, W. H.: Core rewarming by peritoneal dialysis following induced hypothermia in the dog. J. Appl. Physiol., 33:800, 1972.

Shibolet, S., Coll, R., Gilat, T., and Sohar, E.: Heatstroke: Its clinical picture and mechanism in 36 cases. Quart. J. Med., 36:525, 1967.

Zingg, W.: The management of accidental hypothermia. Can. Med. Assoc. J., 96:214, 1967.

40. RADIATION INJURY

Niel Wald

Definition. Radiation energy from sources of ionizing radiation which interacts with human cells, tissues, and organs produces a variety of clinical manifestations, depending on the magnitude and duration of radiation exposure and on the size and function(s) of the body area irradiated. The source of the radiation energy absorbed may be external, such as an x-ray machine, or it may be internal contamination from a radioactive isotope inhaled, ingested, injected, or absorbed through the skin or a wound.

Clinical manifestations of radiation energy absorption may be acute, with or without late sequelae, or they may be delayed and chronic. The acute manifestations include the acute radiation syndrome which typically follows whole body radiation exposure; local tissue or organ injury with little or no systemic manifestations after partial body exposure; and growth and developmental disturbances after exposure of the fetus. The clinical effects of intermittent or constant low level radiation exposure from external or internal sources may present as chronic progressive impairment of certain tissues or organs, or solely as the relatively late appearance of one or another of the long-term sequelae of radiation exposure, such as cancer and leukemia. In addition, any of these forms of exposure which impinge on the gonads may produce germ cell changes or mutations which can cause sequelae in subsequent progeny.

Tissue injury may be produced by cellular interactions with radiations of any part of the electromagnetic spectrum, including the output of the sun, lasers, or microwave equipment. Some of these, such as x-rays, gamma rays, and neutrons, are capable of penetration, and can produce internal tissue damage. Other radiations, such as alpha rays and low energy beta rays, have a very limited range in tissue and are only injurious when given off within the body by incorporated radioactive isotopes. The radiations *emitted* by ionizing radiation sources are quantitated in roentgens (r) of exposure, whereas the radiation energy *absorbed* by the tissues exposed is quantitated in rads. The same absorbed dose delivered at different rates will produce very different effects.

Etiology. Typical radiation injury is caused by exposure to *ionizing radiations.* Since the recognition of man-made radiation by Roentgen in 1895 and of natural radioactivity by Becquerel the following year, occupational and medical exposures have been the most usual sources of radiation injury, the use of nuclear weapons in World War II producing a major addition in human cases of radiation injury. Injury from external sources occurred among the early x-ray workers, the employees of the nuclear weapons project, and the subsequent nuclear energy research and industrial organizations. In addition, unavoidable injury has been produced in some radiation therapy patients through exposure of normal tissues adjacent to the lesion under treatment.

Internal radionuclide exposure resulted in injury to employees of the radium watch dial painting industry in the 1920s. More recently, fallout from nuclear weapons tests has produced some internal radionuclide deposition in the general public. In the medical patient population, the uses of radium as a therapeutic agent and thorium as a diagnostic x-ray contrast medium have resulted in clinical sequelae decades after administration. Also, there have been instances of diagnostic and therapeutic radioisotope misadministration producing acute injury and occasionally causing death.

Incidence and Prevalence. The frequency with which radiation injury occurs is closely related to the availability of sources for radiation exposure and the understanding and care with which they are maintained and used. The largest potential source of radiation casualties is the military use of *nuclear weapons.* The Joint Commission for the Investigation of the Effects of the Atomic Bomb in Japan estimated the incidence of radiation injury in Hiroshima to be about 40 per cent and in Nagasaki about 50 per cent in the injured survivors. In Hiroshima about 30 per cent of the deaths in those who survived longer than one day were ascribed to radiation injury either alone or combined with blast and/or burn damage. In the survivor study population of 113,000, 117 cases of leukemia developed between 1950 and 1966. It is probable that the modern nuclear weapons would exceed these results. In nuclear weapons tests, some 300 people have inadvertently been exposed to local high levels of radioactive fallout, with resultant clinical manifestations in about 25 per cent.

Early peacetime uses of radioactivity led to an initial high incidence of injury. Within seven years of the demonstration of x-irradiation by Roentgen in 1895, some 200 cases of x-ray injury had been reported. After recognition of the hazard, radiation protection standards were developed internationally. There has been a marked reduction in this type of injury, although hand injuries still occur occasionally in industrial radiographers and the users of x-ray diffraction and other analytic equipment in research and development laboratories.

The discovery of natural radioactivity by Becquerel in 1896 led to the purification of radium by the Curies in 1911 and its use in medicine and industry. About 5000 watch dial painters, industrial chemists, and medical patients were involved. A subset of this population, 777 cases, had developed 51 bone sarcomas and 20 carcinomas, mainly paranasal, by 1971. The development of man-made radioactive material during and after World War II led to a nuclear industry population of several hundred thousand workers, but only 97 cases of clinical radiation injury had developed by 1969. Although data collection concerning medical misadministrations of radioactive isotopes designed for diagnostic and therapeutic purposes has not been systematic, several deaths and a number of injuries are known to have occurred in the very large American patient population receiving these materials.

Epidemiology. The manifestations of acute or of late radiation injury are not produced solely by irradiation. It is therefore essential to utilize epidemiologic methodology in order to establish the relationship of the etiologic agent to the clinical symptomatology. Two most helpful features have been the temporal relationship of the exposure to the development of clinical effects and the quantitative dose-response relationship.

The etiologic role of radiation in the clinical syndrome of *acute* radiation injury has been shown in epidemiologic studies of the Japanese atomic bomb survivors, the Marshall Island and Japanese fishermen exposed to fallout from a nuclear weapon test, several groups of radiation therapy patients, and the workers involved in various industrial radiation accidents. Epidemiologic studies relating *late* radiation effects such as neoplastic diseases and life-shortening to radiation exposure have dealt with radiologists and other physicians, the Japanese population under long-term follow-up by the Atomic Bomb Casualty Commission, the radium watch dial painters, therapeutically x-irradiated patients (particularly those receiving thymic irradiation in infancy), and patients receiving radioactive iodine therapy.

Pathogenesis. The basic pathology begins with the interaction of the radiation with tissue within the first second of exposure. The radiation energy in photons or particles penetrating the protoplasm may interact at the atomic level to produce ion pairs. These ions combine radiochemically with cell water, producing free radicals such as H and OH which further react to produce such forms as H_2O_2 and HO_2. These, in turn, may interact with critical molecules of the cell protoplasm such as nucleic acids or enzymes. If the dose is high and interactions are numerous, the cell may be killed directly by the radiation. At lower doses, the ability of the cell to divide may be impaired permanently or temporarily. If the DNA is involved, sublethal damage of this molecule may result in reproduction of the alteration (i.e., mutation) in daughter and descendant cells. Direct cell killing begins with exposures of one or more thousands of rads, in general, although some cells such as lymphocytes and spermatogonia are affected at much lower doses. Those cells which are rapidly dividing and differentiating are most vulnerable. Mitotic arrest occurs after several hundreds of rads and is characterized by continuing function of the existing cells but no new divisions. The continuing synthesis of proteins and enzymes, despite an irreversibly impaired mitotic apparatus, leads to "giant cells" which die after several weeks because their excessive size interferes with nutrition and metabolism. At doses of about 100 rads or more, mitotic delay results from temporary impairment of the mitotic mechanism. At still lower doses transient chromosomal "stickiness" is seen, presumably caused by denaturation of the DNA-histone molecules. Also, beginning at exposures as low as a few rads, are chromosome aberrations, i.e., breaks, deletions, gaps, and abnormal forms such as ring and dicentric chromosomes.

The effects of these cellular abnormalities on the various organs depend on the rate of proliferation of new cells required. In high turnover tissues such as the blood-forming tissue and the gastrointestinal tract, the relatively short life span of the predominant cells leads to rapid depletion before the onset of mitotic recovery and new cell production. In the period of mitotic inhibition of the blood-forming tissue, for example, the consequent depletion of mature cells results in increased probability of infection and hemorrhage. The resultant pathologic manifestations are nonspecific, although the inflammatory changes accompanying infection are deficient in polymorphonuclear cells.

In tissues which have little or no continuous proliferation, such as the liver or brain, this type of radiation injury is not apparent; however, functional impairment may be detected by appropriate means. In very slow turnover tissues, such as the lens of the eye or the thyroid gland, the manifestations of acute radiation effects may require months to years before becoming evident. Also, the small arterioles damaged by local radiation injury may show a compensatory increase in cell production, leading to endothelial thickening, obliterative endarteritis, and extensive fibrosis over a prolonged period of time.

Chromosomal abnormalities produced in injured cells may be reproduced and perpetuated for decades. A long-lived component of the lymphoid cells may even carry the original radiation damage for many years before dividing. Clones of cells with the same specific chromosome abnormality may develop over a period of years as well.

Clinical Manifestations. Clinical manifestations of radiation injury can be subdivided into three major forms: the acute radiation syndrome, acute local radiation injury, and delayed effects. External penetrating irradiation, as well as external and internal radionuclide contamination and local traumatic injury with radionuclide contamination, may produce these manifestations.

Acute Radiation Syndrome. This syndrome is seen typically after exposure of most or all of the body to external sources of penetrating ionizing radiation, although high doses of ^{32}P, ^{131}I, and ^{198}Au have also evoked it. It appears in three major forms, in ascending severity of injury. These are the hematologic, the gastrointestinal, and the central nervous system–cardiovascular forms. Four discernible clinical stages can be recognized, particularly when the severity of injury allows for ultimate survival. These are the initial or prodromal stage which subsides into a latent stage, followed by a stage of manifest or overt illness, and a recovery stage. The duration of each stage is inversely related to the severity of injury.

Typical manifestations of the *hematologic form* are seen after an exposure in the midlethal range (300 rads). Prodromal anorexia, nausea, and possibly vomiting may commence within several hours and generally subside within 48 hours. Transient waves of skin erythema and conjunctivitis may be observed over the same period or longer. The patient may be asymptomatic after the prodromal stage for one to three weeks. Then the increasing inadequacy of the body's defenses against infection and hemorrhage becomes manifest, with development of fever, oropharyngeal lesions, abscesses, petechiae, purpura, and bleeding from body orifices. Other findings include scalp pain and epilation, and recurrent anorexia and nausea accompanied by weakness, fatigue, weight loss, and emaciation. Gradual recovery ensues, beginning about the fifth to sixth week after exposure and requires several months.

The earliest laboratory finding is lymphopenia, reaching absolute lymphocyte levels below 1000 per cubic millimeter within the first 48 postexposure hours. The reticulocytes may disappear in the same time period. A gradual fall in granulocyte counts begins during the first two weeks, reaches a plateau, or even shows an abortive rise, followed by a steep fall to a low point at about 30 days postexposure. The platelet count nadir occurs at the same time, after a more continuous fall. If the individual survives, an abrupt increase in all the cell lines mentioned, except the lymphocytes, will occur within the next week and rapidly reach normal levels. An initial increase in granulocyte count in the first 24 hours may occur on the basis of a nonspecific "alarm reaction," and should not mislead one to exclude radiation injury on this basis. Blood biochemical analyses may show nonspecific indicators of major cell and tissue damage such as creatinuria, increased excretion of DNA breakdown products such as beta-aminoisobutyric acid, deoxycytidine, and various other amino acids. Serum enzyme measurements such as LDG, SGOT, and SGPT may be elevated. Within 24 hours chromosome breakage and abnormal forms can be seen in peripheral blood cytogenetic preparations, with the frequency related to the magnitude of the radiation exposure.

The *gastrointestinal form* is associated with anorexia, nausea, vomiting, and diarrhea within the first few hours after exposure. These may be of sufficient severity to require active treatment but usually subside within 48 hours. A latent period follows which may last only a few days to a week before there is a major recurrence of all the gastrointestinal systems as well as those of infection and hemorrhage as described above. These patients generally die with a fulminating enterocolitis before the full appearance of epilation and other slower developing radiation sequelae.

Laboratory abnormalities in the gastrointestinal form of radiation injury are similar to those of the hematologic form but occur more promptly and with greater magnitude. In addition, the hematocrit may be increased as a result of hemoconcentration caused by fluid loss, which, with hypoglycemia and electrolyte imbalance, results from the loss of a functional intestinal mucosal lining.

In the *central nervous system and cardiovascular form,* immediate nausea, projectile vomiting, and explosive diarrhea are characteristic. These may be accompanied by disorientation, hyperesthesia, ataxia, sweating, prostration, and shock. There may be some improvement after several hours, but alternations develop between evidences of central nervous system hyperexcitability, including convulsions, and CNS depression, such as somnolence and coma. This is accompanied by hypotension which gradually becomes irreversible, as does oliguria, leading to a fatal outcome in 24 to 48 hours.

Laboratory observations in the central nervous system and cardiovascular form of acute radiation injury show marked telescoping of the previously described injury syndromes with abnormalities occurring sooner and with greater severity. Complete lymphopenia and an initial granulocyte level of 30,- to 40,000 may be present within the next few hours. Prompt chromosome examination may show marked increase in chromatid and chromosome aberrations, but as the circulating lymphocytes disappear, it may become difficult to find dividing cells. The biochemical evidences of tissue damage are much more striking in this form of the syndrome. In addition, biochemical evidences of azotemia secondary to hypotension become prominent. Transient hyperbilirubinemia may be observed.

Local Radiation Injury. Localized radiation injury may occur with acute and/or chronic clinical manifestations, depending on the total dose and dose rate with which the exposure takes place.

The early changes result in three major clinical findings: erythema, epilation, and transepidermal injury. *Erythema* comparable to a mild sunburn or a thermal burn of the first degree may appear on exposure to more than 200 to 300 rads. A transient first wave may be present within hours after exposure, associated with hyperesthesia, burning, or itching. The major redness appears two or three weeks later, the interval depending on the dose. In the lower dose range no further changes other than tanning may occur, and medical care is not necessary. A counterpart to this reaction has been described in the conjunctiva and in the anterior chamber of the eye, with inflammatory changes observed promptly after exposure.

Epilation, or loss of hair, may occur after exposure to any form of radiation, beginning with exposures of about 200 to 300 rads. It generally becomes apparent only two or three weeks after exposure. Associated skin or scalp tenderness may occur one or two days preceding the actual hair loss. With doses greater than about 500 rads, epilation may be complete. If the exposure is much greater than 600 rads, hair may not regrow.

Transepidermal injury (dry or wet dermatitis) is comparable to a thermal second-degree burn with erythema, blistering, and pain. Confluent bullae may develop in about one and one-half to three weeks, depending on dose (usually exceeding 1000 rads). These may rupture, leaving open, weeping lesions vulnerable to infection.

With higher doses, probably on the order of 5000 rads, a more serious version of transepidermal injury occurs, in which the lesion resembles a third-degree burn. Pain occurs promptly and is intense. The raw areas may be very slow in healing, or may not heal until surgical resection and skin grafting are performed. Epilation is permanent.

Still higher doses may produce immediate tissue damage to structures below the skin. Such injuries, which have occurred in the abdominal wall, male genitalia, and extremities, are irreversible, requiring surgical excision and further reconstructive management.

Delayed Effects. Delayed effects of radiation exposure are of two varieties: those finally appearing in organs whose cells received the radiation exposure and are relatively slow in responding; and those late effects occurring in organs and tissues in which descendent cells ultimately express the initial radiation injury after a latent period which may be many years in duration. The first type of delayed effect can be seen in the male gonad, for example. Doses as low as 15 rads will produce *impairment in fertility* owing to moderate oligospermia beginning about 50 days after the exposure. Azoospermia will occur with doses of more than 200 to 300 rads for a period of roughly one to one and one half years. Doses of 500 to 600 rads may produce permanent sterility in male or female survivors.

The lens of the eye is another late-responding tissue, with opacities appearing in the posterior subcapsular region in months to several years after exposures of about 200 rads or more. *Cataracts* of the posterior lens may develop in the majority of patients who receive more than 600 rads. The gradual development of *hypothyroidism* several years after exposure of several hundred rads is another example of delayed response. *Skin changes* constitute another late response to either acute injury or repeated low level radiation exposure. There may be loss of the detailed finger-ridge pattern and hair, abnormalities of the fingernails, and dryness of the skin. Localized hyperkeratosis may be seen, as well as breakdown of previously healed but atrophic skin, and, ultimately, neoplastic skin changes may develop in such areas.

In the *fetus* the clinical manifestations will depend largely on its age and the magnitude of exposure. If the exposure takes place in the first one to two weeks, resorption of the conceptus is probable. Between the second and sixth weeks, the effect will be on the particular organs under development at the time. Further along in gestation, there will be more subtle generalized effects ultimately expressed as deficits in growth and development, including microcephaly and mental retardation.

The most common *late effects* of radiation exposure are *neoplastic diseases.* The earliest to appear are the acute leukemias and chronic granulocytic leukemia, with a peak incidence of approximately four to seven years after the radiation exposure. Chronic lymphocytic leukemia is not increased by radiation exposure. Other neoplasms whose induction appears significantly increased by radiation exposure include cancer of the thyroid and salivary glands, lung, bone, and female breast tissues. Internally deposited radionuclides have been associated particularly with malignant neoplasms of bone and reticuloendothelial tissues such as liver, spleen, and lymph nodes. Radium deposition has involved the mastoid bones and those surrounding the paranasal sinuses in particular, whereas internally administered thorium dioxide has produced an increase of hemangiosarcomas of the liver. In addition, a generalized increase in incidence of all forms of cancer has been documented in the Japanese atomic bomb survivors. *Shortening of life expectancy* through somewhat earlier death from all causes has been documented in the radiologist population but not yet in the Japanese A-bomb survivors.

Diagnosis. ***Acute Radiation Syndrome.*** The manifestations of acute radiation injury are not unique to this causative agent. Therefore the diagnosis rests on the history and the evolving clinical pattern defined by time of onset and duration of the clinical signs, symptoms, and laboratory abnormalities, particularly the hematologic changes.

In the absence of an adequate history of radiation exposure, the diagnosis may be elusive. The various manifestations may suggest a wide range of conditions. Prodromes suggest psychoneurosis, food poisoning, or gastrointestinal viral infection; symptoms in the period of manifest illness may mimic aplastic anemia, leukemia, infectious gastroenteritis, typhoid fever, and even mumps (for radiation parotitis). When a radiation exposure history is elicited, hematologic and cytogenetic examinations may be used as well as physical dosimetry data obtained by personnel monitoring equipment, if any, and by reconstruction of the exposure situation, in order to obtain confirmatory and quantitative information concerning the potential severity of the injury. However, it must be kept clearly in mind that the evolving clinical pattern is the final diagnostic criterion for the recognition and management of this form of injury.

Local Injury. Local radiation injury, particularly as it appears on the upper extremities, is often confused with thermal and chemical burns. Differentiating features are absence of waves of erythema in the latter as well as the more severe prolonged pain and slower healing associated with radiation. Recurrent tissue breakdown after healing is also suggestive of radiation injury as opposed to the other possibilities.

Delayed Effects. No clinical characteristics of the late effects of radiation exposure are unique to this etiologic agent.

Radionuclide Contamination. Radionuclides deposited on the surface of the skin may be absorbed, inhaled, or ingested into the body where they may act to produce delayed effects. In order to prevent such sequelae, the recognition of their presence is essential even though no immediate clinical manifestations are present. Such diagnostic procedures must involve close collaboration between the physician and the health physicist, the professional trained to recognize and quantitate radiation exposure in order to prevent deleterious effects of radiation. Radioactivity surveys of the suspected individual with appropriate radiation detection equipment should be carried out. It is most important to collect all urinary and fecal excretions in separate containers until sufficient data of the nature and magnitude of contamination are obtained. Some radionuclides such as radon may be sought in breath samples. An early postexposure blood sample should also be collected and preserved for radionuclide analysis. Finally, it may be necessary to carry out chest or whole body low-level radiation counting in an appropriate facility, i.e., a so-called "whole body counter."

If a traumatic wound is present, radionuclide contamination may be sought by measuring radioactivity of swabs used in cleaning the wound as well as by surveying over the surface with appropriate detectors. If the wound is the sole contaminated area, excreta samples will show whether the contaminant has been absorbed into the body and therefore is sufficiently soluble for circulation and translocation to remote sites from the wound.

Treatment. *Acute Radiation Syndrome.* The treatment of acute radiation syndrome is based on an understanding of its pathophysiology. The prodromal symptoms in the acute radiation syndrome are self-limited, but sedatives and antiemetics may be used if needed. Throughout the syndrome it is important to reduce anxiety by keeping the patient informed about the nature of his injury, the expected transient health impairment, and its anticipated duration and treatment. The prolonged weakness associated with this syndrome even during convalescence may be in some measure secondary to the prolonged anxiety and fear of the unknown often associated with radiation injury.

In the *hematologic form,* the inhibition of mitosis responsible for the overt illness is self-limited. Thus management is directed toward maintenance of the patient through the period in which his defenses against infection and hemorrhage are deficient. This is best achieved by conservative means. The threat of exogenous bacterial and viral infection is reduced by strict reverse isolation of the patient with maintenance of a clean environment by use of a laminar air flow or "life-island" methods. Attendant personnel must be screened for potential pathogens and treated prophylactically if necessary.

Prophylactic oral antimicrobial drugs to clear pathogenic bacterial and fungal organisms from the gastrointestinal tract have been used when the total granulocyte level falls below 1000 per cubic millimeter. Various blood elements may be given to replace deficiencies when needed. Red cells are needed only if significant bleeding has occurred. Fresh platelets should be available for use if significant hemorrhage develops. Their use has been advocated even in the absence of bleeding when the platelet count falls below 10,000 per cubic millimeter. If available in concentrated form, normal granulocytes may be administered in the face of overt infection during the granulocytopenic phase. If not available, in the presence of a clearly life-threatening infection the use of the much greater numbers of granulocytes of patients with chronic granulocytic leukemia has been suggested, because they are capable of phagocytosis. On recovery, it is assumed that the patient's immune system will rid the body of such donor cells.

In the situation in which both biologic and dosimetric indicators suggest the high probability of a fatal outcome, bone marrow transplantation may be warranted. Because such marrow requires about two weeks to correct the deficit in circulating blood cells, such a decision should not be delayed much beyond the first postexposure week. The hazards of a graft reaction by the host if his radiation-induced immunosuppression is not sufficient and of "graft versus host" reaction if it is too long lasting define the narrow boundaries within which therapeutic benefit may be expected. The availability of an identical twin or a very close matching relative on tissue compatibility testing will also influence the decision.

Management of the *gastrointestinal form* of acute radiation syndrome has not been successful thus far in the few human occurrences. Animal studies by Bond and Cronkite suggest that the vigorous and early utilization of adequate anti-infection agents, blood components, nutrients, electrolytes, and fluid may influence mortality favorably.

In the few human instances of the *central nervous system-cardiovascular form,* the progressive hypotension has not been improved by the administration of pressor agents, and the fluid administration involved has augmented the congestive heart failure which has ensued.

Local Radiation Injury. The treatment of local radiation injury is generally similar to that of thermal burn of the same severity. This includes the maintenance of asepsis, eventual removal of devitalized tissue to the degree necessary, and the use of skin grafting to cover nonhealing ulcerations. An additional feature in management is very careful and prolonged observation for possible early neoplastic changes of the skin.

Delayed Effects. Clinical management of the delayed effects of radiation exposure does not differ in any way from the management of similar pathologic conditions not caused by radiation.

Radionuclide Contamination. In the event of an accident in which radionuclide contamination is likely, only urgent first aid should be given and the patient evacuated from the site. Contaminated skin and wounds should be washed promptly, and all excreta collected.

Useful preparations for skin decontamination include soap and water, surgical and laundry detergents, and oxidizing agents. These should be accompanied by brushing and rinsing, with care taken not to abrade the skin.

Contamination of the eyes, nose, and mouth is treated initially with copious water washing as soon as possible. Isotonic irrigants may be substituted as soon as available.

For definitive wound care, the usual surgical principles apply, with modifications only in the aseptic procedures and debridement in order to avoid introduction of skin contamination into the wound. It may also be desirable to give diethylenetriaminepentaacetic acid (DTPA), a chelating agent available from the U.S. Atomic Energy Commission for investigational use, intravenously prior to surgery to minimize the ultimate deposition of any contaminant which may get into circulation during surgery.

If radioactivity measurements of excreta and of the whole body suggest a residual body burden of a larger quantity than seems acceptable on the basis of medical judgment and regulatory agency guides, various treatments may be used to minimize the absorption and enhance the excretion of the radionuclide.

To minimize respiratory absorption, the use of irritants, expectorants, and pulmonary lavage is under current investigation. Inhalation of DTPA aerosol mist is also currently being tested for transuranic isotope contamination.

To minimize gastrointestinal absorption, the simplest measure is to accelerate excretion with a mild laxative. For strontium-90, sodium alginate and aluminum hydroxide gel have been used orally to prevent uptake from the gut. For cesium-137, Prussian blue (ferric ferrocyanide) does the same. To promote excretion of nuclides already within the body and to reduce deposition in target organs, such as bone, a variety of agents are available. For plutonium, americium, yttrium, lanthanum, and fission products, intravenously administered chelating agents are useful, DTPA being the most effective. For strontium, the combination of high calcium intake and acidification of the blood with ammonium chloride has effectively reduced bone absorption.

Prognosis. *Acute Radiation Syndrome.* The estimated short-term radiation exposure which would be lethal for 50 per cent of an untreated human population in 60 days is about 300 rads mean midline absorbed dose. This exposure would be expected to produce the hematologic form of the acute radiation syndrome, with half the exposed population dying within 60 days. However, an accidentally irradiated worker survived an estimated 600 rads absorbed whole body dose, with postexposure treatment, including isogeneic marrow transplantation, by Wald, Thomas, and co-workers, despite tissue damage severe enough to necessitate subsequent amputation of all four extremities; and Thomas et al. have used pre- and postexposure treatment, including isogeneic marrow, successfully in patients with leukemia receiving up to 1600 rads.

Thus it appears that successful management of the hematologic form of acute radiation injury is possible under optimal therapeutic circumstances with great expenditure of medical resources. Clearly, such prognostic optimism would not apply to the large-scale population exposure situation such as occurred in Hiroshima and Nagasaki. Furthermore, even the best clinical management has not yet succeeded in allowing the survival of those few individuals who accidentally have received exposures resulting in major gastrointestinal or central nervous system–cardiovascular damage.

Local Radiation Injury. The outlook for good recovery from local radiation injury depends in part on the adequacy of management of the acute changes, including the removal of devitalized tissue and the prevention of secondary infection. However, the main determinant of the ultimate outcome will be the severity of injury to the underlying blood vessels.

Delayed Effects. The prognosis for the various delayed effects of radiation exposure is similar to that of the same pathology in the absence of such exposure.

The likelihood of a radiation-exposed individual's developing a late effect of the exposure is increased in relationship to the exposure dose. The statistical probability can be assessed for leukemia only on the basis of its occurrence in the population exposed to the atomic bombs in Hiroshima and Nagasaki. There, the increased likelihood is one to two cases per year per million people observed per rad of exposure for a period at least 15 to 20 years after the exposure. Epidemiologic studies of thyroid cancer in patients who received thymic irradiation in childhood suggest a similar incidence. It is not known whether this dose-response ratio holds for all malignant tumors.

Prevention. Since the foregoing discussion has indicated that there are no specific methods of reversing the course of events initiated by radiation exposure, the best measure against radiation injury is prevention. The largest *potential* source of radiation exposure to the general population is the nuclear weapon. It is therefore essential that all measures be taken to minimize the possibility of any human population receiving such an exposure again. Another potential source of population exposure, the widespread and increasing utilization of nuclear energy as a source of electric power generation, has been controlled successfully thus far.

The largest *actual* source of population exposure consists of users of radiation in the healing arts. It is evident that such usage of ionizing radiation has produced untold benefit to the same population. Nevertheless, it is incumbent on the users of medical radiation sources to minimize the exposures needed to obtain the necessary diagnostic information. This requires not only optimal operation of existing equipment by current techniques but also a continuing research and development effort to improve the efficiency of such exposure to allow reduction of exposure while obtaining the necessary biomedical information. Adequate specialized education of all users of radiation sources in the philosophy and methods of radiation protection is another factor in the preventive approach to radiation injury.

Andrews, G. A., Balish, E., Edwards, C. L., Kniseley, R. M., and Lushbaugh, C. C.: Possibilities for Improved Treatment of Persons Exposed in Radiation Accidents. *In* Handling of Radiation Accidents. Vienna, International Atomic Energy Agency, 1969, p. 119.

Basic Radiation Protection Criteria. NCRP Report No. 39, Washington, D.C., National Council on Radiation Protection and Measurements, 1971.

Bond, V. P., Fliedner, T. M., and Archambeau, J. O.: Mammalian Radiation Lethality. A Disturbance in Cellular Kinetics. New York, Academic Press, 1965.

Brent, R. L., and Gorson, R. O.: Radiation exposure in pregnancy. Current Problems in Radiology, Vol. II, No. 5. Chicago, Year Book Medical Publishers, 1972.

Fabrikant, J. I.: Radiobiology. Chicago, Year Book Medical Publishers, 1972.

Ionizing Radiation: Levels and Effects. A report of the United Nations Scientific Committee on the Effects of Atomic Radiation to the General Assembly, with annexes, Vols. I and II. New York, United Nations, 1972.

Manual on Radiation Haematology, Technical Reports Series No. 123, Vienna, International Atomic Energy Agency, 1971.

Michaelson, S. M.: Human exposure to nonionizing radiant energy. Potential hazards and safety standards. Proc. I.E.E.E., 60:389, 1972.
Rubin, P., and Casarett, G. W.: Clinical Radiation Pathology. Philadelphia, W. B. Saunders Company, 1968.
Stannard, J. N.: Toxicology of radionuclides. Ann. Rev. Pharmacol., 13:325, 1973.
The Effects on Populations of Exposure to Low Levels of Ionizing Radiation. Report of the Advisory Committee on the Biological Effects of Ionizing Radiations. Washington, National Academy of Sciences–National Research Council, 1972.
Thoma, G. E., and Wald, N.: The diagnosis and management of accidental radiation injury. J. Occup. Med., 1:422, 1959.
Wald, N.: Radiation injury and its management. *In* Wang, Y. (ed.): Handbook of Radioactive Nuclides. Part IX. Cleveland, The Chemical Rubber Co., 1969, p. 837.

41. ELECTRIC SHOCK

Charles E. Billings

The effects of electricity on the body are determined by a great variety of physical, anatomic, and physiologic factors, and possibly by demographic factors as well. Before going on to a discussion of the effects, it is well to review briefly the most important of these factors.

Physical factors: Ohm's law reminds us that a certain electromotive force or potential, measured in volts, is necessary to permit the flow of a current, measured in amperes, through a conductor having a certain resistance, expressed in ohms. The rule applies whether the conductor is a wire, a volume conductor containing a salt solution, or an interface such as the skin.

Direct currents (DC) exert effects different in some respects from alternating currents (AC); in the latter case, the frequency is very important. In general, the effects of frequencies in the 50 to 60 Hz range are greater than those of AC at very high frequencies. The duration of current flow must also be considered. The electrical properties of shoes, gloves, and clothing through which the current passes are of importance.

Anatomic and physiologic factors: The interior of the body is an excellent volume conductor of low resistance. The skin, however, through which electrical energy usually enters the body, has much higher resistance to the passage of current. Heavily callused, dry skin may have a resistance of several hundred thousand ohms. Thin skin, moist with perspiration, especially if it is lightly abraded to induce hyperemia, may have resistance as low as 1000 to 2000 ohms. Sweating causes marked decreases in skin resistance, both by wetting it and by providing additional conduction pathways to the interior of the body through the glands themselves.

Within the body, current densities are determined by the resistivities of the tissues in the path of current. Most accidental shocks travel either from hand to hand or from hand to foot.

Incidence. Electric currents are used therapeutically; electroconvulsive treatment, cardioversion, and electrical cardiac pacing are their major present uses. In the past, iontophoresis was a method of introducing certain drugs through the intact skin. All these techniques present the danger of overdosage and injury.

Accidental electric shock, with which this chapter is primarily concerned, is encountered most commonly in four settings: industry, the home, lightning strikes, and, increasingly, in medical diagnostic and treatment settings. Each year more than 1000 persons in the United States are killed by electrical injuries, with industrial accidents accounting for more than half the total.

Pathophysiology. Electric currents of sufficient magnitude can cause gross disruption of tissues, especially the brain. More commonly, however, two types of injuries occur. Burns caused by conversion of electrical to thermal energy at sites of relatively high resistance are common, especially in the skin and underlying fat. Interruption of physiologic function may occur, however, especially in neural and neuromuscular tissue, without any obvious anatomic effects in those tissues. Such functional effects in the central nervous system and heart are the major dangers of accidental electric shock.

Clinical Manifestations. The threshold for perception of a direct current is in the neighborhood of 5 mA (range 2 to 13 mA); the predominant sensation is of warmth at the contact site. Much lower thresholds are observed with alternating currents at 60 Hz; the median in one study was below 1.1 mA (range 0.4 to 1.9 mA). Subjects described a tingling sensation at these levels.

Pain thresholds are more difficult to obtain owing to the subjective nature of this symptom. In various studies, ranges of 3 to 10 mA have been found with 60 Hz AC.

As current flow increases beyond these levels, a point is reached at which involuntary muscle spasm is produced. If the current is entering or leaving the body through the hands, the victim is unable to free himself from the electrode. The maximal level of current at which an electrode can be released has been called the "let-go" current by Dalziel et al. They found that mean direct currents of 74 mA (range 61 to 83) and mean alternating currents of 16 mA (range 10 to 22) were maxima in normal subjects. After extensive studies, they concluded that the following were maximal safe current flows through the hands for 99.5 per cent of persons:

	DC	*60 Hz AC*
Men	62 mA	9 mA
Women	41 mA	6 mA

Without question, the most dangerous effect of electric current is its ability to induce ventricular fibrillation. In transverse current flow in animals, about 3 per cent of the current flows through the heart. If the current pathway is parallel to the body axis, however, 9 to 10 per cent of the total current flows through the heart.

There is a relatively short period during the repolarization phase of each cardiac cycle when the heart is extremely sensitive to exogenous electrical stimuli. An electric current of 0.75 mA applied to the surface of the heart during its sensitive period can induce fibrillation. It appears, from extensive studies of this phenomenon, that maximal safe currents for the arm-to-leg pathway are below 100 mA. Currents much above this level, applied for periods longer than one to two seconds, may be expected to induce ventricular fibrillation.

There are other manifestations of electrical injury. An alternating current of several hundred milliamperes passing transversely through the brain rarely causes respiratory disturbances except during the grand mal seizure which results, but such a current traversing the brainstem along a longitudinal pathway will cause respiratory arrest, which may persist for a considerable period of time after interruption of current flow. Thrombotic phenomena in the brain or elsewhere are not uncommon after electrical injury. Still other changes, including burns, cerebral edema, and perivascular hemorrhages, appear to be due to thermal injury rather than to the passage of the electric current per se.

Diagnosis and Treatment. Diagnosis of a serious electrical injury must be immediate, and treatment must begin immediately if the patient is to be saved. Since most electric shock deaths are due to hypoxia secondary to ventricular fibrillation, respiratory arrest, or both, treatment must consist of artificial respiration and closed chest cardiac massage, begun as soon as possible after the current path is interrupted and continued until satisfactory respiratory and cardiac function have returned. This may take several hours. Cardiac defibrillation should be employed if indicated; cardiotonic drugs and other supportive measures may be required. It is most important to realize that even severely shocked patients may have suffered only functional impairment; if hypoxia can be prevented until spontaneous function resumes, they may recover completely.

Complications. Aside from problems caused by severe surface or deep burns (which may require surgical treatment), the most ominous early complication of electrical injury is nephrosis with resultant oliguria or anuria. Cataract formation may occur as late as months after the initial injury; in laboratory animals, this has been observed more frequently after direct current shocks.

Subjects may complain of weakness or paralysis of extremities for many hours after a shock; pain, muscular stiffness, and minor personality changes may persist for months.

Prognosis. There are so many variables in each case of electrical injury that no meaningful data on recovery rates are available. As in the case of ventricular fibrillation from other causes, the likelihood and the completeness of recovery are largely functions of the promptness with which cardiopulmonary resuscitation is begun and of its adequacy thereafter.

Prevention. A word should be said here about primary prevention of electrical injuries, especially in medical settings, in which preventive measures can be controlled by medical personnel. *Any* electrical device, a lamp, electric bed, TV control unit, or patient intercom, poses a very real threat to life. Continuous monitoring of patients in surgical and intensive care units has vastly increased the opportunities for electrical injuries owing to passage of stray currents through monitoring leads attached in ways which minimize skin resistance and maximize the likelihood of internal injury should such currents occur. Cardiac catheters containing sensor leads are another and particularly dangerous source of such injuries.

These catastrophes are totally preventable if, and only if, proper fail-safe protective devices are an integral part of *all* electrical circuits which can involve the body. Protective fuses must be incorporated in all such circuits; adequate grounding of all electrical equipment used in patient areas is mandatory.

Fischer, H.: Pathologic effects and sequelae of electrical accidents. Electrical burns (secondary accidents, renal manifestations, sequelae). J. Occup. Med., 7:564, 1965.

Franco, S. C.: Electric shock and cardiopulmonary resuscitation. Arch. Environ. Health, 19:261, 1969.

Jude, J. R., Kouwenhoven, W. B., and Knickerbocker, G. G.: Cardiac arrest. J.A.M.A., 178:1063, 1961.

Morley, R., and Carter, A. O.: First aid treatment of electric shock. Arch. Environ. Health, 25:276, 1972.

MOTION SICKNESS AND PROBLEMS OF AIR TRAVEL

Harold V. Ellingson

42. MOTION SICKNESS

Manifestations and Occurrence. Motion sickness is a syndrome characterized by pallor, sweating, salivation, and nausea that frequently progresses to vomiting. Prostration may be severe if exposure to precipitating factors is prolonged. It may occur in persons riding in airplanes, ships, automobiles, or trains, or sometimes in children after prolonged or vigorous sessions in playground swings. Among air travelers, the incidence has declined with introduction of newer jet transports that fly at altitudes above the layers of most turbulent air. The disorder still remains a problem among passengers in small aircraft and others flying at low altitudes in stormy or hot weather, when turbulence may be severe.

Etiology. Causative factors are not completely understood. Labyrinthine stimulation resulting from repetitive pitching, rolling, rotating, or up-and-down motion is clearly a most important factor, since persons with nonfunctioning labyrinths are often totally insusceptible to motion sickness, and since incidence and severity are commonly proportional to severity and duration of the motion. Psychic factors also appear to be important. Apprehension undoubtedly predisposes to motion sickness; a few unfortunates feel nauseated on stepping aboard a motionless airplane or a ship at a pier. Some people can tolerate motion without distress until they smell an unpleasant odor such as that of cigar smoke or the vomitus of a fellow passenger. Visceral sensations of motion appear to be contributory, since abdominal restraint reduces incidence of reactions. Visual stimuli apparently may play a part; symptoms sometimes occur in an immobile subject who watches moving pictures depicting motion.

Prevention and Treatment. Prophylaxis may often be achieved by the use of any of a number of drugs, given 30 minutes to an hour before the trip begins. Hyoscine, 0.6 mg, with d-amphetamine, 10 mg, meclizine (Bonine), 25 to 50 mg, cyclizine (Marezine), 50 mg, and dimenhydrinate (Dramamine), 50 mg, are among the most effective agents. For prolonged journeys, the same dose of meclizine or hyoscine-d-amphetamine should be given every 24 hours; doses of cyclizine or dimenhydrinate should be repeated every four to six hours as required. A traveler who senses the onset of an attack may often avert nausea and vomiting by reclining as far as possible, by holding his head firmly against a pillow or head rest, by closing his eyes or fixing his gaze on a point, and by increasing his ventilation with cool air. In treatment, the same drugs mentioned above are useful, though retention may be difficult if vomiting has already occurred. Fortunately, symptoms usually disappear soon after the journey is concluded or motion has ceased. Recovery after prolonged vomiting may be hastened by fluid replacement.

43. PROBLEMS OF AIR TRAVEL

For the normal person, and for most ambulatory patients under a physician's care, air travel is no more trying than is travel by any other means. However, a physician should be informed of factors encountered in flight that may have an influence on his patient's welfare. Besides accepting as passengers many ambulatory patients under the care of physicians, most airlines are prepared to carry litter patients; special litters can be accommodated by adjustment or removal of several seats. In remote areas, private flying agencies sometimes provide air ambulance service to large medical centers. Before a patient travels or is moved by air, the physician should consider the hazards mentioned below and should, if necessary, discuss the case with a medical official of the carrier. The patient's condition, the altitude and duration of the flight, the cabin pressure altitude, and the availability of oxygen in flight all have a bearing on suitability of air travel by, or movement of, a patient. With proper precautions, all but a few patients can safely be carried by air.

Factors to be Considered. Aside from the possibility of motion sickness, the two most important factors to be considered in air travel by patients are reduction in air pressure and reduction in oxygen content of air at altitude. Cabin pressurization in larger and newer aircraft minimizes these changes, but hazards may be present for a few persons.

In pressurized airplanes, cabin pressure is normally maintained at a fixed excess over that of the outside air. The amount of excess varies with the type of aircraft, but the differential is commonly in the neighborhood of 8 pounds per square inch. This gives a cabin pressure that does not fall below that of sea level until the aircraft reaches 22,000 feet. Above this, internal pressure falls until at 40,000 feet the cabin has an "altitude" of 7000 feet above sea level. In older aircraft, pressure differentials are smaller, and cabin pressures on some flights may be equivalent to as much as 9000 feet. Only a few light aircraft are pressurized; these are often flown at 10,000 to 12,000 feet, or even more over mountainous terrain.

Hazards of Reduced Pressure. A bubble of gas trapped within the body will expand as air pressure is reduced. At an altitude of 5000 feet, trapped gas expands to 125 per cent of its sea level volume, and at 10,000 feet to 150 per cent of its sea level volume. Expansion causes pressure on surrounding tissues; this may jeopardize blood supply, and may cause rupture of containing walls.

Persons with *unreduced hernia* should not fly, since if gas is trapped it may expand and interfere with circulation. A *perforating wound of the eyeball or the skull* may allow entrance of a bubble of air that might expand at altitude. Patients with these injuries should not travel or be moved by air until absorption is complete. Patients with *pneumothorax* should not fly until all air has been absorbed. The same caution applies after *pneumoencephalography.* Expansion of abdominal gas causes some distention, and patients who have had *abdominal surgery* should not fly for two weeks after surgery. A patient with a *colostomy* may expect filling of the bag on ascent. Patients with *acute upper respiratory tract disease* may have discomfort in the sinuses or middle ear because of closure of the ostia of the sinuses or the eustachian tube and consequent failure of pressure adjustment during ascent or descent; use of decongestant nose drops or inhalers before flight may avert difficulty. A similar precaution is useful for the patient with *chronic sinusitis* or *allergic rhinitis.* Patients with *lung cavities, abscesses,* or *bullous emphysema* should not fly because of the danger of rupture.

Hazards of Reduced Oxygen. Oxygen content of alveolar air is reduced at increasing altitudes. Though oxygen saturation of the blood is less markedly reduced, patients whose tissue oxygenation is marginal for any reason (whether from impaired pulmonary function, reduced oxygen-carrying capacity of the blood, or impaired tissue circulation) should not fly unless prior arrangement has been made with the airline for oxygen to be continuously available in flight. Patients should not fly after *myocardial infarction* until they are symptom-free with moderate exertion, usually at least six weeks after an attack. Patients with *angina pectoris* that is symptomatic on climbing a flight of stairs should have supplemental oxygen available during flight. *Anemia,* when the hemoglobin is less than 50 per cent, should preclude flight unless oxygen is available. Patients with *developing gangrene* or *carbon monoxide poisoning* should not be moved without supplemental oxygen in flight. Any *pulmonary disease,* when severe enough to cause cyanosis at ground level, to seriously impair exercise tolerance, or to reduce vital capacity below 50 per cent of normal, is a contraindication to flight unless supplemental oxygen is made available.

Sickle cell trait has been the cause of some concern as a possible risk for air travelers and aircrew members. The concern has been based on earlier reports of splenic infarction at moderate altitude, in unpressurized aircraft, or on the ground in persons with sickle cell trait and most commonly after exertion, vomiting, or anesthesia. It should be noted that in no case was the cause-effect relationship with reduced oxygen tension established. Moreover, no reaction attributable to sickle cell trait has been reported from flight in a pressurized aircraft. For prospective passengers in commercial aircraft, screening for sickle cell trait has not been considered warranted. With respect to aircrew members, some airlines in the past have screened prospective employees and have declined to hire those with the sickle cell trait. This policy has been based on the assumption that, if an aircraft accidentally lost its pressurization, the aircrew members might be called upon for physical exertion, possibly rendering themselves vulnerable to splenic infarction. Fears have been allayed by the small number of depressurization incidents in flight, by the uneventful performance of Olympic athletes with known sickle cell trait in Mexico City at an altitude of 2240 meters (7349 feet), and by the documented normal performance of professional football players with sickle cell trait, often at altitudes over 1524 meters (5000 feet). Most airlines no longer screen for sickle cell trait or exclude from employment as cabin attendants those who have it; some, however, do not accept them as pilots. The National Academy of Sciences–National Research Council has recommended that "except for pilots or copilots, persons with the sickle cell trait should not be restricted from flight duty." This exclusion from pilot duty of persons with the trait may be overcautious and unwarranted. At least one major airline accepts pilots with sickle cell trait without question, and has had no incident attributable to this disorder.

Aerial movement is sometimes considered for a patient who has recently suffered from an attack of *poliomyelitis.* In general, such a patient should not be moved by air until his condition has become stabilized. If respiratory paralysis has occurred, the patient who is able to be out of a respirator for 8 to 12 hours a day can usually be moved safely by air. For those requiring a respirator continuously, portable equipment is available that can be carried in aircraft. Such patients should be observed carefully in flight by an experienced attendant, with special attention to the maintenance of normal ventilatory exchange and the avoidance of dehydration, as this tends to make secretions thicker and more difficult to aspirate. If bulbar involvement has caused difficulty in swallowing, a tracheostomy should be performed prior to flight to ensure adequacy of the airway.

Time Zone Changes. Subjective fatigue and delays in adjustment to time zone changes after east-west or west-east travel are matters of common observation. Not only sleeping habits, but more profound cycles of deep body temperature, water and electrolyte excretion, plasma lactic dehydrogenase, and other physiologic measures are involved. The time required for a traveler to "get on schedule" at the destination depends upon many factors, including individual characteristics, the number of time zones passed, the opportunities for rest before and after flight, and, for some, the direction of flight. A traveler to the west is not likely to have trouble in going to sleep at night in the new time zone, but he may have morning insomnia; one traveling several time zones to the east is likely to experience evening insomnia and retarded awakening. If the traveler has a tendency toward insomnia, travel may cause a troublesome accentuation.

Studies have indicated some actual impairment of psychologic performance in the 24 hours immediately after travel through 7 to 12 time zones. Performance has commonly returned to normal after one good night's sleep. Adjustment of sleeping habits and the overcoming of subjective fatigue may take several days; the deeper physiologic cycles require longer periods—from four to eight days for adjustment to a time differential of 7 to 12 zones.

Travelers can minimize problems by giving special attention to rest before and after long flights. If circumstances permit before the trip, the prospective traveler may benefit from modifying his sleep schedules toward those of the destination. If possible, a flight departing in the morning should be chosen. Overindulgence in food and alcohol en route should be avoided. Trusted somnifacients for a few nights after arrival may speed the adjustment. Some experienced travelers recommend that "million dollar decisions" be avoided in the first 24 hours after a long flight.

Other Hazards. Prolonged sitting and inactivity may be hazardous for persons with a history of *thrombophlebitis* or other circulatory disorder of the lower extremities. These patients should be advised to move about frequently during long flights. A patient with a *fractured jaw* treated by fixation should not fly because of the danger of aspirating vomitus in case of motion sickness. If he must fly, a quick-release fixation should be devised.

Common Questions. Physicians are often asked questions about flying. *Normal infants* tolerate air travel well, but feeding should be given during descent, to facilitate aeration of the middle ear by swallowing. *Old age* in itself is no contraindication to flight, if significant disease is not present. *Pregnancy* is no contraindication to flight, but if the mother is near term, the airline may require a physician's statement that delivery is not likely to occur during the flight. There is no evidence that the mild oxygen deficit in the atmosphere is harmful to the fetus. *Hypertension* is not adversely affected by air travel, though preflight sedation may be appropriate. Patients with *communicable diseases* should, of course, not travel when hazards of transmission to others exist. *Patients whose conditions make them objectionable to others,* such as those with urinary incontinence or malodorous discharges, should not travel in the crowded cabins of commercial aircraft. *Mild asthma* is not ordinarily adversely affected by flight. Patients subject to severe asthmatic attacks should carry their tested medications, and should ensure in advance the availability of oxygen if needed. In *epileptics,* oxygen deficiency and hyperventilation attending excitement in flight may precipitate seizures. Persons subject to frequent seizures should have proper medication, including sedation, prior to travel by air and if possible should be accompanied by an attendant. *Psychiatric disorders* require individual evaluation; the likelihood of disturbance or agitation under the minimal stress of travel and the safety and comfort of fellow passengers should be considered. Questions regarding other conditions should be referred to the airline's nearest medical official. Indeed, it is advisable to discuss with the airline's medical official any prospective passenger whose condition might be unfavorably influenced by flight.

Beighton, P. H., and Richard, P. R.: Cardiovascular disease in air travelers. Br. Heart J., 30:367, 1968.

Bergin, K. G.: Transport of invalids by air. Br. Med. J., 3:539, 1967.

Buley, L. E.: Formula for determining rest periods on long distance air travel. Aerosp. Med., 41:680, 1970.

Committee on Medical Criteria: Medical criteria for passenger flying. Arch. Environ. Health, 2:124, 1961.

McFarland, R. A.: Influence of changing time zones on air crews and passengers. Aerosp. Med., 45:648, 1974.

Money, K. D.: Motion sickness. Physiol. Rev., 50:1, 1970.

Murphy, J. R.: Sickle cell hemoglobin (Hb AS) in black football players. J.A.M.A., 225:981, 1973.

National Academy of Sciences–National Research Council. The S-Hemoglobinopathies: An Evaluation of Their Status in the Armed Forces, 1973.

Wood, C. D., and Graybiel, A.: Theory of anti-motion sickness drug mechanisms. Aerosp. Med., 43:249, 1972.

ALTERATIONS IN ATMOSPHERIC PRESSURE

Robert L. Johnson

44. INTRODUCTION

The physiologic and pathologic effects of alterations in atmospheric pressure are governed by the physical behavior of gases. The individual gaseous molecules of the earth's atmosphere have mass and therefore weight owing to the effect of gravity. Atmospheric pressure represents the weight of the mass of air extending upward from the earth's surface. At sea level this amounts to 760 mm of mercury (1.013×10^5 Newtons per square meter, 1013 millibars, 14.7 pounds per square inch, or 1 atmosphere). Atmospheric air (dry) contains 20.94 per cent oxygen, 0.03 per cent carbon dioxide, and approximately 79 per cent nitrogen at all altitudes. However, the partial pressures of the individual gases of the atmosphere, in accordance with Dalton's law, vary directly as the total atmospheric pressure. At sea level, where atmospheric pressure is 760 mm of mercury, the partial pressures of oxygen, carbon dioxide, and nitrogen are 159 (760×0.2094), 2.3 (760×0.0003), and 600 (760×0.79) mm of mercury, respectively, in dry air.

Water, being much denser than air, exerts a much greater pressure. The weight of a 33-foot column of sea water equals that of a like-sized column of air extending through the entire atmosphere. Since water is incompressible, pressure increases in linear fashion with further descent, each 33 feet adding an additional atmosphere of pressure.

The medical problems created by changes in atmospheric pressure may be grouped into direct and indirect effects. The former result from mechanical forces created when pressure differentials develop across the walls of air-containing spaces within the body or upon its surface. Indirect effects result from alterations in partial pressures of the individual gases of the atmosphere.

45. DIRECT EFFECTS OF CHANGES IN ATMOSPHERIC PRESSURE

Gases respond to pressure changes in accordance with Boyle's law. Their volume varies inversely and their density, or molecular concentration, directly as the absolute pressure. The fluids and solids of the human body, being incompressible, transmit pressure freely and thus assume the pressure exerted upon the body's surface. Any alteration in the latter is reflected almost instantly by an identical pressure change in body fluids and tissues. Pressure within air-containing spaces of the body can be maintained equal to external pressure only by appropriate adjustments either of the number of molecules of gas within the space or of the volume of the space. No medical difficulties arise as long as air can pass freely between such spaces and the environment. If additional air cannot enter such a space to increase its pressure during descent, fluids and tissues of the surrounding walls, whose pressure is increasing with increasing ambient pressure, tend to move in to reduce its volume and eradicate the pressure differential. The lining of the walls becomes hyperemic and swollen. Serum or blood may move into the relative vacuum. Conversely, during ascent, pressure within the tissues surrounding the space declines with declining environmental pressure. Unless air can be vented from the space, an increasing pressure gradient creates a distending force against the walls.

The natural air-containing spaces of the body are the paranasal sinuses, the middle ear, the airways and lungs, and the gastrointestinal tract. Small pockets of air may also exist beneath fillings or in diseased teeth. In addition, pockets of air against various surfaces of the body may be produced by goggles, tight-fitting hoods, ear plugs, or wrinkles in diving suits. The middle ear is very susceptible to barotrauma during descent. The sinuses are much less frequently affected, but may also incur barotrauma during ascent. Respiratory infection greatly increases the likelihood of injury. Descent in water may damage tissues beneath air-containing structures closely applied to the surface of the body. All these injuries, including barotitis with ruptured tympanic membranes, tend to heal spontaneously.

The most serious mechanical injuries resulting from pressure changes involve the lungs. If the breath is held during diving, the increasing pressure compresses the thoracic cage to the position of maximal expiration. On further descent air within the lungs can no longer be compressed to counter the increasing external pressure. The relatively negative intrapulmonary pressure results eventually in pulmonary congestion, edema, and hemorrhage, a condition known as "thoracic squeeze." Breathing the denser air at depth through equipment with excessive air flow resistance or breathing through a snorkel tube which is too long may also create a relatively negative pressure within the lungs, leading to similar consequences.

After breathing the denser air at depths, air must be released from lungs during ascent to prevent expanding air from building up sufficient pressure to overdistend or rupture lung tissue; if this occurs, pneumothorax, mediastinal emphysema, or air embolism may ensue. Air embolism has been reported during ascents of as little as 9 feet and is said to be exceeded in frequency only by drowning as a cause of accidental death among divers. Lung tissue distal to a poorly communicating diseased bronchial passage may be similarly damaged even if the diver vents his excess air during ascent. The air traveler with such bronchopulmonary disease, or one who happens to be holding his breath, may be similarly injured during a sudden loss of cabin pressure at high altitude.

Knowledge of the character of the dive, including depth, duration, air supply, and patterns of descent and ascent in relation to symptoms, often simplifies the problem of diagnosing lung injury in divers. Frothy, bloody sputum may be produced in either thoracic squeeze or lung rupture. If the victim has been skin-diving or using a snorkel tube, thoracic squeeze is likely. In a scuba diver, however, the first consideration must be lung rupture with potentially fatal aeroembolism. (The term "scuba" is derived from "self-contained underwater breathing apparatus.") The unconscious diver must be presumed to have aeroembolism or decompression sickness. Either aeroembolism or serious decompression sickness requires treatment by recompression at the earliest possible moment. Transport to a recompression chamber should be by the fastest method available. The gain from prompt treatment far outweighs the potential danger of further decompression during air transportation at low altitudes. Meanwhile artificial respiration by the mouth-to-mouth method should be carried out if necessary, and oxygen should be administered. Placing the victim on his left side may be beneficial if aeroembolism is suspected. Thoracic squeeze usually requires no more than supportive measures.

46. INDIRECT EFFECTS OF CHANGES IN ATMOSPHERIC PRESSURE

Gases in contact with liquids dissolve in direct proportion to their partial pressures and their solubility coefficients. Gases enter and leave the body in response to gradients of partial pressure between blood and alveolar gases. Gradients of partial pressure likewise determine the movement of gases within body fluids.

Only brief mention can be made here of the effects of increases in the partial pressures of nitrogen, oxygen, and carbon dioxide. At 4 atmospheres absolute pressure (100 feet in water), divers or occupants of hyperbaric chambers may show the narcotizing effect of nitrogen. Judgment, thought processes, and motor ability may become impaired and deteriorate with further increases in atmospheric pressure. Fortunately, the symptoms clear rapidly and completely on return to lower atmospheric pressure.

Hypercapnia normally produces subjective distress and stimulation of respiration, but may cause unconsciousness without warning. Scuba divers who restrict their breathing in an attempt to conserve their air supply expose themselves to this potential hazard. Loss of consciousness in skin divers resulting from "shallow-water blackout" is attributed to a large rise in partial pressure of carbon dioxide associated with an inadequate subjective or respiratory response to hypercapnia.

Convulsive seizures and coma may occur with little warning during exposure to high partial pressures of oxygen. The minimal partial pressure of oxygen capable of producing convulsions appears to be less than 2 atmospheres (Po_2 = 1520 mm Hg). Divers breathing air are at little risk of oxygen convulsions. If they use pure oxygen, however, depths greater than 25 feet become hazardous.

Hyperbaric oxygenation is achieved by increasing atmospheric pressure within sealed chambers to levels varying from 2 to 4 atmospheres absolute (Po_2 = 320 to 640 mm Hg). Increased oxygenation of tissues occurs chiefly as a result of increased solution of oxygen in plasma. Hyperbaric oxygenation has been reported to be of value during surgical correction of certain congenital cardiovascular disorders and in the treatment of carbon monoxide poisoning and certain anaerobic infections. Precautions must be taken to protect the patient and medical personnel from all the direct and indirect effects of altered atmospheric pressure.

DECOMPRESSION SICKNESS
(Caisson Disease)

In decompression sickness the manifestations are due to formation of nitrogen bubbles in body tissues and fluids. On exposure to lower atmospheric pressure the partial pressure of nitrogen dissolved in body fluids and tissues exceeds nitrogen partial pressure in the lungs. If this pressure reaches the point where nitrogen evolves from tissues and fluids faster than it can be transported by blood to the alveolar membrane to diffuse into alveolar air, bubbles will form. Bubbles large enough to produce symptoms develop when the partial pressure of nitrogen in tissues rapidly becomes more than twice as great as nitrogen partial pressure in the atmosphere. This situation can arise in a diver whose tissues are saturated with nitrogen at a depth somewhat in excess of 33 feet who surfaces rapidly, or by a flier who rapidly ascends from sea level to higher than 18,000 feet.

The processes of nitrogen diffusion and transport necessary for equilibration between tissues and alveolar air require time. Since nitrogen must be transported by blood, equilibration in highly vascular tissues occurs more rapidly than in those that are poorly vascularized. Fatty tissue is not only poorly vascularized but in addition takes up larger volumes of nitrogen since nitrogen is far more soluble in lipids than in water.

The complete elimination of excess nitrogen from the body after exposure to a lower partial pressure of nitrogen in the atmosphere requires about 12 hours. About 75 per cent of the total is eliminated within 2½ hours, mainly from aqueous solution in plasma and interstitial tissue. The slower component arises mainly from tissues high in lipid content such as fat deposits, bone marrow, and spinal cord.

The total amount and the rate at which nitrogen is taken into solution during a dive will depend not only upon the depth but the time spent at depth. The magnitude of this depth-time factor and the rate of ascent determine whether decompression sickness occurs. Beyond certain depth-time values, it is necessary to ascend in stages with time to allow an adequate amount of denitrogenation to occur before ascending further. Stage decompression is based on never exceeding the 2:1 ratio of alveolar to tissue partial pressure of nitrogen. These general principles also apply in altitude decompression sickness, in which tissues are saturated at 1 atmosphere when ascent begins.

Manifestations. The symptoms produced depend primarily upon the site of bubble formation. The size of the bubbles and their rate of growth influence the severity of symptoms. Although bizarre clinical pictures may occur, certain patterns occur frequently, suggesting a predilection to bubble formation in some tissues and organs. The most common and familiar manifestation is *"bends."* This consists of deep, boring, and usually constant pain in the vicinity of large joints, the knees and shoulders being most frequently involved. Pain may be so severe as to be incapacitating. Most cases of bends occur within the first 30 minutes after decompression, that is, after reaching a critical altitude or after surfacing following a dive in which the depth-time factor was exceeded. Bends in flight disappear completely during descent.

Subjective skin manifestations, usually prickling or burning sensations, termed the "itches" or "creeps," occur rather commonly in fliers. Although objective skin manifestations occur uncommonly, a characteristic pale, cyanotic mottling of the skin sometimes appears, usually over the upper trunk and typically later than bends.

Chokes, believed to be due to bubbles in the pulmonary vasculature, occurs later than bends, and consists of burning retrosternal distress and cough. Relieved at first by shallow breathing, the symptoms progress in severity until coughing becomes paroxysmal and uncontrollable. Recompression by descent produces partial relief, but symptoms may persist for several days. Often associated with cyanosis and syncope, the syndrome has ominous significance because shock and coma may ensue.

Homonymous scintillating *scotomas* are neurologic manifestations of decompression sickness. Although apparently not observed in divers, they are common manifestations at high altitude. They are transient, and frequently disappear while still at altitude.

One or more of the manifestations already mentioned usually precede more serious stages of decompression sickness, which are characterized by neurologic manifestations and sometimes vasomotor instability that may progress to circulatory collapse with cyanosis, shock, and coma. Almost every possible neurologic sign has been observed, including motor paralysis. In altitude decompression sickness, neurologic findings are usually limited to transient paresis and dysthesias. The lower segments of the spinal cord are most frequently involved in divers, and permanent residuals may occur. In decompression sickness a period of apparent recovery from the earlier manifestations may precede the appearance of circulatory collapse and shock. During this latent period vague symptoms can usually be elicited, and signs of instability of blood pressure and heart rate and at least minor focal neurologic signs can be detected. Hemoconcentration, with hematocrit as high as 60 to 70 per cent, is a characteristic finding that presumably results from widespread vascular injury and loss of plasma into tissues.

Treatment. All the varied manifestations of decompression sickness respond rapidly to early and adequate treatment by recompression. Descent from altitude produces sufficient recompression to abolish the early manifestations, but merely retards the appearance of the more slowly developing serious forms of decompression sickness. In such cases widespread bubble formation has presumably already occurred, and descent is entirely analogous to inadequate recompression therapy during which symptoms subside only temporarily. The clinical picture of decompression sickness in divers and fliers might also be expected to differ because of the greater volumes of nitrogen that must be eliminated in divers on decompression.

Divers can prevent decompression sickness by knowing and following established limits for depth and time at depth. Limitations of air supply unfortunately often prevent ascent in stages after depth-time limits have been exceeded. Adequate denitrogenation by breathing 100 per cent oxygen prior to and during ascent is an effective preventive measure in fliers. Divers should avoid the increased hazard of repeating a dive before adequate time at surface to eliminate excess nitrogen from the previous dive. Similarly, fliers who have experienced decompression symptoms during a flight should delay return to even relatively low altitudes because the expansion of bubbles still present in tissues may cause a rapid recurrence of more serious symptoms. The hazard of exposure to altitudes as low as 7000 feet after even safe depth-time dives should be recognized.

Adequate recompression performed at the earliest possible time is the specific therapy for decompression sickness. All other measures are adjunctive. Those reported to be beneficial include oxygen by mask, low molecular weight dextran and standard replacement fluids to correct hypovolemia, heparin in doses of 50 to 100 mg twice daily, and injectable steroids such as dexamethasone, 8 mg initially with diminishing doses every six hours.

Undersea Medical Society: Modern aspects of treatment of decompression sickness. Aerosp. Med., 39:1055, 1968.

OTHER DIVING HAZARDS

Diving, by its nature, either with or without scuba, involves certain respiratory patterns that are potentially hazardous under water. Hyperventilation and breath-holding, for example, may initiate cardioinhibitory and vasodepressor reflexes capable of causing syncope, cardiac arrhythmias, and arrest. Bradycardia, apparently more pronounced than might occur simply from breath-holding and the head-down position, and various cardiac arrhythmias have also been reported during breath-hold diving. Vigorous hyperventilation by skin divers prior to a dive may lead to lowering of arterial PCO_2 sufficient to abolish the stimulus to breathe and may allow dangerous levels of hypoxemia to develop. In addition, compression of air within the lungs during descent may maintain adequate alveolar PO_2 levels despite a diminishing oxygen supply. Distress from air hunger may not occur because alveolar PCO_2 has been reduced by prior hyperventilation. During ascent the expansion of the air remaining within the lungs results in a sharp reduction in PO_2, possibly to levels that result in loss of consciousness before the diver is able to reach the surface, and he may drown unless help is available for prompt rescue and resuscitation. Divers using properly functioning open-circuit scuba are unlikely to experience hypoxia if they restrict their dives to well within the limits of their air supply. The rate of air utilization increases in proportion to the increase in absolute pressure when using open-circuit scuba. Total duration of air supply is, for example, only one third as long at 66 feet as at the surface. Increased utilization from heavy exertion causes a proportionately greater expenditure of air.

The availability of scuba has enabled large numbers of untrained people to enter an unfamiliar and hostile environment previously restricted to trained professional divers. The increasing number of serious diving accidents attests to a general lack of understanding of basic underwater principles. The greatest medical problem is education of those who participate in this sport. Physicians in almost any locality may now be called upon to manage a diving emergency. Excellent publications concerning this subject, such as the United States Navy Diving Manual and others, should be available for this purpose.

Bennett, P. B., and Elliott, D. H.: The Physiology and Medicine of Diving and Compressed Air Work. Baltimore, Williams & Wilkins Company, 1969.

Dewey, A. W., Jr.: Decompression sickness, an emerging recreational hazard. N. Engl. J. Med., 267:759, 812, 1962.

Ferris, E. B., and Engel, G. L.: The clinical nature of high altitude decompression sickness. *In* Fulton, J. F. (ed.): Decompression Sickness, Diver's and Flier's Bends and Related Syndromes. National Research Council, Committee on Medical Sciences. Philadelphia, W. B. Saunders Company, 1951, p. 4.

Lambertsen, C. J. (ed.): Underwater Physiology. Proceedings of the Fourth Symposium on Underwater Physiology. New York, Academic Press, 1971.

United States Air Force: Flight Surgeon's Guide. No. AFP 161–18. Washington, D.C., Department of the Air Force, 1968.

United States Navy: U.S. Diving Manual. NAVSHIPS 0994–001–9010. Washington, D.C., 1968.

HYPOXIA

Hypoxia refers to the reduced partial pressure of oxygen at altitude. It thus represents an indirect effect of altered atmospheric pressure. The clinical manifestations at a given altitude are influenced primarily by duration of exposure, rate of ascent, and individual tolerance. However, the level of physical activity, the degree of health, physical conditioning, altitude acclimatization, and such factors as temperature, wind, and humidity may all modify the response in varying degrees.

The transfer of gases between lung, blood, and tissues depends upon differences in partial pressures. Alveolar air is saturated with water vapor, which exerts a constant pressure of 47 mm of mercury. Carbon dioxide normally contributes about 40 mm of mercury pressure to total alveolar pressure. Although total alveolar pressure is in equilibrium with atomospheric pressure, the space available for oxygen and other components of inspired air is approximately 87 mm of mercury less than existing atmospheric pressure. Mixing of inspired with residual air further reduces alveolar partial pressure of oxygen from that in the atmosphere. The alveolar pressure constantly contributed by water vapor and CO_2 occupies an increasingly large proportion of alveolar pressure as atmospheric pressure declines. At sea level (alveolar Po_2 = 103 mm of mercury) hemoglobin is normally 95 to 98 per cent saturated. Not until altitudes of 10,000 feet (P_B = 523 mm of mercury and alveolar Po_2 = 61 mm of mercury) does hemoglobin saturation begin to fall below 90 per cent. Thereafter saturation declines rapidly with further increases in altitude and decline in alveolar partial pressure of oxygen.

Manifestations. The first important physiologic effect of hypoxia occurs at about 5000 feet, when night vision begins to be impaired. Ventilatory and cardiovascular adjustments are minimal until about 10,000 feet, above which respiratory rate and depth and heart rate increase progressively to increase alveolar Po_2 and cardiac output. Exertional dyspnea may appear, and in some people mental concentration becomes difficult. Vagal cardioinhibitory reflexes may lead to bradycardia and sometimes ectopic cardiac rhythms, and may precipitate syncope. Headache, slight giddiness, and restlessness are common.

Above 15,000 feet some persons experience lassitude and indifference whereas others exhibit increased activity, irritability, euphoria, and other disturbances of affect. The impairment of judgment that begins at these altitudes jeopardizes the safety of fliers and mountain climbers. Cyanosis, loss of peripheral vision, dimming of vision, and variable degrees of muscular incoordination appear at altitudes of around 18,000 feet. Somewhere between this level and 25,000 feet, consciousness can no longer be retained for more than a few minutes. Rapid descent or administration of oxygen is essential to prevent death. If corrective action is taken soon enough, recovery is rapid and complete.

High-flying jet aircraft make it possible for many people of various ages and states of health to be exposed to the potential hazard of sudden hypoxia from rapid decompression. Should cabin pressure be abruptly lost at high altitudes, only a short period of consciousness would be possible with the breathing of ambient air. At altitudes between 30,000 and 45,000 feet oxygen transfer across alveolar walls would be reversed, and the duration of consciousness would shorten progressively from about 1 minute to 15 seconds, or the lung-to-brain circulation time of about 9 seconds plus around 6 seconds from oxygen already present in brain tissue. Rapid donning of oxygen masks and descent of the aircraft would shorten the period of severe hypoxia and minimize the possibility of serious injury.

Lamb, L. E.: Aerospace medicine *In* Dock, W., and Snapper, I. (eds.): Advances in Internal Medicine, Vol. XII. Chicago, Year Book Medical Publishers, 1964, p. 175.

ACUTE MOUNTAIN SICKNESS

This is a clinical syndrome observed in unacclimatized persons usually within a few hours after rapid exposure to high altitude. Individual tolerance varies widely. Some experience symptoms at altitudes as low as 7000 to 8000 feet, although others tolerate altitudes of 14,000 feet with minimal symptoms. There appears to be no way to predict unusual susceptibility, but rapid ascent, physical exertion, and poor physical condition increase the likelihood. Initial symptoms are usually mild to incapacitating headache, exertional dyspnea, malaise, and weakness. Insomnia, anorexia, nausea, vomiting, diarrhea, and abdominal pain may occur. Mental capacity and judgment may be impaired. Inability to sleep is a common problem. Cyanosis of the lips and nail beds, Cheyne-Stokes breathing, and tachycardia are usually present. These manifestations usually subside gradually over a period of several days, but may recur at higher altitudes. In some instances the symptoms are severe and unrelieved except by oxygen or descent to a lower altitude. Gradual ascent with periodic halts of several days to allow acclimatization will prevent or reduce the severity of symptoms. Acetazolamide, given in dosages of 250 mg every eight hours prior to and during exposure to altitude, has been reported to reduce the frequency and severity of symptoms. The mechanism of its effect is not clear, but increased ventilation and alveolar oxygen tension, decreased carbon dioxide tension and serum bicarbonate, and absence of alkalosis were observed in treated subjects. Furosemide, 80 mg every 12 hours, has produced relief of symptoms and signs usually within 48 hours, apparently in association with the induced diuresis.

Forward, S. A., Landowne, M., Follansbee, J. N., and Hansen, J. E.: Effect of acetazolamide on acute mountain sickness. N. Engl. J. Med., 279:839, 1968.

Singh, I., Khanna, P. K., Srivastava, M. C., Lal, M., Roy, S. B., and Subramanyam, C. S. V.: Acute mountain sickness. N. Engl. J. Med., 280:175, 1969.

HIGH ALTITUDE PULMONARY EDEMA

Acute pulmonary edema is an uncommon but serious and sometimes fatal complication of rapid exposure to altitudes above 9000 feet. Hypoxia is considered the primary etiologic agent. Many earlier fatal cases were erroneously diagnosed as pneumonia. Young, unacclimatized persons and acclimatized residents who have sojourned at lower altitudes for a few days or weeks appear most susceptible. Recurrences are common in those who have experienced an attack. Rapid ascent and heavy physical exertion increase susceptibility.

Autopsy findings have included wet lungs congested with serosanguineous edema fluid. Bronchiolar and alveolar edema with hyaline membranes, resembling those seen in hyaline membrane disease of the newborn, over the internal walls of alveoli, alveolar sacs, and alveolar ducts have been characteristic findings. Dilatation of preterminal arterioles and thrombosis of septal capillaries and of small and medium-sized pulmonary arteries have also been observed. The exact pathogenic mechanism is conjectural. A comparative increase in capillary pressure is thought to be responsible for the alveolar edema. In a few cases pulmonary artery pressure has been elevated and electrocardiograms have suggested acute right ventricular overloading. The hyaline membrane formation, not a characteristic finding in death caused by simple hypoxia, has not been explained, but a deficient pulmonary fibrinolysis system has been postulated.

Symptoms usually appear 6 to 36 hours after exposure

to altitude and may be preceded by acute mountain sickness. Exertional dyspnea, weakness, malaise, and a persistent, dry, irritating cough are the characteristic initial symptoms. Later, noisy respiration, rales, cyanosis, orthopnea, and hemoptysis develop. Unless continuous oxygen therapy is carried out or the patient descends to a lower altitude, these symptoms progress, and death occurs. Gradual acclimatization and avoidance of undue physical exertion during the early period of exposure to altitude are important preventive measures.

CHRONIC MOUNTAIN SICKNESS
(Monge's Disease)

Chronic mountain sickness is a clinical syndrome that occurs in residents at high altitudes, usually over 14,000 feet, characterized by loss of tolerance to hypoxia in a previously acclimatized person. The cause is not known, but associated are increased polycythemia, decreased pulmonary ventilation, increased P_{CO_2}, lowered arterial saturation, and impaired sensitivity of the respiratory center as compared with asymptomatic residents at high altitude. Hemoglobin and hematocrit may be increased to as much as 25 grams per 100 ml and 80 per cent, as compared with 21 grams and 60 per cent in native residents. Hyperplasia and hyperactivity of marrow erythroid cells and pulmonary hypertension are greater than in the healthy residents.

The clinical manifestations are similar to those of erythremia. They include marked cyanosis, dyspnea, cough, palpitations, headache, giddiness, muscular weakness, pain in the extremities, sensory and motor changes, and episodic stupor. The condition can be cured only by returning to a lower altitude or to sea level.

Monge also described a less severe form of chronic mountain sickness in mountain residents that he called *subacute mountain sickness.* Many of the symptoms resemble those of acute mountain sickness, but they persist unless the patient descends to sea level or receives oxygen. The marked cyanosis and alveolar hypoventilation of chronic mountain sickness does not occur, and the laboratory findings are like those in asymptomatic natives.

Hultgren, H. N., and Grover, R. F.: Circulatory adaptation to high altitude. Ann. Rev. Med., 19:119, 1968.
Lenfant, C., and Sullivan, K.: Adaptation to high altitude. N. Engl. J. Med., 284:1298, 1971.
Weihe, W. H. (ed.): Physiological Effects of High Altitude. New York, The Macmillan Company, 1964.

47. DROWNING

Charles J. Stahl

Definition. Drowning is a pathologic condition, terminating in death, which may result from the complex biochemical, respiratory, and cardiovascular changes that follow the aspiration of fluid during immersion, or – less commonly – from asphyxia associated with obstruction of the airway.

Etiology. Accidents account for most drownings. The victims are often children or other persons who have not learned to swim. Less frequently, it may result from suicide or homicide. The circumstances for accidental drowning may include the following: (1) disasters such as floods, tidal waves, shipwrecks, and vehicular accidents; (2) hazardous environmental conditions or careless acts while engaged in fishing, aquatic sport, or occupational activities; (3) impaired ability to swim because of pre-existing illness, intoxication, exhaustion, or exposure to cold water; and (4) unintentional falls into water.

Incidence and Prevalence. Nearly 8000 deaths by drowning and approximately the same number of near-drownings occur annually in the United States. This is the third most common type of accidental death. The majority of the victims are young men under 25 years of age. Several million Americans engage in the sport of underwater swimming, using either self-contained underwater breathing apparatus (scuba) or snorkel. When underwater accidents are considered alone, drowning is the most common cause of death. It occurs more frequently than deaths from barotrauma, including air embolism and decompression sickness, discussed in Ch. 44 to 46.

Pathogenesis. Survivors of near-drowning have provided some knowledge of the sequence of events. The victim usually experiences panic at the time of immersion and struggles to reach the surface, unless previously incapacitated by alcohol, drugs, or injury. Breath-holding is common and persists until accumulation of carbon dioxide stimulates the respiratory center. When the victim can no longer restrain the urge to breathe, high pulmonary carbon dioxide and low pulmonary and arterial oxygen tensions are present. Gasping may result in aspiration of water or other liquid. In about 10 per cent of fatal cases, however, it is believed that the victims do not aspirate fluid, but die from asphyxia during reflex laryngospasm or breath-holding. Swallowing of water, vomiting, and coughing may occur. Convulsions precede death in some cases.

The pathophysiologic changes in drowning were poorly understood until the studies with experimental animals reported by Swann and Spafford. They demonstrated that the hemodynamic and biochemical changes during drowning of dogs are affected by the type of fluid encountered. When drowning occurs in *fresh water,* rapid absorption of hypotonic water from the lungs into the circulation results in hypervolemia, hemodilution, and hemolysis. Serum electrolytes are decreased, except for potassium, which increases because of hemolysis. The altered ratio between sodium and potassium, as well as anoxia, may cause ventricular fibrillation in dogs. The mechanism for drowning in *sea water,* however, is probably different. As the result of the aspiration of sea water, salts pass into the circulation and fluids diffuse into alveoli. Serum electrolytes, particularly chloride and magnesium, increase markedly. Hypovolemia, hemoconcentration, and hypoproteinemia, as well as pulmonary edema, occur.

Recent studies of drowning and near-drowning in laboratory animals by Modell indicate that the biochemical and cardiovascular changes are dependent not only upon the tonicity of fluid but also upon the quantity of fluid aspirated. Sea water, volume for volume, is twice as lethal as fresh water, and causes more profound changes in serum electrolytes. The serum electrolytes of animals that survived aspiration of either fresh water or sea water quickly returned to normal concentrations. These studies confirm prior observations by Fuller that life-threatening changes in electrolytes may not occur in human victims of drowning. After near-drowning with aspiration of water by dogs, the most significant changes include hypoxemia, hypercarbia, and acidosis. Pulmonary edema and decreased pulmonary compliance are evident. Fresh water alters or destroys the normal surface-tension properties of *pulmonary surfactant.* Sea water only partially removes surfactant. The pathophysiologic effects are alveolar collapse, uneven ventilation, pulmonary edema, and hypoxemia. At least 20 ml of fresh water per pound of body weight must be aspirated by dogs to cause changes in electrolytes or ventricular fibrillation.

Although the pathophysiologic mechanisms seem less well understood and may differ from experimental findings, clinical evaluations of near-drowning victims indicate that fluid and electrolyte balance are restored rapidly. The majority of human drowning victims aspirate 10 ml of fluid or less per pound of body weight. Hemodilution has not been demonstrated, and hemolysis is uncommon. The changes in serum electrolytes and blood volume are often transient and depend upon the quantity and tonicity of fluid aspirated. Nonspecific electrocardiographic changes occur as the result of hypoxia. Ventricular fibrillation is uncommon in human victims. The initial effect of the aspirated fluid on the alveolar membranes and pulmonary surfactant results in collapse of alveoli, decreased compliance, and shunting of blood through nonventilated alveoli. Subsequently, hypoxia also occurs from the diffusion deficit resulting from pulmonary edema or pneumonia. The hypoxia caused by near-drowning with aspiration in human victims is manifested by arterial hypoxemia and metabolic acidosis.

The pathologic findings of drowning are often nonspecific. White or bloody foam, usually seen in the mouth, nose, and tracheobronchial tree, may not be evident after attempts at resuscitation. The skin of the palms and soles is often wrinkled and pale. These changes are consistent with prolonged immersion, but are not pathognomonic of drowning. Lacerations or incised wounds of skin, without evidence of vital reaction, reflect the effects of tides, collision of the body with underwater obstacles, and postmortem injuries inflicted by sharp objects such as motorboat propellors. Mutilation of a body by aquatic animals is common, particularly about the soft tissues of the face.

The lungs are heavy and edematous. In children, however, the lungs are often pink and distended with entrapped air. Pressure on the cut surfaces of the lungs yields variable degrees of frothy fluid. Foreign material from the aquatic environment, as well as vomitus, is often seen in the mouth, upper airway, and tracheobronchial tree. Depending on the postmortem interval, the pleural cavities contain variable quantities of straw-colored to dark watery fluid, which is a transudate from the edematous lungs. A relatively dry appearance of the lungs, attributed in some cases to death by reflex laryngospasm and closure of the glottis, may also result from agonal absorption and elimination of water from the lungs after cessation of respiration. Water may be found in paranasal sinuses, and hemorrhagic fluid is frequently observed in the middle ear and mastoid air cells. The latter finding is not specific for drowning, as it is also seen in other asphyxial deaths. Diatoms are microscopic unicellular or colonial algae containing silica. The significance of diatoms in the diagnosis of drowning is controversial. They may offer evidence of the aspiration of water when the same types of diatoms are demonstrated not only in the lungs but also in the water in which the body was found. After prolonged immersion in water, the changes of decomposition and the effects of aquatic life obscure the usual anatomic findings, but the pleural spaces may contain unusual amounts of sanguineous, watery fluid. The microscopic findings in the lungs may include pulmonary edema, focal intra-alveolar hemorrhage, disruption of alveoli, and demonstration of diatoms.

In laboratory animals (rats), Reidbord and Spitz observed differences in the ultrastructural changes of lungs in drownings in fresh water from those in sea water. With sea water, cellular swelling and vacuolation, as well as discontinuity of alveolar lining cells, were noted. After drowning in fresh water, the lungs of rats showed endothelial destruction, mitochondrial swelling, and cellular disruption. Histochemical changes were also reported by Spitz. An acute perivasculitis, consisting mainly of neutrophils, was seen in the lungs of rats after drowning in sea water. Similar changes, but to a lesser extent, were seen in fresh-water drowning. The distribution and amount of peroxidase-positive granules in the histologic sections parallel the density of the neutrophilic infiltration around vessels. These experimental studies may serve as the basis for a distinction between drowning in sea water and drowning in fresh water.

Numerous chemical and physical tests have been applied to the diagnosis of drowning. They include tests for concentrations of chloride or magnesium in whole blood, plasma, or serum; specific gravity of plasma; refractive index, electrical conductivity, and osmolarity of blood. None of them is entirely reliable, and all require considerable judgment in interpretation. There is yet no specific laboratory test for the diagnosis of drowning.

Clinical Manifestations. The victim of drowning usually experiences breath-holding and a substernal burning sensation. Loss of consciousness and aspiration of fluid may occur. Most victims have a violent struggle prior to loss of consciousness, but a few people show passive behavior. After rescue, the patient is usually unconscious, flaccid, cold, and cyanotic. Respirations are absent, and the pulse is imperceptible. If the patient is conscious, tinnitus and visual abnormalities are often reported. Frothy fluid may be seen in the nose and mouth, and examination of the chest may disclose signs of pulmonary edema. If a significant amount of water has been swallowed, nausea and vomiting may occur and gastric distention may be evident. Nonspecific electrocardiographic changes are related to the effects of hypoxia. Cardiac arrhythmias such as ventricular fibrillation, as reported for animals, are uncommon in man. Evidence of arterial hypoxemia and metabolic acidosis is provided by studies of gas and pH in blood. Serum electrolyte changes are usually transient and depend on the quantity and tonicity of fluid aspirated. The postimmersion period is sometimes complicated by pneumonia, hemoglobinuria, acute tubular necrosis, or brain damage from prolonged cerebral anoxia.

Diagnosis. When the patient is a victim of near-drowning, other physical causes for disability should be considered, including injury to the cervical cord from a dive into shallow water. In the differential diagnosis of near-drowning, other causes for aquatic accidents, especially air embolism and decompression sickness, must be considered. These untoward effects of barotrauma (see Ch. 45 and 46) are usually associated with underwater swimming, diving, or the use of self-contained underwater breathing apparatus (scuba). Recognition and differentiation from near-drowning are extremely important, as recompression, the appropriate method of treatment, may bring dramatic and lifesaving results.

The diagnosis of near-drowning is usually not difficult after the circumstances are known. Diagnostic studies include chest films, electrocardiograms, electroencephalogram, central venous pressure, serial determinations of arterial gas and pH, and appropriate laboratory tests, including hematocrit, hemoglobin, leukocyte count, serum electrolytes, and serum protein determinations. Respiratory complications, particularly pneumonia, are invariably present when fever, leukocytosis, pulmonary infiltrate on chest x-ray films, and decreased arterial oxygen tension are evident.

When the body of a dead person is found immersed in water, the diagnosis of drowning alone requires exclusion of other possible causes for death. A careful appraisal of the circumstances of death and of findings from pathologic and toxicologic studies and from postmortem chemical and physical tests is required. The role of a pre-existing illness, such as heart disease, as a precipitating factor in drowning depends on demonstration of pathologic features of the disease, as well as careful correlation with the circumstances and consideration of the hazards in the environment occupied by the victim immediately before the fatal incident. In some cases of suicide, particularly in bathtubs, if a concentration of a drug sufficient to cause coma is found in the blood, the investigator should suspect that the victim ingested a lethal dose of the drug, then went into coma, and drowned subsequently. Failure to find evidence of injury, intoxication, or pre-existing disease, as well as evidence that the person was alive during the period of immersion, favors the presumption that death was caused by drowning.

Treatment. Prompt rescue, first aid, and resuscitation offer the best chance for survival of drowning victims. The airway is cleared of any obstructions, and dentures are removed. Resuscitation by artificial ventilation is continued until oxygen is available, spontaneous breathing occurs, or signs of death are evident. If a heart beat or carotid pulse is not detectable, closed-chest cardiac massage, as well as artificial ventilation, is required. As soon as it is available, 100 per cent oxygen, with or without intermittent positive pressure, is administered continuously en route to a hospital. Survival depends not only upon the emergency care but also the prior health of the victim, the duration of immersion, and the amount of water aspirated.

Since there are both immediate and delayed effects of near-drowning, admission to a hospital for intensive pulmonary care is indicated. If the patient survives the first 24 hours, he is likely to recover. Reoxygenation should be started, followed by aspiration of the airway and suction of the stomach. Tracheostomy is rarely necessary. After insertion of an endotracheal tube, 100 per cent oxygen is given with either intermittent positive pressure or positive end-expiratory pressure, as well as with periodic hyperinflation of lungs. The administration of sodium bicarbonate solution intravenously in a dose of 0.3 to 0.4 mEq per pound of body weight is recommended upon admission to the hospital, for a significant number of near-drowning victims have metabolic acidosis associated with hypoxia. Based on serial determinations of gases and pH in the arterial blood, arterial hypoxemia and acid-base concentrations are corrected by effective ventilation, oxygenation, buffers, or bicarbonate. Respiratory stimulants are contraindicated. As indicated, bronchodilators, diuretics, digitalization, or transfusion of whole blood, plasma, or packed red cells are given. The need for antimicrobial drugs is determined by clinical signs and roentgenographic changes, as well as by culture of tracheal secretions. Although the role of steroids in the treatment of near-drowning is uncertain, the intravenous administration of methylprednisolone sodium succinate, 5 mg per kilogram per 24 hours divided into six equal doses, has been proposed. Intensive care is continued as long as necessary to correct hypoxemia and acidosis. As the patient improves, oxygen is given by catheter or mask and reduced in concentration to 40 per cent.

Bucklin, R.: Drowning: A review of the physiological, experimental, and pathological findings. *In* Wecht, C. H. (ed.): Legal Medicine Annual, 1972. New York, Appleton-Century-Crofts, 1972, pp. 93–104.

den Otter, G.: Low-pressure aspiration of fresh water and sea water in the non-anoxic dog. An experimental study on the pathophysiology of drowning. Forensic Sci., 2:305, 1973.

Editorial: Drowning. Lancet, 2:691, 1972.

Edmonds, C.: A salt water aspiration syndrome. Milit. Med., 135:779, 1970.

Edmonds, C., and Thomas, R. L.: Medical aspects of diving. Part 2. Med. J. Aust., 2:1256, 1972.

Fuller, R. H.: The clinical pathology of human near-drowning. Proc. R. Soc. Med., 56:33, 1963.

Modell, J. H.: The Pathophysiology and Treatment of Drowning and Near-Drowning. Springfield, Ill., Charles C Thomas, 1971.

Sladen, A., and Zauder, H. L.: Methylprednisolone therapy for pulmonary edema following near drowning. J.A.M.A., 215:1793, 1971.

48. LEECHES AS AGENTS OF DISEASE (Hirudiniasis)

Philip D. Marsden

The leeches belong to the class Hirudinea of the phylum Annelida. All blood-sucking species of medical importance live in fresh water or are terrestrial. They possess anterior and posterior suckers used for locomotion and attachment; the anterior sucker contains the mouth and cutting plates. When attachment to a host is gained, the skin is quickly perforated, and suction begins until the leech has taken several times its own weight in blood. In sucking blood, leeches secrete an anticoagulant, hirudin, the action of which continues after detachment. Leeches can survive for years without food. They can pass through boot eyelets and the fabric of loosely woven cloth to reach the skin of the host.

Both external and internal forms of hirudiniasis occur. *External hirudiniasis* is due to both land and aquatic leeches. In Southeast Asia particularly, as well as in India, tropical Australia, and parts of South America, land leeches drop in considerable numbers from jungle vegetation onto man. Large numbers may result in considerable blood loss, and even one or two may have a considerable psychologic impact. To remove these leeches, a lighted cigarette, match, or salt applied to the leech will cause it to release its jaws. The wound should be washed in antiseptic and an antibiotic cream or dressing applied; otherwise, secondary infection commonly occurs. The rarer *internal hirudiniasis* is usually due to accidental ingestion of small immature leeches in raw drinking water. They become attached to the buccal mucosa, pharynx, or larynx, and may grow there to produce signs of hemorrhage and obstruction. Manual removal of the leech with forceps may be difficult. An epinephrine nasal spray may induce it to release its hold. In the rare cases of urethral or vaginal involvement, strong salt solution has caused detachment prior to surgical removal.

Protection against aquatic and terrestrial leeches can be in the form of protective clothing or the use of repellents. Some repellents are rather soluble in water and need to be reapplied, but the use of diethyltoluamide in lanolin may overcome this problem.

Chin, T. M.: A further note on leech infestation of man. J. Parasitol., 35:215, 1949.
Mann, K. H.: Leeches (Hirudinea): Their Structure, Physiology, Ecology, and Embryology. Oxford, Pergamon Press, 1962.
Salzberger, M.: Leeches as foreign bodies in the upper passages in Palestine. Laryngoscope, 38:27, 1928.
Walton, B. C., Traub, R., and Newsom, H. D.: Efficacy of clothing impregnants M-2065 and M-2066 against terrestrial leeches in North Borneo. Am. J. Trop. Med. Hyg., 5:190, 1956.

ARTHROPODA OF MEDICAL IMPORTANCE

Philip D. Marsden

49. INTRODUCTION

The phylum Arthropoda is the largest in the Animal Kingdom, containing at least three quarters of a million species. Some classes of arthropods include species of medical importance. These are the Pentastomida (tongue worms), Chilopoda (centipedes), Diplopoda (millipedes), Arachnida (scorpions, spiders, ticks), and Insecta. The latter are especially important. The major characteristic of arthropods is a segmented body that is invested with a rigid or semirigid cuticle of chitin.

The disorders produced by venoms of arthropods are discussed in Ch. 59.

50. PENTASTOMIDA

(Pentastomiasis, Porocephalosis, Porocephaliasis, Linguatulosis, Armilliferosis)

Although the members of the class Pentastomida that occasionally infect man look very much like helminths, in fact they are modified arthropods with rudimentary legs and annulated but not segmented bodies. Two families of medical interest, the Linguatulidae, and the Porocephalidae, contain the genera Linguatula (with flattened adults) and Porocephalus (with cylindrical adults).

Linguatula serrata is found in adult and nymphal stages in the nose and paranasal sinuses of carnivorous animals and as larvae and encapsulated nymphs in herbivorous animals throughout the world. Rarely, human infection with the adult occurs in the lungs. More commonly larvae and nymphs encyst in the mesenteric lymph nodes, liver, spleen, kidneys, and intestinal wall. Infection is acquired by ingesting eggs discharged in the nasal secretions of canines. This parasite is found in 4 per cent of necropsies in Chile. The syndrome of parasitic pharyngitis (halzoun) may be caused by the larvae.

The genus Porocephalus contains 20 species, of which two, *P. armillatus* and *P. moniliformis,* have been found in man in Africa and Asia, respectively. The adult is a parasite of the respiratory tract of snakes (pythons and others) and crocodiles, and the nymph is found in a wide variety of mammals. Humans acquire infection by ingesting pond or drinking water contaminated by snakes or by eating snake meat. The ingested eggs hatch in the intestine, and the larvae bore through the wall to lodge in any viscus, where they undergo nine molts in six months to a year to form infective nymphs. In man the infection usually comes to a blind end, as they have to be ingested by the definitive host. Human infection with encysted larvae or nymphs on the surface of the liver or in the intestinal mucosa, peritoneal cavity, or lung is fairly common in Africa, particularly in the Republic of the Congo. Painful inflammatory lesions may result, or the parasites may be asymptomatic and their resultant calcification give a characteristic crescentic opacity between 4 and 7 mm in size (1.4 per cent of abdominal x-rays, in Ibadan, Nigeria, show this sign).

A recent report describes the findings of encysted nymphs in 45 per cent of autopsies on Malaysian aborigines. A range of lesions was observed from the encysted pentosomal nymph still viable with relatively little reaction, to the formation of a necrotic granulomatous reaction, with death followed by fibrosis and calcification. It is worth noting that this parasite must also be considered because a blood eosinophilia can occur, especially after the death of the larvae. Rarely, the parasite has caused intestinal obstruction, pneumonitis, meningitis, pericarditis, nephritis, and obstructive jaundice.

Burns Cox, C. J., Prathap, K., Clark, E., and Gillman, R.: Porocephaliasis in Western Malaysia. Trans. R. Soc. Trop. Med. Hyg., 63:409, 1969.
Prathap, K., Lau, K. S., and Bolton, J. M.: Pentastomiasis: A common finding at autopsy among Malaysian aborigines. Am. J. Trop. Med. Hyg., 18:20, 1969.
Schacher, J. F., Saab, S., Germanos, R., and Boustany, N.: The aetiology of halzoun in Lebanon: Recovery of *Linguatula serrata* nymphs from two patients. Trans. R. Soc. Trop. Med. Hyg., 63:854, 1969.
Steinbach, H. L., and Johnstone, H. G.: The roentgen diagnosis of Armillifer infection (porocephalosis) in man. Radiology, 68:234, 1957.

51. TICK PARALYSIS

Tick paralysis is a rapidly progressive flaccid paralysis, usually symmetrical, with loss of tendon and superficial reflexes. It follows tick bite and is probably caused by a neurotoxin in tick saliva. Several pathogenic chains have been suggested, including a conduction block in the somatic motor fibers, interference of the monosynaptic pathways, a depolarizing block at neuromuscular junctions, and an actual muscle lesion.

Symptoms may not come on until five to six days after attachment of the tick, when the patient becomes restless and irritable and may have numbness or tingling of the extremities, lips, throat, and face. Difficulty in walking is rapidly followed by inability to stand. Within a day or two there is paralysis of the limbs and trunk muscles, and a bulbar lesion will lead to dysphagia, slurred speech, and impaired vision. Death may result from respiratory failure or aspiration pneumonia. Pain and fever are rare, but there may be local skin change around the site of the bite, and morbilliform rashes have been reported. Providing that the paralysis is not too far advanced, rapid and complete recovery follows removal of the tick, although recovery may take more than a week. The cerebrospinal fluid is normal; bulbar and respiratory failure must be treated symptomatically, and a respirator may be lifesaving. *The paralysis is often confused with poliomyelitis.* In polyneuritis, myelitis, syringomyelia, and spinal cord tumor, sensory loss is usually present. Sensory signs are very rare in tick paralysis. *Like leeches, ticks should not be pulled off* but should be persuaded to detach by the application of a lighted cigarette or carbon dioxide snow to their posterior end.

Children are more frequently affected than adults. In one series of 119 cases, 79 per cent, including all the fatal cases, were in children under 16; two thirds were girls. Late removal of ticks is more probable in children, particularly in girls with long hair, for in these patients 70 per cent of the ticks are attached to the head and neck. There appears to be no correlation between mortality and the proximity of tick attachment to the brain. With rapid overseas travel, this diagnostic problem may confront a physician anywhere in the world. Various tick species are responsible. *Dermacentor andersoni* and *D. variabilis* are the chief offenders in the Rocky Mountains of North America, *Ixodes holocyclus* in Australia, and *Rhipicephalus simus* in Africa. The paralysis occurs in travelers to tick-infested areas who are likely to intrude into tick habitats by camping, picnicking, fishing, or hunting.

Ransmeier, J. C.: Tick paralysis in the eastern United States. J. Pediatr., 34:299, 1949.
Tick paralysis. Br. Med. J., 2:314, 1969.

52. SCABIES

Scabies is the most common skin disease encountered in some parts of the world, and is usually associated with poor living conditions. It is due to infection of the skin by the mite *Sarcoptes scabiei.* Hyperinfections with crusting and pustulation are termed "Norwegian" scabies. Scabies should be considered in every patient who complains of a persistent itch, and this symptom, together with papules, vesicles, and pustules on the extremities and follicular papules on the trunk, should be regarded as being due to scabies until proved otherwise.

The female mite is acquired by sharing a bed with an infected person or by other close personal contact, and in this sense in adults it can be likened to a venereal disease. The mite burrows into cracked and folded regions of the skin, the tunnel being limited to the stratum corneum except at the anterior end. Burrowing is by means of jaws and the sharp cutting edges on the terminal joints of the first two pairs of legs. Both copulation and egg production occur in the burrow, the rarely seen male ranging over the skin in search of the female. About two eggs are produced daily for two months. The hatched six-legged larvae make their own burrows and develop into adulthood in a fortnight. About one month after the establishment of the first burrow the patient begins to itch, probably because he becomes sensitized to acarine products. The scratching limits the population of mites by depriving them of a roof over their heads and crushing them. In experimentally induced infections Mellanby found that the population reached a maximum within three months and varied from 20 to 400 egg-laying females. Examination of nearly 900 men with scabies showed a mean population of 11.3 adult females per man, and more than half the patients harbored five adult acari or fewer.

The skin eruption has two aspects: the burrows which have to be searched for, and the changes resulting from sensitization and secondary infection which are obvious. The burrow of the ovigerous female appears as a narrow, slightly raised white gray or black line. The white shiny dot sometimes seen at one end, which may be associated with a small vesicle, is the site of the mite.

The *burrows* are commonly found on the sides and webs of the fingers, the ulnar border of the hand, the volar aspect of the wrists, the points of the elbows, the axillary folds, the areolae of the nipples in women, the external genitalia in men, the buttocks, and the margins or soles of the feet. The face and scalp are never affected in adults. Sometimes a typical burrow cannot be found. *There is a widespread rash* of follicular papules usually well marked on the abdomen, buttocks, inner sides of the thighs, and axillary folds. Scratch marks, crusted papules, and pustulation demonstrate the effects of scratching. An infected eczema sometimes develops on the fingers and wrists, nipples, or glans penis. Patients who are unable to scratch do not develop such lesions.

The *diagnosis of scabies* is probable if other members of the household are found infected. The mite can be identified by scraping a burrow along its length with the edge of a scalpel blade held at a right angle to the skin. The resultant material is mounted in 10 per cent potassium hydroxide under a coverslip, and microscopy reveals the mite. It has a body shaped like a tortoise with two pairs of legs in front and two pairs behind. The forelegs end in "suckers" and the hindlegs in long bristles. The female is about 400 μ long and coated in short bristles. Eggs or immature forms may also be present.

The typical clinical picture of scabies is subject to a number of variations. In babies the scalp may be affected, which means that the topical preparation must be carefully applied. Clean people usually have few lesions, and scabies may be overlooked in nurses for this reason. A localized eczema may be the presentation, or persistent sepsis of the skin. The amount of itch is very variable. In Norwegian scabies two million mites may be present, and the stratum corneum may be honeycombed with burrows on biopsy. Clinically, Norwegian scabies resembles exfoliative dermatitis. Often itching is absent, and this has been offered as the explanation of this hyperinfective state. However, some of these patients do itch, and other hypotheses attribute this state to topical or systemic corticosteroids or vitamin A deficiency.

The differential diagnosis includes atopic eczema, neurodermatitis, dermatitis herpetiformis, and two conditions considered in Ch. 54, pediculosis and papular urticaria. Papular urticaria is due to the bites of various insects, often fleas or bedbugs, but may also result from bites of various mites, either cheese straw or grain mites or the Sarcoptes of dogs and cats mentioned at the end of this chapter.

The three essential aspects of treatment are to treat all members of the household simultaneously, to use an application that will kill the parasites, and to apply it to the whole skin area. Since the acaricides mentioned below destroy all adults, larvae, and nymphs, but not the eggs, a further treatment should be given after a week. Suitable topical preparations for total body application are as follows: (1) *Benzyl benzoate, 25 per cent emulsion (60 ml for each application).* It is slightly irritating and may cause secondary eczematization and conjunctivitis if it is carried to the eyes. It has a rather penetrating smell, but is a very effective acaricide. (2) *Gamma benzene hexachloride (Gamma BHC) as a 1 per cent cream (25 grams for each application).* This is odorless, nonirritant, and effective against associated pediculosis as well.

A bath before the first application is desirable, and clean underclothes and sheets should be used after it. The itch may persist for some weeks after treatment, and soothing calamine lotion can be prescribed. Oral antimicrobial drugs may be necessary to combat skin infection and should be given concurrently. Most "failures" of treatment are due to unsatisfactory therapy, but it has recently been suggested that there may be benzyl benzoate-resistant Sarcoptes. As scabies is often transmitted in the course of sexual contact, the possibility of an associated venereal disease should be borne in mind. For effective treatment of scabies in a community where it occurs in high incidence, a treatment center is necessary. During World War II in Britain, scabies clinics brought the disease under control, and a scabies order gave personnel powers to enforce treatment. This species of parasite is comprised of a number of physiologic forms specific to the various vertebrate hosts; the disease in man is produced by *Sarcoptes scabiei var. hominis.* Other forms include *S. scabiei var. canis,* the cause of sarcoptic mange. This parasite and the cat mite *Notoedres cati* can cause severe papular urticaria in man although the classic burrow is not seen as these mites are specific to their normal hosts and incapable of burrowing and breeding in man.

Herridge, C. F.: Norwegian scabies (crusted scabies). Br. Med. J., 1:239, 1963.

Lyell, A.: Diagnosis and treatment of scabies. Br. Med. J., 1:223, 1967.

Mellanby, K.: Scabies. New York, Oxford University Press, 1943.

The scabies epidemic. Br. Med. J., 2:193, 1967.

Thomsett, L. R.: Mite infestations of man contracted from dogs and cats. Br. Med. J., 2:93, 1968.

53. MYIASIS (Maggots)

Myiasis may be defined as the infection of vertebrates with the larvae (maggots) of Diptera (flies) which feed on the tissues of the host. The maggots are usually identified by the form of their posterior spiracles, but this may be difficult to define in the early molts. Rearing the larvae to adults makes identification easier, especially with immature stages. Myiasis is a far greater problem in sheep, cattle, and deer than in man, and there is no form of myiasis found exclusively in man. For the purposes of a textbook of medicine, it is permissible to abandon the scientific classification of the responsible species and consider the clinical type of myiasis produced. For a description of the genera of flies, a textbook of entomology should be consulted. Primary myiasis occurs in the absence of debility of the host or tissue injury; this is in contrast to secondary myiasis.

PRIMARY MYIASIS

Furuncular Myiasis

Furuncular myiasis is a good descriptive term, because the skin lesion looks like a boil but in fact contains a maggot which breathes through a hole in the tip of the lesion. When mature, the maggot drops to the ground to pupate. There are two distinct types occurring in Africa and the Americas, respectively. (1) The African Tumbu fly *(Cordylobia anthropophaga).* The eggs are sometimes laid on clothing or else the larvae actively seek the host and burrow into the skin to feed. Multiple lesions are common. The normal hosts are wild rodents. (2) The human botfly *(Dermatobia hominis).* The botfly is found in South America, Central America, and Mexico. The eggs are frequently laid on a hematophagous insect (mosquito or stable fly) by the female and thence transported to the host. The secondarily infected "boil"-like lesion also occurs in other mammals in endemic areas.

The application of petroleum jelly to the lesion to block the spiracles often brings the suffocating larvae wriggling out backward, especially when mature. Immature larvae can be excised, but if possible it is better to let them mature and drop out.

Creeping Myiasis

Creeping myiasis is a form of larva migrans caused by flies of the genera Gastrophilus and Hypoderma. The former larvae do not mature and, being restricted to the stratum corneum, leave an obvious trail. Hypoderma penetrates more deeply and can complete its development in some instances and perforate the skin to escape.

The behavior of these two species is easily understood if their lives in their normal hosts are mentioned. *Gastrophilus,* normally a parasite of Equidae, has a period of migration as a young larva in the tongue epithelium but matures in the lumen of the intestine. *Hypoderma* is classically a parasite of bovids. *H. bovis* migrates via nerve trunks to gain the spinal canal and paravertebral muscle mass, and *H. lineatus* penetrates, migrating via the mucosa of the upper gut and gaining the same muscles via the esophagus. Both cause voluminous subcutaneous paravertebral abscesses, ruining the hide. It is not surprising, therefore, that when man is the host, the larvae may wander widely and even gain the eye, causing blindness.

Ophthalmomyiasis

A painful conjunctivitis can be produced by the first-stage maggots of *Oestrus ovis* hatching from eggs laid by the female near the conjunctiva. Hypoderma maggots may penetrate the globe of the eye. Such maggots can be irrigated from the conjunctiva or mechanically removed.

Other Forms of Primary Myiasis

Genitourinary myiasis owing to Fannia or Calliphora maggots has been rarely reported, the eggs being laid in the vicinity of the urethra. Maggots of these genera and the genera Sarcophaga and Musca have been found in freshly passed stools and can develop in the fecal stream. Tetrachloroethylene is effective. Intestinal myiasis is cosmopolitan and relatively common. In North America the drone fly *(Tubifera tenax)* larvae is the most frequently encountered species. The larvae of *Auchmeromyia luteola* (the Congo floor maggot) are temporary blood-sucking parasites of Africa; the larvae emerge from hiding places at night to suck blood, but after a meal retire to rest.

SECONDARY MYIASIS

Invasion of the body by maggots can occur in very debilitated individuals and in those with destructive or ulcerative lesions. Thus wounds may be infected by maggots of various fly genera, including Wohlfahrtia, Callitroga, and Chrysomyia. Similarly, myiasis of the nose, upper respiratory passages, or ear is caused by the screwworm fly maggots invading infected debilitated tissues. They should be picked out with forceps; otherwise they can penetrate the base of the skull and invade the brain.

PREVENTION

Reduction of screwworms, botflies, and warble fly maggots in sheep and cattle reduces the chances of human infection. This can be done with various dips of insecticides. Auchmeromyia larvae can be killed by dusting houses with insecticides. Clothing should be ironed and not hung out of doors for Cordylobia to lay eggs on it. Repellents and bed nets will reduce the incidence of Dermatobia lesions. The proper control of refuse disposal will reduce the number of blue- and greenbottle flies. It is worth noting that the eradication of the screwworm fly from Curaçao by releasing sexually sterile males is one of the few instances of a successful form of biologic control.

Baumhover, A. H.: Eradication of the screwworm fly: An agent of myiasis. J.A.M.A., 196:240, 1966.
Flew, G. P., and Grundy, J. H.: Infection with *Dermatobia hominis* occurring in British Guiana. J. Royal Army Med. Corp., 113:148, 1967.
Günther, S.: Furuncular Tumbu fly myiasis of man in Gabon, Equatorial Africa. J. Trop. Med. Hyg., 70:169, 1967.
James, M. T.: The flies that cause myiasis in man. United States Department of Agriculture Misc. Publ. No. 631, 1947.
Palmer, E. D.: Entomology of the gastrointestinal tract. Milit. Med., 135:165, 1970.
Zumpt, F.: Myiasis in Man and Animals of the Old World. London, Butterworth and Company (Publishers), Ltd., 1965.

54. ECTOPARASITIC INSECTS (Fleas and Lice)

Both fleas and lice are ectoparasites of man in the sense that they live outside his body on the skin but are dependent on him for food. Lice are more dependent than fleas and cannot survive long if separated from man because they need his body warmth and his tissues for their frequent feedings. Fleas are more exploratory and are capable of fantastic leaps, thus enabling them to transfer easily from host to host. Lice are flattened dorsoventrally, enabling them to hug the surface of the skin, whereas fleas are laterally compressed, enabling them to slip between the upright hairs. Lice have no true metamorphosis in their life cycle, the young resembling the adults, whereas fleas have a conventional true cycle of metamorphosis with larvae and pupae.

Both ectoparasites play important roles in the transmission of human disease. Louse-borne typhus *(R. prowazeki)* and louse-borne relapsing fever *(Borrelia recurrentis)* are mainly transmitted by the body louse, and in conditions of poverty, war, and famine, great epidemics have occurred. Apart from plague, fleas also transmit endemic or murine typhus caused by *Rickettsia typhi (R. mooseri).*

PEDICULOSIS
(Head, Body, and Pubic Lice)

Man provides food and shelter for two genera of lice. *Pediculus humanis var. capitis* infests the head and *P. humanis var. corporis,* the body and clothing. *Phthirus pubis* (crab lice) usually lives in the pubic area, but on occasion extends its range to the axilla, chest hairs, and even the eyebrows and eyelashes. The eggs or nits are found attached to the hairs of the host, and in the case of the body louse are found in clothing. All three lice suck blood frequently and can exist only a short time away from the host. Their saliva produces an *irritant roseate papular dermatitis.* Scratching leads to secondary bacterial infection of the skin with crusting and induration, and pigmentation may be present in severe infestations (vagabond's disease). Enlargement of local lymph nodes is common, especially the posterior auricular group in severe capitis infections. *Phthirus pubis* infestation of the eyelashes leads to blepharitis. The irritant cutaneous lesions suggest the diagnosis, which is confirmed by finding the eggs or adults. The eggs can be combed out of the hair with a fine-toothed comb.

Treatment. In the treatment of head lice an ointment of 1.0 per cent hexachlorocyclohexane in vanishing cream (Kwell) should be rubbed on the scalp thoroughly. This treatment is also effective for pubic lice when the ointment is massaged into the skin of the infested area. Lice and eggs can be removed individually from the eyelashes or eliminated by the application of 0.25 per cent physostigmine ophthalmic ointment. Body lice are destroyed by sterilizing the clothing by heat, using the ointment on infested areas of the body. A 10 per cent DDT in pyrophyllite dusted onto the head, body, and clothing without undressing is highly effective. Lice in Korea and Egypt have developed resistance to DDT, and 1 per cent hexachlorocyclohexane or pyrethrum powder may be substituted for it. The secondary pyoderma should be treated with appropriate antimicrobial drugs.

Prevention. The prevention of lousiness consists primarily in personal cleanliness and the avoidance of infected persons, bedding, and clothes. *Phthirus pubis* is usually transmitted by sexual intercourse. The rise of the "hippies," with their low standards of personal hygiene and tendency to increasing sexual promiscuity, has resulted in an increase in the incidence of crab lice. Lice are quite host-specific; thus, unlike fleas, the lice of domestic animals are not attracted to man.

Ackerman, A. B.: Crabs—the resurgence of *Phthirus pubis*. N. Engl. J. Med., 278:950, 1968.
Buxton, P. A.: Louse: An Account of the Lice Which Infect Man, Their Medical Importance and Control. London, Edward Arnold (Publishers), Ltd., 1939.

FLEAS

Pulex irritans is primarily a human flea. The fleas of the cat and dog (Ctenocephalides) and of the rat and mouse (Xenopsylla) also frequent man. They usually migrate over the body until a tight garter or belt obstructs their passage, and there they proceed to suck blood. Individuals vary greatly in their reaction to the salivary secretion of fleas. Some are unaffected. On those who are severely irritated, raised red edematous lesions are produced (papular urticaria). Fleas are sensitive to applications of DDT.

The control of fleas requires their destruction in the home. Vacuum cleaning of rugs and removal of debris will eliminate adults as well as eggs, larvae, and pupae. Insecticide sprays such as 5 per cent DDT in oil are effective. The living quarters of dogs and cats and the animals themselves should also be treated. As DDT is rather toxic to young cats, a 4 per cent Malathion powder can be used for them. Bird fleas can also cause papular urticaria; hen runs may require treatment, and birds' nests should be removed from under eaves of affected houses.

TUNGIASIS
(Tunga Penetrans)

The common names jigger or chigoe are to be avoided because they are easily confused with chigger, the name given to trombiculid harvest mites. A highly modified flea, *Tunga penetrans,* parasitizes man, pigs, and dogs, as well as a variety of other mammals. It is common in Africa and South America. The adult female is a permanent parasite of the subcutaneous tissues of warm-blooded animals and is embedded in the skin with just the anal pore having access to the exterior. The male copulates with the embedded female, and several hundred eggs are laid, after which the female dies.

The embedded females are most common on the sole of the foot and the root of the nail, where they cause pain. In debilitated people lying in infested huts many lesions may be present, all on one side of the body including the face. Secondary infection commonly results from the severe irritation. Septicemia, thrombophlebitis, tetanus, and gas gangrene may be complications. The swelling containing the ovigerous female is about the size of a pea and may be mistaken for myiasis. However, the lesion is recognized by the tip of the flea's abdomen appearing as a black dot in the center of the lesion.

Embedded females are best removed individually. After cleansing the skin with antiseptic, the opening hole of the flea pustule is enlarged with a sterile needle, and the intact insect can then be enucleated or expelled by gentle pressure. Antimicrobial therapy may be needed for secondary bacterial infection. Prophylaxis with DDT powder to the feet and socks or benzyl benzoate application is effective.

Bolam, M. R., and Burtt, E. T.: Flea infestation as a cause of papular urticaria. Br. Med. J., 1:1130, 1956.

Jelliffe, D. B.: Tungiasis. *In* Simons, R. D. G. P. (ed.): Handbook of Tropical Dermatology. New York, American Elsevier Publishing Company, Inc., 1953, p. 895.

55. ARTHROPODS AS MECHANICAL CARRIERS OF DISEASE

FLIES

The common house fly and its relatives, the stable fly, greenbottle, bluebottle, blow fly, and flesh fly, breed and feed on human and animal feces and garbage. Typhoid fever, bacillary dysentery, amebiasis, and cholera may be transported on the fly's body from feces to man's food, and are found in the feces and vomitus of flies. Poliomyelitis and infectious hepatitis conceivably could also be transmitted in this way. Small flies called eye gnats may act as carriers of pathogens causing acute purulent conjunctivitis and yaws.

Control of flies by spraying breeding habitats with 10 per cent DDT in kerosene is effective. Garbage should be tightly sealed or destroyed to prevent fly access. Houses and particularly food cabinets should be rendered fly-proof. Outdoor privies and septic tanks should be disinfected.

COCKROACHES
(Blattidae)

These common hospital and home insects may serve as mechanical transmitters of intestinal bacteria, virus, or Protozoa by their contact with filth and food. Cleanliness in the kitchen is essential for their control. The following are effective against roaches: Chlordane, 5 to 10 per cent dust; Chlordane, 2 per cent, and DDT, 5 per cent, in kerosene; or Malathion, 2 per cent in oil.

BEDBUGS
(Cimex)

Bedbugs are reddish brown and wingless, and have a disagreeable odor. As with fleas, the bites of bedbugs may result in papular urticaria. Because they suck human blood, they would seem to be likely disease transmitters, but all attempts to demonstrate this have failed. Although in the laboratory they can be infected with numerous human pathogens, they do not appear to transmit them in nature. In small African babies numerous bites are said to have resulted in iron deficiency anemia. A 5 per cent kerosene solution of DDT or 0.1 per cent lindane oil on infested bed frames, furniture, and wall crevices will control this insect. Infested mattresses should be discarded.

56. ARTHROPODS AS INTERMEDIATE HOSTS OF INFECTIOUS DISEASE

The infectious agents for which arthropods serve as vectors and the hosts in which these pathogens can develop are considered elsewhere in this book. In concluding this discussion of arthropods, it is worth emphasizing that for the medical man with biologic interests the field of medical entomology still holds considerable research possibilities and is worthwhile exploring. To aid in this interest some general references are given below.

Busvine, J. R.: Insects and Hygiene. London, Methuen and Company, Ltd., 1951.

Gordon, R. M., and Lavoipierre, M. M. J.: Entomology for Students of Medicine. London, Blackwell Scientific Publications, Ltd., 1962.

Herms, W. B.: Medical Entomology. 5th ed. Revised by M. T. James. New York, The Macmillan Company, 1961.

Horsfall, W. R.: Medical Entomology, Arthropods, and Human Disease. New York, The Ronald Press Company, 1962.

Leclercq, M.: Entomological Parasitology. Translated by G. Lapage. New York, Pergamon Press, Inc., 1969.

Smart, J.: A Handbook for the Identification of Insects of Medical Importance. London, The British Museum, 1965.

VENOM DISEASES

57. SNAKEBITE

Sherman A. Minton, Jr.

Identification, Distribution, and Classification of Venomous Reptiles. Recognition of venomous snakes is difficult, for the only character common to all species is the presence of venom-conducting maxillary fangs. Handbooks for identification of snakes of most geographic areas are available from natural history museums or government agencies. Local information about reptiles is often untrustworthy, and erroneous beliefs are widespread even among educated and professional persons. Harmless reptiles are often believed dangerous; dangerous species may sometimes be considered innocuous. The number of species of poisonous snakes is nearly always greater in tropical countries; nevertheless, certain species may be abundant in temperate regions, e.g., the prairie rattlesnake in the northern Great Plains of the United States. Even in the tropics it is unusual for more than three or four species to be important in a given area.

Following is a brief classification of venomous reptiles:

Lizards. FAMILY HELODERMATIDAE. Two species known as Gila monsters are restricted to parts of Mexico and the southwestern United States. There are venom-conducting teeth in the lower jaw; the venom has local irritant and neurotoxic effects.

Snakes. FAMILY COLUBRIDAE. This family includes most of the world's snakes, about 2500 species. A few hundred, mostly tropical and subtropical, have grooved fangs on the posterior maxillae. The fangs frequently are not engaged in defensive biting. Little is known concerning the venoms, but some are powerfully hemorrhagic. Nearly all rear-fanged snakes are harmless for practical purposes, but bites of the African boomslang (*Dispholidus typus*) and bird snakes (*Thelotornis kirtlandii*) have caused deaths.

FAMILY ELAPIDAE. These snakes have fixed fangs on the anterior ends of the maxillae; the fangs may be followed by solid teeth. The venoms are predominantly neurotoxic and often very potent. Some are also hematotoxic and necrotizing. About 120 species are confined to the Old World, and almost 50 species of coral snakes inhabit tropical and subtropical America.

FAMILY HYDROPHIDAE. These are marine or brackish water snakes characterized by laterally flattened tails and, in nearly all species, by great reduction or absence of enlarged ventral scales. They have fixed, short fangs followed by solid teeth. Their venoms in man act primarily on skeletal muscle, and are often extremely potent but small in quantity. About 50 species inhabit the coastal waters of south Asia, northern Australia, and islands of the southwest Pacific; one species reaches the western coasts of tropical America.

FAMILY VIPERIDAE. Single, large fangs on short and otherwise toothless maxillae rotate, permitting the fangs to be erected or folded against the roof of the mouth. Venoms usually cause local necrosis and hemorrhage, but some are predominantly neurotoxic. One subfamily, *Crotalinae* or pit vipers, is characterized by a deep pit lined with sensitive heat receptors situated between the eye and nostril. There are about 100 species of pit vipers, mostly in the Americas and Southeast Asia. *All dangerous snakes of the Americas except the coral snakes belong in this group.* The other subfamily, *Viperinae,* lacks the sensory pit. There are about 50 species confined to Africa, Asia, and Europe.

Epidemiology. World mortality from snakebite is estimated as 20,000 to 25,000 annually. The greatest number of reported snakebite deaths occur in the Indian subcontinent (10,000 to 12,000 annually); high figures are also reported from Burma, Ceylon, Thailand, and other Southeast Asian countries, Brazil, and other countries in the American tropics. Mortality is believed moderately high in tropical Africa, although reliable figures are not available. Moderate to low incidence is reported from southern Europe, the Middle East, Australia, and New Guinea, the temperate regions of Africa and South America, Japan and associated islands, and the United States (fewer than 20 deaths annually in recent years). Snakebite mortality is very low to nil in northern Europe and Asia, Canada, the West Indies (exclusive of Trinidad), New Zealand, the Malagasy Republic, and Oceania.

High snakebite mortality and morbidity are seen in localities where a dense human population lives in close proximity to dangerous snakes. Some southeast Asian venomous snakes (Indian cobra, kraits, bamboo vipers) are singularly adapted to life in local villages and even in suburbs of large, modern cities. Dangerous pit vipers of the genus Bothrops in Latin America are plentiful in sugar cane and banana plantations; Russell's viper in Southeast Asia often frequents cultivated fields. Local practices in agriculture, irrigation, and construction may provide good refuges for snakes, or may bring about increase in the rodents and lizards that are the food of many venomous snakes.

Snakebite is most common in adult males. The incidence is next highest in children because of their carelessness and curiosity. Adult females are the least frequently bitten. Persons at greatest risk from snakebite are those who deliberately handle or work with venomous snakes, be they scientists, entertainers, or religious zealots. If this small, high-risk group is excluded, snakebite is chiefly a hazard to farmers who till their land by primitive methods, plantation laborers, and those engaged in construction work or brush-clearing by largely manual methods. Practices of fish netting and trapping sometimes expose fishermen to bites by sea snakes and other aquatic species. Recent studies indicate that snakebites in the eastern United States are usually sustained near the victim's home, and involve persons in the 5- to 19-year age group predominantly.

Ethnic factors increasing the incidence of snakebite include types of dress that do not protect the legs and feet, sleeping outdoors on mats on the ground, and religious protection of venomous snakes or their use in rituals.

Control of snakes is best accomplished by indirect means: better construction of dwellings, disposal of rubbish, and control of rodents. Direct control campaigns have not been successful, except in small areas, and may be undesirable as many beneficial snakes are also destroyed.

Properties of Snake Venoms. Snake venoms are slightly viscid fluids, usually pale yellow to amber, occasionally white or colorless. Most medically important species yield 0.1 to 1.5 ml of fluid venom; yields of 5 ml have been reported for large vipers. Snakes may inject the entire content of their venom glands in biting, but usually do not do so. It has been shown experimentally that the Palestine viper injects about 15 per cent of its venom in an average strike, but in some cases may inject up to half the contents of its glands. Sometimes snakes bite without injecting venom.

Venoms dry as platelets, representing 15 to 45 per cent of the original weight of the sample. In this form they are stable for years if kept in sealed vials at cool to moderate temperature.

Average venom yields from representative species of snakes and the estimated fatal doses for man are given in the accompanying table. It should be emphasized that both the amount of venom and its toxicity are subject to wide variation, according to geographic distribution, age, season, and other factors.

Numerous enzymes have been identified in snake venoms. Hyaluronidases, present in most venoms, account for the rapidity of absorption. Proteases cause local inflammation, necrosis, and damage to vascular epithelium. Phospholipase A alters membrane permeability and releases histamine, thus contributing to hemorrhage and shock. Phosphodiesterase may be responsible for some of the hypotensive effect of venoms. Esterases in many viper venoms liberate bradykinin. Mamba venoms are high in acetylcholine. Many snake venoms inactivate complement.

Many snake venoms interfere with the normal process of blood coagulation and may do this by several mechanisms operating either sequentially or simultaneously. In clinical situations, concomitant intravascular coagulation and fibrinolytic activity frequently produce a defibrination syndrome with nonclotting blood.

About 40 polypeptide toxins have been isolated from elapid and sea snake venoms. The structure of many is known, and synthesis of a peptide with the amino acid sequence of cobrotoxin (from Chinese cobra venom) has been accomplished. Most of these toxins have molecular weights of about 7000 and are composed of a chain of 61 to 74 amino acids linked by disulfide bonds. They produce a nondepolarizing neuromuscular block by acting on the postjunctional membrane of the motor endplate. A few (e.g., β-bungarotoxin) are larger molecules that block the neuromuscular junction by reducing acetylcholine output from presynaptic nerve terminals. Others have cardiotoxic and cytolytic activity. Some additional polypeptide toxins have been isolated from rattlesnake and other viperid venoms. In composition and mode of action, they appear to be more diverse than the elapid toxins.

Snake venoms are antigenically complex, those of vipers generally containing more antigens than those of elapids, whereas sea snake and colubrid venoms contain fewest antigens. With some exceptions, venoms of phylogenetically related snakes have similar antigenic

Snake Species	Geographic Distribution	Venom Yield* (mg)	Lethal Dose for Man† (mg)
Beaked seasnake, *Enhydrina schistosa*	Coastal waters southern Asia and northern Australia	10–15	1.5
ELAPIDAE			
North American coral snake, *Micrurus fulvius*	Southern United States	3–5	5
Indian krait, *Bungarus caeruleus*	Most of India and Pakistan	8–12	2
Tiger snake, *Notechis scutatus*	Australia	35–45	3
Mamba, *Dendroaspis angusticeps*	East Africa	75–100	15
Death adder, *Acanthophis antarcticus*	Australia and New Guinea	70–100	10
Indian cobra, *Naja naja*	Southeast Asia to Indonesia and Formosa	150–200	20
Ringhals, *Hemachatus haemachatus*	South Africa	80–120	60
VIPERINAE			
Puff adder, *Bitis arietans*	Most of Africa; southern Arabia	160–200	100
Saw-scaled viper, *Echis carinatus*	Northern and western Africa to northern India and Ceylon	20–35	5
Russell's viper, *Vipera russelli*	West Pakistan to Formosa	150–250	50
Palestine viper, *Vipera xanthina*	Middle East	90–140	60
CROTALINAE			
Cottonmouth moccasin, *Agkistrodon piscivorus*	Southern United States	100–150	100
Fer-de-lance, *Bothrops atrox*	Mexico to Argentina	100–160	50
Jararaca, *Bothrops jararaca*	Tropical South America	40–70	40
Habu, *Trimeresurus flavoviridis*	Ryukyu Is.; closely related species in Formosa and southeastern part of the People's Republic of China	100–300	100
Western diamondback rattlesnake, *Crotalus atrox*	Southwestern United States and northern Mexico	200–300	70
Neotropical rattlesnake, *Crotalus durissus*	Southern Mexico to Argentina	25–40	10
Western rattlesnake, *Crotalus viridis*‡	Western United States and southwestern Canada	90–130	50

*Venom extractions from adult snakes of average size; maximal yields may be two to four times the upper limit of the average range.
†Estimated for an adult of 70 kg.
‡There are 13 other species of rattlesnakes in the United States. At least one species occurs in every state except Maine, Delaware, Alaska, and Hawaii.

makeup, a matter of practical importance in production and use of therapeutic antisera.

Clinical Manifestations. The clinical picture in snakebite is difficult to summarize briefly. Several syndromes are seen.

In the United States, most snakebites are characterized by severe local pain, edema spreading from the bite, painful lymphadenopathy, and local ecchymosis, often with serum-filled blebs. Systemic manifestations include nausea and vomiting, thirst, sweating, and fever rarely exceeding 38° C. If no additional symptoms develop, the prognosis is excellent, although there may be local necrosis occasionally severe enough to require skin grafting. Danger signs include numbness and tingling of the face, pronounced drop in blood pressure, violent muscle spasms or convulsions, hematuria, hematemesis, cyanosis, and difficulty in breathing. Increased clotting time and a drop in hemoglobin indicate severe envenomation. This syndrome is seen after bites of most rattlesnakes, the copperhead and cottonmouth moccasin, and a number of Old World vipers.

Hemorrhagic manifestations dominate the picture in bites by certain Latin American lancehead vipers (Bothrops), *some African and Asian vipers,* particularly the saw-scales (Echis), a few elapids such as the Australian genus Pseudechis, and the rear-fanged boomslang (Dispholidus). Local symptoms resemble those listed in the previous paragraph, but there is usually less edema. Persistent oozing of blood from fang punctures, bleeding gums, fever, and headache are prominent even in mild cases. Ecchymoses may be seen anywhere, particularly at sites of mild trauma. Gross hematuria, hematemesis, hemoptysis, and blood in the feces are common. Prothrombin time and sometimes clotting time are greatly prolonged; return to normal is a favorable prognostic sign. The usual cause of death is massive cerebral, retroperitoneal, or intestinal hemorrhage that may occur as much as 12 days after the bite. Some patients die of anemia and exhaustion, particularly when there is associated scurvy, malnutrition, hookworm disease, or malaria.

Elapid neurotoxins rapidly involve the bulbar centers, causing ptosis, strabismus, slurred speech, and dysphagia with drooling of saliva. Other early symptoms are vomiting, giddiness, muscular weakness, and drowsiness. Respiration is labored; the patient may complain of a sensation of weight on the chest. The temperature is normal or subnormal. Violent abdominal pain sometimes occurs after krait and coral snake bites. General symptoms usually begin within 30 minutes after the bite; sometimes there is a latent period of several hours. Local symptoms vary. Cobra bites usually cause considerable pain and swelling, occasionally followed by necrosis. Bites by many types of elapids cause little immediate local reaction, but pain radiating from the bite may begin after an hour or more. Hemoglobinuria and albuminuria are common. Death usually occurs within 15 hours after onset of systemic symptoms; patients surviving longer generally recover. Despite severe nervous system involvement, permanent neurologic sequelae do not occur.

A somewhat different neurotoxic syndrome accompanies bites by crotamine-secreting tropical rattlesnakes. Local pain and swelling are slight to moderate. The outstanding symptoms are dizziness, intense headache, impairment of vision that may progress to blindness, paralysis of the neck muscles, and respiratory depression. Albuminuria and hematuria are seen, and suppression of urine flow may supervene. The prognosis is poor.

Seasnake bites show little or no local symptoms. After a latent period of 30 minutes to a few hours, the patient complains of muscular pain, stiffness, and progressive weakness. Trismus, ptosis, and loss of tendon reflexes are seen. In severe cases blurring of vision, thirst, vomiting, and difficulty in breathing occur. The urine contains myoglobin, albumin, and erythrocytes, although gross hematuria is rare. Tubular necrosis may be followed by acute renal failure. When symptoms are severe the prognosis is grave, but many seasnake bites are mild, probably because of the small amount of venom injected.

A singular type of envenomation is ophthalmia, caused by the so-called spitting cobras, of which there are two species in Africa and one in Malaysia. Venom is ejected in a fine spray through an opening on the anterior aspect of the fang. On contact with mucous membranes of the eye, it produces violent pain and sometimes temporary blindness. Permanent ocular damage is rare, and systemic symptoms do not occur. Prompt washing with water or other nonirritant fluids is usually adequate therapy; local use of dilute antivenin has been recommended. Venoms of these snakes have the same effect as other cobra venoms if the snake bites rather than spits.

Diagnosis. The diagnosis of snakebite is materially simplified if the snake has been captured or killed and correctly identified. Differential diagnosis involves distinction between (1) snakebite and other injuries, (2) bites of poisonous and nonpoisonous snakes, and (3) minimal envenomation, in which conservative management is indicated, and severe envenomation, which demands more active therapy.

Injuries by objects such as thorns and spines of plants must occasionally be distinguished from snakebite. Usually these are recognized readily by the nature of the wound and lack of progressive symptoms. Differentiation between snakebite and injuries by other venomous animals may be difficult if the patient did not see the animal that injured him, or is too young to give a reliable history. Wounds inflicted by arthropods such as scorpions, centipedes, spiders, and insects are usually smaller than those caused by fangs of snakes and bleed less. Fish spines and teeth of small mammals usually cause deeper, more ragged wounds.

The pattern of puncture wounds will not reliably differentiate bites of poisonous snakes from those of nonpoisonous species. The writer has been bitten hundreds of times by many species of nonpoisonous snakes and sustained injuries ranging from single punctures to six rows of multiple punctures. Bites by poisonous snakes showing a single fang puncture are not rare, and may terminate fatally. Bites in which the palatine and mandibular teeth cause wounds in addition to those made by the fangs are also seen. Nonpoisonous snakebites show very little local swelling, usually bleed freely, and cause little pain. Unfortunately, bites of some dangerous snakes also show little local reaction.

In North American pit viper (rattlesnake, moccasin) bites, the development of more than 30 cm of edema and erythema in the first 12 hours plus any of the more serious symptoms mentioned in the paragraphs on clinical manifestations calls for administration of antivenin and supportive measures. Cases with less edema and mildness or absence of systemic symptoms need only observation and symptomatic therapy. In bites by snakes with hemorrhagic venom, hemoptysis, hematuria, and increased prothrombin time are early evidences of serious poisoning. Early clinical signs of severe neurotoxic poisoning are impaired vision, ptosis, slurred speech, and drowsiness. The presence of trismus, muscle pain on passive movement, and myoglobinuria differentiates severe seasnake bites from mild ones and from injuries by other venomous marine organisms.

Treatment. Therapy in snakebite has four aims: (1) retarding absorption of venom and removing as much as possible by mechanical means, (2) neutralization of venom by immune serum, (3) counteracting specific pharmacologic activities of the venom, and (4) relief of symptoms and prevention of complications.

Local Treatment. Clinical and experimental evidence indicates that appreciable amounts of rattlesnake and other viperine venoms may be removed by incision and suction. A ligature should be applied immediately and tightly a few centimeters proximal to the fang wounds and released for 90 seconds every 15 minutes. It may be moved proximally as swelling increases. Two to four incisions about 1 cm long are made completely through the skin through or near the fang wounds. Suction is applied intermittently over the incisions for approximately one hour after the bite. A breast pump, modified plastic syringe, or the devices in commercial snakebite kits may be used; oral suction should not be used if other means are available. Bracelet or multiple incisions are not advised. If circulation distal to the bite becomes badly impaired, fasciotomy may be necessary.

Incision and suction increase the danger of infection, and oozing of blood from incisions may be a problem after bites by snakes with powerfully anticoagulant venoms. Absorption of some highly neurotoxic venoms is so rapid that incision and suction are ineffective.

After the first hour, the ligature is released. The bitten part should be immobilized 24 to 96 hours.

After acute symptoms of poisoning have subsided, treatment of vesicles and necrotic areas is similar to that advocated for severe burns.

Serum Therapy. Snake venom antisera or antivenins are prepared by hyperimmunization of animals (usually horses) against one or more snake venoms. The antibody-containing fraction of the serum is concentrated by methods used in preparation of bacterial antitoxins. Sometimes the product is lyophilized for greater stability. Antivenins are prepared by approximately 30 laboratories in various parts of the world. Most are intended for treatment of bites by the important venomous snakes of a particular geographic area. Some success has been achieved in preparation of antivenins against entire phylogenetic groups of venoms; e.g., polyvalent Crotalidae antivenin appears to be effective against venoms of most medically important species of pit vipers. There are no international standards for preparation and assay of antivenins. Products differ widely in potency and stability. The toxin-neutralizing capacity is low in comparison with bacterial antitoxins, and large doses are required. An initial dose of 20 to 50 ml diluted with five times its volume of physiologic saline should be given by intravenous drip over a 30 to 45 minute period. More antivenin should be given as the patient's condition dictates. A total of 100 to 150 ml in the first 24 hours may be required in a severe bite. If intravenous injection is not practicable, undiluted antivenin should be given intramuscularly. Infiltration of the bitten area with antivenin gives no advantage, and is contraindicated on fingers and toes. Allergic reactions to antivenin are common, and fatal anaphylaxis has been reported. A skin test for hypersensitivity should be done before administering serum; a positive reaction is contraindication to its use except in very severe cases. In bites by snakes known to be not highly dangerous (the copperhead in the United States, the European viper) or in bites by small snakes of more dangerous species, antivenin should be withheld unless the patient is a small child or there are signs of severe intoxication.

Supportive and Symptomatic Treatment. Except when it is obvious that only a minimal amount of venom has been injected, snakebite victims should be hospitalized at least 12 hours and kept in bed.

Blood transfusion is valuable therapy for bites by snakes with strongly hematotoxic venom. Blood typing should be done at the earliest opportunity, because the action of some venoms may make the procedure difficult. Adjustment of fluid and electrolyte balance is indicated in presence of shock, severe vomiting, hematuria, and albuminuria.

Oxygen is helpful in cases of hypoxia from blood destruction or respiratory impairment from the action of neurotoxins. In the latter, aspiration of secretions from the throat and trachea may be necessary, and the use of a respirator may be advisable. A tracheostomy may be required.

The presence of necrotic tissue, interference with local blood supply, and the toxic action of venoms on leukocytes and other phagocytic cells increase the hazard of infection even in relatively mild snakebites. Antimicrobial therapy should be instituted in most cases. Tetanus prophylaxis with toxoid or antitoxin is advisable; gas gangrene antitoxin is not recommended as a regular measure.

The necrotizing action of some pit viper venoms is reduced by local infiltration of tissue with 20 to 100 ml of 0.1 M ethylenediamine tetraacetic acid (EDTA). This must be done as soon as possible after the bite. Lethal factors of the venom are *not* neutralized by EDTA.

A corticosteroid preparation in doses of 100 to 500 mg of hydrocortisone or its equivalent may have beneficial antihypotensive and anti-inflammatory effects and is also helpful in treatment or prevention of serum reactions. The replacement of antivenin by repeated large doses of corticosteroids is not recommended. Antihistaminics have not proved effective in snakebite therapy.

Pain is often severe in viper bites, and may require codeine or meperidine. Anxiety and fear, sometimes to the point of hysteria, commonly accompany snakebite. Verbal reassurance and a confident attitude on the part of the physician are often more helpful than any medication; nevertheless, light barbiturate sedation is often advisable. An old and much maligned remedy, an ounce or so of whiskey or brandy, may accomplish the same purpose.

Extensive trials of immunization with snake venom toxoid are being undertaken in the Ryukyu Islands, an area of very high snakebite incidence. Preliminary results have been encouraging but not conclusive.

Nonpoisonous snakebites generally require no treatment unless the snake was a python or other large species. Precautions against infection should be taken. The snake's teeth frequently break off in the wound and should be removed. No specific diseases are transmitted by snakes in biting.

Behringwerk Mitteilungen: Die Giftschlangen der Erde, Wirkung und Antigenitat der Gifte. Therapie von Giftschlangenbissen. Marburg-Lahn, N. G. Elwert, 1963.
Minton, S. A.: Venom Diseases. Springfield, Ill., Charles C Thomas, 1974.
Reid, H. A.: Snake-bite in the tropics. Br. Med. J., 3:359, 1968.
Russell, F. E.: Clinical aspects of snake venom poisoning in North America. Toxicon, 7:33, 1969.
U.S. Navy Bureau of Medicine and Surgery: Poisonous Snakes of the World. Washington, D.C., U.S. Government Printing Office, 1968.
Yang, C. C.: Chemistry and evolution of toxins in snake venoms. Toxicon, 12:1, 1974.

58. MARINE VENOMS

Sherman A. Minton, Jr.

Venomous species occur in most phyla of marine animals. Their relative medical importance is increasing with the growing popularity of travel and of aquatic sports and with expanding exploitation of marine resources. Recognition of these animals and knowledge of their habits minimize opportunities for injury.

Most marine animal venoms appear to be proteins; however, quarternary ammonium compounds, epinephrine, 5-hydroxytryptamine, histamine, and other pharmacologically active compounds have been detected. Zootoxicologic properties of these venoms are too diverse for brief summary. Mechanisms of action for most species are poorly understood.

Jellyfish Stings. The pelagic coelenterates known as jellyfish belong to two main groups, the Portuguese men-of-war or bluebottles of the class Hydrozoa and the "true" jellyfish of the class Scyphozoa. Medically important species occur in all oceans; however, more serious stings are reported from Australian and south Asian waters. The venom apparatus consists of tentacles that may be up to 30 meters long and are thickly studded with highly specialized stinging capsules or nematocysts. Their primary function is capture and immobilization of food. Coelenterates never *attack* man; indeed, they are physically incapable of doing so. Injuries usually occur through contact with floating or stranded coelenterates or their detached tentacles. Such contact is followed by intense burning pain and development of linear, erythematous wheals that may progress to vesiculation. Muscular cramps, dyspnea, and nausea may be seen. Local necrosis may follow severe jellyfish stings. A systemic reaction clinically similar to anaphylactic shock may follow stings by sea wasps *(Chiropsalmus* and *Chironex)*; death has occurred three to four minutes after contact. Irukandji sting, caused by the Australian jellyfish *Carukia barnesi,* is characterized by a mild nettling rash followed after 10 to 60 minutes by sweating, cramps, severe myalgia, vomiting, and, sometimes, cough with hemoptysis. Recovery occurs within a day or two.

If tentacles are clinging to the skin, they should not be pulled or rubbed off, as this may discharge additional nematocysts. Prompt application of alcohol to the tentacle will inactivate the nematocysts. If alcohol is not available, the tentacles should be covered with sugar, salt, or dry sand and left alone 15 to 20 minutes before being scraped off. Local application of analgesic cream or spray, preferably one containing an antihistaminic or corticosteroid, may give some relief. Systemic reactions have been successfully counteracted by epinephrine (0.5 to 1 ml subcutaneously) plus 10 ml intravenously of calcium gluconate, antihistaminics, artificial respiration, and oxygen. Antivenin for the sea wasp, *Chironex,* is available from Commonwealth Serum Laboratories, Australia. Morphine or meperidine may be required to control pain.

Cone Shell Stings. Large marine snails of the genus *Conus* inflict injury with a harpoon-like tooth that can be rapidly extruded and is used for capture of prey as well as defense. Nearly all injuries are seen in shell collectors. Mild cases show only local symptoms resembling those of wasp stings. In severe cases, initial pain is followed by numbness, paresthesia, paresis beginning in the region of the injury and occasionally spreading to involve the entire skeletal musculature, sensation of constriction of the chest, dysphagia, visual disturbances, and collapse. Fatalities are on record, nearly all of them ascribed to the large species, *C. geographus,* widely distributed in the warmer parts of the Pacific and Indian Oceans.

The active principle of cone shell venom appears to be a protein-carbohydrate complex. Treatment is symptomatic with support of respiration essential in severe cases.

Miscellaneous Venomous Invertebrates. Spines of sea urchins cause painful injuries; systemic effects are very rare. A species of spiny Australian starfish inflicts a wound followed by bouts of vomiting lasting several days. Various sessile coelenterates such as hydroids, sea anemones, and stinging corals cause nettle-like stinging, sometimes with zosteriform hemorrhagic lesions and necrosis. Abdominal cramps, chills, diarrhea, and leukocytosis with eosinophilia may accompany severe stings. There is no specific treatment for any of these envenomations.

Venomous Fishes. Stonefish (Synanceja), scorpionfish (Scorpaena), lionfish (Pterois), weeverfish (Trachinus), and related species have venom glands associated with spines, especially those of the dorsal fin. Except for the greater weever, these are shallow-water fish particularly common about reefs, where they lie partly buried or concealed in crevices. Here they are apt to be accidentally touched or trodden upon. In open water the fish may adopt a more active defense, swimming so that the venomous spines are presented to an enemy. Skin divers and aquarium keepers have been injured under such circumstances. Fishermen may be injured when removing the fish from nets or traps. Fresh fish in markets may sting the buyer. Similarity of symptoms and of venom activity in laboratory animals suggests common or similar active principles in their venoms. *Synanceja verrucosa,* found from Oceania to the east coast of Africa, appears to be the most dangerous member of this group.

After injury by spines of these fishes, there is local pain that tends to spread and is often followed by hypesthesia or paresthesia at the site of puncture. Victims invariably describe the pain as almost unbearable, and it is regularly accompanied by hyperactivity often manifest by rolling about on the ground. There is severe local swelling, sometimes with formation of blisters and sloughing. Profuse sweating, dyspnea, hypotension, cyanosis, and collapse are seen especially with Synanceja stings; death may occur within an hour. Those who survive a severe sting may complain of weakness, dyspnea, and muscular aches for several weeks.

Immersion of the injured site in water as hot as can be tolerated is the most effective first aid.

Antivenin for Synanceja is available from Commonwealth Serum Laboratories of Australia; it may be expected to have some effect in stings by related species of fishes. The initial intramuscular or intravenous dose of 2 ml may be repeated in severe cases. Infiltration of the wound with emetine hydrochloride solution (65 mg per milliliter) is recommended if antivenin is not available.

Stingrays are widely distributed in warm coastal waters, including mouths of rivers; one family is restricted to fresh water. There are about 30 medically important species; the larger ones are 8 to 10 feet long, and weigh more than 100 pounds. Venom-secreting tissue is in the grooves and sheaths of barbed bony spines on the dorsum of the tail; in large species of rays, the spine may be 35 to 40 cm long. Stingrays typically bury themselves in sand or mud, where they may be stepped upon or grazed by persons diving. The fish lashes with its tail, driving the sting into its victim. Stings of large rays can readily penetrate the abdominal or thoracic wall. The wound is a puncture or laceration often surrounded by a zone of blanching for the first 30 minutes or so; later the area becomes hyperemic and edematous. Pain is severe, and sweating, nausea, weakness, and syncope are common. Muscular twitching, convulsions, irregular respiration, and cardiac arrhythmia indicate severe poisoning. Of 1097 stingray injuries reported in the United States during a five-year period, 62 patients required hospitalization, and two deaths resulted.

First aid for stingray injuries is immediate irrigation with salt water and removal of any fragments of the sting sheath that can be seen. This is followed by soaking in hot water for 30 to 90 minutes, administration of analgesics, and tetanus prophylaxis. Injuries by large rays, particularly when the chest or abdomen has been penetrated, require surgical management. There are no specific pharmacologic antagonists to stingray venom, nor is antivenin available.

Halstead, B. W.: Poisonous and Venomous Marine Animals of the World (3 Vols.). Washington, D.C., U.S. Government Printing Office, 1965–1970.
Keegan, H. L., and MacFarlane, W. V. (eds.): Venomous and Poisonous Animals and Noxious Plants of the Pacific Region, New York, Pergamon Press, 1963.
Nigrelli, R. F. (Ed.): Biochemistry and pharmacology of compounds derived from marine organisms. Ann. N.Y. Acad. Sci., 90:615. 1960.
Russell, F. E.: Marine toxins and venomous and poisonous marine animals. Adv. Marine Biol., 3:255, 1965.

59. VENOMOUS ARTHROPODS

Philip D. Marsden

CHILOPODA
(Centipedes)

Flattened dorsoventrally, centipedes have a single pair of legs to each body segment. They feed on other arthropods, and the appendages of the first segment are modified as poison claws through which venom is injected into the prey. Although not fatal to man, their bite can produce intense fiery pain, and the area at the site of the bite may be inflamed. Regional lymph nodes enlarge, and rarely there are signs of meningism. Treatment consists of analgesics and the use of local anesthetics at the site of the bite. Recurrence of the local edema and arthritis has been noted. Corticosteroids have been helpful.

Haneveld, G. T.: Centipede bites. Br. Med. J., 2:592, 1957.

DIPLOPODA
(Millipedes)

These have a rounded body contour and two pairs of legs per segment. They are vegetarian, but as a defense mechanism they secrete noxious fluids from body pores when attacked. These secretions may produce a vesicular dermatitis in man.

ARACHNIDA
(Scorpions and Spiders)

Scorpionida
(Scorpions, Eight Legs)

Envenomation of man or scorpiasis is common in some tropical areas. About 20,000 cases of scorpion sting occur annually in Mexico, and approximately 5 per cent are fatal, these deaths occurring mainly in small children. There are ten times more deaths from scorpion stings in Mexico than from snakebite. Scorpions are armed with a single curved caudal sting with which they inject their venom and paralyze their prey—usually other arthropods. Scorpions are nocturnal and hide beneath debris during the day.

The effects of envenomation vary with the species. Violent pain may occur at the site of the sting with radiation into the affected limbs. Chills with abundant cold sweats may be associated with severe thirst and vomiting. Venoms may have neurotoxic effects with paralysis and convulsions or cardiovascular effect with myocarditis and tachycardia, or may cause intravascular hemolysis. Death is often due to respiratory paralysis. Pancreatitis and defibrination syndromes have recently been described. Stings by scorpions with neurotoxic venom may not produce much local reaction.

Immediate treatment, as with snakebite, is aimed at delaying absorption of the venom. A tourniquet is applied to the limb and released every 20 to 30 minutes. If available, ice packs should be applied to the site and the patient kept at rest. Specific antiserum is available in some areas and should be given if signs occur in the central nervous system. Phenobarbital may control convulsions. Spraying DDT or benzene hexachloride (BHC) will cut down the scorpion population.

Bartholomew, C.: Acute scorpion pancreatitis in Trinidad. Br. Med. J., 1:666, 1970.
McIntosh, M. E., and Watt, D. D.: Biochemical immunochemical aspects of the venom from the scorpion *Centruroides sculpturatus*. *In* Russell, F. E., and Sanders, P. R. (eds.): Animal Toxins, London, Pergamon Press, 1967, p. 47.
Poon-King, T.: Myocarditis from scorpion stings. Br. Med. J., 1:374, 1963.
Sita Devi, S., et al.: Defibrination syndrome due to scorpion venom poisoning. Br. Med. J., 1:345, 1970.
Whittlemore, F. W., Jr., Keegan, H. L., and Barowitz, J. L.: Studies of scorpion antivenoms: 1. Paraspecificity. Bull. WHO, 25:185, 1961.

Spiders
(Eight Legs, Abdomen Joined to Cephalothorax by a Narrow Waist)

Most spiders possess venom apparatus in the form of a pair of chelicerae terminating in sharp fangs and associated venom glands. The degree of development of this apparatus varies, and the glands contain only a small amount of venom suitable for paralyzing other arthropods. Of the 200 genera described, only eight contain species reported to be poisonous to man. Human fatalities have occurred after the bite of species of Latrodectus, Loxosceles, Phoneutria, and Atrax.

Latrodectus. It is likely that all species in this genus are poisonous to man, but the black widow (*L. mactans*) and the gray widow (*L. geometricus*) are most important. Males have much less venom than the aggressive females. These spiders are represented in most warm parts of the world and occur in the Americas from Southern Canada to Chile. They spin their webs in dark places, often outhouses. In Texas 90 per cent of spider bites occur on the buttocks and genitals because of the tendency to spin webs under lavatory seats in outside privies. The bite may pass unnoticed; two tiny red spots may be seen at the site, or a severe local reaction occurs. The neurotoxic fraction in the venom is a protein of low molecular weight which affects the cord and nerve endings. Absorption is accompanied by pain and numbness in the affected part. In 15 minutes to a few hours generalized agonizing muscular pains appear, together with symptoms of shock. The blood pressure falls, and there are marked sweating, a feeling of weakness and nausea, and labored respiration. The marked rigidity of the muscles of the abdominal wall may simulate tetanus or an acute abdomen. Paralysis and coma may be followed by cardiac or respiratory failure in severe cases.

An intravenous injection of 10 ml of a 10 per cent solution of calcium gluconate administered slowly will relieve muscular spasm. If this fails, a muscle relaxant such as mephenesin can be given. An antivenin is available in some endemic areas where there is a demand for it. It is effective against most species of Latrodectus. The spiders are sensitive to DDT spraying.

Loxosceles. The hairy brown spiders, *L. reclusa*, of the United States and *L. laeta* of Central and South America, occur in houses among furniture. Pain occurs at the site of their bite, followed by erythema, edema, and local necrosis. A rarer cutaneovisceral form is associated with toxic nephritis and hepatitis, the venom being cytotoxic. Local pain and edema decrease after parenteral antihistamine and corticosteroids have suppressed systemic reactions.

Phoneutria. This is a genus responsible for fatalities in children in some South American countries (Chile, Brazil). The venom acts on both the central and peripheral nervous systems.

Atrax. The Australian funnel web spider also produces neurotoxic symptoms.

Editorial: Spider bites. Lancet, 2:509, 1969.
Horen, W. P.: Arachnidism in the United States. J.A.M.A., 185:839, 1963.
Levi, H. W., and Spielman, A.: The biology and control of the South American brown spider *Loxosceles laeta* (Nicolet) in a North American focus. Am. J. Trop. Med. Hyg., 13:132, 1964.
McCrone, J. D., and Hatala, R. J.: Isolation and characterisation of a lethal component from the venom of *Latrodectus mactans*. *In* Russell, F. E., and Sanders, P. R. (eds.): Animal Toxins. London, Pergamon Press, 1967, p. 29.
Smith, C. W., and Micks, D. W.: Comparative study of the venom and other components of three species of Loxosceles. Am. J. Trop. Med., 17:651, 1968.

ACARINA
(Ticks and Mites)

Families in the order Acarina (ticks and mites) are responsible for carrying some important human infections. The family Ixodoidea contains the hard ticks responsible for transmitting the rickettsia of tick typhus. The Argasidae are the soft ticks, some of which transmit tick-borne relapsing fever (*Borrelia duttoni*). The mites are also of medical importance. The family Trombiculidae contains the important genus of red mites, Trombicula, which transmit scrub typhus caused by *Rickettsia tsutsugamushi (orientalis)*. The larvae of other similar mites cause an unpleasant, irritating skin rash (chiggers, red bugs, or harvest mites). About 24 hours after feeding, small red macules appear, and there may be hundreds if infection is severe. The diagnosis is made by finding the six-legged orange red larvae on the skin. BHC dusting powder destroys mites in their habitats and dibutyl phthalate or benzyl benzoate is quite effective for about a week if dusted over clothing. The house mouse mite Allodermanyssus transmits *Rickettsia akari* of rickettsialpox. One other mite, *Sarcoptes scabiei*, which is responsible for one of the most prevalent skin diseases in the world, is considered in Ch. 52. Tick paralysis, a little-diagnosed entity, is discussed in Ch. 51.

STINGING INSECTS

Hymenoptera
(Bees, Wasps, Hornets, Ants)

All stinging insects are included in this order, which contains 60,000 species. The stinging apparatus consists of a modified ovipositor and paired poison glands that discharge into a reservoir – the poison sac. In bees the venom apparatus is usually torn away from the body when the insect is brushed off. The average bee sting contains 0.3 mg of venom. The venom of bees and wasps contains a number of fatty acids and saponin-like substances.

A direct action (increase in vascular permeability at the site of the sting) is associated with the presence of histamine, serotonin, and a particular kinin. In addition to the effect of these substances there is an indirect effect, depending, among other things, on the properties of histamine liberated from the damaged tissues, probably by an enzymatic mechanism. The position of the sting is of great importance. If it occurs in the buccal or pharyngeal mucosa, a serious edema of the glottis and asphyxia may result. If venom is directly inoculated into a blood vessel, rapid absorption can cause syncope and even death.

In parts of Africa and Asia some varieties of bees are especially aggressive, and a number of deaths have resulted from multiple stings. The total number of simultaneous stings necessary for a fatality is about 500. Apart from deaths owing to multiple stings, many fatalities occur in hypersensitive patients, in whom death may occur in one hour owing to anaphylaxis and laryngeal edema. The allergen occurs in all parts of the insect, and hypersensitive patients can be desensitized by injection of wasp and bee extract. In the United States more deaths were caused by stinging insects than by snakes in the period 1950 to 1954. In such allergic states intense pruritus after sting is followed by severe angioneurotic edema and asthma. Severe abdominal pain and convulsion may occur.

Stings should be removed from the wound, with care taken not to express more venom into the wound by squeezing the poison sac. Acute allergic reactions should be treated with 0.5 ml of 1:1000 epinephrine intramuscularly. This can be repeated as often as necessary, together with an intramuscular injection of an antihistamine. Hydrocortisone, 100 mg, should be injected intravenously in patients with severe laryngeal edema; tracheostomy may be lifesaving. Milder reactions can be relieved by black coffee plus 30 mg of epinephrine. Sensitized persons should carry sublingual tablets of isoproterenol and antihistamines and have epinephrine ampules available (see also Ch. 77).

Barnard, J. M.: Cutaneous responses to insects. Types and mechanism of reactions. J.A.M.A., 196:259, 1966.
Beard, R. L.: Insect toxins and venoms. Ann. Rev. Entom., 8:1, 1963.
Mann, G. T., and Bates, M. R., Jr.: The pathology of insect bites: A brief review and report of eleven fatal cases. South. Med. J., 53:1399, 1960.
Shaffer, J. H.: Stinging insects: A threat to life. J.A.M.A., 177:473, 1961.

Ants

Although most ants possess venom apparatus, only a few are capable of injuring man. The Tucandeira ant of the Central American forests possesses a powerful sting that may result in fever for several hours. Allergic reactions to ants have been reported. The fire ant *(Solenopsis saevissima* richteri) has now established itself in the southern United States, and after multiple stinging produces a pustular, markedly erythematous rash caused by a necrotizing toxin solenamine.

Adrouny, G. A.: The fire ant's fire. Bull. Tulane Univ. Med. Fac., 25:67, 1966.
Cavill, G. W. K., and Robertson, P. L.: Ant venom, attractors and repellents. Science, 149:1337, 1965.
Middleton, E.: In combined staff clinic on poisoning by venomous animals. Am. J. Med., 42:118, 1967.

URTICATING INSECTS

A number of moths and butterflies (Lepidoptera) and beetles (Coleoptera) possess urticating qualities and can cause irritant dermatitis and conjunctivitis.

Lepidoptera

The caterpillars of a large number of moths and some butterflies possess urticating hairs or spines singly or in clusters over the body. If such a caterpillar is handled, these penetrate the skin, and venom passes through an opening at the tip. The hairs frequently break and remain in the skin. When the caterpillar pupates, the urticating hairs are frequently present in the cocoon that surrounds the pupa, and are also carried on the wings and body of the adult insect when it emerges.

Dermatitis produced by caterpillars is very widespread. Outbreaks have occurred in Israel and Japan. In 1956, 250,000 cases of dermatitis were estimated on Honshu Island. In Texas 2130 cases of caterpillar stings were reported in 1968. The hairs can be removed by application of adhesive tape. If cellophane tape is used, the hairs can then be mounted on a slide for microscopic examination. Washing the affected area with mild antiseptic should be followed by the application of calamine. Severe urticaria may require parenteral epinephrine and antihistamines. Adult moths have been recorded as producing similar lesions.

Hellier, F. F., and Warin, R. P.: Caterpillar dermatitis. Br. Med. J., 1:346, 1967.
Zaias, N., Ioannides, G., and Taplin, D.: Dermatitis from contact with moths (Genus Hylesia). J.A.M.A., 207:525, 1969.

Coleoptera
(Beetles)

Two families of beetles that contain urticating substances are the Staphylinidae (rove beetles) and the Meloidae (blister and oil beetles). Eight staphylinids of the genus Paederus cause dermatitis, especially in tropical countries. The irritant is present in the coelomic fluid, and when the beetle is crushed on the skin, erythematous blistering and pigmentary lesions occur. Pederin, a powerful vesicating toxin, constitutes 1 per cent of the tiny beetle's body weight. Staphylinids are so small that they are not usually noted in the skin.

Several genera of Meloidae have urticating properties, including Mylabris, Epicanita, and Lytta. *Lytta (Cantharis) vesicatoria* is familiarly known as Spanish fly. These beetles are night-flying and are frequently attracted to artificial light. The urticating substance occurs in the hemolymph, which is extruded through the integument if the insect is disturbed or escapes when the insect is crushed. Large blisters are produced if the insect contacts the human skin, and blindness may occur if the conjunctiva is affected. The pathogenesis of these lesions is explained in a way similar to that of attacks by gaseous vesicants, namely, by a blocking of enzymes of the SH groups. Like these enzymes, cantharidin inhibits glucide metabolism. *It should be noted that cantharidin has no aphrodisiac effect, and that the fatal dose is less than 60 mg.* Topical treatment of the blisters with magnesium sulfate and methyl alcohol packs has been recommended. Other tropical beetles producing vesicants are in the families Paunidae and Oedemeridae.

Two other conditions associated with beetles can be mentioned here.

Scarabiasis is the term used for the presence of adult dung beetles in the stool of man. Certain beetle larvae survive in the fecal stream, notably the meal worms (Tenebrio) ingested in contaminated cereals.

Carpet beetles can be used as an example of harmless insects which may be associated with delusions of parasitosis and the production of a type of dermatitis artefacta. However, there is at least one report of a patient who became sensitized to the varied carpet beetle *(Anthrenus verbasci)* which can be brought into the house on cut flowers.

Armstrong, R. K., and Winfield, J. L.: *Paederus fuscipes* dermatitis. An epidemic on Okinawa. Am. J. Trop. Med. Hyg., 18:147, 1969.
Ayres, S., and Mihan, R.: Delusions of parasitosis caused by carpet beetles. J.A.M.A., 199:675, 1967.
Browne, S. G.: Cantharidin poisoning due to a blister beetle. Br. Med. J., 2:1290, 1960.
Cormia, F. E.: Carpet beetle dermatitis. J.A.M.A., 200:799, 1967.
Giglioli, M. E. C.: Some observations on blister beetle, family Meloidae, in Gambia, West Africa. Trans. Roy. Soc. Trop. Med. Hyg., 59:657, 1965.
Halprim, K. M.: The art of self mutilation. II. Delusions of parasitosis. J.A.M.A., 198:1207, 1966.
Kerdel Vegas, F., and Gothman Yahr, M.: Paederus dermatitis. Arch. Derm., 94:175, 1966.
Rosin, R. D.: Cantharides intoxication. Br. Med. J., 3:33, 1967.
Scarabiasis. J. Trop. Med. Hyg., 70:49, 1967.

Part IV
IMMUNE DISEASE

60. INTRODUCTION

Henry G. Kunkel

Immunology represents one of the most rapidly expanding areas of biology, and many new techniques for the study of alterations in disease have become available recently. This is particularly true at the cellular level, and much has been learned of the lymphocyte which is clearly the key cell involved in both cellular and humoral immunity. The concept of two major types of lymphocytes, T cells (thymus derived) and B cells (bone marrow derived), is firmly established. Alterations in level and defects in these cells are now recognizable.

Immunologic alterations, both at the cellular level and with respect to immunoglobulins (Igs) and antibodies, have been found in a wide variety of different diseases. However, in many instances it has proved uniquely difficult to pinpoint the abnormality as primary in the disease etiology. It is well recognized that similar changes can occur secondarily, particularly as a result of certain viral infections. In some diseases the significance of the immunologic alterations is clear, as for example in the allergic disorders, in thyroiditis, and in certain types of immune deficiency. In other diseases, such as systemic lupus erythematosus (SLE), Graves' disease, acquired hemolytic anemia, and pemphigus, immunologic alterations are present which appear to be involved in the disease process, but their origin and relative significance remain less clear. Finally, there are diseases such as rheumatoid arthritis, ulcerative colitis, and pernicious anemia in which the evidence for an immunologic disorder remains very tentative. Interest has centered in particular on the challenging question of autoimmunity and its possible pathogenic role in many of these disorders. One difficulty which has hampered investigators stems from the gradual realization that the occurrence of autoantibodies is by no means a rare phenomenon limited to specific diseases. Many normal persons appear to possess such antibodies. Some autoantibodies appear to be without harmful effects, and the possibility exists, at least in certain instances, that they may be of benefit.

Examples of widely prevalent autoantibodies that in most situations appear to be without harmful effects are immunoconglutinin or antibody to complement, the anti-gamma globulins frequently termed rheumatoid factors, and the antinuclear antibodies of many different types. All of these have been found in the serum of normal persons as well as in those with a wide variety of microbial diseases. Evidence has been obtained, however, that under certain conditions harmful effects can be produced by certain types of antinuclear and anti-gamma globulin antibodies. Characteristics such as concentration in serum, exact specificity (particularly toward antigens encountered in the serum), and physical properties such as solubility appear to govern this question.

One immunologic mechanism of tissue injury that is coming increasingly to the fore is the direct effect of antigen-antibody complexes from the circulation. This is particularly true of renal injury. Such a process appears to be involved in a number of diseases in which renal injury is manifest such as systemic lupus erythematosus and glomerulonephritis. The antigen reacting with antibody to form complexes may come from external sources such as streptococci and administered drugs, or it may come from autologous tissue breakdown products. The injury from such complexes is not limited to the kidney, a particularly sensitive target organ, but may also involve the blood vessels as a potential mechanism of vasculitis. Platelet damage represents a well documented example; complexes of drugs such as quinidine and its antibody in sensitive individuals adhere to platelets and bring about their destruction.

TYPES OF ANTIBODIES AND THEIR PROPERTIES

Five major classes of human antibodies have been characterized: IgG, IgM, IgA, IgD, and IgE. In addition the IgG class has been divided into four subclasses which differ markedly in biologic properties: IgG 1, IgG 2, IgG 3, and IgG 4. The concentration in serum and some of the special properties of these classes and subclasses are shown in the accompanying table. All these proteins migrate in the gamma-beta area by electrophoresis, with IgG 4, IgA, IgD, and IgE showing the most rapid mobility at pH 8.6. They have been determined quantitatively primarily through the use of specific antisera in radial immune diffusion assays. The five major classes are very distinct antigenically, and specific antisera are readily obtained. The four subclasses of IgG show marked cross-reactions, and it is primarily because of this distinction that they have been termed subclasses.

It is now apparent that all Igs and antibodies consist of two major polypeptide chains, the heavy or H chain and the light or L chain. Both the H and L chains have a variable and a constant area. The variable portions are directly involved in the antibody combining site. The constant areas of the heavy chains differ among the classes and subclasses and are responsible for the different biologic properties shown in the table. Figure 1 illustrates the basic Ig chain structure, showing the variable and constant areas as they apply to IgG 1 immunoglobulins. There are two L-H chain pairs which make up the two antigen combining sites of this type of molecule. Enzymatic splitting of the molecule has proved of great utility in the study of the various properties of antibodies. Papain produces an Fab and an Fc fragment, and each of these is readily isolated. Most of the properties of the different classes and subclasses shown in the table are based on structural differences in the Fc part of the molecule.

As shown in Figure 1, the common IgG globulin is made up of a single four-chain unit. In the case of IgM or 19S Ig as it is sometimes called, a similar four-chain monomeric unit is further polymerized into a macroglobulin consisting of five such units linked by disulfide bonds. The IgA globulin is more variable and sometimes consists of a simple four-chain 7S molecule and in other instances is polymerized to various larger sizes. Less is known about the IgD type, but this also appears to be a

Biologic Properties of Human Immunoglobulins

	IgG 1	IgG 2	IgG 3	IgG 4	IgA	IgM	IgD	IgE
Concentration mg/ml*	9.4	3.2	1.0	0.6	1.9	0.5	0.03	0.0003
Placental transfer	+	+	+	+	0	0	0	0
Complement fixation†	+	±	+	0	0	+	0	0
PCA‡ reactivity	+	0	+	+	0	0	0	0
P-K§ reactivity	0	0	0	0	0	0	0	+
Lymphocyte receptors¶	±	±	0	0	+	+	+	0
Macrophage binding	+	0	+	0	0	0	0	—

*Mean values in adult whites.
†Classic complement pathway.
‡Passive cutaneous anaphylaxis.
§Prausnitz-Küstner.
¶Ig receptors for antigen on the membranes of B lymphocytes.

7S protein made of two light and two heavy chains. The proteins of the IgE class also consist of two light and two heavy chains. However, longer heavy chains are present, making the four-chain molecule considerably larger. These classes differ from each other in carbohydrate content, which plays an important role in solubility differences. They also differ in their ability to cross the placenta, an important property with regard to maternal-infant antibody relationships. The IgM and the IgA show little or no placental passage, in marked contrast to IgG globulin, which in cord blood reaches similar levels to those in maternal serum. A very significant special property of IgA antibodies is their occurrence as the dominant antibody in all external secretions. Saliva, tears, intestinal secretions, colostrum, and other body fluids contain primarily IgA antibodies.

Recently it has been demonstrated that IgD is of special significance on the membrane of B type lymphocytes. It appears that IgD and IgM act as the primary receptors for antigen on the lymphocyte surface.

The total amino acid sequence is now available for a number of Igs and it is clear that marked differences occur in the variable areas of the heavy and light chains,

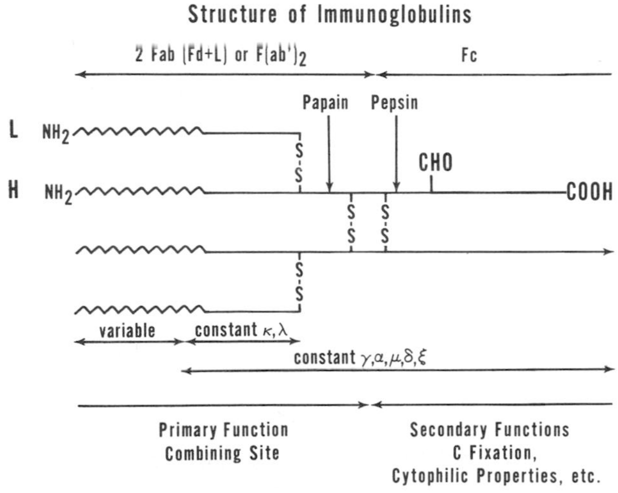

Figure 1. Diagrammatic illustration of the basic structure of the Ig molecule. There are two L chains and two H chains linked by disulfide bonds; the amino terminal ends of the chains are on the left and the carboxy terminal ends at the right. The undulating lines represent the variable portions of both the H and L chains. The sites of cleavage by papain and pepsin to give Fab and Fc fragments are indicated. The Greek letters refer to the kappa and lambda light chains and the heavy chains of the various Ig classes. The position of a carbohydrate side chain (CHO) is shown.

particularly in special regions which have been termed the hypervariable areas. These amino acid substitutions account for the specific combining properties of individual antibodies for antigen. The genetic mechanism by which the huge diversity of antibody molecules is produced with amino acid differences in the hypervariable areas remains unknown. The germ line theory proposes that there are sufficient DNA units in the genome to code for all the different antibodies. The somatic theory, on the other hand, considers a variety of different mechanisms arising during cell development and involving somatic mutations from a very limited number of DNA units.

Antibodies with autospecificity have been found that belong in each of the five main classes of Igs, with the exception of IgD and IgE. Most of the diverse antibodies encountered in the sera of SLE patients are of the IgG type, which goes along with the usual marked elevation in the total serum IgG globulin. A few, however, have been described that fall into the IgM and IgA class, particularly among the antinuclear antibodies. The rheumatoid factors as well as the majority of other anti-gamma globulins are primarily IgM macroglobulins. Most of the cryoglobulins are macroglobulins; this is also true of the cold agglutinins. Decreased solubility in the cold is a general characteristic of the antibodies of high molecular weight. It is known that these antibodies are also very sensitive to sulfhydryl compounds such as cysteine and penicillamine, which act on the disulfide bonds responsible for their polymeric structure. Attempts have been made to utilize this effect for therapeutic purposes, particularly for the cold agglutinin disease, but with limited success thus far. The antibodies of high molecular weight usually fix complement very effectively and as a result produce severe cellular injury when cells are involved as antigens. Many such antibodies are involved in hemolytic reactions of erythrocytes. In other instances the specific properties of macroglobulin antibodies make them more benign. The IgG–anti-IgG complexes found in rheumatoid arthritis sera are readily soluble under most conditions, permitting them to circulate at high concentrations with surprisingly few harmful effects. However, some of the IgG–anti-IgG complexes have been shown to have very harmful effects. This is particularly true in the disorder known as mixed cryoglobulin disease in which severe kidney disease is frequently found.

The skin-sensitizing antibodies or reagins that appear to be responsible for most of the harmful effects in the allergic diseases have many unique properties. The most striking of these is the persistence in the skin for periods of weeks after transfer to normal persons. The demonstration that these properties are characteristics of antibodies of the IgE class has been a significant recent development in immunology. Quantitatively this is a very minor class, representing only approximately 0.05 per cent of the total immunoglobulins of the serum. However, it has become clear that it is specifically involved in histamine release from leukocytes and other cells. The finding of several myeloma proteins of the IgE type has aided greatly in our understanding of the specific characteristics of proteins of this class. Their molecular weight is somewhat higher than IgG proteins and their sedimentation rate is approximately 8S. They are rich in carbohydrate and do not fix complement. It is of particular interest that IgE forming cells are concentrated in the mucosal system of the nose and respiratory tract as well as the regional lymph nodes, raising the possibility that locally formed IgE may be involved in respiratory allergy. Other types of antibodies to allergens are also found in the sera of sensitive patients that do not have the unique skin-sensitizing properties and rapidly diffuse away from the site of the injection. These antibodies, which have been termed blocking antibodies, appear to be typical IgG globulins, in contrast to the reagins. They also combine with antigen and may prevent a reaction with the skin-sensitizing antibody.

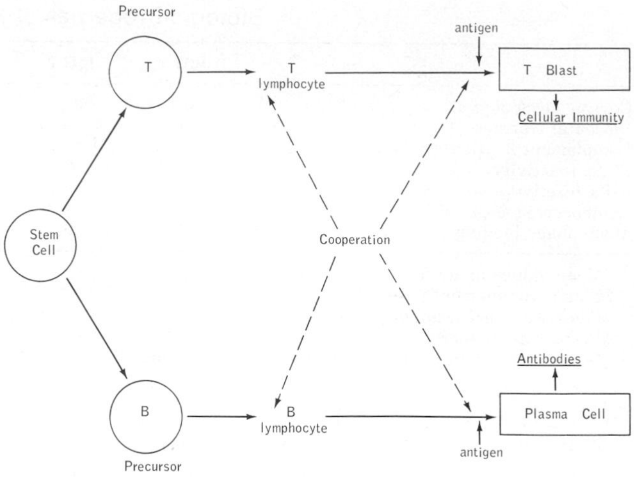

Figure 2. Diagrammatic representation of the development of immunologically active lymphoid cells of the T and B cell types from a common stem cell. Terminal differentiation to plasma cells producing antibodies and to T blasts responsible for cellular immunity follows antigenic stimulation.

LYMPHOCYTES AND OTHER IMMUNOLOGICALLY SIGNIFICANT CELLS

Two major classes of lymphocytes are now well documented which differ strikingly in their biologic properties. The B cell is distinguished by the presence of immunoglobulin receptors for antigen on its surface, and it becomes a plasma cell after stimulation; it is the primary antibody-producing cell. The T cell, on the other hand, plays a number of very different roles. It too has a receptor for antigen on the membrane surface, but the nature of this receptor remains obscure. After stimulation it enlarges to a blast cell that does not produce antibody but produces a wide variety of mediators that are significant in many immunologic processes. One of these has a significant effect on B cells and is the means by which the T cell cooperates with the B cell, thus aiding in the production of antibodies. Another very important function of T cells is their direct participation in cellular immune reactions such as graft rejection. Figure 2 illustrates diagrammatically the pathways that have been envisioned for the evolution of B and T cells from a progenitor stem cell.

A wide variety of other mediators have been described which are released by activated lymphocytes. None of these have been isolated, and it is not clear that they all represent different substances. The best known of these is "transfer factor," which is a low molecular weight dialyzable constituent that appears to transfer delayed hypersensitivity to specific antigens from a positive individual to a negative one; sensitivity to tuberculin, to diphtheria toxoid, and to coccidioidin represent three examples out of many that have been studied. Special interest has centered on "transfer factor" because of its potential value in therapy. Patients with various fungal infections, those with immune deficiency disorders, and even cancer patients have been injected with concentrated material prepared from donor lymphocytes in an attempt to produce a cellular immunity that may aid the immune response of these patients. Evidence has been obtained of therapeutic value for "transfer factor," but the final word on its usefulness is not in.

Migration inhibition factor (MIF) is another mediator released by T cells which has been widely studied. It is released in response to antigen and inhibits the migration of macrophages. This is usually measured by determining the diameter of the ring of macrophages moving out of the end of a capillary tube. It has become a widely used assay for the determination of cellular immunity to specific antigens. Other mediators include interferon, lymphotoxin, chemotactin, and skin reactive factor.

The macrophage clearly plays a key role in cellular immunologic reactions. Many aspects of this role remain poorly understood, but it is evident that a number of the mediators described above affect the macrophage directly and increase its activity against bacterial or other targets. Evidence is available for the release of a variety of enzymes from macrophages after stimulation. In addition, the macrophage has been shown to play an important role in the interaction of antigen with T cells. Some workers view this as a presentation of antigen which otherwise would not activate the T cell.

Another cell type which appears to have broad significance is the K or killer cell. This cell appears to hold a high affinity for antibody and acts in conjunction with antibody to attack target cells, the so-called antibody mediated lympholysis. Little is presently known about this cell and its relation to B cells or macrophages. It is clearly an important cell in tumor rejection in various animal models.

CHARACTERISTICS AND ESTIMATION OF B AND T LYMPHOCYTES

A number of different methods have been developed for differentiating B and T lymphocytes, and some of these provide quantitative results which are of use in assessing these immunologic parameters in diseased individuals. The most characteristic aspect of the B cell is the surface Ig which can be detected readily by a variety of techniques. The most widely used of these is the fluorescent antibody method in which anti-Ig antiserum that is fluorescent is used to stain the Ig on the cell. Figure 3 illustrates the dot-like staining obtained with such an antiserum on the surface of a B cell, whereas a T cell in the same field is entirely negative. This procedure reveals positive staining for Ig on approximately 15 per cent of normal peripheral blood lymphocytes. The Ig is primarily IgM and IgD and has been shown to be synthesized by the B cells. In certain individuals with various disease states, lymphocyte antibodies are found which attach to autologous lymphocytes and give falsely high levels for B cells by the surface Ig staining criterion. Short-term cultures of such lymphocytes aid in distinguishing this type, because the antibody is lost from the surface while the receptor immunoglobulin remains.

Another useful method for determining B cells stems from the presence of a receptor for the third component of complement which is not found on T cells. Red cells that are coated with antibody and complement form rosettes around B cells, and the number of such rosettes is readily quantitated. A third procedure utilizes the B cell characteristic of reacting with the Fc portion of IgG immunoglobulins. This is a weak interaction, and stable binding occurs only when the Ig is aggregated or is in the form of an immune complex. Large aggregates of IgG are readily visualized by a variety of methods attached to B cells specifically. The complement receptor and the Fc receptor procedures give results for B cell levels that are close to those obtained by Ig staining.

The T lymphocyte in the human can be detected by its selective binding of sheep red blood cells to give rosettes. This is a simple and accurate quantitative method that has come into wide use. The explanation for this useful binding procedure remains obscure. Both thymocytes and peripheral blood T cells give the rosettes. Approximately 80 per cent of blood lymphocytes are positive; this figure when added to the B cell population of 15 per cent gives a value close to 100 per cent. Specific antisera that are T cell specific are also available and can be utilized in fluorescent antibody studies or cytotoxic assays to quantitate the T cell population. Results with the antisera usually give a lower percentage figure for blood lymphocytes than is obtained with the rosetting procedure. Specific mitogen stimulation of T cells is also used as an assay of T cell competence. Phytohemagglutinin and concanavallin A are the primary mitogens for this purpose, and the T cell response is measured by determination of the blast cells produced or through the incorporation of tritium labeled thymidine. The advantage of the mitogen procedures is that the functional competence of T cells is determined, rather than just an enumeration of T cells. The disadvantages lie in the difficulty in quantitation and the influence of other cells such as the macrophage in the response.

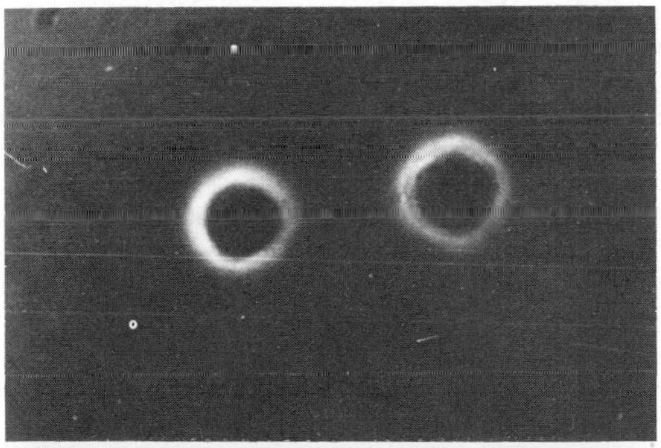

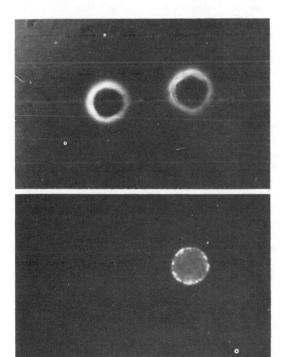

Figure 3. Surface Ig staining by the fluorescent antibody technique of a B type lymphocyte (lower frame). The upper frame shows two lymphocytes by phase contrast microscopy. One lymphocyte of the T type fails to show any Ig.

The *mixed lymphocyte culture* (MLC) reaction is also used as an assay of T cell function. This is usually carried out in a unidirectional system with a known stimulating lymphocyte population that is treated with mitomycin C. The latter reagent prevents these cells from responding but preserves their stimulating potential. The response is measured by the uptake of tritiated thymidine, and cells from different patients can be analyzed in terms of their response. The primary use of the MLC reaction, however, is in histocompatibility testing prior to grafting, in which compatibility is detected through an absence of any response, which is determined primarily by the MLC genes. These appear to differ from the HL-A genes that are separate but closely linked and determine the HL-A antigens that can be determined serologically. Because of the difficulties of the MLC test systems, the different phenotypes are only partially recognized, but their significance for graft survival is clearly recognized.

Alterations in the level and functional capacity of T and B lymphocytes have been found in a wide variety of diseases. The most striking findings are in the immune deficiency disorders (see Ch. 61 to 69), and analyses of the lymphocytes that are present are providing new insight into the basic defects. In Graves' disease and thyroiditis an increase in T cells and a fall in B cells have been demonstrated clearly. Alterations in Hodgkin's disease, leprosy, cancer, and connective tissue disease have been described. However, these studies are only beginning, and their significance remains to be determined. It is of special interest that the leukemic lymphocytes in the vast majority of cases of chronic lymphatic leukemia are of the B cell type; in acute lymphatic leukemia they appear to be of T cell character.

DELAYED TYPE OF HYPERSENSITIVITY

Delayed type of hypersensitivity is clearly a reaction of T cells which have been stimulated by antigen to react against targets such as infectious agents, grafts, and tumors. Antibody is not involved in this phenomenon, and disagreement exists among immunologists concerning the role of macrophages. The term "delayed type of hypersensitivity" arose from the delayed skin response of sensitive subjects to antigen; the reaction does not begin for several hours and reaches a maximum after two or three days. The term "cellular immunity" has also been used, although, as mentioned above, some types of cellular immunity also involve antibodies. Two major types of delayed hypersensitivity have been most widely studied: that induced by infection, and the other, termed contact sensitivity, resulting from exposure to a variety of substances ranging from oily resins of plants to simple chemicals employed for domestic, industrial, and medical purposes. Delayed hypersensitivity to autologous antigens has been difficult to demonstrate in humans, although it can be produced in laboratory animals by immunization with autologous antigens.

Delayed-type hypersensitivity is more strikingly evident in certain specific infections such as tuberculosis, brucellosis, lymphogranuloma venereum, mumps, vaccinia, and some fungal infections. Skin tests that depend on this type of cellular immunity have been utilized in these diseases. Tuberculin reactions have been extensively studied in humans and laboratory animals as a model for the delayed type of hypersensitivity. The skin reactivity to tuberculin can be transferred to normal recipients by means of cells from lymphoid tissue, peritoneal exudate, and peripheral blood. In laboratory animals viable cells are required, but in humans the supernatant fluid of disrupted leukocytes can transfer the reactivity. "Transfer factor," mentioned above in the discussion of mediators, represents the active principle involved.

Graft versus Host Reaction. Another probable manifestation of delayed-type hypersensitivity, or at least cellular immunity, is the graft versus host reaction. This has sometimes been termed "homologous disease." Initially it was largely a disorder of laboratory animals that are able to accept foreign bone marrow or lymphoid cells because they have been irradiated or otherwise treated so that these cells are not rejected. More recently it has been encountered frequently in humans who have received certain grafts, particularly bone marrow. The foreign cells react against various antigens in the host animal, resulting in a variety of clinical manifestations. The skin lesions are most characteristic: edema, erythema, and ulceration, followed by thickening, scaling, and loss of hair. Lesions of the joints and of the heart are also observed and these have aroused considerable interest because of certain similarities to those observed in some of the connective tissue disorders. Hemolytic anemia with a positive Coombs reaction has also been described. The possibility has been raised that in certain human diseases immunologically active cells react against the host in a fashion similar to that of the transferred cells in the laboratory animal experiments. The origin of such cells has been ascribed to some type of failure of tolerance mechanisms or to an alteration of host cells through somatic mutation.

SENSITIVITY TO FOREIGN ANTIGENS

Direct sensitivity to foreign antigens, the most common type of potentially injurious immunologic reaction in man, is usually a result of antigenic stimulation by foreign protein or polysaccharide antigens. These may gain entrance to the body through parenteral, oral, respiratory, or other routes. The classic example is serum sickness, usually resulting from the administration of horse or rabbit immune serum. An Arthus reaction is initiated through the direct union of antigen and antibody in the tissue spaces. Precipitates in and around small blood vessels cause secondary damage to cells, or, when antigen is in excess, soluble complexes are formed that may deposit in certain sensitive organs in the blood vessel walls and cause local inflammatory reactions.

In most of the human allergies such as hay fever and food allergy the exact mode of sensitization to external antigens is not directly apparent. Numerous factors such as heredity, intestinal absorption, respiratory secretion, and even emotional state appear involved. In such sensitive or atopic individuals the reaction to foreign antigens is more commonly of the anaphylactic type. Here the binding of antibody to tissue cells appears to play an important role. Local anaphylaxis results from the association or passive absorption of antibodies to local sites that come in contact with antigen. Not all antibodies have this property, and the IgE class is primarily involved. The antigen in turn reacts with the antibody and alters these cells, which then cause the release of histamine and other pharmacologic mediators into the tissue fluid and circulation. In the skin this gives rise to the wheal and erythema at the site of antigen introduction, as in ordinary prick and scratch diagnostic tests. Hay fever and allergic asthma are local manifestations of such reactions. Extensive urticaria may also represent an expression of local cutaneous anaphylaxis.

The antigens involved in these local allergic reactions are a very diversified group. A number have been isolated and partially characterized. The major allergen of *ragweed pollen* has been found to be a protein of approximately 37,000 molecular weight and represents a very small portion of the extractable solids of the pollen. The biologic activity of the isolated material is very high; as little as 10^{-12} grams cause a positive intracutaneous wheal and erythema reaction in sensitive individuals. A highly active protein has also been isolated from the *timothy hay pollen.* Low molecular weight nonprotein allergens have also been isolated. The best example of these is chloragenic acid, which is the active material from castor beans. Just how this is effective is not clear, but the general hypothesis is that it acts as a hapten and combines with body proteins to become a complete antigen. Similar sensitivity to a wide variety of chemicals, particularly those belonging to the group of nitrogenous aromatic substances, has been observed.

The *drug reactions* represent an analogous type of sensitivity that may become manifest in an extremely variable manner. There is a growing awareness of the possibility that sensitivity to unknown foreign materials may play a role in a variety of diseases that at present remain obscure or have been classified as possibly autoimmune in nature. Particular insight into a variety of mechanisms of immunologic cell injury has been gained from the study of the sensitization caused by drugs, particularly quinidine. In some persons thrombocytopenic purpura is the result of such sensitivity; in others it is a hemolytic anemia. It now appears that this effect is primarily the fortuitous result of the physical characteristics of the antibody produced. If the antibody is of low molecular weight, it forms a type of antigen-antibody complex with quinidine that has a particular predilection for platelets; if it is of high molecular weight, complexes are formed on union with the drug that affect primarily the erythrocytes. Complement is also intimately involved in the different effects. This system illustrates the vagaries involved in the selective action against individual target organs and may be of importance in consideration of disorders of unknown origin such as idiopathic thrombocytopenic purpura and "autoimmune" hemolytic anemia. The possibility of involvement of unknown foreign antigens, particularly haptens, is not excluded.

It has become increasingly evident that many antigens gain entrance into the body via the intestinal tract through the consumption of *food.* This has been demonstrated best for bovine milk proteins, and antibodies to a wide variety of these proteins have been found in the serum of many children and some adults. Clear precipitin reactions between bovine protein fractions and these human sera are readily observed. Usually, apparently, no ill effects result from these antibodies despite the fact that some bovine products that remain antigenic continue to gain entrance into the circulation. However, this is only one example of an antibody response to food products; many others must exist that may have important implications in, for example, certain of the intestinal disorders of unknown origin such as ulcerative colitis.

A somewhat different but very important type of reaction to foreign antigens is that produced by maternal-infant incompatibility in which the foreign antigen is introduced from the fetus. *Hemolytic disease of the newborn* is the outstanding example in which the mother produces antibodies that cause destruction of the erythrocytes in the fetus or newborn. The incompatibility leading to such effects may involve Rh antigens or those of the ABO system. Analogous phenomena have been described for leukocytes and platelets. Cytolytic or cytotoxic reactions occur in which complement is usually but not always necessary to effect the cellular damage. Many other antigens are probably involved in similar maternal-infant incompatibility, but the extent to which they lead to disease is not clear at present. One outstanding example that has become manifest recently is that for genetic types of gamma globulin. A high percentage of infants who lack the genetic gamma globulin character of the mother develop antibodies. These usually appear at approximately the sixth month after delivery and remain throughout the life of the individual. Antibodies to IgA globulins appear to have special significance with regard to transfusion reactions. Most of these appear in individuals who lack all IgA in their serum and probably arise either through maternal immunization or through the administration of blood products.

Another indirect type of reaction to foreign antigens involves antigenic cross-reactions between such antigens and autologous tissues. In this situation an immune response is stimulated by a foreign antigen such as a bacterium, but since a constituent of the organism is antigenically similar to a constituent of the host the immune reaction damages the host tissue. Such cross-reactions have been identified, but the exact role of this mechanism in disease remains to be determined; the possibility exists that presumed autoimmune reactions may be initiated in certain instances by such foreign stimuli. Evidence has been obtained that material from the cell wall of hemolytic streptococci is related antigenically to human cardiac myofibers and the smooth muscle of blood vessel walls. This finding has led to the hypothesis that the cardiac damage of rheumatic fever thus results secondarily from the immune response to the streptococcal infection that preceded it.

SENSITIVITY TO AUTOLOGOUS ANTIGENS

It has become amply clear that many persons develop immunologic reactivity against autologous tissue antigens, but the mechanism by which this sensitivity arises remains obscure. In some instances it may be through the reaction to an unknown foreign organism that contains antigens, particularly polysaccharides, that cross-react with similar polysaccharides in the body tissues. In other instances it may arise through tissue breakdown with release of antigens into the circulation that are ordinarily buried and not subject to the usual tolerance mechanisms. Recent studies in laboratory animals indicate that autologous proteins such as gamma globulin readily become antigenic through slight alteration of the molecule. Antibodies are produced to new determinants not ordinarily exposed but, in addition, as immunization continues, additional antibodies may be produced that involve the native configuration of the protein and will react directly.

One of the best examples of autosensitization in human disease is that found in thyroiditis. There are many features that remain poorly understood, but the evidence is overwhelming that the various degrees of lymphadenoid change in the thyroid gland, particularly in Hashimoto's disease, involve some type of immune reaction against antigens in the thyroid gland. The fact that similar lesions can be produced in laboratory animals by immunization with autologous thyroid antigens lends strong support to such a view. Even in laboratory animals it remains unclear whether some type of cytotoxic antibody or a cellular autoimmunity plays the dominant role in the tissue injury.

In Goodpasture's disease antibodies reactive with autologous antigens of basement membranes have been demonstrated. These react primarily with renal and pulmonary tissues and have been eluted from these diseased organs obtained at autopsy. Clear evidence of a pathogenic role of the basement membrane antibodies in the renal disease of these patients has been obtained. The antibodies eluted from the human kidneys produce glomerulonephritis in monkeys after infusion. The evidence for a role in the pulmonary disease of these patients is more indirect. It has been demonstrated that antibodies eluted from the lung fix to renal glomerular basement membrane, and antibodies eluted from the kidney fix to pulmonary membranes. The origin of these antibodies remains obscure. Similar antibodies also appear to be involved in a few cases of idiopathic glomerulonephritis.

In many blood diseases antibodies occur in the serum that react with autologous cells and in some instances clearly produce disease. The cold agglutinin syndrome is perhaps the clearest from the standpoint of the effect of the abnormal antibody in producing erythrocyte destruction. Anemia, jaundice, and hemoglobinuria can all be traced directly to the action of the cold agglutinin. An "idiopathic" type of the syndrome and one associated with histiocytic lymphoma and lymphocytic lymphoma offer no clues as to the mechanism by which the cold agglutinin was produced. Another type of disease that is usually of shorter duration follows viral or mycoplasmal pneumonia. Paroxysmal cold hemoglobinuria of the Donath-Landsteiner type is closely related and usually is associated with prenatal syphilis, although many nonsyphilitic cases have been reported. The much more common idiopathic, acquired hemolytic anemia of the warm antibody type presents a more obscure picture. Here the relationship of the erythrocyte damage to a variety of red blood cell antibodies is much more tentative. Only in a minority of cases can the antibodies be shown to have a definite specificity. In these instances it is directed against an Rh antigen, usually anti-e. Again no clue is available concerning the origin of these gamma globulins that react with autologous erythrocytes.

Idiopathic thrombocytopenic purpura is another disease in which circulating antibodies react with autologous cells—in this case platelets—and cause disease through the resulting cellular injury. These antibodies have proved surprisingly difficult to detect by conventional immunologic methods, but it is now clear that they are present. The role of leukocyte autoagglutinins as a cause of leukopenia has proved even more difficult to assess. Many of the antibodies reported by early workers have been shown to result from transfusions given to these patients, with the production of isoantibodies. However, most workers still believe that autoagglutinins do occur and are responsible for some cases of leukopenia.

Systemic lupus erythematosus (SLE) is probably associated with a greater variety of antibodies with autospecificity than any other condition. The best known of these are the antinuclear antibodies, certain of which are responsible for the LE cell phenomenon. Special interest has centered on the DNA antibodies because of evidence for an association with disease activity. Antibodies to native double-stranded DNA as well as antibodies specific for the single-stranded form are found in the sera of these patients. Recently antibodies to double-stranded RNA have been detected. It has become evident that antibodies to a wide spectrum of polynucleotides are uniquely present in this disease. Numerous additional antibodies to protein and carbohydrate antigens extracted from the cytoplasm as well as the nucleus of human cells have been described. Some of these appear to be responsible for various secondary manifestations of the disease as, for example, hemolytic anemia. This is associated with a positive Coombs test, suggesting the occurrence of antibodies to autologous erythrocytes. Idiopathic thrombocytopenic purpura, probably involving antiplatelet antibodies, also occurs in these patients. Abnormalities involving blood coagulation have been of special interest to investigators; antibodies to specific clotting factors appear to be involved. The origin of these many antibodies as well as others not discussed remains obscure. Some of them appear to represent a marked elevation of antibodies found at low levels in normal persons, which is compatible with the concept that in SLE a general hyperreactivity of the immune system exists. The high prevalence in females and the familial trend of the disease have not as yet been fitted into the immunologic concepts. Recent work with various strains of mice, particularly the New Zealand NZB strain, has shown that manifestations of a disease with many features resembling SLE occur in a high proportion of the animals. Most striking is the renal disease and the hemolytic anemia. This experimental model shows a marked similarity to the human disease, and the unique antibodies to double-stranded DNA and RNA are present. Studies in these mice have suggested a significant role for secondary viral infections in potentiating various disease manifestations. Whether this also applies to the human disease remains to be proved.

The possibility has been considered that a large number of other diseases in which the cause is unknown may have as their origin some type of autoimmune mechanism. This is particularly true of rheumatoid arthritis, primarily because it is associated with uniquely high incidence and levels of an unusual group of antibodies called rheumatoid factors. These have been clearly demonstrated to be antibodies to gamma globulin and are capable of reacting with autologous gamma globulin. No evidence is available to suggest that the rheumatoid factors play a direct role in the arthritis; however, many workers think they may be indicative of an as yet undefined immunologic reaction. The fact that they are produced at least in part in the synovial tissue of the joints from local accumulation of plasma cells adds some weight to this concept. On the other hand, it has also become clear that the rheumatoid factors could develop as a response to some type of foreign organism. Antibodies to the organism after reaction with the particulate antigen or fragment thereof would form secondary anti-gamma globulins to these antigen-antibody complexes. This possibility has been strengthened by the experimental production of anti-gamma globulins in rabbits after injection of coliform organisms, as well as their appearance in human sera after various types of infection. In bacterial endocarditis, for example, the rheumatoid factors disappear after elimination of the organism with antimicrobial therapy. Similar attempts with such therapy in rheumatoid arthritis patients is without effect on the rheumatoid factors. The accumulated evidence indicates that there must be some profound immunologic stimulus present in the rheumatoid arthritis patient to sustain the rheumatoid factors at the extreme levels often observed and for the prolonged periods in which they are present. The nature of this stimulus remains unknown.

Another disorder showing profound immunologic abnormalities associated with arthritis similar to that in rheumatoid arthritis is Sjögren's syndrome. It also has been considered a possible connecting link between rheumatoid arthritis and SLE. Extreme elevation of gamma globulin similar to that found in SLE patients is observed along with many similar antinuclear and anticytoplasmic antibodies. In addition, the vast majority of these patients have rheumatoid factors, often at extreme levels. Serologically they show the findings of both rheumatoid arthritis and SLE. The lesions observed in the lacrimal, salivary, and other glands of patients with Sjögren's syndrome are highly suggestive of a local immunologic reaction. They closely resemble those observed in the thyroid gland in chronic thyroiditis, in which an immunologic alteration has been more evident.

The immunologic aspects of pernicious anemia are of considerable interest. Antibodies to intrinsic factor have been demonstrated in a large number of cases, and antibodies to the parietal cells of the gastric mucosa are frequently found. These have been revealed by a variety of classic immunologic procedures. In addition, the intrinsic factor antibody inhibits labeled B_{12} absorption in tests in vivo. Many of the antibodies appear to be autoantibodies and are found in untreated cases; others appear to represent antibodies to hog intrinsic factor as a result of therapy. A direct role in the pathogenesis of the disease has not been established, but they at least are important in certain therapeutic considerations.

The serum of patients with myasthenia gravis contains a number of unusual antibodies directed at muscle constituents. These have been demonstrated primarily by fluorescent antibody techniques, a procedure that has proved unusually difficult when dealing with muscle sections. However, precipitating and complement-fixing antibodies have also been found. No direct role for these antibodies in the disease has been demonstrated, but they certainly raise the possibility of an immunologic mechanism. The frequent association of thymic disease with myasthenia gravis is well documented and adds further weight to a possible immune basis for this disease. One of the most important developments in immunology in recent years is the recognition of the profound role of the thymus gland in the development of immunity. It is also known that some infants born of myasthenic mothers have a transient myasthenic syndrome that could be due to placental transfer of antibody.

Antibodies with autospecificity of various types have been found in a variety of other diseases. In ulcerative colitis, antibodies to colon tissue and cellular immunity to colon cells have been described. Patients with liver disease show a wide variety of antibodies to autologous cell constituents. Antibodies reactive with mitochondria are of special interest because of their specific occurrence in primary biliary cirrhosis. They are of diagnostic value, but a pathogenic role remains to be demonstrated. Pancreas antibodies have been described in patients with pancreatitis, and adrenal antibodies in patients with Addison's disease. In all these instances the major possibility that these represent antibodies secondary to tissue breakdown in the disease has not been excluded. As stressed earlier, autoantibodies are far more common than had previously been thought, and any assessment of an injurious role in a specific disease is extremely difficult.

IMMUNE COMPLEX DISEASE

When artificially made antigen-antibody complexes are injected into laboratory animals, they are deposited in a number of organs with resultant tissue injury. By far the most sensitive organ is the kidney, and acute and chronic renal disease has been produced in a number of species by this procedure. The complexes are trapped in the glomeruli and form lumpy deposits along the glomerular basement membrane. These have distinct histologic characteristics by electron microscopy and by fluorescent antibody staining techniques. In human glomerulonephritis similar deposits are frequently observed when these same procedures are utilized. In systemic lupus erythematosus such deposits in the glomeruli are particularly striking, and a large accumulation of additional evidence for antigen-antibody complex mediated renal injury is available.

Extensive studies in a number of different laboratories have demonstrated that DNA-anti-DNA complexes represent one type involved in SLE. Antibodies to DNA aroused considerable interest when they were first described in SLE approximately 17 years ago. However, they were relegated to the position of scientific curiosities, and it has only been recently that their harmful potential has been realized. Antibodies to double-stranded DNA have special significance because double-stranded DNA antigens can appear in the circulation as a result of tissue breakdown; antigen-antibody complexes are formed with fixation of complement and deposition in the most vulnerable organ, the kidney. Elution of antibody from isolated glomeruli of diseased kidneys has proved to be a very effective technique for the detection of antibodies deposited in the kidney. DNA antibody has been found in such eluates at specific concentrations as high as 1000 times those in the serum. DNA antigen has also been demonstrated in the granular deposits observed in the glomeruli. Other, more indirect evidence such as the close clinical relationship among the appearance of DNA antibodies, serum complement depression, and exacerbations of disease has also aided in establishing the significance of the DNA system. Further studies are required to determine the relevance of the many other antibodies in the serum of these patients; some of these, if they can encounter specific antigen, may be involved as well.

Another type of renal disease in which evidence for immune complexes is rapidly accumulating is that associated with various types of drugs. Some of these may present a picture very analogous to that of serum sickness; in others, chronic drug administration may lead to a slowly progressive glomerulonephritis. The latter situation is well illustrated in the case of penicillamine. Numerous instances of nephritis have been reported after long-term administration of this material for the treatment of cystinuria, Wilson's disease, or rheumatoid arthritis. Granular deposits of gamma globulin and complement along the glomerular basement membrane are readily visualized in fluorescent antibody studies which closely resemble those produced in experimental animals by injection of complexes.

The presence of granular and "lumpy" deposits of gamma globulin and complement detected by fluorescent antibody techniques may be well visualized in renal biopsy specimens and have been found in a variety of different conditions such as malaria, bacterial endocarditis, and thyroiditis. Cases of chronic glomerulonephritis of unknown cause frequently show such a pattern. However, supporting evidence for specific antigen-antibody complexes is as yet unavailable for most of these. In poststreptococcal nephritis similar characteristics of complex-induced nephritis are present, and suggestive evidence for streptococcal antigens in the deposits has been obtained.

Eluates obtained from glomeruli isolated at autopsy from kidneys of patients who had subacute and chronic glomerulonephritis have in a number of instances shown high concentrations of gamma globulin. This appears to represent specific antibody, but its nature remains a mystery. The search is on in a number of laboratories for specific antigens that might react with such gamma globulin. Particular attention is being paid to various human viruses, because recent work in laboratory animals has demonstrated complexes of virus and antibody in the kidneys of mice. The task is a difficult one, however, and human tissue antigens, bacterial antigens, and even unknown drugs may be equally reasonable candidates. The possibility also seems likely that multiple antigen-antibody systems are involved in the different cases of idiopathic glomerulonephritis.

Another type of antigen-antibody complex that appears to be involved in some types of renal disease is that composed of IgG globulin and anti-IgG globulin. Such complexes are widely distributed in human sera and reach unusual levels in rheumatoid arthritis. Usually these are quite soluble, but in some patients they precipitate out in the cold as mixed cryoglobulins. Patients with such mixed cryoglobulins show a rather ill-defined clinical syndrome, but renal lesions are common. The components of such complexes along with complement have been identified in the glomeruli of these patients.

Evidence has been obtained that injury to circulating cells, particularly platelets, may be mediated by antigen-antibody complexes. A number of drug-induced thrombocytopenias fall into this category. Particular interest is currently centered on similar mechanisms in the joint inflammation of SLE and rheumatoid arthritis. Gamma globulin complexes are well known in the latter, and high concentrations have been observed in joint fluid, in which they appear to be involved in local complement depletion. Much work remains before a direct cause-and-effect relationship can be established. Lack of an adequate experimental model similar to those available for immunologic renal injury has hampered progress in this field.

Eisen, H. N.: Immunology. *In* Davis, B. D., Dulbecco, R., Eisen, H. N., Ginsberg, H. S., and Wood, W. B., Jr. (eds.): Microbiology. New York, Harper & Row, 1973, pp. 349–595.

Moller, G. (ed.): T and B lymphocytes in humans. Transplant. Rev., 16:3, 1973.

Natvig, J. B., and Kunkel, H. G.: Human immunoglobulins: Classes, subclasses, genetic variants and idiotypes. *In* Dixon, F. J., and Kunkel, H. G. (eds.): Advances in Immunology, Vol. 16. New York, Academic Press, 1973.

Robinson, R. R. (ed.): Immunological aspects of renal disease. Kidney, 3:55, 1973.

Spiegelberg, H. L.: Biological activities of immunoglobulins of different classes and subclasses. *In* Dixon, F. J., and Kunkel, H. G. (eds.): Advances in Immunology, Vol. 19. New York, Academic Press, 1974.

THE PRIMARY IMMUNODEFICIENCY DISEASES

Robert A. Good

61. INTRODUCTION

Knowledge of the lymphoid cells, their functions, and their organization into two separate major immunity systems has advanced rapidly in recent years. Current views are summarized in Table 1. Current understanding of the immunity functions has derived in considerable measure from study of the primary immunodeficiencies of man. In turn, new knowledge and understanding of the relation of structure to function in the lymphoid system have made possible better definition of the several primary immunodeficiencies. A continuing interplay between clinical analysis and advancing basic understanding of immunity and the immunologic apparatus represents a fine model of how progress in medicine can proceed most rapidly to the maximal benefit of man. Consequently, study of the primary immunodeficiencies has had importance to medicine in recent years far beyond the numerical frequency of patients who suffer from these relatively infrequent diseases.

In Table 2 is a listing of those diseases currently recognized by a WHO expert panel as the major primary immunodeficiencies of man. Included in Table 2, as well, is an effort to analyze each of the diseases in terms of its genetic basis and in terms of the types of cells primarily involved in the deficiency. Such an analysis must be recognized as ephemeral because of the rapidity of development of our knowledge and because rapid changes in understanding continue. Nevertheless, for the present these several diseases can be usefully viewed in light of this classification.

62. X-LINKED INFANTILE AGAMMAGLOBULINEMIA

Soon after Bruton initially described agammaglobulinemia in an eight-year-old boy, groups of patients, including multiple cases in several families, were studied in Boston, Minneapolis, and New York. From these studies, one form of agammaglobulinemia could be clearly established as being of sex-linked nature. This form has been called the Bruton type of agammaglobulinemia in recognition of the monumental contribution of the pediatrician who discovered the first of the primary immunodeficiencies and associated disease with absence of gamma globulin in the blood. Bruton's discovery launched a period in which immunology has been maximally influenced by the "experiments of nature" represented by the several forms of primary immunodeficiency.

X-linked agammaglobulinemia is a disease in which fully developed B lymphocytes and plasma cells are absent from blood and blood-forming tissues. Production of immunoglobulins and synthesis and secretion of antibodies are grossly deficient or lacking altogether. Figure 1 represents a characteristic immunoelectrophoretic pattern comparing normal with agammaglobulinemic patients. Figure 2 compares an antigen-stimulated lymph

TABLE 1. The Cellular Basis of Immune Responses

T cell system:	+PHA or Con-A† →	Blast cells	
Thymus-dependent T lymphocytes*	→	Killer cells (e.g., graft rejection)	Cell-mediated immunity
	+antigen →	Soluble lymphocyte factors	
B cell system:			
Thymus-independent, "bursa-equivalent" B lymphocytes	+antigen →	Plasma cell line	Humoral antibody synthesis

*There is evidence that T cells plus antigen can cooperate with B cells to produce antibody.
†Phytohemagglutinin or concanavallin.

TABLE 2

Type	Suggested Cellular Defects			Inheritance		
	B Cells (a)*	B Cells (b)†	T Cells	X-linked	Autosomal Recessive	Other§
X-linked agammaglobulinemia	X	(X)‡		X		
Thymic hypoplasia			X			X
Severe combined immunodeficiency	X	(X)	X	X	X	X
With dysostosis	X	?	X		X	
With adenosine deaminase deficiency	X		X		X	
With generalized hematopoietic hypoplasia	X		X		X	
Selective Ig deficiency						
IgA	?	X	(X)			X
Others		?				X
X-linked immunodeficiencies with increased IgM		X		X		
Immunodeficiency with ataxia telangiectasia		X	X		X?	
Immunodeficiency with thrombocytopenia and eczema (Wiskott-Aldrich syndrome)			X	X		
Immunodeficiency with thymoma	X*		X			X
Immunodeficiency with normo- or hypergammaglobulinemia	X	X	(X)			X
Transient hypogammaglobulinemia of infancy		X				X
Varied immunodeficiencies (largely unclassified and common)	X	X	(X)		(X)	X

*Absent or very low.
†Easily detectable or increased.
‡Some cases with circulation B-lymphocytes without detectable surface Ig have been found.
§Implies multifactorial or unknown genetic basis or no genetic basis.

node from a normal person (*A*) and a stimulated node from an eight-year-old agammaglobulinemic child (*B*). Absence of germinal centers and absence of plasma cells characterize the node of the agammaglobulinemic patient. Plasma cells are not found anywhere in the body. Even the lamina propria of the intestinal tract and exudates of chronic inflammatory processes such as bronchiectasis are devoid of plasma cells in these patients.

Clinically, children with X-linked agammaglobulinemia are normal at birth, but during the second half of the first year of life they begin to have infections with the encapsulated, virulent pathogens such as pneumococci, *Hemophilus influenzae,* and *Pseudomonas aeruginosa.* Infections in these children usually respond well to appropriate drug therapy; but because of lack of humoral immunity, resistance to these infections is minimal. Untreated, the bacterial infections spread rapidly, and recurrent episodes of pneumonia, otitis, sinusitis, dermatitis, meningitis, and osteomyelitis are characteristic. By contrast, these patients seem able to resist well many other infections such as tuberculosis, histoplasmosis, and fungal and viral infections. Herpes, vaccinia, chickenpox, measles, paralytic poliomyelitis, and hepatitis, however, are unusually frequent in these children. Leukemia also occurs with inordinate frequency in these children.

Even though immunoglobulins are virtually absent in serum and antibody synthesis is minimal or absent altogether, cell-mediated immunities, including delayed and contact allergies, are normal. Skin allograft rejection occurs with nearly normal vigor. Specific delayed allergic reactions can be transferred from the agammaglobulinemic child to an immunologically normal person, using large numbers of peripheral blood lymphocytes. Modern techniques for studying the peripheral blood lymphocytes reveal that X-linked agammaglobulinemia may be heterogeneous. The majority of patients with this disease are completely lacking B lymphocytes, as defined by the presence of readily demonstrable immunoglobulins at the cell surface. In these patients T cells are somewhat increased in number, and one finds in the blood a population of lymphocytes whose exact nature is not absolutely clear. The latter may possess receptors for the third component of complement and also receptors for the Fc portion of the IgG molecule. Whether they are incompletely developed B lymphocytes or a separate lymphoid cell remains to be determined.

Diagnosis is established by analysis of the immunoelectrophoretic pattern of serum and by quantitation of each of the several immunoglobulins, using the Manchini radioimmunodiffusion or other suitable immunochemical analyses. IgM, IgA, IgD, and IgE are regularly

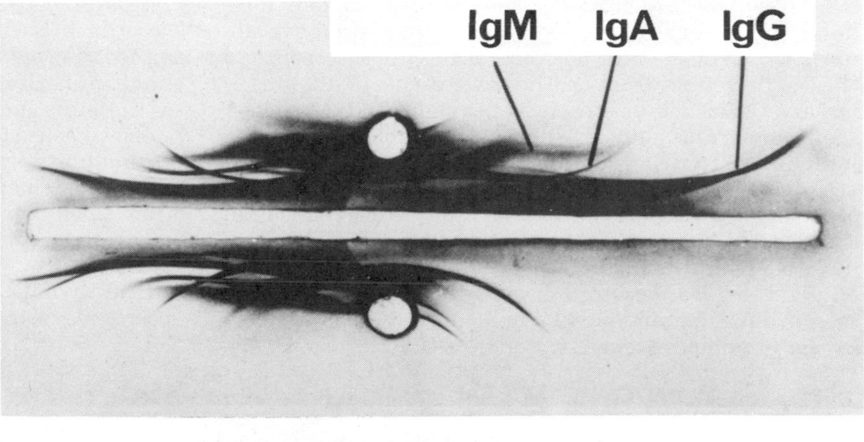

Figure 1. Normal immunoelectrophoretic pattern (above) compared with immunoelectrophoretic pattern from a patient with X-linked infantile agammaglobulinemia. Note absence of demonstrable IgM, IgA, and IgG on the immunoelectrophoretic pattern.

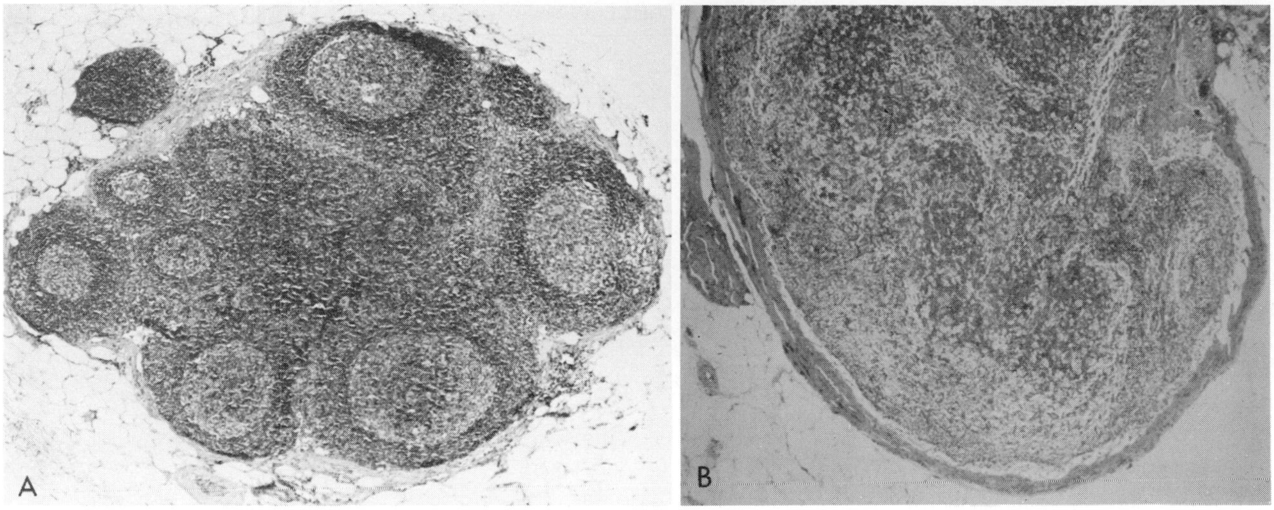

Figure 2. Comparison of normal lymph node *(A)* and lymph node of patient with X-linked infantile agammaglobulinemia *(B)* after antigenic stimulation. Note abundant germinal center formation in the normal node and absence of germinal centers in the stimulated node from the agammaglobulinemic patient.

absent, and IgG is absent or present in extremely low concentrations, 100- to 1000-fold less than that of normal persons.

Treatment involves early detection and intensive and specific treatment of the bacterial infections, as well as prophylaxis using gamma globulin concentrates injected intramuscularly at frequent intervals. We have found 0.3 ml of 16 per cent gamma globulin solution given intramuscularly every two weeks to be a good regimen with which to start prophylactic management. Exudative enteropathy is a common complication and is often due to infestation with *Giardia lamblia.* This infection and the exudative enteropathy can be treated specifically with Flagyl. The usual immunizations may be given, although no antibodies will be formed. Although vaccinia has been tolerated, we recommend that no live virus vaccines be used in any patient with primary or secondary immunodeficiency disease.

63. DiGEORGE'S SYNDROME

Counterpart to patients with X-linked agammaglobulinemia are those born without a thymus who as a consequence lack T lymphocytes in their blood and tissues. Such patients also frequently have no parathyroids. Their ears are often of abnormal appearance, and they have a characteristic facies with prominent forehead and bowed mouth. Frequently they also have abnormalities of the first portions of the great vessels and the outflow tract from the heart. Absence of thymus is not always complete. Absence of thymic shadow on chest roentgenograms and absence of T lymphocytes and T lymphocyte functions on immunologic analysis are characteristic. The stimulated lymph nodes show well developed far cortical areas, and in some cases germinal centers are present. In other cases, germinal centers have been deficient. In all instances, the thymic dependent lymphoid areas are very grossly depleted. Plasma cells are present and may be present in normal numbers in the lymphoid tissues. Absence of thymus and T cells may be incomplete. Treatment of the endocrinopathy requires appropriate use of vitamin D and sterol therapy to raise serum calcium level. The immunodeficiency has now been repeatedly treated successfully, using transplantation of thymus obtained from allogeneic embryos. This form of treatment has in several instances seemed to correct completely the deficiency of T cells and the defects of immunologic functions. Failure of thymus and T cell development of nude mice represents an autosomal recessive defect that seems to be an experimental counterpart of DiGeorge's syndrome. The cause of the human disease is unclear, and a genetic basis has not yet been established for this rare disease. Selective deficiency of thymic and T lymphocyte development without the associated hypoparathyroid or great vessel anomalies has been called Nezelof's syndrome. This disease has also apparently been treated successfully by allotransplantation of fetal thymus.

64. SEVERE COMBINED IMMUNODEFICIENCIES (SCID, Swiss Type Immunodeficiency)

Several different genetically determined primary immunodeficiency diseases in which both T and B lymphocyte systems fail to develop normally have now been described. Each of these diseases is genetically determined. Forms with either autosomal recessive or X-linked inheritance have been defined. Infants with each of these distinct forms of severe combined immunodeficiency disease have very gross deficiencies of both T and B immunity systems. Lymphocyte numbers, generally under 1000 per cubic millimeter, are low but not absent from blood. Both T and B cells are either missing or very much reduced. Levels of all classes of immunoglobulin are low.

The thymus, lymph nodes, and spleen are small and poorly developed. Indeed, these lymphoid organs are often almost completely devoid of lymphoid cells. Antibody production and development of cell-mediated immunities is extremely deficient or absent, and in vitro lymphocyte responses to lectins such as PHA, concanavallin A, and pokeweed mitogen fail to occur. In some of these children, responses of blood leukocytes to stimulation with allogeneic cells have been noted.

If these patients are not treated, they regularly succumb early in life to any of many different forms of infection, i.e., *Pneumocystis carinii,* cytomegalovirus, other viruses, fungi, or low- or high-grade bacterial pathogens. Live virus immunization often leads to lethal infections. Attempts to help these children, or children with DiGeorge's syndrome, by blood transfusion often leads to death from fulminating graft-versus-host disease, because these patients cannot defend themselves against the immunologically competent lymphocytes invariably present in whole blood. If blood or blood products must be given, they should be given only after irradiation of well oxygenated blood with 3000 R or after freezing and centrifugation.

Since both B and T immunity systems are lacking in these children, attempts to correct the immunodeficiency by transplantation of bone marrow have been made. In more than 30 instances, marrow transplantation from an appropriately matched donor has made possible apparently complete restoration of both T and B immunity systems in these children. Whenever definitive markers have been available, it has been possible to establish that the new immunity systems in such marrow-reconstituted children have been derived from the bone marrow cells of the donor. For successful marrow transplantation, a sibling donor selected by HL-A tissue typing and mixed leukocyte culture matching has generally been necessary.

More recently, however, in absence of a matched sibling, a satisfactory matching of an uncle by mixed leukocyte reaction with an SCID child has permitted reconstitution of immunity function. Recently techniques have been developed which promise sufficient matching, even among unrelated persons, to permit reconstitution of the two missing immunity systems in such patients by marrow transplantation with a donor selected from the general population. Definitive diagnosis and immunologic reconstitution of the rare children with this disease are highly technical undertakings that should be done only by those who specialize in this therapeutic approach.

65. SEVERE COMBINED IMMUNODEFICIENCIES WITH ADENOSINE DEAMINASE DEFICIENCY

An autosomal recessive genetically determined disease similar to the severe combined immunodeficiency disorders described in Ch. 64 has recently been found to be associated with absence of adenosine deaminase (ADA) in red blood cells, lymphoid cells, and other cells of the body. Clinical manifestations, immunodeficiencies, cellular defects, and susceptibility to infection in this disease are all similar to those occurring in the X-linked and autosomal recessive forms of SCID, except that, quantitatively, the functional and cellular defects seem more variable in this disease. In the patients with SCID and adenosine deaminase deficiency, however, some lymphoid tissue development does occur and the thymus contains Hassall's corpuscles and has characteristics of an involuted rather than an underdeveloped thymus. Two patients with ADA deficiency and SCID have now been reconstituted by marrow transplantation.

The relationship between ADA deficiency and this form of severe combined immunodeficiency is not yet clear, but it is of great interest that at least one primary immunodeficiency disease can now be associated with an inherited inability to produce an enzyme—adenosine deaminase. Whether the immunodeficiency is due to some toxic product consequent to the enzyme deficiency or whether this enzyme is essential in some crucial step in development of the lymphoid cells remains to be determined. When the immunodeficiency associated with ADA deficiency is corrected by marrow transplantation, the lymphoid cells possess normal amounts of adenosine deaminase, but the red cells continue to lack the enzyme completely.

66. THYMOMA WITH IMMUNODEFICIENCY

More than 50 patients have been studied in which broadly based immunodeficiency, thymoma, and hypogammaglobulinemia have been associated. The first such case provoked the extensive laboratory inquiry which established the major role played by the thymus in developmental immunobiology. Both cellular and humoral immunity functions, and both T and B cell numbers are deficient. Patients are susceptible to a broad range of bacterial, viral, and fungal infections. In one such instance encountered by Siegal et al., normal serum possessed a factor that permitted the patient's lymphoid cells to develop in vitro into B lymphocytes with easily demonstrable surface immunoglobulin. This factor was absent from the blood or serum of the patient with the thymoma-agammaglobulinemia syndrome. Anemia caused by insufficient generation of red blood cells may sometimes be associated. Removal of the thymus tumor which is composed primarily of nonlymphoid spindle-shaped stromal epithelial cells does not correct the immunodeficiency.

67. COMMON VARIABLE IMMUNODEFICIENCY

Among the most frequent forms of primary immunodeficiency disease is that presently called the common variable immunodeficiency. This rather cumbersome term is used as temporary nomenclature for what may indeed be several different diseases. However, in this form the immunodeficiency is variable from time to time in the same patient and from patient to patient in the same family. Inheritance may be autosomal recessive or autosomal dominant. In still other patients the disease is sporadic, and because of its onset later in life has been thought to be acquired. The initial agammaglobulinemic patient described by Bruton probably would now be classified with this group.

Immunodeficiency in these patients is associated with decreased concentrations of all or several immunoglobulins. Antibody production is feeble, and even cell-mediated immunity responses may be decreased. Pneumonia, sinusitis, otitis media, gastrointestinal infection and malfunction, and *Giardia lamblia* infestation are common concomitants. A wide variety of autoimmune phenomena and autoimmune diseases have been frequently encountered. Pernicious anemia, histamine-fast achlorhydria, and gastric cancer occur with high frequency early in life in patients with this syndrome.

The occurrence in these patients of much autoimmunity, autoimmune disease, e.g., Coombs-positive hemolytic anemia, autoimmune thrombocytopenic purpura, pernicious anemia, and many collagen-vascular or mesenchymal diseases, including rheumatoid arthritis and vasculitis, has represented a set of fascinating but perplexing relationships. Sprue-like syndrome with or without giardiasis is frequent.

Diagnosis is made by history of frequent and persistent infections, immunoelectrophoretic pattern, and quantitation of each of the immunoglobulin classes by radial immunodiffusion. Enumeration of T and B lymphocytes is of interest because, in spite of deficiencies in producing immunoglobulins, most of these patients have normal or only slightly reduced numbers of B lymphocytes in the circulating blood. Plasma cells are deficient in the lymphoid tissue in direct proportion to the deficits of antibody production and immunoglobulin levels. In patients possessing normal or increased amounts of IgM who have low levels of IgG and IgA, lymph nodes, spleen, and intestinal lymphatic tissue may be grossly enlarged. Germinal centers may be extraordinarily hypertrophied, suggesting the erroneous diagnosis of follicular lymphoma.

Treatment, as in other forms of primary immunodeficiency, involves early recognition and specific antimicrobial therapy of the frequent bacterial infections. Careful diagnosis and specific treatment of *Giardia lamblia* and fungus infections are also important. Prophylactic administration of gamma globulin concentrates in very large doses, 0.6 ml per kilogram every three to four weeks, is helpful in reducing the frequency of infections in some patients. However, in these patients even more than in patients with Bruton's X-linked infantile agammaglobulinemia, prophylaxis with currently available preparations of gamma globulin is inadequate. More satisfactory prophylaxis has been achieved, using frequent infusions of plasma from carefully selected donors free of history of hepatitis and free of both Australia antigen and antibody to Au antigen. The latter precaution is extremely important, because chronic progressive hepatitis has been an especially difficult and sometimes lethal consequence of administration of blood products to these patients. What is needed are adequate preparations of gamma globulin concentrates that are suitable for intravenous administration.

In addition to the more specific forms of therapy, prophylactic regimens such as those introduced by Mathews for the ideal pulmonary toilet are helpful. Postural and positional pulmonic drainage, breathing exercises, and inhalation therapy have all been helpful in treating and apparently in preventing pulmonary disease in these patients. The autoimmune diseases should be treated as they are in persons of greater immunologic vigor, but with cognizance of the facts that the patients are immunologically compromised and that large doses of adrenal steroids, immunosuppressive agents, and splenectomy can further debilitate the bodily defense.

68. ISOLATED ABSENCE OF IMMUNOGLOBULINS—SELECTIVE DEFICIENCY OF IgA

Selected absence of any of the immunoglobulin classes or subclasses can occur, and such selective deficiencies have already been described for several, e.g., selective absence of IgG 2. However, none of the other immunoglobulins are so frequently lacking from blood as is IgA. The frequency of selective absence of IgA ranges from 1/700 to 1/3000, according to studies of blood bank donors from several parts of the world. Many patients lacking IgA seem to be quite healthy, but a high proportion have severe atopy, autoimmune phenomena, and autoimmune diseases. Respiratory disease is frequent, especially in those patients who possess IgE. Gastrointestinal disease is also frequent, and severe progressive sprue has been reported. Recently Soothill and his associates have observed that classic atopy caused by production of antibody of IgE class occurs especially when the IgA system is slow to develop. One possible basis for the increased frequency of autoimmune phenomena and disease with deficiency of IgA is that the dimeric form of IgA antibodies is transferred across the epithelial barrier onto the gut surface from the site of production in the lamina propria of the gastrointestinal tract. This antibody system normally provides a barrier to absorption of foreign proteins and other antigens, as has recently been shown by Walker and Isselbacher. Consequently, when the local immunity system is lacking or deficient, antigens that are cross-reactive with host constituents can be absorbed and provide excessive stimulation of the systemic immunity systems. This stimulation leads to production of antibodies and immune cells that in some instances cross-react with host constituents, producing autoimmune phenomena and autoimmune disease. Patients lacking IgA frequently develop antibodies to IgA, serum proteins of the bovidae, and many other antigens in food and flora in amounts far in excess of those produced by normal persons. Most patients who fail to produce IgA antibody have in their circulation at least normal numbers of B lymphocytes that produce and have at their surface IgA molecules. For reasons currently poorly understood, these cells do not differentiate to IgA-secreting plasma cells. If these cells could be induced to develop to B cells capable of secreting IgA, these patients might be much improved. Recently Wu et al., using pokeweed mitogen, and Waldmann et al., using blast forms of putative T lymphocytes obtained from patients with Sézary's syndrome (presumably T-cell leukemia), have induced such differentiation of these IgA-producing to IgA-secreting B cells.

69. IMMUNODEFICIENCY DISEASES WITH ATAXIA TELANGIECTASIA AND WISKOTT-ALDRICH SYNDROME

Immunodeficiency diseases also accompany the Wiskott-Aldrich and ataxia telangiectasia syndromes. The former is a disorder of X-linked inheritance that is featured by a clinical triad, including eczema, thrombocytopenic purpura, and increased susceptibility to infection. The immunodeficiency in this syndrome is accompanied by low levels of IgM. These patients form antibody poorly to certain antigens, especially polysaccharide and small protein antigens, and show a progressive deficiency of T cell numbers and functions. The basic genetic fault is unknown, but the patients frequently succumb to infection with any of several viruses, bacteria, or fungi. Nearly 10 per cent of patients with the Wiskott-Aldrich syndrome die of cancer. Usually, but not always, the cancer takes the form of lymphoreticular sarcoma. Bleeding, especially accompanying infection, and intracranial bleeding are also frequent causes of death in these children. Treatment has thus far been unsatisfactory, but platelet transfusions and plasma infusions from selected donors have been helpful in some instances. Patients with *ataxia telangiectasia* also reflect a familial and probably autosomal recessive genetically determined clinical triad of progressive cerebellar ataxia, cutaneous telangiectases, and immunodeficiency. In this disease the thymus fails to develop normally and retains an embryonic appearance. T lymphocytes and T cell functions are regularly grossly deficient, and some 70 to 80 per cent of the patients lack IgA. IgE also is frequently absent from the circulation both in ataxia patients and in healthy family members. These patients are troubled with frequent sinopulmonary infections which seem to relate to the deficiency of IgA but not clearly to the deficiency of IgE.

More than 10 per cent of the patients with ataxia telangiectasia thus far studied have developed malignancies. The malignancics reported are predominantly reticulum cell sarcomas, lymphosarcomas, leukemias, and gastrointestinal cancers. Waldmann recently found that alpha-fetoprotein is present in inordinately high concentration in a majority of patients with ataxia telangiectasia (see also Ch. 446).

70. OTHER PRIMARY IMMUNODEFICIENCIES

Many other forms of immunodeficiency have been discovered in recent years, and the diseases and syndromes associated with them are only now being clarified. For example, selective deficiencies of the components of the complement system are associated with serious immunodeficiency in very high frequency. These deficiencies render the patients susceptible to infection, collagen-vascular diseases, overwhelming pneumonia, or skin and bowel infections, depending on which complement component is lacking. Ongoing studies will define these associations more clearly. It seems fair to predict, however, that deficiencies of each of the specific proteins involved in the defenses of the body will occur and that diseases have been or will be associated with these deficiencies. Such deficiencies will include deficiencies of each immunoglobulin class or subclass, deficiencies of essential lymphokines, complement components, and components of the major effector processes. The latter already include diseases in which malfunction or deficiencies of development of granulocytes occur, as in congenital neutropenia or chronic granulomatous disease. Deficiencies or abnormal function of monocytes or other cells and molecular elements involved in bodily defense are being defined. Each disease will represent an experiment of nature capable of teaching us a new lesson about how the immunity system functions. Each will require treatment, which will be made possible by the advancing knowledge of immunity functions and their organization and development. It is thus to be anticipated that the constructive interplay between clinic and laboratory will continue to produce new knowledge and to test our advancing understanding of the immunologic systems in the bodily defense.

Bach, F. H., and Good, R. A. (eds.): Clinical Immunobiology, Vol. 1. New York, Academic Press, 1972.
Bach, F. H., and Good, R. A. (eds.): Clinical Immunobiology, Vol. 2. New York, Academic Press, Inc., 1972.
Bergsma, D., Good, R. A., and Finstad, J. (eds.): Immunodeficiency in Man and Animals. Stamford, Conn., Sinauer Press, 1974 (in press).
Boder, E., and Sedgwick, R. P.: Ataxia-telangiectasia. *In* Goldensohn, E., and Appel, S. (eds.): Cellular and Molecular Bases of Neurological Disease. Philadelphia, Lea & Febiger, 1973.
Bruton, O. C.: Pediatrics, 9:722, 1952.
Cooper, M. D., Faulk, W. P., Fudenberg, H. H., Good, R. A., Hitzig, W., Kunkel, H. G., Roitt, I. M., Rosen, F. S., Seligman, M., Soothill, J. F., and Wedgwood, R. H.: Meeting report of the Second International Workshop on Primary Immunodeficiency Diseases in Man. St. Petersburg, Florida, February 1973. Clin. Immunol. Immunopath., 2:416, 1974.
DiGeorge, A. M.: Congenital absence of the thymus and its immunologic consequences. *In* Good, R. A., and Bergsma, D. (eds.): Immunologic Deficiency Diseases in Man. New York, The National Foundation Press, 1968, pp. 116–121.
DiGeorge, A. M.: Discussion of paper by M. D. Cooper et al. J. Pediatr., 67:907, 1965.
Dupont, B., Anderson, V., Ernst, P., Faber, V., Good, R. A., Hansen, G. S., Henriksen, K., Juhl, F., Killmann, S. A., Koch, C., Muller-Berart, N., Park, B. H., Svejgaard, A., Thomsen, M., and Wiik, A.: Immunological reconstruction in severe combined immunodeficiency with HI-A incompatible bone marrow graft. Donor selection by mixed lymphocyte culture. Transplant. Proc., 5:905, 1973.
Fudenberg, H., Good, R. A., Goodman, H. C., Hitzig, W., Kunkel, H. G., Roitt, I. M., Rosen, F. S., Rowe, D. S., Seligman, M., and Soothill, J. R.: Primary immunodeficiencies. Report of a World Health Organization Committee. Pediatrics, 47:927, 1971.
Gitlin, D., Janeway, C. A., Apt, L., and Craig, J. M.: *In* Lawrence, H. S. (ed.): Cellular and Humoral Aspects of the Hypersensitive States. New York, Harper & Row, 1959, p. 375.
Good, R. A.: Studies on agammaglobulinemia II. Failure of plasma cell formation in bone marrow and lymph nodes of patients with agammaglobulinemia. J. Lab. Clin. Med., 46:167, 1955.
Good, R. A.: Morphological basis of the immune response and hypersensitivity. *In* Felton, H., et al.: Host Parasite Relationships in Living Cells. Springfield, Ill., Charles C Thomas, 1957, pp. 68–161.
Good, R. A.: Immunodeficiency in developmental perspective. Harvey Lecture Series, 1972. New York, Academic Press, 1973, Vol. 67, pp. 1–107.
Good, R. A., and Bach, H. F.: Bone marrow and thymus transplants: Cellular engineering to correct primary immunodeficiency. *In* Good, R. A., and Bach, F. H. (eds.): Clinical Immunobiology, Vol. 2. New York, Academic Press, 1974, pp. 63–114.
Good, R. A., and Bergsma, D. (eds.): Immunologic Deficiency Diseases in Man. Birth Defects Original Article Series, Vol. 4. New York, The National Foundation Press, 1968.
Good, R. A., and Zak, S. J.: Disturbances in gamma globulin synthesis as experiments of nature. Pediatrics, 18:109, 1956.
Janeway, C. A., and Rosen, F. S.: The gamma globulins. IV. Therapeutic uses of gamma globulin. N. Engl. J. Med., 275:826, 1966.
Lawton, A. R., Wu, L. Y. F., and Cooper, M. D.: The cellular basis of IgA deficiency in humans. Proc. International Symposium on the Immunoglobulin A System. October 23–25, 1973 (in press).
Rosen, F. S., and Janeway, C. A.: The gamma globulins. III. The antibody deficiency syndromes. N. Engl. J. Med., 275:709, 769, 1966.
Soothill, J. F.: Interactions in immunodeficiency. *In* Immunodeficiency in Man and Animals. Stamford, Conn., Sinauer Press, 1974 (in press).
Waldmann, T. A., Broder, S., Suer, M., and Blackman, M.: Regulation of synthesis of immunoglobulins. Proceedings, Sixth Symposium on Plasma Proteins (L. Donato [ed.]). New York, Elsevier Publishing Company, 1974 (in press).
Walker, W. A., Isselbacher, K. J., and Bloch, K. G.: Intestinal uptake of macromolecules: Effect of oral immunization. Science, 177:608, 1972.

71. SERUM SICKNESS

Fred S. Kantor

Definition. Serum sickness is a disease characterized by fever, arthralgia, skin eruptions, and edema which appears after injection of a foreign serum or serum proteins and is dependent upon an immune response of the patient to the injected serum. Hypersensitivity reactions to a variety of drugs may produce an identical illness.

Etiology. With the advent of antimicrobial therapy, the use of serum for the treatment of microbial diseases has declined markedly; the most common cause for "serum sickness" at present is not serum itself but exogenously administered drugs, particularly the antimicrobials. Serum therapy is still used primarily for the neutralization of bacterial toxins such as tetanus and botulinus toxins and also in the form of rabies antiserum.

The incidence and severity of the disease are clearly related to the type of serum preparation as well as to the amount administered. Of patients given prophylactic tetanus antitoxin prepared in horses, approximately 2 to 5 per cent will develop symptoms of serum sickness. The figure is considerably higher for those patients receiving equine rabies antiserum; approximately 16 per cent of these patients develop serum sickness. In general, there is an increasing incidence and severity through childhood, adolescence, and adulthood. Reactions in children are quite mild, lasting from one to four days, whereas in patients over the age of 15, the disease is more frequent and more severe.

Different methods of production of various equine antisera may have a profound effect upon the serum sickness liability of the product. Most tetanus antitoxin preparations involve a peptic digestion which does not impair antitoxic properties while hydrolyzing many of the proteins present in the serum. In contrast, antirabies antiserum is not subjected to peptic digestion because of the great loss of antibody encountered with the enzymatic treatment. The most important factor concerned with the development of serum sickness is the total amount of serum administered. Recommended doses of tetanus antitoxin and rabies antisera vary considerably from time to time; from 5 to 10 ml of tetanus antitoxin may produce serum sickness in 5 to 10 per cent of patients, whereas 80 ml will almost always result in illness. Age and dose relationships in serum sickness resulting from drugs are not as clear cut as with serum or serum proteins. In most cases the drug by itself is not capable of inducing the disease and must combine with a protein of the patient to form a complete antigen or immunogen. In such a situation the genetic potential of the patient of forming complete antigens and producing antibodies to them must be considered in addition to the patient's age and the dose and duration of the drug given.

Mechanism. The essential basis of serum sickness is antigen-antibody interaction. A blood level of circulating foreign protein can be measured in patients shortly after beginning serum treatment. In the early stages the administered protein is catabolized in a manner similar to that seen in the animal from which it came. This is the latent period and usually lasts from four to ten days, during which time the patient develops an immune response that is evidenced by the appearance of antibody directed against the injected protein. As soon as antibody appears, it combines with circulating foreign protein antigen to form soluble complexes. These complexes have a varied fate, depending upon their nature and the ratio of antigen to antibody in the complex. Experimental studies, in the rabbit primarily, have shown a deposition of antigen-antibody complexes beneath the endothelium of blood vessels and within the basement membrane of these vessels. Complexes containing antibodies of the IgM or the IgG classes may initiate fixation and activation of the complement sequence. With localization of complement-containing complexes in the walls of blood vessels, polymorphonuclear leukocytes are attracted to the site and appear to injure the vessel by release of potent enzymes found in their lysosomal granules. The vascular injury mediated by complement and polymorphonuclear leukocytes may lead to thrombosis and hemorrhage, typified by the petechial or ecchymotic rash attendant on serum sickness.

Another manifestation of the interaction of antigen and antibody is the release of potent vasoactive materials such as histamine, serotonin, bradykinin, and slow-reacting substance (SRSA), all of which lead to vasodilatation and leakage of protein and fluid from the vascular space into the tissues, resulting in edema. The disease varies from species to species in laboratory animals. As most of the work has been done in the rabbit, it is pertinent to note that the renal disease, which is a frequent and important aspect of immune complex disease in the rabbit, is often nonexistent or a very mild component in the usual human patient.

Continuation of disease is dependent upon a continual supply of antigen. Removal by the reticuloendothelial system of the immune complexes is signified by a rise in serum antibody directed against the foreign proteins, and reduction of symptoms and signs of illness. Unless the foreign proteins are readministered, the disease is self-limited. During convalescence and for long periods thereafter, antibodies against the foreign proteins are readily demonstrable in the patient's serum. Readministration of foreign antigen promptly leads to formation of immune complexes and clinical manifestations of disease, which continue until antigen is entirely removed from the circulation.

Clinical Manifestations. The onset of disease is often heralded by itching and discomfort, frequently at the site of serum injection. Fully developed serum sickness is a miserable disease. The unfortunate patient lies on his side in bed with a swollen, distorted face, often resulting in closure of both eyes so that he cannot see, with a skin itching all over and often covered with an urticarial or erythematous rash. He is reluctant to scratch his skin because of the pain in all his muscles and joints upon movement, and so he lies quietly in bed suffering from headache, itching, and joint pain. Especially frightening and discomforting is the appearance of neurologic manifestations which may result in weakness of an extremity or a sensory deficit, or occasionally an isolated facial palsy. Compounding the patient's difficulties may be abdominal pain, nausea, and vomiting. Upon examination a generalized lymphadenopathy may be palpated, especially prominent in the regions draining the site of injection of the serum. At that site there may be a local rash with erythema and either urticaria or tenderness, and this may provide a potent clue for the physician as to the nature of the illness. Occasionally, auscultation of the chest reveals a cardiac arrhythmia or a pericardial friction rub. The spleen is usually not palpable. A common manifestation is fever of 38.3 to 39°C (101 to 102° F), and, in addition to the subjective complaints of joint pain, the patient may manifest objective arthritis with swelling, redness, and accumulation of fluid in joints. The skin may show a petechial or purpuric rash in addition to the more common urticarial eruption.

Laboratory Studies. Examination of the blood may reveal a mild leukocytosis, and circulating plasma cells have been observed. The sedimentation rate is usually normal or only slightly elevated. Eosinophilia occurs, but is relatively uncommon. The urine may show slight proteinuria, a few red cells, and occasionally a few casts; but there are rarely significant evidences of renal impairment. Examination of the serum proteins of the patient reveals circulating horse gamma globulins and macroglobulins present early in the disease, and predominantly anti-horse IgA globulin antibodies late in the disease and during convalescence. The development of antibodies to horse alpha-2-macroglobulin in the sera of patients recovering from serum sickness suggests that this component of the equine serum which lacks any antibody value could be deleted in manufacture without impairing the antitoxic benefits of the serum. Serum complement levels are reduced for variable periods during the disease and then return to normal.

Treatment and Prognosis. Very mild symptoms of pruritus and skin rash may be controlled by an antihistamine, such as brompheniramine, 4 mg given every four hours. Epinephrine and sympathomimetic amines have been recommended in the past for the treatment of the urticaria of serum sickness, and salicylates for the treatment of joint pains. However, for all but the mildest symptoms, adrenocortical steroids in the form of prednisone can be given with great safety and efficacy, and the patient need not suffer with less effective medications. As this is a self-limited disease with a natural course of one to three weeks, the usual hazards of steroid therapy are not realized before treatment is stopped. A treatment course of 40 mg per day for four or five days may be sufficient, even for quite severe disease. Symptomatic improvement appears often within hours of the onset of steroid therapy and sometimes is remarkable within 24 hours.

Prevention. Tetanus antitoxin prepared from *human* serum is now commercially available in many parts of the world. When this is available, there is no reason to choose horse serum to obtain antitoxic benefits. When equine sera must be used in treatment, patients should be carefully questioned concerning prior exposure and for allergic symptoms to other horse products, such as horse dander or horsehair, as found in horsehair mattresses. All patients, regardless of history, should be skin tested by production of a minimal wheal (0.01 to 0.02 ml) of a 1:10 dilution of the serum to be tested. After 15 to 20 minutes the skin site is examined for an urticarial wheal, and in its absence treatment may be instituted. If the patient is allergic and the necessity for serum treatment is great, desensitization may be attempted by repeatedly injecting small amounts of serum beginning in dilutions of 1:100 and doubling the tolerated amount about every 15 or 20 minutes until the appropriate dose is achieved. Such treatment is hazardous because of possible anaphylaxis, and the indications for it should be scrutinized carefully.

In patients who have developed serum sickness after tetanus antitoxin, active immunization should be begun during the patient's convalescence from serum sickness. It is generally advisable to immunize against tetanus all individuals who are seen by the physician in connection with unrelated allergic disease and found to be sensitive to horse dander or horse products. The immunization can be accomplished by use of tetanus toxoid.

Occasionally, in the course of serum therapy *an acute anaphylactic reaction* occurs, consisting of sudden vascular collapse, severe pruritus of the face, hands, and feet, often accompanied by bronchospasm and incontinence of stool and urine. Such events must be treated promptly *with epinephrine and not adrenocortical steroids.* A tourniquet should be placed proximal to the injection site of the drug or serum, and 0.2 ml of epinephrine injected into the site of injection which will slow absorption from the site. An additional 0.3 to 0.5 ml of 1:1000 aqueous solution of epinephrine should be given subcutaneously above the tourniquet if the patient has an effective blood pressure. In the absence of adequate blood pressure, the epinephrine must be given intravenously notwithstanding the hazard of production of cardiac arrhythmia, because the drug will not be absorbed from the periphery. After epinephrine administration, diphenhydramine (Benadryl), 50 mg, should be given orally or subcutaneously. The outcome of anaphylactic reactions is usually decided in the first few minutes; rapid restoration of blood pressure with prompt treatment is an excellent prognostic sign. Fatalities are few but tend to occur when the possibility of anaphylaxis is not considered *prior* to the administration of serum or drug so that effective measures are delayed.

Kojis, F. G.: Serum sickness and anaphylaxis. Am. J. Dis. Child., 64:93, 313, 1942.
Kunkel, H. G. (Chairman): Symposium on immune complexes and disease. J. Exp. Med., 134:1s-330s, 1971.
Vaughan, J. H., Barnett, E. V., and Leadley, P. J.: Serum sickness: Evidence in man of antigen-antibody complexes and free light chains in the circulation during the acute reaction. Ann. Intern. Med., 67:596, 1967.
von Pirquet, C., and Schick, B.: Serum Sickness. Baltimore, Williams & Wilkins Company, 1951.

72. DRUG ALLERGY

Fred S. Kantor

The value of therapeutic agents should constantly be weighed against their potential liability. Hypersensitivity reactions must be distinguished from two other untoward effects of drugs. The first is that of intolerance, in which the usual undesirable toxic effects occur at dosages of the drug well below that expected in a normal population. An example of this type of reaction includes visual disturbances and alterations in cardiac rhythm with very small doses of digitalis. The second form of drug reaction to be distinguished from hypersensitivity is that of idiosyncrasy. Whereas intolerance is a quantitative difference, idiosyncrasy is qualitative and is based upon a biochemical alteration in the way the patient handles the drug. Such a reaction does not depend on prior exposure to the drug, is not dose dependent, and does not resemble the other pharmacologic manifestations of the drug. An example of idiosyncrasy is the hemolytic anemia produced in patients with glucose-6-phosphate dehydrogenase deficiency when treated with primaquine. Altered reactivity (von Pirquet combined these two words to produce the word "allergy") on the part of the patient always follows prior exposure, even though this may not be apparent, and its mechanism is related to the hypersensitive state as reflected by delayed hypersensitivity or antibody production.

Incidence. Any drug may produce a hypersensitivity reaction, but some drugs have a much higher liability in this regard than do others. Digitalis and tetracycline have a low liability in producing allergic drug reactions, even though reports of documented cases have appeared. On the other hand, several of the antimicrobials, notably novobiocin, and certain anti-inflammatory agents, such as phenylbutazone, may have a high incidence of drug reaction. In addition to the variations produced by different drugs, equal liability is not shared by all patients for development of drug reactions to a single drug, such as penicillin. Patients with a history of allergic disease or previous drug reactions, as well as patients with certain inflammatory diseases such as lupus erythematosus, are generally thought to be more prone to the development of new drug allergies.

Pathogenesis. Certain therapeutic agents such as insulin are complex protein molecules which are known to be immunogenic. The majority of drugs represent classes of simple chemicals which require complexing with a tissue or serum protein of the patient in order to form an antigenic or immunogenic molecule. Drugs which are highly reactive chemicals usually are the most frequent sensitizers, and conversely the more inert members of the drug armamentarium are of less allergenic potential. Sensitization by means of a simple chemical involves the formation of covalent bonds with host protein which forms a hapten-carrier conjugate. Antibodies and hypersensitivity are directed against the hapten or the hapten and a closely adjacent portion of the carrier molecule, but never to the carrier protein itself. To form a hapten-protein conjugate, the administered drug may have to undergo considerable chemical rearrangement. This may occur during the metabolism of the drug, producing an antigenic determinant which is different from the administered drug. The necessity of chemical rearrangement of the drug to form the allergenic hapten-protein complex predicts difficulty of testing in vitro for drug allergy, because the laboratory must know what the antigenic determinant is.

Drug allergy has been investigated with respect to the antigenic determinant in only a limited number of cases. One of the most recent and extensive investigations has been in the case of penicillin and a derivative, the penicilloyl determinant. This has been labeled the major determinant, and as many as three—and perhaps many more—as yet undescribed chemical rearrangements may account for minor determinants, all of which can produce sensitization in given individuals and produce allergic symptoms upon administration of the drug. It should be borne in mind that not all drug immunization implies drug allergy. A good example of this is that all patients recently treated with penicillin will have developed antibodies directed against the penicilloyl determinant.

Hypersensitive reactions have been divided into *delayed hypersensitivity* and two varieties of immediate hypersensitivity: *wheal-and-flare* and *Arthus reactivity.* Serum sickness, which was discussed in Ch. 71, is an excellent example of an immediate type of hypersensitivity involving complement-fixing antibody and producing reactions to the so-called "Arthus" type.

The other type of immediate hypersensitivity, i.e., wheal-and-flare, is manifested in two major, clinically recognizable situations, urticaria and anaphylaxis. In these cases, the interaction of the drug-protein conjugate with IgE antibodies leads to release of active mediators resulting in vasodilatation and smooth muscle contraction. In this form of reaction, the hapten-protein conjugate and its respective antibody do not enter into the pathogenesis of the reaction but merely cause the release of the vasoactive material which produces the clinical effects. The last type of well-recognized mechanism is that of cellular or delayed hypersensitivity. In this form of immunity, circulating antibody is not important, and the interaction of the drug-protein conjugate is with sensitized cells, causing a release of a variety of biologically active materials which lead to perivascular accumulation of mononuclear cells and the development of induration. The best example of delayed hypersensitivity induced by drugs is skin sensitization resulting from direct contact with a variety of medications. Paradoxically, antihistamines, which have been incorporated into a variety of topical preparations for treatment of itching, burning, or allergic skin conditions, are themselves skin-sensitizing, and by combining with skin proteins form potent sensitizing agents which lead to delayed hypersensitivity and the development of the typical skin lesions of contact sensitivity. A combination of reaction types is often present in typical drug allergy, but one or another of the reaction types usually predominates and treatment is most efficacious when directed against this reaction type.

Clinical Manifestations. Fever may develop immediately after administration of a drug or, more commonly, may increase in a stepwise fashion after the seventh or eighth day of administration. The fever may show a sustained or remittent course and is usually low-grade in the range of 37.8 to 39° C (100 to 102° F), although hectic fevers are often observed, accompanied by constitutional symptoms. In general, the patient appears less ill than would be anticipated from the height of the fever. A drug reaction may mimic the septic picture entirely, but it usually pursues a more indolent course. Cessation of fever within a day or two of discontinuing the offending drug is to be expected. In some cases of fever alone, and if the drug reaction involves other organ systems, such as the skin and the joints, it may take several days, up to a week, for the symptoms to slowly subside. Penicillin, diphenylhydantoin (Dilantin), and barbiturates are frequent causes of drug fever.

Skin Rash. Skin rash as a manifestation of drug allergy may take several forms. A maculopapular, very fine rash appearing in the softer skin of the axillary line and on the extensor surfaces of the extremities and along the trunk may be unnoticed by the patient. Usually, urticarial rashes are reported because they are accompanied by pruritus. Persistent administration of an offending drug causing maculopapular eruptions may lead to confluent erythroderma and subsequent exfoliative dermatitis. Similarly, a rash may progress to an eczematous eruption with weeping papulovesicular lesions and ill-defined patches of erythema and edema, accompanied by intense pruritus. Erythema multiforme-like eruptions may be produced by a variety of drugs and are characterized by the formation of sharply circumscribed lesions that are usually symmetrical in distribution. The individual lesions seem to spread peripherally and clear centrally to form an annular pattern with secondary and tertiary rings evolving into a "target" or "iris" lesion.

Symmetrical lesions of the lower extremities closely resembling typical erythema nodosum may also be caused by drugs, including sulfones, penicillin, and iodides. The term "fixed eruption" is used to describe an erythematous and sharply defined lesion which recurs at the same site and in the same form upon re-exposure to the same drug. Withdrawal of the drug usually leads to healing, but hyperpigmentation of the area involved may remain. Photosensitivity reactions characterized by erythema, edema, and mild scaling are sharply limited to areas exposed to light, and a clue to the examiner may be provided by the **V**-shaped area at the neckline, usually at the site where the collar leaves the skin exposed to light and it becomes involved. Sulfonamides and thiazide derivatives are examples known to engender photoallergic reactions.

Other Organ Systems. Drug allergy is often manifested by reactions involving the hematopoietic system. Sedormid, a once popular sedative, resulted in thrombocytopenic purpura, which was shown to depend upon the presence of drug, a serum factor demonstrated to be antibody, and the presence of platelets. Several other drugs, such as quinine and quinidine, thiouracil, and the anticonvulsant hydantoin group, have been implicated as causes of thrombocytopenic purpura. Hemolytic anemia and agranulocytosis are also common adverse reactions ascribed to drugs. Sulfonamides and thiouracil have caused both types of reaction, but aminopyrine and phenylbutazone produced mainly agranulocytosis. Care should be taken in the interpretation of allergic causality of pathologic events leading to agranulocytosis or hemolytic anemia. One of the outstanding examples of a purported allergic hemolytic anemia was that induced by the fava bean. It was later shown that the presence of an enzyme defect in the red cells of these patients resulted in their shorter life span when exposed to drug and that sensitization in the immunologic sense was not required. Aplastic anemia, involving all the formed elements of the blood, is occasionally associated with drug administration; in particular it is described with chloramphenicol, gold, and the sulfonamides.

Gastrointestinal symptoms are common adverse reactions to the administration of therapeutic agents, but the mechanism of action is rarely allergic in nature. The kidney is involved in periarteritis nodosa caused by drugs. In this disease, antimicrobial drugs, notably the sulfonamides, have been frequently implicated. Interstitial nephritis has been described with the penicillinase-resistant penicillin preparation methicillin in association with hematuria, rash, and marked eosinophilia.

The lupus erythematosus syndrome has been described following ingestion of certain drugs, particularly hydralazine, procainamide, and the hydantoin derivatives. The severity of the syndrome induced by drug ingestion may vary from only a serologic manifestation, such as a positive lupus test, to the full-blown picture of fever, arthritis, polyserositis, and hematologic manifestations. Pulmonary infiltration and eosinophilia (PIE syndrome), peripheral neuritis, and hemorrhagic encephalitis have all been ascribed to allergic drug reactions, and probably represent varieties of allergic vascular injury resident in the particular organs involved. Liver damage has been attributed to treatment with heavy metals, thorazine, and sulfonamides; the evidence supporting the allergic basis of these reactions is meager. In recent times, the introduction of halothane, a potent, widely used anesthetic agent, has led to a series of symptoms, primarily involving liver dysfunction, which in some patients strongly suggest an allergic basis.

GENERALIZED ANAPHYLAXIS. Generalized anaphylaxis as a manifestation of drug allergy is a clinical catastrophe with which the physician must be prepared to deal promptly. The condition is usually initiated by an injected drug, although an orally administered tablet has been reported to produce a fatal reaction. Frequently the initial symptoms are generalized pruritus, particularly on the soles of the feet and the palms of the hands, and the general development of a hyperemia of the skin, particularly about the ears, so that the individual often looks as though he had acquired a recent sunburn. Angioneurotic edema may cause distortion of the face, swelling of the eyelids, and rapid loss of effective plasma volume, leading to vascular collapse and shock. The risk of developing an anaphylactic reaction, particularly to penicillin, is enhanced by the patient's having had a prior, less serious reaction, such as a maculopapular rash.

Diagnosis. Avoidance and challenge is still the best diagnostic means available to the physician, although it is often inadvisable because of the danger to the patient. Certainly in cases of anaphylactic reactions or urticarial eruptions, the challenge to the patient subsequent to the subsidence of the symptoms is not warranted and is extremely dangerous. However, in drug fever, when that condition appears alone, a fractional dose may be administered after the fever subsides to further identify the cause. Unfortunately, laboratory tests performed in vitro have been very disappointing. The basophil degranulation test, lymphocyte stimulation test, skin window technique, and others have been reported with some success from isolated laboratories, but in general they have been found to be difficult to reproduce and have not come into general usage. The necessary information concerning the intermediary metabolites of each drug and the development of specific antigenic determinants is not available for the majority of drugs which cause allergic reactions. Until this information is known, laboratory tests are not likely to be useful in this area. The leukocyte count may be high or low, and therefore not useful; eosinophilia is not a regular occurrence.

Treatment and Prophylaxis. Subsidence of allergic reactions to drugs usually occurs promptly after discontinuance of the drug, often within one or two days, but in many instances prolongation of symptoms for several days and, indeed, in some instances for several weeks and months, is well recognized. Many of our foodstuffs are contaminated with drugs: Chickens are fattened with estrogenic hormones, hogs are fed antimicrobials, and cows, when suffering from mastitis, may be treated with large doses of penicillin which appears in the milk. When strongly suspecting a drug hypersensitivity which fails to subside after cessation of the drug, inadvertent environmental drug administration should be carefully investigated. In general, treatment of the drug reaction should be directed against the altered physiology. In the reactions involving vasoactive substances, the use of a direct vasoconstrictor such as epinephrine may be lifesaving and should be used first, instead of the more glamorous, but less effective, group of adrenocortical steroids. The latter group of agents are very useful in the treatment of the Arthus type of immediate hypersensitivity as manifested by serum sickness and polyarteritis, as well as in many forms of delayed hypersensitivity. Epinephrine should be given in dosages of 0.5 to 1 ml of 1:1000 dilution of aqueous epinephrine, given subcutaneously. Antihistaminics such as diphenhydramine (Benadryl, 50 mg) or brompheniramine (Dimetane, 4 mg) may be administered orally or parenterally, but the intravenous use of diphenhydramine is to be avoided because serious adverse reactions to this medication have occurred. Drug reactions are self-limited diseases, and the use of steroids in these diseases is most efficacious and generally does not impose the usual liabilities of steroid therapy. Accordingly, therapy may be instituted with full doses of 40 to 60 mg a day, and 40 mg a day may be given for three or four days, dropped to 20 mg a day for an additional several days, and discontinued without a long tapering regimen.

Ackroyd, J. F.: Sedormid purpura: An immunological study of a form of drug hypersensitivity. *In* Kallos, P.: Progress in Allergy, Vol. 3. New York, Interscience Publishers, 1952, p. 531.

Chase, M. W.: Hypersensitivity to simple chemicals. Harvey Lectures, 62:169, 1966.

Demis, D. J.: Allergy and drug sensitivity of skin. Ann. Rev. Pharmacol., 9:457, 1969.

DeWeck, A. L.: Drug Reactions. *In* Samter, M. (ed.): Immunological Diseases. 2nd ed. Boston, Little, Brown & Company, 1971, p. 415.

Levine, B. B.: Immunochemical mechanisms of drug allergy. Ann. Rev. Med., 17:23, 1966.

Shulman, N. R.: Mechanism of blood cell destruction in individuals sensitized to foreign antigens. Trans. Assoc. Am. Physicians, 76:72, 1963.

73. ALLERGIC RHINITIS (Hay Fever)

Fred S. Kantor

Definition. Hay fever is the common name applied to allergic rhinitis which recurs each year at a specific season—usually spring or fall. It is characterized by rhinorrhea, sneezing, itching of the eyes, nose, ears, and palate, and edema of the nasal mucous membranes. Nonseasonal allergens, such as feathers and animal danders, may produce year-round disease called perennial allergic rhinitis; vasomotor rhinitis is a "wastebasket" term which designates perennial rhinitis without an identifiable allergic basis.

Etiology and Epidemiology. Susceptible persons exposed each year to airborne pollen of many varieties of plants, particularly trees, grasses, and weeds, develop a "wheal and flare" type of immediate hypersensitivity to protein components of the pollen grains called allergens. The exact hereditable basis of hay fever is still unclear, but clustering of a variety of diseases which involve "wheal and flare" hypersensitivity in certain individuals, and in families, strongly supports the view that such a basis exists. Recent evidence suggests that sensitivity to a particular allergen, such as ragweed, may be dependent upon transmission of a specific immune response gene and therefore might be predictable in an individual before development of the disease.

Drab, colorless plants, unattractive to birds and bees, must depend upon the wind for pollination and release of huge amounts of airborne pollen. In contrast, colorful blossoms and odoriferous plants generally release smaller amounts of heavier, stickier pollen which is not widely disseminated. "Rose fever," a form of allergic rhinitis prevalent in early summer, is a misnomer; while roses are visually in full bloom, it is the pollen from grasses such as timothy, June, and orchard grass which produces the disease.

Ragweed and grass pollen are the most common causes of allergic rhinitis in the United States. Ragweed abounds in the midwestern states, and is prevalent in the eastern and southeastern part of the country. West of the Rocky Mountains and in the dry Southwest, very little ragweed appears. Each area has a distinctive potentially sensitizing flora, and sufferers fleeing from one part of the country to another are often disappointed when symptoms rapidly reappear in their new location. In the northern United States early spring hay fever (April and May) is usually due to tree pollen; the grasses pollinate and produce symptoms in early summer (June and early July) and the ragweed in late summer and early fall. Spores of ubiquitous molds are present throughout the year but increase in numbers at different times because of increased mold growth on decaying vegetation. Spores of Homodendrum peak in number in July, whereas spores of Alternaria increase in the fall, overlapping the ragweed season, and may be the basis of an erroneous diagnosis of ragweed hay fever.

The trees are a varied and an important group; ash, beech, birch, cedar, hickory, maple, oak, sycamore, and poplar all produce important windborne pollen, whereas the less antigenic pollens of the firs and pines are not usual sources of disease. Each species of tree produces an antigenically distinct pollen with a relatively short period of pollination lasting two to four weeks. Hypersensitivity to multiple species of trees with overlapping pollinating periods, and to grasses, molds, and ragweed, may blur the seasonal aspects of the patient's problem and suggest a perennial allergic rhinitis. Unlike the trees, grasses such as timothy, fescue, orchard, redtop, and June (Kentucky bluegrass) share important antigenic determinants and in the extreme South and West may produce year-round symptoms. A careful account of seasonal variations in symptoms coupled with a knowledge of the flora of the patient's locality and the pollinating periods of the indigenous plants is vital to the specific diagnosis and management of this group of diseases. In the British Isles and the European continent, trees and grasses are important causes of pollinosis; allergic travelers would do well to check the season of their proposed trip. Europe has little or no ragweed, so American sufferers may doubly enjoy a late summer European vacation.

Pollen grains are about 20 to 40 μ in diameter, and each species has a distinctive appearance. By collecting grains on a glass slide with a simple timed exposure or with more sophisticated air-sampling devices, pollens may be identified and enumerated. The severity of symptoms of an allergic population will vary with the pollen numbers in an approximate way, but the use of daily radio broadcast pollen numbers as a diagnostic or predictive aid is of little value. The "counts" are derived from samples obtained the previous day, and at different locations and altitudes. Often the patient will ask why he doesn't feel better (or worse) because of the low (or high) pollen count!

Allergic rhinitis may be caused by any inhaled antigen; those often implicated, in addition to plant pollen, are house dust, feathers, fungus spores, and animal danders. Food allergy is often suggested as a basis for inhalant symptoms, but manifestations in the skin such as urticaria or angioneurotic edema (see Ch. 75 and 76) are the rule, and the respiratory tract is an unlikely target organ for this type of hypersensitivity.

Pathogenesis. Sensitization may occur at any time of

life but usually occurs in childhood or adolescence. It is curious that an adult may become sensitized to a pollen to which he has been exposed each previous year of his life; this suggests that factors other than genetic proclivity and exposure are necessary. When pollens impinge upon the nasal mucous membrane, they release a variety of protein antigens called allergens which initiate the immune response. The major allergens of grasses and ragweed have been partially purified and are low molecular weight proteins of relatively low antigenicity. This means that for a given amount of antigen, the immune response in terms of amount and avidity of antibody produced is small. The important point is that this type of antigen in low doses tends to elicit an unusual response characterized by production of reaginic antibody, which is largely or completely of the IgE class. Such antibodies are present in nanogram quantities in serum, and "fix" to the surface of cells so that passive administration will sensitize a particular skin site for weeks. Because of this quality, reaginic antibodies are sometimes called homocytotropic. Contact with the specific allergen will cause "sensitized" cells to release potent vasoactive substances, largely histamine and slow reacting substance of anaphylaxis (SRS-A). These materials cause capillary vasodilatation with leakage of fluid and colloid into the tissues leading to the major symptoms of allergic disease.

Although the symptoms produced by inhalation of pollen are localized to the mucosa with which it comes in contact, the sensitization is systemic. When peripheral leukocytes of sensitive individuals are exposed to allergen in vitro, they release histamine. This reaction affords a rapid measurement of sensitivity, usually expressed in terms of amount of allergen necessary to produce release of 50 per cent of the cellular histamine. It also provides an objective measurement of the efficacy and mechanism of treatment. Production of IgE antibody is not limited to allergic individuals; normal subjects or laboratory animals will develop this class of antibody response after subcutaneous injection of allergens. The presence of extracts of roundworms such as ascaris facilitates production of IgE antibody in an unknown way. Similarly, the nasal route of allergen exposure in an allergic individual facilitates development of IgE antibody. Nonimmunologic factors also play a role in producing what may be called the "inertia" of allergic disease; patients who are well tend to remain well, whereas those who are sick tend to remain sick. Nonspecific irritants of all sorts can cause incapacitating sneezing and rhinorrhea in a patient suffering from allergic rhinitis; these might be tolerated without a sniffle at another time of year. Upper respiratory infections, particularly sinusitis, occur more frequently in the allergic patient owing to edema and obstruction of normal drainage. Similarly, the normal effects of emotional states upon the nasal mucosa are often exaggerated in the allergic patient.

Clinical Manifestations. The abrupt onset of morning sneezing, usually in paroxysms of several sneezes in rapid succession, accompanied by rhinorrhea, itchiness of eyes, palate, and pharynx, are characteristic of allergic rhinitis. Symptoms recur each year at approximately the same time, corresponding to the appearance of the offending pollen in the air. Increased exposure will intensify symptoms: dry, windy days, riding in an open car, and working in a garden are frequently reported to worsen the symptoms. A hay fever sufferer notes that the morning and evening hours are the worst, with a relatively better period during the midday. Mucosal congestion and edema often lead to total blockage of the airway, necessitating mouth breathing. The conjunctivae are red and weepy, and the lids and periorbital tissues may be puffy.

Hay fever is not often accompanied by temperature elevations, and the name is therefore misleading. Fever should alert one to the common complications: sinusitis, otitis, or mastoiditis. Cough, wheezing, and dyspnea are frequent companions of allergic rhinitis. Because pollen grains are too large to affect the terminal bronchioles, it was thought that the allergic reaction in the upper respiratory tract could trigger lower airway obstruction, but recent studies indicate that pollen fragments small enough to reach the bronchioles are present in the inspired air.

Diagnosis. Early in the course, the differentiation of allergic rhinitis from that caused by irritants or infections is difficult, but in retrospect the patient will usually remember similar but milder symptoms at the same time in previous years. The seasonal history is the most important of all clues to correct diagnosis. Allergic rhinitis may be differentiated from viral upper respiratory infections when pruritus of eyes, nose, and pharynx is present, and by the absence of fever, sore throat, and malaise. The nasal mucous membranes appear swollen, pale, and boggy in allergic rhinitis, and red and "angry" in viral infections; but inflammation secondary to sneezing and frequent blowing to clear the nose may blur these differences. Nasal secretions may be obtained by asking the patient to blow his nose into a piece of ordinary wax paper; smears stained with Wright's or Giemsa stains show an abundance of eosinophils in allergic rhinitis, whereas in infectious rhinitis smears reveal polymorphonuclear leukocytes.

Environmental allergens other than pollen are more difficult to diagnose as the basis of allergic rhinitis, but a careful history will often elicit them. Inquiry should be made into the home: How old is it? What is the heating system? What are the floor, wall, and window coverings? What types of pillows, mattresses, quilts, and comforters are used by the patient and by his or her spouse? Frequently the nonallergic marriage partner will sleep on a feather pillow not five inches from the allergic one sleeping on a nonallergenic pillow. The question of what makes symptoms worse or better has a special significance in the allergic history. Often patients can specify a place or activity associated with symptoms which when avoided keeps them symptom-free.

Skin Tests. Since sensitization is systemic, the allergic individual reacts whenever contact with allergen occurs. Injection of minute quantities of allergens into the skin produces a wheal in 10 to 15 minutes in individuals with reaginic antibodies. Unfortunately, the presence of a positive skin test does not prove that the patient's symptoms are related to the allergen provoking the skin response. Often allergic individuals will have multiple positive skin reactions, such as to ragweed and grass allergen, but express symptoms in only one season and not the other. Skin tests are performed as either scratch tests or intradermal injections. Sets of skin test allergens are readily available and are often used indiscriminately. The patient may be tested with 200 to 300 skin tests with confusing results and erroneous diagnosis. A limited number of tests, 10 to 20, including house dust, common animal danders, feathers, common molds, and pollen, should suffice in all but the most difficult cases.

If skin tests are not diagnostic, why do them? They are often helpful in confirming a suspicion based on the history. The degree of skin reactivity in the untreated patient bears an approximate relationship to the degree of sensitivity and the amount of specific IgE antibody. Occasionally a positive skin test will point to a new direction of inquiry; e.g., a positive test to horse dander led to the finding that the patient was sleeping on a mattress with horse hair. Finally, when a decision is made to hyposensitize with allergen injections (see below), the degree of skin test reactivity provides guidance for a starting dosage.

Allergenic materials for testing and treatment are made by extraction of the solid allergen in a neutral buffer; usually a weight-to-volume ratio is employed, such as 1 gram of defatted ragweed pollen extracted with 100 ml of buffer producing 1:100 allergenic extract. In recent years, Kjehldahl analysis has led to standardization of extracts in protein nitrogen units (PNU) per milliliter. One PNU is equal to 10^{-8} gram N.

This "scientific"-sounding quantity may mislead the user, because only a small fraction of the extract contains the allergenic proteins and all the nitrogen is measured. Until the content of specific allergens is assayable, it is likely that the crude weight per volume or PNU per milliliter standard will be used. Extracts prepared in the same manner at different times may have wide variation in the amount of active allergen per milliliter. It is essential to be careful when using a new extract.

Intradermal tests are more sensitive than scratch tests and carry a greater likelihood of causing a constitutional reaction in a highly sensitive individual. Reactions are read after 10 to 15 minutes. A slight but definite wheal is considered 1+; a moderate reaction (wheal 6 to 10 mm) without pseudopods is read as 2+; a wheal of 10 to 15 mm with pseudopod formation is read as 3+; and wheals larger than 15 mm with a wide flare are read as 4+.

The initial intracutaneous tests with pollens should be made with solutions of antigen containing no more than 10 protein nitrogen units per milliliter, and not more than five to ten tests should be done at any one time. A minimal wheal (0.01 to 0.02 ml) is produced in the skin with a 27 needle attached to a tuberculin syringe. If little or no reaction is obtained, subsequent tests may be made with solutions containing 100 units and then 1000 units per milliliter. Reactions less than 2+ at 1000 PNU per milliliter are of doubtful significance in the untreated patient, whereas strongly positive reactions at 10 PNU per milliliter are almost always associated with symptomatic disease. The interpretation of positive reactions must be made in relation to the prevalence of the antigen in the area and the patient's history.

Passive transfer of allergic patient's serum to normal volunteers' skin will sensitize the site to antigenic challenge. Such tests, called P-K reactions (Prausnitz-Küstner), are useful when it is not possible to perform skin tests in young children, or on patients with generalized dermatitis. They are rarely done any more because of the danger of hepatitis and the availability of in vitro tests for histamine release and IgE measurement.

Treatment. Treatment is directed toward avoiding the allergen, modifying the state of hypersensitivity, and ameliorating the symptoms. By far the most effective means is strict avoidance of the offending allergen. When this is due to an increased sensitivity to an animal dander such as that of horse or cat, merely identifying the cause will help greatly in avoidance. Often patients will "hide" their pets from the physician's inquiry because they have a strong suspicion of the offender but hope that something else will be found. Effective filtration of the air within the patient's house is now possible with a variety of electrostatic and barrier-type filters. Dust control and attention to bedding and furniture filling will be rewarding in selected cases.

Treatment with repeated injections of specific allergens has been in vogue for 70 years, and recent studies have confirmed the efficacy of this mode of therapy and given insight to its mechanism. Preseasonal, coseasonal, and perennial administration of allergens all have their proponents, but perennial administration avoids the necessity of building up the dosage each year and results in the same number of patient visits. Increasing amounts of allergen are injected subcutaneously once or twice weekly, starting with a dose shown to be tolerated by skin tests. The goals of hyposensitization are two: production of a nonreaginic (blocking) antibody which can effectively compete with reaginic antibody for allergen, and reduction of the amount of reaginic antibody produced (tolerance induction), thereby decreasing cellular sensitivity to allergen. Addition of serum from a treated individual to sensitized leukocytes in vitro may increase by 100-fold the amounts of allergen necessary for 50 per cent histamine release from these leukocytes.

The increment of allergen injected at each visit is determined by the patient's skin reaction to the previous injection. If redness and swelling exceed the size of a 50-cent piece, the dose should be repeated or lowered until it is better tolerated. Often an increase in sensitivity occurs early in treatment; this may lead to a worsening in symptoms if it coincides with the patient's season. Usually patients are treated for two or more years after maximal benefit has been achieved, at which time hyposensitization is stopped. A proportion of patients will maintain their improvement whereas, in many, a slow return of symptoms during the following year or 18 months is common. Patients should always be advised to remain in the office for 30 minutes after the injection, because the allergen may provoke a constitutional reaction. This is often heralded by reddening of the conjunctivae, nasal swelling, red ears and nose, and a feeling of faintness. Tourniquets should be applied above the injection sites and 0.2 to 0.5 ml of aqueous epinephrine 1:1000 injected above the tourniquet. Such reactions are uncommon. They are usually easily managed in the office or clinic; but if the patient leaves the office immediately after an allergen injection, the reaction at best will be very frightening and might possibly be fatal.

A variety of repository allergen preparations, including mineral oil emulsions, and alum-precipitated allergens, have generated interest because of a putative ability to administer more allergen in fewer injections with less likelihood of systemic reactions. The efficacy and safety of these preparations are still to be determined.

Symptomatic Treatment. Antihistamines are often helpful in ameliorating symptoms of allergic rhinitis. In general they are only partially effective, and patients complain of the soporific side effects. Brompheniramine (Dimetane) and chlorpheniramine (Chlor-Trimeton) are both available in 4 mg tablets and in long-acting preparations containing 8 or 12 mg. Both these preparations seem to have less soporific effects than Benadryl, which should be used only at bedtime. Response to these drugs is often quite variable in different patients, and several preparations should be tried if results are poor or side effects great. Dexamethasone (Decadron), administered locally by a special nasal spray inhaler, delivers 0.1 mg per spray, and it is often efficacious. Its use once on each side twice a day is often all that is necessary during a short pollen season. The local effect without systemic liability makes this therapy attractive. Systemic steroids are very effective but are used rarely because of their considerable side effects. A short course of four to five days of 30 mg per day of prednisone will help a new patient over the worst symptoms before other measures become effective or the peak of the season passes.

A variety of sympathomimetic drugs, such as Neo-Synephrine, 0.5 per cent, phenylephrine, 0.25 per cent, or Privine, 0.1 per cent, have been used intranasally to shrink the nasal mucosa, but the effects are short-lived and all cause a "rebound" swelling of the nasal mucosa which may be a self-propagating disease. These drugs are not recommended in allergic rhinitis. For relief of allergic conjunctivitis accompanying pollinosis, eye drops containing epinephrine (0.025 per cent), or dexamethasone (0.1 per cent drops) may be used for a brief period with excellent relief. Prolonged use of steroid eye drops is not recommended because of corneal thinning and cataract formation.

Ishizaka, K., and Ishizaka, I.: Identification of γF antibodies as a carrier of reaginic activity. J. Immunol., 99:1187, 1967.

Lichtenstein, L. M., Ishizaka, K., Norman, P. S., Sobotka, A. K., and Hill, B. M.: IgE antibody measurements in ragweed hay fever: Relationship to clinical severity and results of immunotherapy. J. Clin. Invest., 52:472, 1973.

Lowell, F. C., and Franklin, W.: A double-blind study of the effectiveness and specificity of injection therapy in ragweed hay fever. N. Engl. J. Med., 273:675, 1965.

Samter, M. (ed.): Immunological Diseases. 2nd ed. Boston, Little, Brown & Company, 1971.

74. VASOMOTOR RHINITIS

Fred S. Kantor

Vasomotor rhinitis is a vague term describing chronic rhinitis without an allergic basis. It is indistinguishable from allergic rhinitis except for chronicity, absence of geographic or seasonal influences, and prevalence of coexistent nasal polyps. Frequently the patient has sought the use of sympathomimetic drugs administered as nose drugs such as Neo-Synephrine or Privine. The problem is compounded by the recurrent rebound rhinitis produced by these agents. Often they are the sole propagating cause of rhinitis which was once allergic or viral in origin, but which has become chronic through the use of these drugs.

The causes of vasomotor rhinitis have been ascribed to bacterial and food allergies, but documentation of these agents is meager and the mechanism is really unknown. Occasionally, a patient with allergies to a variety of ubiquitous substances may present without a clear-cut seasonal environmental history because of the overlapping allergens. These patients may recall a time when their symptoms were seasonal, and skin tests may be helpful in sorting out the problem. In general, however, the bulk of patients with perennial rhinitis at home or away, in summer and winter, will not yield a definite etiologic agent.

Treatment is symptomatic. If nose drops or sprays have been abused, it is useful to discontinue these agents on one side only for a few days and then on the other side so that the patient can breathe through the treated side while the other is recovering from the rebound effects of the drug. Antihistaminics such as brompheniramine (Dimetane), 4 mg every four hours, are sometimes helpful but rarely very successful. Some patients are helped by a nasal dexamethasone spray (Turbinaire) once on each side twice a day. This may produce relief without administering an effective systemic dose and thereby avoid the undesirable side effects.

75. URTICARIA

Fred S. Kantor

Definition. Urticaria, or hives, is an eruption of the skin characterized by elevated, erythematous, sharply demarcated wheals, usually intensively pruritic, lasting hours to days but often recurrent for weeks and sometimes years.

Etiology and Pathogenesis. The characteristic lesion is produced by capillary dilation in the dermis, leading to loss of fluid into the tissues. Swollen collagen bundles, widening of the dermal papillae, and flattening of the rete pegs are seen microscopically. It is useful to divide the causes into immunologic, paraimmunologic, and nonimmunologic categories.

By far the most common *immunologic cause* of acute hives is food allergy. In this circumstance, vasoactive mediators such as histamine, kinins, and slow-reacting substance of anaphylaxis (SRS-A) are released from mast cells, basophils, and other tissues, producing capillary dilation. The release of mediators is typically due to interaction of antigen with circulating, or fixed, reaginic antibody, usually of the IgE variety. This antibody can be passively transferred by the serum of an affected individual to the skin of a volunteer. A wheal is produced at the transfer site upon ingestion of the offending food antigen. This is the classic Prausnitz-Küstner (PK) reaction. Reactions of IgE antibody with antigen are not complement dependent and produce no vascular necrosis. Complement-dependent IgG-antigen interactions may also cause mediator release by cytotoxic action on mediator-containing cells. These reactions may be produced by antibodies directed against cell antigens, such as isohemagglutinins, and may also be due to antibodies directed against foreign antigens in which the antigen or the complex is passively affixed to the cell surface. The urticaria of serum sickness (see Ch. 71) is such an example. The most frequent route of antigen presentation in the production of acute urticaria is oral ingestion. Inhalation uncommonly produces hives, and occasionally contact with allergen on the skin may suffice. People sensitive to animal dander often report that contact with the fur or saliva of the animal may cause hives; patients allergic to bees may develop hives of the lips and mouth upon contact with honey.

The "paraimmunologic" causes are likely to involve similar mechanisms to those of the first category, but the relationship of the antigens and antibodies involved is less apparent. Infection with viruses, bacteria, and fungi may present with hives; hepatitis is a common example. Intestinal parasites, particularly the roundworms, are often associated with hives and eosinophilia. Bites of common insects such as mosquitoes, bedbugs, lice, and other biting insects may produce not only local manifestations but generalized urticaria. Neoplastic diseases, particularly lymphomas of the Hodgkin's variety, and the myeloproliferative diseases are commonly associated with hives. Finally, in the paraimmunologic category are the diseases in which immune complexes have been demonstrated and are thought to play an important etiologic role. In this group, hives are most often associated with systemic lupus erythematosus and dermatomyositis, but the palpable purpura of leukocytoclastic angiitis (Henoch-Schönlein purpura) may first appear as urticaria and then become purpuric.

The nonimmunologic causes of urticaria include physical stimuli such as cold, heat, actinic energy (solar urticaria), and pressure. Cold urticaria may be a familial or sporadic disease in which areas exposed to cold develop urticarial wheals. In about 50 per cent of the sporadic cases, a factor in serum is capable of "sensitizing" normal skin so that a wheal develops when an ice cube is applied to the site. Cold urticaria may be symptomatic of an underlying systemic disease; multiple myeloma, cryoglobulinemia, and syphilis have been reported. The mediators responsible for cold urticaria are presumed to be similar to those released by allergic reactions, but the mechanism of release remains unclear.

Solar urticaria is produced by two spectra of actinic rays of 3100 to 3700Å and 4000 to 5000Å in wavelength. Marked sun exposure in a sensitive individual has led to generalized vascular collapse. Urticaria to sunlight can be passively transferred by serum from individuals who are sensitive to the lower spectrum. The mechanism of mediator release is unknown but, unlike cold urticaria, treatment with drugs and barrier creams is quite effective (see below).

Certain drugs and chemical compounds have the capacity to cause mast cell degranulation directly, resulting in mediator release without an antigen-antibody reaction. Surface-active materials such as saponin, highly negatively charged molecules like polylysines, and many drugs share this property. Common drug examples are morphine, quinine, polymixin B, curare, decholin, hydralazine, and meperidine. Nonimmunologic release of histamine may be the basis of many "drug reactions" which have failed to yield immunologic mechanisms such as the rare reactions to radiographic contrast agents which are iodinated organic compounds. Indeed, the warm "glow" produced by good brandy is probably more a factor of mediator release than alcohol content, as any ethanol sampler can attest.

A special form of urticaria which consists of small, almost papular, wheals surrounded by a large axon flare is called cholinergic urticaria. Affected individuals will produce a similar eruption when injected with small amounts of mecholyl or acetylcholine. The mechanisms are obscure, but clearly emotional stress, exposure to heat, such as a warm bath, or exercise may bring out the eruption.

Urticaria pigmentosa, or systemic mastocytosis, is due to infiltration of the skin by mast cells; it is believed to be a true neoplasm of very slow growth in which the chemical manifestations are much more distressing to the patient than the invasive ones. Areas of infiltration are marked by freckle-like hyperpigmentation which, upon stroking, will produce a typical linear bumpy wheal, because the skin between the accumulation of mast cells does not urticate.

Chronic urticaria implies recurrent lesions for a period of six weeks or more. The clear causal relationship of certain foods to acute urticaria has led to the assumption that the chronic form is due to an extended exposure to an unidentified allergen or urticator. Investigation of such patients yields a single causal factor in very few, and the bulk of these patients defy elucidation of a specific etiologic factor. Many writers have emphasized psychologic factors in chronic urticaria, supporting their arguments with numerous cases of acute urticaria in response to a specific stress—a heavy date, an important examination, or the like. Although these factors must play some role, their magnitude in a particular patient is very difficult to assess.

Clinical Manifestations. Typically, the wheal is 1 to 5 cm in diameter, often irregular, with a blanched center ("target" lesion) and surrounding erythema. The individual lesions are evanescent, often fading within hours. Successive crops appear for the duration of the disease. The lesions tend to appear at pressure points—e.g., the belt line, the brassiere straps, or the garters. Rarely are the soles and palms affected; but when they are, the patient may complain of difficulty in walking. Pruritus is common and sometimes so severe that the patient cannot wait to get home and fling off his or her clothes. When urticaria is due to a single exposure to a food or drug, it usually appears within minutes. An ingestant taken more than 24 to 48 hours before onset is rarely the cause. Occasionally summation of two allergic stimuli may be responsible; e.g., some patients may eat frozen strawberries in winter with impunity, but during the pollen season the same strawberries will cause hives.

Treatment. Acute or sporadic urticaria usually responds well to antihistaminics such as brompheniramine (Dimetane), 4 mg every four hours, or tripelennamine (Pyribenzamine) 50 mg every four hours. If the patient is in acute distress, 0.3 ml of 1:1000 epinephrine subcutaneously will often provide relief until the antihistaminic effect is apparent. In severe or unresponsive cases of sporadic urticaria, four days of prednisone, 40 mg per day may be necessary and very helpful.

In chronic urticaria the cause is rarely evident and therefore hard to remove. Most patients have been treated with antihistaminics without benefit. The use of a rigid elimination diet may not only remove hidden allergens, but more likely may also remove foods such as spices which are direct releasers of histamine. In addition to the elimination diet, liberal doses of brompheniramine (Dimetane), 8 mg every four hours, and hydroxyzine, 10 to 25 mg three times a day, are helpful. After a period of relief, cautious reduction of the drug regimen and addition of selective foods in groups, such as eggs, milk, and milk products, one at a time every three to four days, will often result in cessation of symptoms. The result is frequently a grateful patient on a full diet; the doctor, however, remains perplexed.

Cold urticaria is often refractory to treatment with all the agents mentioned above, and often the patient has to adjust his life style to avoid the cold. In contrast, solar urticaria is readily treated with barrier creams that filter out the actinic energy of the appropriate wave length. Hydroxychloroquine (Plaquenil), 200 mg, once daily or even twice a week, may protect a sensitive person who anticipates sun exposure.

Beall, G. N.: Urticaria: A review of laboratory and clinical observations. Medicine, 43:131, 1964.
Sheffer, A. L., and Austen, K. F.: Urticaria and angioedema. *In* Fitzpatrick, T., Clark, W., VanScott, E., Eisen, A., and Vaughan, J. (eds.): Dermatology in General Medicine. New York, Grune & Stratton, 1971.
Sheldon, J. M., Lovell, R. G., and Mathews, K. P.: A Manual of Clinical Allergy. 2nd ed. Philadelphia, W. B. Saunders Company, 1967.

76. ANGIONEUROTIC EDEMA

Fred S. Kantor

Definition. Angioneurotic edema (angioedema) is characterized by painless swelling in the subcutaneous tissues or submucosa, usually occurring about the face (eyes, lips, tongue), but any part of the body may be involved. Two types are now well recognized: sporadic, transient angioedema, related to giant urticaria but involving deeper vessels, caused primarily by food allergy; and hereditary angioedema, which is transmitted as an autosomal dominant trait and is marked by severe deficiency in function of an inhibitor to the activated first component of complement – C′1 esterase.

Etiology. The causes of the sporadic type are the same as in urticaria (see Ch. 75) and most frequently involve food allergy, although occasionally an inhalant or contactant may be incriminated. In some, emotional factors can trigger an attack. A definite relationship between aspirin ingestion and angioedema has been documented in some individuals. Often asthma and nasal polyps are also associated. Evidence does not favor an immunologic basis for this syndrome, and the mechanism is unknown; the recently reported effect of aspirin upon prostaglandins may provide an important lead.

The lesion of the familial variety is indistinguishable from the sporadic type but is not related to hypersensitivity. Serum from affected persons who are heterozygotes (the trait is dominant) has very low inhibitor activity between attacks and often none measurable during the attack. In a variant of the disease the inhibitor is present but in an inactive form. Deficiency of the inhibitor is due to impaired synthesis, because catabolic rates in affected patients are normal.

Pathogenesis. Sporadic angioedema may be thought of as a variant of giant urticaria, with dilation of subcutaneous instead of cutaneous vessels and leakage of fluid and colloid into the tissues. It is generally believed that interaction of ingested allergens with reaginic antibody causes release of vasoactive mediators, including histamine, slow-reacting substance of anaphylaxis (SRS-A), and, possibly, bradykinins. Because the affected capillaries are deep, redness and intradermal swelling are not features. Respiratory and gastrointestinal symptoms occur rarely; the latter should raise a strong suspicion of hereditary angioedema, because abdominal pain is a common feature of the familial disease.

The relationship of the deficiency of C′1 esterase inhibitor to the attacks of angioedema is a complicated one. Attacks are associated with the presence of active C′1, depletion of its natural substrates which are C′4 and C′2, and elevation of bradykinin levels. In addition to inhibiting C′1 esterase activity, the inhibitor is known to inhibit kallikrein and plasmin. Kallikrein converts a serum alpha globulin to bradykinin; plasmin is a broad tryptic-like enzyme which digests fibrin, may cleave C′3 to produce anaphylatoxin (a vasoactive mediator), and may digest Hageman factor into active fragments which can convert prekallikrein to kallikrein. C′1 esterase inhibitor also reduces the capacity of active Hageman factor or its fragments to convert prekallikrein to kallikrein and to convert plasminogen proactivator to the active form. To sum up: the C′1 esterase inhibitor acts at several places, and its deficiency favors the formation of vasoactive mediators from the complement sequence (C′2a, C′3a) and indirectly from the formation of active plasmin and kallikrein.

Clinical Manifestations. The lesion is a tense, rounded, nonpitting swelling several centimeters in diameter which may last two or three days. In addition to the face, the hands, feet, and genitalia are often affected. In the familial form, laryngeal edema accounts for death in 30 per cent of the patients. Severe abdominal pain, vomiting, and the appearance of an acute intra-abdominal condition is common in the familial type and is an important differentiating feature from the sporadic variety. During abdominal attacks a characteristic pattern of bowel wall edema can sometimes be demonstrated in x-rays of the gastrointestinal tract. Attacks may be initiated after minor trauma such as tooth extraction, supporting the relationship to the clotting mechanism and the role of Hageman factor activation.

Diagnosis. The sudden appearance of profound swelling without trauma or underlying infection is strongly suggestive of angioneurotic edema. Accompanying urticaria or a history of food allergy is helpful, but an inapparent insect bite can sometimes cause swelling of the eyelid or lip and must be considered. The familial form often presents with abdominal complaints accompanying the subcutaneous swelling, and laryngeal edema is also frequently noted. Symptoms of hereditary angioedema may rarely first appear in adult life, and the presence of active C′1 esterase inhibitor should be confirmed in any case involving laryngeal edema or abdominal complaints.

Prognosis. The sporadic variety tends to recur either because all the causative factors are not identified, or, more likely, because the patient "cheats" and samples a forbidden food. The hereditary form of the disease is often fatal in early life, although not before reproductive age.

Treatment. Like urticaria, sporadic angioedema is treated with epinephrine, 0.3 to 0.5 ml, 1:1000, or an aqueous solution containing crystalline epinephrine 1:200 (Susphrine), 0.6 to 0.8 ml, given in conjunction with antihistamines. Brompheniramine (Dimetane), 4 mg, tripelennamine (Pyribenzamine), 50 mg, or diphenhydramine (Benadryl), 50 mg, may be given every four hours. Resolution is slow, because resorption of tissue fluid is required. Prednisone, 40 mg per day, may be given for three to four days in severe or prolonged cases. The patient should be carefully questioned about activities within the 12- to 24-hour period preceding the onset, with special reference to items passing the lips such as food, chewing gum, toothpaste, or aspirin. Usually the patient knows the culprit.

In the hereditary form of disease the aforementioned measures are useless. Poor responses to epinephrine, antihistamine, and corticosteroids are well documented. Some salutary effects of methyltestosterone have been claimed, but recent controlled studies revealed that epsilon-aminocaproic acid (EACA), a potent plasmin inhibitor, prevented or ameliorated attacks when given in doses of 7 to 16 grams per day. The mechanism is unknown. Plasmin may activate C′1, producing the clinical attack, and the drug works by inhibiting plasmin. Infusions of plasma have had only limited trials, because, in addition to providing the inhibitor, plasma contains more substrate for the activated enzymes and could theoretically produce adverse effects.

Fink, A. I., and Gay, L. N.: A critical review of 170 cases of urticaria and angioneurotic edema followed for a period of from two to ten years. Bull. Johns Hopkins Hosp., 55:280, 1934.

Ruddy, S., Gigli, I., and Austen, K. F.: The complement system of man. N. Engl. J. Med. 287:489, 1972.

Thompson, J. S.: Urticaria and angioedema. Ann. Intern. Med., 69:361, 1968.

77. INSECT STINGS

Fred S. Kantor

Allergy to antigens contained in the venom of the Hymenoptera insects (bee, wasp, hornet, yellow jacket) may produce a fatal reaction when an otherwise healthy victim is stung. Often a history is obtained of a previous sting which produced local swelling more extensive and longlasting than usual. The patient may rapidly develop shock with or without respiratory difficulty, urticaria, or angioedema, and prompt treatment is vital. If the site of the sting is known, and on an extremity, a tourniquet should be placed above the site to delay further absorption of venom. Epinephrine, 1:1000, 0.3 to 0.5 ml, should be given subcutaneously. If the patient is in shock, the intravenous route must be used, despite the hazard of arrhythmia, to ensure absorption of the drug. Bees have barbed stingers and leave the stinger and venom sac at the site. These should be removed with a forceps or scraped off with the edge of a fingernail so that the venom remaining in the venom sac is not injected through the stinger into the patient. Antihistaminics and steroids are given as adjuncts to epinephrine as described in Ch. 76.

After the acute episode is controlled and before leaving, the patient should be given an emergency kit which contains two tourniquets (stings may be multiple), forceps, or an eyebrow tweezer, a syringe for epinephrine injection (1 ml, 1:1000), and antihistamine tablets. If restung, the patient is instructed to place the tourniquet above the site, take one antihistaminic tablet (diphenhydramine [Benadryl], 50 mg), and prepare the epinephrine syringe while obtaining help from others. Muscular activity enhances the rate of absorption of venom; the patient should be urged to walk, not run, toward help. Since a generalized reaction may lead to temporary skin-test refractoriness, the patient is urged to return in three weeks for testing and hyposensitization treatment. This is clearly effective in preventing fatal reactions upon subsequent exposure in the majority of patients. Results of treatment and a wider discussion of insect stings may be found in the November, 1973, issue of The Journal of Allergy and Clinical Immunology.

Part V

CONNECTIVE TISSUE DISEASES ("COLLAGEN DISEASES") OTHER THAN RHEUMATOID ARTHRITIS

78. INTRODUCTION

K. Frank Austen

The connective tissue ("collagen") diseases or systemic rheumatic diseases are a group of clinicopathologic entities considered together because of common or overlapping clinical and histologic features. The term "collagen diseases" was introduced by Klemperer for such reasons and not because of any conviction about a common etiology. Each of the major entities within this grouping has prominent nonspecific constitutional manifestations coupled with patterns of organ involvement which determine the clinical designation, i.e., rheumatoid arthritis, rheumatic fever, systemic lupus erythematosus, scleroderma, dermatomyositis, and periarteritis nodosa (polyarteritis nodosa). Except for rheumatic fever (see Ch. 191), these entities are considered in this Part and in Part VI. The common histologic features of the group are widespread inflammatory damage to connective tissues and blood vessels, at times associated with deposition of fibrinoid material. Fibrinoid refers to an amorphous material staining deeply eosinophilic with hematoxylin and eosin, which is deposited along connective tissue fibers and within vessel walls, and most probably represents a nonspecific response of connective tissue to injury. Clinical findings which have been invoked to support a common grouping include cardinal features of more than one entity in the same patient; transitions between one entity and another within the same patient; possible familial aggregation; and serologic abnormalities which may predominate in one entity but have an appreciable incidence in others.

Progressive systemic sclerosis (scleroderma), polymyositis alone or with cutaneous manifestations (dermatomyositis), and systemic lupus erythematosus (SLE) have distinct clinicopathologic and/or serologic features. By contrast, periarteritis nodosa has neither a characteristic morphologic, biochemical, or immunochemical abnormality nor a clinical presentation that is easily distinguished from systemic necrotizing angiitis of other types, including those which may be associated with any of the other connective tissue diseases. It seems pertinent, therefore, to review historically the problem of necrotizing angiitis and to include an operational classification based almost entirely upon clinical considerations. Detailed consideration of the structure and function of the structural proteins, collagen and elastin, ground substance, and cellular elements of connective tissue is presented first.

CONNECTIVE TISSUE

Connective tissues are composed of various combinations of collagen, elastin, proteoglycans, and other less well characterized glycoproteins. The unique proportions and distribution of these individual components give different organs of connective tissue their particular qualities. The proteoglycans and the specific arrangement of collagen fibers at various layers give cartilage its smooth, translucent quality and its toughness with elasticity; in contrast, bone has a lesser amount of proteoglycans and a rigid structure related to mineralization within and around collagen fibers. The lens of the eye is transparent because of the precise planes in which collagen fibrils are laid down. Skin and blood vessels are rich in elastin which confers upon these tissues a capacity for distensibility. Basement membrane, a specialized form of collagen and glycoprotein, separates epithelium and endothelium from their environment in multiple tissues. Only in very rare diseases is a primary abnormality of the connective tissue responsible for symptoms or pathology. However, in all forms of arthritis or vasculitis the connective tissues are the site in which inflammation occurs. Although playing a passive, secondary role in pathophysiology, it is damage to connective tissue that results in the signs and symptoms of disease.

Collagen is synthesized by fibroblasts, chondrocytes, and osteoblasts. Different genes code for synthesis of distinct collagen polypeptides in different organs. Thus skin and bone collagens are triple helical structures with two similar α chain polypeptides (α1 [I]) and one α2 polypeptide chain, whereas cartilage collagen is composed of three α1 (II) chains which have a different primary sequence. Collagen α chains are synthesized on polyribosomes as a procollagen. The pro-α chains of collagen undergo hydroxylation of numerous proline residues to give hydroxyproline and certain lysine residues to yield hydroxylysine; several of the hydroxylysine residues are then glycosylated. Procollagen has an additional peptide attached to the amino terminus which is cleaved off when pro-α chains are released from the cell. The hydroxylated glycosylated collagen molecule then precipitates with other similar molecules in precise register to form collagen fibrils. This precise register gives the 640 to 700 Å periodicity on electron microscopy characteristic of collagen fibrils. After fibril formation an additional change in primary structure of the molecule occurs, that of cross-linking within and between different molecules. Cross-links are derived by oxidation and aldol condensation between lysine, hydroxylysine, and histidine residues on adjacent polypeptide chains of the same molecule and on other molecules as well. Cross-linking makes collagen more stable and may retard its susceptibility to specific collagenases.

Recently synthesized collagen has a more rapid turnover than mature collagen. Since hydroxyproline is present only in collagen and elastin, and since collagen is the most abundant protein in the body, the excretion of urinary hydroxyproline serves as a rough index of collagen turnover. Collagen is degraded by collagenases, present in mesenchymal tissues and in certain epithelial tissues, which cleave through one site on each collagen triple helix. The reaction products uncoil, are thermally denatured at body temperature, and become immediately susceptible to multiple tissue proteases. In rheumatoid arthritis and certain skin and bone diseases, proliferation of cells which synthesize collagenase may result in excessive destruction of collagen.

The so-called "collagen diseases" are not primary diseases of collagen, and there are few examples of true collagen disease. In *dermatosparaxis,* a disease of calves, procollagen is not cleaved to collagen, and the resulting fibrils in the skin lack tensile strength, allowing the animals to become denuded. In humans, a heritable disease with an expression similar to Ehlers-Danlos syndrome occurs in which the enzyme activity which hydroxylates lysine to form hydroxylysine in collagen and other proteins is markedly decreased. In *homocystinuria* an abnormal collagen may be formed because significant quantities of homocysteine inhibit cross-link formation between collagen molecules. Ascorbic acid is one of the cofactors (along with ferrous iron and α-ketoglutarate) essential for hydroxylation of proline and lysine residues in collagen; since poorly hydroxylated collagen forms a less stable helix, this may explain the decrease in tensile strength of healing wounds in ascorbic acid deficiency (scurvy).

Basement membranes provide elastic support and act as a filtration barrier between epithelial and endothelial cells and their environment. The amino acid composition of basement membrane resembles that of collagen except that it has a high concentration of carbohydrate, many sulfur-containing amino acids, and very high concentrations of hydroxylysine relative to other collagens.

Proteoglycans have a role in connective tissue not unlike that of cement in reinforced concrete. The proteoglycans are formed of subunits of disaccharides linked together and joined to a protein core. In articular cartilage this core is a protein with a length of 20,000 to 50,000 Å. The disaccharide chains, many of which are sulfated, have a length of 15,000 to 36,000 Å. Each proteoglycan subunit (core protein plus disaccharide chains) is joined with others to form large aggregates by a link glycoprotein. The physiologic implications of this macromolecular organization are probably related to the excluded volume effect; that is, in connective tissue, they control by virtue of size and domain the passage of other molecules to and from cells. In the polysaccharide component of proteoglycans one of the hexose residues of each disaccharide group is a hexosamine, and the other is a uronic acid or galactose moiety. Proteoglycans are synthesized by mesenchymal tissues by a complicated process involving assembly of the polysaccharide units, sulfation, and covalent linkage to the protein core.

Proteoglycans have a more rapid turnover than collagen and are degraded primarily by acid hydrolases found in lysosomes. Factors such as vitamin A which destabilize lysosomal membranes can result in generalized depletion of proteoglycans from many connective tissues. Proteoglycan destruction is accentuated by products of the inflammatory cells in the connective tissue, but there is no evidence to suggest that there is a primary abnormality of the proteoglycans in the "collagen" diseases. A possible exception may be *degenerative* or *osteoarthritis* in which increased autolysis of proteoglycans by chondrocytes may be an initial factor.

Elastin has covalent cross-links, desmosine and isodesmosine, which are similar to cross-links in collagen and are formed from condensation of lysine residues on different parts of the same chain or other elastin polypeptides. Unlike collagen, which is a rigid rod, elastin is an amorphous random coil aggregate linked by these cross-links; this structure assures its return to an original configuration after it is distorted and gives rise to its elastic properties.

HISTORICAL REVIEW OF ANGIITIS

The term *periarteritis nodosa* was aptly introduced by Kussmaul and Maier in 1866 to designate a morbid process manifested by numerous nodules along muscular-type arteries. Infiltration of the media with polymorphonuclear leukocytes and to a lesser extent eosinophils, plasma cells, and lymphocytes, disruption of the internal elastic lamina, fibrinoid necrosis, and extension to the adventitia and intima are characteristic. Proliferation of the intima leads to partial or total occlusion, and segmental scarring of the entire wall is responsible for the visible and/or palpable aneurysms. It is characteristic of the lesions to be in all stages of evolution from acute to healed. Additional characteristic features of periarteritis nodosa are the sparing of capillaries and veins except for involvement by spread from contiguous arteries, and the absence of involvement of pulmonary arteries despite the location of nodules in the bronchial arteries.

In 1923 Ophüls reported a patient with a periarteritis nodosa–like illness with the additional features of pulmonary vessel lesions, extensive involvement of small arteries and veins, granulomatous vascular and extravascular reactions, and an intense eosinophilic infiltration of vascular and pulmonary parenchymal lesions. The granulomas often included an eosinophilic core of altered collagen and necrotic eosinophils surrounded by radially arranged macrophages, lymphocytes, plasma cells, and varying numbers of polymorphonuclear leukocytes, both neutrophilic and eosinophilic. A detailed study of similar patients in 1951 by Churg and Strauss emphasized the striking clinical feature of severe progressive asthma with peripheral eosinophilia followed by fever, and prompted these authors to term this entity *allergic angiitis and granulomatosis.* Rose and Spencer (1957) also appreciated these unique clinicopathologic features but preferred the term polyarteritis with pulmonary involvement to distinguish this group from classic polyarteritis.

In 1926 von Glahn and Pappenheimer considered that the *arteritis of rheumatic fever* could be distinguished from periarteritis nodosa by the absence of arterial thrombosis (or eosinophils), involvement of small arteries, and minimal fibrinoid necrosis. In the heart, Aschoff bodies represent a key extravascular histologic finding, although the clinical manifestations are predominantly related to rheumatic carditis.

Still another type of necrotizing vascular lesion, originally believed to be limited to the cranial arteries and characterized by the presence of multinucleated giant cells, was recognized by Horton, Magath, and Brown in 1934 and established as a clinical entity by Kilbourne and Wolff in 1946. The process usually involves the innermost layer of the media with predominantly a lymphocyte infiltration, the presence of multinucleated giant cells, fragmentation of the internal elastic lamina, and associated fibrinoid necrosis. The infiltration may extend to involve the adventitia and the intima, leading to intimal thickening with subsequent thrombosis. This entity, *giant cell arteritis,* can be predominantly local—presenting as cranial, especially temporal, or aortic arch (Takayasu's) arteritis—or it may be systemic. The syndrome of polymyalgia rheumatica seems to be associated with a local or systemic form of giant cell arteritis with or without arterial occlusion.

Necrotizing vascular lesions associated with the administration of horse antiserum and the development of clinical serum sickness were described by Clark and Kaplan in 1937. Rich observed similar lesions (1942) which he considered to be periarteritis nodosa not only in cases of serum sickness but also in circumstances of sulfonamide hypersensitivity. However, the more recent and prevailing view proposed by Zeek in 1952 is that hypersensitivity to drugs and serum, termed *hypersensitivity angiitis,* is distinguishable from periarteritis nodosa. Hypersensitivity angiitis involves small arteries, arterioles, and venules in a process of fibrinoid necrosis, occurring in the subendothelial ground substance and extending from the intima to involve the entire vessel wall; the accompanying cellular reaction is pleomorphic with polymorphonuclear leukocyte predominance frequently including eosinophils. Hypersensitivity angiitis often involves the pulmonary system and is characterized by virtually all lesions being at a similar evolutionary stage.

An unresolved issue is whether or not allergic granulomatosis and angiitis as defined by Churg and Strauss encompasses *Wegener's granulomatosis.* This disease, described by Wegener in 1936, is characterized by necrotizing granulomatous lesions of the upper and lower respiratory tract, generalized focal necrotizing lesions of both arteries and veins, and a glomerulitis typified by fibrin thrombi, focal necrosis of tufts, and on occasion a granulomatous reaction. This complex is somewhat similar to allergic granulomatosis and angiitis, but it is noteworthy that Wegener's granulomatosis is not associated with progressive asthma and prominent peripheral eosinophilia and does not exhibit a prominence of eosinophils in the necrotizing lesions. Thus for the present it seems reasonable to list this entity separately; lethal midline granuloma may be a related condition or a local variant. (See Ch. 105.) More recently, variants of Wegener's granulomatosis have been recognized in which the granulomatous reactions are predominantly lymphoid- and sarcoid-like, respectively.

The final category includes miscellaneous entities. Atrophic malignant papulosis, described by Degos in 1954, refers to a characteristic clinical triad associated with necrotizing vascular lesions of the skin, gastrointestinal tract, and brain. Erythema elevatum diutinum is manifested by a chronic erythematous-papular and often purpuric skin eruption with or without systemic signs such as arthritis; it will probably be shifted to the hypersensitivity angiitis group when more information is available. A variety of purely cutaneous vasculitis syndromes have been described, and only time will tell whether these are distinct or are merely limited manifestations of a systemic entity.

OPERATIONAL CLASSIFICATION OF NECROTIZING ANGIITIS

Necrotizing angiitis is a convenient generic term for the entire group of syndromes in which vascular lesions, arterial or venous or both, may involve all three layers of the vessel wall with fibrinoid necrosis and various cellular infiltrates (see accompanying table). The clinical manifestations are caused largely by partial or complete vascular occlusion; the lesions are segmental, and the clinical patterns depend on the size and characteristic distribution of the lesions. Zeek recognized five major syndromes in this group: periarteritis nodosa, allergic angiitis and granulomatosis, rheumatic fever, giant cell arteritis, and hypersensitivity angiitis. With some modification this tabulation continues to be operationally useful.

Rheumatic fever can be placed under a category broadened to include those collagen diseases in which necrotizing vascular lesions are present but are not the most prominent aspect of the entity, i.e., rheumatoid arthritis, scleroderma, dermatomyositis, polymyositis, Sjögren's syndrome, and erythema nodosum. The category of hypersensitivity angiitis is particularly diverse and contains a variety of clinical entities distinguishable on the basis of precipitating events, serologic abnormalities, and relative frequency of involvement of various organ systems—drug reactions, Henoch-Schönlein purpura, serum sickness, systemic lupus erythematosus, mixed cryoglobulinemia (IgG-IgM complexes), hypergammaglobulinemic purpura, C2 deficiency with vasculitis, occasional instances of chronic urticaria, and Goodpasture's syndrome. The problems of any effort at

Necrotizing Angiitis

Periarteritis nodosa (polyarteritis nodosa)

Allergic angiitis and granulomatosis of Churg and Strauss
  ("polyarteritis nodosa with pulmonary involvement")

Connective tissue disease ("collagen disease"), associated with
- Rheumatoid arthritis
- Scleroderma
- Poly- and dermatomyositis
- Rheumatic fever
- Erythema nodosum
- Sjögren's syndrome

Giant cell arteritis

Hypersensitivity angiitis
- Drug reaction
- Henoch-Schönlein purpura
- Systemic lupus erythematosus
- Mixed cryoglobulinemia
- Goodpasture's syndrome
- Hypergammaglobulinemic purpura
- C2 deficiency with vasculitis
- Australian antigenemia with vasculitis

Wegener's granulomatosis and variants

Miscellaneous
- Degos' disease (malignant papulosis)
- Erythema elevatum diutinum

classification are highlighted by the vasculitis associated with Australian antigenemia and designated periarteritis nodosa by some. The clinical manifestations of urticaria, arthralgia, fever, eosinophilia, and azotemia; the pathologic findings of fibrinoid necrotizing lesions of arterioles with deposition of immunoglobulin, viral antigen, and complement; and the serologic presence of circulating immune complexes with hypocomplementemia are entirely consistent with hypersensitivity angiitis. The demonstration of arterial abnormalities by angiography presumably reflects the continuum from periarteritis nodosa to hypersensitivity angiitis under these etiologic circumstances. Separate categories are introduced for Wegener's granulomatosis and for a miscellaneous grouping.

Such an operational classification is a justified interim measure because there are associated implications as to prognosis, treatment, and etiology. A classification based on mechanism is a further goal, and to this end a few cautionary comments about the immunopathologic approach are in order. The fibrinoid in the lesions of systemic lupus erythematosus contains protein residues of nuclear origin, acid mucopolysaccharides derived from altered ground substance, and fibrinogen (or derivatives), immunoglobulins, and complement proteins. These findings are interpreted to mean the presence of immune complexes, consisting of nuclear antigen and antibody, complement fixation, and secondary deposition of fibrinogen and alteration of ground substance. In Goodpasture's syndrome the fibrinoid necrosis of the alveolar wall and in the glomerulus is associated with deposition of complement and immunoglobulins with a specificity against basement membrane. In vasculitis associated with Australian antigenemia, immune complexes with specific antigen have been isolated from the plasma and recognized in tissues along with complement by immunofluorescent studies. Whereas in systemic lupus erythematosus, vasculitis with Australian antigenemia, mixed cryoglobulinemia, and Goodpasture's syndrome the specificity of the antibodies contributing to or responsible for the clinicopathologic manifestations of the disease is known, such is not the case for the other entities shown in the table. Thus, the contribution of immunologic events to their lesions is a matter of speculation. Immunoglobulins and complement have been observed in the glomerular lesions of Henoch-Schönlein purpura, in the vascular lesions of rheumatoid arthritis and of periarteritis nodosa, and in the granulomatous response of allergic angiitis and granulomatosis (often with fibrinogen), but not in Wegener s granulomatosis. Such proteins could deposit nonspecifically owing to trapping, transudation or exudation, or because of aggregation of gamma globulin. Studies should be directed toward determining the specificity of the deposited immunoglobulins. Arguments to favor specific deposition could be based on demonstration of antigen in the lesion, recognition of the antibody specificity following elution, and demonstration that the predominant L chain type or H chain subgroup in the deposit is different from the ratio observed in the circulation. Each of these criteria has been met with regard to the lesions of systemic lupus erythematosus.

Churg, J., and Strauss, L.: Allergic granulomatosis, allergic angiitis, and periarteritis nodosa. Am. J. Pathol., 27:277, 1951.

Frohnert, P. P., and Sheps, S. G.: Long-term follow-up study of periarteritis nodosa. Am. J. Med., 43:8, 1967.

Gocke, D. J., Morgan, C., Lockshin, M., Hsu, K., Bombardieri, S., and Christian, C. L.: Association between polyarteritis and Australian antigen. Lancet, 2:1149, 1970.

Grant, M. E., and Prockop, D. J.: The biosynthesis of collagen. N. Engl. J. Med., 286:194, 242, 291, 1972.

Harris, E. D., Evanson, J. M., Dibona, D. R., and Krane, S. M.: Collagenase and rheumatoid arthritis. Arthritis Rheum., 13:83, 1970.

Kilbourne, E. D., and Wolff, H. G.: Cranial arteritis: Critical evaluation of syndrome of "temporal arteritis," with report of a case. Ann. Intern. Med., 24:1, 1946.

Klemperer, P.: The concept of collagen disease in medicine. Am. Rev. Respir. Dis., 83:331, 1961.

Kussmaul, A., and Maier, R.: Über eine bisher nicht beschreibene eigenthümliche Arterienerkrankung (Periarteritis nodosa), die mit Morbus Brightii und rapid fortschreitender allgemeiner Muskellähmung einhergeht. Deutsch. Arch. Klin. Med., 1:484, 1866.

Liebow, A. A.: Pulmonary angiitis and granulomatosis. Am. Rev. Respir. Dis., 108:1, 1973.

Silbert, J. E.: Biosynthesis of muco-polysaccharides and proteinpolysaccharides. *In* Perez-Tamayo, R., and Rojkind, M. (eds.): Molecular Pathology of Connective Tissues. New York, Marcel Dekker, Inc., 1973.

Wegener, F.: Über generalisierte, septische Gefässerkrankungen. Verh. Deutsch. Ges. Path., 29:202, 1936.

Zeek, P. M.: Periarteritis nodosa: A critical review. Am. J. Clin. Pathol., 22:777, 1952.

79. SYSTEMIC SCLEROSIS (Scleroderma)

Edward D. Harris, Jr.

General Considerations. *Scleroderma* is a disease involving blood vessels and connective tissue. The clinical picture is dominated by symptoms of vascular insufficiency caused by abnormalities in small arterioles and capillaries, and by progressive fibrosis in multiple organs. Most patients have involvement predominantly of the arms and hands with Raynaud's phenomenon and acrosclerosis. The face and upper chest may be affected as well, but it is interesting that the legs and feet are involved less often, and it is rare that diffuse involvement of the entire skin is seen. Associated with the cutaneous manifestations are dysfunctions of certain viscera, particularly the esophagus, lungs, and kidneys.

Localized scleroderma, a term which includes morphea and linear scleroderma, involves the skin exclusively.

The diagnosis of systemic sclerosis is made most often in patients between the ages of 35 and 55. Between three and five new cases per million population appear each year. Only 8 per cent of cases begin in the first two decades of life. The disease is three times more common in females than in males. There is some evidence that black women have a poorer prognosis than white women, and males a poorer prognosis than females.

Pathogenesis and Pathology. *Pathogenesis.* Data are accumulating to indicate that abnormalities in the vascular system are primarily involved in the pathogenesis of this disease. Raynaud's phenomenon with its characteristic blanching and pain followed by suffusion is a very common initial complaint in systemic sclerosis. Patients with Raynaud's phenomenon have been shown to have significantly decreased cutaneous fingertip blood flow compared with that of normal controls when both were cooled to 18°C. In clinically unaffected muscle tissue, patients with scleroderma have been shown to have loss of 80 per cent of the normal amount of capillaries; those remaining capillaries have a diameter increased over normal, swollen endothelial cells, and reduplication of the basement membrane. Surface microvessels of the nail fold in systemic sclerosis are also decreased in number and increased in diameter. Digital arteriograms in patients with Raynaud's syndrome and scleroderma often have shown obstruction of the proper digital arteries, and plethysmography has demonstrated decreased amplitude of reflection of the pulse. There may be a common factor of altered vascular reactivity in the development of Raynaud's phenomenon, depressed sensitivity to cholinergic agonists of the lower esophageal sphincter, pulmonary hypertension, and reduced renal cortical blood flow—all abnormalities associated with systemic sclerosis. Resting venous catecholamine concentrations and urinary catecholamine excretion patterns in scleroderma have been normal.

Studies of the proliferative lesion of scleroderma (the appearance of excessive and inappropriate collagen deposition) have revealed no significant abnormality of physical properties, amino acid analyses, cross-linking, or solubility of collagen. Detailed sequence studies have not been carried out in scleroderma collagen; it is not known whether the thin "beaded" filaments in collagen of scleroderma which resemble "embryonic" fibrils actually do represent $\alpha 1$ (III) collagen—a genetically different type of collagen α chains recently characterized from many soft tissues, including blood vessels and fetal skin.

Numerous studies have indicated that there is an increased rate of collagen synthesis in scleroderma. Increased activity of protocollagen proline hydroxylase has been found in skin biopsies from scleroderma. Medium from cultures in vitro of scleroderma skin fibroblasts has been found to contain significantly more collagen than does medium from control cells. A similar increase in the synthetic rate of sialic acid, a proteoglycan component of connective tissue, has been found. No defect in the collagenolytic system in scleroderma has been reported.

To sum up: A leading yet unproved hypothesis for the development of systemic sclerosis is that a primary abnormality of the small blood vessels causes change in connective tissue sufficient to alter normal patterns of collagen and proteoglycan metabolism.

There is very little evidence that tissue damage in scleroderma is mediated by immune complexes or activation of the complement or kinin systems. Although only rare reports have revealed gamma globulin deposited along renal basement membranes in scleroderma, fibrin as a component of fibrinoid material in walls of small vessels of "scleroderma kidneys" is commonly found.

Pathology. The result of systemic involvement in scleroderma is sclerosis. The *reticular dermis* is usually thickened. It may have a normal collagen-bundle pattern or may show broad, homogeneous, acellular deposits of collagen with indistinct bundle patterns. Other findings include atrophy of the rete pegs of the epidermis, atrophy of the hair follicles and sweat glands, perivascular lymphocytic infiltration, and hyalinization of arterioles. During acute, early phases of the disease, edema may be present in the dermis. The subcutaneous tissue is replaced by thick collagen bundles which bind the dermis to deeper structures. Pathologic changes in the musculoskeletal system include acute and chronic inflammation in the *synovium* with no pannus formation and with more sclerosis than is found in rheumatoid synovium with an equivalent inflammatory response. Fibrin deposits are laid down around *tendons,* and in *muscles* there are a variety of abnormalities, the most common being fibrosis of the perimysium and epimysium, scattered cellular infiltrates, and atrophy and necrosis of muscle fibers similar to that seen in polymyositis.

In the internal organs, microvascular abnormalities (see Pathogenesis), mild inflammation, and edema in connective tissue are followed by increased deposition of fibrous tissue in both appropriate and inappropriate loci. This leads to distortion of the architecture of the tissues affected. In the *lungs,* a relatively low-grade interstitial pneumonitis is followed by interstitial fibrosis, most marked in lower lobes. After this, cyst formation and bronchiectasis may develop. Arteriolar thickening (concentric intimal proliferation or medial hypertrophy) is seen, particularly in those patients with clinical evidence of pulmonary hypertension. In the gastrointestinal tract, the *esophagus* is frequently involved with muscle atrophy and fibrosis. Lesions secondary to reflux of gastric contents are present in 20 per cent. Fibrosis around Brunner's glands in the submucosa of the *duodenum* occurs and can be recognized on specimens obtained by peroral biopsy. Involvement of the *small bowel* begins with patchy subserosal fibrosis and may progress to almost complete replacement of smooth muscle with fibrous tissue and marked thickening of the serosa. The small bowel may develop multiple sacculations, presumably at sites of weakness in the continuity of the wall. Dilation, muscle atrophy, and fibrosis are seen in the *colon;* the fibrosis is irregular, leading to the characteristic sacculations and diverticula. The *heart* is frequently enlarged and may be the only organ weighing more than predicted for the subject's body weight. Small patches of interstitial myocardial fibrosis are commonly found. In very severe cases, as much as 60 per cent of cardiac muscle is replaced by dense, relatively acellular and avascular fibrous tissue. Endocardial or valvular thickening is unusual and is rarely of hemodynamic significance. Fibrinous pericarditis is found quite often, even in the absence of uremia. *Kidneys* in scleroderma are normal in size when renal involvement has not been present clinically. In patients dying with uremia they may be small and frequently have small cortical infarcts. Histologically, intimal proliferation in the interlobular arteries, fibrinoid necrosis of small arteries and arterioles (including the glomerular tufts), and thickening of the basement membrane (the "wire-loop" lesion) may all be present. These changes are similar to those seen in kidneys from patients with malignant hypertension and occasionally may be present in the absence of renal failure or severe hypertension.

Clinical Manifestations and Diagnoses. The disease usually begins insidiously. Raynaud's phenomenon, vague weakness, weight loss, diffuse stiffness and aching, polyarticular arthritis, and diffuse edema of the hands are the most common initial symptoms. If the illness progresses, it generally does so slowly, and is marked by characteristic organ system changes. Rarely, rapid progression to severe cutaneous and visceral involvement may occur in less than six months.

Cutaneous System. The patient with classic, well-developed acrosclerosis presents with taut, thickened, or edematous skin bound tightly to subcutaneous tissues in the hands and fingers. Feet and toes are involved less often than hands, forearms, and neck. Normal skin folds at the knuckles disappear. Chronic recurrent painful ulcerations at the ends of the digits develop, and the fingers themselves may shorten through progressive resorption of the terminal phalanges. Joints become immobilized from tight encasement in thickened skin as well as from contractures of muscles and tendons and palmar fascia. Telangiectasia, increased or decreased pigmentation, and subcutaneous calcification are common. Hair becomes thin, and the skin of the face appears smooth and waxy. The skin around the mouth may constrict, restricting lip movement and preventing adequate dental hygiene. The normal sweating mechanism is often impaired; the involved skin feels leathery and dry and may scale and itch. The CRST syndrome (calcinosis, Raynaud's phenomenon, sclerodactyly, and telangiectasia) and the Thibierge-Weissenbach syndrome (diffuse deposition of insoluble calcium phosphates in subcutaneous tissue in the presence of acrosclerosis) are variants of the cutaneous expression of systemic sclerosis.

Musculoskeletal System. Almost half the patients with systemic sclerosis present with joint pain or develop it during the first year of their illness. Small joints are involved more often than large ones. Joint deformity and immobility in systemic sclerosis do not result from an invasive, erosive synovitis as in rheumatoid arthritis, but are the result of encasement as subcutaneous tissue is replaced by bundles of collagen. Muscle wasting is often severe in areas such as the hands, in which joint mobility is impaired by progressive tightening of the overlying skin.

Gastrointestinal Tract. Of the internal organ systems, the gastrointestinal tract is the one most often involved in systemic sclerosis. *Oral* symptoms include xerostomia and a progressive decrease in the size of the mouth. Sjögren's syndrome is seen often, and the frequency of its association with systemic sclerosis is probably underestimated. Symptoms referable to the *esophagus,* ranging from simple dysphagia to heartburn, nausea, and substernal fullness, are found in 45 to 60 per cent of cases. The dysphagia is related to diminished peristalsis in the lower segments of the esophagus and incompetence of the lower esophageal sphincter. If reflex esophagitis becomes a persistent complication, stricture may develop. There is a very frequent association of Raynaud's phenomenon and decreased esophageal peristalsis, although this association is not limited to patients with scleroderma. Vomiting, abdominal distention, and pain or diarrhea may indicate involvement of the *small intestine.* As in the esophagus, motility of the small bowel is decreased, and there may be malabsorption secondary to intraluminal stagnation with concomitant bacterial overgrowth. Functional bowel complaints secondary to pathologic changes in the *colon* are common. Disease of both large and small bowel may produce a clinical picture identical to paralytic ileus with incomplete obstruction at any level. Pneumatosis cystoides intestinalis (air-filled cysts in the mesentery which may rupture, causing peritonitis) is a rare but striking complication of scleroderma bowel disease.

An association between primary biliary cirrhosis and scleroderma with CRST syndrome is now recognized.

Heart and Lungs. Dyspnea is the most common cardiorespiratory symptom in systemic sclerosis and is present in more than 50 per cent of patients. Fine, dry crackles at the bases of the lung are the first abnormality found on physical examination. In some patients, progression to respiratory insufficiency and death from hypoxemia is related to progressive pulmonary fibrosis. The earliest abnormality of pulmonary function is a decrease in pulmonary diffusion capacity. Those exposed in their occupation to silicate dust have a predilection to develop this form of the disease. Restriction of chest wall expansion by dermal fibrosis around the thorax rarely affects respiratory function. A few patients with severe cystic and fibrotic changes in the lungs have developed multifocal alveolar cell carcinomas.

Signs of elevated pulmonary vascular resistance may develop independent of parenchymal changes in the lungs and lead to cor pulmonale and congestive heart failure.

Replacement of myocardium with fibrous tissue on a primary basis ("scleroderma heart disease") is an occasional cause of heart failure. In addition, impaired cardiac function can be attributed to right ventricular failure secondary to pulmonary hypertension.

Kidneys. The sudden development of malignant hypertension resistant to therapy and uremia progressing rapidly to death is a dreaded complication of systemic sclerosis. Most patients have had skin changes before development of abnormal renal function. Plasma renin is elevated, and renal arteriograms reveal narrowed interlobular arteries and afferent arterioles with focal or generalized loss of the cortical nephrogram. It is rare for patients with this complication to survive longer than four months unless nephrectomy and hemodialysis and/or transplantation are carried out.

Nervous System. Involvement of the nervous system is rare. Facial pain, questionably related to a trigeminal neuropathy, is seen in occasional patients and may be disabling. Significant reduction in mean conduction velocity of peripheral nerves has been reported.

Laboratory Findings. The erythrocyte sedimentation test is elevated in most patients with systemic sclerosis, and a mild anemia of chronic disease may be present. In addition, iron deficiency anemia may result from bleeding from esophagitis, and vitamin B_{12} and/or folic acid deficiency from overgrowth of organisms in an atonic bowel. Hemolysis is unusual, although microangiopathic hemolytic anemia has been described in scleroderma (presumably related to fragmentation of erythrocytes from contact with diseased blood vessels and/or intravascular fibrin). A number of serologic abnormalities link systemic sclerosis to other connective tissue diseases. Mild hypergammaglobulinemia is present in 30 to 50 per cent of patients, rheumatoid factor in 25 to 35 per cent, antinuclear antibodies (often with a speckled or a nucleolar pattern) in sera of 30 to 60 per cent, and LE cells in less than 10 per cent of patients. Urinary hydroxyproline excretion, an index of collagen turnover, has been shown by Rodnan to be greater than normal in some patients, particularly in those with active disease.

The electrocardiogram shows nonspecific abnormalities in almost 50 per cent of patients. The pattern of conduction defects with very low voltage is seen only in those uncommon patients with marked myocardial replacement by fibrous tissue.

Roentgenography. Roentgenograms are important for diagnosis and follow-up evaluation. The findings of soft tissue atrophy, subcutaneous calcinosis, and resorption of the tufts of the terminal phalanges without loss of apparent joint spaces between phalanges are virtually pathognomonic of systemic sclerosis when seen on hand films. The periodontal membrane is occasionally thickened. Upper gastrointestinal films reveal a dilated, atonic esophagus in about 60 per cent of patients. Small bowel studies may demonstrate segmental atony, dilation, and sacculation in the duodenum and jejunum. Linear pneumatosis (air in the wall of the gut) is occasionally seen in flat plates of the abdomen of patients with severe small bowel involvement. Barium studies of the colon reveal wide-mouth, asymmetrical diverticula in 20 to 40 per cent of patients; progression to a dilated, atonic megacolon rarely occurs. In patients with pulmonary involvement, chest roentgenograms reveal a diffuse reticular pattern with a honeycomb appearance in the lower lung fields. Serial films may document progression to a picture of dense interstitial fibrosis amid radiolucent cystic areas.

Differential Diagnosis. When systemic sclerosis presents as persistent symmetrical polyarthritis involving the hands without previous skin changes, it may be impossible to differentiate it from rheumatoid arthritis or systemic lupus erythematosus, or, if the overlying skin becomes edematous or red, dermatomyositis. In fact, "overlap" syndromes combining clinical or serologic manifestations of several of these entities are being described with increasing frequency, and one should avoid hasty classification of any clinical picture that is consistent with more than one of the connective tissue diseases.

Diseases or pathologic findings associated with Raynaud's phenomenon which must be differentiated from scleroderma include occupational trauma; anatomic lesions, e.g., scalenus anticus syndrome and cervical ribs; vasomotor syndromes resulting in disuse atrophy, e.g., Sudek's atrophy or the shoulder-hand syndrome; peripheral vascular arteriosclerosis; heavy metal or ergot poisoning; and hematologic abnormalities, e.g., polycythemia vera, paroxysmal cold hemoglobinuria, and presence of cold agglutinins or cryoproteinemia.

The atrophic changes in the skin in systemic sclerosis must be differentiated from those seen in Werner's syndrome, progeria (Hutchinson-Gilford syndrome), chronic hypostatic edema or myxedema, lichen sclerosus et atrophicus, porphyria cutanea tarda, and/or scleredema. Unlike systemic sclerosis, Werner's syndrome affects the feet more severely than the hands, and has associated with it a high-pitched voice, growth abnormalities, and premature cataracts, arteriosclerosis, and diabetes. Sclerodermatous changes have been reported in skin of patients with progeria, but the dwarf-like stature, characteristic facies, and premature death from coronary insufficiency set this syndrome apart. Porphyria cutanea tarda may have skin changes simulating scleroderma but can be differentiated on the basis of urinary or fecal porphyrin excretion. Scleredema (scleredema adultorum of Buschke) is a brawny edema which appears abruptly, involves skin of the neck and chest initially, and is characterized pathologically by the presence of a material resembling acid mucopolysaccharide diffusely interspersed among collagen bundles in the dermis. This is a self-limited process, perhaps related to a previous bacterial infection, and has a good prognosis. The cutaneous telangiectasia of scleroderma resembles Osler-Weber-Rendu disease (hereditary telangiectasia).

Involvement of viscera in systemic sclerosis can mimic many other illnesses. The abnormalities in pulmonary function and the roentgenographic findings seen are similar to those found in idiopathic pulmonary fibrosis (Hamman-Rich syndrome) and the pulmonary fibrosis of rheumatoid arthritis or advanced sarcoidosis. Scleroderma heart disease must be differentiated from infiltrative cardiomyopathies as well as fibrosis from diffuse coronary artery disease. The dysphagia of scleroderma is completely nonspecific, and disease of the bowel rarely can simulate sprue or any of the malabsorption syndromes, partial intestinal obstruction, or megacolon.

Course Untreated. The course of systemic sclerosis is variable. Those patients with primary acrosclerosis and decreased esophageal motility may have slowly progressive disease with no significant increased probability of early death. Others, particularly patients with pulmonary, cardiac, or renal involvement, may progress rapidly to early death. Renal failure is the cause of death of scleroderma in 20 to 40 per cent of patients. Recent data obtained using life-table methods suggest that there is a 50 to 70 per cent five-year survival. Chances for survival are worse if the patient is a black male, diagnosed over the age of 40 years, with cutaneous lesions of the trunk, pulmonary involvement, and an abnormal electrocardiogram or blood urea nitrogen greater than 40 mg per 100 ml.

Treatment. Patients with acrosclerosis can lead productive and useful lives. The most important goal in therapy is to preserve function in and prevent injury to the hands. Vocational and/or climatic change may be indicated. Hand care must be stressed, including instructions for active and passive exercises that the patient may do himself several times each day in order to prevent further deformity. Early signs of local infection in fingertips must be treated immediately before they progress to large ulcerations. Psychologic support can be of great value in helping a patient adjust to the discomfort and apparently inexorable progression of his disease.

Because so little is known about the underlying defect in scleroderma or its pathogenesis, no specific treatment is available. The one possible exception to this is the use of broad-spectrum antimicrobials in treatment of malabsorption associated with bacterial overgrowth in the upper small intestine. If esophageal motility is decreased, antacid therapy is used liberally to prevent secondary esophagitis and stricture. If stricture develops, bougienage will be needed. Salicylates in pharmacologic doses may decrease clinical signs of inflammation, e.g., elevated sedimentation rates, joint pain, and erythema, which is present in most patients at some time in the course of their disease.

Corticosteroids are ineffective in the treatment of systemic sclerosis; neither the vascular lesions nor the fibrosis are improved by their use. However, there is a subgroup of patients with an overlap syndrome called "mixed connective tissue disease" who present with a variety of symptoms, including Raynaud's phenomenon, arthritis, and skin changes consistent with scleroderma, but with features (including LE cells, leukopenia, inflammatory myositis, and lymphadenopathy) of other connective tissue diseases as well. Many of this group will have high titers of antinuclear antibody in a "speckled" pattern directed against an extractable nuclear antigen (not DNA). In general, this group of patients does not develop renal disease and responds very well to corticosteroid therapy.

Recently, use of intra-arterial reserpine has been advocated to decrease the frequency of Raynaud's phenomenon and potentiate healing of ulcers. Given intra-arterially (0.5 to 1.0 mg), benefit without side effects has been noted up to seven months after a single injection. A decrease in finger vasoconstriction in response to cooling in patients with scleroderma given reserpine in the ipsilateral brachial artery has been documented. The placebo effect of this type of procedure and potential hazards of intra-arterial reserpine must be continually evaluated. Oral reserpine in doses sufficient to relieve symptoms of Raynaud's phenomenon often causes central depression, but when used in small doses (≤ 0.5 mg per day), combined with oral sympathetic or ganglionic blocking agents, may increase capillary blood flow without causing intolerable side effects.

Potassium p-aminobenzoate, ethylenediaminetetraacetic acid, 6-aminocaproic acid infusions, and dimethyl sulfoxide applications have been employed by a number of investigators. D-penicillamine, capable of inhibiting formation of cross-links in collagen and some mammalian collagenases in vitro, has not been of proved benefit in scleroderma. Pilot studies of immunosuppressive therapy are being evaluated; initial results show no clear-cut role for these drugs in systemic sclerosis.

Initial results in few cases in which "scleroderma kidneys" were removed and hemodialysis and/or renal transplantation carried out have demonstrated that life of good quality can be prolonged by these aggressive approaches. It is not yet known whether the transplanted kidneys will develop vascular changes, but it is now clear that patients with systemic sclerosis who develop renal disease need not die from rapidly progressive renal failure.

D'Angelo, W. A., Fries, J. F., Masi, A. T., and Shulman, L. E.: Pathologic observations in systemic sclerosis (scleroderma). Am. J. Med., 46:428, 1969.

Rodnan, G. P.: Progressive systemic sclerosis (scleroderma) and calcinosis. *In* Hollander, J. L., and McCarty, D. J. (eds.): Arthritis and Allied Conditions. 8th ed. Philadelphia, Lea & Febiger, 1972.

80. POLYMYOSITIS AND DERMATOMYOSITIS

H. Richard Tyler

General Considerations. The disorder termed polymyositis refers to an illness first described by Wagner in 1863 in which muscle weakness is the principal clinical feature. Inflammatory, degenerative, and regenerative changes can be seen in the muscles. When skin changes occur and are prominent, the cases are referred to as dermatomyositis. This subgroup was first delineated by Unverricht in 1887. The muscular lesions of dermatomyositis, however, are identical to those seen in polymyositis. Because of the dramatic skin lesions, dermatomyositis was more widely recognized. Appreciation that muscular syndromes are more common than dermatomyositis resulted from the increased use of muscle biopsy and the clinical awareness that an insidious onset and absence of muscle pain are common. If there are changes indicative of nerve damage, the term neuromyositis is occasionally used. Some authors prefer the nonspecific and noncommittal term polymyopathy and identify as separate entities only those cases whose specific cause is known. Others reserve the term polymyositis for cases with evidence of inflammatory changes in muscles. Until the cause of the majority of the cases is more clearly identified, one has to accept the need to reevaluate nomenclature periodically. All these disorders form a large spectrum which ranges from the very acute cases with myoglobinuria to the very chronic localized disorders that mimic muscular dystrophy.

The incidence of the disease has been estimated between 0.1 and 0.6 per 100,000 population, with a prevalence of 6.3 per 100,000. As a cause of acute or subacute muscle weakness in an adult, polymyositis is much more common than muscular dystrophy.

The disease can appear at any age, but it is most common between the ages of 40 and 60. Females are affected about twice as frequently as males. In most instances, no precipitating cause is obvious, but some cases have followed a viral-like illness or the use of antimicrobial drugs. Virus-like particles have been noted in muscle in some cases. Their role in relation to the disease has not been defined. Hypersensitivity has been implicated by some because of the association with malignancy, the frequent relation to a previous infection, and the association with symptoms common to the other collagen diseases.

In most instances, it is not possible to establish a definite etiology. Specific infections (such as toxoplasmosis) may cause a polymyositis, but in most cases there is no evidence of an infectious cause. It has not been possible to demonstrate antimuscle antibodies in these patients. The presence of antimyosin antibody and other antibodies in some patients is nonspecific, as it is also found in patients with muscular dystrophy and neuronal atrophy. It has been possible to produce a myositis in guinea pigs similar to human polymyositis by use of muscle plus Freund's adjuvant. In tissue culture preparations of rat skeletal muscle, "sensitized" lymph node cells from animals previously injected with muscle plus adjuvants destroyed the muscle cells when added to the culture, whereas unsensitized lymph node cells did not. The significance of these experiments for human disease remains uncertain.

Lymphocytes or their products from affected patients have cytotoxic activity toward muscle cells in 79 per cent of cases in one series, suggesting a cell-mediated immune response to muscle antigen. Intramuscular vascular deposits of immunoglobulin and C_3 have been demonstrated, especially in the childhood form of dermatomyositis.

Pathology. Muscle biopsy may show inflammatory cells around vessels and in the interstitium frequently associated with individual muscle fiber necrosis. These necrotic muscle fibers are frequently in various stages of being phagocytized. Attempts at regeneration characterized by basophilic fibers having prominent sarcolemmal nuclei are usually impressive. It should be emphasized that histologic findings vary greatly in the same muscle and between different muscles so that sampling is important. The muscle tissue from the more chronic cases often shows surprisingly little change under the light microscope. This may consist of smaller muscle fibers, which vary significantly in cross-section diameter, associated with proliferation of sarcolemmal nuclei. In the polymyositis associated with Sjögren's syndrome, the muscle may be heavily infiltrated with plasma cells and lymphocytes. In the few studies utilizing the electron microscope, changes such as thickened basilar membranes, myofibrillary degeneration and, rarely, virus particles were seen. These studies have not contributed any new insight into the disease.

In the childhood form of dermatomyositis, there is intense perivascular inflammation with active arteritis and phlebitis. There is often occlusion of vessels with fibrin thrombi and infarction of muscles, nerves, and viscus (Banker and Victor). Other forms of more limited or less intense polymyositic syndromes in children have pathologic changes similar to those previously described.

The three useful laboratory tests, serum enzymes, electromyography, and muscle biopsy, are not always abnormal. Any one or even two may yield normal findings in a particular case. In one series, electromyography was abnormal in 89 per cent and muscle biopsy was confirmatory in 63 per cent. Serum enzymes are usually elevated except in some slowly progressive or chronic cases.

Clinical Manifestations and Diagnosis. The patient usually first notes the insidious development of *weakness in proximal muscles.* The weakness is more common at the hips than in the shoulders. Some weakness in the flexors of the neck is almost always present. Muscle discomfort or tenderness is common but can be completely absent. When present, it is more common in the shoulders, back, and arms than in the thighs. Muscular wasting is a late sign, and when it occurs it is usually in proximal muscles such as the quadriceps. The weakness is out of proportion to the loss of muscle bulk. Reflexes are depressed in proportion to muscle weakness.

The development and the rate of progression of the weakness may show great variations from patient to patient, and even in the same patient at different stages of the illness. Weakness can progress until the patient becomes bedridden, but this is unusual. Contracture of muscles may develop quickly.

A *skin rash* may or may not be present. It usually takes the form of an erythema over the face, shoulders, and arms. It can mimic erythema nodosum, eczema, or exfoliating dermatitis, or can manifest itself by thickened, brawny, edematous skin. On occasion, the skin lesions appear primarily in areas exposed to sunlight. Erythematous, slightly raised lesions occur over bony prominences, i.e., elbows, knuckles, knees, and medial malleoli. These lesions often become scaly and atrophic. Hyperemia around the nail beds is not uncommon. In childhood forms a violaceous suffusion of the upper eyelids, called a "heliotrope" rash, is diagnostic of this disorder. This may also be seen in adults.

Dysphagia, secondary to weakness of pharyngeal muscle and hypotonicity of the upper part of the esophagus, is frequent. About one third of the patients have arthralgias and/or Raynaud's phenomenon. Other visceral manifestations are rare. Many patients have a tachycardia. Electrocardiograms may show nonspecific T wave changes. Interstitial fibrosis and pericarditis have been noted on histologic examination. A transitory pneumonitis has also been reported. Transitional cases with some features suggesting scleroderma have occasionally demonstrated severe gastrointestinal symptoms with malabsorption, severe myopathy, and only slight skin changes. If the muscle weakness comes on acutely with much muscle necrosis, myoglobinuria will occur. This can result in acute renal failure. Polymyositis may also be seen with Sjögren's syndrome.

The *childhood form of dermatomyositis* may be much more pernicious. It starts out with skin changes, anorexia, and fatigue. Weakness, stiffness, and pain in muscles customarily follow. Low-grade fever, dysphagia, contractures, and calcinosis usually develop. A perforated viscus or mediastinitis is often the immediate cause of death.

Course Untreated. The condition can progress to severe disability and death, but most patients either improve spontaneously or proceed to a chronic phase. In earlier series, including patients primarily recognized as having dermatomyositis, case fatality rates of 50 per cent were common. In a later series of adult patients with polymyositis, it was noted that about two thirds were alive after ten years. About 50 per cent of these had complete recoveries, and the rest had some degree of residual disability. Many of the patients in this series had received some steroid therapy.

In a survey by Sheard in which adult cases were accumulated from the literature, tumors were present in nearly 20 per cent, or five times the expected incidence. When polymyositis develops in an adult male, a greater than 50 per cent chance exists that a tumor will be discovered. In another series described by Shy, it was noted that when polymyositis appeared after the age of 50 a *cancer* was found in 71 per cent of males and 24 per cent of females. The muscular weakness may precede the detection of the tumor by two or three years despite diligent search, and in this series all nine males above 50 who were followed for three years or more had an associated neoplasm. In the male, the usual carcinoma is in the lung, stomach, intestine, or prostate; and in the female, in the ovary, uterus, or breast.

Childhood dermatomyositis appears to be a very specific subgroup of polymyositic disorders. It is severely disabling and is associated with a very high fatality rate.

Laboratory Findings. The sedimentation rate is usually elevated, and there may be mild leukocytosis, especially in the acute cases. A number of enzymes which derive from muscle are usually elevated in serum. Creatine phosphokinase and aldolase are the most specific, but lactic dehydrogenase and transaminase (SGOT) are usually elevated also. Serum protein changes occur in about 50 per cent of the patients. These most commonly consist of elevations of the $\alpha 2$ and γ globulins. Rheumatoid factors are positive in 10 to 50 per cent, depending on the series. About 5 per cent will have a positive LE prep. Myoglobinuria is transient and is found only with acute and severe muscular degeneration.

In patients with dysphagia, the roentgenograms often reveal pooling of barium in the vallecular and pyriform sinuses. Hypomotility of the esophagus is present in about one third of the cases. The roentgenograms frequently reveal no abnormalities except the rare deposition of subcutaneous calcification in the childhood form of the disease. Electrocardiograms often show minor abnormalities.

Electromyography is almost always abnormal in the clinically affected muscles. There is excessive irritability of muscle when the needle is initially inserted. The motor units (which are made up of many muscle fibers supplied by a single nerve) often show a loss of amplitude, indicating a reduction in the number of functioning muscle fibers in each motor unit. The mean duration of the units is often shortened. Polyphasic discharges are common, indicating a loss of individual muscle fibers of the unit. Positive denervation waves of 20 to 50 msec and fibrillary potentials are seen, indicating some denervation or separation of a portion of the muscle from its afferent nerve supply. Repetitive discharges of pseudomyotonic firing are not uncommon. When the changes indicating denervation are prominent, the term "neuromyositis" has been used. The electromyogram is useful in indicating which muscles to biopsy. The site of biopsy should be selected to ensure that a proper sampling of abnormal muscle is being taken. It should not be taken at the site of previous electromyographic needle insertion.

Differential Diagnosis. The major causes of weakness, which must be differentiated from polymyositis, are those due to muscular dystrophy and disorders of the peripheral and central nervous system. Muscular dystrophy is usually a familial disorder which is longstanding and can often be traced to childhood. The involvement of proximal muscles and neck flexor weakness would be unusual in most adult forms of muscular dystrophy. In myotonic dystrophy, the only dystrophy which often demonstrates neck flexor weakness, there is a distal weakness of muscles in the extremities. There are also cataracts and myotonia to percussion. Fascioscapulohumeral muscular dystrophy and other proximal dystrophies usually spare neck flexors. All the dystrophies are characterized by family history, significant muscle wasting, and weakness; the deep tendon reflex loss is usually early and prominent. In polymyositis, reflexes are often relatively spared until severe weakness occurs. In some cases it may be impossible to distinguish a dystrophy from polymyositis. The family history may be difficult to verify, and the biopsy in chronic cases may not be characteristic. A few cases of familial polymyositis have been reported.

The weakness in peripheral neuritis tends to be distal, and careful examination usually enables one to find mild sensory loss, autonomic dysfunction, and distal areflexia. Weakness from spinal cord disease has characteristic reflex changes, such as extensor plantar responses and hyperreflexia. Occasionally, motor neuron disease (the primary muscular atrophy variant) presents as a myopathic disorder. Muscle biopsy and EMG usually distinguish between the two conditions. On occasion a subacute variety of Guillain-Barré disease can cause proximal weakness. Elevation of cerebrospinal fluid protein is helpful in establishing this entity and is not seen in polymyositis.

Of the muscular syndromes, the metabolic myopathies most closely mimic the distribution of muscle weakness and the weakness seen with polymyositis. Chronic thyroid myopathy is characterized by its involvement of proximal muscles with significant loss of muscle bulk. The reflexes are usually quite brisk. Although there are no distinctive features, the clinical signs of thyrotoxicosis and the presence of clinical tests to support hyperthyroidism usually make it easy to distinguish this group. The most common myopathy seen today is probably the one induced by excess or chronic use of corticotrophin or steroids. This is especially true of the fluorinated steroids. It is identical to that seen with hyperadrenocorticism. The weakness is primarily proximal, most often involving the pelvic girdle. Early wasting of the quadriceps muscle is especially prominent. Pain and discomfort are unusual. Reflexes usually persist, and severe disabling syndromes are unusual. Muscle biopsy tends to show surprisingly little change, and then only very scattered and in single muscle fibers. These changes are usually much less than one would anticipate from the clinical status of the patients.

Since steroids are often used in the treatment of a number of clinical syndromes, it may be very difficult to establish whether progressive weakness is due to the underlying disease or the steroid treatment. Often one will have to either decrease the steroid dose sharply or increase it significantly to make such judgments. If pain is a significant problem, one must be cautious about the clinical evaluation of weakness or its disappearance with the use of high doses of steroids.

Hyperparathyroidism and hyperinsulinism have rarely been associated with syndromes of muscular weakness and must be separated from idiopathic polymyositis primarily by the associated laboratory findings. Muscle weakness is often associated with osteomalacia.

There are a number of parasitic diseases such as trichinosis and toxoplasmosis which should be considered in acute or subacute syndromes, especially when generalized symptoms and eosinophilia are noted. These are fully discussed elsewhere in this text.

Polymyalgia rheumatica is characteristically associated with significant muscular discomfort and a high sedimentation rate. Changes in serum enzymes or muscle biopsy are usually not present to any significant degree. There are noticeable short-term and even daily fluctuations of symptoms. Significant objective weakness is not common, although complaints of pain and fatigue and feelings of muscular weakness are often voiced by the patient. Although the findings in some are related to those seen with temporal arteritis, the findings in others are very similar to those of some patients seen with epidemic neuromyasthenia.

Treatment. The physician's obvious goal is to eradicate the active disease process, if possible, and improve the functional capacity of the patient. In almost all cases prolonged management and long-term follow-up will be necessary. Often the chronic nature and the severe disability caused by the illness make it essential for the physician to play an active role as a counselor and friend.

Many of these patients achieve significant symptomatic improvement of muscle function when treated with corticotrophin, steroids, or salicylates. The use of immunosuppressive medication has been promising in a few cases. Methotrexate has been used, especially in dermatomyositis. The disorder is rarely "cured," however, and relapses are common, especially if steroids are abruptly withdrawn. Patients may require medication for many years. The initial dose of corticotrophin or steroids should be high (60 to 80 mg of prednisone) and tapered over months. It is useful to monitor serum enzymes during this period, as they often give an early indication of the patient's likely course. Relapses are common when steroids are withdrawn in the first two years, but less frequent if treatment lasts at least three years. When possible, steroids should be used on an alternate-day basis to decrease side effects. When steroid-treated and presteroid series of patients are compared in terms of long-range follow-up, as by Rose and Walton, the group receiving steroid treatment has fared better. Patients with some of the adult forms usually do well. Those with the childhood forms of dermatomyositis usually do not respond satisfactorily to steroids alone.

Banker, B. Q., and Victor, M.: Dermatomyositis (systemic angiopathy of childhood). Medicine, 45:261, 1966.

Pearson, C. M.: Polymyositis. *In* Milhorat, A. T. (ed.): Explanatory Concepts in Muscular Dystrophy and Related Disorders. Amsterdam, Excerpta Medica Foundation, 1967.

Rose, A. L., and Walton, J.: Polymyositis: A survey of 89 cases with particular reference to treatment and prognosis. Brain, 89:747, 1966.

Sheard, C.: Dermatomyositis. Arch. Intern. Med., 88:640, 1951.

Shy, G. M.: The late onset myopathy. World Neurol., 3:149, 1962.

Walton, J. N.: Disorders of Voluntary Muscle. 2nd ed. London, J. A. Churchill, Ltd., 1969.

Walton, J. N., and Adams, R. D.: Polymyositis. Edinburgh, Livingstone, Ltd., 1958.

81. SYSTEMIC LUPUS ERYTHEMATOSUS

Peter H. Schur

General Considerations. Systemic lupus erythematosus (SLE) is a chronic, inflammatory disease of unknown cause affecting skin, joints, kidneys, nervous system, serous membranes, and often other organs of the body. The classic facial "butterfly rash" facilitates diagnosis, although the rash need not be present. The clinical course may be fulminant or indolent, but generally is characterized by periods of remissions and relapses. Patients with SLE develop distinct immunologic abnormalities, especially antinuclear antibodies. A diagnosis of SLE has frequently been established or confirmed by the finding of these antibodies, especially the one causing the LE cell phenomenon.

Lupus, which is Latin for wolf, has been used since about 1230 to describe cutaneous conditions which resemble the malar erythema of a wolf. Numerous publications in the nineteenth century by, among others, Bateman, Biett, Hebra, and Kaposi, described what we know now as lupus of the skin. In 1851, Cazenave first used the term "lupus erythemateux." Kaposi, in 1872, noted the systemic involvement in lupus, and in 1875 noted that the rash resembled a butterfly. Osler described the systemic complications of lupus and noted that they could occur in the absence of skin disease. The clinical recognition of SLE has changed greatly since Hargraves first described the LE cell test in 1948 and since the development of the immunofluorescent antinuclear factor test by Friou in 1957.

Incidence and Etiology. SLE is not a rare disorder. The prevalence rate is approximately 5 per 100,000 population. The disease appears to occur more frequently in blacks than in whites and is rare among Asians. It occurs five to ten times more frequently among females than males and has been diagnosed in patients ranging from 2 to 97 years old. However, the majority of patients are first discovered to have SLE while in their third and fourth decades of life.

The cause of SLE remains unknown. Exposure to sunlight or ultraviolet radiation, viz., sunlamps, often leads to the prompt appearance of the facial butterfly rash or a rash on other exposed skin surfaces. Many other factors, including infections, surgery, and certain drugs, have been shown to be associated with exacerbations of SLE. Recent attention has focused on procainamide, hydralazine, hydantoins, and other drugs which may precipitate a lupus-like illness.

In view of the preponderance of the disease in females, endocrine factors have been thought to influence the development of SLE. The disease tends to remit during the last two trimesters of pregnancy and to relapse post partum. Inhibitors of ovulation can cause an exacerbation of SLE.

Genetic factors may influence the development of SLE in susceptible individuals. Much evidence supports this hypothesis. The high incidence of SLE among females might be considered an X-chromosome-related factor. Connective tissue disorders, dysgammaglobulinemia and autoimmune phenomena are observed frequently among relatives of many patients with SLE. Genetic control of immune responses to certain antigens correlates closely with histocompatibility types in some animals. An association between particular HLA antigens and SLE has been noted, suggesting that SLE patients may hyperreact to some antigens. Additional evidence for a genetic role in SLE comes from studies in certain strains of inbred mice and dogs. NZB and NZW mice develop an illness which includes hemolytic anemia, renal disease, and immunologic abnormalities, and is similar to human SLE. The F_1 hybrid generation, especially the females, develop the illness more frequently, at an earlier age, and with a much higher incidence of autoimmune phenomena.

Lupus erythematosus is characterized particularly by autoimmune phenomena. Patients develop antibodies to many of their own cells, cell constituents, and proteins. The origin of these autoantibodies is as obscure as is the cause of SLE. However, they do appear to represent a loss of tolerance to self antigens. Mice of the NZB strain have been found to lose their tolerance for foreign antigens much more rapidly than do other mice.

A possible viral cause for SLE has also been proposed. Loss of tolerance may be influenced by viral infections. Structures resembling viral nucleocapsids have been found much more frequently in endothelial cells in SLE patients than in normal persons. Antibody titers to certain viruses are elevated in SLE sera, but no one virus has been implicated. The presence, in many SLE patients, of antibodies to double-stranded RNA suggests reaction to an RNA virus (infection). "C" type RNA virus particles have been found in NZB mice; other viruses, including DNA and RNA viruses, can provoke the development of autoantibodies and nephritis in NZB mice. Cell-free filtrates, presumably containing a virus, have been prepared from spleens of dogs with lupus. These filtrates, when injected into normal dogs and mice, induce the formation of antinuclear antibodies; they also activate latent leukemia viruses in mice.

These data suggest that an abnormal immune response in genetically predisposed SLE patients may alter the delicate balance between immunity and tolerance and result in the development of antibodies to intracellular contents released during chronic viral infection or to new antigens in cells which result from viral infection or transformation.

Pathogenesis and Pathology. Many of the manifestations of SLE appear to result from the deposition of antigen-antibody complexes in tissues. Although immune complexes have not been isolated from SLE patients, certain evidence is consistent with their presence. In laboratory animals, when immune complexes are formed in the circulation, serum complement levels fall and nephritis develops. In patients with SLE, especially in those with anti-DNA antibodies, a fall in complement levels is often associated with the development of nephritis. In addition, some patients with serum antibodies to DNA develop fever and nephritis as the antibody disappears and is replaced by free DNA, a sequence which presumably represents immune complex formation and deposition followed by antigen excess. Furthermore, some sera from SLE patients with nephritis, when treated with deoxyribonuclease, have a rise in anti-DNA antibody levels. This fact suggests that DNA has been bound in vivo to the antibody as an immune complex. Using the immunofluorescent technique, immunoglobulins (especially IgG), complement components, and antigens (viz., DNA) have been detected in a granular and lumpy distribution along the renal glomerular basement membrane. After elution of the gamma globulin from the glomeruli, it has been possible to demonstrate that it consists primarily of antinuclear and some anticytoplasmic antibodies. Similar immune complexes have been demonstrated at the dermal-epidermal junction of lupus skin lesions. It is hypothesized that, as the complement system is activated during immune complex formation and deposition, chemotactic factors are released and that damage to normal cells and extracellular tissue is caused both by activated terminal sequences of complement and by lysosomal enzymes released by polymorphonuclear leukocytes.

The pathologic changes of SLE, even in clinically uninvolved organs, are often minor when examined by routine histologic methods. Fibrinoid, an eosinophilic amorphous material, is commonly deposited along tissue fibers and in blood vessels. Fibrin and serum proteins (including immunoglobulins, complement, and DNA) have been detected in fibrinoid and possibly represent deposits of immune complexes. Synovium and serous membranes, including pleura and pericardium, may be edematous and contain deposits of fibrinoid. Vasculitis can involve venules, capillaries, arterioles, and occasionally arteries. Hematoxylin bodies are rounded, hematoxylin-stained masses, roughly the size of nuclei, and are found in areas of inflammation. They are believed to represent in vivo LE bodies analogous to the cytoplasmic inclusions in LE cells.

Skin biopsies may show acute inflammation with liquefaction, degeneration of the basal layer with vacuolization of basal cells, edema of the dermis, and fibrinoid necrosis in the dermis and local blood vessels with cell infiltration. In chronic lesions, hyperkeratosis with follicular plugging is seen.

The spleen is the site of "onion skin lesions," which are characterized by concentric perivascular fibrosis around central and penicilliary arteries.

Libman-Sacks verrucous nonbacterial endocarditis consists of nonbacterial vegetations on the heart valves or chordae tendineae. Fibrinoid is deposited in the superficial connective tissue with infiltration of neutrophils, lymphocytes, and histiocytes. The myocardium may be involved by vasculitis.

Renal lesions are highly variable, from mild to severe. The mildest form of renal lesion consists of deposits of immunoglobulin and complement in the mesangium and along the glomerular basement membrane without any other observable histologic abnormality. The most common renal lesion is focal glomerulitis with minimal increase of cellularity, focal thickening of the capillary basement membrane, and fibrinoid change. In glomerulonephritis, these lesions are more generalized and severe and are usually a mixture of proliferative and membranous changes with hypercellularity of endothelial, mesangial, epithelial, and inflammatory cells, capsular inflammation leading to crescent formation, and focal thickening of the basement membrane. Some kidneys are found to have only a diffuse membranous glomerulonephritis with few cells but considerable thickening of the basement membrane. Basement membrane thickening, when associated with fibrinoid changes, results in the so-called "wire loop" lesions. There may also be hyaline thrombi in glomeruli, focal necrosis, and, occasionally, hematoxylin bodies. Tubular degenerative changes are common.

Clinical Manifestations. The characteristic picture of a patient with well-advanced lupus is one of a young woman with fever, weight loss, arthralgia, a butterfly rash, pleural effusion, and nephritis. With better methods of detection (the antinuclear antibody tests), much larger groups of patients with less obvious and more varied symptoms and signs are being recognized. Most patients complain of some fatigue, arthralgia, rashes, and fever. When specific organs are involved, other symptoms may develop: pleurisy, pericarditis, edema, dyspnea and cough, Raynaud's phenomenon, bleeding, and purpura or seizures. The disease is now considered a chronic illness with periods of remission and activity.

Musculoskeletal System. Most patients complain of pain in their joints (arthralgia) at some time. Commonly the hands, wrists, knees, ankles, and elbows are affected. Arthritis of joints, that is, local redness, swelling, or heat, is observed less frequently than is arthralgia. Although slight deformities at the metacarpophalangeal and proximal interphalangeal joints may occur, major joint swelling with synovial thickening, flexion deformities with subluxations, and deviation are uncommon. It is unusual for joint narrowing or cystic changes such as those seen in rheumatoid arthritis to be found on radiologic examination. The appearance of deforming or destructive joint lesions suggests a diagnosis of an overlap syndrome (rheumatoid arthritis–lupus). Muscle pain is a frequent complaint and is accompanied, occasionally, by proximal muscle atrophy. The bones are rarely affected, but an increased prevalence of aseptic necrosis of the femoral head or condyle has been noted, especially in those patients receiving corticosteroid therapy.

Mucocutaneous Manifestations. The classic "butterfly rash" is seen in less than half the patients with SLE.

TABLE 1. Frequency of Clinical Symptoms in Systemic Lupus Erythematosus*

	Per Cent
Weight loss	62
Fever	83
Arthralgia, arthritis	90
Skin	74
Butterfly rash	42
Photosensitivity	30
Mucous membrane lesions	12
Alopecia	27
Raynaud's phenomenon	17
Purpura	15
Urticaria	8
Renal	53
Nephrosis	18
Gastrointestinal	38
Pulmonary	47
Pleurisy	45
Effusion	24
Pneumonia	29
Cardiac	46
Pericarditis	27
Murmurs	23
EKG changes	39
Lymphadenopathy	46
Splenomegaly	15
Hepatomegaly	25
Central nervous system	32
Psychosis	15
Convulsions	15
Cytoid bodies	11

*Adapted from Dubois, E. L.: Lupus Erythematosus, New York, McGraw-Hill Book Company, 1966; Estes, D., and Christian, C. L.: Medicine, 50:85, 1971; and Fernandez-Herlihy, L.: Lahey Clinic Found. Bull., 21:49, 1972.

There may be only a blush and swelling or a scaly erythematous maculopapular rash on both cheeks and the bridge of the nose after exposure to the sun. This may clear spontaneously, only to recur. Other skin areas, particularly those exposed to the sun, may be involved. The lesions are called "discoid" when they scale, are associated with follicular plugging, and heal with atrophy, scarring (telangiectasia), hyperpigmentation, or hypopigmentation (vitiligo). Discoid lupus per se is not accompanied by systemic complications. Involvement may also occur on the forehead, pinna, and scalp, resulting in alopecia. Patchy hair loss is frequent and usually reversible, but discoid lupus with scarring can lead to permanent partial baldness. In these days of well-fitted hairpieces, alopecia is often undetected on cursory examination. Periungual erythema and telangiectasia are found in about 10 per cent of patients with SLE. Small ulcerations signifying an underlying vasculitis often develop on the fingertips and may progress to gangrene. Raynaud's phenomenon may occur in both hands and feet. Painful ulcers are seen on the buccal mucosa, hard and soft palate, and gums. Purpura and ecchymoses usually reflect an underlying blood platelet and clotting problem, renal insufficiency, or the side effects of corticosteroids. Urticaria and angioedema may be present.

Renal Disease. Kidney involvement is found in about half of SLE patients and usually occurs within two years of the onset of symptoms. Acute nephritis or the nephrotic syndrome may be the presenting manifestation of SLE. The most common abnormality is a mild glomerulitis which is associated with minimal proteinuria or hematuria, or both. This lesion generally responds well to therapy initially, but often recurs in mild form or as even more severe renal involvement. Acute lupus glomerulonephritis occurs less often and is associated with varying degrees of pyuria, hematuria, proteinuria, fluid retention, edema, hypertension, and azotemia. The nephrotic syndrome is associated with variable proteinuria, with fluid retention, and frequently with normal serum cholesterol levels. The finding of pyuria with fever in patients with SLE, especially in young women receiving corticosteroids, may reflect a urinary tract infection rather than lupus nephritis; a renal biopsy may be necessary to make the correct diagnosis.

Most patients recover well from attacks of acute nephritis, with loss of edema and azotemia, but usually some proteinuria and decreased glomerular filtration rate (GFR) persist. Patients have recurrences, and some develop chronic glomerulonephritis with hypertension and proteinuria.

Cardiovascular Manifestations. The endocardium, myocardium, and pericardium are involved in nearly half the patients with SLE. Although electrocardiographic changes, such as nonspecific ST, T wave changes, are not uncommon, clinical myocarditis is seen less frequently. Myocarditis should be suspected when tachycardia is disproportionate to either fever or anemia. Cardiomegaly with congestive failure is rare. Precordial chest pain may be caused by either pleurisy or pericarditis. Careful, frequent auscultation may be rewarded by discovery of a pericardial friction rub. Tamponade or constrictive pericarditis is rare. Libman-Sacks or nonbacterial verrucous endocarditis usually occurs on the mitral valve and is recognized by murmurs which cannot be explained by fever or anemia; but generally this is a postmortem diagnosis. Bacterial endocarditis may develop on a previously damaged valve, especially in patients receiving corticosteroids. Thrombophlebitis may be the first manifestation of SLE. Occlusion of major arteries occurs rarely. Equally rare is pulmonary hypertension.

Pulmonary Involvement. Pleuritic pain is a common complaint and is often the first clue to the diagnosis of SLE. It is generally accompanied by a friction rub and a variable amount of fluid accumulation, but the effusions are often painless. There may be pulmonary infiltrates which are quite difficult to distinguish from those due to infections. The x-ray examination shows bilateral patchy infiltrations which may shift from lobe to lobe. The involvement can progress to atelectasis and to marked pulmonary insufficiency and cyanosis. Most pulmonary symptoms respond well to intensive corticosteroid therapy; but infections must be carefully considered as a cause of the infiltrate.

Neurologic and Psychologic Manifestations. Many patients have read in a dictionary or have heard that SLE is invariably a fatal illness, and this fact understandably leads to great anxiety. Similarly the patient may be told that he or she has arthritis, which leads to ungrounded fears of disabling deformities. These natural fears and anxieties of a chronic illness are complicated frequently by organic neurologic disturbances. The latter manifest themselves as behavioral disturbances, including hyperirritability, confusion, hallucinations, obsessional and paranoid reactions, and frank organic psychosis. The psychosis of SLE may easily be confused with, and in fact is difficult to differentiate from, a steroid-induced psychosis; other symptoms and signs of active SLE usually accompany the organic diease. Organic brain damage most commonly manifests itself as convulsions, which occur in at least 15 per cent of patients. Other less frequent neurologic findings include peripheral neuropathy, hemiparesis, motor aphasia, ptosis, diplopia, and nystagmus.

"Cotton wool spots" are fluffy white exudates (containing cytoid bodies) in the superficial layers of the retina. They are usually associated with some visual disturbance, are present with other signs of active SLE, and are generally reversible.

Gastrointestinal Manifestations. Anorexia, nausea, vomiting, and abdominal pain are common. The cause is obscure, but may be from peritonitis, enteritis, pancreatitis, or a paralytic ileus. Diarrhea and hematochezia have been noted. The liver is often found to be enlarged because of chronic passive congestion, but this is usually transitory. Liver biopsy may be normal or show fatty infiltration and/or fibrosis.

These manifestations in SLE should not be confused with *lupoid hepatitis,* which is a condition primarily of young women with progressive active hepatitis leading to chronic liver disease and failure. Nephritis is said not to occur. Patients have high levels of gamma globulins, positive LE cell preparations, or positive tests for antinuclear factor (ANF); serum complement levels remain normal or elevated.

Lymph Nodes and Spleen. Lymph nodes, characteristically, are enlarged in SLE but are not tender. The enlarged nodes have been mistaken for lymphoma. Splenomegaly, considered very common years ago, is seen now in about 15 per cent of patients.

Menses and Pregnancy. Menses are frequently irregular or heavy, or both. In patients with circulating anticoagulants, bleeding may be profound. Although pregnancy carries some increased risk of miscarriage in the first trimester, most SLE patients without renal disease do well through term. It should be noted, however, that there is a considerable risk of postpartum exacerbation of the disease.

Course Untreated. Until recent years the natural course of untreated SLE was considered to be bleak. The average patient was considered to have but a few months or, at best, a few years to live. Since 1948, this situation has changed for the better. The reason for this improvement lies in the recognition of many cases of mild lupus through the development of very sensitive diagnostic tests (antinuclear antibodies), as well as in the development of improved forms of therapy. The disease in most patients is characterized by periods of remissions and relapses, which may be protracted or brief. The same individuals usually have recurrences of the same symptoms they had previously, such as arthritis, pleurisy, nephritis, or rashes. However, variable symptoms and signs may develop years apart. If nephritis develops, it generally does so early in the course.

The prognosis for patients seems to improve each year, but mortality rates remain high during the first year after diagnosis. Whereas in 1956, patients were given only a 50 per cent chance of surviving four years, today they have a better than 90 per cent chance to survive ten years. Prognosis still remains poor for patients with diffuse proliferative glomerulonephritis or with central nervous system involvement.

Laboratory Findings. *Hematologic.* Anemia occurs in many patients with SLE and is generally mild, normochromic, or normocytic. Anemia may also be due to infection, renal insufficiency, or bleeding. Autoagglutination of red blood cells may be observed. The Coombs test is frequently positive, but severe hemolytic anemia is uncommon. Leukopenia occurs in about one half the patients. The differential cell count is usually normal, although mononuclear cells may be more suppressed than neutrophils. Complicating infections generally result in a rise of the white blood cell count either into the normal or elevated range. Corticosteroid therapy also causes leukocytosis. Thrombocytopenia, with or without purpura, may precede other manifestations of SLE by years or may disappear, leaving other manifestations of the disease. A circulating anticoagulant may be present in as many as 25 per cent of patients with SLE. This anticoagulant, either as antibody to factor VIII or, more commonly, as an inhibitor to the formation of "prothrombinase," results in prolonged clotting and prothrombin times and may be associated with mild or, rarely, severe hemorrhages.

Renal. Renal dysfunction occurs in over half the patients. Most patients have only some impairment of concentrating ability, a few red and/or white blood cells in the urine, and perhaps some proteinuria (< 0.5 gram per day). Active nephritis is defined when there is hematuria (> 5 rc per hpf), pyuria (> 5 wc per hpf), erythrocyte casts, increasing proteinuria, or a decreasing glomerular filtration rate. Hematuria and pyuria are rarely seen in lupus nephritis in remission.

Plasma Proteins. The erythrocyte sedimentation rate is often elevated. Serum albumin levels are low, especially in the nephrotic syndrome. Gamma globulin levels which are elevated in many patients may be low in nephrotics. Cryoglobulins, consisting of immunoglobulins and complement components, have been noted frequently, especially in patients with renal disease.

TABLE 2. Laboratory Abnormalities in SLE*

	Per Cent
Anemia	71
Leukopenia	56
Thrombocytopenia	11
Hemolytic anemia	8
Circulating anticoagulant	2
Rheumatoid factor	19
Biologic false-positive test for syphilis	15
Hypoalbuminemia	50
Hyperglobulinemia	37
LE cell	82
Antinuclear antibodies	96
Anti-double stranded DNA	32
Anti-single-stranded DNA	46
Anti-double-stranded RNA	51
Anti-nucleoprotein	41
Anti-"Sm"	68
Hypocomplementemia	66
CH50	66
C4	64
C3	52

*Adapted from Dubois, E. L.: Lupus Erythematosus, New York, McGraw-Hill Book Company, 1966; Estes, D., and Christian, C. L.: Medicine, 50:85, 1971; and Fernandez-Herlihy, L.: Lahey Clinic Found. Bull., 21:49, 1972.

Abnormal Immunologic Reactions. Biologic false-positive tests (BFP) for syphilis have been noted in about 15 per cent of the patients with SLE, especially in those with circulating anticoagulants. The BFP may be the first laboratory clue to the diagnosis of SLE and may precede symptoms by years. Rheumatoid factors have been found in some patients with SLE, even in the absence of clinical rheumatoid arthritis.

Most characteristic of SLE are the large number of autoantibodies which react with cells and their nuclear and cytoplasmic constituents. Historically of greatest significance is the LE cell phenomenon. The LE cell is formed in vitro as follows: some leukocytes are traumatized and release nucleoprotein (DNA-histone); the nucleoprotein reacts with an IgG antibody; and the complex is phagocytized by the remaining viable leukocytes. The LE cell consists of a leukocyte with a large purple-red homogeneous globulin inclusion body which compresses the nucleus against the cell membrane, leaving only a thin rim of cytoplasm. Because LE cells are not always present in patients with SLE, more sensitive tests have been developed for the detection of various antinuclear antibodies (ANA). An immunofluorescent (IF) technique, employing rodent liver or kidney as the source of nuclei, detects ANA in over 99 per cent of SLE patients. The antibodies may be of IgG, IgA, IgM, IgD, or IgE classes. Circulating DNA and other antigens may rarely block the detection of the ANA. With this immunofluorescent technique, different patterns of nuclear fluorescence reflect antibodies to different nuclear structures. The "homogeneous" or "diffuse" pattern reflects antibodies to nucleoprotein. The "peripheral," "rim," or "shaggy" pattern reflects primarily antibodies to DNA. The speckled pattern reflects antibodies to a group of nuclear proteins, including "Sm" and ribonucleoprotein. A nucleolar pattern has also been observed and appears to represent antibodies to a nuclear RNA.

Antibodies to some antigens, especially to DNA, have also been detected by other methods, including precipitation, diffusion in agar, complement fixation, agglutination, binding (Farr technique), and fluorescent spot test. The titers of antibodies to DNA and, to some extent, to nucleoprotein, double-stranded RNA, and ribosomes, tend to be higher during periods of clinical activity, especially of active nephritis, than during clinical remissions.

Complement levels are depressed in most patients with SLE at some time during their illness, especially when disease activity is present. Markedly depressed complement levels are seen primarily in patients with active lupus nephritis. The low levels reflect in vivo activation and fixation of complement components by circulating immune complexes. Serial determination of whole complement levels (CH5O) or of individual complement components (especially C4 and C3) may be useful in following and managing patients with SLE. "Lupus" has also been seen in some patients with congenital deficiency of C1r or C2.

Diagnosis. The diagnosis of SLE can be made if any four or more of the following manifestations are present, serially or simultaneously, during any interval of observation: butterfly rash, discoid lupus, Raynaud's phenomenon, alopecia, photosensitivity, oral or nasopharyngeal ulceration, arthritis without deformity, LE cells, chronic false-positive STS, profuse proteinuria, cellular casts, pleuritis or pericarditis, psychosis and/or convulsions, or hemolytic anemia, leukopenia, or thrombocytopenia. SLE should also be suspected—especially in young females—with unexplained fever, purpura, easy bruising, diffuse adenopathy, hepatosplenomegaly, peripheral neuropathy, endocarditis, myocarditis, interstitial pneumonitis, peritonitis, or aseptic meningitis.

Patients are frequently first diagnosed as having rheumatoid arthritis, rheumatic fever (especially children), glomerulonephritis, tuberculosis, scleroderma, vasculitis (including periarteritis), idiopathic thrombocytopenic purpura, lymphoma, anemia, or neutropenia. The LE cell is specific for SLE, if rheumatoid arthritis, lupoid hepatitis, or drug reactions can be excluded. Although the LE cell test is quite often negative, the antinuclear factor test is positive in virtually all patients with SLE. The antinuclear antibodies have also been detected in 68 per cent of patients with Sjögren's syndrome, 40 to 75 per cent of patients with scleroderma, especially the speckled pattern, 22 per cent of patients with juvenile rheumatoid arthritis, and 25 to 50 per cent of patients with rheumatoid arthritis, especially the homogeneous pattern. However, the antinuclear factors are present in higher titers in patients with SLE than in other disorders. Antibodies to double-stranded DNA are highly diagnostic of SLE.

TABLE 3. Autoantibodies in SLE

Antinuclear	Nucleoprotein DNA Histone Sm RNA Ribonucleoprotein Residue
Anticytoplasmic	Mitochondria Lysosomes Microsomes Ribosomes Cytoplasmic sap glycoprotein ("Ro") RNA protein
Anti-RNA	Ribosomal RNA Double-stranded RNA (? viral) Single-stranded RNA
Anticell	Red cell White blood cell Platelet
Anticlotting factors	
Antithyroid	
Rheumatoid factor	
Biologic false-positive test for syphilis	

Diagnostic problems always arise in patients with the so-called overlap syndromes, mixtures of signs and symptoms of SLE and other related diseases, such as rheumatoid arthritis, Sjögren's syndrome, scleroderma, and dermatomyositis. These patients are best considered, and treated, for their primary symptoms and complaints.

Drug-Induced Lupus. Drugs that induce lupus can be divided into two categories: drugs that induce lupus in many individuals, and drugs associated with exacerbations of SLE. In the former group are hydrazides (hydralazine, isoniazid), anticonvulsants (Dilantin), and procainamide. Over 50 per cent of subjects taking procainamide develop antinuclear antibodies; about 25 per cent develop symptoms and signs of lupus. Arthralgia, pleurisy with effusion, fever, and weight loss are common features, but renal disease and hypocomplementemia are not seen. Symptoms generally clear in a few weeks after discontinuation of the drug, even though antinuclear antibodies persist for months. Antinuclear antibodies appear less frequently in subjects taking hydralazine. Patients with the hydralazine lupus syndrome may have arthritis, dermatitis, serositis, leukopenia, antinuclear antibodies, and anti-DNA antibodies, but rarely have renal or central nervous system disease. Symptoms usually stop after cessation of the drug. Patients with hydralazine lupus are slow acetylators of the drug. These studies suggest that certain subjects may have a genetic predisposition for developing drug lupus. Other drugs, including penicillin, sulfonamides, and oral contraceptives, are associated with exacerbations of SLE, and rarely cause lupus-like symptoms or antinuclear antibodies in other subjects.

Therapy and Management. As there are no specific remedies for the treatment of the underlying processes of SLE, the main goals of management must be limited to the treatment of acute relapses and prevention of exacerbations. Certain measures are helpful in prevention of relapses. Sunlight, ultraviolet radiation, immunizations, blood transfusions, penicillin, and sulfonamides should be avoided when possible. Surgery or infections may lead to a relapse and may require more aggressive concurrent management of the lupus. In the long-term management of this illness, both patient and physician must learn to recognize those symptoms and signs that herald relapses. Although these symptoms may involve fever and arthralgia in some patients, they may appear as hair loss, mucosal ulcers, pleurisy, weight loss, or simply fatigue in others. Before frank clinical symptoms develop, many patients will develop abnormal laboratory tests such as a reduced level of hemoglobin or serum complement or a reduced white blood cell or platelet count; an abnormal urinalysis or creatinine clearance; or a rising titer of anti-DNA antibodies.

Many of the patients seen in the hospital by physicians or students have severe but not life-threatening disease. By contrast, many of the patients seen in the office have much milder disease. The patient fearing the unknown or having heard the worst must be reassured that a majority of patients have mild to moderate disease and that with proper management many of the more serious complications can now be controlled.

Active disease should be treated aggressively to prevent permanent tissue injury. The general measures to be taken include rest when the disease is active, sunscreens, and physical therapy for muscle weakness and deformities. For those patients on moderate to high dosages of corticosteroids, salt restriction and diuretics may be of benefit. Drugs used for the treatment of SLE include topical steroids, salicylates, antimalarials, corticosteroids, and immunosuppressives. The use of corticosteroids is indicated in most patients with SLE and has improved survival. Dosage should be individualized according to the activity of the disease and side effects. *Immunosuppressives* are best used according to the guidelines of Schwartz and Gowans, whose indications are life-threatening or seriously crippling disease; presence of reversible lesions; failure to respond to conventional therapy or intolerable side effects; no active infection; no hematologic contraindication; meticulous follow-up; and objective evaluation.

The acute erythematous maculopapular rash responds well to the avoidance of sunlight, local application of corticosteroid cream, and the systemic introduction of antimalarials such as hydroxychloroquin. Systemic corticosteroids are rarely warranted. The chronic lesion, or discoid lupus, responds to these same measures to a variable degree. Severe, extensive lesions have been treated with large doses of antimalarials when all else has failed. However, the patient should be cautioned about the relative risks of retinal damage when taking large doses of antimalarials. Arthralgia and arthritis respond well to rest, physical therapy, splinting, salicylates, and antimalarials. Steroids should not be needed.

Fever often responds to rest and salicylates. Antimalarials may be beneficial. Persistent fever not responsive to these measures usually coincides with other signs of activity and responds to moderate doses of corticosteroids. Infections must be excluded.

Pericarditis and pleurisy respond well to rest and corticosteroids. Fluid, if present in moderate amounts, is best removed. Myocarditis should be treated with moderate doses of steroids, fluid restriction, and careful administration of digitalis.

Hemolytic anemia and thrombocytopenia need not be treated unless symptomatic. They generally respond well to steroids. If not, immunosuppressives or a splenectomy may be necessary.

Involvement of the central nervous system responds poorly to treatment. Organic psychosis, in addition, may be difficult to differentiate from a steroid-induced psychosis. Because of the risk of permanent brain damage, large doses of steroids (2 to 3 mg of prednisone per kilogram of body weight per day) are recommended until maximal improvement is achieved, at which time the dosage of steroids is gradually tapered. Immunosuppressives may be necessary.

Mild focal glomerulitis with minimal urinary abnormalities may respond on occasion to bed rest; however, these patients and those with acute glomerulonephritis generally require systemic corticosteroid therapy. Prednisone has been given with good results, according to the following schedule, depending on renal function: blood urea nitrogen (BUN) less than 30 mg per 100 ml, 1 mg of prednisone per kilogram of body weight per day; BUN 31 to 100 mg per 100 ml, 2 mg per kilogram; BUN over 100 mg per 100 ml, 3 mg per kilogram. Patients unresponsive to these regimens may benefit from immunosuppressives. Medication is maintained until hematuria clears and serum complement levels return toward normal; this usually occurs within about three weeks. The LE cells, proteinuria, elevated sedimentation rate, and high titers of antinuclear antibodies may persist. The prednisone dosage is then tapered slowly – 10 mg every five days. Complete blood counts, urinalyses, serum creatinine levels, and serum complement levels are checked weekly to detect relapses; relapses usually respond either to maintaining the dosage at that level or increasing it by 5 to 10 mg of prednisone per day. Many patients can be maintained at a dosage of 5 to 10 mg per day; some can tolerate steroids on alternate days; a few can discontinue steroids and remain asymptomatic. Continued careful monitoring and early treatment of slight relapses may avoid more severe exacerbations.

Patients with chronic membranous glomerulonephritis and nephrotic syndrome respond less well to corticosteroids or immunosuppressives. Some, usually those with normal complement levels, may have fixed proteinuria.

Dubois, E. L., and Tuffanelli, D. L.: Clinical manifestations of systemic lupus erythematosus. J.A.M.A., 190:104, 1964.

Estes, D., and Christian, C. L.: The natural history of systemic lupus erythematosus by prospective analysis. Medicine, 50:85, 1971.

Harvey, A. M., Shulman, L. E., Tumulty, A., Conley, C. L., and Schoenrich, E. H.: Systemic lupus erythematosus: Review of the literature and clinical analysis of 138 cases. Medicine, 33:291, 1954.

Rothfield, N. F., and March, C. H.: Lupus erythematosus. *In* Fitzpatrick, T. B., Arndt, K. A., Clark, W. H., Eisen, A. Z., Van Scott, E. J., and Vaughan, J. H. (eds.): Dermatology in Internal Medicine. New York, McGraw-Hill Book Company, 1971, pp. 1493–1518.

Schur, P. H., and Sandson, J.: Immunological factors and clinical activity in lupus erythematosus. N. Engl. J. Med., 278:533, 1968.

82. PERIARTERITIS NODOSA (Polyarteritis Nodosa)

K. Frank Austen

Definition. Kussmaul and Maier introduced the term periarteritis nodosa in 1866 to designate a morbid process manifested by numerous grossly visible or palpable nodules along the course of medium-sized muscular arteries. The lesions are segmental in distribution, have a predilection for the crotch of bifurcations and branchings, and involve all but the pulmonary arteries. The clinical manifestations are disparate and polymorphic, and result from partial or complete arterial occlusion, hemorrhage, and glomerulitis. In view of the necrotizing nature of the process, involving the entire arterial wall, Ferrari in 1903 suggested the alternate name of polyarteritis acuta nodosa.

The incidence, age distribution, and male-to-female ratio of periarteritis nodosa are difficult to determine because a diagnostic serologic procedure is lacking, and the spotty distribution of lesions makes biopsy uncertain. Nonetheless, the condition has been reported to occur from infancy to old age, with a peak incidence in the fifth and sixth decades of life, and the male to female ratio has been estimated at from 2 to 3:1.

Pathology. The lesions of polyarteritis involve arteries of medium and small caliber, especially at bifurcations and branchings. The segmental process involves the media, with edema, fibrinous exudation, fibrinoid necrosis, and infiltration of polymorphonuclear neutrophils and varying numbers of eosinophils, and extends to the adventitia and intima. Thrombosis and infarction or hemorrhage occur at this stage. Subsequently, the regions of fibrinoid necrosis are replaced by cellular granulation tissue, and the intima proliferates. Finally the involved segment is replaced by scar tissue with associated intimal thickening and periarterial fibrosis. These changes produce partial occlusion, thrombosis and infarction, and palpable or visible aneurysms with occasional rupture.

The glomerulitis is characterized by capillary microthrombi, focal fibrinoid necrosis, polymorphonuclear neutrophil infiltration, and capsular proliferation. With progression, the necrotizing feature of the glomerulitis is less apparent, and the process is difficult to distinguish from glomerulonephritis of other causes.

Clinical Manifestations and Diagnosis. The widespread distribution of the arterial lesions produces diverse clinical manifestations, which reflect the particular organ systems in which the arterial supply has been impaired. In addition, no study including a large number of living patients has or even can limit its patient population to those with classic periarteritis as defined by Kussmaul and Maier. The available studies are likely to include an admixture of patients with allergic angiitis and granulomatosis and hypersensitivity angiitis (see Ch. 78). Among the early general symptoms and signs of periarteritis nodosa are tachycardia, fever, weight loss, and pain in viscera and/or the musculoskeletal system so that the differential diagnosis is of fever of unknown origin. Striking and specific presenting signs may relate to abdominal pain, acute glomerulitis, polyneuritis, or myocardial infarction. Pulmonary manifestations, especially intractable bronchial asthma, would indicate allergic angiitis and granulomatosis rather than classic polyarteritis nodosa.

Renal. Renal involvement in two forms, renal polyarteritis and a glomerulitis, may occur separately or together. Renal polyarteritis was the most common lesion in the postmortem studies of Rose and Spencer (see accompanying table), and in the comparable analysis performed at the Armed Forces Institute of Pathology by Mowrey (1954). Manifestations of the renal involvement include intermittent proteinuria and microscopic hematuria with occasional hyaline and granular casts. The glomerulitis is manifested by marked microscopic and even macroscopic hematuria, proteinuria, cellular casts, and progressive renal failure; survival of the acute phase is followed by progressive hypertension. It is no longer the prevailing view that hypertension precedes or occurs in the initial phase of periarteritis nodosa, but rather that it reflects healing renal polyarteritis, progressive glomerulitis, or both. Such renal involvement is the cause of death in about two thirds of patients with classic periarteritis nodosa and about one third of those with allergic angiitis and granulomatosis.

Incidence of Necrotizing Angiitis in Various Organs at Necropsy*

	Polyarteritis Nodosa (Classic)	Allergic Angiitis and Granulomatosis ("Polyarteritis with Pulmonary Involvement")
	Per Cent	*Per Cent*
Lungs (pulmonary arteries)	0	47
Heart	35	60
Kidneys: Glomerulitis	30	57
Renal polyarteritis	65	60
Stomach and intestines	30	40
Liver	54	37
Pancreas	39	17
Spleen	35	43
Brain	4	3
Periadrenal connective tissue	41	40
Voluntary muscle	20	33

*Reproduced in modified form from Rose and Spencer: Quart. J. Med., 26:43, 1957. There were 54 cases in periarteritis group and 30 with the diagnosis of allergic angiitis and granulomatosis.

Gastrointestinal. Characteristic arterial lesions are commonly found in one or more abdominal viscera. The principal manifestation is pain, especially in the umbilical region or right upper quadrant; anorexia, nausea, and vomiting are less prominent. Impaired arterial supply to the bowel can produce mucosal ulceration, perforation, or infarction with melena or bloody diarrhea. Involvement of appendix, gallbladder, or pancreas can simulate cholecystitis, appendicitis, or hemorrhagic pancreatitis. Liver involvement can range from hepatomegaly with or without jaundice to the signs of extensive hepatic necrosis. Splenomegaly is uncommon. The vasculitis associated with Australian antigenemia and considered by some to be representative of periarteritis nodosa is, of course, characterized by evidence of parenchymal liver disease.

Central and Peripheral Nervous System. Neurologic manifestations are generally late occurrences in the course of periarteritis nodosa, and their particular presentation reflects the specific brain area compromised. Headache, convulsive seizures, papillitis, and retinal hemorrhages and exudates occur with or without localizing signs referable to the cerebrum, cerebellum, or brainstem; meningeal irritation may occur as a result of subarachnoid hemorrhage. Multineuritis multiplex, that is, involvement of several or even many individual nerves at the same or different times, is a common finding and is attributed to arteritis of the vasa nervorum. The peripheral neuropathy is usually asymmetrical with both sensory and motor distribution. The former can be extremely painful, but the latter, with attendant muscular degeneration, has on occasion been so severe as to dominate the clinical presentation.

Articular and Muscular. Arthralgia and myalgia are frequent in polyarteritis nodosa. Arthralgia is migratory, generally without swelling, and apparently due to small localized arterial lesions rather than extensive synovitis. The interpretation of those rare instances of synovitis with deformity and arterial changes of periarteritis nodosa is difficult, but it seems preferable to consider such cases as rheumatoid arthritis. Muscle pain or weakness reflects either direct involvement of the arterial supply or a peripheral neuropathy from involvement of the vasa nervorum.

Cardiac. Polyarteritis of the coronary arteries and their branches has a frequency approaching that of renal polyarteritis, and heart failure is responsible for or contributes to death in one sixth to one half of the cases. The clinical manifestations of cardiac involvement are those of partial or complete arterial occlusion as modified by the superimposition of renal hypertension and an appreciable incidence of acute pericarditis without effusion. Whereas the combination of infarction and hypertension commonly leads to left-sided failure, an occasional patient with allergic angiitis and granulomatosis will present with predominantly right-sided decompensation.

Genitourinary. Involvement of the ovaries, testes, and epididymis is frequent, though usually asymptomatic. Mucosal ulceration in the bladder can occasionally precipitate gross hematuria with dysuria.

Cutaneous. Cutaneous involvement of some form is believed to occur in over 25 per cent of those affected with periarteritis nodosa. The acute cutaneous manifestations of periarteritis nodosa include polymorphic exanthemata—purpuric, urticarial, and multiform in character—and severe subcutaneous hemorrhage, resulting from necrotizing arteritis, with secondary gangrene. Ulcerations and a persistent livedo reticularis are associated with the more chronic stage of the disease. A most characteristic but uncommon finding is cutaneous and subcutaneous nodules; these occur at any time in the disease course. The nodules tend to group, appear in crops, are usually movable, may regress in days or persist for months, range in size from a pea to a walnut, and may cause the overlying skin to become reddened or to ulcerate.

Allergic Angiitis and Granulomatosis ("Polyarteritis with Pulmonary Involvement"). Pulmonary lesions are absent in classic polyarteritis nodosa but almost always precede the onset of polyarteritic lesions in other organs in the process termed allergic granulomatosis and angiitis by Churg and Strauss. Such patients typically present with bronchitis, bronchial asthma, or the findings of pneumonia. The asthma is intractable and associated with a marked peripheral eosinophilia. The pneumonic episodes are transient or progressive and can include hemoptysis or pleuritic pain. The appearance and superimposition of polyarteritis in other organs is followed by a rapid deterioration, respiratory involvement accounting for half the deaths.

Course Untreated. The course of periarteritis nodosa is progressive with destruction of vital organs. Intermittent acute episodes resulting from thrombosis of vital or nonvital structures are prominent. Death is most frequently attributed to renal involvement in cases of classic periarteritis nodosa and to pulmonary lesions in those cases classified as allergic angiitis with granulomatosis. Cardiac failure caused by a combination of infarction and renal hypertension is an additional frequent cause of death in both groups, and acute vascular accidents in the gastrointestinal tract or central nervous system account for much of the remaining mortality. In the retrospective postmortem study of Rose and Spencer, the five-year survival rate was about 10 per cent in classic periarteritis nodosa, and about 25 per cent in allergic angiitis and granulomatosis if onset was dated from the start of respiratory symptoms. The more recent report of the British Medical Research Council in 1960 placed the 54 months' survival rate in polyarteritis nodosa at nearly 50 per cent. A similar survival rate atributed to early steroid treatment has been noted in a Mayo Clinic series in which pulmonary involvement did not appear to influence the prognosis. Rare patients with polyarteritis limited to nonvital sites have been reported to experience an unusually long course or even a lasting remission. The entire issue of prognosis will be influenced by the criteria for entry into a series until the entity of periarteritis is more definitively separated from the more favorable grouping of hypersensitivity angiitis.

Laboratory Findings. Leukocytosis, predominantly polymorphonuclear, is apparent in over 75 per cent of the cases of periarteritis nodosa or allergic angiitis and granulomatosis, eosinophilia often being marked in the latter group. The erythrocyte sedimentation rate is customarily elevated with or without some increase of the globulins. Abnormalities in the urine sediment, especially hematuria and proteinuria, reflect renal involvement. Abnormalities of the electrocardiogram and electroencephalogram are those expected on the basis of arterial occlusive disease or those secondary to the metabolic disturbances of uremia. Lesions apparent on chest roentgenograms are the rule in patients with allergic angiitis and granulomatosis. The findings range from transient or progressive infiltration to consolidation, cavitation, or scarring; upper and lower lobes are involved with equal frequency. As none of these findings is specific, antemortem diagnosis of polyarteritis depends upon biopsy. Since the arterial involvement is segmental and spotty in distribution, it is advisable to obtain tissue from a symptomatic site, and it is essential to section completely the entire specimen. A deep, open surgical biopsy, including subcutaneous tissue and underlying muscle, should be obtained whenever possible from a skeletal muscle exhibiting pain and tenderness. Involvement of the epididymis and testes is sufficiently common to make this a useful biopsy site, if palpation reveals the typical nodularity of segmental vascular lesions. There are insufficient data on needle and surgical biopsies of internal organs, such as liver or kidney, to permit assessment of their usefulness or complications. As an alternative or additional procedure, arteriography of several organs to detect aneurysms of medium-sized muscular arteries may be helpful. Whether or not arteriography will prove definitive depends upon more experience with patients manifesting periarteritis nodosa and other forms of necrotizing vasculitis.

Differential Diagnosis. The differential diagnosis of classic periarteritis nodosa includes all those conditions associated with necrotizing angiitis (see Ch. 78). The absence of pulmonary lesions distinguishes classic periarteritis nodosa from allergic angiitis and granulomatosis. The other connective tissue diseases are recognized by their clinical characteristics even when necrotizing arteritis becomes prominent. For example, cases of rheumatoid arthritis with ulcerating cutaneous lesions and peripheral neuropathy often exhibit prominent rheumatoid nodules and a high titer of rheumatoid factor. Giant cell arteritis, in its limited form, cranial (especially temporal) or aortic arch (Takayasu's) arteritis, or in its disseminated state lacks the glomerulitis, peripheral neuropathy, and cutaneous manifestations notable in periarteritis nodosa. The drug-induced hypersensitivity angiitis group may be difficult to separate on purely clinical grounds, although the history of antecedent drug administration, the frequency of pulmonary involvement, infrequency of gastrointestinal manifestations, and absence of nodules along arteries are useful points. The clinical presentation in Henoch-Schönlein purpura, mostly in children and with a relatively good prognosis, is distinctive. The combination of progressive nephritis and pulmonary hemorrhage seen in Goodpasture's syndrome is unlike polyarteritis nodosa. The findings in the immunoglobulins which accompany active systemic lupus erythematosus or mixed cryoglobulinemia are distinctive; in addition, in the presence of active renal disease both entities manifest a reduced serum complement level not observed in periarteritis nodosa. Necrotizing vasculitis with or without renal disease in C2 deficiency, Australian antigenemia, and hypergammaglobulinemic purpura are differentiated by the unique features responsible for designating the entity.

The key morphologic differences between periarteritis nodosa and other causes of necrotizing angiitis are noted in Ch. 78 and include the absence of extravascular granulomas, sparing of the pulmonary arteries, failure of venous involvement except by contiguous spread, and predilection for medium-sized arteries. For allergic angiitis and granulomatosis the striking granulomatous response excludes all but Wegener's granulomatosis. The prominence of bronchial asthma, peripheral eosinophilia, and the usual absence of necrotizing lesions in the upper respiratory tract permit a tentative clinical distinction between allergic angiitis and granulomatosis (termed by some polyarteritis nodosa with pulmonary involvement) and Wegener's granulomatosis. Additional entities to be considered in the differential diagnosis are certain microbial and occlusive diseases with diverse manifestations, notably chronic meningococcemia, subacute infective endocarditis, trichinosis, certain rickettsial diseases, leptospirosis, and syphilis. A few vascular occlusive diseases, including Degos' disease and thrombotic thrombocytopenic purpura, must also be considered. Necrotizing papulosis of Degos, with its occlusive arterial lesions of the skin, gastrointestinal tract, and brain, is best characterized by the cutaneous manifestations. These lesions typically involve the trunk and extremities, begin as pink to gray papules, undergo central umbilication, and persist for variable periods with depressed (porcelain-like) centers covered with a removable scale and surrounded by a red elevated margin. The absence of both thrombocytopenia and intravascular hemolysis distinguishes periarteritis nodosa from thrombotic thrombocytopenic purpura. Additional points of help in the differential diagnosis of periarteritis nodosa in general are the rarity of Raynaud's phenomenon, the absence of the nephrotic syndrome, and the lack of lymphadenopathy.

Treatment. The therapy of periarteritis nodosa and allergic angiitis and granulomatosis is clearly unsatisfactory. Nonetheless, such patients can remain ambulatory and professionally active for periods of months to years after the clinical onset of the disease. The commonly employed antiinflammatory agents such as salicylates or phenylbutazone have little or no clear effect, and thus corticosteroids have been employed most widely. Large doses, in the range of 40 to 60 mg of prednisone per day, afford symptomatic relief and apparently do improve the one-year survival statistics. On the other hand, the study by the Medical Research Council of England did not reveal a better 54 months' survival period in a steroid-treated group as compared with a control series, whereas early steroid treatment was considered efficacious in the Mayo Clinic series. Experience with antimetabolites, such as azathioprine or cyclophosphamide, is insufficient to allow a conclusion as to their efficacy in periarteritis nodosa. The effect of these classes of compounds and drugs with related activities has been considered beneficial in diverse cases falling within the general classification of necrotizing vasculitis.

Churg, J., and Strauss, L.: Allergic granulomatosis, allergic angiitis, and periarteritis nodosa. Am. J. Pathol., 27:277, 1951.

Collagen Diseases and Hypersensitivity Panel: Report to Medical Research Council. Br. Med. J., 1:1399, 1960.

Mowrey, F. H., and Lundberg, R. A.: The clinical manifestations of essential polyangiitis (periarteritis nodosa) with emphasis on the hepatic manifestations. Ann. Intern. Med., 40:1145, 1954.

Rose, G. A., and Spencer, H.: Polyarteritis nodosa. Quart. J. Med., 26:43, 1957.

Part VI
DISEASES OF THE JOINTS

Charles L. Christian

83. INTRODUCTION

Although the terms "arthritis" and "rheumatism" have similar connotations, the former is restrictive, denoting inflammatory disease of joints. "Rheumatism" embraces a wide variety of illnesses that affect components of the musculoskeletal system: joints, muscles, ligaments, tendons, and bursae. Rheumatic syndromes can be classified as either inflammatory or degenerative, but the pathologic processes are sometimes less distinct than the nomenclature implies. A joint damaged by inflammatory disease is more vulnerable to degenerative influences, and syndromes that appear to be primarily degenerative in nature may be associated with the cardinal signs of inflammation. Musculoskeletal pain and stiffness, although characteristic of rheumatic syndromes, can be significant manifestations of virtually every disease of man. Errors in diagnosis and management result from uncritical elicitation of the medical history, physical signs, and, probably most frequently, from unbalanced interpretations of laboratory data. Hyperuricemia, rheumatoid factors, and antinuclear factors are not disease specific; and radiographic evidence of degenerative joint disease does not constitute proof that pain in an extremity is due to that process.

The accompanying classification of rheumatic disease (table), condensed and somewhat amended from the American Rheumatism Association's recommended (tentative) nomenclature, indicates the diversity of illnesses that can cause manifestations of rheumatic disease.

ARTHRITIS ASSOCIATED WITH KNOWN INFECTIOUS AGENTS

84. BACTERIAL ARTHRITIS

The great majority of cases of bacterial arthritis result from hematogenous spread of infections. Much less frequently, bacterial infection may result from joint aspiration or injection or by spread from contiguous osteomyelitis. In adults, gram-positive cocci (*Staphylococcus aureus, Streptococcus pyogenes, Diplococcus pneumoniae*) and *Neisseria gonorrhoeae* account for most

Rheumatic Disease—Classification

1. Polyarthritis of unknown etiology:
    a. Rheumatoid arthritis
    b. Juvenile rheumatoid arthritis
    c. Ankylosing spondylitis
    d. Psoriatic arthritis
    e. Reiter's syndrome
    f. Others
2. "Connective tissue" disorders (acquired):
    a. Systemic lupus erythematosus
    b. Progressive systemic sclerosis (scleroderma)
    c. Polymyositis and dermatomyositis
    d. Necrotizing arteritis and other forms of vasculitis
3. Rheumatic fever
4. Degenerative joint disease (osteoarthritis):
    a. Primary
    b. Secondary
5. Nonarticular rheumatism:
    a. Fibrositis
    b. Intervertebral disc and low back syndromes
    c. Myositis and myalgia
    d. Tendinitis and peritendinitis (bursitis)
6. Diseases with which arthritis is frequently associated:
    a. Sarcoidosis
    b. Relapsing polychondritis
    c. Schönlein-Henoch purpura
    d. Ulcerative colitis
    e. Regional enteritis
    f. Whipple's disease
    g. Sjögren's syndrome
    h. Familial Mediterranean fever
    i. Others
7. Arthritis associated with known infectious agents:
    a. Bacterial
    b. Rickettsial
    c. Viral
    d. Fungal
    e. Parasitic
8. Traumatic and/or neurogenic disorders:
    a. Traumatic arthritis (the result of direct trauma)
    b. Neuropathic arthropathy (Charcot joints)
    c. Shoulder-hand syndrome
    d. Mechanical derangement of joints
    e. Others
9. Arthritis associated with known or strongly suspected biochemical or endocrine abnormalities:
    a. Gout
    b. Chondrocalcinosis articularis ("pseudogout")
    c. Alcaptonuria (ochronosis)
    d. Hemophilia
    e. Sickle cell disease and other hemoglobinopathies
    f. Agammaglobulinemia (hypogammaglobulinemia)
    g. Gaucher's disease
    h. Hyperparathyroidism
    i. Acromegaly
    j. Hypothyroidism
    k. Scurvy
    l. Hyperlipoproteinemia type II (xanthoma tuberosum and tendinosum)
    m. Hemochromatosis
    n. Others
10. Neoplasms
11. Allergy and drug reactions
12. Miscellaneous disorders:
    a. Pigmented villonodular synovitis and tenosynovitis
    b. Behçet's syndrome
    c. Erythema nodosum
    d. Avascular necrosis of bone
    e. Juvenile osteochondritis
    f. Erythema multiforme (Stevens-Johnson syndrome)
    g. Hypertrophic osteoarthropathy
    h. Multicentric reticulohistiocytosis

cases. (Other areas of this text contain more detailed accounts of the problems and management of sepsis caused by specific bacterial organisms. The emphasis here is on principles of diagnosis and management that are common to all types of bacterial arthritis.)

Certain organisms appear to exhibit a tropism for joints: *N. gonorrhoeae, N. meningitidis, Hemophilus influenzae,* and *Streptobacillus moniliformis.* Host factors associated with debilitating chronic disease, rheumatoid arthritis, sickle cell anemia, hypogammaglobulinemia, and immunosuppressive therapy increase the risk of bacterial arthritis. A problem of increasing frequency is the development of low-grade infection complicating prosthetic joint placement. The recognition of infection may be delayed many months after joint replacement. Organisms of low virulence, especially *Staphylococcus albus,* predominate.

Clinical Manifestations. Although inflammatory signs in a single joint should heighten one's suspicion of bacterial sepsis, the disease may be polyarticular, a pattern that predominates with gonococcal arthritis. Rigor and high temperature, common manifestations of bacterial arthritis, are rare in rheumatoid arthritis and other types of noninfectious joint disease. Inflammatory signs tend to be marked; but in the presence of debilitating disease or treatment with adrenocorticosteroids or immunosuppressive agents, pain, swelling, and erythema may be masked. In patients with chronic rheumatoid arthritis, a preponderance of inflammatory disease in one or a limited number of joints should arouse suspicion of complicating bacterial arthritis.

Diagnosis. Since accurate diagnosis and effective management depend on isolation and characterization of the microbe, the highest priority is to be given to careful and complete bacteriologic studies. Although synovial fluid leukocyte counts in excess of 50,000 per cubic millimeter and reduced synovial fluid glucose content are common manifestations, no level of either is diagnostic of infection. Stained smears of joint fluid may demonstrate bacterial forms in the absence of a positive culture, especially when there has been chemotherapy. Synovial fluid and blood for microbiologic studies should be delivered without delay to the laboratory, preferably by someone involved in the patient's management. In addition to routine aerobic and anaerobic cultures, special media are needed for the isolation of *N. gonorrhoeae.* Obviously, bacteriologic studies of other materials, such as sputum, urine, and cervical exudate, may help to identify the organism causing arthritis.

Radiographic signs indicating loss of articular cartilage or erosion of bone are uncommon during the first week of disease.

Management. Success in management, as in diagnosis, rests with identification of the pathogen. The selection of appropriate antimicrobial agents and recommendations regarding dose and duration of therapy are covered in other areas of this text (see Ch. 268). It should be remembered that bacterial arthritis is usually a part of systemic sepsis and that the involvement of the synovial bursae behaves like a closed space infection. Since there is adequate transport of the commonly employed antibiotics from blood to joint fluid, there are rarely if ever indications for intra-articular therapy. When response to therapy is inadequate, measurement of bactericidal levels of drugs in synovial fluid may be indicated.

The decision whether to drain the joint bursae is influenced by the character of the exudate. When there is gross suppuration, and fluid cannot be easily aspirated with a large-bore needle, surgical incision and drainage are usually performed. When fluid can be aspirated with a needle and syringe, this is the preferred method for periodic decompression. The frequency of aspiration depends upon the extent and rate of reaccumulation. Gross joint destruction and the presence of contiguous osteomyelitis are indications for surgical drainage.

Physical therapy is inappropriate during the acute phase of bacterial arthritis. Maintenance of rest may be facilitated by removable splints. The rate at which gentle passive exercises can be graded into active motion should be tailored to each patient. Even in the absence of structural damage of weight-bearing joints, activity should not be resumed until signs of acute inflammation have subsided. The prognosis for full recovery is good when effective therapy is initiated within a week of the onset.

Gonococcal Arthritis. Gonococcal infection is discussed in Ch. 199. Because of its frequency and somewhat unique manifestations, this form of bacterial arthritis deserves emphasis. It is most common in females and homosexual males whose primary infections, because they are often asymptomatic, are untreated. The manifestations vary, but the most common pattern is migratory polyarthritis associated with tenosynovitis (especially in the hand and foot), followed by a "settling" in one or two joints. Shaking chills often precede or accompany the synovitis. Erythematous skin lesions, which may be macular, vesicular, or pustular (often with a necrotic center), are common in gonococcemia. The same clinical pattern can be associated with *N. meningitidis* and *H. influenzae* infections, although the latter is rare in adults.

Tuberculous Arthritis. The general decline in the frequency of tuberculosis is reflected in the relative rarity of tuberculous bone and joint disease. During the past few decades tuberculous arthritis has been predominantly an adult disease with evidence of pulmonary or disseminated disease frequently lacking. It is usually manifest in a single joint, most commonly hip, knee, or wrist, but any articulation may be affected, and occasionally two or more may be involved. Tuberculous *spondylitis,* predominantly a disease of children, has dramatically decreased in western countries.

Signs of acute inflammation are usually absent. Tuberculous arthritis is most commonly confused with monarticular rheumatoid arthritis. The ultimate differentiation, in a tuberculin-positive subject, often requires synovial biopsy and subsequent histologic and bacteriologic studies. Modern chemotherapy (see Ch. 242) has made surgical procedures (drainage, synovectomy, or fusion) unnecessary except in a rare patient with severe joint destruction.

85. VIRAL ARTHRITIS

Prevailing theories regarding the pathogenesis of rheumatoid arthritis, systemic lupus erythematosus, and related syndromes implicate atypical microbial infection. Although evidence supporting such speculations is indirect, there are well-defined, common viral infections associated with polyarthritis, notably rubella and viral hepatitis. Other viral syndromes associated with arthritis include mumps, infectious mononucleosis, and several arborvirus infections. Polyarthritis resembling acute rheumatic fever or acute rheumatoid arthritis occurs in approximately one third of women with natural or vaccine *rubella* infection. Lower frequencies of this complication are seen in men and children. Rubella arthritis usually follows the onset, or the fading phase, of the characteristic rash. The virus has been isolated from affected joints. The duration of joint inflammation varies from a few days to two weeks, rarely longer. There has been no documentation of chronic arthritis resulting from rubella infection. The management of pain and stiffness, which may be severe, should require nothing more than salicylate therapy.

Transient polyarthritis—more commonly polyarthralgia—is a significant prodromal manifestation of viral *hepatitis*. As with rubella, the pattern of arthritis resembles that of acute rheumatoid arthritis. It is frequently associated with fever and an urticarial skin eruption. These antedate the signs and symptoms of hepatitis by a few days to a few weeks, and have generally receded by the time icterus is apparent. Persistent polyarthritis has not been observed as a complication of viral hepatitis, although a small percentage of individuals with chronic active hepatitis have mild chronic or recurrent synovitis. The role that hepatitis B (Australia) antigen plays in the pathogenesis of the arthritis is not known, but certain manifestations, i.e., depressed serum complement and urticarial rash, are consistent with the hypothesis that immune complexes may be involved. Treatment is symptomatic.

86. OTHER FORMS OF INFECTIOUS ARTHRITIS

Syphilitic Arthritis. Syphilis is discussed in Ch. 246. Syphilitic arthritis, in its various forms, is now rare. A mild chronic synovitis, usually of the knees, may occur at about the age of puberty in patients with prenatal syphilis (*Clutton's joints*). Earlier skeletal manifestations of prenatal syphilis are related to periostitis and osteochondritis. Rheumatic manifestations have been attributed to secondary syphilis, but these, along with gummatous involvement of bones and joints, must have more historical than current importance. The most common rheumatic expression of syphilis, neuropathic arthropathy or Charcot joint, is reviewed in Ch. 97.

Mycotic Arthritis. Any of the invasive *mycoses* such as histoplasmosis, coccidioidomycosis, blastomycosis, and actinomycosis can affect joints, usually by extension from adjacent bone. Their manifestations generally resemble those of tuberculosis. Coccidioidomycosis can also cause the joint inflammation of erythema nodosum (see Ch. 911).

Alpert, E., Isselbacher, K. J., and Schur, P. H.: The pathogenesis of arthritis associated with viral hepatitis: Complement component studies. N. Engl. J. Med., 285:185, 1971.

Davidson, P. T., and Horowitz, I.: Skeletal tuberculosis: A review with patient presentations and discussion. Am. J. Med., 48:77, 1970.

Keiser, H., et al.: Clinical forms of gonococcal arthritis. N. Engl. J. Med., 279:234, 1968.

Schmid, F. R.: Principles of diagnosis and treatment of infectious arthritis. *In* Hollander, J. L., and McCarty, D. J., Jr. (eds.): Arthritis and Allied Conditions. 8th ed. Philadelphia, Lea & Febiger, 1972.

Sharp, J. T. Gonococcal arthritis. *In* Hollander, J. L., and McCarty, D. J., Jr. (eds.): Arthritis and Allied Conditions. 8th ed. Philadelphia, Lea & Febiger, 1972.

Smith, J. W., and Sanford, J. P.: Viral arthritis. Ann. Intern. Med., 67:651, 1967.

87. RHEUMATOID ARTHRITIS

Definition. In 1858 Sir Alfred Garrod introduced the term rheumatoid arthritis for a syndrome which he recognized as distinct from gout and acute rheumatic fever. With only minor exceptions (Garrod included Heberden's nodes as features of rheumatoid arthritis) his description matches the modern definition. The American Rheumatism Association's criteria for "classical, definite, probable and possible rheumatoid arthritis" have led to more consistent reporting in clinical studies, but the diagnosis still rests mainly on exclusion of other causes of synovitis.

Rheumatoid arthritis is a systemic disease of unknown cause. The frequency of extra-articular manifestations justifies the concept of "rheumatoid disease," but in the majority of patients clinical and pathologic findings and disability are the result of chronic inflammation of synovial membranes. There is striking heterogeneity among patients regarding mode of onset, pattern of joint involvement, frequency of extra-articular manifestations, and clinical course. There is a tendency for symmetrical involvement of hands, wrists, and feet. Spontaneous remissions and exacerbations are characteristic. Ten to 20 per cent of patients have complete remissions, whereas the remainder have sustained fluctuating activity. Joint injury results from formation of chronic granulation tissue (pannus), products of proliferative and exudative synovitis; this is capable of altering articular and periarticular structures.

Incidence and Epidemiology. The frequency of rheumatoid arthritis, based on limited population surveys in Europe and North America, is in the range of 1 to 3 per cent. It is two to three times more common in females. The onset is most frequent in the fourth and fifth decades of life, but it may occur at any age. There are no consistent trends relating prevalence to geography, climate, or culture. The apparent relative rarity in tropical climates may reflect the age of indigenous populations and the level of available medical care. Multiple family members in selected kindreds may be affected; but in general, familial patterns (even in monozygotic twins) are not striking.

Pathology. The pathologic elements of chronic synovitis include exudation, cellular infiltration, and the proliferation of granulation tissue. Although polymorphonuclear leukocytes predominate in synovial fluid, the principal infiltrating cells in synovial membranes are lymphocytes. These are often arranged in nodular aggregates, occasionally as true lymphoid follicles with germinal centers. Rarely, the majority of infiltrating cells are plasmacytes. Multinucleated giant cells may be seen. None of the aforementioned histologic features are diagnostic of rheumatoid arthritis.

Pannus, presumably by its content of hydrolytic enzymes, is capable of eroding articular cartilage, subchondral bone, ligaments, and tendons. Products of exudation in synovial fluid may also contribute to cartilage injury. The variable pattern of joint disability (subluxation, loss of motion, or ankylosis) relates to destructive processes in articular and periarticular structures.

Extra-articular manifestations, although clinically evident in a minority of patients, may give rise to widespread pathologic features of rheumatoid arthritis. Many of these appear to result from focal perivascular inflammation. Ten to 20 per cent of patients with rheumatoid arthritis form *subcutaneous or periosteal nodules* over pressure or friction points. The histologic appearance of nodules (central areas of necrosis surrounded by palisading connective tissue cells and an envelope of granulation tissue) is characteristic. In rare instances, the same granulomatous process can occur in multiple organs. More commonly (probably in the range of 50 per cent of cases) there is a mild perivascular infiltration of mononuclear cells in *muscle and peripheral nerves.* An uncommon but significant complication of the disease is the development of diffuse *necrotizing arteritis* with visceral involvement indistinguishable from polyarteritis nodosa. Milder forms of vasculitis, manifested by peripheral neuropathy and *chronic skin ulcers* of the lower extremities, are much more frequent. In such patients chronic inflammation of the sclera is common.

Cardiac pathology is less evident clinically than it is histologically. At necropsy, between one third and one half of rheumatoid patients have evidence of pericarditis (usually healed). Granulomatous lesions resembling rheumatoid nodules rarely may be found in the epicardium, myocardium, valves, and proximal aorta.

Pulmonary lesions, although infrequent, are significant expressions of rheumatoid disease. They include (1) chronic *pleural effusion,* (2) *Caplan's syndrome* (exaggerated pulmonary nodule formation in rheumatoid patients exposed to silica dust), (3) involvement with *granulomatous lesions resembling rheumatoid nodules,* and (4) *interstitial fibrosis.*

The most common patterns of neurologic involvement are peripheral neuropathy and nerve root irritation or myelopathy secondary to vertebral involvement (especially at C1-C2).

Pathogenesis. The role of *inflammation* in the production of articular, periarticular, and extra-articular injury is evident. A variety of lysosomal enzymes, neutral proteases, and synovial collagenase are capable of hydrolyzing constituents of connective tissue, and the role of such enzymes in the induction of tissue injury seems explicit. A more basic question, however, is: What initiates and perpetuates the inflammatory response? In this regard, immunologic theories predominate.

Immunologic Features. Synovial tissue in rheumatoid arthritis often displays histologic features characteristic of lymphoid organs, with prominent collections of lymphocytes and plasma cells (sometimes in the form of germinal centers). Immunoglobulin synthesis has been demonstrated in rheumatoid synovial tissue by immunohistologic and tissue culture studies. There is evidence for a role of immune complexes in the induction of inflammation. Synovial fluid exudate cells and synovial lining cells contain deposits of immunoglobulin and complement. Complement levels in synovial fluid are reduced in a pattern consistent with immune activation, and complexes of immunoglobulins are detectable in joint fluid. Detailed characterization of these has not been accomplished, but in part they consist of rheumatoid factors.

Rheumatoid Factors. Rheumatoid factors are autoantibodies reactive with the Fc portion of IgG. Antigammaglobulin activities are associated with the three major classes of immunoglobulins (IgM, IgG, and IgA), but, because of the enhanced agglutinating property of IgM antibodies, standard tests measure predominantly IgM rheumatoid factors. Rheumatoid factors form soluble complexes with their antigen (IgG). The complexes of IgM rheumatoid factor with IgG have a sedimentation coefficient of approximately 22S, whereas the complexes formed with IgG rheumatoid factors are very heterogeneous, sedimenting in the "intermediate" range between IgG and IgM. These intermediate complexes, which comprise at least part of the complexes measurable in rheumatoid synovial fluid, are capable of reacting with IgM rheumatoid factors to form insoluble aggregates. It is postulated that such complexes in joint fluid, perhaps augmented by their reactivity with IgM rheumatoid factor, activate complement-dependent mediators of inflammation and promote phagocytosis and subsequent release of hydrolytic enzymes. Although this hypothesis is attractive, there are a variety of reasons why one cannot assign an exclusive and primary role to rheumatoid factors in the induction of rheumatoid synovitis. On the basis of current evidence, it is more likely that rheumatoid factors are products of the host response to a more primary event. The nature of this postulated primary event is still unknown, but there is renewed interest in an old concept that microbial disease may underlie the development of rheumatoid arthritis.

Infectious Agents. A number of clinical and pathologic features of rheumatoid arthritis are mimicked by animal models of disease where microbial causes are explicit – in particular, chronic arthritis in swine induced by species of Mycoplasma and by *Erysipelothrix insidiosa.* An interesting aspect of these experimental models is that by the time chronic disease has developed, the inducing microorganism is often not demonstrable. By analogy, if the microbial hypothesis for rheumatoid disease is correct, the generally negative results of efforts to recover microorganisms may thus be explained. Although speculation regarding an infectious cause of rheumatoid disease has been augmented by modern concepts of viral persistence and by studies of animal models, direct evidence in its support is lacking. There have been periodic reports of the isolation of Mycoplasma and bacterial forms and of demonstrations that rheumatoid synovial cells are resistant to infection by exogenous viruses, but these observations still lack confirmation.

Clinical Manifestations. *Mode of Onset.* Usually, rheumatoid arthritis has an insidious onset, often beginning with poorly localized aching and stiffness. These early symptoms may be attributed to "grippe," and the subsequent evolution of frank synovitis may be sufficiently slow that the patient does not seek medical attention for many weeks. A variety of "precipitating" factors have been entertained (trauma, environmental change, infections, and psychologic stress), but none of these is constant in the antecedent history. Most patients manifest symmetrical polyarthritis early in the course of their disease, but a significant number (approximately one third) will have inflammation limited to one or two joints. Occasionally limited expressions of the disease, i.e., monarthritis or even tenosynovitis, may persist for many weeks or months. In contrast to the gradual onset of disease that characterizes the majority, the onset is precipitous in some patients, almost to the hour of a given day.

Symptoms. *Pain,* the dominant symptom, corresponds to the pattern and intensity of joint involvement, whereas *stiffness* is more generalized and is characteristically maximal after periods of physical inactivity. *Morning stiffness* is an almost invariable feature: its intensity and duration can guide one in assessment of disease activity.

The majority of patients experience *constitutional symptoms* such as weakness, increased fatigability, and diminished appetite. Temperature elevation in excess of 37.8° C is uncommon. Higher temperatures should prompt search for superimposed infection, but occasionally temperatures as high as 40° C have no other explanation than active rheumatoid arthritis. Many patients complain of coldness and hypesthesias and paresthesias in the hands and feet (in the absence of signs of nerve entrapment).

Physical Signs. The physical signs of rheumatoid arthritis vary enormously according to anatomic patterns, severity, and stage of disease. The "classic" articular and extra-articular expressions are features of *chronic* rheumatoid arthritis.

GENERAL EXAMINATION. Observations of gait and performance of simple tasks, such as removal of clothing, may reveal evidence of stiffness or specific anatomic patterns of disease. Many, but not all, patients appear chronically ill and undernourished. Generalized lymphadenopathy and splenomegaly are features in some subjects (approximately 10 per cent); rarely this picture is so striking that it mimics lymphomatous disease. Dependent edema not attributable to other causes is an infrequent but significant feature. Easy bruising and increased fragility of skin are common in patients with chronic disease; both are amplified by corticosteroid therapy. Nodules are most commonly found in subcutaneous tissue, but they can occur within the dermis and periosteum. Nodules are characteristically localized over points of pressure or friction, most commonly the extensor surfaces of the proximal forearms. In a bedridden patient they may be found over the posterior aspects of the head, trunk, and spine.

SKELETAL MANIFESTATIONS. The invariable signs of swelling, tenderness, and pain on motion in early cases may seem poorly localized to joints. A common mode of onset, with symmetrical involvement of the distal upper extremities, is diffuse swelling of the hands and wrists. More discrete enlargement of articulations (Fig. 1) may not appear for weeks or months. Warmth is usually evident, especially over the large joints such as the knee, but skin erythema is infrequent. Swelling reflects varying degrees of synovial thickening and proliferation and an increased volume of synovial fluid. From palpation and ballottement, the examiner can usually estimate the relative roles of effusion and synovial proliferation.

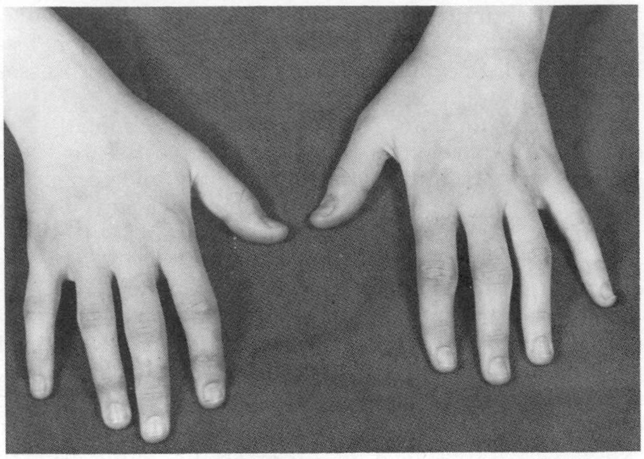

Figure 1. Early rheumatoid arthritis manifest as symmetrical swelling and slight flexion deformities of proximal interphalangeal joints of the hands. Roentgenograms were normal except for evidence of soft tissue swelling.

The characteristic deformities of joints which are products of sustained chronic disease are attributable to a variety of events: loss of articular cartilage, destruction or weakening of ligaments, tendons, and capsular structures, muscle imbalance, and the physical force associated with use of the affected joints (Fig. 2). In addition, there are biologic variations which in some patients favor joint subluxation and instability and in other patients result in bony or fibrous ankylosis.

Muscle atrophy of the affected extremities may be evident within weeks of onset of rheumatoid arthritis. Whether this relates to primary myopathic change or disuse is moot, but rarely an overt myopathy, indistin-

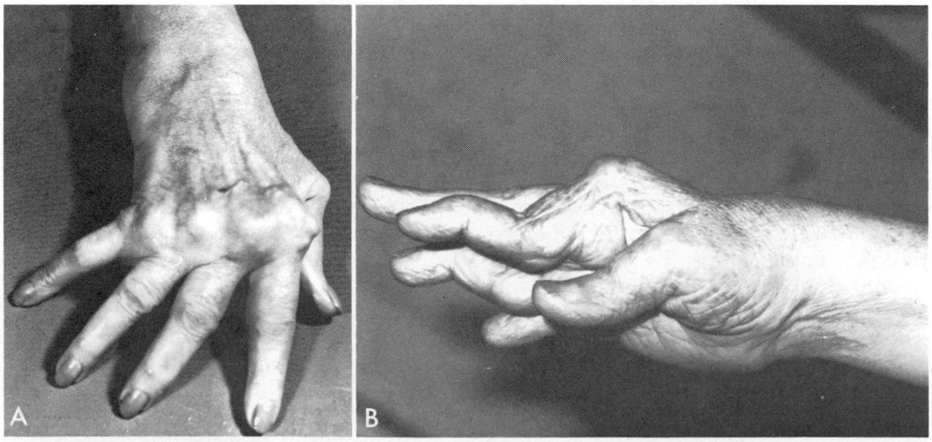

Figure 2. Hand deformities characteristic of chronic rheumatoid arthritis. *A,* Subluxation of metacarpophalangeal joints with ulnar deviation of digits. *B,* Hyperextension ("swan neck") deformities of proximal interphalangeal joints.

guishable from polymyositis, may be a feature of the disease.

Extensions or rupture of synovial bursae beyond the confines of joint capsules can result in features of special importance to the internist. The most common example of this is the communication of joints of the wrists with the tenosynovium of the finger extensors. Popliteal cysts associated with knee synovitis may rupture into the calf and produce an inflammatory reaction that very closely resembles deep vein thrombophlebitis. The sudden onset of this complication, often associated with forceful flexion of the knee, and the intense inflammation help distinguish it from phlebitis, but this differentiation is best accomplished by arthrography. Rarely, extensions from hip synovitis may result in the formation of pelvic or inguinal masses.

EXTRA-ARTICULAR MANIFESTATIONS. Many of the features of rheumatoid arthritis that are associated with diffuse vasculitis have been discussed previously under Pathology. The clinical expressions of vasculitis (neuropathy, chronic skin ulcers, digital gangrene, and rarely visceral arteritis) and the clinical patterns associated with disseminated granulomata (heart, lung, sclera, and dura mater) are invariably features of chronic "classic" disease and are rarely encountered in patients who lack the rheumatoid factor.

For reasons unknown, pulmonary involvement (pleural effusion, granulomatous pneumonitis, and diffuse interstitial fibrosis) is more common in males. Cavitating pulmonary nodules occasionally result in pneumothorax or chronic bronchopleural fistulas. The glucose content of rheumatoid pleural effusions is frequently less than 10 mg per 100 ml.

There are usually no problems in interpretation of neurologic signs related to peripheral neuropathy, nerve entrapment (median nerve involvement at the wrist is common), and radiculopathy. In contrast, the insidious progression of muscle weakness secondary to myelopathy from C1-C2 subluxation can mistakenly be attributed to "arthritis" and associated constitutional symptoms.

Other extra-articular manifestations of rheumatoid arthritis include amyloidosis, keratoconjunctivitis sicca, and Felty's syndrome.

Clinical Course and Prognosis. Statistics regarding the natural history of rheumatoid arthritis are based on studies in large rheumatic disease units where patients are not representative of the entire population of rheumatoid arthritics, i.e., they tend to be patients with more severe and sustained disease. Patients with more remitting patterns of disease are less apt to be entered into prognostic studies. However, even the published figures allow one to present a reasonably optimistic outlook to the patient. After 10 to 15 years of disease, over 50 per cent of patients remain fully employed and only about 10 per cent are completely incapacitated. Ten to 20 per cent of patients have virtually complete remissions; the course followed by the remainder is extremely varied. The average patient with episodic exacerbations and partial remissions will experience gradual progression of deformity and disability. The minority, with sustained disease activity and only slight remissions, may become completely disabled within a few years of onset. The *features associated with a poor prognosis,* in a statistical sense are (1) classic pattern of disease (symmetrial polyarthritis with subcutaneous nodules and high titers of rheumatoid factor), (2) sustained disease of more than one year's duration, (3) onset below age 30, and (4) extra-articular manifestations of rheumatoid arthritis.

Roentgenographic Findings. Early in the disease roentgenograms of affected joints are usually negative except for evidence of soft tissue swelling and joint effusion. Osteoporosis, especially in juxta-articular locations, may be evident within weeks of onset of disease. Loss of articular cartilage, shown by reduction in the apparent "joint space," and bone erosions are rarely evident before several months of sustained disease. Subluxations, dislocations, and bony ankylosis, if they occur, are still later phenomena. Diffuse osteoporosis is common with chronic disease and is heightened with adrenocorticosteroid therapy. The frequency of avascular osteonecrosis, especially of the femoral heads, is also increased with such therapy.

Laboratory Findings. Mild *anemia,* similar to that associated with chronic infection, is common in rheumatoid arthritis. Serum levels of both iron and iron-binding protein are frequently depressed. Anemia is usually normocytic and normochromic, but if there is accompanying iron deficiency, the erythrocytes may be slightly hypochromic and microcytic. Leukocytosis, eosinophilia, and thrombocytosis are occasional laboratory features. (See Ch. 88 for discussion of neutropenia associated with Felty's syndrome.)

The *erythrocyte sedimentation rate* (ESR) is increased above the normal range in virtually all patients with active rheumatoid arthritis. There are a variety of other "acute phase reactants" in the serum which reflect inflammatory activity, but none of them match the simplicity of the ESR or exceed its sensitivity.

Rheumatoid *synovial fluid* is usually turbid with reduced viscosity, increased protein content, and slight reduction of glucose levels relative to the blood. Leukocyte counts (predominantly polymorphonuclear cells) vary between a few thousand and more than 50,000 cells per cubic millimeter. Cells containing inclusions are common, but these may be seen in other types of exudative synovitis. Complement in synovial fluid, relative to protein content, is commonly reduced, a finding usually associated with positive tests for rheumatoid factors.

There are no tests that are specific for rheumatoid arthritis, although the term "rheumatoid factors" has been applied to autoantibodies reactive with IgG (see Pathogenesis above). A variety of test systems are available, but most laboratories utilize the *latex fixation test,* in which polystyrene latex particles coated with IgG are agglutinated by rheumatoid factors. Less commonly applied systems include the *bentonite flocculation test* and a variety of *hemagglutination tests* employing erythrocytes coated with immunoglobulins. The latex fixation test is positive (1:80 titer or higher) in approximately 70 per cent of rheumatoid subjects. Although less than 5 per cent of healthy control subjects are positive, the rheumatoid factor is associated with other connective tissue syndromes, liver disease, and a variety of infectious diseases such as bacterial endocarditis, tuberculosis, syphilis, and leprosy. The frequency of positive tests for rheumatoid factor in the general population increases with age.

Differential Diagnosis. *General.* Differential considerations are numerous and vary according to the pattern of disease. There is seldom confusion in identifying "classic" rheumatoid arthritis, but symmetrical involvement of hand and wrist joints can be a feature of other syndromes (see below). Differentiation is more difficult and complex in patients with early acute polyarthritis or in those with arthritis limited to one or a few joints.

Chronic Polyarthritis. The most common form of chronic arthropathy, degenerative joint disease, is usually quite distinct from rheumatoid arthritis. Minimal inflammatory signs, absence of constitutional symptoms, ESR determinations in the range of normal, and the characteristic radiographic findings usually serve to identify degenerative joint disease. A clinical pattern of degenerative joint disease which has been termed "primary generalized osteoarthritis" (see Ch. 98) may be mistaken for rheumatoid arthritis, especially when there is symmetrical enlargement of interphalangeal joints in the hands. *Bouchard's nodes,* the bony enlargement of proximal interphalangeal joints of the hand (see Fig. 4*B*) are rather frequently misinterpreted as signs of rheumatoid arthritis.

Gout and *chondrocalcinosis* (see Ch. 821 and 97, respectively) may mimic chronic rheumatoid arthritis. The most definitive basis for their identification is polarized light microscopy of synovial fluid.

Other connective tissue syndromes such as *systemic lupus erythematosus* (SLE) and *progressive systemic sclerosis* are infrequently associated with chronic deforming joint change. Their differentiation from rheumatoid arthritis is based on characteristic multisystemic patterns of disease. Certain serologic features of SLE, especially hypocomplementemia and the antibodies to native deoxyribonucleic acid, are rare in rheumatoid arthritis. A few patients, with mixed clinical and laboratory features of two or more syndromes, defy classification.

The majority of patients with arthritis and *psoriasis* are indistinguishable from patients in the spectrum of rheumatoid arthritis. The designation psoriatic arthritis as a separate entity is in part arbitrary, but certain clinical and laboratory features of psoriatic arthritis (see Ch. 92) aid in its differentiation from rheumatoid arthritis.

Rheumatic manifestations of a wide variety of systemic diseases, including sarcoidosis, ulcerative colitis, regional enteritis, Whipple's disease, amyloidosis, acromegaly, chronic infection, and malignancies, can resemble rheumatoid arthritis. This list emphasizes the importance of exclusions in formulating a diagnosis of rheumatoid arthritis.

Acute Polyarthritis. The range of differential considerations for acute polyarthritis includes those listed above plus a variety of disorders that rarely if ever result in chronic joint disease. The most frequent set of diagnostic considerations for acute polyarthritis includes rheumatoid arthritis, acute rheumatic fever, infection, and drug hypersensitivity. Acute arthritis associated with chills and fever should be considered infectious until proved otherwise. The presence of carditis, evidence of recent streptococcal infection, fever, and prompt response to salicylate therapy contribute to the recognition of acute rheumatic fever. Important differentiating features of gonococcal arthritis are prominent tenosynovitis, the cutaneous manifestations, and, most important, isolation of the bacteria from blood or joint fluid. The common viral infections that can resemble acute rheumatoid arthritis are rubella and viral hepatitis. There are other remitting forms of polyarthritis in which viral causes are suspected but not established. A careful clinical history and the recognition of other allergic phenomena will help in the identification of drug hypersensitivity.

Monarthritis or Oligoarthritis. All the conditions listed above under Acute and Chronic Polyarthritis are appropriate to the differential diagnosis of arthritis affecting one or a limited number of joints; but when the pattern of joint involvement is restricted, the most important differential consideration is infection. A complete medical evaluation, including chest x-ray, tuberculin tests, and appropriate microbial studies, is indicated. When there is continued suspicion of bacterial or mycobacterial infection, synovial biopsy may be required.

Management. *Basic Principles.* In the management of rheumatoid arthritis, the physician should keep the following facts in mind: (1) in most patients the disease is chronic; (2) spontaneous remissions occur in almost all patients; (3) the majority of subjects can continue to lead active lives with varying degrees of restrictions; and (4) complications of drug therapy, most notably adrenocorticosteroids, can cause greater morbidity than the underlying disease.

The patient and the doctor must be educated not to expect and seek a short-term solution. The physician can present a reasonably optimistic prognosis, based on knowledge of the natural history of rheumatoid arthritis, and can assure the patient that there are conservative means of ameliorating symptoms and minimizing disability.

There are no specific dietary recommendations; rather, the general nutritional status of the patient and associated medical conditions influence diet selection. Weight reduction, in obese patients, should have high priority. Providing that the diet is well balanced, there are no indications for vitamin supplementation. The anemia of rheumatoid arthritis does not respond to hematinic therapy except to the extent that iron deficiency may be a complicating feature. Rarely the anemia may be so severe as to require transfusion.

Psychologic depression is a common consequence of chronic rheumatoid arthritis. From the physician, the patient needs sympathetic understanding of his problems and a willingness to help solve them. When depression is severe, these efforts may be facilitated by the use of antidepressive medication. If anxiety, restlessness, and insomnia are complicating features, the use of mild sedatives or tranquilizers may be indicated.

A basic program that is applicable to all patients includes (1) rest, (2) employment of salicylates for the relief of pain and suppression of inflammation, and (3) maintenance of joint function by physical measures. Some but not all patients will be candidates for medicinal therapy other than salicylates and/or orthopedic surgical procedures.

REST. Patients and physicians alike tend to be confused by the apparently conflicting goals of rest and exercise. They are not mutually exclusive (see Physical Measures below). It is clear that physical work, applied to an affected extremity, will intensify the synovitis of rheumatoid arthritis. The specific prescription of rest will vary according to the severity and pattern of involvement, but all patients should be directed to respect their symptoms of pain and fatigue and to restrict physical activities to the essentials. Any way that occupational duties can be modified to lighten the work load should be tried, and daytime rest periods are important. Occasionally when symptoms are very severe, hospitalization for attainment of more complete rest is indicated.

EMPLOYMENT OF SALICYLATES. All students of rheumatoid arthritis agree that salicylate therapy is part of the basic management. The majority of patients can tolerate acetylsalicylic acid in doses of 3.6 grams daily or more, if the physician is persistent in his recommendations. When gastrointestinal symptoms complicate therapy, ingestion of the drug with meals or the use of enteric-coated or buffered products may be helpful. When doses of acetylsalicylic acid in the range of 3.6 grams daily are tolerated but rheumatic symptoms are poorly controlled, gradual increase in the dose is warranted. It is too often concluded, on the basis of inadequate trials, that "aspirin was not effective." Measurement of blood salicylate levels is appropriate when there is a question of toxicity or absorption.

PHYSICAL MEASURES. The choice of various heat modalities (warm pool, tank, bath, shower, diathermy, or ultrasound) depends primarily on the areas affected and the availability of services. Diathermy and ultrasound treatments are contraindicated in patients with metal implants. A warm pool permitting exercise under water is optimal for the patient with very severe symptoms, but for most individuals a hot bath or shower will suffice. Morning stiffness and pain will be minimized by ingestion of salicylates followed by a hot bath.

The *goals of an exercise program* are (1) maintenance of motion of affected joints, and (2) prevention of muscle atrophy. Both of these can be achieved without submitting inflamed joints to the task of work. An active exercise program for the lower extremities can maintain motion and strength without heavy weight bearing, allowing the right combination of rest and exercise. The rate of progression from gentle passive exercises, required for the most symptomatic patient, to a more active program will vary according to the pattern of involvement and the response to therapy. In order that the patient avoid assuming a passive dependent role, it is crucial that emphasis be placed on what he or she can do independent of supervision. The average doctor is not sufficiently trained in physical medicine to write detailed prescriptions, but he should be very specific in what his goals are when referring the patient to a physical medicine service. Furthermore, he should review the program periodically with the patient and reinforce its importance in the total management. It is a moot point whether forceful active exercises are appropriate for the distal upper extremities; evidence suggests that heavy work will aggravate hand and wrist deformities. For a patient with acutely inflamed joints, removable splints to achieve rest are helpful, but there are no convincing demonstrations that such devices prevent development of chronic hand deformities.

The role of orthopedic surgery in the management of rheumatoid arthritis is discussed subsequently in this chapter.

Other Antirheumatic Therapy. For the patient whose response to salicylate therapy has not been adequate, several other anti-inflammatory agents can be employed. These include indomethacin, phenylbutazone (and oxyphenbutazone), antimalarial drugs (chloroquine and hydroxychloroquine), and gold compounds. At the time of this writing, several other nonsteroidal anti-inflammatory agents are under evaluation but are not yet licensed for use in the United States. The adrenocorticosteroid drugs are the most potent anti-inflammatory medications available, but their value, for reasons stated below, is limited. Unfortunately all medications employed for the treatment of rheumatoid arthritis, except gold compounds, have in common the property of promoting peptic ulceration.

Among those who specialize in the management of rheumatic disease, there is no uniformity of habit regarding the employment of agents listed above, although the majority, at some time, will institute gold therapy for the patient with sustained rheumatoid arthritis. Codeine and related analgesics may be required on a temporary basis, but their chronic use should be discouraged.

Phenylbutazone is a reasonably potent anti-inflammatory agent, but there is limited enthusiasm for its use in long-term management of rheumatoid disease. In doses of 200 to 300 mg daily, this drug may be helpful in the treatment of intermittent exacerbations. The incidence of serious toxicity (exfoliative dermatitis and hematologic complications) is infrequent but a source of concern. The occasional patient who is helped by long-term therapy should be under close medical supervision and should have periodic blood counts.

Indomethacin, although chemically unrelated to other analgesic and anti-inflammatory drugs, has a pattern of efficacy similar to that of phenylbutazone. Both are more effective in gout and ankylosing spondylitis than in rheumatoid arthritis. In the dose range of 50 to 200 mg per day, a few patients will experience sufficient benefit to warrant its continuation. Gastrointestinal symptoms and vascular headaches are common side effects, but serious complications are rare. Concomitant aspirin therapy appears to diminish gastrointestinal absorption of indomethacin.

Antimalarial compounds such as chloroquine and hydroxychloroquine have moderate anti-inflammatory activity in the treatment of rheumatoid arthritis. Because of the occasional association of irreversible retinopathy, the use of antimalarials has sharply declined.

Although soluble *gold compounds* have been employed in the treatment of rheumatoid arthritis since the 1930s, their mode of action is not known. There is no evidence that they have anti-inflammatory activity; rather, clinical impressions suggest that, in some unknown way, they increase the likelihood of remission. The level of enthusiasm for chrysotherapy varies considerably among rheumatic disease specialists. Some advocate such treatment within weeks of onset of disease; others reserve it for patients who have had sustained disease for several months or more in spite of more conservative therapy. There is a cumulative effect of gold compound administration. Sensitive assays can detect trace amounts many months after discontinuation of therapy. Gold is excreted primarily in the urine. The most common complications are dermatitis and stomatitis. Renal damage, manifested by proteinuria and microscopic hematuria, and hematological dyscrasias (thrombocytopenia and granulocytopenia) are rare but significant complications of chrysotherapy.

The preparations employed are sodium aurothiomalate (Myochrysine) and aurothioglucose (Solganal). Both are administered by deep intramuscular injection at weekly intervals. It is common practice to use small doses (10 to 25 mg) for the first two or three injections, followed by 50 mg at weekly intervals thereafter. Complete blood count and urinalysis should be obtained prior to each injection for several weeks and every few weeks after that as long as therapy is continued. If there is any sign from these tests or from clinical assessment (pruritic rash or stomatitis) of gold toxicity, therapy should be interrupted. If unequivocal evidence of gold toxicity develops, such as severe stomatitis or exfoliative dermatitis or renal or hematologic complications, treatment should not be resumed. In the case of mild, transient skin reactions, it is common practice to reinstitute the medication at reduced levels after the rash has cleared. Experience indicates that remissions, if they occur on gold therapy, will occur during the course of 20 weekly injections (approximately 1 gram total dose). In the absence of improvement during this course, there is no point in continuing therapy. For the patient experiencing a remission, it is recommended that maintenance therapy be continued (50 mg at three- to four-week intervals). The decision as to maintenance therapy in patients who experience only partial remission is more difficult.

Mild gold-induced dermatitis may persist for several weeks or more, but usually requires no therapy other than topical corticosteroids. The most common presentation consists of several scattered, well-circumscribed pruritic lesions associated with mild scaling. The discomfort associated with severe dermatitis may warrant a course of systemic corticosteroid therapy (10 to 20 mg of prednisone daily) or the use of BAL (dimercaprol). Hematologic complications, most commonly thrombocytopenia, are also indications for dimercaprol therapy. Dimercaprol, 2.5 mg per kilogram of body weight, is given every four hours for two days, followed by the same dose twice daily for approximately a week. An alternative means of promoting gold excretion is the employment of penicillamine, although there is less clinical experience to recommend it.

Adrenocorticosteroid Therapy. SYSTEMIC THERAPY. Since the early therapeutic trials of cortisone in 1949, several related compounds with potent anti-inflammatory activity have been introduced. These include prednisone, prednisolone, triamcinolone, methylprednisolone, dexamethasone, betamethasone, and paramethasone. Electrolyte and water-retaining properties, associated with cortisone and hydroxycortisone therapy, are minimal with the newer drugs, but the more serious side effects are common to *all* adrenocorticosteroid preparations (see below). The approximate milligram equivalent of the various drugs that yield comparable pharmacologic effects are cortisone (25 mg), hydrocortisone (20 mg), prednisone (5 mg), triamcinolone (4 mg), methylprednisolone (4 mg), dexamethasone (0.75 mg), betamethasone (0.6 mg), and paramethasone (2 mg).

Because of frequent and potentially life-threatening complications of adrenocorticosteroid therapy, it should not be employed in the management of rheumatoid arthritis until there has been a sustained trial of more conservative therapy. In general, the more experienced the physician is in the management of rheumatoid disease, the more reluctant he is to begin adrenocorticosteroid therapy. The following facts should be pondered before initiating such treatment: (1) adrenocorticosteroid drugs suppress inflammation, but they do not correct or change the underlying process; (2) small doses, in the range of 5 to 10 mg of prednisone, often provide only partial and temporary gains; (3) over periods of months or years, there is a tendency for the dose to increase; (4) once instituted, it is very difficult to discontinue therapy; and (5) the morbidity and mortality associated with long-term adrenocorticosteroid therapy often exceed those of the underlying disease.

In the light of these facts, it is difficult to summarize indications for adrenocorticosteroid therapy of rheumatoid arthritis. If a conservative effort, employing less toxic drugs and physical measures, fails to check progressive disability and if the alternative to adrenocorticosteroid therapy seems to be chronic invalidism, then the former may be indicated. In such cases the daily dose should not exceed 10 mg of prednisone or its equivalent; as little as 5 to 7.5 mg in divided doses may provide some benefit. Although pituitary-adrenal unresponsiveness and other complications of therapy are minimized by alternate-day or single daily dose regimens, most patients with rheumatoid arthritis do not tolerate such programs. Occasionally, sustained disease may be less severe but may compromise the occupational activity of a wage earner or mother of a household. A small dose (5 or 7.5 mg daily of prednisone or equivalent) may allow continuation of employment, but the physician and patient should make the decision deliberately and with full realization of the toxic potential of such therapy.

COMPLICATIONS OF ADRENOCORTICOSTEROID THERAPY. The frequency and severity of *osteoporosis,* a feature of rheumatoid disease regardless of therapy, are increased by adrenocorticosteroid treatment. Compression fractures of vertebral bodies are common. (Detailed discussions of the management of osteoporosis are presented in Ch. 879 to 884). There are theoretic bases for employment of high calcium intake, vitamin D, fluorides, and anabolic steroids, but their efficacy in preventing or reversing osteoporosis is uncertain. Another frequent skeletal complication of adrenocorticosteroid therapy is *avascular osteonecrosis,* most commonly affecting the femoral head.

Although most antirheumatic drugs are associated with *peptic ulceration,* the frequency of this complication is probably highest in patients treated with adrenocorticosteroids. The problem is sometimes compounded, because the signs and symptoms of perforation and peritonitis may be masked by therapy.

Decreased host resistance to acquired or reactivated *infections* is a well-documented feature of adrenocorticosteroid therapy. It is common practice to institute isoniazid prophylaxis of tuberculin-positive patients receiving steroid therapy.

Aggravation of latent or overt diabetes mellitus and psychic disturbances ranging from mild euphoria to frank psychosis are infrequent with the doses of adrenocorticosteroids used in the treatment of rheumatoid arthritis.

Any patient receiving daily adrenocorticosteroid therapy must be assumed to have an *inadequate pituitary adrenal response* to stress. With intercurrent illnesses, or with surgery, the dose should be increased and the patient observed closely for signs of adrenal insufficiency. The same precautions apply to those whose treatment has been discontinued up to two years prior to the stressful illness. The value of intermittent corticotrophin therapy in the amelioration of pituitary adrenal unresponsiveness is unproved.

INTRA-ARTICULAR ADRENOCORTICOSTEROID THERAPY. Several adrenocorticosteroid preparations suitable for intra-articular therapy will temporarily suppress signs and symptoms of synovitis. This mode of therapy is helpful for a patient whose disability relates primarily to disease in one or two joints. With rigorous antiseptic technique, the risk of infection is low. If there is any question of antecedent infection at the time of arthrocentesis, intra-articular steroids should not be administered. The usefulness of intra-articular therapy is dependent upon the duration of symptomatic benefit. Because of clinical suspicions and experimental evidence that steroid compounds are deleterious to articular cartilage, most physicians will not inject a joint more frequently than every four to six weeks.

Immunosuppressive (Cytotoxic) Therapy. Several drugs initially developed for cancer chemotherapy have been applied in the treatment of rheumatoid arthritis. The categories of compounds include alkylating agents, purine and pyrimidine antagonists, and folic acid analogues. There is no basis for concluding that one compound is superior to another in immunosuppressive and anti-inflammatory properties, but the best data with regard to the treatment of rheumatoid arthritis derive from a controlled study of cyclophosphamide therapy. Patients receiving up to 150 mg daily of cyclophosphamide sustained significantly fewer new bone erosions over the period of study. In spite of these observations, the use of immunosuppressive agents is to be viewed as experimental therapy. Acute toxicity, especially myelosuppression, is potentially fatal and, as well, there is concern that immunosuppressive therapy may foster the emergence of primary malignant tumors.

Other Experimental Drugs. *Penicillamine,* in a well-controlled study in England, had moderate efficacy in the suppression of severe chronic rheumatoid arthritis and resulted in reductions of rheumatoid factor titers. As an antirheumatic agent, penicillamine remains in the experimental category, primarily because of potentially serious toxicity (agranulocytosis and nephropathy).

Orthopedic Surgery. Orthopedic surgeons are playing an increasingly important role in the management of rheumatoid arthritis. The value of reconstructive surgery in the rehabilitation of selected subjects is well established. Techniques of arthroplasty and prosthetic joint replacement have improved dramatically during the past decade. The rationale for synovectomy is sound, i.e., the removal of chronic pannus and its destructive potential, but proof of its efficacy is lacking. Disease frequently recurs in regenerated synovium, but the intensity of recurrent inflammation tends to be less. On the basis of current experience, synovectomy is probably warranted for patients with sustained (several months or more) proliferative synovitis affecting knee, hand, and wrist joints.

Cooperating Clinics Committee of the American Rheumatism Association: A controlled trial of cyclophosphamide in rheumatoid arthritis. N. Engl. J. Med., 283:883, 1970.

Duthie, J. R. R., et al.: Course and prognosis in rheumatoid arthritis. Ann. Rheum. Dis., 23:193, 1964.

Freyberg, R. H., Ziff, M., and Baum, J.: Gold therapy for rheumatoid arthritis. *In* Hollander, J. L., and McCarty, D. J., Jr. (eds.): Arthritis and Allied Conditions. 8th ed. Philadelphia, Lea & Febiger, 1972.

Hollingworth, J. W.: Local and Systemic Complications of Rheumatoid Arthritis. Philadelphia, W. B. Saunders Company, 1968.

Ruddy, S., and Austen, K. F.: The complement system in rheumatoid synovitis: I. An analysis of complement activities in rheumatoid synovial fluids. Arthritis Rheum., 13:713, 1970.

Short, C. L., Bauer, W., and Reynolds, W. E.: Rheumatoid Arthritis. Cambridge, Harvard University Press, 1957.

Winchester, R. J., Agnello, V., and Kunkel, H. G.: Gammaglobulin complexes in synovial fluids of patients with rheumatoid arthritis: Partial characterization and relationship to lowered complement levels. Clin. Exp. Immunol., 6:689, 1970.

Zvaifler, N. J.: The immunopathology of joint inflammation in rheumatoid arthritis. *In* Dixon, F. J., and Kunkel, H. G. (eds.): Advances in Immunology. vol. 16. New York, Academic Press, 1972.

VARIANTS OF RHEUMATOID DISEASE

88. FELTY'S SYNDROME

Splenomegaly is observed in approximately 5 per cent of patients with rheumatoid arthritis. Felty originally described a syndrome consisting of rheumatoid arthritis, splenomegaly, and neutropenia. Anemia and thrombocytopenia are occasional features. This syndrome is most common in older individuals who have had longstanding chronic rheumatoid disease. Other extra-articular manifestations of rheumatoid disease such as rheumatoid nodules, chronic skin ulcers, and keratoconjunctivitis sicca are common. Rheumatoid factor tests are invariably positive, and antinuclear phenomena are more common than in uncomplicated rheumatoid arthritis. The indications for splenectomy are influenced primarily by the frequency and severity of infectious complications. Most patients experience hematologic remissions after splenectomy, but relapses occur in many of them.

89. SJÖGREN'S SYNDROME

In 1933 Sjögren called attention to the combination of rheumatoid arthritis, keratoconjunctivitis sicca, and xerostomia. The characteristic ocular and oral mucous membrane involvement may occur in the absence of rheumatic disease. In addition to its association with rheumatoid arthritis, it can be a manifestation of other connective tissue syndromes such as systemic lupus erythematosus, progressive systemic sclerosis, and polymyositis. The sicca complex is clinically manifest in approximately 10 to 15 per cent of patients with rheumatoid arthritis, but pathologic expressions, such as lymphoid infiltration of the minor salivary glands in the lip, are much more frequent. More than 90 per cent of affected patients are women, and most have had longstanding chronic arthritis.

The symptoms related to salivary insufficiency include difficulty with chewing and swallowing, dental caries, and ulcerations of the buccal mucous membranes. Dryness may also involve the upper respiratory tract, larynx, and tracheobronchial tree. In common with Felty's syndrome, patients with Sjögren's syndrome frequently manifest extra-articular features attributed to vasculitis. A small but significant number of patients with Sjögren's syndrome have developed reticulum cell sarcoma or a more benign lymphoproliferative disorder termed "pseudolymphoma." Because lymphomatous complications have occurred primarily in patients with a history of irradiation for parotid gland enlargement, this mode of therapy has been discouraged.

Rheumatoid factor tests are positive in the majority of patients, and antinuclear and a variety of other autoimmune reactants are associated with Sjögren's syndrome.

The treatment is symptomatic. Artificial tears of 0.5 per cent methylcellulose are helpful. Adrenocorticosteroid or immunosuppressive drugs are restricted to those patients with severe disability or life-threatening complications.

Barnes, C. G., Turnbull, A. L., and Vernon-Roberts, B.: Felty's syndrome: A clinical and pathological survey of 21 patients and their response to treatment. Ann. Rheum. Dis., 30:359, 1971.
Shearn, M. A.: Sjogren's Syndrome. Philadelphia, W. B. Saunders Company, 1971.
Whaley, K., Williamson, J., Chisholm, D. M., et al.: Sjögren's syndrome. I. Sicca components. Quart. J. Med., 42:279, 1973.

OTHER FORMS OF POLYARTHRITIS OF UNKNOWN ETIOLOGY

90. ANKYLOSING SPONDYLITIS (Marie-Strümpell Spondylitis, von Bechterew's Syndrome, Rheumatoid Spondylitis)

In this syndrome there is prominent involvement of spinal articulations, sacroiliac joints, and paravertebral soft tissues. Because one third to one half of patients with ankylosing spondylitis manifest synovitis in peripheral joints (especially hips and shoulders), the syndrome was formerly viewed as a variant of rheumatoid arthritis. However, several features of ankylosing spondylitis are distinct from those of rheumatoid arthritis: (1) prominent ligamentous calcification and ossification with a tendency to bony ankylosis; (2) male preponderance; (3) impressive evidence of genetic transmission in selected kindreds; (4) symptomatic benefit with medications, notably phenylbutazone and indomethacin, that are minimally effective in rheumatoid arthritis; (5) absence of rheumatoid factor and rheumatoid nodules; and (6) the association of certain extra-articular manifestations such as iridocyclitis and aortitis.

Etiology. The cause of ankylosing spondylitis is unknown. The disease has been found to be 30 times more prevalent among the relatives of spondylitic patients than among relatives of controls. Recent studies have demonstrated a striking association between ankylosing spondylitis and HL-A 27, but the manner in which this histocompatibility antigen influences pathogenesis is unknown. Infectious causes have long been suspected but never established. Spinal involvement indistinguishable from ankylosing spondylitis is occasionally a feature of Reiter's syndrome, psoriatic arthritis, and inflammatory bowel disease.

Incidence and Prevalence. Ankylosing spondylitis is a common cause of back pain in young men. The male-to-female ratio is approximately 8:1. In an English survey, the incidence of ankylosing spondylitis was 1 in 2000 among the population at large.

Pathology. On the basis of symptoms and early radiographic findings, the disease appears to begin in the sacroiliac joints, with subsequent involvement of zygapophyseal and costovertebral articulations, interspinous ligaments, and paravertebral tissues. The characteristic immobility of the spinal column results from bony ankylosis of zygapophyseal joints and ossification of paravertebral structures. Syndesmophytes, the bony bridges which unite adjacent vertebral bodies, form in the outer lamellae of the anulus fibrosus and adjacent connective tissue fibers. The pathologic character of synovial inflammation is not distinct from that of rheumatoid arthritis. Aortic involvement resembling syphilitic aortitis can result in aortic insufficiency. Iridocyclitis occurs in approximately 25 per cent of patients. The incidence of amyloidosis complicating ankylosing spondylitis is approximately 5 per cent. Rarely, a pattern of pulmonary fibrosis, sometimes associated with cavitation, has been described.

Clinical Manifestations. In the majority of cases the onset of ankylosing spondylitis, usually in the second or third decade of life, is insidious. The initial symptoms are usually low back pain and stiffness; rarely, the first symptoms may relate to involvement of hip, shoulder, or peripheral joints. Symptoms may be sufficiently mild that the patient seeks no medical attention for months. At the other extreme, there may be debilitating pain at the outset, associated with fever, severe fatigue, and weight loss. In most patients, however, constitutional symptoms are not prominent. Pain and stiffness, which are maximal after periods of inactivity, often interrupt sleep in the early morning hours. Radicular and sciatic patterns of pain are common. The pattern and rate of spinal ankylosis are varied. The majority of patients experience gradual cephalad progression of spinal immobility, but the disease may remain confined to the sacroiliac joints and lumbar segments. The development of the poker back type of spinal deformity usually evolves gradually over a period of ten years or more. The majority of patients remain fully employed. Hip involvement, the most common cause of occupational disability, is now amenable to prosthetic surgery.

Physical signs are limited in the early stages of disease. Sacroiliac joint involvement may be evident from palpation of these joints or from orthopedic maneuvers which produce sacroiliac joint movement. Paravertebral muscle spasm and tenderness are common. Physical signs associated with the chronic phase of ankylosing spondylitis relate primarily to spinal immobility. The most accurate estimate of lumbar flexion is accomplished by comparing midline measurements from the sacrum to T-12 in flexion and extension. The normal difference in these two measurements is approximately 3 inches. The presence and progression of costovertebral joint involvement can be documented by measurements of chest expansion.

The most important extra-articular manifestations of ankylosing spondylitis are *iridocyclitis,* occurring in approximately one quarter of patients, and aortitis. The frequency of *aortic insufficiency* has been as high as 4 per cent in some series. *Cardiac conduction disturbances,* most frequently first degree A-V block, occurs in about 10 per cent of cases. *Cauda equina involvement,* a rare but significant complication of longstanding spondylitis, is manifest as urinary or rectal sphincter incompetence and pain and sensory loss in the sacral distribution.

Roentgenographic Findings. Characteristic roentgenographic findings of ankylosing spondylitis involve the following structures: sacroiliac joints, zygapophyseal articulations, vertebral bodies, and paravertebral soft tissues. Changes in the sacroiliac joints are the earliest and most consistent findings. The margins of subchondral bone are blurred, followed by subchondral sclerosis and bony erosions. Progressive narrowing of the interosseous joint space and sacroiliac fusion develop slowly over a period of years. Sclerotic and erosive changes in zygapophyseal and costovertebral articulations are common but less readily demonstrated by x-ray. Alterations in vertebral bodies, loss of anterior concavity, and anterior marginal erosions are features of longstanding disease. Calcification and ossification of the anulus fibrosus and adjacent paravertebral ligaments give rise to the characteristic syndesmophytes that gradually bridge adjacent vertebral bodies. In advanced cases this results in the so-called *bamboo spine.* In addition to sacroiliac joints, other cartilaginous articulations such as the symphysis pubis and sternomanubrial joints may be involved. There is a tendency for ossification of ligaments and tendon insertions. Roentgenographic changes in the hips and shoulders, less commonly in more peripheral joints, are not distinct from those of rheumatoid arthritis, although the incidence of bony ankylosis of the hips is greater in ankylosing spondylitis.

The full set of roentgenographic findings, described above, is a product of many years of progressive disease. In a minority of patients with ankylosing spondylitis, the disease appears to go into remission after involvement of restricted segments of the spine.

Diagnosis. Ankylosing spondylitis should be suspected in anyone, particularly a young male, with persistent or recurrent low back pain and stiffness or recurrent sciatic pain. Although associated phenomena such as elevation of erythrocyte sedimentation rate, thoracic girdle pain, arthritis in the lower limbs, and iridocyclitis will enhance the suspicion, early diagnosis should not be excluded on the basis of normal roentgenograms, because several months or, rarely, a few years may elapse before development of roentgenographic changes. Although degenerative joint disease can result in back pain and loss of spinal motion, this is a problem of later decades of life, and the roentgenographic features are distinct from ankylosing spondylitis. Joint disease identical to ankylosing spondylitis can be a feature of *ulcerative colitis, regional enteritis, Reiter's syndrome,* and *psoriasis.*

Treatment. The highest priority goal in the management of ankylosing spondylitis is the maintenance of a functional posture. It is doubtful that any medication will prevent ankylosis of those spinal segments involved, but the suppression of pain and inflammation is essential before an appropriate physical medicine program can be instituted.

Indomethacin and phenylbutazone are usually more effective than other antirheumatic agents in the control of pain and stiffness, but an initial trial on salicylate therapy (3.6 to 4.5 grams daily) is recommended. For those patients who do not experience sufficient relief of symptoms with salicylates, indomethacin in doses of 100 to 150 mg daily or phenylbutazone (100 to 300 mg daily) is indicated. With control of symptoms, the dose of either indomethacin or phenylbutazone should be gradually reduced to the lowest level that will maintain improvement. With continuous use of phenylbutazone, the risk of hematologic complications should be kept in mind and periodic blood counts obtained. Adrenocorticosteroid therapy is rarely indicated for ankylosing spondylitis. If all other efforts to control progressive disability fail, such therapy may be indicated, as outlined under rheumatoid arthritis (see Ch. 87). Systemic adrenocorticosteroid therapy may be required for the control of iridocyclitis. Although roentgen therapy, directed at areas of involvement, is effective in control of symptoms, this mode of treatment is not recommended because of the demonstrations of chromosomal injury and an observed incidence of leukemia that is ten times greater in patients so treated than in the general population.

For the management of ankylosing spondylitis, emphasis should be given to the institution and maintenance of an exercise program. In order that flexion deformity of the spine be avoided, the patient should sleep on a very firm mattress, preferably without a pillow. There should be a twice daily performance of exercise directed at the maintenance of erect posture, strengthening of paraspinal muscles, and promotion of chest cage motion. A hot bath or shower will often facilitate exercise activity. If physical medicine measures fail to check the progression of flexion deformity, back splints or braces may be tried. In carefully selected individuals with advanced flexion deformity, spinal osteotomy can improve posture, but this is associated with significant risk of neurologic complications. For the patient with severe hip involvement, the most frequent cause of major disability, prosthetic hip replacement offers dramatic relief.

91. JUVENILE RHEUMATOID ARTHRITIS

Although the definition of juvenile rheumatoid arthritis is somewhat arbitrary (onset of disease under age 16), there are clinical features which tend to distinguish it from rheumatoid arthritis in adults. These include high fever, transient morbilliform rash, leukocytosis, uveitis, local growth disturbances, low frequencies of rheumatoid factor and subcutaneous nodules, and a higher incidence of monarticular disease than is observed in adults.

The discussions of etiology, pathogenesis, and pathology of rheumatoid arthritis (see Ch. 87) are relevant to juvenile rheumatoid arthritis except for speculations regarding a pathogenic role of rheumatoid factors.

In approximately 20 per cent of children with juvenile rheumatoid arthritis, the onset is acute and fulminating and is associated with systemic manifestations such as fever, rash, pericarditis, and splenomegaly *(Still's disease).* Occasionally these features may persist for several weeks before synovitis is evident. (A similar systemic pattern of disease has been observed, rarely, in adults.) In approximately half of patients, the onset is polyarticular, resembling rheumatoid arthritis in adults. In one third of juvenile rheumatoid arthritis patients, the onset is monarticular. Many patients in this group continue to have disease limited to one or a few joints, often in an asymmetrical pattern, and manifest no systemic disease except for iridocyclitis (10 to 15 per cent). The frequency of cervical spine and sacroiliac joint involvement exceeds that of adults. Abnormal skeletal growth adjacent to inflamed joints results from varied degrees of accelerated local growth and premature closure of epiphyseal plates.

Leukocytosis in the range of 15,000 to 25,000 is common. Serologic evidence of recent streptococcal infection is found in a third to a half of subjects, adding to the problem of differentiation from acute rheumatic fever. No more than 10 per cent of sera are positive in the commonly employed tests for rheumatoid factor. The frequency of antinuclear antibody is higher than in adults with rheumatoid arthritis. This is especially so in children with iridocyclitis.

Distinctive roentgenographic findings include local growth disturbances (noted above), abnormal periosteal bone accretion, and prominent involvement of cervical zygapophyseal joints.

Differential considerations vary according to the pattern of juvenile rheumatoid arthritis. The systemic form of disease resembles certain infectious syndromes. Recognition of the characteristic morbilliform rash, if it is present, is important in diagnosis. The polyarticular onset of disease, when accompanied by high fever and signs of carditis, is easily confused with acute rheumatic fever. Features of juvenile rheumatoid arthritis that may aid in this distinction are frequent onset of disease under age 5, nonmigratory pattern of polyarthritis, cervical spine involvement, marked leukocytosis, and rash. The immediate suppressive effect of salicylate therapy is less striking in juvenile rheumatoid arthritis than it is in rheumatic fever.

Fifty per cent or more of patients with juvenile rheumatoid arthritis experience complete remissions. The serious consequences of extra-articular involvement relate to carditis, chronic iridocyclitis, and amyloidosis.

Principles of management outlined for rheumatoid arthritis (see Ch. 87) apply to children with chronic arthritis. Contractures and restricted motion of articulations are more common in children than in adults. The patient's parents must be given important roles in the maintenance of a physical medicine program. Aspirin in the range of 90 to 130 mg per kilogram daily is the treatment of choice. Early in the course of the disease, adrenocorticosteroid therapy should be reserved for patients with severe systemic manifestations, such as carditis, that do not respond to salicylate therapy. Periodic ophthalmologic consultation, at approximately six-month intervals, is recommended, since iridocyclitis may be asymptomatic and missed by casual examination. Because of the threat of blindness from sustained iridocyclitis, systemic adrenocorticosteroid therapy may be indicated if this complication is severe and fails to respond to local treatment. In addition to the usual complications and limitations of adrenocorticosteroid therapy, growth retardation, a natural feature of the disease, is augmented by such treatment. The indications for the employment of gold therapy are similar to those presented for rheumatoid arthritis. The dose of gold thioglucose or gold thiomalate is 1 mg per kilogram per week. A course of therapy consists of approximately 20 weekly injections.

92. PSORIATIC ARTHRITIS

The recognition that psoriatic arthritis is a disease entity, as opposed to the coincidental occurrence of two common diseases, i.e., rheumatoid arthritis and psoriasis, is relatively recent. Based on population surveys, approximately 5 per cent of patients with cutaneous psoriasis have chronic arthritis. One quarter to one third of such patients manifest rheumatoid nodules or positive tests for rheumatoid factor, and probably represent cases of coexistence of two diseases. Patients with psoriasis and chronic arthritis are clinically heterogeneous, but some of them manifest sufficiently unique features to justify the term psoriatic arthritis.

Several clinical subtypes of psoriatic arthritis are recognized. The most common pattern is of a scattered asymmetrical involvement of interphalangeal joints of the hands and feet, frequently manifest as "sausage digits" (Fig. 3). Much less common, but recognized by all as "classic psoriatic arthritis" is the exclusive involvement of distal interphalangeal joints. In approximately one quarter of patients with psoriasis there is a symmetrical pattern of arthritis indistinguishable, apart from negative serology, from rheumatoid arthritis. In this group, there is a tendency for severe osteolytic involvement with resorption of bone and telescoping of digits (arthritis mutilans). Approximately 5 per cent of patients with psoriasis and arthritis manifest features identical to those of ankylosing spondylitis, although the roentgenographic character of syndesmophytes tends to differentiate the two syndromes.

It is important to recognize that there may be asynchronous onset of cutaneous involvement and arthritis and that a patient with typical psoriatic arthritis may have minimal or hidden cutaneous involvement. Psoriatic nail involvement occurs in over 80 per cent of patients with psoriatic arthritis, in contrast to only a 30 per cent incidence in patients with uncomplicated psoriasis. Typical psoriatic arthritis, especially spondylitis, may evolve after recurrent attacks of Reiter's syndrome.

The unique clinical patterns of psoriatic arthritis such as bone resorption, asymmetric involvement of interphalangeal joints, and spondylitis are represented in roentgenographic findings. An increased incidence of

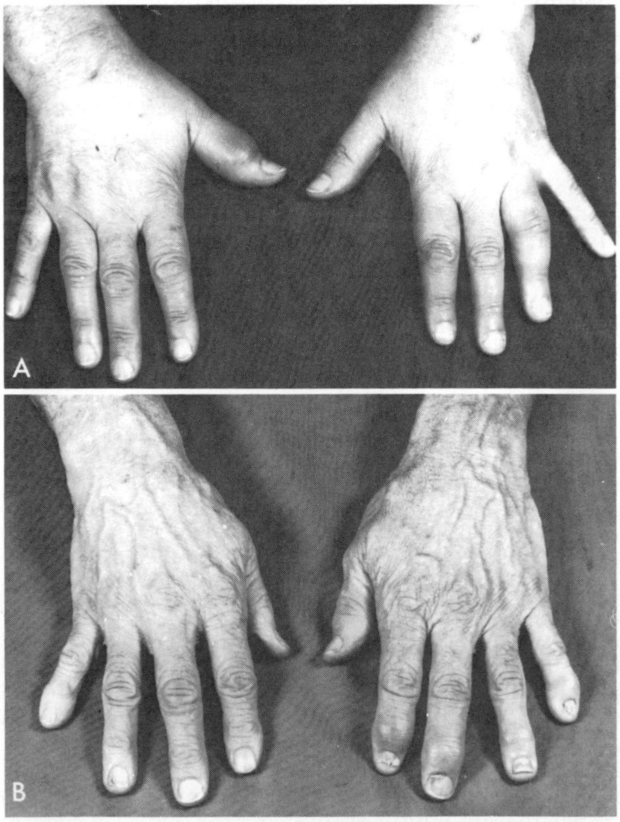

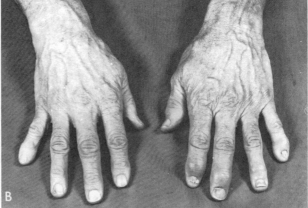

Figure 3. Common patterns of psoriatic arthritis in the hands. *A*, Asymmetrical enlargement of interphalangeal joints of right thumb and left ring finger. *B*, "Classic" involvement of distal interphalangeal joints and nails of digits two, three, and five of left hand.

hyperuricemia in psoriatic patients probably reflects the increased metabolism of skin. Other than the absence of rheumatoid factor in patients with psoriatic arthritis, there are no immunologic, biochemical, or pathologic distinctions from rheumatoid arthritis.

Principles of management of psoriatic arthritis do not differ from those of rheumatoid arthritis. Antimalarial drugs are contraindicated, because they have been observed to provoke exfoliative dermatitis in psoriatic subjects. Reliance should be placed on a basic regimen of salicylates and physical therapy. Adrenocorticosteroid drugs should be employed only as a last resort. For the patient with very severe psoriatic arthritis, immunosuppressive therapy, in spite of its experimental status and considerable toxicity, is probably more appropriate than adrenocorticosteroid therapy.

93. REITER'S SYNDROME

Although the association of arthritis, urethritis, and conjunctivitis was recorded early in the nineteenth century, this triad of clinical manifestations bears the name of the German physician who, in 1916, described a patient with nongonococcal urethritis, conjunctivitis, and arthritis after an episode of diarrhea. Other common manifestations of the syndrome include fever, oral and genital mucous membrane lesions, cutaneous keratosis, and iritis. Most patients are young males; it is rare in women regardless of age.

Etiology. The cause of Reiter's syndrome is unknown, but most attention has focused on infectious causes. Venereal transmission seems apparent in many cases; in others the onset of Reiter's syndrome follows diarrheal illness. In several large epidemics of bacillary dysentery, a small percentage of patients have developed typical Reiter's syndrome, including genitourinary tract involvement. Mycoplasmal and chlamydial species are suspect as etiologic agents. The significance of sporadic isolation of such organisms from synovial fluid or synovial tissue is unknown. In preliminary studies there appeared to be a high association of HL-A 27 with Reiter's syndrome equivalent to that observed with ankylosing spondylitis.

Clinical and Laboratory Manifestations. All the clinical features of Reiter's syndrome may appear simultaneously, but more commonly genitourinary or gastrointestinal symptoms precede the onset of ocular or rheumatic features by several days or a few weeks. Occasionally the classic pattern evolves slowly over weeks or months after the appearance of a single manifestation. Polyarthritis is frequently asymmetrical with predilection for involvement of articulations of the lower extremities, but the pattern of joint involvement can be varied. The majority of patients experience complete remissions within weeks or a few months of onset. A minority (range of 10 per cent) manifest persistence of synovitis in articulations of the extremities or spine and will have disability that parallels that of sustained rheumatoid arthritis or ankylosing spondylitis. Rarely, the clinical picture of chronic or recurrent Reiter's syndrome evolves into typical psoriatic arthritis.

There are no distinctive laboratory features. Peripheral blood leukocytosis is common. Properties of synovial fluid are similar to acute rheumatoid arthritis, although complement levels in joint fluid are invariably high. Roentgenographic abnormalities, equivalent to those associated with rheumatoid arthritis, are found in those patients with sustained synovitis. Periostitis, adjacent to involved joints, is a common but not distinctive feature of Reiter's syndrome.

The most common diagnostic alternative to Reiter's syndrome is *gonococcal arthritis*. The past literature is confusing because of the failure to distinguish these two syndromes and to recognize that gonococcal infection may be coincident to Reiter's syndrome. In a minority of patients, typical mucocutaneous lesions, particularly balanitis circinata and keratoderma blennorrhagica, leave no question regarding diagnosis, but the failure to isolate *N. gonorrhoeae* and the resistance of the manifestations to antimicrobial therapy are the main bases for differentiating Reiter's syndrome from gonococcal arthritis.

Treatment. The management of Reiter's syndrome is similar to that of rheumatoid arthritis. If salicylate therapy in the range of 3.6 to 4.5 grams daily fails to suppress synovitis or constitutional symptoms, phenylbutazone or indomethacin (both in the range of 100 to 200 mg daily) may be beneficial. There is no experience to recommend gold therapy. There are a few reports describing remissions of very severe disease coincident to treatment with immunosuppressive agents; but in the light of their immediate and long-term toxicity, such therapy is considered experimental.

94. PALINDROMIC RHEUMATISM

This term has been applied to a recurring pattern of polyarthritis which results in no permanent joint deformity. The syndrome resembles gout in its acute onset and marked inflammatory signs. Rapid subsidence of signs and symptoms occurs within hours or a few days of onset. The frequency of episodes and the anatomic areas affected are variable, but for individual subjects the pattern of recurrent disease tends to be constant.

Since recurrent polyarthritis can be a feature of many rheumatic syndromes, the term palindromic rheumatism, if it is used at all, requires rigorous exclusion of other causes of synovitis. A significant number of patients, the majority in some series, with palindromic rheumatism eventually manifest typical features of rheumatoid arthritis. Systemic and constitutional symptoms are generally lacking. Since the brief episodes terminate spontaneously, there is no uniformity of opinion regarding response to therapy.

95. INTERMITTENT HYDRARTHROSIS

This term has been applied to the pattern of recurrent joint effusions, usually the knees, in which other inflammatory signs are minimal. The interval between episodes varies from one to a few weeks. In most reports of intermittent hydrarthrosis, there has been female preponderance. Occasionally recurrences correlate with menstruation. The diagnosis of intermittent hydrarthrosis, like palindromic rheumatism, should be restricted to individuals who have been followed long enough to exclude other causes of recurrent synovitis. A significant number of patients will eventually manifest chronic synovitis consistent with rheumatoid arthritis. When discomfort and restricted motion are attributable to joint space distention, simple arthrocentesis may be beneficial; there is no agreement regarding the efficacy of medicinal therapy in suppressing or preventing attacks.

Ansell, B. M., and Bywaters, E. G. L.: Rheumatoid arthritis (Still's disease). Pediat. Clin. North Am., 10:921, 1963.
Calabro, J. J., and Marchesano, J. M.: The early natural history of juvenile rheumatoid arthritis. A ten year follow-up of 100 cases. Med. Clin. North Am., 52:569, 1968.
Kinsella, T. D., MacDonald, F. R., and Johnson, L. G.: Ankylosing spondylitis: A late re-evaluation of 92 cases. Can. Med. Assoc. J., 95:1, 1966.
Moll, J. M. H., and Wright, V.: Psoriatic arthritis. Semin. Arthritis Rheum., 3:55, 1973.
Ogryzlo, M. A.: Ankylosing spondylitis. *In* Hollander, J. L., and McCarty, D. J., Jr. (eds.): Arthritis and Allied Conditions. 8th ed. Philadelphia, Lea & Febiger, 1972.
Schlosstein, L., et al.: High association of an HL-A antigen, W27, with ankylosing spondylitis. N. Engl. J. Med., 288:704, 1973.
Sharp, J. T.: Reiter's syndrome. *In* Hollander, J. L., and McCarty, D. J., Jr. (eds.): Arthritis and Allied Conditions. 8th ed. Philadelphia, Lea & Febiger, 1972.
Williams, M. H., et al.: Palindromic rheumatism: Clinical and immunological studies. Ann. Rheum. Dis., 30:375, 1971.

96. DISEASES WITH WHICH ARTHRITIS IS FREQUENTLY ASSOCIATED

Arthritis may be a significant feature of all of the syndromes listed in this chapter. Discussion here is brief and is limited to rheumatic manifestations of the various disorders. More detailed considerations will be found elsewhere in the chapters devoted to those diseases.

INFLAMMATORY BOWEL DISEASE

The reported incidence of arthritis complicating *ulcerative colitis* and *regional enteritis* (Crohn's disease) has varied, but it is generally in the range of 10 per cent. The most common rheumatic pattern is an asymmetric polyarthritis involving a few joints. In the majority of patients the disease is intermittent and results in minimal joint damage. The frequency and severity of arthritis are generally higher in those subjects with sustained and extensive bowel involvement, but occasionally rheumatic manifestations will antedate the recognition of enteric disease. *Erythema nodosum* and *uveitis* are three to four times more common in patients with enteritis and arthritis than in patients without rheumatic manifestations. In contrast to the generally benign character of rheumatic complications of enteritis, a small number (approximately 10 per cent of those with arthritis) experience a pattern of disease and disability equivalent to rheumatoid arthritis.

The incidence of *spondylitis,* which is indistinguishable from ankylosing spondylitis, in patients with ulcerative colitis and regional enteritis has varied between 2 and 6 per cent. This represents at least a twentyfold increase in the frequency of spondylitis over that in the general population. Clinical, laboratory, or roentgenographic findings do not distinguish spondylitis complicating enteritis from ankylosing spondylitis unassociated with bowel disease, except that male predominance in the former is less striking.

There are no special recommendations regarding the management of arthritis associated with enteritis: the general principles outlined for the treatment of rheumatoid arthritis and ankylosing spondylitis (see Ch. 87 and 90) are appropriate. The main management effort is directed at the intestinal disease. Remissions of arthritis frequently follow surgical resection of diseased bowel, but rheumatic complications rarely affect the decision regarding surgical therapy.

WHIPPLE'S DISEASE

This is a rare syndrome, probably bacterial in cause, characterized by diarrhea, malabsorption, fever, anemia, increased skin pigmentation, and migratory polyarthralgia or polyarthritis. Permanent joint damage is rare.

FAMILIAL MEDITERRANEAN FEVER

Musculoskeletal pain occurs in approximately 7 per cent of patients with this heritable disease. The arthritis is usually monarticular or limited to a few joints; most commonly involved are knees, ankles, hips, or shoulders. Severe pain and tenderness are out of proportion to other modest signs of inflammation. Arthritis, like other manifestations of this syndrome, is usually recurrent, but permanent damage to joints is rare. None of the anti-inflammatory medications have been found to be effective in the treatment of this form of arthritis. Management is limited to analgesics and local physical measures.

SARCOIDOSIS

The most common rheumatic manifestation of sarcoidosis is a transient acute polyarthritis associated with erythema nodosum and hilar adenopathy. Lower extremity joints are primarily involved. At times it is difficult to be certain whether inflammatory symptoms and signs reflect true synovitis or the cellulitis of erythema nodosum. Recovery is uniform. Most patients can be managed with salicylates but, if pain and disability are severe, a course of adrenocorticosteroid therapy may be indicated. Much less common than the acute rheumatic syndrome is chronic granulomatous synovitis that clinically resembles rheumatoid arthritis.

HYPOGAMMAGLOBULINEMIA

A mild polyarthritis, rarely deforming in character, has been observed in as many as one third of patients with congenital and acquired hypogammaglobulinemia. The pattern of joint disease resembles that of rheumatoid arthritis, although other connective tissue syndromes such as systemic lupus erythematosus, systemic sclerosis, and dermatomyositis have been associated with immune deficiency states. A variety of autoimmune phenomena and connective tissue syndromes have been observed in patients lacking IgA, the most common selective deficiency. Regression of arthritis frequently follows institution of gamma globulin therapy.

POLYCHONDRITIS

Relapsing polychondritis is a rare disorder characterized by inflammation and destruction of cartilage. In the majority of patients there is intermittent involvement of cartilage in ears, nose, trachea, pharynx, costochondral junctions, and peripheral joints. With subsidence of inflammation there may be collapse and deforming change of the ears, nose, and laryngotracheal structures. The pattern of joint involvement is usually that of recurrent polyarthritis associated with minimal residual deformity. Other manifestations include fever, iritis, episcleritis, cataracts, deafness, and aortic insufficiency. Aortic involvement, occurring in 14 per cent of reported cases, and involvement of cartilaginous structures of the respiratory tract are the two life-threatening complications of polychondritis. Pathologic studies demonstrate varying degrees of inflammation and loss of cartilage matrix. The cause is unknown. Adrenocorticosteroid therapy has been employed for life-threatening manifestations, but the generally remittent character of the disease makes it uncertain whether any mode of therapy changes its natural history. Aortic involvement has necessitated prosthetic valve replacement in a few reported patients.

BEHCET'S SYNDROME

This syndrome was initially described as a triad (recurrent aphthous stomatitis, genital ulcerations, and iritis), but other manifestations are common: pyoderma, erythema nodosum, erythema multiforme, thrombophlebitis, and polyarthritis. Central nervous system involvement, in a minority of patients, may be fatal. Intermittent or chronic polyarthritis is usually limited to one or a few joints and rarely results in significant deformity. There is a strong suspicion that viral infection underlies the development of Behçet's syndrome, but attempts at microbial isolation have been equivocal or negative. Adrenocorticosteroid therapy is indicated if iritis is severe or if there are neurological manifestations.

HEMOCHROMATOSIS

Joint involvement has been observed in as many as half of patients with idiopathic hemochromatosis. Joint swelling with bony enlargement is particularly common in the small joints of the hands, but other joints may be affected. The clinical and roentgenographic features resemble degenerative joint disease more than rheumatoid arthritis. There is narrowing of the joint space with subchondral erosions and sclerosis. Roentgenographic evidence of chondrocalcinosis is present in a third or more of patients with arthropathy and may account, via crystal-induced synovitis (see Chondrocalcinosis and Pseudogout in Ch. 97), for occasional acute inflammatory manifestations. The management of arthropathy is similar to that described for degenerative joint disease.

ACROMEGALY

The majority of patients with acromegaly develop an atypical form of degenerative joint disease. Increased levels of growth hormone result in hypertrophy of articular cartilage, subchondral bone, and periarticular tissues. Hypermobility of joints, a common manifestation, may contribute to degenerative change. The fingers and knees are most frequently affected. Radiographic features demonstrating overgrowth of bone are pathognomonic. Median nerve entrapment secondary to wrist synovitis is common.

HYPERPARATHYROIDISM

Patients with hyperparathyroidism are subject to a variety of associated rheumatic disorders which may occur singly or in combination. These include (1) hyperuricemia and gouty arthritis, (2) chondrocalcinosis with episodes of calcium pyrophosphate dihydrate crystal-induced synovitis, and (3) degenerative joint disease resulting from deformation of atrophic subchondral bone. Rheumatic symptoms, particularly those associated with chondrocalcinosis (see Chondrocalcinosis and Pseudogout in Ch. 97) may be the first manifestation of hyperparathyroidism.

SICKLE CELL DISEASE AND RELATED HEMOGLOBINOPATHIES

Severe polyarthralgia is a frequent manifestation of the crises of sickle cell disease. Occasionally pain is accompanied by transient joint effusion or other evidence of inflammation. The most common rheumatic symptoms result from avascular osteonecrosis of the femoral head, less commonly of other bony structures. This complication is also associated with sickle cell trait, hemoglobin C disease, SC disease, and sickle cell–thalassemia. In children, periostitis may result in transient diffuse swelling of the hands and feet. Sickle cell disease is associated with an increased incidence of bacterial arthritis and osteomyelitis, especially those caused by gram-negative organisms.

Bluestone, R., et al.: Acromegalic arthropathy. Ann. Rheum. Dis., 30:243, 1971.

Bywaters, E. G. L., Dixon, A. St. J., and Scott, J. T.: Joint lesions of hyperparathyroidism. Ann. Rheum. Dis., 22:171, 1963.

Ferguson, R. H.: Enteropathic arthritis. *In* Hollander, J. L., and McCarty, D. J., Jr. (eds.): Arthritis and Allied Conditions. 8th ed. Philadelphia, Lea & Febiger, 1972.

Hamilton, E., et al.: The arthropathy of idiopathic haemochromatosis. Quart. J. Med., 37:171, 1968.

Hughes, R. A. C., et al.: Relapsing polychondritis: Three cases with a clinicopathological study and literature review. Quart. J. Med., 41:363, 1972.

McEwen, C.: Arthritis accompanying ulcerative colitis. Clin. Orthop., 59:9, 1968.

McEwen, C., et al.: Ankylosing spondylitis and spondylitis accompanying ulcerative colitis, regional enteritis, psoriasis and Reiter's disease. A comparative study. Arthritis Rheum., 14:29, 1971.

O'Duffy, J. D., Carnery, J. A., and Deodhar, S.: Behçet's disease: A report of ten cases, three with new manifestations. Ann. Intern. Med., 75:561, 1971.

Spilberg, I., Siltzbach, L. E., and McEwen, C.: The arthritis of sarcoidosis. Arthritis Rheum., 12:126, 1969.

97. MISCELLANEOUS FORMS OF ARTHRITIS

NEUROPATHIC JOINT DISEASE (CHARCOT JOINTS)

This chronic progressive degenerative arthropathy is a complication of a variety of neurologic disorders. Impairment of proprioceptive and pain sensation deprives the affected joint of the normal protective reactions when exposed to forces of weight bearing and motion. Although any neuropathic process which impairs sensory innervation may underlie neuropathic joint disease, syphilitic tabes dorsalis, in spite of its declining frequency, and diabetic neuropathy are the most common associated conditions. Syringomyelia, myelomeningocele, and congenital indifference to pain are less frequent neurologic bases for neuropathic arthropathy. The distribution of joints affected correlates with the pattern of neuropathy. In tabes dorsalis, the knees, hips, ankles, and vertebrae are frequently involved. In diabetic neuropathy, destructive changes are limited to the distal lower extremities, and in syringomyelia the shoulder and elbow joints are most commonly affected.

Although pain is generally present, discomfort tends to be disproportionately mild relative to signs of joint destruction. Clinical, pathologic, and roentgenographic features of chronic neuropathic joint disease reflect severe degrees of destruction and disorganization of affected joints. In the early cases, the differentiation from other causes of joint derangement depends upon the demonstration of sensory neuropathy.

Management includes immobilization of affected joints and restriction of weight-bearing activities with crutches, splints, and braces. Surgical arthrodesis, although frequently unsuccessful, is indicated in select subjects. Depending on the anatomic pattern and extent of involvement, the application of prosthetic devices after amputation may improve function.

HEMARTHROSIS

Recurrent or chronic hemarthrosis is the most common manifestation of a group of heritable disorders of blood coagulation (see Ch. 796 to 798). Hemarthrosis can be a complication of anticoagulant therapy or trauma in an otherwise normal subject.

In hemophilia, joint bleeding usually begins before the age of five and tends to recur repeatedly during childhood in response to minor injury. The most commonly affected joints are the knees, elbows, and ankles, but any articulation may be involved.

Acute hemarthrosis usually results in marked local inflammatory signs and symptoms which recede within a few days. Approximately half the patients with hemophilia develop chronic deformities in one or more joints. Some of them suffer a chronic progressive synovitis, restricted to one or a few joints, which clinically and roentgenographically resembles rheumatoid arthritis. There may be marked synovial membrane hyperplasia, destruction of articular cartilage, and erosions of subchondral bone. This chronic progressive pattern probably results from a low level of continuous or intermittent bleeding into affected joints. Joint fluid, in the chronic cases, usually contains blood and very high levels of leukocyte-derived proteases. Other musculoskeletal manifestations of hemophilia result from bleeding into muscle and bone. The resolution of large hematomas may cause formation of chronic cysts.

The first principle in management is to prevent trauma, a goal not easily achieved in children. Acute hemarthrosis should be managed by immobilization, analgesic therapy, and the administration of plasma products which contain the appropriate coagulation factor. In the choice of analgesics, it is probably wise to exclude salicylates and other drugs which alter platelet function. If there is marked distention of the joint bursae, aspiration can be accomplished after the defect in coagulation has been corrected. When pain and acute inflammation have subsided, an exercise program directed at restoration of motion should be instituted. For the patient with chronic deforming joint disease, the availability of potent plasma products has permitted application of certain surgical procedures such as synovectomy and arthroplasty.

SCHÖNLEIN-HENOCH PURPURA

Nondeforming polyarthritis, most frequently affecting knees and ankles, is a common manifestation of this syndrome, other features being nonthrombocytopenic purpura, abdominal pain, and glomerulonephritis. The syndrome is rare in adults.

MULTICENTRIC RETICULOHISTIOCYTOSIS
(Lipoid Dermatoarthritis)

This rare disorder usually begins in the middle decades of life and affects females three times more than males. It is characterized by the development of multiple histiocytic nodules in the skin and mucous membranes and severe polyarthritis which may simulate rheumatoid arthritis. The firm reddish-brown or yellow papular nodules are most commonly found on hands, forearms, head, neck, and chest. Mutilating joint destruction, especially in the distal interphalangeal joints, occurs in approximately half the patients with this syndrome. Diagnosis is by demonstration of histiocytes and multinucleated giant cells, containing PAS-positive material, in skin or synovium. Similar infiltrates have been observed in other organs. A few reports of apparent benefit from adrenocorticosteroid or immunosuppressive therapy are difficult to interpret because of the tendency for spontaneous remissions.

HYPERTROPHIC OSTEOARTHROPATHY

This term refers to a syndrome which includes clubbing of fingers and toes, periostitis with new osseous formation at the ends of long bones, arthritis, and signs of autonomic disorders such as flushing, blanching, and profuse sweating. The syndrome occurs with a wide variety of underlying disease states. Less commonly there are hereditary and idiopathic *(pachydermoperiostosis)* forms of disease. The fully expressed pattern is usually associated with intrathoracic disease: lung carcinoma, lung abscess, empyema, bronchiectasis, chronic interstitial pneumonitis, or tuberculosis. Clubbing, usually without periostitis, may be seen with cyanotic heart disease, bacterial endocarditis, biliary cirrhosis, ulcerative colitis, regional enteritis, and thyroid disease.

The distal ends of metacarpals, metatarsals, and long bones of the forearms and legs are most frequently affected. There are inflammatory changes of periosteum, synovial membranes, and periarticular structures. The periosteum is "lifted" by the deposition of new bone matrix and subsequent mineralization. Clubbing results from edema, cellular infiltration, and connective tissue proliferation of the nailbeds.

The production of a humoral substance that mediates increased vascularity and/or connective tissue proliferation has long been suspected as the pathogenic factor in hypertrophic osteoarthropathy, but no such factor has been convincingly demonstrated. Evidence that neural factors are involved derives from observations of striking resolution of signs and symptoms after denervation of the hilum or vagotomy on the same side as the thoracic lesion. Regression of osteoarthropathy has also been observed after resection of pulmonary neoplasms.

Pain, tenderness, and enlargement of the distal portions of extremities may be accompanied by acute polyarthritis that resembles rheumatoid arthritis. The differentiation of the acute polyarthritis syndrome is aided by the recognition of clubbing and roentgenographic evidence of periostitis and intrathoracic disease.

Aside from therapy directed at the associated illness, there is no effective treatment of hypertrophic osteoarthropathy. Symptomatic benefit may be obtained from salicylates, other analgesics, or adrenocorticosteroids.

CHONDROCALCINOSIS AND PSEUDOGOUT

Chondrocalcinosis is defined as the presence of calcium-containing salts in cartilaginous structures of one or more joints. These salts include calcium pyrophosphate, calcium hydroxyapatite, and calcium orthophosphate. The term pseudogout refers to the acute and/or chronic synovitis associated with the appearance of calcium pyrophosphate dihydrate crystals in joint fluid.

There is a tendency to chondrocalcinosis in patients with hyperparathyroidism, alcaptonuria, hemochromatosis, Wilson's disease, and acromegaly, and perhaps with gout as well. There appears to be a significant association of diabetes mellitus with pseudogout, and a familial pattern of chondrocalcinosis has been described. Pseudogout, like true gout, appears to be an expression of crystal-induced synovitis.

The incidence of chondrocalcinosis increases with age. Several clinical patterns have been recognized. The most common is of a progressive arthritis of large joints, especially the knee and hip. This is usually indistinguishable from degenerative joint disease, although superimposed acute inflammatory episodes are common. The intermittent acute pattern of synovitis, which resembles gout, is less common. In a small percentage of patients there is a sustained progressive synovitis that resembles rheumatoid arthritis. Since many patients with calcification of articular cartilage manifest no rheumatic signs or symptoms, the terms chondrocalcinosis and pseudogout are not synonymous.

Attacks of *pseudogout* are usually monarticular; less commonly two or more joints may be involved simultaneously. The knee is the most frequently affected joint. The diagnosis rests on roentgenographic criteria, but proof requires the demonstration of calcium pyrophosphate dihydrate crystals under polarized light microscopy. These crystals usually have rod or rhomboid shapes and show weak positive birefringence.

Roentgenographic evidence of calcification of articular fibrocartilage may be found in many structures, including menisci, intervertebral discs, and symphysis pubis. Since punctate and linear radiodensities may be more evident in asymptomatic joints, suspicion of pseudogout should direct a survey of more than the affected articulation.

The metabolic basis for crystal deposition in chondrocalcinosis is not known. There are speculations regarding inhibition or deficiency of pyrophosphatases in cartilage, synovial tissue, or joint fluid.

Aspiration of an acutely swollen joint is often sufficient therapy in itself. If inflammatory signs are marked, aspiration may be followed by intra-articular adrenocorticosteroid therapy or the oral administration of phenylbutazone.

SYNOVIAL TUMORS

Pigmented villonodular synovitis is the most commonly applied term for a syndrome characterized by villous or nodular growths affecting synovial linings of joints, bursae, or tendons, and a characteristic histopathological picture, i.e., presence of inflammatory granulomas containing hemosiderin and cholesterol crystals and multinucleated giant cells. There is dispute as to whether this condition should be classified as a form of synovitis or as a true neoplasm. Joint involvement is usually monarticular. The knee is most frequently affected, less commonly the hip, elbow, ankle, or foot. Synovial fluid is usually hemorrhagic or xanthochromic. The inflammatory mass frequently invades cartilage, subchondral bone, and periarticular structures. Pigmented villonodular synovitis may affect extra-articular bursae and tendon sheaths or may occur as a localized tumor in only part of a joint. The treatment of choice is synovectomy. Recurrence is uncommon.

Synovial chondromatosis is an uncommon disorder characterized by the presence of multiple foci of cartilage metaplasia in synovial membranes. Bits of metaplastic growths frequently detach and grow as loose bodies in the joint cavity and ultimately become ossified. In the latter state, this condition is referred to as synovial osteochondromatosis. The knee is most commonly affected; the disease is rarely polyarticular. Symptoms include pain, swelling, limitation in motion, and intermittent locking of the affected joint. The treatment is surgical synovectomy.

A variety of benign tumors (lipoma, chondroma, hemangioma, and xanthoma) may affect joints.

Primary malignant tumors are rare. Synovioma is a highly malignant fibroblastic sarcoma which probably originates in periarticular structures. This usually occurs in late childhood or early adult years. The recommended therapy is wide excision (frequently requiring amputation), regional lymph node dissection, and irradiation. With the most aggressive management the five-year "cure" rate is usually less than 50 per cent. Synovial chondrosarcoma is a rare neoplasm that may simulate synovial chondromatosis. Radical excision or amputation is the treatment of choice.

Barrow, M. V., and Holubar, K.: Multicentric reticulohistiocytosis. Medicine, 48:287, 1969.
Eichenholz, S. M.: Charcot Joints. Springfield, Ill., Charles C Thomas, 1966.
Howell, D. S.: Hypertrophic osteoarthropathy. *In* Hollander, J. L., and McCarty, D. J., Jr. (eds.): Arthritis and Allied Conditions. 8th ed. Philadelphia, Lea & Febiger, 1972.
McCarty, D. J., Kohn, N. N., and Fares, J. S.: The significance of calcium phosphate crystals in synovial fluid of arthritic patients: The pseudogout syndrome: Clinical aspect. Ann. Intern. Med., 56:711, 1962.
Moskowitz, R. W., and Katz, D.: Chondrocalcinosis and chondrocalsynovitis (pseudogout syndrome): Analysis of 24 cases. Am. J. Med., 43:322, 1967.

98. DEGENERATIVE JOINT DISEASE (Osteoarthritis)

Early degeneration of articular cartilage probably begins in all subjects by the end of the second decade of life. In the pathologic sense, degenerative joint disease is a "normal" response to aging. If the incidence of degenerative joint disease is estimated by minimal roentgenographic criteria, approximately 90 per cent of the population by the age 40 is affected. Although only a small proportion of those with abnormal roentgenograms are symptomatic, degenerative joint disease is the most common cause of chronic disability.

Degenerative joint disease is sometimes classified as primary and secondary. The latter denotes the acceleration or augmentation of wear by abnormal stresses associated with injuries, obesity, and mechanical joint disturbances. Primary degenerative joint disease, in which there is no abnormal wear or forces, is probably influenced by one or more biochemical abnormalities that impair cartilage metabolism.

Pathology. The earliest lesions of degenerative joint disease are microscopic alterations of articular cartilage. These include diminution of metachromatic material, decreased numbers of chondrocytes, fatty degeneration, alteration of collagen fibrils, and surface irregularities. Later morphologic changes include localized softening of the cartilage with surface flaking and fibrillations. Abrasion of fibrillated cartilage results in progressive loss of cartilaginous surfacing and exposure of subchondral bone.

Subsequent to ulcerations of cartilage, new bone formation occurs at the margin of articular cartilage. These marginal osteophytes are represented in roentgenograms as the characteristic "spurs." Other osseous changes include cysts of varying size beneath the joint surface and remodeling of subchondral bone.

Changes in synovial membranes, including fibrosis, hypertrophy, and occasionally synovitis, appear to be secondary to events affecting articular cartilage. Rarely the pathologic features of inflammation mimic those of rheumatoid arthritis.

Etiology and Pathogenesis. Accepting the likely premise that primary changes in articular cartilage underlie the development of degenerative joint disease, etiologic considerations may relate to the reparative processes of cartilage. In response to injury, the metabolic activity of chondrocytes increases, but their capacity to replicate and form new matrix is limited. Secondary degenerative joint disease occurs when the forces of wear and tear exceed the restricted capacity for repair. When degenerative joint disease develops (frequently in familial patterns) in the absence of abnormal stresses, it is presumed that accelerated degeneration results from one or more biochemical abnormalities affecting cartilage metabolism. Chemical studies of degenerative cartilage have revealed several abnormalities: decreased water and chondromucoprotein contents and alterations in the profile of glycosaminoglycans. Some of these changes could be mediated by the action of lysosomal hydrolases, but the nature of the presumed biochemical defect in degenerative cartilage remains unknown.

Conditions which alter mechanical properties of joints or which affect the osseous support of articular cartilage are numerous. They include obesity, trauma, hypermobility of joints, neuropathy, acromegaly, Paget's disease of bone, hyperparathyroidism, and alterations of articular or periarticular structures by inflammatory joint disease.

Clinical Patterns of Degenerative Joint Disease. Pain is the dominant symptom of degenerative joint disease but, as noted earlier, disease which is roentgenographically moderate to severe may be asymptomatic. Pain is aggravated by joint motion or weight bearing. Transient stiffness after periods of inactivity is common. Loss of articular cartilage and osseous hypertrophy result in bony enlargement and malalignment of joints and crepitation on motion. Mild tenderness to palpation and effusions are common, but other inflammatory signs are usually absent.

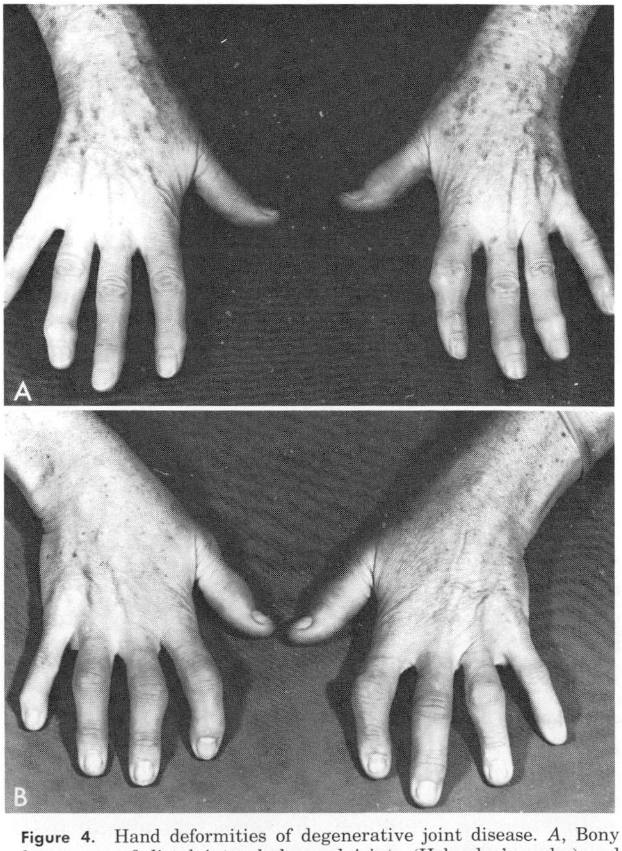

Figure 4. Hand deformities of degenerative joint disease. *A*, Bony enlargement of distal interphalangeal joints (Heberden's nodes) and similar change in one proximal interphalangeal joint (Bouchard's node). *B*, Symmetrical degenerative changes in proximal interphalangeal joints (Bouchard's nodes), a pattern that is frequently mistaken for rheumatoid arthritis.

The present discussion of clinical manifestations of degenerative joint disease is developed largely on anatomic lines, since signs and symptoms reflect regional patterns of involvement.

The Hand. *Heberden's nodes* are bony protuberances at the dorsal margins of distal interphalangeal joints. Early Heberden's nodes have a soft cystic consistency and may be associated with prominent inflammatory signs. The chronic stage of Heberden's nodes, characterized by bony enlargement and angular deformities (Fig. 4*A*), is usually minimally symptomatic. Heredity and sex are prominently involved in the development of Heberden's nodes. They are much more common in women. On the basis of family studies, it has been postulated that a single autosomal gene is involved which is dominant in females and recessive in males.

Patients with Heberden's nodes frequently show degenerative changes in other joints of the hands. The misinterpretation of proximal interphalangeal joint involvement (Bouchard's nodes) as rheumatoid arthritis is a common error (Fig. 4*B*). Metacarpophalangeal joint involvement is rare. Pain on the radial side of the wrist caused by degenerative disease in the first carpometacarpal joint is a frequent manifestation.

Coxarthrosis (Malum Coxae Senilis). Symptoms of *primary degenerative hip disease* usually appear in the later decades of life, but in as many as half the cases there is evidence of antecedent hip disease such as congenital dysplasia, slipped capital femoral epiphysis, or Legg-Calvé-Perthes disease. In addition, a variety of acquired disorders such as rheumatoid arthritis and avascular necrosis of the femoral head may lead to degenerative hip disease. Groin pain on motion or weight bearing is the dominant symptom, and this is often referred to the medial aspect of the thigh or knee. Over a period of months to a few years, the majority of patients become seriously disabled because of pain and restricted motion.

Degenerative Disease of the Knee. Involvement of the knees is the most common source of major disability in degenerative joint disease. Although mild synovitis and effusion may be present, joint enlargement primarily reflects bone proliferation. Crepitation on motion is a consistent finding. Degenerative changes are usually more prominent in the medial compartment of the knee, leading to varus deformity.

An early manifestation of degenerative change in the patellofemoral joint is termed *chondromalacia patellae*. This syndrome of knee pain and mild effusion, usually associated with trauma, is seen predominantly in young adults.

Vertebral Degenerative Joint Disease, Including Herniated Disc Syndromes. Two sets of articulations are present at all levels of the spinal column: the intervertebral discs and the posterior zygapophyseal joints. In addition to these, the cervical spine (between C2 and C7) has articulations between the lateral aspects of adjacent vertebral bodies, usually referred to as *joints of Luschka*. Degenerative changes in joints of Luschka are the most common cause of pain in the cervical area. In lumbar levels degeneration and herniation of the nucleus pulposus of intervertebral discs are usually the bases for symptoms.

CERVICAL SPINE. The close proximity of cervical nerve roots to the joints of Luschka makes them vulnerable to irritation or compression from any derangement in or about the joints. Since the greatest amount of stress in the cervical spine occurs at C4-C5 and C5-C6 levels, degenerative changes in the intervertebral discs and joints of Luschka are most common there. Osteophytic spurs at the margins of joints of Luschka may impinge upon nerve roots as they leave the intervertebral foramina. The pattern of pain and neurologic findings varies according to the level involved: pain is frequently in the supraclavicular and upper trapezius regions but can be referred into the occiput and more distal upper extremity. Discomfort is aggravated by motion of the neck, particularly rotation and lateral bending.

If there is degeneration of the intervertebral discs in the cervical spine, the joints of Luschka provide a barrier against lateral herniation of the nucleus pulposus. The protrusion and subsequent osteophytic reaction may therefore encroach directly on the spinal cord rather than nerve roots. The progression of the resulting cervical myelopathy may be insidious and painless.

LUMBAR SPINE. Symptoms of degenerative disease of the lumbar spine are nearly always attributable to involvement of intervertebral discs. Protrusion or extrusion of degenerated discs is directed posteriolaterally, impinging upon nerve roots or the cauda equina. Although any of the lumbar discs can herniate, this most commonly occurs at L4-L5 and L5-S1. Patients with herniated lumbar discs frequently have a history of mild or recurrent backache prior to development of more acute discomfort. Pain radiates distally into one or the other lower extremity and is aggravated by spinal movement, particularly bending to the side of the pain. There is usually marked paravertebral tenderness and aggravation of pain by straight leg raising. Loss or suppression of the ankle jerk and sensory deficit in the lateral border and sole of the foot and toes suggest L5-S1 root compression. No reflex change, sensory deficit in the lateral leg and mediodorsal aspect of the foot, and weakness of the toe extensors suggest L4-L5 root compression.

Primary Generalized Hypertrophic Osteoarthritis. This is more a concept than a disease: it describes a polyarticular pattern associated with somewhat more inflammatory reaction than is customary with degenerative joint disease. There is usually involvement of the hands, including Heberden's and Bouchard's nodes, along with changes in the first carpometacarpal joints. Women in the middle years of life are most commonly affected, and a familial pattern is prominent. A closely related syndrome of degenerative joint disease has been termed *erosive osteoarthritis*.

Laboratory Findings. There are no specific laboratory abnormalities of degenerative joint disease. The erythrocyte sedimentation rate is usually normal. Synovial fluid is clear and exhibits high viscosity and normal mucin clot test. Leukocyte counts in synovial fluid vary in the range of 200 to 2000 per cubic millimeter. Fragments of cartilage are frequently identified in the fluid.

Roentgenographic Features. Osteophyte formation at the margins of affected joints is the basis for the most striking roentgenographic feature of degenerative joint disease, but earlier and more common findings, resulting from destruction of articular cartilage, are narrowing of the interosseous joint space and subchondral bone sclerosis. Radiolucent cysts, varying in size from a few millimeters to several centimeters, may be seen in periarticular bone.

Degeneration of cervical and lumbar discs results in interspace narrowing. Exostoses at the margins of vertebral bodies may coalesce with adjacent osteophytes, causing fusion at one or more levels. Roentgenographic documentation of intervertebral herniation requires contrast myelography. Disc degeneration is best observed by anteroposterior and lateral roentgenograms. For visualization of osteophytes encroaching on foramina, especially important in the cervical spine, oblique projections are required.

Differential Diagnosis. In their typical expressions, degenerative joint disease and rheumatoid arthritis are easily distinguished. The latter is usually associated with evidence of systemic disease, prominent signs of joint inflammation, and the characteristic symmetrical pattern of disease affecting the hands and wrists. When a patient presents with signs of mild inflammation in one or two weight-bearing joints of the lower extremities, the differentiation between these two syndromes is more difficult. In that setting a normal erythrocyte sedimentation rate, negative rheumatoid factor test, and minimal abnormalities in synovial fluid support the diagnosis of degenerative joint disease. No test singly or in combination can be viewed as diagnostic; even the roentgenographic demonstration of marginal osteophytes may be a secondary change in rheumatoid arthritis. In the most experienced hands, there is a small percentage of patients in whom the diagnosis remains indeterminate.

A common diagnostic error is the interpretation of degenerative changes in proximal interphalangeal joints of the hands as evidence of rheumatoid arthritis (Fig. *4B*). The deformities that characterize Heberden's and Bouchard's nodes may be marked, but this pattern of degenerative joint disease is not associated with prominent signs of inflammation, and the metacarpophalangeal joints and wrist joints are rarely if ever affected.

Important aspects of differential diagnosis involve the recognition of syndromes in which secondary development of degenerative joint disease may occur. These include hemochromatosis, neuropathy, chondrocalcinosis, alcaptonuria, hypermobility of joints (including the Ehlers-Danlos syndrome), mechanical derangements of joints, and a variety of metabolic disorders that affect the support of articular cartilage by subchondral bone.

There should never be confusion in the differentiation of degenerative joint disease of the vertebral column from ankylosing spondylitis. Patients with the latter are almost invariably young men, and the roentgenographic features are distinct from those associated with degenerative joint disease.

Treatment. The management of degenerative joint disease is highly varied, depending upon anatomic patterns and the degree of joint deformity. An optimistic forecast is appropriate for most individuals. Patients should understand that disability can be minimized even though there is no specific remedy. The common statement that "nothing can be done for your kind of arthritis" is a false cliché.

Drugs. No medication has been shown to retard the development or progression of degenerative joint disease. The requirement for analgesic drugs is varied; many patients have so little pain that they require no medicinal therapy. Aspirin in moderate dosage (0.6 gram three to five times a day) is usually helpful for the patient with pain. Sustained salicylate therapy is superior to intermittent or erratic dosage. A common problem in degenerative joint disease, regardless of anatomic location, is the occurrence of intermittent episodes of increased pain which tend to subside spontaneously. For these recurrent episodes, phenylbutazone (100 to 300 mg daily) or indomethacin (75 to 150 mg daily) may be beneficial. Continuous use of drugs other than salicylates is rarely indicated in degenerative joint disease. Some patients with disabling hip pain, however, experience sufficient relief of symptoms with phenylbutazone or indomethacin to warrant maintenance therapy. It is common practice to prescribe muscle relaxants, such as diazepam or carisoprodol, for pain and muscle spasm of vertebral disease, but objective assessment of their efficacy is lacking.

Physical Measures. There are two general goals in the design of a physical medicine program for degenerative joint disease: minimizing the forces of work and weight bearing that apply to affected joints, and maintenance of normal joint alignment and motion. The patient with hip or knee disease should be instructed to avoid unnecessary walking or stair climbing. This recommendation is not inconsistent with the performance of an exercise program (in nonweight-bearing attitude) which can maintain muscle power and joint motion. Quadriceps isometric exercise for degenerative joint disease of the knees is particularly important. There is a powerful rationale for weight reduction for the obese patient with involvement of the spine or lower extremities. The use of a cane or a crutch can reduce forces of weight bearing applied to a symptomatic hip or knee by as much as 50 per cent. In selected patients with an unstable knee, fitting of a brace may be beneficial.

Certain physical measures are selectively relevant to degenerative joint disease of the spine. Patients need to learn to live with the altered mechanics of their spine. With cervical involvement, hyperextension and hyperflexion should be avoided. The patient should sleep supine with no more than one pillow. Most, but not all, patients with cervical radicular pain will be helped by intermittent traction. If this is beneficial, there are inexpensive devices for applying intermittent cervical traction at home. When symptoms are acute, wearing a cervical collar will restrict movement and minimize pain.

The patient with symptomatic degenerative disease of the lumbar spine should sleep on a hard mattress and avoid bending and lifting activities. A program of graded postural exercises is important when pain has subsided. External support provided by a lumbosacral corset will frequently minimize mild chronic symptoms. When lumbar disc herniation results in severe pain or nerve deficit, hospitalization is usually indicated. The majority of such patients will experience a remission of symptoms within a two- to three-week period. Consideration of surgical therapy is appropriate for those patients who fail to respond to conservative management.

Surgical Management. The main anatomic areas affected by degenerative joint disease that are amenable to orthopedic surgical therapy are the hip, the knee, and the vertebral column. Several surgical procedures are appropriate for the patient with debilitating hip pain. These include arthrodesis (if the disease is unilateral), mold arthroplasty, osteotomy, and total joint replacement. In most centers, the last is the preferred procedure. Operative procedures for the knee with degenerative joint disease include debridement, osteotomy, and a variety of prosthetic arthroplasties. If there is reasonable preservation of motion and stability of the maligned knee, tibial or femoral osteotomy is frequently beneficial. When there is a serious disability attributable to malalignment and instability of the knee, one or another prosthetic procedure may be indicated. However, the successes, to date, of knee joint replacement have not been as predictable as have comparable procedures for the hip.

Virtually all orthopedic surgeons agree that surgical procedures for degenerative disease of the spine are appropriate *only* after there has been a systematic and sustained trial of conservative management. If radicular pain is relentless or if there are increasing neurologic deficits from nerve root involvement or myelopathy, surgical correction is warranted.

Armstrong, J. R.: Lumbar disc lesions. 3rd ed. Baltimore, Williams & Wilkins Company, 1965.
Friedenberg, Z. B., and Miller, W. T.: Degenerative disc disease of the cervical spine. J. Bone Joint Surg., 45A:1171, 1963.
Kellgren, J. H., Lawrence, J. S., and Bier, F.: Genetic factors in generalized osteo-arthritis. Ann. Rheum. Dis., 22:237, 1969.
Mankin, H. J.: Biochemical and metabolic aspects of osteoarthritis. Orthop. Clin. North Am., 2:19, 1971.
Sokoloff, L.: The Biology of Degenerative Joint Disease. Chicago, University of Chicago Press, 1969.

99. THE PAINFUL SHOULDER

Because shoulder pain is frequent and due to diverse mechanisms, this subject deserves special attention. Of prime importance is recognition that pain in the shoulder may be referred from disease affecting cervical, intrathoracic, and diaphragmatic areas. Shoulder motion is affected by the action of muscles through a "joint complex" consisting of independent articulations—glenohumeral, acromioclavicular, and sternoclavicular, as well as the scapulothoracic surface relationship. In addition, shoulder function requires movement of gliding surfaces of periarticular structures—the musculotendinous cuff, the subdeltoid bursa, and the long head of the biceps. Any of the syndromes associated with synovitis may be responsible for shoulder pain. The primary concern in this chapter is a group of painful disorders which affect the periarticular soft tissues of the shoulder.

CALCIFIC TENDINITIS AND BURSITIS

The most common cause of shoulder pain results from degeneration of the supraspinatus and infraspinatus tendons. Approximately 3 per cent of people in their middle years have calcific deposits in these rotator tendons. Although the majority of such subjects have few or no symptoms, a significant percentage develop pain because of inflammation of the parietal surface of the overlying subdeltoid bursa. An inflammatory exudate containing calcareous matter may rupture into this bursa. The symptoms may be acute, subacute, or chronic. The acute syndrome is characterized by sudden onset of pain in the shoulder area, often with radiation into the neck and proximal arm. Any motion of the shoulder girdle elicits pain. There is frequently exquisite local tenderness over the anterior and anterolateral aspect of the shoulder joint. Night pain is a prominent feature. Roentgenographic studies usually demonstrate linear calcific deposits in the involved tendon or a more diffuse calcific pattern in the subdeltoid bursa. In most instances acute symptoms abate after a few days, but in a minority subacute discomfort persists for weeks.

The treatment is influenced by the severity and duration of symptoms. Anti-inflammatory agents, such as phenylbutazone or indomethacin, and analgesics are usually sufficient to control acute symptoms. In most patients there is a spontaneous remission of pain and a disappearance of calcific deposits. When the symptoms are very acute, aspiration of calcified material and injection of adrenocorticosteroid preparation may give prompt relief. The prospects of more chronic disability can be minimized by the institution of an active exercise program as soon as the level of discomfort permits. If the patient is not making progress toward regaining normal shoulder motion with a home exercise program, supervised therapy in a physical medicine department is important. A small percentage of patients with refractory pain and persistent roentgenographic findings may require surgical exploration for removal of calcific deposits.

BICIPITAL TENDINITIS

The long head of the biceps originates from the superior surface of the glenoid. It emerges from the glenohumeral bursa to lie in the bicipital groove of the humerus where it is covered by a synovial sheath. The shoulder pain of bicipital tendinitis frequently radiates along the biceps to the forearm, and is aggravated by abduction and internal rotation. Tenderness over the bicipital groove and accentuation of pain with resisted supination of the forearm, with the elbow flexed at 90 degrees, aid in the recognition of bicipital tendinitis. The management is similar to that described for calcific tendinitis: local injection of adrenocorticosteroid preparations, systemic anti-inflammatory agents, and an exercise program. In refractory cases, surgical exploration with tendon transfer usually yields good results.

ROTATOR CUFF TEARS

The same degenerative changes that underlie the development of shoulder tendinitis can weaken the musculotendinous rotator cuff and predispose it to rupture. In most patients with this problem, there is acute onset of shoulder pain after trauma or performance of strenuous work. If the tear is complete, the patient is unable to abduct the arm, but it can be held in abduction, once elevated to 90 degrees, by the action of the deltoid muscle. With incomplete tears, the patient has only mild pain and moderate weakness. The diagnosis of rotator cuff tears can best be established by contrast arthrography. With complete rupture of the supraspinatus tendon, surgical repair is usually warranted. In patients with partial tears, partial immobilization followed by an exercise program is appropriate.

THE SHOULDER-HAND SYNDROME
(Reflex Neurovascular Dystrophy)

This is a poorly understood disorder characterized by pain and stiffness in the shoulder, together with pain, swelling, and vasomotor phenomena in the hand. Involvement of the distal upper extremity is frequently followed by dystrophic change that resembles *Sudeck's atrophy.* The syndrome is presumed to result from reflex sympathetic stimulation analogous to that proposed for causalgia. It principally affects patients above the age of 50 and is often associated with acute illness such as myocardial infarction, trauma to the distal upper extremity, cerebrovascular accident, or pulmonary disease. The significance of associated degenerative change in the cervical spine is uncertain, because of its high frequency in the population at risk. When the disease is bilateral (approximately 25 per cent of cases), the differentiation from acute rheumatoid arthritis may be difficult. There is marked variability in intensity and duration of acute symptoms and extent of dystrophic change. In a small percentage of patients the end result is "frozen shoulder" and dystrophic changes in the hands that resemble those of systemic sclerosis.

There is probably no condition for which aggressive physical therapy is more important than for the shoulder-hand syndrome. An active exercise program, facilitated by analgesic medication, should be instituted as soon as possible. When refractory pain impedes progress in the physical medicine program, a trial of systemic corticosteroid therapy (10 to 20 mg per day of prednisone or equivalent) or stellate ganglion block is warranted.

FROZEN SHOULDER

A minority of patients with any of the shoulder conditions discussed above develop chronic restriction of motion of the glenohumeral joint. When there is no apparent relationship of frozen shoulder to other shoulder disease, such as tendinitis or rotator cuff injury, the condition is sometimes termed *adhesive capsulitis.* This condition may be clinically indistinct from the shoulder-hand syndrome. Pain is generally less severe and less well localized relative to other conditions causing shoulder pain. The most important aspect of management of frozen shoulder is prevention. Early attention to the underlying cause of shoulder pain and the institution of an effective exercise program is nearly always successful in combating the progression of shoulder immobility. Management of the chronic frozen shoulder is much more difficult. Manipulation under general anesthesia followed by intensive physical therapy may be indicated when patients are not helped by conservative management.

DePalma, A. F., and Kruper, J. S.: Long-term study of shoulder joints afflicted with and treated for calcific tendinitis. Clin. Orthop., 20:61, 1961.

Steinbrocker, O.: The painful shoulder. *In* Hollander, J. L., and McCarty, D. J., Jr. (eds.): Arthritis and Allied Conditions. 8th ed. Philadelphia, Lea & Febiger, 1972.

100. NONARTICULAR RHEUMATISM

This term designates a group of painful disorders resulting from involvement of tendons, bursae, and other periarticular structures. Conditions causing shoulder pain are considered separately in Ch. 99.

BURSITIS

Bursae are closed synovial sacs located at sites of friction between skin, ligaments, tendons, muscles, and bones. Trauma is the most common cause of bursitis, but almost any illness characterized by joint synovitis may be associated with involvement of the lining of bursae. Bursae commonly involved include the following: subdeltoid, trochanteric, olecranon, and prepatellar. Septic or gouty bursitis can be documented by appropriate studies of aspirated fluid. Protection of an inflamed bursa from friction and trauma is the most important aspect of treatment, but moderate doses of salicylates, phenylbutazone, or indomethacin may be helpful. Local injection with an adrenocorticosteroid preparation is indicated if symptoms are severe or refractory to other treatments.

TENOSYNOVITIS

Tendon sheaths, like bursae, have synovial linings and can be involved by any process capable of inducing joint synovitis. Tenosynovitis in the hand or foot is a frequent manifestation of gonococcemia. Calcific tendinitis, a common source of shoulder pain, (see Ch. 99) may be associated with marked inflammatory signs resembling acute gout. Focal thickening of the tendon sheath and adjacent tendon can result in "locking or triggering" phenomena. This problem, termed stenosing tenovaginitis, is common in the flexor tendons of the fingers. Involvement of the abductor pollicis longus and extensor pollicis brevis tendons of the thumb *(de Quervain's syndrome)* results in pain and tenderness at the radial aspect of the wrist. There are no generalizations regarding management, since tenosynovitis may be a manifestation of various disease states, including rheumatoid arthritis and other connective tissue syndromes, infection, gout, and hypercholesterolemia. The common form of tenosynovitis, unassociated with systemic disease, will often subside with rest. If symptoms are severe or recurrent, local injections of adrenocorticosteroid preparations are usually effective. Surgical excision of the affected tendon sheath is indicated for those patients with persistent disability.

TENNIS ELBOW
(Epicondylitis)

This common condition is characterized by pain over the lateral aspect of the elbow. Tenderness is localized in the area of the common extensor insertion in the region of the lateral epicondyle. The problem, most common in middle-aged males, is related to sports or occupations that involve repetitive wrist extension or pronation–supination. Pain is accentuated by resisted wrist extension. If symptoms fail to respond to rest, injection of local adrenocorticosteroid preparations is usually successful. For the rare patient with persistent disability, surgical therapy may be needed.

CARPAL TUNNEL SYNDROME

This problem results from entrapment of the median nerve as it passes deep to the transverse carpal ligament of the wrist. Inflammation of the adjacent flexor tendon sheaths, the most common basis for median nerve entrapment, may be a feature of rheumatoid arthritis; but in most patients the tenosynovitis is localized and unassociated with systemic disease. The majority of patients are middle-aged women. The most consistent symptoms are dysesthesia, paresthesia, and hypesthesia in the middle three digits of the hand. Referred pain in the more proximal upper extremity is common. Symptoms are usually intermittent, occurring most frequently during the night. Forced flexion of the wrist or nerve compression locally may induce the characteristic symptoms. In a minority of patients, there is progressive wasting of the muscles of the thenar eminence. Conservative management consists of fitting a removable dorsal splint to hold the wrist in slight extension and the local injection of an adrenocorticosteroid preparation. Surgical release of the transverse carpal ligament is indicated for patients with persistent disability.

TIETZE'S SYNDROME

This mysterious benign disorder is characterized by painful enlargement of the upper costal cartilages. It is usually unilateral and limited to a single costochondral juncture. Occasionally the manubriosternal and sternoclavicular joints are affected. The disease may be recurrent, but remission is the rule. Some patients are concerned that they have cardiac disease; reassurance alone may be sufficient management. If discomfort is severe or recurrent, analgesics, heat, or local infiltration (adrenocorticosteroid or local anesthetic agents) may be beneficial.

FIBROSITIS

This term has been applied to a poorly defined symptom complex which is characterized by pain and stiffness in varying areas, most commonly in the neck, shoulder girdle, and posterior aspect of the trunk. Physical signs except for questionable nodules or thickening of the deep fasciae are lacking, and laboratory and roentgenographic studies are negative. The term fibrositis is based on vague hypothesis and common usage rather than on anatomic abnormalities. Localized areas of tenderness, commonly in the paravertebral areas medial to the scapula, have been termed "trigger points." The syndrome usually begins in the middle years of life. Because the majority of patients appear tense and anxious and have no recognizable objective basis for symptoms, the syndrome is often considered psychogenic. Since pain and stiffness can be manifestations of a variety of musculoskeletal, neurologic, and systemic disorders, the diagnosis of fibrositis requires the exclusion of more defined illnesses. The patient and his physician tend to share an unhappy experience in efforts to control symptoms. The results of strong reassurance, that serious disease is lacking, are variable, as are the results of therapy with salicylates, sedatives, tranquilizers, and muscle relaxants. Temporary relief is occasionally achieved by injection of local anesthetic into tender points or by chilling the overlying skin with ethyl chloride.

Levey, G. S., and Calabro, J. J.: Tietze's syndrome: Report of two cases and review of the literature. Arthritis Rheum., 5:261, 1962.

Phalen, G. S.: The carpal tunnel syndrome: Seventeen years' experience in diagnosis and treatment of 654 hands. J. Bone Joint Surg., 48A:211, 1966.

Swannell, A. J., Underwood, F. A., and Dixon, A. St. J.: Periarticular calcific deposits mimicking acute arthritis. Ann. Rheum. Dis., 29:380, 1970.

Part VII
GRANULOMATOUS DISEASES OF UNPROVED ETIOLOGY

101. INTRODUCTION

Paul B. Beeson

The chapters to follow include a variety of rather uncommon and difficult-to-classify syndromes. These are characterized by long and fluctuating clinical courses, and the affected tissues show the picture of chronic inflammation, usually with formation of granulomas. Sarcoidosis is the most common and best known. The others are comparatively rare, and their natures and classifications are subject to controversy. For the purpose of textbook exposition the best recognized clinical forms have been described as separate diseases. It should be noted, however, that there are shades of similarity and that each of these is thought by some students to be merely a variant expression of one of the other processes, e.g., Wegener's granulomatosis and lethal midline granuloma. Some of these syndromes could well have been discussed with the diseases of connective tissue, as in fact they used to be in former editions. In the present state of knowledge – ignorance is more accurate – the editors have elected to place the descriptions of these syndromes under a heading with a noncommittal title.

102. SARCOIDOSIS

D. Geraint James

Definition. Sarcoidosis is a multisystemic granulomatous disorder of unknown cause most commonly affecting persons in the middle period of life. It is characterized by widespread epithelioid cell granulomas, depression of delayed-type hypersensitivity, and lymphoproliferation. The Kveim-Siltzbach skin test is frequently positive, and there may be abnormal calcium metabolism.

The diagnosis is most securely established when consistent clinicoradiographic findings are supported by histologic evidence of granulomas with minimal necrosis. The course and prognosis are related to abruptness of clinical onset; an acute onset usually heralds a self-limiting course and spontaneous resolution, whereas an insidious onset is often followed by unrelenting progression.

Etiology, Immunology, and Pathogenesis. Since the cause remains unknown, theories abound. Any hypothesis should endeavor to explain certain cardinal immunologic upsets, so it is currently fashionable to try to intertwine possible causal agents with these immunologic abnormalities and produce a working hypothesis of the pathogenesis. It should be remembered that any such theory, however attractive, remains but a tentative bridgehead for a final assault on the still unknown cause. We still do not know whether sarcoidosis is one disease resulting from one cause or a collection of similar reactions to multiple causes. At present most authorities favor the unitarian concept of a single disorder rather than a multicausal syndrome. There are, of course, numerous causes of granulomatous disorders, including infections, chemicals, neoplasms, inhaled allergens, immunologic deficiency states, and at least one inherited enzyme defect (chronic granulomatous disease of childhood). When all these have been excluded, there remains a hard core which we term multisystemic sarcoidosis. It presents in all parts of the world with a similar clinical, radiographic, histologic, chemical, and immunologic pattern, and responds predictably and in similar fashion to treatment. It is this condition which we believe to be one disease resulting from one cause.

Causal Agents. Claims of an infective agent have included human and anonymous mycobacteria, the leprosy bacillus, fungi, viruses, and protozoa. Many organisms provoke a nonspecific granulomatous reaction, but this should not be misconstrued as multisystemic sarcoidosis. Epstein-Barr virus antibody titers of 1:640 and over are significantly more frequent in sarcoidosis than in control subjects. This again should not be misconstrued as evidence of yet another etiologic agent but rather as a reflection of widespread lymphoproliferation, for there may also be raised antibody titers to herpes simplex, rubella, measles, and parainfluenza viruses.

Beryllium and zirconium are known to produce sarcoid granulomas in individuals sensitized to these elements, but other tested elements in the periodic table do not seem to be granulomagenic.

Other agents for which etiologic claims have been made include pine pollen, peanut dust, and clay eating in various parts of the world.

Immunology. The cardinal immunologic upsets in sarcoidosis are threefold: (1) thymus-mediated lymphocyte (T cell) misbehavior, as indicated by depression of delayed-type hypersensitivity; (2) vigorous lymphoproliferation with considerable bursa-dependent (B) mononuclear cell activity; and (3) granuloma formation in all organ systems.

T CELL BEHAVIOR. Depression of delayed-type hypersensitivity is revealed by cutaneous anergy using tuberculin or many other antigens such as dinitrochlorobenzene, and also in vitro by various tests of lymphocyte function. There is a good correlation between in vivo and in vitro anergy in sarcoidosis. Sarcoid lymphocytes show a diminished response to phytohemagglutinin (PHA). When patients recover from sarcoidosis, tuberculin sensitivity returns to what it was before the onset of sarcoidosis. If the T cells were sensitized to tuberculin prior to sarcoidosis, they lose their ability to react with tuberculin during the acute disease but sometimes return to normal with cure. The more obvious the depression of delayed-type hypersensitivity during the acute phase of the disease, the more likely it is to remain depressed. This generalization also applies to in vitro PHA-stimulated lymphoblastic transformation, which may remain below par for many years.

VIGOROUS LYMPHOPROLIFERATION. Whereas there is cutaneous anergy and impaired cellular immunity, the very reverse holds for humoral antibodies, serum immunoglobulins, and other circulating factors in sarcoidosis. At the same time as T cell eclipse, there is vigorous lymphoproliferation, with increased immunoglobulin formation. Simultaneously, there may be significantly increased circulating antibodies to the Epstein-Barr virus, herpes simplex, rubella, measles, and parainfluenza viruses, and an increased antibody response to mismatched blood. The precise immunologic impact which causes this galaxy of high-titer serologic antibodies and profuse immunoglobulins is obscure.

GRANULOMA FORMATION. Granulomas develop in all organ systems at the time of T cell eclipse and lymphoproliferation, possibly reflecting a reaction to circulating immune complexes.

Hypothesis of Pathogenesis. An antigenic insult, whether by one of the aforementioned infective or chemical agents or even by vegetable matter, is met by a reticuloendothelial response in which both thymus-derived (T) cells and plasma (B) cells participate. The T cells are transformed, possibly by undergoing antigenic alteration on their cell surface, and become depleted. Depletion may be due not only to T cell transformation but also to T cell interaction with transformed T cells. Depletion results in depression of delayed-type hypersensitivity, which is recognized by cutaneous anergy and by in vitro lymphocyte transformation tests. At the same time there is vigorous lymphoproliferation, and the B cell response is reflected by an increase in circulating immunoglobulins. During this same phase, transformed T cell circulating immune complexes are probably responsible for such clinical phenomena as erythema nodosum and uveitis. The antigenic insult may be airborne, for bilateral hilar lymphadenopathy is such a frequent mode of onset. The more acute the onset and the more active the reticuloendothelial response, the more likely there will be spontaneous remission with full restoration of T cell function. If this does not occur spontaneously, then it may be induced by corticosteroids, which restore normal T cell function.

The antigen responsible for lymphoproliferation, T cell transformation, and granuloma formation almost certainly resides in Kveim-Siltzbach antigen, possibly linked to and altered by transformed T cells into an immune complex.

Pathology. A granulomatous reaction is the wasteland laid bare by the engagements between indigestible antigen and macrophages, thymus-mediated lymphocytes, and humoral antibodies. Phagocytic cells aggregate into epithelioid and giant cells, which are the hallmarks of a sarcoid granuloma. *Epithelioid cells* are large mononuclear cells about 20 μ in diameter with round or oval nuclei showing a loose chromatin pattern with prominent nucleoli; when stained with hematoxylin and eosin, the cytoplasm is pale, granular, and often vacuolated. *Giant cells* are up to 300 μ in diameter, containing as many as 30 nuclei, usually arranged peripherally. Within these epithelioid and giant cells may be found three types of inclusion bodies – Schaumann, asteroid, and residual bodies – all of which are nonspecific (Fig. 1).

Schaumann bodies are concentrically laminated, deeply basophilic conchoidal bodies, 100 μ in diameter, often with brilliant birefringent crystals. They are made up of calcium carbonate, phosphate, and iron. *Asteroid bodies* are star-shaped lipoproteins, 1 to 5 μ in diameter, with a central core and with radiating, slightly curved spines. They occur in only 2 per cent of patients with sarcoidosis. *Residual bodies* are cytoplasmic lipomucoprotein granules, 1 μ in diameter, and are end-products of activated lysosomes. All three inclusion bodies in turn have been confused with tubercle bacilli and other organisms and parasites.

The granuloma may also contain sparse, inconspicuous plasma cells and a fringe of lymphocytes. Necrosis is minimal in the sarcoid granuloma, and the reticulin fiber framework remains intact in this sparse necrosis. As the lesion ages, reticulin fibers ramify between the epithelioid cells which thicken and become converted into collagen. It loses its outline and becomes a solid amorphous eosinophilic mass of hyaline material.

Williams and his colleagues have shown, by enzyme histochemistry, that the epithelioid cells are identical in the granulomas of sarcoidosis, Kveim-Siltzbach test biopsies, regional ileitis, tuberculosis, swimming pool granuloma, and chronic beryllium disease; all show strong biosynthetic and phagocytic enzyme activity. The epithelioid cells of all these granulomas are metabolically active in synthesizing nucleic acid and attempting to digest extracellular material. Also within this granuloma are the immunoglobulins IgG, IgA, IgM, and IgD,

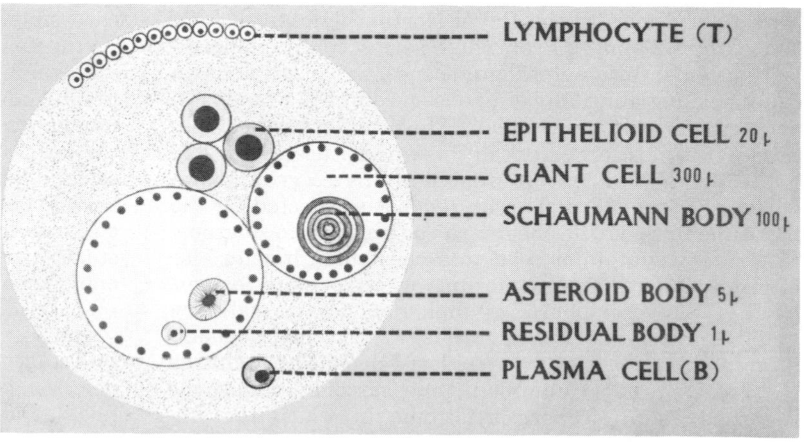

Figure 1. Features of a granuloma.

which can be identified in variable amounts by immunofluorescence.

Epidemiology. Sarcoidosis has a worldwide distribution but is more frequently recognized in sophisticated communities. Mass radiography figures show an over-all prevalence of 20 per 100,000 population in Great Britain, rising to a figure of 120 in Irishmen and 200 per 100,000 in Irishwomen examined in London. In the United States, it is ten times more prevalent in blacks than in whites, regardless of birthplace or residence. The black African appears not yet affected to a significant degree, but this may be due to obscuring tuberculosis or to lessened awareness, or both. It is certainly being recognized more frequently in less sophisticated areas, suggesting that the detection of asymptomatic cases depends on advanced screening techniques.

Irishwomen in London and Puerto Ricans in New York are prone to develop erythema nodosum. Likewise, there is an increased prevalence of sarcoidosis in Martinican subjects living in Paris and in West Indians in Britain. Hormonal factors may play some part, for erythema nodosum caused by sarcoidosis is more common in women of the childbearing years of life, during early pregnancy, and also in women taking oral contraceptives.

Familial sarcoidosis has been reported sufficiently often in various parts of the world to give rise to the suggestion that it is due to a recessive mode of inheritance which finds partial expression in affected homozygotes. Various relationships include brother-sister and mother-son, but father-offspring is exceedingly rare.

Clinical Manifestations. The numerous masquerades of sarcoidosis (Table 1) are reminiscent of syphilis in the days before penicillin. It was always important to remain alert to the possibility of syphilis; otherwise it was occasionally overlooked. The same may now be said for sarcoidosis. Many cases of sarcoidosis remain undetected; instead they are merely termed idiopathic pulmonary fibrosis, hilar adenopathy, iridocyclitis, erythema nodosum, or nephrocalcinosis. Sarcoidosis should always be considered when a middle-aged patient attends several different outpatient clinics, particularly respiratory, ophthalmic, and dermatologic clinics. It is sometimes postulated that the manifestations of sarcoidosis differ in various parts of the world. There are certainly minor differences, but the major patterns of disease which emerge from a comparison of sarcoidosis in London, New York, and Paris are surprisingly similar. This is a retrospective survey of patients attending sarcoidosis clinics at the Mount Sinai Hospital, New York City (Dr. Louis Siltzbach), at the Hôpital Bichat, Paris (Professor J. Turiaf), and ours at the Royal Northern Hospital, London (Tables 2 and 3). From these series, certain generalizations emerge as helpful guidelines. Sarcoidosis has an equal sex distribution, being observed in 302 women (56 per cent) of the Royal Northern Hospital series of 537 patients. It is most prevalent in those under age 40, for 358 of the 537 (67 per cent) presented in this age group, compared with one third over 40. It may be detected for the first time in a routine chest x-ray or because troublesome respiratory symptoms lead to a chest film. It may also present as erythema nodosum or other skin lesions, iridocyclitis, peripheral lymphadenopathy, salivary gland enlargement, or nervous system involvement. Asymptomatic or silent sarcoidosis, detected by routine chest x-ray, is so common that sarcoidosis may be regarded as an iceberg syndrome in which the undiagnosed silent subclinical variant is far more frequent than is realized.

TABLE 1. Modes of Presentation of Sarcoidosis

Chest Physician	Dermatologist	Ophthalmologist
Breathlessness Bilateral hilar lymphadenopathy Pulmonary fibrosis Cor pulmonale	Erythema nodosum Lupus pernio Plaques, scars, keloids Maculopapular eruptions	Iridocyclitis Keratoconjunctivitis sicca Sjögren's syndrome Choroidoretinitis Glaucoma, cataract
Neurologist	**Gastroenterologist**	**Cardiologist**
Cranial nerve palsy Myopathy, neuropathy Space-occupying lesions Meningitis	Hepatic granulomas Splenomegaly Similarity to Crohn's disease	Cardiac arrhythmias Bundle branch block Cardiomyopathy Complete heart block
General Physician	**Rheumatologist**	**Urologist**
Acute rheumatism Lymphadenopathy Parotid enlargement Peripheral lymphadenopathy	Polyarthralgia Bone cysts Dactylitis	Hypercalciuria Renal calculi Nephrocalcinosis Uremia

Physical Examination. General examination of the patient must be thorough (Fig. 2). It is incomplete unless accompanied by a chest radiograph, slit-lamp examination of the eyes, and estimation of the 24-hour urinary calcium. Multisystem involvement is a characteristic feature of sarcoidosis, with intrathoracic involvement in nine tenths of patients, ocular and skin involvement each occurring in about one quarter, and, depending on the series and country, erythema nodosum in up to one third of patients. Involvement of other tissues includes peripheral lymphadenopathy in 29 per cent, the spleen in 12 per cent, neurosarcoidosis in 7 per cent, and salivary gland enlargement or bone cysts in about 6 per cent of patients (Table 3).

Intrathoracic Sarcoidosis. It is convenient to refer to three abnormal chest x-ray appearances:

STAGE 1. Bilateral hilar lymphadenopathy is the earliest and most frequent change, comprising about one half of chest radiographic abnormalities. The right paratracheal chain of lymph nodes is frequently enlarged in this early stage of sarcoidosis and is radiographically visible in at least 25 per cent; hence the popularity of right scalene node biopsy and mediastinoscopy at this stage. Hilar adenopathy is the hallmark of acute early reversible sarcoidosis, and it may be associated with erythema nodosum and acute iritis.

STAGE 2. In one quarter of patients, the chest radiograph shows both bilateral hilar lymphadenopathy and parenchymal mottling of the lungs. The mottling takes the form of localized or disseminated fine miliary or occasionally coarse miliary nodulation, or a fluffy cotton-wool appearance, sometimes with margins sharply circumscribed. Miliary infiltration is a subacute transient stage, usually resolving and certainly changing during one year of observation.

STAGE 3. In one of seven patients, the chest radiograph discloses that the disease has already reached a late stage of diffuse pulmonary mottling on presentation, persisting as coarse or fine reticulation intermixed with nodular densities 1 to 5 mm in diameter. In some in-

TABLE 2. Features of Sarcoidosis Patients in New York, London, and Paris

Features		Mount Sinai Hospital, New York		Royal Northern Hospital, London		Hôpital Bichat, Paris	
		No.	%	No.	%	No.	%
Total		311	100	537	100	329	100
Sex	Women	211	68	302	56	146	45
Race	White	111	36	474	86	277	84
	Negro	146	47	2	<1	3	1
	Caribbean	54	17	33	6	39	12
	Other	–	–	28	5	10	3
Age at presentation (years)	Under 40	221	71	358	67	238	72
	Over 40	90	29	179	33	91	28
Onset	Routine chest x-ray	124	40	119	22	156	47.5
	Respiratory symptoms	59	19	49	9	53	16
	Erythema nodosum	33	11	150	28	22	7
	Other skin lesions	20	6	37	7	14	4
	Ocular symptoms	22	7	53	10	29	8.5
Presenting chest x-ray stage	0	26	8	85	16	20	6
	1	133	43	243	45	123	37.5
	2	108	35	129	24	162	49
	3	44	14	80	15	24	7.5
Skin tests	Positive Kveim-Siltzbach	285	92	384	82	187/243	77
	Negative tuberculin	191	63	246	55	266/329	81
Blood tests	Hyperglobulinemia	158	61	85	34	48/212	22.5
	Hypercalcemia	33	14	57	24	17/249	7
Treatment	Corticosteroids	103	33	185	34	224	68.5
	No steroids	208	67	352	66	89	27
Mortality	Due to sarcoidosis	17	5	25	5	6	1.8
	Due to other causes	9	3	8	1.5	7	2

stances confluence of the mottled areas is noted, pulmonary fibrosis is irreversible, and upward retraction of the lung roots has developed. Bulla formation, gradual enlargement of the right ventricle, and pulmonary hypertension are serious prognostic signs.

Extrathoracic Sarcoidosis. *Ocular lesions* occur in about one quarter of patients. They include acute and chronic iridocyclitis and choroidoretinitis, papilledema, keratoconjunctivitis, conjunctival follicles, and the late complications of cataract and secondary glaucoma. There are certain well-defined ocular syndromes. Acute iritis, erythema nodosum, and bilateral hilar lymphadenopathy have a benign self-limiting course, whereas chronic iridocyclitis with associated lupus pernio or skin plaques, bone cysts, and pulmonary fibrosis are persistent and troublesome. Keratoconjunctivitis sicca with or without parotid and lacrimal gland enlargement mimics Sjögren's syndrome. Parotid gland enlargement, anterior uveitis, and facial nerve palsy are features of Heerfordt's syndrome.

Skin lesions, other than erythema nodosum, are noted in one quarter of patients. They include lupus pernio, plaques, scars, keloids, and transient maculopapular eruptions.

Erythema nodosum is associated with bilateral hilar lymphadenopathy and polyarthralgia. It occurs predomi-

TABLE 3. Frequency of Involvement of Various Tissues in Sarcoidosis in New York, London, and Paris

Organs Involved	Mount Sinai Hospital, New York (311)		Royal Northern Hospital, London (537)		Hôpital Bichat, Paris (329)	
	No.	%	No.	%	No.	%
Intrathoracic	285	92	452	84	300	90
Hilar nodes	241	77	372	70	227	70
Lung parenchyma	152	49	209	40	186	56.5
Peripheral lymph nodes	116	37	153	29	75	23
Eyes	62	20	147	27	37	11
Skin	59	19	135	25	39	12
Erythema nodosum	33	11	167	31	22	6.5
Spleen	57	18	62	12	20	6
Bone cysts	13/139	9	19/475	4	6/165	3.5
Salivary glands	25	8	33	6	21	6
Nervous system	13	4	38	7	14	4

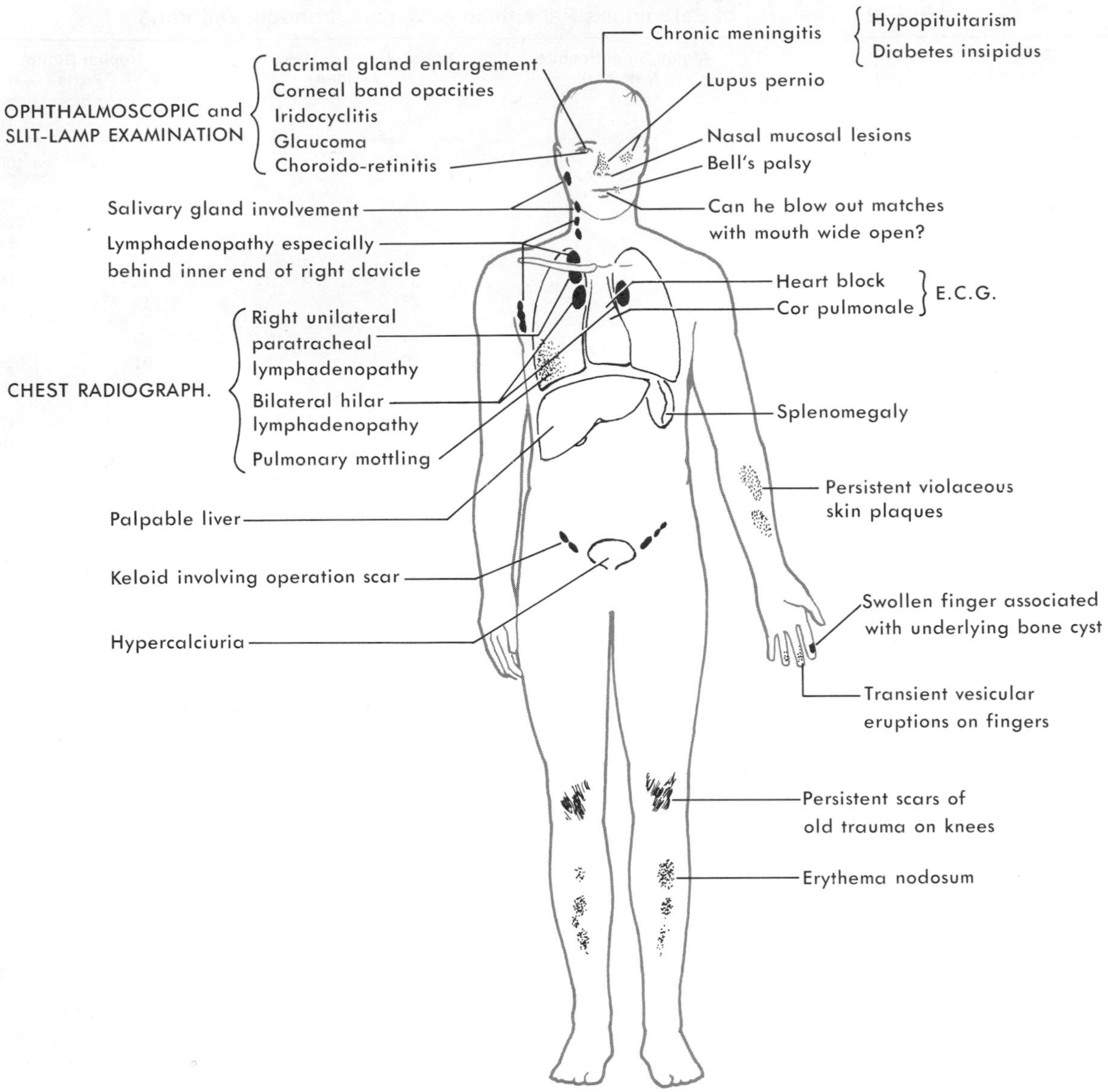

Figure 2. Clinical examination of a patient with suspected sarcoidosis.

nantly in women of childbearing age, often associated with pregnancy or lactation; such patients should be reassured that it is a benign syndrome which will not affect the fetus or leave complications.

Reticuloendothelial system involvement occurs in 215 of 537 patients (40 per cent), comprising peripheral lymphadenopathy in 153 (28 per cent) and splenomegaly in 62 (12 per cent). Splenic enlargement is usually silent, but rarely it may cause hypersplenism or lead to presinusoidal portal hypertension.

Neurosarcoidosis is far less common, occurring in 38 of 537 patients (7 per cent). Facial palsy is a frequent neurologic presentation either alone or with other cranial palsies or with papilledema. Other presentations include peripheral neuritis, myopathy, meningitis, and space-occupying brain lesions.

Bone cysts occur in about 6 per cent of patients; they are most commonly seen in conjunction with chronic skin lesions, so the dermatologist is far more likely than the chest physician to detect them. Bone cysts reflect chronic persistent irreversible sarcoidosis in all systems.

Myocardial sarcoidosis is difficult to recognize clinically. It should be considered if a patient with florid multisystem sarcoidosis develops heart block, bundle branch block, arrhythmias, congestive heart failure, or clinical evidence of cardiomyopathy. Sudden death without previous evidence of a heart lesion may occur in sarcoidosis.

Endocrine involvement in sarcoidosis. The pituitary is more frequently involved than any other endocrine gland, the diagnosis being suggested by the development of polydipsia and polyuria in sarcoidosis without evidence of renal disease. Since 1909, about 60 cases of diabetes insipidus caused by sarcoidosis have been reported. Histologic proof is necessary to distinguish this syndrome from histiocytosis X, in which diffuse infiltration of the lungs coincides with diabetes insipidus. Apart from diabetes insipidus, deficiency of one or more anterior pituitary hormones may occur, comprising gonadotropin, thyroid-stimulating hormone, and adrenocorticotropic hormone in that order of frequency. Hypothalmic involvement may be associated with galactorrhea and raised serum prolactin levels. Adrenal, thyroid, or pancreatic involvement by sarcoidosis is extremely rare.

Special Clinical Situations. Pregnancy. Sarcoidosis is not a contraindication to pregnancy. In fact, patients improve and are able to abandon steroid therapy from the second trimester onward. Chest radiography is unnecessary until after delivery; thereafter it should be performed, because relapse, if it does occur, is more likely during the six months after parturition. The only precaution is to check the serum calcium level, as it is liable to rise with excessive vitamin D intake during pregnancy.

CHILDHOOD. Sarcoidosis is rarely a pediatric problem. In the Royal Northern Hospital series, it was observed in one child under ten years of age and occurred in only 25 of 537 patients (5 per cent) under 20 years of age. When multisystemic granulomas are observed in young children, sarcoidosis should not be considered until the several other causes of granulomatous disorders are excluded, particularly helminth infestation, mycobacterial infection, and chronic granulomatous disease of childhood.

Unusual Features. Fever is not a feature of sarcoidosis, except under certain circumstances. It is commonly associated with erythema nodosum, uveoparotitis (Heerfordt's syndrome), acute meningitis, hypersplenism, and secondary infection complicating end-stage pulmonary fibrosis and nephrocalcinosis. If there is persistent fever in the absence of these features, it is important to consider such alternatives as Hodgkin's disease or Wegener's granulomatosis.

Ulceration, even when a biopsy of the ulcer reveals sarcoid tissue, is not a feature of sarcoidosis, and it is sufficient to raise alternative diagnostic possibilities. A granulomatous nasal or laryngeal ulcer raises the possibility of Wegener's granulomatosis; a leg ulcer in a child might be due to swimming-pool granuloma and an ulcer in the neck due to cat scratch disease.

It should be remembered that all that glitters is not sarcoidosis.

Diagnosis. *Kveim-Siltzbach Test.* Kveim-Siltzbach antigen is a saline suspension of human sarcoid tissue prepared from the spleen of a patient suffering from active sarcoidosis. The antigen, 0.15 ml, is injected intradermally very superficially into the flexor surface of the forearm, and the inoculation site is observed for the development of a visible and palpable nodule during the ensuing six weeks. Any palpable nodule is examined by biopsy, usually one month after the injection, using a Hayes-Martin drill. This core of tissue is serially sectioned for evidence of sarcoid tissue or of a foreign body giant-cell reaction; this decision is made blind, i.e., without knowledge of the clinical picture. A Kveim-Siltzbach test is reported as positive if the intradermally injected antigen produces a nodule in the course of three to six weeks and if this nodule shows evidence of sarcoid tissue, as distinct from a foreign body giant-cell reaction. A parallel may be drawn between it and the beryllium patch test in beryllium disease, the zirconium skin reaction in patients with zirconium deodorant granulomas, and the lepromin reaction in leprosy. All tests are individually specific for their own disease states. That these are delayed hypersensitivity phenomena is suggested by the fact that they occur only in patients who have been in contact with, say, beryllium or zirconium; they are not positive before contact; a positive result can be obtained, using extremely high dilutions of the element; and the reaction is specific.

Several factors influence the Kveim-Siltzbach reaction, which must still be regarded as a crude but most useful biologic test. Potent antigen is essential, and this means that it must be obtained from the spleen of a patient with active sarcoidosis. Another important factor is the histologist's interpretation of the biopsy material, for an inexperienced observer could confuse sarcoid tissue with a nonspecific foreign body giant-cell reaction, particularly if doubly refractile crystals are not sought by polarized light. Finally, the Kveim-Siltzbach test is suppressed by oral corticosteroids, just as any sarcoid tissue is suppressed by these agents. An occasional false-positive result is inevitable with a biologic test of this kind, but a figure of less than 2 per cent is acceptable. The Kveim-Siltzbach test is positive in three quarters of patients with sarcoidosis. It is particularly helpful when histologic confirmation is otherwise lacking or equivocal. It is useful in the differential diagnosis of diffuse pulmonary mottling, uveitis, or erythema nodosum; and it is also worth performing in obscure cases of subacute meningitis or cranial nerve palsies. It is negative in patients with nonspecific local sarcoid-tissue reactions and in all other granulomatous disorders.

It is unfortunate that there is no standardized commercial supply of Kveim-Siltzbach antigen. Various institutes prepare their own antigens from sarcoid spleen or lymph nodes, and it is then necessary to carry out skin tests with these antigens in sarcoidosis and other subjects to assess their specificity. Poor nonspecific antigens are discarded, but a potent specific supply will last for years. Undoubtedly the world's best antigens have been, and continue to be, prepared by Dr. Louis Siltzbach at the Mount Sinai Hospital, New York City. We have a satisfactory one at the Royal Northern Hospital, London, as does Professor J. Turiaf at the Hôpital Bichat, Paris. Dr. Andrew Douglas has recently prepared a promising new specific antigen in Edinburgh, and Dr. Behrend's antigen in Hanover, Germany, is effective and specific. Instead of endeavoring to meet the world's needs, what we are all trying to do is discover the specific granuloma-provoking principle and therefrom produce a standardized synthetic and accurately reproducible agent.

KMIF Test. Efforts are being made to develop in vitro Kveim-Siltzbach tests by investigating the response of peripheral lymphocytes from patients with sarcoidosis and controls to stimulation by Kveim-Siltzbach antigen, using guinea pig macrophages as the indicator cells. The technique is termed the Kveim-induced macrophage inhibition factor (KMIF) test. Sarcoid lymphocytes when stimulated in vitro with sarcoid material produce a macrophage inhibition factor with a migration index of less than 0.8 in three quarters of subjects (positive KMIF test). There is a good correlation with the cutaneous Kveim-Siltzbach test. Also resembling the skin test is the effect of steroid therapy which makes the KMIF test negative.

Tuberculin Reaction. The tuberculin reaction is negative in all conventional strengths in about 60 per cent of patients with sarcoidosis. Those exhibiting some degree of tuberculin hypersensitivity have only weakly positive reactions. Insensitivity to tuberculin and to other antigens such as dinitrochlorobenzene is only relative, and the insensitivity does not appear to be as profound as it is in malignant lymphomatous diseases.

Biochemical Findings. ABNORMAL CALCIUM METABOLISM. Hypercalcemia and hypercalciuria may be short-lived and self-limiting, or they may progress to nephrocalcinosis with excretion of renal calculi and eventual uremia. Hypercalcemia occurred in 10 (13 per cent) and hypercalciuria in 37 (49 per cent) in our series of 75 patients with sarcoidosis in whom simultaneous serum and 24-hour urine calcium levels were determined. Thus hypercalciuria is much more common than hypercalcemia and is the more sensitive index of abnormal calcium metabolism. Fortunately it is usually transient and self-limiting.

HYDROXYPROLINURIA. Hydroxyproline excretion is considerably increased in acute sarcoidosis, returning to normal as the chest x-ray abnormality resolves, whereas excretion is normal in chronic sarcoidosis.

ALKALINE PHOSPHATASE. Elevation of the alkaline phosphatase level is due to hepatic involvement by space-occupying miliary granulomas and not because of bone cysts.

Lung Function Studies. The two most useful practical tests are the single-breath diffusing capacity and the vital capacity. Impairment of the diffusing capacity can be observed even at the early stage of bilateral hilar lymphadenopathy when the lung fields are radiographically clear. The deficit may become more marked because of the natural fall in diffusing capacity with increasing age, and also because of reduction in lung volume and impaired perfusion of ventilated lung. Reduction of vital capacity is also observed with advancing disease.

Immunoglobulins. Serum IgG is elevated in one half, IgA in one quarter, and IgM in one eighth of patients. There is a relative deficiency of IgD associated with the rise in IgM. There is no clear-cut association between clinical patterns of disease and the abnormal immunoglobulin, and certainly none of diagnostic value.

Other Factors. Serum complement activity is increased, haptoglobin is decreased, and cryoglobulins have been identified in serum in erythema nodosum. Serum autoantibodies, including thyroid, gastric, mitochrondrial, and antinuclear factor, are similar in incidence to those found in the normal population.

Monocytes from sarcoidosis patients show an increase in rosette erythrophagocytosis, compared with controls for both IgG and C3 complement receptors, indicating an increase in monocyte phagocytic capacity and membrane receptor function. These observations should help to explain circulating immune complexes in this disease.

Anemia and Eosinophilia. These are not characteristic features of sarcoidosis. When a patient is found to have biopsy evidence of a granuloma and this is associated with anemia and/or eosinophilia, it is necessary to consider disorders other than sarcoidosis in the first instance. If noted in a child, helminthic infestations, such as Toxocara infection, should be considered. If these are the findings in a young male adult, granulomatous Hodgkin's disease should be ruled out before considering sarcoidosis.

Sedimentation Rate. This test is of limited value in the management of sarcoidosis. It is grossly elevated when there is associated erythema nodosum, and its elevation may also reflect raised, abnormal serum immunoglobulin levels. Finally, it is raised when there is secondary infection associated with end-stage pulmonary fibrosis or with nephrocalcinosis.

TABLE 4. Differences Between the Multisystemic Disorder Sarcoidosis and a Nonspecific Local Sarcoid Tissue Reaction

	Sarcoidosis	Sarcoid Reaction
Number of systems involved	Several	Usually one
Age group	20–50 years	Any
Chest radiograph	Abnormal in 84%	Normal
Slit-lamp examination of eyes	Abnormal in 25%	Normal
Tuberculin test	Negative in 66%	Variable
Kveim-Siltzbach test	Positive in 84%	Negative
Calcium metabolism	Abnormal in 20%	Normal
Response to corticosteroids	Good	Variable
Other treatments	Oxyphenbutazone, chloroquine, *p*-aminobenzoate	Depends on cause—anti-infective, immunosuppressive

Comment. The diagnosis is most securely established when consistent clinical and radiographic findings are supported by histologic evidence of noncaseating epithelioid cell granulomas by organ biopsy in more than one system and/or a positive Kveim-Siltzbach test.

When confronted with a patient suspected of having sarcoidosis, certain steps in the management are essential. (1) Seek histologic confirmation of the clinical diagnosis as soon as possible. The patients who are troubled in later years by their disease are almost always those in whom the clinical diagnosis was not supported by histologic confirmation initially, and so treatment was delayed until it was too late to be effective. (2) Make sure that granulomas found in one system are part of the multisystemic disorder and not just a nonspecific local sarcoid tissue reaction. There are several points of differentiation (Table 4)—clinical, radiologic, and immunologic—but the simplest and most secure way of distinguishing them is by the Kveim-Siltzbach test, which is positive in sarcoidosis and negative in local sarcoid tissue reactions. (3) Judge whether the disease is acute or chronic (see Course and Prognosis).

Differential Diagnosis. It should be remembered that there are many causes of nonspecific local sarcoid tissue reactions and other unrelated granulomatous disorders. The disorders with which sarcoidosis is confused depend to some extent on the discipline and interests of the clinician concerned. The chest physician must distinguish it from tuberculosis and extrinsic allergic alveolitis; the gastroenterologist must differentiate it from Crohn's regional ileitis or primary biliary cirrhosis; and the general physician may have to distinguish it from Hodgkin's disease. The modes of presentation of sarcoidosis involve most disciplines (Table 1); it cannot be overemphasized that sarcoidosis is a multisystemic disorder, and the diagnosis should be entertained when the patient is seen to attend many different outpatient clinics, particularly respiratory, ophthalmic, and dermatologic.

Tuberculosis. It is more important to recognize tuberculosis than to overlook sarcoidosis. Now that tuberculosis is becoming less common and sarcoidosis more frequently recognized, there remains considerable confusion, particularly between tuberculin-positive sarcoidosis and tuberculin-negative tuberculosis. There are several distinguishing features (Table 5), and the

Kveim-Siltzbach test may be of crucial help. With steroid therapy the negative tuberculin skin test in sarcoidosis may become positive and the strongly positive tuberculin test in tuberculosis may wane.

Hodgkin's Disease. Disseminated Hodgkin's disease is similar to sarcoidosis from clinical, radiographic, and immunologic standpoints (Table 6), but histology is distinctive. Hodgkin's disease has a male preponderance, and the patient is usually ill with weight loss, fever, pruritus, and anemia, whereas sarcoidosis has an equal sex distribution and the patient is usually asymptomatic and well.

Intrathoracic Hodgkin's disease most frequently involves the upper mediastinum; the subcarinal and posterior mediastinal nodes are seldom involved without enlargement of the upper mediastinal nodes. The hilar nodes tend to fuse with the right cardiac border, whereas in sarcoidosis the right hilar nodes stand away from the right border of the heart.

Primary Biliary Cirrhosis (PBC). Sarcoidosis and PBC are both chronic granulomatous disorders, which may provide superficial confusion to the gastroenterologist who has found hepatic granulomas by aspiration liver biopsy or sarcoid tissue in abdominal lymph nodes at laparotomy. However, the clinical presentations and physical signs are quite different (Table 7). The two most helpful distinguishing tests are the Kveim-Siltzbach test, which is always negative in PBC, and the serum antimitochondrial antibody test, which is negative in sarcoidosis.

Crohn's Regional Ileitis. This is a chronic granulomatous disorder of the intestinal tract. In contradistinction to sarcoidosis, it is almost never multisystemic. Distinguishing features are the over-all clinical picture, radiographic changes, calcium metabolism, serum antireticulin antibodies, and Kveim-Siltzbach test (Table 8).

Extrinsic Allergic Alveolitis. There are several different inhaled antigens which provoke an antigen-antibody reaction and a granulomatous histology in the lower reaches of the bronchi. The prototype is farmer's lung; others include suberosis, bird fancier's, thatcher's, maplebark stripper's, and sequoia tree feller's asthma. The keys to the diagnosis are the occupational history, the clinical picture of asthma, the histology of a granuloma encompassing the inhaled foreign body, the presence of serum precipitins against the provoking inhaled antigen, and the negative Kveim-Siltzbach test (Table 9).

Course and Prognosis. There are two forms of sarcoi-

TABLE 5. Differences Between Sarcoidosis and Tuberculosis

Features	Sarcoidosis	Tuberculosis
Age incidence (years)	20–50	<20 or>50
Fever	Rare	Common
Erythema nodosum	Common	Uncommon
Uveitis Skin involvement Enlarged parotids Bone cysts	Common	Very rare
Ulceration and sinuses	No	Common
Involvement of:		
Pleura Peritoneum Pericardium Meninges Small intestine	Very rare	Common
Caseation	Minimal	Maximal
Acid-fast bacilli	Absent	Present
Tuberculin test	Negative in 55%	Positive in most
Kveim-Siltzbach test	Positive in most	Negative
Hypercalcemia	Yes	No
Hypercalciuria	Yes	No
Calcification	No	Yes
Hilar lymphadenopathy	Bilateral	Unilateral
Pulmonary cavities	Rare, late	Common, early
Ghon focus	No	Yes
Corticosteroids	Helpful	Harmful alone
Antituberculous drugs	Unhelpful	Treatment of choice

TABLE 6. Comparison Between Sarcoidosis and Hodgkin's Disease

Features	Sarcoidosis	Hodgkin's Disease
Age (years)	20 to 50	20 to 40
Sex	Equal	Males, 3:1
Weight loss	Rare	Common
Splenomegaly	Rare	Frequent
Submental lymph nodes	Infrequent	Frequent
Erythema nodosum	No	Rare
Gut symptoms	Absent	Common
Pruritus	Absent	Common
Bone lesions	"Punched out" phalangeal cysts	Sclerotic lesions of spine and pelvis
Sclerotic lesions	No	Mixed sclerotic/osteolytic in 16%
Leukocytosis Lymphopenia Eosinophilia	Absent	May be present
Hilar lymphadenopathy	Bilateral	Bilateral or unilateral
Hilar gland pressure symptoms	No	Yes
Pulmonary infiltration	Common	Uncommon
Pulmonary infiltration followed by hilar adenopathy	Never	Yes
Pleural effusion	Rare	Common
Skin lesions	Distinctive histology	Specific histology with eosinophilia
Secondary infections	Rare	Common
Delayed-type hypersensitivity	Depressed	Depressed
Immunoglobulins	Abnormal	Normal
Kveim-Siltzbach test	Positive	Negative
Histology	Distinctive	Distinctive
Radiotherapy	Unhelpful	Curative
Corticosteroids	Therapy of choice	Helpful
Immunosuppressive regimens	Not indicated	Indicated
Prognosis	Good	Poor

TABLE 7. Features Distinguishing Sarcoidosis from Primary Biliary Cirrhosis

Features	Sarcoidosis	Primary Biliary Cirrhosis
Sex	Equal	Females, 8:1
Decade of onset	3, 4	5
Onset over 40 years	Rare	Frequent
Erythema nodosum	Yes	No
Uveitis	Yes	No
Respiratory	Yes	No
Pruritus	No	Yes, nearly always
Jaundice	No	Yes
Xanthomas	No	Yes
Clubbing	No	Yes (in 25%)
Hepatomegaly	No	Yes (in 100%)
Splenomegaly	Yes (in 12%)	Yes (in 50%)
Skin pigmentation	No	Yes (in 71%)
Steatorrhea	No	Yes
Bilateral hilar lymphadenopathy	Yes	No
Kveim-Siltzbach test	Positive in 75%	Always negative
Depression of delayed-type hypersensitivity	Yes	Yes
Circulating anti-mitochondrial antibodies	No	Yes (in 99%)
Calcium metabolism	Hypercalcemia Vitamin D sensitivity	Hypocalcemia (Steatorrhea)
Raised alkaline phosphatase	Yes, minority	Yes, majority
Raised serum cholesterol	No	Yes, majority
Liver granulomas	Yes	Yes
Corticosteroids	Helpful	Contraindicated
Vitamin D	Contraindicated	Helpful
Cholestyramine	Not necessary	Helpful
Prognosis	Very good	Poor; dead in five years

dosis, acute and chronic, with clear-cut differences in onset, natural history, course, prognosis, and response to treatment (Table 10).

Acute sarcoidosis has an abrupt explosive onset, a high spontaneous remission rate, a predictable response to anti-inflammatory drugs, and a good prognosis. From the onset to complete resolution usually occupies less than two years.

Chronic sarcoidosis has an insidious, ill-recognized onset and progresses inexorably; treatment relieves symptoms but rarely leads to resolution of the fibrotic process, and pulmonary fibrosis, cor pulmonale, secondary cataract formation, and nephrocalcinosis are liable to supervene.

It is important to distinguish acute (transient) from chronic (persistent) sarcoidosis, because their natural history and prognosis vary as greatly as in acute and chronic nephritis or acute and chronic hepatitis.

Undoubtedly the most predictable course and the best prognosis accompany erythema nodosum. It usually subsides within a month of its onset, and accompanying hilar adenopathy will regress in the course of one year. Recurrence and sequelae are rare.

TABLE 8. Differences Between Sarcoidosis and Crohn's Regional Ileitis

Features	Sarcoidosis	Crohn's Regional Ileitis
Histology	Granulomas	Similar
Involvement		
Intestine	Rare	Invariable
Intrathoracic	Yes in 90%	No
Skin	Yes in 25%	Mucocutaneous ulceration extending to involve genitalia
Erythema nodosum	Yes	Yes
Eyes	Yes in 25%	No
Associated ankylosing spondylitis	No	Yes
Complicating		
Malabsorption	No	Yes
Amyloidosis	No	Yes
Peritonitis	No	Yes
Hepatic granulomas	Yes	Yes
Depression of delayed-type hypersensitivity	Yes	Yes
Kveim-Siltzbach test	Positive in 75%	Negative
Abnormal calcium metabolism	Hypercalcemia and hypercalciuria	Hypocalcemia associated with malabsorption
Serum antireticulin antibodies	Negative	Positive in 25%

It is not possible, unfortunately, to define such a clear-cut natural history in other forms of sarcoidosis, except to predict that maculopapular eruptions, conjunctivitis, salivary gland enlargement, Bell's palsy, and peripheral lymphadenopathy usually regress without treatment in the course of one year. On the other hand, chronic iridocyclitis, keratoconjunctivitis sicca, lupus pernio, plaques, and keloids persist unchanged or with minor fluctuations indefinitely.

TABLE 9. Comparison of 95 Patients with Extrinsic Allergic Alveolitis and 68 Patients with Sarcoidosis by Villar (Lisbon)

Features	Extrinsic Allergic Alveolitis	Sarcoidosis
Age	Older	Younger
Erythema nodosum	Absent	Common
Hilar adenopathy	Rare	Frequent
Multisystem	No	Yes
Depression of delayed-type hypersensitivity	Yes	Yes
Kveim-Siltzbach test	Negative	Positive
Serum precipitins	Yes	No
Histology	Granuloma encompassing foreign body	Granuloma
Prognosis	Good if removed from exposure to antigen	Good

TABLE 10. Differences Between Subacute (Transient) and Chronic (Persistent) Sarcoidosis

	Subacute	Chronic
Natural history	Transient	Persistent
Age at onset	Under 30 years	Over 30 years
Onset	Abrupt	Insidious
Skin	Erythema nodosum, maculopapular rash, vesicular eruptions	Lupus pernio, plaques, scars, keloids
Eyes	Conjunctivitis, acute iritis, papilledema, hemorrhages, exudates	Keratoconjunctivitis sicca, chronic uveitis, cataract, glaucoma
Lungs	Hilar adenopathy	Pulmonary mottling
Bone cysts Parotitis Lymphadenopathy Splenomegaly Bell's palsy	Usually transient	Rarely permanent
Histology	Epithelioid and giant cells	Hyaline fibrosis
Calcium metabolism	Hypercalcemia, hypercalciuria	Nephrocalcinosis
Kveim-Siltzbach test	Positive	May be negative
Hydroxyproline excretion	Increased	Normal
Spontaneous remission	Frequent	Rare
Steroid therapy	Abortive effect	Symptomatic relief
Alternative treatments	Oxyphenbutazone	Chloroquine, para-aminobenzoate, phosphate
Recurrence after steroid therapy	Rare	Frequent
Low calcium diet	Unnecessary	May be necessary
Prognosis	Good	Poor

Skin and pulmonary lesions follow a very similar course and likewise parallel each other's response to treatment. Transient skin lesions are usually associated with hilar adenopathy, whereas chronic skin lesions are more likely to be accompanied by pulmonary fibrosis. The former tend to clear without treatment, and the latter fail to do so despite prolonged therapy. Resolution of all types of pulmonary sarcoidosis may be expected in two thirds of patients. It is less likely to be achieved in older patients and in those in whom there is accompanying extrathoracic disease—particularly in bone or skin. The combination of pulmonary and cutaneous sarcoidosis constitutes the hallmark of chronicity, presumably because longstanding fibrosis has supervened. Clearing of the abnormal chest x-ray occurs in only one third of patients with bone cysts, in only one fifth with skin lesions, and in only one sixth in whom bone and skin lesions accompany pulmonary sarcoidosis. The other significant factor influencing the course is treatment by corticosteroids, chloroquine, or oxyphenbutazone (see Treatment).

Complications. Sarcoidosis would remain a relatively benign and unimportant disease but for the development of certain devastating complications, namely, irreversible fibrosis in the lungs and eyes and abnormal calcium metabolism affecting the kidneys. In assessing the prognosis, it is important to assess the degree of functional failure of lungs, heart, eyes, and kidneys. In the practical management of sarcoidosis, it is the physician's duty to diagnose the condition sufficiently early so that effective therapy may prevent these unfortunate sequelae.

The over-all mortality is 8 per cent, comprising a mortality of 5 per cent directly caused by sarcoidosis and the remaining few deaths resulting from unrelated causes. Comparative figures indicate that the patient seems to have the same chance of survival whether he lives in London, New York, or Paris (Table 2).

Two forms of sarcoidosis—acute and chronic, with clear-cut differences in onset, course, and prognosis—have been defined, because this concept is important in the practical management and treatment of the individual patient with sarcoidosis. What we do not know is whether the two forms represent different diseases. The balance of evidence favors two forms of the same disease in which the differences reflect varying interplay between the causative seed and the receptive soil. Acute sarcoidosis is probably triggered by active circulating immune complexes with the development of acute vasculitis and iritis, whereas chronic sarcoidosis is maintained at a slower pace by a fibrotic hyaline reaction on the part of the tissues involved.

Acute and chronic forms of the same disease are well exemplified by beryllium disease, nephritis, and hepatitis.

Treatment. Corticosteroids, the sheet anchor of therapy, are indicated in about one third of patients (Table 2).

Various Preparations of Corticosteroids. The profound influence of corticosteroids on clinical, radiologic, immunologic, and biochemical abnormalities is well established. The range of available preparations for oral administration or topical application is wide; a combination of oral and topical steroid therapy is often the most effective. For instance, iridocyclitis may be brought under control by prednisolone eye drops, particularly if reinforced by one subconjunctival depot injection of hydrocortisone. Likewise, triamcinolone acetonide may be injected directly into the disfiguring skin plaques with great benefit, alone or in conjunction with oral corticosteroids or chloroquine. Oral corticosteroids may contribute several unpleasant side effects, not the least being fluid retention and cushingoid facies. These undesirable sequelae may be overcome by using prednisolone-21-stearoylglycolate (Sintisone) which does not seem to be fluid retaining. When treatment is changed from other steroids to Sintisone, patients appear to lose fluid, the weight drops a little, and mooning of the face lessens. Preliminary evidence would also suggest that it is less likely to cause a rise in intraocular pressure, and thereby less likely to contribute to secondary glaucoma. The potency of one 6.65-mg tablet is approximately equivalent to that of one 5-mg tablet of prednisolone or prednisone. It is particularly indicated for patients who are fluid retainers and for those who have or are likely to develop glaucoma or patients with a family history of glaucoma. Oral steroid therapy in a dose of 30 mg daily for about six months is necessary in one third of patients with sarcoidosis. Indications for treatment are now well established.

Indications for Corticosteroid Therapy. OCULAR INVOLVEMENT. Topical corticosteroids should always be administered for iridocyclitis, in eye drops applied frequently during the day, reinforced with a corticosteroid eye ointment at night. If there is no substantial and continuing improvement during ten days, then the concentration of corticosteroid in the anterior segment of the eye may be increased by a local subconjunctival depot of cortisone. Oral corticosteroids are indicated if local treatment does not lead to a rapid response or if ophthalmoscopy reveals posterior uveitis. In addition, the inflamed iris should be rested by local atropine eye drops to maintain a dilated pupil.

ABNORMAL CHEST RADIOGRAPH WITHOUT SPONTANEOUS IMPROVEMENT IN SIX MONTHS. Bilateral hilar lymphadenopathy is likely to subside without treatment, particularly if it is associated with erythema nodosum. On the contrary, pulmonary infiltration which remains static or worsens during the course of six months is an indication for oral steroids in an effort to prevent irreversible pulmonary fibrosis.

BREATHLESSNESS. If this symptom is present, the disease has already reached a stage of irreversible pulmonary fibrosis or disturbed gas transfer. Steroid treatment provides symptomatic relief but does not influence the grave prognosis at the irreversible stage of breathlessness.

PERSISTENT HYPERCALCIURIA. Steroids will prevent excessive gastrointestinal absorption and excessive urinary excretion of calcium. Calcium metabolism usually reverts to normal within ten days.

DISFIGURING SKIN LESIONS. When lupus pernio or other unsightly lesions distress patients, oral and local corticosteroids may correct the deformity. Unfortunately, small doses of steroids must be continued indefinitely if the cosmetic improvement is to be maintained. In order to minimize the side effects of oral corticosteroids, local intralesional steroids or chloroquine, or both, are helpful alternatives.

NEUROLOGIC INVOLVEMENT. The more acute the presentation, the more likely it is to respond to systemic corticosteroids, which should be administered as soon as the diagnosis has been established. Most patients are aged 20 to 50 years. There is evidence of intrathoracic involvement in 82 per cent, ocular disease in 58 per cent, cutaneous sarcoidosis in 29 per cent, peripheral lymphadenopathy in 26 per cent, parotid enlargement in 16 per cent, and splenomegaly in 10 per cent. This multisystem involvement is a key to the diagnosis of neurosarcoidosis; it is supported by evidence of a positive Kveim-Siltzbach test in 76 per cent and a negative Mantoux status in 60 per cent of patients.

Neurosarcoidosis carries a mortality of 10 per cent, which is twice the over-all mortality of sarcoidosis. Resolution of neurosarcoidosis is more likely to occur in younger patients with an explosive onset such as meningitis. The response to treatment is better (1) with accompanying erythema nodosum than with chronic skin lesions, (2) with acute than with chronic uveitis, and (3) with hilar adenopathy than with old diffuse pulmonary infiltration.

GLANDULAR INVOLVEMENT. Glandular involvement occurs particularly if there is disordered function, e.g., dry eyes caused by lacrimal gland involvement, dry mouth caused by salivary gland enlargement, or hypersplenism resulting from sarcoidosis of the spleen. The indication for treatment is disordered function rather than anatomic enlargement of the gland in question.

MYOCARDIAL INVOLVEMENT. It is easy to include involvement of the heart in a theoretical list of indications for corticosteroid therapy, but much more difficult in practice to recognize myocardial sarcoidosis. It is, of course, suspected and treated when a patient with multisystemic sarcoidosis develops cardiac arrhythmia or bundle branch block.

Other Drugs. Treatment may be necessary when there are contraindications to corticosteroid therapy or when it has proved fruitless. Under these circumstances it is proper to consider treatment with oxyphenbutazone, chloroquine, potassium para-aminobenzoate, or immunosuppressive agents such as azathioprine.

OXYPHENBUTAZONE. In a controlled trial comparing oxyphenbutazone, prednisolone, and a placebo in the management of pulmonary sarcoidosis, both active drugs were significantly better than the placebo. Prednisolone and oxyphenbutazone were equally effective. Although one in six patients showed spontaneous regression of pulmonary sarcoidosis in six months, this trial showed that the number is increased to one in two patients by oxyphenbutazone or prednisolone. Not only does oxyphenbutazone influence the radiologic picture; like corticosteroids, it can also prevent the development of sarcoid tissue, for it may delay the evolution of sarcoid tissue in the Kveim-Siltzbach nodule. Oxyphenbutazone is of value only in acute exudative sarcoidosis and not in the chronic fibrotic form of the disease.

CHLOROQUINE. The way in which chloroquine acts is unknown, but it is helpful in the management of lupus pernio and pulmonary fibrosis. It is of no value in acute sarcoidosis.

POTABA. Potassium para-aminobenzoate is known to have an antifibrotic effect, and it is worth considering in pulmonary fibrosis and lupus pernio caused by sarcoidosis. Three-gram envules should be taken by mouth four times daily for several months. This form of treatment is an effective alternative to corticosteroids and chloroquine, and giving all three in rotation helps to overcome the undesirable long-term complications of steroids and chloroquine.

Immunosuppression. Azathioprine, chlorambucil, and methotrexate have met with mixed success, possibly because patients for such treatment have been incorrectly selected. They have usually been patients with hard-core chronic fibrotic sarcoidosis who have already resisted all other forms of treatment. Azathioprine can be used with advantage in combination with long-term steroids, allowing the dose of the latter to be reduced and thereby minimizing the adverse effects of steroids. Thus far, there have been no trials of the effect of antilymphocytic globulin or of transfer factor in sarcoidosis.

Treatment of Hypercalciuria. Hypercalciuria is swiftly brought under control by oral corticosteroids. If they are contraindicated, then sodium phytate or an oral phosphate preparation is an alternative means of preventing overabsorption of calcium. There is an effective and palatable effervescent phosphate preparation containing 500 mg elemental phosphate and also sodium cellulose phosphate which is recommended as 5-gram doses three times daily with meals. A high chapati diet may also be considered because of its phytate content. Calcitonin has not yet been assessed adequately in sarcoidosis.

Drugs Which Should Not Be Used. Patients with sarcoidosis are peculiarly sensitive to vitamin D, which causes unpleasant symptoms associated with hypercalcemia, hypercalciuria, and elevated blood urea levels. In precorticosteroid days, *calciferol* was often given in sarcoidosis. It is useless, toxic, and obsolete. Vitamin D preparations should be withheld during pregnancy.

Antituberculous drugs have no influence on the course of sarcoidosis and should not be used for the treatment of sarcoidosis. An argument could be made for prophylactic isoniazid along with corticosteroids in countries where there is considerable tuberculosis.

Tuberculin injections had a vogue, especially for sarcoid uveitis, but they are no longer indicated.

Radiotherapy is no longer used even for the lymphoproliferative forms of sarcoidosis.

James, D. G.: The Lettsomian Lectures on "The Granulomatous Disorders." Trans. Med. Soc. Lond., 88:116, 1973.
James, D. G.: Modern concepts of sarcoidosis. Chest, 64:675, 1973.
Jones Williams, W., Pioli, E., Jones, D. J., and Dighero, M.: The Kmif. (Kveim-induced macrophage migration inhibition factor) test in sarcoidosis. J. Clin. Pathol., 25:951, 1972.
Scadding, J. G.: Sarcoidosis. London, Eyre & Spottiswoode, 1967.
Siltzbach, L. E.: Sarcoidosis: Clinical features and management. Med. Clin. North Am., 51:483, 1967.
Siltzbach, L. E.: Proceedings of the Sixth International Conference on Sarcoidosis held in Tokyo, September 1972. In press.
Villar, T. G.: Proceedings of the Sixth International Conference on Sarcoidosis held in Tokyo, September 1972. In press.
Williams, D., Jones Williams, W., and Williams, J. E.: Enzyme histochemistry of epithelioid cells in sarcoidosis and sarcoid-like granulomas. J. Pathol., 97:705, 1969.

103. POLYMYALGIA RHEUMATICA AND CRANIAL ARTERITIS (Temporal Arteritis, Giant Cell Arteritis, Polymyalgia Arteritica)

Paul B. Beeson

The two clinical syndromes of cranial arteritis and polymyalgia rheumatica are described together, because they are often associated and because of the probability that they represent different expressions of one process. The age distribution of patients is almost unique, and the diseases seem to follow similar courses. Most persons affected are more than 60 years of age; occurrence before age 50 is exceedingly rare. Although symptoms may come on quite abruptly and may cause serious incapacity for a time, the natural tendency is toward gradual improvement, with complete subsidence after a period of several months to a few years. The remarkable age incidence and self-limited course must figure prominently in any attempt to determine the nature of these disorders.

POLYMYALGIA RHEUMATICA

Polymyalgia rheumatica is a distinctive kind of muscular rheumatism in old people, more frequent in women than in men. It is characterized by pain and stiffness in the neck, shoulders, and back, and sometimes of the pelvic girdle. Tenderness and true muscle weakness are usually lacking. The stiffness may be particularly troublesome in the morning so that patients are barely able to get out of bed. There may be headache or painful areas over the cranium. Systemic manifestations aside from occasional low-grade pyrexia are not prominent. The patients have a vague sense of malaise simply described as "feeling rotten." Unfortunately these people are too often dismissed with the assumption that symptoms are caused by degenerative processes about which little or nothing can be done.

The distinctive laboratory finding is marked elevation of the erythrocyte sedimentation rate, i.e., more than 80 mm by the Westergren method. Mild anemia is not uncommon, and some hematologists are reporting cases of unexplained anemia in old people which, like the muscular symptoms, respond promptly to steroid therapy. Other laboratory tests are of little help. Muscle biopsy generally reveals no significant inflammatory change even when the tissue is taken from areas which seem to be the site of much pain and stiffness. Blood enzymes which sometimes become elevated in other disorders of muscle are normal in this disease. There may be slight elevation of the alpha 2 globulin. Electromyographic findings are normal. A possible element of autoimmunity is indicated by the observation that lymphocyte transformation occurs in the presence of muscle tissue, especially during acute phases of the symptoms. The affected muscles do not atrophy.

Because of the frequent association of polymyalgia rheumatica with cranial arteritis, and especially because cranial arteritis may cause sudden blindness, some experienced clinicians believe that biopsy of a temporal artery should be carried out in all patients with polymyalgia rheumatica. When this has been done as a routine procedure, the artery has shown the characteristic changes in more than half the cases, regardless of clinical manifestations of arteritis. Others regard this as unnecessary because a trial of steroid therapy, which would be appropriate for cranial arteritis as well as for polymyalgia, will be carried out in any event.

In the differential diagnosis rheumatoid arthritis and degenerative joint disease may present problems; however, careful questioning and examination will show that polymyalgia is a disease of muscles, not joints. Various neoplastic diseases, including multiple myeloma, have to be considered in the differential diagnosis. Similarly the collagen diseases, especially polymyositis, may resemble polymyalgia rheumatica.

Therapy with adrenal steroids is remarkably effective, usually bringing about prompt amelioration of symptoms. It should be begun with a moderately large dose, e.g., 40 to 60 mg of prednisone daily for the first week, with gradual reduction over the next few weeks to a maintenance dose of 7 to 12 mg daily for several months. Some experienced observers recommend at least two years of this low-dose therapy for all patients. There are cases on record in which the symptoms have persisted for as long as ten years. Usually, by occasional trials of reduced dosage and by following the sedimentation rate, the physician can determine when to terminate steroid therapy.

Esiri, M. M., MacLennan, I. C. M., and Hazleman, B. L.: Lymphocyte sensitivity to skeletal muscle in patients with polymyositis and other disorders. Clin. Exp. Immunol., 14:25, 1973.
Fessel, M. J., and Pearson, C. M.: Polymyalgia rheumatica and blindness. N. Engl. J. Med., 276:1403, 1967.
Hamrin, B.: Polymyalgia arteritica. Acta Med. Scand., Suppl. 533, pp. 1–131, 1972.

CRANIAL ARTERITIS

This entity, like polymyalgia rheumatica, occurs only in people past middle age. In a substantial proportion of cases, symptoms resembling those of polymyalgia rheumatica are present weeks or months before the onset of the severe headache which characterizes cranial arteritis. In contrast with polymyalgia rheumatica there is a distinctive histologic lesion in the large and medium-sized arteries of the upper part of the body, especially the temporal vessels.

Cranial arteritis often has an abrupt onset, with severe pain usually in one temple but sometimes in the occipital area, face, jaw, or side of the neck. This may be associated with exquisite hyperesthesia so that the patient dislikes touching the scalp, combing the hair or washing. The pain may have a throbbing character. Pain in the tongue, blanching of the tongue, and even gangrene of the tongue have been described in this disorder, doubtless ascribable to involvement of lingual arteries. Peripheral neuropathy with both sensory and motor components has also been described. When the temporal artery is affected it may be tender, thickened, and nodular. Conversely the vessel may be pulseless and impalpable. The erythrocyte sedimentation rate is elevated, and there may be a substantial fever and polymorphonuclear leukocytosis.

The most feared complication of cranial arteritis is impairment of vision. This may lead to sudden onset of blindness in one or both eyes. The pattern of involvement may be uniocular, resulting from disease of the ophthalmic artery, or occipital, resulting from disease of the vertebral artery. A precise estimate of the frequency of this complication cannot be made because patients with visual symptoms receive special medical attention. The danger is real, and it is generally agreed that all patients with active cranial arteritis should receive steroid treatment for some months, especially to prevent visual loss. There is also suggestive evidence that patients with cranial arteritis are at special risk of certain other vascular accidents, including brainstem strokes and coronary occlusion.

Although it cannot be doubted that the arteries most often affected are branches of the external carotid (accounting for the use of such names as cranial arteritis and temporal arteritis), it should be recognized that other arteries may also be the site of giant cell arteritis. Autopsy has disclosed arteritis in the aorta and even in the hepatic and renal vessels. Instances of aortic aneurysm thought to be due to giant cell arteritis are on record. These may result from an associated pathologic process described under a variety of names such as medial aortopathy.

Steroid therapy should be given according to the plan outlined for polymyalgia rheumatica.

Fauchald, P., Rygvold, O., and Oystese, B.: Temporal arteritis and polymyalgia rheumatica. Ann. Intern. Med., 77:845, 1972.
Marquis, Y., Richardson, J. B., and Ritchie, A. C.: Idiopathic aortopathy and arteriopathy. Am. J. Med., 44:939, 1968.
Wilkinson, I. M. S., and Russell, R. W. R.: Arteries of the head and neck in giant cell arteritis. Arch. Neurol., 27:378, 1972.

104. LETHAL MIDLINE GRANULOMA

Paul B. Beeson

Lethal midline granuloma is a horrid, rare, chronic destructive disease affecting the midline structures of the face and nearly always terminating in death. The process most often affects males aged 20 to 50 and usually begins with symptoms of nasal obstruction with purulent, sometimes bloody discharge. Months or years later the skin of the nose and inner eyelid become red, then necrotic, with the formation of fistulas and with progressive loss of facial tissue. Owing to a tendency to thrombosis of blood vessels it progresses by causing necrosis of hard or soft tissues, leading to destruction of the nasal septum, the hard or soft palate, the paranasal sinuses, and the orbital cavities. There is little tendency for regional lymph nodes to become enlarged, and the process does not ordinarily affect the lungs. Pain and fever are variable. Death may result from inanition, hemorrhage, or sepsis (notably when the destructive process has exposed the meninges).

A disease conforming to the aforementioned description can be caused by several specific infections, e.g., syphilis, yaws, leprosy, mucormycosis, by carcinoma arising in the nose or paranasal sinuses, and by lymphomas. Sometimes, despite prolonged and intensive study including repeated biopsy, the specific causes are identified only late in the disease or at autopsy. Some writers have classified lethal midline granuloma and Wegener's granulomatosis together, but that seems unwarranted. Kassel and his colleagues take the view that most cases of lethal midline granuloma are forms of neoplastic disease, some of which eventually are found to resemble accepted types of lymphoma, others a less easily recognized form which has been called "polymorphic reticulosis." Others, who agree with the neoplastic concept, have suggested the designation "midline malignant reticulosis." They feel that the old term lethal midline granuloma should be used only as a clinical designation for a process which can have several causes.

As might be expected from scattered reports of an unusual clinical disorder probably comprising more than one pathogenetic entity, recommendations as to treatment have varied. Radiation therapy to the affected regions seems the procedure most likely to palliate or arrest the process. Occasional benefits from the use of cytotoxic drugs (cyclophosphamide, methotrexate, chlorambucil) are on record. Steroid hormones do not help. Antimicrobial therapy may be called for from time to time to combat secondary infection by bacteria or fungi.

Eichel, B. S., and Mabery, T. E.: The enigma of lethal midline granuloma. Laryngoscope, 78:1367, 1968.
Fechner, R. E., and Lamppin, D. W.: Midline malignant reticulosis. Arch. Otolaryngol., 95:467, 1972.
Kassel, S. H., Echevarria, R. A., and Guzzo, F. P.: Midline malignant reticulosis (so-called lethal midline granuloma). Cancer, 23:920, 1969.

105. WEGENER'S GRANULOMATOSIS

Paul B. Beeson

The central pathologic lesion in this disease is a granuloma which tends to affect blood vessels, with resulting necrosis of tissue. Lesions usually appear first in the upper and lower respiratory tract, but at some stage an associated generalized vasculitis develops and causes severe damage in the kidneys and other organs.

Persons of both sexes and all ages are affected, but the highest incidence appears to be in mid-adult life. In the "classic" picture, i.e., that which was first identified, the initial involvement is usually in the nose and paranasal sinuses. The patient suffers for months with symptoms of nasal stuffiness and discharge and is treated for recurrent sinusitis or chronic otitis. Later there is extension to the lower respiratory tract, with symptoms and signs caused by single or multiple lesions in the lungs. This may lead to an erroneous diagnosis of neoplastic disease. At some time after this the generalized vasculitis becomes evident, and there may then be rapid deterioration, with manifestations of disease in the nervous system, the gut, the joints, the skin, and subcutaneous tissues. At autopsy there may be destructive lesions in spleen and liver. The most sinister aspect of the disease is its tendency to cause severe damage to the kidneys, and renal insufficiency is the most common cause of death. Hypertension rarely develops despite severe renal disease. After onset of manifestations of disseminated disease the course rarely lasts more than a few months without treatment.

Limited Forms of Wegener's Granulomatosis. Carrington and Liebow have called attention to a group of cases in which the major pathologic change is in the lungs, and in which there is little evidence of disease in the nose or paranasal sinuses, or of generalized vasculitis.

Lymphomatoid Granulomatosis. Liebow et al. have now described another subgroup, which they consider to be related to Wegener's granulomatosis; in this the principal sites of involvement are the lungs, skin, and central nervous system. The histologic findings are those of angiitis with extensive necrosis and an infiltrative process resembling some form of lymphoma. The dominant clinical manifestations are cough, fever, and massive hemoptyses. This form of disease, despite the local "lymphomatoid" appearance, generally does not spread to lymphoid tissues, such as hilar nodes or spleen.

Diagnosis. The diagnosis can be suspected on clinical grounds but can only be made by histologic examination of affected tissue. Routine blood studies, including eosinophil counts, are usually normal. Biopsy from the nasal structures or lung will show the characteristic granuloma with special involvement of arteries and resulting tendency to necrosis. Biopsy of the kidney may show focal necrotizing glomerulitis.

Course. As already mentioned, once there is evidence of dissemination, especially with renal involvement, the downhill course may be rapid. On the other hand, in the "limited forms," some patients have lived several years and in some of them the disease has appeared to go into remission. Generally, however, this still must be regarded as a disease which tends to progress and to end fatally.

Treatment. Most patients are treated with antimicrobials; these may be required from time to time to deal with secondary infections, but certainly do not affect the primary disease. Steroid therapy has been generally disappointing; in fact, some writers regard this as a diagnostic feature. Others recommend that steroids should be given, along with cytotoxic drugs. Although comparative clinical trials have not been carried out, there is now a rather convincing volume of individual case reports which seem to show definite benefit from use of cytotoxic drugs with or without steroids. Several seem to have had an effect, including azathioprine, 2 to 3 mg per kilogram, chlorambucil, 0.2 mg per kilogram, cyclophosphamide, 1 to 2 mg per kilogram, or methotrexate. The last can be given in intermittent intravenous courses, 15 to 50 mg once a week, provided that renal function is reasonably good, and may have the advantage of rapid effect. If remission is obtained, these therapies can sometimes be stopped without reappearance of symptoms, but it is impossible to predict how long remission will last.

Carrington, C. B., and Liebow, A. A.: Limited forms of angiitis and granulomatosis of Wegener's type. Am. J. Med., 41:497, 1966.
Fahey, J. L., Leonard, E., Churg, J., and Godman, G.: Wegener's granulomatosis. Am. J. Med., 17:168, 1954.
Fauci, A. S., and Wolff, S. M.: Wegener's granulomatosis: Studies in eighteen patients and a review of the literature. Medicine, 52:535, 1973.
Leading article: Wegener's granulomatosis. Lancet, 2:519, 1972. (References to cytotoxic drugs in therapy.)
Liebow, A. A., Carrington, C. R. B., and Friedman, P. J.: Lymphomatoid granulomatosis. Hum. Pathol., 3:457, 1972.

106. WEBER-CHRISTIAN DISEASE (Relapsing Febrile Nodular Nonsuppurative Panniculitis, Panniculitis)

Paul B. Beeson

The designation Weber-Christian disease will be used to describe several clinical syndromes which may or may not be variants of the same disease. The feature shared by all is the occurrence of localized inflammatory lesions in adipose tissue. Histologically these show chronic inflammation with mononuclear cell infiltration; sometimes the mononuclear cells are filled with fatty material. Giant cells occur occasionally, and in more acute lesions polymorphonuclear leukocytes may be present. There is a tendency to inflammatory occlusion of small blood vessels, and necrosis is common.

The term *Weber-Christian disease* is usually applied to a clinical syndrome in which the principal involvement is in the panniculus adiposus. Women are affected more frequently than men with this form of the disease. It is characterized by development of multiple tender nodules in the subcutaneous fat, from 5 mm to 10 cm in diameter. The lesions are located principally on the thighs and trunk and in the breasts. They are tender, and there may be some reddening of the skin. Occasionally necrosis of the skin leads to sinus formation with discharge of an oily liquid. The course is usually indolent; crops of lesions develop from time to time over periods of months or years. When the inflammation subsides, there often remains an area of loss of subcutaneous tissue which cause dimpling of skin. Systemic manifestations are usually mild, but may include malaise, low-grade fever, leukocytosis, and eosinophilia. Enlargement of the liver and spleen are reported in some cases. The illness may grumble along for months or several years and then cease.

A more serious expression of this pathologic process has been termed *systemic Weber-Christian disease.* Here there is widespread inflammation affecting not only the panniculus adiposus but similar tissue within the abdominal and thoracic cavities. There may be parenchymatous inflammation, affecting thoracic or abdominal organs, including lungs, pericardium, pleura, bowel, spleen, kidneys, and adrenal glands. At least a dozen cases are recorded in which this form of disease has led to death.

The term *mesenteric panniculitis* has been applied to an obscure disease characterized by inflammation of the mesenteric fat. This has been encountered mainly in males, and reports of the syndrome have appeared principally in surgical journals. Symptoms include recurrent episodes of fever, abdominal pain, nausea, vomiting, and malaise. At operation the mesentery is found to be thickened, with red or yellow patches, and biopsy reveals the characteristic panniculitis, which cannot be differentiated from the lesions of Weber-Christian disease.

Several writers have suggested that these forms of inflammation in the retroperitoneal adipose tissue may represent the initial lesion in at least some cases of retroperitoneal fibrosis.

There is no specific therapy. Considerable relief of symptoms by use of large doses of steroids has been reported, but in other instances this has not proved helpful. Antimicrobial drugs should not be given. The use of immunosuppressive or cytotoxic agents could be considered, especially when there is evidence of systemic extension of the panniculitis.

Milner, R. D. G., and Mitchinson, M. J.: Systemic Weber-Christian disease. J. Clin. Pathol., 18:150, 1965.

Ogden, W. W., II, Bradburn, D. M., and Rives, J. D.: Mesenteric panniculitis. Ann. Surg., 161:864, 1965.

107. FIBROSING SYNDROMES (Multifocal Fibrosclerosis)

Paul B. Beeson

In rare instances the delicate fibrous areolar tissue in certain anatomic regions becomes the site of a chronic low-grade inflammatory process, leading to deposition of dense sclerotic plaques, which may obstruct or limit the movement of adjacent viscera. When the process is in the active phase, there are characteristic findings of chronic or granulomatous inflammation, featured by mononuclear cell infiltration and occasional giant cells. In the end stages the pathologic lesion is simply that of scar tissue so that by the time this process causes clinical manifestations there may be little evidence of the initial inflammatory reaction. As a general rule the process tends to originate in the midline, around the great vessels, and then to spread laterally. At the periphery of the lesion there appears to be an inflammation of fatty tissue; this is gradually converted to a dense fibrous mat, with little or no sign of inflammation. In most cases a clue to the inciting mechanism is lacking, hence the frequent use of the term "idiopathic" in describing the various syndromes. Indubitably this pattern of response may follow different kinds of injury. For example, there is an association between therapy with methysergide and some cases of retroperitoneal fibrosis, and the suggestion has been made that fibrosing mediastinitis can occur as a sequel to infection with *Histoplasma capsulatum*. In a number of instances the disease has developed concurrently with a neoplastic process such as reticulum cell sarcoma or carcinoid tumor.

Although most of these syndromes have been described as separate entities, depending on the clinical manifestations and the interests of the writers who have reported them, it should be emphasized that several anatomic areas may become affected in one person. For example, retroperitoneal fibrosis and sclerosing mediastinitis may be present at the same time. Even more interesting is the report by Comings and his associates of two brothers, offspring of a consanguineous marriage, who exhibited varying combinations of retroperitoneal fibrosis, mediastinal fibrosis, sclerosing cholangitis, Riedel's thyroiditis, and pseudotumor of the orbit. This remarkable constellation of syndromes in two siblings brings up the possibility of a genetic predisposition to disease of this character, but of course does not exclude other precipitating factors, e.g., common exposure to some chemical.

RETROPERITONEAL FIBROSIS
(Periureteral Fibrosis)

In retroperitoneal fibrosis the fibrosing process is most commonly located over the promontory of the sacrum with extension laterally to the ureters and up as high as the level of the second or third lumbar vertebra. Less commonly the lesion develops in other extraperitoneal areas, for example, contiguous with the kidneys, duodenum, descending colon, or urinary bladder.

In some cases there has been an associated vasculitis in the skin and subcutaneous tissues, manifested by the formation of nodules, erythematous discolorations, and ulcerations. Similarly, inflammatory changes in small vessels at the sites of the sclerosis have been noted.

The occurrence of retroperitoneal fibrosis in patients taking methysergide for migraine has been reported with greater frequency than could be due to chance, and that drug must be listed as one etiologic factor. It has also been thought that continued use of amphetamine compounds may evoke this process.

The manifestations of retroperitoneal fibrosis are variable, depending on the anatomic location of the process. Pain is the most common symptom; it is vague and tends to be located in the low back and may be accompanied by symptoms referable to the gastrointestinal tract. The patient is likely to lose weight and have low-grade fever. There may be some anemia and elevation of the erythrocyte sedimentation rate. Although the ureter is the structure most often affected, symptoms referable to the urinary tract are uncommon until obstructive uropathy has led to azotemia and other clinical manifestations of renal insufficiency. The fibrosing process may surround the inferior vena cava, but signs of obstruction of that vessel are uncommon; this contrasts with mediastinal fibrosis in which the most common expression is superior caval obstruction.

Diagnosis of retroperitoneal fibrosis is difficult because of the lack of localizing manifestations. It is most often suggested by the findings at intravenous pyelography: displacement of the ureters toward the midline and evidence of obstruction usually at the level of the pelvic brim. One or both ureters may be affected. Less often a mass can be palpated in the pelvis or on the posterior abdominal wall. Once the presence of a mass has been disclosed, by roentgenography, by palpation, or at laparotomy, the main problem in differential diagnosis lies in distinguishing retroperitoneal fibrosis from retroperitoneal tumor.

Surgical treatment, if employed before there has been

severe renal damage, is often highly successful. Inasmuch as the fibrosing process is seldom invasive, the constricted organ can often be freed by blunt dissection so that normal movement or flow is restored. Relief of ureteral obstruction is usually achieved simply by dissecting this structure free of its fibrous encasement and bringing it out on the anterior surface of the sclerotic mass. Occasionally, however, the obstruction recurs months or years after such treatment. The claim has been made that prolonged steroid therapy may be helpful, but the evidence for this is unconvincing, and prompt surgical relief should be attempted whenever the risk is not very great. Nevertheless, many people who have had experience with this disease recommend that steroid treatment should be employed as an adjunct to surgical measures. When the inferior vena cava is obstructed, surgical relief is technically difficult and risky; here it may be preferable to temporize, in the hope that development of collateral pathways may alleviate the circulatory block.

The long-term outlook is fairly good if the disease is recognized and if its obstructive consequences can be treated suitably by surgical means. Prolonged observations of some successfully treated patients indicate that the disease tends to run its course and subside so that the life expectancy may not be shortened. Most deaths have been caused by renal failure.

MEDIASTINAL FIBROSIS

Taut bundles of collagenous tissue form in the superior and anterior mediastinum with impingement on the aorta, trachea, and pericardium, but the predominant manifestations are those caused by obstruction of the superior vena cava: puffy, suffused appearance of the face and conjunctivae, nonpitting edema of the face, neck, and upper extremities, and distended veins in the neck and upper extremities. The main task in differential diagnosis is to distinguish this relatively benign condition from obstruction caused by tumor. Roentgenographic examination of the chest may reveal little or no abnormality, but angiographic studies will show the obstruction of the superior vena cava and its large tributaries. Thoracotomy may be required for histologic diagnosis.

As already mentioned, some evidence suggests that histoplasmosis may be a cause of mediastinal fibrosis; therefore it should be considered, and when tests for this infection are positive a trial of appropriate chemotherapy seems justified.

Some patients with this syndrome have shown gradual improvement over months or years, presumably because of development of collateral circulation. Attempts to remove the fibrosing tissues from the large veins are technically difficult and hazardous.

SCLEROSING CHOLANGITIS

A diffuse fibrous sheath sometimes envelops the common bile duct, the hepatic ducts, and the gallbladder. The clinical manifestations are pain and tenderness in the right upper quadrant and prolonged, gradually deepening jaundice. Liver function tests reveal changes of extrahepatic biliary obstruction. This condition may progress to death, with the picture of biliary cirrhosis.

Treatment is not very satisfactory. Steroid therapy has rarely seemed to help. It is suggested that prolonged T-tube drainage of the bile ducts may ameliorate the situation until the disease regresses.

FIBROSCLEROSIS IN OTHER ORGANS

Riedel's thyroiditis is a rare form of fibrotic disease affecting the structures in the anterior part of the neck. This differs from Hashimoto's thyroiditis in being equally common in males and females and in the tendency of the fibrotic process to involve not only the thyroid but also its neighboring structures.

Peyronie's disease is a sclerotic induration of the corpora cavernosa of the penis. This disease has been encountered in association with sclerosing processes in other parts of the body.

Pseudotumor of the orbit causes unilateral exophthalmos and is likely to be confused with tumor. It has been seen in association with Riedel's thyroiditis, as well as in other fibrosclerosing syndromes.

Dupuytren's contracture has been thought by some to be another expression of the systemic fibrosclerosing syndromes; however, it is so often independent that the case for similar pathogenesis seems weak.

Alpert, L. I., and Jindrak, K.: Idiopathic retroperitoneal fibrosis and sclerosing cholangitis associated with a reticulum cell sarcoma. Gastroenterology, 62:111, 1972.

Carton, R. W., and Wong, R.: Multifocal fibrosclerosis manifested by vena caval obstructions and associated with vasculitis. Ann. Intern. Med., 70:81, 1969.

Catino, D., Torack, R. M., and Hagstrom, J. W. C.: Idiopathic retroperitoneal fibrosis: Histochemical evidence for lateral spread of the process from the midline. J. Urol., 98:191, 1967.

Comings, D. E., Skubi, K. B., Van Eyes, J., and Motulsky, A. G.: Familial multifocal sclerosis. Ann. Intern. Med., 66:884, 1967.

Glenn, F., and Whitsell, J. C., III: Primary sclerosing cholangitis. Surg., Gynecol. Obstet., 123:1037, 1966.

Hewlett, T. H., Steer, A., and Thomas, D. E.: Progressive fibrosing mediastinitis. Ann. Thorac. Surg., 2:345, 1966.

Salmon, H. W.: Combined mediastinal and retroperitoneal fibrosis. Thorax, 23:158, 1968.

Wagenknecht, L. V., and Auvert, J.: Symptoms and diagnosis of retroperitoneal fibrosis. Urol. Int., 26:185, 1971.

108. EOSINOPHILIC SYNDROMES

Paul B. Beeson

GENERAL CONSIDERATIONS

Many diseases characterized by eosinophilia are dealt with in other areas of this book, for example, parasitic infestations, polyarteritis nodosa, and Hodgkin's disease. In addition there remains a group of poorly understood, uncommon syndromes in which substantial eosinophilia is a striking clinical feature. Some of these will be described in this chapter, and some bibliographic citations are appended. It must be emphasized that these conditions almost certainly comprise a heterogeneous group; doubtless with further study better understanding and more rational classification will be possible.

Despite a considerable amount of investigation there remains a vast ignorance about the role of the eosinophil. In the minds of many people it is merely a granulocyte which stains peculiarly and tends to proliferate when an allergic reaction develops. It resembles the neutrophil in morphology and has similar phagocytic ability, but differs in possessing a peroxidase not found in the neutrophil, in having a crystalline structure (the internum) within its granules, and in its behavior after administration of adrenal cortical steroid. It tends to lodge in tissues that have contact with the environment and to congregate in the neighborhood of antigen-antibody complexes and to ingest them. Although much has been written about the relationship of the eosinophil to histamine, there is no convincing evidence in man that the eosinophil makes histamine, neutralizes histamine, or is subject to a chemotaxis by histamine.

Indubitably the behavior of eosinophils is altered in some allergic states and immune processes. Their number in the circulation increases, and this is almost certainly a reflection of increased production in the marrow. Common factors of many diseases characterized by eosinophilia are constant or repeated exposure to comparatively large quantities of foreign material. Increased production of eosinophils by hematopoietic tissue follows the general pattern of immune responses and is mediated by the lymphocyte.

EOSINOPHILIC PULMONARY SYNDROMES

The term *Löffler's syndrome* is applied to a benign illness usually lasting less than a month, characterized by transient pulmonary infiltrations, low fever, and peripheral eosinophilia. Characteristically the infiltrates are located in peripheral areas of the lungs; when in the apices, the radiologic appearance may simulate that of tuberculosis. Some instances of this are associated with parasitic infestations in which circulating parasites lodge in the lungs, causing inflammatory reactions there. More often, however, the same clinical picture is found in patients who show no sign of parasitic infestation. A somewhat similar clinical picture may develop as a manifestation of sensitivity to nitrofurantoin. In most instances steroid treatment causes prompt amelioration of symptoms and clearing of the infiltrates.

A form of illness which resembles Löffler's syndrome except for longer duration and greater severity has been designated *pulmonary infiltration with eosinophilia* or *PIE syndrome.* This can cause marked disability because of fever, cough, and breathlessness and can persist for some years. Here again there is no clue to the etiology. Steroid therapy should be tried and may bring about improvement, but may have to be maintained for many weeks or months because of the tendency to relapse.

A wide variety of etiologic entities goes by the name *tropical pulmonary eosinophilia.* Doubtless many of these are either parasitic disorders or allergic responses to an inhaled antigen. This term has been used so broadly that it has little more significance than "nephritis" or "dermatitis."

Some patients exhibit pulmonary infiltration and eosinophilia during the course of *bronchial asthma* or *polyarteritis nodosa.* These entities can usually be distinguished from the aforementioned syndromes.

Liebow and Carrington have described a group of patients who had chronic pneumonia characterized by infiltration with eosinophils. They make the point that, although there is usually an increased number of eosinophils in the blood, this is not always true; but on the basis of the lung lesions they use the diagnostic term *eosinophilic pneumonia.* The consistent anatomic feature is an alveolar exudate made up of a mixture of large mononuclear cells and eosinophils. In most cases of this type the etiology cannot be determined; certainly the clinical picture can be caused, among other things, by parasites, fungi, and drugs or other chemical agents.

EOSINOPHILIC SYNDROMES AFFECTING OTHER ORGAN SYSTEMS

Eosinophilic Endomyocardial Disease (Löffler's Endocarditis). Löffler described cases in which there was a marked and prolonged eosinophilia of the blood, associated with increasing cardiac disability. Autopsy in such cases discloses cellular infiltration of the myocardium and a fibrotic process on the parietal endocardium in which eosinophils are prominent. Frequently there is also an eosinophilic infiltrate in other tissues. Therapy with steroids has little or no beneficial effect. Differentiation between Löffler's myocarditis and diffuse eosinophilic collagen disease (see below) is sometimes impossible.

Eosinophilic Meningitis. From countries bordering on the Pacific come case reports of a subacute meningitis characterized by the presence of more than 10 per cent eosinophils in the cerebrospinal fluid. A striking clinical feature is pain and paresthesia in the extremities. There may be palsy of the sixth and seventh cranial nerves. Epidemiologic investigations point to a nematode, *Angiostrongylus cantonensis,* as the causative agent; the infestation seems to be acquired by eating raw or insufficiently cooked snails. The case fatality rate is only about 1 per cent (see Ch. 315).

Eosinophilic Collagen Disease. Many cases have been reported of a multisystemic illness, resembling dermatomyositis, in which there is marked eosinophilia. Muscle and joint pain are common, and the myocardium may be affected (as in Löffler's myocarditis). The kidneys are seldom injured.

Eosinophilic Gastroenteritis. See Part XIV, Section Three.

Eosinophilic Leukemia and the Hypereosinophilic Syndromes. Whether there is such an entity as *eosinophilic leukemia* continues to provoke controversy. Numerous cases have been described under that title. They have been characterized by prolonged clinical course, marked elevation of the eosinophil count in blood and bone marrow, hepatomegaly, splenomegaly, and fatal termination; at autopsy eosinophilic infiltration of various tissues has been noted. Doubt has been expressed about the designation of leukemia in some of these, principally because the eosinophils in the blood and tissues are mature forms; nevertheless some of those reported seem to satisfy conventional criteria for the diagnosis.

Hardy and Anderson believe that it is possible to depict a broad spectrum of hypereosinophilic syndromes extending from the most benign, Löffler's syndrome, to a clinically malignant form often confused with eosinophilic leukemia. This last group is characterized by manifestations of cardiac and pulmonary infiltration as well as marked enlargement of the liver and spleen, and often terminates fatally.

Steroid Treatment in the Eosinophilic Syndromes. In this heterogeneous group of diseases the efficacy of steroid treatment has been variable. Sometimes there has been a prompt and dramatic response, with apparent clinical cure. In others prolonged therapy has been required to suppress the cardiac and pulmonary manifestations. In a further group steroid therapy has had little or no beneficial effect.

Benvenisti, D. S., and Ultmann, J. E.: Eosinophilic leukemia. Ann. Intern. Med., 71:731, 1969.

Hailey, F. J., Glascock, H. W., Jr., and Hewitt, W. F.: Pleuropneumonic reactions to nitrofurantoin. N. Engl. J. Med., 281:1087, 1969.

Hardy, W. R., and Anderson, R. E.: The hypereosinophilic syndromes. Ann. Intern. Med., 68:1220, 1968.

Klein, N. C., Hargrove, L., Sleisenger, M. H., and Jeffries, G. H.: Eosinophilic gastroenteritis. Medicine, 49:299, 1970.

Liebow, A. A., and Carrington, C. B.: The eosinophilic pneumonias. Medicine, 48:251, 1969.

Pierce, L. E., Hosseinian, A. H., and Constantine, A. B.: Disseminated eosinophilic collagen disease. Blood, 29:540, 1967.

Punyagupta, S., et al.: Eosinophilic meningitis in Thailand. Am. J. Trop. Med. Hyg., 19:950, 1970.

Reeder, W. H., and Goodrich, B. E.: Pulmonary infiltration with eosinophilia (PIE syndrome). Ann. Intern. Med., 36:1217, 1952.

Part VIII
MICROBIAL DISEASES

109. INTRODUCTION TO MICROBIAL DISEASES

Walsh McDermott

Microbial diseases are all those produced by a transmissible agent capable of multiplication in living tissue and sufficiently small in its individual units to be visible only by light or electron microscopy. One might question whether a useful purpose is served by including under the one label such diverse entities as diseases produced by protozoa and those caused by the smallest viruses. Certainly at one level of analysis a grouping of this sort is not particularly useful. For this reason, protozoa have been removed from the present Part and, with the helminths, form one of their own (Part IX); general discussions of the rest of the microbial diseases have been placed with the individual subdivisions, such as viral or bacterial diseases. But there is a larger sense in which all these diseases are usefully regarded as a single group separate from and unlike all other diseases. For the nonmicrobial diseases, except for those resulting from undernutrition, are essentially individual, private affairs which, if uncontrolled, represent personal tragedies but seldom have wide public impact. By contrast, a society unable to employ contemporary technology to manage its microbial diseases is condemned to misery; infant and childhood deaths are a commonplace, pregnancy is virtually a permanent way of life for all women from their mid-teens to their mid-forties, and back-breaking toil is the lot of most people. To gain understanding of microbial disease in a scientific and technologic sense is thus an essential prerequisite to the building and maintenance of a modern society.

With that understanding of microbial disease is an appreciation of the tremendous adaptive plasticity of microbes – their great capacity for *change* both in themselves and in the conditions of their parasitism. This ability to adapt to change means that the microbial world is an enduring potential source of new diseases. It also means that there is no real prospect for a world free from microbial diseases, either those of man or of the plants and other animals. Thus if we are to continue our long record of successes in meeting microbial challenges to man, there can be no letup in our search for greater knowledge of the subject at the bedside, in the field, and in the laboratory. Our brilliant successes in the prevention and treatment of so many microbial diseases are not founded on the extermination of the microbe. They are all based on making the environment outside or within the human host a place in which the microbe cannot flourish to its full capacity. To exploit some weak link in the pathogenic chain in this way requires exact scientific and clinical knowledge. The incapacitation of the microbe thus affected may or may not jeopardize its survival as a species. Paleontology has taught us that species or genera have disappeared from this planet. Our systematic study of microbes is not yet of sufficient age to document such extinction of a disease-producing microbe, but there is no reason to doubt that it could occur. There is considerable reason to doubt, however, that it can be produced by the purposeful actions of man. A far greater body of knowledge would be necessary than is now available to produce such purposeful extinction of a microbial species. This is so not only because of microbial adaptability, but also because we have so little ability to identify and successfully interrupt *all* significant ecologic relationships involved. The story of the malaria eradication campaign (see Ch. 271) is a case in point. Whether the situation with smallpox will be any different remains to be seen. In the writer's judgment, it seems most unlikely. "Final victories" in the form of microbial extinction are not to be expected, but neither are they necessary or particularly desirable. Our existing conceptual base and pluralism of practical approaches have yielded an array of triumphs that make our current management of microbial disease one of the finest chapters in the whole history of science for man's benefit. To a considerable extent, however, these practical cures and preventives rely upon the change in hygienic habits in and around the home that come with, or are made possible by, improved socioeconomic status. What is needed now is not only a continued effort in the same direction but also a new massive effort of a different sort. This new effort should be devoted to reviewing those major microbial diseases for which we already have effective technologies, with the object of developing new and quite different methods suitable for wide application in economically underdeveloped regions.

Dubos, R. J.: Man Adapting. New Haven, Yale University Press, 1965, pp. 369–399.
Morrison, R. S.: The concept of eradication and public education. The Pharos, 23:3, 1963.

Section One. VIRAL DISEASES

110. INTRODUCTION TO VIRAL DISEASES

Edwin D. Kilbourne

The thread that binds together such differing diseases as influenza, mumps, smallpox, and yellow fever for common consideration in this section is the tenuous one of viral etiology. All are the result of infection with viruses, and all viruses share in common submicroscopic size and complete and intimate dependence on the cells of the host that they infect. Yet these tiny packages of protein-coated nucleic acid are as different as the diseases discussed in these pages. They vary in size from the 30 mμ RNA-containing particle of yellow fever virus to the 250 mμ antigenically complex particle of smallpox virus, with its DNA core. The relation of design and function of viruses is now being appreciated. Certain myxoviruses, including the influenza and parainfluenza viruses, possess a potent neuraminidase that probably abets their attack on the mucin-coated cells of the respiratory tract. The myxoviruses are fragile and unstable in the environment, whereas the enteroviruses, including poliovirus, can pass unscathed through the barrier of gastric acidity in their journey to the target cells of the small intestine.

Neither structural nor chemical similarity of viruses, however, is any sure guide to the diseases that they may cause. Mumps and parainfluenza viruses are indistinguishable by electron microscopy and even share antigens in common, but one invades the salivary glands, pancreas, or meninges, whereas the other produces mild upper respiratory tract infection or infantile croup. Nor does viral dissimilarity predict dissimilar disease. The structurally amorphous, genetically plastic RNA virus of influenza and the geometrically precise DNA-bearing adenovirus, with its potential for latency, both evoke clinical syndromes that may be difficult to differentiate.

With this caution in mind about the great dissimilarities among viruses and their associated diseases, the common features of viral infections can be considered as useful generalizations.

Most viral infections occur in childhood, at which time any of the 200 obligate human viruses ordinarily produce acute but benign disease or no disease at all. However, the unborn child may be peculiarly vulnerable to the effects of rubella, and the newborn—if unprotected by maternal antibody—may be severely damaged by infection with the ordinarily innocuous virus of herpes simplex. With the exception of the neonatal period, the severity of disease associated with primary or initial viral infections increases with the age of the patient. Poliomyelitis is more frequent and more severe in adult infection; varicella pneumonia is essentially limited to adults; the postpuberal complications of mumps are notorious; and jaundice occurs more frequently in older than in younger patients with infectious hepatitis. It is necessary to emphasize the evidence for greater potential susceptibility of the adult because it may *appear* that the adult is less vulnerable to viral disease, protected as he is by a legacy of immunity to many viruses from his childhood experience with them. This fact of age-related susceptibility is increasingly important as the epidemiologic patterns of viral infections change with changes in man's environment and with the introduction of new vaccines. If a vaccine induces impermanent immunity so that infection is merely postponed, the consequences might be disastrous.

Although firm and enduring immunity attended by persisting humoral antibody follows most viral infections, it is unlikely that antibody formation per se is the essential mechanism of recovery. Interferon, a nonspecific and nontoxic product of virus-infected cells, is more closely related temporally to the decline of virus in tissues and to recovery from infection, but its role in the self-termination of viral infections is still conjectural. Experimental evidence that corticosteroid hormones are inhibitory to interferon synthesis may explain the deleterious effect of these hormones or of stress on certain viral infections of man—notably on the extension of recurrent herpes simplex keratitis or on varicella in children already receiving steroid therapy.

The enduring immunity of viral infections has few exceptions. The frequency of common colds is now explicable as the result of multiple infections with multiple antigenically unrelated viruses; the seemingly transient immunity of influenza reflects the changing nature of the virus itself. For most viral infections there is no indication whether protracted immunity is maintained by recurrent subclinical infection or by persistence of the virus in the host. With a few—varicella-zoster, herpes simplex, and cytomegalic inclusion disease—all associated with herpesviruses which replicate in the cell nucleus, viral genomes undoubtedly persist throughout life in the tissues, and there may be reactivated to produce recurrent disease in the partially immune host. In the growing number of patients who are immunologically crippled with cancer or subjected to chemical immunosuppression for transplantation surgery, such reactivations may occur as new and sometimes terminal diseases.

Evidence is increasing that viruses are involved in a variety of mammalian cancers and also in chronic diseases of the central nervous system. In man, the association of the herpes-like Epstein-Barr virus (EBV) with Burkitt's lymphoma and cancer of the retropharyngeal space is striking, although an etiologic relationship has not been proved. The human papilloma virus (associated with the common wart) is a member of a group of mammalian viruses—the papovaviruses—two of which have recently been proved to be capable of genetic integration with the host cell chromosome in the manner of lysogenic bacteriophages.

The recent direct demonstration of a measles-like virus in patients with subacute sclerosing panencephalitis suggests the awesome potential of common agents of acute infection.

In contrast to the bacterial diseases of man, the viral diseases are relatively insusceptible at present to chemotherapy, but the efficient immunity of natural viral infection can be duplicated with vaccines. The coat proteins of all viruses are antigenic, and it is reasonable to conclude that vaccines could be made for all viruses that can be cultivated in the laboratory. The great number of viral pathogens limits the feasibility of this approach, however, as does our uncertain knowledge of the ultimate potential of these viruses for good or evil. The vaccine itself may be a two-edged sword: if a living virus, it may be contaminated with alien viruses or nucleic acid; if inactivated, it may be poorly antigenic. At its best, however, the vaccine may be the ultimate weapon if eradication of the virus can be effected by substitution in the community of vaccine virus for wild type. A trend in this direction is evident with poliomyelitis.

The intractability of viral infections to chemotherapy is a corollary of the intimacy of virus-host association. To the extent that the viral parasite subverts the host's cellular machinery to its own synthesis, it cannot be interrupted without compromising the host as well. But the recent discovery of new, virus-coded enzymes in infected but not in normal cells suggests the possibility of employing highly selective antimetabolites specifically directed against virus synthesis. Indeed, this effect has already been realized in vitro, and in man limited success in arresting the progression of recurrent herpes simplex keratitis has been achieved even with antimetabolites not specific for virus. Chemoprophylaxis of smallpox and effective therapy of progressive vaccinia have attended the semi-empiric use of isatin β-thiosemicarbazone.

Man may never be free of viruses, but, hopefully, he may gradually replace the plagues of the past with more peaceful coexistence in the future.

VIRAL (AND FILTER-PASSING MICROBIAL) INFECTIONS OF THE RESPIRATORY TRACT

111. THE COMMON COLD (Acute Coryza)

George Gee Jackson

Definition. The common cold is a symptom complex caused by viral infection of the upper respiratory passages. Most precisely, the term applies to afebrile, acute coryza of viral origin. In the broadest sense, the common cold refers to any undifferentiated upper respiratory infection. The terms rhinitis, pharyngitis, laryngitis, and "chest cold" are sometimes used to designate the principal anatomic site of infection. The main difference between the common cold and other viral or bacterial respiratory infections is the absence of fever and the relatively mild constitutional symptoms and signs.

Etiology. Many viruses can cause the common cold. No single strain of virus accounts for more than a small proportion of the illnesses. Among the viruses recently identified, rhinoviruses comprise the largest single etiologic group. Isolates have been made from about 70 per cent of acute coryzal illnesses in young adults and about 35 per cent of common colds in children. The viruses listed in Table 1 comprise six categorical groups that have been etiologically related to the common cold in some investigations. (The coxsackie- and echoviruses listed therein are also considered separately in Ch. 126 to 136.)

The increasing ability to recover viruses and better serologic means for the diagnosis of viral infections have shown that 5 to 10 per cent of common colds are associated with more than one virus, and definite evidence of simultaneous dual infection is not rare. The causative agents of some of the infections have not been revealed by tissue culture methods currently in use. Certain of the more labile or fastidious viruses have been grown only in unusual cultures of human cell strains or in organ cultures of human embryonic trachea. Other viruses can be shown only by the transmission of illness to volunteers. More than 90 antigenically different strains of rhinoviruses are known to cause the common cold syndrome. Well over 100 viruses that can cause mild respiratory illnesses in man may be prevalent in the population at any one time.

TABLE 1. Viruses Sometimes Associated with the Common Cold

Myxoviruses:	
	Influenza A, B, C
Paramyxoviruses:	
	Parainfluenza 1, 2, 3, 4
	Respiratory syncytial
	Measles
Coronaviruses: > two types	
Reovirus 1	
Adenoviruses:	
	Types 1, 2, 5, 6; 3, 4, 7, 14
Picornaviruses:	
	Coxsackievirus A 21, 24
	Coxsackievirus B 3, 4, 5
	Echovirus 7, 8, 11, 15, 19, 20 (others rarely)
	Rhinovirus > 90 types or subtypes

Incidence and Prevalence. The incidence of common colds is related to age and environment. Preschool children have an average of six to twelve respiratory illnesses per year, most of which are common colds. Parents with young children have approximately six viral respiratory illnesses per year, and other adults have two to three per year. Statistics gathered by the United States Public Health Service show that in the winter quarter of the year at least one half of all persons acquire a common cold; 20 per cent of persons have a similar illness in the summer quarter.

The prevalence of common colds is approximately 15 per cent of persons per week during the winter months. Surveillance of a group of student nurses during one winter revealed that individuals had common cold symptoms on 10 per cent of the days. Among industrial employees in the United States, common colds accounted for nearly one million person-years lost from work among an industrial force of 60 million. This amounts to one half of all absences and one quarter of the total time lost. Similarly, acute respiratory illness is highly prevalent among military forces, especially recruits, and is a major cause of disability.

Epidemiology. The common cold is spread by direct person-to-person contact. Under conditions of household association, 10 per cent of adults acquired the disease from an index case. From studies in volunteers, it was shown that some persons became infected and shed virus without having symptoms.

It is a common observation that an increase in the frequency of colds occurs in the winter. Sometimes this has been correlated with sharp changes in the temperature, humidity, or pollution of the air, but the popular belief that cold weather causes common colds cannot be substantiated from epidemiologic observations in the Arctic or tropics or from studies in volunteers. Exposure of volunteer subjects to cold did not activate latent respiratory viruses. The reason for the apparent relation between the season and common colds remains unclear. In the United States, it is usual to observe three waves of common colds per year. One occurs in the autumn a few weeks after the opening of schools, another in midwinter, and a third wave in the spring. The separate epidemics have usually been shown to be due to different viruses, each of which may have its own seasonal epidemiology.

Pathology. The pathologic changes in the mucous membranes of the respiratory passages are edema, hyperemia, transudation, and exudation. The severity of the cytopathic effect is related to the type and virulence of the infecting virus and the extent of infection. Picornaviruses (rhinoviruses and enteroviruses) have been observed to cause more metaplasia and degeneration in smears of exfoliated cells from the nasal turbinates than the myxoviruses. This generalization does not hold for infections of the lower respiratory tract. During the acute phase of infection, protein components of the respiratory secretions are altered, and serum globulins become more abundant. Abnormal soluble substances of cellular origin also can be found. The secretion is rich in glycoprotein. Repair is relatively rapid and, insofar as is known, occurs without residual pathologic damage. Recently, however, inquiry has been made regarding the role of repeated viral respiratory infections in the pathogenesis of later degenerative diseases, such as bronchitis and emphysema.

Viral infection induces swelling and some exudation, but it causes no significant change in the bacterial flora of the nasopharynx. When the inflammatory changes are of sufficient magnitude, channels connecting the paranasal sinuses and middle ear to the airway become obstructed. Suppuration can develop from secondary bacterial growth under these conditions.

Mechanisms of Infection and Immunity. Viruses from infected persons are airborne in droplet spray that is emitted during respiration, talking, sneezing, and coughing. Particles in the size range of 5 to 50 μ are probably the most infectious. Transmission can also be made by hand contact. The nasopharynx is the portal of infection. The incubation period is short, usually one to four days. Proliferation of virus can often be demonstrated within 24 hours after the infection of volunteers. Virus shedding usually precedes the onset of symptoms by one to two days, and the peak excretion occurs a few days later, during the symptomatic phase of the illness. Virus excretion ceases after several days, and symptoms decrease concomitantly. Later studies from the same person as well as attempts to recover viruses from well persons indicate that the carrier state after infection is transient, and the prevalence of asymptomatic chronic carriers is not great. Rhinoviruses have not been recovered from more than 1 to 2 per cent of well persons in populations where colds are occurring.

Host susceptibility or resistance to infection is determined primarily by the immunologic status resulting from recent previous infection with the same or related viruses. Some physiologic functions, such as menses and fatigue, and constitutional factors, such as an allergic diathesis and vasomotor rhinitis, are secondary determinants of host susceptibility. Emotional distress and overconcern with personal health increase symptoms, whereas stoical and ascetic personality traits decrease overt susceptibility. In controlled studies, chilling did not increase the susceptibility of volunteers to infection nor did ventilation with frigid air.

The nasal secretion is the first barrier against infection of the epithelial cells of the respiratory tract. In addition to the mechanical movement of mucus, the secretion contains glycoprotein inhibitors for some myxoviruses that can compete with cell receptors for the virus. Because virus union with inhibitors is reversible whereas cellular infection is not, these inhibitors probably do no more than delay and decrease the multiplicity of infection. Specific gamma globulins of low molecular weight, principally IgA and IgG, also are contained in nasal secretion. The former is primarily the result of local antibody production and plays an important role in immunity from prior infection. The activity of IgG is related to, but poorly correlated with, the height of specific antibody in the plasma. In one study, the gradient between nasal and serum antibody was 1 to 30. During the early stages of infection, before symptoms have begun, there is an easily demonstrable increase of globulins in nasal washings.

Infection with some respiratory viruses stimulates the local production of a protein or proteins referred to as interferon. Noninfected cells exposed to interferon are protected against viral infection. The mechanism offers an attractive thesis for the termination of infection and repair of the mucosa before specific antibody is formed.

A response in serum-neutralizing antibody against the infecting virus is not always sufficiently prompt or of great enough magnitude to permit diagnosis of the causative role of a virus in the infection. Specific immunity against illness from reinfection with the same strain of virus, however, is readily demonstrable in volunteers. This clinical immunity is apparent for a period of about two years after infection. Asymptomatic infections are not entirely prevented. Reinfection in the presence of serum antibody usually results in a modified illness. The specificity of the antibody and its concentration at the site of infection on the surface of the mucosa appear to be critical factors. Although serum antibody reduces infection and illness, it is possible for infection of the respiratory mucosa to occur. In such cases, the acute inflammatory response can be exaggerated, presumably as a result of the local antigen-antibody reaction or hypersensitivity of the persons resulting from earlier infection.

Clinical Manifestations. The common cold is in large part a subjective symptomatic diagnosis. The major symptoms for any individual tend to be repetitive, but they differ appreciably from person to person. Some persons have only "head colds," whereas others complain regularly of pharyngitis or cough as characteristic principal symptoms of their colds. The occurrence of symptoms that 100 young adults described as characteristic of a naturally acquired common cold is shown in Table 2.

The same symptoms occur in volunteers challenged with an infectious virus, and their time of occurrence and duration have been observed. Sneezing, headache, and malaise are the initial symptoms, followed by chilly sensations, sore throat, rhinorrhea, and nasal congestion. The chilly sensations may be associated with some lowering of oral temperature that is sometimes interpreted as the initiating cause in natural colds. Fever of any significant degree is absent. The constitutional symptoms are transient, lasting only one or two days. There is sometimes a lull for a day between the early symptoms and the development of characteristic nasopharyngeal symptoms of a full-blown cold. The dry or sore throat tends to recede as the cold progresses. Nasal discharge is the hallmark of the common cold. At the onset, the secretion is clear, watery, and often profuse. Later, secretions thicken, become mucopurulent, yellow-green, and tenacious. Nasal obstruction is at first an intermittent symptom associated with an exaggeration of the rhythmic physiologic turgescence of the nasal turbinates. Later, the turbinates become swollen and boggy,

TABLE 2. The Syndrome of the Common Cold

Symptoms	Frequency
Severe:	
Nasal discharge	100
Nasal obstruction	99
Moderate:	
Sore or dry throat	96
Malaise	81
Postnasal discharge	79
Headache	78
Cough	76
Mild:	
Sneezing	97
Feverishness	49
Chilliness	43
Burning eyes and mucous membranes	28
Muscle aching	22

encroaching on the nasal lumen, which contains increased secretions. These symptoms ordinarily run their course within a week. As the illness progresses, cough may appear as an increasingly prominent symptom, and persists for one to two weeks. It may be dry or productive of a variable amount of mucoid sputum.

Physical signs are limited to the nasopharynx, the surrounding sinuses, and middle ears. Usually, mild hyperemia, congestion, or both, are all that can be seen, and the deviation from normal may be insufficient to recognize as pathologic.

Hematologic changes have been observed in volunteers when the initial blood values and the time sequence of infection were known. Mild leukopenia with relative lymphocytosis is the initial response, followed after a day or two by a slight leukocytosis with some increase in polymorphonuclear leukocytes. A fall in the hematocrit and rise in the erythrocyte sedimentation rate can also occur. Although the aforementioned changes can be related to the infection in volunteers, their deviation from normal is not great enough to be useful in isolated cases.

Complications of a cold are usually bacterial in origin. They are infrequent and consist of suppuration in the nasopharynx and its contiguous passages. Serous effusion, however, may appear in the middle ear and perhaps in the sinuses.

Diagnosis. The diagnosis of a common cold is made on the basis of history and symptoms. At the peak of the illness, signs of the infection also are apparent. Examination is important for the recognition or exclusion of illnesses of more severe nature that patients may be prone to designate as a cold. The differential diagnosis includes prodromes of other infections and infectious, vascular, allergic, and neoplastic processes in the nose, pharynx, sinuses, or ears. Other serious diseases, such as bacterial endocarditis, tuberculosis, bronchitis, bronchiectasis, and lung abscess have been called "chest colds" because of lack of characteristic symptoms and incomplete examination of the patient by a physician. The diagnosis of common cold therefore should be avoided as a designation for a broad category of respiratory symptoms of diverse causes.

The clinical symptoms do not permit discrimination with regard to the specific viral cause of a cold. The overlap in the symptoms produced by infection with any one of many viruses that cause the common cold is so great as to preclude more than a judgment regarding the general group of viruses to which the etiologic agent might belong. Under the controlled conditions of studies in volunteers, different viruses cause appreciably different syndromes. For each, the clinical manifestations are also related to the dose, size of particle inhaled, and modifications by host factors. The diagnosis of the specific viral cause of a common cold is based on laboratory procedures.

Treatment and Prevention. In considering treatment and prevention of the common cold, the following factors that have been discussed must be kept in mind: (1) The number of antigenically distinct viruses that cause the common cold is large. (2) Except for the time and economic loss, the infection is benign and the duration of severe symptoms is brief. (3) Viral infection does not significantly change the bacterial flora of the nasopharynx, and bacterial complications are infrequent. (4) Infection initiates production of interferon and antibodies that naturally limit the infection. (5) Specific immunity to illness with the same virus exists for one to two years after infection. (6) Reinfection can occur in the presence of antibody in the plasma.

At present there are no antimicrobial drugs of practical effectiveness in man against the viruses responsible for the common cold; hence the use of such drugs is not recommended. Carefully controlled trials with unlicensed drugs in volunteers indicate that effective chemoprophylaxis against the common cold is possible. The development of such products could initiate a more optimistic position regarding drug treatment. Suppurative complications are caused by obstruction more often than by the virulence of local bacteria. Routine antibacterial chemoprophylaxis selects resistant bacterial strains and does not prevent suppurative complications.

Supportive treatment is desirable and helpful. Additional rest in bed, warm clothing, and prevention of chilling increase the patient's comfort. If ventilatory insufficiency, stridor, and anoxemia that may accompany a cold are present, steam inhalation, a decongestant, a bronchodilator, or an expectorant may be indicated. Postural changes can help in the drainage of secretions and the raising of sputum. Because of the diverse causes and syndromes, there is no one regimen to be recommended. Aspirin in a dose of 0.6 gram for an adult or 10 mg per kilogram of body weight for children can reduce headache and malaise. However, it increases virus shedding and should generally be avoided. Oral phenylpropanolamine hydrochloride (15 to 50 mg), inhalation of hexamine vapor, or nose drops with 0.5 per cent ephedrine or phenylephrine shrink the vascular bed of the mucosa and provide temporary nasal decongestion. Nose drops in any oily vehicle should be avoided, and potent vasoconstrictors with transient action and physiologic rebound, such as epinephrine, are not desirable. Increased fluids or hard candy lozenges may be adequate for control of coughing. Cough syrups, such as elixir of terpin hydrate with codeine (64 mg per 30 ml), are more effective if necessary. Antihistamines have no effect on the common cold, except that a person prone to severe inhalant allergy may experience some reduction in the volume of nasal secretion. Large doses of vitamin C (ascorbic acid) have no significant protective effect against viral infections causing the common cold and no appreciable inhibitory effect on rhinoviral colds. Excessive amounts which have been recommended are rapidly excreted in the urine and can cause urinary symptoms owing to the increased acidity of the urine. The numerous compounded remedies, including those with vitamins, bioflavonoids, quinine, alkalinizers, multiple analgesics, antihistamines, decongestants, and tranquilizers, are developed for sales profit in a large market of uninformed and uncritical people and are not for the benefit of the patient or his physician. Their widespread and repeated use invariably leads to cases of fatal hematologic disorders, eruptive or exfoliative dermatitis, and anaphylaxis or other severe idiosyncratic reaction.

Prevention of common colds by quarantine or isolation of cases is without effect because of the number of infected but asymptomatic persons and because virus excretion usually precedes the symptoms. The hygienic collection and disposal of respiratory secretions to reduce airborne dissemination from coughing and sneezing should be encouraged as common courtesies. Interruption of the airborne phase of transmission by increasing space, higher rates of air ventilation, alterations in temperature and humidity, vaporization of disinfectants, and ultraviolet irradiation of overhead air all have been given trials without clearly significant results.

Vaccines for protection against the common cold are not available. Former "cold vaccines" were bacterial suspensions and have no basis for effectiveness. The large number of antigenically distinct viruses augurs numerous difficulties in the production of an effective vaccine. Nevertheless, promising vaccines are being developed for specific groups of viruses.

Andrewes, C. H.: Rhinoviruses and common cold. Ann. Rev. Med., 17:361, 1966.

Badger, G. F., Dingle, J. H., Feller, A. E., Hodges, R. G., Jordan, W. S., Jr., and Rammelkamp, C. H., Jr.: A study of illness in a group of Cleveland families. II. Incidence of the common respiratory diseases. Am. J. Hyg., 58:31, 1953.

Hendley, J. O., Fishburne, H. B., and Gwaltney, J. M., Jr.: Coronavirus infections in working adults: Eight-year study with 229E and OC43. Am. Rev. Respir. Dis., 105:805, 1972.

Jackson, G. G., Dowling, H. F., Anderson, T. O., Riff, L., Saporta, J., and Turck, M.: Susceptibility and immunity to common upper respiratory viral infections—the common cold. Ann. Intern. Med., 53:719, 1960.

Jackson, G. G., Dowling, H. F., Spiesman, I. G., and Boand, A. V.: Transmission of the common cold to volunteers under controlled conditions. I. The common cold as a clinical entity. Arch. Intern. Med., 101:267, 1958.

Johnson, K. M., et al.: Role of enteroviruses in respiratory diseases. Am. Rev. Respir. Dis., 88:240, 1963.

Paul, J. H., and Freese, H. L.: An epidemiological and bacteriological study of the "common cold" in an isolated arctic community (Spitzbergen). Am. J. Hyg., 17:517, 1933.

Tyrrell, D. A. J.: Common Colds and Related Diseases. Baltimore, Williams & Wilkins Company, 1965.

WHO Technical Report Series, No. 408: Respiratory Viruses. Geneva, 1969.

112. RHINOVIRAL RESPIRATORY DISEASE

George Gee Jackson

Etiology. For many decades, attempts were made to isolate the common cold virus. On some occasions, propagation of infectious material was accomplished for a brief period, but the viruses could not be sustained. In 1954, the virus known as 2060 and the closely related JH strain were isolated from adults with acute coryza. These viruses were believed to be enteroviruses and were designated echovirus 28. Soon thereafter, several different workers isolated similar viruses that were designated in the early literature as Salisbury agents, ERC viruses, entero-like viruses, coryzaviruses, muriviruses, and unclassified common cold viruses. Because of common biologic properties, these are all designated now as rhinoviruses. There are approximately 90 different serotypes of rhinoviruses capable of infecting man. They comprise a subclass in the family of picornaviruses, which also includes the coxsackie-, polio-, entero- and echoviruses. These are all small viruses (10 to 30 mμ) of the ribonucleic acid type that are not inactivated by ether. The acid lability (pH 3) of rhinoviruses is probably the reason for their absence from the intestine, and is the major property that distinguishes them from enteroviruses. Rhinoviruses characteristically grow best in tissue cultures held at a reduced temperature (33° C) similar to that found in the nose of man.

Prevalence and Epidemiology. It is likely that rhinoviruses infect persons in all countries and climates. Nearly all adults have evidence of earlier infection with several different serotypes of rhinoviruses. Similar viruses have been recovered from cattle, but transfer from other animals to man has not been shown. In human infections, some serotypes may occur annually, but the occurrence of different serotypes has been haphazard. About 15 per cent of a young adult population will have neutralizing antibody against any one serotype. Infection with rhinoviruses is more prevalent among adults than among children. In persons with colds, one third of adults and 10 to 15 per cent of children have had rhinovirus recovered from the nasal secretion. Infection with these viruses is relatively more frequent in summer, fall, and spring than in midwinter. Rhinoviruses have been recovered in 1 to 3 per cent of well adults observed during epidemic disease. Infection is believed to occur by the airborne route, but transmission can also occur by hand transfer from contaminated surfaces.

Clinical Manifestations and Diagnosis. Rhinovirus infections begin with headache, malaise, chilliness, a dry, scratchy sore throat, and burning nasal membranes and eyes. Nasal discharge and obstruction of the upper air passages rapidly become the dominant symptoms. Cough is a variable and later symptom. Fever is absent or of slight degree and transient. No pharyngeal exudate is observed, but cervical adenopathy can occur. In children, rhinoviruses sometimes cause croup or lower respiratory tract disease. Adults occasionally develop symptoms of lower respiratory disease, and sensitive tests of bronchial clearance are abnormal even if lower respiratory symptoms are minimal or absent. The incubation period is one to three days, and the course of illness is about one week. Rhinovirus appears in the nasal secretion a day or two before the onset of nasal symptoms, and is shed during the period of illness. The pathologic findings and pathogenesis are described in Ch. 111. A rise in neutralizing antibody in the convalescent serum occurs in only about one half of the infections.

Treatment. There is no specific treatment directed against propagation of the rhinovirus. Supportive measures are those given under treatment of the common cold. Quarantine is not necessary. Interferon produced by rhinovirus infection may be a principal factor in the amelioration of the disease. Recently, pretreatment of volunteers by topical administration of high doses of interferon obtained from human leukocytes was shown to reduce infection and illness. Also, the prior administration of a substituted propanediamine, which induces interferon, was effective in reducing infection, illness, and virus shedding. Although these products are not currently available, both are under development. They are attractive because interferon inhibits rhinoviruses without regard to serotype. In similar studies, vitamin C (ascorbic acid) in doses of 3 grams per day by mouth failed to prevent infection and illness. No polyvalent vaccine is available, but experimental vaccines have been effective against a single type of rhinovirus. The large number of distinct serotypes is discouraging to the prospects of developing an effective vaccine unless strains that cause heterotypic responses are found. Immunity to reinfection is quite specific and probably lasts only several months to two years after most infections, although detectable serum antibody may persist longer.

Beem, M.: Rhinovirus infections in nursery school children. J. Pediat., 74:818, 1969.

Bloom, H. H., Forsyth, B. R., Johnson, K. M., and Chanock, R. M.: Relationship of rhinovirus infection to mild upper respiratory disease. J.A.M.A., 186:38, 1963.

Dick, E. C., Blumer, C. R., and Evans, A. S.: Epidemiology of infections with rhinovirus types 43 and 55 in a group of University of Wisconsin student families. Am. J. Epidemiol., 86:386, 1967.

Douglas, R. G., Jr.: Pathogenesis of rhinovirus common colds in human volunteers. Ann. Otol. Rhinol. Laryngol., 79:563, 1970.

Douglas, R. G., Jr., Lindgren, K. M., and Couch, R. B.: Exposure to cold environment and rhinovirus common cold. Failure to demonstrate effect. N. Engl. J. Med., 279:742, 1968.

George, R. B., and Mogabgab, W. J.: Atypical pneumonia in young men with rhinovirus infections. Ann. Intern. Med., 71:1073, 1969.

Hendley, J. O., Gwaltney, J. M., Jr., and Jordan, W. S., Jr.: Rhinovirus infection in an industrial population. IV. Infection within families of employees during two fall peaks of respiratory illness. Am. J. Epidemiol., 89:184, 1969.

Kawana, R., Yoshida, S., Matsumato, I., Kaneko, M., and Wako, H.: Rhinovirus isolated from Japanese children with common cold. Jap. J. Microbiol., 10:127, 1966.

Monto, A. S., and Johnson, K. M.: A community study of respiratory infections in the tropics. II. The spread of six rhinovirus isolates within the community. Am. J. Epidemiol., 88:55, 1968.

Person, D. A., and Herrmann, E. C.: Experiences in laboratory diagnosis of rhinovirus infections in routine medical practice. Mayo Clinic Proc., 45:517, 1970.

Scott, E. J., Grist, N. R., and Eadie, M. B.: Rhinovirus infections in chronic bronchitis: Isolation of eight possibly new rhinovirus serotypes. J. Med. Microbiol., 1:109, 1968.

113. VIRAL PHARYNGITIS, LARYNGITIS, CROUP, AND BRONCHITIS

George Gee Jackson

The same viruses that cause the common cold also cause other syndromes of respiratory illness. Pharyngitis, laryngitis, croup, or bronchitis may be even more characteristic of infection with some of the viruses than acute afebrile coryza. This clinical classification of the illnesses according to the anatomic site of predominant symptoms is the principal (although unreliable) way the physician has of differentiating diseases of different etiology. The mildest infections are those limited to the upper respiratory tract. As progressively more caudal sites are involved, the infections become more severe and cause more constitutional symptoms. *Acute rhinitis* (the common cold) and *nonexudative pharyngitis* nearly always occur without fever, whereas *exudative viral pharyngitis,* which is relatively uncommon among civilians, is a febrile illness. When adenovirus is the cause, *conjunctivitis* is very likely to be a prominent part of the syndrome. With viruses that cause pharyngitis the inflammation may extend into the eustachian tubes and cause *primary* or *secondary otitis media* and *sinusitis.* The lymphoid hyperplasia can include cervical adenitis. *Croup* is a distinctive clinical syndrome resulting from involvement of the larynx with resultant edema and stridor. It is a relatively common manifestation of respiratory viral infection in children. The classes of viruses most often causing croup are the myxoviruses and parainfluenza viruses. Bronchitis, bronchiolitis, and bronchopneumonia are severe manifestations of viral respiratory infection. They cause fever, respiratory difficulties, and symptoms that often require hospitalization of the patient. The course may be quite abrupt, including sudden unexpected death. The occurrence of these different clinical syndromes resulting from infection with some of the viruses responsible for the common respiratory infections is indicated in Table 3. Further details about the illnesses and their management are given in the discussions of the specific viruses.

The spectrum of diseases is caused not only by the fact that viruses are relatively nonspecific in the clinical syndrome produced, but also because the age and status

TABLE 3. Spectrum and Relative Importance of Clinical Syndromes Caused by Different Respiratory Viruses

Virus	Coryza	Pharyngitis (Conjunctivitis) (Otitis)	Croup	Bronchitis	Pneumonia or Systemic Disease
Influenza A, B	++			++	++++
Influenza C	++			+	
Parainfluenza 1, 3	+++	++	+++	+	+++
Parainfluenza 2	+		++++		
Parainfluenza 4	++++	+			
Respiratory syncytial	+++		++	++++	+
Coronavirus	++++	+		+	
Reovirus 1	+				
Adenovirus 1, 2, 5	+	++			+
Adenovirus 3, 4, 7, 14, 21	++	++++		+	+
Coxsackievirus A 2, 3, 4, 6, 8, 10	+	++++	+		++
A 21, 24	++++	+			
Coxsackievirus B 2, 3, 4, 5	+	+	+	+	++++
Echovirus 7, 8, 11, 15, 19, 20 (others rarely)	++	++	+		++
Rhinoviruses	++++	+		+	
Mycoplasma		+			+++

of individuals influence the site and severity of the symptoms. In infants and children, the airway is smaller and the amount of lymphoid tissue is relatively greater than in adults. In the former, croup and bronchitis are more common manifestations of infection with the same viruses that may cause only coryza or pharyngitis in adults. A stronger effect on the amelioration of viral respiratory illness, however, is exerted by the immunologic responses of the host to previous infections.

FACTORS RELATED TO THE MANIFESTATIONS AND PREVALENCE OF VIRAL RESPIRATORY INFECTIONS

The initial infection with a virus may be resolved without establishing solid immunity to reinfection, or if immunity is established, it may be transient. The capacity of many of the respiratory viruses to cause reinfection has now been established. Reinfection in a partially immune host causes different illnesses from the initial infection. Usually the disease is milder on successive reinfections, but the dose of virus, manner of infection, season, presence of dual infection, and other factors may be of more importance. Sometimes, reinfection in the presence of antibody appears to increase the tissue response and exaggerate the symptoms.

In order for a viral infection to maintain a high prevalence of infection, one or more of several conditions is required. Some of these are virologic; others are epidemiologic or immunologic, as exemplified in Table 4. All these mechanisms are found in the case of one or another of the different viruses that cause common respiratory infections. The result is that we experience a continual endemic and cyclic epidemics of viral respiratory disease, with a large number of viruses infecting various sites of the respiratory tree and producing different anatomically designated clinical syndromes. The level of disease is exaggerated by new types of viruses or new exposures of susceptible hosts and is moderated by a progressive buildup of herd immunity developed by aging, naturally acquired infections, and vaccines. Likewise, the clinical syndrome is affected by these viral, epidemiologic, and host conditions. An appreciation of these factors is essential to the understanding of the problem of viral respiratory infections, their treatment, and control.

TABLE 4. Mechanisms That Contribute to the High Prevalence of Viral Respiratory Infection

Mutagenic or recombinant production of new types:
Influenza A, B
Multiple antigenically distinct types simultaneously present:
Rhinoviruses
Virus shedding before recognition of disease (or with asymptomatic infections):
Rhinoviruses, parainfluenza, influenza
Social congregation of infected and uninfected persons:
Rhinoviruses, adenoviruses
Latent infections:
Adenovirus 1, 2, 5, 6; herpes simplex
Inadequate antibody response from infection (children):
Respiratory syncytial, rhinoviruses
Reinfection in the presence of circulating antibody:
Parainfluenza 3, 1; respiratory syncytial
Transient specific immunity from infection or vaccine:
Rhinoviruses, influenza
Lasting immunity but recurrent epidemic disease among susceptibles:
Adenovirus 4, 7; measles

Chanock, R. M., and Parrott, R. H.: Acute respiratory disease in infancy and childhood: Present understanding and prospects for prevention. Pediatrics, 36:21, 1965.
Ferris, J. A. J., Aherne, W. A., Locke, W. S., McQuillin, J., and Gardner, P. S.: Sudden and unexpected deaths in infants: Histology and virology. Br. Med. J., 2:439, 1973.
Foy, H. M., Cooney, M. K., and Maletzky, A. J.: Incidence and etiology of pneumonia, croup, and bronchiolitis in preschool children belonging to a prepaid medical care group over a four-year period. Am. J. Epidemiol., 97:80, 1973.
Glezen, W. P., and Denny, F. W.: Epidemiology of acute lower respiratory disease in children. N. Engl. J. Med., 288:498, 1973.
Hope-Simpson, R. E., and Higgins, P. G.: A respiratory virus study in Great Britain: Review and evaluation. Prog. Med. Virol., 11:354, 1969.
Kevy, S. V.: Current concepts: Croup. N. Engl. J. Med., 270:464, 1964.
Monto, A. S., and Cavallaro, J. J.: The Tecumseh study of respiratory illness. I. Plan of study and observations on syndromes of acute respiratory disease. Am. J. Epidemiol., 94:269, 1971.
Mufson, M. A., Webb, P. A., Kennedy, H., Gill, V., and Chanock, R. M.: Etiology of upper respiratory tract illnesses among civilian adults. J.A.M.A., 195:1, 1966.

114. ADENOVIRAL INFECTIONS

George Gee Jackson

Definition and Etiology. The adenoviruses comprise a distinct group of viruses of the deoxyribose nucleic acid variety. The viral particle has a coat (capsid) consisting of 254 capsomeres arranged in an icosohedron, which is a structure with 20 equilateral triangular faces; it is 60 to 90 nm in size. Most of the capsomeres (240) are six sided, called hexons; the other 12, at the junctions of the triangles are five sided, called pentons. The hexons have a common group-specific antigen characteristic of all adenoviruses. Each type has specific hexon and penton antigens. There are more than 31 specific serotypes among the strains of human origin. Only a few of them cause infections of the respiratory tract. The common types involved are 1, 2, 3, 4, 5, and 7. Types 14 and 21 also have caused acute respiratory illness. Type 8 is the principal cause of epidemic keratoconjunctivitis.

Some early isolates were recovered from surgically removed adenoids grown as tissue culture explants. These were reported as adenoidal degenerative or AD agents. The first strains from respiratory illnesses were designated RI agents. A later name, used briefly, was adenoidal-pharyngeal-conjunctival or APC agents. All the strains are now included under the term adenoviruses.

Incidence and Prevalence. Adenoviruses types 1, 2, and 5 infect virtually all persons early in childhood. They have been associated with febrile pharyngitis, with lower respiratory disease (sometimes fatal), and with gastrointestinal symptoms in infants. In older children and adolescents, adenoviruses, predominantly types 3 and 7 in the United States and 3, 4, 7, 14 and 21 in Europe, cause about 5 per cent of the viral respiratory illnesses. The incidence among college students may be as great as 8 per cent. At military recruit camps, infection with adenovirus types 4 and 7 is highly prevalent. It is often the predominant cause of respiratory illness, and 70 to 80 per cent of all incoming recruits become infected. Among civilian adults, adenoviruses cause only 1 to 3 per cent of respiratory illness.

Epidemiology. Adenoviruses occur in all parts of the

world. Man is the principal reservoir of infection. Many species of animals also are infected with adenoviruses, but these are of different serotypes, and cross-infection between man and animals either does not occur or is rare. Transmission is by person-to-person contact, but spread occurs only when the contact with an infected person is close or prolonged. The incubation period is from three to eight days. Swimming pools have been an effective vehicle for the transmission of adenovirus conjunctivitis. Such epidemics occur in the summer and have been referred to as Greeley disease and pseudomembranous conjunctivitis. As noted above, military inductees often become infected with adenoviruses 4 or 7 in the first few weeks in training and develop the syndrome called acute respiratory disease (ARD) of recruits. Season affects the transmission and symptoms of infection, with incidence of clinical disease being highest in the autumn and winter. Asymptomatic enteric infections are common.

Pathogenic Mechanisms. During the acute infection and for a period of one to three weeks, virus is excreted in the respiratory secretions or in those of the eye, or in both. A high proportion of infected persons have virus in the stool, which may be a source for the spread of infection. Viruria also has been observed during the acute respiratory illness. Adenoviruses replicate in the nucleus of the cell and, when the concentration is high, form crystals of virus. The nuclear chromatin becomes clumped, and the cells may undergo lysis. A most remarkable aspect of adenoviral infections with types 1, 2, 3, and 5 is the capacity of the virus to persist as a latent infection in lymphoid tissue for years after the initial infection. Fifty to 90 per cent of surgically removed adenoids yield adenovirus of one of these types. Whether this provides a source for infection of others or any harm to the host is unknown.

Some of the adenoviruses are capable of producing tumors when injected into newborn hamsters. Among the respiratory strains, some isolates of type 7 and type 3 have been oncogenic in baby hamsters. These studies on the tumorigenicity of adenoviruses also have shown the capacity of adenoviruses to combine within the same envelope (capsid) the oncogenic genome of some other tumor-producing viruses of DNA type, specifically the simian virus, SV-40. Thus under defined experimental conditions, adenoviruses can be oncogenic in their own right or act as a carrier for oncogenic material. There is no evidence that these properties give the virus any oncogenic capacity in man, but the phenomena are of basic biologic importance.

Some adenoviruses have an associated smaller virus (AAV). It is a defective DNA virus which can multiply only in the presence of adenoviruses. The significance of AAV in the pathogenesis of adenoviral infections is not known.

Clinical Manifestations and Differential Diagnosis. Different clinical syndromes produced by adenoviral infections in older children and adults are characteristic. Fever and pharyngitis are the hallmarks; catarrhal otitis occurs frequently, cervical adenopathy is common, conjunctivitis may be present, and a few patients develop pneumonia. The syndromes have been given descriptive names, as follows: (1) acute febrile pharyngitis, (2) nonstreptococcal exudative pharyngitis, (3) acute respiratory disease of recruits, (4) pharyngoconjunctival fever, and (5) adenoviral pneumonia. Any single type of virus among those that cause natural respiratory infections in man can produce the entire spectrum of these clinical manifestations and also the common cold. The age of the patient and the route of inoculation are important. In newborn infants, giant cell pneumonia, myocarditis, and encephalitis have been described. In young children, mesenteric adenitis and intussusception have been reported. Infection with adenovirus types 1, 2, 5, and 6 may occur in the preschool child without any overt illness, whereas type 7 causes severe illness in this age group, with 5 per cent fatality. The former types infect nearly all children, but type 7 infections are infrequent. The common adenoviruses have been associated in a possible interrelated role with *H. pertussis* in whooping cough. Type 11 has been found as a cause of acute hemorrhagic cystitis in children (girls).

Conjunctivitis, when present, is an acute follicular lesion, often unilateral, with marked erythema, suffusion, and narrowing of the palpebral fissure. Keratoconjunctivitis, caused by adenovirus type 8, is a serious infection of the eye with corneal infiltrates; it rarely occurs in pharyngoconjunctival fever. Pharyngeal exudate, if present, is more likely to appear on the pharyngeal wall than as follicular tonsillitis. Cervical lymph nodes are enlarged and firm but less tender than with streptococcal infections. A macular rash that is difficult to distinguish from rubella has been described in a few cases. The leukocyte count is normal or slightly elevated. A prompt antibody response usually accompanies the infection. It can be measured in the serum by complement fixation or virus neutralization tests.

Treatment and Prevention. Treatment is supportive and with few exceptions recovery occurs without sequelae, excluding those of type 8 keratoconjunctivitis. Immunity to reinfection is demonstrable, but second infections have been observed with types 1, 2, 3, and 5. These types cause latent infections, and it is possible that later episodes represent an activation or recrudescence of the latent infection. Reinfection, if it occurs, usually causes mild illness.

Vaccine administration can elicit protective antibody and effectively prevent specific adenovirus infections. Live, enteric-coated, oral adenovirus vaccines of types 4 and 7 have been extensively evaluated in military recruits at stations where the incidence of infection and disease is high. Given prophylactically, it stimulates antibody, prevents specific adenovirus illness, and reduces pharyngeal infection after natural exposure by about two thirds. In epidemic situations mass immunization with live virus vaccine promptly interrupts the epidemic. Use of the vaccine is not recommended for civilians because of the low incidence and sporadic occurrence of infection with adenovirus types 4 and 7 among them.

No adenovirus vaccines are available commercially.

Becroft, D. M.: Bronchiolitis obliterans, bronchiectasis, and other sequelae of adenovirus type 21 infection in young children. J. Clin. Pathol., 24:72, 1971.

Bell, J. A., Rowe, W. T., Engler, J. I., Parrott, R. H., and Huebner, R. J.: Pharyngoconjunctival fever. Epidemiological studies of a recently recognized disease entity. J.A.M.A., 157:1083, 1955.

Brandt, C. D., Kim, H. W., Vargosko, A. J., Jefferies, B. C., Arrobio, J. O., Rindge, B., Parrott, R. H., and Chanock, R. M.: Infections in 18,000 infants and children in a controlled study of respiratory tract disease. I. Adenovirus pathogenicity in relation to serologic type and illness syndrome. Am. J. Epidemiol., 90:484, 1969.

Chou, S. M., Roos, R., Burrell, R., and Gutmann, L.: Subacute focal adenovirus encephalitis. J. Neuropathol. Exp. Neurol., 32:34, 1973.

Dudding, B. A., Top, F. H., Jr., Winter, P. E., Buescher, E. L., Lamson, T. H., and Leibovitz, A.: Acute respiratory disease in military trainees. The adenovirus surveillance program, 1966–1971. Am. J. Epidemiol., 97:187, 1973.

Fox, J. P., Brandt, C. D., Wasserman, F. E., Hall, C. E., Spigland, I., Kogon, A., and Elveback, L. R.: The virus watch program: A continuing surveillance of viral infections in metropolitan New York families. VI. Observations of adenovirus infections: Virus excretion patterns, antibody response, efficiency of surveillance, patterns of infection, and relation to illness. Am. J. Epidemiol., 89:25, 1969.

Hamory, B. H., Couch, R. B., Douglas, R. G., Jr., Black, S. H., and Knight, V.: Characterization of the infectious unit for man of two respiratory viruses. Proc. Soc. Exp. Biol. Med., 139:890, 1972.

Klenk, E. L., Gaultney, J. V., and Bass, J. W.: Bacteriologically proved pertussis and adenovirus infection. Possible association. Am. J. Dis. Child., 124:203, 1972.

Levy, J. L., Jr.: Etiology of "idiopathic" intussusception in infants. South. Med. J., 63:642, 1970.

Manalo, D., Mufson, M. A., Zallar, L. M., and Mankad, V. N.: Adenovirus infection in acute hemorrhagic cystitis. A study in 25 children. Am. J. Dis. Child., 121:281, 1971.

McCormick, D. P., Wenzel, R. P., Davies, J. A., and Beam, W. E., Jr.: Nasal secretion protein responses in patients with wild-type adenovirus disease. Infect. Immun., 6:282, 1972.

115. RESPIRATORY SYNCYTIAL VIRAL DISEASE

George Gee Jackson

Definition and Etiology. Infection with respiratory syncytial virus (RS) causes epidemic acute respiratory disease. The illnesses are rather acute in onset and may be mild or severe. Since its recognition in 1956 as an infection of man, RS has produced regular epidemics of influenza-like respiratory disease.

Respiratory syncytial virus is a paramyxovirus that resembles influenza and parainfluenza viruses in its structure and many biologic characteristics. It is serologically distinct from them, does not agglutinate erythrocytes as they do, and does not cause lesions in eggs or common laboratory animals. The virus was first isolated from chimpanzees and was designated chimpanzee coryza agent (CCA). The name respiratory syncytial virus is descriptive of the cytopathic effect of the virus in infected tissue cultures. Only one type of the virus is known; some isolates have shown minor differences when tested against specific immune serum, but these appear clinically insignificant with regard to man.

Epidemiology. Respiratory syncytial virus has been recovered at several locations in the United States and elsewhere; it is likely that it has worldwide distribution. The epidemiologic pattern of infection lies somewhere between the epidemicity of influenza A and the endemicity of the parainfluenza viruses. Usually there are sharp, well defined limits to each epidemic. In the interepidemic period, the virus is detected much less frequently, but RS virus has been isolated from illnesses in every month of the year. Epidemics recur at intervals of 8 to 16 months. These have appeared simultaneously in geographically widely separated locations. During an epidemic, a large proportion of the population may experience infection, even persons who have had prior infection and have residual serum antibody. The pattern of the epidemic spread is characteristic of airborne or direct contact transmission. The incubation period is three to seven days.

Incidence and Prevalence. The high prevalence of infection is indicated by the fact that 70 per cent of infants at birth have appreciable amounts of maternal antibody against RS virus. During the first few months of life this declines, and between 3 and 12 months about 35 per cent develop antibody as a result of natural infection. By five years of age, 95 per cent of children have been infected. The incidence of infection with RS virus varies because of its epidemicity, but it makes a significant contribution in the production of serious respiratory diseases of children. Among hospitalized pediatric cases, RS infection has been found to be etiologic in approximately 20 per cent. In this respect, it ranks ahead of the parainfluenza viruses or adenoviruses and is also more prevalent than influenza. In the first year of life, RS virus is the single most frequent clinical infection causing lower respiratory illness and is a major cause of death in this age group. Among adults, the incidence is less well documented because of the milder nature of the disease, but an increase in hospital admission of adults with lower respiratory disease occurs during periods of RS virus infection.

Pathogenesis. Infection causes inflammation of the respiratory mucosa with a tendency for necrotizing bronchiolitis, bronchiolar obstruction, focal atelectasis, and patchy pneumonia. Infants and adults with chronic bronchopulmonary disease are especially at risk of fatal or severe illness. Bacterial pneumonia can be a complication. The annual epidemiologic recurrences of disease, the reisolation of virus from the same children in successive years, and investigations in adult volunteers have all emphasized the importance of reinfections with respiratory syncytial virus. The pathogenesis of the reinfections is not antigenic differences among strains. The studies in volunteers show convincingly that the presence in the serum of neutralizing antibody against the challenge strain does not prevent reinfection or illness. The high prevalence and importance of RS virus in the causation of respiratory disease appears to reside in this capacity to produce reinfections with clinical symptoms.

Clinical Manifestations. Fever and bronchiolitis are the characteristics of infection in children. Rhinitis and pharyngitis are usually present. Otitis may occur. In one study, pneumonia was shown roentgenographically in more than two thirds of the cases. Croup may develop, but it is relatively infrequent. The average maximal temperature is 39° C, but in individual patients it may reach 40.5° C. Ordinarily, fever lasts for three days. Dyspnea, cough, and wheezing are obvious symptoms. Tachypnea, rhonchi, and crepitant rales are present on examination. A few of the patients are cyanotic. The leukocyte count is elevated to between 10,000 and 20,000 per cubic millimeter in many cases. This clinical syndrome cannot be distinguished with certainty from epidemic influenza. Ordinarily, there is more rhinitis, and the onset is less abrupt. A fatality rate of 2.5 per cent has been estimated for hospitalized patients. Sudden death of infants and young children in their cribs at home after mild respiratory symptoms has been suspected by epidemiologic association to be of RS etiology.

In about two thirds of the documented cases there is a less severe syndrome, which has been diagnosed in outpatient clinics. These patients have fever, but they have fewer constitutional symptoms than those who are hospitalized. Rhinitis and pharyngitis are relatively more prominent. Cough is frequent, but rales and rhonchi are scarce.

Among adults with prechallenge antibody, the clinical manifestation of infection is acute coryza. At least, this is the conclusion reached from studies in volunteers and by isolation of RS virus from patients with common colds. An analysis of proved cases in adults admitted to a hospital in one study, however, indicated that persons with chronic bronchitis (one half of the cases studied) had an acute exacerbation of bronchitis; in one fourth of them infection caused bronchopneumonia, and in one fourth it produced the influenza syndrome with severe constitutional symptoms. Thus the entire spectrum of viral respiratory illness is produced in adults by RS virus.

Diagnosis. The suspicion of RS virus infection is based upon clinical and epidemiologic observations. The diagnosis can be made by virus isolation from the respiratory secretions or by serologic tests. Respiratory syncytial virus is recovered by the inoculation of secretions into cultures of a human epithelial cell line or diploid cell strain. The specimens must be fresh or collected and frozen in a stabilizing medium, because of the extreme sensitivity of the virus to freezing and thawing. Several days are required before the virus becomes apparent in the tissue culture and can be identified; hence virus isolation is not of immediate value in the diagnosis of an ill patient. The use of specific immunofluorescent antibody to recognize viral antigens in nasopharyngeal secretions has been recommended for rapid diagnosis.

Serodiagnosis can be made by either complement-fixation (CF) or neutralization tests, using paired sera collected as early as possible after the onset of illness and again after two to three weeks. A fourfold or greater rise in the serum antibody titer is regarded as diagnostic of infection.

Treatment and Prevention. Careful assessment of respiratory competence, close observation, and supportive care are important, especially in children, in view of the relative severity of the involvement of the lower respiratory tract. Anticipation of the possible need for tracheostomy (to reduce respiratory dead air space and assist in the removal of secretions) and mechanical assistance with ventilation in occasional patients is wise. Antimicrobial drugs have no effect on the RS virus or on the outcome of the usual infection. Isolation of the patient from other susceptible contacts should be done during hospitalization, but the spread of infection in the community is not controlled by isolation procedures.

The annual occurrence of epidemic infection and the clear demonstration of reinfections, often with equally severe second episodes, might suggest that immunoprophylaxis would have little effect on the infection. On the other hand, the mildness and lower frequency of infections in adults are circumstantial support for the development of immunity. The antigens of the RS virus are labile and poorly antigenic. Use of investigational inactivated vaccine that produced nonprotective levels of serum antibody augmented the clinical severity and fatality of subsequent infection. Similarly, the high fatality among infected infants in the first few months of life, when maternal antibody is demonstrable, suggests that passively acquired antibody may have a paradoxical aggravating effect. Attenuated, temperature-sensitive mutants that can be given as live virus vaccines into the respiratory passages are being developed. Perhaps the larger amount of viral antigen and repeated doses that can be given in this way will induce protection.

Beem, M.: Repeated infections with respiratory syncytial virus. J. Immunol., 98:1115, 1967.

Berglund, B.: Respiratory syncytial virus infections in families. A study of family members of children hospitalized for acute respiratory disease. Acta Paediatr. Scand., 56:395, 1967.

Cradock-Watson, J. E., McQuillin, J., and Gardner, P. S.: Rapid diagnosis of respiratory syncytial virus infection in children by the immunofluorescent technique. J. Clin. Pathol., 24:308, 1971.

Fransen, H., Sterner, G., Forsgren, M., Heigl, Z., Wolontis, S., Svedmyr, A., and Tunevall, G.: Acute lower respiratory illness in elderly patients with respiratory syncytial virus infection. Acta Med. Scand., 182:323, 1967.

Hilleman, M. R.: Respiratory syncytial virus. Am. Rev. Respir. Dis., 88:181, 1963.

Hornsleth, A., and Volkeit, M.: The incidence of complement-fixing antibodies to the respiratory syncytial virus in sera from Danish population groups aged 9-19 years. Acta Pathol. Microbiol. Scand., 62:421, 1964.

Jacobs, J. W., Peacock, D. B., Corner, B. D., Caul, E. D., and Clarke, S. K. R.: Respiratory syncytial and other viruses associated with respiratory disease in infants. Lancet, 1:871, 1971.

Kapikian, A. Z., Mitchell, R. H., Chanock, R. M., Shvedoff, R. A., and Stewart, C. E.: An epidemiologic study of altered clinical reactivity to respiratory syncytial (RS) virus infection in children previously vaccinated with an inactivated RS virus vaccine. Am. J. Epidemiol., 89:405, 1969.

Mufson, M. A., Levine, H. D., Wasil, R. E., Mocega-Gonzalez, H. E., and Krause, H. E.: Epidemiology of respiratory syncytial virus infection among infants and children in Chicago. Am. J. Epidemiol., 98:88, 1973.

Sommerville, R. G.: Respiratory syncytial virus in acute exacerbations of chronic bronchitis. Lancet 2:1247, 1963.

Urquhart, G. E., and Gibson, A. A. M.: RSV infections and infant deaths. Br. Med. J., 3:110, 1970.

116. PARAINFLUENZA VIRAL DISEASES (Croup)

George Gee Jackson

Definition. Infection with parainfluenza viruses is a common and recurrent cause of respiratory illness. Croup is a prominent syndrome in children, but the spectrum of illness varies from the common cold to pneumonia and systemic illness.

Etiology. Parainfluenza viruses are members of the myxovirus family. They closely resemble influenza virus but differ from it serologically and in some biologic respects. Four distinct types of parainfluenza viruses are recognized that cause infections in man. They are closely related to one another and have some characteristics in common with mumps, measles, and respiratory syncytial virus. Types 2 and 4 differ somewhat from types 1 and 3 in the clinical illnesses produced and in their epidemiology.

Parainfluenza viruses were first designated as hemadsorption or HA viruses, owing to their property of causing erythrocytes to adsorb and stick to infected cells in tissue cultures. Type 2 was recovered from cases of croup and initially was called the "croup-associated" or CA virus.

A strain of parainfluenza type 1, the Sendai virus, was first isolated in mice and called influenza D. Mice and other rodents were then recognized to have natural infection with parainfluenza viruses. The Sendai and other animal strains of parainfluenza type 1 have slight serologic differences from strains of human origin. A simian myxovirus (SV-5) is commonly found in monkey kidney tissue cultures, occasionally in eggs and other tissues. It resembles parainfluenza type 2; virus isolates from cattle with shipping fever (SF-4) were found to be parainfluenza type 3.

Incidence and Epidemiology. Few, if any, persons escape infection and reinfection with the different types of parainfluenza viruses. Most children develop antibody from infection with parainfluenza type 3 before the age of four years. By the time they enter school, 70 per cent of children have antibody against more than one type. Among older children and adults, nasopharyngeal reinfection with types 1 and 3 is common regardless of the presence of serum antibody. Reinfection with parainfluenza viruses accounts for an appreciable proportion of common colds and upper respiratory illnesses in adults.

Parainfluenza types 1 and 3 are endemic and cause illness in all seasons of the year. A study in Glasgow, Scotland, indicated that infections in the autumn were usually type 1 and those in the summer type 3. The former tended to have a biennial epidemic cycle; the latter had annual endemicity. All types can cause epidemics of respiratory disease in the winter season. Together, the parainfluenza viruses cause about 40 per cent of all cases of croup. A greater proportion of infections with types 1 and 2 cause croup, but because of its greater prevalence and transmissibility, type 3 is a more common cause of the croup syndrome. Type 3 virus spreads easily from person to person. It infects virtually all contacts who have no antibody and reinfects many persons with a demonstrable level of antibody in the serum. Type 1 virus does not spread as efficiently as type 3, but is nevertheless highly transmissible. Type 2 infection has been less prevalent and more episodic in its occurrence than either types 1 or 3. Infections caused by type 4 have been entirely sporadic and infrequently recognized.

Although many animal species have a high incidence of infection with the parainfluenza viruses, spread to man from these sources has not been well established.

Clinical Manifestations. The clinical syndrome of croup in children is the most common characteristic of infection with parainfluenza viruses. Involvement of the trachea and bronchi also increases the amount of mucous secretions which can become inspissated and cause additional respiratory obstruction. Type 3 infections may be symptomatically more severe and cause more lower respiratory tract disease. Although croup is the most distinctive syndrome, parainfluenza virus infections cause rhinitis or pharyngitis more than twice as often as croup, and bronchitis, bronchiolitis, or pneumonia at least as frequently as croup. Over-all, croup is a symptom in fewer than 10 per cent of infections.

The initial infection with parainfluenza viruses produces more severe disease than reinfection and produces fever of 39 to 40° C in about three fourths of the cases. Among adults, parainfluenza viruses cause mostly upper respiratory tract disease, predominantly the common cold or afebrile coryza. About one third of patients with reinfection will have fever. In dual viral infections, a parainfluenza virus has been recognized as a common member of the pair with a resultant increase in the severity of the symptoms.

Diagnosis. Clinical differentiation of the type of parainfluenza viral infection and even the differentiation from other viral infections of the respiratory tract cannot be made with confidence. The virus can be isolated from nasopharyngeal secretions during the illness and for a brief period thereafter. This is the most certain and may be the only way to identify the specific type of parainfluenza virus involved. Serologic responses are often heterotypic owing to the nearly universal infection of persons with type 3 early in life and the common infection with types 1, 2, and mumps viruses. A rise in antibody against one of these viruses does not permit confidence in a strain-specific diagnosis.

Treatment. The treatment is supportive, as described for the common cold. The croup syndrome may be very acute, and cause respiratory insufficiency requiring urgent and decisive management. A comfortably warm, draft-free environment with high humidity (steam) is recommended for reducing laryngeal stridor. Maintenance of an adequate airway is essential. Antimicrobial drugs are usually contraindicated. Vaccines have been produced for types 1, 2, and 3, and their antigenicity has been shown, but their effectiveness in the prevention of natural infection has not been convincing.

Banatvala, J. E., Anderson, T. B., and Hocking, E. D.: Parainfluenza infections in the community. Br. Med. J., 1:537, 1964.

Chanock, R. M., Parrott, R. H., Johnson, K. M., Kapikian, A. Z., and Bell, J. A.: Myxoviruses: Parainfluenza. Am. Rev. Respir. Dis., 88:152, 1963.

Gardner, S. D.: The isolation of parainfluenza 4 subtypes A and B in England and serological studies of their prevalence. J. Hyg. (Camb.), 67:545, 1969.

Herrmann, E. C., Jr., and Hable, K. A.: Experiences in laboratory diagnosis of parainfluenza viruses in routine medical practice. Mayo Clinic Proc., 45:177, 1970.

Kim, H. W., Vargosko, A. J., Chanock, R. M., and Parrott, R. H.: Parainfluenza 2 (CA) virus: Etiologic association with croup. Pediatrics, 28:614, 1961.

LaPlaca, M., and Moscovici, C.: Distribution of parainfluenza antibodies in different groups of population. J. Immunol., 88:72, 1962.

Lennette, E. H., Jensen, F. W., Guenther, R. W., and Magofin, R. L.: Serologic responses to parainfluenza viruses in patients with mumps virus infection. J. Lab. Clin. Med., 61:780, 1963.

McLean, D. M., Bach, R. D., Larke, P. B., and McNaughton, G. A.: Myxoviruses associated with acute laryngotracheobronchitis in Toronto, 1962–63. Can. Med. Assoc. J., 89:1257, 1963.

Miller, W. S., and Artenstein, M. S.: Aerosol stability of three acute respiratory disease viruses. Proc. Soc. Exp. Biol. Med., 125: 222, 1967.

Mogabgab, W. J., Dick, E. C., and Holmes, B.: Parainfluenza 2 (CA) virus in young adults. Am. J. Hyg., 74:304, 1961.

Parrott, R. H., Vargosko, A., Luckey, A., Kim, H. W., Cumming, C., and Chanock, R. M.: Clinical features of infection with hemadsorption viruses. N. Engl. J. Med., 260:731, 1959.

Pierson, M., deLavergne, E., Gelgenkrantz, S., and Worms, A. M.: Aspect clinique et épidémiologique de quelques cas d'infection à myxovirus Parainfluenza III (EA 102). Arch. Gesamte Virusforsch., 13:257, 1963.

Starke, J. E., Heath, R. B., and Curwen, M. P.: Infection with influenza and parainfluenza viruses in chronic bronchitis. Thorax, 20:124, 1965.

Von Euler, L., Kantor, F. S., Hsuing, G. D., Isaacson, P., and Tucker, G.: Studies of parainfluenza viruses: I. Clinical, pathological, and virological observations. Yale J. Biol. Med., 35: 523, 1963.

Wenzel, R. P., McCormick, D. P., and Beam, W. E.: Parainfluenza pneumonia in adults. J.A.M.A., 221:294, 1972.

117. INFLUENZA

Edwin D. Kilbourne

Definition. Influenza is an acute, contagious disease that is usually attended by fever and prostration and is ordinarily benign in outcome. The headache, myalgia, and asthenia that characterize the disease are severe out of proportion to the symptoms originating from involvement of the respiratory tract – the primary and perhaps exclusive site of infection with the causative virus.

History. Epidemics of respiratory disease similar to modern influenza have been recorded through the centuries. Since the year 1510 there have been 31 pandemics described. The calamitous nature of these epidemics may have led to the naming of the disease by the Italians as an "influenza" or influence of the heavenly bodies or perhaps as an "influenza di freddo" (influence of the cold).

In 1933 the isolation of a virus in ferrets by Smith, Andrewes, and Laidlaw established the specific infectious etiology of the disease, and led rapidly to accurate definition of its epidemiology and clinical variations. The virus isolated in 1933 is now known as influenza A virus.

A second type of virus was isolated independently in 1940 by Francis and by Magill (influenza B virus). In 1950 influenza C was isolated from a patient in nonepidemic circumstances by Taylor, and later was shown by Francis and his associates to be the cause of epidemic disease.

The discovery by Burnet (1940) that the influenza viruses could be cultivated readily in the chick embryo led directly to simplified methods of studying influenza and to the development of an inactivated viral vaccine. Hirst's discovery (1941) that the virus could agglutinate erythrocytes in vitro (hemagglutination) (also noted by McClelland and Hare in 1941) provided not only a new technique for basic virology but a practical method for the precise measurement of virus and antibody.

In 1941 Horsfall and associates published the first evidence of protection of man against influenza by a vaccine containing inactivated influenza A virus. The Commission on Influenza of the Armed Forces Epidemiological Board has demonstrated the feasibility of mass immunization, and has developed the vaccines now in standard use.

Etiology. Influenza is a consequence of infection with certain *myxoviruses* that have common physical, chemical, and biologic properties. These viruses comprise three groups (A, B, and C), which are completely unrelated antigenically, do not induce cross-immunity to one another, and have different epidemiologic characteristics. Four major subgroups of influenza A viruses have been identified since discovery of the virus in 1933, one having replaced the other in chronologic succession. Serologic studies defined a virus that first appeared in swine in 1918 (HswN1) as the probable cause of the notorious human pandemic of that year. Influenza A virus subtypes are defined on the basis of antigenic analysis of their two outermost proteins. These biologically active glyoproteins (hemagglutinin [H] and neuraminidase [N]) are the primary determinants of immunity and mutate independently, as was clearly evident in the replacement of H2N2 by H3N2 (Hong Kong) virus in 1968 (see accompanying table). The hemagglutinin (H) is responsible for binding the virus to the cell; antibody to this protein therefore neutralizes the virus and is the major determinant of immunity. The viral neuraminidase (N) is instrumental in release of virus from cells; antineuraminidase antibody is not neutralizing, but limits viral replication and therefore the course of infection. As external spike-like projections from the viral envelope, H and N are in immediate contact with host antibody during infection and therefore are under selective pressure (see Epidemiology). Beneath these "spikes" the virus particle is bounded by a lipid bilayer derived from the host cell (Fig. 1). Just beneath the lipid layer the core of the particle is surrounded by the M or membrane protein. The nucleoprotein (NP) occurs in helical form in association with the viral RNA. The internal M, NP, and P proteins (of undefined location and function) are common to all influenza A viruses and do not differ significantly in antigenic nature from one subtype to the other. Type-specific A, B, or C categorization of virus thus depends on serologic reactions (usually complement-fixation) mediated by these internal antigens.

The viral genome within comprises segments of RNA (totaling 3.9×10^6 daltons) capable of reassortment during infection to provide an unusually high frequency of genetic recombination. Isolated viral RNA(s) is not infectious, because it does not constitute the message. Transcriptase is necessary for viral replication. It is not known which of the viral proteins described above has transcriptase function.

Influenza B and C viruses have been less thoroughly studied, but appear to be structurally similar to influenza A viruses. Little antigenic variation of influenza C virus has been remarked, and antigenic variation of influenza B virus has been of lesser magnitude than that observed with influenza A. However, a new variant that appeared in 1972 (prototype strain B/Hong Kong/5/72) is markedly different from earlier strains and appears to be emerging to predominance.

The influenza viruses are of medium size (approximately 850 Å in diameter), and by conventional electron microscopy they appear spherical or filamentous in form, with spike-like projections.

Epidemiology. The arbitrary designation of the three types of influenza virus as A, B, and C coincides fortuitously with their relative rank as causes of severe epidemic disease. Influenza B and C viruses have been associated chiefly with sporadic epidemics in children and young adults, notably in school or other institutional populations. Most adults carry antibodies to these viruses, probably as the result of recurrent subclinical infection. There is no evidence that pandemics of influenza B or C have occurred.

Major Subtypes of Influenza: Antigenic Variations in Hemagglutinin (H) and Neuraminidase (N) of the Virus in Relation to Pandemic Severity of Influenza*

Year of Appearance	Virus		Former Designation	Change in	Extent of Change	Result
1918	Hsw	N1	(Swine)	?	?	Pandemic (severe)
192?	H0	N1	(A_0)	H N	++ +	No evident pandemic
1947	H1	N1	(A_1)	H N	++ +	Pandemic (mild)
1957	H2	N2	(A_2)	H N	+++ +++	Pandemic (severe)
1968	H3	N2	(HK)	H N	+++ 0	Pandemic (moderate)

*Modified from Kilbourne, E. D.: J. Infect., Dis., 127:478, 1973.

Vertical connecting lines indicate antigenic relatedness (i.e., shared antigenic determinants). Double lines indicate close similarity. H0N1 is new subtype designation for A_0, etc. Plus signs indicate grading of extent of antigenic change from immediately preceding viral subtype. The severity of the subsequent pandemics appears to be related to the degree of antigenic change in the virus.

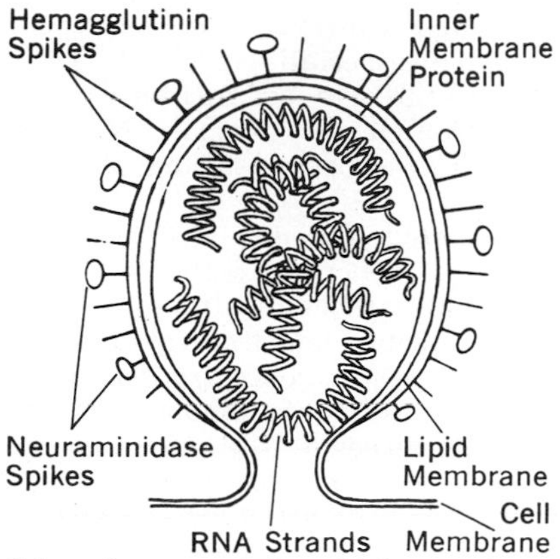

Figure 1. Schematic representation of influenza virus particle as it buds from the plasma membrane of the infected cell, incorporating host lipid and carbohydrate in the process. The surface proteins, hemagglutinin, and neuraminidase are subject to mutations that permit the virus to escape previously established immunity. (Reprinted, by permission, from Kilbourne, E. D.: Man's adaptable predator. Natural History, 82:72, 1973. Copyright © The American Museum of Natural History, 1973.)

Discussions of influenza are usually concerned with the influenza A viruses, for these are the important and apparently more mutable viruses that cause widespread epidemic and pandemic disease. The complicated and still puzzling epidemiology of influenza A is most conveniently considered by separate discussions of the *pandemic, epidemic,* and *endemic* infections—all attributable to the same virus under different conditions.

Pandemic Influenza. The isolation of a virus of the influenza A group from the pandemic of 1957 established that pandemic influenza was etiologically linked with the less extensive epidemic disease from which viruses had been recovered during the 1933–1956 period.

Influenza A virus is an obligate human parasite which is transmitted directly from man to man under conditions of close interhuman contact, presumably via the respiratory tract. With *human* viruses survival of the virus appears to depend on its serial transmission from man to man.

When a major antigenic change in the virus occurs—perhaps as a reciprocal of high immunity in the general population—this mutation may be so extreme that acquired immunity in the population to previously existing influenza A viruses is inadequate to prevent infection or disease initiated by the new virus, which replaces the older virus completely. Under these conditions, people of all ages and in all places are susceptible to influenza, and a worldwide epidemic or pandemic may ensue (Fig. 2). The source of the markedly different strains of virus that suddenly appear to initiate pandemics is unknown. Direct mutation from the antecedent virus seems unlikely in view of the magnitude of change in H and N antigens. Therefore recombination in nature of human and animal influenza A viruses has been proposed to explain the recurrent decennial introduction of apparently novel viruses into the human population.

The incubation period of influenza is only 24 to 48 hours, so that, once progressive spread begins, the impact on the community is sudden and devastating. Both the incidence and the severity of illness are highly variable and are influenced by age, pregnancy, and pre-existing chronic disease and by such environmental factors as crowding and season of the year. Morbidity is usually first noted among schoolchildren, then in young adults, and finally in older, less active, and presumably less exposed members of the community. Infection of the aged is more frequently followed by bacterial pneumonia. As a consequence, a "second wave" of increased community mortality may coincide with the delayed appearance of influenza in this age group—*at a time when influenza is no longer apparent in the community* by the usual criteria of absenteeism from school or industry.

Specific immunity to influenza develops rapidly after infection, but it may decline within one or two years so that recurrence of infection and disease from the same antigenic type of virus may occur *under conditions of heavy exposure* as in military barracks or boarding schools. On the other hand, the steady decline in community morbidity after the initial pandemic wave obviously points to the acquisition of immunity of some durability by most of the population.

Interpandemic "Epidemic" Influenza. Influenza occurs in its characteristic acute epidemics in the early months of the year in the north temperate zone. In a par-

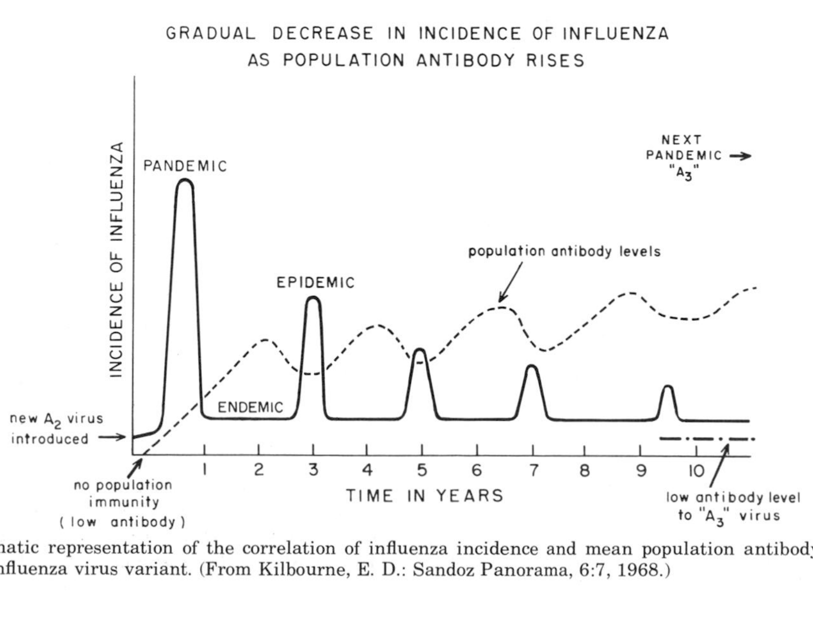

Figure 2. Schematic representation of the correlation of influenza incidence and mean population antibody levels after introduction of a new influenza virus variant. (From Kilbourne, E. D.: Sandoz Panorama, 6:7, 1968.)

ticular community the epidemic usually comes and goes within a month, rising to a peak in 12 to 14 days, and subsiding almost as rapidly. Although the case fatality rate is less than 1 per cent, the presence of influenza may be detected by a sudden increase in unspecified total mortality in the community. This mortality occurs at both extremes of age, and is occasioned principally by the bacterial pneumonias that may complicate influenza in the very young and very old.

Epidemics of influenza A have been demonstrated to occur every year since discovery of the virus, but communities are usually spared recurrence for two or more years after an epidemic.

After a pandemic, the frequency and extent of epidemics gradually abate with the development of population immunity to the new virus. Minor antigenic variations of the virus may be detected during this time, but at least a decade seems to be required for change sufficient to establish a truly "new" subtype (Fig. 2).

Endemic Influenza. The interepidemic survival of influenza virus has long been a puzzle in view of the fragility of the virus and its apparently obligate restriction to human hosts. It has become increasingly clear, however, that influenza virus infections may occur continuously within the population, either as sporadic instances of disease that are not recognized as influenza or as clinically inapparent infections. As more and more members of the population develop immunity, infections without disease become more and more frequent and serve to maintain the virus in the community. Such infections are recognized by serologic studies.

Pathology and Pathogenesis. The primary lesion of influenza is a necrosis of the ciliated epithelium of the respiratory tract. In the uncomplicated infection epithelial damage is probably confined to the upper and middle portion of the respiratory tract, the trachea being the most strikingly involved. Early in infection the necrotic ciliated cells are desquamated, leaving intact the basal cell layer. On about the fifth day of illness regeneration begins in the basal layer with the development of undifferentiated "transitional" epithelium, which may simulate metaplasia. After two weeks ciliated cells may again be seen.

When influenza is complicated by bacterial pneumonia, the pathologic findings are variable and depend on the nature of the secondary invader. However, *primary influenza virus pneumonia* presents a characteristic picture. The lungs are dark red, heavy, and edematous. The trachea and bronchi contain bloody fluid, and the mucosa is hyperemic. Microscopy shows ciliated epithelium to have been lost from the trachea, bronchi, and bronchioles, but evidence of epithelial regeneration may be seen. In the submucosa, focal hemorrhage, edema, and slight leukocytic infiltration may occur. Capillary thrombosis with focal leukocytic exudate has been described. The alveolar spaces contain neutrophilic and mononuclear cells admixed with fibrin and edema fluid. Intra-alveolar hemorrhage is common in the lower lobes. The alveolar septa may be thickened, and acellular hyaline membranes may line alveolar ducts and alveoli.

Pathologic changes attributable to influenza occur only rarely outside the respiratory tract. There are no physiologic or biochemical changes in the patient that are pathognomonic of influenza. Although "leukopenia" is often stated to be characteristic, total leukocytic counts in the uncomplicated disease may vary from 2000 to 14,000 cells per cubic millimeter, and are usually in the normal range. However, *lymphocytopenia* is commonly detectable, especially in the first four days of illness. The erythrocyte sedimentation rate may be moderately elevated or normal. No characteristic changes occur in the bacterial flora of the respiratory tract.

The Complicated Disease. In primary influenza viral pneumonia, *leukocytosis* is the rule, even in the absence of bacterial pathogens, although the erythrocyte sedimentation rate may not be elevated. *Serum glutamic oxaloacetic transaminase concentrations* are elevated in proportion to the severity of pulmonary involvement and may exceed 60 units per milliliter. *Oxyhemoglobin saturation* is reduced to 46 to 85 per cent. *Partial pressure of* CO_2 is elevated, and the *pH of arterial blood* is lowered. The *proteinuria* and elevated *blood urea nitrogen* concentrations that may be noted are the results of fever and dehydration and do not reflect primary renal damage. No notable changes in *serum electrolytes* or in *blood clotting* occur.

Clinical Manifestations. Infection with influenza virus may be asymptomatic, may be attended only by slight fever, or may result in the "typical" prostrating disease that identifies epidemics. This disease is remarkably constant in its expression from year to year, and the uncomplicated case of pandemic influenza does not differ from the "three-day fever" of nonpandemic outbreaks. The higher fatality rates associated with the 1918 pandemic were usually attributable to secondary bacterial pneumonia. Significant variations in the disease caused by any of the A or B subtypes of virus have not occurred. Influenza C appears to be a less severe disease, but it has not yet received adequate study.

Patients with influenza almost invariably *cough,* although this symptom may not be bothersome or even noted by the patient. The cough is brief and spasmodic, and usually not productive of sputum. Other symptoms related to the destruction of respiratory epithelium are *substernal burning pain* (from the trachea), *dryness or soreness of the throat,* and *nasal obstruction and discharge.* Neither sore throat nor evidence of rhinitis is particularly prominent in influenza. Slight *pharyngeal injection* may be noted. *Epistaxis* is rare, but is valuable diagnostically when it occurs. *Conjunctival burning and injection* are common.

In 5 to 10 per cent of patients with uncomplicated disease, crepitant or musical *rales, roughened breath sounds,* or *pleural friction rub* may be detected. Such signs rarely persist for more than one or two days. *Chest pain* may accompany the friction rub, or more often is substernal and referable to the trachea.

The prostrating effects of influenza are associated with *fever, chilly sensations* (seldom with rigors), *headache,* and *myalgia. Fever* usually exceeds 38° C and may reach 41° C. It is usually abrupt in its onset and decline and lasts for only two to five days in the absence of complications. *Headache* is often frontal and is of the throbbing sort associated with fever; its severity is proportional to the degree of fever. *Extraocular myalgia* is a characteristic but not universal complaint that may be elicited only by examination. *Myalgia* may be generalized or confined to the back or lower extremities. *Gastrointestinal symptoms* are uncommon, and occur more often in patients with pre-existing gastrointestinal disease.

In sum, the picture of uncomplicated influenza is that of a patient with flushed face and reddened eyes who lies flat in bed and coughs occasionally with a dry spasmodic cough. He moves about fitfully, complaining of headache or backache. By contrast, the rare patient with influenza virus pneumonia (see below) sits erect, is extremely anxious and agitated, gasps for breath, and manifests *cyanosis* of the lips and nailbeds.

Course and Complications. In both pandemic and epidemic influenza the disease, although acute and prostrating, is brief, so that it is uncommon for any symptom to last beyond seven to ten days, and fever usually subsides earlier (Fig. 3). A protracted *postinfluenzal asthenia* has been emphasized in some reports. It is not clear to what extent secondary bacterial infections or psychogenic factors contribute to the state. Nevertheless, the alerting of the patient to the possibility may save some apprehension during the convalescent period. *Encephalitis* and *myocarditis* have been described infrequently as complications of influenza, and have rarely been well documented or associated with virus isolation from the brain or heart.

The important and potentially lethal complications of influenza derive from infection of the lung, either with the influenza virus itself or with bacterial pathogens. The pulmonary complications of influenza may be considered as (1) *primary influenza virus pneumonia,* (2) *combined influenza virus and bacterial pneumonia,* and (3) *influenza complicated by secondary bacterial pneumonia.* All three types of complication are more frequent in patients with pre-existing cardiac or pulmonary disease or in women late in pregnancy. The aged, in whom apparent or inapparent chronic disease is more frequent, are also understandably more vulnerable to pulmonary complications of influenza. Neurologic complications have been temporally associated with influenza, as with other respiratory viral infections. Evidence for a clearcut causative role of the virus in such sequelae is lacking. Recently, Reye's syndrome in children (see Ch. 397) has occurred with increased frequency after influenza epidemics, especially influenza B.

Primary Influenza Virus Pneumonia. Primary influenza virus pneumonia is a severe disease that is usually fatal. Within 24 hours of the onset of typical symptoms of influenza, the patient experiences high fever (39.5 to 40° C), a cough productive of bloody sputum, and profound dyspnea and anxiety. Cyanosis is notable, and poor air exchange is indicated by the generalized pulmonary findings, which include suppression of breath sounds, expiratory wheezing, and diffuse, moist rales. Signs of consolidation are absent. Chest roentgenograms disclose diffuse bilateral nodular infiltrates that radiate outward from the hilum, sparing the lung periphery.

The patient almost always dies within five to ten days of the onset of illness after a course characterized by unremitting fever, progressive pulmonary involvement, and terminal vascular collapse (Fig. 4). Antibacterial drugs, oxygen, bronchodilators, and corticosteroids are usually unavailing.

Pathogenic bacteria are not recoverable from the sputum, blood, or lung during life or post mortem, and influenza virus is demonstrable in high concentrations in the lung.

Primary influenza virus pneumonia is restricted almost invariably to patients with pre-existing cardiac or pulmonary disease or pregnancy. Still more specifically, the victim usually has rheumatic cardiovascular disease and mitral stenosis. The predilection of this complication for the patient with mitral stenosis suggests that hemodynamic factors such as pulmonary hypertension are more important in its pathogenesis than general debility or the absence of specific immune mechanisms.

There appears to be a graded spectrum of severity of the disease caused by influenza virus, so that, intermediate between the uncomplicated case with transient rales and the fatal virus pneumonia, occasional instances of "mild segmental influenza virus pneumonia" have been described.

Combined Influenza Virus and Bacterial Pneumonia. In patients with primary influenza virus pneumonia, infection with bacterial pathogens may supervene. In such patients the characteristic and dramatic onset of the virus pneumonia may be attended or closely followed by such symptoms of bacterial pneumonia as *productive cough, shaking chills,* or *pleuritic pain.* Signs of focal consolidation may be engrafted upon the diffuse pulmonary findings of the viral infection. Pneumococcus, Staphylococcus, *Hemophilus influenzae,* or, more rarely, group A streptococci may be demonstrated by culture of lung, blood, or sputum. In 1957–1958, pneumococcus and Staphylococcus were the most frequent bacterial invaders.

The host setting and course of the combined infection are basically the same as in the pneumonia associated with influenza virus infection alone.

Influenza Complicated by Secondary Bacterial Pneumonia. Bacterial pneumonia, characterized by focal consolidation, may occur after influenza in previously healthy persons as well as in the ill and infirm. This complication is further distinguished from influenza virus pneumonia by (1) the lag between influenzal symptoms and the appearance of pneumonia, sometimes with brief interval of freedom from symptoms; (2) the presence of focal and not diffuse pulmonary involvement; and (3) the absence of influenza virus in throat washings, but the presence of bacterial pathogens in the sputum. This "late" type of pulmonary complication is by far the most common.

Diagnosis. In the context of an epidemic, influenza may easily be distinguished from other acute respiratory diseases, although diagnosis of the isolated case may be difficult. In its typical form influenza is characterized by relatively high fever, which sets it apart from the syn-

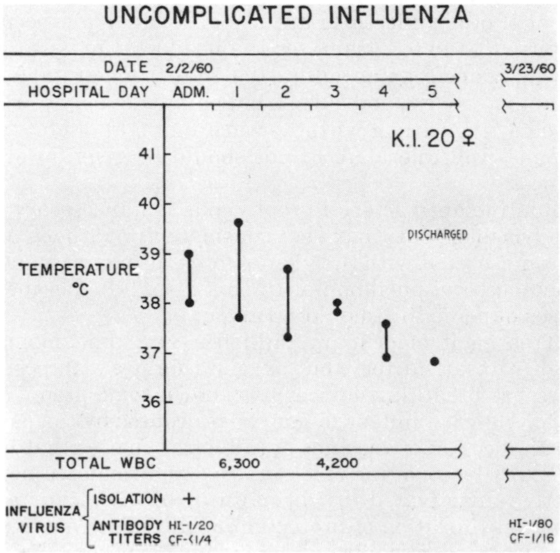

Figure 3. (From Kaye, D., et al.: Am. Rev. Respir. Dis., 85:9, 1962.)

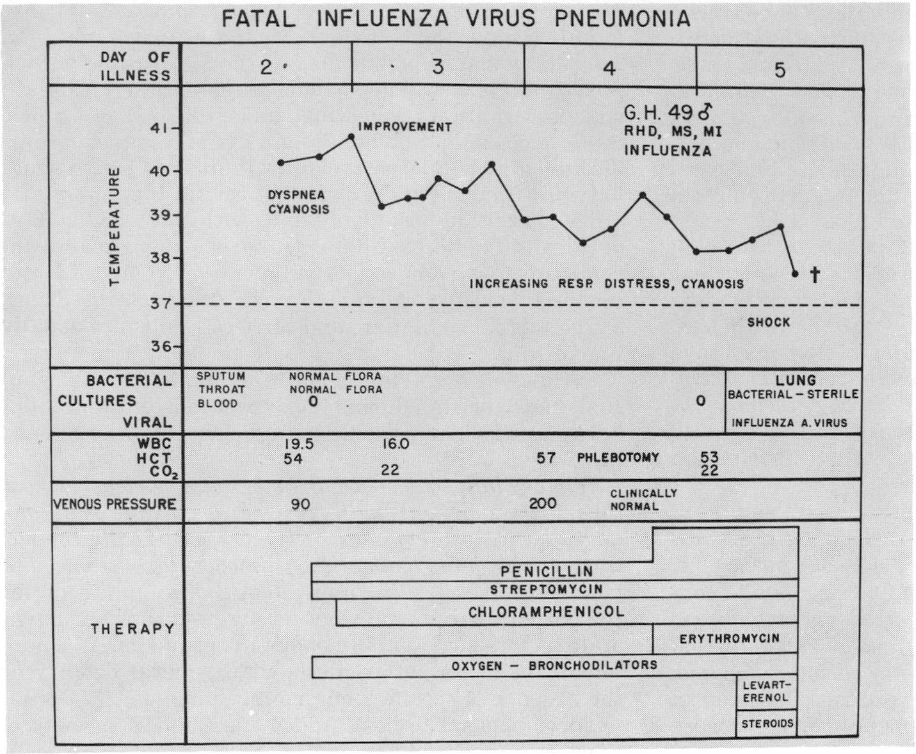

Figure 4. (From Kaye, D., et al.: Am. Rev. Respir. Dis. 85:9, 1962.)

drome of the *common cold.* With the common cold, nasal symptoms predominate, but they are usually minor in influenza. *Adenoviral infections* are the most difficult to distinguish from influenza, but, in general, fever and prostration are less, onset is less sudden, and sore throat and laryngitis are more prominent in adenoviral disease. One of the clinical forms of respiratory syncytial viral disease may closely mimic influenza. The aching, febrile, minor illnesses associated with infection by various arbo- or enteroviruses may also simulate influenza but are notably unattended by cough, although sore throat may occur. In *streptococcal pharyngitis,* the greater frequency of vomiting, the predominance of sore throat, and the occurrence of cervical adenitis and leukocytosis are helpful in differential diagnosis. *Primary atypical pneumonia* is usually distinguishable clinically from influenza virus pneumonia by its more gradual onset, purulent sputum, and indolent, ordinarily benign course.

The *definitive diagnosis* of influenza depends upon isolation of the virus from throat washings or sputum and the demonstration of an increase in specific humoral antibodies. Viral isolation is most successful in the first two to three days of illness and is best accomplished by the intra-amniotic inoculation of chick embryos. Primary cultures of mammalian cells may also be used but are less satisfactory. If virus grows to high enough titer on the first passage, isolation and identification of the agent may be accomplished within 48 to 72 hours of inoculation of the specimen. Recently, fluorescent antibody staining of exfoliated nasal epithelial cells has been applied as a quick and specific diagnostic test.

Antibody may be detected in the patient's serum by neutralization, hemagglutination-inhibition, or complement-fixation tests as early as eight to nine days after the onset of illness, but maximal response is evident only after 14 days. The diagnosis cannot be made with a single serum specimen because of the prevalence of antibody in the population; rather an *increase* in antibody titer of fourfold or more must be demonstrated by the study of two or more serum specimens obtained early in illness and in convalescence.

Prognosis. The prognosis is ordinarily favorable in this brief and self-limited disease. However, the severity of the disease is a reciprocal of host susceptibility, and the outcome may be fatal in those with prior cardiac or pulmonary disease. The prognosis is also influenced by the prevalence of potential respiratory bacterial invaders in the community and the prospects for their control.

Treatment. There is no specific treatment for influenza. The general measures used in the symptomatic treatment of other infections are useful, including especially aspirin (0.3 to 0.6 gram) for the headache, malaise, and myalgia, and codeine sulfate (0.016 to 0.064 gram) for irritability, cough, and substernal pain. Diet may be regulated by the patient with the warning that high fat foods are not well tolerated. Fluids should be given in abundance.

Routine antibacterial prophylaxis is unnecessary and inadvisable, but may be considered for those with chronic disease with the view of forestalling the sequel of pneumococcal pneumonia. In this case, full therapeutic doses of penicillin should be given.

Treatment of primary influenza viral pneumonia is highly unsatisfactory, but oxygen therapy with positive pressure breathing devices has shown some promise.

Prevention. Influenza may be prevented by the parenteral injection of vaccines of influenza viruses that have been produced in the chick embryo and rendered noninfective (inactivated) by formalin or ultraviolet irradiation. The duration of protection usually does not exceed one year under conditions of epidemic exposure. Present vaccines are principally *bivalent* in that they contain the contemporary influenza A virus (Hong Kong) component and also lesser amounts of influenza B antigen. These newer vaccines have been purified by density gradient centrifugation or chromatography and are far less toxic than preparations of the past. A so-called "hemagglutinin" vaccine contains antigens of the disrupted virus. It is of low reactogenicity, but may be less immunogenic than vaccines made from whole virus.

In experimental field trials amantadine hydrochloride has had a chemoprophylactic effect in influenza, as evidenced by lower infection rates and less severe illness in subjects who received the drug shortly before exposure to the infection. After infection, antibody titers were lower in drug-treated subjects, presumably reflecting a decreased antigenic stimulation from reduced viral replication. The drug is presumed to act by inhibiting virus penetration and not intracellularly on virus replication. Some evidence suggests that amantadine may have a slight therapeutic effect if given soon after the initiation of infection. Central nervous system toxicity may limit the usefulness of this compound in older people.

Because protection provided by influenza vaccine is transient, immunization of the general population is not feasible. The vaccine is useful in three special situations: (1) to reduce *morbidity* in groups essential for the community life, such as policemen, physicians, and the military; (2) to reduce *morbidity* in groups particularly subject to the occurrence of epidemics, as in boarding schools, institutions, and military camps; and (3) to prevent disease and hence reduce *mortality* in those peculiarly vulnerable to the effects of infection, especially those with chronic cardiac and pulmonary disease. In these groups, especially the latter, vaccine should be administered annually in the autumn.

Live virus vaccines for influenza are in use in the Soviet Union, but are still under experimental evaluation in the United States.

International Conference on Hong Kong Influenza. Bull. W.H.O., 41:335, 1969.

Kilbourne, E. D.: The molecular epidemiology of influenza. J. Infect. Dis., 127:478, 1973.

Louria, D. B., Blumenfeld, H. L., Ellis, J. T., Kilbourne, E. D., and Rogers, D. E.: Studies on influenza in the pandemic of 1957–1958. II. Pulmonary complications of influenza. J. Clin. Invest., 38:213, 1959.

Smith, W., Andrewes, C. H., and Laidlaw, P. P.: A virus obtained from influenzal patients. Lancet, 2:66, 1933.

VIRAL DISEASES THAT MAY INVOLVE THE CENTRAL NERVOUS SYSTEM

For a detailed description of these diseases, the reader is referred to Ch. 387 to 403.

VIRAL DISEASES CHARACTERIZED BY CUTANEOUS LESIONS

118. MEASLES (Moribilli, Rubeola)

Edwin D. Kilbourne

Definition. Measles is an extremely contagious, febrile disease of high morbidity characterized by rash and catarrhal inflammation of the eyes and respiratory tract. It is principally a benign disease of children, but may afflict with equal frequency persons of any age not previously immunized by infection or vaccination.

Etiology. Measles is caused by a medium-sized RNA *paramyxovirus* approximately 1400 Å in diameter. The virus is of a single antigenic type and resembles other paramyxoviruses (e.g., parainfluenza and mumps viruses) in structure and biologic activity, except that it lacks a neuraminidase. Thus measles virus is an enveloped, lipid-containing virus that is released from the infected cell by budding evagination. The virus bears external spikes that contain a hemagglutinin capable of agglutinating erythrocytes of certain primates. Hemolytic and fusing activity is dissociable from the virus particle. In contrast to the genome of influenza viruses, the RNA is not segmented and high frequency genetic recombination of the virus does not occur. Antigenic variation of the virus has not been noted. Measles virus is antigenically and biologically related to the viruses of canine distemper and bovine rinderpest.

Measles virus replicates most readily in primary cultures of human embryonic tissue or primate kidney cells. However, adaptation of virus to a variety of primary or continuous mammalian and avian cell cultures has been achieved. (Vaccine viruses are propagated in chick embryo cells.)

Subhuman primates have long been known to be susceptible to measles; recently, propagation of the virus in the brains of mice, hamsters, and ferrets has been achieved, demonstrating its neurotropic potential.

Prevalence and Epidemiology. Measles is a disease of cosmopolitan distribution, endemic in all but isolated populations. It may occur at any time of the year, but most outbreaks are in the late winter and early spring, with a peak at the end of April. The disease recurs in epidemic cycles at two- to three-year intervals in most civilized communities that have been studied. This epidemic periodicity is best explained as a result of the introduction of new susceptibles into the population by birth or ingress from other areas. When the proportion of nonimmunes reaches a certain crucial concentration (45 to 50 per cent), disease and coincident dissemination of virus may occur to produce an epidemic. It is likely that virus is introduced from sources external to the involved population, probably by incoming susceptibles. Isolated communities such as the Faröe Islands (Panum) are infrequently attacked by measles, at which times manifest illness appears in virtually all persons not previously infected. In Greenland, a country not known to have been invaded previously by the disease, an epidemic resulted in overt measles in 99.9 per cent of the indigenous population (Christiansen et al.)

Throughout most of the world, measles is a disease of children; most adults possess acquired immunity. Beyond the age of ten more than 90 per cent of the population have specific antibody. Although the peak attack rate coincides with the beginning of school (age six) in technologically advanced societies, it occurs between the ages of two and three in most developing countries. Morbidity and mortality rates do not appear to be influenced by sex or race. Case fatality rates are highest in children less than five years of age, and are also relatively high in the aged. Congenital infection has occurred.

There is no evidence that the virus may vary in virulence in nature. The oft-cited and notorious virulence of the disease in primitive, isolated, or crowded populations may be explained as a corollary of (1) more prevalent infection of feeble and aged adults, (2) poor environmental conditions, (3) inadequate medical care, and (4) secondary bacterial infections. A strikingly increased mortality rate is observed in areas such as West Africa in which protein-calorie malnutrition is prevalent. Because measles virus per se rarely induces fatal disease, it is evident that fatalities attributable to measles may vary in incidence according to the prevalence of bacterial pathogens and the resistance of the population to their presence.

Communicability. Measles is one of the most contagious of infections. Demonstration of virus in nasopharyngeal secretions is in accord with epidemiologic evidence that infection is disseminated and acquired by the respiratory tract. Close physical proximity or direct person-to-person contact is the usual requisite for infection.

Immunity. An unmodified attack of measles is usually followed by lifelong immunity. This observation is in accord with the observed persistence of both complement-fixing and neutralizing antibodies after infection and the relatively high titer of antibodies present even in older persons. The mechanism of persistent immunity after measles is undefined. Although persistence of infective virus after infection seems not to occur, the internal nucleocapsid of measles virus or a closely related variant is demonstrable years after infection in the brain and peripheral lymph nodes of those rare individuals afflicted with subacute sclerosing panencephalitis (SSPE) (see Ch. 401). Thus the potential for viral persistence exists, and in those afflicted with SSPE, antibody levels to measles virus are higher than in those who have experienced uncomplicated measles.

A more likely explanation for the persistent immunity in measles is the maintenance of such immunity by subclinical exogenous reinfection. Careful studies of isolated or closed populations after administration of live virus vaccine have demonstrated a more rapid decline of antibody titer than in populations in which measles virus is circulating. Anamnestic antibody response in the absence of disease has been shown in immune contacts of patients with measles. Thus achievement of eradication of the virus may be compromised as vaccination (see below) is more and more effective in curtailing the circulation of the wild virus; then the booster immunization provided by natural reinfection will become inoperative, and repeated vaccination in the same subject may be required. Passively transferred maternal antibody protects the young infant from measles but also reduces the possibility of effective immunization by live virus vaccines at that age.

Pathology and Physiologic Responses. Pathologic changes in fatal measles usually represent the compound effect of viral and secondary bacterial infection. Pneumonia is almost invariably present; it is most frequently interstitial, but may produce purulent exudate within the alveoli. More representative are changes of the uncomplicated viral disease within the tonsillar, nasopharyngeal, and appendiceal tissue removed during the prodrome. These changes consist of subepithelial round cell infiltration and the presence of multinucleated giant cells. The latter are so characteristic that skilled pathologists have predicted the development of rash from their presence in surgical specimens. Similar cells are commonly observed in tissue cultures infected with measles virus. Cytoplasmic and nuclear inclusions may be seen in epithelial cells. The lesions clinically apparent as Koplik's spots derive from inflammatory mononuclear cell infiltration of buccal submucous glands and necrosis of focal vesicular lesions of the mucosa. Rash is the result of proliferation of capillary endothelial cells in the corium and the coincident exudation of serum, and occasionally erythrocytes, into the epidermis. Viral microtubular aggregates within nuclei and cytoplasm of syncytial giant cells of skin lesions and Koplik's spots attest to the direct role of the virus in the production of these lesions.

No consistent or characteristic physiologic aberrations are observed with measles. The transient hemoconcentration and albuminuria found with other febrile diseases may occur. A normal total leukocyte count or leukopenia is observed throughout the febrile period. Initially, the leukopenia is occasioned by a decline in lymphocytes on the first day of fever; subsequently, granulocytopenia ensues as well. The incubation period is characterized by neutrophilia, and convalescence by a relative lymphocytosis. Measles virus has been isolated from the leukocytic fraction of blood, and is propagable in suspensions of leukocytes in vitro. A false-positive serologic test for syphilis may be observed.

Hormone-Like Effects of Measles Infection. Several striking physiologic effects of measles, although poorly understood, mimic the influence of corticotrophin or the adrenal corticosteroids. These are transient suppression of the tuberculin reaction (observed also with measles vaccines), improvement in eczema and allergic asthma, delay in wound healing, and the induction of remissions in leukemia, Hodgkin's disease, Burkitt's lymphoma, and lipoid nephrosis. Whether these effects are directly attributable to the virus or are hormonally mediated is not known. In recent in vitro experiments, addition of measles virus to human lymphocytes depressed the usual proliferative response of such cells to phytohemagglutinin P or antigen.

Clinical Manifestations. After an incubation period that averages 11 days, measles becomes clinically manifest with symptoms of fever, malaise, myalgia, and headache. Within hours *ocular symptoms* of photophobia and burning pain are evidenced by conjunctival injection, tearing, and exudate in the conjunctival sac. Concomitantly, or soon thereafter, *catarrhal inflammation of the respiratory tract* is manifested by sneezing, coughing, and nasal discharge. Less commonly, hoarseness and aphonia may reflect laryngeal involvement. In this prodromal stage of one to four days' duration, petechial lesions of the palate and pharynx or tiny white spots on the buccal mucosa (*Koplik's spots*) may herald the appearance of skin rash. The white lesions described by Koplik characteristically occur lateral to the molar teeth, and typically are mounted on red areolae of injected mucosa, which may coalesce to form a diffuse red background. Not invariably present, they constitute a valuable, if not pathognomonic, diagnostic sign. The enanthem may involve other mucous membranes such as the vaginal lining. It may "overlap" the subsequent appearance of the cutaneous rash by one to three days. Rarely, a transient, erythematous exanthema may occur in the prodromal period.

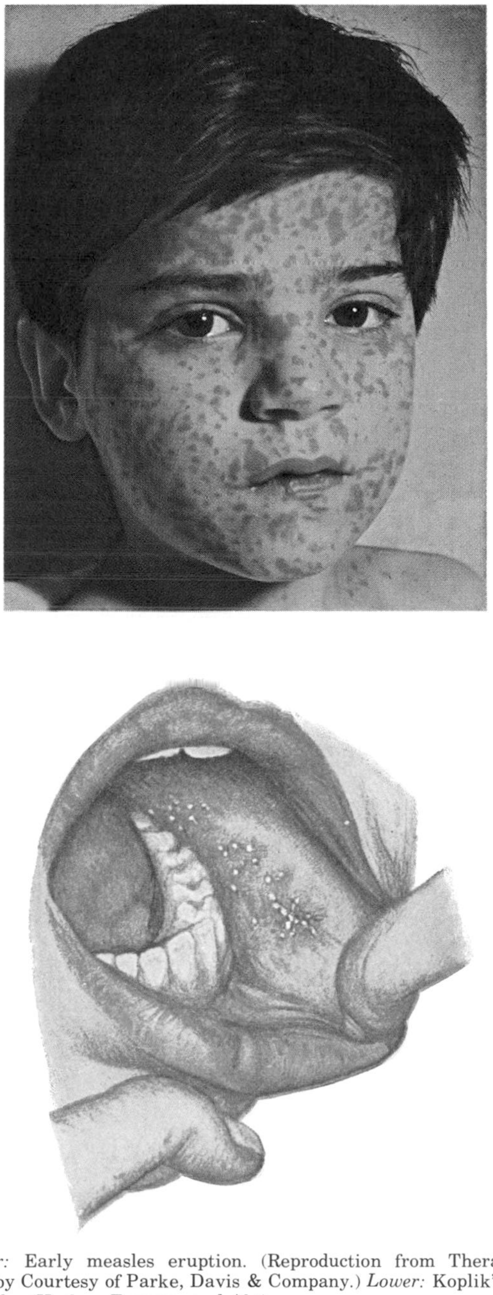

Upper: Early measles eruption. (Reproduction from Therapeutic Notes, by Courtesy of Parke, Davis & Company.) *Lower:* Koplik's spots in measles (Hecker, Trumpp, and Abt).

The *rash* of measles follows the prodromal symptoms by two to four days, occasionally as late as seven days. It first appears behind the ears or on the face as a blotchy erythema, spreads downward to cover the trunk, and finally is manifest on the extremities. The hands and feet may escape involvement. Initially, the eruption consists of discrete, reddish-brown macules that blanch with pressure. Subsequently, these lesions become slightly elevated, tend to coalesce, and may develop a hemorrhagic, nonblanching component. Rash is sometimes very extensive in children with protein-calorie malnutrition, and skin lesions associated with kwashiorkor may develop at the site of the exanthem. The rash fades in the order of its appearance; its disappearance about five days after onset is attended by a fine, powdery desquamation that spares the hands and feet. At its maximum the exanthema usually marks the termination of malaise and fever in the uncomplicated illness.

The *fever* of measles is commonly of the typhoidal, progressively rising type, and falls by lysis. It persists for about six days, and frequently reaches 39.5° C. In the adult, fever may follow rather than antedate the catarrhal symptoms. Throughout the febrile period, productive *cough* and auscultatory evidence of bronchiolitis may be evident. These manifestations may persist after defervescence, and cough is often the last symptom to disappear. It is probable that bronchopulmonary symptomatology is an integral part of the primary viral infection; roentgenographic evidence of pulmonary involvement is frequently seen in the uncomplicated disease in the absence of leukocytosis and obvious bacterial infection.

Complications. It is difficult to distinguish between those complications directly attributable to the virus of measles and those resulting from secondary bacterial infections. The persistence or recurrence of fever and the occurrence of leukocytosis are presumptive evidence of the usual bacterial sequelae of *otitis media* or *pneumonia.* The pneumonia resembles other forms of viral pneumonia and is often caused solely by a specific reaction to the measles virus. Superimposed bacterial infection is common, however, and accounts for most of the severe or fatal cases. Pneumococcus, *Streptococcus hemolyticus, Staphylococcus aureus,* and *Hemophilus influenzae* are the usual secondary invaders. The incidence of bacterial complications is increased by crowding, debility, and the prevalence of bacterial pathogens in the population. Bacterially engendered sequelae may be unduly frequent in crowded contagious disease hospitals.

Serious complications directly related to the measles virus are rare. *Laryngitis* of sufficient severity to embarrass respiration has been observed, and may warrant tracheostomy. *Electrocardiographic abnormalities* may be found in as many as 30 per cent of children, but clinical evidence of cardiac disease is meager in such cases. *Abdominal pain* or *diarrhea* may be related to invasion of lymphoid tissue of the appendix or Peyer's patches. These symptoms may lead to unnecessary surgery before the appearance of the typical rash. The frequency of stomatitis and gastrointestinal symptoms is greater in malnourished children in tropical areas and may reflect coincident bacterial and parasitic infection.

Encephalomyelitis. A rare (0.1 per cent) but serious consequence of measles is a demyelinating encephalomyelitis that may appear from 1 to 14 days after the onset of infection. This complication is associated with a recurrence of fever, and headache, vomiting, and stiff neck. Stupor and convulsions occasionally follow. Localizing neurologic symptoms may or may not be present. Death ensues in about 10 per cent of patients; about half of survivors suffer permanent residuals of varying severity. Measles virus has been recovered from the brain of a patient with fatal measles "postinfectious" encephalitis six weeks after onset of measles. Recently, abnormal electroencephalograms were recorded in 51 per cent of children with measles *without evidence of encephalitis.* In some of the children the abnormal encephalographic findings were persistent. As noted above, the presence of virus has been demonstrated in patients with subacute sclerosing panencephalitis.

Other late sequelae of measles are thrombocytopenic purpura and exacerbation or activation of pre-existing pulmonary tuberculosis.

Giant-Cell Pneumonia. In children with severe disease involving the recticuloendothelial system (especially leukemia), measles virus may induce an interstitial pneumonia characterized by giant cells and intracellular inclusion bodies. The disease is usually fatal; if the patient survives, persistence of virus and poor antibody formation are evident in convalescence. The pneumonia may occur in the absence of rash so that its etiologic relation to measles may be unsuspected.

Measles Modified by Vaccine or Antibody Administration. Attenuation of the natural disease by antibody prophylaxis may result in an illness of lessened severity comparable with the milder infection of the maternally immunized newborn. Fever alone may be observed, but some degree of exanthema is usually apparent. Koplik's spots may not appear. In general, the course is truncated and relatively uncomplicated. Similar attenuated disease may occur in children partially immunized with inactivated viral vaccine.

Unfavorably Modified Measles—A New Disease. After administration of inactivated measles vaccine (no longer in general use), infection of vaccinees with either live measles vaccine or wild-type natural measles virus led to the development of a new syndrome characterized by dermal hypersensitivity to measles virus and an atypical (petechial, vesicular, or urticarial) rash atypical in distribution. In some cases pulmonary complications occurred. The exact mechanism of this reaction is unknown, but it is almost certainly a manifestation of delayed hypersensitivity to the viral proteins engendered by alum-precipitated inactivated viral vaccine. No such sequelae have followed use of live virus vaccine (see below).

Diagnosis. The experienced layman can diagnose typical measles. The querulous, bleary-eyed child, his face blotched and his nose crusted with exudate, presents a characteristic, if miserable, picture as he breathes openmouthed between paroxysms of sneezing and coughing. The severity of the catarrhal symptoms distinguishes the disease from other eruptive fevers. In the prodromal period the diagnosis should be suggested by (1) fever higher than that of the usual common cold, (2) known measles in the community, and (3) Koplik's spots on the buccal mucosa.

Differential diagnosis (see accompanying table) includes consideration of rubella, scarlet fever, exanthema subitum, infectious mononucleosis, secondary syphilis, drug eruptions, and infection with certain coxsackie- and echoviruses. Of value in excluding these possibilities are the milder course and pinker rash of rubella, the sore throat and leukocytosis of scarlet fever, and serologic tests for infectious mononucleosis and syphilis. The rash of exanthema subitum does not appear until the termination of fever. Fever, enanthema, and catarrh are uncommon with the cutaneous manifestations of drug hypersensitivity.

Specific Diagnosis. Specific diagnosis depends on the isolation of measles virus from throat washings, blood, or urine by inoculation of various types of tissue culture with materials obtained during the first five days of illness. Increase in specific antibody may be detected as early as the first or second day of rash by the complement-fixation test. Antibody is also demonstrable by neutralization and hemagglutination-inhibition procedures.

Presumptive diagnosis may be made if giant cells are detected in stained smears of nasal exudate in the preeruptive period.

Prognosis. Uncomplicated measles is rarely fatal, and complete recovery from the disease is the rule. Fatalities are almost always the result of secondary streptococcal or pneumococcal pneumonia, occurring principally in children below the age of five who become infected after the dissipation of passive neonatal immunity. Mortality in developing countries may be 250 times that observed in the United States or northern Europe. Case fatality rates are also high in elderly and tuberculous patients. Congestive cardiac failure is a common cause of death in patients over 50 years old.

Antimicrobial drugs effective against the usual secondary invaders have reduced the case fatality rate of measles sharply. The incidence of otitis media and pneumonia may be lowered by the prophylactic use of penicillin or a tetracycline early in illness.

Encephalitis occurs as frequently in mild as in severe measles (i.e., about one in a thousand cases). However, the incidence of neurologic sequelae after administration of attenuated live virus vaccine is only one in a million.

Treatment. There is no specific treatment for measles.

Symptomatic Therapy. In the absence of complica-

A Guide to the Differential Diagnosis of Measles

	Conjunctivitis	Rhinitis	Sore Throat	Enanthem	Leukocytosis	Specific Laboratory Tests Available
Measles	++	+	0	+	0	+
Rubella	±	±	±	±	0	+
Exanthema subitum	±	±	0	0	0	0
Enterovirus infection	0	±	±	0	±	+
Scarlet fever	±	±	++	0	+	+
Infectious mononucleosis	0	0	+	0	±	+
Drug rash	0	0	0	0	0	0

0 Not usually present; no test available.
± Variable in occurrence.
\+ Present; test available.
++ Present and severe.

tions, bed rest is the essence of treatment in this usually benign, self-limited disease. Codeine sulfate (0.015 to 0.06 gram) is useful in the amelioration of headache and myalgia and is effective in the management of cough. Aspirin (0.3 to 0.6 gram) may be employed for its analgesic and antipyretic actions. Diet should be unrestricted. Bright light is not an ocular hazard, but photophobia may require darkening of the patient's room.

Antimicrobial Prophylaxis. The course of uncomplicated measles is not influenced by antimicrobial therapy. In common practice the incidence of serious bacterial infections is not sufficient to justify the routine prophylactic use of antimicrobials. Certain special circumstances may warrant full therapeutic dosage with penicillin or the tetracyclines in anticipation of the potentially fatal sequelae of pneumococcal or beta-hemolytic streptococcal infections. These circumstances include treatment of the chronically ill, the very young, or the aged, and the treatment of patients under crowded conditions that foster the increase and dissemination of pathogenic bacteria, as may occur in contagious disease hospitals. If careful observation of the patient is possible, rational therapy is based on the prompt recognition and etiologic definition of complications, followed by initiation of the appropriate antimicrobial drug in proper dosage.

Prevention. *Vaccination.* Highly effective vaccines are now available for the prevention of measles. Most are derived from the Edmonston strain of measles virus isolated in the laboratory of Dr. John Enders. This strain, although it proved very effective in early trials as a live virus vaccine, produced febrile and other reactions (attenuated measles) with such high frequency that it has been supplanted by *"further attenuated" (live virus) vaccines* that are almost as effective as the original vaccine in inducing immunity. These live virus vaccines produce immunity by infection, and therefore need be given only as a single injection. They induce antibody response of somewhat lesser magnitude than that following natural infection. In children over one year of age, seroconversion after vaccination is 90 to 97 per cent. Although a gradual fall in antibody titer occurs in the absence of exposure to wild type virus (see Epidemiology; Immunity), serum antibody is demonstrable in most individuals eight to ten years after a single administration of vaccine. Reinfection with disease has occurred in a small fraction of vaccinated subjects under epidemic conditions. The vaccine virus is not contagious.

Live virus vaccine is given as a single parenteral injection to persons more than one year of age. The coincident injection of standardized *measles immune globulin* (0.01 ml per pound of body weight) at a different site will greatly reduce the incidence of fever and other symptoms. If *live "further attenuated" vaccine* is used under the same conditions, gamma globulin is unnecessary.

Contraindications to live virus vaccine include pregnancy, leukemia and other systemic malignant diseases, active tuberculosis, and administration of resistance-depressing drugs such as corticosteroids and antimetabolites.

Inactivated vaccine produces impermanent immunity and unfavorably alters response to later infection. It therefore is no longer recommended (see Complications, above).

Eradication of measles through administration of live virus vaccines is a scientifically reasonable possibility. The introduction of immunization in the United States in 1963 led to a decrease in annual incidence of from 4,000,000 to 250,000 cases in five years. However, a subsequent resurgence of disease was undoubtedly attributable to underutilization of vaccine in susceptible groups, particularly nonwhite populations in impoverished circumstances. The reinstitution of Federal funds for measles vaccine in 1971 reversed the upward trend of disease in the following year.

Christiansen, P. E., et al.: An epidemic of measles in southern Greenland, 1951. Acta Med. Scand., 144:313, 430, 450, 1952–53.

Enders, J. F., Katz, S. L., Milovanovic, M. V., and Holloway, A.: Studies on an attenuated measles-virus vaccine. I. Development and preparation of the vaccine: Technics for assay of effects of vaccination. N. Engl. J. Med., 263:153, 1960.

Koplik, H.: The diagnosis of the invasion of measles from a study of the exanthema as it appears on the buccal mucous membrane. Arch. Pediat., 13:918, 1896.

Linnemann, C. C., Jr.: Measles vaccine: Immunity, reinfection and revaccination. Am. J. Epidemiol., 97:365, 1973.

Panum, P. L.: Observations Made During the Epidemic of Measles on the Faröe Islands. Delta Omega Society, 1940.

Tyler, H. R.: Neurological complications of rubeola (measles). Medicine, 36:147, 1957.

119. RUBELLA (German Measles)

Edwin D. Kilbourne

Definition. Rubella is an acute, benign, contagious disease of children and young adults. The cardinal manifestations of the illness are a pale pink rash and posterior cervical lymphadenitis. Paradoxically, this mild disease is one of the few viral infections convincingly associated with the genesis of fetal abnormalities. When infection is acquired in utero, it often results in generalized disease of the infant and protracted excretion of virus after birth. Accordingly, recognition and prevention of the disease are matters of far-reaching consequence.

Etiology. Rubella virus is a small, spherical RNA virus with a mean diameter of 550 to 600 Å. The particle is ether sensitive—an attribute of lipid-containing enveloped viruses. The virus develops by budding from marginal and intracytoplasmic membranes. Classification of the virus is uncertain at present, but similarities of structure and development to certain group A togaviruses (including the infectious nature of its isolated RNA) have been noted. (There is no evidence of arthropod transmission.) Thus the virus is clearly unrelated to the virus of measles.

The virus agglutinates the erythrocytes of newly hatched chicks—a characteristic that permits measurement of both virus and antibody. Rubella virus replicates with the production of cytopathic effects in a number of commonly employed cell culture systems, including African green monkey and human diploid cells. Virus replication and production of embryopathic effects similar to those in humans have been experimentally induced in rats.

Incidence and Epidemiology. Accurate information on the incidence of rubella is not available, but approximately 80 per cent of young adults have specific hemagglutination-inhibiting (HI) antibodies against the virus. The mildness and brevity of clinical signs of rubella may confound the diagnosis and reporting of many instances of infection. Studies of the experimental disease lend support to prior clinical evidence that infection may occur without rash, and indicate a further diagnostic pitfall. It can be said, however, that the disease is seen on every continent, may occur in epidemic form, and has its highest incidence in the early spring. The disease is less frequently acquired in childhood than measles, as is attested by serologic studies and by the fact that rubella is more common than measles in young adults. The higher incidence of infection in younger age groups in institutional outbreaks argues against a greater susceptibility of the adult. It is probable that rubella is spread by the respiratory route by close and sustained personal contact. The usual infection is contagious during the period of prodromal symptoms and for as long as seven days after the appearance of rash. However, it is now recognized that the infant with congenitally acquired infection may excrete virus for months after birth and is contagious during this time. The epidemiologic implications of this fact—first established in the large epidemic of 1963–1964—are yet to be determined. There is evidence that the newborn may be unusually contagious, and that although he may have no obvious stigmata of infection, yet he may be shedding virus.

Immunity is lasting. HI antibodies have been demonstrated 30 years after initial infection. Authenticated second attacks are rare, and require serologic documentation because of the nebulous nature of the clinical syndrome. *Subclinical* reinfection demonstrated by increase in IgG serum antibody has been documented with increasing frequency as better serologic methods and increased surveillance have become available. Reinfection occurs most commonly in crowded populations in which the density of infection and probably of spread are high. It is important to note that most such reinfections are not associated with viremia and thus probably pose little threat in pregnant women. As in many other infections, IgM response serves to distinguish primary from reinfection. Presumably, as in measles, inapparent infections may boost immunity throughout life. Immunity that follows artificial immunization with live virus vaccine is of a lesser degree. (See Prevention, below.)

Pathology. Death from uncomplicated postnatally acquired rubella is unknown. Histologic changes characteristic of the disease have not been demonstrated. The onset of disease is attended by leukopenia resulting from a decrease in both lymphocytes and neutrophils. After five days, absolute lymphocytosis is manifest. The total leukocyte count is normal at the tenth day.

Congenital Rubella. Necropsies of fetal and infantile victims of maternal infection have shown a variety of embryonal defects related to developmental arrest involving all three germ layers. Those defects most consistently associated with maternal rubella are microcephaly, cataract, patency of the ductus arteriosus, and defects of the interventricular septum. However, recent studies have revealed a wide spectrum of tissue damage in association with virologically proved disease of varying severity. In some infants hepatic and renal degeneration and myocardial necrosis without inflammation have been noted, whereas in others thrombocytopenia and purpura may be the sole abnormality. It has been proposed that the generalized visceral involvement and characteristic residua of the disease may result from a sequence of platelet damage, intravascular coagulation, and thrombosis. Another theory holds that the smaller size of the rubella-infected infant and some abnormalities may reflect inhibition of multiplication of embryonic cells by the virus.

Clinical Manifestations. *Postnatally Acquired Rubella.* Fourteen to 21 days after exposure to the infection, the onset of rubella is evidenced by symptoms variable in their occurrence and severity. Cough, sore throat, and coryza may initiate the illness, but are often absent; headache, malaise, and myalgia may precede the eruption, especially in young adults. Commonly, fever and obvious enlargement of posterior cervical nodes antedate the appearance of the rash. Fever, when present, rarely exceeds 38° C and seldom persists beyond 48 hours. Injection of the bulbar conjunctivae may be noted. Palpable, tender, and occasionally visible lymphadenopathy involves postauricular and suboccipital nodes with sufficient frequency to be an important diagnostic sign. Generalized peripheral lymphadenitis, and, more rarely, splenomegaly, may occur.

The exanthema of rubella is usually apparent within 24 hours of the first symptoms as a faint macular erythema that first involves the face and neck. Characterized by its brevity and evanescence, it spreads rapidly to the trunk and extremities, sometimes leaving one site even as it appears at the next. The pink macules that constitute the rash blanch with pressure and rarely stain the skin. Rubella virus has been isolated from the skin lesions. Diffuse erythema on the second day of rash may closely simulate scarlet fever. The eruption has vanished by the third day. Rubella may occur without rash. An enanthema has been described that is inconstant in form and occurrence, and lacks the premonitory significance of the Koplik spots of measles. The lesions consist of red macules that usually involve the soft palate.

Complications. Recovery is almost always prompt and uneventful, although relapse occurs with greater frequency than in most viral diseases (5 to 8 per cent). Secondary bacterial infections rarely occur. Rare complications are arthralgia, neuritis, gingivitis, thrombocytopenic purpura, and increased capillary fragility. Heart block has been described. A *meningoencephalitis* of short duration may occur one to six days after the appearance of rash. Its incidence is estimated at 1 in 6000 cases, and it is fatal in approximately 20 per cent of those afflicted. Rubella encephalopathy is not associated with demyelinization (in contrast to other postviral encephalitides). Survivors may have electroencephalographic abnormalities, but intellectual function seems to be preserved.

Congenital Rubella. The fortuitous coincidence of the development of cell culture systems for the isolation of rubella virus and the occurrence of a global epidemic of rubella (in 1963–1964) demonstrated that the classic ocular and cardiac "teratogenic" effects of rubella are but isolated manifestations of a continuing and persisting fetal infection. It is now clear that congenital transplacental infection of the fetus occurs as a consequence of maternal infection (which may or may not be clinically evident), usually in the first trimester of pregnancy. Virus is demonstrable in placental and fetal tissues obtained by therapeutic abortion at that time. If pregnancy is not interrupted (and spontaneous abortion is uncommon), fetal infection persists, and upon delivery of the infant, virus is recoverable from the throat, urine, feces, conjunctivae, bone marrow, and cerebrospinal fluid of the living infant and from most organs at autopsy. About 10 to 15 per cent of infants born to mothers infected in the first trimester of pregnancy have stigmata of infection readily recognizable in the first year of life. These include *cardiac lesions, cataracts, glaucoma, microphthalmia,* and *esophageal atresia.* Most infants in whom virus is detectable do not have evidence of disease at birth or may simply have a lower than normal birth weight. In others, disease of intermediate severity has been recently recognized. Most prominent of the newly observed manifestations is *thrombocytopenic purpura,* which disappears soon after birth. *Hepatosplenomegaly* may persist for months. Other signs include *corneal clouding, fullness of the fontanels, lesions of the long bones,* and *electroencephalographic abnormalities.*

A most striking finding has been the persistence of virus in the pharynx, gastrointestinal tract, and cerebrospinal fluid for as long as one year after birth (9 per cent). Infective virus was present in a congenital cataract after three years, and in the urine of a victim of congenital rubella 29 years after her birth. This evidence of continuing viral synthesis occurs coincidentally with circulating antibody (initially of maternal origin) and originally suggested a form of "immunologic tolerance" to the virus. However, it has been shown that the character of the antibody changes during the first year from IgG (presumably maternal) to IgM, indicating a primary response of the infant to the persisting viral antigen. Studies of older infants and children with stigmata of congenital rubella show them to be free of demonstrable virus and to possess the IgG immunoglobulins that characteristically persist after other viral infections. The defect in host response that is responsible for viral persistence has not yet been defined.

Diagnosis. Rubella may be diagnosed clinically with assurance only during an epidemic. It may be difficult to distinguish from mild or modified measles, infectious mononucleosis, or scarlet fever. Distinction from measles may be made on the basis of pinker, nonstaining rash, the milder course, and the lesser catarrh of rubella. Sore throat is a more prominent complaint in scarlet fever; the course of infectious mononucleosis is often more protracted, and splenomegaly is more frequent than in rubella. Specific diagnosis of rubella is made by isolation of the virus in any of several cell culture systems, or by demonstration of neutralizing, hemagglutination-inhibiting, or complement fixing antibody response during infection. The high incidence of dermatoglyphic abnormalities (50 per cent) and increased percentage of chromosome breaks described in patients following congenital rubella may prove to have diagnostic value when studied further.

Prognosis. Complete recovery from postnatally acquired rubella is almost invariable. The rare deaths attributable to rubella follow the infrequent complication of meningoencephalitis. Infection in pregnancy constitutes a hazard to the fetus but not to the mother.

Treatment. There is no specific treatment for the disease. Few patients suffer discomfort severe enough to warrant symptomatic medication. Headache and myalgia may be controlled by aspirin; bed rest is advisable for the duration of the fever.

Prevention. *Passive Immunization. Administration of gamma globulin to the pregnant woman may only mask her symptoms of infection yet not protect the fetus from viral invasion.* Its use may thus only obscure the picture and confound decision about the need for therapeutic abortion. Hence the practice seems inadvisable and is now seldom carried out.

Active Immunization. Rubella may be prevented in children and adults by the parenteral administration of attenuated live virus vaccines either produced in duck embryo cell cultures and derived from passage of virus in African green monkey kidney cells or derived from primary rabbit cell kidney passage. Seroconversion rates after immunization are approximately 95 per cent. As with other live virus vaccines, serum antibody titers are lower than those that follow natural infection. However, antibody persists for at least four years after vaccination, but the permanence of vaccine-induced immunity must still be established by further observation. Natural infection of individuals immunized with vaccine is not uncommon, although such infection is usually asymptomatic. In children, vaccination is attended by little, if any, reaction; but in women, rash, malaise, arthralgia, and mild, acute arthritis occur frequently, the incidence being directly related to age. For this reason, and in order to induce "herd immunity" to depress circulation of the virus, it is currently recommended in the United States that immunization be carried out principally in childhood. However, since the epidemic threshold—at least in semiclosed populations—is low (between 4.7 and 8.4 per cent), containment of the disease by mass immunization may prove difficult. A high level of vaccine-induced immunity in elementary school children (83 per cent) failed to prevent the spread of rubella in one community. Despite the higher reaction rates in adults, it seems advisable to immunize adolescent girls or women of childbearing age for whose unborn children rubella may have tragic consequences. Of this population, only seronegative individuals should be immunized, and contraception (when appropriate) should be carried out for at least three months after vaccination. The inadvertent administration of vaccine to pregnant women has demonstrated that attenuated vaccine viruses can infect the fetus and thus have the *potential* for teratogenesis.

Cooper, L. Z.: Rubella: A preventable cause of birth defects. *In* Bergsma, D. (ed.): Birth Defects: Original Article Series, Vol. IV, No. 7, Intrauterine Infections. The National Foundation, December, 1968, pp. 23–35.

Gregg, N. M.: Congenital cataract following German measles in the mother. Trans. Ophthal. Soc. Austral., 3:35, 1941.

Horzinek, M., Maess, J., and Laufs, R.: Studies on the substructure of togaviruses. Arch. Gesamte Virusforsch., 33:306, 1971.

Leedom, J. M., Wilkins, J., Portnoy, B., and Salvatore, M. A.: Important assumptions, extrapolations, and established facts which underlie the use of live rubella virus vaccines. Am. J. Epidemiol., 92:151, 1970.

Proceedings of the International Conference on Rubella Immunization. Am. J. Dis. Child., 118, July 1969.

120. EXANTHEMATA ASSOCIATED WITH ENTEROVIRAL INFECTIONS

Edwin D. Kilbourne

Infection with any of a number of enteroviruses may be associated with erythematous, macular eruptions. In some patients occipital and cervical lymphadenopathy may be noted, so that the infection may closely simulate rubella. However, differential diagnosis is aided by the frequency of a vesicular ulcerative enanthem and aseptic meningitis in patients with enteroviral disease and also by its summertime occurrence. Those enteroviruses most frequently associated with rash are the group A coxsackieviruses 9 and 16, and (quite fortuitously) echoviruses bearing the same numerical designations (i.e., echovirus 9 and echovirus 16). The eruptions associated with the coxsackieviruses may include small vesicles, especially notable with coxsackievirus A16 (hand, foot, and mouth disease). Echovirus 16 and coxsackievirus B5 produce eruptions that mimic roseola infantum. Rash seems to be more common in children than in adults.

Lerner, M. A., Klein, J. O., Cherry, J. D., and Finland, M.: New viral exanthems. N. Engl. J. Med., 269:678, 1963.

Wenner, H. A., and Lou, T. Y.: Virus diseases associated with cutaneous eruptions. Prog. Med. Virol., 5:219, 1963.

121. VARIOLA AND VACCINIA

C. Henry Kempe

INTRODUCTION AND HISTORY

Immunization against the dread disease of smallpox is perhaps the most widely applied immunization procedure currently in use. Over the past 150 years it has demonstrated its effectiveness beyond question. The vaccinia virus *(Poxvirus officinale),* which is in effect a laboratory strain carried for many generations in a variety of laboratory animals, differs from the newly isolated virus of cowpox *(Poxvirus bovis),* which was originally employed by Jenner (1798) and his predecessors for the immunization of man against the smallpox virus *(Poxvirus variolae).*

Smallpox was described in detail by Rhazes in the tenth century, and had been described previously by Galen in the second century. Spread from Asia to Europe and North Africa occurred in the Middle Ages, and the disease was prevalent in the sixteenth century. At approximately the same time the disease was introduced into the West Indies by African slaves and from there into Mexico and South America. The best studied epidemics are those in the eighteenth century in England when over 90 per cent of the cases occurred in children under ten years of age and when smallpox accounted for one third of all deaths in children. Smallpox occurred in epidemic form less frequently in North America until 1752 when over 30 per cent of the inhabitants of Boston, Massachusetts, were affected and the mortality rate was over 30 per cent (Creighton, 1894). In 1721 deliberate inoculation of smallpox as protection against the natural disease was introduced in England. It consisted of the inoculation of pustular material by puncturing the skin. This resulted in a febrile disease after an eight-day incubation and a general eruption on the ninth day. The mortality rate from this procedure was 1 to 2 per cent, and it is stated that 17 of 897 inoculated persons died from the disease (Woodville, 1796). Needless to say, modified infection did give rise to highly virulent natural disease in susceptible contacts. In 1738 variolation was successfully used in Charleston, South Carolina, with material that had been allowed to dry. With better care of the patients, the death rate was somewhat reduced; it was thought to be about one or two out of 500, whereas the mortality from the naturally acquired smallpox was 10 to 20 per cent. Variolation was followed by inoculation of cowpox after widespread acceptance of Jenner's studies published in 1798. In truth, this practice had been current among a number of colleagues of Jenner's at a previous time, and he made no claim to originality. Jenner, however, did play a decisive role in popularizing this method of protection against smallpox, and variolation was outlawed in England in 1840. It is possible that the endemism of smallpox in England during the eighteenth century was due to the practice of variolation rather than to natural epidemic occurrence.

VARIOLA
(Smallpox)

Etiology. Smallpox virus is readily visible with any microscope equipped with darkfield illumination or by phase contrast microscopy. With electron microscopy, the smallpox virus resembles elementary bodies of vaccinia virus. The elementary bodies are small, brick-shaped structures with a diameter of about 200 $m\mu$. They can be demonstrated by direct examination of smears of early skin lesions. The virus is very resistant to drying, and living virus can be demonstrated from scabs kept at room temperature for over three years. Virulent virus has survived on clothing of patients and on bedclothes of hospitalized patients, and has caused the disease in laundry workers who were not protected.

Incidence. In 1967, when an intensified eradication program was begun, there were 42 countries reporting a total of 131,000 cases of smallpox. Since it is likely that only about 5 per cent of cases were actually reported, it is estimated that at least 2,500,000 cases occurred in 1967 in 30 countries that had endemic smallpox and in 12 others that experienced importations. In contrast, in 1972, 19 countries reported 65,000 cases at a time when reporting had been vastly improved.

By 1973 only five countries had endemic smallpox – Ethiopia, Sudan, India, Bangladesh, and Pakistan – whereas 14 others had cases as a result of importations.

In South America, Brazil was the last country to become smallpox free. It seems likely now, after 450 years, that smallpox has been eliminated from the Western Hemisphere. In Asia, on the other hand, the difficulty of eradication is still a serious problem.

Epidemiology. The principal natural reservoir of smallpox is thought to be the patient suffering from the disease. The patient is not infective until the third day of the clinical disease, that is, one day before the maculopapular phase of the skin eruption is noted. Contacts may be allowed at large until they actually become ill, because they are not infective during the early pre-eruptive febrile disease.

Intensive efforts are currently being made to determine a possible nonhuman host, the most likely of which is the nonhuman primate. The surprising and significant animal reservoirs of yellow fever and malaria, which have materially affected the eradication campaign for those two diseases, have, understandably, also been of concern to those working in the field of smallpox.

In 1970, 13 cases of pox infection occurred in humans in areas of Africa which had been free of smallpox for two years or more (Foege, 1973). In ten of these, the illness was typical smallpox; all but one of these patients had not been vaccinated. No human source of infection was discovered, but none of over 100 unvaccinated close contacts subsequently contracted the disease. Virus was isolated and appeared indistinguishable from monkeypox virus isolated among outbreaks in captive monkeys, but there was no illness among monkeys in the area (Ladnyr, 1973). Therefore although it is possible that monkeypox can cause a clinical illness resembling smallpox in man, its infectivity appears to be low.

Pathology and Pathogenesis. It is likely that the site of entry of the smallpox virus is the upper respiratory tract and, possibly, the eye. In the 12-day incubation period the virus probably multiplies in the regional lymphoid tissues. The fact that no patient is infectious during the incubation period suggests that in this interval an open lesion does not exist in the respiratory mucosa. In the unmodified case, a massive viremia occurs at the onset of the fever, and remains during the first two or three days of the pre-eruptive phase. In this way the virus localizes in the mucous membranes and in the skin as well as in the internal tissues. After the virus disappears from the blood and the skin eruption appears, the patient feels better, and the temperature tends to decrease. Antibodies are noted in the blood as early as the fourth day of the disease. The virus multiplies in the epithelial cells of the skin while being relatively protected from the action of circulating antibody so that cell destruction continues for some time. When pustulation occurs, the temperature tends to rise again, probably because of the absorption of the toxic products of cell necrosis. It is of interest that patients become infectious on the third day of the disease, probably because saliva has been contaminated through the early mucosal lesions noted in the pharynx and mouth. Skin lesions become infective after the superficial corneal layer has been severely damaged. Scabs remain infectious throughout the illness and until their separation during the third to fourth week of illness. The pitting is generally confined to the face, even in severe cases, and is due to destruction of sebaceous glands followed by organization and subsequent shrinking of granulation tissue and fibrosis. In cases of hemorrhagic smallpox numerous blood cells are present in the corium. *Cytoplasmic inclusions* are characteristic of infection with the vaccinia-variola group of viruses. Inclusion bodies can be shown best in epithelial cells, particularly of the involved skin and mucous membranes. Skin scrapings stained with hematoxylin and eosin show the inclusion to be round or oval homogeneous masses, either basophilic or acidophilic, located in the cytoplasm fairly close to the nucleus. The appearance of the inclusion bodies varies with the stage of infection but also with the method of fixation and staining, and this suggests that they consist of masses of elementary bodies. Intranuclear inclusions have also been described, but these are not invariably seen. With antimicrobial therapy, pathologic changes from bacterial complications are not found, and bacterial cultures, in this situation, are usually sterile.

Clinical Manifestations. The incubation period of smallpox is generally 12 days. The illness begins with intense malaise and high fever lasting for four to six days. There is intense prostration, and the clinical impression is often that of dengue. Severe headache, photophobia, and, occasionally, vomiting are noted. A small number of patients show a prodromal or "toxemic" rash, most easily noted in the groins, the axillae, and the flanks. On the fourth day the *focal rash* occurs, the fever diminishes slightly, and the patient feels much better, just at a time when the first macular skin lesions begin to form. The focal rash usually occurs first on the mucosa of the mouth and pharynx, the face, or the forearms, and it then spreads to the trunk and legs. A feature of variola is the fact that lesions in any one area are all at the same stage of development, whereas in varicella they are in all stages. The initial rash is macular and quickly becomes papular. Within two days the papules have developed into vesicles and these, within a few hours, become cloudy and pustular. On the eighth or ninth day from the beginning of the rash, drying and crusting begin. From three to four weeks from the onset of the disease, scabs have generally fallen off, leaving pigment-free skin, frequently with some scarring or pitting. The eruption is characteristically more severe on the face and the distal parts of the arms and legs, and less severe over the trunk and abdomen. The groins and axillae may be entirely spared. This centrifugal distribution is distinct from the characteristic rash of varicella, which tends to be centripetal. Lesions are generally found on the palms of the hands and the soles of the feet, a situation uncommonly seen in varicella of childhood, although these parts are often involved in the adult form. Fever generally recurs during the pustular stage, but the temperature returns to normal as the lesions become crusted. The characteristic pustular lesions of smallpox are round, raised, and tense, with a tendency to central depression as they begin to dry out. Clinical classification of disease from the mildest form (variola sine eruptione) to modified, to confluent, to malignant confluent, to hemorrhagic indicates degrees of severity of smallpox influenced in part by age, state of immunity, and state of hormonal balance. It is of great interest that women within a short time of term, either before or after delivery, tend to have a much more severe disease than those not pregnant.

In cases modified by vaccination or transplacental immunity in the first few months of life, the rash may be scant and the evolution of lesions may be very quick. *Regardless of how mild an index case of smallpox may be, the susceptible infected contacts suffer unmodified disease,* and overlooked early cases are frequently the cause of severe epidemics. Permanent scarring or pitting may result even in the absence of purulent infection of lesions with secondary bacterial pathogens (staphylococci and streptococci) in patients who have deep lesions and serious disease.

In previous years, the bacterial complications were incriminated as the principal cause of death, particularly after the pustular phase had commenced. It is now known that the mortality rate is chiefly related to the amount of virus present in the blood during the viremic phase that occurs in the first two days of the disease before any eruption is noted. It has been shown that if the amount of virus in the blood is so great that the whole blood of the patient in the viremic pre-eruptive phase can be used as the antigen in the complement-fixation test, the patient will almost surely die, although death may be delayed for nine or ten days. Patients who do die in the first week of illness often show evidence of heart failure and terminal pneumonia. Even in the absence of any antimicrobial therapy, the lungs are often sterile, indicating that the pneumonia is caused by the smallpox virus itself. The majority of deaths occur, however, in the pustular stage toward the end of the second week of the disease. Occasionally an encephalitis has been described that is indistinguishable from that associated with measles, varicella, or smallpox vaccination and tends to occur between the eighth and sixteenth days of disease.

Infection in Utero. No congenital anomalies have been described in infants of mothers infected with smallpox, but abortion is common because of the frequent bleeding that occurs during the toxemic phase. Infection of the fetus in utero may occur during the viremic phase in the mother; if this occurs near the end of pregnancy, the child will show clinical disease within a few days after birth. Infection has also been shown to occur at the time of birth if the disease is still active in the mother. There are two reports of smallpox in babies infected in utero a few days before birth, although the mothers showed no signs of the disease (Bancroft, 1904; Lynch, 1932).

Variola Minor. In the twentieth century, a milder clinical form of smallpox became prevalent in this hemisphere. It was recognized in Brazil in 1910, when a widespread outbreak of this mild form of the disease was recorded with a mortality of only 1 per cent. To this mild type of smallpox the name alastrim—variola minor—was given. Similar mild forms of the disease were recognized in South Africa, and it is now accepted that alastrim probably existed in Jenner's day side by side with variola major, the mortality of which has remained steady at about 30 per cent.

The vast majority of epidemics seen in this century in North America and Europe have been due to variola minor. Thus there were 12,000 cases in 1927 in England and Wales and over 48,000 cases in 1930 in the United States. In the 1930's, with the widespread application of smallpox vaccination in infancy, smallpox began to decrease in the United States. An important factor in this decrease was the better preservation of smallpox vaccine with the wider availability of refrigerators. It is likely that more potent vaccines and widespread improvement of health services also contributed to the decline in the number of cases. The two types of disease (variola major and variola minor) appeared to be distinct with a markedly different mortality for the two. At present there would appear to be no evidence that an outbreak of alastrim gives rise to cases of classic variola major, although the two types may produce coexistent separate outbreaks, as they apparently did in Detroit in 1924.

There is complete cross-protection for these two infections as there is from vaccinia. The clinical picture is similar in the prodromal or pre-eruptive phase to that of variola major, but hemorrhagic and toxic cases are almost never seen. The lesions tend to be more superficial and develop more rapidly; the total illness is shorter than in classic variola major. There may be no secondary fever during the pustular stage.

Differential Diagnosis. Smallpox is easily diagnosed, particularly during an epidemic period. More difficult to diagnose is the first and unsuspected case in those countries where smallpox is not endemic. This is particularly true if the first case is hemorrhagic. In this situation meningococcemia, a bleeding diathesis as a part of a blood dyscrasia, or typhus may be the suspected diagnosis. Very mild smallpox, modified by previous vaccination or alastrim, may be thought to be varicella, a drug eruption, or erythema multiforme. Except after known exposure, the clinical diagnosis cannot be made with certainty during the febrile phase, because the picture is indistinguishable from that of dengue, enteroviral infections, and other febrile diseases. In the eruptive phase, the most useful clinical points to remember are (1) the centrifugal distribution of lesions; (2) the fact that in a given area all the lesions are at the same stage of development; (3) the fact that there is a relative progression of eruptions from the face and arms to more recent lesions on the arms or legs; (4) the presence of a severe, febrile, three-day pre-eruptive disease; and, on occasion, (5) a known contact at least 12 days previously.

Laboratory Tests. Laboratory diagnostic procedures are of great value in quickly establishing the diagnosis of smallpox in the first case that appears in a community. These consist of (1) light microscopic or electron microscopic demonstration of viral particles in stained smears of vesicular fluid, (2) serologic or fluorescent demonstration of viral antigen in materials from cutaneous lesions, (3) isolation of virus from such materials, and (4) detection of antibodies in the serum early in the eruptive phase. The results of such tests are particularly helpful in differentiating varioloid from varicella and the hemorrhagic forms of the disease from other conditions (see Ch. 388). A detailed description of these procedures may be found in the 1969 article by Downie and Kempe.

Treatment. No specific treatment for smallpox is currently available, although a number of promising antiviral drugs are under study. Penicillin and broader-spectrum antimicrobials have been used in the prevention and treatment of bacterial complications. There is suggestive clinical evidence that secondary late bacterial complications, including pneumonia and staphylococcal involvement of skin and bones, are decreased by the use of antimicrobial therapy. But even with such therapy the mortality rates have not been reduced below 25 per cent in most outbreaks of variola major. Good nursing care and maintenance of fluid and electrolyte balance are essential. Convalescent smallpox serum and vaccinia-immune gamma globulin have been used in the treatment of severe cases without any evidence of success.

Prevention of Smallpox. *Management of Recently Exposed Persons.* The use of vaccinia-immune gamma globulin (see below) has been successful in the prophylaxis of smallpox and has reduced the incidence after known contact fourfold in control trials (Kempe et al., 1956, 1961). This compares with approximate six-, four-, 3.5-, and twofold reductions in attack rates in methisazone-treated groups reported in the studies of Bauer (1963, 1969) doValle (1965), Rao (1969), and Heiner (1971), respectively. In Heiner's study only the vaccinated contacts showed significant reduction in attack rates (twofold), and no difference in mortality or morbidity was noted between tested and placebo groups.

Community Control. There is no evidence that we owe our freedom from smallpox in the United States to routine vaccination. Compulsory routine vaccination was discontinued in Great Britain in the late 1950's, and 90 per cent of the population has either never been vaccinated or not vaccinated in the past ten years. Since 1969 there have been 12 smallpox importations into England, but the experience with secondary cases, deaths, and generations of cases until control has been no different in that country than in Germany, which has a far higher level of immunity in its population. Public health policy in the United States long held that high immunity levels are vital, and that an 80 per cent vaccination rate would give "herd protection." This has been thoroughly discredited, because importations have caused repeated outbreaks even though as many as 90 per cent of the population in an area were vaccinated. Only one third of the adults in the United States have been vaccinated in the past ten years, and fewer than 20 per cent of them in the last three years. Individuals who have not had a recent successful vaccination can be infected and may have a difficult-to-diagnose case, but they can, nevertheless, transmit the infection in its most virulent form, as has, in 1973, been shown again in the case of the English laboratory worker who had a greatly modified case of smallpox but still was able to transmit the infection in a fatal form to two contacts. There has been no smallpox in the United States since 1949, because we have been fortunate in not having the virus introduced rather than because our population is adequately protected. If variola major had been introduced, secondary cases would have resulted; but their number would have depended on early versus late diagnosis, prompt versus delayed ring vaccination of contacts, and careful immunologic survey and case finding, as well as the presence of a high level of immunity in our hospital staff personnel. In 1964, because of the persistent concern with the number of serious complications of smallpox vaccination, we recommended the discontinuation of nonselective routine vaccination of American children. *Selective* vaccination as a general policy has been endorsed in 1971 by all major public health and professional groups, except for the American Medical Association. Vaccination is now limited to (1) hospital personnel, (2) travelers to endemic areas, and (3) contacts of those with proved cases of smallpox. If the global eradication programs now underway should not be successful, it will be necessary to remain constantly alert that foreign quarantine procedures and selected traveler surveillance are maintained at a high level, and that adequate measures are taken, from both the clinical and laboratory points of view, in making the proper diagnosis at the earliest possible time.

With currently available techniques, an importation of smallpox and the development of some secondary cases in an unprotected population will, even with failures in early diagnosis, not result in any greater number of deaths than have occurred in the past 40 years from universal infant vaccination itself.

Control of Infected Persons, Contacts, and Environment. All cases should be reported to the local health authority, and patients should be isolated in a hospital until all crusts have disappeared. All oral, nasal, fecal, and urinary discharges and articles associated with patients should be disinfected by burning, high-pressure steam, or boiling. All contacts at home, place of work, or elsewhere should be vaccinated or revaccinated with a potent product and kept under daily surveillance for 16 days from the time of last contact. Any fever during surveillance calls for prompt isolation until smallpox can be excluded. The patient's source case should be sought assiduously. Adults with chickenpox or patients with hemorrhagic or pustular lesions of the skin need careful review for possible errors in diagnosis.

Epidemic Measures. In an epidemic the measures to be taken are as follows: (1) All smallpox patients and suspects should be isolated in hospital until they are no longer infectious. (2) All contacts should be carefully listed, vaccinated, and kept under surveillance for 16 days. (3) A public statement of the situation should be made by all available methods, and all possible contacts should be urged to be vaccinated. Potent vaccine should be provided and arrangements made for early vaccination of inner-ring and outer-ring contacts. (4) The use of vaccine, immune gamma globulin, and chemoprophylaxis with N-methylisatin B-thiosemicarbazone for close household contacts should further decrease the number of secondary cases. (5) Mass immunization of the entire population of a community or larger area is an emergency measure to be used only when an outbreak has given evidence of material spread.

International Measures. The World Health Organization and countries adjacent to the one in which an outbreak occurs should be notified by telegram of the existence of any cases of smallpox. At all times, the measures applicable to ships, aircraft, and land transport arriving from smallpox areas should be enforced, as specified in International Sanitary Regulations. It should be noted that evidence of protection by successful vaccination or revaccination (within a period of three years) is a widely enforced requirement for entry to the United States for *travelers from endemic countries but from no others.*

Vaccination vs. Chemoprophylaxis. Vaccination remains the best method of prevention for any individual likely to be exposed through travel in the smallpox-endemic regions of Asia or Africa. To be fully effective, successful revaccination every three years or, better, each year is recommended.

Upon exposure to a case of smallpox, vaccination and revaccination should be supplemented by chemoprophylaxis with methisazone, 3 grams given twice only 12 hours apart. For children three to ten years old, 1.5 grams twice only should be given, and for infants under three years of age, 0.75 gram twice only. Vaccination after exposure is generally inadequate to prevent disease, but should be done because in an epidemic situation subsequent repeat exposures may occur. The use of vaccinia-immune gamma globulin also markedly reduces clinical incidence and severity when used in full doses of 10 ml intramuscularly once for adults and 5 ml intramuscularly once for children under 12 years. Vaccinia-immune globulin and methisazone can and should both be given, when available, for a limited number of known contacts, such as may occur in aircraft exposures and to family contacts. A common but harmless side effect of methisazone is emesis. If vomiting occurs less than one hour after the dose, the full dose should be repeated with an antiemetic such as dimenhydrinate (Mavezine or Dramamine). Alcohol is strictly contraindicated because of the similar structure of methisazone and of the antialcoholic Antabuse.

WHO and health agencies of member countries in which there is endemic smallpox successfully depend on vaccination alone and concentrate on the elimination of specific smallpox foci, attempting to break the transmission chain rather than to rely on mass vaccination campaigns, which had been the time-honored method of eradication in the attempts at eradication in the past. It is believed that, particularly in Africa and Asia, it is much more efficient and economical to try to interrupt transmission at a time of low seasonal incidence of smallpox. Current strategy consists of an attempt to contain outbreaks of smallpox by the early detection and containment of cases so as to reduce smallpox incidence as quickly as possible, rather than the institution of mass vaccination.

In an outbreak in central Java in 1969, when more than 95 per cent of the 23,000,000 inhabitants in the province bore vaccination scars, almost 1700 cases of smallpox nevertheless occurred, 85 per cent of them developing in persons who had never been successfully vaccinated. In other words, in a population in which only 5 per cent were unimmunized, continued transmission was readily possible—definite evidence that "herd immunity" does not work. The incredible success obtained in West and Central Africa, and parts of Indonesia and Ethiopia, is entirely due to this change of strategy based on early detection of outbreaks and the establishment of trained teams to investigate and contain them. Case-finding requires a reporting network which had to be developed. The use of freeze-dried potent vaccine replaced liquid vaccine in all WHO programs. A very useful tool for case-finding is the WHO photo recognition card often given to schoolchildren, who proved to be one of the most fruitful sources of information in remote villages in

Asia and Africa. The schoolchild through recognition cards, visits to the principal markets which are held every week in different locations, and searching out through walking from village to village are the three bases for case-finding which lead to case identification and subsequent vaccination.

VACCINIA
(Vaccination)

Smallpox vaccine commonly in use is prepared from the vaccinia lesions on the skin of inoculated calves or sheep or from the allantoic membranes of chick embryos. All currently used smallpox vaccine contains infective virus, and all successful vaccinations are deliberately induced mild viral infections. It is thought that within one year after primary vaccination the chance of an attack is reduced to one one thousandth of that in the unvaccinated; within three years, to one two hundredth; within ten years, to one eighth, and within twenty years, to one half; after twenty years there is little if any protection against infection. However, the mortality in smallpox patients successfully vaccinated many years before is less than in the unvaccinated. There is no question that regular revaccination induces a high degree of immunity even with very massive exposure to the disease. Targeted vaccination and surveillance with case-finding in the remaining endemic areas of Asia and Africa will, in time, reduce the susceptible population below that necessary to permit the survival of the pathogenic virus.

Recommended Program for Vaccinations in the United States. We can look forward to the time when the present eradication program will have eliminated smallpox as a threat to man. At that time, vaccination will no longer be necessary, and jennerian vaccinations will then be a matter of only historic importance. Until this is achieved, however, smallpox vaccination will continue to be necessary for those at risk, namely, travelers to endemic areas and those who, by their occupation, are likely to come into contact with such travelers. These include hospital personnel and those involved with transportation services, as well as those in the armed forces.

Contraindications to Vaccination. Primary *routine* vaccination is no longer performed on North American infants, but even *selective* vaccination is generally contraindicated in infant patients who fail to thrive; in persons with dysgammaglobulinemia, blood dyscrasias, eczema, or other dermatitides; in the presence of radiation or other immunosuppressant therapy; in those exposed to infectious diseases; or in unvaccinated siblings of children with eczema. In the eczematous child, vaccination can be performed safely with attenuated vaccine when travel to endemic regions is contemplated. If exposure is likely, elective vaccination of the eczematous child *should* be performed, because the eczema vaccination in this situation is only 1 in 150 and the mortality is zero. Vaccination or revaccination is absolutely contraindicated for adult patients with neoplastic diseases, including Hodgkin's disease, lymphomas, and other conditions involving the prolonged use of corticosteroids, nitrogen mustard, or radiation therapy.

When travel outside the limits of the United States to nonendemic areas is contemplated, vaccination is no longer required for re-entry into the United States. At most, telephonic health surveillance for 14 days after reentry to the United States may be required. This is much to be preferred to life-threatening disease from vaccination. Vaccination has not been carried out by the Quarantine Service when the patient's physician has presented written evidence that the procedure should not be performed. If such a person must travel to an endemic area, the use of vaccinia-immune gamma globulin should be considered so as to provide temporary protection and to act as a substitute for the use of vaccination with live vaccinia virus.

Recommended Vaccination Techniques. To minimize the risk of unnecessary complications, the following practices are recommended:

Age for Primary Vaccination. In nonendemic areas, primary vaccination is not routinely done or is performed when the child is over two years of age. There are no conclusive data indicating the exact period when complication rates are minimal. The presence of some transplacental maternal immunity, provided that the mother has been vaccinated, may be desirable in modifying the primary vaccination reaction, and vaccination may be carried out in the first months of life. Vaccination of newborn infants has been done without complications (Kempe et al., 1952). However, in such cases in endemic areas, revaccination should be performed after an interval of six months. If primary vaccination is delayed for several months, children who are at increased risk, such as those suffering from the Swiss type of agammaglobulinemia, will have been readily identified by their clinical course and will therefore not become casualties of smallpox vaccination. The 1966 experience in the United States fails to show a higher risk of postvaccinia encephalitis for the two-to-ten age group (Neff et al., 1968), but some European authors have stressed that the first years of life may be a safer period. The case mortality for encephalitis is certainly highest among the youngest children (Berger, 1964; Coneybeare, 1948; Muller, 1946; Neff, 1968).

Site for Vaccination. Primary vaccination and revaccination are best performed on the outer aspects of the upper arm, over the insertion of the deltoid muscle or behind the midline. Reactions are less likely to be severe on the upper arm than on the lower extremity or other parts of the body. With proper technique, resultant scars are small and unobtrusive.

Preparation of the Vaccination Site. With a clean skin, the best preparation is none at all. The use of chemical skin cleaners may leave a residue that contains virus-inactivating material, and vigorous physical cleansing of the site may create minute abrasions that then can become sites of secondary vaccinia eruptions, with resultant involvement of a comparatively large skin area.

Vaccination Technique. Regardless of age, primary vaccination should be performed with no more than two or three pressures with the side of a needle. These pressure points should be as close together as possible, and should be made only at one site. With the highly potent vaccines currently in use, more numerous pressure points are not necessary and certainly should not be utilized for a nonimmune person. When children or adults are to be revaccinated after a lapse of more than five years, the same small number of pressure points should be used. For revaccination within a five-year period of those persons known to have had a major reaction, the full complement of 30 strokes can safely be used (Leake, 1946).

Vaccination Reaction. The description of the reactions after vaccination or revaccination should follow the criteria recommended by the Expert Committee on Smallpox of the World Health Organization. A successful primary vaccination is one that on examination after seven to ten days presents a typical jennerian vesicle. If this is not present, vaccination must be repeated with fresh vaccine and a few more strokes of the needle. The successful revaccination is one that on examination one week (six to ten days) later shows a vesicular or pustular lesion *or* an area of definite palpable induration and congestion surrounding a central lesion; this lesion may be a scab or an ulcer. These reactions are termed *major reactions;* all others should be called *equivocal reactions.*

A major reaction indicates virus multiplication with consequent development of immunity. An equivocal reaction may merely represent an allergic response, which could be elicited by inactive vaccine or poor technique in someone who had been sensitized by earlier vaccination; or the equivocal reaction may result from sufficient immunity to prevent virus multiplication. Since the allergic response cannot be readily differentiated from the one caused by true immunity, another vaccination should be performed, using a different lot of vaccine if there is the possibility that the first was of weak potency, and the procedure should be completed with an additional number of pressures. The site should be examined one week later; if the result is again equivocal, revaccination should be repeated, using a full 30 pressures as recommended by Leake. For the sake of expediency, an equivocal reaction to revaccination with a minimal insertion may be followed by vaccination at two sites, not less than 2 inches apart, using known potent vaccine. This method will make a third return unnecessary in almost all instances.

In summary, successful smallpox vaccination consists of the production of a major reaction. When potent vaccine and good technique are used, repeated inability to produce a major reaction can be assumed to be due to solid immunity from previous immunization.

Frequency of Vaccination. Revaccination is essential to reinforce the immunity conferred by previous vaccination. This not only maintains a high level of immunity against smallpox, but minimizes the risk of complications on revaccination. To maintain adequate immunity against smallpox, revaccination should be carried out at approximately five-year intervals. Those persons at some increased risk, such as hospital and public health personnel, members of the armed forces, and those working at port or airline offices, as well as shipping personnel, should be revaccinated at least once every three years. When exposure to smallpox is probable, by travel or residence in a smallpox-endemic area, annual revaccination is desirable.

Complications of Vaccination. With the abandonment of universal routine vaccination of infants in 1971, complications in the United States have markedly decreased. Life-threatening complications of primary vaccination include eczema vaccinatum, postvaccinial encephalitis, and vaccinia gangrenosa (progressive vaccinia). The principal danger after revaccination is vaccinia gangrenosa, a condition in which the impairment of the patient's immune mechanism permits the continuing multiplication of the vaccinia virus. Vaccinia gangrenosa is seen in seemingly normal subjects as well as in those suffering from dysgammaglobulinemia, Hodgkin's disease, leukemia, blood dyscrasias, and other conditions in which corticosteroid therapy or ionized irradiation has been administered therapeutically. The presence of these conditions is an absolute contraindication to vaccination.

Human vaccinia-immune globulin has been shown to be effective in the prevention and treatment of eczema vaccinatum and has also been used extensively in the treatment of other complications, in which it also produces a significant reduction in mortality. Vaccinia-immune globulin reduces the incidence of postvaccinial encephalitis. In the Royal Netherland Army, 53,630 of 106,174 recruits received hyperimmune vaccinia-immune gamma globulin, and the remaining 52,544 recruits received a placebo. In the group treated with gamma globulin, 3 cases of postvaccinial encephalitis occurred in contrast to 13 cases in the control group. There was one fatality in each group. Gamma globulin failed to have an effect on the severity and duration of the encephalitis produced by the vaccination, and it was not effective in treatment. There is evidence that transplacental maternal immunity is also effective in modifying the course of primary vaccination; significant reactions are rarely reported in very young infants whose mothers have been vaccinated in the past. In cases of vaccinia gangrenosa, the simultaneous use of vaccinia-immune globulin and N-methylisatin beta-thiosemicarbazone appears to be of value. The therapeutic dose of the drug is 200 mg per kilogram orally initially, followed by 50 mg per kilogram every six hours for three days. After an interval of three days, another three-day course may be required. Adequate early treatment of the complications of smallpox vaccination can materially reduce the morbidity and mortality. Through the Center for Disease Control in Atlanta, Georgia, a group of experts is available for telephone consultation (day: [404] 633-3311; night: [404] 633-2176). When such consultation is used in conjunction with vaccinia-immune globulin and chemotherapeutic agents, effective diagnostic and therapeutic aids are available for all.

Bauer, D. J., St. Vincent, L., Kempe, C. H., Young, P. A., and Downie, A. W.: Prophylaxis of smallpox with methisazone. Am. J. Epidemiol., 90:130, 1969.

Downie, A. W., and Kempe, C. H.: Variola and vaccinia viruses. *In* Lennette, E. H. (ed.): Diagnostic Procedures for Viral and Rickettsial Diseases. New York, American Public Health Association, 1969, Chap. 25.

DoValle, L. A. R., DeMelo, P. R., De Salles Gomes, L. F., and Proença, L. M.: Methisazone in prevention of variola minor among contacts. Lancet, 2:976, 1965.

Heiner, G. G., et al.: Field trials of methisazone as a prophylactic agent against smallpox. Am. J. Epidemiol., 94:435, 1971.

Kempe, C. H., et al.: The use of vaccinia hyperimmune gamma globulin in the prophylaxis of smallpox. Bull. WHO, 25:41, 1961.

Kempe, C. H., et al.: Smallpox vaccination of eczema patients with a strain of attenuated live vaccinia (CVI-78). Pediatrics, 42:980, 1968.

Neff, J. M.: Complications of smallpox vaccination. I. National Survey in the United States, 1963. N. Engl. J. Med., 276:125, 1967.

Rao, A. R., et al.: Chemoprophylaxis and chemotherapy in variola major. I. An assessment of CG 662 and Marboran in prophylaxis of contacts of variola major. Indian J. Med. Res., 57:477, 1969.

WHO Expert Committee on Smallpox: Second Report, Publication 393, World Health Organization Technical Report Series. Geneva, World Health Organization, 1968.

For more detailed lists of references see the following:

Dixon, C. W.: Smallpox. London, J. & A. Churchill, Ltd., 1962.

Downie, A. W.: Smallpox. *In* Horsfall, F. L., Jr., and Tamm, I. (eds.): Viral and Rickettsial Infections of Man. 4th ed. Philadelphia, J. B. Lippincott Company, 1965.

122. ORF (Ecthyma Contagiosum, Contagious Pustular Dermatitis)

Clayton E. Wheeler, Jr.

Orf is a worldwide viral infection of sheep and goats that is occasionally transmitted to the skin of man. The disorder occurs most often in sheepherders and shearers, meat porters, butchers, veterinarians, technicians engaged in vaccine manufacture, and children or adults caring for pet lambs.

The virus is a round-ended, brick-shaped particle that measures 260 by 160 mμ and is classified with the paravaccinia viruses. Inoculation into the glabrous skin of sheep produces erythematous macules in three or four days, followed by pustular, granulomatous, papillomatous, and crusted phases. Healing occurs in four to six weeks. Infected animals show crusted, warty, or granulomatous lesions about the lips, nose, and eyelids that have occasioned the term "scabby mouth." The agent proliferates in primary tissue cultures of human amnion, monkey kidney, and bovine testis, in which a characteristic appearance is produced. Neutralizing and complement-fixing antibodies have been demonstrated in the blood of recovered animals and man.

Human lesions are usually single and appear most often on the hands, fingers, forearms, or face. There is often a history of trauma at the site of the lesion, followed in four to eleven days by the appearance of a red macule or papule. In a week or two this becomes a multiloculated vesicle from which little fluid can be expressed upon incision. In the next two weeks the surface becomes white and sodden, a crust usually forms, and a granulomatous reaction often develops. Healing takes place with little or no scar formation in four to six weeks. Mature lesions are 1 to 4 cm in diameter, elevated, dome-shaped, plateau or tumor-like, and well demarcated from normal skin. Regional lymphangitis or lymphadenopathy may occur as part of the viral infection or as a result of secondary bacterial involvement. Erythema multiforme is an uncommon complication. Persistent, giant orf has been observed in an immunosuppressed individual.

Microscopically, proliferation, ballooning, and reticular degeneration of epidermal cells, multilocular vesiculation, and pseudoepitheliomatous hyperplasia may be found. A granulomatous reaction is present in the dermis.

Treatment is symptomatic and is directed toward prevention or cure of secondary bacterial infection. Vaccination with live virus provides effective control in animals but it is not practicable in man.

Leavell, U. W., Jr., McNamara, M. J., Muelling, R., Talbert, W. M., Rucker, R. C., and Dalton, A. J.: Orf: Report of 19 human cases. J.A.M.A., 204:657, 1968.

Nagington, J., Newton, A. A., and Horne, R. W.: The structure of orf virus. Virology, 23:461, 1964.

Nagington, J., and Whittle, C. H.: Human orf. Isolation of the virus by tissue culture. Br. Med. J., 2:1324, 1961.

Savage, J., and Black, M. M.: Giant orf of finger in a patient with lymphoma. Proc. R. Soc. Med., 65:766, 1972.

123. MOLLUSCUM CONTAGIOSUM

Clayton E. Wheeler, Jr.

Molluscum contagiosum is an infection of the skin, and occasionally of the conjunctiva, with the largest of the true animal viruses. The viral particle is oval or brick shaped and measures approximately 300 by 220 mμ. It does not grow in the skin or cornea of animals or in tissues of the chick embryo, and its growth in tissue culture is questionable, although a cytopathic effect occurs, and interferon production is induced. Experimental inoculation of ground, filtered molluscum material into human skin is followed by a new lesion at the inoculation site in 14 to 50 days. Studies of immunity are fragmentary, although there is suggestive evidence for the development of complement-fixing antibodies and cutaneous sensitivity of the delayed type.

The pathologic change is confined to the epidermis, which grows into the dermis as multiple, closely packed, pear-shaped globules. Epidermal cells undergo characteristic degeneration as they progress from the basal layer to the surface, where they form a cavity at the center of the growth. Cellular degeneration is produced by intracytoplasmic growth of viral particles that form huge inclusions. These enlarge and distort the cell and crowd the nucleus to one side. Inclusions contain large amounts of deoxyribonucleic acid and stain deeply with hematoxylin and eosin.

This common disorder is worldwide and usually affects children. The disease is autoinoculable and mildly contagious, but the source of the infection and method of spread are often unknown.

Lesions are most often seen on the trunk, face, arms, or genital areas, although they occur almost anywhere. Conjunctival infection may result in epiphora, discharge, conjunctivitis, or keratitis. Lesions may be solitary, few and localized, numerous and generalized, or eruptive in association with atopic dermatitis or immunosuppressive therapy. They vary in size from barely visible to 0.5 cm or larger. They are usually discrete, but they may be grouped or form plaques or tumor-like masses. Characteristic papules are skin colored or slightly pink, pearly, circumscribed, elevated, firm, rounded, or semiglobular, and present central umbilication from which a curdlike material can be expressed. Inflammation is usually absent, but it may develop from irritation or secondary infection. Systemic infection with the virus is unknown.

The clinical appearance of the papules and the expression of a gelatinous central core usually suffice for diagnosis. The microscopic picture is diagnostic. Molluscum contagiosum is most often confused with nevi, warts, epithelioma, pyogenic granuloma, folliculitis, and other forms of pyoderma. Cure can usually be accomplished by curettage or light electrodesiccation. Spontaneous involution is not uncommon.

Lynch, P. J.: Molluscum contagiosum venereum. Clin. Obst. Gynecol., 15:966, 1972.

Postlethwaite, R.: Molluscum contagiosum. A review. Arch. Environ. Health, 21:432, 1970.

Sturt, R. J., Muller, H. K., and Francis, G. D.: Molluscum contagiosum in villages of the West Sepik district of New Guinea. Med. J. Aust., 2:751, 1971.

124. FOOT-AND-MOUTH DISEASE (Aphthous Fever)

Walsh McDermott

Foot-and-mouth disease is a viral infection of animals, chiefly cattle, which occurs in man only with great rarity. Infection, when it does occur in man, presumably results from direct contact with the agent either in the laboratory or from handling the tissues or body fluids of infected animals. The disease in man is characterized by a short incubation period followed by the appearance of a febrile illness with vesicular lesions of palms, soles, and the oropharyngeal mucosa. Neurologic involvement has not been reported, and the disease is self-limited. There is no treatment of established value; the tetracycline drugs have yielded inconclusive results in the treatment of laboratory animals. Prevention of the disease in man has not been extensively studied, for man generally has a high degree of resistance to the infection. Spread among cattle is presumably by the airborne route. An effective vaccine for use in cattle has been developed. As in influenza, however, there are many types and subtypes of foot-and-mouth (FMD) virus, and it is believed that for optimal effectiveness the homologous viral strain, i.e., the "epidemic" strain, should be present in the vaccine.

Annotations: Spread of foot-and-mouth disease. Lancet, 2:580, 1969.

Flaum, A.: Foot-and-mouth disease in man. Acta. Pathol. Microbiol. Scand., 16:197, 1939.

Hyslop, N. St.G., Davie, J., and Carter, S. P.: Antigenic differences between strains of foot-and-mouth disease virus of type SAT 1. J. Hyg. (Camb.), 61:217, 1963.

125. MUMPS

Dorothy M. Horstmann

Definition. Mumps is an acute contagious viral infection, most commonly manifested by nonsuppurative swelling of the parotid glands. Other salivary glands, the testes, pancreas, and central nervous system are among the various organs that may also be involved.

Historical Note. Hippocrates described mumps in the fifth century B.C. Because of its characteristic manifestations, it was one of the earliest diseases to be recognized as a clinical entity. A classic description was written by Hamilton (1790), who was the first to stress the importance of orchitis as a complication. He also noted that central nervous system signs sometimes accompany the parotitis, but it was early in the twentieth century before clinicians recognized meningoencephalitis as a relatively frequent manifestation. In 1940 Wesselhoeft called attention to the occurrence of oophoritis and pancreatitis, and later others reported involvement of many organs and tissues. Not until 1934 did Johnson and Goodpasture prove the viral etiology of mumps by reproducing the disease in monkeys inoculated with filtrates of infective human saliva. The virus was adapted to growth in hens' eggs in 1945 by Habel, and by Levens and Enders, who demonstrated its hemagglutinating properties. Enders and his associates also described the appearance of dermal hypersensitivity and of complement-fixing (CF) antibodies after mumps. The availability of a skin test and of serologic tools allowed the demonstration that infection with mumps virus can occur without parotitis and not infrequently without any signs at all. Immunization with a killed virus vaccine was tried in the 1950's with limited success. In 1966 Bunyak and Hilleman developed a highly effective live attenuated mumps virus vaccine, prepared in chick embryo tissue culture, which is currently widely used.

Etiology. Mumps is an RNA virus, a member of the myxovirus family that includes the influenza and parainfluenza viruses. These agents all have the property of agglutinating chicken, human, and other erythrocytes. In monkeys, mumps virus induces parotitis, and in suckling mice or hamsters it may cause fatal meningoencephalitis. The virus multiplies in embryonated chick embryos and in a variety of tissue culture cells. For primary isolation (usually from saliva), eggs or preferably cell cultures derived from monkeys or humans are used. In tissue cultures the presence of the virus is recognized either by the appearance of cytopathic changes or by means of the hemadsorption test, which depends on the ability of the virus-infected cells to adsorb guinea pig erythrocytes. In infected cultures these are seen firmly attached to the cell sheet, whereas in control tubes the erythrocytes float in the media. The specificity of the reaction is established serologically, using the hemadsorption inhibition test. Mumps virus is associated with soluble (S) and viral (V) complement-fixing (CF) antigens and a skin test antigen. Infection induces CF, hemagglutination-inhibiting, and neutralizing antibodies.

Epidemiology. Mumps is a common disease, endemic all over the world. It occurs throughout the year, but there is a seasonal prevalence, with a regular increase in cases in winter and spring. Epidemics are frequent, large outbreaks tending to have a seven- or eight-year cycle. The disease incidence is the same in both sexes, but males are more prone to develop central nervous system complications. Most cases occur between the ages of 5 and 15 years; young adults are nevertheless sometimes susceptible, as evidenced by epidemics in military camps and schools.

The only known reservoir of infection is man. In experiments in volunteers, Henle et al. showed that the virus may be present in the saliva from two to six days before the occurrence of parotid swelling, and as long as seven to nine days after onset. *Transmission* is thought to be by direct contact, air-suspended droplets, or fomites contaminated with saliva. Rather more solid contact appears to be necessary for transmission of mumps than is the case with measles or chickenpox.

Although it is a common disease, only about 60 per cent of the adult population gives a positive history, in contrast to more than 90 per cent for measles. The difference is due in part to the frequency of inapparent infection with mumps virus. About 50 per cent of those with a negative history give a positive serologic test, indicating previous silent infection. One experience with mumps virus appears to confer lifelong immunity.

Pathogenesis and Pathology. The widespread involvement of glandular and other tissues in the body indicates that mumps is a systemic infection. The virus apparently enters and multiplies first in the upper respiratory tract; it then invades the bloodstream, and localizes in the salivary as well as other glands and in the central nervous system. The parotids are one of many target organs, the greater frequency with which they are involved being simply a reflection of greater sensitivity.

Limited observations on pathologic specimens indicate that the reaction in the parotid gland is a nonspecific inflammatory one, which is not extensive. The testes and pancreas also demonstrate inflammatory and degenerative changes. Lesions induced by the virus in the central nervous system are of two types: those induced by direct viral invasion, resulting in a primary encephalitis; and the demyelination characteristic of postinfectious encephalitis. Mumps virus has been shown to cause hydrocephalus in laboratory animals, and there is some evidence that this lesion may also occur rarely in man.

Clinical Manifestations. The incubation period is 17 to 21 days, usually 18; extremes of 12 and 35 days have been reported. In most cases, pain and swelling in the parotid region are the first signs of the disease, although occasionally in adults pain in the testicle may be the initial symptom. Rarely, meningitis appears first, followed later by parotitis. In more severe cases, there is often a prodromal period, sometimes lasting as long as two or three days, with fever, malaise, headache, chills, sore throat, earache, and tenderness along the region of the parotid ducts.

Parotid swelling is first observed below the ear, usually obliterating the hollow between the mastoid process and the ascending ramus of the lower jaw. The gland increases in size over a two- to three-day period, but there is great variation in the degree of swelling; in mild cases it may be scarcely apparent, but in severe ones the associated edema may eventually spread superiorly to the eyes, posteriorly to the mastoid region, and inferiorly below the chin and over the anterior aspect of the neck. For the first two days, unilateral involvement is the rule, but eventually both glands are affected in about 70 per cent of cases. The skin over the swollen parotids is not usually reddened, but is tense and tender on pressure. Not infrequently the submaxillary and sublingual glands are also affected. Involvement of the sublingual glands can result in swelling of the tongue, with attendant painful swallowing. Presternal pitting edema is also occasionally present, apparently because of obstruction of the lymphatics by the enlarged salivary glands.

The patient seldom suffers severe pain except on movement of the jaws, e.g., in talking or chewing. If Stensen's duct becomes partially occluded as the gland swells, there is sharp pain on taking food or an acid drink, which stimulates the secretory mechanism. Because this occurs only with partial occlusion of the duct, it is not a constant sign. The papillae at the opening of Stensen's or Wharton's duct may be reddened, but this also is inconstant.

Constitutional symptoms vary greatly and may be virtually absent. They are especially mild in children, but tend to be more severe in adults, in whom the incidence of extraparotid lesions is higher. Fever varies with the extent of involvement, ranging between 38 and 39.5 C in full-blown, uncomplicated cases, but going as high as 40.5 and 41° C if orchitis, meningoencephalitis, or both develop.

The duration of parotid swelling and fever is dependent upon the extent and severity of the process. Usually the temperature is normal within five days, and swelling has disappeared by seven to ten days. A peculiar tendency to relapse with recurrence of parotid swelling has been noted in buglers, horn players, and others whose occupations involve similar exertion.

Neurologic Manifestations. The incidence of *aseptic meningitis* varies widely in different epidemics, but can be as high as 25 per cent. Serial examination of the cerebrospinal fluid indicates that the cell count is elevated in approximately one half of all cases of mumps. Clinically evident neurologic involvement may occur preceding, simultaneously with, or after parotitis. It affects males three to five times more commonly than females, and may be the only manifestation of the infection. The clinical picture of headache, fever, stiff neck, and lethargy is similar to that in other forms of viral meningitis, but the cerebrospinal fluid findings may differ in several respects. Thus cell counts tend to be higher; 500 to 1000 cells, predominantly lymphocytes, are common, and occasionally even several thousand are present. The pleocytosis in mumps is also more prolonged, and may persist for several weeks. Glucose levels below 40 mg per 100 ml have recently been reported in 10 to 20 per cent of cases. The protein levels are moderately elevated. *Encephalitis,* whether resulting from direct attack by mumps virus or occurring as postinfectious encephalitis, is rare.

Other rare neurologic complications include permanent nerve deafness, either unilateral or bilateral; labyrinthitis; polyneuritis, sometimes affecting the facial or trigeminal nerves; disturbances in accommodation; optic neuritis, iritis, and iridocyclitis; and possibly hydrocephalus.

Orchitis. Orchitis is rare before puberty. After puberty, its incidence varies, but is usually about 25 per cent; there is considerable variation in different epidemics. Testicular involvement is most often unilateral, but may be bilateral, one following the other by one to nine days. The onset is commonly between the fifth and tenth days of illness, as the parotid swelling is subsiding. In mild cases there may be nothing more than discomfort, with tenderness and slight fever. In others, onset is abrupt, with a chill, fever to 40° C or higher, nausea, vomiting, sweats, backache, prostration, and severe testicular pain. Swelling of the testicle may be moderate, or the gland may rapidly reach three to four times normal size, in which case it is excessively hard, tender, and so painful that even 0.030 gram of morphine is not always effective. In severe cases, the epididymis, spermatic cord, or tunica vaginalis may be involved, and straw-colored hydrocele fluid sometimes collects.

In mild cases the testicle may be normal in four days, although in the most severe, it may require three or four weeks before all evidence of inflammation has disappeared. Some degree of atrophy, apparently caused by pressure necrosis, occurs in about a third to a half of all cases of orchitis, *but in most instances it is unilateral. Even when both testes are involved, the distribution of the inflammatory reaction and loss of functional tissue are apt to be spotty, and seldom result in sterility.*

Oophoritis. Oophoritis occurs occasionally in adult females, but it may be more frequent than suspected, as mild forms are difficult to recognize. High fever, chills, lower quadrant or back pain, and palpable ovarian enlargement have been described. Sterility resulting from mumps oophoritis is virtually unknown.

Pancreatitis. Pancreatitis has been estimated to occur in less than 10 per cent of cases. Severe epigastric pain, vomiting, diarrhea or constipation, and fever are characteristic; abdominal tenderness and muscle spasm may be marked.

Other Organs. More rarely, other glands or organs are involved, particularly in adults. The following have been reported as complications of mumps: prostatitis, bartholinitis, and mastitis (in both males and females); involvement of the thyroid, thymus, and lacrimal glands; splenomegaly; and hepatitis. Transient abnormalities of renal function occur frequently, but persistent nephritis is unusual, although fatal cases have been reported. Polyarthritis, occurring ten days to two weeks after onset, is a rare complication. Myocarditis, accompanied by precordial pain or heart block, has been described. Serial electrocardiograms on patients with mumps have revealed some abnormality in as high as 15 per cent, although very few patients show clinical evidence of myocarditis.

Diagnosis. Sudden onset of parotitis in a previously healthy patient with a negative history of mumps presents no diagnostic problem. Other causes of parotid swelling are suppurative parotitis, an acute bacterial infection in which there is marked tenderness, the skin over the gland is red and hot, and pus can often be expressed from the duct; preauricular and anterior cervical lymphadenopathy; and salivary calculi obstructing the duct and giving rise to recurrent parotitis. Chronic enlargement of the gland occurs with tumors, Mikulicz's disease, and uveoparotid fever of sarcoidosis.

Mumps infection in the absence of parotitis is often difficult to recognize. Orchitis can be due in rare instances to infection with other viruses such as coxsackievirus B, echovirus, and lymphocytic choriomeningitis virus. A variety of viral agents cause aseptic meningitis or meningoencephalitis that cannot be distinguished clinically from central nervous system involvement caused by mumps. In such situations specific laboratory tests are necessary to establish the etiology. Mumps virus can be isolated from saliva, urine, and, in meningitis, from the cerebrospinal fluid. More commonly, confirmation of the diagnosis is based on the demonstration of a significant rise in antibody titer (either complement-fixing or hemagglutination-inhibiting) when acute and convalescent serum samples are tested. If only a single convalescent specimen is available, the presence of a high titer is suggestive of recent infection. The *skin test* is of no value in diagnosis, because dermal hypersensitivity usually does not develop until three to four weeks after onset; it is less reliable than serologic tests in determining immune status.

Routine laboratory tests frequently indicate a relative lymphocytosis in uncomplicated parotitis; with orchitis, pancreatitis, or aseptic meningitis, the total leukocyte count often reaches 15,000 to 20,000, with a high percentage of polymorphonuclear cells. The blood amylase is usually elevated as a result of parotitis and is therefore not a reliable indication of pancreatic involvement.

Prognosis. Complete recovery is the rule, and mortality is virtually nil. A few fatal cases of encephalitis have been reported; bilateral testicular atrophy with resultant sterility (see above) and permanent nerve deafness are rare residua.

Treatment. Bed rest and symptomatic therapy are all that can be offered. For parotid pain, aspirin or codeine is effective. Some patients find an ice bag applied to the parotid region comforting, but others prefer heat. The headache associated with meningitis may be relieved by lumbar puncture. If orchitis is mild, no special treatment is required; if severe, meperidine (Demerol) (0.05 to 0.1 gram) or morphine (0.01 to 0.015 gram) may be necessary to control the pain. Local support and provision of warmth by means of a nest of absorbent cotton are more effective than an ice bag to the scrotum. Corticosteroids relieve the pain but do not appear to alter the duration of illness, nor do they protect against the subsequent development of atrophy. They are not indicated in mild cases, but in severe ones hydrocortisone, 10 mg per kilogram per day, may be given for three to four days.

Prevention. A live attenuated mumps virus vaccine, grown in tissue cultures of chick embryo cells, was licensed in 1968. To date, more than 10 million persons have been immunized in the United States. The vaccine is available as a monovalent preparation or combined with measles and rubella vaccines. It is given subcutaneously, causes virtually no clinical reaction, and induces antibody conversions in more than 95 per cent of susceptibles. The serum titers are lower than those that follow natural infection, but they have persisted satisfactorily for the six-year period over which antibodies have been tested. Vaccinees have been shown to be resistant to mumps when subsequently exposed to siblings with the disease.

The vaccine may be given to persons of any age over 12 months; it is not recommended for infants under one year because of the possible presence of residual maternal antibody which interferes with the development of active immunity. Immunization is recommended particularly for boys approaching puberty who give no history of mumps. If the vaccine is given after exposure, it is unlikely that it will protect. However, it may be given under these circumstances so that if contact infection failed to develop in a susceptible subject who was exposed, he will be protected when he next meets the virus.

Mumps vaccine should not be given to persons with allergy to egg proteins or to neomycin. It is contraindicated for those with any disease that results in compromised immune mechanisms and for patients on immunosuppressive therapy. Since the vaccine contains live virus, it should not be given during pregnancy.

Henle, W., and Enders, J. F.: Mumps virus. *In* Horsfall, F. L., Jr., and Tamm, I. (eds.): Viral and Rickettsial Infections of Man. 4th ed. Philadelphia, J. B. Lippincott Company, 1965, pp. 755–768.

Johnstone, J. A., Ross, C. A. C., and Dunn, M.: Meningitis and encephalitis associated with mumps infection. A 10-year survey. Arch. Dis. Child., 47:647, 1972.

Reed, D., Brown, G., Merrick, R., Sever, J., and Feltz, E.: A mumps epidemic on St. George Island, Alaska. J.A.M.A., 199:113, 1967.

Roseman, R. D.: Mumps orchitis. Clin. Proc. Children's Hospital, Wash. D. C., 14:239, 1958.

Weibel, R. E., Bunyak, E. B., Stokes, J., Jr., and Hilleman, M.: Persistence of immunity following monovalent and combined measles, mumps, and rubella vaccines. Pediatrics, 51:467, 1973.

ENTEROVIRAL DISEASES

Albert Z. Kapikian

126. COXSACKIEVIRUSES, ECHOVIRUSES, AND NEWLY RECOGNIZED ENTEROVIRUSES: INTRODUCTION

The coxsackieviruses, groups A and B, echoviruses, and polioviruses comprise the enterovirus subgroup of the picornaviruses of humans. It has been proposed recently that newly recognized serotypes of the enterovirus subgroup be designated simply as enteroviruses rather than as members of a specific enterovirus subgroup (i.e., polio-, coxsackie-, or echovirus) on account of overlapping properties among certain enterovirus strains. In this system, the first newly recognized serotype has been designated enterovirus 68 in order to avoid confusion with enterovirus numbers proposed previously, and, in addition, because 67 enteroviruses, comprised of 3 polio-, 30 coxsackie-, and 34 echoviruses, had already been described (1 coxsackievirus and 3 echoviruses have been reclassified [see below]). Previously recognized serotypes of the polio-, coxsackie-, and echoviruses would not be affected by this proposal, for they would retain assigned subgroup and number designations. In addition to the enterovirus subgroup, picornaviruses of humans include two other subgroups: the rhinoviruses (described in Ch. 112), and the unclassified picornaviruses representing those viruses that cannot be classified with certainty into the proper subgroup. The picornaviruses are grouped on the basis of certain common biochemical and biophysical properties, such as small size (15 to 30 nm), ribonucleic acid (RNA) core, and resistance to inactivation by ether. The term picornavirus was chosen to signify two of these properties: "pico" implying small, and "rna" referring to the nucleic acid type.

COXSACKIEVIRUSES

The isolation of the first of the group A coxsackieviruses during a study of a small poliomyelitis outbreak was reported by Dalldorf and Sickles in 1948. Suspensions of fecal specimens from two patients with paralytic poliomyelitis were found to cause paralysis in suckling mice, with widespread degeneration of the skeletal musculature. Since polioviruses were not known to cause illness in suckling mice and since these newly recovered agents (unlike the polioviruses) produced no illness in monkeys, it was assumed that a new agent distinct from the polioviruses had been isolated. As neither the anatomic lesions nor the range of symptoms induced by infection with this agent in man was known, it was suggested that the virus be called "Coxsackie virus," because the first strains were isolated from residents of Coxsackie, New York. The following year, additional types, including the first of the group B coxsackieviruses, were isolated. In the ensuing years, numerous other group A and B coxsackieviruses were isolated; at this writing, there are 23 group A coxsackieviruses (numbered A1 to A22 and A24) and 6 group B coxsackieviruses (numbered B1 to B6). Coxsackievirus A23 is omitted because it has been reclassified as echovirus type 9.

The coxsackieviruses are divided into groups A and B on the basis of differences in lesions induced in suckling mice. In this animal the group A viruses characteristically produce flaccid paralysis with widespread degeneration of skeletal musculature and no other lesions, whereas the group B viruses produce fewer and less severe skeletal muscle lesions, but produce in addition encephalitis, fat necrosis, pancreatitis, hepatitis, and myocarditis; clinically, group B–infected suckling mice develop tremors, spasticity, and spastic paralysis. All group B coxsackieviruses (and polio- and echoviruses [except echovirus 21]) grow readily in monkey kidney cell cultures, but none of the group A coxsackieviruses (with the exception of A9) are capable of consistently growing in these cultures.

ECHOVIRUSES

The first echoviruses were isolated in the early 1950's as a result of the introduction of cell culture techniques as an efficient tool for the isolation and study of polioviruses. During the course of studies attempting to isolate poliovirus from fecal specimens in cell cultures, agents were found that not only were not neutralized by either poliovirus or coxsackievirus antisera, but also were incapable of inducing illness in suckling mice or in monkeys. These new "human enteric" or "orphan" viruses were later termed enteric cytopathogenic human orphan viruses (echo), because they were isolated predominantly from the lower alimentary tract, caused cytopathogenic changes in monkey and human cell cultures, and were recovered from humans. Moreover, they had neither been associated etiologically with disease in humans nor shown to be pathogenic in selected laboratory animals. The term "orphan" was suggested because of this lack of etiologic association with disease.

The echoviruses were numbered from 1 to 34. Currently, 31 serotypes are recognized as types 10, 28, and 34 and have been reclassified. Type 10 was found to be considerably larger in size than other echoviruses and was reclassified as reovirus type 1; type 28 was found to possess certain properties (such as inactivation at pH 3) not shared by other echoviruses and was reclassified as rhinovirus 1A; and type 34, although nonpathogenic in suckling mice, was found to be antigenically related to coxsackievirus A24 and was therefore reclassified as a strain of coxsackievirus A24.

NEWLY RECOGNIZED ENTEROVIRUSES

Enteroviruses 68, 69, and 70 are the most recent additions to the enterovirus subgroup and are classified according to the new system described above because of overlapping properties among certain enterovirus strains. For example, one strain of enterovirus 68 induces characteristic group A coxsackievirus lesions in suckling mice, whereas three other strains of this serotype do not. In addition, among the classified coxsackie- and echoviruses, certain strains of coxsackievirus A24 are not pathogenic in suckling mice, whereas the prototype strain is; and certain strains of echovirus 9 are pathogenic in suckling mice, whereas the prototype strain is not.

DISEASES DUE TO COXSACKIEVIRUSES, ECHOVIRUSES, AND NEWLY RECOGNIZED ENTEROVIRUSES

A definitive presentation of diseases caused by coxsackie- and echoviruses is difficult, because these agents have been isolated from an ever-increasing list of specific diseases and clinical syndromes. The mere isolation of the virus from a patient's throat or anal swab and/or the demonstration of serologic evidence of infection is not sufficient evidence to establish an etiologic relationship between the virus and the patient's illness. Isolation of virus from blood, cerebrospinal fluid (CSF), or diseased tissue is more meaningful evidence for an etiologic association than the above, but even more meaningful evidence may be obtained from controlled epidemiologic studies. The establishment of an etiologic association is especially difficult with the coxsackie- and echoviruses. These viruses not only commonly cause subclinical infections but also are frequently shed in the stools for several weeks after either subclinical or clinically apparent infection. Therefore an isolation could occur by chance during various periods of illness or well-being. Only those specific diseases or clinical syndromes in which either satisfactorily controlled epidemiologic studies have established the etiologic relationship between coxsackievirus, echovirus, or newly recognized enterovirus infections and an illness, or in which virus isolations have been made from blood, CSF, or diseased tissue will be presented in the following discussions (see accompanying table).

Epidemiology. Coxsackie- and echoviruses are widely distributed throughout the world. They are found most commonly in human feces, but may also be found in the oropharynx or in nasopharyngeal washings; in patients with aseptic meningitis these agents may also be recovered from the CSF. They are resistant not only to the common antimicrobial drugs such as penicillin, streptomycin, and the tetracyclines, but also to many of the commonly used antiseptics such as 70 per cent alcohol, 5 per cent Lysol, and 1 per cent quaternary ammonium compounds. The occurrence of these infections is not influenced by sex or race. They have been isolated from all age groups, but it is apparent that in most instances infants and children are most susceptible to infection. The prevalence of these agents in surveys of presumably normal infants and children has ranged from less than 5 per cent to 50 per cent, depending on the location of the survey. Season appears to be an important factor in the epidemiology of coxsackie- and echovirus infections, for the majority of infections occur during the summer and early autumn months. The incubation period may vary widely, but usually ranges from 1 to 15 days. Recently, enterovirus 70 and a strain related to coxsackievirus A24 have been recovered from the conjunctiva during outbreaks of acute conjunctivitis; these outbreaks have had some unusual epidemiologic characteristics (see below).

Diseases Caused by Coxsackieviruses, Echoviruses, and Newly Recognized Enteroviruses

Coxsackieviruses group A, types 1–22, 24:
Herpangina (types 2, 3, 4, 5, 6, 8, 10, 22)
"Hand, foot, and mouth disease" (types 5, 16)
Acute lymphonodular pharyngitis (type 10)
Aseptic meningitis (types 1, 2, 4, 5, 7, 9, 10, 14, 16, 22, 24)
Epidemic exanthemata (type 9)
"Common-cold like" (type 21)
Acute undifferentiated respiratory or nonrespiratory illnesses (all types listed above with clinical syndromes)
Acute hemorrhagic conjunctivitis (epidemic conjunctivitis) (type 24)
Coxsackieviruses group B, type 1–6:
Epidemic pleurodynia or Bornholm disease (types 1–5)
Aseptic meningitis (types 1–6)
Myocarditis of newborn infants (types 1–5)
Myocarditis and pericarditis of infants beyond newborn period, children, and adults (types 1–5)
Orchitis (types 1–5)
Acute undifferentiated respiratory or nonrespiratory illnesses (types 1–6)
Echovirus types 1–9, 10–27, 29–33:
Aseptic meningitis (types 1–9, 11, 12, 14–19, 21, 22, 25, 30, 31, 33)
Epidemic exanthemata (types 9, 16)
Diarrhea (type 18, possibly types 6, 7, 14, 19)
Acute undifferentiated respiratory or nonrespiratory illnesses (all types listed above with clinical syndromes, plus type 20)
Enterovirus types 68–70:
Acute hemorrhagic conjunctivitis (epidemic conjunctivitis) (type 70)

As shown in the table, these viruses produce a broad spectrum of clinical manifestations, ranging from inapparent infection and mild undifferentiated respiratory or nonrespiratory illnesses to severe illnesses with varying involvement of the central nervous system. Illnesses associated with these agents are described in Ch. 127 to 136.

PREVENTION OF COXSACKIEVIRUS, ECHOVIRUS, AND NEWLY RECOGNIZED ENTEROVIRUS INFECTIONS

The ability to produce effective inactivated and live poliovirus vaccines offers hope that such vaccines can also be produced for the other enteroviruses. However, at present, the need and demand for such vaccines have not been determined.

127. HERPANGINA

Definition. Herpangina is a specific infectious disease characterized by the presence of small papulovesicular lesions on the anterior pillars of the tonsillar fauces and the soft palate; it occurs frequently in outbreaks among infants and children during the summer and early autumn.

History. It was first described in 1920 as a distinct clinical syndrome by Zahorsky in a report of 82 cases of "herpetic sore throat"; he subsequently suggested that this "peculiar throat disease . . . the clinical features of which are sufficiently clear to separate . . . from other diseases of the mouth and throat" be named "herpangina." Two other outbreaks of illness resembling herpangina were reported in 1939 and 1941.

Etiology. Herpangina was not described again until 1950 when Huebner et al. described studies in which certain group A coxsackieviruses were recovered from 32 of 37 herpangina patients, and on the basis of epidemiologic evidence an etiologic association was suggested. Numerous clinical and epidemiologic reports from many parts of the world have confirmed an etiologic relationship between certain group A coxsackieviruses and herpangina (see table). Reports have appeared recently relating certain group B coxsackievirus and echovirus infections temporally with herpangina-like syndromes; further epidemiologic studies are needed to elucidate the role of the group B coxsackieviruses and echoviruses in the pathogenesis of herpangina-like syndromes.

Epidemiology. Herpangina is a common infectious disease occurring frequently in outbreaks, but also sporadically, in most parts of the world predominantly during the summer and early autumn. Although it occasionally occurs in adults, the highest incidence is found in infants and young children. Multiple cases in a family are frequently observed. Spread is from person to person with an incubation period of about four days. Subclinical infections as well as illnesses without the characteristic herpanginal lesions commonly occur in family members infected with the same serotype as that recovered from the herpangina case. Immunity to the infecting type appears permanent, but recurrent attacks occur as a result of infection with a different serotype.

Pathology. The pathologic process of herpangina in man is not known, as no deaths have been reported.

Clinical Manifestations. The illness is characterized by a sudden elevation of temperature (37.8 to 40.5° C) and the development of the characteristic throat lesions in association with variable systemic signs and symptoms. In a study of 69 group A coxsackievirus-positive infants and children with herpangina, 89 per cent developed a fever which lasted an average of two days with a range of one to four days; 5 per cent of patients with temperature elevations developed febrile convulsions. Anorexia, dysphagia, or sore throat was evident in 70 per cent, vomiting in 38 per cent, abdominal pain in 21 per cent, and headache in 16 per cent (Parrott and Cramblett, 1957). The disease is characterized by the presence of discrete 1 to 2-mm grayish papulovesicular pharyngeal lesions on an erythematous base. These lesions, which gradually progress to slightly larger ulcers, may appear on the anterior pillars of the tonsillar fauces, the soft palate, the uvula, and the tonsils, and are usually present for four to six days after the onset of illness. In one herpangina case in a seven-year-old girl, small ulcers were also observed on the labia and skin near the genital region (Mitchell and Dempster, 1955). White blood cell counts usually reveal no characteristic abnormality; cerebrospinal fluid examinations have been normal.

Diagnosis. In a typical case, careful, repeated examination of the oral cavity and pharynx should facilitate the diagnosis. Herpangina can be differentiated from acute infectious gingivostomatitis resulting from infection with herpes simplex virus, because the lesions in the latter disease are located on the gums, lips, tongue, or buccal mucous membrane. In acute infectious gingivostomatitis, lesions may also be found on the anterior pillars of the faucial tonsils or soft palate (as in herpangina), but almost always occur in association with similar lesions in the anterior portions of the mouth. In addition, gingivostomatitis caused by herpes simplex virus infection occurs sporadically in all seasons of the year. In recurrent aphthosis the lesions do not usually occur in the pharynx and are not generally accompanied by fever. Herpangina should also be differentiated from "hand, foot, and mouth disease" and acute lymphonodular pharyngitis, both of which are described below.

Prognosis and Treatment. Herpangina is a self-limited disease, with complete recovery occurring usually within four to six days. There is no specific therapy for the coxsackievirus infection. Treatment is supportive and symptomatic.

128. HAND, FOOT, AND MOUTH DISEASE (Vesicular Stomatitis and Exanthem)

An outbreak in Toronto of a new clinical syndrome caused by coxsackievirus A16 was reported in 1958 (Robinson et al.). Observed mostly in infants and children, and occasionally in young adults, the new syndrome was characterized by vesicular and ulcerative lesions of the mouth and oropharynx or fauces and a vesicular eruption involving the hands, feet, and legs. In 1960 the term "hand, foot, and mouth disease" was first used to describe a similar outbreak in England (Alsop et al.). Coxsackievirus A5 has also been found to be associated with sporadic cases (Flewett et al., 1963).

129. ACUTE LYMPHONODULAR PHARYNGITIS

An outbreak in Kentucky of a new clinical syndrome caused by coxsackievirus A10 was reported in 1962 (Steigman et al.). Observed chiefly in children, the illness was characterized by lesions on the uvula, anterior pillars, and posterior pharynx. The lesions were raised and discrete, whitish to yellowish in color, solid and not vesicular, and surrounded by a 3 to 6 mm zone of erythema. Patients experienced fever, headache, and sore throat, with symptoms lasting 4 to 14 days. The incubation period was estimated at 5 days.

130. EPIDEMIC PLEURODYNIA OR BORNHOLM DISEASE (Epidemic Myalgia, Devil's Grip)

Definition. Epidemic pleurodynia or Bornholm disease is a specific acute infectious disease of viral etiology, characterized by the sudden onset of severe abdominal and/or chest pain, fever, and headache. It occurs most often in the summer or early autumn, frequently in outbreaks, but may also occur sporadically.

History. Numerous outbreaks of this disease were described in early medical literature. Windorfer relates that Hannaeus described an outbreak occurring in Schleswig-Holstein in 1732. In 1872, Daae and Homann each reported an epidemic in Drangedal, Norway. Two years later Finsen, using the term pleurodynia, described outbreaks in 1856 and 1865 in Iceland. In 1888, Dabney provided the first description of such an outbreak in the United States; a patient described the severe chest pain as the "devil's grip"—a term subsequently applied on occasion to designate this disease. Hanger, McCoy, and Frantz reported 16 cases in 1923 and called the syndrome epidemic pleurodynia. Sylvest in 1930 described an outbreak on Bornholm, a Danish island in the Baltic; in 1933 he wrote a classic monograph "Epidemic Myalgia," in which he reviewed the world literature and presented detailed case histories of 93 patients with the disease in Bornholm and Copenhagen; the designation Bornholm disease was frequently applied following Sylvest's descriptions.

Etiology. The group B coxsackieviruses are recognized as the etiologic agents of epidemic pleurodynia or Bornholm disease. In 1949 Curnen, Shaw, and Melnick recovered a group B coxsackievirus from the feces of a 14-year-old boy with acute pleurodynia; in addition, they reported the occurrence of illnesses resembling pleurodynia in several laboratory personnel working with this virus. Subsequently, numerous studies appeared relating temporally epidemic pleurodynia and group B coxsackievirus infections (see table in Ch. 126).

Epidemiology. Outbreaks of Bornholm disease have been reported from most parts of the world. It is noteworthy that they generally occur in the summer and early autumn. Although all age groups can be affected, children and young adults experience the highest incidence. Intrafamilial spread is common, multiple cases in a single family being observed frequently; however, absence of intrafamilial spread should not exclude the diagnosis. In one large study, about one third of the patients developed the illness as single cases in a household (Warin et al., 1953). Although both large outbreaks and sporadic cases have been described, epidemic pleurodynia is not a common disease in that it is not generally prevalent each summer and early fall, but rather occurs in sharp outbreaks confined to geographically limited areas. The mode of transmission is probably by person-to-person contact, with an incubation period of about two to five days.

Pathology. The specific pathologic manifestations in humans are unknown, as no deaths have been reported.

Clinical Manifestations. Epidemic pleurodynia is characterized typically by the sudden onset of abdominal and/or chest pain, fever, and headache. The spasmodic abdominal or chest pain which may range from mild to extremely severe and which is often aggravated by respiration and movement is the most characteristic feature. In a report on 22 patients with epidemic pleurodynia who had a mean age of 25 years, Huebner et al. described the sensation of difficult breathing as particularly striking, and cited some characteristic descriptions of this symptom: "I can't breathe," "pain cut off my breath," "can't get a real long breath," and "it hurts to breathe." In a study of 114 patients hospitalized with epidemic pleurodynia in Boston, Finn et al. reported that the typical severe paroxysmal pleuritic type of pain was often described as "smothering," "stabbing," "knifelike," "catching," and "like a vise around the lower ribs." It is noteworthy that, although the onset of pain is typically the initial symptom, in the Boston study about one quarter of the patients had prodromal symptoms one to ten days before the onset of pain—symptoms such as "head cold," headache, anorexia, and myalgia.

Review of several outbreaks reveals that the location of the characteristic pain in infants and young children tends to be more abdominal than thoracic, whereas in older children and adults it tends to be more thoracic than abdominal. For example, in the 1949 Boston study in which almost three quarters of the patients were between 10 and 30 years of age, the characteristic pain was located in the chest alone in 48 per cent, in the chest and abdomen in 37 per cent, and in the abdomen alone in 14 per cent. In contrast, in a 1953 Birmingham, England, study of 104 hospitalized children whose average age was 5½ years, the characteristic pain was located in the abdomen alone in 81 per cent, in the abdomen and chest in 11 per cent, and in the chest alone in 9 per cent (Disney et al.). Similar findings were reported in a South African outbreak in which 32 (80 per cent) of 40 children had abdominal pain alone, 4 both abdominal and chest pain, and 4 chest pain alone (Patz et al., 1953).

In the Boston study the chest pain was located "over the lower ribs and for varying distances up the chest, usually on the lateral aspect but not infrequently over the front and back" except in six patients whose thoracic pain was limited to the substernal region only; about one third of patients with chest pain experienced referral of such pain to one or both shoulders, one or both scapulae, the interscapular region, or the neck. Among those with abdominal pain, approximately three quarters experienced epigastric or upper abdominal pain; it was noteworthy that in two patients the site of pain was in the right lower quadrant. Other symptoms among the total group included moderately severe or severe headache (44 per cent), cough (33 per cent), anorexia (26 per cent), nausea (24 per cent), chilly sensations (21 per cent), chills (18 per cent), "head cold" (16 per cent), vomiting (16 per cent), sore throat (12 per cent), and diarrhea (7 per cent). Physical examination revealed that 95 per cent were febrile (37.2 to 40° C) with a mean temperature of 38.3° C; the fever lasted a mean of 3½ days with a range of 1 to 14 days. Recrudescences of fever after the temperature had returned to normal or nearly normal were common. The pulse rate was proportional to the temperature. Visible splinting of the chest was observed commonly, especially during paroxysms of pain. In addition, a pleural friction rub confined to the lower half of the chest was heard in about one quarter of all cases. Localized tenderness to pressure was found in about one quarter of cases and was usually confined to those areas of the chest where pain was present. Tenderness confined to the abdomen (in 29 per cent), or tenderness in both abdomen and chest (in 9 per cent) were the most common abdominal findings, although "splinting and rigidity of the upper abdominal area were not infrequently present, especially when the pain was severe" (Finn et al.). In the Birmingham children's study, generalized abdominal tenderness was present in 34 per cent and right iliac fossa tenderness in 13 per cent (Disney et al., 1953). Roentgenographic examinations of the chest have revealed no characteristic abnormalities. The white blood cell count is usually within normal limits; occasionally a moderate leukopenia, leukocytosis, or eosinophilia may be present. The majority of patients are well within one week of onset, but longer periods of illness are not unusual. It is noteworthy that not infrequently relapses may occur a few days or more than one month after recovery.

Complications. Complications of epidemic pleurodynia occur relatively infrequently and include orchitis, aseptic meningitis, and pericarditis. Cases of group B coxsackievirus myocarditis of newborn infants have occasionally been reported during outbreaks of epidemic pleurodynia. It is noteworthy that myocarditis has only very rarely been reported as a complication in a patient with epidemic pleurodynia; however, the possibility should be borne in mind.

Diagnosis. A clinical diagnosis is usually not difficult once the presence of an epidemic is known. However, during the early stages of an outbreak or when a sporadic case is encountered, it may be quite difficult, if not impossible, to make the correct diagnosis. A vivid illustration of this difficulty is provided by a children's hospital study in which it was found that, until the house staff and other medical personnel in the community became aware that a pleurodynia outbreak was occurring, admission diagnoses on children eventually shown to have epidemic pleurodynia included the following: acute abdomen, possible appendicitis, possible duodenal ulcer, pyelonephritis, pneumonia, pleurisy with pneumonia, rheumatic fever, pain of unknown origin, trauma (fractured rib), myositis (influenzal), collagen disease, tuberculosis, and intussusception (Bain et al., 1961). Symptoms of common duct obstruction, pancreatitis, coronary occlusion, and intestinal infections may also be mimicked by epidemic pleurodynia.

Laboratory Findings. Laboratory diagnosis of group B coxsackievirus infection is made by isolation of the virus from throat washings or stools during the early phase of illness and by demonstrating a rise in neutralizing antibody against one of the group B coxsackie viruses in paired acute and convalescent phase sera. Unfortunately results of such tests become available too late to be of assistance in making a diagnosis in the acute case.

Treatment and Prognosis. There is no specific therapy for the coxsackievirus infection. Treatment is supportive and symptomatic. Recovery is usually complete and follows after variable periods as noted above. However, some patients may experience lingering aftereffects of tiredness and weakness, with a gradual return to normal health.

131. CARDIAC MANIFESTATIONS OF COXSACKIEVIRUS INFECTIONS

MYOCARDITIS NEONATORUM

(Epidemic Myocarditis of Newborn; "Acute Aseptic Myocarditis")

Group B coxsackieviruses were first recognized as a cause of severe, often fatal myocarditis in the newborn infant in the mid-1950's when investigators in South Africa, the Netherlands, and the United States reported 14 fatalities among 20 newborns who developed the disease from 3 to 21 days after birth (Montgomery et al., 1955; Javett et al., 1956; van Creveld and De Jager, 1956; Verlinde et al., 1956; Kibrick and Benirschke, 1956). Isolation of a group B coxsackievirus from the myocardium in six fatal cases provided firm evidence of an etiologic association. In most cases infection undoubtedly occurred soon after birth; however, in several it may have occurred in utero. It was noteworthy that outbreaks of other syndromes etiologically associated with group B coxsackieviruses (such as Bornholm disease, "summer grippe," and aseptic meningitis) were occurring concurrently in the general population.

The onset of the disease is typically acute and is characterized by dyspnea, cyanosis, pallor, and tachycardia. Some patients may have a fever, and in others the temperature may be subnormal. Vomiting and coughing attacks may also be present. Initially the disease may be mistaken for pneumonia, but symptoms of cardiac decompensation with enlargement of the heart and liver soon appear. Significant cardiac murmurs are not usually present. The electrocardiogram shows evidence of severe damage to the myocardium. In fatal cases the infant rapidly develops severe prostration and circulatory collapse. Pathologic examination of the heart reveals both a diffuse and focal infiltration of lymphocytes, polymorphonuclear leukocytes, plasma cells, and reticulum cells. In some areas the striations of the myocardial fibers are distinct but in others degeneration and necrosis may be present. Encephalitis, meningitis, and lesions in the lungs, liver, pancreas, spleen, kidneys, adrenal glands and pituitary glands may also be present in newborns with myocarditis. There is no specific therapy for coxsackievirus infections. Treatment is supportive and symptomatic (see Ch. 580). Individuals suspected of having group B coxsackievirus infections (based on epidemiologic, clinical, or other evidence) should, of course, be denied access to maternity and nursery units; medical personnel suspected of having such infections should also be denied access to such units. In addition, appropriate quarantine measures should be taken if a patient in a maternity or nursery unit develops an illness suggestive of a group B coxsackievirus infection.

MYOCARDITIS AND PERICARDITIS IN INFANTS BEYOND THE NEWBORN PERIOD, IN CHILDREN, AND IN ADULTS

Cases of myocarditis and pericarditis in infants beyond the newborn period, in children, and in adults have also been found to be associated with group B coxsackievirus infections. In addition to occurring as a distinct clinical entity, pericarditis may also occur as a complication of Bornholm disease. Myocarditis has only rarely been reported as a direct complication of Bornholm disease, but the possibility should be borne in mind.

It is not possible at this time to estimate the relative importance of the coxsackieviruses in the over-all etiology of myocarditis or pericarditis; epidemiologic and laboratory studies are needed to answer this important question (see Ch. 571 to 576 and Ch. 580).

132. "ASEPTIC MENINGITIS" DUE TO COXSACKIE- AND ECHOVIRUSES

Coxsackie- and echoviruses are important causes of aseptic meningitis in infants and children, as numerous serotypes have been implicated etiologically with this syndrome (see table). The epidemiology, clinical manifestations, and diagnosis of aseptic meningitis caused by coxsackie- and echoviruses (and other agents as well) are presented in Ch. 389.

It is noteworthy that sporadic cases of paralytic illness resembling paralytic poliomyelitis have been associated temporally with certain coxsackie- and echovirus strains (especially coxsackievirus A7, which also causes neuronal lesions in monkeys); in addition, sporadic cases of encephalitis have been associated with these viruses. Further epidemiologic studies are needed to elucidate the role of these viruses in the pathogenesis of such illnesses.

133. EXANTHEMATA AND "ASEPTIC MENINGITIS WITH RASH" DUE TO COXSACKIE- AND ECHOVIRUSES

In 1954 Neva et al. described the isolation of a new virus, later classified as echovirus 16, from patients with a mild exanthematous illness. The same virus was recovered during a similar outbreak occurring three years later, and it was suggested that the disease be called "Boston exanthem," because the first outbreak had occurred in and around that city. The illness, which affected infants and children, and adults as well, was characterized by several days of fever and a macular or maculopapular rash which usually appeared soon after the fever and other signs and symptoms had subsided; no central nervous system (CNS) manifestations were observed. It is noteworthy, however, that echovirus 16 was also recovered during the Boston outbreak from hospitalized patients with aseptic meningitis without rash (Kibrick et al., 1957).

In the mid and late 1950's numerous outbreaks of aseptic meningitis with rash caused by echovirus type 9 were observed in many parts of the world; in a few of the outbreaks an exanthem was not present. In typical outbreaks the clinical manifestations may vary widely from a very mild illness to the classic aseptic meningitis syndrome with or without rash. The eruption, which is characteristically macular or maculopapular, usually appears during the febrile period and occurs most often in infants and young children.

Coxsackievirus A9 has also been found to be a cause of an illness characterized by fever and a maculopapular or vesicular eruption with or without signs of CNS involvement; CNS involvement without rash may also occur. "Hand, foot, and mouth disease" has been associated etiologically with coxsackievirus A16 and A5 infections and is discussed in Ch. 128. In addition, it is noteworthy that various other coxsackie- and echovirus serotypes have been associated with sporadic cases or small outbreaks of exanthematous illnesses.

134. ACUTE UNDIFFERENTIATED RESPIRATORY AND NONRESPIRATORY ILLNESS DUE TO COXSACKIE- AND ECHOVIRUSES

Most of the coxsackie- and echovirus serotypes that are etiologically related to specific or severe illnesses such as aseptic meningitis, epidemic pleurodynia, herpangina, various exanthemata, myocarditis, and pericarditis have also been shown to be capable of producing mild acute undifferentiated febrile or afebrile respiratory or nonrespiratory illnesses that are indistinguishable from such illnesses caused by other agents (see table in Ch. 126). These mild illnesses are the most common clinical manifestations of coxsackie- and echovirus infections in infants and children, and are frequently described as "summer grippe." It is of interest that these nonspecific illnesses occur with greater frequency than the specific ones and often in the total absence of any concomitant occurrence of the more specific illness usually regarded as characteristic of these viruses.

Coxsackievirus A21 (Coe) virus has been shown to be the etiologic agent of an upper respiratory illness in an outbreak in a military population in which the agent was shed by 32 (26 per cent) of 122 patients with respiratory illness and by only 6 (6 per cent) of 108 of the controls (Bloom et al., 1962). A "common cold syndrome" was the most frequent illness observed, a fever of at least 37.8° C occurring in 14 of the virus-positive patients; fever in 5 of the 14 patients reached 38.9° C. Studies of this agent with volunteer subjects have also shown its ability to induce a characteristic upper respiratory illness (Parsons et al., 1960). It is of interest that coxsackievirus A21 was isolated much more frequently from throat swabs than from anal swabs in both the naturally occurring and artificially induced illnesses. Coxsackievirus A21 does not appear to be a major cause of upper respiratory illnesses in civilian populations. In volunteer studies, echovirus types 11 and 20 have been shown to be capable of inducing mild undifferentiated illnesses in adults (Philipson, 1958; Buckland et al., 1959, 1961).

135. COXSACKIE- AND ECHOVIRUSES IN DIARRHEAL DISEASES OF INFANTS

The relative importance of the coxsackie- and echoviruses in the etiology of gastroenteritis and epidemic diarrhea in infants and young children is difficult to determine at this time and awaits further epidemiologic studies, although it appears that these agents are not major causes of viral gastroenteritis. In 1958 epidemiologic data were presented on the etiologic association of echovirus type 18 in an epidemic of summer diarrhea which was not severe and which occurred in 12 premature and 5 older full-term infants in a hospital in New York City (Eichenwald et al.).

Controlled studies among infants and young children under four years of age conducted in Cincinnati demonstrated that enteroviruses were recovered approximately 2.5 times more frequently from patients with diarrhea than from controls (48 per cent versus 20 per cent) (Ramos-Alvarez and Sabin, 1958). Echoviruses were recovered approximately six times more often from children with diarrhea than from controls (31 per cent versus 5 per cent), whereas the recovery of polioviruses and coxsackieviruses was about the same in the diarrhea and control groups. Echovirus types 6, 7, and 14 were isolated from the majority of echovirus-positive children. In a controlled study of infants and children with diarrhea in the summer and fall in Mexico, it was found that echovirus infections occurred 8.5 times more often in diarrheal patients than in controls (Ramos-Alvarez and Olarte, 1964). Two other controlled studies (one in Texas, the other in Scotland) have failed to demonstrate statistically significant differences in the recovery rate of enteroviruses from infants and children with and without diarrhea (Yow et al., 1963; Sommerville, 1958). The recovery rate of echoviruses was greater in the diarrheal patients than in the controls in both studies, although the differences were not statistically significant. It is noteworthy that recent studies have indicated that "reovirus-like" viruses may be major etiologic agents of diarrhea of infants and children (Bishop et al., 1973, 1974; Flewett et al., 1973; Middleton et al., 1974; Tan et al., 1974; Cruickshank et al., 1974; Sexton et al., 1974; Kapikian et al., 1974; Bruce White et al., 1974). In addition, other recent studies have shown that a 27 nm "parvovirus-like" particle (Norwalk agent) was associated with a community outbreak of viral gastroenteritis (Kapikian et al., 1972, 1973; Dolin et al., 1972). Additional studies should aid in assessing the relative importance of different virus groups as etiologic agents of gastroenteritis.

136. ACUTE HEMORRHAGIC CONJUNCTIVITIS (Epidemic Conjunctivitis)

Acute hemorrhagic conjunctivitis is a recently described clinical entity which occurred in parts of Africa in 1969–1971, and in parts of Asia in the early 1970's, afflicting large numbers of people—predominantly adults—and spreading in pandemic fashion (Lancet, 1973). A small outbreak occurred in England in 1971; no cases have been reported in North and South America, Australia, or New Zealand. Certain epidemics have been associated etiologically with either of two distinct enterovirus serotypes—enterovirus 70, the more prevalent strain, and a strain related to coxsackievirus A24 (Mirkovic et al., 1974; Schmidt et al., 1974). The disease, which is highly contagious, is estimated to have an incubation period of about 24 hours and is characterized by a sudden swelling of the eyelid, and "redness," congestion, and pain in the eye, with excess lacrimation (Kono et al., 1972). Subconjunctival hemorrhage, which may vary from minute petechiae to large hemorrhagic areas, is the most characteristic symptom in most outbreaks. In the Singapore epidemics, however, subconjunctival hemorrhage was not as prevalent as in other outbreaks (Lim and Yin-Murphy, 1971). Complete recovery usually occurs within two weeks of onset. Corneal involvement is rare. It should be noted that during an outbreak of acute hemorrhagic conjunctivitis in India, radiculomyelopathy, predominantly lumbar, was observed infrequently as a complication; viral studies were not reported from this outbreak (Bharucha and Mondkar, 1972; Wadia et al., 1972).

Acute Haemorrhagic Conjunctivitis. Lancet, 1:86, 1973.

Dalldorf, G., and Melnick, J. L.: Coxsackie viruses. *In* Horsfall, F. L., Jr., and Tamm, I. (eds.): Viral and Rickettsial Infections of Man. 4th ed. Philadelphia, J. B. Lippincott Company, 1965, p. 474.

Finn, J. J., Jr., Weller, T. H., and Morgan, H. R.: Epidemic pleurodynia; Clinical and etiologic studies based on one hundred and fourteen cases. Arch. Intern. Med., 83:305, 1949.

Horstmann, D. H.: Viral exanthems and enanthems. Pediatrics, 41:867, 1968.

Huebner, R. J., Beeman, E. A., Cole, R. M., Beigelman, P. M., and Bell, J. A.: The importance of Coxsackie viruses in human disease, particularly herpangina and epidemic pleurodynia. N. Engl. J. Med., 247:249, 1952.

Kibrick, S.: Current status of Coxsackie and echoviruses in human disease. Progr. Med. Virol., 6:27, 1964.

Melnick, J. L.: Echoviruses. *In* Horsfall, F. L., Jr., and Tamm, I. (eds.): Viral and Rickettsial Infections of Man. 4th ed. Philadelphia, J. B. Lippincott Company, 1965, p. 513.

Rosen, L., Melnick, J. L., Schmidt, N. J., and Wenner, H. A.: Subclassification of enteroviruses and echo type 34. Arch. Gesamte Virusforsch., 30:89, 1972.

Weller, T. H., Enders, J. F., Buckingham, M., and Finn, J. J., Jr.: The etiology of epidemic pleurodynia: A study of two viruses isolated from a typical outbreak. J. Immun., 65:337, 1950.

POLIOMYELITIS

See Ch. 392.

ARTHROPOD-BORNE VIRAL FEVERS, VIRAL ENCEPHALITIDES, AND VIRAL HEMORRHAGIC FEVERS

(Arboviruses and Arenaviruses)

137. INTRODUCTION

Karl M. Johnson

Arthropod-borne viruses (arboviruses) are defined on an epidemiologic basis. Thus any virus is an arbovirus if it actually multiplies in one or more arthropods and if it is biologically transmitted to vertebrates with sufficient frequency by arthropods to make this an important means of virus survival. More than 300 distinguishable agents have been tentatively so classified. Many have similar physical and chemical properties and could reasonably be placed within families on this basis as well; others have fundamental properties relating them to animal virus groups not generally associated with recognized arthropod transmission.

Immunologic properties are currently used to cluster individual arboviruses. Viruses having such relationships are included in groups that historically began with A, B, and C; thereafter, the name of the first virus to be discovered was used to designate the group. Originally virus names were derived from antecedent diseases, e.g., yellow fever, dengue, and equine encephalitides. Later, geography in combination with disease syndrome was favored, providing names such as St. Louis encephalitis and Colorado tick fever. Finally, there are many geographically named arboviruses for which no clinical syndromes have been defined, either because they rarely infect man or because they have not been associated with morbidity of dramatic proportions.

About 90 arboviruses are known to infect man, and most of these have been shown to produce illness. With rare exceptions, such as dengue and urban yellow fever, these are zoonoses in which man is an accidental host of no apparent importance in the fundamental natural history of the virus.

Clinical syndromes produced by arboviruses share the common properties of fever and myalgia accompanied by viremia. Beyond that, classification is inevitably arbitrary, because the same virus can induce a wide variety of patterns in different patients, and different viruses have been linked to remarkably similar syndromes. Emphasis is given here to the often infrequent but spectacular severe diseases some of the agents evoke. Thus individual descriptions are placed in one of the following groups: (1) *fevers of a relatively undifferentiated type,* with or without rashes, usually benign; (2) *encephalitides,* often severe and with significant case fatality rates; and (3) *hemorrhagic fevers,* also frequently severe and fatal.

The largest number of viruses have been associated exclusively with milder, undifferentiated disease. The majority of these are encountered most commonly in tropical and semitropical countries (see table in Ch. 140). The classic clinical prototype is *dengue.* Those to be described represent but a small sample. Of these, *Chikungunya, Mayaro, O'nyong-nyong,* and *Ross River* are group A viruses, *dengue* and *West Nile* belong to group B, and the remainder are unclassified or are in the *sandfly fever* group. Although each gained entry to this book because of its proved epidemic disease potential for man, clinical differentiation even during epidemics is generally difficult; epidemiologic and laboratory methods are more important. When more than one such virus is simultaneously endemic, the latter techniques are essential.

All arboviruses conspicuously associated with encephalitis and hemorrhagic fever are included. In the case of the latter syndrome, all but one of the viruses belong to antigenic group B. Yellow fever is listed among the hemorrhagic fevers because many cases do not display the "classic" picture of jaundice, but manifest gastrointestinal hemorrhage (black vomit), epistaxis, and melena with fatal shock and thus fit this description better than either of the other two arbovirus clinical syndromes. Arenavirus-caused hemorrhagic fevers, although not arthropod borne, are described here because of their clinical similarity to those induced by arboviruses and because they are zoonotic infections.

It should be emphasized that all these viruses frequently provoke only mild clinically undifferentiated infections. Thus specific virologic diagnostic tests are of fundamental importance in sporadic infections as well as during epidemics. Specific diagnosis of all arboviral disease depends upon isolation of virus and/or detection of a homologous antiviral immune response. In many parts of the world malaria is first sought in acute febrile disease with or without neurologic manifestations. The findings of such parasites, however, may not solve the problem; it should be remembered that either a simultaneous arbovirus infection or a drug-resistant parasite may account for the lack of response to supposed specific chemotherapy.

Virus isolation, together with an antibody rise to that agent between acute and convalescent phase sera from the patient, provides nearly incontrovertible evidence for an etiologic association between virus and disease. Blood is the best source of virus for all the diseases here described except for Venezuelan equine encephalitis which may be gotten from pharyngeal swabs at least as readily. *Such specimens should be obtained on the very first day the patient is seen,* because viremia rarely persists for long into the encephalitic period. Since antibodies are often present at the end of the first week of symptoms, it is important to obtain the acute phase serum specimen for serologic diagnosis at this time. A convalescent serum obtained 10 to 30 days after onset will usually reveal an increase in specific antibodies when measured by the complement-fixation (CF), hemagglutination-inhibition (HI), or neutralization test. No more than 10 ml of blood need be obtained for any of these specimens unless special studies are contemplated. Materials for virus isolation should be kept chilled, or frozen at temperatures of at least $-60°$ C if shipment for testing involves great distances.

Hammon, W. McD., and Sather, G. E.: Isolation and identification of arthropod-borne-viruses. *In* Lennette, E. H., and Schmidt, J. J. (eds.): Diagnostic Procedures for Virus and Rickettsial Diseases. 4th ed. New York, American Public Health Association, 1969, pp. 227–280.
Horsfall, F. L., Jr., and Tamm, I. (eds.): Viral and Rickettsial Infections of Man. 4th ed. Philadelphia, J. B. Lippincott Company, 1965.
Taylor, R. M. (ed.): Catalogue of Arthropod-Borne Viruses of the World. Washington, U.S. Government Printing Office, 1967.

UNDIFFERENTIATED FEVERS

138. DENGUE

Karl M. Johnson

Definition. Dengue is an acute, febrile, self-limited infectious disease caused by an Aedes mosquito-borne dengue virus. Malaise, prostration, and pain of muscles and joints are characteristic, accompanied by lymphadenopathy, leukopenia, and one or two episodes of exanthem. Typically an illness of about one week is followed by one or more weeks of depression and weakness.

Etiology. Four distinct immunologic subtypes of dengue virus have been recovered from patients. These agents produce partial cross-immunity such that a primary infection will protect against another subtype only for a few months, although homologous immunity is of long duration. Sequential infection with any two subtypes, however, appears to confer long-term clinical protection against infection with any of the remaining two subtypes.

Epidemiology. Man and certain Aedes mosquitoes are the essential links in the recognized natural virus cycle. Size of human populations and ecologic factors affecting the mosquito vector and multiplication of virus in that host are of prime importance. Thus the disease has occurred in all continents and many islands, but only in "summer-like" temperatures where there are large numbers of *Aedes aegypti, Aedes albopictus,* or *Aedes scutellaris* mosquitoes. Since infection is usually clinically apparent in adults and frequently inapparent in children, various combinations of human and Aedes ecology may produce nearly silent continuous endemic infection, repeated seasonal epidemics, or massive outbreaks affecting populations previously free of dengue for many years.

Viremia adequate for mosquito infection is present just prior to and for the first three days of illness. An infected mosquito requires eight to twelve days to become infective at warm temperatures. Such a mosquito is infective for life and may transmit the virus to one or more susceptible persons on whom it feeds or probes. The incubation period in man is five to six days.

Aedes aegypti, by far the most important vector, breeds, rests, and feeds in or near human habitations. It is primarily attracted to man, biting in daylight and twilight. These attributes make it an ideal virus vector and explain why dengue is principally an urban disease. In rural areas other Aedes species such as *A. albopictus* may transmit infection, but their habits and relatively sparse human populations render explosive epidemics uncommon.

No extrahuman virus reservoir has been conclusively documented, but there is suggestive evidence that monkeys and forest mosquitoes may be capable of virus maintenance.

Pathology. Since dengue is rarely if ever fatal, the only information available is that from biopsy of the skin rash. Such lesions consist of endothelial swelling, perivascular edema, and mononuclear infiltration of small vessels. Petechiae are characterized by extravasation of blood without significant inflammatory reaction.

Clinical Manifestations. Dengue in adults is typically sudden in onset with rising temperature and only minor chilliness, headache, and fatigue. By the second day temperature is frequently 40° C, headache with ocular or retrobulbar pain is severe, and the patient complains of back pain, generalized myalgia, and aching joints. During this interval there is a diffuse blushing of the face and upper trunk, sometimes accompanied by a fleeting *erythematous macular* or *pinpoint rash* of the limbs. General lymphadenopathy is usually apparent, but hepato- or splenomegaly is rare. The leukocyte count at this stage is apt to be essentially normal.

At about the third to fifth day a *maculopapular* or *scarlatiniform rash* appears, beginning on the trunk and spreading in centripetal fashion. This generally lasts at least three days, becomes itchy as it fades, but rarely desquamates. The fever is generally of five to seven days' duration, sometimes with a fall at about the fourth day, giving a saddleback curve. The second bout of fever is often more severe, accompanied by relative or absolute bradycardia and by leukopenia. Monocytes, lymphocytes, and segmented leukocytes all decrease in absolute numbers, although there may be an absolute increase in immature polymorphonuclear cells. A few small petechiae may appear, especially on the lower extremities.

Dengue in young children is definitely a milder disease; recent longitudinal population studies in cities of endemic virus activity confirm an impression formed down the years by the paucity of description of pediatric cases during epidemics. Clinical manifestations may also vary with infecting subtype. Halstead retrospectively documented that volunteer studies done nearly 50 years ago in the Philippines employed subtype 1 and 4 viruses, the disease associated with the latter being milder and less "classic" than that caused by the former.

Diagnosis. During sharp epidemics occurring in places where ecologic factors are compatible, clinical diagnosis of many cases of average severity will usually be correct. But several other arboviruses as well as rubella may be the cause. Thus laboratory confirmation of a *few* cases during an epidemic and of *every* case when the pattern is sporadic is important. Travel history during the previous ten days is essential whenever dealing with a suspect case in areas where the disease is rare.

Virus may be isolated from blood or serum of patients early in the course of illness by inoculation of suckling mice, Aedes mosquitoes, or cell cultures. Serologic diagnosis is also possible, using acute and convalescent (two weeks) sera, but is frequently complicated by previous infection with one or more viruses of arbovirus group B. A laboratory competent to execute and interpret tests for a number of different arboviruses is required.

Treatment and Prognosis. There is no specific therapy. Bed rest is indicated, as well as the usual supportive measures to maintain fluid and electrolyte balance and alleviate discomfort. Secondary bacterial infection is uncommon but should be anticipated and appropriately treated. Except in severely debilitated persons, the prognosis is uniformly excellent. Final recovery is complete, although temporary depression and lassitude are common during convalescence, and patients should not be rushed back to normal occupations.

Prevention. Vaccines for dengue viruses are not generally available, although experimental work on the problem continues. Individual protection is difficult, because mosquito attacks occur during daytime, and continuous use of repellent is not practical. Community protection is possible through effective control or eradication of the Aedes vector. Patients should be protected from mosquitoes during the first five days of illness in order to prevent further virus transmission, and space-spraying of buildings frequented by patients should be done to eliminate mosquitoes possibly infected prior to the diagnosis of the disease.

139. WEST NILE FEVER

Karl M. Johnson

Definition. West Nile fever is an acute febrile mosquito-borne illness marked by headache, lymphadenopathy, and a macular skin eruption. It is generally self-limited, although rare cases of mortality caused by encephalitis occur in aged persons. The disease is caused by a group B arbovirus.

Etiology. West Nile virus is a small ribonucleic acid–containing virus belonging to an antigenic complex within the B group of arboviruses, which includes *Japanese B*, *Murray Valley*, and *St. Louis encephalitis* viruses, as well as *Ilheus* virus. Immunologic relationships are shared to a somewhat lesser degree with *yellow fever* and *dengue* viruses. Immunologic cross-protection is readily demonstrable experimentally among members of this antigenic complex. Despite the fact that such closely related viruses are frequently distributed geographically in a discontinuous manner, reflecting a long process of evolutionary segregation, West Nile and *Japanese B* viruses have been repeatedly recovered from the same mosquitoes in the same localities in southern India.

Epidemiology. Millions of people have been infected with West Nile virus, which is endemic in many parts of Africa, the Middle East, Southwest Asia, and southern Europe. Continuous human migration into Israel over the past 30 years has resulted in repeated epidemics among adults. Elsewhere the disease is mainly an affliction of children. Annual summer epidemics are correlated with seasonal peaks in populations of culicine mosquitoes. In Egypt and Israel, *Culex univittatus* is the principal epidemic vector. Much lower levels of virus transmission occur in winter when the suspected vector is *Culex pipiens.*

In ecologic terms, West Nile virus is one of the least evolved arboviruses. In addition to moquitoes, it multiplies in, and can be experimentally transmitted by, the bite of various species of hard and soft ticks. It has been recovered from Argas and Hyalomma ticks in nature. Although the primary natural virus cycle appears to comprise mosquitoes and wild birds, virus or antibody has been detected in rodents, camels, cattle, horses, and monkeys.

The incubation period in man is about three to six days. Most infections are clinically apparent. A number of documented laboratory infections suggest that the agent also can be transmitted by the respiratory route.

Clinical Manifestations. Sudden onset of fever, lasting three to six days, is accompanied by photophobia, myalgia, and chilling. Nausea and vomiting may occur early in the febrile period. A saddleback fever curve is seen in a minority of patients, and there is usually a definite leukopenia with absolute reduction of polymorphonuclear cells by the third day of illness. At about this time a fine *maculopapular* rash is observed on the trunk and occasionally on the extremities. It is more common in children than in adults, is *nonirritating,* and fades rapidly without desquamation. Lymphadenopathy is often demonstrable at the time the patient is first seen.

Although mild meningismus is demonstrable in a minority of patients and may be accompanied by increased cells and protein in the cerebrospinal fluid, clinical encephalitis is not a feature of West Nile infection except in a handful of very old patients. Pathologic studies were not done in the few fatal cases reported. Convalescence is generally uneventful, although older patients may complain of generalized weakness for several weeks. No permanent sequelae have ever been observed.

Diagnosis. Clinically this disease is so similar to dengue that laboratory diagnosis is essential in all cases. Virus isolation is by far the best hope, and blood specimens obtained as late as the fourth symptomatic day yield a reasonably high percentage of strains when inoculated into suckling mice or the yolk sacs of embryonated eggs. Serologic diagnosis may also be attempted with the usual paired serum samples, but previous infection with related group B arboviruses, including 17D live yellow fever vaccine, may render interpretation of results extremely difficult beyond the confirmation that infection was due to a mosquito-borne member of this large antigenic group.

Treatment and Prevention. Management of patients is completely symptomatic. Complications are unusual, and the only reason to keep patients under observation after the rash has faded is to ensure the collection of appropriate diagnostic specimens in situations in which knowledge of the specific cause of illness may have public health implications.

Although there is an impression that prior infection with related group B viruses may lessen the symptomatology of West Nile fever, this has not been rigorously established. Inactivated or attenuated West Nile virus has been used in combination with other group B agents in experimental attempts to produce broad-spectrum immunity to this virus group. Such vaccines are not ready for general use. Thus mosquito control and individual protective measures against mosquito bite represent the only available means of prevention of this infection. Since the main epidemic mosquito vectors are not concentrated around human dwellings and since infection rarely causes severe human disease, expensive systematic mosquito control systems have not often been mounted.

140. FEVERS CAUSED BY GROUP A ARBOVIRUSES: CHIKUNGUNYA, O'NYONG-NYONG, MAYARO, AND ROSS RIVER

Karl M. Johnson

Definition. Chikungunya, O'nyong-nyong, Mayaro, and Ross River fevers are acute nonfatal diseases caused

Etiologic and Epidemiologic Features of Undifferentiated Arbovirus Fevers

Fever	Virus	Vector(s)	Vertebrate Host(s)	Geographic Distribution	Human Epidemiologic Features
Dengue	Group B (4 types)	*Aedes aegypti*	Man	Tropics and subtropics; Old and New World	Varies from continuous endemic to repeated epidemic pattern based on human-Aedes population cycles
West Nile	Group B	Culex mosquitoes Argas, Hyalomma ticks	Wild birds	Mediterranean basin, Middle East, Soviet Union, Southwest Asia	Continuously endemic (tropics) to annually epidemic in Mediterranean climates
O'nyong-nyong	Group A	*Anopheles funestus, Anopheles gambiae*	Man	East Africa	Singular massive epidemic; malaria control may affect pattern
Chikungunya	Group A	*Aedes aegypti, A. africanus,* Culex mosquitoes	Man, monkeys?	Africa, Southern Asia, Philippines	Basically similar to dengue
Mayaro	Group A	Haemagogus, Psorophora mosquitoes	Monkeys, marsupials	Northern South America and Central America	Endemic, forest-associated infection; localized outbreaks during forest destruction
Ross River	Group A	Culex, Aedes mosquitoes	Wild mouse	Eastern Australia	Endemic infction in subtropical north; summer-fall epidemics farther south
Rift Valley	Ungrouped	Aedes, Culex mosquitoes	Large wild and domestic animals	East and South Africa	Sporadic rainy season transmission to man; mainly contact infections during livestock epizootics
Colorado tick	Bluetongue group	*Dermacentor andersoni* tick	Ground squirrels, chipmunks	Rocky Mountains of North America	Sporadic and focal summer infections during recreational and occupational activity
Sandfly	Phlebotomus fever group (15 types)	Phlebotomus, Lutzomyia sandflies	Man, monkeys, small wild mammals	Mediterranean basin, eastward to southern Asia; forests of tropical America	Annual seasonal transmission to children; epidemic whenever large numbers of susceptible adults introduced; forest-associated infections in American tropics.

by an antigenically related, geographically dispersed complex of group A arboviruses. Maculopapular rashes and arthralgia are common features of these infections, which occur in Africa, Southeast Asia, tropical America, and Australia.

Epidemiology. Each of these viruses has caused epidemic disease in human populations. Perhaps the most dramatic was that due to O'nyong-nyong in East Africa from 1959 to 1962, when an estimated two million persons of all ages were affected. The important mosquito vectors of each disease are listed in the accompanying table. Chikungunya virus is often transmitted by *Aedes aegypti;* because of the rash and minor hemorrhagic phenomena associated with infection, this agent has at times been considered responsible for cases of hemorrhagic fever during outbreaks basically caused by dengue virus infection. O'nyong-nyong virus is the only known arbovirus transmitted principally by anopheline mosquitoes. Sylvan maintenance cycles involving arboreal mosquitoes and monkeys have been postulated for Mayaro and Chikungunya viruses. Epidemic behavior of these agents is far from understood. Irregularly occurring outbreaks during warm rainy months are the rule. There is strong circumstantial evidence that Chikungunya virus has moved steadily eastward into Asia from Africa during the last 25 years, employing a simple cycle composed of man and *Aedes aegypti* mosquitoes. The incubation periods of these agents in man vary from about two to twelve days. Clinical attack rates are high in relation to those for infection, with the exceptions of Ross River and Mayaro viruses, which induce mild or inapparent infection in children.

Clinical Manifestations. Onset is typically abrupt, and arthralgias or rashes are more likely to be the chief complaints than are headache and fever. Fever is usually mild, and is virtually absent with Ross River virus. Chikungunya virus frequently induces a saddleback fever curve, but the second episode, in contrast to dengue, is usually less severe. Arthralgias may or may not be symmetrical in distribution and usually involve terminal joints most severely. The maculopapular rashes are generally irritating, distributed over the trunk and extensor surfaces of the extremities, and may appear early or late in the course of the first week of symptoms. Leukopenia is a common feature of these diseases, and cervical lymphadenitis is frequently reported in cases caused by O'nyong-nyong and Ross River viruses.

Diagnosis. All these viruses except Ross River can be recovered readily from the blood of patients during the initial three days of illness. Standard serologic techniques are highly reliable in making specific diagnosis, provided a second serum specimen is obtained 10 to 14 days after onset of symptoms. Differentiation of O'nyong-nyong and Chikungunya viruses in East Africa may present problems. Malaria, rubella, enterovirus infection, and other nonviral causes of acute arthralgia must be considered in the differential diagnosis of individual cases.

Treatment and Prognosis. Treatment is symptomatic, and prognosis is uniformly excellent, although polyarthritis may persist or recur over an interval of several weeks to months. Corticosteroid therapy is contraindicated for joint pain in adults, at least until the third week, when hormonal antibodies have appeared. Children possibly infected with Chikungunya virus in areas where *Aedes aegypti* and dengue viruses are endemic should be hospitalized, because it is impossible to differentiate this disease from the prodrome of the dengue shock syndrome.

141. COLORADO TICK FEVER

Gordon Meiklejohn

Definition. Colorado tick fever is an acute, tick-transmitted viral disease which occurs throughout the Rocky Mountain area and is characterized by a biphasic febrile course and leukopenia.

Etiology. Colorado tick fever virus is an arbovirus which has not yet been shown to be related to other members of this group. The virus has been isolated from a wide range of ticks and a number of small mammals in the Rocky Mountain area. Only the wood tick, *Dermacentor andersoni,* is important in transmission. Cases occur throughout the Rocky Mountain area, including western Canada and the eastern parts of California and Oregon.

Epidemiology. The disease occurs in the spring and summer when tick exposure is common. The reservoir of the disease is in small mammalian hosts which infect the larvae or nymphs of ticks. The ticks maintain the virus over the winter months, and the adult tick then transmits the virus to other small mammals or to man.

Pathogenesis. Viremia can be detected at the time of onset of fever and persists throughout the febrile course. The virus may persist in, or in association with, the red blood cells for long periods.

The disease is characterized by a profound leukopenia and occasionally thrombocytopenia which is usually greatest during the second febrile episode. Pathologic data on the disease in man are meager because there have been only two reported fatal cases. In those instances, the pathologic changes were those of an extensive hemorrhagic diathesis associated with encephalitis.

Symptoms and Clinical Course. The onset is usually sudden, with chilly sensations, malaise, and fever. Muscle aching and pain about the joints are common manifestations, along with headache and backache. In children, anorexia, nausea, and vomiting are common. The disease is characteristically biphasic. The first episode of fever usually lasts two or three days, after which the temperature returns to normal. After a day of normal temperature, the fever again rises, and the second cycle usually approximates the first in length. Rashes are uncommon, but a small proportion of patients have petechial or macular rashes. Involvement of the central nervous system with meningitis or, less frequently, encephalitis may occur, especially in children. Patients who develop encephalitis have findings similar to those infected with other arboviruses, such as disorientation, coma, and convulsions. Hemorrhagic manifestations, including epistaxis and gastrointestinal bleeding, occur very infrequently and are most commonly seen in patients with encephalitis.

Diagnosis. The diagnosis is based on a history of tick exposure during the preceding three to seven days, followed by a biphasic febrile course with leukopenia. During the first febrile episode, the disease cannot be differentiated from many other acute febrile illnesses, including Rocky Mountain spotted fever during the first day or two of that illness before a rash becomes obvious. The differentiation between these two diseases is extremely important, because early treatment of Rocky Mountain spotted fever with tetracycline will abort the illness and cure the patient. Laboratory procedures to confirm the diagnosis include viral culture from blood, demonstration of viral antigen on red cells by fluorescent antibody techniques, and serologic tests with paired serum specimens.

Prevention. Protection against ticks by appropriate clothing or repellents is possible but usually impractical. Experimental vaccines have shown promise but are not currently available.

Prognosis. The disease almost invariably runs a benign course and produces a lifelong immunity. The rare exception is the patient who develops either an encephalitis or a hemorrhagic diathesis.

Treatment. Treatment is symptomatic. When the patient is seriously ill and the diagnosis of Rocky Mountain spotted fever is entertained, it is advisable to give tetracycline in doses of 2.0 grams per day. If the patient has Rocky Mountain spotted fever, the temperature usually falls to normal within 48 hours, whereas the course of Colorado tick fever is not altered by this regimen.

142. RIFT VALLEY FEVER

Karl M. Johnson

Definition. Rift Valley fever is a febrile illness of short duration characterized by headache, myalgia, prostration, photophobia, and leukopenia. It is the only such arbovirus infection accompanied by significant complications which are ocular. The virus is mosquito borne, enzootic in wild game animals, epizootic in domestic livestock, and restricted geographically to East and South Africa.

Etiology. Rift Valley virus is a 30 to 50 nm, ribonucleic acid–containing arbovirus antigenically unrelated to any other known agent. Historically it was the second disease-producing, mosquito-borne virus ever described, the first being yellow fever.

Epidemiology. The virus was initially recovered from sheep in East Africa. Subsequent investigations showed that infection was common among large wild mammals of the region, and that virus was naturally present in a variety of mosquito species of the genera Aedes, Culex, and Erethmapodites, many of which are now known to feed primarily on wild game. After seasonal rains which lead to high mosquito populations, the virus spills over from this wild cycle, causing epizootics with high mortality in sheep, cattle, and even fowl. The agent is pantropic in these animals, the most striking lesion being a severe necrotizing hepatitis, reminiscent of yellow fever in man.

Human infection can be acquired in at least two ways: by mosquito bite, which is usually associated with big-game hunting or with ranching activity, and by direct or aerosol contact with the virus through the handling of tissues of affected livestock, or working with the agent in the laboratory. More human disease has been associated with the latter than the former transmission mechanism. This virus is so infectious to man, and of such potential economic hazard to the livestock industry, that it is now prohibited in the United States, even for experimental purposes.

Clinical Manifestations. After an incubation period of three to six days, onset of symptoms is usually abrupt, with fever, photophobia, and severe generalized headache. There may be severe prostration, myalgia, nausea, and vomiting. Epigastric pain is a frequent complaint. Temperature oscillates between 38 and 40° C, is often "saddleback" in evolution, and may persist up to one week. Leukopenia is common, as is a relative bradycardia. Skin eruptions are almost never observed, although minor hemorrhages in skin and from mucous membranes are infrequently present. Convalescence is usually, although not always, uneventful.

Complications. These consist of a *central serous retinopathy* with an associated *central scotoma.* The fundus shows exudates involving the macula that may be secondary to thrombosis of vessels. Whether such lesions represent direct viral damage or result from an immunopathologic reaction to infection is not known. The exudates usually shrink and disappear over the course of several weeks, but in a minority of patients *retinal detachment* has ensued.

Diagnosis. This is above all a disease of place and of particular human activity. A history is more valuable than any other procedure. Blood obtained during the first three days of illness almost always contains virus which is lethal when inoculated into mice. Serologic diagnosis of this infection is also definitive, because interpretation of antibody responses in paired sera is never compromised by heterologous reactions with any other agent.

Treatment and Prevention. Management of patients, as for other arthropod-borne fevers, is symptomatic. Serial examination for retinal complications should be done, and continued rest is indicated for persons in whom such lesions occur. Since the ocular complications appear to have an acute episodic rather than a subacute or chronic allergic pathogenesis, corticosteroids are of no benefit in their management.

Prevention of infection is principally through individual anti-mosquito measures. A live attenuated vaccine has been used in animals and man in South Africa, but this has more recently been replaced for human use among persons at high risk of infection, such as veterinarians, by a formalin-killed preparation which appears to confer complete clinical protection for at least two years.

143. SANDFLY FEVER

Karl M. Johnson

Definition. Sandfly fever is a self-limited viral disease consisting of fever, headache, and myalgia. Leukopenia and conjunctival injection are characteristic. It occurs during the warm season in the littoral of the Mediterranean Sea and eastward through Asia Minor, Pakistan, and northern India. Sporadic cases have been recognized in tropical America.

Etiology. Although the classic syndrome in the Old World is caused by two antigenically related viruses, Sicilian and Neapolitan, recent ecologic studies in various parts of the world have led to the recovery of at least 15 distinct but related agents from phlebotomine sandflies. These are now referred to as members of the Phlebotomus fever group of arboviruses. Many can be isolated in suckling mice or hamsters, but cell cultures, especially an African green monkey continuous cell-line (Vero), appear to be uniformly susceptible to infection with cytopathic effect.

Epidemiology. The vector of classic sandfly fever is *Phlebotomus papatasii,* and the only known vertebrate host is man. The fly has a very short flight range, stays close to ground level, and breeds best during warm dry periods in small collections of organic debris beneath stones, in masonry cracks, and in other protected sites. It has a short life span, probably not more than three weeks, but because of its small size it can readily penetrate the usual barriers of screens or netting which exclude mosquitoes. Serial man-fly transmission probably accounts for much of the virus activity during the season of peak fly populations, but transovarial transmission by the vector appears to be an important mechanism for long-term virus survival in view of the repeated recovery of virus in nature from nonbiting male sandflies.

Although antibodies have been found in forest-dwelling rodents and especially arboreal mammals in tropical America, equivalent isolation rates of some serotypes from male and female flies strongly suggest that the transovarial mechanism is a basic biologic adaptation for maintenance of viruses of this antigenic group.

Human disease patterns are determined by geographic and ecologic distribution of vector and virus. In highly endemic areas most infections occur during childhood and are rarely recognized in epidemic form. Epidemics in such regions are generally the result of introduction of large numbers of susceptible adults, such as during wars and national immigration.

Pathogenesis. Since there are no fatalities, the pathology of this disease in man is unknown. Experimental studies in man, however, disclosed that after intracutaneous inoculation the incubation period is three to six days. Viremia is brief, usually being confined to the day prior to and that of the onset of symptoms. Postinfection immunity is type specific and is clinically complete for at least two years. It may be lifelong.

Clinical Manifestations. Inapparent infection during experimental studies was rare. Onset is sudden, and peak fever is usually attained in the first 24 hours, subsiding after two to four days. It is accompanied by headache, myalgia, photophobia and ocular pain, and definite conjunctival injection. There may be erythema, but not a true eruption, over the face and upper trunk. Constipation and diarrhea sometimes occur. Bradycardia is not a feature of this disease, although the typical viral leukopenia is common. Cerebrospinal fluid remains normal. A few patients experience a second bout of fever and symptoms during the second week of evolution, but convalescence is otherwise uneventful and complete.

Diagnosis, Treatment, and Prevention. Epidemiologic history represents the best clue to diagnosis. Virus isolation and serologic procedures may be carried out but serve principally to exclude other possible causes such as dengue and influenza. Management of patients is purely symptomatic. No vaccine is generally available, but DDT and other insecticides have proved highly effective in control of the classic Phlebotomus vector.

Anderson, C. R., Downs, W. G., Wattley, G. H., Akin, N. W., and Reese, A. A.: Mayaro virus: A new human disease agent. II. Isolation from blood of patients in Trinidad, B.W.I. Am. J. Trop. Med. Hyg., 6:1012, 1957.

Barnett, H. C., and Suyemoto, W.: Field studies on sandfly fever and Kala-azar in Pakistan, in Iran, and in Baltistan (Little Tibet). Trans. N.Y. Acad. Sci., Sec. II, 23:609, 1961.

Clarke, J. A., Marshall, I. D., and Gard, G.: Annually recurrent epidemic polyarthritis and Ross River virus activity in a coastal area of New South Wales. I. Occurrence of the disease. Am. J. Trop. Med. Hyg., 22:543, 1973.

Doherty, R. L., Barrett, E. J., Gorman, B. M., and Whitehead, R. H.: Epi-

demic polyarthritis in Eastern Australia, 1959–1970. Med. J. Aust., 1:5, 1971.
Eklund, C. M.: Natural history of Colorado tick fever virus. J. Lancet, 82:172, 1962.
Emmons, R. W., and Lennette, E. H.: Immunofluorescent staining in the diagnosis of Colorado tick fever. J. Lab. Clin. Med., 68:923, 1966.
Florio, L., Stewart, M. O., and Mugrage, E. R.: The etiology of Colorado tick fever. J. Exp. Med., 83:1, 1946.
Halstead, S. B., Nimmannitya, S., and Margiotta, M. R.: Dengue and chikungunya virus infection in man in Thailand, 1962–1964: II. Observations on disease in outpatients. Am. J. Trop. Med. Hyg., 18:972, 1969.
Hotta, S.: Twenty years of laboratory experience with dengue virus. I. Epidemiology–past and present. *In* Sanders, M., and Lennette, E. H. (eds.): Applied Virology. Sheboygan, Wisc., Ellis Corporation, 1965, pp. 228–256.
Robinson, M. C.: An epidemic of virus disease in Southern province, Tanganyika Territory in 1952–1953. I. Clinical features. Trans. R. Soc. Trop. Med. Hyg., 49:28, 1955.
Sabin, A. B., Philip, C. B., and Paul, J. R.: Phlebotomus (pappataci or sandfly) fever. A disease of military importance. Summary of existing knowledge and preliminary report of original investigations. J.A.M.A., 125:603; 693, 1944.
Schrire, L.: Macular changes in Rift Valley fever. S. Afr. Med. J., 25:926, 1951.
Shore, H.: O'nyong-nyong fever: An epidemic disease in East Africa. III. Some clinical and epidemiological observations in the Northern province of Uganda. Trans. R. Soc. Trop. Med. Hyg., 55:361, 1961.
Silver, H. K., Meiklejohn, G., and Kempe, C. H.: Colorado tick fever. Am. J. Dis. Child., 101:30, 1961.
Spigland, I., Jasinska-Klingberg, W., Hofshi, E., and Goldblum, N.: Clinical and laboratory observations in an outbreak of West Nile fever in Israel. Harefuah, 54:275, 1958.
Taylor, R. M., Work, T. H., Hurlbut, H. S., and Rizk, F.: A study of the ecology of West Nile virus in Egypt. Am. J. Trop. Med. Hyg., 5:579, 1956.
Tesh, R. B., Chaniotis, B. N., Peralta, P. H., and Johnson, K. M.: Ecology of viruses isolated from Panamanian phlebotomine sandflies. Am. J. Trop. Med. Hyg., 23:258, 1974.
Weiss, K. E.: Rift Valley fever. A review. Bull. Epizoot. Dis. Afr., 5:431, 1957.
Wisseman, C. L., Jr.: The ecology of dengue. *In* May, J. M. (ed.): Studies in Disease Ecology. New York, Hafner Publishing Company, 1961, Chap. 2, p. 15.

ARTHROPOD-BORNE VIRAL ENCEPHALITIDES

Karl M. Johnson

144. INTRODUCTION

The arthropod-borne viral encephalitides comprise a group of clinically similar diseases induced by a variety of small viruses containing ribonucleic acid. Although infection usually occurs through the bite of an infectious arthropod, some of the agents are also transmitted by contact through mucous membranes, by aerosol, and by ingestion. In general, arthropods become infectious only after an extrinsic incubation period of one week or longer, which may be modified further by environmental temperature. Once infectious, however, such vectors remain so for long periods, in many cases for life. Encephalitis is usually an infrequent manifestation of human infection, but the agents to be considered all cause this dramatic and life-threatening syndrome with sufficient frequency that the term has been included as an integral part of viral nomenclature. This exposition is designed to provide the physician with the key clues necessary to aid him in sorting the variables involved in diagnosis and prognosis of infection, and to suggest areas where ignorance rather than understanding characterizes the state of knowledge concerning these diseases and their clinical management. Because of the very real public health significance attached to the occurrence of even a single case of some of the encephalitides, the importance of specific diagnosis of arboviral encephalitis cannot be overstressed.

It is possible to subdivide these diseases in a variety of ways. They are distributed nearly worldwide, occurring in both temperate and tropical climates; they are caused by different viruses, some of which are antigenically related; they are transmitted by mosquitoes or ticks; they cause central nervous system (CNS) disease predominantly in adults or in children; and they may or may not clinically affect domestic livestock.

Pathogenesis and Pathology of Arboviral Encephalitis. After deposition in the skin, virus may multiply locally and spread via lymphatics to cells of the reticuloendothelial system localized in lymph nodes, small vessels, and other organs such as spleen. In vitro studies suggest that macrophages are inherently susceptible to virus replication but that lymphocytes are resistant unless "blast transformed." Release of virus from such cells leads to viremia and widespread dissemination to other organs. Clinical symptoms and pathologic changes in many of these organs suggest that vascular endothelial cells are regularly damaged, but no direct or indirect visualization of virus in such cells in man has yet been achieved.

Although myocarditis, focal hepatic necrosis, and damage to lungs and kidneys may occur, the hallmark of these agents is their ability to induce damage to the brain. Despite some variation from virus to virus, a basic similarity exists in the gross and microscopic pathology of arbovirus-induced encephalitis. Brains are minimally edematous grossly with occasional small hemorrhages. Microscopic edema and hyperemia are present in the leptomeninges and cortex. There are small hemorrhages in many parts of the brain, sometimes with small arteriolar thrombi. Most striking of all are conspicuous collections of mononuclear, occasionally polymorphonuclear leukocytes around small vessels, the so-called "perivascular cuffs." Neuronal lesions are often focal and reveal nuclei and cytoplasm in various states of degeneration. Microglial and polymorphonuclear accumulations often present a picture of focal nodules. These lesions are most common in the gray matter, midbrain, basal nuclei, brainstem, and cerebellum, although some of the viruses induce destruction of anterior horn cells of the upper spinal cord.

Leukocytes and modest increases in protein concentration in cerebrospinal fluid are almost always seen. Although polymorphonuclear cells may be slightly more numerous early in the course of disease, there is always an evolution to a pleocytosis. It is of interest also that clinical encephalitis is almost always marked by a moderate leukocytosis rather than the leukopenia so characteristic of undifferentiated and primary hemorrhagic fevers produced by arboviruses.

A central question is how much of the CNS damage produced by these arboviruses is due to direct virus-induced destruction of neurons and how much may be the result of immunologically mediated injury to small vessels and/or neurons. In most instances virus is difficult to recover at autopsy from the brain, and it is not readily obtained from cerebrospinal fluid either. This has been explained in the past on the basis that antiviral antibodies are usually present at death in fatal encephalitis such that in vivo or in vitro neutralization obscures the real sequence of events. Although some neuronal destruction almost certainly occurs, the clinical course in the majority of patients who make rapid and nearly complete recovery and the pathognomonic *mononuclear* perivascular cuffs strongly point to an immune-induced inflammatory lesion as a major contributor to disease. What is wanted are new investigations of general and local immunologic reactions in patients with these diseases. The problem is of more than theoretical interest, because an elucidation of pathogenesis might well lead to a rationale for employment of therapeutic measures which present wisdom must continue to regard as potentially more harmful than helpful.

Clinical Manifestations. The shifting, protean neurologic manifestations seen in arbovirus encephalitis suggest a mixture of permanent neuronal damage and temporary central dysfunction secondary to intermittent anoxia and edema. This pattern accounts also for the observed wide range of convalescent behavior and permanent sequelae.

The temperature course is frequently bizarre, indicating an anoxic effect on central thermoregulatory function. Indeed, persistent high fever is the most ominous clinical sign, and *external artificial control of temperature may be the most important measure available* for the management of the severely ill patient.

Although statistically significant differences in the frequency of specific neurologic symptoms and signs of encephalitis caused by individual arboviruses are slowly emerging, it remains evident that the range provoked by each agent is quite broad. Symptomatology in the individual patient rarely provides assurance as to the specific etiologic agent. Unexplained differences in patterns correlated with human age, however, are sometimes striking. Thus death caused by St. Louis encephalitis virus (SLE) is almost invariably restricted to the elderly, as though the vascular reserves available to cope with an acute inflammatory anoxia were compromised. By contrast, CNS disease and death caused by Venezuelan equine encephalitis virus (VEE) are observed almost exclusively in children. Major upper motor neuron destruction leading to permanent paralysis is largely attributable to Japanese B and Russian spring-summer encephalitis viruses. Sophisticated clinical investigation of all these diseases is nearly nonexistent. More work such as that of the Dallas group who measured cerebral blood flow and certain hormonal functions in patients with St. Louis encephalitis virus is urgently needed.

Differential Diagnosis. The most common disease clinically indistinguishable from arbovirus encephalitis is that caused by *herpes simplex* virus. Previous clinical herpetic infection and the fact that this disease occurs throughout the year may offer clues to its recognition (see Ch. 390).

Enteroviruses and *leptospira* may produce disease which mimics arboviral encephalitis, and the seasonal pattern is often coincident. Indeed mixed arboviral and enteroviral epidemics are not infrequently recognized.

Meningitis and rarely encephalitis caused by *mumps* virus may also be confused with that caused by arboviruses (see Ch. 125).

Postinfectious or *postvaccinal* encephalitis after measles, rubella, or varicella infection or inoculation with rabies or vaccinia vaccines must always be considered in such cases. History is the key to these diagnoses (see Ch. 118 to 121 and Ch. 396).

Rabies and *lymphocytic choriomeningitis* viruses can also resemble arboviral encephalitis. History of animal bite usually establishes the former diagnosis, but the latter must usually be separated by viral diagnostic procedures.

An assortment of acute febrile encephalopathies marked by hypoglycemia, diarrhea, convulsions, and coma, with or without visceral pathologic changes, has been described. These syndromes of undetermined etiology generally do not induce significant cerebrospinal fluid pleocytosis, nor do they display the marked central inflammatory changes so typical of arbovirus infection.

Bacterial and *fungal meningitides* can usually be distinguished by reduced sugar, high protein, and a mixture of cells, as well as by presence of stainable organisms in cerebrospinal fluid. Not uncommonly, however, incompletely treated bacterial meningitis may present a real diagnostic challenge.

Tumors and *abscesses* are usually separable by strong localization of neurologic signs, by absence of high fever unless septicemia is present, and by suitable tests to document abnormal space-filling lesions. *Toxic encephalopathies* must be thought of. History and chemical determinations are the best aids to establishment of such diagnoses.

It should thus be apparent that competent microbiologic diagnostic facilities are essential to establishing the specific diagnosis, and that such competence must extend beyond the arboviruses per se.

145. WESTERN EQUINE ENCEPHALITIS

Etiology. Western equine encephalitis (WEE) virus was the first such agent to be recovered from equines and humans. Isolated from an encephalitic horse in 1930 by Meyer, this agent represents the prototype for arboviruses immunologically collected into group A by Casals. The agent produces inapparent infection, mild febrile illness, or clinical encephalitis in both equines and humans.

Epidemiology. This virus, as well as its immunologic relatives, eastern equine encephalitis (EEE) and Venezuelan equine encephalitis (VEE), is limited in distribution to the Western Hemisphere. Virologic and serologic studies have disclosed seasonal mosquito-bird activity cycles in many areas of the United States and Canada and in parts of southern and eastern South America as well. It is not present in tropical Middle America. In North America clinical infection of man has been recognized in the Mississippi drainage basin, the Great Plains, and the valleys between the western mountains. In most of these regions the mosquito vector is *Culex tarsalis,* and a variety of small birds appear to provide the principal blood virus source for mosquito infection. Equines and humans are frequently infected, as disclosed by population surveys for specific antibodies, but do not develop viremia of sufficient concentration to serve as hosts for further amplification of the basic cycle. Seasonal temperature fluctuations play a decisive role in disease transmission, exerting effects on mosquito population, on virus incubation period in mosquitoes, and on migratory behavior of birds. Thus WEE is a disease of summer and early fall.

Experimental work has shown that WEE virus may persist during winter in hibernating snakes, and claims for such a mechanism in nature have been made but are as yet not generally accepted as valid. Human attack rates are highest in young adult males and in infants less than one year old. This pattern is due to the strong geographic localization of WEE virus and to the fact that agricultural irrigation projects vastly increase the breeding habitat available for *Culex tarsalis.* Incubation period of infection in man is generally five to ten days. Mortality among patients with encephalitis may reach 10 per cent.

Clinical Manifestations. A two- to four-day prodrome of fever, headache, and myalgia commonly precedes the appearance of CNS signs in children; adults more often experience abrupt onset of stiff neck and drowsiness with fever and muscle aching. Clinically, CNS disease is almost always more severe in children, who, in addition to the hallmark signs of disorientation, somnolence, and coma, often suffer convulsions, abnormal reflexes, and flaccid or spastic paralyses. Fever lasts for a week or more, but rarely for two, and ranges from 39 to 40° C. Higher temperatures are prognostically ominous and should be reduced by external means.

Clinical improvement at the end of the febrile period is often dramatic in adults, most of whom make uneventful recoveries without residual motor or psychologic residua. Children, especially the very young, are not so fortunate; more than half of them are left with permanent damage, producing mental retardation, emotional instability, or spastic paralyses.

Although leukopenia may be present early in the course of illness, a mild leukocytosis with polymorphonuclear cells predominating is more common. Cerebrospinal fluid is clear, contains normal sugar concentration but moderately increased protein, and nearly always shows a mild pleocytosis.

Diagnosis. Encephalitic signs occurring in both children and adults during summer should immediately raise suspicion of an arboviral causation. The major differential is similar disease caused by enteroviruses. Specific laboratory diagnosis is required in both instances.

Although WEE virus has been recovered on occasion from brain tissue of patients dying during the first week of disease, isolation of the agent from blood or cerebrospinal fluid is difficult even during the initial three days of symptoms. Specific diagnosis thus depends on demonstration of increasing anti-WEE antibody titers in sequentially collected sera. A specimen should be obtained and frozen as part of the initial examination of the patient, because such antibodies often appear during the first week of symptoms. The second serum can be taken 10 to 14 days later. Although single convalescent sera are of limited usefulness in areas where WEE infection is common, detection of specific antibodies of the IgM class is good evidence for very recent infection. This test is of proved utility in cases occurring among infants who have residual IgG antibodies from their immune mothers.

Treatment. Control of high fever and maintenance of water and electrolyte balance are the essential measures in management of patients. When necessary, reduction of fever should be by use of external chilling techniques rather than by use of analgesics such as aspirin. Continuous care should be taken to see that a patient's airway and normal respiratory function are maintained.

Convalescence is usually prolonged and should never be forced. Children should be thoroughly examined at intervals up to a year after acute encephalitis in order to detect those who may require psychiatric or special educational and motor therapy.

Prevention. During epizootics or epidemics the prime objective is to prevent mosquitoes from biting babies. Houses should be screened; cribs, bassinets, and carriages should be covered by fine mesh netting. Transmission of WEE virus can also occur in utero; thus *pregnant women* should be specially protected against mosquito attack by restricting outdoor activity, by using repellents, and by use of residual and knockdown insecticides within and near their homes.

Community-wide organized control programs to reduce mosquito populations are important in areas where repeated epidemics have occurred. Based on combinations of insecticide and management of irrigation water, the value of such measures has been documented in California, Colorado, and Texas.

Epizootics of WEE in equines frequently precede human epidemics. An effective formalin-killed chick embryo virus vaccine is now used to protect horses, thus reducing the "sentinel" value of this species as a warning of an impending epidemic. The vaccine is not licensed for use in human medicine.

146. EASTERN EQUINE ENCEPHALITIS

Etiology. Eastern equine encephalitis (EEE) virus is a group A arbovirus which produces severe encephalitis and death in a high proportion of equine and human infections. It was first isolated in 1933 by Ten Broeck and Merrill and has been shown to be the most common cause of summertime epizootic-epidemic arboviral encephalitis in the eastern United States. Most outbreaks have occurred along the seaboard from northern Florida to Canada. Sporadic disease outbreaks also have been documented in some of the Caribbean islands during the fall. An antigenically distinguishable EEE virus variant is present in Middle and parts of South America. To date this variant has been associated with acute neurologic disease in equines but not in man.

Epidemiology. Basic elements in the natural cycle of EEE virus in North America are the mosquito *Culex melanura* and a large number of species of small wild birds. Although reminiscent of WEE epidemiology, that of EEE differs significantly owing to the fact that *Culex melanura* distribution is strongly localized to a series of coastal fresh water hardwood swamps. Virus activity in these swamps occurs each summer, commencing later as one moves from south to north. Two possible mechanisms may account for this seasonal chain; either the virus overwinters in each swamp by infection of vertebrates (hibernating turtles as well as contact infections among rodents have been proposed), or the Culex-bird cycle is maintained through the winter in the most southerly swamps where frost is unusual. In the latter case spring migration of birds could provide the means for reintroduction of virus into northern swamps each year. Southward fall bird migration definitely seems to account for the Caribbean outbreaks because EEE-infected migrants have been detected in the southern United States and on the islands, and virus strains recovered during these autumnal epizootic epidemics were identified antigenically as North American rather than South American in origin.

Epizootics in equines and in exotic gallinaceous birds such as pheasants, chukar partridges, and Pekin ducks usually precede by one to three weeks the appearance of human encephalitis. Evidence has accumulated indicating that accessory mosquito vectors such as the saltmarsh *Aedes sollicitans* and the widely dispersed *Aedes vexans* may be important in transmission of virus to these abnormal hosts. As with WEE virus, equines and humans are of no or very limited significance as hosts for further mosquito infection. Disease patterns observed in game-bird farms strongly suggest, moreover, that direct contact infection is important in the epizootics which at times devastate these exotic species.

Although EEE infection of wild birds is usually not symptomatic, the reverse is true for horses and humans. More than half of equine infections are clinically overt, and mortality among such animals may approach 90 per cent. Serologic surveys among human populations resident very close to the fresh-water swamps have revealed individuals with specific antibodies and no history or stigmata of encephalitis. Nevertheless, it is probable that clinical encephalitis occurs in a high proportion of human North American EEE infections. Mortality among hospitalized patients runs to 50 per cent or higher, and many survivors have residual neurologic dysfunction regardless of age.

Clinical Manifestations. The incubation period is assumed to be about seven to ten days, after which there is sudden onset of high fever, headache, conjunctivitis, nausea, and vomiting. This pattern, particularly common in adults, progresses rapidly from drowsiness to delirium and coma. There is stiff neck and irritability, at times accompanied by positive Kernig's sign, absent or hyperactive reflexes, and muscle spasticity in the extremities, often asymmetrical. Patients, if conscious, may be unable to speak or swallow. Excessive salivation is common. The disease terminates fatally within the first two weeks, usually within seven days, or shifting signs of deep CNS involvement may continue for several weeks, the patient gradually returning to consciousness. Serial neurologic examination usually discloses which centers and nerve supplies have sustained permanent damage.

Polymorphonuclear leukocytosis which can reach 50,000 cells per cubic millimeter is characteristic. During the first days of disease the CSF, usually under considerable pressure, also contains such cells in numbers up to 1000. Protein is elevated; as illness progresses, the cells become predominantly mononuclear.

A diphasic disease pattern is often seen in children. After a day or two of fever, headache, and gastrointestinal upset, followed by two or three days of clinical improvement, there is fulminating onset of high fever, vomiting, delirium, convulsions, and coma. There may be intermittent or persistent opisthotonos, generalized rigidity, and localized paralyses. Circulatory stasis or mechanical obstruction leads to clinical cyanosis, especially in the very young.

Convalescence is slow, and during this time neurologic residua become apparent. There may be permanent damage to cranial nerves, as to those regulating muscle function of one or more extremities. Mental or emotional deterioration, or both, may be so severe as to require permanent institutional care.

Diagnosis. Although EEE virus can be isolated from the brains of persons who die during the first week of illness, little success attends attempts to recover the agent from blood or CSF specimens during the acute illness. Sera taken during the first seven days of disease may contain neutralizing and hemagglutination-inhibiting antibodies for EEE virus. If so, the diagnosis is likely, because such substances are rarely found in the general population. A second serum obtained at about 14 days usually shows rising titers of specific antibodies.

Treatment. There is no specific chemotherapy, and there is no evidence that passively administered anti-EEE antibodies alter the course of clinically apparent disease. Thus management is that of any desperately ill patient: careful control of fluid and electrolyte balance, constant maintenance of a patient's airway, and external treatment of direct life-threatening hyperthermia. Secondary bacterial infections, if they occur, generally appear after the most acute primary phase of disease, and are those attendant to mechanical maintenance of respiratory and urinary function, physical inactivity, and bed sores. Physiotherapy to minimize paralytic contractures should begin after the febrile period.

Prevention. The principles are similar to those for WEE infection. There is a killed virus vaccine for equine, but not human, use. Since the ecology of EEE virus is centered in natural rather than man-modified habitats, organized mosquito-control efforts directed specifically at annual disease prevention are not economically feasible. Insecticides, however, are of some value both near residences and in accessible areas of mosquito-virus activity whenever a human epidemic exists or is threatened by the appearance of an epizootic.

Convalescent human plasma has been used to prevent disease after inadvertent direct exposure to EEE virus in laboratory workers. It is of unproved value and appears to be of no help unless given within 24 hours of the accident.

147. VENEZUELAN EQUINE ENCEPHALITIS

Etiology. Venezuelan equine encephalitis (VEE) virus is a group A arbovirus which causes fatal CNS disease in equines and an acute influenza-like syndrome in humans. During large epidemics cases of encephalitis are seen in young children, but the incidence of neurologic signs in this age group rarely exceeds 1 to 3 per cent of infections.

First isolated from horses by Kubes and Rios during a 1938 epizootic in Venezuela, the virus was not associated with human disease until several years later. Investigation of arbovirus ecology in tropical America during the past three decades has resulted in the recognition of several antigenic subtypes of VEE virus which differ in pathogenicity for equines and possibly humans and which have distinct cycles of maintenance and transmission. Taken together, VEE viruses have killed more equines and produced more human illness in the Western Hemisphere than any other arbovirus.

Epidemiology. Enzootic VEE virus cycles have been carefully studied in Trinidad, Colombia, Panama, Brazil, Mexico, and the United States (Florida Everglades). Virus activity was always focal, localized to shaded fresh-water swamps or to slow-moving bodies of water where floating water lettuce plants, *Pistia*, were common. The vector mosquitoes in each instance were members of the taxonomically complex subgenus *Culex melanoconion*. Small rodents, or in some cases water birds, are the principal vertebrate hosts. These animals develop high levels of virus in blood without significant mortality. Humans resident near or entering such enzootic foci suffer overt clinical infection, because the mosquito vectors are opportunistic rather than highly specialized blood feeders.

For some time it was thought that such enzootic foci were the sources for the periodic equine-human VEE outbreaks that swept large parts of Venezuela, Colombia, Ecuador, and Peru. But antigenic analysis of virus strains from all countries where VEE occurs together with experimental studies in horses has disclosed that enzootic VEE viruses were never involved in epizootics. Such strains, although capable of infecting and inducing cross-immunity, produced no encephalitis or sufficient viremia to infect mosquitoes when inoculated into equines. In contrast, antigenically distinct epizootic virus strains are highly pathogenic for equines, and induce truly dramatic viremias in them. Many genera and species of mosquitoes are thus infected and capable of further transmission of virus to equines, humans, and other vertebrates. Unlike the related WEE and EEE viruses, then, the equine is the single major host responsible for amplification and dissemination of the classic VEE strains. At present no mechanism has been discovered to account for interepizootic maintenance of such viruses in nature. Epizootics of VEE typically take place in rural tropical regions characterized by climates having a pronounced dry season. Cattle raising is the dominant land use, and outbreaks most often occur after the advent of the rainy season. Although human-mosquito transmission chains are possible, the timing of human disease one to two weeks after appearance of equine encephalitis suggests that epidemic VEE in man is mainly a spillover from the fulminant equine-mosquito cycle. At times nearly all equines and large fractions of rural human populations are infected during such outbreaks. Many thousands of human infections, most of them clinically apparent, can thus occur in a few weeks.

A unique outbreak occurred recently in Central America, with the apparently exotic epizootic virus finally reaching into southwestern Texas during the summer of 1971.

All subtypes of VEE virus are highly infectious for humans and other vertebrates when administered via the respiratory route. Thus many laboratory infections have been recorded.

Clinical Manifestations. Onset of illness is typically abrupt, patients frequently reporting the exact time of appearance of severe headache, chills, fever, and explosive vomiting and diarrhea. These symptoms ensue two to four days after infectious mosquito bite but can occur within 24 hours after exposure to highly infectious aerosols. Conjunctival injection and mild sore throat are present early in the clinical course, and myalgia is usually intense. Fever often reaches 40° C. In general the first day of symptoms is the worst, and the fever curve shows daily evening peaks which regress to normal after three to five days. Mild somnolence is common, but severe neurologic signs are seen in only a small percentage of cases, nearly always among children. Individual cases may thus be readily confused with influenza, acute infectious or toxic gastroenteritis, or leptospirosis.

During the first day of illness blood leukocytes are usually normal or slightly increased in numbers, with a strong shift toward polymorphonuclear dominance and a conspicuous eosinopenia. There follows a definite leukopenia, and by the fourth or fifth day a relative lymphocytosis is usual. Normal total and differential values are re-established by about the tenth day.

Nuchal stiffness is unusual, and the CSF generally shows no cells or a very mild pleocytosis with normal protein. Children exhibiting more serious neurologic signs, including abnormal reflexes, spastic paralyses, convulsions, and coma, usually experience a biphasic febrile course with the second fever spike associated with CNS signs. Epilepsy, paralyses, tremors, hallucinations, and emotional instability may persist as permanent sequelae of infection in children, and occasional cases of residual epilepsy and intention tremors have been cited among adults.

Most fatalities occur in children under five years of age. Autopsies revealed gross and histologic changes similar to those seen with other arboviruses causing encephalitis, but in addition were noteworthy for the presence of scattered gross focal hemorrhages in brain, heart, and lungs.

Diagnosis. Since clinical presentation of VEE infection is rarely overtly encephalitic, the diagnosis will be missed unless it is considered in a patient with high fever, respiratory symptoms, and gastrointestinal upset who resides in or has recently visited either an enzootic focus or an epizootic area of tropical America. Virus can be recovered with ease, however, from either blood or throat swab specimens taken during the initial 72 hours of symptoms. Since patients are potentially infectious for humans and mosquitoes during this phase, the importance of establishing the cause is obvious. Paired serum samples obtained early in illness and about 10 days later will reliably reveal rising levels of specific anti VEE antibodies.

Treatment. There is no specific treatment. Analgesics and external chilling may be required to control hyperthermia. Life-threatening fluid and electrolyte imbalance may result from vomiting and diarrhea in children and must be alertly detected and corrected. Patients frequently complain of lassitude and inability to concentrate mentally for one to four weeks after fever has subsided, but convalescence is otherwise usually uneventful.

Prophylaxis. Formalin-inactivated vaccines have been used to protect equines in South America for 30 years. The potency of these products is borderline at best, and the frequent persistence of live VEE virus in them may well have been the cause of subsequent major epizootics. An experimental live attenuated vaccine, strain TC-83, has been used with success in immunizing laboratory personnel at high risk of aerosol infection. This vaccine, which produces febrile reactions in up to 20 per cent of adult recipients, has not been tested in children or pregnant women. It has been associated with birth defects when inoculated into pregnant rhesus monkeys and seems unlikely ever to be generally safe for human protection.

Nevertheless, this vaccine is the single most important tool available for interdiction of human VEE epidemics. Most mosquitoes acquire virus from equines, and it has been shown that mass vaccination of equines prevents further viremic infection of these animals within three days. Once horse infections cease, transmission to man generally comes to an end within a short interval as infected mosquitoes die. Insecticides are useful in killing infected mosquitoes when temporally combined with equine vaccination.

Since patients are potentially infectious, precautions should be taken to prevent them from mosquito bite. Although medical personnel attending patients are potentially at risk of acquiring the disease by aerosol, the infrequent occurrence of significant coughing during VEE infection may explain the absence of well-documented instances of such transmission.

148. CALIFORNIA ENCEPHALITIS

Definition. California encephalitis is an acute CNS disease which occurs during summer in many areas of the United States and is caused by one or more antigenically related viruses of the California arbovirus complex.

Etiology. The original virus strain of this antigenic complex was recovered from *Aedes dorsalis* and *Culex tarsalis* mosquitoes in the San Joaquin Valley of California in the 1940's. Serologic studies showed this agent to be associated with a few cases of childhood encephalitis previously thought clinically to be caused by WEE or St. Louis encephalitis viruses.

In 1960 the La Crosse strain was recovered from the brain of a six-year-old child who died of encephalitis. Although very few other isolates have been made from man, antigens prepared from the La Crosse agent have been used in recent years to document many cases of acute CNS disease in different regions of the United States.

At least six antigenically related California arboviruses have been recovered from a variety of mosquitoes and wild vertebrates in the United States. Related agents are known from tropical America, Europe, Africa, and Asia. One variant is annually active in the far north of western Canada and Alaska.

Epidemiology. Frequent epidemics of California encephalitis have been documented in Wisconsin, Indiana, and Ohio, and sporadic cases are on record from North Carolina and Florida. It is probable that the disease occurs over a much wider area of the midwestern and southern United States, but is not diagnosed because specific serologic tests are not generally employed and because cases often appear sporadically in a large number of small rural communities.

The La Crosse virus is transmitted principally by tree-hole breeding mosquitoes of the genus Aedes. Small mammals such as rabbits, chipmunks, and squirrels provide sources of virus for new mosquito infection, but the basic mechanism of virus maintenance is probably transovarial transmission of virus through the various life stages of the mosquito. This behavior was recently proved for *Aedes triseriatus,* the first known instance of insect maintenance of a mosquito-borne arbovirus.

More than 90 per cent of human cases of encephalitis occur in persons 15 years old or under. Males are more often affected than females, probably because exposure to the virus is most frequently related to the outdoor recreational pursuits of camping, fishing, or hunting in woodlands where infected day-biting Aedes mosquitoes are present. Although mortality from California encephalitis has not been established, it is low, not exceeding 5 per cent. Serologic studies also show that human infection with these viruses is far more common than clinical encephalitis.

Clinical Manifestations. Although not accurately known, the incubation period is probably between five and ten days. Onset of symptoms is typically insidious, with mild fever and headache for several days. As these symptoms increase, the headache usually becomes frontal, and the complaints are sometimes ascribed by patient or relatives to a minor traumatic incident. Mental confusion may or may not precede the sudden occurrence of convulsions, which may be the only overt sign of CNS disease on admission to hospital. Coma may supervene, and meningeal signs are occasionally seen, but shifting deep neurologic signs such as paralyses and reflex changes are rarely observed.

Mild to severe leukocytosis is characteristic of the acute stage of illness, counts sometimes reaching 30,000 per cubic millimeter. Cerebrospinal fluid is clear under moderate pressure and contains up to several hundred leukocytes, predominantly polymorphonuclear early, becoming mononuclear as illness progresses.

Fever generally subsides by lysis after a course of less than two weeks. Motor and sensory neurologic sequelae have not been observed, but emotional and learning dysfunction has been noted in children several months after physical convalescence is complete.

Diagnosis. The differential diagnosis of importance is that between viral encephalitis and post-traumatic *subdural hematoma.* Favoring the former are season of occurrence, history of forest exposure, the presence of leukocytosis, a clear cerebrospinal fluid, and the absence of localizing neurologic signs.

Specific diagnosis of California encephalitis must be made serologically, no isolate having yet been obtained from blood or excretions of acutely ill patients. Thus a fourfold or greater increase in CF, HI, or neutralizing antibodies between acute and early convalescent serum specimens provides the only confirmation of etiology.

Treatment and Prophylaxis. Management of patients is completely symptomatic. Hyperthermia and respiratory failure, although unusual, are the dangerous signs that must be detected and corrected without delay. No vaccine is available, nor has any experimental work been reported in this direction. Mosquito control is virtually impossible on a large scale because of the specialized breeding habits of the vector species. Protective clothing, nets, and repellents are the only effective measures available to individuals entering the woodlands where infected mosquitoes are present.

149. ST. LOUIS ENCEPHALITIS

Definition. St. Louis encephalitis (SLE) was the first recognized and is the most important arboviral encephalitis in the United States. It occurs sporadically and in major outbreaks during late summer and fall, afflicting rural populations in the West and urban-suburban communities elsewhere in the nation.

Etiology. St. Louis encephalitis virus is a group B arbovirus, most closely related antigenically to Japanese B and Murray Valley encephalitis viruses. It occurs only in the Western Hemisphere.

Epidemiology. The causative virus was first recovered from fatal cases during a major outbreak of encephalitis in St. Louis in 1933. Since that time sporadic cases and outbreaks of varying intensity have occurred in rural Washington and California, and in suburban and urban areas of Florida, Texas, the lower Ohio Valley, Pennsylvania, and New Jersey. Presence of virus is indicated by antibodies and/or isolation of virus strains from wildlife in Mexico, Central America, South America, and several Caribbean islands.

The basic virus cycle leading to human outbreaks involves birds and certain Culex mosquitoes. Although the possible mechanisms for virus survival during winter are not precisely known, they include reintroduction by northward migrating birds, recrudescent infection in nonmigratory birds, persistence of infected adult mosquitoes, and persistent infection in hibernating bats. The principal mosquito vector in the western United States is *Culex tarsalis,* especially abundant in irrigated agricultural areas. The vectors of urban-suburban epidemics elsewhere in the country are *C. pipiens, C. quinquefasciatus,* and *C. nigripalpus.* The virus has been recovered from many different mosquitoes in tropical America, many of them strongly arboreal in activity pattern, but it is not clear which are the most important in ecologic terms.

Although the distribution of SLE virus in the United States overlaps to a considerable degree with that of both EEE and WEE viruses, two important epidemiologic features distinguish the former from the latter group A viruses. First, although all three agents "spill over" from birds to horses, only EEE and WEE cause equine disease. Second, because the extrinsic incubation period in the mosquito is longer for SLE than for the equine viruses, St. Louis encephalitis always occurs later in the summer and is not found as far north (Canada) as the group A encephalitides.

Clinical Manifestations. Acute disease probably occurs in no more than 1 to 2 per cent of St. Louis encephalitis virus infections. Usually the course is benign, comprising a few days of fever and pronounced headache followed by complete recovery. More severe disease is occasionally seen in young children and occurs in a substantial number of adults more than 40 years of age. After an incubation period variously estimated at up to two weeks, there is acute onset of fever and altered sensorium. Convulsions are more common in children than in adults. The most common neurologic signs are stiff neck, tremors of the hands and face, dysdiadochokinesia, and nystagmus. Cranial nerve abnormalities are found in about 20 per cent of cases. Myalgia, photophobia, and conjunctival suffusion are common, and acute urinary symptoms with unexplained mild pyuria and increased blood urea nitrogen concentration occur in nearly one fourth of patients.

White blood cell counts are usually normal to moderately elevated, and increased numbers of immature polymorphonuclear leukocytes may be found early in the course. Although an occasional patient has no cells in the cerebrospinal fluid on admission to hospital, all eventually are found to be positive, the total number of leukocytes rarely exceeding 500. Although some polymorphonuclear cells may be present at the beginning, later examinations reveal only lymphocytes. Cerebrospinal fluid protein is typically increased, but rarely exceeds 100 mg per 100 ml.

Diagnosis. Given appropriate season and place, the differential diagnosis of St. Louis encephalitis virus infection centers on other arboviruses and enteroviral meningitis in children and on *acute cerebrovascular accidents* in the elderly. An infectious cause may not even be considered in the latter group until a cluster of cases demands explanation. The virus itself has never been recovered from blood or cerebrospinal fluid of patients, and only rarely from brains of persons who die during the first week of illness. Specific diagnosis is thus dependent upon serologic testing of paired sera. The most practical technique is that of complement fixation, although the neutralization test provides the most definitive result if the early acute specimen is recovered before significant levels of antibody have been produced.

Treatment and Prognosis. Treatment is purely symptomatic. Persistent fever above 40° C is an ominous sign and should be vigorously controlled. About 10 to 25 per cent of adults with acute encephalitis die, most of them from complications of underlying diseases. Such deaths generally occur after the first 10 days of illness when most of the neurologic manifestations have subsided. Hyponatremia is a frequent problem in management of the acute phase of disease, and in some cases has been ascribed to a partial persistent elaboration of antidiuretic hormone. Convalescence is often quite prolonged, and long-term examination of patients reveals frequent persistence of personality changes and emotional disturbance. Motor deficits are uncommon.

Prevention. There is no specific vaccine. Surveillance of seasonal mosquito-avian activity patterns of the virus in endemic regions is valuable as a guide to the timing of measures designed to reduce populations of vector mosquitoes. Emergency use of insecticides against adult mosquitoes during urban-suburban epidemics is probably of considerable help in reducing morbidity.

150. JAPANESE B ENCEPHALITIS

Definition. Japanese B encephalitis is a severe arbovirus disease which occurs in eastern Asia. Summer-fall outbreaks occur in Siberia, Korea, Japan, Taiwan, and other Pacific islands. Continuous endemic virus transmission has been proved or is suspected in Southeast Asia, the Philippines, and East Indies.

Etiology. The causative agent is a group of B arbovirus closely related antigenically to St. Louis, Murray Valley, and West Nile viruses. Unlike these agents, however, Japanese B virus is pathogenic for certain monkeys and equines, and has been shown to induce abortion or stillbirth in pregnant sows, a fact of major economic significance to the porcine industry of Japan and Taiwan.

Epidemiology. The basic cycle of infection in both temperate and tropical areas is mosquito-vertebrate-mosquito. In temperate areas the primary vector is *Culex tritaeniorhyncus,* and the important vertebrate hosts are herons, egrets, and pigs. Virus is detected in a given locale annually, first in mosquitoes in July, and then in birds and pigs within a few weeks. Epidemics of encephalitis occur later, in August and September, and by November virus has apparently disappeared. Winter survival has not been elucidated. Epidemics tend to be larger in alternate years for reasons not clearly understood.

In tropical areas virus transmission is less strongly seasonal, and although the basic cycle is similar to that of temperate zones, other vectors such as *C. gelidus* in Malaysia, Thailand, and Vietnam and *C. annulirostris* on Guam are important. Regardless of area, the ratio of inapparent to disease-associated infections in man is very high. Annual infection rates in children may reach 10 per cent, but only 1 in 300 to 500 infections results in clinical disease. This ratio apparently declines with increasing age, one case of encephalitis occurring per 25 infections in American troops.

Clinical Manifestations. Japanese B infection is similar to that of St. Louis encephalitis virus in the high frequency of inapparent infection or mild illness, in onset, and in the signs or symptoms of central nervous system disease. But urinary tract symptoms and signs are less common, and the over-all severity of neurologic disease is more severe in Japanese B infections. Children commonly evidence paralysis of the face or extremities. Adults tend toward bilateral paresis without sensory changes. Sensorial changes, spastic rigidity, cerebellar signs, and coma are frequent in adults. The fever usually peaks four or five days after onset, then slowly subsides. Relative bradycardia is often seen, accompanied by a modest transient leukocytosis. Cerebrospinal fluid pressure is often increased moderately, and pleocytosis and increased protein are invariably present.

Diagnosis. Although epidemiologic considerations may strongly suggest it, specific diagnosis requires a variety of virologic procedures. Isolation of virus from blood has been reported but is uncommonly achieved. Virus or, more often, fluorescent antigen can sometimes be demonstrated in brain tissue of fatal cases. Serologic diagnosis offers the best possibility of establishing the cause, but in many areas of Southeast Asia and India this is often confounded by the prior presence of antibodies to other related group B viruses. In Japan, where fewer such problems exist, it has been shown that primary infection induces early IgM antibodies reactive in neutralization and HI tests only, whereas IgG antibodies reactive in CF test are detectable eight or more days after onset of disease. Depending on the timing of serum specimens, diagnosis may thus require use of any or all three procedures. Detection of specific IgM HI antibodies has increased the precision of diagnosis in areas where related group B viruses are endemic.

Treatment and Prognosis. Intensive supportive care is mandatory and is all that is available. Artificial control of hyperthermia is frequently required. Anticonvulsant drugs may be needed, although prognosis in such cases is generally poor. The mortality rate varies from about 30 per cent for those under 20 years of age to nearly 80 per cent in older persons. Severity of clinical disease is directly correlated with quantitative antibody response. It has also been shown that early appearance of IgG antibodies was more common in persons who had received one dose of inactivated vaccine or who were more than 50 years old. Correlation of disease severity with early IgG immune response has not yet been reported.

Permanent sequelae are most common in children under age ten, severe residual damage generally being reserved for the very young. These changes run the gamut of upper motor paralyses, cerebellar syndromes, personality changes, and mental deterioration frequently requiring permanent institutional care.

Prevention. Formolized vaccine has been widely used in Japan and, providing that two or more doses are given, is credited with significant protection. A live attenuated vaccine has been tried in pigs in an effort to prevent annual amplification of the natural virus cycle; but although individual animals can be thus protected, the suppression of vaccine virus replication by passively acquired antibodies and the rapid turnover of this economically exploited species in Japan effectively preclude large-scale use of this measure. Specific vector control is not practical either, although modernization of rice culture techniques with attendant increased use of insecticides has apparently reduced peak mosquito vector populations in both Japan and South Korea, and is credited with significant reduction in epidemic disease transmission in recent years.

151. MURRAY VALLEY ENCEPHALITIS

Murray Valley encephalitis is similar to Japanese B encephalitis in pathogenesis and clinical features, and is caused by a very closely related virus. Diagnosis requires laboratory studies similar to those for other group B encephalitides.

The disease almost certainly was recognized in 1917–18 when an epidemic of 134 cases, then called *Australian X disease,* occurred in the Murray and Darling River valleys of Victoria and New South Wales. Virus strains isolated at the time were lost. Sporadic cases occurred during the next three decades, but the present designation was established during an outbreak of some 40 cases in 1951, more than a third of them fatal. This time the virus was recovered and completely characterized. Many inapparent human infections were detected. Endemic infection is maintained in a bird-mosquito cycle in Northern Australia and New Guinea, and it has been postulated that the virus is intermittently brought south by migratory birds, where an amplifying cycle involving domestic fowl, waterbirds, and *Culex annulirostris* mosquitoes produces epidemic disease, most commonly among children. An epidemic early in 1974 promises further elucidation of this disease in the Murray Valley.

152. TICK-BORNE GROUP B ARBOVIRUS DISEASES: RUSSIAN SPRING-SUMMER ENCEPHALITIS, LOUPING ILL, KYASANUR FOREST DISEASE, OMSK HEMORRHAGIC FEVER

Definition. The tick-borne complex of group B arboviruses cause mild to severe febrile illness with frequent neurologic abnormalities and in two instances (Kyasanur Forest disease [KFD] and Omsk hemorrhagic fever [OHF]) acute hemorrhagic manifestations. These agents are distributed throughout Eurasia (KFD, OHF, Russian spring-summer encephalitis [RSSE]) and Great Britain (louping ill). Powassan virus occurs in Canada and the western United States but has so far caused only a single recognized case of human disease.

Etiology. The group B tick-borne arboviruses constitute an antigenic complex readily distinguishable from most mosquito-borne group B agents, and separable into several closely related subtypes. With the exception of RSSE and OHF, which overlap geographically, these viruses are found in distinct regions of the world. Suckling mice and a variety of cell cultures have proved most satisfactory for virus isolation, and a complete range of serologic techniques is available for differential classification. Hemorrhagic pneumonia is induced in muskrats by inoculation of OHF virus, encephalitis with occasional hemorrhagic diathesis follows administration of KFD virus to langur and bonnet monkeys, and varying clinical encephalitis occurs upon intracerebral inoculation of monkeys, sheep, and goats with the remaining members of the complex.

Epidemiology. The viruses persist in discrete geographic foci by interchange between wild and domestic vertebrates and ixodid ticks, principally of the genera Ixodes, Dermacentor, and Haemaphysalis.

Many vertebrates, including rodents, birds, bats, sheep, goats, and cattle, experience clinically silent viremic infection. The capacity of the tick vectors to transmit virus transovarially has been experimentally documented, thus providing a fundamental mechanism for winter survival of some of the viruses. Persistent infection of hibernating species such as bats and hedgehogs has also been demonstrated. In the case of OHF and KFD viruses, respectively, viremia and overt fatal infection occur naturally in muskrats and monkeys, and major epizootics among these animals often precede or accompany outbreaks in man.

In addition to tick transmission, RSSE infection in man may be acquired through *drinking raw milk* of infected goats. Tick-transmitted infection may result from factors affecting residence, occupation, or recreation. Residents of rural forested areas, particularly agricultural, veterinary, and forest workers, are at highest risk. Seasonal disease patterns reflect temperature-dependent tick activity, with peaks ranging from late spring to autumn, depending on the tick and the geographic locality. Some of the agents can also apparently infect man by the respiratory route, as evidenced by winter outbreaks among trappers and skinners of muskrats (OHF) and by aerosol-associated laboratory infections (OHF, KFD).

Clinical Manifestations and Pathology. Onset is typically abrupt after an incubation period of three to twelve days. The pattern is frequently diphasic except for OHF, the initial phase consisting of fever, headache, myalgia, gastrointestinal disturbances, and, in KFD, mild to moderate hemorrhages from the nose and intestines. Leukopenia is common during this phase which lasts five to ten days.

The second phase usually begins with high fever and severe headache. Louping ill is usually mild to moderate in over-all severity, but RSSE infection tends to be progressively more severe from Europe to Far Eastern Asia. Although serous meningitis is the most common form over-all, infection in the easternmost part of the Soviet Union is frequently grossly encephalomyelitic, with transient or permanent flaccid paralysis, nystagmus, deafness, and somnolence. Bulbospinal disease is the most serious, resulting in neck and shoulder paralysis or even death. The second phase of KFD also is predominantly neurologic, although severity is usually moderate. Moderate leukocytosis and cerebrospinal fluid pleocytosis and elevated protein are characteristic of this phase. The latter abnormalities have been shown to persist in louping ill for weeks after apparent clinical recovery.

Pathologically the lesions produced by these viruses are generally similar to those observed with other arbovirus encephalitides or hemorrhagic fevers (inflammatory vasculitis in brain or focal capillary hemorrhages without inflammation). But not infrequently RSSE virus produces neuronal damage in the cervical cord reminiscent of poliomyelitis, and the viruses of OHF and KFD induce a focal hemorrhagic bronchopneumonia with occasional necrotic foci in the liver and gastrointestinal tract.

Diagnosis and Treatment. Specific diagnosis, in contrast to disease caused by most mosquito-borne encephalitides, can often be made by isolation of the virus from blood during the initial febrile phase, or from brain in rapidly fatal infection. Serologic diagnosis is even more reliable, although access to all three common techniques is necessary to establish the cause in some instances. With the exception of RSSE-OHF, anamnestic responses to infection with related agents are usually not a problem. Treatment is symptomatic. Blood loss in OHF and KFD is rarely sufficient to warrant transfusion.

Prognosis and Prevention. Louping ill virus infection has not caused fatalities or permanent neurologic sequelae. Far eastern RSSE, in contrast, has a fatality rate of more than 15 per cent and leaves many survivors with permanent paralysis of an arm or the shoulder girdle. Soviet workers also claim that 3 to 5 per cent of paralytic patients follow a chronic progressive course that develops into clonic spasms, epilepsy, and death. Strong indirect evidence for chronic virus persistence in the brain of one patient during a period of 14 years with final deterioration and death has been obtained by Japanese workers. Fatality rates do not exceed 5 per cent for KFD and OHF, and there are no permanent sequelae associated with these diseases.

Soviet workers have administered formolized mouse brain RSSE vaccine to thousands of persons with reported good results. Work proceeds in that country on a live attenuated vaccine. Otherwise, protection is largely individual against tick bite, consisting of adequate clothing and insect repellents. Aerial spraying of insecticides has been tried on a large scale for tick control in parts of Russia but has been abandoned as too expensive.

Anderson, S. G., et al.: Murray Valley encephalitis in the Murray Valley, 1956 and 1957. Med. J. Aust., 2:15, 1958.

Blaskovic, D., and Nosek, J.: The ecological approach to the study of tick-borne encephalitis. *In* Melnick, J. L. (ed.): Progress in Medical Virology. Vol. 14. Basel and New York, S. Karger, 1972, pp. 275–320.

Eklund, C. M.: Human encephalitis of the western type in Minnesota in 1941: Clinical and epidemiological study of serologically positive cases. Am. J. Hyg., 43:171, 1946.

Feemster, R. F.: Equine encephalitis in Massachusetts. N. Engl. J. Med., 257:701, 1957.

Finley, K. H.: Post-encephalitis manifestations of viral encephalitides. *In* Fields, W. S., and Blattner, R. L. (eds.): Viral Encephalitis. Springfield, Ill., Charles C Thomas, 1958, pp. 69–94.

Grabow, J. D., Mathews, C. G., Chun, R. W. M., and Thompson, W. H.: The electroencephalogram and clinical sequelae of California arbovirus encephalitis. Neurology, 19:394, 1969.

Hart, K. L., Keen, D., and Belle, E. A.: An outbreak of eastern equine encephalomyelitis in Jamaica, West Indies. I. Description of human cases. Am. J. Trop. Med. Hyg., 13:331, 1964.

Hilty, M. D., Haynes, R. E., Azimi, P. H., and Cramblett, H. G.: California encephalitis in children. Am. J. Dis. Child., 124:530, 1972.

Johnson, K. M., and Martin, D. H.: Venezuelan equine encephalitis. *In* Brandly, C. A., and Cornelius, C. E. (eds.): Advances in Veterinary

Science and Comparative Medicine. Vol. 18. New York, Academic Press, 1974, pp. 79–115.
Lincoln, A. F., and Sivertson, S. E.: Acute phase of Japanese B encephalitis. Two hundred and one cases in American soldiers, Korea, 1950. J.A.M.A., 150:268, 1952.
Matthews, C. G., Chun, R. W. M., Grabow, J. D., and Thompson, W. H.: Psychological sequelae in children following California arbovirus encephalitis. Neurology, 18:1023, 1968.
Parkin, W. E., Hammon, W. McD., and Sather, G. E.: Review of current epidemiological literature on viruses of the California arbovirus group. Am. J. Trop. Med. Hyg., 21:964, 1972.
Quick, D. T., Thompson, J. M., and Bond, J. O.: The 1962 epidemic of St. Louis encephalitis in Florida. IV. Clinical features of cases occurring in the Tampa Bay area. Am. J. Epidemiol., 81:415, 1965.
Southern, P. M., Jr., Smith, J. W., Luby, J. P., Barnett, J. A., and Sanford, J. P.: Clinical and laboratory features of epidemic St. Louis encephalitis. Ann. Intern. Med., 71:681, 1969.
Venezuelan Encephalitis: Washington, D.C., Pan-American Health Organization Publication Number 243, 1972, pp. 416.
Wallis, R. C.: Recent advances in research on the eastern encephalitis virus. Yale J. Biol. Med., 37:413, 1965.
Weaver, O. M., Haymaker, W., Pieper, S., and Kirland, R.: Sequelae of the arthropod-borne encephalitides. V. Japanese encephalitis. Neurology, 8:887, 1958.
Webb, H. E., and Rao, L.: Kyasanur Forest disease: A general clinical study in which some cases with neurological complications were observed. Trans. R. Soc. Trop. Med. Hyg., 55:284, 1961.
White, M. G., Carter, N. W., et al.: Pathophysiology of epidemic St. Louis encephalitis. Ann. Intern. Med., 71:691, 1969.

VIRAL HEMORRHAGIC FEVERS

153. INTRODUCTION

Karl M. Johnson

The viral hemorrhagic fevers form a group of acute diseases in which bleeding is a prominent clinical manifestation. These diseases occur in distinct parts of the world, are caused by ribonucleic acid–containing viruses, and may be transmitted to man by mosquitoes, by ticks, or by direct contact with excreta of virus-infected rodents (see table on opposite page). Despite its longstanding fame as a cause of acute hepatocellular necrosis, *yellow fever* is included under this heading because of its recognized ability to induce gastrointestinal hemorrhage and a shock syndrome similar to that seen with other viruses of the group.

After a variable period of a few days to one to three weeks, during which virus multiplies in lymphoid cells and produces a viremia, hemorrhagic fever patients experience fever, myalgia, and other nonspecific symptoms. Bleeding ensues, generally near the end of the febrile period, and although usually not sufficient per se to account for it, such hemorrhage is the harbinger of a clinical crisis dominated by hypovolemic shock. In at least two instances, epidemic hemorrhagic fever and dengue hemorrhagic fever, there is evidence that shock is caused by a widespread capillary vascular lesion in which plasma protein escapes the circulation much faster than erythrocytes. Thrombocytopenia and deficits in various circulating hemostatic factors are frequently present, but it is not clear whether they are etiologically related to this condition.

How the hemorrhagic syndrome is produced thus remains a mystery. No evidence for a direct virus-induced lesion of capillary endothelium has been obtained to date. Disseminated intravascular coagulation (DIC) has been shown in a few instances and postulated in others. But even assuming that DIC occurs, we have no clear idea about the vital pathophysiologic triggers for this chain reaction. Certain facts suggest, however, that altered immunologic function may be important in the pathogenesis of hemorrhagic fever. First, the pathology of such viral disease, unlike that associated with arboviral encephalitis, is characterized by the absence of inflammatory tissue reaction. Second, the high evidence of secondary bacterial infections and the delay of specific humoral antibody response observed in arenavirus-caused disease and Crimean hemorrhagic fever implies a direct suppression of B-cell lymphocyte function. Finally, there is the possibility that antigen-antibody complexes may be important in the genesis of some of these conditions. Available data include long incubation period, leukocytosis, and acute, reversible renal insufficiency in epidemic hemorrhagic fever; the temporal association between hemorrhagic disease and secondary dengue virus infection together with reduction of circulating complement components is even more suggestive. As for the arboviral encephalitides, elucidation of the operative variables is important. Clinical management of disease and vaccine development appear to offer more hope of averting fatal infection than does interruption of the nonhuman natural virus cycles.

154. YELLOW FEVER

Wilbur G. Downs

Definition. Yellow fever is an acute viral disease characterized by sudden onset, prostration, moderately high fever, and a pulse rate slow in relation to temperature. Severe cases are often characterized by vomiting of altered blood, albuminuria (sometimes massive), and jaundice, and may progress to collapse and death. The disease is endemic in tropical rain forest regions of Africa and South America. There are two epidemiologic types of the disease. When the virus is transmitted from man to man by the domestic mosquito, *Aedes aegypti,* it is called *urban yellow fever,* but when it occurs in a forest environment and is transmitted to man by some forest mosquito, usually in the absence of *A. aegypti*, it is called *sylvan* (or *jungle*) *yellow fever.*

Etiology and Epidemiology. Yellow fever is a group B arbovirus, is small, $38 m\mu \pm 5 m\mu$, and readily passes Berkefeld V and N and Seitz filters. Unadapted virus exhibits both viscerotropic and neurotropic characteristics. Viscerotropism is manifested by involvement of liver, kidneys, and heart, and neurotropism by infection of cells of the central nervous system. By successive brain-to-brain passage in mice, the virus becomes adapted and manifests more neurotropism, losing its viscerotropic properties almost entirely. Prolonged passage of the virus in chick embryo tissue culture has produced an attenuated strain, 17D, widely used as a vaccine.

Man is universally susceptible to the virus, and characteristic symptoms and lesions of yellow fever in man are reflections of its viscerotropism. Certain monkey species, including *Macacus rhesus* and Alouatta species, are very susceptible to infection and usually die, whereas other species – for example, Cebus species – may be readily infected but usually recover. Albino mice,

Viral Hemorrhagic Fevers: Etiologic and Epidemiologic Considerations

	Causative Agent	Vector(s)	Vertebrate Host(s)	Geographical Distribution	Epidemiologic Features of Involvement of Man	Control	Remarks
Yellow fever (urban)	YF virus–a group B arbovirus	*Aedes aegypti* in cities	Man	Human populations (usually urban) in tropics of South and Central America and Africa	Person-to-person passage by *Aedes aegypti*	*Aedes aegypti* control; vaccination	Sylvan YF can spread to cities
Yellow fever (sylvan)	YF virus–a group B arbovirus	*Haemagogus* mosquitoes in New World; *Aedes* species in Africa	Monkeys of several genera and species	Forests and jungles of South and Central American and West, Central, and East Africa	Man infected by exposure in jungle (i.e., woodcutters, hunters, etc.)	Vaccination	Human cases sporadic and unpredictable; disease often a "silent" endemic in forests
Dengue hemorrhagic fever	Dengue viruses of four types; group B arboviruses	*Aedes aegypti*	Man (involvement of other primates has been postulated)	Tropical and subtropical cities of Southeast Asia and Philippines	Small children usually involved in cities where *Aedes aegypti* densities are high	*Aedes aegypti* control; mosquito repellent, screens, etc.	Disease may represent an immunologic over-response to a sequential infection with a different dengue strain
Omsk hemorrhagic fever	Two distinguishable subtypes of HF virus	Ticks of genus *Dermacentor*	Small rodents and muskrats	Omsk region of USSR; northern Roumania	People exposed in fields and wooded lands.	Tick repellents and protective clothing	
Kyasanur forest disease	KFD virus–a group B arbovirus	Ticks of several species in genus *Haemaphysalis*	Monkeys (Rhesus and langur) and small rodents and birds	Mysore State, India	People exposed in fields and wooded lands	Tick control; tick repellents and protective clothing	Monkey mortality signals epidemic activity
Argentine hemorrhagic fever	Junin virus, an arenavirus LCM-related	None proved; mites suspected	Small rodents: Akodon; *Calomys laucha, musculinus*	Argentina: NW of Buenos Aires extending west to Province of Cordoba	Field workers at harvest time are particularly at risk	Rodent control in fields	Infected rodents contaminate environment with urine
Bolivian hemorrhagic fever	Machupo virus, an arenavirus LCM-related	None recognized	Small rodent, *Calomys callosus*	Beni Province of Bolivia	Residents of small, rodent-infested villages and homes; 1971 nosocomial outbreak in Cochabamba, Bolivia	Rodent control in villages; full isolation in hospital patient care	High mortality in man
Lassa fever	Lassa virus, an arenavirus LCM-related	None required	Small rodent; *Mastomys natalensis*	West Africa: Nigeria, Liberia, Sierra Leone	Residents of small rodent-infested villages; dramatic nosocomial outbreaks	None known; possibly rodent control	High mortality in man
Crimean hemorrhagic fever	CHF-Congo virus; an ungrouped arbovirus	Ticks of several genera	Larger domestic animals implicated; also African hedgehog	Southern USSR, Bulgaria, East and West Africa	Cowhands and field workers in USSR; nosocomial outbreaks reported	Tick control relating to livestock; full isolation in patient care	Human disease important in USSR; importance to man in Africa not known
Korean hemorrhagic fever (hemor. nephroso-nephritis)	Not known; virus suspected	Not known	Possibly small mammals	Korea; northern Eurasia to and including Scandinavia	Rural or sylvan exposure (military, forest occupations, farmers)	None	A baffling epidemiologic and clinical entity

especially of the Swiss strain, are highly susceptible to the neurotropic element of virus strains recovered from nature, provided they are inoculated intracerebrally.

In urban yellow fever, the *A. aegypti* mosquito transmits the virus by biting a human host during the initial period of viremia and later biting a susceptible person. An extrinsic incubation period of nine to twelve days in the mosquito must elapse before the mosquito can transmit infection by bite.

In sylvan yellow fever, man acquires his infection through the bite of some mosquito other than *A. aegypti.*

Since 1934 no large epidemics of urban yellow fever have been reported from the Western Hemisphere. In Africa, in areas contiguous to the rain forest areas where sylvan yellow fever is endemic, there are still frequent epidemics of urban yellow fever. The announcement of urban yellow fever, *A. aegypti*-transmitted, in a seaport or airport brings strict international quarantine regulations into effect.

There is no evidence that yellow fever has ever been present in the Orient.

Pathology. Yellow fever produces characteristic lesions in the liver of man. There are necrosis and necrobiosis of the parenchymal cells, most evident in the midzones of the lobules, with normal or much less involved cells around the central and portal veins. The necrosis is scattered and irregular rather than massive and uniform. Scattered among the necrotic cells are Councilman bodies, parenchymal cells that have undergone eosinophilic hyaline necrosis. There are also fatty changes in the parenchymal cells. The liver lobules are not collapsed. Pathologic changes in the kidneys are seen mainly in the tubules, with extensive damage to the epithelium and with lumina containing debris, casts, and basophilic concretions.

Clinical Manifestations. Most attacks of yellow fever are mild and show few if any of the classic symptoms. The only symptoms may be fever and headache, both of short duration. The epidemiologic implications of this disease make diagnosis of great importance, and it is essential to maintain a high index of suspicion with regard to undiagnosed fevers (vernacular terms: "PUO," "FUO," "flu," etc.) in regions where yellow fever is known to be, or can be suspected of being, endemic.

The incubation period is from three to six days. The onset is sudden, often with a chill, and without prodromal symptoms. The first stage of the disease, which lasts about three days, is the *period of infection.* The symptoms are feverish feeling, severe headache, backache, pain in the legs, and prostration. The face is flushed, and the eyes are injected; there is photophobia. The tongue is bright red at the tip and edges. There is no jaundice at the onset of illness. The temperature rises abruptly to about 40° C, sometimes higher. The pulse rate may rise to 90 or 100 initially, only to become increasingly slow in relation to the temperature (Faget's sign). The pulse is strong and full during this stage. Nausea and vomiting are the rule, as are epigastric distress and tenderness. Constipation is to be expected. A progressive leukopenia, sometimes pronounced, has frequently been observed early in the disease. The sudden development of intense albuminuria about the third or fourth day is characteristic.

After a short remission, the *period of intoxication* begins about the fourth day. The remission in fever is often indefinite or absent, and it may be accompanied by a deceptive temporary improvement. In this period, lassitude and depression may replace restlessness and agitation. Headache may diminish, and jaundice gradually develops. Although jaundice is always present in severe cases, it is usually not so intense as the name of the disease would indicate. Various hemorrhagic manifestations are evident. The gums are swollen and bleed easily, either spontaneously or when pressed; the nose may bleed. There may be petechiae in the skin. Hemorrhages from the stomach, intestine, or uterus, or subcutaneously, may be massive. The pulse rate falls progressively and may go below 50 per minute. Even in otherwise mild cases there may be dilatation of the heart and low blood pressure as evidence of myocardial damage. Vomiting may be frequent and distressing, and the vomitus in this stage usually contains altered blood, whence the name "el vomito negro" often applied to the disease in Latin America. The amount of albumin in the urine rises, often to 3 to 5 grams per liter, sometimes much higher. Fatal cases often exhibit hiccup, copious vomiting of altered blood, tarry stools, and anuria. Coma may last two or three days, or death may be immediately preceded by a short period of wild delirium. Death occurs most frequently from the sixth to the ninth day.

When there is recovery from a severe case, the temperature is likely to reach normal by the seventh or eighth day. Convalescence begins then and progresses rapidly to complete recovery with rapid disappearance of the albuminuria. Relapses do not occur, and there are no sequelae. Complications are rare. A lifelong immunity follows the attack, whether it be mild or severe.

A feature of yellow fever is the great variation in the degree to which different organs are affected. With much renal involvement there may be no cardiac symptoms, and vice versa. In mild and moderate cases there is little or no albuminuria, jaundice, or hemorrhage.

Diagnosis. In a severe illness with "black vomit," intense albuminuria, jaundice, and melena, as a group or in combinations, yellow fever must be suspected. Diseases that must be differentiated from severe yellow fever include hepatitis, carbon tetrachloride poisoning, other jaundices, malaria, and typhoid. In mild cases, which have been confused with dengue and influenza, clinical diagnosis is notoriously inaccurate. The necessary laboratory procedures are highly specialized. The isolation of virus in mice, rhesus monkeys, or certain tissue cultures from serum of the acutely ill patient or from serum or liver of a deceased patient, affords convincing diagnosis. Specialized procedures are needed for the identification of the isolate. Serologic tests on paired acute-phase and convalescent serums, using techniques of complement-fixation, hemagglutination-inhibition, and virus neutralization, can also give positive diagnosis. Although the tests must be done in a specialized laboratory, nevertheless under primitive conditions the serum specimens can be collected and submitted to such a laboratory.

For postmortem diagnosis, specimens of liver and other tissues should be preserved in 10 per cent formalin for histologic examination. Virus recovery can be attempted from such tissues if small pieces are placed in 50 per cent glycerol-saline and shipped, under refrigeration if possible, to a laboratory.

Prognosis. Early in the disease the prognosis should be guarded, because sudden changes for the worse may occur. If early symptoms are mild, rapid recovery is probable. Some patients with severe disease will recover, but symptoms of hiccups, copious black vomit, melena, and anuria imply a very grave prognosis.

The over-all average case fatality rate is less than 10 per cent, and rates of less than 5 per cent have been observed in epidemics involving completely susceptible populations. Rates based on hospitalized cases may be higher.

Treatment. There is no specific treatment. A patient should be moved as little as possible and should be kept quiet in bed. Heroic efforts to get a patient from some remote area to a district hospital should be discouraged. The severe headache and body aches may require relief with an analgesic. The heart should be watched carefully throughout the illness and into early convalescence.

Water should be given in adequate amounts, parenterally if necessary. Easily assimilated food should be given to the extent that the patient will tolerate. Milk in moderate quantities can be recommended. When vomiting has ceased and the temperature is down, full diet may be given. Full activity should be resumed only gradually.

Prevention. If a case of yellow fever is treated in a place in which vector mosquitoes exist, the patient must be kept under a bed net or in a mosquito-proof room during the first four days of illness.

Vaccination is essential for persons who intend to visit yellow fever endemic areas and for the people resident in such areas. Yellow fever is notorious for existence in endemic areas with no overt signs of its presence, and despite negative reports of the weekly international epidemiologic bulletins relative to a given area, vaccination for persons going to an endemic area must be stressed.

Two strains of living virus have been used extensively for immunization of man. The 17D vaccine, developed by Rockefeller Foundation workers, is prepared in chick embryos and is inoculated subcutaneously. The French neurotropic vaccine, developed by Institut Pasteur workers, is prepared from mouse brains suspended in gum arabic solution and is given by scarification. With either strain, an effective immunity to yellow fever is readily induced. The 17D vaccine is currently recommended, because it produces fewer undesirable reactions, particularly in small children. Vaccination ordinarily gives protection in a week, and the consequent immunity has been shown to last at least ten years. An urban epidemic can be stopped by mass vaccination of the population combined with vigorous anti-*aegypti* measures.

155. HEMORRHAGIC FEVER CAUSED BY DENGUE VIRUSES

Karl M. Johnson

Definition. These hemorrhagic fevers of Southeast Asia and India are acute, infectious, urban, mosquito-borne diseases caused by dengue viruses. Endoepidemic in pattern, dengue hemorrhagic fever is clinically defined as a dengue disease that worsens two or more days after onset, and is characterized by hypoproteinemia and one or more hemostatic abnormalities such as thrombocytopenia, prolonged bleeding time, or elevated prothrombin time. The dengue shock syndrome consists of hemorrhagic fever plus shock (hypotension or a pulse pressure of 20 mm Hg or less) and hemoconcentration (hematocrit at least 20 per cent greater than convalescent value). Chikungunya virus infections fulfilling these criteria are rarely encountered.

Etiology. All evidence suggests that these diseases are caused by each of the four recognized dengue virus subtypes. How they produce such disease is still not clear. A current hypothesis is that severe dengue disease is produced by an immunologic reaction that occurs in some individuals experiencing a second dengue infection. However, in a 1972 outbreak on Niue Island, Oceania, several hemorrhagic cases were seen in children with no possibility of prior dengue infection.

Epidemiology. These hemorrhagic fevers were first seen in epidemic proportions in Manila and Bangkok (1954) and in Singapore (1960). Other outbreaks have been reported from Malaysia, South Vietnam, India, Indonesia, and Oceania. In Bangkok age-specific rates in children have reached 7 to 8 per 1000. In most outbreaks cases occur only in children, principally below the age of 8 years; otherwise, the epidemiology of infection leading to dengue hemorrhagic fever is basically similar to that associated with ordinary dengue fever; outbreaks occur during the rainy season in large urban centers where *Aedes aegypti* is well established. Halstead has proposed that dengue hemorrhagic fever is an immune disease, brought on usually by a second (but not a third) dengue virus infection in a previously sensitized host. The syndromes have not been observed in many places where dengue is or has been prevalent, including the New World and many parts of Southeast Asia, Australasia, and Oceania.

Pathology. Autopsy data are scant. The chief abnormalities include generalized vascular congestion and dilatation with edema and multiple focal hemorrhages in most organs, mild to moderate pleural effusion and ascites, mononuclear cell infiltration of interstitial tissues and alveolar walls of lungs, focal myocardial congestion, and a decrease in mature lymphocytes with proliferation of mononuclear forms in the germinal centers of lymph follicles.

Necrosis is unusual, and no specific damage of the blood vessels has been observed. Perivascular infiltration by mononuclear cells is common, but there is no evidence for significant vasculitis or for platelet or thrombin thrombosis of vessel walls. About one third of cases show evidence of globulin on endothelial surfaces and the walls of arterioles. The bone marrow often shows maturation arrest of megakaryocytes, and sometimes there is marked generalized cellular hypoplasia with rapid restoration to normal after emergence from shock.

Pathologic change in the liver, although generally inconspicuous, consists of focal lesions and varies greatly in degree of severity. These lesions are of particular interest, because occasionally Councilman bodies and other changes characteristic of yellow fever are observed.

Pathogenesis or Mechanism of Disease. The pathogenesis is as yet poorly understood. The vascular congestion, dilatation, and increased permeability lead to the extensive edema and hemorrhage observed in the gastrointestinal tract, the skin, and other tissues. The cause of these vascular changes is unknown, but they result in loss of plasma volume and associated electrolyte disturbances. Platelet deficiency probably plays a role in the hemorrhages. Bleeding time is usually prolonged, prothrombin times are somewhat prolonged, clot retraction is poor, and the blood fibrinogen is slightly reduced. None of these changes is very profound. The circulatory collapse and shock observed appear to be far in excess of what might be expected from the extent of loss of edema fluid and blood. The adrenal changes suggest exhaustion of steroid reserve. Death in some cases has been accompanied by severe hyperkalemia.

Clinical Manifestations. The onset is that of a dengue infection, usually abrupt, with fever. Nausea and vomiting are common. The throat appears injected, and there may be a dry cough. About the second or third day petechiae appear, usually first on the face or distal portions of the extremities but sparing the axillae and chest. The tourniquet test may be conspicuously positive before petechiae appear. Purpura and large ecchymoses as well as other manifestations of bleeding tendency are occasionally prominent. There may be severe abdominal pain and tenderness. About the third or fourth day, vomiting may produce copious coffee-ground material. Melena also is not uncommon, but gross bleeding from the intestines is rare. Shock is likely to occur in severe cases about the fourth day, and this critical state lasts about 12 to 24 hours. At this time the temperature falls to normal, the blood pressure and pulse pressure are low or unmeasurable, and the limbs are cool and present a purple or brownish mottled appearance. Perspiration is frequently profuse. The face and hands appear edematous. Restlessness and apprehension are conspicuous as the patient enters shock. This state of shock is entirely out of proportion to the apparent loss of blood. Thrombocytopenia is noted during this period, and bleeding time is prolonged. Leukocytes remain at approximately normal levels, but are elevated in number in serious cases more frequently than they are depressed. The total and differential leukocyte counts are not those observed in dengue. Although the numbers of both immature and mature polymorphonuclear cells are decreased, there is an increase in lymphocytes and sometimes in monocytes.

Diagnosis. Hemorrhagic fever begins as an extension of a classic dengue infection, and the early dengue syndrome intergrades into the milder and atypical manifestations of the later hemorrhagic syndrome. The diagnosis in a febrile child acutely ill for only two or three days is rendered highly probable by the presentation of petechiae, purpuric lesions, and unusual ecchymosis of the skin with most prominent distribution on the extremities and face, together with melena, thrombocytopenia, and a relatively normal leukocyte count. In a milder case or at an earlier stage, the tourniquet test may be of great assistance in detecting unusual capillary fragility. The rapid development of circulatory collapse and shock during the fourth to sixth day, associated with the aforementioned findings, differentiates this from most other exanthematous diseases. Meningococcemia and the Waterhouse-Friderichsen syndrome need careful consideration. Thrombocytopenic purpura can be expected to have an entirely different onset and is usually not associated with fever. Laboratory methods available for diagnosis are those described for dengue fever.

Treatment. There is no specific therapy, but case fatality rates can be greatly reduced by skillful management directed toward combating shock. Close monitoring of pulse, respiration, and blood pressure during the course of treatment is essential for at least 48 hours, because shock can occur and recur. Oxygen should be administered if there is cyanosis or labored breathing. Hypovolemia should be treated by administration of lactated Ringer's solution or 5 per cent glucose in normal saline, on the basis of 20 ml per kilogram of body weight, administered rapidly. In profound or unresponsive shock, plasma or a plasma expander (dextran in normal saline) can be given at the rate of 20 ml per kilogram of body weight. When signs improve, 5 per cent glucose in normal saline or in lactated Ringer's solution should be given at the rate of 10 ml per kilogram per hour, and continued until vital signs are normal. Acidosis should be corrected with sodium bicarbonate as necessary.

Whole blood should be given only if blood loss is known to be large. Administration of whole blood to a patient with elevated hematocrit may result in heart failure. Paraldehyde or chloral hydrate may be required for children who are markedly agitated. Salicylates administered during the febrile period may cause bleeding and acidosis, and they should not be given to febrile patients during a hemorrhagic fever outbreak. Pressor amines, alpha-adrenergic blocking agents, and steroids have not been demonstrated to be of value in treatment.

Prognosis. Death is almost always associated with shock, and rarely occurs after the sixth day of illness. Case fatality rates among hospitalized patients have ranged from 5 to 50 per cent, depending to a large extent upon the condition of patients on admission and the facilities available for treatment. Careful management should be able to save all but the 5 or 10 per cent of patients admitted in a moribund state. Residual effects have not been observed, and, in contrast to primary dengue, recovery is usually prompt and complete seven to ten days after onset. Mental depression is seldom observed.

Prevention. The control of this hemorrhagic fever is the same as that for dengue, and consists of mosquito control or protection from mosquito bites and isolation of the patient from mosquitoes. No vaccine is available, and if the immunologic theory of causation is confirmed, vaccines as presently conceived would be specifically contraindicated.

156. CRIMEAN HEMORRHAGIC FEVER

Karl M. Johnson

Definition. Crimean hemorrhagic fever (CHF) is an acute febrile disease, often marked by severe hemorrhage and high mortality, occurring in the Soviet Union and Bulgaria.

Etiology. The CHF agent is an arbovirus first isolated from human blood specimens in 1967. It is pathogenic for suckling mice and grows in several types of cultured cells. This virus is indistinguishable from Congo virus of Africa in CF and neutralization tests. Strains from Eurasia and Africa are thus referred to as CHF-Congo virus.

Epidemiology. CHF-Congo virus is naturally transmitted by several species of hard ticks belonging to the general Hyalomma, Rhipicephalus, Amblyomma, and Boophilus. Active foci of infection with transmission to man exist in the lower Don and Volga river basins and the Central Asian republics of Kazakstan and Uzbekistan of the Soviet Union. A single tick isolate has been reported from Pakistan. Few human cases have been recognized in Africa. The disease occurs most frequently among adults who are heavily exposed to ticks while working among cattle. Cases begin to appear in April and reach a peak during summer months. Proved or presumed vertebrate hosts for the virus include cattle, goats, hares, rooks, and hedgehogs. Transovarial tick transmission is suspected but not yet proved. Nosocomial human infections have occurred repeatedly in Central Asia, suggesting transmission by aerosol. The incubation period is estimated at about one week.

Clinical Manifestations. Onset is typically abrupt with high, unremittent fever, chills, headache, and myalgia. There may be hyperemia of the upper trunk and neck, conjunctival effusion, vomiting, and diarrhea. Hepatomegaly is noted in about half the cases; splenomegaly is uncommon. Pronounced panleukopenia is almost invariably present, as is thrombocytopenia. Bleeding begins on about the fourth day of illness. Petechiae appear in the oral mucosa and skin, at times presenting as frank *purpura hemorrhagica.* Nose, gums, and intestinal tract are the most common sites of bleeding, and in this disease above all other viral hemorrhagic fevers, blood loss per se may be life threatening. Stiff neck, hyperexcitability, or coma occurs in about 10 per cent of cases and these are grave prognostic signs. The cerebrospinal fluid, however, contains no leukocytes or increased protein. There may be proteinuria and microscopic hematuria, but renal function is rarely compromised. The fever and bleeding generally resolve by lysis at about the eighth day. Hypovolemic shock with a paradoxical rising hematocrit may appear just prior to the end of fever and is the most common cause of death.

Diagnosis. Virus can be gotten easily from blood of patients during the first few days of illness. Specific CF and neutralizing antibodies appear in the sera of most patients 30 to 60 days after onset of symptoms.

Treatment and Prognosis. Therapy is symptomatic. Management of fluid, electrolyte, and erythrocyte balance forms the continuous clinical challenge. Shock is a grave problem and should be anticipated and treated as outlined in Ch. 157. Whole blood transfusion may be necessary. Intercurrent bacterial infection is very common, especially pneumonia. Mortality in the Soviet Union ranges from 20 to 50 per cent. Patients surviving the acute illness generally recover completely, albeit quite slowly. Several instances of mono- or polyneuritis persisting for several months have been recorded.

Prevention. There is no vaccine yet available; thus avoidance of the disease in endemic foci depends on personal measures designed to prevent tick bites.

157. HEMORRHAGIC DISEASES CAUSED BY ARENAVIRUSES: ARGENTINE AND BOLIVIAN HEMORRHAGIC FEVERS AND LASSA FEVER*

Karl M. Johnson

Definition. Argentine and Bolivian hemorrhagic fevers and Lassa fever are acute diseases caused respectively by Junin, Machupo, and Lassa viruses. Clinically, the diseases share the common features of fever, severe myalgia, leukopenia, hemorrhagic manifestations, shock, and (excluding Lassa fever) neurologic abnormalities.

Etiology. The three viruses are serologically and morphologically related, and related to lymphocytic choriomeningitis virus, in a grouping designated as arenaviruses.

Geographical Distribution, Incidence, and Prevalence. Argentine hemorrhagic fever is localized to the provinces of Córdoba and Junin in northern Argentina, where several hundred to several thousand cases occur annually, principally in agricultural field hands, in the harvest months. Bolivian hemorrhagic fever has been reported only from Beni province of Bolivia, between the rivers Mamore and Branco, with the exception of a hospital outbreak in Cochabamba, Bolivia, in 1971, traceable to contact with a person from Beni province. Infections are seen in inhabitants of certain of the small towns, as well as in rural populations. Lassa fever has been reported from Nigeria, Liberia, and Sierra Leone, and hospital outbreaks account for most of the cases reported. Case fatality rates are estimates in the usual absence of prompt and specific diagnosis, but may be as high as 50 per cent in hospitalized cases of Lassa, and 10 to 20 per cent for the South American diseases.

Epidemiology and Probable Mode of Transmission. The viruses have been isolated from wild rodents: Junin, most commonly from *Calomys musculinus, Calomys laucha,* and also *Akodon arenicola;* Machupo, from *Calomys callosus;* and Lassa, from *Mastomys natalensis.* An attractive current hypothesis is that infection is acquired by direct human contact (ingestion, inhalation, or entrance through mucous membranes or skin breaks) with virus-containing rodent excreta. For all three agents, persistent infection in rodents has been demonstrated, with viremia readily detectable for months. A similar pattern of chronic virus infection in rodents has been described for lymphocytic choriomeningitis virus.

Pathology. Few cases have received full study. Findings include irregularly focal diapedesis and capillary hemorrhage without much evidence of inflammatory reaction. Gross hemorrhages may be seen in the mucosa of the stomach and intestines and in the brain. Pulmonary infection, probably intercurrent, is frequently seen.

Clinical Manifestations. Although as many as half of all etiologically confirmed cases appear as acute undifferentiated fevers, the findings and clinical cause of "full-blown" Argentine and Bolivian infections are so nearly identical as to justify joint description. The same holds for Lassa fever. Onset is usually gradual, with increasing fever, headache, diffuse myalgia, and anorexia. By the third day the temperature may be 39.5 to 40.5° C, with severe myalgia, particularly in the lumbar regions (or legs in Lassa fever). Conjunctival injection is present, a flush involving the upper trunk and face is frequently observed, and there may be a relative bradycardia. Beginning about the fourth day, scattered fine petechiae may appear on the face and neck, about the pectoral girdle, and/or in the buccal mucosa or palate. Aphthous ulcers of the oral mucosa have been a noteworthy feature of Lassa infections. The Rumpel-Leede test is frequently positive. Frank hemorrhages from one or more sites, including the stomach, intestines, nose, gums, and uterus, accompanied by microscopic hematuria, may occur. Hemorrhagic phenomena are not a common feature of Lassa infections. Although hemorrhage per se is rarely the precipitating cause, a hypotensive crisis frequently develops between the sixth and eighth days, coincident with a rapid return of temperature to normal after five or more days of sustained fever. Patients surviving this stress for 48 hours generally make slow but complete recovery.

Perhaps a fifth of the patients with the Bolivian or Argentinian disease develop neurologic signs. These are quite characteristic, and begin on about the fifth or sixth day with a fine intention tremor of the tongue. This may become so severe as to render speech unintelligible and to preclude oral ingestion of solid or even liquid food. If so, gross intention tremors of the extremities usually appear, occasionally accompanied by an intermittent nystagmus. Such patients often become delirious, and may experience generalized clonic and tonic convulsions. The cerebrospinal fluid appears normal, however, and contains neither leukocytes nor virus. Convalescence is marked by weakness and signs of autonomic nervous system lability such as postural hypotension, spontaneous flushing and blanching of the skin, and episodes of diaphoresis.

Neurologic findings have not been described for Lassa fever, but a state of mild euphoria during the initial several days of fever has been noted, as well as blurring of the sensorium and semicomatose state in later stages of the illness. Some Lassa fever patients have shown electrocardiographic evidence of myocardial involvement.

Transient loss of scalp hair and typical Beau's lines in the nails, particularly those of the fingers, are observed in a majority of cases several weeks after subsidence of

*The author wishes to express his thanks to Dr. Wilbur G. Downs for his considerable assistance in the preparation of this chapter, particularly with reference to the material on Lassa fever.

the high, sustained fever. Many patients are not able to resume full activity for at least one month after illness.

Leukopenia is almost invariably present, and cell counts may be as low as 1000 per cubic millimeter by the fourth or fifth day. All elements are reduced nearly equally, and there is often a mild to moderate thrombocytopenia during the first week. Usually the peripheral blood picture returns to normal rapidly after defervescence, although there may be transient relative lymphocytosis and mild anemia. During the latter portion of the febrile period, progressive increase in hematocrit similar to, but usually milder than, that of hemorrhagic nephrosonephritis (q.v.) is frequently observed. At about the same time, moderate proteinuria is common, although renal function is rarely compromised seriously, and frank azotemia and hyperkalemia are almost never present.

Diagnosis. The presence of high fever, severe myalgia, and leukopenia should arouse immediate suspicion of viral hemorrhagic fever within the known endemic areas of its occurrence. Potential intimate contact with wild rodents in a rural or semirural setting serves to strengthen the likelihood of this diagnosis. Since these findings and all others described cannot be relied upon to differentiate the disease clinically from other infections such as yellow fever, typhoid and paratyphoid fevers, typhus, malaria, and leptospirosis, specific identification of cases depends upon laboratory confirmation. Virus can sometimes be isolated from blood, throat washing, and urine during the febrile period. At autopsy splenic tissue almost always yields the agent. Serologic detection of infection is a reliable method if paired acute and convalescent serums are employed. Both group-reacting complement-fixing antibodies and virus type-specific neutralizing antibodies appear in three to four weeks and reach peak values in seven to ten weeks after the onset of illness.

These three agents have been responsible for several fatal laboratory infections, and work with the viruses should be carried out only with strictest precautionary measures, and complete isolation from other laboratory activities, in special high-risk laboratories.

Treatment. In the absence of any specific therapy, successful treatment presents an acute challenge in the science and art of physiologic management. Patients require complete rest and maximal comfort. Mild sedatives and analgesics should be judiciously used. Careful measurement of fluid intake and output is mandatory. The electrolyte balance should be checked regularly; marked underhydration and overhydration are to be avoided, because these conditions appear to compromise the patient's ability to weather the hypotensive crisis. Daily hematocrit determinations and examinations of urine for protein are the most valuable tests for anticipating and managing this problem. Frequent measurement of blood pressure is also important, because many patients enter the shock phase with persistent relative bradycardia and warm, dry skin. Raising the foot of the bed may suffice to stabilize the pressure at levels adequate to preserve vital urinary output. If not, careful administration of human plasma or concentrated albumin (not whole blood) is indicated. In one instance of a Lassa infection, administration of plasma from a recovered patient appeared to be effective. Great care should be exercised in administering plasma or other fluids intravenously during shock, because intractable pulmonary edema is readily induced. Complications, particularly bacterial infections, should be anticipated and promptly treated. Convalescence should never be hurried.

Prognosis. Although the case mortality may exceed 20 per cent, there is no single finding early in the disease that aids prognosis in the individual case. In general, the very young and the very old, as well as those who do not receive medical attention prior to the sixth day of disease, are subject to the highest risk. The onset of severe shock and neurologic abnormalities are both ominous prognostic signs, and at least half the patients exhibiting these signs succumb. The prognosis in Lassa fever is even poorer in diagnosed cases.

Prevention. Effective elimination of intimate human contact with certain wild rodents represents the only proved method for prevention of disease. This may be achieved by maintaining sound standards of personal and environmental hygiene. Campaigns to eliminate rodents, repair buildings, and clean rubbish near dwellings are highly successful when the disease is acquired mainly from peridomestic animals. There is insufficient evidence at present to warrant recommendation of systematic measures to control attacks by any potential arthropod vector.

Hospital outbreaks involving hospital staff have provided most of the Lassa fever cases to date. There has been a recent hospital outbreak of Machupo virus in Cochabamba, Bolivia. Such outbreaks can be extremely dangerous to personnel and demoralizing to hospital operation.

158. EPIDEMIC HEMORRHAGIC FEVER: HEMORRHAGIC NEPHROSONEPHRITIS

Karl M. Johnson

Definition. Epidemic hemorrhagic fever is an acute disease of unknown cause that occurs in northeastern Asia and, in milder form, in northern European U.S.S.R., Scandinavia, Czechoslovakia, Rumania, and Bulgaria. It is characterized by fever, prostration, vomiting, proteinuria, hemorrhagic manifestations, shock, and renal failure.

History. The disease was first described in the far east of the Soviet Union in the 1930's, with suggestive history as far back as 1913. An epidemic in United Nations troops in Korea, beginning in 1951, attracted much attention.

Etiology. Soviet investigators detected a filtrable virus, by parenteral inoculation of serum or urine of patients prior to the fifth day of illness into human volunteers. Despite repeated claims, no agent has yet been established in any other experimental host system.

Epidemiology. The disease is rural, characterized by isolated cases widely separated in place. Environmental exposure in forests or fields near forests is invariably noted. Person-to-person transmission does not occur. Soviet workers believe that the disease is transmitted directly from asymptomatically infected rodents to man by means of virus-contaminated rodent excreta. Some outbreaks in Europe have coincided with population "explosions" of the redbacked vole *(Clethrionomys glareolus)*, involving invasion by rodents of fields, barns, and even houses.

Pathology. Profound, protein-rich retroperitoneal edema is characteristic of early death in shock, but not of later deaths. Changes in various organs apparently have a similar pathogenesis and consist of widespread, often focal, congestion and hemorrhage, sometimes accompanied by necrosis, without significant inflammatory response. The "pathognomonic" lesion is found in the kidneys, which appear swollen and, when incised, exhibit extreme hemorrhagic congestion sharply localized to the medulla. Gross congestion or hemorrhage derived from dilated, congested small blood vessels is also found frequently in the right atrium, the pituitary, and the stomach, and less often in intestines, adrenals, lungs, and central nervous system. Liver and spleen are usually not grossly involved. Petechial hemorrhages may occur in the skin, heart, adrenals, brain, and serous surfaces.

Clinical Manifestations and Pathologic Physiology. The following description is based on the minority of patients (about 20 per cent) who exhibit the more severe form of disease, which can be divided into five clinical phases. All patients, however, have fever, proteinuria, and isohyposthenuria.

The febrile phase lasts three to eight days and is characterized by fever, malaise, a flush over the face and neck, and injection of the eyes and palate. Toward the end of this period, petechiae occur, blood platelets decrease, traces of protein appear in the urine, and the hematocrit begins to rise.

The hypotensive phase develops suddenly during defervescence and lasts one to three days. Shock is insidious with warm dry extremities and initially no increase in pulse rate. The dominant feature is a reduction in effective blood volume owing to a loss of plasma from the vascular system. Hematocrit values may reach 70 per cent, and erythrocytes are sequestered in dilated capillaries. Nausea and vomiting are common, as are back and abdominal pain, the latter having occasioned ill-advised exploratory laparotomy in misdiagnosed cases. Heavy proteinuria and oliguria progressing to acute renal failure occur during this interval. Capillary hemorrhages are most prominent at this time also, and blood leukocytes, earlier normal or reduced, now show a leukemoid reaction.

The oliguric phase begins as the sequestered plasma returns to the vascular system and the hematocrit falls. Deaths during this three- to five-day interval are due to pulmonary edema, hyperkalemia, and shock secondary to dehydration or secondary pulmonary infections. Some patients become hypertensive and display a reactive hypervolemic syndrome that responds to phlebotomy. Biochemical abnormalities associated with renal failure appear at this time.

The diuretic phase, lasting for days or weeks, usually initiates clinical recovery but is fraught with problems in clinical management. Diuresis of 3 to 8 liters daily and isohyposthenuria lead to an extremely brittle situation with respect to hemodynamics and salt balance. Hypokalemia and hypernatremia can be problems. Shock may occur, and bacterial pulmonary infections are common. Nearly a third of all deaths occur during this phase.

Convalescence requires three to twelve weeks and is marked by gradual return of appetite, strength, and urinary concentrating ability.

Diagnosis. In the absence of any specific test, the diagnosis must be made on clinical evidence and should be suspected when an acute febrile illness associated with the characteristic flush and petechiae occurs in a subject who has been in an endemic area. The subsequent developments such as hypotension or shock, increased hematocrit, thrombocytopenia, oliguria, and renal failure assist in establishing the diagnosis, but proteinuria and isohyposthenuria developing near the time of defervescence are the most useful diagnostic signs.

Prognosis and Treatment. Because antimicrobial drugs, convalescent serum, hormones, and other agents are entirely ineffective, the management of hemorrhagic fever must be supportive and based on an understanding of its physiologic and biochemical characteristics and on frequent clinical observations. Adequate sedation with barbiturates or opiates is frequently required for restlessness. Contrary to the practice in other febrile diseases, fluid intake must be limited because any excess will simply leak out of damaged capillaries and increase edema and symptoms. When intravenous fluid is required, it usually should be 10 per cent dextrose in water, and must be given very slowly. If shock fails to respond to simple measures such as shock blocks, then concentrated (salt-poor) human serum albumin to restore plasma volume may be required. Treatment in the oliguric phase is that of acute renal failure, with careful control of electrolytes and particular attention to hyperkalemia. If oliguria persists, hemodialysis or peritoneal dialysis is indicated. Soviet workers have so treated 60 severe cases and report only three deaths. The chief problem of the diuretic phase is one of careful matching of fluid and electrolyte intake against the brisk urinary output, so as to avoid excessive dehydration and shock, on the one hand, and hypervolemia and pulmonary edema, on the other. Electrolyte abnormalities are still a problem, especially potassium deficiency. Over-all mortality under optimal conditions seldom surpasses 5 per cent.

Prevention. Preventive measures are based on the assumption that the disease is transmitted by rodents with or without the aid of an associated arthropod vector. Vigorous rodent control measures, as well as dipping of clothing in acaricidal solutions and the individual use of insect repellents, are recommended in endemic areas during seasonal periods of disease activity.

Barnes, W. J. S., and Rosen, L.: Fatal hemorrhagic disease and shock associated with primary dengue infection on a Pacific island. Am. J. Trop. Med. Hyg., 23:495, 1974.

Bokisch, V. A., Top, F. H., Jr., Russell, P. K., Dixon, F. J., and Muller-Eberhard, H. J.: The potential pathogenic role of complement in dengue hemorrhagic shock syndrome. N. Engl. J. Med., 289:996, 1973.

Casals, J., Henderson, B. E., Hoogstraal, H., Johnson, K. M., and Shelokov, A.: A review of Soviet viral hemorrhagic fevers, 1969. J. Infect. Dis., 122:437, 1970.

Casals, J., Hoogstraal, H., Johnson, K. M., Shelokov, A., Wiebenga, N. H., and Work, T. H.: A current appraisal of hemorrhagic fevers in the U.S.S.R. Am. J. Trop. Med. Hyg., 15:751, 1966.

Frame, J. D., Baldwin, J. M., Jr., Gocke, D. J., and Troup, J. M.: Lassa fever, a new virus disease of man from West Africa. I. Clinical description and pathological findings. Am. J. Trop. Med. Hyg., 19:670, 1970.

Groot, H., and Bahia Ribiero, R.: Neutralizing and hemagglutination-inhibiting antibodies to yellow fever 17 years after vaccination with 17D vaccine. Bull. WHO, 27:699, 1962.

Halstead, S. B., et al.: Observations related to pathogenesis of dengue hemorrhagic fever. Yale J. Biol. Med., 42:261, 1970.

Hammon, W. McD., Rudnick, A., Sather, G., Rogers, K. D., and Morse, L. J.: New hemorrhagic fevers of children in the Philippines and Thailand. Trans. Assoc. Am. Physicians, 73:140, 1960.

Johnson, K. M., Halstead, S. B., and Cohen, S. N.: Hemorrhagic fevers of Southeast Asia and South America: A comparative appraisal. *In* Melnick, J. L. (ed.): Progress in Medical Virology, Vol. 9. Basel/New York, S. Karger, 1967, pp. 105–158.

Mertens, P. E., Patton, R., Baum, J. J., and Monath, T. P.: Clinical presentation of Lassa fever cases during the hospital epidemic at Zorzar, Liberia, March–April 1972. Am. J. Trop. Med. Hyg., 22:780, 1973.
Sabattini, M., and Maiztegui, J. I.: Fiebre hemorrágica argentina. Medicina (Buenos Aires), 30: Supp. 1, 111, 1970.
Simpson, D. I. H., Knight, E. M., et al.: Congo virus: A hitherto undescribed virus occurring in Africa. Part I. Human isolation—clinical notes. East Afr. Med. J., 44:87, 1967.
Smithburn, K. C., et al.: Yellow Fever Vaccination. Geneva, World Health Organization Monograph Series No. 30, 1956.
Smorodintsev, A. A., Kazbintsev, L. I., and Chudakov, V. G.: Virus Hemorrhagic Fevers (Y. Halperin, translator). Washington, D. C., Office of Technical Services, U. S. Department of Commerce, 1964.
Strode, G. K. (ed.): Yellow Fever. New York, McGraw-Hill Book Company, 1951.
Symposium on Epidemic Hemorrhagic Fever. Am. J. Med., 16:617, 1954.

VIRAL DISEASES CHARACTERIZED BY PROTRACTED, RECURRENT, OR LATENT INFECTION

These diseases are discussed in detail in Ch. 398 to 403.

VIRAL DISEASES (PRESUMPTIVE)

Paul B. Beeson

159. CAT SCRATCH DISEASE

The essential feature of cat scratch disease is lymphadenitis, usually limited to one anatomic region, developing as a sequel to accidental injury of the skin. In two thirds of the reported cases there has been a history of scratch or bite by a cat.

Epidemiology. The disease occurs in all parts of the world, most often in winter. Children are affected more frequently than adults. Although injuries by cat claws or teeth are the most common form of skin injury, other puncture wounds, by wood splinters, thorns, and metallic objects have appeared to be responsible at times. Cats thought to have caused human infection show no sign of illness, do not react to the cat scratch antigen, and probably merely convey the causative agent on claws or teeth. "Epidemics" of cat scratch disease, though reported, are difficult to evaluate because they may simply reflect special interest and awareness of certain physicians. There are, however, several reports of more than one case developing in a family over a period of a few months.

Etiology. Although this disease has the features of a specific infection, efforts to demonstrate a causative bacterium, fungus, or filterable virus have met with failure. Perhaps the most impressive evidence for viral etiology is in a report of electron microscopic examination of affected lymphatic tissue, in which herpes-like viral particles were observed. Serologic investigations have failed to yield evidence pointing to Epstein-Barr virus. The hypothesis has been offered that the clinical manifestations result from an immunologic reaction; hence the inciting agent may no longer be demonstrable at the time the patient seeks medical help. Several groups of workers have reported serologic evidence that the causative agent is related to viruses of the psittacosis–ornithosis–lymphogranuloma venereum–trachoma group, but the proportion of patients exhibiting such positive serologic reactions has varied considerably, and, furthermore, patients with cat scratch disease do not react to intradermal injection of antigens prepared from this group of viruses.

Pathogenesis. An indolent or subacute inflammatory lesion develops at the site of primary inoculation in approximately one third of cases. It becomes clinically evident one to several weeks after the injury. Lymphadenitis, the hallmark of the disease, appears a few days later. Initially this takes the form of a granulomatous inflammation, sometimes containing giant cells. In cases of some duration microabscesses can nearly always be found; in about one fourth of cases these coalesce to form a grossly evident abscess.

Clinical Manifestations. The site of inoculation is most likely to be on the hand, forearm, or face. It may exhibit one or more erythematous papules. Less frequently there is vesicle formation going on to rupture and production of a small eschar. The lesion usually heals without scar formation. The lymph nodes most frequently affected are in the epitrochlear, axillary, or cervical groups, but when the injury has been on the legs the inguinal nodes may be the site of the disease. The process varies in clinical severity and acuteness, sometimes smoldering for weeks with enlarged and tender nodes, at other times progressing more quickly to pronounced swelling, with redness and edema of the overlying skin. There may be fluctuation, and in rare instances the skin undergoes necrosis, permitting discharge of exudate. The usual course is for the swelling and tenderness gradually to subside in two to eight weeks. Systemic manifestations are not prominent, although young children sometimes have high fever for a few days. The erythrocyte sedimentation rate may be elevated; there is often a moderate leukocytosis, and sometimes mild eosinophilia. Transient morbilliform rashes may accompany the adenitis; occasionally lesions are developed which have the appearance of erythema nodosum. Pulmonary and arthritic manifestations are extremely rare, perhaps only coincidental. Development of osteolytic lesions near the adenitis has been described.

The most serious complication is *encephalitis,* evidenced by fever, delirium, cranial nerve palsies, and pleocytosis in the cerebrospinal fluid. The encephalitis usually subsides without residual damage. When the primary lesion affects the conjunctiva, the preauricular nodes are affected, giving the clinical picture of *Parinaud's oculoglandular syndrome.*

It has been suggested that cat scratch disease may present as *mesenteric lymphadenitis,* because positive skin tests have been associated with that clinical picture. The presumption is that the portal of entry in such cases is the intestine.

Diagnosis. The diagnosis is based largely on the clinical circumstances, i.e., a subacute lymphadenitis limited to one region with or without suppuration, with or without a primary skin lesion distal to the node, and history of cat scratch or bite or of some comparable trauma to the skin. Several other processes must be considered in the differential diagnosis. Among infections are tuberculosis, infectious mononucleosis, tularemia, lymphogranuloma venereum, and sporotrichosis. Hodgkin's disease may cause difficulty, because the granulomatous picture in the lymph node of cat scratch disease may bear some resemblance to that of Hodgkin's disease; but the presence of microabscesses usually serves to differentiate these.

The Hanger-Rose test appears to be relatively specific for cat scratch disease. This employs an "antigen" prepared from the purulent matter aspirated from nodes of other patients, in a manner comparable with that formerly employed for lymphogranuloma venereum (Frei test). The exudate is diluted 1 to 5 in saline, and sterilized by heating at 60° C for one hour on two occasions. After intradermal injection of this material, the reaction is read at 24 to 48 hours. A positive result consists of induration 5 mm or more and erythema 10 mm or more in diameter. Unfortunately test material is not available commercially.

Treatment. There is no evidence that antimicrobial therapy, including tetracycline, is of value. Bed rest is advisable when fever and general malaise are present. If fluctuation becomes evident in the affected lymph node, it is recommended that the pus be aspirated (and used for the preparation of skin test antigen). Incision of an abscess is inadvisable, because sinus formation with prolonged drainage sometimes results, but biopsy of intact nodes seems safe in the presuppurative stage.

Daniels, W. B., and MacMurray, F. G.: Cat scratch disease. Report of one hundred sixty cases. J.A.M.A., 154:1247, 1954.
Kalter, S. S., Kim, C. S., and Heberling, R. L.: Herpes-like virus particles associated with cat scratch disease. Nature, 224:190, 1969.
Lyon, L. W.: Neurologic manifestations of cat scratch disease. Arch. Neurol., 25:23, 1971.
Warwick, W. J.: The cat scratch syndrome, many diseases or one disease? Prog. Med. Virol., 9:256, 1967. (This useful review lists nearly every publication up to 1966.)

160. NONBACTERIAL GASTROENTERITIS (Epidemic Nausea, Epidemic Vomiting, Winter Vomiting Disease, Epidemic Diarrhea)

Acute illnesses characterized by nausea, vomiting, and diarrhea are among the most common of human ailments, especially in children of school or preschool age. This pattern of indisposition has many of the characteristics of infectious disease: occurrence in epidemics, short incubation period, sudden onset, fever, brief course, and complete recovery. Indeed, these features may also be manifestations of gastrointestinal infections by recognized pathogens: Salmonella, *Entamoeba histolytica,* Shigella, and the enteroviruses. Furthermore, especially in young children and in travelers, such illness may be attributed to colonization of the bowel by strains of "normal" gut flora, a mechanism thought by some to be involved in the extremely serious syndrome known as infant (or "weanling") diarrhea. There remains, however, a large residue of gastroenteritis in which no microbial etiologic agent can be indicted, and it is generally assumed that as yet unidentified viruses are responsible. Progress in this connection has been made, both in the United States and in Britain. Competent groups of workers have succeeded in transmitting the illness to volunteers by oral administration of bacteria-free fecal filtrates. It seems likely that the causative virus or viruses will soon be characterized (see Ch. 135).

The presenting symptom may vary in different epidemics; this has given rise to reports of "epidemic nausea," "epidemic vomiting," and "epidemic diarrhea." Nevertheless in nearly all of them the clinical descriptions show that the allied symptoms were also present. In some epidemics, especially those affecting schoolchildren, hysteria appears to have played a role in determining the prominence of various symptoms.

The onset is abrupt, usually with nausea and vomiting, followed within a few hours by diarrhea. In young children there may be rise of body temperature, but fever is less common in older persons. The illness usually begins to subside within 24 hours, and recovery is established by the second to fourth day.

In the majority of cases the illness is easily dealt with at home; indeed, the best management could be characterized as masterful inactivity. Bed rests and sips of water or carbonated drinks are sensible therapy during the acute phase. Neither antimicrobial drugs nor purges should be given. If diarrhea is exceptionally troublesome, diphenoxylate hydrochloride (Lomotil), 5 mg every 4 to 6 hours, or paregoric may be used. In rare instances admission to hospital may be advisable so that fluids and electrolytes can be given parenterally.

Clarke, S. K. R., et al.: A virus from epidemic vomiting disease. Br. Med. J., 3:86, 1972.
Dolin, R., et al.: Transmission of acute infectious nonbacterial gastroenteritis to volunteers by oral adminstration of stool filtrates. J. Infect. Dis., 123:307, 1971.
Jordan, W. S., Jr., Gordon, L., and Dorrance, W. R.: A study of illness in a group of Cleveland families. VII. Transmission of acute nonbacterial gastroenteritis to volunteers: Evidence for two different etiologic agents. J. Exp. Med., 98:461, 1953.
Leading Article: Viruses of vomiting. Br. Med. J., 4:442, 1972. (Useful references.)

161. EPIDEMIC NEUROMYASTHENIA (Iceland Disease, Benign Myalgic Encephalomyelitis)

Between 1934 and 1960, several epidemics were reported of symptoms resembling those of poliomyelitis.

The acute phase was often followed by a prolonged period of disability, with headache, muscular weakness, fatigue, and mood depression.

Most outbreaks have occurred in summer, and about half of those reported have involved hospital personnel, especially student nurses. In all instances the attack rate has been much higher in women. Sporadic cases have been reported, but the diagnosis is difficult in the absence of an epidemic.

Severe generalized headache is nearly always a prominent complaint at the onset, and frequently there are pain and stiffness of the neck. Generalized tenderness of the muscles is common, and they frequently exhibit a characteristic of rapid fatigue and loss of motor power on repeated contraction. In perhaps 40 per cent of affected persons, areas of muscle weakness or paralysis appear during the first two weeks. These may be in the trunk or the extremities, and the pattern of involvement often changes from day to day. Cranial nerve signs, bladder dysfunction, and paresthesia may also be noted. In most cases complete recovery of neurologic function occurs within four to eight weeks, but relapses and exacerbations are common during the next few months.

Fever is inconspicuous or absent. The cerebrospinal fluid is usually normal, and routine tests of blood and urine reveal nothing of significance.

A striking feature of this illness is the prolonged period of disability after subsidence of the acute phase. Particularly troublesome are the behavioral manifestations of irritability and mood depression, which together with easy fatigue may interfere with normal living for months and even years after the acute episode. In this stage the subject may present a picture of hysteria or of simple neurasthenia.

Deaths have not been reported; therefore nothing is known of the pathology.

Extensive laboratory investigations failed to yield evidence of participation of any known pathogenic microorganism; nevertheless, the presumption had seemed warranted that it was an infectious disease. However, McEvedy and Beard have cast doubt on the likelihood of an infectious etiology. They carefully reviewed the reports of 15 recorded outbreaks, with special attention to the well-documented epidemic among nurses at the Royal Free Hospital, London. They suggest alternatively that these epidemics represented psychosocial phenomena: either mass hysteria among the subjects or altered medical perception. Their analysis and argument are persuasive, but the question remains unanswered.

Acheson, E. D.: The clinical syndrome variously called benign myalgic encephalomyelitis, Iceland disease and epidemic neuromyasthenia. Am. J. Med., 26:569, 1959.

Dillon, M. J., Marshall, W. C., Dudgeon, J. A., and Steigman, A. J.: Epidemic neuromyasthenia: Outbreak among nurses at a children's hospital. Br. Med. J., 1:301, 1974.

McEvedy, C. P., and Beard, A. W.: Concept of benign myalgic encephalomyelitis. Br. Med. J., 1:11, 1970.

Section Two. RICKETTSIAL DISEASES

162. INTRODUCTION

Edward S. Murray

The rickettsial diseases are caused by a family of microorganisms (Rickettsiaceae) that have characteristics common to both bacteria and viruses. They are now considered to be more like bacteria, because among other characteristics they (1) possess metabolic enzymes, (2) have cell walls, (3) utilize oxygen, and (4) are susceptible to broad-spectrum antimicrobial drugs. They resemble viruses by virtue of the fact that they grow only within living cells. These microorganisms were named "rickettsiae" to honor Dr. H. T. Ricketts, who died in 1910 while investigating the etiology of epidemic typhus and Rocky Mountain spotted fever.

The rickettsial diseases are grouped together because they possess a number of common characteristics. (1) The etiologic agents are similar in size and shape and can be seen as pleomorphic coccobacillary forms under the light microscope. (2) All rickettsial organisms occur under natural conditions in either fleas, lice, ticks, or mites, and these arthropods are in all cases except Q fever the primary means by which the diseases are transmitted to man. (3) All rickettsiae take on a characteristic red color with the Gimenez stain. (4) In all rickettsial infections except Q fever and rickettsialpox, agglutinins are produced to either the OX-19 or OX-K strains of the bacillus *Proteus vulgaris* (Weil-Felix reaction). (5) The characteristic pathologic lesion is a widespread peripheral vasculitis. (6) All are acute infectious diseases characterized clinically by fever, headache, and a rash (except Q fever, which has no rash). Finally, as previously noted, all rickettsial diseases in the early stages are readily susceptible to optimal doses of broad-spectrum antimicrobial drugs, e.g., chloramphenicol and the tetracyclines.

All rickettsial organisms, except the antigenically heterogenic strains of scrub typhus, produce complement-fixing antibodies. Data from these tests when combined with results of Weil-Felix reactions and clinical and epidemiologic features constitute definitive criteria for the diagnosis of each disease.

The immunity produced by any one of the rickettsial diseases is usually of long duration. Although the members of one group confer either partial or complete immunity to diseases caused by other members of the same group, there is, in general, no cross-immunity between groups. A minor degree of cross-immunity does exist, however, between some members of the typhus and spotted fever groups.

Since incubation periods for all the rickettsial diseases vary from 2 to 14 days, any of the rickettsial diseases can appear in air travelers reporting ill in any part of the world.

TABLE 1. Summary of Certain Important Epidemiologic and Clinical Characteristics of Rickettsial Diseases

	Epidemiologic Features			Usual Incubation Period (Days)		Rash	
Disease	Geographic Occurrence	Usual Mode of Transmission to Man	Reservoir		Eschar	Distribution	Type
Typhus group							
Primary louse-borne typhus	Worldwide	Infected louse feces rubbed into broken skin or as aerosol to mucous membranes	Man	12 (8-15)	None	Trunk to extremities	Macular, maculopapular
Brill-Zinsser disease	Worldwide	Recrudescence months or years after a primary attack of louse-borne typhus	–	–	None	Trunk to extremities	Macular, maculopapular
Murine typhus	Scattered pockets, worldwide	Infected flea feces rubbed into broken skin or as aerosol to mucous membranes	Rodents	12 (6-14)	None	Trunk to extremities	Macular, maculopapular
Spotted fever group							
Rocky Mountain spotted fever	Western Hemisphere	Tick bite	Ticks, rodents	6 (2-12)	None	Extremities to trunk; palms and soles	Macular, maculopapular, petechial
Tick typhus	Mediterranean littoral, Africa, Asia	Tick bite	Ticks, rodents	12 (7-18)	Frequent	Trunk, extremities, face, palms, soles	Macular, maculopapular, petechial
Rickettsialpox	USA, USSR, Korea	House mouse, mite bite	Mites, mice	12 (9-24)	Usually present	Trunk, face, extremities	Papular, vesicular
Scrub typhus	Japan, SW Asia, W and SW Pacific	Mite bite	Mites, rodents	11 (6-21)	Frequent	Trunk to extremities	Macular, maculopapular, evanescent
Q fever	Worldwide	Inhalation of dried dusts from environment of infected animals	Ticks, mammals	14 (9-20)	None	None	None

163. THE TYPHUS GROUP

Edward S. Murray

The typhus group is made up of three diseases: *epidemic louse-borne typhus fever, Brill-Zinsser disease* and *murine flea-borne typhus fever.* Clinically and pathologically, these three illnesses are very similar. Differences occur only in the intensity of the symptoms and signs, the severity of the course, and the case fatality rate. Epidemiologically, however, the three members of the typhus group are very different, and hence will be described under separate headings.

EPIDEMIC LOUSE-BORNE TYPHUS FEVER

(Classic, Historic, Human, European Typhus; Jail Fever, War Fever; Camp Fever; Fleckfieber [German]; Typhus Exanthématique [French]; Tifus Exantemático, Tabardillo [Spanish]; Dermotypho [Italian])

History. It is probable that typhus fever has afflicted mankind since ancient times. Although the plague of Athens in 430 B.C. is believed to have been epidemic typhus (MacArthur, 1954), the account of Fracastorius in 1546 is the earliest medical record that describes typhus fever with sufficient accuracy to permit its definite identification. Despite the work of Fracastorius, typhoid and typhus fevers were usually regarded as one entity by physicians until 1837, when Gerhard in Philadelphia clearly differentiated the two disorders on the basis of the important clinical and pathologic differences. Even today, however, confusion in terminology persists in those parts of Europe where *typhoid* fever is called "typhus abdominalis."

Typhus fever has played a major role in the history of the past four centuries. It followed in the wake of wars, famines, and human misfortunes. It often has had a more decisive effect on military campaigns than the actual battles themselves, a subject admirably treated by Zinsser in his book, *Rats, Lice and History.* Typhus epidemics in eastern Europe and Russia between 1918 and 1922 are estimated to have caused 30,000,000 cases and at least 3,000,000 deaths. Millions of cases occurred again during World War II in Nazi prison camps, in the Eastern European combat zone, among Yugoslav partisan forces, and in North Africa.

Etiology. In 1916 da Rocha Lima showed that typhus was caused by the microorganism that he named *Rickettsia prowazekii.* This organism has a protean morphology with coccobacillary forms predominating. However, the most typical form is a diplobacillus which has slightly pointed ends with a transparent band between the two bacilli. The organism takes on a characteristic red color when stained by the Gimenez method (Hoeprich). *R. prowazekii* possesses a soluble antigenic moiety which is shared also by *Rickettsia mooseri,* the other member of the typhus group.

R. prowazekii is readily killed by common antiseptics and dies in a few hours if exposed to room temperature. It remains viable for several days in blood at +5° C. Hence, a specimen of blood from a suspected case of typhus can be held for a day or more in a refrigerator pending isolation procedures. Organisms remain viable for several months in dried louse feces, and have survived for over 20 years when quick frozen in an alcohol bath and stored at –60° C.

Living *R. prowazekii* organisms contain a toxin that is lethal for mice as well as a substance that is hemolytic for the red blood cells of many animals.

Transmission. The role of the human body louse in the transmission of typhus was first demonstrated experimentally by Nicolle, Comte, and Conseil in 1909. A few years later mechanisms of transmission were precisely worked out by Wolbach, Todd, and Palfrey (1922) in their classic experiments in Poland on the etiology of typhus fever.

Man and the louse are the only known natural hosts of *R. prowazekii*. There is no passage of *R. prowazekii* organisms from one louse vector generation to the next via the egg. Furthermore, there is no confirmed evidence of an animal reservoir (Ormsbee). The chain of typhus infection starts when *R. prowazekii* appears in a patient's blood during the febrile period. A louse becomes infected during one of its frequent blood meals. The rickettsiae multiply in the cells lining the gut of the infected louse. First these cells become greatly distended and then burst, discharging myriads of microorganisms into the gut where they invade other lining cells or pass out in the feces. The disease is invariably fatal to the louse owing to the ultimate complete destruction of its intestinal epithelium. Transmission of rickettsiae from an infected louse to a new human host can occur by several mechanisms. When a louse takes a blood meal, it makes a small puncture wound in the skin, defecating at the same time. The louse bite is irritating, causing the patient to scratch and thus rub infected feces into the wound. It is also possible for one to become infected if dried infected louse feces gain access to the mucous membranes of the eye or respiratory tract. In an epidemic the spread of typhus from patient to patient and community to community is clearly related to the temperature preferences of the louse. Lice choose a 29° C environment which they find in the folds of the garments of a healthy man. Here they live and lay their eggs. Lice tend to leave a typhus patient when his temperature rises to 40° C or higher. Also, they quickly abandon a corpse in search of a warm host. Transmission of typhus from man to man occurs only by means of the louse; hence, once deloused and bathed, a typhus patient cannot transmit the disease.

Pathology. The microscopic pathology of typhus is characteristic. Rickettsiae multiply in the endothelial cells lining the small blood vessels. Endothelial proliferation and perivascular infiltration lead to thrombosis and leakage. Such vascular lesions when they occur in the skin produce the rash, whereas lesions in the meninges most probably account for the highly characteristic rickettsial headache. The myocardium is also a frequent focus of vascular lesions. Gangrene is directly related to thrombosis of capillaries, small arteries, and veins in affected areas (McAllister).

Clinical Manifestations and Course. The incubation period is approximately ten days to two weeks. Prodromata of vague malaise and headache are not uncommon, especially in vaccinated individuals. The *onset* is usually abrupt, and the patient can frequently state the exact hour when his illness began. The major clinical signs and symptoms are fever, headache, and rash. The fever may rise to 39 to 40° C the first day, or it may take two or three days to reach this level. However, once the temperature reaches 40° C it tends to remain at this level or higher with only slight fluctuations until altered by treatment or recovery. A remittent (or widely fluctuating) temperature is not characteristic of untreated typhus except very late in the disease or in vaccinated persons.

The headache is characteristic. It is intense, persists night and day, and is intractable to all efforts at alleviation. The rash makes its appearance on the fourth to sev-

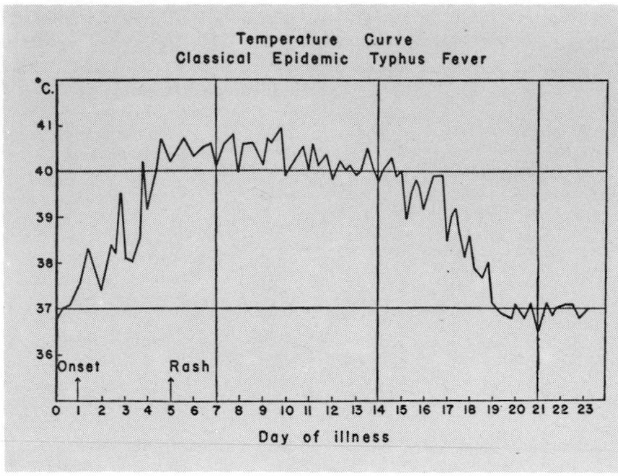

Temperature curve in a case of classic louse-borne typhus. (From Horsfall, F. L., Jr., and Tamm, I. [eds.]: Viral and Rickettsial Infections of Man. 4th ed. Philadelphia, J. B. Lippincott Company, 1965.)

enth day of illness and consists at first of pinkish macules that fade on slight pressure. These discrete macules usually appear first on the upper trunk in the axillary area. In the course of one or two days the rash spreads over the entire body, usually sparing the face, palms, and soles which are involved only rarely. The macules soon become darker, fixed, and maculopapular. In severely ill patients the rash may progress to petechial, hemorrhagic, or confluent forms.

Patients often have a slight cough without sputum as in mycoplasmal pneumonia. An accompanying patchy pulmonary consolidation is more often diagnosed roentgenographically than by physical examination. Respirations may be increased out of all proportion to findings in the chest.

At first the pulse rate is slow in relation to the temperature, but by the end of the first week it becomes rapid (110 to 140), weak, and frequently undulating or irregular. The blood pressure is usually low, and there may be brief episodes of severe hypotension. Conjunctivitis and flushing of the face are frequent findings. The spleen is palpable in about half the cases. Renal insufficiency of varying degree is a common occurrence. During the acute phase, deafness and ringing in the ears are common complaints, as is also myalgia of the back and legs.

In fatal cases the terminal period is usually characterized by a profound stupor, peripheral vascular collapse, and severe renal failure. In cases without complications, the temperature begins to drop rapidly by lysis between the thirteenth and sixteenth days of illness. Recovery of normal mental and physical powers is remarkably rapid, although the patient may not regain his full strength for two to three months.

Typhus Fever in Previously Immunized Persons. The symptoms and clinical course of typhus are greatly modified as a consequence of prior active immunization. The illness may consist merely of a mild headache and fever of several days' duration. Most patients, however, go on to develop a transient macular rash and suffer from a relatively severe headache and fever for about a week. Complications are rare; mortality has not been reported, and the diagnosis can be established only by serologic or isolation studies.

Typhus Fever Modified by Specific Treatment. If specific treatment is begun early, the clinical course of typhus is usually arrested at whatever stage is present when treatment begins. The temperature usually drops to normal within 36 to 72 hours, and the major clinical signs and symptoms (including the rash) disappear soon thereafter. However, weakness of a greater or lesser extent almost always persists for days or weeks after recovery. On the other hand, if the disease is allowed to progress untreated beyond the eighth or ninth day, treatment becomes less and less effective. In such cases clinical recovery will depend largely upon the extent of vascular damage produced in the heart, brain, and kidneys before therapy was begun.

Diagnosis. *Clinical Diagnosis.* Before the characteristic rash appears, it is impossible to assert on clinical grounds alone that a patient is suffering from epidemic typhus. The early stages of a number of acute infectious diseases closely resemble the first few days of epidemic typhus—for example, smallpox, relapsing fever, malaria, typhoid fever, meningococcal infection, yellow fever, and several of the other rickettsial diseases. Of major help in the differential diagnosis is the characteristic maculopapular typhus rash that begins on the upper trunk and extends centrifugally to the extremities. The rash may be evanescent in children as well as in mildly ill adults. It is also difficult to recognize in dark-skinned subjects.

Laboratory Diagnosis. SPECIFIC SEROLOGIC TESTS. Complement-fixing antibodies first appear in the serum of patients between the seventh and twelfth days of the disease. Soluble antigens that are commercially available detect group antibodies common to both murine and epidemic typhus. In most instances epidemiologic considerations such as geographic location and type of vector involved (flea or louse) will suffice to distinguish between these two diseases in the typhus group. When confusion in diagnosis arises, specific washed antigens (available in special rickettsial laboratories) can be used to differentiate between murine and epidemic typhus. In performing the complement-fixation test it is important to use 4 to 8 units of either type of antigen employed in order to detect the early IgM type of antibodies. Evidence has accumulated over the years indicating that serologic cross-reactions frequently occur between the typhus and Rocky Mountain spotted fever groups of diseases. Hence clinicians must evaluate any serologic results along with clinical and epidemiologic data before arriving at a final diagnosis.

Other special serologic tests that can be used in laboratory diagnosis include immunofluorescence (Elisberg), mouse toxin neutralization, and rickettsial agglutination. Agglutination can also be carried out using sheep or human group O erythrocytes sensitized with a serologically active fraction derived from rickettsiae treated with ether, heat, and alkali (erythrocyte-sensitizing substance or ESS). These special tests are available in rickettsial research laboratories, but are rarely if ever needed to establish a diagnosis.

Persons recovered from typhus regularly show significant antibody titers in their sera for years after an attack of the disease. Hence for definitive diagnosis it is important to demonstrate a rise or fall in antibody titer related to the acute or convalescent period of the clinical disease.

WEIL-FELIX TEST. The Weil-Felix reaction, although nonspecific, is of great value in indicating the strong probability of a typhus infection. The test is positive in over 90 per cent of bona fide cases of primary epidemic typhus. The basis for the Weil-Felix reaction is related to the fact that a certain antigenic component found in some rickettsiae is shared by various strains of *Proteus vulgaris.* Thus *R. prowazekii* can stimulate antibodies that will agglutinate the OX-19 strains of Proteus. Since low levels of Proteus OX-19 antibody are present in many healthy individuals, diagnostic significance is only attached to titers of 1 to 160 or greater. Such titers are usually demonstrable between the seventh and eleventh days after onset of typhus. The rapid slide method which can be carried out in only three to five minutes is quite satisfactory when performed with controls. Occasionally agglutinins develop for the OX-2 Proteus strains but none for OX-K. Proteus OX-19 antibody titers also develop in other rickettsial diseases, notably murine typhus and Rocky Mountain spotted fever.

ISOLATION OF RICKETTSIAE FROM THE PATIENT. The laboratory diagnosis of typhus may be made by inoculating blood from a patient into a susceptible species such as the guinea pig or chick embryo if facilities are available for the further manipulation required to establish the identity of the microorganisms thus obtained.

Prognosis. The prognosis in untreated cases is closely correlated with age. In children under ten years the disease is usually mild, and fatalities are uncommon. In adults the mortality ranges from 10 per cent in the second and third decades of life to more than 60 per cent in those over 50. However, active immunization and the use of specific therapy greatly affect mortality figures.

In the absence of specific treatment, the appearance of renal insufficiency is an early sign that a patient's illness will be severe or fatal. The extent and severity of the typhus rash is also roughly indicative of the severity of the disease. Complications such as pneumonia or gangrene of the skin are likewise serious prognostic signs. A fall in systolic blood pressure to values below 80 mm or mercury for a few hours or longer may cause damage from which the patient may not recover, even though the blood pressure rises after the period of severe hypotension.

Treatment. Chloramphenicol or the tetracyclines are highly effective when given early and in adequate dosage. The clinician must decide on the basis of his own preference which drug he will use. Recent reports suggest that doxycycline is an effective drug in the treatment of rickettsial infections.

Prompt and optimal specific therapy is urgent. A maximally effective rickettsiostatic blood level of drug should be obtained at the earliest possible moment. Since large doses of chloramphenicol are well absorbed from the gastrointestinal tract, this drug may be preferred in gravely ill patients. For chloramphenicol the following dosage schedule is considered optimal: Therapy is begun with an initial loading dose of 50 mg per kilogram of body weight, followed by a daily dose of 50 mg per kilogram of body weight divided into three or four equal doses during each 24-hour period. For an adult this schedule would amount to approximately 5 grams of chloramphenicol given over the first 24-hour period (an initial loading dose of 3 grams followed by 0.5 gram every six hours). This dosage of chloramphenicol for the first 24 hours of illness is higher than that recommended in bacterial diseases. However, a large body of experience in using high initial doses of this drug in treating rickettsial diseases fully justifies such a schedule.

Since large single doses of tetracyclines are irregularly absorbed from the gastrointestinal tract, a loading dose of these drugs is not indicated. The daily recommended dose of the tetracyclines is calculated on the basis of 25 mg per kilogram of body weight. Treatment is more effective if the daily dose is divided and administered at intervals of three or four hours rather than on a six- to eight-hour schedule.

As the temperature approaches normal, the daily dosage of the antimicrobial being administered can be cut in half and then continued for two or three more days. Relapses are uncommon even when treatment is begun as early as the first or second day of illness.

Intravenous preparations of chloramphenicol and tetracyclines are available, and should be used in critically ill patients when oral medication is not possible because of vomiting or uncooperativeness. For adults, 1 gram of chloramphenicol sodium succinate in glucose or saline solution can be given intravenously, followed by 500 mg every four to six hours. Intravenous tetracycline can be administered in glucose or saline solution, 1 gram initially, followed by 500 mg every six hours. Intravenous therapy should be discontinued as soon as the patient is able to take the drug by mouth.

Penicillin and streptomycin have very little, if any, effect. Their use should be considered only when secondary bacterial infections develop for which they are specifically indicated. The sulfonamides may have a harmful effect, and are contraindicated. Steroid therapy has been used by some clinicians in severely ill patients. Carefully controlled hormone therapy may be of practical value in patients first seen late in the course of illness at a time when supplemental antitoxemia measures could be lifesaving.

Special nursing care is of utmost importance. Comatose patients should be turned frequently to prevent decubitus ulcers and hypostatic pneumonia. Vomiting necessitates small frequent feedings. Sedatives should be used with care so that the course of the disease is not obscured. Excessively high temperatures should be controlled by alcohol sponging.

It should be kept in mind that because of the widespread endothelial damage in epidemic typhus, as well as in all the other rickettsial diseases, a severely ill patient may be even more desperately ill than he appears. Therefore all laboratory and other manipulative measures that disturb and exhaust him should be reduced to a minimum. The antimicrobial drugs are rickettsiostatic only; hence the patient's own defense and recuperative powers are major factors in his recovery.

Prevention. Two highly effective measures, immunization and louse control, are available for the prevention and control of typhus. Both are applicable to an individual as well as a community. Killed typhus vaccines produced from yolk sacs of infected chick embryos have been widely used. Immunization with killed vaccines does not fully protect against infection. However, when vaccinated individuals do contract typhus, the course of illness is shorter and milder, and fatalities have not been reported. An experimental living attenuated "Strain E" typhus vaccine (Fox) is under trial in the United States, the USSR, and Africa. Moderately severe illness has occurred in a small percentage of those inoculated with minimal immunizing doses of this vaccine. However, the prompt development and prolonged duration of the immunity resulting from a single dose of Strain E vaccine indicates that under certain circumstances this vaccine may be found to play a useful role in typhus control.

Louse control with DDT and the newer developed insecticides offers a powerful weapon against typhus epidemics. Both infected and noninfected lice can be eliminated almost completely by mass delousing of a population. A major factor in the efficacy of DDT is the persistence of its lethal effect on lice for two to four weeks after being dusted into garments.

Recent reports indicate that in several areas lice have become partially resistant to DDT. Other insecticides such as malathione or lindane may have to be used under these circumstances.

BRILL-ZINSSER DISEASE AND THE CARRIER STATE

History. In 1898 Nathan Brill in New York described sporadic cases of a typhus-like illness with fever, headache, and a maculopapular rash which occurred characteristically in immigrants from Russia and Poland. The disease was clearly distinguishable from typhoid, because the Widal test was negative. However, the illness was not typical of typhus, as all cases were sporadic with no spread to family or other contacts.

Over the next three decades many clinicians in the large cities of the eastern United States reported cases that were referred to as Brill's disease. In 1912 Anderson and Goldberger demonstrated by cross-immunity tests in monkeys that Brill's disease was a form of typhus, and for a period thereafter Brill's disease and murine typhus were confused with each other. However, by 1931 murine typhus was clearly defined as a flea-borne disease and Brill's disease remained an isolated syndrome of unknown etiology.

In 1934 Hans Zinsser carried out extensive epidemiologic studies on 538 cases of Brill's disease occurring in New York and Boston. Almost invariably patients were immigrants from eastern Europe where louse-borne typhus was prevalent. This led Zinsser to postulate that the syndrome represented a relapse of a prior typhus infection. He reasoned that man was a carrier and through the medium of recrudescent "Brill's disease" cases served to maintain the disease between epidemics. Over the next two decades Zinsser's hypothesis was widely accepted. To acknowledge the contributions of the two scientists whose observations revealed the interepidemic reservoir of typhus, the syndrome was renamed Brill-Zinsser disease.

Typhus, the Carrier State, and Recrudescence. Clinical and epidemiologic features of Brill-Zinsser disease are consistent with the view proposed by Zinsser that it represents a relapse or recrudescence of a primary louse-borne typhus infection suffered at some time in the past. This makes Brill-Zinsser disease analogous in many ways to a relapse of malaria occurring years after an original malarial attack. Zinsser's hypothesis has received additional confirmation recently from laboratory studies in which normal lice were fed on patients during the acute phase of Brill-Zinsser disease. From these lice microorganisms were isolated that proved to be identical to *R. prowazekii*—the etiologic agent of primary louse-borne typhus.

Brill-Zinsser disease, however, differs from primary louse-borne typhus in a number of respects. (1) Clinically the disease is shorter, milder, and frequently without a rash. This picture is consistent with the fact that the syndrome represents an *R. prowazekii* infection in an individual already partially immune. (2) No louse vector or exogenous source of the infection is apparent. (3) The majority of patients give a history of having suffered an attack of primary louse-borne typhus in the past. But it is the serologic data that provide the most sharply distinguishing characteristics of these two disease entities caused by the same organism. In primary louse-borne typhus the acute phase antibodies are IgM in type, whereas the antibodies in Brill-Zinsser disease are from their very earliest appearance of the IgG class. These differences are characteristic of the primary and secondary immune response.

An interesting feature of the Brill-Zinsser syndrome is the frequent absence of a significant Weil-Felix reaction.

TABLE 2. Distinguishing Characteristics of Primary Louse-Borne Typhus and Brill-Zinsser Disease

	Primary Louse-Borne Typhus	Brill-Zinsser Disease
Epidemiologic		
Past history of typhus	No	Yes
Occurrence of cases	Epidemic	Sporadic
Seasonal occurrence	Winter-spring	Year round
Transmission	By infected lice	Occurs in absence of lice
Clinical		
Duration of fever	12-18 days	7-11 days
Rash	Regularly present	Frequently absent or evanescent
Mortality	10-50% depending on age	Rare
Laboratory		
Specific antibody rise	Slow – begins 7th to 10th day, maximum 15th to 20th day	Rapid – begins 4th to 5th day, maximum 9th to 11th day
Type of immunoglobulin response during acute phase	Primary – IgM	Secondary – IgG
Weil-Felix reaction	Regularly present in titers of 1/160 or higher	Frequently absent (see text)
Cross-reacting specific *R. mooseri* antibodies in acute phase	No	Yes

In fact the reaction is almost always negative when a Brill-Zinsser disease relapse occurs within the first few years after the primary attack at a time when immunity from the original illness is presumably still quite high. As the interval between the original attack and the recrudescence lengthens, positive Weil-Felix reactions occur more frequently. The Weil-Felix reaction is usually also negative in those who develop primary louse-borne typhus after prophylactic vaccination, as well as in typhus patients who receive antimicrobial therapy very early in the course of their illness.*

Brill-Zinsser disease has now been reported from many parts of the world. Wherever it has been recognized, it has always occurred in individuals who were born or had lived for some time in an area where louse-borne typhus occurs in epidemic form – particularly the countries of eastern Europe. Brill-Zinsser disease also occurs in eastern Europe itself. In this area, particularly in Bosnia, Yugoslavia, small family epidemics of primary epidemic typhus in children have been described in which a direct relationship could be traced from the children's infection to an adult recrudescent case of Brill-Zinsser disease that occurred several weeks earlier in the same family.

The epidemiologic significance of Brill-Zinsser disease cases is clear. They indicate the existence of carriers with latent infection who constitute the interepidemic reservoirs of typhus. Thus in a community where louse infestation is prevalent, when a latent carrier relapses and becomes an overt Brill-Zinsser disease case, the scene is then set for a possible epidemic of louse-borne typhus.

Pathology. The findings in Brill-Zinsser disease are the same as those described under Louse-Borne Typhus.

*Weil-Felix reactions are related to the fact that certain Proteus organisms share a common antigen with certain of the rickettsiae. Because the amount of this common antigen in each individual rickettsia must be extremely minute, a relatively large mass of rickettsiae may be required to stimulate the Proteus agglutinins. The partially immune status of a Brill-Zinsser disease patient as well as that of a typhus-vaccinated individual may prevent the rickettsial mass in the blood and tissues from obtaining the necessary level to evoke a Proteus response. Likewise, early antimicrobial treatment may reduce the likelihood of a Proteus response by contributing to an early and rapid elimination of rickettsiae from the infected individual.

Diagnosis. The clinical diagnosis of Brill-Zinsser disease should be considered when a fever of unknown origin with an intense persistent headache occurs in a patient who has lived at some previous time in an area where louse-borne typhus occurs in epidemic form. A macular or maculopapular rash, if present, is of additional help in diagnosis.

The diagnosis can be confirmed in the laboratory by employing the complement-fixation test. A negative Weil-Felix test in the presence of rising CF antibodies is highly suggestive of Brill-Zinsser disease rather than primary louse-borne typhus, because more than 95 per cent of cases of the latter disease show a significant rise in Proteus OX-19 agglutinins. However, it should be kept in mind that the Weil-Felix test may be positive in Brill-Zinsser disease if the period elapsed between the original and the recrudescent attack is ten years or longer. The demonstration of only the IgG class of antibodies in the early acute phase of illness is highly diagnostic of Brill-Zinsser disease.

Prognosis and Treatment. Statements in the paragraphs on Prognosis and Treatment of Louse-Borne Typhus apply to Brill-Zinsser disease as well.

Control of the Interepidemic Typhus Reservoir. The factors that precipitate an attack of Brill-Zinsser disease are unknown, and methods to prevent recrudescent attacks have not yet been discovered. However, the spread of infection from recrudescent Brill-Zinsser disease cases to nonimmune contacts can be curtailed. When Brill-Zinsser disease occurs in an area such as the United States where louse infestation is extremely rare, no spread of the disease will occur, and no measures are required beyond treatment of the Brill-Zinsser disease itself. However, when Brill-Zinsser disease cases occur in a community where louse infestation is prevalent, one practical method of control is the "fire brigade" technique. This consists of a surveillance network throughout the community organized to report promptly the occurrence of a Brill-Zinsser disease case or the first ensuing cases of primary louse-borne typhus. A centrally based control team should then be available to come in with insecticides to eliminate all lice in the environment, including lice on all contacts near and far.

TABLE 3. Complement Fixation and Weil-Felix Reactions in Rickettsioses

Group	Disease	Rickettsial Complement Fixation (CF)*			Weil-Felix (WF) Agglutination*		
		Group Antigen Type			Proteus Strain		
		Typhus	RMSF	Q Fever	OX-19	OX-2	OX-K
I	Primary louse-borne typhus	+++	±	0	+++	+	0
	Brill-Zinsser disease	+++	±	0	0 or +++	0	0
	Murine typhus	+++	±	0	+++	+	0
II	RMSF	±	+++	0	+++†	+++†	0
	Tick typhus	0	+++	0	+++†	+++†	0
	Rickettsialpox	0	+++	0	0	0	0
III	Scrub typhus	0	0	0	0	0	+++
IV	Q fever	0	0	+++	0	0	0

*+++ = Strong reactions in CF 1:40 to 1:280.
Strong reactions in WF 1:160 or greater.
\+ = OX-2 reactions relatively weaker than OX-19.
0 = Negative at 1:5 dilution in CF.
Negative at 1:40 dilution in WF.
± = Recent evidence indicates that frequent cross-reactions occur between the typhus group and Rocky Mountain spotted fever (see text).
†In RMSF or tick typhus, agglutinins to either OX-19 or OX-2 or both can be present in either high or low titer.

MURINE FLEA-BORNE TYPHUS FEVER
(Endemic Typhus, Rat Typhus, Flea Typhus, Urban or Shop Typhus of Malaya)

History. Murine typhus fever probably has occurred for centuries as a sporadic or endemic disease, but only since 1931 has it been clearly distinguished from classic epidemic louse-borne typhus. During the early part of this century in the United States murine typhus was confused with Brill's disease. However, in 1926 Maxey, after extensive investigation, concluded that the typhus occurring in the southeastern United States must have a reservoir other than man, and he mentioned mice and rats specifically. He further suggested that fleas, mites, or ticks could be the vector. Mooser, in 1928, observed a basic difference in behavior of certain strains of typhus rickettsiae in the tissues of guinea pigs. Dyer and colleagues isolated typhus rickettsiae from rat fleas in Baltimore (1931), and Mooser, Zinsser, and Ruiz Castaneda found the agent in rats in Mexico City. Mooser subsequently named the disease "murine typhus" to indicate its presence as a natural infection of rats. Reports showing the worldwide distribution of murine typhus rapidly accumulated. In the United States the incidence of the disease was increasing up to 1946. The rapid decrease in incidence since that time has been attributed, in part, to vigorously applied control measures.

Etiology. The etiologic agent, *Rickettsia mooseri,* is similar to *Rickettsia prowazekii* in metabolic, biochemical, and staining characteristics; however, in size, *R. mooseri* is slightly smaller and more uniform. *R. mooseri* and *R. prowazekii* are classed together in the typhus group by virtue of the fact that they possess a common soluble antigenic moiety.

Epidemiology and Transmission. Rats infected with murine typhus are found scattered throughout the world in circumscribed areas. In the United States reservoirs of the disease are found along the southern Atlantic seaboard and in states bordering on the Gulf of Mexico. Other known areas of infection are Mexico, South America, the Mediterranean littoral, and Manchuria. However, the disease is widespread, occurring elsewhere in such areas as Ethiopia, Malaysia, and Australia.

Murine typhus is maintained in nature as a mild infection of rats, and is transmitted from rat to rat by the rat louse or by the rat flea, *Xenopsylla cheopis.* A flea becomes infected while feeding on a rat during the acute phase of an infection. The rickettsiae multiply in the flea without causing any damage to the host. Once infected the flea continues to discharge rickettsiae in its feces for the remainder of its life; however, infected female fleas do not transmit *R. mooseri* via their eggs to the next generation of fleas. Man usually acquires the disease when bitten by an infected flea. Rat fleas generally prefer to feed on rats, but they will attack man if rats become scarce. At the same time that an infected flea sucks blood it deposits feces that are teeming with rickettsiae. These may be rubbed into the flea bite wound or, as dried aerosol of feces and microorganisms, they may gain access to the body through the mucous membranes of the conjunctivae or respiratory tract. Infection of man is an accidental occurrence and is not related to the maintenance of the disease in nature.

Pathology. Information on the pathology of murine typhus is limited, because death from this form of typhus is rare. It is usually assumed that the lesions are essentially the same as those in louse-borne typhus.

Clinical Manifestation and Course. The incubation period of murine typhus lasts from six to fourteen days. The symptoms are similar to those of louse-borne typhus, the principal differences being that murine typhus is milder and shorter, the rash is less extensive and persists for shorter periods, there are fewer complications, and the case fatality rate is lower.

Diagnosis. *Clinical Diagnosis.* The diagnosis of murine typhus may be suspected when a patient has a sustained fever of several days' duration accompanied by headache, generalized aches and pains, and a macular or maculopapular rash appearing on the fifth or sixth day after onset of fever. The rash is first noted on the trunk and later spreads to the extremities; the face, palms, and soles are rarely involved. Since murine typhus is present in many of the areas where Rocky Mountain spotted fever (RMSF) occurs, it is helpful to remember that the rash of RMSF first appears on the wrists and ankles, rapidly spreads up the extremities to the trunk, and regularly involves the palms and soles. The patient with murine typhus usually gives a history of activities that have brought him into contact with places where rats are numerous. However, there is often no definite recollection of a flea bite.

It is impossible on clinical evidence alone to distinguish an ordinary case of murine typhus from a case of Brill-Zinsser disease or a mild case of louse-borne typhus. Epidemiologic and laboratory data will almost always be required to arrive at a definitive diagnosis.

Laboratory Diagnosis. Both the complement-fixation and Weil-Felix tests are employed in the laboratory to confirm the clinical suspicion of a murine typhus infection. Rising antibodies to the soluble typhus group antigen indicate either a primary louse-borne typhus, Brill-Zinsser disease, or murine typhus infection. From the time of onset Brill-Zinsser disease antibodies are IgG in type. In contrast, the antibodies produced in the acute phase of murine and louse-borne typhus are characteristically IgM. One may have to resort to specific washed rickettsial antigens to distinguish between louse-borne and murine typhus. In murine typhus as in primary louse-borne typhus 4 to 8 units of antigen are required to obtain optimal fixation of complement during the acute phase of illness.

The Weil-Felix test employing Proteus OX-19 strains is regularly positive in murine typhus. Isolation of *R. mooseri* from patients may be accomplished early in the course of the disease by inoculating blood into guinea pigs, mice, or chick embryos. (See Laboratory Diagnosis in Louse-Borne Typhus.)

Prognosis. Even when untreated, murine typhus is usually a mild disease with fatalities occurring only in the elderly. The use of specific therapy further reduces the duration and severity of the disease.

Treatment. Treatment of murine typhus is similar to that for louse-borne typhus. However, the usual mildness of murine typhus permits more leeway in a therapeutic regimen. For example, tetracycline can be used as the preferred drug, thus avoiding the greater potential toxicity of chloramphenicol.

Prevention and Control. Measures to prevent and control murine typhus depend upon limiting the rat population. The first step is to reduce the flea population of rat colonies by dusting rat runs with DDT or its equivalent. After this, rat populations are reduced by poisoning, trapping, eliminating rat harborages, and rat-proofing buildings.

A vaccine has been produced and demonstrated to be effective. However, its use is hardly justified in view of the clinical mildness and sporadic nature of the disease.

Elisberg, B. L., and Bozeman, F. L.: Serologic diagnosis of rickettsial diseases by indirect immunofluorescence. Arch. Inst. Pasteur Tunis, 43:193, 1966.

Fox, J. P., Montoya, J. A., Jordan, M. D., Cornojo Ubillus, J. R., Garcia, J. L., Estrada, M. A., and Gelfand, H. M.: Immunization of man against epidemic typhus by infection with avirulent *Rickettsia prowazeki* (strain E). Arch. Inst. Pasteur Tunis, 36:449, 1959.

Gear, J. H. S.: Rickettsial vaccines. Br. Med. Bull., 25:171, 1969.

Hoeprich, P. D. (ed.): Infectious Diseases. New York, Harper & Row, 1972.

MacArthur, W. P.: The Athenian plague: A medical note. Classical Quarterly, 4:171, 1954.

McAllister, W. B.: The pathology of louse-borne typhus fever from the epidemic of 1943-5 in Egypt. Nav. Med. Res. Inst., Proj. NM 007 017 (X-696), Rep. No. 1, 25 January 1949.

Murray, E. S., O'Connor, J. M., and Gaon, J. A.: Differentiation of 19S and 7S complement-fixing antibodies in primary versus recrudescent typhus by either ethanethiol or heat. Proc. Soc. Exp. Biol. Med., 119:291, 1965.

Murray, E. S., and Snyder, J. C.: Brill-Zinsser disease: The interepidemic reservoir of epidemic louse-borne typhus fever. Proceedings Sixth International Congress of Microbiology, Rome. 4, Section 11, 31-44, 1953.

Ormsbee, R. A., Burgdorfer, W., Peacock, M., and Hildebrandt, F.: Experimental infections of *R. prowazeki* among domestic livestock and ticks. Am. J. Trop. Med. Hyg., 20:117, 1971.

Proceedings of the International Symposium on the Control of Lice and Louse-borne Diseases. Washington, D.C., December 4–6, 1972. Pan American Health Organization Scientific Publication No. 263.

Smadel, J. E.: Status of the rickettsioses in the United States. Ann. Intern. Med., 51:421, 1959.

Snyder, J. C.: The typhus fevers. *In* Horsfall, F. L., Jr., and Tamm, I. (eds.): Viral and Rickettsial Infections of Man. 4th ed. Philadelphia, J. B. Lippincott Company, 1965, Chapter 50.

Wolbach, S. B., Todd, J. L., and Palfrey, F. W.: The Etiology and Pathology of Typhus. Cambridge, Mass., Harvard University Press, 1922.

Zdrodovskii, P. F., and Golinevich, H. M.: The Rickettsial Diseases. New York, Pergamon Press, 1960 (in English).

Zinsser, H.: Rats, Lice, and History. Boston, Little, Brown and Company, 1935.

164. ROCKY MOUNTAIN SPOTTED FEVER (Spotted Fever, Tick Fever, Tick Typhus [England], Fiebre Manchada [Mexico], Fiebre Petequial [Colombia], Febere Maculosa [Brazil])

Herbert L. Ley, Jr.

Definition. Rocky Mountain spotted fever is a relatively severe, self-limited rickettsial infection transmitted to man by various species of hard ticks. The disease is characterized by fever, headache, bone and muscle pains, and a generalized rash that frequently may become petechial or hemorrhagic.

Etiology. The disease is caused by *Rickettsia rickettsi (Dermacentroxenus rickettsi),* the prototype rickettsia of the spotted fever group of organisms. These include, in addition to *R. rickettsi,* the agents of rickettsialpox, north Asian tick-borne rickettsiosis, and African and Queensland tick typhus, all of which are distinctive among rickettsiae in their ability to multiply in the nucleus as well as in the cytoplasm of mammalian and tick cells. All these agents share an antigen common to the group, and each possesses an individual species-specific antigen as well. Serologic differentiation among members of the group has been complicated by the shared antigen; specific antisera, prepared in mice, are useful in laboratory identification of the individual members of the group. All the tick-borne rickettsioses of the Western Hemisphere have proved, to date, to be caused by *R. rickettsi,* regardless of the country of origin or the local name given the disease. The incubation period of the disease may vary from 2 to 14 days; severe illnesses appear to be associated with short incubation periods.

Distribution and Incidence. Rocky Mountain spotted fever is limited in distribution to North and South America. The disease was first described in the United States in Montana at the turn of the century, and for some time was thought to be limited to that area. Beginning in the 1930's, the disease was recognized in the eastern United States, Canada, Mexico, Brazil, and Colombia. Incidence and mortality data are difficult to obtain outside the United States, but in this country an average of 300 cases has been reported annually for the ten-year period from 1950 to 1959, with an average mortality rate of 6 per cent. During the 1960's about 300 cases have been reported annually in the United States, approximately half occurring in the Atlantic seaboard states from Delaware to Florida.*

Epidemiology. Rocky Mountain spotted fever is widely disseminated in nature and is principally a disease of ticks and small mammals. Man is rarely involved except when he intrudes into the "silent" wild cycle of disease. The hard ticks involved in transmission, the Ixodidae, feed on small mammals during their development through the larval and nymphal stages to tick adulthood. Once infected with *R. rickettsi* the tick may transmit the rickettsiae to its progeny transovarially or to man and other animals by feeding upon them. Thus the tick is both a vector and a reservoir of infection. The species of tick involved in the disease cycle varies according to geographic area. In the northern United States, the rabbit tick, *Haemaphysalis leporis-palustris,* rarely bites man, but appears to be responsible for maintaining the disease among rabbits and small mammals. Human infection in the United States is most commonly acquired in the West from *Dermacentor andersoni* (the wood tick), in the East from *Dermacentor variabilis* (the dog tick), and in the South from *Amblyomma americanum* (the Lone Star tick). Many other species of hard ticks have been implicated in transmission of the disease in Central and South America. Under laboratory conditions soft ticks of the genus Ornithodorus are also capable of transmitting the agent, but appear to be unimportant as vectors in nature. Among the animals believed to be involved in the natural cycle of disease are squirrels, rabbits, porcupines, chipmunks, weasels, several species of feral rats and mice, and, perhaps most important from the human viewpoint, dogs. All these animals have been shown to be susceptible to infection with *R. rickettsi;* the disease produced is usually mild and limited in duration but is associated with a rickettsemia sufficient to infect ticks feeding on the animal at the time.

Although it was once considered that the western form of the disease was more serious than the eastern, the higher mortality rates in the western United States appear to be a reflection of a much higher average age among patients. Formerly the disease was one of the adult male in the West and of children of both sexes in the eastern United States. In recent years more than half the patients reported nationally have been less than 15 years of age. As might be expected, the disease has a striking seasonal pattern in which nearly 90 per cent of all cases occur during the period from May through September.

Pathology and Physiologic Responses. Histopathologically, the disease is an endangitis, starting in the endothelial cells and extending into the smooth muscle of the vessel walls. Rickettsiae may be demonstrated in the lesions by appropriate stains. Thrombi are formed at the points of inflammation and lead to areas of focal necrosis and hemorrhage. The major organ systems involved are the skin, subcutaneous tissues, and the central nervous system, although mononuclear cell infiltration may also be found in the lungs, heart, liver, and spleen. Except for the rash, gross findings at autopsy are minimal.

Clinical laboratory findings in the milder cases are usually limited to a moderate leukocytosis. Peripheral vascular collapse, the most serious consequence of the disease, may result from the pooling of blood in the damaged capillaries and from loss of water, electrolytes, and proteins into the extravascular space. Patients having this complication will show a decrease in hematocrit, blood chloride, and serum protein levels, and an increase in serum nonprotein nitrogen levels. Thrombocytopenia has also been observed in severe illnesses.

Clinical Manifestations. Headache and fever, frequently accompanied by mild chills, appear as initial symptoms of infection 2 to 14 days following contact with ticks. Within the first day of fever the patient usually complains of pains in the bones, joints, and muscles, photophobia, and increasing prostration. Initial physical examination usually reveals only flushing of the skin, conjunctival injection, and minor respiratory signs referable to a dry cough. By the second day the fever usually rises to 40 to 40.5° C and stays at that level until the end of the second week. Between the second and sixth days of fever a generalized macular rash develops that resembles the eruption of measles. Initially the rash blanches with pressure, but after 24 to 48 hours the eruption frequently becomes petechial or, in the more severe cases, hemorrhagic. In mild illnesses, or in previously vaccinated persons, the rash may be minimal. Central nervous system symptoms in the form of agitation, insomnia, delirium, or coma usually appear by the end of the first week of fever. It is during the second week of fever that the most critical circulatory and pulmonary complications of the disease occur. Gangrene of the extremities or other dependent parts and pneumonia are sometimes seen in untreated patients. Fever usually abates by the end of the second week, and full recovery commonly takes several weeks or months in untreated patients.

Diagnosis. Rocky Mountain spotted fever should always be considered in the differential diagnosis of a febrile illness with rash occurring in the months of May through September in the United States. The most common initial diagnosis of illness for patients subsequently found to have Rocky Mountain spotted fever is measles, despite the fact that measles usually does not occur during the period when Rocky Mountain spotted fever is most common. As in all the rickettsial diseases, the initial diagnosis must be made solely on clinical grounds because confirmatory laboratory tests are of no assistance until relatively late in the illness. The symptoms, physical findings, and history of exposure in an area known to harbor ticks must be weighed carefully by the physician, and, if the diagnosis is considered probable, treatment should be initiated. Two other rickettsial diseases, rickettsialpox and murine typhus, may mimic mild cases of Rocky Mountain spotted fever. Fortunately both respond equally well to treatment appropriate for Rocky Mountain spotted fever.

Laboratory confirmation of the clinical diagnosis may be obtained by isolation of *R. rickettsi* from the blood during the first week of illness. *Isolation studies in guinea pigs or embryonated eggs should be attempted only by laboratories equipped for such work because of the danger of infection of laboratory personnel.* More commonly, laboratory diagnosis depends upon serologic tests with paired serum samples, the first obtained as early as possible during illness and the second about the fifteenth to twenty-fifth day of disease. These tests utilize either the Weil-Felix Proteus OX-19 and OX-2 agglutination reactions or the complement-fixation test with yolk sac antigen. In the agglutination test, positive results may be

*Source: Morbidity and Mortality Weekly Report, Communicable Disease Center, United States Public Health Service.

obtained with either or both of the OX-19 or OX-2 antigens; approximately 15 per cent of patients may show no rise in Weil-Felix titers even though complement-fixation tests are positive.* A fourfold or greater rise in titer with the complement-fixation test is considered confirmatory.

Treatment and Prognosis. Until 1945 treatment of Rocky Mountain spotted fever was limited to supportive therapy; mortality rates were 20 per cent or greater. In 1945, para-aminobenzoic acid (PABA) was shown to be effective in treatment, producing defervescence in approximately three days and reducing mortality virtually to zero. By the early 1950's, chloramphenicol and the tetracyclines replaced PABA in the treatment of this disease because the newer antimicrobial drugs were equally effective as PABA and far better tolerated. In the majority of patients, headache and other symptoms abate within 24 to 48 hours, and fever disappears within three to four days after beginning therapy with 25 mg per kilogram per day of the tetracyclines or 50 mg per kilogram per day of chloramphenicol, given in four divided doses by mouth. With either regimen, treatment should be continued for 24 to 48 hours after the patient becomes afebrile. The physician must weigh the disadvantages of gastric irritation or the dangers of use in renal insufficiency associated with the tetracyclines against the risks of blood dyscrasias with chloramphenicol. In general, because of the greater seriousness of the toxicity to chloramphenicol, tetracycline is the preferred therapy. For patients too ill to take oral medication, parenteral preparations must be used; when these are necessary, the patient will also require intravenous fluids to correct electrolyte or fluid abnormalities. Corticosteroids may also be of help for severely ill patients.

The most important step in treatment is early diagnosis; no amount of drug therapy can modify the course of the disease in the patient who is admitted in extremis. Heroic measures such as corticosteroid therapy and parenteral administration of antimicrobials are completely unnecessary if the diagnosis is made and treatment begun early in the course of the disease. Early treatment will also prevent sequelae such as brain or heart damage, which have been observed in patients who have been treated late in their illness.

Prevention. Although protective vaccine is available, its use has descreased markedly in recent years, presumably because effective antimicrobial therapy is now available. Nevertheless, use of the vaccine is appropriate for selected persons who may be exposed to the danger of infection in remote areas in which medical treatment may be difficult or impossible to obtain.

Because ticks cannot transmit infection to man without having been attached for several hours, a degree of protection can be achieved by careful examination of one's person and careful removal of attached ticks on a twice daily schedule. Considerable difference of opinion exists regarding the safest method of removal. The use of a lighted cigarette or the application of kerosene, both highly regarded in some circles, appears to have the disadvantage that agonal responses of the tick may cause actual expression of rickettsiae into the wound. Another method appears to be preferable: the tick is grasped by the head and thorax with a pair of fine forceps and pulled gently but firmly until the mouth parts are extracted from the skin. The third category of control measures is directed against the tick vector of the disease. The use of clothing impregnated with tick repellents provides significant protection to those who must travel through tick-infested areas. When groups of people may be exposed to ticks in summer camps or recreational areas, the selective use of residual insecticides, such as DDT, dieldrin, or lindane, has proved effective in limited areas in reducing tick populations.

*See Ch. 163 for discussion of the Weil-Felix reaction.

Lackman, D. B., Bell, E. J., Stoenner, H. G., and Pickens, E. G.: The Rocky Mountain spotted fever group of rickettsias. Health Lab. Sci., 2:135, 1965.

Ricketts, H. T.: Contributions to Medical Science by Howard Taylor Ricketts, 1870–1910. Chicago, University of Chicago Press, 1911, p. 278.

Wisseman, C. L., Jr. (ed.): Symposium on the Spotted Fever Group of Rickettsiae. Medical Science Publication No. 7, Walter Reed Army Institute of Research. Washington, D.C., U.S. Government Printing Office, 1960.

Woodward, T. E., and Jackson, E. B.: Spotted fever rickettsiae. *In* Horsfall, F. L., Jr., and Tamm, I. (eds.): Viral and Rickettsial Infections of Man. 4th ed. Philadelphia, J. B. Lippincott Company, 1965, p. 1095.

Zdrodovskii, P. F., and Golinevich, H. M.: The Rickettsial Diseases. New York, Pergamon Press, 1960, p. 277.

165. TICK-BORNE RICKETTSIOSES OF THE EASTERN HEMISPHERE

*Herbert L. Ley, Jr.**

Definition. The three diseases that constitute this group, i.e., *African tick typhus, North Asian tick-borne rickettsiosis,* and *Queensland tick typhus,* are caused by rickettsiae that are closely related to one another and to the agent of Rocky Mountain spotted fever. Each is transmitted by the bite of an ixodid tick.

African tick typhus *(Boutonneuse fever)* may be regarded as the prototype of the group. It is the most widely distributed geographically, occurring throughout the African continent, in those parts of Europe and the Middle East adjacent to the Mediterranean, Black and Caspian Seas, and in India. Boutonneuse fever is a mild to moderately severe febrile illness of a few days' to two weeks' duration. It is characterized by a primary lesion that develops at the site of the infected tick bite and a generalized maculopapular erythematous rash that appears about the fourth day. As in Rocky Mountain spotted fever, agglutinins against Proteus OX-19 (Weil-Felix reaction) usually appear during convalescence, as do specific complement-fixing antibodies against the rickettsial organisms.

History, Distribution, Etiology, and Epidemiology. Boutonneuse fever was first recognized in 1910 in Tunisia by Conor and Bruch. During the next several decades the occurrence of similar diseases was noted in Africa, Europe, and the Middle East; these were given various local names. However, it was not until modern serologic methods employing specific rickettsial antigens were applied that *Rickettsia conori* was shown to be the etio-

*Ch. 164 to 169 have been written to replace articles on the same subjects prepared for previous editions by the author's former teacher and colleague, the late Dr. Joseph E. Smadel. Thus, Dr. Smadel's many contributions to these subjects understandably permeate the whole section. For this chapter on Tick-Borne Rickettsioses, however, the present author found it inadvisable to do more than make trivial changes and update the references so that, to all intents and purposes, it is as it was originally prepared by Dr. Smadel.

logic agent for a single widely disseminated disease, African tick typhus. Queensland tick typhus caused by *R. australis* was established as an entity during World War II. Although the rickettsial nature of North Asian tick-borne rickettsiosis was demonstrated in 1938, only in recent years has its etiologic agent, *R. siberica,* been clearly differentiated from other members of the spotted fever group of organisms.

The etiologic agents of the three diseases of the Eastern Hemisphere are all members of the spotted fever group of rickettsiae. Together with *R. rickettsi* and *R. akari* they possess common group antigens that are readily demonstrated by agglutination and complement-fixation procedures. In addition, type-specific antigens characterize each member of the spotted fever group; these are demonstrated by similar in vitro serologic procedures employing specially purified antigens. *Rickettsia conori, R. australis,* and *R. siberica* may be differentiated from one another and from *R. rickettsi* and *R. akari* by complement-fixation tests using antisera from mice, by cross-vaccination tests performed in guinea pigs, or by cross-neutralization tests using the mouse lethal toxin obtained from each agent and homologous antisera. Experimental infection of animals with one member of the spotted fever group of rickettsiae induces appreciable resistance to infection with other members.

For the most part, the *epidemiology* of the three tick-borne rickettsioses of the Eastern Hemisphere resembles that of spotted fever in the Western Hemisphere. Thus, the rickettsial agents are maintained in nature by cycles involving ixodid ticks and small wild animals; man, if he intrudes into the cycles, serves as a dead end in the chain of transmission. Boutonneuse fever in the Mediterranean area has a more domesticated and urbanized pattern. Here, another cycle is also involved with the brown dog tick as the vector and the dog as the animal host.

Pathology. In fatal cases, which are few and usually limited to the aged and debilitated, the findings are similar to those in Rocky Mountain spotted fever except for the presence of the *tache noire,* the black button-like necrotic primary lesion that is generally found on the surface areas of the body ordinarily covered by clothing. The basic pathologic changes are found in the small blood vessels (see Ch. 164).

Symptoms, Laboratory Findings, and Diagnosis. The three tick-borne rickettsioses that occur in different parts of the Eastern Hemisphere resemble one another closely. After an incubation period of about five to seven days, the disease begins with fever, headache, malaise, and conjunctival injection. The primary lesion, which is present in most cases at the onset of fever, consists of a small ulcer 2 to 5 mm in diameter with a black center and a red areola; the regional lymph nodes are enlarged. The generalized erythematous maculopapular rash appears about the fourth day and quickly involves most of the body, including the palms and soles and often the face. In severe cases the rash becomes hemorrhagic. Fever abates during the second week. The prognosis is good except in the aged and debilitated. Complications and sequelae are unusual.

The laboratory findings of greatest importance are those derived from the Weil-Felix and rickettsial complement-fixation tests. Agglutinins against Proteus OX-19 develop during the second week and complement-fixing antibodies appear shortly thereafter.

Diagnosis is established by the clinical picture, including the *tache noire,* the geographic location, and positive serologic reactions. In the differential diagnosis the typhus fevers, meningococcal infections, and measles must be considered.

Treatment. Adequate information is available to indicate that treatment with the broad-spectrum antimicrobial drugs is as effective in patients with African tick typhus as in those with other rickettsioses (see Ch. 164 for details of therapy). Presumably, these measures are also applicable to the other two tick-borne rickettsioses of the Eastern Hemisphere.

Prophylaxis. Prevention of human disease is based on avoiding the bites of infected ticks. In Ch. 164 are set forth details regarding personal prophylaxis, including the use of chemical insect repellents, and for reduction of tick population by measures involved in terrain control. Experimental vaccines prepared from formalin-treated yolk sac tissue infected with each of the Eastern Hemisphere rickettsiae under discussion are effective in animals, but commercial vaccines for human use are not available.

Bozeman, F. M., Humphries, J. W., Campbell, J. M., and O'Hara, P. L.: Laboratory studies of the spotted fever group of rickettsiae. *In* Wisseman, C. L., Jr. (ed.): Symposium on the Spotted Fever Group of Rickettsiae. Medical Science Publication No. 7, Walter Reed Army Institute of Research. Washington, D.C., U.S. Government Printing Office, 1960, p. 7.

Freyche, M. J., and Deutschman, Z.: Human rickettsioses in Africa. Epidemiol. Vital Stat. Rep., WHO 3:161, 1950.

Woodward, T. E., and Jackson, E. B.: Spotted fever rickettsiae. *In* Horsfall, F. L., Jr., and Tamm, I. (eds.): Viral and Rickettsial Infections of Man. 4th ed. Philadelphia, J. B. Lippincott Company, 1965, p. 1095.

Zdrodovskii, P. I., and Golinevich, H. M.: The Rickettsial Diseases. New York, Pergamon Press, 1960, p. 292.

166. RICKETTSIALPOX

Herbert L. Ley, Jr.

Definition. Rickettsialpox is a mite-borne rickettsial disease, mild and self-limited, which is characterized by an initial eschar-like lesion and a fever of a week's duration accompanied by headache, backache, and a generalized papulovesicular rash.

Etiology. The disease is caused by *Rickettsia akari,* a member of the spotted fever group of rickettsia. Although *R. akari* possesses an antigen in common with *Rickettsia rickettsi,* it is most closely related to *Rickettsia australis,* the agent of North Queensland tick typhus. The organism is transmitted to man, with an incubation period of 10 to 24 days, by the bite of the mouse mite, *Allodermanyssus sanguineus.*

Incidence and Distribution. The incidence of the disease is difficult to determine. In the first three years after the disease was described in 1946, 500 cases were reported in the United States, most of them from New York City. Reporting of the disease has decreased markedly since that time. It is likely that small numbers of cases continue to occur without being reported because the disease is one in which national reporting is not required. The disease has been reported from Boston, West Haven, Connecticut, New York, Philadelphia, Pittsburgh, and Cleveland in the United States, and from the U.S.S.R.

Epidemiology. When the disease was first described in 1946–1947, in a New York apartment housing project, the investigators demonstrated the presence of the agent in both the commensal mouse, *Mus musculus,* and its mite ectoparasite, *A. sanguineus,* both of which were present in large numbers. The single piece of information that was missing from the initial study was the manner in which the disease agent, *R. akari,* entered the mouse and mite populations. The subsequent isolation from a field mouse in Korea of a rickettsial agent indistinguishable from *R. akari* suggests that the agent may be widely distributed among feral rodents and their ectoparasites. If this view is correct, the disease may be expected to occur in areas of expanding suburbia where man and commensal populations of domestic mice come into contact with feral mice and their ectoparasites.

Pathology. Because rickettsialpox is a benign infection with no reported deaths, pathologic examination has been limited to biopsy material. The initial lesion or eschar resembles the eschars of scrub typhus and boutonneuse fever. The skin lesion of the early rash is characterized by perivascular infiltration with mononuclear cells. During the later stages of the rash when vesiculation occurs, the histologic changes are highly characteristic and consist of necrosis of the superficial epithelial cells, leading to an intra-epidermal vesicle. Clinical laboratory findings are limited to a minimal leukopenia during the febrile period.

Clinical Manifestations. The first sign of infection is the initial lesion or eschar, which appears approximately a week before onset of fever. Most patients are unaware of the small papule that develops at the site of the infecting mite bite, or if they note it, they interpret it as a "pimple." The lesion begins as a small papule that enlarges slowly to 0.5 to 1.5 cm in diameter, develops a central vesicle, and finally forms a dark crust without pustulation. Except for the lack of itching, tenderness, or pustulation, the lesion resembles that of a primary vaccinia reaction, and usually leaves a small scar. When searched for carefully, the initial lesion will be found in over 90 per cent of cases.

About a week after the appearance of the initial lesion, fever of an intermittent type develops, with chills or chilly sensations and drenching sweats. After approximately a week the fever gradually subsides. The early febrile period is characterized by headache, photophobia, marked lassitude, and muscle pains, including backache. Beginning on the first to fourth days of fever a maculopapular rash appears, which develops into a vesiculopapular rash. The vesicles are firm, sometimes surrounded by erythema, and on drying form a dark crust that falls off without leaving a scar. In contrast to chickenpox, the rash appears on many areas of the body at almost the same time and does not itch; it is absent from the palms and soles.

Physical examination during the febrile period yields little additional information. An enlarged spleen or lymphadenopathy will be found in only a few cases. The differential diagnosis very early in the disease should include measles, chickenpox, and smallpox; with the appearance of the vesicles only the latter two diseases need be considered. The presence of an initial lesion, the more superficial position of the vesicle, and the persistence of the papular base throughout the period of rash argue strongly for rickettsialpox rather than chickenpox. Smallpox lesions resemble those of rickettsialpox, but progress to pustules. In addition, the constitutional symptoms of most patients with smallpox are considerably more severe than those of patients with rickettsialpox.

Diagnosis. The clinical characteristics of the disease are so distinctive that in most patients a presumptive diagnosis may be made on clinical grounds. Chickenpox in adults poses the most difficult diagnostic problem. Laboratory confirmation of the diagnosis is possible by isolation of the agent from blood obtained during the acute phase of illness and also by complement-fixation tests on paired specimens of serum. Because the agent of rickettsialpox is closely related to that of Rocky Mountain spotted fever, complement-fixation tests may be performed with antigen prepared from either organism. A fourfold or greater rise in antibody titer may be expected in patients with rickettsialpox when the acute phase specimen is collected early in the febrile period and the convalescent specimen is collected three to four weeks after onset of disease. The Weil-Felix agglutination reaction is of no diagnostic value in rickettsialpox.

Treatment and Prognosis. The disease may be so mild in some patients that no specific treatment may be indicated. When therapy is desirable, the tetracyclines may be used in oral doses of 25 mg per kilogram per day for three or four days. Response to treatment is rapid; most patients become afebrile in 24 to 36 hours. Relapses of infection have not been reported. The course of the disease is benign and the prognosis is excellent.

Control. The principal target of preventive measures is the mite vector of the disease, *A. sanguineus,* which may be controlled by the use of residual insecticides (DDT or dieldrin) in areas of mouse harborage. Vector control should be achieved prior to initiating mouse control measures to avoid further dispersal of the mites in their search for food. No vaccine is currently available.

Dolgopol, V. B.: Histologic changes in rickettsialpox. Am. J. Path., 24:119, 1948.

Greenberg, M., Pelliteri, O., Klein, I. F., and Huebner, R. J.: Rickettsialpox—a newly recognized rickettsial disease. II. Clinical observations. J.A.M.A., 133:901, 1947.

Lackman, D. B.: A review of information on rickettsialpox in the United States. Clin Pediatr. (Phila.), 2:296, 1963.

Roueché, B.: The alerting of Mr. Pomerantz. *In* Roueché, B.: Eleven Blue Men. Boston, Little, Brown and Company, 1954, p. 48.

167. SCRUB TYPHUS (Tsutsugamushi Disease, Mite-Borne Typhus, Japanese River Fever, Tropical Typhus, Rural Typhus)

Herbert L. Ley, Jr.

Definition. Scrub typhus is a mite-borne rickettsial disease that occurs in Southeast Asia and adjacent areas and is characterized by fever, headache, lymphadenopathy, conjunctival injection, a maculopapular rash, and, in most patients, a distinctive eschar or skin lesion.

Etiology. The disease is caused by *Rickettsia tsutsugamushi (R. orientalis),* a group of rickettsial agents that produces a single distinctive clinical syndrome in man, but is characterized by extreme variation in antigenic composition of organisms isolated in different geographic areas and even in adjacent foci of the disease within the same country. All strains of *R. tsutsugamushi* can be propagated in mice and embryonated eggs; some strains will also produce disease in the guinea pig. Because of antigenic variation in the organisms, complement-fixing antibodies produced in response to infection in man appear to be specific only for the infecting or closely related strains. Nevertheless, all strains of *R. tsutsugamushi* have the potential of stimulating Weil-Felix Proteus OX-K agglutinins in man.

Distribution and Incidence. The disease occurs in a roughly triangular area of Southeast Asia and adjacent countries approximately 5,000,000 square miles in extent. The western apex of the triangle is located in Pakistan, the northern in north Japan, and the southern in the north coastal areas of Australia. It is impossible to obtain reliable data on the incidence of the disease among the indigenous populations of the area. However, World War II provided numerous examples of explosive outbreaks of the disease in military units in the Asiatic-Pacific area. In one such outbreak among British troops in Ceylon, 756 patients were hospitalized with scrub typhus as a result of a four-day jungle training exercise. American forces operating on the islands of Owi and Biak experienced over 1000 cases of the disease in less than two months. During the period from 1942 to 1945, nearly 16,000 cases of the disease occurred in American, British, and Australian troops alone. At present the disease is reported sporadically among the people of Southeast Asia and becomes a major medical problem only when development projects or recreational activities bring groups of people into contact with foci of the disease in nature.

Epidemiology. Like Rocky Mountain spotted fever, scrub typhus is principally a disease of rodents and their ectoparasites that is propagated in a "silent" cycle in nature, involving man only when he unwittingly comes into contact with the mites that transmit the disease. A variety of rodents, chiefly rats and feral mice, have been shown to be infected in nature. The disease in these animals is relatively mild but is associated with a rickettsemia that provides an opportunity to infect mites feeding on the animals during their illness. In some areas ground birds have also been implicated in the disease cycle in nature. The vector mite in most areas is a species of the genus Leptotrombiculidium highly adapted to the local ecology, although mites of the genus Schongastia have been shown to transmit the agent in the less important jungle cycle of the disease. The mite vectors are free-living, feeding upon vegetation and insect eggs, except in their larval stage, during which they must obtain a meal of tissue fluid from a vertebrate host in order to complete their maturation to the adult stage. The mites are not only capable of transmitting *R. tsutsugamushi* to their vertebrate host during this feeding but are also capable of transmitting the agent to their offspring transovarially. Thus the mite is both a vector and a reservoir for scrub typhus, just as is the tick for Rocky Mountain spotted fever. The highly specific ecologic requirements for propagation of the mite in terms of temperature, humidity, and food sources, coupled with its limited range of locomotion, lead to the formation of "mite islands," highly localized in terms of both geographic and seasonal distributions. In some exceptional areas, such as Malaysia, the mite population is present throughout the year. More commonly, the mites are highly seasonal in appearance, and are most numerous during the warm, moist months of the year, although one focus of infection in southern Japan is characterized by a winter peak of mite population. The seasonal distribution of scrub typhus understandably parallels the distribution of the mite vector. Man exposes himself to infection by transferring mites from vegetation to his body; most infections have followed contact with grassy "scrub" areas or straw cut from them. The disease may occur elsewhere because infected mites have been found in other habitats.

Pathology. As with the other rickettsioses, the basic lesion is one of inflammation of the walls of the small blood vessels with perivascular infiltration of mononuclear cells. Pneumonitis and a diffuse myocarditis with mononuclear infiltration of the myocardium are frequently observed at autopsy. Gross pathologic findings are usually limited to enlargement of the spleen, lymphadenopathy, and the cutaneous eschar of the disease.

Clinical Manifestations. The initial symptoms of the disease, frontal headache and temperature of 40 to 40.5° C, follow the infecting mite bite by 6 to 21 days. Physical examination at onset reveals only generalized lymphadenopathy, conjunctival injection, and, in most Caucasian patients, the developing eschar. This skin lesion, absent in most Asian patients, appears first as a small papule at the site of the mite bite and enlarges during the first few days of fever to approximately 1 cm in size. On this papular base a multilocular vesicle develops that evolves into the flat, black eschar characteristic of the disease. Regional lymph nodes draining the area of the eschar may become painful, and may enlarge to the size of an acorn. About the end of the first week of fever a generalized macular rash appears, which may last only a few hours or may develop to a livid maculopapular eruption of a week's duration. In untreated patients complications such as pneumonitis, encephalitis, and cardiac failure occur late in the second week of fever; if the patient survives, defervescence begins about the fifteenth day of fever.

Diagnosis. Early diagnosis of the disease must be based on the clinical findings and the history of exposure in an endemic area. Laboratory confirmation of the diagnosis is based on isolation from blood of the agent in mice or on a rise in Weil-Felix OX-K agglutinins in serum during the course of illness. If the acute specimen is obtained before the tenth day of fever and the late specimen is obtained during the third week of illness, fourfold or greater rises in Weil-Felix OX-K titers will be observed in almost all untreated patients and in three fourths of those receiving antimicrobial therapy. Because of strain variation in the etiologic agent, the complement-fixation test is unsatisfactory in the laboratory diagnosis of the disease. Clinical laboratory data are of little assistance in diagnosis; patients usually show only a moderate leukopenia. The differential diagnosis of the disease should include leptospirosis, typhoid fever, dengue, murine typhus, and malaria.

Treatment. The tetracyclines are the therapeutic agents of choice for scrub typhus at oral dosage levels of 25 mg per kilogram per day. Chloramphenicol has also been used at oral dosage levels of 50 mg per kilogram per day. Both drugs carry with them some risk of toxicity, but the nature of the major risk with chloramphenicol (aplastic anemia) is such that its use is distinctly less preferable. Drug therapy may be discontinued 24 hours after defervescence, which usually occurs within 36 hours after beginning therapy. Relapses have been observed in patients treated during the first week of fever; continuation of therapy through the fourteenth day of disease, or the administration of single 3.0 gram oral doses of drug on the seventh and fourteenth days after cessation of the initial course of antimicrobial therapy will prevent recrudescences of infection. The relapses occur because the antimicrobial drugs are not eradicative.

Prognosis and Mortality. Before effective treatment was available, mortality from scrub typhus was appreciable, varying from 5 to 40 per cent. Early antimicrobial therapy has essentially limited deaths from the disease. If the patient is treated in the first week of illness he is usually ready to resume full activity in several weeks.

Prevention. Preventive measures are directed at minimizing contact of man with the mites transmitting the disease. The application of residual miticides such as dieldrin or lindane to large areas of terrain will permit safe continuation of operations in rubber plantations and similar industrial activities that bring workers into contact with areas previously known to be the source of numerous infections. When area miticide application is impracticable, as in military operations, the use of clothing impregnated with mite repellents provides significant protection against infection.

Audy, J. R.: The ecology of scrub typhus. *In* May, J. M. (ed.): Studies in Disease Ecology. New York, Hafner Publishing Company, Inc., 1961, p. 389.

Sheehy, T. W., Hazlett, D., and Turk, R. E.: Scrub typhus: A comparison of chloramphenicol and tetracycline in its treatment. Arch. Intern. Med., 132:77, 1973.

Smadel, J. E.: Influence of antibiotics on immunologic responses in scrub typhus. Am. J. Med., 17:246, 1954.

Smadel, J. E., and Elisberg, B. L.: Scrub typhus rickettsia. *In* Horsfall, F. L., Jr., and Tamm, I. (eds.): Viral and Rickettsial Infections of Man. 4th ed. Philadelphia, J. B. Lippincott Company, 1965, p. 1130.

Tamiya, T. (ed.): Recent Advances in Studies of Tsutsugamushi Disease in Japan. Tokyo, Medical Culture Inc., 1962.

Traub, R., and Wisseman, C. L., Jr.: Ecological considerations in scrub typhus. Bull. WHO, 39:209, 1968.

168. TRENCH FEVER (Five-Day or Quintana Fever, Shin Bone Fever, Volhynian Fever)

Herbert L. Ley, Jr.

Definition. Trench fever is a self-limited louse-borne rickettsial disease characterized by intermittent fever, generalized aches and pains, negligible mortality, and multiple relapses.

Etiology and Epidemiology. The disease is caused by *Rickettsia quintana,* a rickettsial agent that grows extracellularly in the louse intestine and is excreted in louse feces. Transmission takes place by rubbing louse feces into skin abrasions or into the bite wound left by the louse. The incubation period of the disease may vary from 5 to 38 days, but is usually two to four weeks. The disease was a major military problem during World War I, when an estimated 1,000,000 cases occurred in western Europe. It was not seen in epidemic form again until World War II when 80,000 cases were reported in eastern Europe. Recent studies have demonstrated the disease in endemic form in Mexico. During epidemics man is clearly the principal reservoir. He may also be the major long-term reservoir because the disease agent has been isolated from asymptomatic patients years after their initial infection.

Pathology and Clinical Manifestations. Because the disease has a negligible mortality, information on the histopathologic changes is limited. Biopsy studies reveal only perivascular inflammation, principally in the form of lymphocytic infiltrations. The presenting symptoms of the disease are recurrent fever, severe weakness, headache, dizziness, back and leg pains (particularly in the shins), and photophobia. Physical and laboratory examinations are not remarkable except for slight enlargement of the spleen and liver, areas of cutaneous tenderness distributed over the body, and a moderate leukocytosis. A transient rash of erythematous macules or papules occurs in about 70 per cent of patients. The patient's fever may rise as high as 40.5° C in an irregular fashion with intervals of nearly normal temperature between peaks of fever. The fever may last for only four or five days in the more fortunate patients. In others, the initial pyrexia may be followed after five or six days of normal temperature by one to eight relapses of fever similar to the initial episode. In still other patients, the initial fever may decline, shading into relapses without a true afebrile period, producing a "saddleback" or "typhoidal" fever curve.

Diagnosis. The most important fact supporting the diagnosis of trench fever is a history of contact with lice within the incubation period of the disease. Xenodiagnosis—the feeding of clean uninfected lice on a patient suspected of having the disease—is a useful diagnostic aid. The lice are examined a week after feeding on the patient for the presence of rickettsiae in the lumen of the gut. The technique of cultivation of *R. quintana* on blood agar containing 10 per cent of fresh blood has also been used diagnostically. Recently developed serologic tests appear promising in the diagnosis of the disease. The differential diagnosis of the disease should include leptospirosis, dengue, malaria, relapsing fever, and the typhus fevers.

Treatment and Prognosis. Although the tetracyclines and other antimicrobials may be expected to be as effective in the treatment of trench fever as in the treatment of the other rickettsial diseases, in the absence of epidemics of trench fever no reliable information about their efficacy is available. Because the disease has a negligible mortality, the long-term prognosis is excellent. Even without treatment the majority of patients are able to return to full activity within one to two months after onset, although a few continue to experience recurrences of the symptoms of infection for months or years.

Prevention. The only practicable method of control of trench fever is the elimination of the louse vector of the disease by dusting clothing with residual insecticides. Ten per cent DDT powders proved highly effective for louse control during the World War II period, but the development of DDT resistance in lice in many parts of the world has forced the use of 1 per cent lindane or 1 per cent malathion powders. For additional comments on louse control, see Ch. 163.

Trench Fever: Report of Commission on Trench Fever. American Red Cross Medical Research Committee. London, Oxford University Press, 1918.

Varela, G., Vinson, J. W., and Molina-Pasquel, C.: Trench fever. II. Propagation of *Rickettsia quintana* on cell-free medium from the blood of two patients. Am. J. Trop. Med., 18:708, 1969.

Vinson, J. W., Varela, G., and Molina-Pasquel, C.: Trench fever. III. Induction of clinical disease in volunteers inoculated with *Rickettsia quintana* propagated on blood agar. Am. J. Trop. Med., 18:713, 1969.
Warren, J.: Trench fever rickettsia. *In* Horsfall, F. L., Jr., and Tamm, I. (eds.): Viral and Rickettsial Infections of Man. 4th ed. Philadelphia, J. B. Lippincott Company, 1965, p. 1161.

169. Q FEVER

Herbert L. Ley, Jr.

Definition. Q fever is a self-limited rickettsial infection characterized by fever, headache, and constitutional symptoms, associated, in approximately half the patients, with a pneumonitis. It is unique among the rickettsial diseases of man in that human infection is most commonly acquired by inhalation of the agent rather than by contact with an arthropod vector.

Etiology. The disease is caused by *Coxiella burnetii,* a rickettsial agent having the general biologic characteristics of this class of microorganisms but possessing, in addition, a resistance to desiccation and to exposure in dusts and soils that is unique among the rickettsiae. The organism may be propagated in embryonated eggs and in mice, hamsters, and guinea pigs, and has frequently infected laboratory personnel engaged in isolation studies on clinical material. Both patients and animals develop agglutinating and complement-fixing antibodies for the agent. On the other hand, *C. burnetii,* unlike most of the other rickettsiae, does not stimulate the production of Weil-Felix Proteus agglutinins in man.

Incidence and Distribution. The true incidence of the disease in the human population is impossible to determine because the majority of infections are undiagnosed. Isolated serologic surveys have revealed that many persons exposed to infection in sheep and cattle ranches, abattoirs, meat packing plants, or wool processing plants present serologic evidence of past infection. More detailed investigation of animals and arthropods on a worldwide basis has shown *C. burnetii* to be ubiquitous in distribution except for the countries of Denmark, Finland, Ireland, the Netherlands, Norway, and Sweden. In the United States the disease, first recognized in the states of Montana and California, is now recognized as prevalent in most of the states in which sheep and cattle are produced. Small numbers of cases have been reported for most of the remaining states.

Epidemiology. The epidemiology of the disease is complex because it involves two major patterns of transmission. The first pattern, described in Australia, is a disease cycle in wild animals with transmission of the agent from animal to animal by a tick vector. Although the species of animal and arthropod vary from country to country, such a cycle has been demonstrated in Australia in two forms, bandicoot-tick-cattle and kangaroo-tick-sheep. In both these cycles the agent can be transmitted indefinitely as an inapparent infection in the wild reservoir (bandicoot or kangaroo) by ticks, but it may also be transmitted laterally by arthropod to a domestic animal in close contact with man. In these and similar cycles recognized in other parts of the world, *C. burnetii,* like the other rickettsial agents of human disease, is vector-transmitted.

However, Q fever patients rarely give a history of tick bite. Human infection with the agent has now been shown to occur almost exclusively by a second transmission pattern capable of sustaining itself independently of the wild animal cycle. The reservoirs of infection in the second pattern are animals domesticated by man, principally cattle, sheep, and goats, in which *C. burnetii* produces only an inapparent or mild infection. In sheep, Q fever organisms are excreted in very large numbers in placental tissue, and to a lesser degree in birth fluids, milk, and feces. In the cow, and probably the goat, excretion occurs mainly through the placenta and milk. *With all infected animals, the period of parturition is associated with the formation of a primary infectious aerosol, easily demonstrated by air-sampling studies.* Such aerosols infect other cattle in the herd and also the human population in direct contact with the animals. Further, because contaminated clothing, wool, hides, bedding, and soil may be the source of secondary aerosols, *the infections may be transmitted via these vehicles at considerable distances from the infected cattle;* in certain circumstances these distances are measurable in miles. The unique resistance of *C. burnetii* to prolonged exposure in nature contributes to the spread of the agent by such infectious microenvironments. Within California, where the local epidemiology of the disease has been studied in great detail, sheep are the major reservoir for human infection in the northern part of the state and cattle in the southern part. In the latter area milk may be a vehicle of infection if consumed raw. Although the pulmonary route is the most important portal of access of the agent to man, the transmission of the rickettsia from man to man by this method is rare, despite the occurrence of an infectious pneumonitis in some patients.

Pathology. Because the mortality rate is low, postmortem studies have been limited. In those patients having a pneumonitis, the histopathology is similar to that seen in the viral pneumonias and psittacosis. Recent studies in patients have directed attention to hepatic pathology during the acute phase of the disease, demonstrable both in biochemical abnormalities of liver function (elevated cephalin-cholesterol flocculation, alkaline phosphatase, and thymol turbidity tests) and in histologic abnormalities in biopsy specimens (focal inflammation and granulomas). Q fever endocarditis, producing valvular vegetations from which rickettsiae may be isolated, has also been described.

Clinical Manifestations. After an incubation period of 9 to 20 days after respiratory exposure, most patients complain of an abrupt onset of fever, headache, muscle pains, and severe malaise. The temperature may rise as high as 40° C and remain elevated, with considerable fluctuation, for one to three weeks. Occasionally, patients may suffer a prolonged fever of several months' duration. In contrast to the other rickettsial infections, there is no rash. In approximately half the patients there is roentgenographic evidence of pneumonitis, manifested clinically as a slight, nonproductive cough developing in the second week of fever.

Diagnosis. Q fever should always be suspected in a patient having a febrile illness for which no obvious cause can be found. If the patient's occupation brings him into contact with sheep, cattle, or goats, or byproducts such as wool or hides, particular care should be exercised to exclude Q fever from consideration. The presence of Q fever should be suspected in any patient in whom the differential diagnosis includes viral pneumonia, psittacosis, primary atypical pneumonia, pulmonary mycotic disease, or comparable infections. Furthermore, recent data would also support consideration of Q fever in the differential diagnoses of endocarditis and of hepatitis with or without jaundice.

Diagnostic laboratory studies usually must be limited to serologic studies because of the extensive history of accidentally acquired laboratory infections resulting from attempts at isolation. Either complement-fixation or agglutination tests may be employed, and with either test a fourfold or greater rise in titer of antibody may be expected to occur between the first and fourth weeks of illness. Recent reports have emphasized the importance of both strain and phase variation in the selection of antigens for diagnostic use.

Treatment and Prognosis. The tetracyclines or chloramphenicol are both effective in treatment of acute infections with *C. burnetii,* but because of the nature of chloramphenicol toxicity, the tetracyclines are definitely to be preferred. The dosage of antimicrobial given should be the same as that for epidemic typhus or Rocky Mountain spotted fever. The mortality is low (1 per cent or less), even in untreated patients, and is lower still in those treated with antimicrobial drugs. Therapy should be continued for approximately one week even though the patient usually becomes afebrile within 48 hours. Patients occasionally may experience relapses after treatment, and when this complication occurs additional drug therapy should be administered. Prognosis is less favorable for the rare patient in whom Q fever endocarditis develops. In some of these patients the disease has been reported to have been unresponsive to antimicrobial therapy, although favorable results have been reported in one patient treated with trimethoprim and sulfamethoxazole.

Prevention. Experimental lots of yolk-sac vaccines have been effective in prevention of clinical disease in volunteers experimentally infected via the respiratory route. Because this vaccine is not commercially available, control measures are limited to minimizing exposure to the agent. In particular, milk from cattle, sheep, and goats in endemic areas should be pasteurized or boiled before use. Because rickettsiae are excreted in the sputum and urine of patients, these materials should be disinfected by autoclaving to prevent secondary infection in hospitals.

Freeman, R., and Hodson, M. E.: Q fever endocarditis treated with trimethoprim and sulphamethoxazole. Br. Med. J., 1:419, 1972.

Grist, N. R.: Q fever endocarditis. Am. Heart J., 75:846, 1968.

Johnson, J. E., and Kadull, P. J.: Laboratory-acquired Q fever: A report of fifty cases. Am. J. Med., 41:391, 1966.

Ormsbee, R. A.: Q fever rickettsia. *In* Horsfall, F. L., Jr., and Tamm, I. (eds.): Viral and Rickettsial Infections of Man. 4th ed. Philadelphia, J. B. Lippincott Company, 1965, p. 1144.

Powell, O. W.: Liver involvement in "Q" fever. Aust. Ann. Med., 10:52, 1961.

Tigertt, W. D., and Benenson, A. S.: Studies on Q fever in man. Trans. Assoc. Am. Physicians, 69:98, 1956.

170. BARTONELLOSIS (Carrión's Disease, Oroya Fever, Verruga Peruana)

Herbert L. Ley, Jr.

Definition. Bartonellosis is an insect-borne microbial disease limited to South America. It is characterized by two distinctive clinical stages. The first of these (Oroya fever) presents a severe febrile infection associated with a marked anemia, bone and joint pains, bacteremia, and an appreciable mortality. The second stage (verruga peruana) is more benign and is distinguished by the appearance of a generalized eruption of hemangiomatous papules and nodules.

Etiology. The disease is caused by *Bartonella bacilliformis,* a small gram-negative pleomorphic bacillus that may be cultivated readily in enriched bacteriologic media. The disease is transmitted to man by the bite of sandflies of the genus Phlebotomus, with development of the characteristic symptoms of Oroya fever after an incubation period of two weeks to three months.

Prevalence and Distribution. Although a number of epidemics of the disease have been reported, it is more commonly seen as sporadic cases among populations of Peru, Colombia, and Ecuador, and is restricted within these countries to those who live at altitudes of 1500 to 9000 feet on both slopes of the Andes. In general, the distribution of the disease coincides with the ecologic zones supporting populations of Phlebotomus.

Epidemiology. In Peru the disease is transmitted by *Phlebotomus verrugarum,* a night-biting sandfly. The biting habits of the vectors in the other countries are similar, although the species of Phlebotomus involved in transmission in the other areas are not conclusively identified. The principal reservoir of the disease appears to be man; no additional animal reservoirs have as yet been implicated in nature. Reports of cultivation of the agent from apparently healthy persons suggest that as much as 10 per cent of infections may be subclinical. Persons convalescent from the disease are known to have a low-level bacteremia for months or years, providing frequent opportunities for infection of the disease vector.

Pathology and Physiologic Responses. In the Oroya fever stage of illness the causative organism may be found in peripheral blood smears stained with Giemsa or Wright's stain as well as in the reticuloendothelial cells of the viscera and lymphatics. In the blood the parasite is found both free in the plasma and adhering to the erythrocytes. The parasitization of the erythrocytes causes an increased mechanical fragility and also an increased sequestration of the cells in the spleen and the liver. A hypochromic and macrocytic anemia develops rapidly during the febrile period, erythrocyte counts decreasing within a period of only a few days to levels of one million to two million cells per cubic millimeter. The bone marrow is hyperplastic, with an abundance of nucleated erythrocytes. The pathologic findings secondary to the anemia are absent in the verruga stage of infection. The histopathology of the skin lesions is that of dilation of the capillaries and proliferation of the vascular endothelial cells that may be shown to contain the causative agent.

Clinical Manifestations. The presenting symptoms of patients with Oroya fever are intermittent high fever, painful muscles and joints, tender enlarged lymph nodes, and the systemic symptoms and prostration of a severe anemia. These symptoms may persist from several weeks to several months in untreated patients, half of whom may die within the first three weeks of fever. If the patient survives, gradual convalescence is punctuated, after a few days to a month, by the appearance of the cutaneous lesions of the second phase of the disease. The verrugae may persist for a month to a year in untreated persons, but mortality is negligible. Occasional patients may experience only the fever and anemia without the skin manifestations or only the cutaneous lesions without the initial fever. Although these two aspects of the infection were once thought to be different diseases, there is no doubt that both syndromes are manifestations of infection with the same organism. The current interpretation that the skin lesions are an expression of developing immunity in the patient is supported by the observation that second attacks of the disease are exceedingly rare even in highly endemic areas and that the attacks are almost always caused by verruga rather than by Oroya fever.

Diagnosis. In endemic areas the diagnosis can usually be made on the basis of clinical findings. In the acute stage of Oroya fever both blood smears and blood culture usually reveal the presence of the agent. As the patient progresses toward the verruga stage of infection, or with treatment, the organism becomes more difficult to demonstrate.

Treatment and Prognosis. The prognosis in the untreated patient depends upon both the nature and the severity of his infection. Mortality in the Oroya fever phase of the disease may exceed 50 per cent, particularly when the infection is complicated by concurrent attacks of malaria, amebiasis, tuberculosis, salmonellosis, or other diseases. The disease responds well to treatment with penicillin, streptomycin, chloramphenicol, and the tetracyclines. Chloramphenicol is favored by many South American clinicians because of the frequency of concurrent salmonella infections, but the risks of its potentially more serious toxicity must be weighed against the fact that the other drugs mentioned are therapeutically effective. In general, as in the rickettsial infections, the tetracyclines are the preferred form of antimicrobial therapy for bartonellosis. When the broad-spectrum antimicrobials have been used, oral doses of 1 to 2 grams per day have been used for a period of a week or more with excellent results. Patients become afebrile in 24 to 48 hours, and, if they receive transfusions, recover strength rapidly. Although the mortality of the verruga stage of infection is less than 5 per cent, antimicrobial therapy is desirable to hasten the disappearance of the skin lesions.

Prevention. Control measures are directed principally against the Phlebotomus vector. Because the insect is a night feeder and moves by a series of short "hops" between surfaces, the application of a residual insecticide to the exterior and interior of doorways, windows, and other avenues of entry to human habitation is effective. Where insecticide application is impracticable, bed nets or insect repellents provide significant protection. Control of breeding of the vector is difficult, but may be undertaken when it is otherwise impossible to prevent contact of the vector with man. No protective vaccine is available. Patients need not be isolated in hospital wards if the vector is absent because the disease cannot be transmitted by person-to-person contact.

Reynafarje, C., and Ramos, J.: The hemolytic anemia of human bartonellosis. Blood, 17:562, 1961.

Urteaga, B. O., and Payne, E. H.: Treatment of the acute febrile phase of Carrión's disease with chloramphenicol. Am. J. Trop. Med., 4:507, 1955.

Weinman, D.: The Bartonella Group. *In*: Dubos, R. J., and Hirsch, J. G. (eds.): Bacterial and Mycotic Infections of Man. 4th ed. Philadelphia, J. B. Lippincott Company, 1965, p. 775.

DISEASES CAUSED BY CHLAMYDIAE

171. TRACHOMA AND INCLUSION CONJUNCTIVITIS

Ernest Jawetz

Definition. Trachoma and inclusion conjunctivitis are chronic infectious diseases of the eye and genital tract, caused by closely related microorganisms and exhibiting overlapping spectra of clinical manifestations and epidemiologic patterns. These range from mild and self-limited to severe and blinding eye disease, with or without involvement of the genital tract.

Etiology. The agents of *trachoma and inclusion conjunctivitis* (TRIC agents) are members of the psittacosis–lymphogranuloma venereum–trachoma group. Formerly these agents were considered viruses; now they are called *chlamydiae.* They are nonmotile, gram-negative, obligate intracellular parasites which multiply in the cytoplasm of their host cells by a distinctive developmental cycle. Chlamydiae differ from viruses in many important respects: they possess both RNA and DNA; they multiply by binary fission; they possess bacterial types of cell walls and ribosomes; they produce a variety of metabolically active enzymes; and their growth can be inhibited by several antibacterial drugs. It is probable that chlamydiae are closely related to gram-negative bacteria, but lack some significant mechanism for the production of metabolic energy so that they are restricted to an intracellular existence.

TRIC agents can infect epithelial cells of conjunctiva, cornea, urethra, and cervix of man and monkey, but do not replicate in most other tissues of the body. The infective particle ("elementary body") is a sphere with a diameter of 250 nanometers (millimicrons) and stains purple with Giemsa's or red with Macchiavello's stain. The infective particle is taken into the host cell by phagocytosis and, after replication, results in the development of an inclusion body. This is an oval or crescent-shaped mass of "elementary bodies" embedded in a matrix of glycogen, lying in the cytoplasm of an epithelial cell often adjacent to the nucleus. Inclusion bodies can be stained brightly with specific immunofluorescence.

TRIC agents can be grown in the yolk sac of embryonated eggs and in X-irradiated cells in culture. The growth of TRIC agents is markedly inhibited by tetracyclines, sulfonamides, erythromycins, penicillins, and chloramphenicol, but not by aminoglycosides. Therefore aminoglycosides can be used to suppress bacterial contaminants in clinical specimens and to aid in isolation of TRIC agents in the laboratory.

TRIC agents share with other chlamydiae a heat-stable group antigen. These are lipopolysaccharides detectable by complement-fixation tests. In addition, species- or strain-specific antigens have been detected in the cell wall. Infected persons may develop antibodies to both types of antigens in serum and tears. By immunofluorescence tests specific antigens and antibodies can be identified. Thus genital TRIC isolates often fall within certain antigenic groups (D, E, F, etc.), whereas ocular TRIC isolates from endemic trachoma areas often fall within other groups (A, B, C). At least nine specific antigenic groups have been identified to date. There exist cross-reactions between the specific antigens of the chlamydiae of lymphogranuloma venereum and of certain TRIC agents. However, to date there is no specific laboratory characteristic that can always differentiate isolates of trachoma from isolates of inclusion conjunctivitis agents.

TRIC agents can persist in man for years, with or without symptoms and signs of infection. Subclinical infection can be activated by trauma, corticosteroid administration, and perhaps bacterial superinfection. The development of scarring and blindness in some endemic trachoma regions is attributable to a large extent to recurrent bacterial infections of the eye, especially with Hemophilus or Neisseria.

Prevalence and Epidemiology. Since antiquity, trachomatous infection was recognized in the Mediterranean basin and in the Orient. Today, trachomatous eye disease is very prevalent in Africa and Asia. It has been estimated that up to 400 million persons may be infected with TRIC agents, and up to 20 million may be economically blinded as a result. Trachoma flourishes in areas that are hot and dry, and that have a shortage of available water and poor hygienic customs. In such areas endemic levels are high, and initial infection commonly occurs in early childhood. In certain parts of the world, e.g., in North Africa, virtually the entire population is infected with TRIC agents before reaching adulthood. The high prevalence of bacterial superinfection in such populations undoubtedly contributes to the severity of eye disease and to its causing widespread blindness. In parts of the United States, e.g., Indian reservations of the Southwest, endemic TRIC infection is relatively common, but it rarely leads to major visual impairment, perhaps because bacterial superinfection is infrequent. Throughout the world sporadic cases of ocular TRIC infection occur, often with a clinical picture resembling trachoma. It is probable that some of these originate in genital infections rather than in contact with ocular trachoma.

Active cases of ocular TRIC infection shed the infective agent in desquamated conjunctival cells, conjunctival exudate, or tears. The infectious agent may be transmitted by fingers, fomites, and perhaps flies. Patients with early active infection probably shed more infective TRIC agent, and thus are more infectious for contacts than are those with chronic infection. However, even patients with longstanding scarred eye disease, and without signs of current activity, may shed TRIC agent and thus serve as a source of infection.

These comments concern ocular TRIC infection, particularly typical endemic trachoma. *Typical inclusion conjunctivitis* has a radically different epidemiologic pattern. Inclusion conjunctivitis is fundamentally an infection of the adult human genital tract, transmitted as a venereal disease. In the female the TRIC agent grows mainly in the transitional epithelium of the cervix. These cells may contain typical inclusions, and occasionally a mild cervicitis is present. In the male, genital infection may produce ("nonspecific") *urethritis,* as the TRIC agent replicates in urethral epithelium. In both sexes, adult genital tract infection and proctitis are often asymptomatic. Adults may transfer genital secretions to their own or other eyes by fingers, by fomites, and—occasionally—in swimming pools. The infection may pass from the cervix of the infected mother to the eye of her newborn during passage through the birth canal. The newborn infant may then develop eye disease between 5 and 14 days after birth.

The epidemiologic patterns described for typical trachoma and typical inclusion conjunctivitis may be mixed. Thus the genital tract of women in endemic trachoma regions may harbor TRIC agents, and these may produce either inclusion conjunctivitis or clinically typical trachoma in the offspring. Genital isolates from adults in nonendemic areas may, upon inoculation into the eye, give rise to disease resembling either inclusion conjunctivitis or trachoma.

Pathology and Pathogenesis. TRIC agents invade mainly the epithelium of the conjunctiva, cervix, and urethra. The earliest sign of infection is the appearance of inclusion bodies within epithelial cells and neutrophil infiltration of the epithelium of mucous membranes. Subepithelial infiltration with plasma cells and lymphocytes and the development of lymphoid follicles then follow. In the cornea, epithelial keratitis is often accompanied by the formation of subepithelial opacities. Blood vessels from the limbus, accompanied by fibroblasts, may invade the cornea to form a pannus. Progression of the inflammatory process leads to necrosis and scar formation in the conjunctiva. In classic trachoma, these changes occur more markedly in the upper half of the conjunctival sac and cornea; in inclusion conjunctivitis, more markedly in the lower conjunctiva. Inflammatory changes, lymphoid infiltration, necrosis, and scar formation have also been observed in TRIC agent infection of cervix and urethra.

Classic inclusion conjunctivitis of the newborn is an acute purulent conjunctivitis; in the adult it is a follicular conjunctivitis. However, all pathologic changes from limited follicular conjunctivitis to full-blown "trachoma" with scars and pannus may follow inoculation of genital isolates into the adult eye.

Classic, chronic, severe trachoma in hyperendemic areas progresses to marked lid deformation and loss of vision. As a result of cellular infiltration and scarring near the lid margins, the tarsal plate is bowed and the lid margins inverted (entropion), and some eyelashes turn inward (trichiasis), rubbing against the cornea with each lid movement, and aggravating corneal opacification. The scarring may destroy tear function, with resulting keratinization of corneal epithelium.

TRIC agents exhibit a pronounced tendency to persist in infected tissues for years even in the absence of signs of active disease, and this predisposes to relapses and to chronicity.

Clinical Manifestations. In experimental human infection with TRIC agents the incubation period is from two to seven days. *Inclusion conjunctivitis* of the newborn usually begins between the fifth and fourteenth days of life (whereas gonococcal ophthalmia usually begins two days after birth). The incubation period of naturally occurring trachoma is uncertain because the onset is often insidious, particularly in children. Early symptoms of TRIC infection are those of irritation, lacrimation, and mucopurulent discharge. The earliest physical signs are conjunctival hyperemia, mucopurulent discharge, papillary hypertrophy in infants, and follicular hypertrophy in adults.

Typical *trachoma* in children and adults begins as a follicular conjunctivitis, most noticeable in the conjunctiva of the upper lid and the tarsal plate. There are epithelial keratitis and subepithelial corneal infiltration, followed by gradual corneal vascularization from the upper limbus downward. This evolves into a dense fibrovascular pannus extending over part, or all, of the cornea, grossly impairing vision. Linear or stellate scars appear on the conjunctiva. Progressive scarring of the subepithelial tissues leads to deformation of the tarsal plate, resulting in entropion, trichiasis, and further corneal damage. These changes often follow secondary bacterial infection, which may also produce corneal ulceration and accelerate loss of vision. Typically there are no systemic symptoms or signs of infection, and the eye is the sole involved organ.

Typical *inclusion conjunctivitis* of the newborn presents as an acute purulent conjunctivitis with papillary hypertrophy but little involvement of the cornea. Over a period of weeks or months this tends to regress spontaneously and eventually heal without any scars or with only fine linear conjunctival and corneal scars and minimal, if any, pannus. In the adult, inclusion conjunctivitis is an acute mucopurulent conjunctivitis, often accompanied by preauricular adenopathy. Follicular hypertrophy is most noticeable in the conjunctiva of the lower lid, and tends to persist for weeks or months, occasionally accompanied by epithelial keratitis and subepithelial corneal infiltrates. Some adults with chronic inclusion conjunctivitis develop a limited pannus and a few scars of conjunctiva and cornea.

Adult genital TRIC infection usually precedes the eye involvement. Adult *cervicitis* and *urethritis* either are asymptomatic or produce only slight discharge and discomfort. This so-called nongonococcal urethritis forms as much as half of the acute urethritis in the male seen in venereal disease clinics (see Ch. 199).

All intermediate stages between minimal self-limited inclusion conjunctivitis and typical progressive trachoma can occur as a result of infection with TRIC agents of either ocular or genital origin. The typical, severe trachoma that leads to blindness and is seen in hyperendemic areas occurs probably as a result of longstanding infection with many relapses of TRIC agent activity, hypersensitivity reactions, and repeated bacterial superinfections. Conversely, the self-limited inclusion conjunctivitis of the newborn may be characteristic of a first infection, without hypersensitivity reaction, and without bacterial complications in an immunologically immature host. The basis for different clinical patterns of mild or severe disease seen in different areas of the world is not clearly understood.

Diagnosis. The traditional criteria for the diagnosis of trachoma are the triad of follicular hypertrophy, most prominent on the upper tarsal conjunctiva, pannus, and conjunctival scars. The last two signs may be detected only by biomicroscopic examination (slit lamp).

The diagnosis of inclusion conjunctivitis rests on finding typical inclusions in a purulent conjunctivitis of the newborn or in a follicular conjunctivitis of the adult. There should be only minimal vascular invasion of the cornea. Examination of the adult genital tract may reveal cervicitis and urethritis with moderate discharge and inclusions in epithelial cells. Proctitis may be present.

Among laboratory tests for TRIC infections, the demonstration of typical intracytoplasmic inclusions in conjunctival or genital cells is most widely used. Specific immunofluorescent stain is more sensitive than Giemsa stain. Polymorphonuclear leukocytes are often prominent in scrapings that contain TRIC inclusions. Isolation of TRIC agents in embryonated eggs or in irradiated cell cultures remains a specialized laboratory procedure. Serologic tests can support the diagnosis only if a rise in complement-fixing or immunofluorescence antibodies occurs during acute disease. The cytologic appearance of expressed follicular material may be helpful. Among follicular diseases of the conjunctiva, only TRIC infections (especially trachoma) produce the necrotic changes in follicles that are evidenced by the presence of many macrophages engorged with cell fragments.

Differential Diagnosis. In differential diagnosis of ocular TRIC infections, adenovirus infections, herpetic keratoconjunctivitis, folliculosis of children, chronic follicular conjunctivitis (Axenfeld type), reactions to allergens and irritating chemicals, and certain bacterial infections must be considered. Some of these entities may coexist with TRIC infections, and repeated competent ophthalmologic examinations and elaborate laboratory assistance may be required to establish a correct diagnosis. The demonstration of morphologically typical inclusions by immunofluorescent or Giemsa stain is most helpful in the diagnosis of TRIC infections, when combined with efforts to isolate viruses or bacteria of possible etiologic significance.

The single most difficult differential diagnosis may be between ocular trachoma and oculogenital inclusion conjunctivitis, as described above. This differentiation requires epidemiologic considerations, clinical and laboratory examination of the genital tract, and—if a TRIC agent has been grown—a "typing" of the isolate by immunofluorescent tests. At times the eye lesions of trachoma and of oculogenital inclusion conjunctivitis in the adult cannot be distinguished. The most important differential diagnosis of inclusion conjunctivitis of the newborn is chemical or bacterial conjunctivitis.

Treatment and Prognosis. TRIC agents are susceptible to several antibacterial drugs. Tetracyclines and sulfonamides have been most widely used in treatment. Tetracycline suspensions or ointments can cling to the conjunctiva for prolonged effect. Ophthalmic topical tetracycline preparations have been administered in various dosage schedules for several months in chronic endemic trachoma. Sometimes there was clinical improvement, but often active disease recurred, and the over-all efficacy of topical tetracyclines in chronic TRIC infections is being questioned. In inclusion conjunctivitis of the newborn, there is a strong natural tendency toward healing. The administration of topical tetracycline two to four times daily for three weeks further accelerates healing.

Oral tetracycline hydrochloride, 1 to 2 grams in three divided daily doses, or doxycycline, 2.5 to 4.0 mg per kilogram in a single daily dose, or oral trisulfapyrimidines, 4 grams daily in divided doses for five to six weeks, often suppress signs of activity in chronic trachoma of adults. However, these treatment regimens often fail to eradicate the infectious agent. By contrast, in acute TRIC infections these oral drug regimens alone, or combined with topical tetracycline, may result in permanent cure. This is probably true for both eye infections and genital tract infections, providing that they are of short duration.

In areas of hyperendemic trachoma, mass treatment

must be applied to early infection of children and must be repeated at intervals in order to control TRIC infection before scarring occurs. No conclusive evidence exists that mass drug treatment can eradicate trachoma from a population, but repeated courses of drug treatment are probably beneficial by reducing the reservoir of infection, by temporarily suppressing TRIC agent and clinical activity in the patient, and by controlling bacterial superinfection.

Drug therapy has no influence on established scars or pannus. Surgical correction is required in serious entropion or trichiasis. Topical corticosteroids and caustics have no place in therapy.

Prevention. Endemic trachoma is favored by ignorance, poverty, and cultural patterns that oppose hygienic improvement and medical treatment. In addition, the sheer lack of water available for washing seems to be important.

The most potent preventive measures include efforts to increase the total supply of water, simple cleanliness such as frequent hand washing, avoidance of common towel or common eye pencil, and measures to reduce flies. It is also important to detect mild, early infection in young children in endemic areas and to apply effective drug treatment repeatedly. This prevents the blinding progression of the disease, and probably reduces the infective reservoir. Detection and treatment of adults who already suffer visual impairment can probably reduce the source of infection for children.

Prevention of genital TRIC infections requires the control of sexual promiscuity, early diagnosis and effective treatment of cases and sexual contacts, and prolonged follow-up to establish that the genital or ocular infection is not relapsing. Effective treatment of pregnant women with genital TRIC infection can prevent inclusion conjunctivitis in the newborn. The usual instillations into the eye of the newborn (silver nitrate or penicillin) do not prevent inclusion conjunctivitis. A newborn baby with inclusion conjunctivitis should be isolated to prevent spread to others.

Experimental vaccines against TRIC infections have been prepared. In field tests no vaccine has given unequivocal protection against infection, or against progression of disease. Work is continuing in the hope of developing preparations of greater immunogenicity.

However, natural infection engenders only minimal protection against reinfection. The most that could be expected of artificial immunization is an attenuation of the disease resulting from infection. The best current hope for control of TRIC infections rests on a combination of public health measures and drug treatment.

Dunlop, E. M. C., Jones, B. R., Darougar, S., and Treharne, J. D.: Chlamydia and non-specific urethritis. Br. Med. J., 2:575, 1973.

Dunlop, E. M. C., Vaughan-Jackson, J. D., Darougar, S., and Jones, B. R.: Incidence of chlamydiae in nonspecific urethritis. Br. J. Vener. Dis., 48:425, 1972.

Jawetz, E.: Chemotherapy of chlamydial infections. *In* Garattini, S., Goldin, A., Hawking, F., and Kopin, I. J. (eds.): Advances in Pharmacology and Chemotherapy. Vol. 7. New York, Academic Press, 1969, pp. 253–282.

Jawetz, E., Hanna, L., Dawson, C., Wood, R., and Briones, O.: Subclinical infections with TRIC agents. Am. J. Ophthal., 63:1413, 1967.

Jones, B. R.: Ocular syndromes of TRIC virus infection and their possible genital significance. Br. J. Vener. Dis., 40:3, 1964.

Moulder, J. W.: The relation of the psittacosis group (Chlamydiae) to bacteria and viruses. Ann. Rev. Microbiol., 20:107, 1966.

Thygeson, P.: Trachoma Manual and Atlas. U.S. Department of Health, Education and Welfare, U.S. Public Health Service Publication No. 541, Revised 1960.

Wang, S. P., and Grayston, J. T.: Immunologic relationship between genital TRIC, lymphogranuloma venereum, and related organisms in a new indirect immunofluorescence test. Am. J. Ophthalmol., 70:367, 1970.

172. LYMPHOGRANULOMA VENEREUM

Ernest Jawetz

Definition. Lymphogranuloma venereum (LGV) is an acute and chronic venereal disease with prominent systemic manifestations, caused by a chlamydial agent closely related to trachoma and inclusion conjunctivitis (TRIC) agents. LGV produces early genital lesions followed by enlargement and suppuration of regional lymph nodes and a variety of febrile systemic manifestations. Late results are prominent inguinal draining sinuses in men and fibrosing proctitis and rectal strictures in women and homosexual males.

Etiology. The chlamydiae of LGV resemble TRIC agents (see Ch. 171) in many respects, including the formation of compact intracytoplasmic inclusions with a glycogen matrix, inhibition of growth by sulfonamides, and antigenic features. All LGV chlamydiae carry the chlamydial group reactive antigen. Specific antigens have been defined by immunofluorescence, thus permitting classification of LGV isolates into three specific antigenic types. These antigens cross-react with type-specific antigens of certain TRIC agents. LGV chlamydiae differ from TRIC agents in growing more readily in cell cultures and in several animal tissues.

Prevalence and Epidemiology. LGV is transmitted almost exclusively by sexual contact. The genital tract and rectum of chronically infected persons serve as reservoirs of infection. The highest incidence of the disease has been reported from subtropical and tropical areas, but the infection occurs all over the world. Definitive serologic surveys of LGV infection by appropriate specific methods have not been performed.

Pathogenesis and Pathology. A primary vesicular or ulcerative lesion develops at the site of inoculation one to four weeks after infection. The chlamydiae spread rapidly to regional lymph nodes which become enlarged and inflamed. From the penis or vulva the spread is mainly to inguinal and iliac nodes. From the vagina or rectum the spread is mainly to perirectal and pelvic nodes. The involved nodes become matted and suppurate and may discharge pus through multiple sinus tracts.

During the stage of early, active lymphadenitis, the chlamydiae may become widely disseminated by the bloodstream and may reach various organs, including the central nervous system. In the late, chronic stages of infection, fibrosis, obstruction, and strictures develop. Lymphatic obstruction may lead to elephantiasis of external genitalia (penis, scrotum, vulva). Chronic proctitis may lead to progressive rectal strictures, with obstruction of the bowel lumen and fistula formation.

The histologic appearance of involved lymph nodes shows acute and chronic inflammation, suppuration, and fibrosis, but is not specific or diagnostic of LGV.

Clinical Manifestations. Several days to several weeks

after exposure, a small, evanescent papule or vesicle develops on any part of the external genitalia, anus, or rectum. The lesion may ulcerate, but usually—especially in women—it remains unnoticed and heals in a few days. Soon thereafter the regional lymph nodes enlarge and tend to become matted and often painful. In males, inguinal nodes are most commonly involved both above and below Poupart's ligament, and the overlying skin often turns purplish as the nodes suppurate and eventually discharge pus through multiple sinus tracts. In females, the perirectal nodes are prominently involved with proctitis and bloody mucopurulent anal discharge. This is also seen in homosexual males.

During the stage of active lymphadenitis, there are often marked systemic symptoms, including fever, headaches, meningismus, conjunctivitis, skin rashes, nausea and vomiting, and arthralgias. Rarely is there meningitis, arthritis, or pericarditis. Unless effective antimicrobial therapy is instituted at that stage, the chronic inflammatory process progresses to fibrosis, lymphatic obstruction, and rectal strictures. The lymphatic obstruction may lead to elephantiasis of the penis, scrotum, or vulva. The chronic proctitis of women or homosexual males may lead to progressive rectal strictures, rectosigmoid obstruction, and fistula formation.

Diagnosis. LGV must be considered in every case of enlarged, matted, tender inguinal lymph nodes, active proctitis, draining inguinal or perianal fistulas, and rectal strictures. It must be distinguished from inguinal adenopathy of any cause, including pyogenic infection of lower extremities, plague, tularemia, chancroid, granuloma inguinale, syphilis, and inflammatory or neoplastic lesions of the rectum. A clinical impression of LGV can be supported by the demonstration of the chlamydiae, a skin test, or a meaningful serologic response, but histologic appearance of biopsied tissue is not specific.

Material from fluctuant suppurating nodes may be obtained by aspiration or biopsy. When inoculated into x-irradiated cell cultures, into embryonated eggs, or, by intracerebral injection, into mice, LGV chlamydiae can sometimes be isolated. Only rarely can chlamydial inclusions be seen in stained smears of such material.

The skin test (Frei test) consists of the intradermal injection of LGV antigens, prepared in embryonated eggs, and a suitable control of egg material. The test is considered positive if an indurated area or papule—at least 6 mm larger than the control site—develops in 48 hours. Reactivity to chlamydial group antigen develops within 3 to 8 weeks after LGV infection and may remain positive for life. This delayed hypersensitivity reaction may be positive after *any* chlamydial infection. A negative skin test cannot exclude LGV infection. Skin tests with commercial antigens are sometimes negative even when LGV chlamydiae are isolated from pus, or when the serologic response unequivocally proves a chlamydial infection. Thus the Frei test is of only limited value in the diagnosis of suspected LGV infection. Early antimicrobial drug treatment may interfere with the development of a positive skin test and antibody response.

The complement-fixation (CF) test with heat-stable group reactive antigen is at present the most generally available test for LGV and other systemic chlamydial infections. In the presence of inguinal adenopathy or proctitis, a rise of antibody titer in sera taken two to three weeks apart strongly supports the diagnosis of LGV. In untreated LGV patients, the CF titer is often 1:64 or more, and such a high titer in a single serum from a patient with a compatible clinical picture also supports the diagnosis. With effective treatment the titer declines. Persisting high antibody titers suggest chronic persistent infection. Indirect immunofluorescence tests for antibodies to LGV antigens are as sensitive as and more specific than CF tests but are not generally available.

Other abnormal laboratory findings are less helpful. The white blood cell count is often elevated during lymph node suppuration or proctitis, sometimes with a relative monocytosis. Total serum proteins may be elevated with a reversed albumin-globulin ratio. Gamma globulin, cryoglobulins, rheumatoid factor, and IgM are sometimes significantly increased in serum.

Treatment. The growth of LGV chlamydiae can be inhibited by sulfonamides, tetracyclines, and some other antimicrobials. Full systemic doses of a soluble sulfonamide (e.g., trisulfapyrimidines USP, 6 to 8 grams daily) or of a tetracycline (e.g., tetracycline HCl, 2 to 4 grams daily) are administered for three to four weeks as early in the course of LGV infection as possible. LGV acquired since 1967 in Southeast Asia has responded more regularly to tetracycline than to sulfonamides. In some patients, two or three courses of treatment are required. Supportive therapy consists of bed rest, compresses to inflamed areas, analgesics, and aspiration of fluctuant sites. Treatment is guided by the subsiding of constitutional symptoms and of lymph node swelling, closure of fistulas, and resolution of proctitis. If the infection is eradicated, the serum antibody titer drops markedly over a period of six to eight months.

Prognosis. Although the acute illness in early LGV is usually self-limited, the chronic complications resulting from lymphatic blockade or rectal stricture are debilitating and often require surgical correction. It is important therefore to prevent these late complications by early diagnosis and prolonged or repeated treatment. Death from LGV uncomplicated by bacterial superinfection is very rare. There may be an increased incidence of anorectal carcinoma in persons with anorectal chronic LGV.

Prevention. Since LGV is generally acquired as a venereal disease, all measures applicable to the prevention of venereal diseases are pertinent. No active immunization is available.

Abrams, A. J.: Lymphogranuloma venereum. J.A.M.A., 205:59, 1968.

Jawetz, E.: Chemotherapy of chlamydial infections. Adv. Pharmacol. Chemother., 7:235, 1969.

Management of Chancroid, Granuloma Inguinale, and Lymphogranuloma Venereum in General Practice. U.S. Public Health Service, Publication No. 255. Washington, D.C., U.S. Government Printing Office, 1968.

Schachter, J., Smith, D. E., Dawson, C. R., Anderson, W. R., Deller, J. J., Hoke, A. W., Smart, W. H., and Meyer, K. F.: Lymphogranuloma venereum. Comparison of the Frei test, complement fixation test, and isolation of the agent. J. Infect. Dis., 120:372, 1969.

Sigel, M. M.: Lymphogranuloma Venereum. Coral Gables, University of Miami Press, 1962.

173. PSITTACOSIS
(Ornithosis, Parrot Fever)

David E. Rogers

Definition. Psittacosis is a specific infection of birds produced by the obligate intracellular bacteria, *Chlamydia psittaci.* When transmitted to man, this agent can produce asymptomatic infection, a transient influenza-like illness, or serious pneumonic disease characterized by high fever, headache, cough, myalgia, pulmonary infiltrates, and a significant mortality. Because it is now recognized that many species of birds other than the order Psittaciformes transmit psittacosis, *ornithosis* has been suggested as a more accurate title. Usage has made psittacosis the accepted term for the human disease.

History. In 1879, Ritter, a Swiss physician, described seven cases of an unusual pneumonia that occurred after contact with tropical birds. Morange, in 1894, established the parrot as a vector and termed the disease *psittacosis* after the Greek *psittakos* (the parrot). During 1929–1930 a serious epidemic of pneumonia occurred in Europe and America after shipments of infected South American parrots. This epidemic led to clearer recognition of psittacosis as a human disease. The etiologic agent was demonstrated to be a filterable agent by Bedson, Western, and Simpson in 1930. Subsequent studies have shown that over 90 species of birds can harbor the agent, and its worldwide distribution has been documented. Reported cases in the United States have declined since 1960, probably as a consequence of requiring tetracycline treatment of imported psittacine birds.

Etiology. *C. psittaci* is an obligate intracellular parasite. It is morphologically and serologically related to lymphogranuloma venereum and to a number of mammalian agents producing pneumonitis, meningoencephalitis, and abortion in their native hosts. To date, these agents have not been shown to produce human disease. Because of their large size (250 to 400 mμ), possession of both RNA and DNA, a demonstrable cell wall containing muramic acid, division by binary fission, and their susceptibility to chemotherapeutic agents known to inhibit bacterial enzyme systems, these agents have recently been reclassified as bacteria. Parrots and parakeets are the most common carriers and until recently represented the major source of human infection. With better control of psittacine disease in aviaries, other birds now contribute more human infections, and cases have resulted from contacts with turkeys, pigeons, ducks, chickens, pheasants, finches, and other fowl. Although individuals of both sexes and all ages are susceptible, overt clinical infections in children are uncommon. Persons working with birds are at greatest risk of infection, and there is an increased incidence of psittacosis in pet shop employees, pigeon handlers, and poultry workers.

The agent is present in the blood, tissue, and discharges of infected birds. It is hardy and can withstand drying. Although the avian disease can be fatal, infected birds frequently show only minimal evidence of illness, such as ruffled feathers, lethargy, and failure to eat. Birds having active infections are most likely to transmit the disease, but asymptomatic carriers are common, and birds that recover can shed transmissible agent for many months. In general, human psittacosis acquired from psittacine birds or turkeys has been more severe than that acquired from pigeons, ducks, chickens, or pheasants. Bird ectoparasites can harbor the agent and may serve as a source of reinfection for domestic flocks. Antimicrobials incorporated in bird foodstuffs may not eradicate psittacosis from infected parrots or parakeets but can render them less infectious for man.

Psittacosis is generally acquired by the respiratory route through inhalation of infected dried bird excreta, more rarely by handling the feathers and the tissues of infected birds. On rare occasion the disease may be acquired through an open lesion or the bite of a bird. Mouth-to-beak intimacies have led to infection in man. Small epidemics have been attributed to aerosols of dust laden with dried excreta. Cases have been reported after only brief exposure to birds. There is some evidence that the incubation period may be shortened by a large inoculum. Person-to-person transmission of psittacosis, although rare, has been documented. These cases of "human" strain psittacosis have been severe, with high mortality.

Pathology. In birds, the principal sites of disease are the liver, spleen, and pericardium. In man, the lung is most commonly involved. The psittacosis agent generally gains access to the human body via the respiratory route, and then rapidly enters the blood and produces systemic disease involving the lungs and the reticuloendothelial tissues. The agent can be isolated from the blood and sputum during the first two weeks of illness, and has been found in the spleen in fatal cases. The mature pulmonary lesion is a lobular pneumonitis. The process is initiated by inflammation and progressive edema of the alveolar cells. Exudation is often accompanied by small hemorrhages. Polymorphonuclear leukocytes appear early in the process. Later inflammatory exudates show lymphocytes and large numbers of mononuclear leukocytes within the alveoli and interstitial spaces. The mucosa of the trachea and bronchi generally remains intact but is edematous and invaded with mononuclear cells. Thick, gelatinous plugs of mucus may fill major and minor bronchi and may account for the severe cyanosis and progressive anoxia seen in fatal cases. Foci of necrosis may occur in more severely affected areas of the lung and are sometimes associated with capillary thrombi. The process is generally most severe in dependent bronchopulmonary segments. Vasculitis and thrombosis may account for many findings. Large monocytes and macrophages containing cytoplasmic inclusion bodies, which may represent the agent (LCL bodies), are characteristic of psittacosis infection. Hyperplasia and monocytic infiltration of pulmonary and hilar lymph nodes and splenic enlargement with occasional areas of focal necrosis may occur. Rarely the liver may show intralobular focal necrosis and swollen Kupffer cells containing the psittacosis elementary bodies. Changes in the myocardium, pericardium, meninges, brain, adrenals, and kidneys have been reported.

Clinical Manifestations. Wide variations can occur in the clinical picture. The incubation period ranges from 7 to 15 days but may occasionally be longer. Asymptomatic infection or mild influenza-like infections probably are the rule. Moderate or severe infections, although less frequent, are more commonly diagnosed. The onset of illness may be insidious, but it often starts with chills and a fever that rises slowly from initial levels of 38 or 39 to 39.5 to 40.5° C during the first week of illness. The pulse may be slow relative to the height of the fever. Headache is severe. Malaise, anorexia, severe myalgias, particularly in the neck and back, and arthralgias are common. Cough is generally prominent but may be delayed until late in the first week. Small amounts of mucoid sputum with occasional blood streaking are the rule, and pleuritic pain is rare. Changes in mentation are often seen. Delirium or stupor may occur in severe cases toward the end of the first week, and is usually associated with severe pulmonary involvement, cyanosis, and other evidences of anoxia. Other neurologic manifestations are uncommon. Nausea and vomiting are frequent. Epistaxis may occur early in the course of the illness. A macular rash resembling that seen in typhoid has occasionally been described. Jaundice and progressive nitrogen retention have been reported in severe cases. Severe dyspnea, tachypnea, tachycardia, cyanosis, jaundice, delirium, and stupor are all poor prognostic signs.

The physical findings of pneumonia are often sparse. Chest roentgenograms may reveal evidence of infiltrates not detected at the bedside. Examination may reveal only fever, painful muscle groups, an elevated respiratory rate, and a relative bradycardia. Fine, crepitant rales may be heard in localized areas over the lungs. Frank percussion or auscultatory changes suggestive of true consolidation are less common. Pleurisy with effusion can occur but is unusual. Mild hepatomegaly is frequent. A palpable spleen has been noted in a substantial number of patients. An erythematous pharynx may be noted. In rare instances there may be signs of pericarditis or myocarditis. In prolonged, severe illness, thrombophlebitis and pulmonary infarction have been reported as late complications.

Patients with mild cases may recover in 7 to 8 days. More severe infections may last 12 to 21 days without specific treatment. Fever is ordinarily sustained or remittent, and when accompanied by bradycardia, resembles the fever seen in untreated typhoid infections. Defervescence is generally slow, and a prolonged convalescence is common. Relapses have been reported even after appropriate treatment. Secondary bacterial infections are rare.

Laboratory Findings. Simple laboratory studies are not helpful in establishing a diagnosis. The leukocyte count is usually normal, but leukopenia or low-grade leukocytosis ranging to over 20,000 cells per cubic millimeter may occur. The erythrocyte sedimentation rate is generally elevated. Proteinuria is common during the febrile period. Chest roentgenograms generally show soft patchy infiltrates radiating outward from the hilum, which tend to be more prominent in dependent lobes or segments. Occasionally diffuse miliary, nodular, or frank lobar distribution of infiltrates is seen.

A specific diagnosis can be made only by isolation of the agent or by serologic studies. The agent is present in the blood and sputum during the first two to three weeks, but isolation is hazardous, and should not be attempted except in special laboratories. Diagnosis is generally made by a fourfold rise in complement-fixing antibodies against a heat-stable group antigen prepared from psittacosis agent grown in eggs. Paired acute and convalescent sera should always be tested. A significant change in antibody titers is generally present by the twelfth to fourteenth day of disease; the titers are usually maximal by 30 days, then slowly disappear. Treatment can delay or suppress antibody response. There is considerable cross-reaction between antigens prepared from psittacosis and lymphogranuloma venereum viruses. False positive complement-fixation tests may occur with Q fever or brucellosis. Cutaneous hypersensitivity to the Frei antigen may develop during psittacosis.

Differential Diagnosis. Specific diagnosis of psittacosis is of extreme importance because of its potential severity (reported fatality rates range from 5 to 40 per cent), its response to antimicrobials, and the public health significance of psittacosis infection. All cases should be reported to the local health department. The syndrome of viral pneumonia accompanied by protracted high fever, unusually severe headache, and relative bradycardia should suggest psittacosis. Often a history of contact with birds is the only clue to diagnosis and may be elicited only by repeated questioning of the patient and family. When pneumonic symptoms are prominent, psittacosis must be differentiated from viral pneumonias, mycoplasmal pneumonia, influenza, Q fever, tuberculosis, histoplasmosis, coccidioidomycosis, bacterial pneumonia, and other processes that produce pulmonary infiltrates. If pneumonic symptoms are not prominent, psittacosis can be confused with other systemic febrile illnesses such as typhoid fever, brucellosis, infectious mononucleosis, infectious hepatitis, miliary tuberculosis, or the viral meningoencephalitides.

Treatment. The tetracyclines are the drugs of choice, and early diagnosis and initiation of treatment may be lifesaving. After institution of therapy with 2 to 3 grams daily, both fever and symptoms are generally controlled within 48 to 72 hours, although the response may be indolent. Although the disease apparently responds to penicillin in doses above 2 million units daily, tetracycline remains the drug of choice. Treatment should be continued for at least 10 days. The high fever and progressive anoxia secondary to extensive pulmonary involvement in severe cases may require appropriate measures directed at these problems.

Favour, C. B.: Ornithosis (psittacosis). Am. J. Med. Sci., 205:162, 1943.
Harding, H. B.: The bacteria-like chlamydiae of ornithosis and the diseases they cause. CRC Crit. Rev. Clin. Lab. Sci., 1:451, 1970.
Meyer, K. F.: The ecology of psittacosis and ornithosis. Medicine, 21:175, 1942.
Schaffner, W., Drutz, D. J., Duncan, G. W., and Koenig, M. G.: The clinical spectrum of endemic psittacosis. Arch. Intern. Med., 119:433, 1967.
Wilson, G. S., and Miles, A. A.: The psittacosis-lymphogranuloma group. *In* Wilson, G. S., and Miles, A. A. (eds): Topley and Wilson's Principles of Bacteriology and Immunity. 5th ed. Baltimore, Williams & Wilkins Co., 1964, vol. 2. pp. 2246–2267.

Section Three. MYCOPLASMAL DISEASES

Robert B. Couch

174. INTRODUCTION

The mycoplasmas (formerly called pleuropneumonia-like organisms, PPLO) are the smallest free-living organisms. They share a number of properties with bacteria, e.g., growth outside the host cell, susceptibility to antimicrobial drugs, generation of metabolic energy, reproduction by fission, and possession of both RNA and DNA. In contrast to bacteria, they do not possess a cell wall. The mycoplasmas are commonly confused with L-forms of bacteria, because L-forms also lack a cell wall

The Human Mycoplasmas

Species	Usual Site of Occurrence
M. pneumoniae	Respiratory tract
M. salivarium	Oropharynx
M. orale 1	Oropharynx
M. orale 2	Oropharynx
M. orale 3	Oropharynx
M. fermentans	Oropharynx and genital tract (rarely detected)
M. hominis	Genital tract
T-mycoplasmas	Genital tract

and their colonial morphology resembles that of mycoplasmas. However, L-forms are related to their bacterial parents and are unrelated to the mycoplasmas.

Members of the genus Mycoplasma cause a variety of diseases in animals. These include sinusitis, pneumonia, arteritis, arthritis, and neurologic disease. Because of these varied pathologic states in animals, it has been proposed that many inflammatory diseases of man of unknown etiology are caused by mycoplasmas. In this regard, extensive efforts to incriminate mycoplasmas in the etiology of rheumatoid arthritis have thus far been inconclusive. At present, eight species of human mycoplasmas have been identified. Only one species, *Mycoplasma pneumoniae,* has been clearly shown to produce disease in man, and the disease is essentially limited to the respiratory tract. Two species have been incriminated as causing disease of the male and female urogenital tract, and the other known species appear to be commensals. Nevertheless, because of the variety of animal diseases described, it would be surprising if some other human diseases are not caused by mycoplasmas.

The eight species of human mycoplasmas and their usual anatomic site of occurrence are shown in the accompanying table. *M. pneumoniae* is a significant cause of acute respiratory disease, including pneumonia (see Ch. 175). *M. salivarium* and *M. orale* 1 are common inhabitants of the oropharynx, particularly if oral hygiene is poor. *M. orale* 2 and 3 are uncommon inhabitants of the oropharynx, and *M. fermentans* has on rare occasions been recovered from the oropharynx and genital tract. None of the latter 5 species have been shown to cause human disease. *M. hominis* and the T-mycoplasmas (so called because of the "tiny" colonies produced on agar medium) have been collectively called the genital mycoplasmas and have been incriminated as etiologic agents in several disease syndromes (see Ch. 176).

175. PNEUMONIA AND OTHER RESPIRATORY DISEASES CAUSED BY M. PNEUMONIAE

Definition. Pneumonia is the most severe manifestation of respiratory infection with *Mycoplasma pneumoniae.* Bronchitis, pharyngitis, and asymptomatic infections are frequently seen, particularly in young children; pneumonia occurs predominantly among older children and young adults. The disease responds to treatment with the tetracyclines and erythromycins.

History. A pneumonia that was unlike lobar pneumonia of *Diplococcus pneumoniae* was recognized in the 1930's. Extensive bacteriologic studies failed to reveal a specific etiology in many of these cases, and Dingle and Finland in 1942 applied the term primary atypical pneumonia to this group of nonbacterial pneumonias. In 1943 the discovery that cold hemagglutinins developed in the sera of many of the patients provided a useful diagnostic test. During World War II the Armed Forces Commission on Acute Respiratory Disease described many of the clinical and epidemiologic characteristics of an atypical pneumonia, retrospectively identified by serologic tests as caused by infection with *M. pneumoniae.*

The causative agent was first isolated by Eaton in cotton rats, and subsequently was shown to infect hamsters and chicken embryos. It is filterable and for this reason was considered to be a virus for many years. In 1957, Liu reported an immunofluorescent test for antibody, using sections of infected chicken embryo bronchi for antigen, and Chanock in 1961 reported that the organism was the cause of most cases of pneumonia associated with the development of cold hemagglutinins. Subsequent to these studies and the demonstration that the organism was a Mycoplasma, it was given the name *Mycoplasma pneumoniae.*

Etiology. *Mycoplasma pneumoniae* can readily be distinguished from the seven other known human species of Mycoplasma. The organism is about 200 nm in size. It will grow aerobically or anaerobically on artificial media, but the medium must be enriched with 20 per cent horse serum and yeast extract. The small granular colonies grow embedded in the surface of the agar, and are best detected by microscopic examination. Tentative identification procedures utilize the fact that *M. pneumoniae* ferments glucose, exhibits hemadsorption, hemolyzes guinea pig and sheep red blood cells, and is resistant to methylene blue. Final identification requires serologic procedures.

Analysis of the lipids of *M. pneumoniae* has partially explained some of the serologic responses noted in this infection. The protective antigen appears to be a glycolipid contained in the membrane of the organism. A phospholipid which reacts with some Wassermann-positive sera has been identified, and cross-reactions with glycolipids of Streptococcus MG and the I antigen of human erythrocytes probably account for these occasional serologic responses. The anti-tissue antibodies noted in this infection may have a similar explanation.

Epidemiology. *M. pneumoniae* infection is endemic in large populations, but numerous localized outbreaks have occurred in schools and military populations. There is no periodicity such as occurs with influenza and no seasonal prevalence as with bacterial and viral respiratory illnesses.

The basic epidemiologic unit is the family, where the infection is often introduced by five- to nine-year-old schoolchildren. Infection spreads slowly but will ultimately involve 80 to 90 per cent of family members who are not immune. Though most common in young school-age children, the very young, adolescents, and young adults frequently acquire the infection. It is rare above age 50 when serum antibody is almost universally present.

Roentgenographic evidence of pneumonia occurs in 30 to 50 per cent of infected family members, but studies in the military have suggested that less than 10 per cent of infections result in pneumonia. This disparity may be accounted for by the finding that illness is more likely to occur and to be more severe with advancing age.

Pathogenesis. *M. pneumoniae* is a primary pathogen of the respiratory tract that is spread by close and frequent contact between infected and susceptible persons. The organism can be recovered from sputum and throat swab specimens two to three days prior to onset of illness. Thereafter, the concentration of organisms in secretions rises to the time of occurrence of illness and remains high for four to six days. After illness subsides, the agent may persist in respiratory secretions for several weeks in a considerable percentage of cases, and positive cultures frequently occur after antimicrobial treatment.

The organism grows on the ciliated border and between respiratory epithelial cells. All evidence indicates that it does not invade lung parenchyma. It has been suggested that the peroxide produced by the organism might produce cell damage; more recently it has been suggested that the illness may be a result of hypersensitivity to the organism or one or more of its products.

Resistance to infection has been shown to correlate with presence and magnitude of serum antibody, and this mechanism may also influence recovery from illness. Antibody is detectable in respiratory secretions, and recent data suggest that resistance more closely correlates with this antibody than with serum antibody. The association between antibody and resistance probably accounts for prevalence of the infection in younger age groups, as most adults have detectable serum antibody. Nevertheless, reinfection with mild illness has been shown to occur.

Pathology. From the limited studies available, it is apparent that a great variety of pathologic findings may occur in pneumonia, including patchy or confluent bronchopneumonia, interstitial pneumonia, and lobar pneumonia. Pleuritis with a small pleural effusion may be present, but significant pleural effusion is rare. Gross pathology usually reveals patchy areas of lung infiltration and inflamed bronchial and bronchiolar lumina containing mucoid and occasionally purulent exudate. Microscopic sections reveal mononuclear peribronchial and peribronchiolar infiltrates with edema and mononuclear cell infiltration of neighboring alveolar septa. Mucosal cell lining of respiratory passages usually remains intact, and polymorphonuclear cell infiltration is prominent only if necrosis and sloughing of the mucosal cell lining occur. No pathologic alterations have been described in other areas of the body.

Clinical Manifestations. Infection may be manifested by pneumonia, tracheobronchitis, pharyngitis, or bullous myringitis. Pneumonia is the most serious and best described syndrome. The incubation period to onset of illness is about three weeks, most cases occurring in 15 to 25 days.

Pneumonia. The onset of pneumonia is usually insidious, with malaise and headache as prominent symptoms. For a period of two to three days these symptoms increase in severity, and feverishness, myalgias, and sore throat may also occur. Cough is usually not prominent until two to three days after onset of illness. It is either nonproductive or productive of small amounts of mucoid sputum that occasionally contain flecks of blood. *Despite the delayed appearance of cough, it becomes the dominant respiratory symptom in mycoplasmal pneumonia, and its absence or the occurrence of only mild cough makes a clinical diagnosis questionable.* In some cases cough occurs early, and patients may exhibit the paroxysms, substernal discomfort, and tracheal tenderness characteristic of acute tracheobronchitis. Headache is commonly reported as the most distressing symptom in an adult. Ear discomfort, owing to myringitis, mild nasal symptoms, and prominent sore throat may also occur, especially in the younger age groups. Substernal or diffuse chest discomfort on inspiration is common, but typical pleuritic pain is rare.

Patients usually do not appear seriously ill. Tachypnea, dyspnea, and cyanosis are rare and are not seen unless pulmonary involvement is extensive or other disease is present. The degree of fever is variable, but fever is present in virtually all cases of pneumonia.

Physical examination usually reveals mild nasal obstruction and discharge and mild to moderate injection of the posterior pharynx. Mild injection of the tympanic membranes is commonly seen, and about 15 per cent of patients will exhibit frank myringitis, some of whom will develop blebs or bullae. Hemorrhage into the blebs or bullae is common, and these patients usually complain of severe ear pain. Tender cervical lymphadenopathy is a common finding, particularly when pharyngitis is also present.

Findings on chest examination may be minimal, and roentgenographic findings that seem out of proportion to physical findings frequently occur. Auscultation of the chest may reveal rhonchi and wheezes over the involved area of the lung owing to mucus in large bronchi and bronchioles, and fine to medium moist rales may also be heard. In the occasional patient with more extensive disease, signs of consolidation may be detected.

Tracheobronchitis. Tracheobronchitis alone may occur from infection with *M. pneumoniae* and is more common than pneumonia. The onset and clinical picture are little different from that described for pneumonia, and a significant proportion of cases clinically diagnosed as tracheobronchitis will exhibit infiltration when x-rays are obtained. The cases in which the chest x-rays are normal tend to be less severe.

Pharyngitis. Pharyngitis frequently accompanies the tracheobronchitis and pneumonia caused by *M. pneumoniae;* however, pharyngitis alone may also occur. The onset and constitutional manifestations are similar to those described for pneumonia, but sore throat appears early and persists as the predominant symptom. Mild nasal symptoms and some cough may also occur. Pharyngeal examination may reveal a diffusely erythematous pharynx with or without pharyngeal and tonsillar exudate, or only mild pharyngeal congestion may be present. Tender cervical lymph nodes frequently accompany pharyngitis.

Ear Disease. Myringitis, occasionally accompanied by blebs or bullae, is most commonly seen in association with disease of the respiratory tract; however, it has also been reported as an isolated disease occurrence. Such patients complain of ear pain which on occasion may be severe.

Roentgenographic Findings. No roentgenographic changes can be considered typical of mycoplasmal pneumonia. Infiltrates are usually unilateral, confined to a lower lobe, and more prominent near the hilum. Frequently a single segment is involved, but on occasion the infiltrate may be extensive and lobar or may involve more than one lobe. Small pleural effusions are not uncommon.

Laboratory Findings. In pneumonia and the other mycoplasmal respiratory diseases, the leukocyte counts are usually within normal limits and rarely exceed 10 to 15,000 per cubic millimeter. Differential counts usually reveal slight neutrophilia with counts of 60 to 85 per cent neutrophils. During the period of acute illness lymphopenia may be seen. The erythrocyte sedimentation rate is usually elevated. Urinalysis is within normal limits except for occasional albuminuria, which may be attributed to fever. Gram stain and culture of sputum usually reveal normal flora.

Course and Complications. The clinical course is variable and is best described for pneumonia. Illness on occasion may be severe, but very few deaths from pneumonia have occurred. Fever is variable in duration, lasting from three days to two weeks. Fever usually subsides by lysis, and when this occurs, slow but progressive improvement in the cough, malaise, and lethargy ensues. However, symptoms may persist for three to six weeks. Roentgenographic abnormalities frequently persist for two to four weeks.

The most common pulmonary *complication* is relapse soon after clinical recovery. This appears to occur in about 10 per cent of cases, and the disease may involve the same or a different lobe of the lung. Cases of residual pleural abnormality have also been reported. Clinically significant intravascular hemolysis in association with demonstrable cold hemagglutinins occurs in a small percentage of cases. Such patients exhibit cold hemagglutinin titers of 1:500 or greater and also have demonstrable hemagglutinins at room temperature. Hemolysis usually occurs when fever subsides or chilling of peripheral tissues occurs.

M. pneumoniae has been associated with central nervous system and cutaneous manifestations. The former patients have had psychosis, meningitis, meningoencephalitis, or radiculopathy. A variable number and type of cell have been noted in the cerebrospinal fluid. Skin manifestations have included urticaria, vesiculopustular eruptions, maculopapular eruptions, erythema multiforme, and erythema nodosum, although many patients were simultaneously receiving drugs, so that causation is not certain. A reported association with Stevens-Johnson syndrome is perhaps of special significance as these cases are frequently preceded by respiratory symptoms and accompanied by pneumonia. Evidence of *M. pneumoniae* infection should be sought in such cases.

Hemorrhagic bullous myringitis (see under Clinical Manifestations), bronchiectasis, pericarditis, myocarditis, Guillain-Barré syndrome, arthritis, and thrombocytopenic purpura have also been reported as complications of *M. pneumoniae* infection.

Diagnosis. Early diagnosis can be made only by clinical means. The presence of marked headache, lassitude, myalgias, definite nasopharyngeal findings, and nonproductive cough suggests nonbacterial pneumonia. Absence of the usual features of bacterial pneumonia, such as sudden onset, shaking chills, pleuritic pain, and purulent or bloody sputum, offers important support for the diagnosis. Other causes of pulmonary infiltration such as tuberculosis, mycotic infection, pulmonary infarction, and malignancy must be considered.

Among the causes of nonbacterial pneumonia that may mimic mycoplasmal pneumonia are psittacosis and Q fever, for which an exposure history should be sought, and adenoviral and influenzal pneumonias, which are usually more acute in onset and occur primarily during recognizable epidemics. If the age of the patient is 5 to 30 years and other similar cases have occurred in a family, diagnosis is more certain, but the only clinical finding that makes mycoplasmal pneumonia almost a certain diagnosis is the additional presence of myringitis with a bleb or bulla on the tympanic membrane.

Isolation of *M. pneumoniae* may be accomplished from sputum or throat swab specimens. Either enriched solid or special liquid medium may be used, although identifiable isolations are not usually detected for at least five days after inoculation, and 14 to 21 days of incubation may be required.

The cold hemagglutinin test is generally available and useful. Sera of about 50 per cent of patients with *M. pneumoniae* pneumonia will develop this autoantibody which agglutinates human red blood cells when reacted in the cold (4° C). It is more likely to occur in more severely ill patients, and usually appears toward the end of the first week or the beginning of the second week of illness. *Serum for this test should be separated from red blood cells before refrigeration.* Positive direct Coombs tests and an occasional false positive serologic test for syphilis may occur.

A variety of serologic procedures have been described for detecting rise in specific serum antibody titer to *M. pneumoniae* between acute and convalescent sera. Complement fixation is the most available procedure and will demonstrate a rise in titer in 75 to 80 per cent of cases. Growth inhibition is a more sensitive and specific method and is preferred, but it requires experience with cultivation techniques which is not widely available.

Treatment. Tetracycline and its derivatives and erythromycin have been shown to hasten the disappearance of fever, rales, and cough in treated cases of pneumonia. Since definitive diagnosis is not possible within the first few days after onset of illness, decisions regarding administration of antimicrobials must be made on clinical grounds. Patients presumed to have mycoplasmal pneumonia should receive tetracycline or its equivalent in doses of 0.25 gram every six hours. Erythromycin in doses of 0.5 gram every eight hours appears to be an acceptable alternative. Incomplete relief of cough, occasional relapse, and continued shedding of the organism frequently follow six- to eight-day courses of treatment with these antimicrobials. It is possible that continuing treatment for two to three weeks will provide more complete recovery, and therefore this duration of treatment is recommended. The additional use of antipyretics, antitussives, intermittent positive pressure breathing, oxygen, and the like is determined by individual needs.

It is recommended that all patients with bullous myringitis be treated with erythromycin or tetracycline for 10 to 14 days. Treatment of patients with pharyngitis and tracheobronchitis on a routine basis is not recommended unless the organism has been isolated, because these illnesses are indistinguishable by clinical techniques from the great majority of acute respiratory illnesses caused by viruses. However, if protracted illness occurs and *M. pneumoniae* has been isolated, the antimicrobials listed above may be used.

Prevention. No established method is presently available to prevent *M. pneumoniae* infection. Patients in the acute stage of pneumonia should probably be isolated and attempts made in the home to prevent close contact with ill individuals. There is no vaccine currently available.

Chanock, R.: Mycoplasma infections of man. N. Engl. J. Med., 272:1257, 1965.

Couch, R.: *Mycoplasma pneumoniae. In* Knight, V. (ed.): Viral and Mycoplasmal Infections of the Respiratory Tract. Philadelphia, Lea & Febiger, 1973, pp. 217–235.

Dingle, J. H., and Langmuir, A. D.: Epidemiology of acute respiratory

disease in military recruits. Am. Rev. Respir. Dis., 97 (Supplement):1, 1968.
Hayflick, L. (ed.): The Mycoplasmatales and the L-phase of Bacteria. New York, Appleton-Century-Crofts, 1969.
Mufson, M., Manko, M., Kingston, J., and Chanock R.: Eaton agent pneumonia: Clinical features. J.A.M.A., 178:369, 1961.

176. GENITOURINARY DISEASE CAUSED BY MYCOPLASMAS

Etiology. *Mycoplasma hominis* and T-mycoplasmas may cause genitourinary disease. *M. hominis* typically produces colonies on agar with the often-described "fried-egg" appearance. Colonies are usually 200 to 300 μ in diameter and are best visualized by microscopy. This colony size contrasts to that of the T-mycoplasmas, which is 10 to 30 μ in diameter. On agar medium *M. hominis* grows well under aerobic conditions, whereas T-mycoplasmas grow best anaerobically. Both grow well in broth, and tentative identification procedures employ the preferential metabolism of arginine by *M. hominis* and the fact that T-mycoplasmas possess a urease system and grow best in an acidic medium. The T-mycoplasmas are antigenically heterogeneous, and the number and significance of types and subtypes has not yet been delineated. A recent report suggests that *M. hominis* is also antigenically heterogeneous.

Epidemiology. The genital mycoplasmas may be recovered from the distal urethra of both the male and female and the vulva, vagina, and cervix of the latter. Presumably because of intimate association with mucosal surfaces, specimens that contain epithelial cells are superior to urine or secretion specimens for isolation tests.

Infants may become colonized with genital mycoplasmas at birth, presumably acquiring them from the birth canal. The frequency of recovery of organisms decreases for the first year or two of life, and most individuals then remain free of genital mycoplasmas until puberty. Mycoplasmas then reappear, and frequencies are directly proportional to extent of sexual activity and promiscuity, suggesting the possibility of the disease being acquired venereally.

Despite the fact that genital mycoplasmas are commonly recovered from the urogenital tract, disease is uncommon. This suggests a low order of pathogenicity for these organisms.

Clinical Manifestations. *Nonspecific Urethritis.* The syndrome of dysuria, urgency, and frequency of urination with urethral discharge and without evidence of gonococcal infection has been called nonspecific or nongonococcal urethritis. A negative urine culture for bacteria and absence of prostatitis if the patient is a male are essential supportive findings. Patients with postgonococcal urethritis in which the gonococcus disappears but symptoms of urethritis remain are also included in this category of patients. The urethritis may be caused by a T-mycoplasma but apparently not by *M. hominis*.

Pelvic Inflammatory Disease. Patients with lower abdominal pain and fever who exhibit tenderness on movement of the cervix and in the adnexal areas are usually designated as having pelvic inflammatory disease. In most instances acute or subacute salpingitis is present, although tubo-ovarian abscesses or pelvic abscesses elsewhere may present similar findings. *M. hominis* may cause the disease in many of these cases.

Cervicitis and vaginitis as separate disease entities may occasionally be caused by *M. hominis,* although the data are inconclusive in this regard.

Mycoplasmal Disease in Pregnancy. Both *M. hominis* and the T-mycoplasmas have been recovered from the uterus, amnion, and fetus. Infection is more likely to occur with *M. hominis* than with T-mycoplasmas and to occur during therapeutic or spontaneous abortion, or when premature rupture of the membranes has occurred. Blood cultures are occasionally positive, and such patients exhibit fever and serum antibody responses. The frequency and significance of *M. hominis* infection of the uterus and products of conception are uncertain, but it seems probable that *M. hominis* is responsible for some cases of septic abortion and puerperal infection.

Postpartum fever in patients with normal pregnancy and delivery may occasionally be caused by invasion of the bloodstream with *M. hominis* or T-mycoplasma. The frequency of such cases attributable to mycoplasmas is probably low.

Treatment. All mycoplasmas are susceptible to the tetracyclines. *M. hominis* is susceptible to lincomycin and resistant to erythromycin, whereas the converse is true for the T-mycoplasmas. Patients with nonspecific urethritis should receive tetracycline or its equivalent in doses of 0.25 gram every six hours for five to seven days. Although T-mycoplasmas are also susceptible to erythromycin, results of treatment have been somewhat better with tetracycline. When erythromycin is used for therapy of nonspecific urethritis, patients should receive 0.5 gram every eight hours for five to seven days. Relapse and/or reinfection occurs in about 20 per cent of patients within three months. Second courses of the drug are frequently beneficial, but the sexual contacts of such patients should be examined for T-mycoplasmas. Recurrent nonspecific urethritis is an indication for urologic evaluation for structural abnormality of the urethra.

Since pelvic inflammatory disease may be caused by gonococci, *M. hominis,* and perhaps other bacteria, and since the site of disease is not accessible for obtaining culture specimens, antimicrobial therapy directed toward the specific cause is often not possible. In nonhospitalized patients tetracycline has been reported to be effective treatment. In most instances of postpartum fever caused by mycoplasmas, spontaneous cure without specific antimycoplasmal therapy occurs. Patients considered as candidates for treatment should receive tetracycline in doses noted above.

McCormack, W. M., Braun, P., Lee, Y. H., Klein, J. O., and Kass, E. H.: The genital mycoplasmas. N. Engl. J. Med., 288:78, 1973.

Section Four. BACTERIAL DISEASES

177. INTRODUCTION

Walsh McDermott

For the past few decades the problems presented by bacterial and mycotic diseases have presented themselves in two different forms depending upon the nature of the society. In the economically underdeveloped parts of the world, the individual diseases have presented in classic form, each occupying its traditional niche in the over-all pattern. By contrast, in nations with highly developed health services, the familiar bacterial diseases have by no means disappeared, but their menace has been largely nullified by vaccines and by prompt and appropriate antimicrobial therapy. For example, one hears that lobar pneumonia "has largely disappeared." In actuality is *has* become much less prominent, not because its major cause, pneumococcal infection, is any less frequent, but because with prompt chemotherapy the early pneumonic lesion is halted in its progress well short of the confines of the lobe. It is the same old pneumonia, but it is no longer "lobar." Expressed differently, without any change in the annual incidence of pneumococcal infection or disease, the annual incidence of *serious problems* from this cause has substantially diminished. In place of such clinical problems there are now essentially new menaces in the serious systemic disease produced by *E. coli*, Proteus, Pseudomonas, Candida, and other microbes that were formerly regarded as essentially harmless inhabitants of man. The disease caused by staphylococci and tubercle bacilli can likewise be regarded as being partially of this sort, in that the microbes can subsist harmlessly in the tissues for considerable periods between eruptions as destructive disease. In effect these new clinical patterns represent *endogenous microbial disease*—clinical entities that appear almost exclusively in people with some temporary or sustained lowering of local or general defenses. Because of the resulting changes in the tissue environment, disease-producing microbes are evoked from the dormant or latent state. Generally speaking, these changes in the internal milieu represent a direct or indirect consequence of our modern therapies. They are the unsought-for effects of practical therapeutic gains that in themselves represent great scientific achievements. The practices involved include the use of corticosteroids and immunosuppressants; the suppression of customary microbial flora by drugs, thus compromising the protection to the host afforded by *bacterial interference;* surgical procedures, e.g., subtotal gastrectomy or splenectomy that can reduce previously acquired host resistance; and the longer survival of many patients despite protracted, severe, and ultimately fatal illness.

This increasing ability to alter man's internal environment has had the effect that virtually no microbial species today can be considered nonpathogenic, for in appropriate circumstances virtually any can give rise to disease. All these mechanisms unleash what are, in effect, "new" microbial diseases. There are other "new" diseases that may have been similarly unleashed or may have merely become easier to recognize by virtue of the selectivity of drug action. The separation of "atypical" pneumonia from bacterial pneumonia by the introduction of sulfonamide back in the 1930's and the growing importance of "atypical" mycobacteria as disease agents are cases in point. What is happening was biologically predictable, and the changing nature of the situation may be expected to continue.

To be capable of staying with this change the physician must know considerably more about the behavior of microbes, as they cause disease and are exposed to drugs within an otherwise normal or a compromised host, than he had to master only one or two decades ago. This knowledge is of two sorts: certain concepts and principles related to the microbe-drug-host interactions, and a body of knowledge sufficient to permit him to make microbiologically relevant diagnosis on clinical grounds. Knowledge of the latter sort is presented in the individual chapters that follow. For discussion of host defenses and their behavior during administration of immunosuppressive drugs, the reader is referred to Ch. 60 to 70 and Ch. 771 to 775. Endogenous microbial disease itself is discussed in Ch. 178, whereas the concepts and principles related to microbe-drug-host interactions are considered in Ch. 267 and 268.

McDermott, W.: Inapparent infection. The Dyer Lecture. Public Health Rep., 74:485, 1959.
Rogers, D., et al.: Infections in the altered host. *In* Year Book of Medicine, 1972, 1973, 1974. Chicago, Year Book Medical Publishers.

178. HOSPITAL-ASSOCIATED INFECTIONS: ENDOGENOUS MICROBIAL DISEASE

Jay P. Sanford

A startling metamorphosis has occurred in the disease pattern presented by microbes in the highly industrialized countries as contrasted with the classic pattern in most of the economically underdeveloped world. The nature of this pattern is illustrated by the data of Rogers, based upon a comparison of life-threatening infections demonstrated at necropsy in a group of patients who were hospitalized in 1938–1940 and a group who were hospitalized in 1957–1958 (see accompanying table). It

Changing Pattern of Life-Threatening Microbial Diseases at Necropsy (%)

	Year of Study	
Etiology	*1938–1940*	*1957–1958*
Pneumococci, streptococci, tubercle bacilli	20	2
Staphylococci	8	8
Gram-negative bacilli (aerobic)	4	11
Mycotic	1	4
"Hospital-associated infections"	7	54

should be noted that, although infections caused by *D. pneumoniae, Strep. pyogenes, and M. tuberculosis* had dropped significantly, there had been a concomitant two and a half-fold increase in infections caused by aerobic gram-negative bacilli, especially Enterobacteriaceae and Pseudomonadaceae, and a fourfold increase in those caused by fungi. Over-all, infections were either the major or a significant contributory cause of death in 28 per cent of patients hospitalized in 1938, but remained the major or a significant contributory cause of death in 14 per cent of patients hospitalized in 1958, at a time when antimicrobial drugs, corticosteroid agents, and other therapeutic modalities were available. The problem is essentially summarized by the observation that in 1938 most patients were admitted to hospitals with infection, less than 10 per cent being hospital associated, whereas by 1958 over 50 per cent of the life-threatening infections were acquired while the patient was hospitalized originally for a noninfectious problem. *Current studies in community hospitals suggest that about 5 per cent of patients who are admitted to general hospitals will acquire an infection while hospitalized.*

This metamorphosis in the pattern of infectious diseases reflects the impact of control and better management of infections caused by more virulent or invasive microorganisms and the introduction of medical practices which compromise the antimicrobial defense mechanisms of the patient. The organisms currently responsible for hospital-associated infections often were considered as "saprophytes" which were present in the environment or the "normal flora" of the patient. The antimicrobial defense systems include local mechanisms which depend upon the integrity of skin and mucosal barriers, the occurrence of bacterial interference, the inflammatory defense mechanisms which are evoked when the local defenses have been breached, and immune mechanisms, both humoral antibody (B lymphocyte-mediated) and cellular (T lymphocyte- and macrophage-mediated).

This change in the pattern of hospital-associated infections is well illustrated by the sequence of infections which have occurred in patients with extensive thermal burns with the progressive application of control measures and therapy. Before the introduction of penicillin G, group A streptococci were a leading cause of infection in the burned patient; subsequently, staphylococci became the leading cause of death. With better control of contact transmission of staphylococci and the development of more effective antistaphylococcal drugs, the staphylococci were superseded by aerobic gram-negative bacilli, such as *Pseudomonas aeruginosa, Serratia marcescens,* and *Providencia stuartii.* These organisms are the major problem in most burn centers today, but where control has been achieved, burn wounds have become infected with fungi such as members of the genus Mucor and viruses such as *Herpesvirus hominis* (simplex). This susceptibility of the burned patient is not only the consequence of the loss of the integumentary barriers; these patients also have a defect in granulocyte responsiveness and depression of cellular immunity.

The common hospital-associated infections include *urinary tract infections,* these usually being associated with the use of indwelling urethral catheters; *pneumonia,* which often may be attributed to the use of contaminated ventilatory therapy equipment; *cellulitis, phlebitis, and bacteremia* associated with the use of indwelling venous and arterial cannulas or improperly sterilized intravenous fluids; and *postsurgical wound infections.* These four categories of infection account for about 85 per cent of hospital-associated infections. The causative microorganisms include both bacteria and fungi such as *Candida spp.* Most of these causative organisms are present in the external environment of the patient and are delivered by contact transmission or through contaminated materials such as contaminated "disinfectants." Control of many of these infections can be accomplished by meticulous attention to good nursing practices. However, knowledge is lacking in many basic areas, such as the question as to why "sick" patients lose their ability to resist colonization of the skin and oropharynx with aerobic gram-negative bacilli, even if they have not received antimicrobial drugs.

In addition to these hospital-associated infections, there is a broad category of infections which are increasing in frequency both in hospitalized and in nonhospitalized patients. These infections occur in patients whose antimicrobial defenses are severely impaired and in whom the causative microorganisms not only include the usual "pathogens" such as staphylococci and hospital-associated microorganisms such as Pseudomonas, but also include the patient's endogenous microorganisms such as *Clostridium perfringens;* organisms in the environment which are of very low virulence such as *Aspergillus spp.;* and viral and parasitic agents whose epidemiology still is poorly defined – for example, infections caused by cytomegaloviruses and *Pneumocystis carinii* in the renal transplant patient on immunosuppressive therapy. These infections are termed "opportunistic" infections and are often caused by microorganisms considered as "saprophytes" or "commensals."

Advances in biomedical engineering and in the chemotherapy of malignant disease have blurred the traditional boundaries between pathogens and nonpathogens. Today physicians must consider virtually all microorganisms as capable of producing human disease in the patient whose antimicrobial defenses are compromised and who is placed in an environment which often is contaminated; hence we learn of infections caused by *Serratia marcescens,* a nonpathogen used as a marker organism 20 years ago, *Bacillus subtilis,* and even *Erwinia spp.,* a "coliform" of tulips.

Curry, C. R., and Quie, P. G.: Fungal septicemia in patients receiving parenteral hyperalimentation. N. Engl. J. Med., 285:1221, 1971.

Eickhoff, T. C., Brachman, P. S., Bennett, J. V., and Brown, J. F.: Surveillance of nosocomial infections in community hospitals. I. Surveillance methods, effectiveness, and initial results. J. Infect. Dis., 120:305, 1969.

Kunin, C. M., and McCormack, R. C.: Prevention of catheter-induced urinary-tract infections by sterile closed drainage. N. Engl. J. Med., 274:1155, 1966.

Pierce, A. K., and Sanford, J. P.: Bacterial contamination of aerosols. Arch. Intern. Med., 131:156, 1973.

Rogers, D. E.: The changing pattern of life threatening microbial disease. N. Engl. J. Med., 261:677, 1959.

PNEUMONIA

179. INTRODUCTION

Walsh McDermott

To discover that a pneumonia, i.e., an intrapulmonary process of some sort, is present in an adult patient is no very difficult feat; neither is that knowledge particularly helpful unless two further steps can be taken. These are detection of evidence that the disease is indeed microbial in origin and not an infarct or neoplasm, and identification of the specific microbe or kind or microbe that is involved. Every aspect of management—the choice of treatment, the complications to be watched for, and the hour-by-hour prognosis—depends on the nature of this information. To obtain it accurately *and in proper time* requires that the physician be wholly familiar with the various ways in which each one of the microbial pneumonias expresses itself. Some of these—for example, plague pneumonia—he may never see. Yet he must know at least enough about plague pneumonia so that he could avert its terrible consequences for others should he ever encounter a case. Other forms of pneumonia encountered relatively rarely arise as complications of some familiar microbial disease such as measles or tuberculosis or streptococcal disease. Occasionally, well-known viruses such as influenza or chickenpox cause pneumonia, or the physician may be asked to see a patient with psittacosis. In the compromised host, necrotizing pneumonias caused by Pseudomonas and other gram-negative bacilli are being recognized increasingly as one form of the endogenous microbial disease mentioned in the preceding two chapters. Most of the time, in an adult patient the physician is dealing with *mycoplasmal pneumonia* or with *one of three bacterial pneumonias,* pneumococcal, staphylococcal, or some other form of necrotizing pneumonia in an obviously altered host. This narrowing of the probabilities does not really lighten the seriousness of making the correct choice. The most effective treatment for pneumococcal pneumonia is utterly without value in Klebsiella pneumonia; a choice of therapy based on a diagnosis of mycoplasmal pneumonia when the patient actually has staphylococcal pneumonia could result in a fatality.

As *staphylococcal pneumonia* is so closely related to viral influenza, it is discussed both under staphylococcal disease (Ch. 195) and under influenza (Ch. 117). *Mycoplasmal pneumonia* is discussed in Ch. 175; the other major bacterial pneumonias, *pneumococcal, Klebsiella,* and the other *necrotizing pneumonias,* are presented in Ch. 180 to 183. Klebsiella pneumonia, although infrequent, is of great importance because of its potential severity and the ease with which it can be misdiagnosed. The pneumonias caused by the individual viruses and by rickettsial (and chlamydial) agents are considered in earlier chapters of Part VIII. Pneumococcal pneumonia is the most important of all pneumonias, not only in numerical terms, but because in large measure, and especially in its complications, it is the prototype of all the bacterial pneumonias.

180. PNEUMOCOCCAL PNEUMONIA

*Edward W. Hook**

Definition. Pneumococcal pneumonia is an acute bacterial infection of the lungs caused by *Streptococcus pneumoniae* (the pneumococcus) and characterized clinically by an abrupt onset, rigor, fever, chest pain, cough, and bloody sputum. Bacterial pneumonia occurring in otherwise healthy persons is usually caused by the pneumococcus.

Bacteriology and Immunology. The somatic portion of the lancet-shaped pneumococcal cell is gram positive. In its virulent form (smooth, S), the pneumococcus has an outer capsule consisting of a high molecular polysaccharide polymer that is specific for each serologic type. In addition to the type-specific capsular antigen, there is a species-specific carbohydrate in the cell wall, known as the "C" substance. The capsule of pneumococcus acts as an armor against phagocytic cells and thus contributes significantly to the pathogenicity of the organism. Pneumococcal variants having no capsules (rough, R strains) are essentially avirulent. Antibody to the type-specific carbohydrate promotes phagocytosis by combining with the highly polymerized polysaccharide of the capsular gel. The pneumococcus also produces hyaluronidase, a hemolysin that causes greenish discoloration around colonies on blood agar, and autolytic enzymes that, when activated, render the organism gram negative and eventually cause its dissolution.

Pneumococci grow rapidly on a variety of bacteriologic media. Blood agar and beef infusion broth containing 0.5 per cent dextrose and 5 to 10 per cent blood or serum are the media most commonly used. On blood agar virulent strains form circular, glistening, dome-shaped colonies that are alpha hemolytic. Because of the great quantity of capsular polysaccharide formed by type 3 pneumococcus, its colonies are more mucoid and usually much larger than those of other types. Unlike the alpha-hemolytic Streptococcus, pneumococcus is soluble in bile, sodium deoxycholate, and other surface-active agents, is highly sensitive to ethyl hydrocuprein chloride (optochin), and is mouse virulent.

The extraordinary virulence of pneumococci for mice may be made use of in isolating the organisms from sputum. The technique usually used consists in injecting intraperitoneally 0.5 ml of sputum previously emulsified by having been drawn repeatedly into a tuberculin syringe. When virulent pneumococci are present, the mouse usually dies within 48 hours, and a pure culture of the organism can be isolated from the heart's blood. Since other bacteria in the sputum do not ordinarily produce fatal infections in mice, the animal serves as a convenient and highly sensitive differential "culture medium" for the isolation of pneumococci.

More than 82 different serologic types of pneumococci have been identified by agglutination tests with specific antiserums or by the quellung test. The latter is based upon the fact that when pneumococci come in contact with homologous anticapsular serum, a capsular precipitin reaction and swelling occur, rendering the capsule easily visible under the microscope.

Anticapsular antibody usually appears in the blood of patients with pneumococcal pneumonia between the fifth and tenth days of the disease. In some untreated patients, its appearance coincides with recovery; in others no such relation is demonstrable. Specific polysaccharide, which has diffused away from the bacteria, can often be identified in the urine and blood. Using counterimmunoelectrophoresis, circulating polysaccharide

---

*Dr. W. Barry Wood, the author of this chapter for many years, died on March 9, 1971. Dr. Hook has revised the chapter but has retained much of the original material.

can be detected in the blood of one third to one half of patients with pneumococcal bacteremia but much less often in the absence of demonstrable bacteremia. The technique may have diagnostic usefulness because it can give specific diagnostic information in about one hour. Patients frequently continue to excrete the capsular carbohydrate in the urine for days and even weeks after recovery.

Epidemiology. Pneumococcal pneumonia may occur at any season, but it is most common during the winter and early spring, when viral respiratory infections are most prevalent.

The types of pneumococci that most commonly cause pneumonia in adults are types 1, 3, 4, 5, 7, 8, 12, 14, and 19. Together, these nine types account for about three quarters of all cases. The most common types encountered in childhood pneumonias are 1, 6, 14, and 19.

Pneumococci, particularly of the higher types, are frequently present in the respiratory tracts of normal subjects. Ordinarily the prevalence of carriers of highly pathogenic types is relatively low, except for type 3, which is a common inhabitant of the normal pharynx. Nevertheless, there is evidence that normal carriers play a more important role in the dissemination of infective types than do patients ill with pneumonia. Occasionally, in relatively closed communities, high carrier rates of pathogenic types are encountered. In such circumstances the occurrence of widespread viral disease of the respiratory tract may result in an epidemic of pneumococcal pneumonia. Except for these rare epidemics, most of which occur in hospitals or custodial institutions, the disease is sporadic. Pneumococcal pneumonia occurs frequently in patients with multiple myeloma or hypogammaglobulinemia.

Pathogenesis and Pathology. The lung is the only major viscus of the body exposed to air. As the atmosphere, particularly in congested places, contains many pathogenic bacteria, it is remarkable that pneumonia is not more common. The failure of normal subjects to acquire acute bacterial pneumonia as an airborne infection is due to efficient defense barriers of the lower respiratory tract. These include (1) the epiglottal reflex, which prevents aspiration of infected secretions; (2) the sticky mucus that lines the bronchial tree and to which airborne organisms adhere; (3) the cilia of the respiratory epithelium, which keep the mucus moving constantly toward the pharynx at the rate of 1 to 3 cm per hour; (4) the cough reflex, which serves to propel mucus or foreign bodies out of the lower tract; (5) the lymphatics that drain the terminal bronchi and bronchioles; (6) phagocytic cells, especially alveolar macrophages that are ever present in the normal alveoli; and (7) opsonins and specific antibody. In addition, the alveoli themselves are relatively dry and thus offer a poor medium for growth of bacteria that succeed in reaching them. Acute bacterial pneumonia results only when the defense barriers of the normal respiratory tract fail.

The thesis that bacterial pneumonia usually results from aspiration of infected secretions from the upper respiratory tract is strongly supported by both experimental and clinical observations. Rats infected with pneumococci in the nasopharynx regularly exhibit pulmonary lesions only when subjected to experimental procedures involving chilling of the body, anesthesia, administration of morphine, or alcoholic intoxication, all of which are predisposing factors in human pneumonia and have been shown in laboratory animals to slow the epiglottal reflex and thus to facilitate aspiration. Experimental pneumonia can best be produced by intrabronchial inoculation of organisms suspended in mixtures of gastric mucin or starch having viscosities similar to that of mucus. Viral infection of the upper respiratory tract in man usually precedes the onset of acute bacterial pneumonia by several days. Not only is the volume of secretion from the nasopharynx greater than normal during viral infections such as the common cold, but also the number of pathogenic microorganisms in the secretions is significantly increased. Thus the stage is set for aspiration of infected mucus. That such aspiration often occurs at the onset of pneumonia in man is suggested by the usual sites of initial involvement of the lung. The earliest lesions of bacterial pneumonia usually appear in those parts of the lungs into which aspirated fluid is most likely to drain. Whereas most airborne bacteria are caught on the sticky surfaces of the bronchial tree and never reach the alveoli, organisms contained in thin nasopharyngeal secretions are readily carried into the alveoli by the liquid mucus. The latter, like Lipiodol, cannot all be ejected by ciliary action, and much of it penetrates to the farthest reaches of the bronchial tree, where it establishes the initial focus of infection.

Other factors known to predispose patients to acute bacterial pneumonia include exposure to noxious gases and anesthetics, cardiac failure, influenza viral infection of the lungs, and trauma to the thorax. A feature common to all these conditions is the accumulation of fluid in the alveoli. Harford (1950) has shown that the dry lungs of normal mice are able to rid themselves of large numbers of inspired bacteria, whereas lungs containing fluid are readily infected. This observation suggests that pulmonary edema, by providing a suitable culture medium for the bacteria, may facilitate the establishment of active infection within the alveoli. Influenza also causes destruction of the ciliated columnar epithelial cells lining the tracheobronchial tree, thus interfering with function of cilia. In addition, influenza virus also apparently inhibits phagocytosis.

Pneumococcal pneumonia may also occur as a complication of bronchogenic carcinoma, chronic pulmonary disease, such as bronchiectasis or lung abscess, or any process that produces obstruction of a bronchus.

Splenectomy carries an increased risk of severe bacteremic infections which are predominantly although not exclusively pneumococcal in etiology. The clinical course is often fulminant, frequently associated with evidence of diffuse intravascular coagulation and a high mortality rate. Although it appears that even healthy adults with post-traumatic splenectomies show increased susceptibility, the risk is greatest in infants and young children, in patients with underlying diseases which compromise reticuloendothelial function, and during the first postsplenectomy years. The mechanism of this relationship is unknown, but it appears that the spleen is important in removing encapsulated bacteria in the absence of antibody.

Children with sickle cell anemia and other sickle cell hemoglobinopathies also seem especially vulnerable to severe pneumococcal infections, especially meningitis. The pneumococcus, not *Hemophilus influenzae,* is the most common cause of bacteremia and meningitis in patients with sickle cell anemia. The causes of this relationship are probably multiple and include deficient pneumococcal opsonizing activity, functional asplenia in some instances and actual splenic atrophy in others, and impaired phagocytic and killing capacity of reticuloendothelial cells.

In patients with severe pneumococcal disease with bacteremia and pneumonia or extrapulmonary sites of infection in cerebrospinal, pleural, or peritoneal fluids, the frequency of underlying disease exceeds 50 per cent.

Early Lesion. Once the infection has gained a foothold within the alveoli, the lesion evolves in a characteristic manner. The first response of the lung to bacterial invasion is an outpouring of edema fluid into the alveoli which serves to "float" organisms into new alveoli through the pores of Kohn and terminal bronchioles.

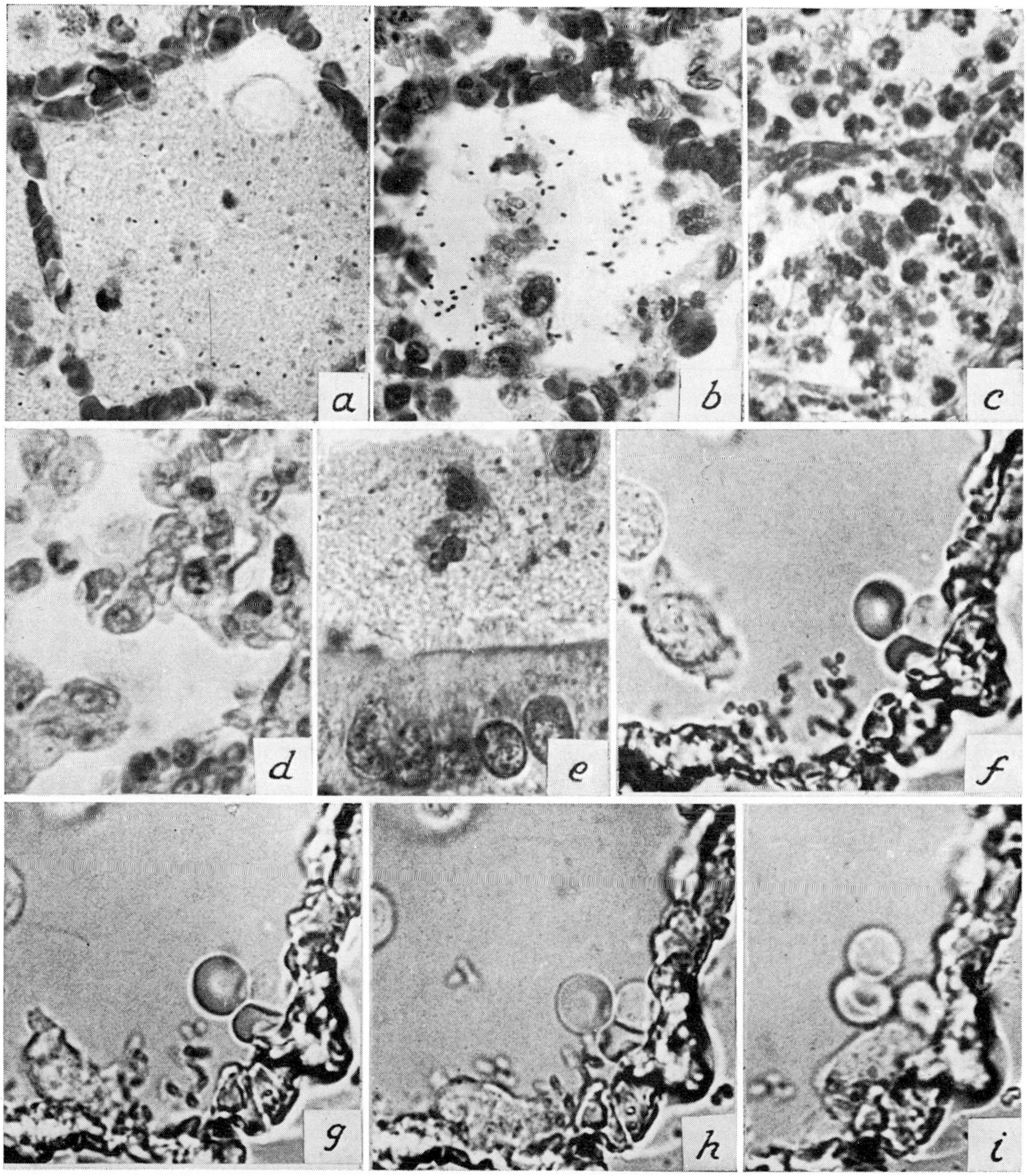

a, Pneumococci in edema-filled alveoli at margin of spreading pneumonic lesion (×800).
b, Beginning stage of polymorphonuclear exudation in zone of early consolidation. Note leukocytes in alveolar capillaries, some in process of diapedesis (×800).
c, Leukocytic exudate (still predominantly polymorphonuclear) in inner zone of advanced consolidation. Pneumococci have been phagocytized and destroyed (×800).
d, Alveolar macrophage reaction characteristic of late stage of resolution (×800).
e, Pneumococci in edema fluid contained within lumen of a large bronchus. Such infected bronchial fluid causes spread of pneumonia to other lobes of the lungs (×1250).
f–i, Surface phagocytosis of encapsulated microorganisms in formalin-fixed rat lung (×1250). Bacteria shown in these photomicrographs are klebsiella, but same results have been obtained with pneumococci.
f, Polymorphonuclear leukocyte is seen approaching bacteria near alveolar wall. Time 12:30.
g, Leukocyte has reached alveolar wall and is about to trap organisms against the tissue surface. Time 12:31.
h, Cell has trapped some of the encapsulated bacteria against the wall and is in the process of phagocytizing them. Time 12:32.
i, Having ingested several of the organisms, the leukocyte is moving up the alveolar wall. Time 12:35.
(Photomicrographs from studies on experimental pneumonia. W. B. Wood et al.: J. Exp. Med., Vol. 73; and Smith and Wood: *ibid.,* Vol. 86.)

Centrifugal spread of infection occurs. After the outpouring of edema fluid, polymorphonuclear leukocytes and some erythrocytes accumulate in the infected alveoli, first in small numbers but later in such quantities as to fill each alveolus and thus render the area completely consolidated. Once the infected alveoli become crowded with leukocytes, phagocytosis of bacteria takes place, and the invading organisms are destroyed. Macrophages appear in the exudate, and resolution begins only after most of the organisms have been ingested.

Spreading Lesion. Three stages in the inflammatory reaction account for the distinguishing histologic features of the spreading pneumonic lesion. In the outermost portion there appears an "edema zone" in which the alveoli are filled with acellular serous fluid containing bacteria. Inside the edema zone a second zone may be identified in which there are signs of early consolidation with leukocytes in most of the alveoli. Here phagocytosis is often noted. Still more centrally a third transition to a "zone of advanced consolidation" is noted where the alveoli are packed with cells and where beginning resolution may be evident.

All stages of inflammation can be found in a spreading lesion. In the most recently invaded areas at the periphery, edema and hemorrhage predominate, causing "red hepatization," whereas in the older, more central parts of the lesion, dense consolidation with leukocytes accounts for the characteristic color of "gray hepatization."

Not all pneumococcal pneumonia causes lobar consolidation. Lesions may be patchy in distribution and concentrated particularly about the bronchi. Because a clear-cut distinction between pneumococcal bronchopneumonia and lobar pneumonia cannot always be made even by the pathologist, and because management of the two conditions is the same, it is rarely important for the clinician to differentiate them. The etiology rather than the anatomy of the lesion determines therapy.

Interlobar Spread. The spread of the pneumonic process may be stopped by the pleural boundaries of the lobe. Often, however, the infection spreads to other lobes of the lungs by flow of infected edema fluid from bronchi of the involved lung into the bronchial tree of a new lobe.

Bacteremia. Bacteremia is common during the course of pneumococcal pneumonia, particularly when the infection is fulminating. The fact that organisms appear in the thoracic duct in experimental pneumonia before they appear in the systemic circulation suggests that the bacteria reach the bloodstream via the lymphatics. Blood cultures are positive in 20 to 30 per cent of patients with pneumococcal pneumonia. The prevalence of bacteremia increases with age, and is more common with type 2 pneumonia and less common with type 3 pneumonia than with other pneumococcal types.

Invasion of Pleura and Pericardium. The exact mechanism whereby pneumococci invade the pleura or pericardium is not known. As the lymphatics at the periphery of the lung drain outward toward the pleura, it is possible that pleural invasion results from lymphangitic spread. When infection of a pleural or pericardial cavity occurs, there results an outpouring of serous fluid followed by the deposit of fibrin. Leukocytes accumulate in the infected cavity, and, if infection persists, a purulent focus results. The pus in such cavities is at first thin but later becomes thick and stringy as a result not only of fibrin formation but also of the precipitation of deoxyribonucleic acid derived from the nuclei of disintegrating leukocytes. Finally, the thick fibrinous pus becomes walled off, forming loculated foci of chronic suppuration.

Similar purulent foci may occur in the meninges, peritoneum, or joints, as a result of hematogenous spread. Acute vegetations on the endocardium of the heart valves are sometimes encountered. Children with nephrotic syndrome are more prone to pneumococcal peritonitis than normal children. Pneumococcal peritonitis also occurs as a complication of hepatic cirrhosis with ascites.

Mechanism of Recovery. SURFACE PHAGOCYTOSIS. Owing to the antiphagocytic properties of their capsules, fully encapsulated, virulent pneumococci are resistant to phagocytosis when suspended in a fluid medium devoid of opsonins. In the presence of relatively immovable cellular surfaces, however, as in the alveoli, leukocytes are able to trap the encapsulated organisms and ingest them without the aid of opsonizing antibody.

HEAT-LABILE OPSONINS. Leukocytes in vivo are also assisted, right from the start of infection, by heat-labile opsonins that are present in normal plasma. These opsonins, which gain access to acute inflammatory exudates, are immunologically polyspecific, i.e., they act on all sorts of bacteria, in contrast to the monospecific anticapsular antibody that is eventually generated. Their opsonizing action on pneumococci has been shown to involve multiple components of the complement system, including C3. Its cleavage product, C3b, appears to act as a ligand between the organism on which it is deposited and the surface of the phagocyte.

ANTICAPSULAR OPSONINS. Most patients with pneumococcal pneumonia who survive long enough eventually generate an excess of monospecific anticapsular antibody. The process usually takes five to ten days. These newly formed immunoglobulins not only agglutinate the pneumococci in the edema zone of the lesion and thereby inhibit their spread, but also act as potent accessory opsonins and further increase the efficiency of phagocytosis.

MACROPHAGE REACTION. The exact role of the "macrophage reaction" in the recovery process is not entirely clear. Because the appearance of macrophages in the alveolar exudate coincides in general with the disappearance of organisms from the lesion, it has long been assumed that these large mononuclear phagocytes take an active part in destroying the bacteria, and in the final analysis tip the scales in favor of the cellular defenses of the host. Studies relating to experimental lymphadenitis cast some doubt upon this assumption. The "macrophage reaction" in a regional lymph node draining an area of active infection can be artificially initiated at any stage of the nodal inflammation by merely cutting the afferent lymph vessels bringing bacteria to the node. Thus it appears that macrophages accumulate in the exudate only when the active stimulus of direct bacterial invasion has been eliminated. If this interpretation is correct, the polymorphonuclear leukocytes may be looked upon as the "shock troops" that play the major role in controlling the infection, whereas the macrophages serve primarily to remove the particulate debris from the resolving exudate and thus promote clearing of the lesion.

RESOLUTION. One of the most remarkable features of pneumococcal pneumonia is the completeness with which it resolves. Even when several lobes are completely consolidated, recovery usually results in restoration of the entire pulmonary parenchyma to its normal state within a few weeks. Not all the processes that take part in this dramatic resolution have been identified, but they include (1) the action of cytolytic enzymes upon disintegrating leukocytes; (2) transport of cells from the lesion via lymphatics; and (3) phagocytosis and digestion of cellular debris by macrophages. The rarity with which tissue necrosis occurs in pneumococcal pneumonia, despite the violence of the inflammatory response, appears to account for the completeness of the healing. Occasionally recovery proceeds more slowly than usual and leads to "delayed resolution." The factors responsible for delaying the removal of exudate from the lesion in such cases are not known. In rare instances, as the result of irreversible damage to the pulmonary parenchyma, resolution fails to take place altogether, and the lesion becomes the site of intense fibroblastic activity that leads to permanent scarring or "organized pneumonia."

Infection with type 3 pneumococcus may occasionally lead to pulmonary necrosis and abscess formation. This pneumococcus has a large capsule that interferes with phagocytosis and accounts, at least in part, for its extraordinary pathogenicity.

SUPPURATIVE EXTRAPULMONARY FOCI. Suppurative pneumococcal lesions, which usually occur in such extrapulmonary sites as the pleura, pericardium, meninges, joints, mastoids, or accessory sinuses, resolve much less readily, even with intensive chemotherapy, than does uncomplicated pneumococcal pneumonia. In such areas of suppuration, phagocytosis appears to be relatively inefficient, because trapping of bacteria by leukocytes in the exudate is inefficient and many of the leukocytes in the exudate are not viable. Although a drug like penicillin may reach the organisms in a purulent focus, it may not destroy them, because pneumococci do not multiply rapidly in pus of long standing, and "resting" bacteria are not susceptible to the bactericidal action of penicillin. In fact, suppurative pneumococcal lesions may respond satisfactorily only when chemotherapy is combined with some form of drainage that removes the bulk of the necrotic exudate.

Clinical Manifestations. *Symptoms.* Victims of pneumococcal pneumonia are often seriously ill when first seen. The degree of prostration may be such that an adequate history can be obtained only from the family. The story of a mild nasopharyngitis preceding by several days the onset of major symptoms is frequently elicited. The first distressing symptom is usually a shaking chill, lasting for several minutes to a half hour. More than 80 per cent of patients with pneumococcal pneumonia experience one or more chills during the earliest stages of the disease. The initial rigor is often so violent as to cause the bed to shake and the patient's teeth to chatter. It is followed in about one case in three by vomiting. The initial chill usually coincides with bacterial invasion of the lung and marks the onset of fever. Several chills may occur at the start of pneumococcal pneumonia, but repeated attacks of rigor late in the disease suggest an extrapulmonary complication such as empyema, pneumonia caused by some other bacterium, or administration of antipyretics.

CHEST PAIN. In approximately 70 per cent of cases, severe chest pain occurs at the onset and may even precede the rigor. The pain, which is "stabbing" in character and exaggerated by cough and respiration, is caused by inflammation of the pleura resulting from the characteristically peripheral location of the initial lesion. There may be local tenderness in the chest wall at the site of the pleurisy. When the diaphragmatic surfaces of the pleura are affected, the pain may be referred either to the corresponding side of the lower chest wall and upper abdomen or to the shoulder. The patient may gain some relief from the knifelike pain by lying on the affected side, thereby splinting that half of the thorax.

COUGH. A cough may be absent at the onset, but usually is a prominent symptom during the course of the disease. Stimulation of the cough reflex results from irritation of the lower respiratory tract and from accumulation of mucus and exudate within the bronchial tree. Approximately 75 per cent of patients raise diffusely bloody or "rusty" sputum in contrast to "blood-streaked" sputum. The thorough mixing of the blood appears to be due to the fact that bleeding occurs directly into the alveolar exudate and thus constitutes an integral part of the inflammatory response to the infection. When the sputum is particularly sticky or jelly-like, type 3 pneumococcus or Klebsiella should be suspected, because both these organisms produce an inordinate amount of capsular polysaccharide that causes the exudate to be highly viscous.

FEVER AND TOXEMIA. Constant features of the disease are fever and toxemia, with the temperature usually ranging between 39.5 and 41° C. During the febrile period complaints of malaise, anorexia, weakness, myalgia, and general prostration are extremely common. Pneumococcal pneumonia may occasionally progress with great rapidity, and the general condition of the patient may deteriorate alarmingly within a few hours.

Physical Signs. Patients with well-established pneumococcal pneumonia appear acutely ill. There is moderate to severe respiratory distress. The nostrils dilate with each inspiration. Paroxysms of hacking cough, often productive of bloody or rusty sputum, occur during the examination. The chest pain, which is usually unilateral, may be so severe as to interfere with the patient's breathing and coughing; in these circumstances grunting expiration results. The location of the pain indicates immediately the approximate site of at least part of the lesion. The patient occasionally appears apprehensive and may even be delirious.

The temperature, pulse rate, and respiratory rate are usually elevated by the time the patient seeks the aid of a physician. The temperature should be taken by rectum, because oral measurement with the subject breathing rapidly through the mouth is likely to be inaccurate. The pulse pressure is characteristically widened, as in any high fever.

The skin is usually hot and moist, with beads of perspiration visible on the face and forehead. Cold extremities may indicate impending shock. Herpetic blisters are frequently noted about the mouth. The lips, mucous membranes, and nail beds are often cyanotic as a result of blood passing through poorly aerated lung. The cyanosis may be exaggerated by lowered respiratory exchange associated with rapid shallow breathing, often resulting from pleural pain. Icterus of the sclerae should be carefully looked for because of the prognostic significance of overt jaundice in pneumonia.

The ears should always be examined with an otoscope to exclude the presence of active otitis. Tenderness over a mastoid process or over an accessory nasal sinus should also be noted. The presence of exudate in the pharynx or over the tonsils suggests the possibility of streptococcal or adenoviral pneumonia. Definite nuchal rigidity may indicate pneumococcal meningitis, a serious complication of pneumonia. The neck veins must be carefully examined to detect the presence of increased venous pressure caused by complicating congestive heart failure. Deviation of the trachea constitutes an important sign of either atelectasis (toward the involved side) or pleural effusion (away from the involved side).

EXAMINATION OF THE CHEST. Diminished respiratory excursion or a slight inspiratory lag of one side of the chest often reveals the site of the principal lesion. A localized area of tenderness in the chest wall, noted during percussion, may be one of the earliest signs of pleural invasion. Careful percussion and auscultation do not always reveal signs of consolidation. In early cases, particularly, there may be no conclusive physical signs. Lesions at a distance from the chest wall are difficult to outline by percussion. When consolidation is extensive, the typical findings of dullness to percussion, bronchial or tubular breath sounds, and fine crackling rales are easily elicited, except in the presence of complicating bronchial obstruction or extensive pleural effusion. A coarse "leathery" friction rub is frequently audible in the region of consolidation.

Examination of the heart may be difficult because of loud respiratory sounds. An apical systolic murmur is frequently heard during high fever and is often of no significance. Diastolic murmurs, on the other hand, arising from either the mitral or aortic valve, are usually indicative of underlying organic heart disease or complicating pneumococcal endocarditis. A pericardial friction rub often constitutes the first sign of spread of the pneumococcal infection to the pericardial cavity. Ventricular premature contractions are not uncommon in the presence of any moderate or severe infection.

ABDOMINAL DISTENTION. Distention of the abdomen is frequently encountered. When tympany is noted in the left axilla and left upper quadrant, acute gastrectasia should be suspected. Occasionally, the examiner will note rigidity and even tenderness in one or both upper quadrants of the abdomen, suggesting a subdiaphragmatic lesion. This sign is usually due to referred pain resulting from involvement of the parietal pleura over the outer part of the diaphragm.

The neurologic examination is rarely abnormal in pneumococcal pneumonia except in the presence of meningitis or brain abscess. Digital examination of the rectum may be postponed if the patient is acutely ill, but in women a sufficiently complete pelvic examination should be performed to exclude the possibility of an infected abortion, which may lead to metastatic bacterial pneumonia.

Laboratory Findings. As in most acute bacterial infections, the total leukocyte count in pneumococcal pneumonia is elevated, and there is a "shift to the left" in the differential count. The number of leukocytes in the peripheral blood during the active infection usually ranges from 15,000 to 40,000 per cubic millimeter; counts above 40,000 are occasionally encountered. Leukopenia (with a "shift to the left") is observed in fulminating pneumococcal infections, particularly in the presence of bacteremia and in alcoholics.

Although the presence and location of the pulmonary lesion can usually be determined by physical examination, confirmatory roentgenographic evidence is often helpful. Both posteroanterior and lateral views of the chest should be taken. Pneumococcal infection of the lungs usually begins in the right middle lobe or in one of the lower lobes. The pulmonary process is limited to a single lobe in the majority of patients. In fact, it is not unusual for the process to be limited to a single pulmonary segment. In the series of Austrian and Gold, collected since the introduction of antimicrobial drugs, fewer than one third of the patients with pneumococcal pneumonia and bacteremia had more than a single lobe involved. Bulging interlobar fissure may be observed occasionally in pneumococcal pneumonia, although it is much more characteristic of Friedländer's pneumonia.

Whenever the diagnosis of pneumococcal pneumonia is suspected, the patient's blood should be cultured. Anaerobic as well as aerobic cultures are recommended to ensure detection of pneumonia caused by a microbe other than pneumococcus. A blood culture positive for pneumococci provides important information regarding both etiology and prognosis.

Pneumococci are usually present in sputum, nasopharynx, and material aspirated from the trachea. Sputum for smear and culture may be difficult to obtain, but this usually can be accomplished by urging the patient to cough, or a paroxysm of cough can be induced by passing a nasal catheter into the trachea. If a sputum specimen cannot be obtained, a nasopharyngeal culture should be collected, because there is a high positive correlation between specific pneumococci isolated from cultures of the nasopharynx and from the sputum of patients with pneumococcal pneumonia. Transtracheal aspiration or lung puncture is not indicated for the diagnosis of bacterial pneumonia in the usual patient.

The sputum in pneumococcal pneumonia shows large numbers of gram-positive, lancet-shaped diplococci in association with polymorphonuclear leukocytes. Gram-positive cocci which are not pneumococci are frequently observed in sputum smears and account for the poor correlation of results of studies to identify pneumococci on Gram-stained sputum smears and on sputum cultures. Omniserum, a pool of antibody against 82 pneumococcal types, can be used for definitive identification of pneumococci in sputum. The results of the quellung reaction using omniserum correlate with the results of cultures in about 90 per cent of cases. Because the carrier rate of pneumococci in the general population may be quite high, positive identification of pneumococci in sputum or nasopharynx does not establish a definitive diagnosis of pneumococcal pneumonia.

Other laboratory examinations that may be of value in the management of the patient include blood electrolyte and urea determinations.

Clinical Course. During the course of the disease the patient should be examined carefully once a day. More frequent physical examinations may unduly exhaust an acutely ill subject. The common complications of pneumococcal pneumonia should be specifically looked for during each examination, particularly when fever persists.

Defervescence. The fever of untreated pneumococcal pneumonia either may terminate abruptly by "crisis" five to ten days after onset or may gradually subside by lysis. When effective antibacterial therapy is used, a dramatic crisis may occur within 24 hours, or the fever may persist for several days. Physical signs in the chest may also change, coarse sticky rales of resolution replacing the fine crepitant rales and tubular breath sounds of consolidation. Complete clearing of the pulmonary lesion may occur within a few days, but usually the auscultatory signs of resolution persist for a week or more after defervescence. If resolution is not complete within 21 days, it is arbitrarily classified as delayed. The promptness of defervescence and the speed of resolution are in general inversely proportional to the age and extent of the lesion at the time treatment is begun.

Crisis marking the start of recovery must be differentiated from the "pseudocrisis" occasionally noted at the onset of shock or at the time of interlobar spread of the infection. Although the temperature may fall precipitously during a pseudocrisis, the pulse rate remains elevated, and the patient's general condition fails to improve.

Relapse. Relapse may occur in pneumococcal pneumonia when chemotherapy is discontinued too soon. If fever, tachycardia, and other signs of active infection recur while the patient is still receiving penicillin therapy, it may usually be assumed that a previously unrecognized purulent complication of the pneumococcal infection (such as empyema) exists, that a drug-resistant secondary invader has gained a foothold in the lung, or that hypersensitivity of the patient to penicillin has caused the development of drug fever.

Complications. *Pleural Effusion.* The most common specific complication of pneumococcal pneumonia is pleurisy with effusion. In somewhat less than 10 per cent of cases, fluid can be demonstrated in the pleural cavity by either physical or roentgenographic examination. Such effusions are usually small, and, when sterile, are rarely of significance. They result from inflammation of the pleura overlying the lesion in the lung. Occasionally they may be of sufficient volume to cause respiratory embarrassment and necessitate thoracentesis. Whenever pleural effusion is detected in a patient who has failed to respond promptly to treatment, a thoracentesis should be performed in order to determine whether the fluid is infected and thus represents an early empyema.

Empyema. Empyema, though less common than sterile pleural effusion, is far more serious. Before the advent of chemotherapy, the incidence of this complication was approximately 5 per cent. With the use of penicillin, empyema is much less common (less than 2 per cent). Its presence is indicated by continued fever (often irregular), persistent leukocytosis, and signs of pleural effusion. Localized tenderness is frequently noted in the chest wall overlying the site of the lesion. The exudate in the pleural cavity may become loculated by thick, fibrinous adhesions. When the lesion is confined to an interlobar fissure or is located in the thoracic "gutter" adjacent to the spine, it may be detectable only by roentgenographic methods. Repeated exploratory thoracenteses, done preferably with the help of fluoroscopy, may be required to prove the presence of empyema. Its detection is of the greatest importance, because, once discovered, it is amenable to proper therapy, whereas, if left untreated, it may eventually drain exteriorly through the chest wall *(empyema necessitatis)* or rupture into a bronchus and cause a bronchopleural fistula. Rarely, empyema heals spontaneously, causing calcification of the pleura.

Meningitis and Endocarditis. Two serious complications of pneumococcal pneumonia that are often associated with one another are endocarditis and meningitis. Pneumococci usually localize on the aortic valve, producing aortic insufficiency. The development of pneumococcal endocarditis is rare at present. Equally serious is *pneumococcal meningitis* resulting from blood-borne metastasis to the meninges. About 20 per cent of cases of pneumococcal meningitis develop secondary to pneumococcal infection of the lung. The meningitis is characterized by the presence in the pia-arachnoid of a heavily infected exudate, which may cause subarachnoid block or may lead to localized subarachnoid abscesses. Unless vigorous therapy is instituted promptly, the prognosis is hopeless. Even when treatment is intensive, the patient may fail to recover, or may sustain permanent damage to the brain.

Pericarditis. Like the other complications of pneumococcal pneumonia, pericarditis has also become relatively rare since the introduction of potent antimicrobial drugs. When the pericardium is invaded, the patient usually experiences precordial pain, and a leathery friction rub may be heard over the heart. Pericardial effusion usually results, causing a "dampening" of the heart sounds. If the fluid is sterile, the condition is benign, unless so large a volume accumulates as to cause cardiac tamponade. Empyema of the pericardium, on the other hand, is a serious complication requiring prompt and vigorous treatment. Pericardiocentesis is mandatory to establish the diagnosis of purulent pericarditis.

Other Specific Complications. Still rarer specific complications include peritonitis and pyogenic arthritis. Occasionally the pulmonary lesion of pneumococcal pneumonia fails to resolve even after many weeks, and finally is replaced by fibrous tissue.

Nonspecific Complications. Acute dilatation of the stomach (gastrectasia) and *paralytic ileus* occur particularly in patients suffering from anoxia and severe toxemia and give rise to gaseous distention of the abdomen (tympanites) that causes discomfort and often increases respiratory embarrassment. *Shock,* likewise, is a complication of severe toxemia and indicates a serious prognosis. *Congestive heart failure* occurs frequently as a complication of severe pneumonia in patients with underlying heart disease. As congestive heart failure is an important predisposing factor in bacterial pneumonia, it is not surprising that they are often associated, and obviously both must be treated. The diagnosis of congestive heart failure in the presence of pneumonia may at times be difficult, but should be considered in any patient with abnormal distention of neck veins, peripheral edema, an enlarged tender liver, and elevated venous pressure. Pulmonary signs of congestion may be unreliable, particularly if the pneumonia is bilateral.

Jaundice, the pathogenesis of which is controversial, may be related to lysis of erythrocytes in pneumonic lesions, depressed liver function resulting from anoxia, or focal hepatic necrosis consequent to the pneumococcal infection. Pneumococcal pneumonia may also precipitate hemolysis and jaundice in persons with glucose-6-phosphate dehydrogenase deficiency. The presence of prominent icterus usually indicates a poor prognosis, and may be associated with chronic liver disease, e.g., cirrhosis. As in any bedridden patient, *phlebothrombosis* may occur during pneumonia. Its early presence should suggest the possibility that the pulmonary lesion is due to infarction of the lung rather than to primary pneumonia. *Herpes labialis* occurs in at least 10 per cent of patients with pneumococcal pneumonia.

Differential Diagnosis. Pneumonia resulting from organisms other than pneumococcus may at times be difficult to differentiate from pneumococcal pneumonia. Only by bacteriologic study of the sputum can pneumonia caused by *Klebsiella pneumoniae* (Friedländer's bacillus), *Staphylococcus aureus,* or *group A Streptococcus* be identified. *Tuberculous pneumonia* rarely causes the acute prostration characteristic of coccal infection. *Mycoplasmal pneumonia* and other infections of the lungs, such as psittacosis and Q fever, do not often cause shaking chills, diffusely bloody sputum, severe pleural pain, or a marked leukocytosis, although they may at times be confused with acute bacterial pneumonia. *Tularemic pneumonia* and pneumonia caused by *H. influenzae,* especially common in young children, must also be considered. When the diagnosis is in doubt, repeated examinations of the sputum should be made, using both the Gram and "acid-fast" stains.

The most important noninfectious processes that must be differentiated from pneumococcal pneumonia are *pulmonary infarction* and *atelectasis.* Pulmonary infarction may be exceedingly difficult to differentiate from pneumonia. The dyspnea, pleural pain, hemoptysis, fever, physical signs of pulmonary consolidation, roentgenographic findings, and leukocytosis are all in keeping with an acute infection of the lungs. Frequently, however, the initial symptom is intense pleural pain of sudden onset; shaking chills rarely occur; there is no preceding history of respiratory infection; the fever is usually not high; frank hemoptysis is common; pulmonary signs, when present, appear early; and the total leukocyte count rarely reaches 20,000 per cubic millimeter. Moreover, although the chest signs develop rapidly in pneumococcal pneumonia, they appear right away with a pulmonary infarct. A combination of perfusion and ventilation scans may serve to differentiate infarction from pneumonia.

When a pulmonary infarct becomes infected, as sometimes happens, differentiation from primary bacterial pneumonia may be extremely difficult. Although in such cases the patients should receive antimicrobial treatment as in pneumonia, recognition of the infarction is of importance because of the need for anticoagulant therapy.

Pulmonary atelectasis, resulting from bronchial obstruction, not only may simulate pneumonia but often leads to serious infection of the lung if the bronchial obstruction is not relieved. Aspiration of mucus during or after surgical anesthesia is a common cause of atelectasis. Dyspnea, cough, chest pain, splinting of one side of the thorax, dullness to percussion, and suppressed breath sounds may all suggest primary pneumonia. Fever and leukocytosis also are noted when infection is present. As pulmonary atelectasis may be relieved by forced coughing and postural drainage or, if necessary, by bronchoscopy, it is important to differentiate it from primary pneumonia. Occasionally, sufficient shift of the mediastinum occurs to make the diagnosis obvious. Collapse of a segment of the lung may also result from chronic bronchial obstruction caused by bronchogenic carcinoma or aortic aneurysm.

Subdiaphragmatic infection may be confused with pneumonia. Subdiaphragmatic abscess, liver abscess, or other infections in the upper abdomen may extend to the diaphragm and produce local inflammation, small collections of pleural fluid, chest pain, and atelectasis secondary to decreased respiratory excursions. Conversely, pneumococcal pneumonia may simulate intra-abdominal disease. Pleurisy may result in pain referred to the abdomen so as to suggest acute appendicitis or cholecystitis.

Even when the diagnosis of pneumococcal pneumonia is established beyond doubt, the possibility of a second underlying lesion of the lung must be borne in mind. Chronic obstructive pulmonary disease or lung abscess may lead to repeated attacks of bacterial pneumonia and often becomes evident only after the pneumonic consolidation has resolved. Bronchogenic carcinoma, as well as pulmonary tuberculosis, must also be looked for in the follow-up examination.

Treatment. The treatment of pneumococcal pneumonia may best be discussed under three headings: (1) antibacterial therapy, (2) supportive measures, and (3) the treatment of complications. Before the advent of effective antibacterial therapy, supportive treatment was of the greatest importance. The introduction, first, of antipneumococcal serum and, later, of sulfonamides, penicillin, and the other antimicrobial drugs has so altered the management of pneumococcal pneumonia that today supportive treatment is rarely crucial, and serious complications are only occasionally encountered.

Antibacterial Therapy. PENICILLIN. Penicillin is at present the drug of choice in the treatment of pneumococcal pneumonia. All strains of the organism isolated in the United States and most other areas of the world are extremely susceptible to penicillin, and most are inhibited in broth by concentrations of less than 0.02 μg per ml. However, pneumococci relatively resistant to penicillin have been isolated frequently in New Guinea and rarely in Australia. The minimal inhibitory concentration of benzylpenicillin for these strains is 0.1 to 2.0 μg per ml. These strains are also relatively resistant to the penicillinase-resistant penicillins and cephalosporins, but are fully sensitive or only slightly resistant to ampicillin.

The effectiveness of antimicrobial treatment is due in part to the natural resistance of the host, which accounts for the destruction of a large proportion of the invading bacteria. Host resistance, which results primarily from the activity of phagocytic cells in the lung, when combined with the bacteriostatic and bactericidal effects of drug therapy, controls promptly all but the most malignant pneumonia. Even with no treatment at all, approximately seven of every ten patients with pneumococcal pneumonia eventually recover, but some will have experienced a very severe illness before recovery has occurred.

Antipneumococcal therapy should be initiated promptly, therefore, in order to halt the spread of the infection both locally and through the bloodstream. An effective method is to give aqueous procaine penicillin G intramuscularly in a dose of 300,000 units at 12-hour intervals. Some authorities recommend the administration of aqueous penicillin G by the intramuscular route in doses of 300,000 units several times during the first 24-hour period of observation in addition to the procaine penicillin. In the presence of shock, penicillin should be given intravenously. Treatment should be maintained for at least one week or until the temperature has been normal for 72 hours; if treatment is discontinued too soon, relapse of the infection occurs.

Penicillin may also be given by mouth. However, in a serious infection such as pneumococcal pneumonia, it is inadvisable to rely on oral penicillin therapy in acutely ill patients. In fact, parenteral therapy throughout probably provides the greatest margin of safety. If parenteral therapy is not feasible or advisable throughout the period of therapy, procaine penicillin G can be given parenterally initially and penicillin V can then be given orally after defervescence. When oral penicillin V is used, it should be given in a dosage of at least 250 mg every six hours.

Response to penicillin therapy is often dramatic. Bacteremia, when present at the start of treatment, clears within a few hours. A crisis, characterized by rapid defervescence and a striking subsidence of symptoms, occurs in less than 48 hours in approximately half the patients. The others experience a more gradual recovery, the temperature falling by lysis over a period of four to seven days. Frequently a secondary rise in temperature occurs after the crisis. This elevation is usually low-grade and subsides spontaneously within a few hours, or at most a few days.

When a patient's pneumonia fails to respond satisfactorily to penicillin therapy, three possible explanations should be considered: (1) that the patient is suffering from a serious complication such as empyema, endocarditis, meningitis, or pulmonary suppuration (possibly secondary to bronchogenic carcinoma); (2) that the primary infection is of nonpneumococcal origin and is due to an agent that is resistant to the action of penicillin, e.g., a penicillin-resistant strain of Staphylococcus or Klebsiella; or (3) that drug fever has developed as a result of penicillin hypersensitivity. Occasionally, patients will respond initially to treatment only to have unmistakable signs of persistent pneumonia subsequently develop, in spite of continued therapy. This sequence of events is usually due to the presence of a mixed infection, the initial response to treatment resulting from control of penicillin-susceptible organisms, and the relapse occurring as a result of persistence of a penicillin-resistant species. Re-examination of the sputum and modification of the antimicrobial therapy are immediately indicated. Patients with underlying chronic pulmonary disease are particularly prone to such mixed infections.

Persons giving a history of having had a penicillin reaction in the past should, of course, not be treated with penicillin.

OTHER ANTIMICROBIAL DRUGS. Cephalothin or cefazolin can be used as effective alternatives to penicillin for parenteral therapy in patients hypersensitive to penicillin. Patients hypersensitive to penicillin sometimes show cross-sensitivity to cephalosporins; a cutaneous scratch test with the cephalosporin to be used should probably be performed in these patients to determine whether the drug can be used as an alternative to penicillin. Cephalothin should be administered in doses of 1 gram every four hours by the intramuscular or intravenous route, and cefazolin should be given in doses of 0.5 gram every six hours. Erythromycin in doses of 250 mg every six hours by the oral route is also adequate for treatment of patients with a history of penicillin allergy, provided they are not severely ill. Methicillin, cloxacillin, and nafcillin are also effective in the treatment of pneumococcal pneumonia. Tetracyclines should not be used in treating pneumococcal infections unless the organism is known to be susceptible. The prevalence of tetracycline-resistant pneumococci has increased greatly in recent years, now exceeding 5 per cent in many areas of the world. Pneumococci are relatively resistant to gentamicin, and pneumococcal pneumonia has been shown to progress during the administration of this drug.

Supportive Treatment. Patients suffering from pneumococcal pneumonia should be kept at bed rest, and visitors to the sick room should be limited to the immediate family. Pleural pain, if mild, may be treated with codeine sulfate (30 to 60 mg) orally. A tight chest binder may relieve pain but is inadvisable because it inhibits effectiveness of cough. Hypoxemia should be treated with oxygen administered by nasal catheter or by mask. Acetylsalicylic acid should not be used, because it interferes with the utilization of the fever curve to evaluate response to therapy.

FLUID AND ELECTROLYTES. During the acute state of pneumococcal pneumonia, considerable fluid is lost from the body, chiefly through the skin as the result of high fever. Dehydration may develop rapidly and, if severe, may become a contributing factor in the development of shock. Intravenous fluids and electrolytes may be required to control dehydration. When hydration is adequate, the specific gravity of the urine should remain below 1.020. Pneumonia may occasionally lead to the syndrome of inappropriate secretion of antidiuretic hormone.

DIET. Many patients with pneumococcal pneumonia are too ill to tolerate a full diet and should receive only liquids during the height of the fever. Fruit juices, ginger ale, and soups are well tolerated. After the crisis a regular diet may be prescribed.

The patient should be kept in bed until the temperature is approximately normal and should be observed closely until the pneumonic lesion has resolved. As already emphasized, all patients should be subjected to a follow-up roentgenographic examination three to four weeks after recovery.

Treatment of Complications. SHOCK. Patients with peripheral vascular collapse (shock) resulting from severe pneumococcal pneumonia usually respond poorly to the accepted forms of antishock therapy. The prognosis is almost invariably grave when this complication develops. Oxygen therapy should be begun immediately, even if cyanosis is absent. The central venous pressure should be used as a guide for fluid replacement. The use of corticosteroids has not been demonstrated to be of value.

ABDOMINAL DISTENTION. Decompression is indicated if distention is severe. Acute gastric and ileal dilatation is best managed with the use of gastric suction; a rectal tube may be indicated if colonic distention is a problem.

DELIRIUM TREMENS. Delirium tremens may sometimes be difficult to control in patients with a history of chronic alcoholism. Restraints may be required. The safest sedative to control hyperactivity in these patients is diazepam (Valium) in a dose of 0.066 mg per kilogram every four to six hours.

EMPYEMA AND PERICARDITIS. The treatment of choice for empyema and purulent pericarditis is systemic antimicrobial therapy and surgical drainage. Injection of penicillin into the pleural or pericardial cavity is not required. Repeated needle aspirations are occasionally effective but do not provide effective drainage in most patients.

The treatment of the remaining two major complications of pneumococcal pneumonia, namely endocarditis and meningitis, is discussed in Ch. 192 and 201.

Prognosis. The case fatality rate in untreated pneumococcal pneumonia ranges from 20 to 40 per cent. The widespread use of sulfonamide drugs in the late 1930's resulted in a lowering of the fatality rate among treated patients to approximately 10 per cent. Penicillin therapy has lowered the rate still further. At present approximately 95 per cent of patients with pneumococcal pneumonia recover when properly treated with penicillin.

The prognosis in pneumococcal pneumonia is influenced adversely by each of the following: (1) old age (and also infancy), (2) late treatment, (3) infection with certain types of pneumococci (particularly types 2 and 3), (4) involvement of more than one lobe of the lung, (5) leukopenia, (6) occurrence of bacteremia, (7) jaundice, (8) the presence of complications (notably shock and meningitis), (9) pregnancy (particularly in the third trimester), (10) the presence of other disease such as heart disease or cirrhosis of the liver, and (11) alcoholic intoxication and delirium tremens. Through a consideration of these factors a rough estimate may be made of the severity of the infection in each case, and therapy may be modified accordingly.

Even with the most intensive penicillin treatment, a significant number of patients will die of pneumococcal pneumonia. A recent study, for example, has revealed that in patients destined, at the onset of illness, to die within five days (because of complicating disease, old age, etc.), penicillin therapy has little if any effect. Similarly, the case fatality rate in type 3 pneumococcal pneumonia with bacteremia still exceeds 50 per cent regardless of treatment.

Prevention. Because pneumococcal pneumonia is not highly contagious and usually responds promptly to early therapy, prophylaxis constitutes less of a problem than in many other infectious diseases. It is estimated that only one in every 500 persons of all ages in the United States may be expected to contract the disease in any one year.

Although pneumococcal pneumonia can undoubtedly be prevented (or at least aborted) in many patients by the intensive treatment of every upper respiratory tract infection with antimicrobial drugs, their use for this purpose should be avoided. The possible inconvenience to the patient of hypersensitivity reactions and the danger of favoring drug-resistant strains of bacteria outweigh the advantages to be gained in preventing such a relatively uncommon and readily treatable disease as pneumococcal pneumonia. Some authorities do recommend penicillin prophylaxis for children with sickle cell anemia less than three or four years of age whose circulating erythrocytes contain Howell-Jolly bodies as an indicator of splenic hypofunction.

During recent years Austrian has redirected attention to the possibility of specific immunization as a means of preventing pneumococcal infection. During World War II, MacLeod and colleagues showed in controlled experiments in man that pneumococcal polysaccharides are effective antigens, evoking the formation of antibody that persists for years and that confers type-specific immunity to pneumococcal infection. Austrian has proposed immunization of that portion of the population at greatest risk with the types of pneumococci that are most often responsible for disease. Austrian's recent data, reported in 1972, show that 62 per cent of 2000 cases of pneumococcal bacteremia in adults were caused by six types (1, 3, 4, 7, 8, 12), that 70 per cent of 100 bacteremias in the pediatric age group were caused by six types (1, 6, 14, 18, 19, 23), and that 70 per cent of 300 isolates from otitis media in children were caused by seven types (1, 3, 6, 14, 18, 19, 23). Since high risk groups can be identified and a large proportion of infections are caused by a few pneumococcal types, studies on the value of immunization are indicated and are in progress. Whether effective immunization of certain groups by polysaccharide vaccines will be followed by an increasing occurrence of infections with other pneumococcal types is unknown but is a definite possibility.

Patient Isolation. The cross-infection rate in pneumococcal pneumonia is low, and patients receiving chemotherapy are probably not highly infectious. Isolation is not indicated in the usual patient.

Austrian, R.: Current status of bacterial pneumonia with especial reference to pneumococcal infection. J. Clin. Path. [suppl.] 21:93, 1968.

Austrian, R.: Pneumococcal infections in sickle cell anemia. Am. J. Dis. Child., 123:614, 1972.

Austrian, C. R., and Austrian, R.: Pneumococcal pneumonia (lobar pneumonia). *In* Tice's Practice of Medicine. Hagerstown, Md., W. F. Prior Company, 1959, Vol. 1, p. 1.

Austrian, R., and Gold, J.: Pneumococcal bacteremia with especial reference to bacteremic pneumococcal pneumonia. Ann. Intern. Med., 60:759, 1964.

Bisno, A. L.: Hyposplenism and overwhelming pneumococcal infection – a reappraisal. Am. J. Med. Sci., 262:101, 1971.

Coonrod, J. D., and Rytel, M. W.: Detection of type-specific pneumococcal antigens by counterimmunoelectrophoresis. II. Etiologic diagnosis of pneumonia. J. Lab. Clin. Med., 81:778, 1973.

Heffron, R.: Pneumonia with Special Reference to Pneumococcus Lobar Pneumonia. New York, Commonwealth Fund, 1939.

Kauffman, C. A., Watanakunakorn, C., and Phair, J. P.: Purulent pneumococcal pericarditis. A continuing problem in the antibiotic era. Am. J. Med., 54:743, 1973.

Lukems, J. N.: Hemoglobin S, the pneumococcus and the spleen. Am. J. Dis. Child., 123:6, 1972.

Wood, W. B.: Studies on the Cellular Immunology of Acute Bacterial Infections. The Harvey Lectures, Series 47, 1951–52.

Wood, W. B., and Smith, M. R.: An experimental analysis of the curative action of penicillin. J. Exp. Med., 103:487, 1956.

KLEBSIELLA AND OTHER GRAM-NEGATIVE BACTERIAL PNEUMONIAS

Jay P. Sanford

181. INTRODUCTION

The combination of improved identification of gram-negative bacilli by diagnostic laboratories and the increased frequency of their isolation from clinical specimens has resulted in a striking increase in recognition of various gram-negative bacilli as serious human pathogens. Previously, procedures for the identification of gram-negative bacilli were primarily designed to enable rapid detection of Salmonella and Shigella from fecal specimens and Klebsiella from sputum specimens, with a lumping of the remaining organisms as "coliforms." Today, members of three families of aerobic gram-negative bacteria (Enterobacteriaceae, Pseudomonaceae, and Achromobacteraceae) have been recognized as potential pulmonary pathogens. The family Enterobacteriaceae is composed of numerous interrelated bacilli, all of which are gram-negative, are nonsporing, grow on ordinary media, and rapidly ferment glucose. The following genera are included in the family: Shigella, Escherichia, Salmonella, Arizona, Citrobacter, Edwardsiella, Klebsiella, Enterobacter (formerly Aerobacter), Hafnia, Serratia, Proteus, and Providence. Whereas the Enterobacteriaceae have received considerable attention, the nonfermenting aerobic gram-negative bacilli are being recognized with increased frequency. Organisms that fall into this category include *Pseudomonas aeruginosa, P. maltophilia, P. pseudomallei, P. cepacia, P. stutzeri, Acinetobacter lwoffi* (previously *Mima polymorpha*), *Acinetobacter anitratus* (previously *Herellea vaginicola* and *Achromobacter anitratus*), *Moraxella spp., Alcaligenes spp., Flavobacterium spp.,* and *Aeromonas hydrophilia.*

Pulmonary infections associated with the small aerobic gram-negative bacilli belonging to the genera Bordetella, Brucella, Hemophilus, Pasteurella and Yersinia and nonsporulating anaerobic gram-negative bacilli, e.g., Bacteroides, Fusobacterium, Dialister, will be discussed elsewhere. Infections caused by *Pseudomonas pseudomallei* (melioidosis) are presented in Ch. 220.

182. PNEUMONIA DUE TO KLEBSIELLA PNEUMONIAE (Friedländer's Pneumonia)

In 1882, Friedländer first cultivated the organism now designated as *Klebsiella pneumoniae* from the lungs of patients who had died of pneumonia. Although he considered it to be the etiologic agent in most cases of pneumonia, four years later the pneumococcus was described and established as the predominant etiologic agent in lobar pneumonia. Consequently for many years *Klebsiella pneumoniae* (Friedländer's bacillus) was thought to be only a secondary invader. It is now recognized that a small but definite percentage, 0.5 to 5.0 per cent, of primary pneumonias are due to *Klebsiella pneumoniae.* This historical background is of interest because it reflects the current disagreements regarding the role of other gram-negative bacilli as primary pulmonary pathogens.

Pathogenicity. Klebsiella may persist in the oropharynx of normal persons, although the prevalence is low, 1 to 6 per cent. There is no tendency for contacts to acquire the organism from a carrier, and Bloomfield was unable to implant organisms in the pharynx of healthy volunteers. Yet the prevalence in pharyngeal cultures increases to 8 to 23 per cent in hospitalized subjects. Pulmonary infections arise most likely from the inhalation or aspiration of organisms from the oropharynx during circumstances when the major pulmonary antibacterial defense mechanisms, the mucociliary blanket, or alveolar macrophages are compromised.

The pathogenesis of experimental Klebsiella pneumonia is similar to that of encapsulated type 1 pneumococcal pneumonia. The outer margin of the spreading lesion is characterized by an edema zone in which the alveoli are filled with fluid containing many bacteria (see illustration in Ch. 180). The organisms multiply freely in the fluid, and are carried mechanically into adjacent alveoli through the pores of Kohn. Phagocytosis is noticeable only in the central zone of consolidation where alveoli are packed with leukocytes, thus allowing "surface phagocytosis." Three differences in experimental Klebsiella pneumonia in comparison with type 1 pneumococcal pneumonia are (1) greater numbers of Klebsiella in the areas of consolidation, (2) destruction of alveolar walls, and (3) organization with fibroblastic activity.

Klebsiella pulmonary infections are usually classified as primary, i.e., infection developing in a patient without underlying disease, or secondary. The demarcation between primary and secondary is often indistinct, as classic primary Klebsiella pneumonia usually occurs in patients with underlying conditions such as alcoholism, chronic obstructive airways disease (emphysema-fibrosis), or diabetes mellitus. Operationally, infections may be considered as primary if Klebsiella organisms are isolated from specimens obtained when the patient first seeks medical aid. The designation "secondary" is then applied to those infections that either represent superinfection of an underlying infection or are opportunistic in origin.

Predisposing Factors. In patients with primary pneumonia, males heavily predominate (80 to 90 per cent), most infections occurring in middle-aged and older patients (average age being the mid-50's). The most common co-existing disease is alcoholism (66 per cent). The few series in which alcoholism is not frequent are drawn from predominantly black populations. Both chronic bronchopulmonary disease and to a lesser extent diabetes mellitus appear to predispose patients to Klebsiella pneumonia.

Pathology. The involvement in fatal primary Klebsiella pneumonia is most often lobar, but may be lobular or a combination of the two. An upper lobe is most commonly involved. The pleural surface is covered by a fibrinous exudate and adhesions form early. Empyema is appreciably more frequent than in pneumococcal pneumonia, probably occurring in one fifth to one quarter of cases. Microscopically in the acute stage, the alveolar walls are congested. Usually the alveoli are filled with an exudate composed of a mixture of polymorphonuclear and mononuclear cells, with a predominance of the former. In rare cases, mononuclear cells may predominate. There is often necrosis of alveolar walls, with abscess formation. Other findings at autopsy may include extrapulmonary sites of dissemination, e.g., pericarditis or meningitis. Evidence of alcoholic hepatosis and alcoholic cirrhosis is common.

Clinical Manifestations and Course. Based upon clinicobacteriologic findings, Klebsiella infections can be classified as primary or secondary (as defined under Pathogenicity, above); pure or mixed, depending upon whether klebsiellae are isolated as the predominant organism or associated with other organisms, especially other gram-negative bacilli; and acute or chronic.

Primary Klebsiella Pneumonia. The "classic" clinical pattern is that of acute primary Klebsiella pneumonia. As with pneumococcal pneumonia, the onset is usually sudden (90 per cent), associated with cough productive of sputum (90 per cent), pleuritic chest pain (80 per cent), and true rigors (60 per cent). Early prostration is a usual feature. Occasionally the acute onset is preceded by an undifferentiated upper respiratory infection and cough. Rarely epigastric pain and vomiting are the initial symptoms. The characteristic sputum has been described as a nonputrid homogeneous thick mixture of blood and mucus, often brick red in color, which is sufficiently thick to be expectorated with difficulty. This typical sputum is seen in one quarter to three quarters of patients. In some patients the sputum is thin, resembling currant jelly, although in most it is either blood tinged or rusty. Frank hemoptysis may occur. On examination, patients appear acutely ill, febrile, dyspneic, and often cyanotic. Although temperatures are often said to be less than those observed with pneumococcal pneumonia, two thirds are between 39 and 40° C. Tachycardia coincides with the fever. Chest examination typically reveals signs of pulmonary consolidation; there may be loss of lung volume as manifested by decreased size and expansion of the involved hemithorax and diaphragmatic elevation. Auscultation may reveal suppressed breath sounds with few rales, even with advanced consolidation. Involvement of more than one lobe is frequent (in two thirds of patients) with a predilection for upper lobes.

Laboratory and Roentgenographic Findings. Peripheral leukocyte counts range from marked leukopenia to leukocytosis, leukopenia and neutropenia being poor prognostic signs. In one quarter of patients the total leukocyte count may be in the normal range. On sputum culture, either gram-negative bacilli other than Klebsiella or pneumococci often may be isolated. A mixed sputum flora containing other gram-negative bacilli such as *Pseudomonas spp.* is especially common in secondary infections. In the prechemotherapeutic era, blood cultures were positive in about 15 per cent of cases during the course of the illness. At present, a pulmonary source is still often incriminated in patients with Klebsiella bacteremia. This is unusual in other types of gram-negative bacillary bacteremia, in which the urinary tract usually represents the major primary source.

The roentgenographic features are variable, and include massive lobar consolidation, lobular involvement, lung abscess formation with either multiple small thin-walled or large abscess cavities, and residual parenchymal fibrosis. Bulging of a fissure, sharp advancing borders of the infiltrates, and abscess formation occur with greater frequency than in other types of pneumonia. The pneumonic infiltrate is relatively dense, but shadows of similar density are seen with other types of pneumonia. Bronchopneumonic distribution is less usual but can occur, and even bilateral perihilar infiltrates are reported. The diagnostic usefulness for any given roentgenographic configuration has been questioned; however, in many instances a correct diagnosis can be suggested from the roentgenogram.

Complications. Rapid destruction of pulmonary tissue with suppuration or residual fibrosis occurs in as many as half of the surviving patients. Necrosis may occur within 24 to 48 hours, and abscess formation may be recognized within four days. Other less common pulmonary complications include pleural effusion and pneumothorax. In the past, activation of quiescent pulmonary tuberculosis has been reported.

The course of illness is not marked by an unusual propensity for extrapulmonary manifestations, but they can occur, and include pericarditis, meningitis, gastroenteritis, erythematous skin rashes, and nonsuppurative polyarthritis.

Prognosis and Treatment. In the pre-antimicrobial era, the case mortality of Klebsiella pneumonia ranged from 51 to 97 per cent. With the advent of drug therapy, the various tetracycline derivatives, streptomycin, and chloramphenicol were found to have an excellent in vitro effect, and clinical use resulted in a marked decrease in mortality in most series. In some series, the mortality remains nearly 50 per cent; in these there has been a predominance of severely ill alcoholic patients, although good results have been reported even in this group. Analysis of the mode of death frequently reveals inadequate removal of tenacious pulmonary secretions to be a significant factor. The correlation of bloodstream invasion and fatality is frequently close.

In vitro studies reveal the majority of strains of Klebsiella to be susceptible to cephalothin, cefazolin, chloramphenicol, colistimethate, gentamicin, kanamycin, polymyxin B, and tobramycin. The antimicrobial regimen of choice is often varied according to the gravity of the acute clinical situation and the extent of underlying problems. In less seriously ill patients, cephalothin or gentamicin is preferable, but in patients with life-threatening infections combination therapy, e.g., cephalothin or cefazolin and kanamycin, gentamicin, or tobramycin, is usually employed. Meticulous measures directed at supportive care, maintenance of clear airways, adequate but not excessive ventilation and oxygenation, adequate fluid and electrolyte replacement, and often control of delirium tremens are essential.

183. PNEUMONIA DUE TO AEROBIC GRAM-NEGATIVE BACILLI OTHER THAN KLEBSIELLA PNEUMONIAE

The large number of bacterial species other than *Klebsiella pneumoniae* that belong to the families Enterobacteriaceae, Pseudomonaceae, and Achromobacteraceae are considered together because of the similarities in their abilities to produce pulmonary infection.

Until recently the over-all frequency of pneumonia caused by gram-negative bacilli other than Klebsiella received relatively little attention. Between 1963 and 1965, 4.3 per cent of all pneumonias of patients admitted to the Detroit General Hospital were caused by gram-negative bacilli (82 episodes, 78 of which were classified as primary). In 1967–1968, of 292 patients admitted to Grady Memorial Hospital (Atlanta) with pneumonia, the disease in 167 could be attributed to specific bacterial pathogens; of these, 33 (20 per cent) were due to gram-negative bacilli. Among these gram-negative bacillary pneumonias, the following organisms were encountered: *Klebsiella pneumoniae, Enterobacter aerogenes, Escherichia coli, Pseudomonas spp.,* Bacteroides, Proteus, *H. influenzae,* and Achromobacter. In addition, in many hospitals other gram-negative organisms such as nonpigmented *Serratia marcescens* are being encountered, especially in hospital-associated secondary pneumonias. It appears that collectively gram-negative bacilli other than Klebsiella may be more prevalent than Klebsiella in causing both primary pneumonia and secondary hospital-acquired pneumonias.

Predisposing Factors. As with primary Klebsiella pneumonia, in primary pneumonias caused by these other agents, older males are more often affected. Underlying disease conditions occur in almost all patients; these include heart disease, alcoholism, renal disease, diabetes mellitus, and chronic bronchopulmonary disease, especially cystic fibrosis. Primary gram-negative bacillary pneumonia may be more common during the summer.

Infections most frequently occur in patients who are receiving inhalation therapy that incorporates reservoir nebulization and who are also receiving antimicrobial therapy. Adrenocortical steroids, immunosuppressive agents, cytotoxic chemotherapy, and tracheostomy may also be predisposing factors. However, such infections may occur in patients who are not receiving inhalation therapy, as these organisms are ubiquitous and appear with increased frequency in seriously ill patients.

Pathology. On microscopic section, bronchopneumonia with confluent microabscesses is seen. The intra-alveolar inflammatory exudate is mixed polymorphonuclear leukocytic and mononuclear. With infection caused by *E. coli* and Pseudomonas, however, the cellular infiltrates may consist predominantly of mononuclear cells admixed with fragmented pyknotic nuclei of necrotic neutrophils. At a later stage, alveolar spaces are filled with a deeply basophilic granular material containing large macrophage-like cells and dense colonies of gram-negative bacilli.

When caused by Pseudomonas, in the areas of an abscess there is often focal hemorrhage. The dominant microscopic lesion is that of alveolar septal necrosis. In association with these necrotizing lesions, necrosis of arterial walls and secondary thrombosis of vessels have been encountered when the Pseudomonas pneumonia was of bacteremic origin or associated with nebulization therapy equipment. With the primary Pseudomonas pneumonia reported by Tillotson and Lerner, the vascular involvement was not a feature. *Pseudomonas cepacia* was also associated with a necrotizing granulomatous pneumonia. With the other non-Klebsiella gram-negative bacilli, alveolar septal necrosis is not a usual feature.

Clinical Features and Course. The clinical features are generally similar to those observed in patients with primary Klebsiella pneumonia, except that hemoptysis is unusual.

In patients with Pseudomonas pneumonia, apprehension, toxicity, confusion, and progressive cyanosis are characteristic. Relative bradycardia may occur. Alteration in diurnal temperature patterns with the peak temperature in early morning was noted by Tillotson and Lerner. The physical signs over the thorax are not characteristic. The development of empyema is common (22 to 80 per cent). Roentgenograms reveal bilateral bronchopneumonic infiltrates, usually lower lobe, that often are nodular and may undergo necrosis with abscesses which may be small but are often greater than 1 cm in diameter. A pattern of interstitial infiltration may be seen.

Primary *E. coli* pneumonia tends to present as a bronchopneumonic process in the lower lobes. The pulse is proportional to the temperature. Early findings include rales without consolidation. Empyema formation is less common than with Klebsiella or Pseudomonas.

Proteus species also produce a clinical picture similar to Klebsiella, with fever, chills, dyspnea, pleuritic chest pain, and cough productive of purulent sputum. Signs of consolidation are usual. Roentgenograms reveal dense infiltrates in the posterior segment of an upper lobe or superior segment of the right lower lobe. Progression to lung abscess or empyema is common.

Serratia infections, which are almost always secondary, have been associated with the clinical oddity "pseudohemoptysis" owing to the red pigment prodigiosin produced by some strains of *Serratia marcescens.* Other features may include abscess formation or empyema, or both.

Clinical experience with the other bacterial genera such as Hafnia, Flavobacterium, Mima, and Herellea, is limited, but other characteristics suggest that their clinical features are similar to secondary Klebsiella infections.

Laboratory Findings. The usual laboratory findings such as leukocyte counts are of little help, being either normal or moderately increased. Cultures of sputum are only of moderate help, because these organisms are frequently present as commensals in patients who are receiving antimicrobial therapy or in those who are critically ill. Specimens collected by the transtracheal technique in which neutrophils are present and gram-negative bacilli are stained and cultured are most helpful in making a diagnosis. With empyema, thoracentesis with staining and culture of the fluid will confirm the diagnosis and facilitate the selection of optimal therapy.

Prognosis and Treatment. Prognosis varies with the type of organism as well as with the underlying condition of the patient. Mortality rates in the range of 80 per cent are not uncommon with Pseudomonas pneumonia, whereas they may be lower with the other organisms.

The antimicrobial regimen of choice may be selected according to antimicrobial susceptibilities anticipated in a given community but must be confirmed by tests on an individual patient's organism. In general, *Pseudomonas aeruginosa* and *Enterobacter aerogenes* are most susceptible to carbenicillin, colistimethate, gentamicin, polymyxin B, and tobramycin. In contrast, *Pseudomonas cepacia* may be susceptible only to chloramphenicol. *E. coli* is susceptible to the same agents as *Ps. aeruginosa,* and in addition most strains are susceptible to cephalothin or cefazolin. *Serratia marcescens* and the indole-positive *Proteus spp.* are most susceptible to gentamicin and tobramycin. As with Klebsiella pneumonia, in pneumonias caused by these other gram-negative bacilli, meticulous attention to supportive care is as important as the antimicrobial therapy.

Bloomfield, A. L.: The fate of bacteria introduced into the upper air passages. V. The Friedländer bacilli. Bull. Hopkins Hosp., 31:203, 1920.

Hyde, L., and Hyde, B.: Primary Friedländer pneumonia. Am. J. Med. Sci., 205:660, 1943.

Jervey, L. P., Jr., and Hamburger, M.: The treatment of acute Friedlaender's bacillus pneumonia. Arch. Intern. Med., 99:1, 1957.

Johanson, W. G., Pierce, A. K., Sanford, J. P., and Thomas, G. D.: Nosocomial respiratory infections with gram-negative bacilli. Ann. Intern. Med., 77:701, 1972.

Manfredi, F., Daly, W. J., and Behnke, R. H.: Clinical observations of acute Friedländer pneumonia. Ann. Intern. Med., 58:642, 1963.

Pennington, J. E., Reynolds, H. Y., and Carbone, P. P.: Pseudomonas pneumonia. Am. J. Med., 55:155, 1973.

Pierce, A. K., Edmondson, E. B., McGee, G., Ketchersid, J., Loudon, R. G., and Sanford, J. P.: An analysis of factors predisposing to gram-negative bacillary necrotizing pneumonia. Am. Rev. Respir. Dis., 94:309, 1966.

Pierce, A. K., Sanford, J. P., Thomas, G. D., and Leonard, J. S.: Long-term evaluation of decontamination of inhalation-therapy equipment and the occurrence of necrotizing pneumonia. N. Engl. J. Med., 282:528, 1970.

Rose, H. D., Heckman, M. G., and Unger, J. D.: *Pseudomonas aeruginosa* pneumonia in adults. Am. Rev. Respir. Dis., 107:416, 1973.

Sullivan, R. J., Dowdle, W. R., Marine, W. M., and Hierholzer, J. C.: Adult pneumonia in a general hospital. Arch. Intern. Med., 129:935, 1972.

Tillotson, J. R., and Lerner, A. M.: Characteristics of pneumonia caused by *Escherichia coli.* N. Engl. J. Med., 277:115, 1967.

Tillotson, J. R., and Lerner, A. M.: Characteristics of nonbacteremic pseudomonas pneumonia. Ann. Intern. Med., 68:295, 1968.

STREPTOCOCCAL DISEASES

184. INTRODUCTION

Gene H. Stollerman

Streptococci constitute a large heterogeneous group of gram-positive bacteria that are very common parasites of man. Their name derives from their growth in liquid media as chains of globular bacteria. Classification of streptococci has been confusing, because a single species may cause a variety of diseases and because several kinds of streptococci can often be cultured from the same site of infection.

CLASSIFICATION

The modern classification of streptococci is based upon Lancefield's identification of the group-specific cell wall "C" carbohydrate antigens which are present in beta-hemolytic streptococci and in some nonhemolytic species as well.

Group A Infections. The most important human streptococcal pathogen, *Streptococcus pyogenes,* can be identified as containing group A carbohydrate with specific rabbit antiserum to the carbohydrate cell wall antigens, and thus can be distinguished from other beta-hemolytic streptococci which are also frequently isolated from the respiratory tract of man. Diseases caused by group A streptococci will be considered in detail in Ch. 185 to 191 and in Ch. 610. Streptococci belonging to other serogroups that are of importance to man will be mentioned briefly here.

The traditional classification of streptococci by their properties of hemolysis on the surface of blood agar plates is clinically useful. It helps to distinguish hemolytic streptococci, to which the more virulent species belong, from the alpha-hemolytic *Streptococcus viridans* ("green" streptococci), the predominant normal flora of the upper respiratory tract, and the nonhemolytic streptococci which include the *enterococci,* a common inhabitant of the gastrointestinal tract.

Beta-hemolytic streptococci are those that produce a completely clear zone around the colony as a result of the formation of either extracellular hemolysin, streptolysin O and streptolysin S, or both. Classification of streptococci based on the type of hemolysis they produce, however, is unsatisfactory for many reasons. Many species belonging to specific serologic groups may be nonhemolytic, such as group D. On the other hand, some enterococci belonging to the usually nonhemolytic group D may produce beta hemolysis, or some apparently nonhemolytic colonies may become alpha hemolytic upon prolonged incubation. Beta hemolysis is therefore primarily useful in the first step of the identification of group A organisms which are, with only rare exceptions, consistently hemolytic.

Group B Infections. The group B organisms are classically represented by the species *Streptococcus agalactiae.* They were well known for many years as the cause of bovine mastitis but produced human disease rarely. Until recently, little attention was paid to group B organisms in man, although it was known that they could colonize the vagina and genitourinary tract and were occasionally found in the upper respiratory tract as well. In fact, between 5 and 10 per cent of hemolytic streptococci isolated from man were identified in many studies as group B. In the past decade, however, group B streptococci have been reported with increasing frequency as a cause of perinatal infections. In the preantibiotic era, group A streptococci were the common agent of puerperal fever. Since the early 1960's, however, group B streptococci have emerged as a major cause of puerperal infection and as a cause of neonatal sepsis, with or without meningitis.

The frequency with which group B streptococci are recovered from the female genital tract (and the male genitourinary tract as well) appears to be increasing, and cervicovaginal carrier rates in normal pregnant women vary from 3 to 6 per cent. In some studies, approximately one third of infants born to such carriers have contracted serious group B infections. Group B organisms also seem to be causing bacteremic complications of pyelonephritis in both men and women more often than heretofore, especially in diabetics and other compromised hosts. These infections have remained susceptible to penicillin so far.

Group D Infections. This group includes *Streptococcus faecalis,* often referred to as *enterococcus* because of the frequency with which it is found in the human gastrointestinal tract. Enterococci may also be cultured from the oropharynx and, although usually nonhemolytic, some strains can produce beta or alpha hemolysis. *S. faecalis* is an exceptionally hardy organism which can resist heat (62° C for 30 minutes), grow well at room temperature, multiply in hypertonic media (6.5 per cent sodium chloride), and grow in the presence of 0.05 per cent sodium azide.

Enterococci are often isolated from the blood in bacterial endocarditis and from the urine in urinary tract obstruction. The precise role of these organisms in the pathogenesis of pyelonephritis has not been fully evaluated. They can be associated with suppurative abdominal lesions, especially after bowel surgery.

The failure of some laboratories to distinguish the enterococci from other streptococci often leads to inappropriate therapy in serious infections. These organisms may also be recovered from the respiratory tract and may be regarded mistakenly as penicillin-resistant group A streptococci. This error occurs most often during the post-treatment follow-up study of cases of group A streptococcal sore throat and may lead to needless overtreatment in an attempt to eradicate the organisms from the pharynx. It cannot be emphasized too strongly that enterococci do *not* cause pharyngitis and tonsillitis.

Streptococci of Other Groups. Strains of groups C, E, G, H, K, and O are isolated from the respiratory tract of man but are of little clinical significance. "Human" group C strains may occasionally cause illnesses that resemble those of group A, but such infections are relatively rare. Moreover, as far as is known, only group A organisms cause rheumatic fever. Group G may occasionally cause mild infections, but these are relatively infrequent and are uncomplicated. Groups A, C, and G all elaborate in vivo antigenically similar streptolysin O, streptokinase, hyaluronidase, and erythrogenic toxin.

Alpha-Hemolytic Streptococci ("Green" Streptococci). The alpha-hemolytic streptococci are often referred to collectively as the *viridans group.* They have never been satisfactorily classified. Their colonies are surrounded by a narrow zone of incompletely hemolyzed red cells (some red cells are spared for unknown reasons). Green discoloration of the colonies occurs owing to the formation of an unidentified reductant of hemoglobin. The degree of "greening" varies with the animal source of blood and is best brought out by sheep red blood cells which differentiate most clearly beta from alpha hemolysis.

Streptococcus viridans is the predominant normal flora of the upper respiratory tract and is generally nonpathogenic except as a cause of subacute bacterial endocarditis. *Streptococcus salivarius* is one of the most commonly encountered of these species.

The term *nonhemolytic* Streptococcus is confusing because it is often used to include any Streptococcus that is not beta hemolytic, and because many nonhemolytic species (including the common *Streptococcus faecalis*) possess the same group-specific cell wall antigens as certain hemolytic strains. The organisms of the nonhemolytic group are generally of low pathogenicity for man and, like alpha-hemolytic streptococci, are of concern to physicians primarily as causative agents of subacute bacterial endocarditis. They may multiply and cause inflammation in traumatized or diseased structures and wounds and in obstructed sinuses, bronchi, and urinary and biliary tracts.

Anaerobic Streptococci. The varieties of streptococci considered above are facultative anaerobes. Microaerophilic streptococci which are *obligate* anaerobes do exist, however, and cause human disease. They are usually nonhemolytic and have not been systematically classified. These organisms are found in the mouth, bowel, and female genital tract. Their virulence is low and they tend to multiply in necrotic or frankly gangrenous lesions, producing a foul odor such as may be noted in lung abscesses or intrauterine infections. They may cause very extensive necrotizing wound infections. Although most anaerobic streptococci are susceptible to antimicrobial drugs, the lesions in which they are found usually require adequate surgical drainage as well as chemotherapy.

185. GROUP A STREPTOCOCCAL INFECTION

Gene H. Stollerman

History. Many of the clinical syndromes caused by group A streptococcal infection were recognized for many years before the discovery of *Streptococcus pyogenes* by Rosenbach in 1884. Thus Sydenham is often stated to have described scarlet fever, but the early accounts are inadequate and inexact. Certainly clinical recognition of scarlet fever, of tonsillitis and pharyngitis without a skin rash, of erysipelas, and of puerperal sepsis date back for many centuries before the modern era of bacteriology. Significant understanding of streptococcal infections, however, began with the discovery by Schottmüller, in 1903, that certain strains produce hemolysis on blood agar. Brown, in 1919, defined this reaction in greater detail and coined the descriptive terms that are still in use.

The streptococcal cause of scarlet fever and tonsullitis was known by 1895. The more modern work of the Dicks and of Dochez (1925) resolved the temporary issues raised concerning the possible role of other pharyngeal bacteria in scarlet fever, and Bloomfield clearly defined the streptococcal etiology of most cases of tonsillitis. The serologic classification of the organism into groups by Lancefield and into types by Lancefield and Griffith by 1935 and the introduction of the antistreptolysin O titer by Todd (1932) to identify streptococcal infection immunologically led to the modern era of the clinical bacteriology, immunology, and epidemiology of streptococcal infections and their nonsuppurative sequels, acute rheumatic fever (ARF) and acute glomerulonephritis (AGN).

The great epidemics of streptococcal disease in the armed forces in World War II supplied an enormous volume of clinical material for the clearer definition of the epidemiology of group A streptococcal disease and of the effect of penicillin therapy and prophylaxis upon the prevention of rheumatic fever and glomerulonephritis. The current era has been one of precise chemical definition of the structure and antigenic composition of Streptococcus and the pathophysiology of the cellular and extracellular antigenic and nonantigenic products it produces. Of particular interest has been the demonstration of immunologic cross-reactivity of streptococcal products with tissues of the heart and of the skin and the demonstration of complement-fixing immune complexes in the glomeruli of patients with acute nephritis.

The recent intensive studies of group A streptococcal skin infections have clarified the roles of these organisms in impetigo and secondary pyodermas and have pointed out the difference in the serotypes that produce such infections from those that produce pharyngitis alone. Such studies have sharpened the distinction between three populations of group A streptococci: (1) those that infect the throat but not the skin and that cause acute rheumatic fever (ARF) but not acute glomerulonephritis (AGN); (2) the streptococcal pharyngeal strains that cause AGN but not ARF; and (3) the pyoderma strains that primarily affect the skin but may also be found in the throat, and that cause AGN but apparently little or no ARF. The persistent enigma of the pathogenesis of ARF and of AGN continues to stimulate studies that unfold the remarkable complexity and variation of *Streptococcus pyogenes.*

Pathogenesis. The two most common sites of infection with streptococci in man are the nasopharynx and the skin. Most of our knowledge of the host-parasite relation is based on studies of the former, whereas streptococcal skin infection received little attention until recently. A growing interest in the role of streptococcal pyoderma in acute glomerulonephritis has led to increasing awareness of many distinctive features that set skin infections apart from those of the upper respiratory tract. In the ensuing discussion, some of these will be pointed out, and the specific clinical features of skin infections will be considered separately.

Strains of group A streptococci may vary greatly in infectivity or virulence. During epidemics of pharyngitis, most strains isolated from the throats of patients who are acutely ill contain relatively large amounts of the type-specific surface antigen, M protein. More than 60 antigenically distinct types of M protein have been differentiated so far. This substance has particular importance in the pathogenesis of group A streptococcal infection because immunity is type specific, that is, dependent upon antibody to the homologous type of M protein. Such antibodies tend to persist for many years after infection. For this reason, repeated infections with strains of different M types occur during the lifetime of most persons, but reinfection with the same M serotype is very rare unless the type-specific immune response is suppressed by penicillin therapy.

The production of large amounts of M protein is correlated with the ability of Streptococcus to resist phagocytosis. A hyaluronic acid capsule, which may attain very large size in some epidemic strains and produce large mucoid colonies, also contributes to the organism's resistance to phagocytosis, particularly in certain laboratory animals such as mice. Rapid passage of group A streptococci through mice usually results in increase in M protein production by group A strains and frequently in an increased size of the capsule. Interestingly, strains that form mucoid colonies (large capsules) are rarely if ever found in the skin. In the presence of homologous anti-M antibody, virulent group A streptococci are rapidly and efficiently destroyed by human blood phagocytes. This phenomenon forms the basis for the so-called bactericidal test for the presence of circulating type-specific anti-M antibody. It is not yet clear to what extent cross-immunity exists to strains of streptococci less virulent than those that are rich in M protein and that are highly encapsulated. Strains of group A organisms lacking both these virulence factors are readily phagocytized and destroyed by human and animal blood. It is possible that with increasing age and number of previous streptococcal infections, the human host acquires greater resistance to all but the most virulent strains of group A streptococci. This may account, in part, for the striking age incidence in the epidemiology of human group A streptococcal pharyngitis and streptococcal pyoderma. It also may account for the progressive tendency, betweeen infancy and childhood, for nasopharyngeal inflammatory reactions to become more and more focalized and intense. Certainly, immediate and delayed skin allergy to streptococcal products becomes increasingly frequent and severe during childhood and adolescence. Indeed, the widespread incidence of immediate and delayed allergy to streptococcal products has seriously hampered the development of effective vaccines against streptococcal M protein preparations.

The portion of highly purified M protein which is not the type-specific determinant is, instead, a determinant common to most if not all M proteins and has been called "M-associated" or "non-type-specific M" protein. Both cellular and humoral hypersensitivity to this antigen(s) is intense in man, and antibodies prepared to it can cross-react with streptococcal protoplast membranes and with the sarcolemma of myocardial tissues.

Other somatic protein antigens of the streptococcal surface which are of clinical significance are the so-called T proteins of group A streptococci. Although these play no part in virulence, they are useful antigenic markers of streptococci, particularly when the latter have dissociated to less virulent strains with the loss of their M protein marker. The T antigens include a number of immunologically distinct proteins which resist digestion by proteolytic enzymes. Antisera prepared against these antigens can identify the T type of trypsin-digested whole streptococci by a slide agglutination method. This method has proved particularly useful in identifying pyoderma streptococci (see below) which could not be serotyped with available anti-M sera because these organisms contained M proteins of hitherto unidentified types. Thus the T type pattern of a streptococcal strain is a useful marker in following its epidemiology, especially when its M protein marker is unknown or not present. There is little difficulty in M-typing the strains isolated from most outbreaks of acute streptococcal respiratory infection, but it is seldom possible to identify an M antigen in more than 50 per cent of any large and unselected collection of cultures. This is generally not due to the absence of M antigen but to the difficulty of preparing anti-M antisera to some types and the apparent large number of M proteins which still remain unidentified.

No definite biologic property has been defined for the *"C"-carbohydrate group A antigen.* The antigenic determinant of group A polysaccharide has been shown to be composed of repeating units of a dimer of N-acetyl glucosamine and rhamnose. Antibodies against this somatic antigen are not readily demonstrated in man by conventional antibody tests, but recent studies employing radioactive-labeled antigen have identified very persistent antibodies to group A polysaccharide in the sera of patients with rheumatic heart disease. The *mucopeptide* (peptidoglycan) which forms the backbone of the streptococcal cell wall cross-reacts with the structurally similar mucopeptides of many other bacteria and produces many of the same biologic reactions as the endotoxins of gram-negative bacteria.

In the course of human infections, group A organisms produce a great variety of antigenic extracellular products, such as streptolysin O, streptokinase (fibrinolysin), hyaluronidase, nicotinamide adenine dinucleotidase (NADase), several deoxyribonucleases (DNAses), and proteinases. The antibody responses to many of these substances are useful in diagnosis (see below), and some of these products undoubtedly contribute to the pathologic features of streptococcal infection. For example, the breakdown of fibrin and nucleic acids by streptokinase and the DNAses, respectively, produces the characteristic thin pus of streptococcal infections and, with hyaluronidase, may aid the organisms' rapid spread through tissues, as observed in streptococcal cellulitis and lymphangitis. The erythrogenic toxin causes the typical erythema of scarlet fever (see below). The pathogenic role of other toxins is not yet clearly understood.

With the virtual disappearance of diphtheria in the United States, the group A Streptococcus is the only significant bacterial organism that commonly causes primary sore throat, that is, that can invade the normal tissues of the pharynx. Because nasal and throat carriage of these organisms is very common, virulent streptococci may be inoculated into open wounds or skin abrasions, producing rapidly spreading *cellulitis* and *lymphangitis* or *erysipelas;* they may contaminate the denuded postpartum endometrium to produce puerperal sepsis; they may secondarily infect the lungs to produce a *streptococcal pneumonia* after viral respiratory diseases such as influenza. Therefore group A streptococci have always been a major cause of sepsis and suppurative complications. In addition, certain so-called *nonsuppurative complications* such as *rheumatic fever, glomerulonephritis,* and *erythema nodosum* may follow streptococcal infection by pathogenic mechanisms that are not yet clear, although delayed allergy to bacterial antigens is the probable mechanism in erythema nodosum. In addition, anaphylactoid or Schönlein-Henoch purpura may follow streptococcal infection (in addition to other infectious agents), representing, presumably, another form of immunologic disorder to infection with this agent. The relation of streptococcal antigens to the pathogenesis of ARF and AGN is discussed in Ch. 191 and 610.

Epidemiology. Quantitatively, upper respiratory infections, including scarlet fever, pharyngitis, and tonsillitis, are the most important forms of group A streptococcal infection. Illness in these categories occurs most frequently in children from 5 to 15 years of age, but younger and older persons are also highly susceptible to infection. The key to the understanding of the epidemiology of streptococcal infection is an appreciation of its mode of transmission. Transmission of group A streptococcal infections occurs as a result of direct contact between infected persons or healthy carriers and susceptible persons. Significant extrahuman or animal reservoirs of these organisms do not exist, although occasional outbreaks caused by contamination of an article of food, often milk, have occurred. In general, however, streptococci dissociate rapidly outside the human host, and organisms recovered from clothing, bedding, or house dust, although identifiable as group A, have been found to be noninfective when inoculated into the throats of human volunteers. Children, among whom infection is commonplace and healthy carriers are abundant, are primarily responsible for the spread of streptococcal disease. The introduction of an untreated, infected five-year-old into a family will be followed by pharyngeal infection of more than half of his siblings and a significant number of adults in the household. The spread of an M-typable, virulent strain of group A Streptococcus through a family occurs much more readily than that of non-M-typable organisms. The problem of control of hemolytic streptococcal disease is complicated by the fact that a very large proportion of infections by these organisms is either exceedingly mild or completely inapparent. Persons with this type of "subclinical" infection are fully capable of disseminating the streptococci, but will not necessarily come under the care of a physician who could apply modern chemotherapy, eradicate streptococci from the pharyngeal tissues, and eliminate the possibility of transmission of the disease.

Epidemiologic factors such as climate, season, and geography are important primarily as they affect close contact of individuals. For example, military recruit populations, particularly when mobilized in large camps in cold climates and crowded housing conditions, provide the most ideal circumstances for the rapid passage of the organism from individual to individual, and such populations give rise to some of the most severe epidemics on record. Streptococcal disease is most severe in civilian populations when poverty and poor housing promote the most crowded living conditions.

In the temperate zones of the United States pharyngeal streptococcal infections vary strikingly with the season of the year. The peak incidence occurs between December and May, and only rare sporadic infections appear during the hot summer months. In recent family studies of a large metropolitan area in the northern part of the United States, it was estimated that a streptococcal infection occurs approximately once every three to four years during childhood and adolescence, and that in a middle class population in this metropolis only about 2 per cent of all respiratory illnesses that occurred were due to group A streptococcal infection.

The epidemiology of *scarlet fever* is the same as that of other group A streptococcal infections except that the strains producing the infection seem to be lysogenized by a bacteriophage that induces the production of erythrogenic toxin in a manner entirely analogous to diphtheria organisms that produce diphtheria toxin. Thus the epidemiology of scarlet fever is essentially that of any other strain of group A Streptococcus that does not produce the erythrogenic toxin. This explains the mild sporadic cases of scarlet fever, the severe epidemics of streptococcal pharyngitis *without* any scarlet fever cases, and the localized outburst of scarlet fever in a single concentrated population such as a school or institution.

The epidemiology of streptococcal pyoderma is strikingly different from that of streptococcal pharyngitis in several respects. Seasonal occurrence of the two is quite disparate in temperate climates: pharyngitis is more common and intense in cold weather, whereas streptococcal pyoderma occurs often in the late summer and early fall. The close indoor contact during the colder months may facilitate respiratory spread, whereas increased exposure of the uncovered skin to minor trauma and insect bites may favor skin infection during the warmer months. Although, geographically, epidemic streptococcal pharyngitis is more common in temperate or cold climates and streptococcal pyoderma in hot or tropical climates, exceptions are not uncommon in both diseases.

Streptococcal pyoderma affects an even younger age group than pharyngitis, occurring most often in children of preschool age and in infants. Transmission of streptococcal pyoderma may be aided mechanically by insects, particularly flies, that are attracted to skin lesions. Poverty and filth, as well as crowding, are major predisposing factors. Patients with streptococcal pyoderma often harbor the same organisms in the throat that colonize the skin.

The Contrasting Epidemiology of Acute Rheumatic Fever and Acute Glomerulonephritis (see accompanying figure). Students of the nonsuppurative sequels of group A streptococcal infection have long been impressed with the extreme rarity with which ARF and AGN occur in the same patient at the same time, and the antecedent infection is considered, therefore, to be due to a strain that is *either* "rheumatogenic" *or* "nephritogenic," but not both! Simultaneous appearance of both sequelae has not been a feature of the reported experience of large numbers of patients with either disease in severe epidemics in which a single streptococcal strain could be identified as the cause (Rammelkamp, 1953). The route of infection also seems to differentiate rheumatogenic from nephritogenic strains. Acute rheumatic fever seems to be almost always, if not exclusively, a complication of a pharyngeal infection. Acute glomerulonephritis occurs after *either* skin or pharyngeal infection. Although skin strains often parasitize the throat, the best known rheumatogenic pharyngeal strains do not seem to parasitize the skin.

The strains which belong to the M serotypes that have clearly caused pharyngitis followed by rheumatic fever are those commonly encountered in the throats of children in the cities of the temperate zones of the United States and western Europe and include, among others, 1, 3, 5, 6, 14, 18, 19, and 24. *All* strains containing these M

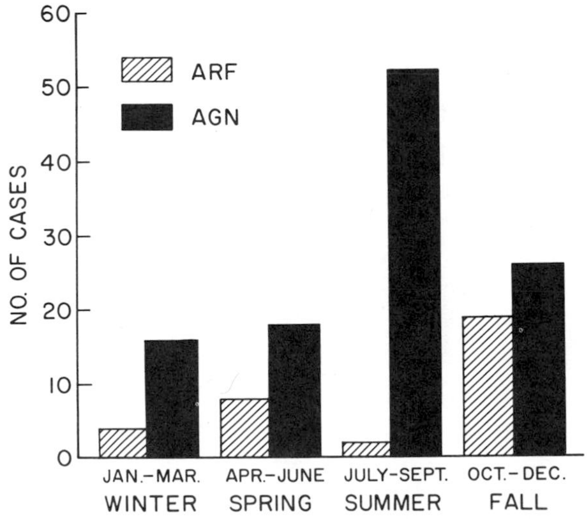

Seasonal distribution of acute rheumatic fever (ARF) and acute glomerulonephritis (AGN) admissions at City of Memphis Hospitals, September 1965–August 1968. (After Bisno, A. L., Pearce, I. A., Wall, H. P., Moody, M. D., and Stollerman, G. H.: N. Engl. J. Med., 283: 561, 1970.)

antigens are not necessarily non-nephritogenic, and from time to time sporadic cases of AGN have appeared which seemed to be due to strains representing some of these serotypes (types 1, 3, and 6).

The identification of M type 12 organisms as the major pharyngeal serotype that has been associated with AGN (Rammelkamp et al., 1952) is of interest because this M serotype is perhaps the most common one encountered in the throats of schoolchildren, and yet AGN does not appear consistently in populations harboring this strain. Thus not all members of a given M serotype are necessarily nephritogenic.

The recent attention to the bacteriology of skin strains of streptococci has revealed them to contain M and T proteins of types hitherto unrecognized (types 49 and 52 to 60). Although AGN has occurred in association with most of the strains in these categories, no specific M or T antigen per se has been related to this complication.

The factors of infection determining the attack rate of rheumatic fever are also quantitative. The attack rate may vary from as low as 0.3 per cent after very mild, sporadic streptococcal infections associated with strains of low virulence to as high as 3 per cent or greater after infections with highly virulent strains of group A streptococci. The two factors that appear to have most influence on the frequency with which rheumatic fever follows a streptococcal infection are (1) the duration of convalescent carriage of the strain after the infection, and (2) the magnitude of the immunologic response associated with the infection. Thus patients with relatively feeble antistreptolysin O responses may show an attack rate of rheumatic fever of considerably less than 1 per cent, whereas those with the most vigorous streptococcal antistreptolysin O responses may suffer attack rates of rheumatic fever as high as 5 to 10 per cent. The acquisition of streptococci in the throat and their subsequent carriage *without* immunologic response has not been associated with reactivation of rheumatic fever in rheumatic subjects, nor do primary attacks of rheumatic fever occur very often without a well defined immune response. The epidemiology of rheumatic fever is therefore a reflection of the prevalence and severity of group A streptococcal pharyngitis.

CLINICAL SYNDROMES OF GROUP A STREPTOCOCCAL INFECTION

Gene H. Stollerman

186. STREPTOCOCCAL SORE THROAT

The classic syndrome described as most typical of group A streptococcal infection in older children and adults is as follows:

Symptoms. Sudden onset of sore throat, sometimes associated with abdominal pain and nausea, especially in children, and accompanied by constitutional symptoms of malaise, headache, and feverishness.

Signs. Redness and edema of the throat, and particularly the presence of an *exudate* on the tonsils or tonsillar fossae; enlargement and particularly *tenderness* of the anterior cervical nodes, and fever of 38.2° C or greater. Helpful laboratory data, other than results of throat culture, include leukocytosis greater than 12,000 leukocytes per cubic millimeter.

Although this classic syndrome is, indeed, associated with group A streptococcal infection, the full clinical picture develops in a minority of patients with pharyngitis, except during epidemics. Much more common in clinical practice is the patient with some, but not all, of the aforementioned signs and symptoms. It is not unusual for mild streptococcal disease to be associated with *nonexudative* pharyngitis, and, conversely, for viral infections, particularly adenovirus, to produce purulent tonsillar exudate and a syndrome indistinguishable from streptococcal tonsillitis. Hemolytic streptococci are the only significant *bacterial* cause of nonexudative pharyngitis. Many viral infections may mimic this clinical state, making the study of upper respiratory infection without bacteriologic control most difficult.

Streptococcal respiratory infection is not accompanied by significant cough or by coryza. The presence of either of these manifestations should suggest a different cause. Rhinorrhea does occur, especially in young children, who frequently develop suppurative sinusitis.

Scarlet Fever. The disease is clinically similar in almost all respects to tonsillitis and pharyngitis caused by nonscarlatinal strains of group A streptococci. Its name, however, comes from the presence of a skin rash caused by the erythrogenic toxin produced by scarlatinal strains. The erythrogenic effect of the toxin on the skin can be neutralized by antitoxin. This is the basis of the diagnostic *Schultz-Charlton reaction.* The injection of 0.1 ml of scarlet fever antitoxin, or of 0.2 to 0.3 ml of convalescent human serum, into an area where the rash is florid will be followed by blanching around the site of injection in 8 to 12 hours. Streptococcal antitoxin is no longer readily available, and usually clinical and bacteriologic studies suffice for diagnosis.

The enanthem of scarlet fever includes a tongue that may be bright red with large papillae (raspberry tongue) or coated with the red papillae protruding (strawberry tongue). These manifestations of the disease are rarely seen in adults. The rash usually appears on the second day of the disease. It consists of a diffuse, bright scarlet erythema with many points of deeper red. The distribution is variable, but the trunk and inner aspects of the arms and thighs are most often affected. In many cases the rash is clearly seen only in the axillae and groins. The face is flushed and red, but a pale area, the *circumoral pallor,* is often seen around the mouth. The palms and soles are not erythematous. Petechiae and occasionally ecchymoses are observed, especially in severely ill patients. The application of a tourniquet to the arm for five minutes will be associated with the appearance of large numbers of petechiae distal to the obstruction in nearly all cases. This is the *Rumpel-Leede* sign; it is not specific for scarlet fever. The erythema disappears usually by the sixth to the ninth day of infection in association with the return of the temperature and the throat to normal. Desquamation of the skin is characteristic of scarlet fever, and it begins as a fine scaling of the face and body that is usually completed during the second week. About this time the extensive and characteristic desquamation of the palms and soles starts and continues for one to two weeks. Often the diagnosis is made retrospectively in patients who show this desquamation after a sore throat and in whom the scarlatinal rash may have been overlooked. Eosinophilia may be a feature of scarlet fever, especially during desquamation, and is sometimes striking (up to 20 per cent).

The course and clinical features of scarlet fever vary greatly with the severity of the disease. Many mild cases are observed in which constitutional symptoms and sore throat are minimal, fever is low grade and of short duration, and the rash is evanescent. A florid eruption is sometimes seen in persons in whom all other evidences of the disease are slight, indicating that the reaction to the erythrogenic toxin per se is not primarily responsible for the systemic manifestations of scarlet fever. Again, the situation is comparable to that in diphtheria. A mild sore throat with a strain that is a potent toxin-producer may result in a clinical picture dominated by the effects of the exotoxin. Conversely, severe pharyngeal infection may be present with a strain that is a relatively mild toxin-producer, and the clinical manifestations resulting from the toxin may be slight.

Course of Steptococcal Pharyngitis. The course of untreated hemolytic streptococcal pharyngitis in older children and adults is benign. Seventy-five per cent of patients are afebrile within 72 hours after onset, but sore throat, abnormal signs in the pharynx, and tender adenitis may persist for two or three days after the return of the temperature to normal. Although the whole process is shortened by appropriate antimicrobial therapy by 24 to 48 hours, it is not always easy to distinguish the treated from the untreated patient. An acute pharyngitis that *fails to respond* to adequate penicillin therapy is virtually never due to group A streptococcal infection. On the other hand, the course of viral pharyngitis is often also very brief, and a spontaneous defervescence in 24 to 48 hours may mislead the clinician who has treated the patient into believing the patient has had a therapeutic response to penicillin therapy. In severe streptococcal infections, leukocytosis, when present in the acute stage, may persist in more than one half of untreated patients for a week or more, but this disappears more quickly after the institution of antimicrobial therapy. The erythrocyte sedimentation rate returns to normal in 80 per cent of patients by the third week.

Group A streptococci tend to persist in the pharynx for long periods after recovery if antimicrobial therapy has not been employed. In general, the more virulent the strain, the longer and more consistent is the duration of convalescent throat carriage. Under epidemic conditions, 80 per cent of untreated patients may carry the infecting strain for as long as four weeks. On the other hand, sporadic and mild streptococcal infections among schoolchildren studied in recent years are not as frequently associated with such prolonged throat carriage.

Streptococcal pharyngitis in infants and small children lacks an acute and well defined onset, has rhinorrhea as a dominant manifestation, is rarely associated with high fever, and runs a protracted and indeterminate course. The physical signs in the throat are nondescript, and usually do not permit an accurate clinical diagnosis. Suppurative complications such as otitis media and cervical lymphadenitis occur frequently.

The change of the pharyngeal response after the first few years of life to an explosive onset with fever, sore throat, and exudative pharyngitis may be a reflection of the sharp increase in delayed hypersensitivity (cellular immunity) that appears after the first or second year of life as a result of repeated infection with different types of group A streptococci. It is noteworthy that rheumatic fever is very rare before heightened cellular and humoral immunity to the Steptococcus occurs, whereas acute glomerulonephritis is common.

Diagnosis of Steptococcal Pharyngitis. Streptococcal tonsillitis and pharyngitis in its typical form needs to be differentiated from diphtheria, nonstreptococcal exudative pharyngitis (usually adenovirus), and infectious mononucleosis. When streptoccal infection is nonexudative, however, it cannot be differentiated (in the absence of scarlet fever) from a variety of viral agents producing an identical clinical picture. Cough, coryza, and rhinorrhea (in adults) make a nonbacterial disorder more likely. Unfortunately therefore the clinical diagnosis of the kind of streptococcal pharyngitis that now occurs most commonly as a sporadic infection in civilian communities is usually a crude guess. It is possible, however, to *exclude* the diagnosis of streptococcal disease in considerably more than half the patients studied for sporadic pharyngitis by the use of throat cultures. The incidence of throat cultures positive for beta-hemolytic streptococci decreases progressively with age in patients with sporadic acute respiratory diseases in civilian communities. In several large cities in the northern sections of the United States, surveys have shown that less than 5 per cent of adults who had routine cultures for upper respiratory infections harbored group A streptococci in their throats. It is obvious therefore that without bacteriologic confirmation, the clinical diagnosis of viral versus streptococcal pharyngitis is quite unsatisfactory.

Before any antimicrobial therapy is administered, swabs should be passed through the mouth under direct vision, using a good light, and rubbed over the tonsils and posterior pharynx. The swab should be streaked directly, with a minimum of delay, on sheep blood agar plates of low dextrose content. After incubation overnight, the number of hemolytic streptococci present should be recorded in a roughly quantitative manner. These organisms will be very numerous in nearly all cases if they are the cause of the infection. The presence of a few does not provide convincing evidence that they are responsible for the illness, because 5 to 10 per cent of the general population are nasopharyngeal carriers of these organisms. Serologic grouping and typing of the isolated organisms are usually not necessary for routine clinical diagnosis. Because all group A streptococci are susceptible in vitro to discs containing less than 0.02 unit of bacitracin, some laboratories determine the bacitracin susceptibility of hemolytic streptococci routinely. A hemolytic Streptococcus resistant to such low concentrations of bacitracin is virtually never a group A Streptococcus. On the other hand, approximately 5 per cent of non-group A hemolytic streptococci are also susceptible to this low concentration.

Immunologic Diagnosis of Streptococcal Pharyngitis. The immunologic diagnosis of group A streptococcal infection is of no value in the treatment of the acute illness, because an antibody response will not usually be detected until 10 to 20 days after the onset of the disease. Measurement of antistreptolysin O, antihyaluronidase, antistreptokinase, anti-NADase, or anti-DNAse B is of great value in determining whether or not there has been preceding streptococcal pharyngitis in patients with possible rheumatic fever or glomerulonephritis. The presence of low titers of such antibodies during convalescence virtually excludes recent streptococcal disease except in patients who have been intensively treated early in the illness. Helpful in excluding the diagnosis of recent streptococcal infection is a hemagglutination test which employs red blood cells sensitized with all the streptococcal extracellular antigens contained in a crude filtrate of a group A culture (Streptozyme). When human sera are reacted with such cells, an increase in antibody to any of these numerous antigens can be detected readily, and low titers therefore denote freedom from recent streptococcal infection. It should be noted that streptococcal pyoderma does not produce an equally strong immune response to all streptococcal antigens. In particular, antistreptolysin O and anti-NADase are increased relatively infrequently, whereas anti-DNAse B and antihyaluronidase, particularly the former, are better indicators of recent streptococcal pyoderma. The clinician should be aware that elevated serum levels of streptococcal antibodies may persist for long periods of time after an immune response has occurred. Such elevated serum levels do not necessarily imply an unfavorable prognosis, and are not an indication for additional prolonged antimicrobial therapy.

The Value of Throat Cultures in Deciding When to Treat. There may be some difficulty in interpreting the significance of a throat culture weakly positive for hemolytic streptococci when streptococcal disease is mild and sporadic. Such a positive culture may represent the acquisition of a strain temporarily in the pharynx that does not actually invade the deeper tissues of the host, does not produce a significant immune response, and does not lead to acute rheumatic fever. Such a positive culture may also represent the convalescent carriage of an infection that occurred several weeks previously and may bear no relation to subsequent acute symptoms of viral pharyngitis from which the patient may now be suffering. The physician's problem in deciding which patient with pharyngitis to treat with antimicrobial drugs will be clarified if he obtains throat cultures routinely in all such patients whom he examines. By doing this he becomes alert to the epidemiology of the infections he encounters. A throat culture negative for beta-hemolytic streptococci will exclude a great many patients from unnecessary and promiscuous use of expensive antimicrobial drugs. In outbreaks of exudative pharyngitis, negative throat cultures in a succession of patients will immediately reveal the nonstreptococcal nature of the disease encountered. Conversely, a succession of strongly positive cultures leaves little doubt that a local outbreak of streptococcal pharyngitis is in progress.

When exudative pharyngitis is associated with a throat culture heavily seeded with beta-hemolytic streptococci, there is little argument with the general recommendation for prompt and adequate antimicrobial therapy. Moreover, when a succession of such cases is observed, the practitioner is immediately alerted to the need to culture material from the throats of asymptomatic contacts to prevent the spread of an epidemic. It is with the sporadic cases of nonexudative pharyngitis that are associated with positive throat cultures that some argument has been raised as to the need to employ intensive penicillin therapy in the regimens recommended for the prevention of rheumatic fever (see below). In some populations and under some conditions, such intensive treatment may not be necessary. At present, however, these conditions have not yet been sufficiently defined to justify broad generalizations. Until further studies define more precisely the risk of withholding or modifying chemotherapy of such infections, it is safer to err on the side of overtreatment and thus to ensure the prevention of passage of streptococcal strains through a population. Indeed, with the assistance of the throat culture, all contacts of patients with well diagnosed exudative streptococcal pharyngitis may be studied for acquisition of potentially dangerous strains, and those identified as carriers may be treated. The consequence of such practice would undoubtedly have a profound influence on the epidemiology of streptococcal infection and therefore upon the incidence of rheumatic fever and glomerulonephritis.

Complications of Pharyngitis. Suppurative and nonsuppurative complications may follow untreated streptococcal tonsillitis and pharyngitis.

Suppurative Complications. *Peritonsillar abscess* or *quinsy sore throat* is an interesting and infrequent complication of streptococcal tonsillitis. Its exact pathogenesis is unknown. Suppuration extends through the capsule of the palatine tonsil into the loose connective tissue of the neck. This is associated with formation of brawny edema of the affected side with movement of the tonsil toward the midline of the throat. An abscess eventually forms and drains in untreated cases, *but the pus does not regularly contain streptococci.* It is probable that the initial streptococcal infection does not cause this lesion directly, but may permit other organisms such as anaerobic gram-negative bacilli of the Bacteroides group and anaerobic nonhemolytic streptococci to gain a foothold in the affected tissues. The onset of this complication is marked by an abrupt increase in soreness and swelling of the neck, and often by increased fever and malaise. The involved tonsil and anterior pillar are greatly swollen, the cervical nodes are large and tender, and eventually a fluctuant mass may be felt in the affected area with the gloved finger. Complications of peritonsillar abscess arise when the infection extends further into the neck or leads to the development of suppurative thrombophlebitis. Peritonsillar abscess is only rarely seen today, because severe hemolytic streptococcal tonsillitis is often treated early in its course with effective antimicrobial agents.

Direct extension of hemolytic streptococci from the locus in the throat to the surrounding tissues may result in certain suppurative complications. Paranasal sinusitis, otitis media, mastoiditis, suppurative cervical adenitis, and impetigo are the most common, and will occur most frequently in untreated children less than four years old. It has been demonstrated that otitis media occurring early in the course of streptococcal respiratory infection is caused by the same serologic type that was present in the throat at the onset. A similar complication that develops after the first week is likely to be the result of a reinfection, and a different type will be recovered from the purulent exudate. Bacteremia was once observed rather frequently during the course of streptococcal respiratory infection and was often associated with metastatic lesions in the joints, bones, and elsewhere. Such cases are now almost unknown, even if antimicrobial therapy is withheld. Similarly, there has been a nearly complete disappearance of group A streptococcal meningitis. Pneumonia has always been a surprisingly uncommon complication of streptococcal upper respiratory infections. Tender cervical adenitis is regularly present and is not to be regarded as a complication unless the lymph nodes become very large and fluctuant. All the various suppurative streptococcal complications may be prevented by early and adequate antimicrobial therapy. Response to similar management is excellent if any such complications should develop in an untreated patient.

Nonsuppurative Complications. The principal nonsuppurative complications of streptococcal disease, acute rheumatic fever (ARF), and acute glomerulonephritis (AGN), are discussed in Ch. 189 (ARF) and in Ch. 610 (AGN).

187. STREPTOCOCCAL SKIN INFECTIONS

STREPTOCOCCAL PYODERMA

Clinical Features. Aside from secondary infections of wounds or burns, group A streptococci can cause at least two kinds of skin infection, *pyoderma* and *erysipelas.* These differ markedly in clinical appearance, in epidemiology, in pathogenesis, and perhaps in the strains of streptococci causing infection. The term streptococcal pyoderma includes all kinds of streptococcal skin infections, other than erysipelas, many of which are secondary infections. The term *impetigo,* or *impetigo contagiosa,* describes what often appears to be a *primary* infection, is initially and transiently vesicular, and presents as crusted, nonscarring lesions in its later stages.

The initial lesion of streptococcal impetigo is a papule that develops rapidly into a vesicle with a small surrounding area of erythema. The vesicles are often missed clinically because of their evanescence and rapid transformation into pustules with thick, amber-colored crusts that appear to be "stuck on" the skin. Aside from occasional itching and burning, the lesions are not painful unless they become deep seated. Regional lymph nodes are commonly involved even without extensive local cellulitis. Often an apparently innocuous lesion may yield large numbers of group A streptococci in cultures taken beneath dried crusts, and such indolent-appearing lesions can produce full-blown acute glomerulonephritis. Bacteremia, which is rare in streptococcal pharyngitis, occurs more frequently with skin and wound infections, and occasionally scarlet fever has been reported. Superficial streptococcal skin infections often pursue a chronic course of weeks or months, and their onset is often difficult to establish. A deeply ulcerated form is known as *ecthyma.*

Contagiousness of streptococcal skin infections is evident from the tendency of multiple cases to occur in a family and from their tendency to occur in epidemics. The importance of antecedent skin trauma is apparent in the epidemiology of streptococcal pyoderma (see above). Its preponderance in the summer when insect bites and trauma to exposed parts of children are most common, especially in populations in which poverty results in poor hygiene, neglect, flies, and crowding, suggests the conditions for maximal opportunity of invasion of the skin by virulent strains. Because of the frequency, especially in children, of such minor skin trauma as mosquito bites, abrasions, burns, eczema, scabies, and pediculosis, it is often difficult to determine whether or not group A streptococci invade the unbroken skin. In epidemic conditions owing to particularly virulent strains, the clinical appearance of the lesions often suggests direct invasion, but it is virtually impossible to exclude minute and transient antecedent trauma.

Diagnosis. The frequency with which staphylococci colonize the skin makes contamination of skin lesions with these organisms almost the rule. Cultures of lesions more clearly considered streptococcal pyoderma are frequently also associated with staphylococci, and the relative role of each organism in the etiology of impetigo has caused much confusion and controversy. Although the issue is not entirely settled, current evidence suggests that impetigo can be divided on clinical, bacteriologic, and epidemiologic grounds into two basic forms: a bullous type, in infants, which forms thin, varnish-like crusts and is primarily staphylococcal in origin, and a vesicular type, which develops thick "stuck-on" crusts and is primarily streptococcal in etiology. Whereas the classic bullous impetigo caused by staphylococci yields a pure culture of phage Type 71 organisms, the early vesicular stage of streptococcal impetigo may yield pure cultures of group A streptococci, but in the purulent and crusted stages large numbers of staphylococci may be present also. The latter are of a variety of phage types suggesting secondary colonization.

Skin cultures of pyodermas should be made after careful cleansing of the surface of the lesions with gauze soaked in sterile warm water, avoiding antiseptics, soaps, and detergents that kill or suppress the more fastidious streptococci and favor the survival of the more adaptable Staphylococcus. Often the removal of crusts and careful culture of the serous exudate beneath will yield large numbers of hemolytic streptococci in almost pure culture. Sheep blood agar plates incubated anaerobically or in 10 per cent CO_2 favor the growth of streptococci.

The higher numbered M and T serotypes associated with pyoderma strains of group A streptococci set them apart from the primarily pharyngeal strains, although it should be noted that throat carriage of the "skin strains" may be high in populations in which much pyoderma is present, especially during the summer months.

The weak antistreptolysin O response to pyoderma strains should be borne in mind, and anti-DNAse B or antihyaluronidase titers should be measured when studies of the immune response to these streptococcal infections are indicated (see above), as in the diagnosis of poststreptococcal AGN.

ERYSIPELAS

This form of group A streptococcal skin infection has special characteristics and may be considered in greater detail. Erysipelas usually involves the face and head, but may affect any area of the body. Other than an occasional case of a group C strain that has been recognized, erysipelas is caused by group A streptococci. The precise way in which the bacteria are introduced into the skin in primary facial erysipelas has not been determined. Large numbers of group A streptococci are fairly constantly present among the nasopharyngeal flora of patients with early erysipelas. It may be that the primary infection is a nasopharyngitis from which the organism is transferred to the skin.

After reaching the face, the streptococci may enter the skin through minute abrasions that are not recognizable after the disease is well established. In surgical and wound erysipelas, it is probable that streptococci are introduced into the traumatized areas from external sources, usually the nose and throat of attendants and other patients. The epidemiology of facial erysipelas differs somewhat from that of group A streptococcal infection in the affected age groups. This disease, when large numbers of cases were observed in the past, was rather common in infancy, rare between the ages of six and thirty, and predominantly a disorder of middle age. There has been no explanation for this discrepancy in age distribution.

Erysipelas usually begins as an abrupt onset of fever with a shaking chill. A history of preceding acute or subacute upper respiratory infection is obtained in about one third of adult cases and more frequently in infants. Very early in the disease a definite zone of redness and edema of the skin appears, most frequently around the bridge of the nose or around a surgical incision, traumatic wound, area of dermatitis, or the newly severed umbilical cord. Facial erysipelas is usually self-limited if no antibacterial therapy is administered. Under these circumstances, the temperature remains at a high level for four to ten days and then falls by lysis or crisis. During this interval a local process involves a large part of the face. As the lesion develops and spreads from the central focus, the skin is red, hot, edematous, and glistening. Blebs are frequently formed. The advancing edge of the lesion is sharply defined and slightly elevated. Great swelling occurs when the infection involves the eyelids.

The disease may involve one or both sides of the face, and usually remains active and spreading until the cheeks and eyelids are affected. Very often the inflammatory process does not extend over the bony prominences, and is limited to the area between the mandible, the malar eminence, and the hairline. In certain cases the ear is included, but spread to the scalp and trunk is rare except in infants.

Untreated *erysipelas of the trunk or extremities,* which usually occurs in infants or persons who have undergone surgery or have been injured, is a more malignant disease. Large areas of skin are often involved rapidly, prostration frequently occurs, and death is a common event. In this form of the disorder it is often possible to observe the characteristic recovery of the skin first affected while the process advances elsewhere. Healing of the skin requires one to two weeks after the temperature has returned to normal.

188. HEMOLYTIC STREPTOCOCCAL PNEUMONIA

Group A hemolytic streptococci were once responsible for 3 to 5 per cent of cases of bacterial pneumonia, but this form of the disease is now rarely seen. It usually appears as a complication of influenza or other viral respiratory infection or in persons with underlying pulmonary disease. It is almost never observed as a sequel to streptococcal tonsillitis and pharyngitis or scarlet fever.

The pneumonic process is lobular in distribution in the lung. Empyema develops in 30 to 40 per cent of untreated cases. It is present early in the illness and is characterized by the formation of large amounts of thin fluid. Bacteremia is demonstrable in 10 to 15 per cent of the cases of streptococcal pneumonia. The demonstration of large numbers of hemolytic streptococci in the sputum by cultural methods, or the isolation of these organisms from the blood or pleural fluid, is required for diagnosis.

189. TREATMENT OF GROUP A STREPTOCOCCAL INFECTION AND CHEMOPROPHYLAXIS OF NONSUPPURATIVE COMPLICATIONS

Gene H. Stollerman

The management of the various group A streptococcal illnesses should include those general measures that are applied in all acute infections. Bed rest, light or liquid diet if pharyngeal discomfort is present and severe, and adequate but not excessive fluid intake are indicated.

Most important is the prompt institution of appropriate antimicrobial therapy, which has four goals: (1) the prompt control of the acute suppurative process in the respiratory tract or elsewhere, (2) the prevention of suppurative complications, (3) the prevention of nonsuppurative complications, and (4) the elimination of the carrier state and the prevention of transmission of the organism to others. The third and fourth goals will be fully attained only if the organism is permanently eradicated from the tissues. This can best be accomplished by the administration of penicillin. Sulfonamides are not effective either in eradicating the carrier state or in preventing an immunologic response, and thus do not prevent nonsuppurative complications. Erythromycin is an acceptable second choice to penicillin in the presence of allergy to penicillin. Tetracycline-resistant group A streptococci have been described with increasing frequency, and this drug is therefore an unreliable choice. It is essential that treatment in full doses be given over a period of at least ten days, regardless of which of the effective drugs is used.

Group A streptococci are among the most susceptible of all bacteria to the action of penicillin. The range of susceptibility for all strains of this serologic group is extremely narrow, between 0.01 and 0.04 unit per milliliter of culture. Moreover, no penicillin-resistant strains of group A streptococci have been demonstrated.

Duration of exposure to penicillin is the most important factor in therapy. Prolonged exposure to small concentrations of penicillin therefore is just as effective as a more intensive form of treatment of group A streptococcal pharyngitis. A single intramuscular injection of 600,000 units of benzathine penicillin provides blood levels that are barely detectable but that persist for about ten days; 1.2 million units results in levels that persist for at least two to four weeks or more. Such doses cure streptococcal pharyngitis, terminate carriage in the throat, and prevent rheumatic fever with optimal efficiency. Shorter-acting penicillin salts, such as aqueous procaine penicillin, must be administered still more often (usually daily for ten days) in a dose of 300,000 or 600,000 units intramuscularly to accomplish the same results. In the treatment of streptococcal pharyngitis, combinations of aqueous, procaine, and benzathine penicillin have no advantage over a single injection of benzathine penicillin G alone if a dose of at least 600,000 units or, preferably, 1.2 million units of the latter is employed.

If given orally, penicillin G must be administered in doses of 200,000 to 250,000 units four times daily for ten days. Thus, penicillinemia of about ten days' duration, regardless of the choice of preparation, is necessary to ensure bacteriologic cure. Sulfonamides are ineffective in preventing rheumatic fever when used to treat streptococcal pharyngitis. They do not suppress the immune response, do not terminate pharyngeal carriage of streptococci, and thus do not reduce the attack rate of subsequent rheumatic fever. They may be used, however, as continuous prophylaxis to *prevent* new infections (see below).

PREVENTION OF RHEUMATIC FEVER

Although the more promptly penicillin therapy is instituted, the more effective is prevention of subsequent rheumatic fever, there is no harm in delaying therapy for 24 hours to await report of a throat culture. It has been shown that the incidence of acute rheumatic fever can be partially reduced by treatment instituted as long as nine days after the onset of pharyngitis. When the patient has been seen within the first day or two of his infection, withholding treatment for one day more has not proved to constitute a risk. One exception to this statement involves the patient with a history of rheumatic fever. In such a patient, the prevention of rheumatic recurrence is not always possible unless treatment is instituted at the first clinical sign of streptococcal infection. In such a patient, any delay of therapy entails the risk of reactivation of the disease. Certain features of the chemoprophylaxis of rheumatic fever are also presented in Ch. 191.

Patients with more serious streptococcal infections, such as streptococcal pneumonia, severe wound infections with sepsis, or suppurative complications of ordinary respiratory infection, should receive 600,000 units of procaine penicillin G per day intramuscularly for several days until the illness is well controlled, when a shift to a single dose of benzathine penicillin or to oral penicillin may be made. The response of extrapharyngeal suppurative complications of streptococcal infection to penicillin is good, and recovery without surgical intervention is the rule, with one exception. Sterilization of abscesses in well-established suppurative cervical adenitis is most difficult. Incision and drainage is usually required in such cases unless spontaneous rupture occurs. As in all situations of antimicrobial therapy in the presence of pus and necrosis, prolonged therapy for as long as several weeks may be required when adequate debridement is not possible. For patients allergic to penicillin, erythromycin is recommended in doses of 1 gram per day, which may be given in four divided doses for a period of ten days. Severely ill patients may receive 500 mg of erythromycin twice daily intravenously for a short time until they are able to accept the drug by mouth.

PREVENTION OF GLOMERULONEPHRITIS

As in rheumatic fever, initial attacks of glomerulonephritis can be prevented by prompt and adequate penicillin treatment of streptococcal pharyngitis. However, the latent period between streptococcal infection and glomerulonephritis is generally shorter than for rheumatic fever. Therefore glomerulonephritis is not as efficiently prevented by treatment of the antecedent streptococcal infection with penicillin as is rheumatic fever. When the clinician is aware of the appearance of other cases of acute glomerulonephritis or rheumatic fever in the population he attends, he should treat sore throat promptly and vigorously and should be more energetic than ever in obtaining throat cultures from the contacts of his patient.

The treatment of streptococcal pyoderma has been studied far less methodically than pharyngitis and has varied widely in practice. The principles guiding the treatment of pyoderma may be somewhat different from those of pharyngitis in which prevention of rheumatic fever requires thorough eradication of group A streptococci. Unlike pharyngeal infections, topical treatment of skin infections may be adequate for mild cases of impetigo. Whether or not parenteral antimicrobial drugs are used, the removal of crusts and cleansing of the affected skin surfaces with soap seems to be an important part of the treatment of streptococcal pyoderma. In patients with extensive, persistent, or recurring impetigo, intramuscular benzathine penicillin is the treatment of choice.

190. PROPHYLAXIS OF STREPTOCOCCAL INFECTION

Gene H. Stollerman

Mass Prophylaxis. Mass prophylaxis is the term applied to the treatment of an entire population, both healthy and affected persons, to interrupt or prevent an epidemic, impending or in progress. This has been done frequently in military populations when epidemic streptococcal pharyngitis and its aftermath of rheumatic fever or glomerulonephritis have appeared. Occasionally, similar measures have been taken against local epidemics in schools or institutions. A single injection of 1.2 million units of benzathine penicillin G intramuscularly has proved extremely effective for this purpose because it (1) is therapeutic in those actually infected, (2) terminates pharyngeal carriage, and (3) protects against the acquisition of new infections for four to five weeks.

Unfortunately, no form of immunization is of avail. However, alert medical practitioners who will promptly detect and adequately treat streptococcal infections, a good system of public health reporting of rheumatic fever and acute glomerulonephritis, and good facilities for routine use of throat cultures should reduce extensive epidemics of streptococcal disease to a rarity. This should so alter the spread of streptococcal infections as to diminish the virulence and epidemicity of the Streptococcus and thereby continue the present trend in the decline of nonsuppurative complications of streptococcal disease.

Tonsillectomy has been employed prophylactically in the past, but is now known to be useless for this purpose, as it does not prevent infection by hemolytic streptococci. Subsequently acquired streptococcal respiratory illnesses may be less severe, but the frequency of occurrence of nonsuppurative complications is not reduced.

Continuous Chemoprophylaxis. Continuous chemoprophylaxis against group A streptococci has proved to be highly effective in preventing recurrences of rheumatic fever (see below) and may be attained by one of three regimens listed here in order of their apparent efficacy and practicability:

1. Benzathine penicillin G in a single injection of 1.2 million units will provide protection for about 30 days. The disadvantages and discomfort of this regimen have to be weighed against the susceptibility to rheumatic recurrences of the individual patient. Those with rheumatic heart disease, those who have had a recent attack of rheumatic fever, and those exposed to an environment in which the incidence of streptococcal infection is frequent deserve the most effective protection. For such patients, benzathine penicillin by injection monthly is recommended.

2. Sulfonamide in daily administration by mouth of 1.0 gram of sulfadiazine or one of the other sulfapyrimidines provides satisfactory prophylaxis, but failures will occur. Toxic reactions may be observed during the first 60 days of continuous treatment. These have been rare, however, with the small doses of sulfadiazine that have been employed extensively.

3. Oral penicillin in doses of 200,000 (125 mg) units of penicillin G has been employed widely for prevention of streptococcal infections. This regimen has not been any more effective, however, than the daily dose of 1.0 gram of sulfadiazine. Indeed, 200,000 units of penicillin *twice* daily has not proved as yet to be clearly superior to the single dose. It is possible that the oral dose of penicillin may have to be increased to nearly therapeutic proportions to be more effective than sulfonamides, and this would increase further its expense and impracticability.

Franciosi, R. A., Knostman, J. D., and Zimmerman, R. A.: Group B streptococcal neonatal and infant infections. J. Pediatr., 82:707, 1973.
Lancefield, R. C.: Current knowledge of type-specific M antigens of group A streptococci. J. Immunol., 89:307, 1962.
Parker, M. T., Bassett, D. C. J., Maxted, W. R., and Arneaud, J. D.: Acute glomerulonephritis in Trinidad: Serologic typing of group A streptococci. J. Hyg. (Camb.), 66:657, 1968.
Rammelkamp, C. H., Jr.: Epidemiology of Streptococcal Infections. Harvey Lectures, Series 51, 1955–56. New York, Academic Press, 1957, p. 113.
Rheumatic Fever Committee, American Heart Association: Prevention of rheumatic fever. Circulation, 43:983, 1971.
Seegal, D., and Seegal, B. C.: Facial erysipelas: A study of 281 cases treated at the Massachusetts General Hospital from 1870–1927. J.A.M.A., 93:430, 1929.
Siegel, A. C., Johnson, E. E., and Stollerman, G. H.: Controlled studies of streptococcal pharyngitis in a pediatric population. I. Factors related to the attack rate of rheumatic fever. N. Engl. J. Med., 265:559, 1961.
Stetson, C. A., Rammelkamp, C. H., Jr., Krause, R. M., Kohen, R. J., and Perry, W. D.: Epidemic acute nephritis: Studies on etiology, natural history, and prevention. Medicine, 34:431, 1955.
Stollerman, G. H.: Factors determining the attack rate of rheumatic fever. J.A.M.A., 177:823, 1961.
Stollerman, G. H.: Rheumatogenic and nephritogenic streptococci. Circulation, 43:915, 1971.
Stollerman, G. H., and Pearce, I. A.: The changing epidemiology of rheumatic fever and acute glomerulonephritis. Adv. Intern. Med., 14:201, 1968.
Uhr, J. W. (ed.): The Streptococcus, Rheumatic Fever and Glomerulonephritis. Baltimore, Williams & Wilkins Company, 1964.
Wannamaker, L. W.: Infections of the throat and skin. N. Engl. J. Med., 282:23, 78, 1970.
Wannamaker, L. W., and Matsen, J. M. (eds.): Streptococci and Streptococcal Diseases. New York, Academic Press, 1972.
Wood, H. F., Feinstein, A. R., Taranta, A., Epstein, J. A., and Simpson, R.: Rheumatic fever in children and adolescents. III. Comparative effectiveness of three prophylaxis regimens in preventing streptococcal infections and rheumatic occurrences. Ann. Intern. Med., 60 (Suppl. 5):31, 1964.

191. RHEUMATIC FEVER

Richard M. Krause

Definition. Rheumatic fever is an uncommon, but by no means rare, delayed sequel of an upper respiratory tract infection caused by group A hemolytic streptococci. The pathogenesis remains obscure. Multiple focal aseptic inflammatory lesions are the basis for the acute manifestations, which may include migratory arthritis, carditis, chorea, erythema marginatum, and subcutaneous nodules, as well as a number of less prominent signs and symptoms. Recurrences of rheumatic fever are common after an untreated streptococcal infection in patients with a previous history of this disease. The acute disease is of limited duration, but the carditis may lead to permanent valvular damage. It is for this reason that extensive studies have been concerned with methods to prevent first attacks as well as recurrences of rheumatic fever. Prevention can be achieved only by the prompt detection, diagnosis, and treatment of streptococcal pharyngitis.

Etiology and Pathogenesis. Despite the decline in recent years in the incidence of rheumatic fever, interest in the disease is unabated because of its unique relationship to streptococcal infections. All the available evidence indicates that only group A streptococcal infections of the upper respiratory tract lead to rheumatic fever. Further, the two episodes are separated by a latent period during which the signs and symptoms of either illness are commonly absent. Although streptococci may be present in the throat from the onset of pharyngitis to the onset of rheumatic fever, there is no satisfactory evidence that foci of living streptococci contribute to the occurrence of rheumatic inflammatory lesions. Thus rheumatic fever appears to be a reaction to the streptococcal infection, and not a continuation of the infectious process.

The epidemiologic, clinical, and laboratory evidence for the association between streptococcal infections and rheumatic fever deserves special comment. Numerous epidemiologic studies have described a temporal relationship between these two diseases. Prior to the days of penicillin, an epidemic of scarlet fever in a closed population, such as a boarding school, was followed in two to four weeks by an uncommonly high incidence of rheumatic fever. But the certain relationship between the two diseases was only established once there had been major advances in the bacteriology of streptococci. The advent of methods to delineate the antigenic structure of the group A Streptococcus and the immune response to the various streptococcal antigens permitted the identification of the group A Streptococcus as the only pathogen that causes the pharyngitis leading to rheumatic fever. The serologic methods to detect antibodies to streptococcal antigens played an especially important role in establishing this relationship. With such methods, it was possible to determine for the first time that nearly every patient with rheumatic fever had a preceding streptococcal sore throat. This was not always evident from the results of throat cultures taken at the onset of rheumatic fever. Although group A streptococci may persist in the throat during the interval between streptococcal pharyngitis and rheumatic fever, it is not uncommon for repeated cultures of the pharynx to be negative for these organisms.

The most persuasive argument in favor of a relationship between streptococcal pharyngitis and acute rheumatic fever stems from the treatment schedules that have been devised to prevent primary as well as recurrent attacks of rheumatic fever. In brief, it is clear that adequate antimicrobial therapy of streptococcal pharyngitis will prevent a subsequent attack of rheumatic fever.

Once the bacteriology of streptococcal pharyngitis was clarified, the recurrent nature of rheumatic fever was no longer a mystery. Almost all serologic types of group A hemolytic streptococci are apparently capable of causing a pharyngitis that can lead to rheumatic fever (the possible exceptions to this rule are some of the recent new types of streptococci that have been most prominently isolated from skin lesions, some of which are associated primarily with the occurrence of acute nephritis). Because immunity to streptococcal infections is M-type specific, infection with one type results in no significant protection against the many other types. Thus, it is common for a child to experience several different streptococcal infections during the school years, and this, in turn, makes possible repeated attacks of rheumatic fever. A child who has had an attack of rheumatic fever retains a special susceptibility to repeated attacks in subsequent years. However, the reason for this special susceptibility remains to be explained.

Although most, if not all, serologic M types of group A streptococcal infections of the pharynx can lead to rheumatic fever, it should be stressed that only 3 per cent or less of all patients who do not receive adequate antimicrobial therapy for a streptococcal infection will develop subsequent rheumatic fever. Epidemiologic evidence indicates that rheumatic fever occurs only after streptococcal pharyngitis, but not in association with streptococcal skin infections, e.g., impetigo. It is conceivable that the response to the pharyngeal infection is qualitatively and quantitatively different from the response to skin infections. It is known, for example, that the antibody response to streptolysin O is more likely to be elevated after pharyngeal infections than after skin infections, whereas the antibody response to DNAse B occurs with high frequency after infection at either site. Thus it is conceivable that the special consequences of a pharyngeal infection set the stage for the occurrence of rheumatic fever.

The selective occurrence of rheumatic fever in only a few people with pharyngitis argues for the importance of host factors in addition to the infectious process in the pathogenesis of rheumatic fever. It is possible that the accumulative effects of repetitive streptococcal infections in any one individual are a factor that increases the risk. Young children under the age of three have streptococcal pharyngitis, but rheumatic fever is uncommon in this age group. Throughout the remainder of childhood repetitive streptococcal infections lead to delayed hypersensitivity to streptococcal products, but such hypersensitivity is not commonly present in children less than three years of age. It is after the age of four that rheumatic fever is most common in children. The possible importance of genetic factors in predisposition has been suggested. Although it has been observed that rheumatic fever may occur in families, no clear-cut genetic pattern has been found. In a study of monozygotic twins, less than one fifth were concordant for rheumatic fever. Unsatisfactory and inconclusive though these studies are, the selective occurrence of rheumatic fever in only a few of all those infected with streptococci suggests that predisposing factors work in conjunction with the infectious process to produce rheumatic fever, but the nature of such contributory causes has remained obscure.

Although the central role of streptococcal infections in the etiology of rheumatic fever is now established beyond question, the mechanism by which the hemolytic streptococci initiate the disease process is unknown. For convenience, evidence can be marshaled for the support of three different theories of pathogenesis. Each of these theories is less than satisfactory.

The most currently attractive hypothesis is that rheumatic fever is a consequence of an immunologic response or hypersensitivity reaction, or both, to streptococcal antigens. An immunologic mechanism is suggested by the intriguing parallel between the latent period of serum sickness and rheumatic fever. Patients who develop rheumatic fever appear to have an exaggerated antibody response to streptococcal antigens. Such patients commonly, but not always, have a higher antistreptolysin O response than those who do not develop this complication after streptococcal pharyngitis.

The arguments suggesting that autoimmunity may be of importance in pathogenesis cannot be recorded in detail here. The occurrence of autoantibodies that react with mammalian muscle in the sera of patients with rheumatic fever in concentrations greater than in the sera of patients who do not develop this complication has been emphasized. What remains to be determined is the source of antigenic stimulus for this autoantibody and the pathologic significance of such autoantibody. Because this autoantibody cross-reacts with a streptococcal antigen, it has been argued that these antibodies are only another manifestation of the immune response to the preceding streptococcal infection. It is also possible, however, that the host's own tissues were so altered by the toxic processes at the time of the infection that altered tissue antigens became the stimulus for autoantibody production. In addition to the controversy over the source of the stimulus that gives rise to these autoantibodies, there is the additional controversy over their pathologic significance. It is unknown if they participate in the genesis of the inflammatory lesions in a manner similar to the autoantibodies to nucleic acid which appear to be intimately associated with the inflammatory lesions of lupus erythematosus.

Another possible explanation for the pathogenesis of rheumatic fever is that the inflammation is a direct consequence of the deleterious effects of streptococcal toxins produced at the time of the infection. Despite the marked toxicity of certain streptococcal products, such as streptolysin O and S, there is little evidence for or against the importance of toxins in pathogenesis.

It remains to mention the possible role of persistent foci of the infecting Streptococcus in the pathogenesis of rheumatic fever. Aside from several earlier bacteriologic reports prior to the era of antimicrobial drugs, there is little bacteriologic evidence for a direct infection of the heart valves, the myocardium, or other organs involved in rheumatic fever. Nevertheless, because the prevention of rheumatic fever requires the successful and complete eradication of the infecting Streptococcus from the pharynx by drug therapy, the view lingers that persistence of the infecting Streptococcus in some form may be a factor in the disease process.

Epidemiology. It is obvious from what has been said that the epidemiology of acute rheumatic fever and the epidemiology of streptococcal pharyngitis are clearly interrelated. The incidence of the two diseases is related. Any environmental or host factor that enhances the occurrence of streptococcal pharyngitis will enhance the occurrence of rheumatic fever. Streptococcal disease is most common between the ages of five and fifteen years, with a peak incidence between six and eight years, and this is the age group with the highest attack rate of rheumatic fever. Although adults have fewer streptococcal infections than children because of acquired immunity and less exposure to streptococci, the special circumstances of military service or close association with children enhance the risk of higher attack rates for adults.

As is the case for most other respiratory diseases, the occurrence of streptococcal pharyngitis fluctuates widely with the seasons. The occurrence of acute rheumatic fever parallels such fluctuations. The peak occurrence falls in the late winter and early spring months, although not uncommonly the number of cases increases sharply for a brief period shortly after the onset of school in the early fall.

Classic epidemiologic studies indicate that rheumatic fever occurs most commonly in the temperate zones. But recent scattered reports from Africa, India, and countries of Southeast Asia suggest that rheumatic heart disease is by no means rare in these areas. Why acute rheumatic fever has been unrecognized in these regions remains to be determined, but it is conceivable that the disease is modified there so that the manifestations are less typical than the classic picture that defines the illness in the United States and Europe. In this connection it has been noted that the southern United States has had a low incidence of acute rheumatic fever, but at autopsy the population has a prevalence of rheumatic heart disease similar to that seen in the north. It is conceivable that, for unknown reasons, the manifestations of the acute disease are blunted in the south as well as in subtropical and tropical regions of the world.

Socioeconomic factors, such as overcrowding, either in tenement areas or in army barracks, that favor the spread of streptococcal disease also favor the occurrence of rheumatic fever. There is no evidence for differences of susceptibility because of race or sex, although chorea and mitral stenosis are more common in females, and aortic insufficiency is more common in males.

A number of factors have undoubtedly been responsible for the decline in the occurrence of rheumatic fever and rheumatic heart disease in the past several decades. Not the least of these are improvements of socioeconomic conditions and the treatment of streptococcal infections with penicillin. Certainly antimicrobial therapy has had a major impact on the prevention of recurrent attacks of rheumatic fever, and such cases have shown a precipitous decline. Less well documented is the decline in first attacks. Indeed, long-time students of the disease have commented on the persistent occurrence of first attacks in the largé cities of the United States, and suggest that the over-all decline in cases stems primarily from the prevention of recurrences and less from the prevention of first attacks. Recently it has been estimated, for example, that no less than 200 cases of acute rheumatic fever occurred in the city of Cleveland during one year.

For the United States at large, the yearly incidence of first attacks of rheumatic fever has been estimated at about 50,000 to 100,000 children, but for a variety of reasons such estimates are unsatisfactory. The disease is not reportable in all states and, in addition, without unequivocal pathognomonic signs and symptoms that clearly establish diagnosis, the disease is both over- and underreported. Some idea of the continued occurrence of rheumatic fever in the population can be obtained by the examination of schoolchildren, college students, and military recruits for the prevalence of rheumatic heart disease. Among schoolchildren, the prevalence is between 0.7 and 1.6 per 1000. The prevalence for freshmen college students and servicemen is between 6 and 9 per 1000.

Clinical Manifestations. The most striking clinical manifestations are due to arthritis, carditis, and chorea. Each sign and symptom of rheumatic fever may be either mild or severe, and the severity of each may vary independently. Thus severe carditis may be associated with minimal or no evidence of arthritis, and vice versa. Because the manifestations of rheumatic fever at first glance appear so variable, and because no single set of manifestations is typical for rheumatic fever, the Jones criteria have been devised as a guide to aid in the differential diagnosis. The signs and symptoms that comprise the Jones criteria are listed in the accompanying table. Use of these criteria for guidance in differential diagnosis will be discussed later.

Although a history of a preceding streptococcal pharyngitis is common, this infection may have been so mild as to have escaped medical attention. Indeed, a number of patients can recall no recent sore throat. The

Clinical and Laboratory Manifestations of Acute Rheumatic Fever

Major Manifestations	Minor Manifestations
1. Carditis	1. Clinical
2. Polyarthritis	a. Previous rheumatic fever or rheumatic heart disease
3. Chorea	b. Arthralgia
4. Erythema marginatum	c. Fever
5. Subcutaneous nodules	2. Laboratory
	a. Acute phase reactions, erythrocyte sedimentation rate, C-reactive protein, leukocytosis
	b. Prolonged P-R interval
	plus

Supporting evidence of preceding streptococcal infection (increased ASO or other streptococcal antibodies, positive throat culture for group A Streptococcus, recent scarlet fever)

The Jones criteria (revised) have been employed as a guide in the diagnosis of rheumatic fever, but this scheme has not received universal acceptance. The presence of two major manifestations, or of one major and two minor manifestations, indicates a high probability of the presence of rheumatic fever *if supported by evidence of a preceding streptococcal infection.* The absence of the latter should make the diagnosis doubtful, except in situations in which rheumatic fever is first discovered after a long, latent period from the antecedent infection, e.g., Sydenham's chorea or low-grade carditis.

Adapted from the recommendations of the Committee of The American Heart Association (Circulation, 32:664, 1965.)

interval between the pharyngitis and the onset of rheumatic fever has been termed the latent period. This is a period of one to four weeks, and during this time the patient usually appears entirely well. On some occasions, however, laboratory examination will reveal evidence of disease activity.

The onset of rheumatic fever, with characteristic signs and symptoms, is usually sudden, but it may be insidious. In the latter case, diagnosis depends on observation of the clinical course and the interpretation of laboratory data. Usually the first symptoms are fever and joint pain. Fever may be high and sustained in severe cases, but more frequently it is moderate and often low grade. Sore throat is not uncommon, even though examination reveals minimal evidence of acute inflammation. Epistaxis occurs commonly both at the onset and throughout the acute stage of the disease, and in some cases results in serious loss of blood. In children, severe abdominal pain is not uncommon, and vomiting may occur. Localization of such pain in the right lower quadrant with fleeting signs of peritoneal inflammation may suggest the diagnosis of appendicitis.

Arthritis. The arthritis in rheumatic fever may involve multiple joints, but a characteristic feature is that the inflammation occurs and subsides in the joints first affected, only to occur in others that were initially spared. This phenomenon has been termed migratory polyarthritis. The large joints of the extremities are most frequently affected, but all are potentially susceptible. Arthritis can occur in the hands, feet, or spine, or in such joints as the sternoclavicular and the temporomandibular.

The manifestations of arthritis may be either mild with vague discomfort in the joints of the extremities, or severe. Acutely inflamed and swollen joints are commonly very painful. In mild cases there may be no objective evidence of arthritis. When arthritis is severe, the skin over the joint shows local redness and heat, the joint is swollen, and fluid is obviously present within the joint cavity. Passive or active movement of the joint is extremely painful. The fluid in such cases is turbid and contains inflammatory leukocytes, but is sterile on bacteriologic culture.

Although uncommon, the arthritis may not affect multiple joints. Experienced clinicians have observed the occasional case in which arthritis may persist for prolonged periods in only one joint, with minimal evidence of arthritis in the others.

There is usually a difference between the pattern of arthritis in children and that in adults. Frank arthritis is less common in children between four and six years of age. Only mild joint pains may be noted, or merely vague localized aching in the extremities. It is this type of complaint that has been referred to in the past as "growing pains." Such symptoms and low-grade fever suggest a mild illness, but examination of the heart may reveal severe carditis. It bears repetition that rheumatic fever can occur without any evidence of joint involvement whatever.

Carditis. Palpitation and precordial chest pain or discomfort are common symptoms. If the carditis is severe, symptoms of cardiac failure may occur in addition to those of rheumatic fever. The final and definitive diagnosis of carditis depends upon the physical, roentgenographic, and electrocardiographic examinations.

The carditis may be mild or severe. In mild cases, tachycardia, persistent during sleep, may be the only sign suggesting carditis. Persistent bradycardia has been well documented in rheumatic fever, but it is far less common than tachycardia. In the more severe cases, generalized cardiac enlargement frequently occurs, often associated with a diffuse precordial impulse.

On auscultation, the heart sounds in the apical area may be muffled, indistinct, and of poor quality. The second sound in the pulmonic area is usually greatly accentuated in comparison with the second aortic sound. Gallop rhythm may occur, and is usually an indication of serious myocardial disease. The sounds may seem distant if precordial effusion is present, and the pericarditis may produce a to-and-fro friction rub (see Ch. 571 to 576).

The most common cardiac murmur during the acute phase of the initial attack of rheumatic fever is a blowing systolic murmur best heard in the apical area. Such murmurs are caused by dilatation of the valve rings as a result of general dilatation of the heart. Less commonly, soft diastolic murmurs are heard along the left sternal border in the third and fourth interspaces. It is difficult to determine whether inflammation of the valve leaflets contributes significantly to these murmurs in all cases. As the murmurs may disappear permanently on recovery, their final significance cannot be determined except by repeated examinations during and after convalescence. Mitral stenosis and aortic stenosis are late manifestations of cardiac damage that do not develop until months or years after the initial or repeated attacks.

Disturbances of the conduction system are a common feature of rheumatic carditis. Although certain irregularities, such as second degree heart block, can be recognized clinically, the electrocardiogram is the best method to detect all potential conduction system disturbances. One of the most commonly observed electrocardiographic changes is the prolongation of the P-R interval. In some cases, the Wenckebach phenomenon is observed. Further delay in conduction may lead to drop beats, with the occurrence of couplets and triplets. Finally, complete dissociation is indicated by an independent rhythm for both the ventricles and the atria. Atrial fibrillation is uncommon during the acute attack.

In addition to these conduction abnormalities, the electrocardiogram may show T wave changes, such as inversion of the T wave in one or more leads. When pericarditis is present, elevation of the S-T segment is observed initially. Late in the course, the configuration of the T wave simulates that seen in coronary disease.

Although cardiac enlargement, when present, is usually detectable on physical examination, the dilatation of the various chambers of the heart is more accurately determined by roentgenography of the chest. It is not uncommon for dilatation to arise rapidly when severe myocarditis is present.

The recurrence of active rheumatic fever should be suspected in patients with chronic rheumatic heart disease when the character of the murmurs changes over a short period of time. Cardiac failure may occur, but the carditis associated with recurrent rheumatic fever in such cases poses several diagnostic problems, because the manifestations of acute rheumatic carditis are superimposed on those of chronic valvular disease. Furthermore, the status of the pre-existing heart disease is often unknown. When there is evidence of advanced valvular deformity, any final assessment of the extent of cardiac damage must await convalescence from the acute attack.

Erythema Marginatum. *Erythema marginatum* or *circinatum* of the skin is one of the characteristic manifestations of acute rheumatic fever and occurs in 10 to 20 per cent of the childhood cases. It is a multiform type of erythema, and consists of roughly circular lesions that may be distributed over the extremities, the trunk, and sometimes the face, and that spread centrifugally, leaving a clear center. The lesions tend to coalesce so that, although individual areas are iris-like, the larger areas are serpiginous in outline. The erythema blanches on pressure and may be evanescent, disappearing and later reappearing at the same sites. The lesions are usually not elevated, although in some cases a slight papular quality may be detected. Most commonly, no discomfort is associated with the lesions. Erythema marginatum is uncommon in other diseases.

Subcutaneous Rheumatic Nodules. These lesions are one of the physical findings that lend strong support to the diagnosis of rheumatic fever, but in recent years they have occurred less commonly than was the case in the past. They are firm, insensitive nodules that occur over the bony prominences of the various joints and tendons of the extremities, the spine, and the back of the head. They are loosely attached to the underlying tissue, and the skin is freely movable over them. If the joint can be flexed without undue pain, the nodules are more readily apparent because of the tension of the skin. If nodules are numerous, they may occur in a symmetrical distribution. The nodules are more frequently encountered in the more severe cases of rheumatic fever with serious cardiac involvement.

Sydenham's Chorea. Chorea may occur in combination with other symptoms of rheumatic fever, but it is commonly seen as the sole manifestation of the disease. This phenomenon is explained by the fact that chorea tends to make its appearance late in the course of rheumatic fever. The onset may be delayed for as long as six months after the initiating streptococcal infection, although the delay is usually less than this. Patients with chorea may have had an easily recognizable preceding attack of arthritis and carditis, and, indeed, may have been hospitalized with it, only to have the chorea occur as a late manifestation at a time when all other evidence of any inflammatory process had disappeared. When the onset of chorea is delayed and the other manifestations of rheumatic fever have abated, the laboratory findings are often normal. It is not uncommon for chorea to occur in patients who can recall no earlier illness. It seems likely that such individuals had an attack of acute rheumatic fever in the recent past which was so mild that it escaped clinical detection. It is for this reason that patients with so-called "pure chorea" may develop rheumatic heart disease.

The onset of chorea is usually insidious, and the parents of the child with chorea may first note increased awkwardness and a tendency to spill food or drop objects that is attributed to carelessness. Even the appearance of involuntary purposeless movements of the extremities may be discounted as nervousness. However, with further progression of the disease, the irregular and uncontrollable movements become obvious. They may become extensive, and may involve not only the hands, feet, arms, and legs, but the tongue and facial muscles. The severity may range from no more than minimal involuntary movements observed only by close inspection, to violent, continual activity, totally incapacitating the patient and requiring protection from self-injury. In moderate cases, interference with all coordinated activity, such as writing and eating, is common. On occasion, chorea may be limited to one side of the body. The disease appears to affect females somewhat more frequently than males.

Miscellaneous Clinical Manifestations. Rheumatic pneumonitis may occur, but this is difficult to detect clinically, particularly if there is superimposed heart failure. Rheumatic pneumonia has seldom been seen in recent years, probably because the disease process itself appears to be much more mild than in former times. Such few cases as do occur are in patients with severe rheumatic fever.

Erythema nodosum is less common than erythema marginatum. The dull, red nodular lesions occur most frequently on the extensor surfaces of the extremities in various sizes from less than 1 cm to several centimeters in diameter. They are extremely tender on pressure, and the pain is aggravated by movements of the extremities. These lesions occur in patients in whom there is little or no other clinical evidence to suggest acute rheumatic fever. They have been seen in association with a number of infections, including tuberculosis, as well as streptococcal pharyngitis. For these reasons, the presence of erythema nodosum is not considered a major sign for the diagnosis of rheumatic fever.

Laboratory Findings. *Hematology.* There are no characteristic abnormalities of the leukocyte differential count that are indicative of rheumatic fever. Leukocytosis is common, but not always present, with a total count from 12,000 to 24,000 per cubic millimeter. This is associated with an increase in the percentage of polymorphonuclear cells.

A moderate degree of anemia is generally seen, which is normochromic with proportional decreases in the hemoglobin concentration and the erythrocyte count. The anemia usually persists for as long as the rheumatic process is active. The most severe anemias are obviously encountered in patients who have an associated blood loss owing to epistaxis.

Urinary Findings. Some proteinuria and an increase in the number of red and white cells in the urine are common during the acute phase of the disease. However, it is seldom that these abnormalities are as great as those characteristically encountered in acute glomerulonephritis. When this is the case, simultaneous acute nephritis and rheumatic fever must be considered, but such a combination is a most uncommon event.

Evidence for a Prior Streptococcal Infection. The most important laboratory information for establishing the diagnosis of rheumatic fever is data that substantiate the prior occurrence of streptococcal pharyngitis. The detection of group A beta-hemolytic streptococci by a throat culture is helpful in this regard, but of greater usefulness is the serologic detection of antibodies that are indicative of a previous streptococcal infection.

Because the streptococci that caused the initial infection may persist for many weeks in the pharynx in those instances in which antimicrobial therapy was not given or was inadequate, a throat culture may detect the infecting group A streptococci at the time of the onset of rheumatic fever. But such a finding is only suggestive of a preceding streptococcal pharyngitis and is not an unambiguous indication of it. This stems from the fact that 5 to 30 per cent of the healthy population may carry group A streptococci in the pharynx during the respiratory disease season. Thus the recovery of this organism from a patient may be an inadvertent finding and not indicative of a preceding streptococcal sore throat. Nevertheless, the throat culture is helpful, and should be obtained in all cases. When the patient has a negative throat culture, it is frequently possible to isolate the group A streptococci from other members of the family. Such a finding is indicative of a recent intrafamilial spread of streptococci.

The most helpful information that is indicative of a recent streptococcal infection is obtained with tests that detect serum antibodies to streptococcal antigens. The most widely employed test is the antistreptolysin O determination. As with all antibody tests, the detection of an antibody rise over a one- to three-week interval is the only unequivocal evidence for the recent occurrence of a streptococcal infection. If a patient is seen in the first few days after the onset of rheumatic fever, the antistreptolysin O titer at that time may be less than the titer seen several weeks after onset of rheumatic fever. Not uncommonly, however, the titer has reached a maximal plateau so that it is not possible to detect a progressive increase in titer. When this is the case, the antistreptolysin O titer should be at least 250 units in adults and at least 333 units in children over five years of age to be acceptable as an indication of a previous streptococcal infection. Obviously, a certain proportion of the individuals in the normal population have had a recent streptococcal infection at any one time, and they will have antistreptolysin O titers similar to these.

Approximately 15 to 20 per cent of the patients with rheumatic fever and nearly all patients who exhibit only chorea have a low or borderline low antistreptolysin O titer. In such instances, it is helpful to employ another antibody test. The anti-DNAse B test is becoming widely accepted as a second antibody test, and it is a useful means to obtain additional evidence for the occurrence of a previous streptococcal infection. When both these antibody tests are used, it is possible to obtain antibody evidence for a preceding streptococcal infection in almost all cases of rheumatic fever.

One other serologic test should be mentioned because it may be used more widely in the future. It has been noted that nearly all patients with rheumatic fever have readily detectable serum autoantibodies that react with muscle tissue, including heart, whereas the concentration of these antibodies is very much less or absent in sera of patients with other rheumatic diseases. Such findings suggest that this antibody test may have clinical usefulness for the differential diagnosis of rheumatic fever.

Other Laboratory Tests. An elevated sedimentation rate and a positive C-reactive protein are present in rheumatic fever, but these findings are nonspecific indicators of inflammation, and they cannot be used to differentiate rheumatic fever from other diseases. However, a normal C-reactive protein and a normal sedimentation rate are helpful in excluding active rheumatic fever. In patients with mild symptoms, such as vague arthralgia and lassitude, if the sedimentation rate and the C-reactive protein are normal, active rheumatic fever is unlikely.

Diagnosis and Differential Diagnosis. A history of severe sore throat in the recent past, migrating polyarthritis, carditis, fever, and an elevated antistreptolysin O titer is such a classic combination of signs and symptoms that the diagnosis can seldom be questioned. But the problem is often not as straightforward as this. The various major manifestations of rheumatic fever that have been described above are considered to be part of the same disease because they occur together with a frequency that far exceeds chance. Because they may occur singly or in various combinations in any individual patient, the diagnostic criteria originally proposed by Jones have been suggested as a guide to diagnosis. These criteria are listed in the table. Any combination of these criteria can occur in patients with other disorders. It is for this reason that stress is placed on supporting evidence for a preceding streptococcal infection. When this is the case, the diagnosis is weighed in favor of rheumatic fever and against the other connective tissue disorders that may mimic it.

The designations major and minor for the various criteria are based on the diagnostic importance of the particular findings. The major ones are more indicative of rheumatic fever than the minor. The occurrence of two major manifestations is strong presumptive evidence for rheumatic fever. Only one major manifestation and any combination of the minor suggest possible rheumatic fever. In any case, if evidence is lacking for a preceding streptococcal pharyngitis, the possibility of other diseases must be kept in mind.

In many ways the most useful purpose of the criteria is their value in reducing overdiagnosis. For example, not uncommonly, patients, after streptococcal infections, may have vague pains in the extremities, an increased sedimentation rate, and a borderline temperature elevation. Careful follow-up of such patients has not revealed the delayed occurrence of rheumatic heart disease. Therefore the diagnosis of rheumatic fever should be made with caution and only with clear evidence of one or more of the major manifestations. When the diagnosis is in doubt, because the symptoms are of such a mild nature, treatment with aspirin and steroids should be withheld until the signs and symptoms are unmistakable. Early treatment of a questionable case may so depress the disease activity that clear-cut clinical signs and symptoms do not develop.

In the early stages, during the acute onset, *rheumatoid arthritis* and *systemic lupus erythematosus* may mimic rheumatic fever. Indeed, if the streptococcal antibody tests are elevated, the diagnosis may be in question unless the special diagnostic tests for the other diseases are clearly positive. Usually as time progresses, the special distinctive clinical features of rheumatoid arthritis and lupus serve to exclude the diagnosis of rheumatic fever. On occasion, at the onset, Still's disease may be confused with rheumatic fever, but again the clinical course will aid in differentiating the two.

Subacute bacterial endocarditis can occur in persons with valves previously damaged by rheumatic fever, and it often presents a clinical picture that is not readily distinguishable from a rheumatic recurrence. Vague pains in the extremities are more common than overt arthritis, but these symptoms together with fever and debility in a known rheumatic patient are sufficient to suggest a rheumatic recurrence. The difficulties are increased by the fact that in some cases it is not possible to recover the offending organism in a blood culture. The characteristic petechiae and painful septic emboli of endocarditis are helpful in differential diagnosis (see Ch. 192).

The so-called *benign idiopathic pericarditis*, which is apparently not rheumatic in origin, is indistinguishable in the acute phase from those cases of rheumatic fever in which pericarditis is the major detectable manifestation.

The diagnosis of idiopathic pericarditis is dependent primarily on elimination of other possibilities and on the subsequent course of the disease, which is characterized by complete recovery without residual damage. Thus the final conclusion is often reached only in retrospect, and must remain somewhat uncertain because rheumatic pericarditis with minimal involvement of the myocardium and endocardium could conceivably behave in a similar fashion.

Fever, arthritis, and positive acute phase reactants may also occur in bacterial arthritis, serum sickness, subacute bacterial endocarditis, sickle cell anemia, and acute aleukemic leukemia. In such cases in which confusion exists, only a careful assessment of the clinical course, physical examination, and laboratory findings will exclude rheumatic fever.

Persistent monarticular arthritis, without other major manifestations of rheumatic fever, is usually not due to rheumatic fever, and osteomyelitis or local injury must be considered.

Therapy. There is no specific treatment for rheumatic fever. Therapeutic measures are devised to promote, or at least hopefully not to hinder, the natural healing processes. Bed rest is always prescribed, and most students agree that it should continue for as long as there is unequivocal evidence of disease activity. It is not at all clear that absolute bed rest without bath privileges is essential. Nevertheless, hospitalization has an advantage over home care because the degree of activity is more readily supervised. This is particularly true because aspirin and steroids will generally eliminate all painful manifestations, and the patient sees no necessity for remaining at rest and in bed. A program for a progressive increase in recreational and occupational therapy has important psychologic value and should be an integral part of the long-term bed rest management. Schooling should not be neglected during this time. Hospital or home visit teaching programs, or both, are available in many cities, and instruction should be begun as soon as the acute manifestations of the disease are brought under control by anti-inflammatory therapy.

After the first few weeks of bed rest in patients without carditis, gradual ambulation can be started. In patients with carditis, this is usually delayed until six to ten weeks after onset of the disease. As long as the presence of carditis is suspected, even though masked by treatment, ambulation should not be started. During the period of bed rest, the patient is permitted a number of activities in increasing amounts, such as sitting up in a chair, occupational therapy, and schoolwork.

The period of bed rest is a good time for patients of all ages to be informed about the nature of the illness and the optimistic prospects for an active, long life. The need for a continuous program to prevent streptococcal pharyngitis should be discussed in detail. It is at this time, also, that patients with more severe forms of heart disease should be advised that some curtailment of normal physical activity may be necessary during convalescence. But pessimism is not warranted. All too often, patients are left with the impression that their useful, active life is at an end. This is almost invariably not the case.

It is recommended that all patients with acute rheumatic fever be treated with a course of penicillin to eliminate the hemolytic Streptococcus from the pharynx. This is recommended even if the throat culture does not reveal group A beta-hemolytic streptococci, because these organisms may persist in areas where they remain undetected, such as the interior of the tonsils. Parenteral penicillin is the drug of choice unless there is a history of allergy to it. Three hundred thousand units of penicillin G once a day in children and twice a day in adults for ten days is an effective dose. A single dose of 1.2 million units of long-acting benzathine penicillin is preferred by many, as the one injection facilitates administration. Oral penicillin, 200,000 units four times a day, also for ten days, is acceptable therapy, but requires careful supervision in order to be sure that all doses are taken without fail. If there is a history of penicillin allergy, the drug of choice is erythromycin. The dose is 250 mg four times a day for ten days. Sulfonamide in any form should never be used. After completion of the ten-day course of penicillin or erythromycin, a continuous prophylaxis regimen should be started to prevent reinfection with group A streptococci and to reduce the risk of recurrent attacks of acute rheumatic fever (see Ch. 189).

Aspirin and Steroid Therapy. Most patients respond rapidly to either steroid or aspirin therapy. After one or two weeks, arthritis and fever have disappeared, and the acute phase reactants frequently have returned to normal, or nearly so. On occasion, neither fever nor arthritis responds to full aspirin dosage, and steroids are required to control the disease. Most clinicians favor use of steroids in nearly all patients with carditis. It is certainly indicated in patients with severe carditis and pancarditis. Some prefer to withdraw the steroid treatment after several weeks and continue treatment by substituting aspirin. Others continue steroid therapy for the full course. The arthritis in nearly all patients responds readily to aspirin alone. The evidence remains equivocal for the beneficial effect of steroid therapy in preventing the development of permanent rheumatic heart disease, even though there is apparent clinical improvement in the acute carditis when steroids are used.

It should be stressed again that when full and adequate treatment eliminates all the clinical manifestations of the disease, including laboratory abnormalities, the underlying disease process is still continuing unabated for its natural course. If the drugs are withdrawn before the process is at an end, the disease with all its clinical manifestations will recur. Duration of therapy is discussed below.

The daily dose of aspirin is 60 mg per pound of body weight. The actual total dose per day varies from 3 grams in young children to 10 grams in adults. It is preferable to give this total amount in at least six divided doses. Aspirin should be given throughout the 24-hour day, at least during the early stages of the disease. Individual variation in the efficacy of absorption or excretion of the drug and in its therapeutic effectiveness requires readjustment of the dose in many cases. The aim is to give the minimal dose that results in full control of symptoms and to avoid serious toxic side reactions because of overdosage. Studies on the concentration of salicylates in the blood have shown that optimal therapeutic effect usually requires at least 25 mg per 100 ml of serum. The optimal therapeutic range is between 25 and 35 mg per 100 ml of serum. Levels greater than the upper limit are associated with toxicity. When aspirin is given in conjunction with the prednisone, it is frequently necessary to give a daily dose of aspirin larger than that recommended above in order to achieve the therapeutic salicylate level. Furthermore, as aspirin is continued upon the withdrawal of prednisone, less aspirin is frequently required to maintain an adequate serum salicylate level.

The most common toxic manifestations of aspirin therapy are nausea, vomiting, and gastric distress. Tinnitus and partial but temporary impairment of hearing usually occur only at full therapeutic dosage. Hyperpnea frequently results from central stimulatory action in respiration and can lead to alkalosis. It is uncommon to see the more severe metabolic disturbances of acute salicylate toxicity.

In practice, nausea and vomiting are the most frequent complications that result from starting aspirin. This can be minimized if the initial daily dosage is below the optimum and is then gradually increased over a period of a few days. Attempts to achieve full and optimal salicylate levels within 24 hours often result in severe nausea and vomiting. In such cases it may be difficult to reach an effective therapeutic level of salicylate, and in such instances steroids afford an alternative therapeutic approach. The use of sodium bicarbonate to reduce gastric irritation is not recommended, as it increases the excretion of salicylate and interferes with the maintenance of an anti-inflammatory concentration of the drug in the blood. If a portion of the aspirin is given as enteric-coated pills, some degree of gastric irritation can be eliminated.

Prednisone is the recommended steroid because a low salt diet and added potassium are usually not required. There is no firm agreement on the dosage of this drug. The usual procedure is to begin with a relatively large daily dose until activity of the disease appears to be under control, and then to reduce the dosage to the minimal amount that will maintain the full effect. In the experience of many, the total daily dosage of 0.5 mg per pound given in divided doses is adequate to bring the signs of inflammation, including fever, rapidly under control. Almost all signs and symptoms are suppressed in two or three days. It is at this point that the daily dose may be reduced. After two or three weeks of steroid therapy, some prefer to shift to aspirin, particularly for those patients without carditis. The advantage of this is that most side effects of prolonged steroid therapy, such as the mild manifestations of Cushing's disease, are avoided. Prolonged use of steroid therapy may lead to complications, such as infections, growth retardation, gastric ulcers, and toxic psychoses.

The treatment of chorea is symptomatic. There is no evidence that either steroids or aspirin have any influence on the symptoms of chorea. The usual case lasts from two weeks to several months, but in rare instances it may persist longer. Many patients show improvement when bright light, noise, and undue activity are eliminated from their bedroom. In some cases, measures must be taken to prevent self-injury from violent chorea movements, including tongue-biting. Phenobarbital and other sedatives may be helpful.

Duration of Therapy. The duration of therapy bears some relationship to the severity of the acute manifestations. The disease process in the typical mild case without carditis subsides in three to four weeks. When severe arthritis and carditis are present, the natural course lasts two to three months. Such estimates for the duration of the disease can be used to determine the termination of therapy, recognizing, however, that disease activity in the occasional case may persist for many months. Laboratory tests such as determination of the sedimentation rate and the C-reactive protein assume normal values during the course of adequate therapy. For this reason, they cannot be used to determine the duration of therapy.

Many clinicians prefer to withdraw either aspirin or steroid therapy gradually over a period of one or two weeks. After withdrawal, a clinical "rebound" is commonly seen. This may be so mild that only the acute phase reactants indicate its occurrence, but not uncommonly clinical manifestations are present. These may be mild or severe, and include fever, arthritis, and tachycardia. Usually the rebound subsides in five to ten days without use of anti-inflammatory drugs. The occurrence of positive C-reactive protein, an elevated sedimentation rate, and an elevated white count, without significant clinical manifestations, is not sufficient grounds for reinstituting therapy. But progressive clinical severity and particularly the emergence of severe carditis may require reinstitution of therapy. In such instances, it is assumed that the natural duration of the disease has yet to run its course. In practice, if therapy must be reinstated because of the emergence of carditis, the drugs are continued for another three to four weeks.

If no significant rebound occurs, ambulation should begin, and usually full activity, except vigorous exercise, may be permitted three to four weeks after the termination of therapy. If persistent rheumatic heart disease is present, the permissible level of physical activity is determined by an assessment of its severity.

Prevention. Prior to the days of antimicrobial drugs, measures were not available to prevent recurrences of rheumatic fever. Now properly supervised continuous chemoprophylaxis is effective in preventing these recurrences, and it should be employed for all patients with a well-documented history of rheumatic fever or unequivocal evidence of rheumatic heart disease. Prophylaxis prevents streptococcal pharyngitis and therefore the recurrences of rheumatic fever.

A detailed consideration of drug regimens for prophylaxis has been presented in Ch. 189. Intramuscular benzathine penicillin, 1.2 million units each month, is the preferred drug and route of administration. Such a route of administration does not leave open to question the degree of patient compliance, as is the case with orally administered penicillin.

The duration of antimicrobial prophylaxis should be extended through childhood. In the case of adolescents and adults, it should not be terminated as long as the patient is associated with population groups that have high attack rates of streptococcal infections, such as military recruits, schoolchildren, medical personnel, and school teachers. Because of the risk of additional valvular damage during a recurrence, prophylaxis should be continued for life for all patients with definite rheumatic heart disease. Contrary to popular belief, people in late middle age can have a recurrence of rheumatic fever after streptococcal pharyngitis.

Epidemiologic studies clearly indicate that streptococcal disease spreads in the home and in the school. The physician must be alert to the occurrence of streptococcal pharyngitis in the family and the school of the patient on prophylaxis. This is a potential risk to the patient, and strict compliance with the prophylaxis must be urged. If streptococcal disease occurs in the family, it should be treated with adequate antimicrobial drugs.

For a number of reasons, the prevention of first attacks

of rheumatic fever is difficult to achieve. Prompt recognition and treatment of streptococcal pharyngitis is hampered in a number of cases by the fact that the symptoms are so mild that the patient does not see a physician. Not uncommonly, when the patient is seen by a doctor, the disease is misdiagnosed or the antimicrobial therapy prescribed is inadequate. For example, the tetracyclines should never be used to treat streptococcal pharyngitis, because 25 to 40 per cent of all group A streptococci are now resistant to this family of drugs.

The occasion arises when special measures are needed to control epidemics of streptococcal pharyngitis in a school or a community or in an army recruit camp. Several unexpected cases of rheumatic fever in a short period of time in a small population group should alert the physician to the possibility that there is a serious streptococcal epidemic in the community in question. Methods to curtail such epidemics have been described in Ch. 190.

Prognosis. Recovery from the acute attack is the rule. Death at this stage is very rare, even in cases of severe carditis, because of the anti-inflammatory effects of steroid therapy. The disease process in mild cases of rheumatic fever without carditis usually subsides in two to four weeks, and the patient usually makes a complete recovery. When carditis is present, the disease usually persists for six weeks to three months. Patients with carditis during the acute attack may progress to valvular rheumatic heart disease. This is less common in patients without carditis, but absence of carditis during an acute attack is unfortunately not an absolute guarantee against the development of subsequent valvular deformity.

Chronic disability and death owing to rheumatic heart disease are related to recurrent attacks. In former years, before antimicrobial therapy, patients who had had rheumatic fever usually suffered recurrences. Additional valvular deformity was the frequent outcome of each recurrence. As a result, a progressive severity of rheumatic heart disease was common. In current times the prognosis is more optimistic. Progressively severe valvular deformity after an initial attack, if recurrences are prevented, appears to be much less common than in former times, but this point requires further epidemiologic study. The efficacy of adequate chemoprophylaxis in the prevention of recurrences is clearly documented. In one study more than two thirds of the patients with a history of rheumatic fever who were not on prophylaxis had one or more recurrences over an eight-year follow-up period. If prophylaxis is adequately supervised and the drug is taken without fail, a recurrence is an extremely uncommon event.

Kuttner, A. G., and Mayer, F. E.: Carditis during second attacks of rheumatic fever: Its incidence in patients without clinical evidence of cardiac involvement in their initial rheumatic episode. N. Engl. J. Med., 268:1259, 1963.

Lendrum, B. L., Simon, A. J., and Mack, I.: Relation of duration of bed rest in acute rheumatic fever to heart disease present 2 to 14 years later. Pediatrics, 24:389, 1959.

Markowitz, M., and Gordis, L.: Rheumatic Fever. 2nd ed. Philadelphia, W. B. Saunders Company, 1972.

McCarty, M.: Missing links in the streptococcal chain leading to rheumatic fever: The T. Duckett Jones Memorial Lecture. Circulation, 24:488, 1964.

United Kingdom and United States Joint Report: The natural history of rheumatic fever and rheumatic heart disease: Ten-year report of a cooperative clinical trial of ACTH, cortisone, and aspirin. Circulation, 32:457, 1965.

Wood, H. F., and McCarty, M.: Laboratory aids in the diagnosis of rheumatic fever and in evaluation of disease activity. Am. J. Med., 17:768, 1954.

Zabriskie, J. B., Hsu, K. C., and Seegal, B. C.: Heart-reactive antibody associated with rheumatic fever: Characterization and diagnostic significance. Clin. Exp. Immunol., 7:147, 1970.

192. INFECTIVE ENDOCARDITIS (Bacterial Endocarditis, Prosthetic Valve Endocarditis)

Paul B. Beeson

GENERAL CONSIDERATIONS

In the group of diseases to be considered here, an infective agent colonizes a focus in the heart (or much less commonly in a large vascular channel elsewhere), producing a disease characterized by fever, heart murmur, splenomegaly, embolic manifestations, and bacteremia. This clinical state is of special importance because it almost invariably leads to death unless recognized and treated properly.

In common clinical parlance the term *bacterial endocarditis* is usually employed. The adjective "bacterial" is inadequate inasmuch as the same clinical disease can be caused by fungi, rickettsiae, or spirillar organisms; hence "infective" appears more nearly correct and is gaining in popular usage. The word "endocarditis" is itself misleading, because most of the endocardial surface remains unaffected, and the lesion is more or less restricted to a focus on a cardiac valve leaflet. In rare instances the same form of infection develops at the site of coarctation of the aorta or in a large arteriovenous fistula.

It is customary, and indeed helpful, to speak of either "acute" or "subacute" infective endocarditis. There are major differences between these two forms, and the practice of lumping them together has been responsible for inexactness and confusion. The important differences between acute and subacute endocarditis are shown in the accompanying table.

Having emphasized the difference between the two groups, a qualification must now be entered, because there are borderline cases with both acute and subacute features. Thus infections caused by such organisms as enterococcus or one of the fungi may be difficult to classify. Nevertheless it seems preferable to emphasize,

Differences Between Subacute and Acute Infective Endocarditis

	Subacute	Acute
Causative agent	Normally noninvasive, usually *Strep. viridans*	Capable of primary invasion, e.g., *Staph. aureus*
Pre-existing valve damage	Usually present	May not be present
Other foci of infection by same organism	None	Nearly always
Duration if untreated	Months to 1 to 2 years	Days to weeks
Response of infection to appropriate chemotherapy	Majority cured	Less than half cured

rather than to blur, the division between subacute and acute infective endocarditis.

A special new category of infective endocarditis has been created by cardiac surgery, namely, that engrafted on prosthetic devices.

SUBACUTE INFECTIVE ENDOCARDITIS

Definition. As a rule this form of illness begins insidiously and pursues a long clinical course lasting several months. The causative agent survives only in the endocardial vegetations, and consequently there are no other foci of infection either prior to or after the establishment of the focus. Deaths are due to heart failure, renal failure, embolism, or hemorrhage.

Age and Sex Incidence. The disease is comparatively uncommon before puberty, but may be encountered at any later period of life. It is by no means a rarity in advanced age, when recognition may be especially difficult. The incidence is higher in males.

Microbiology. Literally hundreds of different microbes have been reported as the causative agents in this illness. Most of them are commensals that seem incapable of invading other parts of the body and are pathogenic only when growing in the privileged sanctuary of an intravascular vegetation. Despite the long list of possibilities, the *viridans streptococci* are by far the most common causes of this infection, accounting for 50 to 80 per cent of the reported cases. These organisms are normally present in the mouth and intestine. Classification of the viridans group is unsatisfactory, but the variety called *Streptococcus sanguis,* characterized by the production of dextran, is the one most commonly encountered in infective endocarditis. Other streptococci which may cause the disease include group D or enterococcus and some microaerophilic organisms. Second to the streptococci are *Staphylococcus epidermidis* or *albus;* other well known causes include *diphtheroids* and *Hemophilus spp.* The list of possible etiologic agents is not confined to bacteria, but also includes the *rickettsiae of Q fever,* some spirillar organisms resembling *Spirillum minus,* and a number of *fungi. Viruses* have not been implicated as yet, although the coxsackievirus agents have been shown capable of producing endocardial lesions in laboratory animals. There has been much interest in the possibility that *L forms* of bacteria can be the etiologic agents, and indeed some have been recovered from valve leaflets in patients who had received penicillin therapy, but there is no clear evidence yet that these can be the primary causes of the disease.

It is accepted that organisms become established in some sort of pre-existing nidus on a heart valve, having been carried there in the circulating blood. The frequency with which various microbes are encountered in this disease does not seem to parallel the frequency with which various species enter the bloodstream. For example, *Streptococcus sanguis* is not the predominant organism among the streptococci found in the mouth, although it is the most common single cause of endocarditis. In those cases that arise after instrumentation of the urinary tract, enterococcus is far more important than the coliform bacteria which are the most common organisms in bacteremia associated with urinary tract infection. As a matter of fact, one of the striking features of this disease is the comparative rarity of infections caused by coliform bacteria. Conceivably this may be related to their susceptibility to lysis by the combined action of complement and antibody without requiring assistance from phagocytes. Another possible factor may be the surface properties of different organisms, whereby some are more likely than others to adhere to a small mass of platelets.

Pathogenesis. In infective endocarditis the organisms find shelter in a structure which develops on a heart valve (or elsewhere in the circulatory system), which provides them with optimal growth conditions as well as protection from phagocytic cells. In a sense one should look on this infection as comparable to that which sometimes develops in the presence of a foreign body or mass of necrotic tissue, in that phagocytes cannot reach the parasite.

It is known that bacteria gain access to the bloodstream fairly commonly: for example, during dental treatment or even vigorous chewing, cleansing of the teeth, parturition, or at the time of urethral instrumentation. In the vast majority of instances such bacteremias are asymptomatic and harmless, but when a suitable nidus is available within the cardiovascular system, circulating microorganisms may stick to it and find conditions there which permit their survival. The original nidus for such growth could be a tiny platelet thrombus on a roughened surface. Angrist, who has studied this question extensively, has offered evidence that the pre-existing lesion is probably so-called *nonbacterial thrombotic endocarditis.* He feels that lesions of this type may, when colonized during an episode of bacteremia, be converted into the vegetation of bacterial endocarditis. Studies of experimental endocarditis in rabbits have shown that such lesions are indeed very susceptible to infection; bacteria lodging there multiply in a manner comparable to that observed under optimal conditions in vitro. Sequential studies of such lesions appear to show that, when the population of bacteria on the surface of a small lesion reaches a certain point, it stimulates the laying down of a covering blanket of platelets and fibrin. Beneath such "blankets" bacterial colonies develop, safe from phagocytes.

Subacute infective endocarditis usually affects valves which have already been damaged. In the past, rheumatic valvulitis was the factor in about 70 per cent, and congenital defects were responsible for another 10 per cent. Syphilitic valvulitis is only rarely complicated by bacterial endocarditis, and perhaps the cases in which this has been reported simply represent the coincidence of syphilis and infective endocarditis. With the present diminishing prevalence of rheumatic heart disease, a higher proportion of cases of infective endocarditis seems to occur in middle-aged and elderly people who have not previously been known to have a valvular defect. In them one presumes that changes associated with aging may render the valve susceptible. The disease is much more common on the left side than on the right. The approximate percentages in autopsied cases are as follows: mitral, 85; aortic, 55; tricuspid, 15; and pulmonic, 1. More than one valve may be affected.

The tendency of subacute bacterial endocarditis to develop in some valve areas and to spare others has excited much speculation. Vegetations are usually found on the downstream side of a leaflet where there is a regurgitant stream. Rodbard points out that the dynamics of flow in such areas during the regurgitant phase would provide little or no lateral pressure; this could either interfere with nutrition of surface tissues or create a situation in which platelets and fibrin could collect, thus offering protection to circulating bacteria. Factors identified by Rodbard are (1) a high pressure source (left ventricle, aorta); (2) a narrow orifice (insufficient valve, ductus arteriosus); and (3) a low pressure chamber beyond the orifice (atrium, ventricle during diastole, and pulmonary vein). This fits with the frequent development of endocarditis on the mitral and aortic valves or in small ventricular septal defects, coarctation of the aorta, ductus arteriosus, or peripheral arteriovenous fistula, and with the rarity of endocarditis on the roughened aorta or in association with atrial septal defect or a large ventricular septal defect. Also in line with this concept is the tendency of subacute bacterial endocarditis to occur in patients with comparatively mild heart disease without failure and without atrial fibrillation. In the presence of the latter complications, decreased pressure gradients and flow rates would perhaps be less favorable to the initiation of a lesion. The concepts of Rodbard and Angrist are thus compatible, and they comprise the most acceptable explanations currently available for development of this unique infection.

After infection has been established on a heart valve or other intravascular focus, steady and continuous *bacteremia* usually ensues. Study of the dynamics of this bacteremia, whereby samples of blood were withdrawn simultaneously from different parts of the circulatory system, has shown that the apparent constancy of the bacteremia is due to an equilibrium between steady replenishment of the arterial blood with fresh organisms and their removal from blood passing through organs containing reticuloendothelial tissue. The notable characteristic of this constant bacteremia is absence of metastatic foci of infection. Most of the organisms must be filtered from the blood and destroyed in reticuloendothelial tissue; those that lodge elsewhere are prey to phagocytes and do not seem capable of establishing infection.

The distinguishing feature of subacute bacterial endocarditis is its chronicity and durability. This lesion, caused by microorganisms incapable of persisting in or infecting other tissues, becomes responsible for a progressive disease, nearly always fatal unless treated with antimicrobial drugs. The host responds with formation of antibodies which react with the infecting organism. Capillaries do not extend into all areas of the vegetation; consequently, comparatively few phagocytic cells can reach the nests of bacteria. It appears therefore that bacteria can colonize superficial portions of the vegetations, safe from phagocytosis, yet capable of drifting out into the circulating blood at a comparatively even rate. Their presence in the vegetation doubtless provides a stimulus to further deposition of fibrin and platelets, causing a gradual enlargement. The lesion may at the same time lead to erosion of the underlying structures, with destruction or perforation of the valve leaflet and worsening of a pre-existing insufficiency.

Pathology. The *vegetation* is composed of masses of platelets, fibrin, and bacteria. In the deeper areas next to the endocardium there may be beginning organization and some capillary blood supply. Attempts at healing may be seen—endothelialization of the surface and organization of the deeper parts. Bacteria are never found in the deeper parts of the vegetation; they tend to be distributed in discrete colonies lying just beneath the surface of the vegetation, adjacent to the moving blood.

Other features of the disease may be attributed either to the bacteremia or to embolization of fragments of vegetation. Enlargement of the *spleen* with follicular hyperplasia is doubtless an example of acute splenic tumor developing in response to continued bacteremia or to antigen administration. The spleen may also be the site of infarction by emboli from the vegetations. The *kidney* may be infarcted grossly or may show evidence of multiple small emboli ("flea-bitten kidney"); there may also be glomerulitis. The last-named lesion has received much study lately. It appears to be an example of immune complex disease, and is probably the factor responsible for renal failure in some longstanding cases, as it is doubtful that embolic injury is ever sufficient to result in renal insufficiency. Major embolization may affect the *brain* and *mesentery*. Myocardial infarction caused by emboli in the coronary vessels is an occasional event, especially in patients with endocarditis on the aortic valve; more commonly the heart shows focal myocarditis, which is probably caused by multiple small emboli. *Mycotic aneurysms* may develop in the walls of large or medium-sized arteries, usually at sites of bifurcations, also occasionally at the base of the aorta. They are thought to result from embolization in vasa vasorum. They are especially dangerous when in the cranial cavity, where rupture may produce manifestations of subarachnoid or intracerebral hemorrhage. Rupture elsewhere can cause severe localized pain and swelling.

Manifestations. In well over half of all cases the disease begins without an identifiable predisposing factor. Some patients give a history of a respiratory infection at about the time the cardiac infection seems to have begun, but this may represent only the coincidental occurrence of a common ailment or erroneous interpretation of early nonspecific symptoms. In 5 to 10 per cent of cases there is a history of dental extraction or other manipulation within three weeks of the onset. In an even smaller proportion of cases the illness has been preceded by urologic instrumentation or by parturition. Opinions differ about the role of dental sepsis, but probably gingival or peridental infection adds to the hazard.

The *onset* in most cases is subtle, with malaise and low-grade fever; patients usually think they have "the flu." Occasionally there is a more dramatic beginning, with greater initial prostration or with an embolic accident. *Fever,* although present in nearly every case, is variable in extent, sometimes not more than 0.5° C above normal; in other cases there may be hectic variations accompanied by chilliness and sweating. In addition to malaise, other accompaniments of fever such as fatigue, weight loss, and anorexia may be noted.

Heart murmur is present in nearly all cases of subacute endocarditis. Percentages as high as 98 or 99 have been reported, but this is too high. There is no cardiac murmur if the vegetations are outside the heart, as in coarctation or infected arteriovenous fistula. Occasionally, even when the infection is on a valve leaflet, auscultation may reveal nothing early in the illness, but a murmur may be detected later. This seems especially common in middle-aged men with aortic valve endocarditis. Right-sided endocarditis, too, is especially noted for the absence of heart murmur. Changing murmurs are often said to be characteristic of subacute bacterial endocarditis; actually the day-to-day changes are often simply caused by fluctuations of body temperature and heart rate. However, the abrupt appearance of an aortic diastolic murmur is of great significance. Infected patent ductus arteriosus may be accompanied by significant changes in character of the murmur from time to time. *Pericardial friction rubs* are notably rare in this disease. *Splenomegaly* is present in about 80 per cent of cases, but the organ seldom becomes greatly enlarged. It may be tender after infarction. *Clubbing of the fingers and toes* develops in at least half the longstanding cases, but nowadays, with early recognition and effective therapy, this physical sign should not have time to develop.

Findings in the *skin* and *mucous membranes* may be helpful in diagnosis, especially late in the course. *Petechiae* appear on any part of the body. These are small, are red or purple, and do not blanch on pressure. It may help to mark the locations of red spots and to inspect them again after a day or two, an interval in which petechiae should fade. Petechiae in the conjunctiva or oral mucosa are especially easy to recognize and not likely to be confused with any other lesion. Sometimes they have white centers. Small areas of hemorrhage may be seen in the ocular fundi. Hemorrhages in the nail beds usually have a linear distribution near the distal end, hence the name "splinter hemorrhages." These can be helpful diagnostic signs, but it must be emphasized that *they are by no means pathognomonic of bacterial endocarditis.* They often occur in patients with other chronic diseases of the heart and lungs, apparently caused by dissemination of tiny thrombi, and they can frequently be found in people who do manual work. *Osler's nodes* are acute, tender, barely palpable nodular lesions in the pulps of the fingers and toes. There may be reddening of the overlying skin. They tend to appear abruptly and then to subside within a few days. *Pallor* caused by anemia is present when the disease has existed for a few weeks or longer. Older descriptions of the disease mention a *café-au-lait color of the skin.* This is rarely seen today; it may have been related to longstanding untreated infection with renal decompensation. *Neurologic manifestations* are common, and may constitute the chief complaint, especially in older patients. Cerebral embolism may simulate an ordinary stroke. Less commonly there may be encephalopathy, meningitis, or convulsions. Peripheral neuropathy has been reported.

The *blood picture* is not distinctive in bacterial endocarditis. Mild normochromic anemia, without reticulocytosis, develops in patients untreated for more than a few weeks. The leukocyte count is moderately elevated or in the high normal range because of increase in granulocytes. *Abnormal histiocytes* may be found in the peripheral blood in this disease, especially when the specimen examined is the first drop of blood obtained by puncture of an ear lobe. The characteristic cells are bizarre in appearance and may contain erythrocytes or other leukocytes. Their demonstration has occasionally been helpful in diagnosis.

Dramatic clinical events may follow lodgment of large emboli in arteries throughout the body, and these can occur some days after institution of appropriate treatment. *Cerebral* or *coronary* embolism may cause *cerebral* or *myocardial infarction. Splenic infarction* is manifested by tenderness and sometimes by pain on respiration. *Renal infarction* is usually asymptomatic but may reveal itself by the sudden appearance of hematuria. Embolism of the *mesenteric arteries* can cause severe abdominal pain, ileus, distention, and melena. Occlusion of a distal artery may result in *gangrene* of a digit, the tip of the nose, or the ear.

Heart failure is a frequent and important complication that merits discussion under manifestations of bacterial endocarditis. The mechanism of failure may be either further impairment of valvular efficiency or injury to the myocardium. The former may be due to perforation of a valve cusp or leaflet or from rupture of a papillary muscle or chorda tendinea. It is especially likely when the aortic valve is affected; here there may be sudden intensification or alteration in character of the regurgitant murmur, accompanied within hours by evidence of worsening circulatory status. The myocardium may be injured by multiple small emboli or by larger ones affecting whole segments of the coronary circulation. In any event the development of signs of heart failure during the acute or convalescent stage of bacterial endocarditis has grave prognostic significance. Deciding when to resort to cardiac surgery because of this complication is an important aspect of modern management.

Rheumatic Manifestations. Pains in muscles and joints are fairly common in bacterial endocarditis. Occasionally there are swelling and heat in one or more joints that may be difficult to differentiate from an exacerbation of rheumatic fever; indeed the conditions can probably coexist.

Mild or moderate *proteinuria* is common, and microscopic *hematuria* is a useful diagnostic finding; needle biopsy of the kidney has revealed active lesions of glomerulitis even when urinalysis showed nothing. In untreated cases, death may result from *renal failure;* this is rare now except when the true nature of the underlying disease is unrecognized. As already mentioned, the serious form of kidney damage is that which resembles glomerulonephritis morphologically. Interestingly, renal function may improve after institution of effective antimicrobial therapy.

ACUTE INFECTIVE ENDOCARDITIS

In this kind of endocarditis the course is generally more fulminating than in the subacute form. The determining factor is the kind of etiologic agent. Here we are dealing with microorganisms that are recognized pathogens. The most common is *Staphylococcus aureus,* but many others may produce the same clinical disease: *β-hemolytic streptococcus, pneumococcus, gonococcus, Pseudomonas, Proteus, Brucella, Bacteroides, Candida,* and *Histoplasma.*

This type of infection of a heart valve often develops secondary to infection elsewhere, e.g., meningitis, pneumonia, or septic thrombophlebitis such as that which may arise at the site of an indwelling catheter. As a consequence, the existence of bacterial endocarditis must be recognized in the setting of an acute microbial disease. On the other hand, it may come on without evidence of a pre-existing focus. Whatever the beginning, metastatic infections are frequent elsewhere, especially in the lungs, kidneys, meninges, and joints.

This disease can exhibit all the clinical manifestations already described in the subacute form. Although more frequent on the left side of the heart, the proportion of tricuspid valve infections is greater: 25 to 50 per cent in different reported series. Two physical findings seen only in acute endocarditis are the *Janeway lesion* and the *Roth spot.* The first is a painless red-blue lesion a few millimeters in diameter, found on the palm or sole. The second is in the optic fundus: an oval pale area near the disc, perhaps a quarter the area of the disc, surrounded by hemorrhage. Acute endocarditis frequently develops in patients with no pre-existing valvular disease; consequently there may be no murmur at the onset. However, damage to the valve and adjoining structures is likely to occur, and perforation of an aortic cusp or rupture of a chorda tendinea may cause sudden appearance of signs of aortic or mitral insufficiency. Another frequent lesion is *myocardial abscess in the valve ring area*—a complication with grave prognostic significance.

Since a heart murmur may not be present at the onset, and since significant foci of infection may be evident elsewhere, the existence of endocarditis may not be obvious. Its possibility must always be kept in mind, especially when appropriate antimicrobial therapy fails to bring about clinical improvement within a few days. Patients must be examined frequently for the appearance of a murmur or signs of heart failure.

The treatment and prognosis of all forms of infective endocarditis will be dealt with in one section. Nevertheless, it is worth emphasis here that antimicrobial therapy in acute endocarditis is substantially less effective than in the subacute forms. Furthermore the need for cardiac surgery is more likely to arise in acute than in subacute bacterial endocarditis.

PROSTHETIC VALVE ENDOCARDITIS

As the number of operations to implant prosthetic valves in human hearts has increased, a new, third category of infective endocarditis has been created. This can take either the acute or the subacute form. The vegetations are most often found along the line of suturing of the device; they may spread on to adjacent endothelium or on to the device itself.

The reported incidence of endocarditis as a complication of prosthetic valve surgery has varied from as low as 1 per cent to as high as 6 per cent. The variation is doubtless related to differences in the length of follow-up after the operative procedure, in operative techniques, in materials employed, and in the kind of prophylactic antimicrobial therapy. The risk of infection appears far higher with aortic than with mitral valve replacement; in one series 17 per cent of aortic valves became infected, in contrast to only 1.5 per cent of mitral valves.

There are probably at least three modes of infection in prosthetic valve endocarditis. In some cases microbes may be implanted during the operative procedure, from air, circulatory pumps, and the like. Prophylactic therapy at the time of surgery doubtless diminishes the frequency of such infections but cannot be expected to bar all possible invaders. Second, during the postoperative period, infection can establish itself on the prosthesis secondary to a suppurative process elsewhere, e.g., sternal infection, empyema, or infection around a venous catheter. Finally, endocarditis may originate "spontaneously" at any time after surgery as a chance event in a transient bacteremia, as has been described in discussing the genesis of subacute infective endocarditis. It is reasonable to assume that the risk of endocarditis in persons with prostheses is at least as great as in patients with rheumatic or congenital heart disease. If that is correct, we can expect this form of endocarditis to become increasingly common as patients live longer after cardiac surgery.

The bacteriology of prosthetic valve infections is variable, and may include pathogens as well as commensals. In those instances which appear to have had their onset at the time of surgery, the organisms have been mainly *Staphylococcus epidermidis* and diphtheroids. Those developing secondary to sepsis elsewhere have most commonly been due to *Staphylococcus aureus,* but other pathogens such as Pseudomonas and Proteus and Candida also constitute a threat. Among late cases, i.e., those becoming evident more than two months after surgery, *Staphylococcus epidermidis* and *Streptococcus sanguis* are particularly important.

SPECIAL SITUATIONS

Infected Arteriovenous Fistula. Perhaps 20 such cases have been reported. The infecting organism in most of them has been a viridans streptococcus. In about a third of reported cases, bacterial endocarditis has later developed on the aortic valve. Presumably the fistula, by causing circulatory strain, has rendered the valve liable to infection. This seems analogous to the observations of Lillehei on susceptibility to endocarditis in dogs with surgically induced arteriovenous fistulas.

Chronic Hemodialysis. Numerous reports have appeared of infective endocarditis as a complication of chronic hemodialysis for renal insufficiency. In some there has been an obvious pre-existing septic process, such as the site of the shunt. The infecting organisms in such cases have been *Staphylococcus aureus,* Candida, or Pseudomonas. In several others the causative organism has been a viridans streptococcus; this suggests an analogy with the cases developing in association with arteriovenous fistula, just described.

Heroin Addiction. Acute bacterial endocarditis is one of the hazards of heroin addiction, for the drug is usually self-administered intravenously with little or no aseptic technique. There appears to be a special likelihood of tricuspid endocarditis. Because of the resulting embolization, the principal clinical manifestations may be pulmonary (pleuritic pain, cough, hemoptysis, and multiple shadows in radiogram). Heart murmur may not be detected. The clinical impression is thus likely to be that of pneumonia with septicemia. The most common infecting organism is *Staphylococcus aureus,* and other possibilities include enterococcus, Candida, and such gram-negative bacilli as Pseudomonas or Proteus. The bacteriology of the endocarditis of heroin addiction must vary according to local mores: in Detroit there are many Pseudomonas infections, whereas in New York City *Staph. aureus* is by far the most frequent cause.

Pneumococcal Endocarditis. In some instances pneumococcal endocarditis has appeared to be associated with chronic alcoholism and malnutrition. The possible coexistence of endocarditis should always be considered in pneumococcal meningitis, and Austrian has estimated that endocarditis will be found in a quarter to a third of patients with pneumococcal meningitis. Rupture of the aortic valve cusp is likely to occur in this disease, and it is almost invariably followed by severe heart failure.

Enterococcal Endocarditis. Middle-aged or elderly men with urologic disease and women in the child-bearing period are at special risk of enterococcal infection; hence, there is little question that instrumentation of the urogenital tract is an important pathogenetic event. The clinical features are intermediate between the subacute and acute forms, because there is a tendency to metastatic suppurative foci, especially splenic abscess.

Gonococcal Endocarditis. Two distinctive features have been reported. About half the patients show an unusual kind of fever; a double rise and fall during each 24-hour period. This has not been characteristic of any other form of endocarditis, and an explanation is lacking. The second noteworthy feature is evidence of hepatic dysfunction. The liver is conspicuously spared in most kinds of endocarditis, but jaundice is relatively common when gonococcus is the infecting organism.

Bacteroides Endocarditis. Portals of entry include the respiratory, gastrointestinal, and genitourinary tracts. The clinical picture is one of acute bacterial endocarditis, and septic thrombophlebitis may be a feature. Some strains are penicillin sensitive, and in them the prognosis is better.

Fungal Endocarditis. The clinical features in fungal endocarditis may be those of either acute or subacute bacterial endocarditis. In some the valvular involvement has been only one aspect of an overwhelming septicemic process, but in the majority the endocarditis has been the central lesion. One notable characteristic is embolic occlusion of large arteries; this may be related to the bulkiness of vegetations induced by fungi. The most frequent fungal infections are by Candida or Histoplasma, but a few cases of infection with Aspergillus, Blastomyces, Coccidioides, Cryptococcus, and Mucor have also been reported.

Q Fever Endocarditis. This kind of infection should be thought of, and tested for, in patients with the clinical manifestations of subacute infective endocarditis, in whom blood cultures yield no growth, and in whom a trial of penicillin therapy fails to cause clinical improvement. The majority of reported cases have been in males with aortic insufficiency, and the progress has been slow. Serologic tests for *Rickettsia burnetii* should reveal antibodies in high titer. Some apparent cures have been reported by use of tetracycline, chloramphenicol, or co-trimoxazole, plus valve replacement.

Diagnosis. The possibility of bacterial endocarditis must always be kept in mind, because it is a curable disease, yet fatal if unrecognized. Unexplained fever lasting more than a week in a patient with a heart murmur imposes on the physician an obligation to consider the likelihood of bacterial endocarditis *and to draw blood cultures.* Delay until the appearance of such "cardinal" manifestations as clubbing of the fingers, splenic enlargement, anemia, changing murmurs, and petechiae is inexcusable.

Firm diagnosis can be achieved only by demonstration of bacteremia, which is possible in about 95 per cent of cases. As already discussed, bacteremia, if present at all, is usually a fairly steady, continuous process. Cultures are not more likely to be positive at a particular time of day or when the patient's body temperature is high or low. The best practice therefore is to draw four to six samples of blood for culture during the first day or two. Blood from the antecubital vein is as likely to yield positive cultures as arterial blood or bone marrow. If the patient had been receiving antimicrobial therapy, it may be necessary to stop treatment and wait a few days before obtaining the cultures. If an organism with unusual growth requirements is suspected, special culture media may have to be employed.

Diagnosis is considerably more difficult in abacteremic cases. It is impossible to say why, in a small proportion of cases, bacteria rarely gain access to the bloodstream, in contrast to the more common state of affairs when they are demonstrable almost continuously. Some agents cannot be demonstrated by the usual blood culture techniques; for example, cases caused by the Rickettsia of Q fever will be identified only by testing specifically for serologic evidence of this infection. Likewise in some cases of fungal endocarditis the organisms may not show up in blood cultures; in such situations help may be obtained from serologic tests or by demonstrating the organism in biopsy of another tissue. At any rate, the clinician must recognize the existence of this type of case and must weigh the indications for proceeding with a "blind" trial of antimicrobial therapy, as described later under Treatment.

Differential Diagnosis. Subacute infective endocarditis is one of the most familiar causes of prolonged fever of obscure origin. When bacteremia can be demonstrated, the diagnosis is relatively easy; it is the abacteremic cases that present the main difficulty. A treatise on the differential diagnosis of this disease could be of great length; here it is possible only to mention some of the most common diseases with which infective endocarditis can be confused.

Systemic lupus erythematosus may present many of the findings of bacterial endocarditis, e.g., fever, heart murmur, anemia, hematuria, arthralgia, and petechiae. A positive LE test or demonstration of antinuclear factor and negative blood cultures are the usual criteria for differentiation. Therapeutic trials of antimicrobial drugs and of steroids may give assistance.

It may be extremely difficult to distinguish between *acute rheumatic fever* and infective endocarditis. Erythema marginatum, pericarditis, and severe disabling arthritis would point toward acute rheumatic fever. Changing titers of antibody to beta-hemolytic streptococcal antigens would also favor that disease.

Sickle cell disease can cause fever, anemia, heart murmur, arthralgia, and abnormal kidney function. Demonstration of sickling or of abnormal hemoglobin should clarify the issue.

Atrial myxoma can mimic infective endocarditis. There may be fever, arthralgia, changing heart murmur, petechiae, splinter hemorrhage, and embolic manifestations. Several patients with this rare disease have been treated for infective endocarditis – a fatal clinical error in view of possible surgical cure.

Nonbacterial thrombic endocarditis is a common finding at autopsy in people who have suffered long wasting illnesses, especially lung cancer. It is now well accepted that embolization by pieces of these structures can occur, with manifestations of infarction, in spleen, kidney, and brain. Thus these patients may have heart murmur, fever, and embolic manifestations.

Drug reactions resulting in fever and anemia can resemble infective endocarditis. The finding of eosinophilia would help to differentiate such reactions from endocarditis, and the results of discontinuing drug therapy will resolve the issue.

Other well-known causes of obscure febrile illness such as *miliary tuberculosis* and *lymphoma* or *other neoplasms* may cause confusion if the patient happens to have a heart murmur.

The differential diagnosis in *acute bacterial endocarditis* includes various major acute infectious processes such as pneumonia, meningitis, pyelonephritis, and biliary tract infection. In these, the existence of endocarditis may be overlooked because of the prominence of local manifestations.

Prosthetic valve endocarditis developing soon after the surgery may be exceedingly difficult to identify. The differential diagnosis includes various kinds of postoperative sepsis and postcardiotomy and postpump syndromes as well as drug fever. When it develops two or more months after operation, the picture is likely to be that of subacute infective endocarditis, and here the correct diagnosis should be reached more easily.

Treatment. *General Considerations.* Bacterial endocarditis stands out among infectious diseases as the one in which cure depends on use of drugs capable of killing bacteria without assistance of phagocytes. The difficulty doubtless stems from the protection that is offered when microbes grow in a mass of platelets and fibrin that cannot be penetrated by phagocytes. Ample clinical experience has shown that the bacteriostatic antimicrobial drugs, such as sulfonamides, tetracycline, and chloramphenicol, seldom cure this infection. Although their administration may result in clinical improvement and sterile blood cultures, relapse occurs each time treatment is terminated. *The penicillins are by far the most valuable agents,* and it should be said that when the infecting organism is not killed by a member of this family, or when the patient is so allergic that one dare not give penicillin, the chances of successful result are reduced. Nevertheless, cures have resulted from treatment with several other bactericidal drugs, including the cephalosporins, neomycin, kanamycin, vancomycin, gentamicin, carbenicillin, and colistin. In a few cases fungal infection has been cured with amphotericin B or 5-fluorocytosine.

The place of streptomycin as an adjunct to penicillin therapy deserves special consideration. There can be no question of its value in combination with penicillin in the treatment of enterococcal infections, and there are also reports which show a similar enhancement of the efficacy of vancomycin. Authorities disagree on the need for streptomycin when dealing with infections caused by microorganisms highly sensitive to penicillin. Certainly, literally thousands of these have been cured by treatment with penicillin alone. There is reason to argue, however, on the basis of in vitro tests as well as studies of experimental endocarditis in rabbits that bacterial killing proceeds more rapidly and more completely with combined treatment than with penicillin alone. Because of this, and in view of the minimal risk of toxicity from streptomycin in the dose recommended, it seems reasonable to combine streptomycin therapy with penicillin as a general rule.

A second requirement for success is prolonged therapy. Unlike most infections, in which an antibacterial effect sufficient to tip the balance in favor of the host will suffice, the cure of bacterial endocarditis seems to depend on the ability of the drug to sterilize the vegetation unaided by host defenses. Therefore opportunity must be provided for every germ present to enter a phase of growth in which it is susceptible to killing by the agent or agents being used. Perhaps also some time is required for erosion of the surface of the vegetation, exposing the nests of bacteria that lie embedded there so that they can be carried off to other tissues for destruction. A few cures have been reported in cases treated for only ten days, and hundreds of patients have been successfully treated in 14-day courses. On the other hand, there is ample experience to demonstrate that treatment should extend for far longer periods in certain kinds of cases, as will be described subsequently.

The question of combining antimicrobial therapy with anticoagulant or fibrinolytic agents to inhibit further deposition of fibrin and platelets on the vegetations has often been raised. There is little evidence to show that this is beneficial; and indeed it adds a serious hazard of fatal hemorrhage, usually intracranial, from mycotic aneurysms. Therefore *this form of treatment is to be avoided* if possible. The risk is great enough to call for cessation of anticoagulant treatment for such indications as atrial fibrillation or deep vein thrombosis, but perhaps it must be accepted in patients with prosthetic valves.

Certain considerations influence the decision on how soon to begin therapy once the diagnosis seems probable and blood cultures have been obtained. Because excessive delay in instituting treatment undoubtedly permits further damage to heart valves and opportunity for serious embolic accidents, there is a tendency to commence antimicrobial therapy immediately. Indeed, when the clinical course is acute and the causative microorganism is probably a pathogen, or when the aortic valve is affected, it is advisable to begin treatment without delay, using the best guess as to appropriate drugs and doses, and making changes later when laboratory results are available. On the other hand, waiting until the diagnosis has been confirmed by blood culture, so that chemotherapy can be based on secure knowledge of the etiology, also has advantages. When the clinical manifestations are mild, and viridans streptococcus infection seems likely, there is comparatively little danger in waiting until the diagnosis can be confirmed by blood culture. Sensitivity tests can then provide information on the best drug to use and the proper dosage.

When bacteremia has been demonstrated, the organism should be kept viable in the laboratory until conclusion of treatment, because further tests to confirm or improve the efficacy of the treatment regimen may be desired. It is useful to test the patient's serum during treatment for bactericidal effect on the causative organism. For probability of favorable clinical result, bacterial killing by a dilution of 1 to 8 or greater is desirable.

It is generally believed that antimicrobials should be administered parenterally in this disease, although some successes have been obtained by giving penicillin orally. It would be essential in this situation to ascertain that suitable levels in body fluids are being attained, by testing the antibacterial activity of the patient's serum from time to time during the course of therapy.

Penicillins. Even when penicillin appears to be the drug of choice, the necessary dosage may vary considerably. When the etiologic agent is a viridans streptococcus, sensitive to 0.05 μg per milliliter or less, therapy consisting of 2 million units of penicillin daily, given parenterally at six-hour intervals, is sufficient. For strains less sensitive to penicillin, e.g., 0.05 to 1.0 μg per milliliter, considerably larger amounts of penicillin, up to 10 or 20 million per day, may be required, and it is common practice to add probenecid, 0.5 gram four times a day, to retard penicillin loss via the kidneys. In cases of enterococcal infection, one is dealing with an organism generally exhibiting a considerable resistance to penicillin, i.e., 5 or more μg per milliliter. Here the requirement is for large daily doses of penicillin, and the need for streptomycin as an adjunct is unquestioned. The amount of penicillin required may be 20 million to 100 million units daily, together with 1.0 gram of streptomycin per day, in four doses. Quantities of penicillin of this magnitude must be given by continuous intravenous infusion because of the pain caused by intramuscular injection. Ampicillin may be better than penicillin G in some enterococcal infections; streptomycin should be given here, too.

When the causative organism is a penicillinase-producing organism, especially *Staphylococcus aureus*, cure may be effected by use of a semisynthetic penicillin such as oxacillin. The dose is 4 to 18 grams daily intramuscularly or, with less pain, intravenously.

Occasionally the patient is so allergic to penicillins that their administration would threaten his life. Attempts may be made to suppress the allergic manifestations by steroid therapy, but this can lead to most serious difficulty. Here it may be preferable to try another bactericidal drug.

Other Antimicrobials. When the causative organism is not sensitive to one of the penicillins, or in the rare event that the patient is impossibly allergic to drugs of this family, it becomes necessary to treat with other agents.

The *cephalosporins* are valuable assets in this situation, and a substantial number of patients have been successfully treated with them. In view of the need for prolonged treatment with large doses, the best-tolerated method of administration is cephaloridine or another analogue by continuous intravenous drip, in a dose of 1 to 3 grams every six hours.

Vancomycin treatment has also succeeded against a number of gram-positive organisms, including the enterococcus; it must be given intravenously, 0.25 to 0.5 gram every six hours.

In *gram-negative bacterial endocarditis* the drugs mentioned so far may all be ineffective, but cure may be achieved with other agents. The choice must be made with the aid of detailed laboratory tests, but the following are among the most likely possibilities: *kanamycin*, 10 to 20 mg per kilogram of body weight, intramuscularly or intravenously, every eight hours; *gentamicin*, 50 to 100 mg per kilogram of body weight, intramuscularly or intravenously, every eight hours; *carbenicillin*, 10 to 30 grams per day, by continuous intravenous infusion. The last-named agent can be given with either of the first two, though not in the same vehicle. It is necessary to be on the alert for signs of toxicity with gentamicin or kanamycin, especially to kidney or eighth nerve; nevertheless, their use even to the point of serious injury may be justified when nothing else seems able to cure the infection.

Treatment of *prosthetic valve endocarditis* by chemotherapy alone is rarely successful, and there is a growing tendency to combine it with surgery, as discussed subsequently. There may be some advantage to be gained by a preliminary course of chemotherapy for a few weeks, on the assumption that surgery will be technically easier if inflammation of surrounding tissues has been lessened by control of active infection. However, worsening of the circulatory status is an overriding indication to proceed with surgery immediately.

In rare instances, resistant cases of bacterial endocarditis have been handled successfully by use of unusual combinations of antimicrobials, e.g., rifampicin and erythromycin; or tetracycline, chloramphenicol, and streptomycin. Laboratory guidance concerning combinations of drugs is difficult, and the results are somewhat unreliable because of the changing concentrations that take place in the patient's body fluids. Perhaps the best guide is to test the bactericidal effect of the patient's serum while he is under treatment.

The chemotherapy of the various mycotic infections is discussed in Ch. 255 to 266.

Treatment of abacteremic cases is difficult because there is no guide to the selection of drugs and dosages. In view of the probability of gram-positive infection, a reasonable program of treatment is the following: Begin with 10 million units of penicillin and 1 gram of streptomycin daily. If the patient's condition improves and his temperature level falls during the next 72 hours, continue with this program. If there is no evidence of clinical effect in three days, raise the dose of penicillin to 100 million units daily, and continue treatment for three days. If there is still no sign of benefit, discontinue penicillin and streptomycin and try oxacillin, 12 grams daily for four days. If this does not appear to be effective, change to vancomycin, 2 grams daily, by continuous intravenous drip, for another four days. If the causative agent is a gram-positive bacterium, one of the foregoing plans of treatment should have produced some sign of improvement. Because the possibility of gram-negative bacterial infection must also be considered, one could then try the effects of kanamycin, gentamicin, or carbenicillin, in the doses already described. If all these fail, the possibility of infection by something like *R. burnetii*, Candida, or Aspergillus must be given special consideration.

In the decision on *duration of antimicrobial drug treatment*, some variation is permissible and proper. There is no convincing clinical evidence that all cases must be treated for several weeks; on the other hand, it seems prudent in some instances to continue therapy for three or more months. As stated earlier, therapy must be maintained for many days, no matter how prompt the clinical response. At present the minimal time for any treatment is thought to be two weeks. This would be reasonable in a case in which all the auguries are favorable, e.g., *Streptococcus sanguis* sensitive to less than 0.05 μg of penicillin per milliliter, short duration of illness before therapy is begun, prompt defervescence after institution of treatment, and patient under 50 in good general health. Contrarily, in dealing with infection of a prosthetic valve by *Staphylococcus aureus*, one would be ill advised to think of discontinuing treatment in less than two months, regardless of apparent clinical response. In some instances, with indolent but stubborn infections of prostheses by, say, *Staphylococcus epidermidis*, oral treatment with a semisynthetic penicillin has had to be maintained for two or more years and even then has succeeded only in suppressing bacterial growth.

At the conclusion of a planned course of therapy, if the infection has been eradicated, the patient's temperature should be normal, the spleen should have diminished in size, and he should be free of complaints. After cessation of therapy he should be watched for signs of recurring infection. Blood cultures should be obtained during the first week, and at two weeks and six weeks. If there has been no return of symptoms by the end of six weeks and if blood cultures have remained negative, it is safe to assume that cure has been accomplished. Second attacks of bacterial endocarditis are by no means rare, whereas relapse of the original infection after a free interval of six weeks would be unlikely. Prophylactic chemotherapy to prevent development of a second infection is not advisable, because it may cause the next infection to be associated with a more resistant organism.

Surgical Measures. Even before the advent of modern chemotherapy, a few cures of this disease were achieved by closure of an infected arteriovenous fistula or patent ductus arteriosus. Simply by obliterating the vascular channel in which the vegetation was placed, the infection has been caused to burn itself out. This point is worth bearing in mind even in the "chemotherapy era," as it may encourage the undertaking of radical surgical treatment in emergency situations.

Prosthetic valve implantation during the active phase of infective endocarditis has now become fairly common practice, and the indications for it are becoming better defined. Review of recent experience at the Henry Ford Hospital showed that surgery had been employed in 15 per cent of cases of infective endocarditis. There are two main indications for surgery: (1) *Insufficiency of the valve resulting from damage caused by infection.* This may result from injury to a natural leaflet, or a paraprosthetic leak caused by infection at the suture line. Aortic valve infection is especially dangerous from this standpoint. The delicate leaflets are subject to erosion or perforation, and such damage may throw the patient into very severe pump failure which cannot be controlled by digitalis and diuretics. Sometimes it becomes necessary to operate within hours because of a shocklike state. This is a desperate situation, but nothing is gained by delaying surgery in the hope that the patient's condition can be improved by medical measures. The likelihood that viable microorganisms may still be present should not argue against operation. The surgeon may be able to remove some infected tissue when implanting the new valve, and if circulatory efficiency is improved, there may then be time for chemotherapy to cure the infection: (2) *Inability to cure the infection with drugs alone.* In some cases the removal of an infected prosthesis and its vegetations, with the placement of a new one, together with intensive chemotherapy, has served to eradicate a previously intractable infection. In acute tricuspid endocarditis caused by Pseudomonas the entire valve has been excised, with subsequent cure by chemotherapy, and the patients have been described as hemodynamically stable one or two years later even without their tricuspid valves.

Prophylaxis. *Care of the Teeth.* It is a general impression that the incidence of *Streptococcus viridans* endocarditis is lower in edentulous persons than in subjects with teeth. This has led to an extreme view in some clinics that teeth should be removed as a prophylactic measure in all patients with valvular heart disease. The majority opinion, however, is that otherwise healthy teeth should not be sacrificed. Nevertheless, it is reasonable to recommend that special attention be given to oral hygiene in patients with valvular heart disease, and that indications for extraction be interpreted liberally.

Chemoprophylaxis When Bacteremia Is Anticipated. In view of the indubitable role of manipulations likely to produce transient bacteremia in the origin of some cases of bacterial endocarditis, it has become accepted practice to "protect" persons with valvular or congenital heart disease by giving a short course of antimicrobial drug therapy at the time of such procedures. This is recommended in all textbooks and is the subject of special educational programs by national heart associations in many countries. The specific recommendations have been based on the probable infecting organisms and their in vitro sensitivities. It must be pointed out, however, that these are based only on what seems to be a good idea, for the efficacy of such prophylaxis has never been proved. There are, in fact, a number of reports of endocarditis caused by penicillin-sensitive organisms after tooth extraction despite the fact that penicillin had been given according to one of the "approved" regimens. Actual proof of value of such therapy would be almost impossible to achieve by clinical experiment, because the risk of endocarditis, even in patients with valvular heart disease who must have tooth extraction, is very small – perhaps one in several hundreds.

Recently a suitable experimental model for producing endocarditis in rabbits after a single intravenous injection of bacteria has permitted for the first time an evaluation of current recommendations for chemoprophylaxis. This has revealed that dosage schedules comparable with those recommended for clinical use are rarely successful in preventing development of endocarditis in the test animals. Giving the antimicrobial drug just before or just after the bacterial inoculum does not affect the result. Tetracycline, commonly recommended for use after genitourinary manipulations, is worthless even though the therapy is maintained for seven days. Penicillin, to be effective, must be given in large dosage, and a bactericidal level maintained for some hours. The effectiveness of penicillin is enhanced when streptomycin is given with it. Vancomycin appears to be excellent, even with a single injection, but has the drawback of intravenous administration.

On the basis of present information derived from the animal work, the following is here recommended: (1) *For dental extraction:* in order of probable efficacy, (a) penicillin G, 1,000,000 units intramuscularly, plus 0.5 gram of streptomycin intramuscularly; (b) vancomycin, 1.0 gram intravenously; (c) penicillin G, 2,000,000 units, plus procaine penicillin, 600,000 units intramuscularly. All can be given immediately before or immediately after the procedure. (2) *For urethral or gynecologic procedures:* ampicillin, 1 gram, plus streptomycin, 0.5 gram, intramuscularly, just before and six hours after the procedure.

Chemoprophylaxis at Time of Cardiac Surgery. Cardiac surgeons are likely to have their own views about this, but at present a reasonable scheme would be 1 gram each of ampicillin and oxacillin intramuscularly or intravenously every 6 hours for 10 to 14 days, beginning just before surgery.

Prognosis. Most reports of series of cases of infective endocarditis treated with modern chemotherapy indicate that the infection can be eradicated in 60 or 70 per cent of cases; a few have claimed success in as high as 80 per cent. Both figures are far too high for acute bacterial endocarditis, in which a 25 to 30 per cent recovery rate would be felt to be a considerable achievement. It must also be emphasized that eradication of infection is not the whole story, because a significant proportion of patients have nevertheless suffered additional cardiac injury, either by valve damage or by coronary artery embolization. In some of these the valvular defect can now be alleviated surgically. Aside from circulatory insufficiency, a few patients are permanently disabled by cerebral embolism. As an over-all figure, including both acute and subacute cases, it may be said that somewhat less than 50 per cent of treated patients will be well and free of cardiac failure five years later. Such results are remarkably good, however, when viewed in the light of the almost certain fatal outcome without chemotherapy and surgery.

The following factors indicate a poor outlook: (1) *Insusceptibility of the causative organism* to penicillin and other bactericidal drugs. Results are likely to be less favorable in infections caused by staphylococci, gram-negative bacteria, enterococci or fungi. (2) *Heart failure,* appearing during treatment. This is likely to resist supportive therapy and may lead to death within a few weeks or months. It carries with it the added risk of surgery if the failure is due to valvular insufficiency. (3) *Aortic valve involvement.* The likelihood of serious valvular damage and intractable failure seems much greater when the aortic valve is one of those infected. (4) *Old age.* The death rate is high in all forms of endocarditis after the age of 60. (5) *Abacteremic disease.* In most reports the survival rate for abacteremic patients is about half that for bacteremic patients. Diagnosis is likely to be delayed and treatment begun later. Without laboratory aid the treatment must be by guesswork and evidence of clinical response; this means further delay before an effective program is hit upon. (6) *Infection of a prosthetic device.* Chemotherapy seldom eradicates infection established on a prosthesis. (7) *Delay in institution of therapy.* Failure to think of the possibility of this diagnosis may lead to loss of precious days or weeks. The common practice of prescribing a broad-spectrum antimicrobial such as tetracycline for any patient with fever may lead to serious delay.

Angrist, A. A.: Pathogenesis of bacterial endocarditis. J.A.M.A., 183:249, 1963.

Arbulu, A., Thoms, N. W., and Wilson, R. F.: Valvulectomy without prosthetic replacement. J. Thorac. Cardiovasc. Surg., 64:103, 1972.

Black, S., O'Rourke, R. A., and Karliner, J. S.: Role of surgery in the treatment of primary infective endocarditis. Am. J. Med., 56:357, 1974.

Dreyer, N. P., and Fields, B. N.: Heroin-associated infective endocarditis. Ann. Intern. Med., 78:699, 1973.

Durack, D. T., and Beeson, P. B.: Experimental bacterial endocarditis: I. Colonization of a sterile vegetation. Br. J. Exp. Pathol., 53:44, 1972.

Durack, D. T., and Petersdorf, R. G.: Chemotherapy of experimental streptococcal endocarditis. I. Comparison of commonly recommended prophylactic regimens. J. Clin. Invest., 52:592, 1973.

Griffin, F. M., Jr., Jones, G., and Cobbs, C. G.: Aortic insufficiency in bacterial endocarditis. Ann. Intern. Med., 76:23, 1972.

Gutman, R. A., Striker, G. E., Gilliland, B. C., and Cutler, R. E.: The immune complex glomerulonephritis of bacterial endocarditis. Medicine (Baltimore), 51:1, 1972.

Kerr, A., Jr.: Subacute Bacterial Endocarditis. Springfield, Ill., Charles C Thomas, 1955.

King, L. H., Jr., Bradley, K. P., Shires, D. L., Jr., Donohue, J. P., and Glover, J. L.: Bacterial endocarditis in chronic hemodialysis patients. Surgery, 69:554, 1971.

Kristinsson, A., and Benthall, H. H.: Medical and surgical treatment of Q-fever endocarditis. Lancet, 2:693, 1967.

Lerner, P. I., and Weinstein, L.: Infective endocarditis in the antibiotic era. N. Engl. J. Med., 274: 323, 388, 1966.

Nastro, L. J., and Finegold, S. M.: Endocarditis due to anaerobic gram-negative bacilli. Am. J. Med., 54:482, 1973.

Quinn, E. L., Madhavan, T., Salahuddin, N., Cox, F., and Fisher, E.: The increasing role of surgical therapy in bacterial endocarditis. Surg. Clin. North Am., 52:1467, 1972.

Reyes, M. P., Palutke, W. A., Wylin, R. F., and Lerner, A. M.: Pseudomonas endocarditis in the Detroit Medical Center, 1969–1972. Medicine, 52:173, 1973.

Rodbard, S.: Blood velocity and endocarditis. Circulation, 27:18, 1963.

Rosen, P., and Armstrong, D.: Nonbacterial thrombotic endocarditis in patients with malignant neoplastic disease. Am. J. Med., 54:23, 1973.

Slaughter, L., and Morris, J. E.: Prosthetic valve endocarditis. Circulation, 47:1319, 1973.

Westenfelder, G. O., Paterson, P. Y., Reisberg, B. E., and Carlson, G. M.: Vancomycin-streptomycin synergism in enterococcal endocarditis. J.A.M.A., 223:37, 1973.

STAPHYLOCOCCAL INFECTIONS

F. Robert Fekety

193. INTRODUCTION

Staphylococci are the most common cause of suppurative skin infections of man. They also cause bacteremia and serious infections of lungs, pleura, endocardium, meninges, muscles, bones, joints, and other viscera. Troublesome staphylococcal infections have been recognized with increasing frequency since antimicrobial drugs were introduced. Pathogenic staphylococci are ubiquitous in our environment and are constituents of our normal flora. Some strains are resistant to many of our most useful antimicrobial drugs and increase in prevalence when they are used. Hospitalized patients are frequently exposed as well as being highly susceptible to this organism. They are particularly likely to develop these infections and to have great difficulty in handling them.

Bacteriology. Staphylococci are spherical gram-positive cocci that grow well on simple laboratory media, both aerobically and anaerobically. Grapelike clusters of organisms are seen in stained smears from cultures; small irregular clusters, pairs, and short chains are seen in smears of pus. When gram-positive cocci are seen *within* leukocytes in smears, it is very likely that they are staphylococci, since other cocci are usually killed and digested soon after phagocytosis, but staphylococci are not.

Staphylococci are the most important pathogens in the genus Micrococcus, which also includes many saprophytes. Pathogenic staphylococci *(Micrococcus pyogenes, Staphylococcus pyogenes)* are noteworthy for their metabolic and biochemical versatility. Two species can be tentatively identified by lipochrome pigment production on agar: *S. aureus* is characteristically golden yellow, and *S. epidermidis* (formerly *S. albus*) is white. Differentiation according to pigment production is unreliable, because *S. aureus* often grows as white colonies on primary isolation. Cream-colored, orange, golden, or lemon-yellow colonies of *S. aureus* are also seen. *S. aureus* is the most important pathogenic Staphylococcus.

Pathogenic staphylococci usually produce a variety of toxins with hemolytic, necrotizing, leukocidal, vasospastic, or lethal properties. They are also capable of fermenting mannitol and other sugars. They produce a number of other potentially important extracellular substances, including lysozyme, catalase, enterotoxin, exfoliatoxin, fibrinolysin, hyaluronidase, lipase, nuclease, beta lactamase, phosphatase, deoxyribonuclease, protease, and coagulase (a plasma-clotting substance). The pathogenetic role of these toxins and enzymes is still uncertain, but coagulase production and mannitol fermentation correlate best with pathogenicity for man. By convention, coagulase-positive mannitol-fermenting staphylococci are called *S. aureus.* The tube coagulase test is more reliable than the slide test, which measures bound coagulase (clumping factor).

Coagulase-negative and mannitol-negative isolates are called *S. epidermidis. S. epidermidis* does not often cause infection of man unless susceptibility is increased or there is a nidus of infected foreign material, such as an intracardiac prosthesis or an intravascular plastic catheter or shunt. However, such appropriately susceptible hosts are now commonplace in hospitals. Consequently, these opportunistic organisms are being recognized more and more frequently as the etiologic agents in serious infections, and *they can no longer be dismissed automatically as contaminants whenever they are isolated from cultures of blood or other specimens.*

Pathogenesis. Abscess formation is the characteristic feature of staphylococcal infection. When staphylococci lodge in susceptible tissues and begin to multiply, an acute inflammatory reaction rapidly ensues. Thrombosis of small blood vessels occurs, and fibrin is deposited in the lesion, which becomes avascular, necrotic, and surrounded by a fibroblastic wall. The tissues become hypertonic, edematous, congested, tense, and painful. The center of the lesion gradually liquefies, forming the characteristic thick, creamy yellow pus which is slightly acidic and comprised mostly of dead organisms, leukocyte debris, and proteinaceous substances. Further evolution of the lesion is slow, even under drug therapy, until it drains, after which it usually begins to heal. Thus antimicrobial drugs do not affect undrained abscesses very much.

Granulomatous reactions are occasionally seen at sites of chronic staphylococcal infections. These may contain masses of staphylococci resembling "sulfur granules," and can be confused with actinomycosis (staphylococcal botryomycosis). Granulomas are also characteristic of staphylococcal lesions in association with the leukocytic deficiency syndromes, such as the chronic granulomatous disease of childhood.

Very little that is conclusive has been established about the mechanisms of the pathogenicity of staphylococci. There are obvious but unproved clinical implications for the dermonecrotic, lethal, and leukocidal toxins. Fibrin products of coagulase activity may help to wall off the lesion and protect the organism from granulocytes, but the resultant fibrin network may also enhance surface phagocytosis. The pathogenetic role of hyaluronidase, fibrinolysin, hemolysins, and the other extracellular products is entirely speculative. The factors important in promoting phagocytosis and intracellular killing of the organism are incompletely understood.

Some of these substances that may be involved in pathogenesis have been used as antigens in experimental vaccines, but immunization as a means of enhancing resistance to staphylococci has met with little success. Most adults possess serum antibodies to a number of staphylococcal antigens, but high titers of these antibodies have not correlated well with protection from disease. Protein A, a component of staphylococcal cell walls, nonspecifically binds antistaphylococcal antibodies at the Fc fragment instead of appropriately at the Fab fragment. This reversed attachment of immune globulins appears to render them functionally ineffective, and may be the explanation for the observation that neither vaccination nor the disease seems to result in immunity despite the production of large amounts of antibody. In addition, there is some evidence that hypersensitivity reactions to antigenic products of the microorganism may deleteriously influence local susceptibility to infection. Additional studies are required if safe and effective vaccination against staphylococci is to become possible.

Epidemiology. Pathogenic staphylococci are normally acquired by a high percentage of healthy infants within a few days or weeks of birth. Most healthy humans harbor virulent staphylococci in the anterior nares or on the skin, either occasionally or consistently. Clinical disease occurs in exposed persons or asymptomatic carriers when local or general resistance is decreased or when the exposure is heavy. Staphylococci are abundant in our environment and can survive in dust for long periods, but implantation of large numbers of staphylococci derived from air and other exogenous sources seems an uncommon explanation for disease. To produce skin infections experimentally in healthy persons, more than a million pathogenic staphylococci must be inoculated, and no significant differences have been demonstrated between strains derived from lesions or from healthy mucous membranes. The experimental evidence that certain strains of pathogenic staphylococci are especially virulent is inconclusive, but the epidemiologic evidence suggests that this factor may be important in nursery outbreaks and in recurrent furunculosis. Factors that increase host susceptibility to relatively small numbers of ordinary staphylococci thus seem of great importance in explaining the high frequency of staphylococcal disease.

Although numerous conditions are known to predispose to staphylococcal disease, the mechanisms causing the organism to become invasive in these patients are not well understood. Skin infections usually begin about hair follicles, sebaceous glands, or at sites of wounds, abrasions, or foreign body penetration. Greasy substances, oils, sunburn, and other conditions causing blockage of the ducts of cutaneous glands predispose to infection. In some cases infection results because of massive multiplication of the organism within exudates or devitalized tissues. Burns, surgical wounds, and dermatitic lesions frequently become secondarily infected with staphylococci. Sutures enhance local susceptibility to staphylococcal infection, possibly because bacteria can multiply within their interstices as in a protected sanctuary or because a tight suture may reduce local blood flow and thus impair cellular or humoral defense mechanisms. Furthermore, the inflammatory response to sutures may lower local resistance. Similar mechanisms may explain infection at the site of other foreign bodies, such as prosthetic devices and intravenous catheters. Diabetics seem to have an increased frequency of cutaneous staphylococcal infections, possibly because their acute defensive inflammatory responses may be delayed and deficient (especially during ketoacidosis), because of vascular disease and gangrene, and because of the frequent exposure that diabetics have to hospitals and medical procedures that increase the risk of infection. The chronic granulomatous disease of childhood is characterized by serious infections with catalase-positive organisms such as staphylococci, because the granulocytes of the affected individuals are unable to generate sufficient hydrogen peroxide to permit intracellular bactericidal mechanisms to operate normally. Other congenital or acquired conditions characterized by defective leukocyte formation and frequent staphylococcal infections have recently been described. Malnutrition and a wide variety of serious chronic debilitating diseases predispose to serious staphylococcal infection. In some cases this may be attributable to treatment with antimicrobial drugs that encourage overgrowth of pathogenic staphylococci. In others it may be the consequence of therapeutic efforts or disease processes adversely affecting cellular or humoral defense mechanisms. Neoplasms, uremia, extensive operations, and treatment with adrenal steroids and cytotoxic or immunosuppressive agents predispose to serious staphylococcal infection. Influenza, measles, diabetes mellitus, and cystic fibrosis predispose to staphylococcal pneumonia. Newborn infants are hypersusceptible to this organism, and are subject to severe spreading skin infections and primary staphylococcal pneumonia with pneumatocele formation.

Because of their ubiquity, versatility, and resistance to antimicrobial drugs, staphylococci have become a major cause of serious infections in highly susceptible persons who tend to congregate in hospitals. Bacteriophage typing of staphylococci has contributed to understanding the modes of transmission of these infections. Man is the major source of the organism. Patients and personnel in hospitals are more commonly asymptomatic carriers of the organism than are those without hospital contact. The organism is most often found in the anterior nares, in intertriginous areas of hair, and on the hands. Carriers and infected patients readily contaminate their environment, and staphylococci can be isolated from air, dust, floors, mops, blankets, clothing, dressing carts, and other fomites. The usual habitat of *S. epidermidis* is the skin and mucous membranes of man and animals.

Studies in nurseries for the newborn have shown that transmission of the organism occurs primarily via the hands of personnel who either are carriers or have recently handled infected or colonized newborns. The spread of organisms from heavily colonized infants via the airborne route ("cloud babies") may occur, but this seems much less frequent than transmission via hands. Postoperative wound infections are more frequent in nasal carriers and often appear to be attributable to strains carried by the patient prior to operation (endogenous infection). Infected patients or personnel are also important sources of strains causing wound infections (exogenous infections); the usual mechanism is contact spread via hands. Transmission via air, environment, or fomites is a less common route of wound infection. All these mechanisms contribute to the perpetuation of the reservoir of staphylococci in the hospital and to the spread of organisms to personnel and highly susceptible patients.

Most authorities believe that special attention in hospitals to measures such as isolation and frequent handwashing with antiseptics in order to prevent the spread of staphylococci is worthwhile. Infected patients can shed large numbers of bacteria into the environment and should be isolated unless the infection is at a closed site (e.g., blood, meninges). Personnel with clinical infections should not have contact with susceptible patients. The indiscriminate use of antimicrobial drugs favors the transmission and survival of drug-resistant strains. Few surgical patients deserve chemoprophylaxis, for there is little evidence that prophylaxis is capable of preventing staphylococcal infection. Because so many persons are asymptomatic carriers of pathogenic staphylococci, it is not practical to exclude all of them from contact with susceptible persons in hospitals. Actually, healthy carriers of ordinary strains seem unlikely to acquire new and potentially more dangerous strains, which is probably an example of *bacterial interference.* However, it may be necessary during outbreaks to exclude carriers of *especially dangerous* staphylococcal strains (as demonstrated by *both* bacteriophage typing and clinical experience) from nurseries, delivery rooms, and operating rooms.

Treatment. Although antimicrobial therapy has markedly improved the prognosis in serious staphylococcal infection, it must be emphasized that surgical drainage of abscesses and removal of infected foreign bodies are not only equally important, but may be the only way to achieve a cure. Patients with staphylococcal infections usually respond relatively slowly to drug therapy, and despite optimal treatment the mortality rate is high in persons with compromised defense mechanisms. Although antimicrobial therapy is considered elsewhere in detail (Ch. 267 and 268), there are certain points that should be stressed here.

Appropriate cultures and drug-susceptibility tests should always be obtained to confirm the diagnosis of serious staphylococcal disease and to guide therapy. Although many antimicrobial drugs are now available for treating these infections, the often unpredictable susceptibility of the organism narrows the initial choice to only a few. Bactericidal penicillin analogues are preferred unless the patient is allergic to them. Because most strains causing infection in the hospital and also in the community are resistant to penicillin G and ampicillin, the choice should be limited to drugs that are not significantly inactivated by staphylococcal penicillinase. Toxic-appearing patients with serious infections are best treated parenterally. Methicillin, oxacillin, nafcillin, cephalothin, and cefazolin are recommended for serious infection. Used properly, they seem to produce equally good therapeutic results. Many if not most experts still prefer methicillin, but nafcillin has become increasingly popular because it is the most active derivative and rarely causes nephritis or other serious side effects. The cephalosporins are especially useful with mixed infections because of their relatively broad spectrum. Cephaloridine should rarely be used because of its nephrotoxic potential in doses greater than 4.0 grams per day. Cefazolin is a well-tolerated new cephalosporin preparation providing good serum antistaphylococcal activity, and is preferred over the other cephalosporins for intramuscular use. Cephalothin should be avoided in treating central nervous system staphylococcal infections, because its less active desacetyl metabolite tends to accumulate in the cerebrospinal fluid.

For oral therapy of less serious infections, cloxacillin, dicloxacillin, and the more expensive cephalexin are suitable and equally efficacious when given orally in proper amounts. Oxacillin and nafcillin are not recommended, because their oral absorption is too erratic.

The penicillinase-resistant penicillin analogues are also adequate for the treatment of infections caused by more sensitive organisms such as penicillin-susceptible staphylococci, pneumococci, and group A beta streptococci when the dosages commonly recommended for staphylococcal disease are used. It is *not* necessary to add penicillin G to the regimen when these organisms are suspected of playing a role in the illness. However, many persons prefer to use both penicillin G and methicillin or nafcillin initially and switch to the more active drug when the nature of the etiologic agent becomes clear. If the organism is susceptible to it, penicillin is preferred, because it is usually the most active drug as well as the most convenient and inexpensive one to administer. Penicillin V is better than penicillin G for oral therapy of staphylococcal infections because of its better absorption.

If the patient is allergic to penicillin, all the semisynthetic penicillins should be avoided. Vancomycin, clindamycin, gentamicin, cephalothin, cefazolin, or cephalexin are suitable substitutes. Allergic cross-reactions between penicillin and the cephalosporins have been observed. Kanamycin, erythromycin, and bacitracin are occasionally useful. Tetracyclines, including minocycline, and chloramphenicol are less frequently employed because of frequent drug resistance, fear of toxicity, or lack of bactericidal action.

Because of the numerous suitable antimicrobial agents and variable clinical situations, only general guidelines for dosage and duration of treatment of staphylococcal infections can be given here. A delay in initiating appropriate therapy is often deleterious. Severe infections respond slowly and require large doses given for long periods. Relapses are common if therapy is terminated too early, especially if the lesion has not drained or foreign bodies are not removed. It is unusual for the organism to become resistant to the penicillin derivative during therapy. Endocarditis and other serious infections are usually treated for at least four to six weeks. In serious infections, parenteral therapy is preferred because of the desirability of ensuring the maintenance of high concentrations of the antimicrobial in blood and tissues. In order to maintain adequate serum antistaphylococcal activity, the interval between intravenous doses of penicillins and cephalosporins should not exceed four hours in critically ill patients, and the drugs should not be given rapidly as an "intravenous bolus."

Although methicillin-resistant strains of *S. aureus* have been encountered frequently in Europe, they are not common in the United States. Faulty drug-susceptibility discs occasionally result in their spurious detection. Methicillin-resistant organisms usually show multiple resistance to other semisynthetic penicillins and cephalosporins. Resistant strains grow better at 30 than at 37° C and in high salt media. They may be recognizable only after prolonged incubation (48 hours) in the presence of methicillin or oxacillin, presumably because the isolates contain only a small proportion of resistant clones. Most laboratories do not employ these special conditions routinely. These organisms seem less virulent than methicillin-susceptible staphylococci, but they have occasionally been of clinical importance. Wide misuse of the new penicillins will probably result eventually in an increase in the prevalence of these strains. Vancomycin, gentamicin, clindamycin, or a combination of kanamycin or gentamicin with cephalothin or methicillin has been recommended for treatment of infections with these organisms.

Cephalosporins, vancomycin, gentamicin, and the macrolides are the most active drugs against *S. epidermidis*. These coagulase-negative organisms are often surprisingly resistant to methicillin and the other semisynthetic penicillins.

194. CUTANEOUS STAPHYLOCOCCAL INFECTIONS

FURUNCLES

A furuncle (boil) is an acute circumscribed staphylococcal abscess of the skin and subcutaneous tissues. The term folliculitis refers to pustular furuncles involving hair follicles. Folliculitis is common in persons with oily skin, poor hygiene, or occupational exposure to cutting oils. Deep folliculitis of the beard area is known as *sycosis barbae.* Patients with multiple or recurrent furuncles are said to have *furunculosis,* but otherwise normal adults commonly experience an average of five or six furuncles per year.

Furuncles are most common on the face, neck, buttocks, thighs, perineum, breasts, and axillary skin. Most furuncles begin at the base of a hair follicle and take three to five days to evolve. Itching or pain may be the earliest symptom. As the center of the lesion becomes necrotic and hypertonic, fluid is drawn into the furuncle and it swells, thinning the overlying erythematous skin. Spontaneous drainage usually occurs soon thereafter. A hard core of necrotic debris is sometimes extruded from the center of the abscess. Relief of pain and onset of healing are usually rapid after drainage occurs, although erythema and swelling may persist for several weeks. A furuncle may regress without draining and form a "blind boil" that is indolent and prone to exacerbation after minor local trauma.

When the sebaceous glands of the face and upper back are extensively involved with furuncles, the condition is referred to as *pustular acne vulgaris. Juvenile acne* is not caused by staphylococci, but these organisms may secondarily infect acne lesions.

Furuncles involving blocked apocrine sweat glands *(hidradenitis suppurativa)* frequently become chronic. This troublesome infection tends to spread to other local sweat glands and hair follicles and leads to interconnecting draining sinuses and extensive scarring. Lesions occur in the axillary, perianal, and genital areas. Hydradenitis is difficult to cure with antimicrobial drugs and drainage alone. Excision of the involved tissues and skin grafting are frequently necessary and usually successful.

Although systemic symptoms and bacteremia are unusual with an ordinary furuncle unless the lesion is squeezed or manipulated, asymptomatic bacteremia related to a furuncle is probably fairly common. Furuncles are believed to be important in the pathogenesis of endocarditis, osteomyelitis, pyarthrosis, and other metastatic infections developing after hematogenous dissemination of the organism. Septic thrombophlebitis caused by local extension of infection is another serious complication of furuncles. Lesions in the middle third of the face are especially dangerous, because they may spread intracranially via emissary veins and cause cavernous sinus thrombophlebitis.

CARBUNCLES

A carbuncle is a large furuncle or an aggregate of interconnected furuncles. Carbuncles often drain through multiple skin openings. They represent an acute suppurative inflammation of subcutaneous tissues extending between hair follicles in clefts along fibrous and adipose tissues. They occur where the skin is thick (such as the back of the neck), possibly because thick skin promotes internal and lateral extension rather than external drainage. Carbuncles may attain the size of lemons, and are often associated with extreme pain, chills, fever, leukocytosis, malaise, prostration, bacteremia, and sometimes death.

IMPETIGO

Impetigo is a superficial primary pyoderma caused by group A beta streptococci, *S. aureus,* or both. It is most common in infants and children. It begins as macules and progresses to vesicles and bullae, which rupture, releasing a cloudy yellow fluid which forms crusts, and reveal a weeping denuded area. Central healing occurs, and the lesions may become chronic and resemble fungal infections. The lesions are superficial, rarely larger than 2 cm, and they spread by autoinoculation. Streptococci are usually responsible for these lesions, but there is good evidence that staphylococci of bacteriophage type 71 may be involved in some cases.

THE SCALDED SKIN SYNDROME

An association of bacteriophage group II staphylococci with exfoliative dermatitis has been recognized in three distinct but related clinical entities. (1) *Generalized exfoliative dermatitis (scalded skin syndrome, pemphigus neonatorum, Ritter's disease, staphylococcal toxic epidermal necrolysis)* is severe and characterized by generalized painful erythema, formation of bullae, and shedding of the upper epidermis in large sheets. The focus of infection may be at a distant site. The disease is usually seen in newborns but has been recognized in adults, and is often confused with pemphigus. (2)*Bullous impetigo* is a localized form of the scalded skin syndrome in which the infection occurs at the site of the lesion. (3) *Staphylococcal scarlet fever* is a mild variant of the generalized scalded skin syndrome and is clinically similar to streptococcal scarlet fever. A localized infection is the usual focus of toxin production. Antibodies to the streptococcal erythrogenic toxin do not seem to be cross-reactive.

These three clinical variants appear to represent the spectrum of a disease process with a common etiology—the exfoliative exotoxin produced by group II staphylococci (especially types 3A, 3C, 55, and 71). The disease has been duplicated in a laboratory model. The characteristic lesion consists of intraepidermal cleavage through desmosomes of the stratum granulosum. Other forms of toxic epidermal necrolysis can be distinguished because they show necrosis of the entire epidermis with cleavage near the dermoepidermal junction.

TREATMENT OF CUTANEOUS INFECTIONS

Some authorities believe that furuncles and pustules can be aborted at early stages by the administration of an antimicrobial drug or by the local application of an antiseptic such as alcohol. Once drained, small lesions require no further therapy, but they should be kept covered with a dressing or zinc oxide ointment to help prevent contamination of other sites. More severe lesions require local and systemic therapy. Rest, heat, and elevation of the affected site tend to relieve pain and minimize spread of the infection. Warm compresses hasten maturation of the lesion, but care should be taken to ensure that they do not cause maceration of the skin. Incision should be delayed until frank suppuration and fluctuance are detectable, because early incision is ineffective and may promote local extension and bacteremia.

Antimicrobial drugs should be given if the furuncle is large, on the face or neck, or accompanied by lymphadenitis, fever, or other systemic reaction. They should also be given if the patient has diabetes or another underlying disease predisposing to complications, or if surgical incision is to be performed. Oral therapy with a penicillin analogue, erythromycin, or clindamycin is usually satisfactory. Therapy should be continued until signs of active inflammation have disappeared; a week is usually sufficient. Gamma globulin, adrenal steroids, and vaccines are of no proved value.

Impetigo responds rapidly to treatment with appropriate systemic antimicrobial therapy, but topical bacitracin ointment may be adequate in mild cases.

PREVENTION OF CUTANEOUS INFECTIONS

Furuncles are difficult to prevent, because the patient usually continues to be susceptible and the organism is ubiquitous. However, measures that protect the skin and minimize contact with the organism may be worth the trouble they entail. Predisposing conditions should be treated or eliminated. Skin irritants and abrasive tight clothing should be avoided. The fingernails should be kept short, and frequent handwashing should be stressed. Draining lesions should be considered highly contaminated and kept covered. Daily bathing and shampooing with antiseptic soap may be useful. Very rarely it may be possible to treat carriers with antimicrobial drugs for several weeks or months and eliminate the organism and thus prevent recurrences. Antimicrobial ointments or 2 per cent hexachlorophene cream may be applied several times daily to susceptible areas or to the anterior nares to suppress the organism. It is sometimes possible to get rid of a troublesome organism by intentionally inducing nasal carriage with a relatively nonpathogenic species after the more virulent Staphylococcus strain has been suppressed by drug therapy (bacterial interference). The 502A strain of *S. aureus* has been employed for this purpose in patients with recurrent furunculosis. Small numbers of organisms of the 502A strain have been used to intentionally colonize the umbilicus and nares of newborn infants in order to prevent acquisition of more dangerous strains. Outbreaks in nurseries have been terminated in this way. Minor but definite infections have been caused in infants and adults by strain 502A, and its use is still experimental. Staphylococcus vaccines, toxoids, and bacteriophage lysates are of no proved value in prevention, and irradiation to produce atrophy of sebaceous glands is not recommended.

195. STAPHYLOCOCCAL PNEUMONIA

Staphylococci cause less than 5 per cent of all bacterial pneumonias, except during influenza epidemics, but the disease is especially important because of its high mortality rate (up to 50 per cent) (see Ch. 179).

In so-called primary staphylococcal pneumonia, the organisms gain access to the lung via the tracheobronchial tree. Primary staphylococcal pneumonia is most often seen in infants; in children with cystic fibrosis or measles; in adults with influenza; or in debilitated, hospitalized persons being treated with antimicrobials, steroids, cancer chemotherapy, or immunosuppressants.

The diagnosis of primary staphylococcal pneumonia in adults with serious underlying diseases is often difficult. High spiking fever, multiple chills, cyanosis, rapidly progressive dyspnea, chest pain, and the production of thick, creamy yellow, salmon-colored, or reddish-yellow sputum should lead to the suspicion of staphylococcal pneumonia. Peripheral vascular collapse and marked signs of toxicity should also cause one to suspect the diagnosis in patients with pulmonary filtrates. Staphylococcal pneumonia developing in association with influenza or an underlying debilitating illness characteristically begins with a sudden and marked worsening of the illness, accompanied by prostration, cyanosis, tachypnea, bloody or purulent sputum, and high fever. Fever, cough, sputum production, dyspnea, and chest pain may be minimal during early stages of staphylococcal pneumonia. In infants the sudden development of pneumothorax, pneumatoceles, or empyema is a characteristic feature. Necrosis of lung tissue and formation of multiple abscesses is characteristic in adults.

Hematogenous or *secondary staphylococcal pneumonia* is seen most frequently in narcotic addicts with endocarditis and in others with bacteremia from a primary focus elsewhere. Secondary staphylococcal pneumonia is characterized by multiple peripheral infiltrates resembling embolic lesions which progress to necrosis and abscess formation, with a high frequency of pleuritic pain, empyema, and pneumothorax, and infrequent signs of consolidation. The signs of septicemia frequently overshadow the pulmonary disease in these patients.

The physical signs in patients with staphylococcal pneumonia are highly variable. A toxic appearance and low-grade fever may be the only detectable manifestations, particularly when the pneumonia is in a central location or interstitial, which is common. Patchy bronchopneumonia with multiple small abscesses is another common presentation, and can be detected by the presence of either coarse or fine rales. Dullness to percussion is not an early sign, and signs of frank consolidation are rarely found. Pleural effusion and empyema are frequent, but the fluid is commonly loculated in intralobar fissures and may not be readily detected or aspirated.

The leukocyte count is usually elevated to between 15,000 and 25,000 per cubic millimeter. A leukocyte count greater than 15,000 in an adult with influenza should raise the question of a secondary bacterial pneumonia. Chest roentgenograms show patchy infiltrates, most often near the hilum, multiple cavities, and pleural effusions. The Gram-stained smear of the sputum usually shows polymorphonuclear leukocytes and large numbers of clustered gram-positive cocci. When cocci are seen within leukocytes in sputum, staphylococcal pneumonia is the presumptive diagnosis. The blood culture is *not* often positive unless the pneumonia is secondary to staphylococcal bacteremia originating at some other site.

Differential Diagnosis. All other forms of pneumonia must be considered. The distinction from pneumonia caused by gram-negative organisms is especially important in patients developing pneumonia in the hospital. A carefully performed Gram stain of a good sample of sputum is the keystone of choosing initial therapy, and may be helpful in interpreting subsequent culture reports. Abscess formation, salmon-colored sputum, and an appropriate setting for the development of staphylococcal pneumonia are helpful clues.

Since drug-resistant staphylococci frequently colonize the respiratory tract soon after the administration of antimicrobial drugs, one should not diagnose staphylococcal pneumonia solely on the basis of a sputum culture revealing rare or moderate numbers of the organism in someone under treatment for other pulmonary infections.

Prognosis. Even under the best of circumstances, the case fatality rate for pneumonia is 15 to 20 per cent. Higher fatality rates are seen in very young infants and in elderly debilitated patients. As this pneumonia is characterized by necrosis of lung parenchyma, recovery is usually slow. Improvement after the initiation of therapy is often not evident for 48 to 72 hours, and the illness usually lasts three to four weeks. Convalescence may be markedly prolonged when empyema is present. Bronchiectasis is frequently a consequence of staphylococcal pneumonia.

Treatment. Once the diagnosis is tentatively established, vigorous antimicrobial therapy by the parenteral route should be initiated promptly. Methicillin, oxacillin, nafcillin, cephalothin, or cefazolin, in doses of at least 1 gram every four to six hours, are preferred and equally good. The organism should be considered resistant to penicillin and ampicillin until it is demonstrated to be susceptible. If the organism is susceptible, penicillin G (20 million units intravenously per day) is the drug of choice. If the patient is allergic to penicillin, vancomycin (0.5 gram intravenously every six to eight hours), gentamicin, or clindamycin (600 mg four times per day) may be used. Therapy should be continued for 10 to 14 days or more after the patient shows a definite clinical response. The clinical response is usually very gradual. When empyema is present, it may be helpful to administer antimicrobial drugs directly into the pleural cavity, and proteolytic enzymes may be instilled to help thin the exudate. Surgical drainage of empyema with a chest tube is usually required, because the pus is often loculated or too thick for needle aspiration. Oxygen, bronchodilators, expectorants, fluids, and other supportive measures are important.

196. STAPHYLOCOCCAL OSTEOMYELITIS

Staphylococcus aureus is the etiologic agent in the majority of instances of primary or hematogenous osteomyelitis. The disease is becoming uncommon and is readily cured if treated early with appropriate antimicrobial drugs. Bacteremia occurring from a skin infection which may be no more serious than a furuncle is the usual inciting event. Secondary staphylococcal osteomyelitis is related to penetrating trauma, surgery, or a contiguous focus of infection. It is also seen in patients with diabetes mellitus or peripheral vascular disease after local cutaneous infections.

Hematogenous staphylococcal osteomyelitis is primarily a disease of children, adolescents, and intravenous drug abusers. It is more frequent in boys. It usually begins in the metaphyseal area of the diaphysis near the epiphyseal plate, and is uncommon after epiphyseal closure. The metaphysis is a weak spot in growing bones. It has a terminal blood supply subject to bacterial embolization and thrombosis. The capillary and venous networks in this area are extensive, and strains and other minor injuries readily result in hematomas which afford a nidus for bacteria. Furthermore, the capillaries in this area are deficient in phagocytic lining cells. The most common sites of involvement are the lower femur, upper tibia, ankle, wrist, or hip, but any metaphyseal area can be involved. The vertebrae are more commonly involved in adults, particularly narcotic addicts. As the infectious process develops in the metaphysis, the arterial blood supply is usually compromised because it is terminal and encased in rigid bony canals. Thromboses and vascular insufficiency develop and lead to necrosis of bone. An early radiologic sign of the inflammatory process is decalcification or rarefaction of bone caused by hyperemia and injury to osteoclasts. If the infection is untreated, a sequestrum of necrotic bone will separate in six to eight weeks. Treatment with antimicrobial drugs has practically eliminated this result. In pyogenic osteomyelitis it is characteristic for the periosteum to react to the infection by forming a layer of reparative bone (osteosclerosis) called the involucrum. Reactive bone formation is much less common in tuberculous osteomyelitis, unless the process has been going on for more than six months.

The infection tends to spread along the diaphysis or outward to the subperiosteal space where an abscess often forms, particularly in children. From there the infection may extend and involve nearby joints. This is seen in about 10 per cent of cases, and is more frequent when the hip or shoulder bones are infected. It is uncommon for the infection to enter the joint by crossing the epiphyseal plate barrier in children, but this is not unusual in adults. In addition, sterile joint effusions are not uncommon when there is an osteomyelitic focus nearby.

If not treated early or adequately, the infection tends to become chronic, with recurrent exacerbations, metastatic lesions, the formation of draining sinuses, and extensive scarring, eventually requiring surgical debridement and saucerization of bone. Amyloidosis occasionally develops after longstanding osteomyelitis.

Staphylococcal infections of vertebrae and intravertebral discs are especially frequent in intravenous drug addicts. They are also seen after pelvic and urinary tract infections. The patients usually complain of back pain accentuated by straining or coughing, pain radiating down the leg, or abdominal pain. *Paravertebral abscesses* are a frequent complication. Narrowing of the disc space, erosion of the vertebral end plates, and bridging of the disc space by new bone formation are important radiologic findings. The condition may be mistaken for tuberculous spondylitis, but osteophytic bridging or isolated involvement of the vertebral arches or processes is unusual in tuberculosis. Acute endocarditis is an occasional complication of staphylococcal vertebral osteomyelitis.

High fever, chills, and throbbing pain in the bone are the early signs of osteomyelitis. Local muscle spasm, splinting, or limping are the early local signs. Redness, swelling, and warmth are seen later. Bacteremia is frequent in osteomyelitis, and the patient may appear delirious and critically ill. The systemic signs and symptoms may overshadow the local manifestations. Leukocytosis and anemia are common. Rarefaction of bone is the earliest radiologic sign, but may not appear until 10 to 14 days after onset. Periosteal reaction with new bone formation is seen after the disease has been present for at least a month. Bone scans, using radioactive strontium or fluorine, can localize the lesion prior to x-ray changes. They are particularly useful in drug addicts who present with fever and vague somatic complaints referable to the lower back.

Rheumatic fever, traumatic lesions, leukemia, scurvy, pyogenic arthritis, hemoglobinopathies, Ewing's tumor, and other neoplasms should be considered in the differential diagnosis of osteomyelitis.

Treatment. With appropriate treatment, death from acute osteomyelitis is rare, and progression to chronic osteomyelitis is not likely. Mixed infection with other organisms, such as Pseudomonas, is seen fairly often. Empirical treatment without the aid of exudate or operative specimens of bone for culture and histologic study is hazardous and should be avoided. Since early treatment is important, therapy directed against the Staphylococcus should be started as soon as cultures have been obtained when this organism appears likely. Intensive parenteral therapy should be given initially. One of the penicillins, cephalosporins, or clindamycin is recommended. Gentamicin is useful in addicts when Pseudomonas as well as Staphylococcus is suspected. Immobilization is important. Some evidence of a clinical response should be noted within four days. It may be necessary to aspirate the subperiosteal abscess, or to drain it surgically. Vigorous treatment should be continued for at least three or four weeks. Ideally, oral therapy should then be continued for two or three months. Radiologic signs of the infection may never become apparent if treatment is given early. Although small sequestra usually absorb spontaneously, larger pieces of dead bone require surgical removal, especially if there is a slow or incomplete clinical response. Operative removal of foreign bodies is frequently necessary to achieve a cure in secondary osteomyelitis.

With chronic osteomyelitis, antimicrobial therapy should be given, and sequestrectomy, saucerization of infected bone, and removal of sinus tracts should be performed. Only rarely will such patients respond to drug therapy alone. Closed irrigation with antimicrobial agents is occasionally a useful adjunct to surgery.

197. STAPHYLOCOCCAL BACTEREMIA AND ENDOCARDITIS

Bacteremia may occur with any localized staphylococcal infection, but is relatively uncommon with minor postoperative wound infections and pneumonia, unless of hematogenous origin. Carbuncles and other serious skin infections; infected intravascular shunts, catheters, and other foreign bodies; endocarditis; and osteomyelitis are the most common foci causing bacteremia. Staphylococci bacteremia is frequent in patients with marked granulocytopenia or serious chronic debilitating diseases. It is usually associated with hectic fever, temperatures to 40° C or more, repeated shaking chills, and marked systemic toxicity. Widespread metastatic abscesses may develop in kidneys, lungs, bone, skin, brain, meninges, myocardium, and other viscera. The case fatality rate with staphylococcal bacteremia is 50 per cent when there is predisposing underlying disease, and about 20 per cent when there is not.

Bacteremia with coagulase-negative staphylococci sometimes pursues an indolent course for many weeks with remarkably few clinical manifestations. Bloodstream infections with these organisms are usually seen after ventriculoatriostomy shunting or cardiac surgery with insertion of prostheses. A proliferative and membranous glomerulonephritis and the nephrotic syndrome may be seen as a result of chronic *S. epidermidis* bacteremia in patients with infected shunts, and prompt improvement in the renal disease may follow removal of the shunt.

Endocarditis frequently complicates staphylococcal bacteremia from another site. The disease is usually of the acute, malignant, or ulcerative type with *S. aureus*, but a form indistinguishable from that caused by *S. viridans* is occasionally seen, especially when *S. epidermidis* is responsible. The illness usually has an acute onset, with shaking chills, high fever, changing cardiac murmurs, cutaneous pustules and petechiae, splinter hemorrhages, metastatic abscesses, hematuria, progressive anemia, and marked leukocytosis. Thrombocytopenia and disseminated intravascular coagulation may be seen. Normal heart valves may be infected and destroyed in just a few days. Abscess of the myocardial valve ring occurs frequently and should be suspected when serious arrhythmias develop.

The distinction between endocarditis and bacteremia originating from another focus may be difficult. Continuous bacteremia suggests endocarditis or other intravascular focus; intermittent bacteremia suggests an extravascular focus.

Acute staphylococcal endocarditis in heroin addicts is characterized by frequent involvement of the tricuspid valve. Multiple septic pulmonary emboli and infarcts with abscess formation and empyema are the usual presenting manifestations. The classic peripheral cutaneous manifestations of endocarditis such as splenomegaly, Osler's nodes, and splinter hemorrhages may be lacking in right-sided endocarditis, but blood cultures are usually positive. Cerebral manifestations relative to abscess formation, embolization, meningitis, and subarachnoid hemorrhage are frequent. Panophthalmitis is occasionally a complication. A murmur from the tricuspid lesion is usually present but often overlooked initially until pulmonary emboli call attention to its presence. Other clues to tricuspid involvement are atrial or ventricular diastolic gallops along the lower left sternal border and the external jugular vein, or a short soft murmur along the lower left sternal border which is increased with inspiration (Carvallo's sign) and with the patient standing.

Acute proliferative glomerulonephritis of the immune complex type may develop during the course of staphylococcal endocarditis and is sometimes confused with an allergic reaction to drugs used in treatment.

Treatment. Even with appropriate therapy, staphylococcal bacteremia still has a mortality rate of almost 50 per cent. Patients over the age of 50 have a particularly poor prognosis. Parenteral therapy is necessary, and the regimen must be bactericidal. Therapy for bacteremia should be continued for no less than four weeks, and preferably for six to eight weeks if it is believed that the patient has endocarditis as well as bacteremia. In doubtful cases, therapy should be given for six to eight weeks. Surgical treatment of the focus of infection is important to consider, and early replacement of damaged valves may be necessary if there is severe or intractable heart failure. When the site of infection is an intravascular foreign body, the infection is rarely cured until the foreign material is removed. However, infected cardiac prostheses are not usually replaced until at least one course of intensive treatment has proved unsuccessful, because 5 to 10 per cent of these infections may be cured with medical therapy alone.

MISCELLANEOUS INFECTIONS

Staphylococci are commonly found in *nose* or *throat* cultures, but they do not cause pharyngitis or tonsillitis, except rarely in patients with agranulocytosis or leukemia. Their presence usually represents nothing more than colonization, and does not by itself justify treatment with antimicrobial drugs.

Staphylococcal pyarthrosis represents a diagnostic and therapeutic challenge in adults. It may occur after orthopedic surgery or in association with osteomyelitis. Skin ulcers and contaminated intra-articular injections or aspirations are often important in pathogenesis. Rheumatoid factor may bind antistaphylococcal antibodies, and may contribute to lowered resistance. Joint infection should be suspected in all patients with rheumatoid arthritis who show an apparent exacerbation of joint disease with fever, pain, effusion, and leukocytosis. Chills favor the diagnosis of septic arthritis over rheumatoid disease. Joint fluid aspiration is essential for early diagnosis. Immobilization, repeated aspiration, surgical drainage when indicated, and appropriate antimicrobial drugs are the treatment.

Staphylococcal meningitis is uncommon. It is usually the result of penetrating trauma, local surgery, or bacterial endocarditis. Therapy must be vigorous. If the organism is known to be susceptible to penicillin G, 24 to 30 million units should be given daily by the intravenous route. If it is resistant to penicillin G or of unknown susceptibility, methicillin (12 to 24 grams per day), oxacillin (12 grams per day), or nafcillin (12 grams per day) may be used. Cephalosporins are not recommended. If gentamicin is used, it should be given intrathecally (5 mg) as well as by the usual routes. Bacitracin (5000 to 10,000 units in 5 to 10 ml of sterile saline) has also been used successfully intrathecally as supplemental therapy.

Primary spinal epidural abscess is a neurosurgical emergency in which prompt recognition and treatment are indicated to prevent permanent spinal cord damage. It is sometimes seen in narcotic addicts in association with vertebral osteomyelitis. The process is usually acute, is located dorsally in the lower thoracic or lumbar regions, and is most often caused by staphylococci. Fever, localized spinal tenderness, and rigidity of the spine are followed by root pain, localized weakness, progressive paresthesias, sphincter changes, and evidence of spinal cord compression. The lumbar spinal fluid usually is under reduced pressure and shows pleocytosis, but may be normal. Myelography localizes the lesion, but is seldom necessary. Antimicrobials are merely adjuncts to treatment, for total recovery depends on early diagnosis followed by prompt surgery, usually laminectomy, and drainage (see Ch. 384).

Staphylococcal pericarditis usually occurs after bacteremia, often in association with osteomyelitis or endocarditis, with formation of focal myocardial abscesses and spread to the pericardium. The Staphylococcus is the most frequent cause of purulent pericarditis. Treatment consists of antimicrobial therapy and pericardiocentesis, but if rapid improvement is not noted, open surgical drainage should be instituted.

Staphylococcal parotitis is seen in debilitated adults who become dehydrated and receive inadequate mouth care. Extensive edema, erythema, and tenderness are seen in the parotid area, and pus may be seen oozing from Stensen's duct. The patient usually has a high fever and disorientation. Shock and death are common. Irradiation of the gland may be a useful adjunct, but appropriate antimicrobial therapy and supportive care are more important.

Staphylococcal (tropical) pyomyositis is a relatively common disease of indigenous residents of hot, humid tropical areas. It is occasionally seen in temperate climates, where it is usually misdiagnosed. Bacteremia resulting from minor superficial lesions is followed by abscess formation beneath the deep fascia of skeletal muscles, especially in the leg. Local trauma may be important in determining the site of the infection. There is diffuse swelling of the limb, but usually no fluctuance or regional adenopathy. The skin may become tense and cellulitic, but is often normal. Fever may be minimal during the first week of illness. The diagnosis is frequently made at operation, at which time multiple abscesses are found to have coalesced and extended between muscle fasciculi and within fascial compartments. It is uncommon for osteomyelitis to coexist. Staphylococci of bacteriophage group II are usually implicated. Surgical drainage and antimicrobial therapy are efficacious.

198. STAPHYLOCOCCAL GASTROENTERITIS AND ENTEROCOLITIS

The enterotoxins produced by staphylococci are an important cause of acute epidemic gastroenteritis or food poisoning. The toxin is formed prior to ingestion of contaminated and usually improperly refrigerated or stored food (see Ch. 22).

Staphylococci are normal inhabitants of the intestines, although their presence is not usually recognized unless selective media are used. They may increase during antimicrobial therapy, and patients may concomitantly experience mild diarrhea. Much more rarely the organisms cause acute necrotizing pseudomembranous enterocolitis. Most common after abdominal surgery, shock, or antimicrobial therapy or in leukemia, this syndrome has a high mortality rate. Locally produced enterotoxin is thought to be responsible for the manifestations of the disease. Symptoms include abdominal pain, distention, ileus, fever, diarrhea, bloody stools, electrolyte depletion, dehydration, and shock. Gram stain of the stool reveals leukocytes and large numbers of cocci in sheets and clumps, and establishes the diagnosis. Vancomycin given by *mouth* is useful in treatment; a dose of 1.0 gram hourly for four doses and then every four hours has been used. Parenteral therapy with another appropriate drug may also be given. Oral neomycin is no longer recommended, because many staphylococci in hospitals are resistant to it. Shock and electrolyte imbalance should be treated vigorously with appropriate fluids.

Andriole, V. T., and Lyons, R. W.: Coagulase-negative Staphylococcus. Ann. N.Y. Acad. Sci., 174:533, 1970.

Banks, T., Fletcher, R., and Ali, N.: Infective endocarditis in heroin addicts. Am. J. Med., 55:444, 1973.

Boyle, J. D., Pearce, M. L., and Guze, L. B.: Purulent pericarditis: Review of literature and report of eleven cases. Medicine, 40:119, 1961.

Cohen, J. O. (ed.): The Staphylococci. New York, Wiley-Interscience, 1972.

Elek, S. D.: Staphylococcus Pyogenes. Edinburgh, E. & S. Livingstone, Ltd., 1959.

Fekety, F. R.: The epidemiology and prevention of staphylococcal infection. Medicine, 43:593, 1964.

Keys, T. F., and Hewitt, W. L.: Endocarditis due to micrococci and *Staphylococcus epidermidis*. Arch. Intern. Med., 132:216, 1973.

Levin, M. J., Gardner, P., and Waldvogel, F. A.: "Tropical" pyomyositis. N. Engl. J. Med., 284:196, 1971.

Lillibridge, C. B., Melish, M. E., and Glasgow, L. A.: Site of action of exfoliative toxin in the staphylococcal scalded skin syndrome. Pediatrics, 50:728, 1972.

Mailbach, H. I., Strauss, W. G., and Shinefield, H. R.: Bacterial interference: Relating to chronic furunculosis in man. Br. J. Dermatol., 81: Suppl. 1, 69, 1969.

McCloskey, R. V.: Scarlet fever and necrotizing fasciitis caused by coagulase-positive hemolytic *Staphylococcus aureus*, phage type 85. Ann. Intern. Med., 78:85, 1973.

Shinefield, H. R., Ribble, J. C., Boris, M., and Eichenwald, H.: Bacterial interference: Its effect on nursery acquired infection with *Staphylococcus aureus*. Am. J. Dis. Child., 105:646, 1963.

Van Prohaska, J., Mock, F., Baker, W., and Collins, R.: Pseudomembranous (staphylococcal) enterocolitis. Surg. Gynecol. Obstet., 112:103, 1961.

Waldvogel, F. A., Medoff, G., and Swartz, M. N.: Osteomyelitis: A review of clinical features, therapeutic considerations and unusual aspects. N. Engl. J. Med., 282:198, 260, 316, 1970.

Watanakunakorn, C., Tan, J. S., and Phair, J. P.: Some salient features of *Staphylococcus aureus* endocarditis. Am. J. Med., 54:473, 1973.

Waxman, A. D., Bryan, D., and Siemsen, J. K.: Bone scanning in the drug abuse patient: Early detection of hematogenous osteomyelitis. J. Nucl. Med., 14:647, 1973.

DISEASES CAUSED BY NEISSERIA

199. GONOCOCCAL DISEASE

Donald Kaye

Definition. Gonorrhea is an infection of the mucous membrane of the urethra and genital tract caused by *Neisseria gonorrhoeae*. Involvement of the pharynx and rectal mucosa is common. Infection is almost always the result of sexual contact. After invasion of mucosal sites, gonococci may spread and cause infections such as arthritis, tenosynovitis, perihepatitis, endocarditis, and meningitis.

Etiology. *N. gonorrhoeae* is a gram-negative coccus that was first described by Neisser in 1879 in exudates from patients with gonorrhea. In stained smears of exudates the organisms appear as diplococci with flattened or slightly concave adjacent sides and resemble a pair of kidney beans. A considerable portion of the organisms in exudates are within polymorphonuclear leukocytes.

Gonococci grown in laboratory media assume an oval or spherical form, and single cocci and clumps of cocci may be found in addition to diplococci. *N. gonorrhoeae* can be distinguished from other Neisseria by its ability to ferment glucose but not maltose or sucrose.

Primary isolation of the gonococcus is difficult. The organism is fastidious in its growth requirements, and is susceptible to toxic substances that are present in many media. Blood, serum, ascitic fluid, or other agents must be added for enrichment, as growth will usually not occur on plain agar. Blood is commonly used, and the medium is heated (chocolate agar) to reduce the deleterious effect exerted by certain amino acids toxic to the gonococcus. Commercial media are available that satisfy the various growth requirements of *N. gonorrhoeae.* Most strains require an atmosphere of 2 to 10 per cent carbon dioxide. Colonies of *N. gonorrhoeae* are round, gray-white, and translucent. Overgrowth with other bacteria occasionally occurs in cultures of exudate from the urethra, vagina, and cervix and is frequent in cultures from the pharynx and rectum if nonselective media are used.

All Neisseria produce an oxidase that can be used for tentative identification of colonies of *N. gonorrhoeae* (colonies turn purple on exposure to 1 per cent para-aminodimethylaniline monohydrochloride). With cultures from the genital tract, the combination of colonies of typical morphology composed of gram-negative diplococci and a positive oxidase test is strong presumptive evidence of the presence of *N. gonorrhoeae.* However, other Neisseria and members of the tribe Mimeae resemble *N. gonorrhoeae* both in colonial morphology and microscopic appearance and give a positive oxidase reaction (*Mima polymorpha* var. *oxidans* is the only Mimeae that is oxidase positive). Therefore cultures that are presumptively positive for *N. gonorrhoeae* should be confirmed by fermentation reactions or by fluorescent antibody techniques.

Thayer-Martin selective medium, containing vancomycin, sodium colistimethate, and nystatin, permits growth of *N. meningitidis* and *N. gonorrhoeae* but inhibits growth of many other bacteria frequently found in specimens from urethra, cervix, vagina, rectum, and pharynx. Growth of other Neisseria and of *Mima polymorpha* var. *oxidans* is inhibited.

Incidence and Prevalence. There has been an increase in the reported incidence of gonococcal infections in recent years. However, the true incidence and prevalence of gonorrhea are unknown because of problems in diagnosis, antimicrobial therapy by nonmedical persons, incomplete reporting by physicians, and the presence of many undetected asymptomatic female carriers. It has been estimated that over 2 million new cases of gonorrhea occur annually in the United States. The magnitude of the problem of asymptomatic gonorrhea in females may be demonstrated by the fact that there is about a 5 per cent prevalence of asymptomatic gonorrhea in pregnant women.

Gonorrhea is a disease of the sexually active, and most cases occur in patients 15 to 24 years of age. Gonorrhea rates are higher among military personnel, migrant groups (such as itinerant laborers and seafarers), homosexuals, and prostitutes. In surveys 10 to 33 per cent of prostitutes have gonorrhea.

Epidemiology. *N. gonorrhoeae* is a parasite of man; it does not cause disease in animals. Gonorrhea is almost always acquired from sexual contact, exceptions are gonococcal conjunctivitis (which occurs primarily in infants) and vulvovaginitis. Conjunctivitis results either from passage of the infant through an infected genital tract (ophthalmia neonatorum) or from contamination after birth. Vulvovaginitis is an infection of the genital tract of infants and preadolescent girls that results from direct contact with infected adults or, rarely, can be spread by contact with towels or linens contaminated with gonococci.

Repeated attacks of gonorrhea are common; therefore individual attacks seem to confer little or no immunity. However, individual variation in susceptibility to infection has been demonstrated after inoculation of *N. gonorrhoeae* into the urethras of male volunteers. Trauma to the urethra probably increases susceptibility to gonorrhea. After an episode of acute gonorrhea, *N. gonorrhoeae* may remain in the genital tract for months. Chronic asymptomatic carriers of the gonococcus are important in the epidemiology of gonorrhea because they are difficult to detect and therefore are rarely treated. It has been common knowledge that most women with gonorrhea are relatively asymptomatic, but only recently has it been appreciated that as many as 10 per cent of males with gonorrhea seen in a venereal disease clinic may be asymptomatic (Pariser).

Pathogenesis and Pathology. *N. gonorrhoeae* are unable to penetrate stratified squamous epithelium, but penetration and infection of columnar and transitional epithelium readily occur. In males the urethra is attacked first, resulting in purulent urethritis and involvement of the urethral glands. Direct spread of infection may result in prostatitis, epididymitis, or seminal vesiculitis. During stages of healing, stricture formation may occur. Gonococcal proctitis in the male is almost always the result of rectal intercourse.

In the female, urethritis is mild and transient. Bartholin's and Skene's glands and glands of the cervix may become infected with or without involvement of the urethra. Contiguous spread of infection can cause salpingitis. Proctitis may result from contiguous spread or rectal intercourse. Gonococcal salpingitis is usually bilateral and may cause pyosalpinx and formation of a tubo-ovarian abscess. The inflammation tends to heal with fibrosis and adhesions that may produce obstruction of the fallopian tubes and sterility. Ascent of infection to the fallopian tubes often occurs during or just after menstruation. Although endometrial infection is usual when *N. gonorrhoeae* invades the fallopian tubes, it is not serious and tends to subside promptly. The vagina does not become infected in adults, probably because of the presence of squamous epithelium with many layers of cells and the lack of glands.

Conjunctivitis is the most common manifestation of gonococcal disease in infants. It is a destructive inflammation of the eye and before the use of antimicrobial agents frequently caused blindness. Between one year of age and pubescence, gonococcal infection is rare in males but causes vulvovaginitis in females. The increased susceptibility to gonococcal infection of the immature vaginal mucous membrane in contrast to the resistance of the mucosa of adults is probably explained by the thin mucous membrane present prior to adolescence.

Gonococcal infection of the pharynx is common and results from oral-genital contact. Gonococcal pharyngeal infection has been demonstrated in up to 20 per cent of homosexual men and 20 per cent of women practicing fellatio who had gonococcal infection at any site. In 3 to 4 per cent of these patients, only pharyngeal cultures were positive for gonococci (Pariser; Wiesner et al.).

Occasionally invasion of the blood occurs and *N. gonorrhoeae* may disseminate and produce infection at distant foci. Joints are the most frequent extragenital sites of localization, but tenosynovitis, endocarditis, meningitis, skin lesions, and infection at other foci may also occur.

Dissemination of gonococcal infection is more common in women than in men and is probably more common in homosexual males than in heterosexual males. This is probably explained by the fact that men with gonococcal urethritis are usually symptomatic and therefore are treated promptly, greatly decreasing the chances of dissemination of infection. In contrast, women with gonorrhea and males with gonococcal proctitis or pharyngitis (almost always homosexuals) are usually asymptomatic and are therefore unlikely to be treated. Although asymptomatic urethritis is relatively uncommon in men with gonorrhea, there seems to be a disproportionately high incidence of these men among males with disseminated gonococcal infection. The source for dissemination may be the genital tract, rectum, or pharynx. It has been estimated that dissemination of gonococcal infection occurs in up to 3 per cent of women with gonorrhea and is most prone to occur during pregnancy or during or just after menstruation.

Clinical Manifestations. *Gonorrhea in the Male.* The incubation period of gonococcal urethritis in the male is usually two to eight days. There is sudden onset of dysuria, urgency, and frequency associated with mucoid urethral discharge that rapidly becomes purulent and profuse. Gonococcal urethritis usually does not cause fever, but prostatitis, seminal vesiculitis, or epididymitis is frequently associated with fever. Acute urinary retention may result from involvement of the prostate. Rectal examination reveals tenderness of the affected organ in the presence of prostatitis or seminal vesiculitis. Epididymitis causes severe pain and tenderness of the epididymis.

Untreated gonorrhea subsides over a period of weeks, but a small amount of mucoid discharge from the urethra may continue to be found each morning for months. Gonococci may persist, usually in the prostate. Urethral stricture is a common sequela of untreated urethritis, especially after recurrent attacks of gonorrhea. Epididymitis can result in sterility.

Gonorrhea in the Female. In females the disease may begin with dysuria, urgency, and frequency after an incubation period of two to eight days. However, the urethritis is frequently of short duration and often is mild or completely asymptomatic. Cervicitis gives rise to a mucopurulent discharge that varies from scant to profuse. Involvement of Skene's ducts or Bartholin's glands is common, and abscess formation may occur. Gonococci can be isolated from the rectum in 20 to 50 per cent of women with gonorrhea, and occasionally can produce symptomatic proctitis. In 5 per cent of women with gonococcal infection only the anorectal culture contains gonococci. The duration of symptoms from an untreated infection that remains localized in the lower genital tract is usually no longer than a month or two. However, the patient may remain a carrier of the disease for many months.

Salpingitis is manifested by acute onset of fever and lower abdominal pain. Physical examination usually reveals lower abdominal tenderness, pain on movement of the cervix, and tenderness of the adnexa (with or without palpable masses). Acute pelvic inflammatory disease tends to recur, and pelvic pain and fever are present intermittently. Sterility is common.

Extragenital Gonococcal Infection. PROCTITIS. Gonococcal proctitis is usually asymptomatic but may be manifested by anal discharge, burning rectal pain, blood and pus in the stools, and pain on defecation.

PHARYNGITIS. Gonococcal infection in the oropharynx can probably cause symptomatic pharyngitis, tonsillitis, and gingivitis but is usually asymptomatic.

ARTHRITIS. Arthritis is the most common form of clinically recognized disseminated gonococcal infection; it usually occurs within one to three weeks after initial infection in the genital tract or may follow pharyngeal or rectal infection. Onset may be gradual with migratory polyarthalgias leading to frank arthritis in one or more joints, or it may be sudden with hot, swollen, and extremely painful joints. Fever and leukocytosis are usually present. Over 75 per cent of patients have polyarthritis. The joints that are most commonly involved are the knees, ankles, and wrists, but any joint may be involved, including the spine and sternoclavicular and temporomandibular joints. *Tenosynovitis,* which is rarely observed in other types of pyogenic arthritis, is common in gonococcal arthritis and most often occurs about the wrists and ankles. The skin lesions associated with gonococcal bacteremia are also frequently present.

N. gonorrhoeae can be isolated from joint fluid in only 25 to 50 per cent of cases. The fluid ranges from serous to frankly purulent, has the protein content of an exudate and usually contains increased numbers of leukocytes that are mainly polymorphonuclear. Muscle wasting about the joint and permanent deformity may result. Some authorities have described two types of arthritis produced by the gonococcus: (1) polyarticular arthritis, usually with no or small effusions that tend to be sterile, often associated with bacteremia and skin lesions, and (2) frank pyogenic arthritis (often involving one joint from which gonococci can frequently be isolated) without bacteremia or skin lesions. The first type has been attributed by some to hypersensitivity, but it seems more likely that it represents the initial or bacteremic phase during which organisms localize in joints. Frank pyogenic arthritis may occur after a clinically apparent or inapparent bacteremic phase. Sterility of the joint fluid in patients during the bacteremic phase may be due to taking cultures early in the disease, before microorganisms in the joint have sufficient time to proliferate.

GONOCOCCAL BACTEREMIA. Gonococcal bacteremia can produce a syndrome with recurrent episodes of fever, skin lesions, arthralgia or arthritis, mild to severe constitutional symptoms, and intermittently positive blood cultures. This syndrome occurs with infection in the genital tract, rectum, or pharynx, and, if untreated, can recur over a period of months or even years. The rash usually appears during the first day of symptoms and may recur with each episode of fever. The rash is found on the distal part of the extremities and consists of scanty pin-point erythematous macules that rapidly become maculopapular, vesiculopustular, and frequently hemorrhagic. Bullae can form. The mature lesion is elevated, has a dirty gray necrotic center, and is surrounded by erythema. It heals in three to four days. Gram-negative cocci can often be seen in stains of fluid from the lesions, but cultures for *N. gonorrhoeae* are usually negative. Immunofluorescent studies on the exudate from the pustules demonstrate *N. gonorrhoeae* in a high percentage of patients. Identical skin lesions may be seen in patients with meningococcemia, which can present an indistinguishable clinical sydrome.

GONOCOCCAL ENDOCARDITIS. Gonococcal endocarditis is extremely rare at present. In most patients, previously normal valves are attacked. The valves on the left side of the heart are involved most often, but valves on the right side are affected with a higher frequency than with endocarditis caused by other bacteria. A double daily temperature elevation (double quotidian) is common in patients with gonococcal endocarditis.

PERIPHEPATITIS [FITZ-HUGH–CURTIS SYNDROME]. Perihepatitis is a rare complication in women with gonococcal pelvic inflammatory disease and results from direct spread of gonococci from the pelvis to the upper abdomen. It is manifestated by fever, upper quadrant pain (usually right upper quadrant), tenderness and spasm of the abdominal wall, and occasionally a friction rub over the liver. During the acute stage the gallbladder temporarily may not be visualized on cholecystography; this can lead to an erroneous diagnosis of cholecystitis. The patient often has a recent history of pelvic pain or vaginal discharge, and physical examination may reveal evidence of pelvic inflammatory disease. *N. gonorrhoeae* can frequently be demonstrated in the cervical or vaginal discharge.

The symptoms respond to antimicrobial therapy. The untreated disease subsides after one to four weeks of fever and abdominal pain, leaving "violin-string" adhesions between the anterior surface of the liver and the anterior abdominal wall. Recently this syndrome was reported in a male, probably caused by lymphatic or hematogenous dissemination.

Diagnosis. In the male the combination of urethritis and the presence of intracellular gram-negative diplococci in smears of exudate from the urethra is strong presumptive evidence of gonorrhea. Confirmation is obtained by culture or, if available, fluorescent antibody studies. Anorectal cultures should be obtained in homosexual males.

For routine screening, cervical cultures will detect the vast majority of females with asymptomatic gonorrhea. Gonorrhea should be suspected in any female contact of an infected male. Similarly the asymptomatic carrier state should be suspected in asymptomatic male contacts of symptomatic females or asymptomatic females detected by routine cultures. In the female with suspected gonorrhea, cultures of exudate from the cervix and anorectal area should be obtained in addition to urethral cultures.

Pharyngeal cultures for *N. gonorrhoeae* should be obtained from homosexual males and females practicing fellatio. In all patients with suspected disseminated gonococcal infections, cultures of the pharynx and anorectal area should be obtained in addition to genital tract cultures.

Gonococci die within hours if allowed to dry. Therefore exudates should be inoculated as soon as possible on Thayer-Martin medium or on a suitable transport medium for *N. gonorrhoeae.* Transgrow, a commercially available antibiotic-containing medium, is packaged in a bottle with an increased carbon dioxide tension, and is preferred for transporting specimens containing gonococci or meningococci to central laboratories.

With use of fluorescent antibody it is frequently possible to make a definite identification of *N. gonorrhoeae* in exudate within one hour of obtaining a specimen.

Genital tract infection with the chlamydiae of inclusion conjunctivitis may occur in both sexes, and in the male can present as urethritis. Strictly speaking, it is the genital infection that is primary, with the conjunctivitis representing a secondary involvement. This disease is a common finding in venereal disease clinics where its incidence may approach that of gonococcal urethritis in the male. Since the discharge in the chlamydial infection is not grossly purulent, it is seldom confused with acute gonorrhea, but it can resemble gonococcal urethritis at the time of onset of post-treatment relapse. The chlamydial form of urethritis is discussed in Ch. 171. It is not established whether this infection is responsible for any cases of *Reiter's syndrome,* or whether the latter represents a separate entity (see Ch. 93.)

Salpingitis. Acute salpingitis must be differentiated from appendicitis and tubal pregnancy. The presence of bilateral tenderness in the adnexa with or without masses, a history of recent sexual intercourse followed by urethritis or vaginal discharge, and demonstration of gonococci on cervical smear are strongly suggestive of gonococcal salpingitis. When it is impossible to differentiate acute salpingitis from appendicitis or tubal pregnancy, the diagnosis must be established at laparoscopy or laparotomy.

Arthritis; Blood-Borne Lesions. The diagnosis of gonococcal arthritis or bacteremia with skin lesions should be suspected in a patient with the appropriate clinical syndrome, especially if there is a recent history of urethritis or vaginal discharge. Tenosynovitis is suggestive of disseminated gonococcal infection. Isolation of *N. gonorrhoeae* from the genital tract, rectum, or pharynx is supportive evidence, and demonstration of gonococci in skin lesions, blood, or joint fluid is confirmatory. The serum complement-fixation test for gonococci may be of aid in suggesting gonococcal arthritis, especially if titers are rising. However, this test is not well standarized. Other serologic tests which look promising are currently under investigation.

When stains and cultures of joint fluid are negative for gonococci (50 to 75 per cent of cases), it is frequently difficult to differentiate gonococcal arthritis from Reiter's syndrome (nonbacterial urethritis, conjunctivitis, and arthritis). The problem in differential diagnosis is compounded by the fact that patients with Reiter's syndrome may have concomitant gonococcal urethritis. Urethritis and arthritis in a female suggest gonococcal arthritis, because this disease is more common in females, whereas Reiter's syndrome is rare in females. The presence of tenosynovitis and response to antimicrobial therapy strongly imply gonococcal arthritis. Patients with Reiter's syndrome frequently have prolonged courses with recurrences and do not respond to antimicrobial therapy. Keratodermia blennorrhagica (a symmetrical eruption with a predilection for the soles, palms, and genitals) occurs in Reiter's syndrome and is probably not associated with gonococcal arthritis. After an initial polyarthritis in Reiter's syndrome, ankylosing spondylitis may develop.

Gonococcal arthritis can often be differentiated from acute rheumatic fever, rheumatoid arthritis, and gout by the absence of carditis, lack of rheumatoid factor in serum, and failure to respond to colchicine, respectively.

When *N. gonorrhoeae* cannot be isolated from the joint, the response to penicillin therapy is often the strongest confirmatory evidence of gonococcal arthritis.

Treatment and Prognosis. Penicillin is the drug of choice for all gonococcal infections. Prior to 1954 a single injection of 300,000 units of penicillin cured almost all cases of gonorrhea. In recent years gonococcal strains of increased resistance to penicillin (requiring up to 2.0 μg per milliliter for inhibition) have constituted as much as 50 per cent or more of all isolates. Concomitantly there has been a striking increase in the incidence of failure of therapy with 600,000 to 2,400,000 units of penicillin. It must be stressed that penicillin remains the drug of choice for gonorrhea but that much larger doses are required than in previous years. If the trend in increasing resistance to penicillin continues, the point will soon be reached at which the doses of penicillin required will preclude the use of parenteral penicillin for routine therapy of uncomplicated gonorrhea.

N. gonorrhoeae organisms have also been becoming more resistant to tetracycline. Although the level of resistance to tetracycline is not yet of clinical importance in the United States, more resistant strains are being isolated in certain areas of the Far East. The same strains of *N. gonorrhoeae* that are relatively resistant to penicillin also tend to have increased resistance to tetracycline and ampicillin but not to spectinomycin.

The current recommendations of the Venereal Diseases Branch of the Center for Disease Control for treatment of uncomplicated gonorrhea (urethral, cervical, pharyngeal, or rectal) in men or women or in patients with known exposure to gonorrhea are as follows:

Aqueous procaine penicillin (4.8 million units) should be administered intramuscularly at one visit (two sites of injection) together with 1 gram of oral probenecid preferably 30 to 60 minutes before the penicillin; or 3.5 grams of oral ampicillin simultaneously with 1 gram of probenecid. When penicillin or ampicillin is contraindicated, alternate regimens are: spectinomycin, 2 grams in one intramuscular injection; or tetracycline hydrochloride orally, 1.5 grams initially, followed by 0.5 gram four times a day for four days (9 grams) for both men and women.

Spectinomycin (Wiesner et al.) and ampicillin do not seem to be effective in eliminating *N. gonorrhoeae* from the pharynx. With this exception, the cure rates with these regimens are over 90 per cent in the United States. Aqueous procaine penicillin and spectinomycin have the important advantage of one-visit parenteral therapy which guarantees absorption of the total course of treatment. A major advantage of the procaine penicillin regimen (although clearly more painful) is that it will cure incubating syphilis (Schroeter et al.). The advantage of the tetracycline regimen is that it will usually prevent postgonococcal urethritis in males (see below).

Urethritis should subside within two to three days after therapy. A watery urethral discharge may persist in males for weeks despite elimination of gonococci and usually requires no treatment (postgonococcal urethritis or nongonococcal urethritis). Several studies have demonstrated that postgonococcal urethritis can usually be prevented by use of tetracycline for therapy of gonorrhea and that postgonococcal urethritis will usually respond to tetracycline treatment.

Relapse of gonorrhea occurs most commonly during the first week after treatment. Therefore to evaluate cure, a culture should be obtained one week after therapy and, if possible, at two more weekly intervals. In homosexual males and in females, anorectal cultures should be obtained as well as cervical cultures to evaluate cure of genital tract gonorrhea. If relapse occurs (and relapse is often difficult to differentiate from reinfection), the patient may be retreated with one of the alternative regimens, preferably spectinomycin.

Causes of failure of therapy, other than infection with gonococci relatively resistant to penicillin, are failure to distinguish between relapse and reinfection; failure to identify nongonococcal urethritis, e.g., Reiter's syndrome or infection with chlamydiae; and possibly the presence of penicillinase-producing bacteria at the site of infection.

Patients with gonococcal prostatitis, seminal vesiculitis, epididymitis, salpingitis, arthritis, perihepatitis, or the syndrome of gonococcal bacteremia with skin lesions should be treated with bed rest and 10 to 20 million units of aqueous penicillin G intravenously each day. Patients who are allergic to penicillin may be treated with tetracycline, 0.5 gram orally four times a day; cephalothin in doses of 6 to 12 grams intravenously each day may be used in pregnancy. The duration of therapy should be seven to ten days (two weeks for arthritis) or longer until signs of infection have subsided and cultures become negative. Response to therapy usually occurs within two to three days. However, arthritis frequently responds more slowly, and it may take seven to ten days for the patient to become afebrile. Recent evidence suggests that gonococci that are relatively resistant to penicillin are less likely to cause disseminated infection (i.e., are less virulent), and that after several days of intravenous penicillin therapy the course can be completed with oral ampicillin in treatment of disseminated infection.

In acute gonococcal disease in the genital tract, surgery is indicated only for drainage of abscesses. However, in the chronic stage in some female patients it may become necessary to remove involved pelvic organs. In gonococcal arthritis, pus should be aspirated by needle when possible, but occasionally surgical drainage of the joint becomes necessary. Injection of penicillin into the joint is not indicated. Physiotherapy should be started during the period of convalescence to promote return of function of the joint.

For gonococcal endocarditis or meningitis, 20 million units of aqueous penicillin G should be administered parenterally each day (four to six weeks for endocarditis and two weeks for meningitis).

About 3 per cent of patients with gonorrhea may be in the incubation period of syphilis. The doses of procaine penicillin recommended for therapy of uncomplicated gonorrhea will cure incubating syphilis but will not cure established syphilis. Therefore serologic tests for syphilis should be performed prior to initiation of therapy in all patients treated for gonococcal infections. If the serologic test is positive, therapy for syphilis must be initiated. If the serologic test is negative, no follow-up tests are required if procaine penicillin is used to treat the gonorrhea. Ampicillin, spectinomycin, and tetracycline in the doses recommended for gonorrhea have not been shown to abort incubating syphilis. Therefore serologic tests for syphilis should be obtained monthly for four months after therapy for gonorrhea with these regimens.

Prevention. Use of a condom provides a high degree of protection for the uninfected partner. Past experience has indicated that prophylactic use of oral penicillin in a dose of 250,000 units within two to three hours after exposure markedly decreases the incidence of infection. Sexual partners of patients with gonorrhea should be identified and treated as quickly as possible to prevent further spread of disease.

The instillation of 1 per cent silver nitrate (Credé method) or an antimicrobial drug into the eyes of the newborn has largely eradicated gonococcal ophthalmia neonatorum.

Barr, J., and Danielsson, D.: Septic gonococcal dermatitis. Br. Med. J., 1:482, 1971.

Brown, W. J.: Trends and status of gonorrhea in the United States. J. Infect. Dis., 123:682, 1971.

Holmes, K. K., Counts, G. W., and Beaty, H. N.: Disseminated gonococcal infection. Ann. Intern. Med., 74:979, 1971.

Martin, J. E., Jr., and Lester, A.: Transgrow, a medium for transport and growth of *Neisseria gonorrhoeae* and *Neisseria meningitidis*. HSMHA Health Rep., 86:30, 1971.
Owen, R. L., and Hill, J. L.: Rectal and pharyngeal gonorrhea in homosexual men. J.A.M.A., 220:1315, 1972.
Pariser, H.: Asymptomatic gonorrhea. Med. Clin. North Am., 56:1127, 1972.
Schroeter, A. L., Turner, R. H., Lucas, J. B., and Brown, W. J.: Therapy for incubating syphilis. Effectiveness of gonorrhea treatment. J.A.M.A., 218:711, 1971.
Sparling, P. F.: Antibiotic resistance in *Neisseria gonorrhoeae*. Med. Clin. North Am., 56:1133, 1972.
Venereal Diseases Branch, State and Community Services Division, Center for Disease Control: Recommended treatment schedules for gonorrhea. Ann. Intern. Med., 76:991, 1972.
Vickers, F. N., and Maloney, P. J.: Gonococcal perihepatitis. Report of three cases with comments on diagnosis and treatment. Arch. Intern. Med., 114:120, 1964.
Wiesner, P. J., Tronca, E., Bonin, P., Pederson, H. B., and Holmes, K. K.: Clinical spectrum of pharyngeal gonococcal infection. N. Engl. J. Med., 288:181, 1973.

200. MENINGOCOCCAL DISEASE

Harry A. Feldman

Definition. Meningococcal infections may affect the upper and lower respiratory tracts, blood (meningococcemia), central nervous system (meningococcal meningitis, cerebrospinal fever, spotted fever, or epidemic cerebrospinal meningitis), joints (arthritis), heart, pericardium, eyes, skin, urethra, and other organs, singly or in any combination in a given patient. First recognized in 1805 by Vieusseux in Geneva and in 1806 by Danielson and Mann in Massachusetts, meningococcal meningitis, the best known form, occurs sporadically and as localized or widespread epidemics.

Etiology. *Neisseria meningitidis,* a gram-negative coccus, variable in size and occurring singly or as biscuit-shaped diplococci, was established as the causative agent by Weichselbaum in 1887. Metabolically fastidious, the organism grows best on enriched culture media at 37° C in an atmosphere of increased CO_2. Mueller-Hinton or meat infusion broths, or agar containing 10 per cent of blood (rabbit, sheep, or horse), or human ascitic fluid are excellent. Chocolate agar is especially good for initial isolation. Incorporating the vancomycin and colistin with or without nystatin (Thayer-Martin agar) makes this especially useful for isolation from throats or other areas of marked contamination. Cultures incubated in an atmosphere of 5 to 10 per cent carbon dioxide grow more luxuriantly, improving the isolation rate. Meningococci are very susceptible to chilling or drying, so all cultures should be inoculated and incubated promptly. Some meningococcal strains are exquisitely susceptible to sulfonamides so that media inoculated with specimens from such patients should have para-aminobenzoic acid (5 mg per 100 ml) added to them.

Identification of meningococci is based on morphology, Gram staining, fermentation of glucose and maltose but not sucrose, and immunologic reactions. The four classic immunologic groups, A, B, C, and D, have been expanded to include X, Y, Z, 29-E, and W-135. The most common are A, B, C, and Y. Group D is so rare that such identification is almost suspect. The groups are usually identified by their agglutination with specific antisera. A and C organisms are encapsulated so young cultures quell (capsular swelling) with specific antisera. This reaction is especially useful for the rapid, precise identification of such meningococci in cerebrospinal fluid, but requires potent antisera. Subgroups of B and C have been described, but the techniques are complex and the results are mainly of epidemiologic significance.

Lipopolysaccharides or "endotoxins" in purified form have been prepared from meningococci. Although these are toxic for animals and probably play significant roles in the pathogenesis of human disease, this remains to be defined. A true, group-specific exotoxin has not been demonstrated.

Epidemiology. Any discussion of the epidemiology of meningococcal infections is complicated by the multiplicity of serogroups. Sporadic infections may be seen almost constantly in all areas. Major epidemics are generally caused by Group A organisms and seem to occur in 20- to 30-year cycles. For example, during World Wars I and II there were massive civilian and military outbreaks which persisted for several years. Groups B and C produce lesser outbreaks, usually in the intervening years. The remaining groups are usually detected in carriers or sporadic cases, with Group Y the most frequent. Thus the over-all picture is that of high waves about every 20 to 30 years and lower ones in the interims. There are localized exceptions to this generalization. Detroit had a major Group A epidemic in 1929, with 724 cases reported in an eight-month period and a general mortality rate of 50 per cent. In infants, however, the mortality rate was 84 per cent, and in those over 40 years, 72 per cent. Santiago, Chile, had a severe Group A epidemic in 1941 to 1942 with 5885 cases; of these, 15.9 per cent were fatal. The contrasting mortality rates probably reflect the effectiveness of sulfonamide treatment.

In recent years the most devastated area has been that portion of Africa which lies below the Sahara and north of the Equator. This "meningitis belt" now averages about 10,000 cases per year with about 1200 deaths, but from 1939 to 1962 it reported 593,738 cases with 102,956 (17 per cent) deaths! In earlier outbreaks in the same area, as many as 85 per cent of cases were fatal. Here, as in South Africa, Group A organisms continue to predominate. The latter has also produced major outbreaks recently in Morocco, Finland, and Canada, but has been detected only rarely in the United States.

Infants and children are most frequently affected, about 60 per cent of cases occurring in those under 15 years. Military recruits for some unknown reason are especially vulnerable. About 80 per cent of their cases occur within the first 90 days of service, most often in the first month. The incidence of both cases and carriers is usually higher in males. Race and color do not seem to influence either incidence or susceptibility, but socioeconomic level does. The higher rates reported among blacks in certain urban areas probably reflect increased poverty with its concomitant crowding. The exact incubation period is often nondeterminable, but the range is probably one to ten days. There are a few instances in which this seems to have been longer—about three weeks.

The portal of entry of meningococci is the upper respiratory tract, and transmission from person to person occurs by direct or intimate contact, by airborne droplets, or by articles contaminated with fresh secretions from the respiratory tract. Mouth-to-mouth resuscitation has resulted in several cases in physicians, and in one instance nasopharyngeal carriage followed a kidney transplant from a donor who had died of meningococcemia. Yet even during severe epidemics, the majority of clinical infections seem to be unrelated to others, so that case-to-case spread is usually impossible to trace. Posterior nasopharyngeal culture surveys during outbreaks may demonstrate as much as 90 per cent of the population to be carriers of meningococci, constantly or intermittently, without clinical evidence of disease. Although the carrier rate often is less than 5 per cent during interepidemic periods, much of the population may harbor meningococci at some time, because the respiratory tract flora is constantly undergoing change.

Group A meningococci and, to a lesser extent, Group B and C strains have been the usual causes of epidemics in the past. Organisms of these groups were highly susceptible to sulfonamides so that such drugs were exceedingly effective for both the treatment of cases and mass prophylaxis. This changed in 1963 when sulfonamide-resistant Group B meningococci were noted to be prevalent. Subsequently, markedly resistant Group C strains were detected, and more recently, and perhaps even more disturbing, sulfonamide-resistant Group A strains first were isolated during an epidemic in North Africa, and subsequently in the "belt" below the Sahara, South Africa, Greece, Finland, Norway, Canada, Australia, and Southeast Asia. This phenomenon is now so widespread that all cases must be considered to be due to sulfonamide-resistant strains unless specifically proved to be otherwise. The same holds for carrier strains and for those of the other, less frequent, serogroups.

The physician is often concerned with the question of whether family members or other contacts of meningococcal patients are at excessive risk from this disease. Fortunately, secondary cases are unusual, but they do occur. In the Detroit epidemic of 1929, 4 per cent of cases were in affected households. In the Santiago epidemic of 1941–1942, the over-all secondary attack rate was 2.5 per cent. Because most of these follow within ten days (many four days) of the index case, they are often considered to be co-primaries. Acceptance of this concept leads to another control approach which will be dealt with subsequently (see Prevention). Household *carrier* rates, on the other hand, are high. In several studies of families of meningococcal patients, 45 to 50 per cent were found to be carrying organisms of the same group as the patient. These figures provide some justification for the anxieties of both families and physicians when cases occur which, unfortunately, cannot be resolved by the relatively simple procedure which was possible when sulfonamide-susceptible strains were the rule.

Pathogenesis and Pathology. In meningococcemia the essential lesion is vascular, with endothelial damage, inflammation of vessel walls with necrosis and thrombosis, and focal hemorrhages into cutaneous, subcutaneous, submucosal, and synovial tissues. In rapidly extending meningococcemia the Waterhouse-Friderichsen syndrome is often present. This is usually but not necessarily accompanied by bilateral adrenal hemorrhages.

Involvement of the central nervous system is characterized by acute purulent meningitis, although, if suspected early, there may be only hyperemia. Some degree of encephalitis usually accompanies the meningitis. When treatment is delayed or ineffective, permanent damage to some cranial nerves is to be expected.

The pathogenesis of meningococcal infections is usually initiated by the colonization of the posterior nasopharynx and adjoining structures by bacteria entering through the upper respiratory passages. Symptoms and signs of an acute upper respiratory infection may result, although this is not accepted by all observers. Invasion of the bloodstream follows, but this may be relatively asymptomatic. The resulting dissemination of the meningococci leads to metastatic lesions in skin, meninges, joints, eyes, ears, lungs, pericardium, urethra, and in other organs and tissues. The sites of these localizations determine the symptoms and signs that follow.

We are totally at a loss to explain why meningococcal infections are so limited and innocuous in some individuals and so extensive and overwhelming in others. No microbe can kill more quickly; deaths have been observed within several hours after the first symptom.

Chemical alterations reflecting the severity of the meningococcal infection may be profound. Their cause is not known, but it is assumed that to some degree they are endotoxic in origin. They may be furthered by the release of various substances from damaged tissue cells. Hemorrhagic manifestations may be owing to direct vascular damage because of a Shwartzman-like reaction, to thrombocytopenia, or to both. Other changes are those found in acute sepsis: fever, dehydration, reduction in blood volume, altered acid-base balance, and negative nitrogen balance. In severely ill patients, cyanosis, circulatory collapse, and other signs of shock appear, probably the result of the combined actions of bacterial endotoxins and tissue anoxia. Alterations suggestive of acute adrenal insufficiency, low serum sodium, elevated potassium, low chloride, and hypoglycemia may be present and are consistent with absent or diminished cortical secretion by damaged adrenal glands. There is no evidence that adrenal insufficiency as judged by the degree of excretion of corticosteroids in fulminating infections per se occurs independently of glandular destruction.

Clinical Manifestations. A sequential development of clinical manifestations of meningococcal infections can be discerned from a number of cases, but any one patient may present with symptoms and signs of advanced diffuse illness. The usual sequence consists of infection of the upper respiratory tract, bacteremia, septicemia, meningitis, and/or other metastatic localization. One stage will appear to dominate, giving the appearance of mild illness, grave illness, or none.

Infection of the Upper Respiratory Tract. The upper respiratory tract is the most frequent site of meningococcal infection. Most patients have no or inconsequential symptoms so that the organism is detectable only by culture of the posterior nasopharynx. Whether symptoms result from such colonization is contested by many observers, because descriptions of this stage usually have been derived from military recruits who also are subject to many viral and mycoplasmal respiratory infections. On the other hand, many but not all patients with meningococcal illnesses give histories of preceding or concurrent nasopharyngitis.

Meningococcemia. Bacteremic meningococcal infections may vary from acute fulminating illnesses of a few hours' duration to indolent, chronic infections lasting days, weeks, or, rarely, months. Symptoms may be relentlessly progressive or intermittent, with relapses and recrudescences at different times.

MILD OR SUBACUTE MENINGOCOCCEMIA. The most common form of meningococcemia is that of a relatively mild, acute, or subacute infection. Prodromal symptoms are frequently absent except for those of a mild upper respiratory infection in some. Onset is usually sudden, with fever, chilliness or frank chills that may be recurrent, malaise, myalgia, and apathy. The presenting symptoms may be any combination of these, but frequently the initial complaints are those of recurrent fever, rash, arthralgia, acute mono- or polyarthritis, nausea and vomiting, and conjunctivitis. The symptoms may regress or persist if the disease progresses. Fever may be remittent and irregular with spikes to 39 or 39.5° C. The pulse rate is proportionate to the fever. Respirations are usually normal or only slightly increased except when pneumonia or pleurisy is present.

The most striking feature on physical examination is the rash, which occurs often. It appears soon after onset, is variable (the severest is petechial or purpuric), measuring from 1 or 2 mm to 1 cm or more in diameter, and is pink to reddish blue (see accompanying figure). Early in the disease there may be a generalized, mottled erythema which appears dusky in slightly cyanotic patients. Light pink macules resembling the "rose spots" of typhoid, wheals, or nodules like erythema nodosum may appear before petechiae and ecchymoses. *Careful search in good daylight may be necessary to detect early lesions.* Occasionally, vesicular, pustular, or bullous lesions are present. Superficial or deep ulcerations may result from petechiae, especially when coalescent. These are sometimes very extensive and ultimately may require grafting. *The rash often appears first on the wrists and ankles,* but any area may be involved, including the conjunctivae and the mucous membranes. Hemorrhagic lesions fade to a brown, rusty color three or four days after their appearance; if new crops appear, often after chills, multiple skin lesions may be present at the same time. This is more likely when treatment is delayed or unsuccessful.

Other physical findings, including splenomegaly, are inconstant. Herpetic lesions of the lip are found in about 10 per cent of the cases. Unless meningismus develops, symptoms referable to the central nervous system are absent, although those resulting from metastatic localizations are usually self-evident, depending upon their site.

The firm diagnosis is established with laboratory aids. Leukocytosis up to 40,000 cells per cubic millimeter with 80 to 90 per cent neutrophils is almost always present. In overwhelming cases, gram-negative intracellular diplococci may be seen within leukocytes in stained smears from capillary blood, buffy coat, or directly from skin lesions. A blood culture positive for meningococci furnishes final etiologic proof. It should be emphasized that several cultures of the blood may be necessary to detect meningococci and that growth of the organism in liquid medium may be slow. Other laboratory examinations are either normal or compatible with any febrile illness.

The subsequent course is dependent on therapy, although some patients with very mild disease recover spontaneously after several weeks or months. Any of the complications and sequelae of meningococcal infections may develop.

ACUTE FULMINATING MENINGOCOCCEMIA. This differs from the milder form in the rapidity with which it progresses and in its overwhelming character. The onset is usually abrupt and quite dramatic, with a shaking chill, severe headache, dizziness or vertigo, collapse, or unconsciousness. Patients with massive purpura, low blood pressure, rapid, quiet respiration, and overwhelming bacteremia are said to have the Waterhouse-Friderichsen syndrome. They are often clear mentally. Their extensive rash (see figure) involves skin and mucous membranes as well as internal organs such as skeletal muscle and, classically, the adrenal glands. Leukopenia is another indicator of the gravity of the patient's condition. Body temperature may be subnormal, normal, or slightly elevated. Within a few hours there may be circulatory collapse with intravascular coagulation. Often there is a consumptive coagulopathy (see Ch. 201).

Others may have the encephalitic form, which is characterized by rapidly developing coma, rapid stertorous

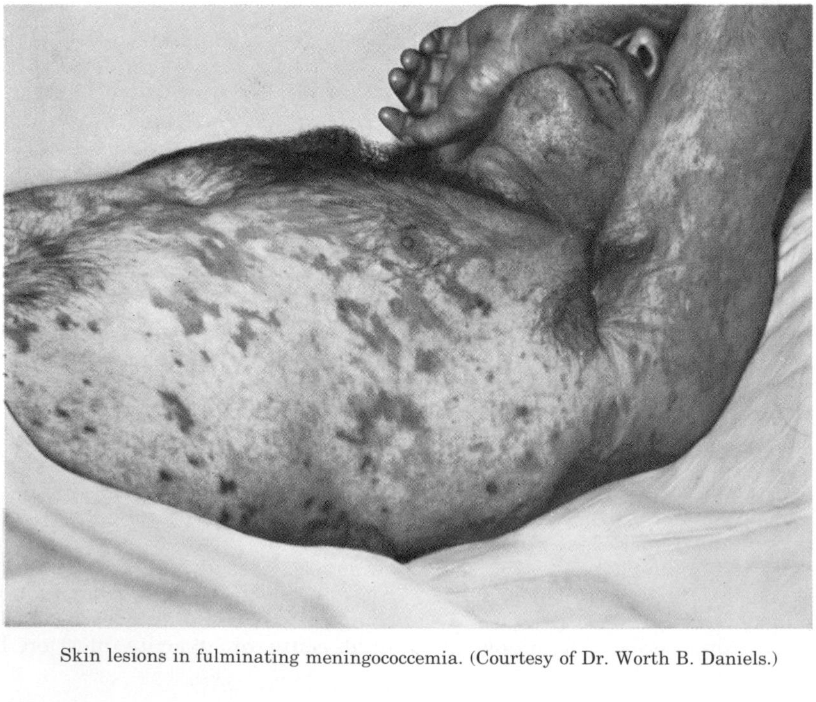

Skin lesions in fulminating meningococcemia. (Courtesy of Dr. Worth B. Daniels.)

breathing, a petechial but not massive purpuric rash, and normal blood pressure. Some may present with a combination of encephalitis and adrenal involvement with early deep coma, purpura, and low blood pressure. Occasionally, the pituitary gland, like the adrenals, is damaged by hemorrhage. These severe illnesses are often rapidly fatal. It is in the attempt to prevent or to reverse this rapid course that so much emphasis is placed upon early, intensive treatment.

CHRONIC MENINGOCOCCEMIA. Chronic meningococcemia is an uncommon form of meningococcal disease in which episodes of fever of a few days' duration recur at intervals of days, weeks, or more rarely, months. Chills and arthralgic symptoms are frequent, but rash may be absent or evanescent. Repeated cultures of the blood may be necessary before meningococci are recovered. Failure to suspect, recognize, and treat chronic meningococcemia may result in meningitis or endocarditis.

Meningitis. Although it constitutes only a relatively small percentage of the total number of meningococcal infections, meningitis is the most characteristic and important manifestation. The onset and symptoms are often indistinguishable from those of a generalized infection; in some, meningeal involvement seems to predominate. In others, both groups of symptoms appear almost simultaneously, but there may be great variations in their intensity and severity. In addition to the signs of sepsis and the rash, patients with meningitis have evidence of inflammation of the meninges: pain in the neck and back on forward flexion of the head, stiff neck, retraction of the head or severe opisthotonos, Kernig's and Brudzinski's signs, hyperesthesia, hyperirritability, and exaggerated reflexes. Unequal reflexes are unusual, but may be present. Involvement of the cranial nerves, when present, may result in strabismus and deafness. The increased intracranial pressure may lead to severe headache, nausea, vomiting, dilated or irregular pupils, engorgement of the fundal veins, choking of the discs, irregular slow pulse, and moderately elevated blood pressure. Cheyne-Stokes or Biot's respiration may appear. As the disease progresses, restlessness and irritability may be followed by delirium or by generalized or jacksonian type convulsions; the patient may become greatly depressed, somnolent, and finally stuporous and comatose. In infants the signs of meningitis may be no more than refusal of feedings, vomiting or regurgitation, diarrhea, irritability, and fever. Convulsions and bulging of the fontanelles, when present, are extremely useful signs.

LABORATORY FINDINGS IN MENINGITIS. The cerebrospinal fluid is under increased pressure and varies from clear to frankly purulent. The cell count is elevated, often to thousands per cubic millimeter, mostly neutrophils. Gram-negative intra- and extracellular diplococci can be seen in variable numbers in stained smears of the sediment. The total protein in the cerebrospinal fluid is increased, and its sugar content is usually reduced. Meningococci may be grown from the fluid by proper cultural methods. Fluid obtained early in meningitis may have few or no cells and no reduction of its glucose content, but cultures nonetheless will often be positive.

COURSE OF MENINGITIS. Extremely variable, the course is greatly influenced by therapy. In untreated cases the temperature is erratic, and symptoms progress to early death or to chronic meningitis with severe sequelae or delayed death.

Complications of Meningococcal Infections. The complications of the different forms of meningococcal infections include intercurrent infections, metastatic localizations, and permanent damage to the central nervous system. These may appear during the acute stage or subsequently. Intercurrent infections of the respiratory tract with other agents may occur. Bacteremic or metastatic complications include conjunctivitis, panophthalmitis, otitis, purulent mono- or polyarthritis, pneumonia, pleurisy, pericarditis, myocarditis, endocarditis, orchitis, epididymitis, jaundice, hepatorenal failure, transient albuminuria and hematuria, and adrenal hemorrhage with necrosis. Infection of the central nervous system may produce transient or permanent paralyses, hemiplegia, neuroradiculitis, encephalitis, encephalomyelitis, altered cerebration, convulsions, cranial nerve damage, cerebral thrombosis, and brain abscess. Organization of exudate in the ventricular channels and the subarachnoid space may mechanically obstruct the flow of cerebrospinal fluid, producing hydrocephalus. The accumulation of subdural fluid of high protein content, which when encapsulated resembles a subdural hematoma, is fairly frequent in infants and young children. Recurrent meningitis caused by meningococci or other bacteria is usually due to structural defects of bone resulting from trauma or other causes which sometimes require surgical repair. Complications resulting from therapy can be avoided or minimized, if anticipated.

Permanent sequelae may result from almost any complication; the most frequent are deafness, ocular palsies, blindness, changes in intellectual ability, psychoses, and hydrocephalus.

Diagnosis. The specific diagnosis of meningococcal disease depends primarily upon differentiation from other acute systemic and meningococcal infections. Final confirmation of the diagnosis requires bacteriologic identification of the causative organism as a meningococcus. During an epidemic, especially in a recruit military camp or a closed population, all cases of fever with abrupt onset, of prostration with or without fever, of petechial or purpuric rash, of drowsiness or coma, and of meningitis should be treated vigorously as meningococcal infections whether or not organisms are found in initial smears and cultures.

Meningococcal infections in their early stages may resemble any acute systemic infection. In sepsis caused by pyogenic organisms such as staphylococci, streptococci, or pneumococci, there may be a preceding upper respiratory infection, recurrent fever, malaise, arthralgia, and leukocytosis. A rash similar to that of severe meningococcemia and even signs of the Waterhouse-Friderichsen syndrome occasionally may be present in such cases. Final proof is accomplished by isolation of the offending organisms from the blood, joint fluid, sputum, and so forth. Meningococcal infections must also be differentiated from the acute exanthemata, typhus (both endemic and epidemic), typhoid and other enteric fevers, subacute bacterial endocarditis, rheumatic fever, brucellosis, and others.

Diagnosis of Meningitis. The diagnosis of meningococcal meningitis requires differentiation from meningismus, other bacterial meningitides, viral meningoencephalitis, myeloencephalitis resulting from bacterial toxins (tetanus, botulinus) or chemicals, and noninfectious problems such as subarachnoid or cerebral hemorrhages or thrombosis, diabetic coma, and uremia. In most cases of meningococcal meningitis, the diagnosis is readily established by the specific identification of the organism; in others the etiology may not be determinable when the patient is first seen, but a number of helpful procedures can be carried out. The usual medical history should be obtained, but a careful inquiry should be made into recent localized infections, especially of the ear, and trauma to the head, because these predispose to secondary bacterial meningitides, more likely to be caused by *H. influenzae* or pneumococci.

Physical examination should include a thorough search for diseases of the eyes and upper respiratory passages, sinuses, and ears and for evidence of injury to the head, in addition to careful general and neurologic examinations. A complete blood count should be made and cultures of the blood and posterior nasopharynx obtained. Any suspected localized areas of infection likewise should be cultured. Urinalysis and determinations of serum electrolytes and the blood nonprotein nitrogen may aid in the differential diagnosis and help to indicate precautions to be observed in therapy. In seriously ill, if not in all patients, blood coagulation analyses should be performed to determine the presence of a consumptive coagulopathy. Bleeding from the upper gastrointestinal tract ("stress ulcers") should be suspected in the very sick, especially those in shock.

Lumbar puncture should be performed as soon as possible and before specific treatment is instituted. After determining the initial pressure, fluid should be removed slowly until the pressure is reduced to an approximately normal level. The dynamics of the cerebrospinal fluid can then be estimated by jugular compression for evidence of block or sinus thrombosis. Examination of the cerebrospinal fluid should include the following: gross appearance, total and differential cell counts, determination of sugar (compare with blood level) and protein, and cultures and examination of Gram-stained smears. If organisms are seen, they can often be identified tentatively from their appearance and precisely with proper and *potent* antisera by a positive direct quellung test if of Group A or C.

A presumptive diagnosis can usually be made from the Gram-stained smear, the differential cell count, and the sugar content of the cerebrospinal fluid. Caution should be exercised in the interpretation of smears, because even experienced personnel may be misled by overdecolorized or dead gram-positive diplococci or other bacteria. Final identification depends on serogrouping organisms from culture. The leukocytes are almost entirely neutrophils in purulent meningitides, except syphilitic or tuberculous. In the latter, as in viral infections (mumps, herpes, coxsackieviruses, echoviruses, and others), mononucleated cells predominate except in their early stages. The sugar content is usually low in bacterial meningitis and normal in viral infections. In meningismus the fluid is usually normal. The proportion of erythrocytes to leukocytes is similar to that in whole blood in cases of subarachnoid hemorrhage. The history, other physical findings, and special laboratory tests should help to differentiate myeloencephalitides resulting from toxins or chemicals.

Treatment. During the past 30 years, Groups A, B, and C meningococci have been responsible for almost all meningococcal infections regardless of their clinical forms. Until about 1963 practically all meningococcal strains were exquisitely susceptible to the sulfonamide drugs, whether in carriers or cases. For these reasons, the sulfonamides were the agents of choice for both treatment and prophylaxis. They are still excellent, providing that one is certain that the patient or carrier has a sulfonamide-susceptible organism. Without suitable tests of the homologous strain, this assumption is no longer permissible.

Since sulfonamide-resistant Group A, B, C, and Y strains are now commonplace, the treatment of patients requires penicillin G in massive dosage. For adults, this means 20,000,000 units per day intravenously or 1,000,000 units every two hours intramuscularly. The latter should not be used for patients in, or on the verge of, shock. When the 20,000,000 unit dose is used intravenously, it is best to divide it into four or more doses per day rather than to administer it by continuous drip. Doses in children should be reduced in accordance with pediatric therapeutic principles.

Ampicillin may be used as an alternative, although an occasional patient does not seem to respond adequately to this drug. Close observation of the patient's course will alert the physician to this problem, should it arise. The dose should be at least 150 mg per kilogram per day for children and 10 to 12 grams per day for adults, parenterally, divided into six to eight doses.

In patients known to be truly allergic to penicillin, chloramphenicol is the alternative drug of choice. The use of this drug imposes precautions of its own. These can be managed, but close watch should be kept on the hematopoietic system and the drug withdrawn immediately if a complication appears. Thus far, no meningococci resistant to penicillin or chloramphenicol have been identified. If the patient's organism is found to be susceptible to sulfonamide, treatment can be altered accordingly. *Cephalothins and lincomycin should not be used, because therapeutic failures have followed their administration.*

Patients with meningococcal disease are usually more dehydrated than they appear. Care should be taken to ensure a daily urine output of more than 1000 ml. Treatment should be continued at least until all signs and symptoms have been normal for a minimum of two days and preferably for five. It may be stopped abruptly. Relapse occurs occasionally and requires prompt treatment.

Patients with fulminating meningococcemia or meningitis, or both, should be started on therapy as soon as the diagnosis is suspected and specimens obtained, without waiting for bacteriologic confirmation. Penicillin should be given by vein. (Patients allergic to penicillin are best treated with chloramphenicol.) The central venous pressure should be monitored and corrected as necessary. Disseminated intravascular coagulation when diagnosed should be managed as in any other disease state (see Ch. 201). Norepinephrine, intravenously, may be required to maintain blood pressure. Steroids are clearly required if there is evidence of adrenal collapse; such patients are managed as are those with acute adrenal insufficiency. Otherwise, there is no good evidence that steroids are of any positive value. These severely ill patients are the most likely ones to bleed from gastric lesions ("stress ulcers") which require special handling, contraindicating steroids. Intravenous infusions will be required to correct dehydration, but an excess should be avoided. Oxygen therapy should be instituted and maintained as long as cyanosis or dyspnea is present. Blood transfusions have not been shown to be of significant value in this type of circulatory failure.

Certain laboratory tests such as hematologic examinations should be repeated as aids in monitoring the patient's course. This is especially true for patients admitted with severe leukopenia or thrombocytopenia. Their reversal is of considerable prognostic importance. Blood cultures should be repeated if the fever persists or returns, for continued bacteremia suggests the presence of endocarditis or other metastatic localization. Repeat lumbar punctures are indicated if there is persistent increased intracranial pressure, failure to respond to adequate therapy, or relapse of meningitis.

Symptomatic and supportive treatment is essential for patients with meningococcal infections. Sedation should be minimal, yet sufficient to assure adequate rest but not to interfere with the assessment of the patient's course. Approximately one month of convalescence is required for complete recovery in most cases and even more for those with severe illnesses.

The treatment of complications of meningococcal infections is primarily that of the underlying disease. Should fever or signs of meningeal irritation reappear, then the most probable causes are recurrence of infection with the meningococcus because of inadequate treatment, drug fever, or superinfection with another organism. In such circumstances, the cerebrospinal fluid and blood should be re-examined and cultured. If the meningococcal infection has relapsed, intensive treatment should be reinstituted and maintained until the patient has fully recovered.

Prognosis. The prognosis in meningococcal infections has improved enormously because of the efficacy of the sulfonamides and penicillin. In untreated cases of meningococcemia and meningitis the mortality formerly varied from 20 to 90 per cent, averaging about 70 per cent. The introduction of serum therapy reduced this to about 50 per cent. With the sulfonamides the case fatality rate has been reduced to 5 to 10 per cent, depending upon age and complicating conditions. The recent recognition of sulfonamide-resistant meningococci has not altered this significantly, because cases can be treated as successfully with penicillin. Age is perhaps the most important factor in prognosis, for the greatest mortality, despite adequate therapy, occurs in those less than two or more than 40 years old. In the U. S. Army during World War II, the over-all mortality was slightly less than 5 per cent and, in some series, even below 1 per cent. More than 90 per cent of these cases were caused by sulfonamide-susceptible Group A strains. In addition to a most favorable age distribution in the Army, the excellent physical condition of patients, early diagnosis, and the prompt institution of effective therapy were probably responsible for this remarkable recovery rate. The prognosis is still poor in fulminating cases with abrupt onset, extensive cutaneous lesions, and circulatory collapse. In spite of rapid, intensive therapy, such cases frequently terminate fatally. Relapses, recurrences, and complications have been greatly reduced by specific treatment so that the prognosis for total recovery is generally good. *The most frequent permanent sequelae despite adequate treatment* are deafness, cranial nerve paralyses, mental deficiency, and, less often, blindness and hydrocephalus. These are all relatively uncommon and usually result from treatment delays for whatever cause.

Prevention. Prophylaxis as applied to meningococcal infections during the past 30 years represented an outgrowth of the World War II experience which demonstrated not only that sulfadiazine rapidly cured meningococcal disease but also that the nasopharyngeal carrier state was reversed soon after such treatment was begun. After several successful trials in military recruits, a policy was adopted whereby small amounts of sulfadiazine were administered simultaneously to all members of recruit training centers, schools, ships, and similar groups upon the recognition of a predetermined number of cases. This resulted in an immediate reduction in carriers, accompanied by a sharp decrease in cases. Thus was reflected the interaction of a susceptible organism with an effective drug when administered to a total population at risk.

Because of the fears often generated by the diagnosis of meningitis, the same sulfadiazine regimen was adopted for general use by physicians and health departments to treat family and hospital (staff) contacts of sporadic cases. But the "secondary" cases which occasionally occur in households usually begin within 96 hours or less of that of the index patient, suggesting that they are co-primary rather than secondary. Sometimes this interval is as long as 7 to 10 days. It would seem then that if *disease* is to be prevented under such circumstances, therapeutic rather than "prophylactic" medication is needed. Unless the causative strain is known to be sulfonamide susceptible, it must be assumed to be resistant, requiring penicillin for treatment with dosage in the therapeutic range. If taken orally, this will require 8 million or more units per day in young or older adults. Suitably reduced doses should be prescribed for children. Either oral or parenteral regimens for streptococcal prophylaxis provide *no* protection for meningococcal infections.

The recommendation for meningococcal disease is really for *intervention* rather than *prevention.* Alternatively, one can observe closely (including nasopharyngeal cultures) and treat immediately upon the appearance of any symptoms. But over-all, the risk is very low and should not induce the hysteria which so often accompanies the hospital admission or diagnosis of a case of meningococcal meningitis. The isolation of patients after 24 to 48 hours of adequate therapy is not indicated.

Although the foregoing is suitable for the immediate contact or family, it is not applicable to a population group such as in a camp, school, or mental institution. In such instances the objective is to rapidly reduce the overall carrier level to a point where transfer is impeded, decreasing the case rate. Again, sulfonamides are the most effective drugs for this purpose, but only when the causative organisms are susceptible. Penicillin, in contrast to sulfonamides, often fails to eliminate the carrier state, even in therapeutic doses. Both rifampin (600 mg daily for five days) and minocycline (200 mg, then 100 mg twice daily for five days), singly, sequentially, and together, have been used for this purpose in military units and in modified dosage in an elementary school population. Meningococcal carrier rates are reduced quite effectively, but resistance to rifampin does occur and increases with reuse. Some toxic effects have been noted, especially in children, so that additional experience will be required for further definition. Caution with regard to the widespread use of rifampin in populations with high tuberculosis rates is probably well advised because of possible increased resistance among tubercle bacilli. At no time should either rifampin or minocycline be used for the treatment of actual cases of meningococcal disease.

There is considerable reason for optimism regarding meningococcal vaccines. Potent group-specific polysaccharides have been prepared from meningococci of

Groups A and C, but not yet from B. After very careful graduated trials, Group C meningococcal polysaccharide vaccine was made a routine for all American military recruits in single subcutaneous doses of 50 μg. Disease caused by this serogroup has all but been eliminated from that population. Currently, field trials with Group A polysaccharide vaccine are under way, and the early results are encouraging. The duration of protection has not yet been established, nor has either effectiveness or usefulness been defined in children. Measurable responses to polysaccharide vaccines are quite different and less in children (especially under two years) than adults. No polysaccharide vaccine has been licensed, and thus such vaccines are not yet available for general use.

Artenstein, M. S., Gold, R., Zimmerly, J. G., Wyle, F. A., Schneider, H., and Harkins, C.: Prevention of meningococcal disease by Group C polysaccharide vaccine. N. Engl. J. Med., 282:417, 1970.

Evans, R. W., Glick, B., Kimball, F., and Lobell, M.: Fatal intravascular consumption coagulopathy in meningococcal sepsis. Am. J. Med., 46:910, 1969.

Feldman, H. A.: Neisseria infections other than gonococcal. *In* Bodily, H. L., Updyke, E. L., and Mason, J. O. (eds.): Diagnostic Procedures for Bacterial, Mycotic and Parasitic Infections. 5th ed. New York, American Public Health Association, Inc., 1970.

Feldman, H. A.: Meningococcal Infections. *In* Stollerman, G. H. (ed.): Advances in Internal Medicine. Vol. 18. Chicago, Year Book Medical Publishers, 1972, pp. 117–140.

Gotschlich, E. E., Goldschneider, I., and Artenstein, M. S.: Human immunity to the meningococcus. V. The effect of immunization with meningococcal Group C polysaccharide on the carrier state. J. Exp. Med., 129:1385, 1969.

201. BACTERIAL MENINGITIS

Robert G. Petersdorf

Definition. Meningitis is an inflammatory process involving the coverings of the central nervous system. Bacteria, viruses, spirochetes, parasites, and fungi may be the offending pathogens. This chapter is concerned with meningitis caused by bacteria other than meningococci and mycobacteria; these are discussed in Ch. 200 and 236, respectively.

Etiology. With the exception of *Mycobacterium tuberculosis,* the three most common microorganisms causing meningitis are *Diplococcus pneumoniae, Neisseria meningitidis,* and *Hemophilus influenzae.* The meningitis caused by *H. influenzae* is usually of type B and occurs uncommonly after the age of 6 and rarely after 12. When it occurs in adults, a deficiency in immune globulins, a parameningeal focus, or head trauma should be suspected. Meningococcal disease is found in both children and adults, but is rare after the age of 50. Pneumococcal meningitis is most common in infancy and old age. Other, less common pathogens are *Staphylococcus aureus,* which is usually found in association with epidural or brain abscess, in thrombosis of the cavernous sinus, or after cranial trauma and neurosurgical procedures; *Escherichia coli,* a common offender in meningitis in newborns; and other enteric organisms, including Proteus species, Klebsiella-Enterobacter, Paracolon, Salmonella, and Pseudomonas. Infection with Pseudomonas has followed lumbar puncture, spinal anesthesia, and the establishment of shunting procedures to relieve hydrocephalus. Gonococcal meningitis, which is quite indistinguishable from meningococcal infections, is being reported with increasing frequency. The group A Streptococcus, formerly a common offender, is now a relatively rare cause of meningitis, although enterococci and anaerobic streptococci continue to be isolated, primarily from patients with brain abscess and meningitis. Rarer organisms include *Listeria monocytogenes,* a small gram-positive rod resembling nonpathogenic diphtheroids; *Mima polymorpha,* a pleomorphic gram-negative organism that is difficult to differentiate on Gram stain (but not culture) from *H. influenzae* and *N. meningitidis;* and *Cl. perfringens* and *Past. multocida.*

Incidence. The precise incidence of bacterial meningitis is difficult to determine, because, except for meningococcal infections, meningitis is not reportable. There appears to be a decrease in incidence of all forms of meningitis except perhaps for *H. influenzae.* However, the mortality rate has remained relatively constant. This may reflect the susceptibility of aged or "poor risk" patients to meningeal infections. Like many infections, most forms of bacterial meningitis are more prevalent among individuals of low socioeconomic status.

Pathology. There is considerable variation in the pathologic picture, depending in part on the duration of the disease, the infecting organism, the resistance of the host, and the type and duration of therapy. Although bacterial meningitis is usually localized to the subarachnoid space, infections caused by viruses, spirochetes, parasites, and fungi are commonly complicated by cerebritis or encephalitis. In bacterial meningitis, grossly purulent exudate is present over the cortical and basal surfaces of the brain, and may invest the spinal cord as well. The pus is often localized to the cerebellopontine angles. Cortical phlebitis with its consequences of vascular congestion, thrombosis, and infarction may be prominent findings. Microscopically, exudate consisting of several hundred layers of polymorphonuclear leukocytes is present over the surface of the brain and in the ventricular system, where the pus may produce noncommunicating hydrocephalus. Occasionally, the exudate penetrates the arachnoid, forming a subdural empyema. Although migration of inflammatory cells into subjacent neuronal tissue and necrosis of nerve cells may occur, in general, the meninges provide remarkable protection to the neurons, which are usually spared from the inflammatory process and invasion by bacteria.

Pathogenesis. The routes by which microorganisms penetrate the blood–cerebrospinal fluid barrier and establish infection in the subarachnoid space have not been clearly defined. In a number of instances, bacterial meningitis follows infection of the middle ear, mastoid, paranasal sinuses, and trauma or surgery to the face and head. In these instances, it seems likely that bacteria enter through a rent in the leptomeninges or that infection in a neighboring focus may render the meninges more permeable to microorganisms. Pneumococci, streptococci, staphylococci, and (more rarely) *H. influenzae* and gram-negative enteric bacilli have been implicated in this type of meningitis. Meningococci, which are usually carried in the nasopharynx, have been assumed to ascend to the meninges via the small venules and via arachnoid sheaths investing the olfactory nerves and accompanying them through the lamina cribrosa. However, there is no direct evidence for this route of infection in man. It has been postulated that infection emanating from distant foci, such as pneumococcal meningitis that follows pneumonia, or infection without a primary focus, is blood borne. In laboratory animals, bacteremia is not associated with meningitis unless the meninges are subjected to microtrauma (in the form of needle puncture) at the height of bacteremia. It is conceivable that this situation exists in man and that a microscopic defect in the meninges is a prerequisite for entry of bacteria from the blood. Occasionally, meningitis follows the rupture of a brain abscess. Anaerobic streptococci, enterococci, staphylococci, mixtures of bacteria, and actinomycetes may be isolated under these circumstances.

Clinical Manifestations. *History.* Most patients with meningitis report fever, lethargy, confusion, headache, vomiting, or stiff neck. The mode of onset may vary. Some patients rapidly develop headache, confusion, and loss of consciousness within 24 hours; they usually do not have antecedent respiratory symptoms. Others complain of headache, fever, and stiff neck associated with otitis, rhinorrhea, sore throat, or cough for one to seven days prior to the appearance of the full clinical picture. Still others have symptoms referable to the respiratory tract for several weeks before meningitis sets in. *Cough* is a common symptom in pneumococcal meningitis which is often accompanied by pneumonia; *earache* often antedates infection with *H. influenzae,* and a *sore throat* may precede neisserial meningitis. Other symptoms of bacterial meningitis include backache, weakness, dizziness, ataxia, photophobia, and generalized myalgias. Additional clues are a history of sickle cell disease, a common accompaniment of pneumococcal meningitis in children; previous or recent infection or surgery involving the nose, throat, or sinuses; head trauma; recent lumbar puncture or spinal anesthesia; and close and intimate contact with a patient who has a meningococcal infection.

Physical Findings. Most patients demonstrate the signs of meningeal irritation, i.e., stiff neck and positive Kernig or Brudzinski signs. Patients without these signs are often very young, very old, or severely obtunded. A *petechial eruption* is relatively rare in meningitis caused by bacteria other than meningococci unless bacterial endocarditis is present. There may be physical signs of pneumonia, particularly in patients with pneumococcal meningitis, and evidence of aural infection may also be found. Often, however, a primary focus (otitis, mastoiditis, sinusitis, pneumonia, or empyema) is not apparent on physical examination and should be carefully sought by other means, because failure to eradicate the primary focus may result in failure of therapy or post-treatment relapse. Although intracranial pressure is characteristically elevated, papilledema is rare. When it is encountered in the course of acute bacterial meningitis, it should call to mind the possibility of subdural empyema, brain abscess, or venous sinus thrombosis. The level of consciousness in most patients with meningitis may vary from confusion and mild lethargy to deep coma. About 10 to 15 per cent are remarkably alert. In approximately 50 per cent, however, other signs of neurologic damage develop during the course of infection. These include major motor seizures, hemipareses, which are often transient and probably postictal, signs of diffuse central nervous system damage (bilateral Babinski signs and fixed, mid-stage pupils), or paresis of the second, third, sixth, seventh, and eighth cranial nerves.

Associated Disease. With the exception of epidemics of meningococcal meningitis, which are usually confined to closed environments such as army camps or schools, bacterial meningitis occurs sporadically, usually in a setting of some associated disease. Pharyngitis antedates meningitis in many patients with meningococcal and Hemophilus infection. Otitis with or without mastoiditis, although much rarer nowadays than 20 years ago, remains an important precursor of Hemophilus and pneumococcal meningitis, which is also frequently associated with pneumonia. Pneumonitis is also often present in meningitis caused by gram-negative pathogens. A number of patients with pneumococcal meningitis have multiple myeloma; patients with this neoplasm are generally prone to recurrent pneumococcal infections. A similar propensity has been described for children with sickle cell disease. In addition to the common meningeal pathogens, meningitis in patients with diabetes mellitus is likely to be caused by uncommon organisms such as Klebsiella-Enterobacter, and *Staphylococcus aureus.* Enteric bacteria not uncommonly are seen in meningeal infections among patients with leukemias or lymphomas. Cranial trauma may precede meningitis by several days and occasionally months or years; in such instances *D. pneumoniae,* hemolytic *Staph. aureus,* or coliform bacteria are usually the offending organisms. Cranial osteomyelitis may intervene between head trauma and the development of meningitis. Patients undergoing shunt procedures for relief of hydrocephalus tend to have infections with bacteria that are ordinarily not pathogenic such as *Staphylococcus epidermidis* or micrococci; gram-negative enteric bacterial and Pseudomonas meningitis also complicate shunting procedures. Occasionally, subcutaneous or mucosal infections such as furunculosis, decubitus ulcers, omphalitis in neonates, and endometritis precede leptomeningitis.

Rare Types of Meningitis. MIMA POLYMORPHA MENINGITIS. *Mima polymorpha* is a gram-negative pleomorphic bacillus that is easily confused on Gram stain with members of the Neisseria group and *H. influenzae.* It can be separated from these organisms, however, by cultural and serologic techniques. Meningitis caused by *Mima polymorpha* closely resembles meningitis caused by the more common pathogens and cannot be differentiated from them on clinical grounds. Separation of mimae from Neisseria is of more than academic importance because mimae may be resistant to penicillin and sulfonamides and respond only to the tetracyclines.

LISTERIA MENINGITIS. The most common clinical illness caused by Listeria is meningitis, and any patient with clinical and laboratory evidence of meningeal infection said to be caused by a diphtheroid should be assumed to harbor Listeria in the cerebrospinal fluid. Clinically, the illness cannot be distinguished from meningitis caused by other bacteria (see Ch. 222).

OTHER ORGANISMS. Bacteria that have caused infections usually in patients with antecedent head trauma or neurosurgical procedures include *Cl. perfringens* and *Past. multocida,* although any organism can occasionally produce infection in this setting.

Recurrent Meningitis. Recurrent bouts of meningitis are most frequently related to remote as well as to recent head trauma. The individual episodes are usually caused by the same bacterial species that are associated with meningitis occurring in the absence of trauma, except that pneumococci of higher serologic types are isolated most commonly, and may account for 80 per cent of these infections. Bouts of meningitis may be separated by an interval of several years. Cerebrospinal fluid rhinorrhea owing to a defect in the cribriform plate is often associated with recurrent meningeal infection. These patients also usually have evidence of a recent or remote skull fracture involving the frontal bone. All patients with repeated bouts of meningitis should be subjected to vigorous search for a communication between the subarachnoid space and the nasopharynx. This should include laminagrams of the frontal and ethmoid bones, and instillation of radioiodinated albumin or a dye such as indigo carmine intrathecally, followed by testing for these substances in nasal secretions. Testing these secretions with glucose oxidase (Dextrostix) may give a positive test, connoting CSF rhinorrhea.

Rarer situations predisposing to recurrent meningeal infections include chronic mastoiditis or petrositis, congenital abnormalities of the cranial vault, and congenital dermoid sinus tracts. Ventriculomastoid shunts aimed at relief of hydrocephalus are also complicated by recurrent infections, which are often heralded by otitis media. Recurrent bouts of meningitis have been reported in children who have undergone splenectomy; this does not appear to be true of adults. Nor is there evidence that the incidence of meningitis is increased in children with hypo- or dysgammaglobulinemia.

Infections with Multiple Organisms. Meningitis caused by two or more organisms occasionally occurs in infants, young children and neonates, who may develop brain abscesses after surgery or birth trauma. *H. influenzae* is usually one of the organisms, and has been found in conjunction with *N. meningitidis, D. pneumoniae,* group A Streptococcus, and *E. coli.* In adults infections with multiple organisms most commonly follow rupture of a brain abscess into the subarachnoid space, and streptococci, staphylococci, and gram-negative enteric pathogens may all be isolated from the same specimen of cerebrospinal fluid.

Complications of Bacterial Meningitis. *Disseminated Intravascular Coagulation.* This syndrome, which is also called consumptive coagulopathy, is manifested by multiple petechiae, ecchymoses, purpura, bleeding from other surfaces, hypotension progressing to shock, and gangrene of distal extremities (see Ch. 200).

Although fulminant meningococcemia (with or without meningitis) is an important cause of disseminated intravascular coagulation (DIC), other gram-negative infections (particularly when accompanied by endotoxin shock), pneumococcal bacteremia in asplenic patients, Rocky Mountain spotted fever, disseminated herpes and congenital rubella, and falciparum malaria are among the other infectious causes of this syndrome. (See also Ch. 801.)

Clinical manifestations of DIC are due to the consumption of platelets and clotting factors and the anticoagulant effects of fibrin degradation products, leading to actual or potential bleeding; the deposition of fibrin, resulting in capillary thrombosis and ischemic infarction; and the distribution of red cells, leading to microangiopathic hemolytic anemia. Treatment should be directed at the underlying meningococcal infection.

Temporal and Cerebellar Herniation. These complications are commonly found in fatal meningitis, and may be recognized by distinct respiratory, ocular, and motor signs that indicate loss of diencephalic, midbrain, pontine, and medullary function in an orderly rostral-caudal sequence. In the presence of these signs, repeated lumbar punctures should be avoided.

Endocarditis. Endocarditis, most often involving the aortic valve, is found in 10 to 15 per cent of fatal cases of pneumococcal meningitis. Pneumonia is also frequent in this setting. Rheumatic or congenital valvular disease may antedate development of endocarditis, but frequently normal valves are involved. Staphylococci and coliform organisms and gonococci may also be the cause of the endocarditis-meningitis syndrome. Endocarditis may be difficult to detect clinically but should be seriously considered in patients with meningitis, pneumococcal, staphylococcal, gonococcal, and coliform bacteremia, and heart murmurs. The appearance of an aortic diastolic murmur when none was present previously is diagnostic of endocarditis in this setting.

Purulent Arthritis. Purulent arthritis may complicate pneumococcal, meningococcal, and staphylococcal meningitis. In general, it responds to antimicrobials, although aspiration of synovial fluid may be necessary.

Subdural Effusions. Subdural effusions have been a frequently reported complication of Hemophilus meningitis, but may also follow other types of meningitis in children. Prolonged unexplained fever, confusion despite adequate antimicrobial therapy, and convulsions after the apparent subsidence of infection are classic manifestations of accumulating subdural fluid that is usually sterile. Aspiration of this fluid, which may need to be repeated, results in relief of symptoms.

Neurologic Residua. Residual damage to the nervous system occurs in 10 to 20 per cent of patients, and is most common after pneumococcal meningitis in adults and *H. influenzae* meningitis in children. *Deafness* remains the most common sequel of pyogenic meningitis; hemiparesis, convulsive disorders, and dementia are seen occasionally.

Diagnosis. *General Considerations.* The diagnosis of bacterial meningitis is not difficult, provided a high index of suspicion is maintained. Meningeal infection should be considered in every patient with a history of upper respiratory illness interrupted by vomiting, headache, lethargy, confusion, or stiff neck. When first seen, some of these patients present only with low-grade fever, mild headache, or occasional emesis. Nevertheless, the possibility of meningeal infection must be carefully considered. In patients with pneumonia it is particularly dangerous to ascribe confusion to age or "toxemic" depression. Meningitis may be present in addition to pulmonary infection, and the dosage of antimicrobial drug used to to treat pneumonia is often inadequate to control meningeal infection. The susceptibility of alcoholics to pneumococcal meningitis cannot be emphasized too strongly, and may be related to the high prevalence of pneumonia in this group. Fever and confusion in these patients should not be attributed to alcoholic intoxication, delirium tremens, or hepatic encephalopathy unless the cerebrospinal fluid has been examined.

Two unusual types of recurrent meningitis may mimic bacterial infection, at least initially. *Mollaret's meningitis* consists of recurrent febrile attacks, malaise, headache, and meningeal signs accompanied by a marked polymorphonuclear inflammatory reaction in the CSF. Attacks last two to three days and subside spontaneously. *Behçet's syndrome* is characterized by recurrent oral and genital ulcerations and relapsing ocular lesions along with meningitis. Other neurologic abnormalities may include cranial nerve palsies, seizures, hemiparesis, extrapyramidal signs, and chronic brain syndromes.

Cerebrospinal Fluid. The cerebrospinal fluid should be examined in any patient with evidence of meningeal irritation. In patients with papilledema or other evidence of elevated cerebrospinal fluid pressure, lumbar puncture should be performed with care, employing a small-gauge needle. Papilledema does not constitute a contraindication to lumbar puncture in patients in whom the diagnosis of meningitis is suspected. The cerebrospinal fluid pressure is usually elevated, and the gross appearance of the fluid may vary from slight turbidity to gross pus. The fluid should be centrifuged immediately, and the sediment stained by Gram's method and cultured on blood and chocolate agar under increased CO_2 tension and anaerobically in thioglycollate. Some common pitfalls encountered in Gram staining include washing the organisms off the slide, decolorizing gram-positive bacteria, and interpreting particles of stain as bacteria. Nevertheless, carefully performed Gram stains are accurate in 90 per cent of cases in which organisms are seen. Pneumococci are more easily identified than meningococci. Although immunofluorescent techniques have been used to expedite the diagnosis in a variety of bacterial meningitides, they appear to be no more accurate than a well-performed Gram stain. The cause of pneumococcal, meningococcal, and *H. influenzae* meningitis may be determined by counterimmunoelectrophoresis. However, this technique requires potent antisera for accurate results.

The number of cells in the cerebrospinal fluid is always elevated and varies between 100 and 100,000 per cubic millimeter. Initially, polymorphonuclear leukocytes predominate; these are replaced by lymphocytes as the inflammatory process progresses. Early in the infection one may find a plethora of bacteria with only a few cells. This is particularly true in pneumococcal and staphylococcal infections.

A low cerebrospinal fluid sugar is the hallmark of bacterial meningitis, and distinguishes it from the viral meningitides. Usually the value is below 40 mg per 100 ml and may be close to 0. Patients who have diabetes mellitus or who are receiving intravenous infusions of glucose may have falsely high glucose values. However, the ratio of blood to cerebrospinal fluid sugar in these patients is always higher than the normal value of 1.5 to 1. For example, a cerebrospinal fluid sugar of 150 mg per 100 ml in the presence of a blood sugar of 500 mg per 100 ml is highly significant. The information obtained from blood sugar, which should be obtained routinely at the time of initial lumbar puncture, is frequently critical.

The protein content of the cerebrospinal fluid is generally elevated and may be as high as 800 mg per 100 ml. Higher values are usually obtained in pneumococcal meningitis than in infections with other pathogens. The development of subarachnoid block is usually heralded by very high CSF protein values (800 to 1500 mg per 100 ml).

Other Cultures. Blood cultures should be obtained routinely in patients suspected of having meningitis; they are positive in approximately 50 per cent of cases. Occasionally, when the cerebrospinal fluid cultures are negative, the blood cultures may provide the only clue to the etiologic agent. Nose, throat, and ear cultures may not reflect the meningeal pathogen and are misleading too often to be of more than ancillary value in diagnosis.

Roentgenographic Studies. All patients with meningitis should have roentgenograms of the chest, skull, mastoid, and paranasal sinuses as soon as their condition permits. Frequently these provide the clue to the portal of entry of the pathogen. Eradication of these foci with antimicrobial therapy or surgical drainage may be essential for control of the meningeal infection. When a mass lesion is suspected, brain scan and arteriography should be performed.

Other Laboratory Tests. Most patients with meningitis are sufficiently ill to warrant determination of blood urea nitrogen and serum electrolytes, particularly because water intoxication and severe hyponatremia are not uncommon. Blood sugar should be determined routinely (best in conjunction with determination of the cerebrospinal fluid sugar). Lactic dehydrogenase and its isozymes are elevated in bacterial meningitis. Most of this increase is due to a rise in fractions representing leukocytes, but a rise in LDH isozyme fractions emanating from brain occurs only in patients who die or who are destined to develop neurologic sequelae.

Prognosis. Untreated meningitis is almost always fatal. Antimicrobial therapy has dramatically improved the outlook for patients with meningeal infections. However, except for recurrent pneumococcal meningitis in which the prognosis is remarkably good, the mortality in adequately treated pneumococcal meningitis remains between 10 and 70 per cent, and 50 per cent of infections with staphylococci and gram-negative enteric bacilli are lethal. On the other hand, the mortality rate associated with meningococcal and *H. influenzae* meningitis is less than 10 per cent. In addition to the difference in prognosis engendered by different microorganisms, factors that adversely influence outcome include (1) improper or delayed diagnosis, usually a consequence of falsely attributing confusion or delirium to "toxemic" depression of the central nervous system or hepatic encephalopathy; (2) fulminating infection with rapid loss of consciousness; (3) bacteremia; (4) old age or the neonatal period; (5) certain underlying and complicating illnesses, including bacterial endocarditis, brain abscess, diabetes mellitus, and pneumonia; and (6) development of coma, localizing neurologic signs, and convulsions.

Treatment. *Choice of Therapy.* Antimicrobials are the mainstay of therapy in bacterial meningitis and should be administered parenterally at the earliest possible moment. If the Gram stain of the cerebrospinal fluid reveals the causative microorganism, specific treatment may be instituted from the beginning. However, if microscopy of the stained smear has been inconclusive, the initial therapy must be sufficiently broad to be fully effective against the most reasonable possibilities. For example, purulent meningitis in an adult without evidence of an overt portal of entry is most apt to be pneumococcal or meningococcal; in a young child, *H. influenzae* must also be considered. Primary staphylococcal meningitis would be rare in a previously healthy adult, but should be considered in a long-hospitalized patient, particularly if neurosurgery has been performed.

Penicillin is the drug of choice for pneumococcal and meningococcal meningitis, and should be administered parenterally in a dosage of 10 to 20 million units a day. For patients who are sensitive to penicillin, chloramphenicol in dosage of 4.0 to 6.0 grams per day should be used. The cephalosporins enter even the inflamed meninges poorly and should not be used for the treatment of meningitis.

There is still considerable debate whether *H. influenzae* meningitis should be treated with chloramphenicol (4.0 to 6.0 grams a day) or ampicillin (6.0 to 12.0 grams a day). Both drugs are probably equally effective, but ampicillin has the additional advantage of being bactericidal for pneumococci and meningococci. Use of this agent should, for all practical purposes, eliminate multiple drug therapy in "undiagnosed meningitis." A few "ampicillin failures" have been reported in children with *H. influenzae* meningitis. These were probably related to inadequate dosage or poor absorption of the drug, although a few resistant strains of *H. influenzae* have been reported. Staphylococcal meningitis should always be treated with one of the penicillinase-resistant penicillins, e.g., methicillin, oxacillin, or nafcillin in dosage of 6.0 to 12.0 grams parenterally. For the rare cases of meningitis caused by the Enterobacteriaceae or Pseudomonas, gentamicin in dosage of 5 mg per kilogram parenterally plus 4 to 8 mg intrathecally is the regimen of choice.

In patients with mastoiditis, an infected ventriculomastoid shunt, or cranial osteomyelitis, surgical attack on these primary foci while the patient is receiving appropriate antimicrobial therapy is indicated, but may be postponed until the acute meningeal episode is over.

Duration of Therapy. The duration of antimicrobial therapy in meningitis cannot be prescribed categorically. The cerebrospinal fluid should be examined every 24 to 48 hours during the early days of therapy, but once the patient is recovering, the intervals between lumbar puncture may be as long as a week, and numerous examinations of the CSF are rarely necessary. In the absence of extrameningeal foci, a seven- to ten-day course of antimicrobial therapy should suffice.

Other Measures. If there is evidence of increased intracranial pressure, and supratentorial or cerebellar herniation, therapy with mannitol, urea, or dexamethasone should be instituted. Adrenal cortical hormones also have been used as an adjunct to antimicrobial therapy, but have not resulted in noteworthy improvement. They should never be used unless the etiologic organism has been clearly identified and the appropriate drug is being administered. There have been some enthusiastic reports about proteolytic enzymes in the treatment of pneumococcal meningitis, but these agents have not been evaluated in sufficient detail to recommend their general use.

Other supportive therapy includes administration of adequate but not excessive parenteral fluids and anticonvulsants when indicated. Sedation should be employed with caution, even for delirious patients; of the many agents available, paraldehyde continues to be safe and effective.

Barrett, F. F., Taber, L. H., Morris, C. R., Stephenson, W. B., Clark, D. J., and Yow, M. D.: A 12 year review of the antibiotic management of *Hemophilus influenzae* meningitis. J. Pediatr., 81:370, 1972.

Beaty, H. N., and Oppenheimer, S.: CSF lactic dehydrogenase and its isoenzymes in infections of the central nervous sytem. N. Engl. J. Med., 279:1197, 1968.

Carpenter, R. R., and Petersdorf, R. G.: The clinical spectrum of bacterial meningitis. Am. J. Med., 23:262, 1962.

Coonrod, D. J., and Rytel, M. W.: Determination of aetiology of bacterial meningitis by counterimmunoelectrophoresis. Lancet, 1:1154, 1972.

Hand, W. L., and Sanford, J. P.: Post-traumatic bacterial meningitis. Ann. Intern. Med., 72:869, 1970.

Harter, D. H., and Petersdorf, R. G.: A consideration of the pathogenesis of bacterial meningitis: Review of experimental and clinical studies. Yale J. Biol. Med., 32:280, 1960.

Mangi, R. J., Kundargi, R. S., Quintiliani, R., and Andriole, V. T.: Development of meningitis during cephalothin therapy. Ann. Intern. Med., 78:347, 1973.

Oppenheimer, S. J., O'Toole, R. D., and Petersdorf, R. G.: Bacterial meningitis: *In* Shy, G. M., Goldensohn, E. S., and Appel, S. H. (eds.): The Cellular and Molecular Basis of Neurological Disease. Philadelphia, Lea & Febiger (in press).

Rahal, J. J.: Treatment of gram-negative bacillary meningitis in adults. Ann. Intern. Med., 77:295, 1972.

Rapaport, S. I.: Defibrination syndromes. *In* Williams, W. E., Beutler, E., Erslev, A. J., and Rundles, R. W. (eds.): Hematology. New York, McGraw-Hill Book Company, 1972.

Snyder, S. N., and Brunjes, S.: *H. influenzae* meningitis in adults. Am. J. Med. Sci., 250:658, 1965.

Swartz, M. N., and Dodge, P. R.: Bacterial meningitis—a review of selected aspects. N. Engl. J. Med., 272:725, 779, 842, 898, 954, 1003, 1965.

202. HEMOPHILUS INFLUENZAE INFECTIONS

Walsh McDermott

Although principally a pathogen for young children, *H. influenzae* may occasionally cause serious disease in the adult. In addition, the microbe is frequently present as a secondary "invader" in chronic obstructive lung disease and has played a similar role in the past in epidemics of presumed viral influenza. Virtually all severe primary infections are caused by serotype b, although other types may be present in the secondary "invader" role. The microbe is recognized as the most frequent cause of purulent meningitis in children; it is also the cause of a form of croup known as *obstructive laryngitis with epiglottitis.* Both conditions are quite serious. The *meningitis* is described in Ch. 201. The *laryngitis/epiglottitis* presents quite a characteristic picture. The onset is sudden and the course fulminating. Mild fever and dysphagia develop during an apparently innocuous respiratory infection. Dyspnea starts abruptly, and laryngeal obstruction requiring tracheotomy develops. High fever develops along with laryngeal redness and edema, and when the tongue is pressed downward, the enlarged, distorted, red, and edematous epiglottis is easily seen.

The diagnosis of an *H. influenzae* infection can be made rapidly by microscopy of Gram-stained smear or the demonstration of capsular swelling (quellung) of bacterial cells found in the appropriate biologic fluid. For initial culture, chocolate agar incubated in a candle jar may be used. Further cultural studies may be necessary of autoclaved blood agar, or yeast agar extract.

Therapy of the laryngitis/epiglottitis in children should be prompt and should include tracheostomy and appropriate antimicrobial therapy. Treatment of the meningitis is discussed in Ch. 201. Ampicillin, tetracycline, and chloramphenicol are all effective agents. As it has not been possible to demonstrate the superiority of any one drug in clinical trials (Nelson et al., 1972; Barrett et al., 1972), it seems advisable to use ampicillin.

Another disease caused by Hemophilus is *chancroid,* which is a localized venereal disease caused by *H. ducreyi.* It is characterized by painful, nonindurated ulceration involving the genitalia, accompanied by enlargement and suppuration of regional lymph nodes. Early syphilis often occurs simultaneously with chancroid. Tetracycline and erythromycin are both quite active against *H. ducreyi;* they have the disadvantage that conceivably they could mask a concurrent initial syphilis. Careful attention must be paid to the possibility of syphilis; otherwise, sulfadiazine should be used in the treatment of chancroid.

H. parainfluenzae, another member of the Hemophilus species, is an occasional cause of bacterial endocarditis.

Nelson, K. E., Levin, S., Spies, H. W., and Lepper, M. H.: Treatment of *Hemophilus influenzae* meningitis: A comparison of chloramphenicol and tetracycline. J. Infect. Dis., 125:459, 1972.

203. WHOOPING COUGH (Pertussis)

Stephen I. Morse

Definition. Whooping cough is an acute respiratory illness that classically affects infants and young children. The etiologic agent is usually *Bordetella pertussis;* occasionally *B. parapertussis* and rarely *B. bronchiseptica* produce a similar syndrome. The descriptive name derives from a distressing, prolonged inspiratory effort that follows paroxysmal coughing. Whooping cough is still responsible for a significant number of deaths in infants in areas where pertussis immunization is not practiced.

History. The disease was first recorded in the middle of the sixteenth century by Moulton and by DeBaillou. Whether whooping cough was indigenous to Europe or had been transported there in the preceding century is uncertain. Sydenham applied the name "pertussis" to any illness accompanied by violent coughing, but the term became restricted to the epidemic disease that was a well-recognized clinical entity by the middle of the eighteenth century. In 1900 Bordet and Gengou observed coccobacilli in the sputum of a child with whooping cough, but it was not until 1906 that they were able to culture the organism. Many years passed before the Bordet-Gengou bacillus was universally accepted as the etiologic agent of whooping cough. *B. pertussis* undergoes marked biologic and morphologic changes on prolonged cultivation, thereby accounting for the difficulties in establishing the etiologic role of the agent and the inconstant protective effect of immunizing preparations. Although the mortality rate of whooping cough in the United States began to decline in the early part of this century, the incidence in young children did not significantly decrease until after the use of prophylactic vaccines became widespread.

Etiology. When first isolated, *Bordetella pertussis* is a minute, nonmotile, weakly staining, gram-negative coccobacillus, 0.5 to 1.0 μ in length. Capsules can be demonstrated by special procedures, and bipolar metachromatic granules are present. The complex medium containing blood originally employed by Bordet and Gengou is still often used for cultivation. Primary isolates, phase I organisms, will not grow on conventional laboratory media, but will do so after prolonged passage. At the same time colonial morphology changes, marked pleomorphism of individual cells is evident, and there is an alteration in antigenic composition. The change from phase I to phase IV has been likened to the smooth to rough transition of other microbes. Only phase I organisms are virulent, and only phase I organisms provide effective immunizing material.

Members of the Bordetella genus were formerly regarded as species of Hemophilus. However, the Bordetella group does not have the strict requirement for X and V growth factors, and they are antigenically distinct. The addition of blood to Bordet-Gengou medium is required for the growth of phase I organisms, but the blood acts to neutralize bactericidal substances, probably fatty acids, rather than to provide nutrients. Charcoal, starch, or ion exchange resins can be substituted for blood.

B. pertussis produces a heat-stable toxin (endotoxin) and a heat-labile toxin. A role of toxins in the development of disease has not been demonstrated. A hemagglutinin has also been isolated. The capsular material does not swell in the presence of antiserum. A species agglutinogen has been recognized as well as agglutinating factors that differ between strains. Serotyping is therefore a useful epidemiologic tool. The role of the interaction between the organism and phagocytes has not been defined, although the presence of antisera appears to increase uptake of *B. pertussis* by leukocytes.

Remarkable biologic effects are induced in laboratory animals by the injection of killed phase I organisms. These include development of heightened sensitivity to histamine and serotonin; increased susceptibility to anaphylaxis and to experimental allergic encephalomyelitis; increased antibody production, including reaginic antibody, in response to heterologous antigens; and hyperleukocytosis and hyperlymphocytosis. The factors responsible for these reactions have not been characterized fully.

It should be emphasized that none of the cellular components or products of *B. pertussis* has been shown to be of central importance in the pathogenesis of whooping cough.

Approximately 5 to 10 per cent of clinical whooping cough is caused by *B. parapertussis.* The animal pathogen *B. bronchiseptica* is responsible for a very minor percentage of cases. These organisms can be differentiated from *B. pertussis* by appropriate further bacteriologic or serologic procedures. It has recently been suggested that adenoviruses, alone or in concert with *B. pertussis,* may play an etiologic role in some cases of whooping cough.

Incidence and Epidemiology. In communities of susceptibles the family attack rate is 80 to 90 per cent, which is extremely high for a bacterial disease, approaching that seen in varicella or measles. Transmission is by droplet infection. Carriers of *B. pertussis* are found infrequently, and the reservoir is therefore unknown. Disease usually occurs in late winter in the northern climates and in late spring in southern zones, but there is great variation.

The mortality rate from whooping cough has fallen since the turn of this century owing to improved supportive therapy. The incidence of whooping cough, however, did not change until after the 1940's, when immunization of young children became standard practice. In the five-year periods 1926–1930, 1936–1940, 1956–1960, and 1965–1969, the fatality rate per thousand cases in the United States was 39.1, 19.4, 6.8, and 5.9, respectively. In the same time frames, the number of reported cases was 909,705; 956,262; 146,989; and 32,329, respectively. The majority of deaths, over 70 per cent, occur in children under one year of age, with the preponderance in infants under the age of six months.

Neither immunization against pertussis nor natural disease provides lifelong protection. In the case of artificial immunization, an attack rate greater than 50 per cent has been reported when the interval after immunization exceeds 12 years, a rate no different from that in unimmunized individuals of the same age. Thus in the face of routine immunization, it is possible that pertussis will become primarily a disease of older children and adults.

Pathology. Interpretation of pathologic material obtained at autopsy is difficult because of the common presence of complicating respiratory infections. Lesions caused by *B. pertussis* are found principally in the bronchi and bronchioles, but changes are also seen in the nasopharynx, larynx, and trachea. Masses of bacteria are intertwined with the cilia of the columnar epithelium together with mucopurulent exudate. There is also necrosis of the midzonal and basilar epithelium with infiltration of polymorphonuclear leukocytes and macrophages. Peribronchial accumulation of lymphocytes and granulocytes produces the picture of interstitial pneumonitis. Secondary atelectasis and localized emphysema are common. The alveoli in uncomplicated whooping cough do not contain exudate.

Clinical Manifestations. After an incubation period of 7 to 16 days, symptoms appear. It is customary to divide the clinical course into three stages, each of two weeks' duration, but variation is frequent, particularly in the immunized community.

Catarrhal Stage. Whooping cough begins with symptoms indistinguishable from those of a mild viral upper respiratory infection or common cold. Sneezing is frequent, the conjunctivae are injected, and a nocturnal cough appears. The temperature may be slightly elevated at this time. Infectivity is greatest during the catarrhal stage.

Paroxysmal Stage. Seven to 14 days after onset, the cough becomes more frequent, diurnal, and then paroxysmal. In a typical paroxysm there is a series of 15 to 20 short coughs of increasing intensity, and then with a deep inspiration the air is drawn into the lungs, making the "whoop." A tenacious mucus plug is usually expelled, and vomiting frequently follows the spasmodic episode. Paroxysms may occur as often as every half hour, and are accompanied by signs of increased venous pressure. The conjunctivae are deeply engorged; there is periorbital edema; and petechial hemorrhages, particularly about the forehead, as well as epistaxis are common. During the attack the infant may be cyanotic until the crowing whoop occurs. In between paroxysms the child usually feels well though justifiably apprehensive.

Physical examination of the chest is usually unremarkable, although scattered rhonchi may be heard. The chest roentgenogram sometimes reveals hilar and mediastinal nodal enlargement. The presence of fever immediately suggests the development of a secondary infectious process.

Convalescent Stage. Gradually the paroxysms become less frequent and less intense, vomiting ceases, and slow recovery ensues. Often for many months even a mild, unrelated respiratory infection will be manifested by a return of paroxysmal cough and whoop.

It is important to recognize those patients with whooping cough in whom variation from the pattern frequently occurs. In young infants the paroxysms and the whoop are often absent; instead, choking spells and apneic periods may be the major manifestations. Second attacks of whooping cough as well as disease occurring in previously immunized individuals often present simply as an upper respiratory illness or bronchitis.

Complications. Complications may be related to the primary disease or to secondary events. Alterations in acid-base balance occur as a result of metabolic alkalosis when vomiting is severe. Recurrent vomiting can also lead to malnutrition. Anoxemic manifestations are seen when ventilation is markedly impaired. Central nervous system changes can result from cerebral anoxia or hemorrhages consequent to the elevated venous pressure. Rarely, cortical degeneration occurs, but the exact pathogenesis of the encephalopathy is unknown. A serous meningitis with lymphocytosis of the cerebrospinal fluid has been described. Localized areas of emphysema and atelectasis generally return to normal after the disease has run its course, and pneumothorax and interstitial emphysema are infrequently seen.

The major cause of death in whooping cough is complicating pneumonia or bronchopneumonia caused by other bacteria or viruses. In addition, secondary bacterial otitis media occurs frequently.

Diagnosis. There is little difficulty in making the clinical diagnosis of whooping cough in a patient who, after a variable period of coryzal symptoms, develops paroxysmal coughing with a terminal inspiratory whoop. Toward the end of the catarrhal stage, or early in the spasmodic phase, leukocytosis often occurs. In contrast to the leukocytosis found in most bacterial diseases, the predominating cell type is the mature small lymphocyte. Characteristically the leukocyte count ranges from 15,000 to 30,000 per cubic millimeter, and 80 per cent of the cells are small lymphocytes. However, the leukocyte count either may be normal or may reach a level greater than 100,000 per cubic millimeter. Polymorphonuclear leukocytosis suggests a secondary bacterial complication.

Difficulty in recognizing whooping cough occurs in the catarrhal stage, in abortive or mild cases, and in young infants. Epidemiologic awareness may suggest the possibility, but microbiologic identification of the organisms is required. During the early stages of whooping cough *B. pertussis* can be isolated from approximately 90 per cent of patients. By the third or fourth week of illness the organism can be recovered in only 50 per cent of cases, and in the convalescent stage it is unusual to obtain a positive culture.

Adequate specimens and appropriate media are essential if bacteriologic diagnosis is to be efficient. *Specimens are best obtained by pernasal swab rather than by the cough plate method.* A sterile cotton swab wrapped about a flexible copper wire is passed through the nares, and mucus is obtained from the posterior pharynx. The swab must not be allowed to dry out because *B. pertussis* is readily killed by desiccation. As quickly as possible the specimen is plated onto fresh Bordet-Gengou medium, to which penicillin has been added to prevent overgrowth of adventitious organisms. Incubation is at 35° C, and although the trained observer can recognize the small, bisected pearl colonies of *B. pertussis* within 48 hours, at least 72 hours of growth is usually required. Presumptive identification can be made by agglutination tests with appropriate antisera. It is virtually impossible to distinguish between Bordetella species on primary isolation except by serologic means.

A fluorescent antibody staining procedure that can be applied directly to clinical specimens as well as to organisms grown in culture is now in more general use.

Serologic procedures are of little help in the diagnosis of whooping cough because a rise in titer of most antibodies does not occur until at least the third week of illness.

It is difficult to distinguish abortive or mild cases of pertussis from tracheobronchitis caused by other agents except by bacteriologic means. On the other hand, paroxysmal coughing may be associated with pulmonary lesions such as allergic bronchitis, atypical pneumonia, or cystic fibrosis.

Treatment. Mild cases of pertussis require only supportive treatment. Specific therapy of severe whooping cough has been disappointing despite the in vitro susceptibility of *B. pertussis* to various antimicrobial agents and the protective effect of passively administered antibody in experimental disease.

Antimicrobials. A number of antimicrobial drugs have significant in vitro activity against *B. pertussis.* Agents that readily eradicate the organisms in human disease may shorten the course of the illness if given in the catarrhal or early paroxysmal stages. In the established paroxysmal stage the organisms can also be readily eliminated by antimicrobials, but the course of the illness is unaltered. Even in the paroxysmal stage the use of drugs is justified in order to render the patient noninfectious.

Erythromycin, oxytetracycline, and chloramphenicol are more effective in eliminating organisms than ampicillin. On the basis of drug safety and efficacy either erythromycin or tetracycline is the drug of choice. The daily dose for each is 50 mg per kilogram of body weight given in four divided doses. The organism is eliminated after a few days of therapy, but because bacteriologic relapse may occur, treatment should be continued for ten to fourteen days.

Immunotherapy. Hyperimmune human gamma globulin is often used in therapy of unimmunized patients, particularly small infants. The usual dose is 1.25 or 2.5 ml intramuscularly for three successive days.

Supportive Therapy. Particularly in the young infant, supportive measures combined with careful nursing care are of paramount importance. Specific attention must be devoted to the maintenance of proper water and electrolyte balance, adequate nutrition, and sufficient oxygenation. Constant alertness for the presence of secondary infectious complications such as pneumonia is required, and appropriate therapy should be promptly instituted upon discovery.

Prevention. The great communicability of whooping cough, particularly during the first few weeks of illness, makes it desirable to isolate the patient for four to six weeks, or, ideally, until cultures are negative. Unfortunately, the diagnosis is usually not made until the end of the catarrhal stage, and by then spread of the disease has already occurred. Exposed susceptibles should be isolated from social groups until it is determined whether disease is present. Unimmunized contacts, especially infants, should receive 2 to 4 ml of hyperimmune gamma globulin intramuscularly, the dose to be repeated in five days. Those young children who have not received a booster dose of vaccine in more than a year should receive an injection upon exposure.

Recent studies have suggested that erythromycin may be effective in prophylaxis against pertussis in exposed, susceptible persons.

Active Immunization. The fall in incidence of whooping cough in the very young is directly related to widespread immunization with suitable, killed suspensions of *B. pertussis.* The highest risk of serious morbidity and mortality is in the young infant. Women of childbearing age generally do not have significant levels of protective antibody in their sera, and consequently the newborn are not protected by maternal antibodies. Therefore active immunization is begun as early as is commensurate with the production of a satisfactory immune response. At present, it is recommended that the infant receive three injections of pertussis vaccine at one-month intervals beginning at 6 to 12 weeks of age. Each injection provides four NIH* units. The NIH unitage is based upon the ability of a vaccine to protect mice against a standard intracerebral infection. The pertussis suspension is usually incorporated into a triple vaccine with alum-precipitated diphtheria and tetanus toxoids (DPT). Booster injections are given one, three, and five years after completion of the initial course. Administration of pertussis vaccine to those over six years of age is not generally recommended because of an apparent increased incidence of untoward reactions. However, low doses have been administered to adults without incident. There is no protection against parapertussis.

*National Institutes of Health.

As previously noted, immunization does not confer lifelong protection. Approximately 80 per cent of those vaccinated within four years of exposure will be protected, whereas 80 to 90 per cent of a matched unimmunized group with similar exposure will contract pertussis. However, as the time after immunization increases, the attack rate in both groups approaches 50 per cent.

Instances of "vaccine failure" have usually been shown to be due to the use of preparations of low potency. However, it has recently been suggested that a change in the dominant serotype causing disease, unrepresented in certain vaccine preparations, may be of importance. This controversial point is under study.

Local reactions as well as fever may occur after injection of pertussis vaccine. The exact incidence of the more severe complication of encephalopathy is uncertain, but both fatalities and residua have been reported. The occurrence of neurotoxicity appears to be decreasing as more refined immunizing suspensions are used, and certain soluble extracts of *B. pertussis* may prove to be effective without engendering serious side effects. Despite the small, but real, incidence of neurologic complications of pertussis immunization, the risk still seems far less than the hazards of whooping cough in the young child. Nevertheless, in infants with a personal or family history of convulsions or other neurologic disorders, pertussis immunization should be deferred, or very small doses should be cautiously administered. Care should also be exercised in the immunization of children with a family history of an allergic diathesis.

Klenk, E. L., Gaultney, J. V., and Bass, J. W.: Bacteriologically proved pertussis and adenovirus infection. Am. J. Dis. Child., 124:203, 1972.

Kurt, T. L., Yeager, A. S., Guenette, S., and Dunlop, S.: Spread of pertussis by hospital staff. J.A.M.A., 221:264, 1972.

Morse, S. I.: The Hemophilus-Bordetella group. *In* Davis, B. D., Dulbecco, R., Eisen, H. N., Ginsberg, H. S., and Wood, W. B., Jr. (eds.): Microbiology. 2nd ed. Hagerstown, Md., Harper & Row, 1973.

Pittman, M.: *Bordetella pertussis*—bacterial and host factors in the pathogenesis and prevention of whooping cough. *In* Mudd, S. (ed.): Infectious Agents and Host Reactions. Philadelphia, W. B. Saunders Company, 1970.

Preston, N. W., and Stanbridge, T. N.: Efficacy of pertussis vaccines: A brighter horizon. Br. Med. J., 3:448, 1972.

204. GRANULOMA INGUINALE

Walsh McDermott

Granuloma inguinale is an indolent granulomatous and ulcerative disease usually localized to the genitalia and caused by a pleomorphic coccobacillus, *Donovania granulomatis,* the so-called "Donovan body." When grown on artificial medium, the organism develops a large capsule that reacts immunologically with klebsiella capsular material. *Donovania granulomatis* also resembles *K. pneumoniae* in morphology. Presumably, the infection is customarily transmitted during coitus or other close bodily contact, and the degree of communicability appears to be relatively low. The lesion tends to be single, and may rarely appear on surfaces of the body other than the genitalia. Systemic infection, notably with the production of arthritis or osteomyelitis, has been reported. Usually, the lesion appears on the genitalia or in the perianal area as a relatively painless nodular infiltration that soon breaks down, leaving a sharply demarcated ulcer with friable granulation tissue at the base. On histologic examination, the lesion appears well vascularized and is the site of considerable cellular infiltration, especially with polymorphonuclear leukocytes and monocytes. In appropriately stained tissue scrapings, the causative microbe, *Donovania granulomatis,* may be seen situated principally within the monocytes, although smaller numbers of extracellular microorganisms can usually be identified. The lesion spreads by direct extension, it is highly destructive to the skin and subcutaneous tissue, and secondary infection with other microorganisms is common. Rarely, if sufficiently extensive, the process may cause elephantiasis of the genitalia.

There is nothing particularly characteristic about the lesions of granuloma inguinale, and the early lesion is indistinguishable from those produced by *T. pallidum, H. ducreyi,* or other processes that involve the genitalia. The diagnosis can be established only by appropriate microbiologic techniques, and these should be employed whenever the physician encounters a genital lesion (or an indolent ulceration elsewhere) that is not clearly caused by some other process. Microscopy of deep scrapings or impression smears from the lesion of granuloma inguinale stained by the Wright method usually reveals *Donovania granulomatis* within the monocytes. The ease with which the microorganisms can be detected varies to some extent with the age of the lesion. In a relatively old lesion, the scrapings should be made from the depth of the lesion, and an extensive search of the smears may be necessary. The microorganisms can also be cultured in medium containing chick embryo yolk by methods originally developed by Anderson and her associates. Antigen prepared from capsular material of *D. granulomatis* has been employed in a complement-fixation reaction and in a cutaneous reaction, but these have not yet been developed to the point of general application.

Granuloma inguinale has been successfully treated with streptomycin and the tetracyclines. As initial therapy, tetracycline should be employed in a total daily dosage of 2.0 grams administered by mouth in divided doses for a two-week period. In unusually extensive lesions it may be necessary to continue the treatment for a longer period in order to attain complete healing. If relapse occurs or the lesions appear refractory to tetracycline treatment, streptomycin should be administered intramuscularly in a total daily dosage of 2.0 grams in divided doses for a two-week period.

No detailed studies are available concerning the prevention of granuloma inguinale. It seems likely, however, that thorough washing of the genitals with soap and water immediately after sexual intercourse has a significant influence in reducing the probability of infection.

Anderson, K., Goodpasture, E. W., and DeMonbreun, W. A.: Immunologic relationship of *Donovania granulomatis* to granuloma inguinale. J. Exp. Med., 81:41, 1945.

Davis, B. D., Dulbecco, R., Eisen, H. N., Ginsberg, H. S., and Wood, W. B., Jr.: Microbiology. New York, Hoeber Medical Division, Harper & Row, 1970, Chap. 36.

Sheldon, W. H., Thebaut, B. R., Heyman, A., and Wall, M. J.: Osteomyelitis caused by granuloma inguinale. Am. J. Med. Sci., 210:237, 1945.

205. DIPHTHERIA

Heonir Rocha

Diphtheria is an acute infectious disease caused by a bacillus, *Corynebacterium diphtheriae.* The infection usually localizes in the pharynx, larynx, and nostrils and occasionally in the skin, and gives rise to both local and systemic signs. The latter are related to the production of a potent soluble exotoxin elaborated by the microorganisms multiplying at the site of infection.

Etiology. *Corynebacterium diphtheriae* is a gram-positive, nonsporulating, nonmotile pleomorphic bacillus, which grows best aerobically and does not form gas. In stained smears diphtheria bacilli are frequently club shaped in appearance and are arranged in palisade form. The most common media used to isolate the bacilli are Löffler's and potassium tellurite agar. By the appearance on tellurite agar and the ability to ferment starch and glycogen, three distinct types of colonies can be identified: *gravis, mitis,* and *intermedius.* All three types can produce the same powerful toxin, which is a complex protein, with a molecular weight of 64,000, produced by bacterial cells infected with a lysogenic bacteriophage. In so-called avirulent diphtheria strains no parasitism with bacteriophages can be demonstrated, and the bacilli fail to produce toxin. The amount of toxin produced depends on genetic and nutritional factors. The ability to produce toxin under laboratory conditions is not entirely related to potential for causing severe disease, because several virulent strains are poor toxin formers.

It is usually said that the *gravis* strain is more frequently associated with epidemic diphtheria; also, that the case fatality rate associated with any epidemic is determined by the proportion of cases infected with the *gravis* or *mitis* types. However, these views are not generally accepted. Although there seems to be a trend toward more severe infection with the *gravis* and *mitis* types, without question the same clinical picture can be produced by all three types.

Epidemiology and Immunity. Diphtheria has a worldwide distribution, its natural incidence being greatest in temperate climates. The disease occurs predominantly in poor socioeconomic conditions where inadequately immunized hosts and crowding are common. It exhibits a tendency to be most prevalent in autumn and winter but can give rise to epidemics at any time of year.

The human host is the only significant reservoir of *Corynebacterium diphtheriae,* which is transmitted directly or indirectly from one person to another. The usual habitat of *Corynebacterium diphtheriae* is the respiratory tract. The organism can multiply in the mucous membranes of the respiratory tract (pharynx or nares) of immunized hosts without giving rise to clinical disease. The transmission of diphtheria is mainly via droplets, although fomites and dust may have a minor role. Milk has been shown to be a vehicle of infection in rare instances. Duration and closeness of contact are the important factors in transmission. In some tropical areas the skin has been implicated as a major reservoir of *Corynebacterium diphtheriae* infection.

Immunity against the disease depends basically upon the existence of antitoxin in the blood of the host, which is formed in response to direct stimulation of diphtheria toxin either by artificial immunization or by clinical or subclinical infection. Infants under the age of six months are normally protected by passive immunity received through the placenta from immune mothers. Adults are usually protected by artificial immunization or subclinical infection. It has been suggested that cutaneous diphtheria may be the main method whereby natural immunization is acquired in tropical countries.

A relatively simple way to gain valuable information concerning a patient's immune status is obtained by observing the reaction after the intradermal injection of 0.1 ml of diluted, highly purified diphtheria toxin (Schick test). A positive reaction is interpreted to mean that the patient is susceptible to the disease; a negative reaction indicates that the levels of antitoxin exceed 0.03 unit per milliliter and that the host is not likely to acquire the clinical disease.

The maximal age incidence of diphtheria lies in the period of two to six years. The disease is an unusual occurrence in adults in endemic areas. However, recently in the United States, approximately 25 per cent of the cases occurred in persons 15 years of age or older.

Pathogenesis. The most serious consequences of *Corynebacterium diphtheriae* infection are the result of production and absorption of an extremely active and damaging exotoxin. The organisms multiply on epithelial cells at the infected site (usually pharynx), secreting the specific toxin which produces local signs and is absorbed, producing a systemic illness. The initial cytotoxic effect of the toxin is in tissues immediately adjacent to the bacterial growth, resulting in necrotic changes. As a consequence, an exudate which tends to coalesce is formed during the initial 24 to 48 hours. This fibrinous exudate contains leukocytes, necrotic epithelial cells, red blood cells, and the growing diphtheria bacillus. The exudate forms a tough membrane (so-called pseudomembrane) which is firmly attached, with a white shiny center and a gray or brownish periphery. If this membrane is forcibly removed, bleeding occurs. Occasionally it extends throughout the tracheobronchial tree, forming a cast. Edema of soft tissues subjacent to the membrane may be intense. These local lesions when present in the larynx can result in encroachment of the airway with varying degrees of respiratory obstruction.

From the local site of production the soluble toxin is disseminated by the blood and lymphatics and can produce degenerative changes in the heart, nervous system, and kidneys. The diphtheria toxin is regularly lethal to the affected cells. It becomes adsorbed to the cell membrane, penetrates into the cell, and alters the protein synthesis by interfering with the transfer of amino acids from RNA to the growing polypeptide chain. As a result, the cell degenerates and dies. Specific antitoxin may neutralize even adsorbed toxin, but does not prevent the chain of events once the toxin penetrates the cell.

Diphtheria infection may be localized infrequently in wounds, buccal mucosa, vagina, and conjunctiva. These extrarespiratory locations usually give rise to milder disease with much less systemic illness.

Clinical Manifestations. The incubation period of diphtheria varies from one to seven days, but is most commonly two to four days. *The clinical picture* depends upon the anatomic location of the lesions and the severity of the toxic process. The most common localization of infection is the oropharynx.

Faucial diphtheria is the most common clinical form and includes the most toxic forms. In a typical case the onset is usually sudden, with low-grade fever (37 to 38° C), malaise, and mild sore throat. The pharynx is only moderately injected, and a thick tonsillar exudate is frequently seen. This exudate usually spreads from one tonsil to the other and may invade the pillars, uvula, and soft palate. Moderate tonsillar as well as cervical lymph node enlargement is usually present.

In some cases the membrane or exudate is limited to the tonsils *(tonsillar diphtheria)*, and toxic manifestations are inconspicuous. In other cases, there is spread of the original process to the uvula, posterior pharyngeal wall, and posterior nasal mucosa *(nasopharyngeal diphtheria)*, sometimes with massive cervical lymphadenopathy (bullneck appearance) and signs of toxemia. In this clinical form the child is pale, lethargic, prostrated, restless at times, and extremely weak. The pulse is rapid and thin; heart beats become muffled; respiration is labored and frequently noisy. This state of toxemia may result in death within a few days if the condition remains untreated. Finally, in some patients the infection spreads downward to the larynx, producing a clinical picture of progressive laryngeal obstruction *(laryngeal diphtheria)*. When the larynx is involved, the first symptoms are hoarseness, dyspnea, a brassy cough, and an increasing expiratory and inspiratory stridor. In a few instances laryngeal involvement may be the first sign of infection.

As the obstruction progresses, dyspnea becomes more severe, bronchial secretions accumulate, the accessory muscles of respiration come into full play, and there are supra- and infrasternal retraction at each stridulous breath. If obstruction is not relieved, the patient becomes extremely restless, anxious, and cyanotic, and the condition then merges into severe exhaustion and a comatose stage.

In some cases the infection is basically localized in the anterior nasal area *(anterior nasal diphtheria)*. Clinically it is manifested by bilateral serous or serosanguineous discharge which causes crusted lesions on the upper lip. Small rounded ulcers, some of them covered with a whitish exudate, are usually seen in the anterior part of the nasal septum. Constitutional symptoms are lacking, and this process is chiefly important because of its epidemiologic implications. It is frequently undiagnosed in an endemic area, and may be an important source of spreading the disease.

Other parts of the body may be the site of primary or secondary diphtheric lesions, the most commonly described being the skin. *Cutaneous diphtheria* takes the form of chronic nonhealing ulcers, sometimes covered with a grayish membranous exudate. It seems probable that these ulcers, mainly described in the tropics, have a complex etiology. Treatment with antitoxin alone usually gives disappointing results. Involvement of the conjunctiva, vagina, or ear by *Corynebacterium diphtheriae* has been rarely reported.

Diagnosis. In most instances of diphtheric oropharyngeal infection, a presumptive diagnosis must be made on clinical grounds, without awaiting laboratory confirmation, because therapy should be started at once.

The clinical manifestations which should arouse suspicion of *nasopharyngeal diphtheria* are (1) insidious onset of a painless pharyngitis associated with an exudate (usually localized or predominantly in one tonsillar area); (2) association of a faucial exudate with insidious and progressive signs of laryngeal obstruction, or with a serous or serosanguineous nasal discharge; and (3) the presence of faucial exudate with marked cervical adenopathy and signs of toxicity (prostration, tachycardia, marked pallor).

For laboratory diagnosis, a swab from the suspected site should be promptly inoculated on a Löffler slant, a tellurite plate, and a blood agar plate. Identification of the etiologic agent can be made after overnight incubation on the basis of colony formation, cellular morphology, and sometimes fermentation reactions. Immunofluorescence techniques have been tried for the rapid diagnosis of diphtheria. For reliable results the specimen has to be incubated four hours before applying the fluorescent antibody technique. Slides prepared directly from throat swabs are unsatisfactory. The fluorescent antibody technique is not of value for the identification of toxigenic strains.

Several conditions may be confused with diphtheria, especially during an epidemic bout. This is the case, for instance, with streptococcal pharyngitis. In this condition there is usually high fever (39 to 40°C) with frequent chills, the throat is fiery red, the exudate is thin and easily removable, and swallowing is painful. Other pharyngeal infections which may be accompanied by an exudate are adenoviral exudative pharyngitis, infectious mononucleosis, Vincent's angina, and angina of agranulocytosis. Rhinitis associated with diphtheria must be differentiated from rhinitis of simple colds and from foreign bodies in the nostrils. The distressful laryngeal manifestations of diphtheria should be differentiated from acute laryngotracheobronchitis.

Complications. The most important complications of diphtheria are related to the cardiovascular and nervous systems. They are most frequently associated with the severe forms of the disease.

Although electrocardiographic changes have been described in a high percentage (25 per cent) of cases of diphtheria, clinically manifest myocarditis is less common. The onset of myocarditis is often insidious, appearing in the second or third week of the infection. Characteristically, the patient exhibits a weak rising pulse with distant heart sounds and a profound weakness and lethargy. When heart failure ensues, the patient becomes dyspneic, with marked pallor and epigastric pain, and he develops cardiac enlargement and an apical diastolic gallop. The most common electrocardiographic changes are T wave flattening or inversion, bundle branch block or intraventricular block, and several types of disorders of rhythm (premature contraction and atrial fibrillation).

Diphtheria myocarditis, particularly when associated with heart block, carries an extremely poor prognosis. Despite vigorous treatment, including steroids and digitalis, the mortality rate is very high. Glucagon has also been tried but is ineffective.

Nervous system involvement is manifested by cranial nerve or peripheral nerve paralysis. The most common form of cranial nerve palsy is paralysis of the soft palate, which is suspected by the development of nasal regurgitation of fluid upon attempted swallowing. Nasal speech may be present but is frequently slight. This condition is mild, and recovery usually occurs within two weeks. Ciliary paresis and oculomotor paralysis (affecting both sides) make up the next most common form. Rarely, facial, pharyngeal, or laryngeal paralysis is observed.

Peripheral neuritis, usually affecting the limbs, may appear from about the fourth to the eighth week. It varies greatly in extent but is frequently manifested by weakness in the dorsiflexors of the feet, accompanied by decreased or absent tendon reflexes in the lower extremities. Less commonly, the upper limbs, the neck, and the trunk may be involved. The prognosis is good. Diphtheric polyneuritis has been described after cutaneous diphtheria.

It must be emphasized that recovery from the complications of diphtheria is nearly always complete insofar as can be determined by clinical examination. It has been suggested that a lowering of cardiac reserve can persist in some cases, but this assumption needs further documentation.

Treatment. The most important act in the treatment of diphtheria is to administer antitoxin as soon as the diphtheria is suspected on clinical grounds without awaiting laboratory confirmation. Admittedly this practice will result in the unnecessary use of antitoxin in some cases. But this is of little consequence in view of the considerable improvement in prognosis in severe forms of the disease when antitoxin is administered early and in adequate amounts.

Opinions vary as to what constitutes an efficient dose. It is usually accepted that in mild or moderate cases a dose of 20,000 to 40,000 units, injected intramuscularly, is enough. In severe cases, 50,000 to 100,000 units is the recommended dose, half of it being given by slow intravenous infusion. As the antitoxin is a horse protein, precautions should be observed to avoid severe hypersensitivity reactions (anaphylaxis). It is mandatory to inquire if allergy to horse serum is known, and to perform a conjunctival or intracutaneous skin test with a 1:10 saline dilution of the antitoxin. If a positive reaction is obtained by either method, desensitization with increasing doses of antiserum is recommended. Epinephrine must be at hand before antitoxin is administered by any route.

As the *Corynebacterium diphtheriae* is susceptible to several antimicrobials, these drugs have been used routinely, in addition to antitoxin, in cases of diphtheria. Penicillin G is still the drug of choice, and is usually given as procaine penicillin, 400,000 units intramuscularly every 12 hours, for a period of 10 to 12 days. Erythromycin, also very active against the diphtheria bacillus, is an alternative drug and is recommended in a dosage of 30 to 40 mg per kilogram of body weight for a similar period. In suspected cases, these drugs must not be administered without the antitoxin, because they may mask the infection and thus may make it impossible to establish a laboratory diagnosis.

Bed rest is essential in all patients during the acute phase of the disease; this can vary in completeness and duration, depending on the degree of toxicity and the presence of cardiac involvement. In any event, the patient's return to activity should be carefully guided by the physician. Complications such as dehydration, shock, and congestive heart failure should be promptly diagnosed and properly treated.

In cases exhibiting marked toxicity and in patients with severe laryngeal involvement and/or shock, corticosteroids (prednisolone, 3 to 5 mg per kilogram of body weight per day) have been advocated along with the antitoxin and antimicrobials. Cases of laryngeal obstruction may require emergency tracheostomy and careful postoperative aspiration to avoid complications. Such patients need special nursing for safety.

Patients with diphtheria should be isolated, preferably in hospital. Before their discharge from isolation, cultures from throat and nose (or local lesion) should be taken, and at least two consecutive negative cultures should be obtained.

Prevention. Diphtheria may be effectively prevented by *active immunization.* The primary course of immunization should be administered within the first year of life, preferably between the third and sixth months. Of the preparations available, *fluid toxoid* and *alum-precipitated toxoid* are the most commonly used. The primary course of fluid toxoid consists of three intramuscular injections (0.5 ml, 1.0 ml, and 1.0 ml) at weekly intervals (one to three weeks). For immunization with the alum-precipitated toxoid, two 1-ml intramuscular injections administered at intervals of one to two months are enough. Despite its greater antigenic potency, the alum-precipitated toxoid also has a greater sensitizing ability, and may induce sterile local abscesses at the injection site owing to the irritating effect of the alum upon tissues. Both fluid and alum-precipitated toxoid are excellent immunizing agents, conferring immunity to at least 90 per cent of those receiving a primary course. After this immunization in infancy, one stimulating dose should be given one or two years later, and another given at the time the child enters school.

Diphtheria toxoid has been combined with immunizations against tetanus and pertussis and should be given within the first year of life. All children under eight years of age who are not immunized are susceptible to diphtheria and should be actively immunized without preliminary Schick testing. In older children and adults, before immunization with toxoid, a sensitivity test should be done. The development of a local reaction within 48 hours of the intracutaneous injection of 0.1 ml of 1:10 dilution of toxoid in normal saline *(Moloney test)* is a warning that toxoid should be administered cautiously in multiple small diluted doses.

Passive immunization against diphtheria may be rapidly conferred by subcutaneous inoculation of 1500 units of diphtheria antitoxin. This procedure should be limited to persons peculiarly at risk of infection, such as nonimmunized children heavily exposed to an infected case. The protection is limited to a period of two to three weeks, and active immunization with a toxoid preparation should be started at the same time. Human diphtheria antitoxin is not yet available.

Treatment of Diphtheria Carriers. Whenever diphtheria is common, carrier rates are high. In approximately 15 to 20 per cent of cases, the cultures will remain positive for as long as one month after the disease, but they will subsequently become negative in most instances. Erythromycin in a dosage of 30 to 40 mg per kilogram of body weight has been found effective for treatment of carriers. Tonsillectomy and adenoidectomy have also been advocated to eliminate the carrier state.

Belsey, M. A., Sinclair, M., Roder, M. R., and LeBlanc, D. R.: *Corynebacterium diphtheriae* skin infections in Alabama and Louisiana. N. Engl. J. Med., 135:135, 1969.

Bray, J. P., Burt, E. G., Potter, E. V., Poon-King, T., and Earle, D.: Epidemic diphtheria and skin infections in Trinidad. J. Infect. Dis., 126:34, 1972.

McCloskey, R. V., Eller, J. J., Green, M., Mauney, C. V., and Richards, S. E. M.: The 1970 epidemic of diphtheria in San Antonio. Ann. Intern. Med., 75:495, 1971.

McCracken, A. W., and Mauney, C. V.: Identification of *Corynebacterium diphtheriae* by immunofluorescence during a diphtheria epidemic. J. Clin. Pathol., 24:641, 1971.

Naiditch, M. J., and Bower, A. A.: Diphtheria: Study of 1433 cases observed during 10-year period at Los Angeles County Hospital. Am. J. Med., 17:229, 1954.

Scheid, W.: Diphtherial paralysis. An analysis of 2292 cases of diphtheria in adults, which included 174 cases of polyneuritis. J. Nerv. Ment. Dis., 116:1095, 1952.

Tasman, A., and Lansberg, H. P.: Problems concerning the prophylaxis, pathogenesis and therapy of diphtheria. Bull. WHO, 16:939, 1957.

CLOSTRIDIAL DISEASES

206. INTRODUCTION

Emanuel Wolinsky

The clostridia are spore-forming anaerobic gram-positive bacilli that for the most part lead a saprophytic existence in nature. The may be found in large numbers in the intestinal tracts of humans and animals, and in the soil. They are capable of producing disease by virtue of their elaboration of powerful exotoxins, but special conditions must be present in the tissues to allow the organisms to germinate, proliferate, and elaborate toxins. The mere presence of clostridia in the wound or on the surface of the body is not significant. Most clostridial disease is caused by *C. perfringens,* although occasionally *C. novyi (oedematiens), septicum, sordellii (bifermentans), histolyticum,* and *fallax* may be human pathogens.

The pathologic states attributable to clostridial infection cover a wide range of severity and localization, from the relatively benign wound infection to the highly fatal gas gangrene; from transient bacteremia to life-threatening septicemia; from relatively mild food poisoning to necrotic enteritis; and from pleural empyema to purulent meningitis. The neurotoxic disease caused by *C. tetani* is discussed below, and that caused by *C. botulinum* is discussed in Ch. 23.

BACTERIOLOGY

All the clostridia owe their pathogenicity to the elaboration of exotoxins that have enzymatic activity. Four major toxins and eight minor ones have been described and given Greek letters. The most important of them is the alpha toxin, which is a lecithinase capable of splitting lecithin in the red cell envelope and causing severe hemolysis. Many of the species of clostridia have been separated into types according to their ability to elaborate specific exotoxins. *C. perfringens* may be divided into five or six toxigenic types; Type A elaborates more alpha toxin than any other type or species and is by far the most important variety of Clostridium in human disease, particularly gas gangrene.

207. CLOSTRIDIAL MYONECROSIS (Gas Gangrene)

Emanuel Wolinsky

The clostridial gas gangrene is best called *clostridial myonecrosis* because the outstanding feature is rapidly progressive muscle necrosis with relatively little inflammatory reaction, and because other organisms can produce skin and subcutaneous gangrene with gas formation. The disease most often arises from traumatic or surgical wounds in which anoxic conditions prevail as a result of ischemia or crushed muscle. Battle wounds of World Wars I and II supplied plentiful case material for study; gas gangrene occurred in approximately 10 per cent of World War I wounds and in 1 per cent of those that occurred in World War II. In civilian practice the rate of gas gangrene among 188,000 major open wounds has been estimated to be 1.8 per cent. The rate of contamination or local infection of open wounds, on the other hand, amounts to 30 to 80 per cent. The soil is the usual source of the clostridia in exogenous infection, the intestine or biliary tract in autogenous infection.

Pathogenesis. The factors that predispose to the invasion of muscle by the bacilli with the subsequent elaboration of exotoxins are related to lack of oxygen and lowering of the oxidation-reduction potential of the tissues. These factors are (1) impaired local vascular supply owing to vessel trauma or pressure from foreign bodies, casts, or tourniquets; (2) presence of metallic bodies, clothing, or dirt in the wound; (3) presence of necrotic tissue or hemorrhage; and (4) growth of aerobic microorganisms in the wound.

Under these circumstances the bacilli can multiply anaerobically and elaborate toxins, which diffuse out and damage surrounding muscle, which in turn becomes colonized with the bacilli. Thus the disease spreads rapidly to surrounding muscles and gains momentum. The severe generalized toxemia remains poorly explained. Alpha toxin is not found in the blood, and it is postulated that a toxic factor that acts on certain vital centers or enzymes is produced by the interaction of clostridial toxin with infected muscle.

Clinical Manifestations. The clinical picture of gas gangrene is dominated by rapidly progressive toxemia and shock. After a relatively short incubation period of one to four days the patient suddenly exhibits restlessness and anxiety; the temperature and pulse rate begin to rise and the blood pressure to fall. He is noted to be pale and sweating. The wound becomes painful and markedly swollen. Some hours later, after progression of the signs and symptoms, a thin brownish exudate begins to ooze from the wound, and a small amount of crepitus may be noted in the surrounding tissues. A bronze discoloration starts at the edge of the wound and progresses outward. Blebs filled with purplish fluid may appear. An odor characterized as "mousy" or "sickly sweet" is described by many observers. By this time the patient may be anuric and in irreversible vascular collapse. When the muscle is exposed by incision, it appears to be "cooked" or dead—it does not bleed when cut or retract when pinched. Smears from *involved muscle* show many large gram-positive rods and no other organisms, but very few pus cells. Smears and cultures from the *wound exudate* at the surface may reveal other organisms in addition to the clostridia, especially in grossly contaminated wounds. Roentgenograms reveal the presence of gas in and around muscle bundles in the form of fernlike, lacy patterns. Untreated, fully developed clostridial myonecrosis is almost always fatal.

Myonecrosis must be differentiated from clostridial and nonclostridial *crepitant cellulitis,* from *anaerobic streptococcal myonecrosis,* and from *physical* and *chemical* causes of gas in the tissues. *Clostridial cellulitis* (anaerobic cellulitis, local gas gangrene, epifascial gas gangrene, or gas-forming fasciitis) is a gas-forming infection of connective tissue mainly localized to subcutaneous areas with spread in fascial planes, but healthy muscle is not involved. It arises as a result of clostridial infection of tissue already necrotic from ischemia or trauma. The onset is gradual, and toxemia, pain, and swelling are less than in gas gangrene. A large amount of gas is distributed in the form of large bubbles along the fascial planes, but not in the muscle. Incision will show that the muscle is viable, and smears from muscle tissue away from the open wound will not reveal organisms.

Nonclostridial crepitant cellulitis is similar to clostridial cellulitis, except that the infection is associated with other organisms usually in a mixed flora consisting of two or more of the following: aerogenic coliforms (*E. coli,* Klebsiella, Enterobacter), anaerobic streptococci, Bacteroides, and gamma streptococci. In many cases this mixed bacterial flora in gas-forming cellulitis includes clostridia; these cases do not appear to differ in prognosis from those in which clostridia are absent.

Anaerobic streptococcal myonecrosis was described by MacLennan in infected war wounds from the Middle East in 1948, but there have been few reports since then. Other organisms, especially group A streptococci and *Staph. aureus,* were always found with the primary agent, and 3 of 19 patients had anaerobic streptococcal bacteremia.

Simple contamination of wounds with clostridia is not uncommon. The organisms, usually in association with a mixed flora, exist as saprophytes on necrotic tissue and debris and do not invade further. Clostridia may also be found in localized collections of purulent material in wounds, or in a collection of foul-smelling brownish fluid known as a "gas abscess" or a "Welch abscess." Drainage will usually suffice to bring these conditions under control. There is not always a clean-cut distinction among the various pathologic states described above, nor is it clear how often one can recognize an orderly progression in the severity of clostridial invasion from simple contamination to full-blown myonecrosis.

Diagnosis. The diagnosis of gas gangrene is essentially a clinical one. Upon first suspicion of the disease, dressings and casts must be removed and the wound or suspected area thoroughly inspected. Roentgenograms may help to show the fine bubbles of gas distributed in and around muscle bundles. Incision should be made into

TABLE 1. Classification of Histotoxic Clostridial Disease

Traumatic
- A. Wound infection (war and civilian)
  1. Simple contamination
  2. Localized (purulent or "gas abscess")
  3. Gas-forming cellulitis
  4. Myonecrosis
- B. Uterine infection (postabortion and postpartum)
- C. Burns, panophthalmitis, brain abscess, etc.

Nontraumatic
- A. Postoperative (abdominal, amputation)
- B. Postinjection
- C. Spontaneous
  1. Localized (pneumonia, empyema, cholecystitis, myonecrosis)
  2. Septicemic (malignant disease, intestinal lesion)
- D. Bacteremia without hemolysis or sepsis (from decubitus ulcer, gangrenous extremity, uterus)

TABLE 2. Gas-Forming Soft Tissue Infections

	Clostridial Myonecrosis	"Anaerobic" Cellulitis	Streptococcal Myonecrosis
Onset	Sudden	Gradual	Gradual
Toxemia	Extreme	Slight	Slight
Pain	May be severe	Slight	Gradually increasing
Swelling	Marked	Slight	Marked
Skin color	Bronze	No change	Erythematous
Exudate	Thin, brown	Thin, bloody; later purulent	Profuse, thin seropurulent
Gas	Little, in muscle	Profuse, large bubbles in fascial planes	Little, in muscle
Muscle	Dead, "cooked," healthy muscle invaded	Not involved	Initially edematous, then hemorrhagic
Bacteriology	Mixed flora from exudate or open wound; from muscle aspirate pure gram-positive rods	May be pure clostridia or mixed flora from exudate or subcutaneous tissue; no organisms in muscle aspirate	Anaerobic streptococci, along with Group A Streptococcus, *Staph. aureus, etc.*, from exudate and muscle
Prognosis	Serious	Good	Good
Treatment	Radical surgery, penicillin, antitoxin, hyperbaric oxygen	Surgical drainage and debridement, appropriate antimicrobials	Surgical drainage and debridement, penicillin

the muscle so that the characteristic appearance may be appreciated. At the same time a specimen of muscle may be examined by Gram stain and by anaerobic cultural techniques. Slides may also be made for staining by the fluorescent antibody technique (Clark et al., 1969). Smears and cultures from the exudate around the wound surface may be misleading. Tables 1 and 2 summarize the most important findings for the differential diagnosis.

Treatment. Treatment must be prompt and vigorous. Most important is thorough *debridement* and *excision* of all devitalized tissue and dead muscle. Hopelessly involved extremities usually need to be amputated except perhaps under the influence of hyperbaric oxygen. It is said that if any infected muscle is left behind, it will prevent cure. General *supportive measures* should include intravenous fluids and blood, other measures to combat vascular collapse and shock, and peritoneal dialysis when necessary. *Antimicrobial* treatment is given to prevent bloodstream invasion and to suppress further spread of infection. Penicillin is the drug of choice given in large doses of 10 to 20 million units per day intravenously. Erythromycin may be substituted in patients allergic to penicillin. In a recent study it was found that 11 per cent of clostridial strains were resistant to tetracycline. *Antitoxin* is recommended, especially during the first few hours of the disease, in the hope of neutralizing any free toxin in the body fluids, although its usefulness is doubtful because the exotoxins are very rapidly bound to cells. The recommended dose is 40 thousand units of trivalent or pentavalent antitoxin intravenously at once and 20 to 40 thousand units repeated at four- to six-hour intervals. The usual precautions for horse serum must be observed. *Hyperbaric oxygen* at 3 atmospheres has been recommended by some as a dramatically successful mode of therapy that should take precedence over immediate surgical treatment and antitoxin. It is said that debridement may be deferred until systemic toxicity has been relieved and demarcation between necrotic and viable tissue is clear. In this way loss of tissue may be minimized and amputation sometimes avoided. If a suitable chamber is not available locally, it is probably unwise to delay surgical extirpation in favor of a long journey.

Treatment of "anaerobic" cellulitis and streptococcal myonecrosis need not be so radical. Usually wide excision and debridement along with supportive measures and appropriate antimicrobials will suffice. A Gram-stained smear of wound exudate and muscle aspirate will help one to decide whether penicillin alone should be given (for pure Clostridium or Streptococcus) or whether antistaphylococcal or anticoliform agents should be added or substituted. For the former, one should use a semisynthetic penicillinase-resistant penicillin (methicillin, nafcillin, or cephalothin) to initiate treatment; for the gram-negative bacilli one can add tetracycline, gentamicin, or kanamycin.

Prevention. The prophylactic use of antitoxin and antimicrobials at the time of injury does not prevent gas gangrene. Careful attention to good surgical technique is most important. All devitalized tissue must be excised and vascular supply left intact. Care must be taken with tourniquets and casts to prevent undue ischemia. Plaster of Paris itself may be contaminated with clostridia.

UTERINE INFECTION

Postabortion and postpartum clostridial infections of the uterus are still important causes of serious disease in obstetrics. At least 5 per cent of women harbor clostridia in the vagina as simple contaminants. Fulminant infection usually follows criminal abortion or prolonged and difficult labor, and presents a clinical picture similar to that seen in traumatic gas gangrene. Unlike wound gas gangrene, however, uterine infection is frequently accompanied by clostridial sepsis leading to jaundice, hemolysis, hemoglobinemia, hemoglobinuria, and renal shutdown. As in wound infection, there may be various grades of clostridial involvement, from simple contamination to secondary invasion of necrotic matter in the uterus or a dead fetus to true invasion of intact uterine muscle producing myonecrosis or "physometra." Clostridial infection must be differentiated from the more slowly progressive uterine infection produced by anaerobic streptococci and Bacteroides which commonly leads to pelvic thrombophlebitis and septic pulmonary infarcts.

Treatment is essentially the same as that outlined above, except that a decision must be made quickly on whether to do a hysterectomy or merely to empty the uterus. Evidence for uterine perforation or necrosis will call for the more radical procedure. Antimicrobial therapy should probably include clindamycin or chloramphenicol in addition to penicillin to control Bacteroides.

POSTOPERATIVE GAS GANGRENE

Nontraumatic gas gangrene that follows surgical operations is probably the most common variety of the disease in civilian hospitals today. Of 42 cases of *C. perfringens* infection reported from a single hospital, 18 followed operations and 10 were secondary to trauma (Pyrtek and Bartus, 1962). Most of these infections involve the abdominal wall after biliary or intestinal surgery, or the leg or hip after amputation or correction of hip fractures, although the complication has been described after many other kinds of surgical procedures. Recent investigation in England indicated that most of these infections were sporadic and autogenous in origin, probably as a result of fecal contamination of the skin. Parker called attention to the importance of adequate preoperative sterilization of the skin with sporicidal agents and the advisability of giving prophylactic penicillin from a few hours before operation to one week after to those patients at greatest risk from postoperative clostridial infections—elderly patients who will have hip surgery or thigh amputations.

208. OTHER CLOSTRIDIAL DISEASES

Emanuel Wolinsky

SEPTICEMIA

Clostridial septicemia occurs rarely from traumatic wound gangrene, occasionally from postoperative gas gangrene, and commonly from uterine infection. In addition, nontraumatic or spontaneous clostridial septicemia has been described from such conditions as acute cholecystitis, perforated peptic ulcer, ulcerating carcinoma of the colon, acute pancreatitis, diverticulitis, appendiceal abscess, decubitus ulcer, and gangrenous limbs. Septicemia may occur in terminal cancer patients from portals of entry such as ulcerations of the respiratory or alimentary tracts. A study of 21 patients suffering from various malignant diseases who had septicemia caused by *C. septicum* has been reported (Alpern and Dowell, 1969). As a result of septicemia, infection may localize in the pleura, myocardium, endocardium, and meninges. Benign clostridial bacteremia without hemolysis was observed in a series of 20 patients, all of whom survived (Rathbun, 1968).

MISCELLANEOUS FORMS

Pneumonia and empyema may be associated with clostridial infection, usually as a result of aspiration of contaminated material from the mouth or the stomach, but occasionally by way of the bloodstream. Penetrating injuries may lead to serious clostridial infections of the eye, brain, and meninges. Severe gas gangrene may result from injections into the buttock or thigh, presumably from inadequately sterilized skin. In at least one instance the organism was also isolated from cotton sponges soaked in alcohol.

209. CLOSTRIDIAL GASTROENTERITIS

Emanuel Wolinsky

Clostridial food poisoning has been the second most common variety reported to the Communicable Disease Center, representing 16 per cent of the total outbreaks and 34 per cent of the cases. There is no seasonal preference, and the most common vehicles have been beef and turkey products. *C. perfringens* type A may be recovered from the stools of patients and from the suspected food product. The disease is characterized by a short incubation period, acute onset, absence of fever, and a relatively benign course. The outbreaks are self-limiting, and the disease is not spread to other people directly. Evidence points to an infection rather than an intoxication as the primary mechanism of the disease. *Enteritis necroticans* ("Darmbrand") was first described shortly after World War II in Germany. Other outbreaks occurred in North Germany and the Rhineland; then the disease apparently vanished. The disease was characterized by severe diarrhea, collapse, high mortality, and patchy hemorrhagic necrosis of the small bowel. It was originally attributed to a new type of *C. perfringens* called type F, but these organisms are now considered to be members of type C. It corresponds in many ways to certain clostridial enterotoxemias of animals.

Altemeier, W. A., and Culbertson, W. R.: Acute non-clostridial crepitant cellulitis. Surg. Gynecol. Obstet., 87:206, 1948.

Ayliffe, G. A. J., and Lowbury, E. J. L.: Sources of gas gangrene in hospital. Br. Med. J., 2:333, 1969.

Bornstein, D. L., Weinberg, A. N., Swartz, M. N., and Kunz, L. J.: Anaerobic infections—Review of current experience. Medicine, 43:207, 1964.

Cabrera, A., Tsukada, Y., and Pickren, J. W.: Clostridial gas gangrene and septicemia in malignant disease. Cancer, 18:800, 1965.

MacLennan, J. D.: The histotoxic clostridial infections of man. Bact. Rev., 26:177, 1962.

Parker, M. T.: Postoperative clostridial infections in Britain. Br. Med. J., 3:671, 1969.

Roding, B., Groenveld, P. H., and Boerema, I.: Ten years' experience in the treatment of gas gangrene in hyperbaric oxygen. Surg. Gynecol. Obstet., 134:579, 1972.

Unsworth, I. P.: Gas gangrene in New South Wales. Med. J. Aust., 1:1077, 1973.

210. TETANUS

Alexander Crampton Smith

Tetanus, often called "lockjaw," is a disease of the nervous system characterized by intense activity of motor neurons resulting in severe muscle spasms. It is caused by an exotoxin of *Clostridium tetani.*

History. Tetanus has caught the imagination of physicians since Hippocrates, and this is probably in part due to the horrifying nature of the clinical picture in the established untreated case. The presence of the causative organism in soil was demonstrated by Nicolaier, who produced tetanus in animals by soil injections. The Clostridium was isolated in pure culture in 1899 by Kitasato, and in 1892, Nocard immunized horses by injections of antitoxic horse serum. Passive immunization after wounding saved many lives in World War I, and active immunization with toxoid almost eliminated tetanus in the allied armies in World War II. Curare was first suggested as having an application in the treatment of tetanus in 1811, but as curare in sufficient dosage to abolish the spasms of severe tetanus will certainly paralyze the muscles of ventilation, the large-scale use of curare had to wait almost 150 years until intermittent positive pressure ventilation (IPPV) through a cuffed tracheotomy tube was introduced into the treatment of tetanus in Denmark in 1953 (Bjørnboe et al.).

ETIOLOGY AND PATHOGENESIS

Clostridium tetani is a gram-positive actively motile bacillus, which in its spore-bearing form has a characteristic "drumstick" appearance. Spores may develop at either end of the bacillus, giving a "dumbbell" appearance. It is a strict anaerobe, and spores will not germinate in the presence of even the smallest amount of oxygen. An oxidation-reduction potential of + 0.01 volt or less at pH 7 is required if germination is to take place. The Clostridium grows well on laboratory media at 37° C, and growth occurs slowly at 22° C. Vegetative bacilli are readily killed by antiseptics and by heat, but spores are highly resistant to antiseptics and, to a certain extent, are resistant to heat. To kill most spores, boiling for one hour is necessary, but the most resistant may require boiling for four hours. Autoclaving for ten minutes at 120° C may, however, be relied on to sterilize contaminated objects. *Clostridium tetani* is commonly found in soil and in the feces of domestic animals and humans. Presumably by contamination with soil and feces, spores can be recovered from dust and clothing; in suitable surroundings like dried earth, spores will survive for many years.

Clostridium tetani produces two exotoxins, *tetanospasmin* and *tetanolysin,* and of these tetanospasmin is the neurotoxin which produces the typical muscle spasms of tetanus. It is extremely potent, each milligram of crystallized toxin containing 50 to 75 million mouse lethal doses. This extreme toxicity may be the reason why an attack of tetanus does not confer immunity, as it is postulated that the fatal dose of tetanus toxin is less than the amount required to provoke an immune response. Tetanolysin can cause hemolysis on blood agar plates, but does not seem to play any significant part in the pathologic process caused by the Clostridium.

There have been differences of opinion about the site of action of tetanospasmin and about the route by which it spreads, but it now seems firmly established that the toxin acts in the spinal cord and the brainstem and that it spreads centrally along motor nerve trunks and up the spinal cord. Tetanus will follow the intravenous injection into animals, but the route by which toxin in the blood enters the nervous system is not clear. Toxin injected intramuscularly apparently spreads not only by passing up motor nerves but also by absorption into the blood, and it has been suggested that vascular spread is the more important route in generalized tetanus. Payling Wright surveyed the evidence for neural and vascular spread, but research, notably with radioactive isotopes (Fedenec, 1967), is continuing.

EPIDEMIOLOGY

The incidence of tetanus is difficult to establish because it is not a notifiable disease in many countries. The total world deaths each year, however, probably exceed 160,000, and if the average crude fatality rate is about 45 per cent (and it may be much higher), there must be more than 350,000 cases in the world every year. Tetanus is thus still a major public health problem in developing countries. The organism is found in soil and human and animal feces, and tetanus is common in warm climates and in rural areas that are highly cultivated and consequently have a large population of men and animals. Agricultural workers, in whom injuries may easily be contaminated with the Clostridium, are particularly at risk. *Clostridium tetani* can also be found in urban areas, but the degree of contamination is not high, and it is likely that the increased standards of living and hygiene which urbanization implies also contribute to a lower incidence of tetanus in cities. Further evidence of the importance of education and hygiene is the absence of neonatal tetanus in countries where obstetric hygiene is good, compared with the high incidence in countries where dung is sometimes used as a dressing for the umbilical stump.

PREVENTION OF TETANUS

Before Injury

Active Immunization. The U.S. Public Health Service Advisory Committee has stated that the need for active immunization against tetanus is universal and that such immunization is the only way by which tetanus may be eliminated as an important health problem. There is little doubt that active immunization with adsorbed tetanus toxoid will convey a remarkably high degree of immunity. LaForce et al. (1969) have calculated that the incidence of tetanus in the under-ten age group in the United States of America was about 3.8 per 100 million. This underscores the excellent results obtained by active immunization of American and British military personnel in World War II.

In the United Kingdom, the recommended course of injections is three doses of adsorbed toxoid in a mixed vaccine, one injection at six months of age, and two others, with six to eight weeks between first and second and six months between second and third. A "booster" is advised at school entry and another at 15 to 19. Thereafter, "booster" doses should be given at ten-year intervals. The American Academy of Pediatrics suggests three injections of toxoid no less than one month apart in infancy, a reinforcing dose about twelve months later, and a fifth or "booster" injection on entering school. Subsequent routine toxoid "boosters" should be administered at intervals of approximately ten years.

After Injury

Prevention of Contamination. Simple measures that prevent contamination can contribute significantly to the prevention of tetanus, and the effect of attention to treatment of the umbilical stump on the incidence of neonatal tetanus is a good example of the effectiveness of simple hygiene. The aim of surgery in prophylaxis is to remove all dead tissue and foreign bodies from a wound. This will not only remove spore-bearing material, but will also deny the spores the anaerobic conditions necessary for their growth. As Adams et al. suggest, it is probably realistic to recognize a "tetanus-prone" wound. Such wounds include deep penetrating puncture wounds in which anaerobic conditions are likely to exist and surgical exposure is difficult or impossible. Tetanus-prone wounds also include wounds heavily contaminated with soil or manure, wounds with dead or devitalized tissue or retained foreign bodies, and wounds seen more than six to eight hours after infliction.

Active Immunization. In the United Kingdom a "booster" dose of toxoid is recommended if an injury occurs more than three years after the completion of the last course or more than three years after a "booster." If the wound is judged to be "tetanus prone," a "booster" should be given. The American Academy of Pediatrics recommends that an emergency injection of toxoid should be given if injury occurs more than one year after the last "booster." In spite of this, it has been suggested (Peebles et al., 1969) that if there is a valid history of an accepted immunization program, special tetanus boosters on admission to camps, schools, and colleges and emergency injections at times of injury are unnecessary and should be abandoned to minimize toxoid reactions. If a wounded patient's immune status is in doubt, he should be regarded as unimmunized, and other means of preventing tetanus should be used. If passive immunization with antitoxin is chosen, active immunization should be commenced at the same time with an injection of toxoid in another limb. Antitoxin will not influence active immunization conferred by a full course of adsorbed toxoid.

Passive Immunization. The use of passive immunization by means of antitoxin has probably resulted in the saving of many lives. The absence of a controlled trial precludes certainty, but circumstantial evidence is very strong. Animal experiments show that antitoxin given soon after inoculation with tetanus will protect against the disease, and Bruce (1920), reviewing 1458 cases of tetanus occurring in World War I, showed that the incidence of tetanus, after prophylactic antitoxin was available in large quantities, fell from 9 per 1000 wounded to 1.4 per 1000 wounded. Other improvements in surgical care could have been contributory, but it seems likely that antitoxin was an important factor in the decrease in incidence.

Antitoxin has two disadvantages, both relative. The antitoxin commonly used is produced by the active immunization of horses, first with toxoid and then with tetanus toxin. If a patient has had a previous injection of horse serum, he may develop antibodies against horse serum proteins very soon after an injection of prophylactic equine antitoxin. This will result in immune elimination of the subsequently injected equine antitoxin so that protection is absent or incomplete. This elimination may be accompanied by sensitivity reactions, either local redness and swelling of the injected limb or generalized serum sickness. If circulating antibodies are present, immune elimination may be very rapid and may be accompanied by fatal anaphylaxis. The dose of equine antitoxin for prophylaxis is 1500 units, but prophylactic antitoxin should not be given if either local or general reactions follow the subcutaneous injection of a test dose of 75 units. Epinephrine, 1 per 1000, should always be available whenever equine antitoxin is given; in cases in which antitoxin is indicated and either a history of previous injections of horse serum or a reaction to a test dose has been elicited, prophylaxis with human antitetanus immunoglobulin, 250 units, will be more effective and much safer.

Chemoprophylaxis. Antimicrobial drugs can inhibit the multiplication of *Clostridium tetani* and kill the vegetative form of the organism. By killing aerobic organisms coexisting with the Clostridium, antimicrobial drugs can prevent multiplication by denying the Clostridium the conditions favorable to its growth; they have no effect, however, on tetanus toxin. Because of the dangers of passive immunization, some centers in the United Kingdom have largely abandoned the use of antitoxin in favor of chemoprophylaxis, and at least one of these has provided data showing no increase in the incidence of the disease. Although the efficacy of chemoprophylaxis is not yet certain, it seems clear that in certain circumstances it may provide an alternative to prophylaxis by antitoxin.

For effective chemoprophylaxis certain criteria must be fulfilled: the organism must be susceptible to the drug chosen, and the patient must not be sensitive to the drug. *Clostridium tetani* is susceptible to a variety of drugs, including penicillin, tetracycline, and erythromycin, so that it is probably not difficult to make a suitable choice for a particular patient. Chemoprophylaxis must be started early. Smith (1964) has shown that in mice inoculated with tetanus spores, chemoprophylaxis was effective if it was started four hours after inoculation but not if started eight hours after inoculation. The time interval in humans is not established, but it is suggested that in injuries seen later than six hours after infliction, some other form of prophylaxis should be chosen. Antimicrobial therapy must be continued for a sufficient time to ensure that tetanus spores cannot survive, and this means for at least five days.

PATHOGENESIS

If tetanus is to supervene, the Clostridium must be introduced into human tissue, and the disease may follow a trivial or a serious injury. In countries with good medical services, serious wounds receive effective treatment, and tetanus is usually avoided. Apparently minor wounds then become a common cause of the disease, but in quite a high proportion of cases no responsible injury can be identified. The site of action and method of spread of the exotoxin have been mentioned, but it is rather surprising that no unequivocal evidence of recognizable pathologic lesions caused by tetanus has yet been forthcoming even after careful postmortem studies.

CLINICAL FEATURES AND CRITERIA OF SEVERITY IN TETANUS

The criteria of severity may be established in two ways: from the history and from the symptoms and signs.

From the History. The severity of an attack of tetanus is related to the incubation period (the period from injury to the first sign of tetanus) and the onset period, described by Cole (1940) as the period from the first sign to the first generalized spasm. If the former is less than 9 days and the latter less than 48 hours, the attack of tetanus may be expected to be severe. The length of the onset period is, in general, the more reliable guide to the expected severity of the attack.

From the Symptoms and Signs. *The Mild Case.* Tetanus usually presents with rigidity of muscles, and this rigidity may be severe enough to cause pain. The patient with mild tetanus may have "local tetanus" in which rigidity affects only one limb, or the patient may have mild generalized rigidity. Stiffness of the jaw muscles causes trismus, and stiffness of the facial muscles may cause a change of expression. Stiffness of the muscles of the neck and back may cause discomfort or even pain on attempted flexion of the spine.

The Moderate Case. The patient has more severe generalized rigidity. Trismus is pronounced, the mouth can hardly be opened, and rigidity of the muscles of the face may cause the sneering "risus sardonicus." Opisthotonos may be pronounced, but more typically the stiffness of the antagonist muscles makes the patient lie "at attention" in bed, and the muscles of back and abdomen are hard to the touch. Patients with moderate tetanus may show mild exacerbations of this generalized rigidity as "reflex spasms." These spasms may arise spontaneously or more commonly as a result of stimuli. The important difference, however, between the patient with mild and the patient with moderate tetanus is the presence or absence of dysphagia. Spasm of the pharyngeal muscles makes swallowing difficult, and the patient coughs or splutters while drinking. This will predispose to the inhalation of pharyngeal contents and is the diagnostic characteristic of the moderate case.

The Severe Case. The patient who represents a severe case is distinguished from the patient with a moderate case by the presence of reflex spasms that may be of appalling intensity. If the spasms are untreated opisthotonos becomes extreme, and the intense muscle spasm may fracture vertebrae. Spasm of the laryngeal muscles, the diaphragm, and the intercostals prevents ventilation, and cyanosis occurs. The occurrence of reflex spasms that cause cyanosis and cannot be controlled except by powerful relaxants such as curare is the characteristic feature of the severe case of tetanus.

Patients with severe tetanus may also show a group of signs that have often been described but have been attributed by workers in Oxford to overactivity of the sympathetic nervous system (Kerr et al.). Many patients sweat profusely and, in some, oxygen uptake and carbon dioxide output are increased. In some patients most severely affected, extreme peripheral vasoconstriction develops with a glove-and-stocking distribution and a sharp line of demarcation between warm skin and cold skin. Hyperpyrexia may also develop, and probably reflects the inability of the vasoconstricted patient to lose heat. The most striking features of this syndrome, however, involve the cardiovascular system. Sinus tachycardia occurs and may progress to multifocal ventricular ectopic beats. The blood pressure is generally elevated, and superimposed on this elevation are peaks, often associated with spasms or stimuli, in which the systolic pressure may reach 300 mm Hg, and the diastolic 150 mm Hg. The syndrome may progress to hypotension that does not respond to pressor agents.

Perhaps fortunately, patients with severe tetanus often remember little of their illness and have failed to remember such bizarre incidents as a Union Jack being waved in the ward during the playing of "Rule Britannia." Electroencephalography shows a sleep pattern, with arousal during stimulation such as tracheal aspiration.

DIAGNOSIS

The diagnosis of the established case of tetanus is all too easy, and strychnine poisoning is the only condition which is truly similar to established tetanus. Trismus may occur from dental infections, and the author has seen one case of hysterical tetanus. More recently, overdose with the phenothiazine group of drugs has been confused with tetanus, but the movements in this condition usually include grimacing and jaw movements in which the jaw is opened widely.

CAUSES OF DEATH IN TETANUS

One of the most remarkable features of tetanus is that when patients recover, even from the most severe forms of the disease, they recover completely. It would therefore seem reasonable to study the causes of death carefully in tetanus so that by avoiding them the natural tendency of the disease toward recovery may be exploited. In a survey in Oxford, the causes of death in 18 of 82 patients were bronchopneumonia, 4; pulmonary embolus, 3; technical failure, 2; coincidental causes, 5; and no identifiable cause of death, 4.

Bronchopulmonary complications of tetanus are becoming less common now that the management of patients receiving IPPV through a tracheostomy tube is better understood, and it is likely that chest complications will become still less common in the future. In general on the writer's service, pulmonary embolus is not a common cause of death in patients with other diseases treated by tracheostomy and IPPV. However, the difference in the incidence of pulmonary embolus between *patients with tetanus* requiring treatment with curare and IPPV and patients *with other diseases similarly treated* is so striking that anticoagulants are now used in patients with tetanus severe enough to merit treatment in this way. The incidence of technical failure underlines the complexity of treating the fully paralyzed patient; the coincidental causes of death apparently had nothing to do with the main disease. No identifiable cause of death could be found in four patients who had all displayed a syndrome suggestive of sympathetic overactivity. Careful study of patients with similar symptoms and signs admitted subsequently has reinforced our belief that in some patients with severe tetanus the sympathetic nervous system is as grossly uninhibited as is the motor nervous system (Prys-Roberts et al.).

TREATMENT

There are certain forms of treatment required by all patients with tetanus.

Control of Rigidity and Reflex Spasms. Drugs to control rigidity vary with the severity of the case. *Barbiturates* have been used for many years, and in mild or even moderate cases are useful, but the amount of barbiturate necessary to obtund severe reflex spasms would cause coma. *Chlorpromazine* has proved antispasmodic properties in tetanus and is a sedative. It also is useful in mild and moderate cases, but has been shown by a clinical trial (Adams, 1958) to be no more effective than barbiturates, and like the barbiturates is inadequate to obtund the spasms in the severest cases. It may be used in doses of up to 50 mg intramuscularly every four to six hours. *Mephenesin* is a centrally acting muscle relaxant that has been used extensively in the treatment of tetanus with good results, especially in moderate cases, but it must be given frequently and in large doses. The effect of a dose as large as 1 gram can be observed to have diminished significantly in one hour, and this dose, continued at hourly intervals, is close to that which will paralyze ventilation. If it becomes necessary to give paralyzing doses of mephenesin to control rigidity or reflex spasms, it is clearly not the drug of choice. Mephenesin is a local anesthetic and must be given by nasogastric tube. If given intravenously, except in extremely dilute solutions, it will cause hemolysis and hemoglobinuria. *Diazepam* is currently popular and has been used in mild and moderate cases in doses from 10 mg every four hours intramuscularly, to 600 mg intravenously per day. Like the other drugs mentioned above, it will not control the spasms of the severest case, and it is probably unwise to use very large doses. The severity of the case should be admitted and treatment changed to curare and IPPV. *Curare* and similar powerful relaxants will completely abolish the reflex spasms of the severest case of tetanus, but will also paralyze the muscles of ventilation. It is therefore necessary in addition to apply IPPV through a cuffed tracheostomy tube. Curare can be given intramuscularly in doses from 15 to 30 mg.

Wound Excision. Wound excision has been discussed under Prevention and seems a logical course of action if the causal injury can be identified. It has been suggested that excision of the wound is ineffectual in established tetanus because all the exotoxin produced by the organism has been fixed by the nervous system before symptoms and signs develop. Francis (1914) inoculated animals with tetanus and killed them when symptoms and signs began. He was able to recover many thousands of mouse lethal doses of toxin from the site of the inoculation, and this would seem to make the case for wound excision unassailable. A careful search should be made for foreign bodies in any wound excised, and excision should probably be conducted under cover of antitoxin.

Chemotherapy. Antimicrobial therapy has also been discussed under Prevention. As a therapeutic measure all patients with tetanus should have large doses of penicillin or another active antimicrobial for a sufficient time to ensure that the Clostridium cannot survive. This should be for at least five days.

Antitoxin. The advisability of using equine antitoxin as a therapeutic measure has been a controversial matter for many years. There is some, but not clear-cut, evidence that the use of equine antitoxin reduces mortality in established tetanus. On general grounds, however, the work of Francis cited above suggests that toxin is still being produced at the time when symptoms and signs begin, and hence it would seem reasonable to neutralize any accessible toxin. Therapeutic antitoxin is subject to the same objections and hazards as prophylactic antitoxin, and its dangers must be balanced against the possible gain by its use. A suitable dosage regimen, including subcutaneous, intramuscular, and intravenous injections, should be designed to uncover sensitivity if present, and to avoid anaphylaxis. Ten thousand units intravenously is a suitable dose, but up to 100,000 units has been used. If a history of previous injections of horse serum can be obtained, or if a sensitivity reaction occurs, equine antitoxin should not be used. If available, human antitoxin in the same dose is more effective and much safer.

Mild Tetanus

The patient with mild tetanus needs only these general measures, including a relaxant and sedative such as diazepam. The patient should be encouraged to drink water under supervision every two hours in the early stage of the disease when it may be progressing. If a patient coughs or splutters while drinking, dysphagia is present, and the patient moves into the moderate group.

Moderate Tetanus

The patient with moderate tetanus differs from the mild case by the presence of dysphagia. He needs the general measures applicable to all patients with tetanus, but in addition he must have a tracheostomy and have a cuffed tracheostomy tube inserted into the trachea to make inhalation of pharyngeal contents impossible. The operation is performed under general anesthesia with a cuffed endotracheal tube in situ so that the operation may be careful and unhurried. A cuffed tracheostomy tube should be inserted through a high U-shaped incision into the trachea so that the tube lies easily in the trachea where it is approximately parallel to the skin. If the tracheostomy is high, there is sufficient distance between the tracheostome and the carina to make it unlikely that the tube will enter the right main bronchus. The wound should not be covered and should be cleaned frequently with a mild antiseptic. It is necessary to aspirate secretions from the trachea, and disposable gloves should be worn during this procedure, not only to prevent contamination of the trachea with organisms carried on the aspirating catheter, but also to avoid contamination of the tracheostomy wound. The patient with moderate tetanus must be fed by nasogastric tube, and may require large amounts of fluid to offset excessive sweating. A high calorie diet of about 3000 calories a day is necessary, but too much protein should not be given. Patients with moderate tetanus may have a considerable degree of muscle rigidity and may even have occasional mild reflex spasms. Diazepam in divided doses of up to 400 mg intravenously per day has a considerable effect on the rigidity of tetanus without interfering with ventilation. In spite of treatment, muscular rigidity is painful and uncomfortable, and the patient should be turned every two hours to lessen this discomfort and avoid pressure sores.

Severe Tetanus

The patient with severe tetanus differs from the patient with moderate tetanus in that he has frequent reflex spasms that cannot be controlled by muscle relaxants other than curare, and needs to be paralyzed with curare or another powerful relaxant. Curare may be given by intramuscular injection of 15 to 30 mg; if the patient must be paralyzed, there seems little to be gained by withholding the drug. At Oxford the nurses are instructed to give a further dose of curare when reflex spasms become obvious, and 400 mg of curare per day has been necessary. The high incidence of pulmonary embolus in patients with severe tetanus has led to the use of anticoagulants in patients severely enough affected to require treatment with curare and IPPV. Anticoagulants are not, however, used within 24 hours of tracheostomy. The treatment of a paralyzed patient with IPPV is complex, and appropriate monographs should be consulted (Adams et al., 1969; Spalding and Crampton Smith, 1963). The patient cannot breathe, and IPPV must be applied through the cuffed tracheostomy tube. It has become common practice in recent years to ventilate with a large tidal volume at a slow rate, for example, with a tidal volume of 1 liter and a rate of 12 to 14 per minute. An artificial dead space is introduced between ventilator and patient so that rebreathing of expired air may bring the tension of carbon dioxide in the arterial blood to about 30 mm Hg. Large tidal volumes seem to contribute to the health of the lungs, but the patient must also be turned every two hours to promote lung drainage, the inspired air must be fully humidified and at body temperature, and chest physiotherapy three times a day is indicated. Frequent chest films are necessary, and tracheal aspiration must be carried out with aseptic precautions. The patient cannot drink and must be fed by nasogastric tube or by vein if absorption fails. Patients with severe tetanus sweat profusely and may need large quantities of fluid, but the urine specific gravity is not always a good guide to hydration, and the patient should be weighed daily. It is not uncommon to observe a patient seriously ill with tetanus who is having a large fluid intake and gaining weight, but who still produces a high specific gravity urine. Later in the disease a diuresis may occur, and the patient may lose weight abruptly. A patient with severe tetanus needs 3000 calories per day, but too much protein is not advised, even though the patient, being functionally denervated by curare, may show muscle wasting. Urine is voided normally, but manual extraction of feces may be necessary. The patient cannot communicate, and sedation is probably indicated for patients paralyzed with curare. Withdrawal of sedation in severely ill patients may, however, disclose that the patient is unconscious.

Some patients most severely affected by tetanus develop a syndrome suggesting sympathetic overactivity. The cardiovascular component of this syndrome, tachycardia, arrhythmias, and hypertension, should be treated with beta- and alpha-adrenergic blockers (Prys-Roberts et al.). If it is thought necessary to administer a beta blocker intravenously, this should be done with great caution. Propranolol in 0.2 mg aliquots to a total of 2 mg has been successfully used to control arrhythmias and severe tachycardia. Control can sometimes be maintained by intragastric propranolol, 10 mg every eight hours, but larger doses may be required. In some cases, when hypertension is not severe, control of the heart rate may be all that is necessary, but if the blood pressure is elevated, alpha-adrenergic blockade is also indicated. Bethanidine, 5 mg by nasogastric tube every two hours, has been used successfully, and as this drug acts at postganglionic nerve endings, an overdose could be counteracted by pressor agents. The receptors, however, remain susceptible or perhaps hypersensitive to circulating catecholamines, and other combinations of antihypertensive drugs may be more effective. The author is aware of a patient successfully treated with propranolol, reserpine, and bethanidine. It is important not to reduce the heart rate to a point at which the cardiac output fails, because the depressed heart is working against an increased peripheral resistance. Moderate control of heart rate should be effected with a beta blocker, but hypertension when the heart rate is 100 or less must be controlled by alpha blockade.

In summary, in *a mild case* the patient needs (1) wound excision, (2) human or equine antitoxin, (3) penicillin or another appropriate antimicrobial drug, and (4) a centrally acting relaxant and sedative drug, such as diazepam.

In *the moderate case* the patient needs in addition (5) tracheostomy and the insertion of a cuffed rubber tracheostomy tube to separate the pharynx from the trachea and to make inhalation of foreign material impossible, and (6) nasogastric tube feeding.

In *the severe case* the patient needs in addition (7) virtually complete paralysis with curare or another powerful relaxant and IPPV, (8) anticoagulant drugs, and (9) if sympathetic overactivity is present, treatment with alpha- and beta-adrenergic blockers.

PROGNOSIS

The patient with mild tetanus will almost certainly survive whether treated or not. The patient with moderate tetanus, if untreated, is at risk from inhalation of foreign material. Repeated episodes of this kind may lead to fatal pneumonia. The patient with moderate tetanus, if treated, should not die except from causes unrelated to the primary disease. The patient with severe tetanus who is having reflex spasms severe enough to cause cyanosis will certainly die if untreated. Even with treatment, the severity of the illness and the complexity of the therapeutic regimen make the outlook uncertain. In the United Kingdom in 1967, even in the best centers the mortality in patients with tetanus severe enough to indicate treatment with curare and IPPV varied between 10 and 40 per cent. Over-all mortality in the best hands is often still as high as 20 per cent, and at the extremes of age the mortality may be higher. It is paradoxical that in advanced countries where the immunization programs are efficient, mortality in the cases that do occur is high, not only because unimmunized patients are generally at the extremes of age, but also because patients who escape the immunization programs tend to have a poor physical status. Tetanus is becoming increasingly common among drug addicts.

Adams, E. B., Laurence, D. R., and Smith, J. W. G.: Tetanus. Oxford, Blackwell Scientific Publications, 1969.

Bjørnboe, M., Ibsen, B., and Johnson, S.: Et tilfaelde af tetanus behandlet med curarisering, tracheostomi of overtryksventilation med kvaelstofforilte og ilt. Ugeskr. Laeger., 115:1535, 1953.

Kerr, J. H., Corbett, J. L., Prys-Roberts, C., Smith, A. C., and Spalding, J. M. K.: Involvement of the sympathetic nervous system in tetanus. Br. Med. J., 2:236, 1968.

Prys-Roberts, C., Corbett, J. L., Kerr, J. H., Smith, A. C., and Spalding, J. M. K.: Treatment of sympathetic overactivity in tetanus. Lancet, 1:542, 1969.

Wright, G. P.: Neurotoxins of *Clostridium botulinum* and *Clostridium tetani.* Pharmacol. Rev., 7:413, 1955.

ANAEROBIC BACTERIA

211. DISEASE DUE TO NONSPOREFORMING ANAEROBIC BACTERIA

Sydney M. Finegold

Definition. Essentially every type of infection may be caused by nonsporeforming anaerobes. No organ or tissue of the body is immune to infection with these organisms. The majority of anaerobic infections involve two or more anaerobes, but infection with a single species of anaerobe does occur. Aerobic or facultatively anaerobic organisms may also be present in mixed infections. In mixed anaerobic infections, clostridia may be found together with nonsporeforming anaerobic bacilli and cocci. There are a number of unique features associated with certain clostridial infections, however, and it is convenient to consider these infections separately (see Ch. 206 to 210). Actinomycosis may also show distinctive clinical features; this disease (also often a mixed infection) is discussed in Ch. 224.

Etiology. The nonsporulating anaerobic bacteria are distributed widely throughout the body as indigenous flora. Numerically, they are the dominant flora on the various mucosal surfaces.

The anaerobic gram-negative bacilli and the anaerobic cocci are the major etiologic agents in anaerobic infections. They are encountered at least 15 times as frequently as clostridia. Gram-positive nonsporeforming anaerobic bacilli are encountered less commonly.

Anaerobic Gram-Negative Bacilli. The anaerobic gram-negative bacilli found in human infections belong to the genera Bacteroides and Fusobacterium, the former being encountered with much greater frequency. *Bacteroides fragilis* is the most commonly seen of all anaerobes. It is of added importance because it is the most resistant of the anaerobes to antimicrobial compounds. The subspecies of *B. fragilis* recovered most often from infections are, in order, *ss. fragilis, ss. thetaiotaomicron,* and *ss. vulgatus. B. fragilis,* like other gram-negative anaerobic rods, stains poorly. The staining is usually irregular, with bipolar staining (and a central clear or light area) especially common. There is a variable amount of pleomorphism. Two other Bacteroides species seen relatively often, though rarely as single infecting agents, are *B. melaninogenicus* (coccobacilli) and *B. oralis* (morphologically similar to *B. fragilis*). *Fusobacterium nucleatum,* the fusiform bacillus, is the most frequently found of the fusobacteria. This organism is long and thin, with tapered ends; they are often in pairs end to end. Long filaments may also be noted. Granules (sometimes gram-positive) may be seen. *F. necrophorum,* formerly commonly encountered, is now seen much less. Other species of Fusobacterium seen include *F. mortiferum* and *F. varium,* the latter being relatively resistant to antimicrobials. Medically important fusobacteria other than *F. nucleatum* tend to be highly pleomorphic, with long filaments containing central swellings, large, free round bodies, and considerable irregularity of staining.

The spirochetes of the genus Treponema, also gram-negative anaerobes, which are part of the indigenous flora, are very likely not pathogenic, judging from experimental studies. The old terms "fusospirochetal infection" and "Vincent's infection" are therefore no longer appropriate.

Anaerobic Cocci. The anaerobic cocci include gram-positive streptococci (Peptostreptococcus), gram-positive cocci in pairs or masses (Peptococcus), and gram-negative cocci (Veillonella, Megasphaera, Acidaminococcus). The anaerobic cocci are not usually pleomorphic, but many are smaller than facultative streptococci. Veillonella are tiny cocci in masses. As a group, anaerobic cocci are found in human disease almost as often as are the gram-negative anaerobic bacilli. The most commonly encountered species include *Peptostreptococcus anaerobius, intermedius,* and *micros* and *Peptococcus magnus, asaccharolyticus, prevotii,* and *variabilis.*

The microaerophilic cocci and streptococci are a very poorly characterized heterogeneous group. They are best defined as organisms which tolerate reduced oxygen tension (18 per cent oxygen) – with or without added carbon dioxide. Most of these are probably actually facultative streptococci. These organisms are encountered in serious infections with some frequency, not uncommonly in pure culture. They are considered with the obligate anaerobes, because they will often be overlooked unless good anaerobic techniques are used for transporting and culturing clinical specimens.

Gram-Positive Nonsporeforming Anaerobic Bacilli. The most commonly encountered gram-positive anaerobic nonsporeforming bacilli belong to the genus Eubacterium, particularly *E. lentum, E. alactolyticum,* and *E. limosum.* Gram-positive anaerobic bacilli in general destain readily and may appear gram-negative. Eubacterium strains may be filamentous. Propionibacterium strains, chiefly *P. acnes,* are seldom involved in infections of significance other than endocarditis (in patients with pre-existing valvular disease or artificial heart valves) or other infections related to implanted artificial prostheses. *Bifidobacterium eriksonii* is another well-established pathogen. Actinomyces may also be involved in infections without the distinctive clinical features of actinomycosis.

Features of Infections Due to Various Organisms. There are differences in the types of infection involving various anaerobes related to differences in their distribution in the body as normal flora. Thus the anaerobic cocci are encountered more often in oral and pulmonary infections and in female genital infections than in intra-abdominal disease. *Bacteroides fragilis,* which is the dominant member of the colonic flora, is involved in intra-abdominal infection commonly but is less frequently involved in dental infections or lung abscess. Aside from these differences, all the nonsporeforming anaerobes may be involved in any of the infections to be discussed in this chapter. Furthermore, the clinical picture is basically the same in these conditions regardless of the specific flora involved. Minor exceptions include distinctive odors related to end-products of metabolism (e.g., butyric acid produced in large amounts by Fusobacterium strains), the occasional formation of soft granules resembling sulfur granules by Fusobacterium, and the production of black color in blood-containing exudates by *B. melaninogenicus.*

Relative Importance of Various Organisms in Mixed Infections. It is difficult to determine the role of each species recovered from a mixed anaerobic infection and to assess the relative importance of the anaerobes and aerobic or facultative bacteria in mixed infections. Quantitative culture techniques may help. A small number of patients with pulmonary and intra-abdominal mixed infections of mild to moderate severity have been treated with agents active only against the anaerobes and have done well. This suggests that the anaerobes may have been the key pathogens.

Incidence and Prevalence. Anaerobic infections are the most frequently overlooked or misdiagnosed of all bacterial infections. Fortunately, the introduction of simplified anaerobic cultural procedures and an increased awareness of anaerobes and their importance on the part of bacteriologists and clinicians are beginning to overcome the problem.

Good data on the incidence of anaerobes in various infections are not always available. One big problem has been a tendency to overlook anaerobes in mixed cultures when one or more aerobic or facultative forms are present. Problems in specific identification have interfered with accurate determination of the involvement of particular organisms in various anaerobic infections.

A major reason for the lack of good information is the fact that most published studies focus on only clinical aspects or bacteriologic features, but not both. Nevertheless, there are studies supporting the view that anaerobes are common causes of infection. Some years ago Stokes (1958) found anaerobes in over 10 per cent of 4737 positive cultures of clinical specimens. Lodenkämper and Stienen (1955) detected 690 anaerobic infections in an eight-year period. Mattman et al. (1958) found anaerobic cocci in 45 per cent of 437 positive cultures from hospitalized patients. Recently, Martin et al. (1972) isolated 601 anaerobes from clinical specimens in an eight-month period.

Several recent studies have combined good clinical and bacteriologic analysis to yield reliable information on the incidence of anaerobes in certain infections. Thus Heineman and Braude (1962) have shown that anaerobes are the dominant cause of brain abscess. Bartlett and coworkers (1972, 1973) have established that lung abscess and aspiration pneumonia are most often due to anaerobes and that these organisms are important causes of necrotizing pneumonia and of empyema. Several groups have data to indicate that at least half to two thirds of cases of intra-abdominal abscess and of peritonitis involve anaerobes. Very likely over half of all cases of pyogenic liver abscess also involve these organisms. Rotheram and Schick have demonstrated that anaerobes are the most prevalent pathogens in postabortal sepsis. Other types of infections in which anaerobes play an important role include chronic otitis media and sinusitis, gingivitis and other oral infections, dental infections, bronchiectasis, other pulmonary infections, breast abscess, appendicitis, diverticulitis, abdominal wound infections, puerperal sepsis, various other obstetrical and gynecologic infections, ischiorectal and perirectal abscess, infected pilonidal sinuses, gas-forming cellulitis, necrotizing fasciitis, and septic thrombophlebitis.

Pathogenesis or Mechanisms. Anaerobic bacteria basically are saprophytic members of the indigenous flora. Under certain conditions, however, they may invade and produce disease.

A simplistic definition of anaerobic bacteria would be bacteria which cannot survive in the presence of air. However, it is well known that a number of anaerobes generally regarded as fairly fastidious will tolerate 2 to 8 per cent oxygen in the atmosphere, and a number of these organisms will tolerate considerably more. A more important factor determining whether or not the environment is suitable for growth of anaerobic bacteria is the oxidation-reduction potential of the medium. This is a measure of the tendency of the system to give up electrons and is usually expressed as the Eh value in millivolts. The Eh of a system is a function not only of its inherent reducing tendency but also of its hydrogen ion concentration, the Eh becoming more negative as the hydrogen ion concentration decreases.

One of the major defenses of the body against infection by anaerobes is the normal Eh (+120 mv). Lowering of the redox potential permits anaerobic growth in tissues, even those exposed to air. Lowered oxidation-reduction potential results from impaired blood supply, tissue necrosis, and growth of facultative bacteria in a wound. Thus vascular disease, epinephrine injection, cold, shock, edema, trauma, surgery, presence of a foreign body, malignancy, gas production by microorganisms, and aerobic infection all may predispose to anaerobic infection. The predisposition of diabetics to anaerobic infection is undoubtedly related at least partially to impaired blood supply and lowering of Eh. The association of malignancy (particularly of the colon, the bronchus, and the uterus) and anaerobic infection is well established; at times, anaerobic infection may be the first clue to the malignant process.

Certain toxins such as collagenase, hyaluronidase, deoxyribonuclease, and proteinases account for the virulence of some anaerobic infections.

The septic thrombophlebitis seen commonly in anaerobic infections may relate to production of heparinase by anaerobic bacteria. This lesion may lead to metastatic infection and helps account for the difficulty in eradicating anaerobic infections. Tissue destruction and abscess formation are also common manifestations of anaerobic infection.

Previous antimicrobial therapy is a not uncommon background for anaerobic infection. Preoperative "bowel preparation" with oral neomycin often results in a residual anaerobic flora, as many anaerobes tolerate even the very high concentrations achieved in the bowel lumen with such therapy. The popular combination of gentamicin plus cephalothin (given parenterally) may lead to anaerobic superinfection, particularly with *Bacteroides fragilis.*

Conditions which predispose to infection in general (malnutrition, severe debilitating disease, corticosteroid and other immunosuppressive therapy, granulocytopenia) also facilitate anaerobic infection.

Aspiration and poor dental hygiene are common background factors in anaerobic pulmonary infection.

The unique involvement of only certain subspecies of *B. fragilis* in infection is probably related to resistance to normal serum bactericidal factors (Casciato et al., 1973). Under anaerobic conditions the granulocyte phagocytic bactericidal system may not function efficiently.

Clinical Manifestations. For the most part the manifestations of anaerobic infection are those of the basic process (e.g., peritonsillar abscess, cholangitis, endometritis). Tissue necrosis, abscess formation, and septic thrombophlebitis are common with anaerobic infection, as are a foul odor and gas in tissues or in discharges.

Tonsillitis, Ludwig's Angina. Exudative tonsillitis (Vincent's angina) used to be a common anaerobic infection, usually caused by *Fusobacterium necrophorum.* The local tonsillar infection undoubtedly still occurs but is rarely recognized as an anaerobic process. The dreaded Ludwig's angina (cellulitis of the submandibular space), probably an anaerobic infection in most cases, is also uncommon now.

Bacteremia, Endocarditis. In recent years, bacteremia caused by anaerobes has dominated clinical reports on anaerobic infections. Most likely this is because anaerobes are much more likely to be present in pure culture in bacteremia than in other sources of anaerobic infection, and consequently it is much easier to isolate the offending organism. On the other hand, it is clear that anaerobic bacteremia is relatively common. At both the Mayo Clinic and the Oschsner Clinic, bacteroides are the second most common isolates from blood cultures. The primary sources of anaerobic bacteremia at present are gastrointestinal and gynecologic infections. Less common sites include infected decubitus ulcers and other wounds. Gram-negative anaerobic bacilli possess endotoxin, and septic shock and disseminated intravascular coagulation have been described in the course of anaerobic bacteremia.

In large series of endocarditis, only 1 to 2 per cent of positive blood cultures have yielded anaerobes as a rule. As high as 15 per cent, however, were sterile in the presence of strong clinical or pathologic evidence of endocarditis. Our experience is that approximately 10 per cent of cases of endocarditis are caused by anaerobic or microaerophilic cocci. The main portals of entry for anaerobes in bacterial endocarditis are the mouth, the gastrointestinal tract, and, to a lesser extent, the genitourinary tract. The incidence of pre-existing heart disease is lower in the case of anaerobic endocarditis, and there is evidence to indicate that embolization may be more common in the case of the disease involving anaerobes.

Pleuropulmonary Infection. Anaerobic pulmonary infection is commonly overlooked. Unfortunately, even when suspected, it has often not been confirmed by proper culture of appropriate specimens. Coughed sputum culture is unsatisfactory because of the presence of anaerobes as normal upper respiratory tract flora. The clinical course of anaerobic pulmonary infection ranges from incidentally discovered infection to fulminant infection. Most patients present with a smoldering illness. The most common underlying condition is a predisposition to aspirate caused by altered consciousness or dysphagia. Important clues to anaerobic etiology are aspiration, pulmonary necrosis, indolent course, and foul-smelling sputum or pus. The principal types of anaerobic pulmonary infection are lung abscess, necrotizing pneumonia, and pneumonia without necrosis; many patients have an associated empyema.

Anaerobes are probably second only to the pneumococcus as causes of pneumonia in hospitalized patients, because aspiration pneumonia is a common event.

Intra-abdominal Infection. Anaerobes are a prime cause of peritonitis and intra-abdominal abscess and are involved in virtually all cases of complicated appendicitis or diverticulitis.

Anaerobes (especially nonsporeformers) play a relatively minor role in gallbladder infection.

Genitourinary Tract Infection. Various urinary tract infections may involve anaerobes, but these organisms are not common causes of such infection. Factors predisposing to anaerobic urinary tract infection are stones, malignancy, obstruction, and previous renal tuberculosis.

A large variety of female genital tract infections involve anaerobic bacteria. Clostridia cause the most serious female genital tract infections, but infections in this system are much more commonly produced by nonsporeforming anaerobic bacteria. Predisposing conditions include pregnancy, the puerperium (particularly with premature rupture of the membranes, prolonged labor, or postpartum hemorrhage), abortion (spontaneous or induced), malignancy, radiation, surgery, cauterization, stenosis, uterine fibroids, and old gonococcal salpingitis.

Skin, Soft Tissue, and Muscle Infection. These infections include such entities as cellulitis, pyoderma, infected cysts, infection of decubitus and other ulcers, abscesses, bacterial synergistic gangrene, chronic undermining ulcer of Meleney, necrotizing fasciitis, bite infection, noma, and tropical ulcer. Anaerobes are common infecting agents in hidradenitis suppurativa. Subcutaneous abscesses involving anaerobes are seen in narcotic addicts who are "skin-poppers."

Anaerobic (gas-forming) cellulitis is an acute soft tissue infection, seen particularly in diabetics and commonly ascribed to coliforms. Although gas-producing nonanaerobes may be involved, it is our experience that anaerobes predominate. Muscle is not involved, but it is essential that clostridial myositis be ruled out. This differentiation may require surgery which, in any case, is important therapeutically.

Anaerobic streptococci may produce a myositis simulating "gas gangrene," but the infection is much less severe. Rarely, Bacteroides may be involved in a mild form of myositis.

Bone and Joint Infection. Osteomyelitis caused by anaerobes is probably overlooked often. Anaerobes are relatively common in infected diabetic ulcers of the foot with bony involvement.

There are a number of well-documented cases of purulent arthritis caused by anaerobes, chiefly gram-negative bacilli. Predisposing factors include underlying joint disease and local or systemic corticosteroid therapy. Any joint may be affected, but there is a peculiar susceptibility of the sternoclavicular and sacroiliac joints.

Diagnosis. *Clues Suggesting Anaerobic Infection.* Features indicating the likelihood of anaerobic infection include foul or putrid odor, infection located near mucosal surfaces (particularly with manipulation of the associated organs), tissue necrosis, gas in tissues or discharges, infection associated with malignancy or other tissue-destructive process, endocarditis with negative routine blood cultures, infection related to the use of aminoglycoside antimicrobials (by any route) and/or broad-spectrum penicillins or cephalosporins, septic thrombophlebitis, infection after bites, black coloration or red fluorescence under ultraviolet light of discharges or lesions (*B. melaninogenicus* infection), unique morphology on Gram stain of exudate, and failure to obtain growth on routine culture (particularly when organisms are seen on Gram stain of exudate).

Specimen Collection. The major consideration is to avoid "contaminating" a specimen with normal flora, because anaerobes are prevalent as indigenous flora.

Expectorated sputum is not suitable for anaerobic culture. Bronchoscopically obtained specimens are also not suitable, because the instrument becomes "contaminated" during insertion; however, fiberoptic bronchoscopy through a nasotracheal tube may prove to be satisfactory. Transtracheal needle aspiration or direct lung puncture is the optimal method of obtaining specimens.

In the case of uterine infection, the patient must be positioned to provide maximal exposure. The cervical os is decontaminated. Then material is obtained from the uterine cavity by syringe or swab technique, using great care to avoid normal vaginal flora. Rough quantitation of growth may help to distinguish between infecting organisms and normal flora, because a certain degree of contamination may be inevitable in this situation.

In the case of abscesses, unbroken skin or mucosal surface is decontaminated, and pus is removed with a syringe. This is preferable to using a swab on a portion of an exposed lesion.

Voided midstream urine may contain anaerobes from the urethral flora; therefore percutaneous suprapubic bladder aspiration is necessary.

Specimen Transport. Proper transport of specimens to the laboratory is crucial for recovery of anaerobes which may be present. Since some anaerobes are tolerant to oxygen contact, a laboratory which isolates such organisms as *B. fragilis* and *C. perfringens* may not realize that it is overlooking more demanding anaerobes. Many anaerobes responsible for clinical infections do not tolerate oxygen exposure well, so that special transport methods are needed to ensure their survival. Various means for proper anaerobic transport include the following:

1. Syringe technique—eliminate all air from specimen in syringe and needle and then stick needle into a sterile rubber stopper.
2. Gassed-out tubes—inject specimen into butyl rubber-stoppered tube which has been gassed out with oxygen-free CO_2. Commercial vials of this type are available.

Treatment. *General Aspects.* Surgical aspects of therapy are extremely important. Drainage of collections of pus and excision of necrotic tissue are commonly necessary, and in minor infections they may be all that is required. Obstructions must be relieved.

Anticoagulant therapy or venous ligation may be indicated in patients with septic phlebitis. Treatment of shock and disseminated intravascular coagulation, when they occur, and general supportive measures are important aspects of therapy.

Local use of hydrogen peroxide or zinc peroxide is useful. Hyperbaric oxygen therapy is not indicated in infection with nonsporeforming anaerobes.

Antimicrobial Therapy. In vitro susceptibility tests, properly performed, serve as a good guide to drug therapy of anaerobic infections. Standardized disc susceptibility tests are available for most anaerobic bacteria but are most satisfactory with organisms which have been identified. Use of a disc test without measurement of zones of inhibition, or application of standards which were developed for aerobic and facultative organisms, yields completely undependable results. Conventional tube or plate dilution tests with incubation in an anaerobic jar are reliable. Patterns of susceptibility to selected drugs are noted in the accompanying table.

Penicillin is active against most anaerobes other than *Bacteroides fragilis;* however, this organism is the anaerobe most commonly isolated from infection. Certain strains of anaerobic cocci require as much as 8.0 μg per milliliter for inhibition, and occasional strains of *Fusobacterium varium* are resistant to penicillin. Dosage of penicillin G should be at least 6 to 8 million units daily in the case of seriously ill patients or infection with relatively resistant strains. Ampicillin and cephaloridine are usually comparable to penicillin G, but several other penicillins and cephalosporins are less active. Some agents in these classes may be useful because very high blood levels are achieved safely or because of their resistance to beta lactamases.

Tetracycline is no longer valuable in many geographic areas, because many strains of anaerobes of all types are now resistant. Two new tetracycline derivatives, doxycycline and minocycline, are more active in vitro but have not yet been studied extensively clinically.

Lincomycin, erythromycin, and vancomycin are active against certain anaerobes; more information is needed, however, on the validity of in vitro tests with these drugs, and they are not approved by the Food and Drug Administration for use in anaerobic infections.

Chloramphenicol is active against all anaerobes, with only rare strains resistant, and is very effective clinically. It penetrates the central nervous system well. However, because of its serious and unpredictable toxicity, it should be reserved for seriously ill patients and used only until bacteriologic data indicate that a less toxic drug would be suitable. Nevertheless, chloramphenicol is the drug of choice for serious anaerobic infection of uncertain cause. Initial dosage of chloram-

Susceptibility of Anaerobes to Selected Antimicrobial Agents

	Microaerophilic and Anaerobic Cocci	*Bacteroides fragilis*	*Bacteroides melaninogenicus*	*Fusobacterium varium*	Other Fusobacterium Species	Eubacterium
Penicillin G	++++	+	++++	+++*	++++	++++
Clindamycin	+++	+++	+++	++	+++	+++*
Metronidazole†	++	+++	+++	+++	+++	?
Chloramphenicol	+++	+++	+++	+++	+++	+++

++++ Drug of choice.
+++ Good activity.
++ Moderate activity.
+ Poor or inconsistent activity.

*A few strains are resistant.
†Experimental for anaerobic infections.

phenicol in such a patient should be 40 to 50 mg per kilogram of body weight daily; once the patient has shown a good response, 30 mg per kilogram per day should be adequate.

Clindamycin (7-chlorolincomycin) has broad activity against anaerobes, with only *Fusobacterium varium*, among the nonsporeformers, commonly resistant. However, a number of strains of Clostridium other than *C. perfringens* are not uncommonly resistant. At the time of this writing it would be regarded as one of the drugs of choice for nonsporeforming anaerobic infections, except in very serious infections in which the nature of the infecting organism and its susceptibility to clindamycin are not yet known. Oral dosage for adults is 150 to 450 mg every six hours, and parenteral dosage is 600 to 2700 mg per day (in two to four equal doses), depending on the severity of the infection. Daily doses as high as 4.8 grams have been given intravenously to critically ill patients.

Metronidazole has broad activity against anaerobic microorganisms and is consistently bactericidal versus *Bacteroides fragilis* and other anaerobes. Its use for anaerobic infections is still on an experimental basis.

Although it is true that *Bacteroides fragilis* infections are more common below the diaphragm and that most anaerobes recovered from infections above the diaphragm are penicillin susceptible, there is too much overlap for practical application of this knowledge in the individual case—particularly if the patient has a serious infection. For example, *B. fragilis* is part of the infecting flora of 20 to 25 per cent of anaerobic pulmonary infections. It has also been recovered from such infections as sinusitis, mastoiditis, and brain abscess.

Therapy with antimicrobial agents in anaerobic infections must be intensive and prolonged. These infections have a considerable tendency to relapse.

Prognosis. In general, infection with nonsporeforming anaerobes carries a relatively good prognosis, provided the diagnosis is suspected and confirmed early and appropriate therapy instituted promptly. To some extent, of course, the prognosis varies with the site and extent of the lesion. Brain abscess is still a very serious infection with a significant mortality (50 per cent). The over-all mortality in anaerobic pulmonary infections is 15 to 20 per cent, with a distinctly higher mortality in the case of necrotizing pneumonia (greater than 30 per cent). The mortality in liver abscess varies greatly from series to series, depending primarily on whether or not cases were discovered ante mortem and on how early they were picked up. On the whole, the mortality is in the range of 25 to 50 per cent. The mortality in sepsis caused by nonsporeforming anaerobes is 30 per cent. In patients with endocarditis caused by gram-negative anaerobic bacilli, mortality is also 30 per cent, but it is higher in cases caused by *Bacteroides fragilis* than in those caused by other, more sensitive gram-negative anaerobic bacilli. The mortality in endocarditis caused by anaerobic cocci is not significantly different from that caused by facultative streptococci. The availability of a number of effective drugs has permitted a reduction in mortality and morbidity resulting from anaerobic infection.

Prevention. The major principles in prophylaxis are avoidance of conditions which reduce the redox potential of the tissues and avoidance of the introduction of anaerobes from the indigenous flora into sites where they may set up infection. Discriminate use of antimicrobial drugs will minimize anaerobic superinfection.

Early appropriate therapy of anaerobic infections will prevent metastatic infection.

Precautions to minimize the possibility of aspiration will be helpful in preventing anaerobic pulmonary infection. Good surgical technique (e.g., minimal devitalization of tissue, use of closed methods of resection) will prevent postoperative anaerobic infections.

Bartlett, J., and Finegold, S. M.: Anaerobic pleuropulmonary infections. Medicine, 51:413, 1972.

Finegold, S. M., and Rosenblatt, J. E.: Practical aspects of anaerobic sepsis. Medicine, 52:311, 1973.

Goldsand, G., and Braude, A. I.: Anaerobic infections. D. M., November 1966.

Marcoux, J. A., Zabransky, R. J., Washington, J. A., II, Wellman, W. E., and Martin, W. J.: Bacteroides bacteremia: A review of 123 cases. Minn. Med., 53:1169, 1970.

Rotheram, E. B., Jr., and Schick, S. F.: Nonclostridial anaerobic bacteria in septic abortion. Am. J. Med., 46:80, 1969.

Saksena, D. S., Block, M. A., McHenry, M. C., and Truant, J. P.: Bacteroidaceae: Anaerobic organisms encountered in surgical infections. Surgery, 63:261, 1968.

TYPHOID FEVER AND SALMONELLOSIS

212. TYPHOID FEVER*

Abram S. Benenson

Definition. Typhoid fever is an acute, often severe illness caused by *Salmonella typhi* and characterized by fever, headache, apathy, cough, prostration, splenomegaly, maculopapular rash, and leukopenia. Typhoid fever is the classic example of enteric fever caused by salmonellae.

Incidence and Prevalence. Typhoid fever is a disease of major importance in areas of the world that have not attained high standards of public health. A progressive decrease in incidence of typhoid fever has occurred in the United States since 1900, but sporadic cases and limited outbreaks continue to occur. About 400 cases per year have been reported in recent years; over a third of these were in persons under 15 years of age, and in about 10 per cent the patients were under 5 years. About 40 per cent of these infections were acquired in other areas of the world, but most were acquired in the United States from food contaminated by chronic typhoid carriers. In the United States more than 3000 chronic typhoid carriers are under supervision by health departments, but the actual number of chronic carriers is probably considerably higher. Typhoid fever will continue to occur on a limited scale in countries with high standards of public health because of the frequency of typhoid in other areas of the world, the magnitude of intercontinental travel, and the existence of reservoirs of chronic carriers.

*In the two previous editions the chapter on Typhoid Fever was written by Dr. Edward W. Hook. Significant portions of that chapter are included in the present version prepared by Dr. Benenson, who joins with the Editors in expressing indebtedness to Dr. Hook.

Epidemiology. The ultimate source of infection with *S. typhi* is man, either a patient with typhoid fever or a typhoid carrier. The patient with typhoid excretes large numbers of *S. typhi* in feces or urine, and viable bacilli may also be present in vomitus, respiratory secretions, or pus. Chronic enteric carriers, the most important source of infection, often excrete 10^6 or more viable bacilli per gram of feces. The typhoid bacillus can survive for weeks in water, ice, dust, and dried sewage. Water containing typhoid bacilli has been responsible for many outbreaks in the past; it may be contaminated directly by excreta containing *S. typhi* or by excreta washed down from remote sites by rain or introduced by faulty sanitation or plumbing. Foods may be contaminated by dirty hands or water contaminated by *S. typhi* and occasionally by contaminated dust. Flies are excellent mechanical vectors for the transmission of infection. Oysters and other shellfish may be infected in polluted tidal waters. In areas where typhoid fever is common, the incidence usually increases during the summer.

Pathogenesis. The portal of entry of *S. typhi* is almost always the gastrointestinal tract. In studies with human volunteers, bacilli were recovered from the stools within 24 hours after the organisms were swallowed; within a few days the stool usually became negative. The bacilli penetrate the intestinal epithelial lining without causing appreciable inflammation, and apparently enter the small lymphatics, reaching the mesenteric lymph nodes where they enter mononuclear cells within which they multiply. Although transient bacteremia may occur, the involvement of the reticuloepithelial cells in a proliferative process in liver, spleen, bone marrow, and other lymph nodes may be the response to circulating endotoxin. The incubation period represents the period for significant intracellular multiplication; its length is inversely proportional to the number of organisms ingested. When the symptoms do appear, there is a bacteremia; this has been considered to cause the clinical manifestations, although asymptomatic bacteremias have been observed not infrequently. Incidental to the systemic dissemination of bacilli, hepatomegaly occurs frequently, and infection of the biliary tract occurs regularly. Typhoid bacilli multiply in bile, with subsequent seeding of the intestinal tract with millions of bacilli. Infection of the gallbladder is usually asymptomatic, although symptoms of cholecystitis occasionally do develop.

The similarity of many manifestations of typhoid fever to the events observed after the intravenous injection of purified endotoxin of *S. typhi* suggests that the clinical picture is produced by these endotoxins. Both typhoid fever and injected endotoxin produce headache, chills, fever, anorexia, abdominal discomfort, myalgia, thrombocytopenia, and leukopenia. The specific pathologic findings of typhoid fever can be produced in the rabbit by intravenous administration of the purified endotoxin. Tolerance to the pyrogenic action of endotoxin is present during the convalescent phase of typhoid fever, and vascular hyper-reactivity to epinephrine or norepinephrine (exaggerated blood pressure rise after intravenous injection and local hemorrhagic lesions after intradermal injection) appears during the febrile phase of the disease and persists into convalescence. Both the development of tolerance and the vascular hyper-reactivity can be produced by endotoxin and strongly suggest that endotoxin does play an important role in human typhoid fever. However, volunteers made tolerant to endotoxin prior to challenge with *S. typhi* develop a clinical disease indistinguishable in severity and incubation period from that of controls, an observation apparently in conflict with the hypothesis that endotoxin released during infection is responsible for the early fever and other manifestations.

The infective dose of *S. typhi* is influenced by many factors. Epidemiologic data suggest that a few organisms, possibly 10 or 100, could initiate infection. Among human volunteers, 50 per cent developed overt disease after the oral ingestion of 10^7 viable *S. typhi* organisms of a strain containing the Vi antigen. When the same dose of non-Vi strains was administered, only 26 per cent developed disease, indicating the potential influence of different bacterial strains. Animal studies with *S. enteritis* have indicated that alteration in intestinal flora may increase susceptibility; pretreatment of human volunteers with streptomycin was followed by clinical disease in one of four volunteers given 1000 typhoid bacilli, a dose which produced no clinical disease in 14 untreated volunteers.

Pathology. A granulomatous proliferation of mononuclear cells with the formation of ill-defined nodular masses of reticulohistiocytic elements, principally in the mesenteric lymph nodes and spleen, together with a marked reactive follicular hyperplasia of lymphoid tissue, characterizes the pathology of typhoid fever. Hypertrophy of the lymphoid tissue of the small intestine, especially of the Peyer's patches in the terminal ileum, is followed by superficial coagulation necrosis; this sloughs to form an ulcer usually confined to the mucosa and submucosa. Erosion of blood vessels results in hemorrhage; extension of the ulcer into the muscularis and serosa leads to intestinal perforation. The liver is enlarged, and areas of focal granulomatous lesions form by the third week. Focal necrosis is also found in spleen, cardiac muscle, and lymph follicles. Bronchitis is common, and pneumonia caused by *S. typhi* or *Diplococcus pneumoniae* is not unusual.

Clinical Manifestations. The incubation period usually is eight to 14 days but varies from five days to five weeks. The duration of illness in an untreated case of average severity is about four weeks. The onset is usually gradual and associated with anorexia, lethargy, malaise, headache, general aches and pains, and fever. During the first week there is a gradually increasing remittent fever. Dull, continuous headache is a prominent symptom in almost all cases. About two thirds of the patients have a nonproductive cough, and epistaxis occurs in about 10 per cent. The majority of patients have vague abdominal pain or discomfort. Constipation is frequent and more common than diarrhea, which occurs in only about 20 per cent of the patients. During the second week of illness the fever shows less of a tendency to remit and is often sustained at around 40° C. During this phase patients are often severely ill with marked weakness, abdominal discomfort, and distention. Mental dullness is prominent, and delirium may occur. Diarrhea is more common during the second week than during the first, and stools may contain blood. As the illness extends into the third week, the patient continues to be febrile and becomes increasingly exhausted and weak. Patients without complications usually begin to improve during the third and fourth weeks. The fever gradually begins to decline, and the temperature may be normal by the end of the fourth week.

The physical signs vary with the stage of the disease.

During the first week fever and slight abdominal tenderness may be the only findings. However, during the second and third weeks findings characteristic of typhoid fever may develop. The patient appears acutely ill with a dull, expressionless, lethargic face. The mental state varies within wide limits from normal to frank mental confusion and delirium. The pulse is often not as fast as might be expected to accompany the degree of temperature present. Rhonchi or scattered moist rales may be present as a manifestation of bronchitis. The majority of patients have slight abdominal tenderness, most pronounced on the right side and in the upper abdomen. Abdominal distention may be severe. A soft spleen can be palpated in about three fourths of the patients. Maculopapular skin lesions appear during the second or third week of illness in about 80 to 90 per cent of patients with typhoid fever. These "rose spots" are 2 to 5 mm in diameter, blanch on pressure, are located predominantly on the upper abdomen or anterior chest, and are sparse, usually not exceeding 20 in number. The skin lesions last for two to four days and then disappear, but may be followed by fresh crops. The signs of illness subside as fever diminishes. Convalescence is slow; a month or more is often required to regain normal status.

Variation in the typical course described in preceding paragraphs is common. The illness may be mild and last only a week or may be prolonged, with a febrile course as long as eight weeks.

Laboratory Findings. Normochromic anemia develops during the course of the disease. Anemia may be aggravated by blood loss in stools. Leukopenia is frequent, and is characterized by a relative decrease in the number of polymorphonuclear leukocytes and an absence of eosinophils. Thrombocytopenia is common. Albuminuria is common during the febrile period of the disease. Feces often give a positive reaction for occult blood during the third and fourth weeks of illness.

S. typhi can be isolated from the blood in about 90 per cent of patients during the first week of disease and in about 50 per cent at the end of the third week; positive blood cultures are infrequent after the fourth week. The bacilli may persist in the bone marrow after blood cultures are negative. *S. typhi* can be isolated from feces at any stage of illness, but the greatest incidence of positive results is obtained during the third to fifth week when 85 per cent of the patients have positive cultures. Many reports indicate that typhoid bacilli can be cultured from the urine in about 25 per cent of those with typhoid fever during the third and fourth weeks of illness. Care should be taken in collection of urine to avoid contamination with feces containing typhoid bacilli.

The frequency of positive stool cultures begins to decrease rapidly about six weeks after onset of illness; two or three months after onset only 5 to 10 per cent of patients continue to excrete bacilli. Other patients become negative for typhoid bacilli during subsequent months, but approximately 3 per cent continue to excrete organisms for periods in excess of one year, becoming chronic enteric carriers. This occurs approximately three times more frequently when the disease occurs in an adult than in a child, and approximately two to three times as often among women than men. Many carriers give no past history of typhoid fever. Chloramphenicol therapy has not reduced the frequency of the chronic carrier state; among chloramphenicol-treated women in Chile a chronic carrier state existed in 2.3 per cent of those who had been under 15 years old at time of disease versus 25 per cent among those who had been 35 years old or older. There was increased likelihood of the carrier state when the disease was more severe, when there was a relapse, when therapy was delayed, and when there were symptoms of gallbladder disease. Organisms persist in the gallbladder or biliary tract and enter the intestinal tract in large numbers in bile, resulting in as many as 10^6 or more virulent organisms per gram of feces. Chronic carriers will continue to excrete organisms for many years, usually for life, unless measures are taken to terminate the carrier state.

An increase in titer of agglutinins against the somatic (O) antigens and flagellar (H) antigens of *S. typhi* (Widal reaction) usually occurs during the course of typhoid fever, reaching a peak during the third week of illness. A fourfold or greater increase in titer in the absence of typhoid immunization during the previous four to six weeks should be considered highly suggestive of infection. In occasional cases there is no increase in agglutinins during the course of typhoid fever. The use of the agglutination reaction as a diagnostic test should always be subordinated to direct cultural demonstration of the causative organism.

Complications. *Intestinal hemorrhage* and *perforation* may occur during the second or third week of illness. Severe hemorrhage occurs in about 2 per cent of patients, although gross blood in feces is present in 10 to 20 per cent of cases, and a positive test for occult blood is even more common. Intestinal perforation, usually in the lower ileum, develops in about 1 per cent of cases and is the most serious of all complications of typhoid fever. The first signs of hemorrhage or perforation may be a sudden drop in temperature and an increase in pulse rate. Often, however, one or more episodes of bleeding will precede a perforation. The perforation is usually associated with acute abdominal pain, tenderness, and rigidity, which are most marked in the right lower quadrant of the abdomen. Signs of peritonitis develop rapidly after perforation, and temperature returns to febrile levels. Thrombophlebitis, particularly of the femoral vein, pneumonia, and cholecystitis occur in a small proportion of patients. Other complications include osteomyelitis, meningitis, and localized infection of almost any organ. Alopecia was a well known sequel of typhoid fever in the preantimicrobial era. The incidence of abortion is increased when typhoid fever occurs during pregnancy, especially during the first trimester.

Relapse. One or two weeks after defervescence illness may recur with signs and symptoms similar to those during the initial illness, including bacteremia. Relapse occurs in 8 to 10 per cent of patients with typhoid fever who do not receive antimicrobial therapy and in 10 to 20 per cent of patients treated with chloramphenicol. The relapse is usually milder than the initial episode but may be severe, even fatal. Manifestations may last as long as three weeks during a relapse. Second and third relapses have been described.

Diagnosis. The diagnosis of typhoid fever can often be suspected on the basis of the clinical picture. Definitive diagnosis is established by isolation of the organism from blood or feces, or, occasionally, from sputum or purulent exudates. A fourfold or greater increase in agglutinin titers, in the absence of recent immunization, provides confirmatory evidence of infection. However, when the rise in antibodies is only against the O antigen, infection with other salmonellae in Group D, which share common somatic antigens (IX, XII), must be considered.

Since in the early stages the patient frequently appears ill, is highly febrile, and has a leukopenia and no localizing signs, the differential diagnostic possibilities include many diseases. Prominent among these are systemic infections with other salmonellae, disseminated tuberculosis, malaria, leptospirosis, brucellosis, shigellosis, murine typhus fever, tularemia, Rocky Mountain spotted fever, acute bronchitis, influenza, and pneumonia caused by viruses or *Mycoplasma pneumoniae*. Central nervous system manifestations may suggest meningitis or encephalitis. Certain nonmicrobial diseases associated with fever and abdominal complaints, such as Hodgkin's disease, may also be confused with typhoid fever. Herpes labialis is rare in typhoid fever, and its presence should lead to a consideration of other diagnoses.

Prognosis. The fatality rate prior to effective antimicrobial therapy varied among different socioeconomic and age groups but was around 10 per cent. Death was usually associated with profound toxemia, intestinal perforation, intestinal hemorrhage, or intercurrent pneumonia. The fatality rate since the introduction of chloramphenicol is 1 or 2 per cent when facilities are available for appropriate supportive care.

Treatment. Chloramphenicol has been employed successfully in the management of typhoid fever since 1948 and is still the antimicrobial agent of choice. However, in 1972 and 1973, typhoid bacilli isolated in Mexico, Kerala (India), Saigon, and Bangkok were resistant to chloramphenicol, tetracycline, streptomycin, and sulfonamides; all but a few were susceptible to ampicillin. Thus isolates should be tested for drug susceptibility, especially if infection may have been acquired in these areas or if the response to therapy is disappointing. Chloramphenicol is given orally in doses of approximately 50 mg per kilogram per day in four divided doses until the temperature is normal; thereafter, the dose may be reduced to 30 mg per kilogram per day. Chloramphenicol therapy should be continued for a total of two weeks. Response to treatment is not rapid. Patients usually show subjective improvement after one or two days, but the temperature does not return to normal until three to five days after the beginning of therapy. Hemorrhage and perforation may develop during chloramphenicol therapy, even in afebrile patients. Treatment of relapse is the same as for the initial episode. Chloramphenicol may result in suppression of agglutinin response in patients treated during the early phase of typhoid fever.

Ampicillin is also effective in the treatment of typhoid fever. As mentioned above, ampicillin is particularly valuable for treatment of infections with chloramphenicol-resistant strains, but the response appears to be slower with ampicillin than with chloramphenicol. If ampicillin is used in the treatment of typhoid fever, a total daily dose of 150 to 200 mg per kilogram of body weight should be administered intravenously in four divided doses until the patient is afebrile, and should then be continued orally for a total of two weeks of therapy. With highly susceptible strains, 40 mg per kilogram per day intramuscularly may suffice.

Typhoid organisms whose multiple-drug resistance is due to the prevalent R factor, a plasmid transferable to other enterobacteria, retain their susceptibility to a variety of other antimicrobial drugs, none of which have yet been evaluated for effectiveness in treatment of typhoid fever. Several studies have suggested that trimethoprim-sulfamethoxazole is comparable to chloramphenicol in treatment of typhoid, and that it was effective in the management of chloramphenicol-resistant infections. The use of prednisone or drugs with similar activity should be considered for patients with severe toxemia and pyrexia. Prednisone should be given in a dose of 60 mg per day in four divided doses for the first day, 40 mg during the second day, and 20 mg on the third day; corticosteroid therapy should be discontinued after the third day. In patients treated with prednisone, temperature returns to normal or occasionally decreases to hypothermic levels within hours, and the toxic state rapidly ameliorates. Prednisone should be administered only in conjunction with appropriate antimicrobial therapy, and under these conditions it does not increase the risk of complications.

Perforation, although previously managed by surgical means, is now usually treated conservatively without surgical intervention. When perforation occurs, the antityphoid drug therapy should be continued, and additional antimicrobial drugs administered to control multiplication of intestinal flora in the peritoneal space. Transfusion is required for large hemorrhages.

Patients with typhoid fever are unusually sensitive to the antipyretic effect of salicylates and may develop profound hypothermia after small doses. Tepid sponge baths are effective in lowering temperature and should be used instead of salicylates. Laxatives and enemas should not be used because of the danger of inciting intestinal perforation or hemorrhage.

Treatment of Carriers. Cholecystectomy results in termination of the chronic enteric carrier state in about 85 per cent of cases. When the organism has been shown to be susceptible to it, ampicillin, in a total dose of 6 grams per day given orally in four equal doses for a period of six weeks, combined with probenecid, will apparently terminate the carrier state in most patients without gallstones and with normal gallbladder function as indicated by cholecystogram. Ampicillin occasionally terminates the carrier state in persons with evidence of gallbladder disease or gallstones, but the proportion of apparent cures is less than 25 per cent. Penicillin G in doses of 12 million units or more daily combined with probenecid for 14 days has also been successful in terminating the carrier state in some persons. Chloramphenicol has not been shown to be effective in the treatment of the chronic carrier state and should not be used in this situation.

Prophylaxis. Controlled field trials have shown that typhoid vaccine is effective in reducing the incidence of disease, and that acetone-killed and dried vaccine was more effective than the heat phenol product. Protection has not been correlated with any specific antibody response. The immunity is relative and can be overcome by exposure to a large number of organisms; no protection could be demonstrated in healthy volunteers against an oral dose of 10^7 organisms, a dose known to produce disease in 50 per cent of normal subjects. Immunization should be considered for inhabitants of areas where the incidence of the disease is high, for travelers to these areas, and for persons working with *S. typhi.* A course of immunization consists of two subcutaneous injections of 0.5 ml of vaccine separated by four or more weeks. Booster doses should be given at three-year intervals if exposure continues. Local discomfort and fever frequently follow administration of the vaccine; these can be alleviated by an antipyretic. Booster doses of the heat phenol vaccine can be inoculated intradermally in doses of 0.1 ml with less systemic reaction. The acetone-killed and dried product, however, should *not* be injected intradermally, because it produces local pain and tenderness more marked than after subcutaneous injection.

Patients with typhoid fever should remain in isolation during hospitalization. Persons known to be carriers should not be permitted to work as food handlers; members of their households should be immunized against the disease.

Second attacks of typhoid fever have been observed, but as a general rule one attack confers lifelong immunity comparable to that elicited by the inactivated vaccine.

Armijo, R., Pizzi, A., and Lobos, H.: Prevalence of typhoid carriers after treatment with chloramphenicol. Bol. Of. Sanit. Panam., 62:295, 1967.

Ashcroft, M. T., Singh, B., Nicholson, C. C., Ritchie, J. M., Sobryan, E., and Williams, F.: A seven-year field trial of two typhoid vaccines in Guyana. Lancet, 2:1056, 1967.

Cvjetanovic, B., and Uemura, K.: The present status of field and laboratory studies of typhoid and paratyphoid vaccines. Bull. WHO, 32:29, 1965.

Dinbar, A., Altman, G., and Tulcinsky, D. B.: The treatment of chronic biliary Salmonella carriers. Am. J. Med., 47:236, 1969.

Hornick, R. B., Greisman, S. E., Woodward, T. E., DuPont, H. L., Dawkins, A. T., and Snyder, M. J.: Typhoid fever: Pathogenesis and immunologic control. N. Engl. J. Med., 283:686, 739, 1970.

Huckstep, R. L.: Typhoid Fever and Other Salmonella Infections. Edinburgh, E. and S. Livingstone, Ltd., 1962.

Lawrence, R. M., Goldstein, E., and Hoeprich, P. D.: Typhoid fever caused by chloramphenicol-resistant organisms. J.A.M.A., 224:861, 1973.

Marselis, J. G., Jr., Kaye, D., Connolly, C. S., and Hook, E. W.: Quantitative bacteriology of the typhoid carrier state. Am. J. Trop. Med. Hyg., 13:425, 1964.

Overturf, G., Marton, K. I., and Mathies, A. W., Jr.: Antibiotic resistance in typhoid fever. N. Engl. J. Med., 289:463, 1972.

Robertson, R. P., Wahab, M. F. A., and Raasch, F. O.: Evaluation of chloramphenicol and ampicillin in Salmonella enteric fever. N. Engl. J. Med., 278:171, 1968.

Stuart, B. M., and Pullen, R. L.: Typhoid: Clinical analysis of three hundred and sixty cases. Arch. Intern. Med., 78:629, 1946.

Woodward, T. E., and Smadel, J. E.: Management of typhoid fever and its complications. Ann. Intern. Med., 60:144, 1964.

213. SALMONELLA INFECTIONS OTHER THAN TYPHOID FEVER

Edward W. Hook

Definition. The genus Salmonella consists of more than 1700 serotypes and variants. These organisms with a few exceptions are primary pathogens for animals that are readily transmitted to man. The outstanding exception is *S. typhi,* which is a parasite only of man and does not cause disease in lower animals in nature.

Human infection with Salmonella may be expressed as *acute gastroenteritis, enteric fever* (paratyphoid fever), *bacteremia,* or *localized metastatic infection* at almost any site. The clinical syndromes resulting from Salmonella infection cannot always be sharply differentiated and sometimes overlap.

Transient *asymptomatic infection* of the intestinal tract is also common with most serotypes. A *chronic carrier state* may occur occasionally after infection with Salmonella other than *S. typhi,* and is characterized by prolonged excretion of the organism in feces or urine.

Typhoid fever is considered in a separate chapter (see Ch. 212) because of its historical identity, the host specificity of the pathogen, and the wealth of data on basic and clinical aspects of the disease. This separation is unrealistic to the extent that an illness closely resembling typhoid fever can result from infection with other salmonellae, and *S. typhi* can on occasion produce all the clinical syndromes described for the other Salmonella serotypes.

Etiology. Salmonellae are gram-negative, aerobic, nonsporing rods that grow readily on simple culture media. Presumptive identification of salmonellae involves relatively simple biochemical and agglutination reactions, but definitive identification of serotype depends on precise analysis of the somatic (O) and flagellar (H) antigens of the organism. Subdivision of certain serotypes, for example *S. typhimurium,* can be achieved by bacteriophage typing. Specific identification of all isolates is desirable, especially for epidemiologic reasons, and can be obtained through local, state, or federal health agencies.

Salmonella serotypes most frequently isolated from human infections in the United States during 1972 were, in descending order of frequency, *S. typhimurium, S. newport, S. enteritidis, S. infantis, S. heidelberg, S. saintpaul, S. thompson, S. derby, S. oranienburg,* and *S. javiana.* These ten serotypes accounted for about 66 per cent of the total Salmonella isolates from man during 1972. *S. typhimurium* is the serotype most frequently isolated year after year, usually accounting for 20 to 30 per cent of the total.

Incidence and Prevalence. Salmonellae are widespread among members of the Animal Kingdom in all parts of the world. Virtually all domestic and wild animal species have been shown to harbor these organisms, and infection rates range from 1 per cent to more than 40 per cent. For example, in certain studies salmonellae have been isolated from 41 per cent of turkeys, 7 to 50 per cent of swine, and 24 per cent of apparently healthy cattle.

In 1972, 26,110 isolations of Salmonella from humans were reported in the United States. The annual incidence of reported isolations has remained approximately constant since 1963, the first full year of operation of the Salmonella Surveillance System in the United States. The true incidence of human salmonellosis is probably much higher than the number of reported cases.

The prevalence of asymptomatic human carriers of salmonellae in the general population has been estimated to be about 0.2 per cent. The carrier state in the vast majority of these people is transient and probably represents persistence of organisms in the stools after asymptomatic or mild intestinal infection. The transient carrier state is more frequent in persons whose occupations provide opportunity for contact with Salmonella in foods, such as professional food processors or abattoir workers, than in the general population.

Epidemiology. Man almost always acquires Salmonella infection by the oral route. Any item of food or drink can be contaminated directly or indirectly with viable bacilli from infected animals or man and can serve as a source of infection. Although the role of human carriers in the spread of salmonellosis must not be minimized, the majority of infections of man in the United States are related to the enormous reservoirs of salmonellae in lower animals.

The greatest single source of human disease is poultry products, including chickens, turkeys, ducks, and eggs. Other animal meats, especially pork, beef, and lamb, also serve as sources of infection. Salmonellae on meats or other foods contaminate utensils, tables, and other items in the processing plant, market, or kitchen, and may be transferred from these items to previously uninfected foods. A significant proportion (1 to 58 per cent) of raw meat purchased in retail markets is contaminated with salmonellae.

Eggs or egg products are common sources of Salmonella infection. The bacilli may be found on the external surface of the eggshell, between the shell and the shell membranes, or in yolks of eggs from hens with ovarian infection. The incidence of infection of eggs is low, but pooling of large numbers for freezing or drying increases the possibility of contamination of large quantities of materials. Prepared food mixtures containing dried eggs have been implicated many times in outbreaks of Salmonella infection.

Sterilization of contaminated foods is not always achieved by cooking. Viable salmonellae contaminating large birds such as turkeys, especially if the fowl is stuffed, may persist despite the baking process, and organisms in eggs occasionally survive frying, scrambling, or boiling in the shell.

The numerous byproducts of the meat-packing industry, such as bone meal, fertilizer, domestic animal food, and fish meal, often contain salmonellae and may serve as sources of infection, especially among lower animals. Finally, in considering potential sources of infection, household pets, including dogs, cats, birds, and turtles, should not be overlooked; all have been shown to harbor salmonellae.

Direct transmission from man to man without food as the intermediate source does occur. Person-to-person transmission appears to be a relatively common mode of spread in hospital outbreaks, especially those occurring in nurseries or pediatric wards. For example, salmonellae may be introduced into a nursery by a newborn infected at birth from an infected mother and then spread to other babies by nursery attendants. Several nursery and hospital outbreaks have also been described in which infection appeared to be perpetuated by airborne spread of salmonellae.

S. choleraesuis bacteremia has been reported in immunologically compromised patients who received platelet transfusions from a donor with chronic intermittent bacteremia secondary to minimally symptomatic osteomyelitis.

Pathology. Death from Salmonella gastroenteritis occurs primarily in infants, the aged, and persons with underlying diseases. The intestinal mucosa is red and swollen and often shows petechial hemorrhages. The pathologic findings in paratyphoid fever are qualitatively similar to those of typhoid fever, although the involvement of Peyer's patches is less prominent and ulcerations are much less frequent. Intestinal lesions are usually absent in patients with Salmonella bacteremia, and the findings are similar to those of any acute generalized infection. Blood-borne salmonellae may localize in almost any organ, producing single or multiple suppurative lesions.

Pathogenesis. Multiplication of salmonellae in the intestinal tract is associated with invasion of mucosal cells of the small intestine, inflammation of the intestinal mucosa, and symptoms of gastroenteritis. Gastroenteritis is a true infection of the mucosa; ingestion of a large number of dead bacilli will not produce the disease. An enterotoxin analogous to that produced by *Vibrio cholerae* and certain other enteric pathogens has not been demonstrated.

Salmonellae multiplying in the intestinal tract occasionally gain access to the blood, producing transient bacteremia or localized infections that can serve as sources of persistent bacteremia. The pathogenesis of enteric or paratyphoid fever is similar to that of typhoid fever.

The prevalence of salmonellae in foods for human consumption makes it almost inevitable that man come in contact with these organisms relatively frequently. The outcome of such exposures depends on many factors, especially the characteristics of the Salmonella serotype, the number of bacteria ingested, and the status of the host.

Every serotype of Salmonella has the capacity to produce asymptomatic infection, acute gastroenteritis, bacteremia with or without localized infection, or paratyphoid fever. However, some serotypes are much more likely to produce certain of these clinical syndromes than others. For example, *S. anatum* usually produces inapparent infection or gastroenteritis and only rarely invades the blood. In contrast, *S. choleraesuis* only occasionally produces gastroenteritis or inapparent infection but is a common cause of bacteremia or metastatic infection. Differences in pathogenicity are observed not only between serotypes, but also between strains of the same serotype.

Limited information is available on the number of organisms required to produce salmonellosis in man. Experiments in volunteers suggest that a large number (approximately 10^5 to 10^6) of viable salmonellae are usually required to produce gastroenteritis in normal adults. A transient carrier state may follow ingestion of inocula 10 or 100 times smaller than those required to produce disease.

The resistance of the host also plays a major role in determining the wide range of responses from no disease to rapidly fatal illness observed in human salmonellosis. Local factors in the stomach and intestine may be the first lines of defense. It is known that salmonellae are rapidly killed at pH of 2, a level readily attained in the stomach, and that concomitant administration of certain antacids reduces the challenge dose of organisms required to initiate infection under experimental conditions. It has been established that major gastric surgery, including subtotal gastrectomy, gastroenterostomy, and/or vagotomy, predisposes to Salmonella gastroenteritis. The mechanism of this effect is unknown, but may be related to reduced bactericidal acitivity of gastric juice or altered intestinal flora. It has been shown in experimental Salmonella infections of mice that the microbial flora of the normal intestine exerts a protective action by suppressing multiplication of salmonellae. In these studies alteration of intestinal flora by antimicrobial drugs increased susceptibility to infection with *S. typhimurium* 100,000 times, and resistance was restored by re-establishing the normal enteric flora. Prior antimicrobial therapy also enhances susceptibility of man to symptomatic intestinal infection with salmonellae.

The incidence of severe Salmonella infections is increased in patients with certain underlying diseases. Another process, such as hepatic cirrhosis, lupus erythematosus, leukemia, lymphoma, or neoplasm, is present in one third to one half of patients with Salmonella bacteremia. These conditions are associated with a general depression of resistance to microbial invasion, and secondary infection is not unexpected. However, in a few diseases—acute bartonellosis, sickle cell anemia, and, perhaps, malaria—there appears to be a predisposition to infection with salmonellae that exceeds any general susceptibility to other bacterial species. The acute hemolytic phase of bartonellosis is complicated by the development of Salmonella bacteremia in as many as 40 per cent of cases. Patients with sickle cell anemia and other sickle hemoglobinopathies are unusually susceptible to invasion of the blood by Salmonella, and there is a strong tendency for localization of infection in bone. In fact, Salmonella species, not staphylococci, account for the vast majority of instances of osteomyelitis in patients with sickle cell anemia. Osteomyelitis is probably related to the localization of organisms in the areas of ischemia and necrosis of bone so common in sickle cell anemia; this is but one example of the striking tendency of salmonellae to localize at sites of pre-existing disease. Localization of salmonellae has been reported in vascular aneurysms, bone compressed by aortic aneurysms, hematomas, areas of infarction, and a variety of cysts and neoplasms.

Clinical Manifestations. *Salmonella Gastroenteritis.* Symptoms of gastroenteritis develop 8 to 48 hours after ingestion of contaminated food. The relatively long incubation period represents the time required for multiplication and invasion by the organism. Nausea and vomiting are common initial manifestations and are rapidly followed by colicky abdominal pain and persistent diarrhea, occasionally with mucus or blood. Nausea and vomiting are rarely severe or protracted. An initial chill is not unusual, and fever of 38 to 39° C is common. Symptoms usually subside in two to five days, and recovery is uneventful.

Considerable variation in the severity of Salmonella gastroenteritis is observed, even among patients infected at the same meal. Some patients have a mild afebrile disease with a few loose stools, whereas others have high fever and 30 to 40 liquid stools per day. Severe diarrhea occasionally occurs in an afebrile patient. Abdominal pain may be intense, localized, and associated with rebound tenderness, suggesting appendicitis or some other acute intra-abdominal process. Symptoms of gastroenteritis persist in some patients for as long as two weeks.

The leukocyte count is usually normal, and blood cultures are sterile in almost all cases. The causative organism can be isolated from the feces of almost all patients during the acute illness. About 50 per cent of the patients continue to have stool cultures positive for salmonellae at two weeks after onset of gastroenteritis, but only 15 per cent remain positive at the end of the fourth week. A small proportion of patients continue to excrete organisms after two months, but in most of these the cultures become negative in the next six months. The period of excretion of organisms in stool tends to be longer in infants than in older children or adults. The term "chronic enteric carrier" should be reserved for the patient shown to have persistently positive stools with the same Salmonella species for one or more years.

Enteric or Paratyphoid Fever. Salmonellae other than *S. typhosa* may produce an illness with all the features of typhoid fever, including prolonged sustained fever, respiratory and gastrointestinal symptoms, rose spots, leukopenia, and positive blood, stool, and urine cultures. Although paratyphoid fever may be clinically indistinguishable from typhoid fever, it is usually milder with a shorter course and a lower mortality rate. The organisms most likely to produce this syndrome are *S. paratyphi A, S. paratyphi B,* and *S. choleraesuis.* Paratyphoid fever is occasionally preceded by manifestations of Salmonella gastroenteritis.

Bacteremia. Salmonellae also produce a clinical syndrome that is characterized by chills, prolonged intermittent fever, anorexia, and weight loss. The characteristic features of typhoid or paratyphoid fever, such as rose spots, sustained fever, and leukopenia, are absent. Patients with this form of illness usually have no gastrointestinal complaints, and, indeed, stool cultures are usually negative for the causative organism despite its presence in blood. The leukocyte count is normal in most cases.

A prolonged febrile illness lasting weeks or months and characterized by weight loss, anemia, hepatosplenomegaly, and bacteremia with salmonellae, including *S. typhosa,* has been described in South America and the Middle East in patients with schistosomiasis. The organisms apparently find a protected environment for multiplication within the gut of the worm. Eradication of the worms may also result in cure of the bacterial infection (see Ch. 296).

Localized Disease. Signs of localized infection appear in many cases of Salmonella bacteremia. Abscess formation may occur at almost any site, or bronchopneumonia, empyema, endocarditis, pericarditis, pyelonephritis, osteomyelitis, or arthritis may develop. Meningitis is a focal manifestation more common in newborns and infants than in adults. Patients with localized infections usually have striking polymorphonuclear leukocytosis as high as 20,000 to 30,000 cells per cubic millimeter of blood.

Diagnosis. Salmonella gastroenteritis must be differentiated from other acute diarrheal diseases, especially shigellosis, invasive and enterotoxigenic *Escherichia coli* infection, staphylococcal food poisoning, and enteritis produced by viral agents. A short incubation period, absence of fever, and prominence of nausea and vomiting are characteristic of staphylococcal food poisoning, whereas tenesmus, dysentery, and numerous fecal leukocytes suggest a diagnosis of shigellosis. However, differentiation on the basis of clinical information alone is difficult, especially in sporadic cases, and definitive diagnosis depends on isolation of the causative organism from the stool.

In patients with enteric fever, blood cultures are usually positive early in the course of the disease, and feces and urine become positive somewhat later. In patients with Salmonella bacteremia, the organisms can be isolated from blood, or in some cases from pus or exudate from localized infection.

Patients with salmonellosis may show during the course of illness a fourfold or greater increase in titer of agglutinins against the causative organism or closely related species. However, agglutination tests performed in the ordinary clinical laboratory are usually not helpful in diagnosis, because only a limited number of Salmonella antigens are used.

Treatment. The most important aspect of the management of patients with Salmonella gastroenteritis is prompt correction of dehydration and electrolyte disturbances. Diphenoxylate hydrochloride with atropine (Lomotil), paregoric, or small doses of morphine may be used to relieve abdominal cramps and diarrhea if contraindications do not exist. There is no convincing evidence that antimicrobial drugs, including chloramphenicol, ampicillin, or trimethoprim combined with sulfonamide, reduce the duration of illness or the period of excretion of organisms in the stool. In fact, recent studies indicate that the period of excretion of salmonellae in the stool during convalescence after symptomatic intestinal infection is actually longer in patients who have been treated with antimicrobial drugs during the acute illness than in patients who have received no antimicrobial therapy.

In Salmonella bacteremia, paratyphoid fever, or localized infections of bones, joints, meninges, and other sites, chloramphenicol is the drug of choice and should be administered in divided doses of about 50 mg per kilogram per day for at least two weeks. Four to six days may be required for defervescence in favorable cases and even longer in patients with localized infection. In patients with localized infections, it may be necessary to continue antimicrobial therapy for four to six weeks, and surgical drainage of collections of pus may be required. Salmonellae persisting in tissues during chloramphenicol therapy may be responsible for relapse after the antimicrobial is discontinued. Relapse is not related to the emergence of chloramphenicol-resistant strains during therapy, and clinical response to a second or third course of therapy usually differs in no way from the first.

Ampicillin has also been shown to be effective in treating paratyphoid fever, but the response to ampicillin is slower than the response to chloramphenicol. Ampicillin is also often effective in the treatment of other systemic Salmonella infections if the causative organism is susceptible to this drug. Ampicillin is preferred over chloramphenicol for patients requiring prolonged therapy. Approximately 10 to 20 per cent of the *S. typhimurium* strains isolated in the United States and a somewhat higher proportion in England are resistant to ampicillin. Ampicillin resistance is mediated by transferable resistance determinants or R factors, and is uncommon among serologic types other than *S. typhimurium.* Strains of Salmonella resistant to chloramphenicol do occur but are not common, with the exception of *S. typhi* in Mexico, Vietnam, and certain areas of India. Nevertheless, the physician must remain alert to the possibility of chloramphenicol resistance among nontyphoidal strains.

Excretion of salmonellae in stool after clinical or subclinical infection ceases spontaneously in almost all patients; the convalescent carrier state is not an indication for antimicrobial therapy. Chronic enteric carriers of salmonellae other than *S. typhi* are managed as are typhoid carriers.

Prognosis. The case fatality rate in Salmonella gastroenteritis rarely exceeds 1 or 2 per cent, and probably averages about 0.3 per cent. Fatalities occur almost entirely in infants, the aged, and persons with major underlying disease. The case fatality rate in the more serious systemic infections is high; it approaches 20 per cent in *S. choleraesuis* bacteremia.

Prevention. Every effort should be made to prevent the spread of salmonellae among the population by the excreta of patients with acute illness and convalescent or chronic carriers. Patients with acute illness should be isolated, and convalescent or chronic carriers should not be employed as food handlers and should practice strict personal hygiene.

The control of salmonellosis among animals and prevention of spread of infection to man present many problems. Progress is being made in developing methods of detection and control of salmonellosis in domestic animals and in improving hygienic conditions in food-processing and food-dispensing establishments.

Aserkoff, B., and Bennett, J. V.: Effect of therapy in acute salmonellosis on salmonellae in feces. N. Engl. J. Med., 281:636, 1969.

Bauer, H.: Growing problem of salmonellosis in modern society. Medicine, 52:323, 1973.

Bennett, I. L., Jr., and Hook, E. W.: Infectious diseases (some aspects of salmonellosis). Ann. Rev. Med., 10:1, 1959.

Center for Disease Control: Salmonella Surveillance Annual Summary, 1972. Issued November 1973. Atlanta, Georgia.

Musher, D. M., and Rubenstein, A. D.: Permanent carriers of nontyphosa salmonellae. Arch. Intern. Med., 132:869, 1973.

Rhame, F. S., Root, R. K., MacLowry, J. D., Dadisman, T. A., and Bennett, J. V.: Salmonella septicemia from platelet transfusions. Study of an outbreak traced to a hematogenous carrier of *Salmonella choleraesuis*. Ann. Intern. Med., 78:633, 1973.

Wahab, M. F. A., Robertson, R. P., and Raasch, F. O.: Paratyphoid A fever. Ann. Intern. Med., 70:913, 1969.

OTHER BACTERIAL INFECTIONS

214. ENTERIC BACTERIAL INFECTIONS

Calvin M. Kunin

Definition. The wide variety of microorganisms commonly found in the gastrointestinal tract, particularly the gram-negative, nonsporulating bacilli, have become increasingly important in clinical medicine. They are the principal organisms found in infections of the abdominal viscera, peritoneum, and urinary tract, as well as being frequent secondary invaders of the respiratory tract, burned or traumatized skin, and sites of decreased host resistance and instrumentation. Currently, they are the most frequent cause of life-threatening bacteremia. Infections with these organisms will be considered together because of their common habitat in the gut and on mucous surfaces, the similarity of epidemiologic and pathogenic characteristics, and the common approach used in diagnosis, treatment, and prevention.

Bacteriology. The gastrointestinal flora is exceedingly complex. The large intestine contains about 10^{10} to 10^{11} organisms per gram of contents. Of these, 90 to 95 per cent are obligate anaerobes. Most common are the gram-negative bacilli, Bacteroides and Fusobacterium, gram-positive bacilli, including Bifidobacterium, Eubacterium, and Corynebacterium species, and a wide variety of anaerobic streptococci. Other anaerobes include the gram-positive spore-forming rods of the clostridia species and gram-negative cocci, Veillonella. Enterococci are also present. The well-known aerobic gram-negative rods, which are members of the family Enterobacteriaceae, account for only 5 to 10 per cent of the total flora. These include the most common, *E. coli,* as well as the Klebsiella-Enterobacter group, Proteus, Providencia, Edwardsiella, Serratia, and, under pathologic conditions, Salmonella and Shigella. Pseudomonas is an entirely unrelated species, and is usually found in only small numbers in the bowel. Various yeasts are also found in lesser numbers in the normal large intestine.

Although the human gastrointestinal tract is usually considered to be colonized in the anatomic regions proximal to the cardia of the stomach and distal to the ileocecal valve, recent studies have demonstrated organisms in the jejunum and almost always in the ileum. Moderate changes in the diet do not affect the ratio of predominant bacteria in the feces, but antimicrobial therapy has a strong selective effect and is the single most important reason for the increasing emergence in human infection of these heretofore unusual organisms.

All the microorganisms of the gastrointestinal tract are potentially pathogenic under conditions of altered host resistance. The major diagnostic problem is to differentiate superficial colonization from actual tissue invasion.

Endotoxin. The gram-negative bacteria of the gastrointestinal tract produce disease by invasion of tissue and by release of a pharmacologically active lipopolysaccharide from the cell wall, known as endotoxin. Endotoxins from a wide variety of unrelated species behave quite similarly, regardless of the inherent pathogenicity of the microorganism from which they are derived or their antigenic structure.

In the intact microorganism they exist as complexes of lipid, polysaccharide, and protein. The biologic activity seems to be a property of a lipid and carbohydrate portion. The cell wall of gram-negative bacteria may be roughly divided into three regions. The outermost region contains the chains of specific sugars which characterize the O-specific antigens and determine individual serotypes within a species. This is linked to a core polysaccharide which is of similar structure among related groups of bacteria. This is in turn linked through 2-keto-3-deoxyoctonate trisaccharides to the major lipid component termed lipid A. Evidence has now accumulated to indicate that all the properties of endotoxin may be accounted for by this complex lipid substance. Lipid A is a polymer containing glucosamine disaccharide units linked through pyrophosphate bridges and esterified with lauric, palmitic, and myristic acids. Perhaps the most important finding in recent years is that lipid A is immunogenic and will induce antibodies which cross-react among the gram-negative bacteria. Animal studies reveal that antibody prepared against the active component of endotoxin will protect against challenge from heterologous gram-negative bacteria. The frequency of shock and death in patients with gram-negative bacteria appears to be lower in individuals with initially high titers of cross-reacting antibody to the Re or core lipopolysaccharide (lipid A) component. These findings hold promise for development of immunoprophylaxis and therapy.

When inoculated intravenously, the endotoxins cause fever, leukopenia, circulatory collapse, capillary hemorrhages, necrosis of tumors, and the Shwartzman phenomenon. Noteworthy is the remarkable tolerance that develops after repeated injections of endotoxin. For example, the first intravenous injection in man of as little as 0.01 ml of typhoid vaccine will give rise to a violent response, with chill and high fever; yet after 10 to 14 daily injections of increasing quantities, the subject can accept 25 ml or more without symptoms and with only a slight rise in temperature. This state of tolerance is not obviously dependent on specific antibodies; it extends to endotoxins of unrelated bacterial strains. The clinical features of gram-negative bacteremia resemble the reaction of laboratory animals or man to intravenous injection of purified endotoxic preparations, and may well represent a direct "pharmacologic" response to bacterial endotoxin. In other types of infectious process there is reason to doubt that such phenomena as fever, leukocytosis, and leukopenia are direct effects of endotoxin liberation.

The phenomenon of endotoxin tolerance may explain the remarkable tendency of the symptoms of pyelonephritis to subside spontaneously. By contrast, endotoxin tolerance is not a feature of experimental typhoid fever, but, rather, volunteers infected with this organism have been shown to be hypersensitive to its effects. Endotoxin tolerance is currently under intensive study because of the presumed important pathologic effect of this substance. The often conflicting observations on tolerance to the fever-producing property of endotoxin now appear to be due to the fact that multiple phenomena are operating simultaneously. Endotoxin is believed to be pyrogenic by inducing macrophages (monocytes, Kupffer and related cells) to release a protein, termed endogenous pyrogen. This protein is carried in the circulation to the temperature-regulating nuclei in the hypothalamus, producing an alteration in thermoregulation. Frequent, repeated doses of endotoxin are thought to exhaust the cells' capability of releasing this substance. More prolonged exposure is believed to induce antibodies which block the action of endotoxin.

Antibodies. Antibodies reacting with most Enterobacteriaceae can be demonstrated in sera of normal animals and man, probably because of the continual production of antigen in the gastrointestinal tract. Gram-negative bacteria contain a wide variety of antigenic determinants. The best studied include the H or flagellar antigens which are heat-labile proteins present in motile strains. They have not been shown to be of pathogenetic significance. Some of the enteric bacteria contain K or capsular polysaccharides (they are particularly prominent among Klebsiella, but are not confined to this group). These surface slime layers interfere with phagocytosis and may be important in imparting virulence to encapsulated strains. They appear to account for invasiveness but not toxicity. The *Enterobacteriaceae* share a common antigen (CA). Antibody to core lipopolysaccharide, described above, is currently thought to be the key determinant of resistance to endotoxin damage. Antibodies to the O or somatic antigens of *E. coli* have been most extensively studied. Very low titers are present in human newborns, presumably because they are mostly of the high molecular weight IgM variety, and do not readily pass the placenta. Human colostrum is rich in O antibody, but this is not absorbed during breast feeding. Colonization of the digestive tract, however, is soon accompanied by appearance of a wide variety of antibodies in serum, which contains virtually all the *E. coli* O antibodies by one year of age. It is likely that the great susceptibility of the newborn to overwhelming gram-negative bacterial sepsis is related to lack of maternal antibodies.

As a rule, most strains are susceptible to opsonization and lysis by the combined effects of antibody and complement. Some strains, however, seem insusceptible to lysis in vitro. Nonetheless, this system may be of great importance in preventing strains from invading and persisting in the blood.

Tests for Endotoxemia. A remarkably sensitive test for endotoxemia has been developed, based on the finding that small amounts will cause gelation of lysates of amebocytes of the horseshoe crab. The test must be currently considered primarily as a research test, because, although it is commonly positive in gram-negative bacteremia, this is not always true, and a positive test does not correlate well with the outcome of infection. Since endotoxemia does not require living organisms, the test may be positive in the absence of detectable bacteremia. A less sensitive test is based on the enhanced cutaneous vasoconstriction that follows intradermal injection of the patient's serum into rabbits given endotoxin intravenously. This test must also be considered as investigational. Perhaps the most important aspect of these tests is that they offer strong evidence that endotoxin is indeed often present in the blood of patients with gram-negative sepsis.

THE ROLE OF ENTERIC BACTERIA IN PYOGENIC INFECTIONS OF THE ABDOMINAL CAVITY

The mixed flora of the intestinal tract participate in infections that originate from lesions of the bowel, such as appendicitis, cholangitis, diverticulitis, and perforation (from ulcerative colitis, ileitis, or carcinoma). These may lead to subdiaphragmatic, hepatic, and pelvic abscesses, which are frequent causes of fever of unknown origin in the patient recovering from abdominal surgery or trauma to this region. Because enteric bacteria grow luxuriantly in both aerobic and anaerobic media and therefore are likely to predominate in cultures, their relative importance tends to be exaggerated. There is good reason to believe that anaerobic bacteria – bacteroides, clostridia, and anaerobic streptococci – play more important roles in this kind of process. It should be pointed out here that a "fecal" odor of pus, though often ascribed to coliforms, is doubtless caused by associated anaerobic bacteria. Anaerobic bacteria are usually present as mixtures of two or more species. They should be suspected when there is foul pus and when organisms can be visualized microscopically but fail to grow under routine conditions.

OTHER INFECTIONS CAUSED BY THE ENTERIC BACTERIA

Gastroenteritis. A significant proportion of cases of gastroenteritis occurring in the neonatal period of life appear to be caused by enteric bacteria. About ten serologic strains of *E. coli* have been identified with this capability; they are spoken of as enteropathogenic strains. Outbreaks of diarrhea among adults, particularly travelers abroad, have been associated with enterotoxigenic strains of *E. coli.* Sporadic epidemics with invasive strains have been reported after ingestion of imported cheese. Certain strains of Proteus and Pseudomonas have at times also been held responsible for similar illness.

Meningitis and Brain Abscess. During the first four weeks of life, purulent meningitis is frequently caused by members of the enteric group of bacteria. Such cases occur sporadically in nurseries, and may be associated with infection of any other tissue of the body. Infants with meningoceles are especially liable to enteric bacterial meningitis. In adults, such infections are rare, but may occasionally be seen as complications of gram-negative bacteremia or in association with other diseases affecting host resistance, e.g., diabetes mellitus or lymphoma (see Ch. 201). Nontraumatic brain abscess is frequently due to infection by multiple species of anaerobic organisms similar to those found in the gastrointestinal tract. The sites of origin include chronically infected ears, sinuses, lung, abdomen, and pelvis.

Bacteremia in Hepatic Cirrhosis. Occasionally persons with cirrhosis of the liver develop an acute febrile illness and are found to have bacteremia caused by one of the enteric organisms, usually *E. coli.* Occasionally these patients have signs of peritonitis, but in most of them the event comes "out of the blue" without evidence of localized sepsis anywhere. The illness is short and self-limited or responds to appropriate chemotherapy. Speculation as to its pathogenesis has included the possibility of shunting bacteria away from the filtering action of the liver, impairment of humoral or cellular defense mechanisms, or complement inactivation owing to high blood ammonia. In actuality a satisfactory explanation is lacking at present.

Surface Infection. Enteric bacteria, particularly Proteus and Pseudomonas, are commonly recovered from the surfaces of burns, varicose ulcers, decubitus ulcers, tracheostomy sites, and the like. Generally, these organisms appear to play no pathogenic role, and satisfactory healing may proceed regardless of their presence. They can at times result in fulminant gram-negative sepsis, particularly in the patient with severe burns. The exudate from the sinus of a chronic osteomyelitis or chronic otitis media often contains Proteus as the dominant organism. Otitis of the external auditory canal owing to Pseudomonas may give troublesome local symptoms, especially in swimmers.

Perirectal Abscess. This is an important complication in patients with marked granulocytopenia. Rectal examination should be carefully performed in such patients, particularly when they develop fever and perianal pain.

Abscesses at Sites of Subcutaneous Injections. Rarely, enteric bacilli cause abscesses in subcutaneous tissue at sites of hypodermic injections, notably in diabetic subjects who inject their own insulin. These are sometimes characterized by gas formation, and they thus arouse fear of more serious clostridial infection, whereas, in fact, they are usually of minor clinical importance.

Metastatic Infections. Despite the frequency with which enteric bacteria succeed in invading the blood, metastatic localization of infection is rare. There are, however, occasional instances of such suppurative lesions as arthritis and panophthalmitis in patients with bacteremia originating in acute pyelonephritis. Of special interest in this regard is osteomyelitis of the spine. This is usually seen in men with prostatic disease, chronic cystitis, and posterior urethritis. Possibly the method of spread here is by way of septic emboli to the spine through the vertebral venous plexus.

Superinfection. Enteric bacteria frequently predominate in the bronchial secretions of patients under treatment with large doses of penicillin or broad-spectrum antimicrobial agents. In most instances, this is not of significance and simply represents emergence of unaffected bacterial strains after the suppression of the primary pathogens. Transtracheal aspiration, followed by gram stain and culture of the secretions, is a useful method to distinguish between colonization of the pharynx versus true infection of the lower respiratory tract. It is not an indication for cessation or change in antimicrobial therapy unless there is clinical evidence of tissue invasion by the newly emergent organism. Primary gram-negative bacterial pneumonia often superimposed on viral influenza, however, does occur and may be exceedingly difficult to manage.

GRAM-NEGATIVE BACTEREMIA

Bacteremia caused by gram-negative bacilli has become a problem of greater relative importance since the advent of penicillin and better control of gram-positive coccal infections. Urinary tract infection accounts for about two thirds of all cases of blood invasion by the enteric bacteria. Other causes include surgical disease of the gastrointestinal tract, infections developing at the site of "cut-downs" and intravenous catheters, postpartum or postabortal sepsis (including the so-called "placental bacteremia"), and infection of wounds, ulcers, burns, and internal prosthetic devices such as heart valves. Sometimes there is a clearly apparent precipitating factor such as cystoscopy, surgical or obstetrical procedure, or manipulation of an infected wound.

These bacteremias have clinical characteristics closely resembling the recognized biologic effects of gram-negative bacterial endotoxins. Onset of symptoms may occur with a shaking chill and rise in temperature of 38 to 40.5° C. There is an initial leukopenia, but after 6 to 12 hours usually there is leukocytosis. An *important and highly significant accompaniment is circulatory embarrassment with lowering of the blood pressure.* This may be manifested only by some alteration in the patient's state of consciousness, and the skin may continue to feel warm, although sometimes the skin is cold and clammy. Occasionally patients slip into a shocklike state without much elevation of temperature; hence infection of this kind must always be taken into consideration in evaluation of peripheral circulatory failure. Petechial hemorrhages and purpura are not common. Some patients, however, do develop the syndrome of disseminated intravascular coagulation (DIC). This phenomenon is not unique to gram-negative bacteremia and may be due to such diverse causes as rickettsial and gram-positive bacterial infections. The most common findings are reduced platelet count, low factor V levels in plasma, and fibrin split products in serum. Serum complement is low only in the most seriously ill patients. There are diminution in urine output, increase in proteinuria, and often a rise in nonprotein nitrogen of the blood. The cardiac output may be unpredictably low, normal, or elevated. Some patients show shifts in acid-base balance in the direction of metabolic acidosis, whereas others have compensatory hyperventilation. The pH of the blood, however, often remains normal. Lactic acidosis is common in severely ill patients. It is characterized by a marked anion gap with low levels of both serum bicarbonate and P_{CO_2}. These findings are often confusing, particularly if they occur in patients with complicating problems such as pulmonary or renal insufficiency or congestive heart failure. Serum lactate levels are helpful in sorting out these factors. Much depends on the nature of the underlying disease and the renal reserve. The outlook is grave, being influenced by age, associated disease, and evidence of shock. When obvious signs of circulatory collapse are present, the fatality rate may be as high as 75 per cent.

UNIQUE FEATURES OF PSEUDOMONAS INFECTIONS

Pseudomonas infections, although often similar to those caused by other gram-negative bacteria, sometimes have unique characteristics. As already mentioned, this organism frequently appears in necrotic tissue, as in ulcers, burns, or draining sinuses. Usually such colonization is of little clinical significance, and mere removal of necrotic tissue may cause it to disappear. Nevertheless, under certain circumstances, especially in chronically debilitated persons or in patients with agranulocytosis or acute leukemia, severe sepsis may be produced by this class of bacteria.

Pseudomonas is notoriously resistant to antimicrobial therapy; hence it tends to emerge as the dominant microorganism after eradication of other bacteria by drugs, and it may then be responsible for the phenomenon of superinfection, as in the bronchopulmonary infections that may complicate prophylactic chemotherapy of chronic lung disease.

Because Pseudomonas commonly occurs in tap water, and because it may be resistant to antiseptics used in sterilizing instruments, it is likely to be carried into the body by such procedures as cystoscopy. Furthermore, most of the reported instances of meningitis after lumbar puncture have been associated with this organism.

Tissue invasion, most often seen in patients with leukopenia or relapse in leukemia, is characterized by necrotizing vasculitis with bacterial invasion of the walls of arteries and veins. This leads to a distinctive necrotic skin lesion (called ecthyma gangrenosum) that is found most commonly along the axillary folds or in the anogenital area, but may also develop on any part of the body. It may begin as a vesicle that later becomes necrotic. The typical lesion of ecthyma gangrenosa is a round, indurated ulcer with a black center that varies from a few millimeters to several centimeters in diameter.

TREATMENT OF ENTERIC BACTERIAL INFECTIONS

General Principles. The major clinical problems in management of enteric bacterial infections are (1) differentiation of superficial contamination that often requires no treatment from true or potential tissue invasion, (2) early recognition and drainage of abscesses, (3) anticipation of the role of anaerobic bacteria that cannot be readily cultured, and (4) early recognition of bacteremic shock. *Many of these infections are preventable,* particularly those arising from instrumentation of the urinary tract, intravenous catheters and contaminated fluids, suction, and ventilation equipment. *Every physician must consider elimination of such sources of contamination as one of his prime responsibilities.*

Gram-Negative Bacteremia. The presence of gram-negative organisms in the blood should alert the physician to search for a site of origin such as intravenous or urinary catheters and abdominal or perirectal abscesses. Removal of devices and drainage of abscesses should be done as soon as possible. Antimicrobial therapy should be guided as often as possible by in vitro drug-susceptibility tests because of the remarkable ability of enteric bacteria to develop resistant strains. Among the aminoglycoside antimicrobials, gentamicin and kanamycin are most reliable, followed by streptomycin. Rapid emergence of resistant strains is a major problem with streptomycin. It should rarely be used alone. The so-called broad-spectrum drugs such as tetracycline and chloramphenicol are also useful against the Enterobacteriaceae, as are ampicillin and cephalothin. They are most often effective when not previously used in the patient, because emergence of resistant strains is common. Drug susceptibility tests are essential to guide the choice of drugs. Large doses of penicillin G are effective against many of the gram-positive and some gram-negative anaerobes. Chloramphenicol, clindamycin, and occasionally tetracycline are useful for Bacteroides, whereas Pseudomonas will generally respond only to drugs such as polymyxin B or colistin methane sulfonate (polymyxin E) and gentamicin. Carbenicillin is a new semisynthetic penicillin that may be of considerable value in treatment of Pseudomonas, Enterobacter, and Proteus infections. The problems are the large doses required, development of resistance, tendency for sodium overload (4.7 mEq per gram), and high cost. It should be reserved for clearly established infection caused by a susceptible organism. It is generally advisable to use two and sometimes more agents, including gentamicin, in severe gram-negative sepsis, particularly when bacteriologic identification is delayed.

Antimicrobial therapy in severe gram-negative sepsis is often a guessing game, but it can be approached with a reasonable rationale rather than, as is often the practice, merely by giving large doses of the most currently popular antimicrobial drugs. It should be remembered that gram-negative bacteremia is more common than is usually suspected and is often transient and without complication. For example, bacteremia may occur after gastrointestinal endoscopy, urinary instrumentation, and manipulation of the bowel during surgery. These events often go undetected, or there is a single temperature rise and no further complications. Antimicrobial therapy probably plays little role in management of these transient episodes. The main problem is caused by the release of endotoxin. Endotoxin is not affected by antimicrobial drugs. Judgment will therefore have to be made to determine whether there is an infected site which requires treatment.

The site of origin of the infection, the underlying illness of the patient, and prior receipt of antimicrobial agents are key determinants in planning therapy. For infection arising in the urinary tract in a patient not previously on chemotherapy, relatively safe drugs such as ampicillin, tetracycline, or a cephalosporin should be effective. For patients previously receiving multiple antimicrobials, gentamicin is preferred. Mixed anaerobic infections in patients with a perforated abdominal organ or a brain abscess should receive large doses of aqueous penicillin G plus chloramphenicol. Clindamycin also shows great promise as an effective agent for the anaerobic intestinal flora. A cephalosporin may be substituted for penicillin G in the allergic patient, although cross-sensitization has been described. Acute cholecystitis is often associated with *E. coli* in the gallbladder. Ampicillin or tetracyclines or chloramphenicol are recommended as the first drug, provided they have not been used previously. Gentamicin should be added if the course is complicated. Pneumonia caused by gram-negative bacteria is usually overdiagnosed. It is best established by transtracheal aspiration or culture of the blood, pleural fluid, and, occasionally, percutaneous lung aspiration. The clinician must distinguish this from the superficial gram-negative bacterial colonization of the oropharynx which commonly accompanies debility or antimicrobial therapy. It almost uniformly occurs in patients with tracheostomies and usually should not be treated. In addition, patients with debility or difficulty in clearing secretions will often aspirate the oral contents and develop a mixed anaerobic infection of the lung. This problem is best treated with large doses of penicillin or clindamycin rather than with drugs used for aerobic gram-negative infections. True gram-negative pneumonia (as defined above) should be treated with the most potent agents, depending in part on drug susceptibility tests. Gentamicin is probably the single most effective agent. Cephalosporins are useful for Klebsiella; ampicillin tends to be more effective for Enterobacter, whereas gentamicin alone or with carbenicillin is useful for Pseudomonas. Gram-negative sepsis in patients with burns or leukemia is often due to Pseudomonas and should be treated with gentamicin and carbenicillin. The subject of antimicrobial therapy is considered in greater detail in Ch. 267 and 268.

Management of bacteremic shock is complex, requiring corrective measures designed to improve cardiac function, tissue perfusion, and electrolyte imbalance, particularly acidosis. This requires monitoring of the central venous pressure by a well-placed catheter in the superior vena cava or right atrium in an attempt to achieve a pressure of about 8 to 12 cm of water, and following the dynamics of pressure changes as fluid replacement is given. Replacement fluids include blood, dextran, and saline solutions. Drugs such as isoproterenol may be used to increase cardiac output and improve tissue perfusion; vasopressors such as metaraminol should be used sparingly except in severe shock. High doses of corticosteroids are widely used, but their efficacy has not been established by controlled studies. Heparin may be useful in the syndrome of disseminated intravascular coagulation.

Blair, E., Wise, A., and MacKay, A. G.: Gram-negative bacteremic shock. J.A.M.A., 207:333, 1968.
Editorial: Consumption coagulopathy in septicemic shock. N. Engl. J. Med., 279:884, 1968.
Moore, W. E. C., Cato, E. P., and Holdeman, L. V.: Anaerobic bacteria of the gastrointestinal flora and their occurrence in clinical infections. J. Infect. Dis., 119:641, 1969.
Steinhauer, B. W., Eickhoff, T. C., Kislak, J. W., and Finland, M.: The Klebsiella-Enterobacter-Serratia division. Clinical and epidemiologic characteristics. Ann. Intern. Med., 65:1180, 1966.

215. SHIGELLOSIS

Leighton E. Cluff

Definition. Shigellosis is an enteric infection with one of the species of Shigella bacilli, which may be asymptomatic or may cause dysentery.

Bacillary dysentery is usually a self-limited, acute illness characterized by diarrhea with mucous-bloody feces, tenesmus, fever, and abdominal colic and tenderness. Symptomless infected persons and those convalescing from dysentery may harbor Shigella in the stool for several days, serving as a source of infection for others. The infection is worldwide and is most common among persons living in crowded unhygienic circumstances. Man is the principal host to the microorganism, and the infection is usually transmitted from person to person, directly or indirectly.

History. Dysentery has been recognized for centuries. Delineation of dysentery attributable to Shigella, however, was not possible until 1896, when epidemic diarrhea in Japan was shown by Shiga to be caused by a specific microorganism.

Association of the bacillus isolated from feces of patients with the disease was possible by demonstration of rising titers of specific serum agglutinins in a significant proportion of patients. Subsequently, Flexner, Boyd, and Lentz identified other species of Shigella bacilli responsible for dysentery in man. From the beginning, dysentery has been a nemesis to encamped military troops, persons living in unhygienic conditions, and patients in mental institutions. It has occasionally caused epidemic disease in hospitals, nurseries, and schools. Currently, Shigella infection is responsible for a significant proportion of diarrheal disease particularly among children and older persons living in crowded urban areas. There was a progressive increase in the number of infections identified in England and Wales after 1940. Over 40,000 cases were noted in 1960.

Etiology. Strains of Shigella can be characterized antigenically, and there are four serologic groups responsible for disease in man. These are usually identified as serotypes of *Shigella dysenteriae* (shiga), *Shigella flexneri, Shigella boydii,* and *Shigella sonnei.* Another group, formerly referred to as *Shigella alkalescens,* may also produce enteric infection in man, but biochemically and antigenically it is more closely related to coliform bacilli.

The shigellae are gram-negative, slender, nonmotile, nonsporulating bacilli, which on primary isolation resemble coccobacilli. They are aerobic and facultative anaerobic, growing readily on relatively simple media at 37° C. They can be selectively grown in the presence of various bile salts (SS and desoxycholate media), thereby being distinguished from most coliform bacilli. Species and strains of Shigella can be identified by carbohydrate fermentation and antigenic analysis with specific antiserum. As with other enteric pathogens, Shigella bacilli do not ordinarily ferment lactose.

Epidemiology. Shigellosis is most common in tropical countries under unhygienic, crowded conditions, but is endemic throughout the world.

Young children appear to be more susceptible than adults to bacillary dysentery, but the disease is less common in the first six months of life than in older infants and children. Eighty per cent of children under nine years of age infected with Shigella will develop dysentery, whereas only about 50 per cent of infected older persons develop illness. Under the age of 20 years the frequency of shigellosis in males is greater than in females, but over the age of 20 years the reverse is true. Nevertheless, the case fatality rate is higher in men at all ages. In some countries bacillary dysentery has its peak incidence in summer months, often after heavy rains, whereas in other areas, such as the United States, the highest incidence may be in winter, spring, or autumn. The months when shigellosis is particularly prevalent in tropical and semitropical countries correspond with the time of year when flies are prevalent. Shigella may be found in the intestinal tracts of flies having contact with infected human feces, but carriage of the bacilli on the insect's feet is probably the means by which it may spread infection. In countries with a high standard of sanitation flies play an inconsequential role in transfer of infection.

Infection is usually transmitted by patients with dysentery, ambulatory persons convalescing from the disease, or asymptomatic carriers. Inadequately washed hands or contaminated inanimate articles are the principal means of transmission. The seats of toilets may become contaminated during flushing and serve as a source of infection. Epidemics of shigellosis have been related to milk, ice cream, and other foods and water contaminated by the hands or feces of infected persons. Shigella in dust has also been incriminated in outbreaks of bacillary dysentery. These sources of infection are also important in perpetuation of endemic infection. Outbreaks of shigellosis in winter usually spread from an infected person in a school or institution to other persons. Secondary cases may result in extension of the disease to other schools or institutions such as hospitals or nurseries. Relapsing disease, reinfection, and chronic infection may enable perpetuation of infection among patients in nursing homes and inmates of mental hospitals. In this setting, outbreaks are often not explosive.

Endemic and epidemic shigellosis is commonly characterized by isolation of several different serologic types of Shigella. Major outbreaks caused by a single serotype are rare, but small outbreaks may be attributable to a single serologic type.

Shigella dysenteriae (shiga) is an uncommon cause of infection in Britain, Europe, and North America, but is responsible for a significant proportion of cases in Asia. *Shigella sonnei* is the prominent cause of bacillary dysentery in countries where personal contact and endemic infection, rather than poor sanitation and unhygienic conditions, are responsible for spread of the disease.

After infection, the bacilli may be isolated from feces or rectum for only a week or slightly longer. Rarely does carriage of the bacilli persist as long as three months. Carriage of *Shigella dysenteriae* (shiga), however, persists longer than with other species, and carriage of *Shigella flexneri* may be intermittent during convalescence from infection. Generally, however, persistent carriers of *Shigella dysenteriae* remain ill, whereas carriers of *Shigella flexneri* are well. Convalescence from infection caused by *Shigella sonnei* is not associated with prolonged excretion of the bacilli in feces except in the very young and very old.

Although Shigella infection is largely confined to human beings, primates have been shown occasionally to be a source of infection in man. Shigella survive in eggs, oysters, clams, and shrimp for many days, but these serve as sources of infection only when contaminated by infected persons and their excreta.

Pathogenesis and Pathology. Shigella species possess an endotoxin similar to that of other gram-negative bacteria, but it seems unlikely that it plays a significant role in the pathogenesis of bacillary dysentery. *Shigella dysenteriae* (shiga) produces an exotoxin that can exert a deleterious effect upon the nervous system and may affect the intestinal epithelium like cholera enterotoxin and cause diarrhea. The occurrence of paralytic manifestations in dysentery produced by this species may be attributable to the exotoxin.

Bacillary dysentery is infrequently associated with bacteremia, and the infection is confined to the intestinal mucosa, occasionally invading mesenteric lymph nodes. Morphologic lesions are most frequently observed in the colon, occasionally involving the terminal ileum. Ulceration of the mucosa develops, with intervening inflamed membrane but no undermining of the ulcer edges as in amebic dysentery. The bowel wall is infiltrated with granulocytes, there is edema of the submucosa, and occasionally the involvement may extend to the serosa. If ulceration is not extensive, healing occurs without scarring, but when it is severe, fibrosis and even stenosis of the bowel may develop.

Clinical Manifestations. Patients with shigellosis may have simple self-limited diarrhea, acute gastroenteritis, true dysentery, or no symptoms of illness. It has been proposed that bacillary dysentery may occasionally be responsible for chronic colitis, but it has been difficult to establish this relationship with certainty.

The incubation period of dysentery is usually about 48 hours, but it may be shorter. The illness begins abruptly with abdominal cramps, pain relieved by defecation, and watery diarrhea. This is followed promptly by the development of tenesmus, feverishness, and passage of mucous stool, occasionally containing blood. Abdominal tenderness, most pronounced in the lower quadrants, is found, and the bowel is hyperactive on auscultation. The temperature rarely rises very high, except in children, in whom it may become 40° C or more. Without treatment the illness persists for a few days and then subsides.

Acute gastroenteritis, associated with nausea, some vomiting, and diarrhea, is seen particularly in outbreaks of infection by *Shigella sonnei.*

Shigella dysenteriae (shiga) infection is often more severe than that caused by the other species. The fever may be higher, hypotension develops more frequently, and the intestinal symptoms are more intense. Recovery may be delayed, and debility may persist for several weeks. Peripheral neuritis more commonly complicates infection by *Shigella dysenteriae.*

Conjunctivitis, iritis, and nystagmus are occasional complications of bacillary dysentery, appearing between the first and second weeks of disease. Nonsuppurative arthritis may also develop. Fluid and electrolyte depletion may be considerable, particularly in infants and children, producing severe dehydration and acidosis. Potassium deficit may be recognized, particularly as the patient's fluids are replenished. Convulsions develop occasionally in children, but appear to be correlated to the degree of fever.

At times, bacillary dysentery seems to have been precipitated by onset of measles, and almost half the cases may be accompanied by infection with enteropathic viruses, including adenovirus, echovirus, poliovirus, and coxsackievirus. The association of a virus with the disease, however, does not influence its clinical manifestations. The frequency of serious underlying disease in persons with shigellosis is not as common as in salmonellosis. Massive intestinal bleeding occurs in severe bacillary dysentery when there is extensive intestinal necrosis and ulceration.

Diagnosis. Isolation and identification of Shigella in the stool or from swab culture of the rectal mucosa are the only means of establishing the diagnosis of shigellosis. The serum agglutinin titer will rise in about half the patients with bacillary dysentery, but it is not ordinarily useful for diagnostic purposes. Shigella survive in feces for only a short while. Therefore feces should be promptly cultured, or the specimen should be collected in a 30 per cent glycerol-saline solution for preservation. Examination of the feces microscopically in bacillary dysentery will usually reveal a large number of granulocytes, comprising about 90 per cent of all cells, apart from erythrocytes. As convalescence begins, mononuclear cells become predominant. Specific immunofluorescence techniques have been developed for the rapid detection of Shigella in feces. This test agrees with cultural results in over 90 per cent of instances.

Viral enteritis caused by echovirus, coxsackievirus, and poliomyelitis virus may be epidemic and may be confused with shigellosis. Fever is uncommon, however, in viral enteritis unless there is severe dehydration, and the feces contain no blood or pus. *Staphylococcal enterocolitis* develops usually in hospitalized patients undergoing abdominal surgery who have received antimicrobial therapy. *Amebic dysentery* usually has a gradual onset, the diarrhea is ordinarily not severe, there is often little or no fever, and microscopic examination of the feces will reveal a predominance of mononuclear cells. Sigmoidoscopy reveals undermined ulcers with normal intervening mucosa. *Salmonellosis* is more often accompanied by nausea and vomiting at onset and occasionally by a chill and very high fever. Blood cultures are often positive. *Staphylococcal food poisoning* and many forms of viral gastroenteritis are more prominently associated with nausea and vomiting than with diarrhea.

Treatment. Sulfonamides were effective in treatment of shigellosis when they were first used. Resistant bacilli emerged, however, and sulfonamides are not now considered to be the most effective drugs for the infection. Resistance of Shigella to multiple antimicrobials has been induced by episomal transfer from other enteric bacilli. Conceivably, therefore, drug-susceptible Shigella may become drug resistant from other drug-resistant bacilli in the intestinal tract.

Tetracycline has been an effective drug against Shigella, but resistant strains have been identified. A few strains of Shigella are resistant to chloramphenicol. Colimycin and neomycin are almost always effective in vitro, but a few strains resistant to ampicillin have been found. Streptomycin given orally has been used to treat shigellosis, but strains resistant to this drug have also been identified. Cephalothin and massive doses of penicillin G may be effective.

At present, ampicillin in a dosage of 2 or more grams orally each day in divided doses for five days is the preferred agent in treatment of shigellosis in adults. Tetracycline or (in very serious circumstances) chloramphenicol may be effective alternatives if either the microorganism is resistant to ampicillin or the patient is allergic to the penicillins. Oral streptomycin, 0.5 gram twice daily, is also recommended in Great Britain.

Fluid and electrolyte replacement should be given to the patient who is in collapse or who is dehydrated. Diphenoxalate hydrochloride and atropine (Lomotil) and opiates such as paregoric or morphine may alleviate the abdominal discomfort and tenesmus but should be used cautiously.

Prognosis. The mortality rate in untreated bacillary dysentery is about 0.1 per cent or less, but it may be higher during famine or starvation. In addition, the fatality rate with dysentery caused by *Shigella dysenteriae* (shiga) is higher than with that attributed to other Shigella. Death rarely occurs when appropriate treatment is prescribed.

Dammin, G. J.: The pathogenesis of acute diarrheal disease in early life. Bull. WHO, 31:29, 1964.

Gordon, J. E., Behar, M., and Scrimshaw, N. S.: Acute diarrheal disease in less developed countries: I. An epidemiological basis for control. Bull. WHO, 31:1, 1964.

Levine, M. M., et al.: Pathogenesis of *Shigella dysenteriae* (Shiga) dysentery. J. Infect. Dis., 127:261, 1973.

Ramos-Alvarez, M., et al.: Diarrheal disease of children. The occurrence of enteropathogenic viruses and bacteria. Am. J. Dis. Child., 107:218, 1964.

Reller, L. B., et al.: Shigellosis in the United States, 1964–1968. J. Infect. Dis., 120:393, 1969.

Watanabe, T.: Infective heredity of multiple drug resistance in bacteria. Bact. Rev., 27:87, 1963.

216. CHOLERA
(Asiatic Cholera)

Leighton E. Cluff

Definition. Cholera is a specific infectious disease of man caused by *Vibrio cholerae*. It is characterized by diarrhea with fluid and electrolyte depletion, occurring endemically and epidemically in Asia and occasionally pandemically.

Etiology. In a classic study in 1857, Snow described an outbreak of cholera in London and incriminated contaminated water as the source of disease. In 1883, Koch identified *Vibrio cholerae* in the feces of a large number of patients with cholera. The cholera vibrio is a comma-shaped, gram-negative, flagellated, and motile microorganism that grows aerobically on nutrient media at 37° C, preferentially at an alkaline pH. There are two biotypes of *Vibrio cholerae*, the "classic" and the El Tor. The El Tor strain is hardier than the classic strain, persists longer in nature and in man, is more resistant to chemical agents, is hemolytic, and is antigenically separable from the classic strain. *V. cholerae* can be differentiated from noncholera vibrios by its fermentative, hemolytic, pathogenic, and antigenic reactions.

Incidence and Prevalence. Cholera is endemic in India, Burma, Pakistan, Thailand, and a few other areas in Asia. It has occurred in epidemics throughout the world. Prior to the nineteenth century, cholera was unknown outside India, but during that century it was observed sporadically and as an epidemic in Europe, England, Russia, and North America. In the twentieth century, cholera has largely disappeared from the Western Hemisphere and Europe but continues to occur endemically and epidemically in Asia, primarily along the Ganges River in India and in Pakistan. The pandemic of cholera extending from 1898 to 1907 was responsible for at least 370,000 deaths in India. A current pandemic, attributable to the El Tor strain, began in 1961 in Indonesia and has spread through most of Asia, the Middle East, Africa, and recently (1972–1973) into Western and Eastern Europe.

Epidemiology. Only man is naturally infected with *V. cholerae*. The infection is transmitted most commonly by contaminated water, but it can be transmitted by contamination of fresh leafy or root vegetables and fruit fertilized with human feces or with water containing the microorganism. *V. cholerae* has been isolated from flies, roaches, and other insects, but these may be an unimportant source of contagion. Doctors and nurses caring for patients with cholera rarely contract the disease, suggesting that direct contact under hygienic conditions is an uncommon mode of transmission of the infection. Cholera is primarily a disease of persons who live in poverty or who have poor standards of living and sanitation. The case-infection ratio in classic cholera is about 1:7, but in El Tor cholera this ratio can be 1:25 or 1:100. Asymptomatic infected persons who travel may establish new foci of cholera. *V. cholerae* does not survive long in fresh water, but can survive for long periods in sea water, particularly along beaches contaminated with human sewage.

Outbreaks of cholera usually appear during dry, hot weather preceding a rainy season. The reason for this seasonal occurrence of cholera is unexplained. Although sporadic cases may occur throughout the year, there are rare chronic carriers of *V. cholerae*, as there are of typhoid bacilli, and the principal reservoir of the organism in interepidemic periods is unclear. In endemic areas around river basins, *V. cholerae* can be isolated from the water throughout the year, although most cases of cholera occur seasonally.

Pathology and Pathogenesis. Recent studies of cholera indicate that the small intestine is most severely involved. The gastrointestinal epithelium remains intact, even in the acute phase of the disease, but there are mononuclear cell inflammation of the mucosa, vascular congestion, and goblet cell hyperplasia. This acute stage may be followed by increased "turnover" of the epithelial cells. These morphologic changes are similar to those seen in nonspecific diarrhea but do not explain the clinical features of the disease. Chronic atrophic gastritis may precede and persist after the infection. It is likely that nutritional and other chronic affections of the intestine and stomach are predisposing causes of cholera. Occurrence of the disease in impoverished and malnourished persons further suggests this possibility. A cholera-like disease has been produced in dogs by feeding them vibrio with bicarbonate.

The cholera vibrio produces an enterotoxin which is responsible for the disease manifestations. The enterotoxin is a heat-labile protein with a molecular weight of 10,000 to 90,000 which binds to intestinal epithelium, initiating intense secretion of isotonic fluid, but does not interfere with absorption of glucose and electrolyte. One step in this sequence is activation of adenyl cyclase–producing cyclic AMP and providing the energy for ion secretion and water transport into the gut lumen.

The primary difficulty in cholera is severe fluid and electrolyte depletion. The feces contain mucus, epithelial debris, large quantities of water, sodium, potassium, and bicarbonate, but little plasma protein. There is no significant loss of albumin into the intestines, as illustrated by the failure of intravenously injected Evans blue dye to appear in the feces.

Clinical Manifestations. Cholera begins as an acute diarrhea with abdominal pain. Vomiting may appear early, but is not prominent. Fever and chills are usually absent. The oral and axillary temperature may be depressed, whereas the rectal temperature may be elevated slightly above normal. Over a few hours the diarrhea increases in severity, and the volume of feces may be as great as 15 to 20 liters in 24 hours. Initially, the feces are bile stained, but as the diarrhea worsens, the feces become watery, mucoid, and odorless, and occasionally may contain blood. The feces of patients with cholera may resemble rice water or starch water and may contain cellular debris and masses of cholera vibrios. The patient becomes rapidly dehydrated, the skin is cold and withered, and the face becomes drawn. As dehydration increases, the patient becomes stuporous, comatose, hypotensive, and cyanotic, and may die in shock. Urine output decreases, mouth and eyes become dry, but lacteal and sweat secretion may persist. Muscular cramps may be severe. Thirst is intense, and the ingestion of fluid rarely induces vomiting. Recovery ordinarily is prompt after replacement of fluid and electrolytes, but the patient may continue to have anuria or oliguria and may die in renal failure. The renal insufficiency may be attributable to hypokalemia, shock, or reduced renal blood flow owing to dehydration.

With severe dehydration the hematocrit, leukocyte

count, and specific gravity of the plasma rise. The plasma sodium chloride and total serum protein are increased above normal. The plasma potassium may be slightly elevated or normal, although potassium depletion is severe. Metabolic acidosis is usually severe.

In cholera the fecal sodium and chloride concentrations are increased above normal, as is fecal osmolarity, but these are consistently lower than the plasma values. Fecal potassium and carbonate concentrations, however, are higher than those of the plasma. These electrolyte changes in cholera resemble those in other diarrheal disease, but are more severe.

Many patients with cholera are anemic before onset of the disease; therefore the rise in hematocrit with dehydration may not be demonstrable. Infection by El Tor vibrio often causes no symptoms or mild diarrhea difficult to distinguish from other acute enteric illnesses.

Diagnosis. In endemic areas and during epidemics, cholera is easily recognized clinically. Sporadic cases must be differentiated from other diarrheal diseases such as typhoid fever, bacillary dysentery, amebiasis, other forms of intestinal parasitism, viral enteritis, staphylococcal food poisoning, and chemical poisoning. The epidemiologic and fulminant characteristics of cholera, however, are helpful diagnostically. Bacteriologic and immunologic identification of *V. cholerae* from the feces is usually possible. Microscopic examination of the feces may reveal masses of the microorganism. *V. cholerae* may be cultured from the feces of patients convalescing from cholera, but ordinarily disappears within a few days or a few weeks.

Strains of *Escherichia coli* and other enteric organisms may elaborate an enterotoxin similar to that of cholera vibrio and cause a cholera-like illness. Cholera-like diarrhea also can be caused by *Clostridium perfringens,* Salmonella, and Shigella.

Many patients with cholera will have a positive serologic test for *V. cholerae* antibodies on the day of onset of disease. Serum antibody titers, measured by hemagglutination or vibriocidal assay, however, rise to maximal levels in about seven days after onset of cholera. Vibriocidal titers fall rapidly after illness.

Other Vibrio Infections. Noncholera vibrios are widespread in surface water throughout the world and have been associated with diarrheal disease. *Vibrio fetus* produces disease in human beings but is primarily an infection of cattle causing septic abortion, and can be differentiated serologically from *V. cholerae.* Man is infected after occupational exposure to diseased animals or animal products. *V. fetus* infection of man does not produce diarrhea, but is responsible for bacteremia, abortion, pneumonia, endocarditis, thrombophlebitis, and an illness resembling acute brucellosis.

Treatment. The treatment of cholera is correction of the fluid and electrolyte depletion attributable to the severe diarrhea. Urine output and the patient's clinical appearance are indices of hydration if the patient does not have renal failure. The degree of hydration can be estimated clinically. The hemoglobin or hematocrit determination may be misleading because of pre-existing anemia. When the patient is first seen, the blood electrolyte determinations also may be unreliable as indices of the degree of electrolyte depletion and dehydration. Plasma protein concentration, and particularly plasma specific gravity, can serve as an index for administration of fluids and electrolyte.

A good replacement solution for intravenous administration to adults contains 133 mEq sodium, 98 mEq chloride, 13 mEq potassium and 48 mEq bicarbonate, prepared by addition of 5 grams sodium chloride, 4 grams sodium bicarbonate, and 1 gram potassium chloride to 1 liter sterile, pyrogen-free distilled water. In hypotensive adults the initial infusion should be given rapidly (50 to 100 ml per minute) until a strong radial pulse is restored. Subsequently, fluids are infused in quantities equal to fecal losses, measured preferably by having the patient on a "cholera cot" (a cot with a centrally placed hole to collect feces). If fluid loss cannot be accurately determined, fluid should be given to maintain radial pulse, blood pressure, and skin turgor. Overhydration can be avoided by observation of neck veins and auscultation of lungs. In children, sodium loss is less, and potassium loss is greater than in adults. Therefore the intravenous fluid used for replacement should be different (94 mEq sodium, 15 mEq potassium).

Many liters of fluid will be needed (25 or more) until the administration of fluid is no longer required. The cholera patient, even if in shock and comatose when first seen, will often be able to take oral feeding after four hours. At that time potassium, as juices or in other form, may be fed. Otherwise, if the diarrhea continues for more than 24 hours, the intravenous fluids should contain 10 mEq of potassium per liter. Oral fluid therapy of cholera patients is effective in adults and children. The fluid may contain 100 mEq sodium, 10 mEq potassium, 70 mEq chloride, 40 mEq bicarbonate, and 120 mM per liter glucose, with an osmolarity of 327 mOsm per liter.

Tetracycline given orally (40 mg per kilogram per day) or in a dosage of 100 mg per liter of intravenous fluid and administered in a total dosage of 250 to 500 mg during the first day of treatment shortens the period of diarrhea and decreases the requirement for fluid replacement. This is associated with a hastening of the disappearance of *V. cholerae* from the feces. Advances in understanding the action of cholera enterotoxin indicate the possibility that an antagonist of adenyl cyclase or an agent lowering intracellular levels of cyclic 3′5′ adenosine monophosphate may reverse the disease.

Prognosis. The case mortality rate from untreated cholera in persons 10 to 20 years of age is 50 per cent; in persons over 50 it is 70 per cent. Death is more common among those less than 10 years of age than among patients between 10 and 20 years of age. Almost invariably, death can be prevented if the fluid, electrolyte, and alkali therapy is begun early in the illness and if there is no serious associated disease or renal failure.

Prevention. Cholera can be eliminated by improved standards of living, public health, and sanitation. In those parts of the world where water supply and sewage disposal are controlled effectively, cholera no longer occurs.

There is a killed bacterial vaccine for immunization against cholera that provides some temporary protection. It may be useful in reducing the incidence of the disease in endemic areas. A toxoid of cholera enterotoxin is being evaluated and may add to the effectiveness of cholera vaccine in protection against the disease. Administration of cholera vaccine is no longer a requirement for entrance into the United States from cholera endemic areas.

Barua, D., and Burrows, W.: Cholera. Philadelphia, W. B. Saunders Company, 1974.

Carpenter, C. C. J.: Cholera: Diagnosis and treatment. Bull. N.Y. Acad. Med., 47:1192, 1971.

Gangarosa, E. J.: The epidemiology of cholera, past and present. Bull. N.Y. Acad. Med., 47:1140, 1971.
Hendrix, T. R.: The pathophysiology of cholera. Bull. N.Y. Acad. Med., 47:1169, 1971.
Holmgren, J., et al.: Experimental studies on cholera immunization. Infect. Immun., 5:662, 1972.
Mahalanabis, D., et al.: Oral fluid therapy of cholera. Johns Hopkins Med. J., 132:197, 1973.
Phillips, R. A.: Asiatic cholera. Ann. Rev. Med., 19:69, 1968.
Snow, J.: Snow on Cholera. The Commonwealth Fund. London, Oxford University Press, 1936.

217. PLAGUE*

Fred R. McCrumb, Jr.

Definition. Plague is an acute or chronic disease of wild and commensal rodents transmissible among these lower animal hosts and to man through the bite of infected ectoparasites. The infection in man is acute and frequently fulminant and usually is characterized by abrupt onset of high fever, lymphadenopathy near the site of exposure, bacteremia, and prostration. Secondary or embolic pneumonia may result in direct respiratory spread of the disease from man to man. Thus two clinical types of human infection are recognized: *bubonic plague,* characterized by either regional lymphadenopathy or bacteremia wherein organisms invade the blood by way of the lymphatics and produce overwhelming sepsis, and *primary plague pneumonia.*

Etiology. *Yersinia pestis* (formerly *Pasteurella pestis*) is a nonmotile, aerobic gram-negative bacillus that grows readily but slowly on artificial media. Small, convex dewdrop colonies become grayish and present a surface appearance like that of beaten copper after 48 hours' incubation at 37° C on blood agar. Virulent organisms are sticky because of the presence of a protein capsule. In liquid media, a surface pellicle and stalactites are characteristic. *Y. pestis* is highly virulent for a variety of laboratory animals. The microorganisms may be seen on microscopy of suitably stained node impressions, peritoneal exudate, and peripheral blood of these hosts as coccoid or large ovoid "safety-pin" bacilli. This bipolar staining is best demonstrated with Giemsa or Wayson's stain, and may be conspicuous in lymph node aspirates and sputum of infected human beings. The organism is destroyed quickly by sunlight and common chemical disinfectants and is noninfectious after 15 minutes at 55° C. *Y. pestis* may survive for several weeks in dry flea feces and human sputum, and may be kept viable and virulent in the frozen state for months. Although streptomycin-resistant mutants have been encountered in experimental plague infections, all naturally occurring human strains of *Y. pestis* studied to date are inhibited in vitro by low concentrations of streptomycin, chloramphenicol, and the tetracyclines.

Incidence and Prevalence. The first adequate description of widespread disease deals with an outbreak of plague in the Egyptian port of Pelusium in 542 A.D. During the next 50 years, plague spread widely into Asia and Europe and it has been estimated that 100 million people perished at that time. Plague assumed catastrophic proportions again during the fourteenth century when it appeared not only in Europe and the Middle East but also in China and India. Pneumonic plague was prominent in this pandemic, which, for unclear reasons, became known as the "Black Death." In Europe alone, 25 million, or one fourth of the population, succumbed. The spread of plague resulted in the establishment of numerous widely distributed permanent natural foci among wild rodent populations.

During recent years, human plague has occurred in Vietnam, Burma, Indonesia, India, Iran, the Malagasy Republic, Central and South Africa, the United States, and several countries of South America. There has been a continuing decline in the incidence of human plague, however, and, in many instances, this decrease in incidence is unquestionably spontaneous. Certain endemic areas are characterized by a constant low human case rate resulting from sporadic infections that occur as a result of man's accidental contact with wild rodent foci. In the United States between 1908 and 1974, some 145 human plague infections associated with wild rodents were distributed over 15 western states. Under certain circumstances, however, such as those now prevailing in Vietnam, plague continues to reach epidemic proportions.

Epidemiology. The ecology of plague varies from one region to another, and the extent to which man is affected by enzootic infections is determined in part by the proximity of human and rodent habitations and the bionomics of rodent ectoparasites. Although ticks and lice are capable of transmitting *Y. pestis* to susceptible animals, practically speaking, the important vectors are fleas. Occasionally man contracts plague by handling the carcass of an infected animal. Epidemics of plague usually arise from infected commensal rats such as *Rattus rattus* and *Rattus norvegicus,* the causative organism being transmitted to man by *Xenopsylla cheopis,* the common rat flea. There is general agreement that natural foci of plague infection among so-called wild rodents (mice, field rats, gerbils, ground squirrels) account for the persistence of this disease in endemic areas. In some instances, man's intrusions into natural foci may result in outbreaks of human plague, and there is ample evidence of an interchange of fleas between commensal and wild rodent species. Flea-borne plague in man is usually of the bubonic variety, and as such does not represent a serious risk to other human beings. By contrast, plague pneumonia secondary to bacteremia may initiate a series of direct transmissions to susceptible contacts in whom the disease is manifest by a fulminant primary pneumonia. Primary pneumonic plague may spread among a susceptible human population with alarming rapidity.

Age and sex distribution of plague is dependent upon the nature of rodent foci and the habits of the human population at risk. Thus domestic rat plague will be distributed evenly among both sexes of all ages when the home is infested with rat fleas. When field rodents constitute the source of infection, the disease will occur predominantly among field workers.

Pathology. Evidence of infection is usually not present at the portal of entry into the skin, although a small pustule is observed in a few patients with bubonic plague. Similarly, lymphatics leading to regional nodes are grossly normal. The primary bubo is usually enlarged, exquisitely tender, and surrounded by a broad zone of subcutaneous edema. There is an intense hemorrhagic inflammatory reaction with infiltration of polynuclear cells. As the inflammation progresses, necrosis and suppuration of the bubo occur. There is a characteristic gelatinous edema of contiguous connective tissue along with dilatation of small blood vessels. Occasionally, infection of the oropharyngeal mucous membrane will lead to tonsillar or mediastinal reaction of the type seen in lymph nodes. Pathologic changes noted in other organ systems can be ascribed to small blood vessel disease, as evidenced by hemorrhages in serous membranes and gastrointestinal mucosa. In addition, degenerative

*The assistance of Colonel Dan C. Cavanaugh, MSC, in the revision of this chapter is gratefully acknowledged.

changes of renal tubular epithelium and parenchymal cells of the liver are frequent. There may be slight enlargement of the liver and spleen. Vascular congestion of the meninges is accompanied by cerebral edema.

Secondary or embolic plague pneumonia is characterized by perivascular foci of inflammatory cells and colonies of *Y. pestis.* As the disease progresses, distinction from primary plague infection of the lung is less obvious, and both may show gradation from lobular pneumonia to lobar consolidation. It is not unusual for several lobes to become involved within a period of 24 to 48 hours. In all instances, reaction in the lung is intense, there being cellular infiltration, gross hemorrhage, and copious exudation of watery sputum. There is overwhelming growth of plague bacilli in the lung that can be readily demonstrated in impression smears of cut lung surface. Bronchial lymph nodes are usually enlarged and hyperemic.

Pathogenesis. After the ingestion of plague bacilli, the proximal digestive tract of the flea becomes obstructed as organisms multiply in the proventriculus. Refeeding results in regurgitation of the freshly ingested human blood as well as *Y. pestis* into the feeding site. Organisms are then carried to regional lymph nodes, where a local inflammatory reaction leads to the formation of a bubo. In most instances, bacteremia occurs early in the disease and may assume enormous proportions in fulminant infections. Plague pneumonia is associated with the production of infectious droplets and respiratory spread of *Y. pestis.* Epidemiologic studies suggest that intimate contact is a prerequisite to successful respiratory transmission of this organism, and the nature of the primary lung lesion favors spread by particles of small size.

Although much has been said about intoxication in human plague infection, evidence of specific toxin activity in human beings is wanting. Extraction of virulent and attenuated strains of *Y. pestis* has revealed the presence of a water-soluble toxic substance that is highly lethal for Swiss mice. Although this material is antigenic in laboratory animals and antibodies may be demonstrated in the sera of patients recovered from plague, its role in the pathogenesis of plague has not been established. However, a classic gram-negative endotoxin has been identified in the plague bacillus, and Shwartzman-like reactions have been described in severe cases.

Clinical Manifestations. Most plague infections make their appearance abruptly with high fever, tachycardia, malaise, and aching of the extremities and back. Temperature usually rises to 39.5 to 40° C within a few hours of onset, and the patient has the general appearance of profound illness, with flushed face and anxious expression. As the disease progresses, delirium may become a prominent feature of the clinical syndrome, and anxiety gives way to depression.

Bubonic Plague. The incubation period in bubonic plague varies from one to six days in most instances and progresses to fulminant bacteremia, death ensuing within three to five days of the onset of symptoms. The case fatality in untreated bubonic plague is variously estimated at 60 to 90 per cent. Regional lymphadenopathy or buboes of flea-borne plague are found in the groin in more than 50 per cent of patients with this form of the disease. Femoral and inguinal buboes are followed in frequency by axillary and cervical node involvement. The site of infection is influenced by the nature of exposure to vectors, there being a high frequency of lower extremity exposure among working adults and axillary and cervical buboes among children exposed as they sleep in a flea-infested dwelling. The involved node may not be greatly enlarged but is invariably painful and exquisitely tender. Within a few hours, there is periadenitis with edema of surrounding tissue. Buboes may involute slowly or suppurate with discharge of necrotic material in patients who survive the acute phase of infection. When bacteremia progresses relentlessly, the clinical picture is one of overwhelming sepsis, and death is associated with peripheral vascular collapse.

Plague Pneumonia. Plague pneumonia acquired as a result of respiratory spread of *Y. pestis* is even more fulminant, untreated patients rarely surviving for more than three days. The disease is characterized by an explosive onset of high fever, tachycardia, tachypnea, and restlessness. Flushing of the skin, conjunctival suffusion, and anxious expression are common. Headache and myalgia may be severe, but are inconstant. During the early phase of illness, the paucity of signs is disproportionate to the obvious severity of the infection. Cough may be absent until six or more hours have passed. Subjective symptoms referable to the chest may be absent, or the patient may complain of pleural pain or dull substernal oppression. Physical signs of pneumonitis may be lacking at this time; however, as the disease progresses, rales, suppressed breathing, and impaired percussion appear. Signs of consolidation are not encountered frequently until after therapy has been instituted. The general clinical state rapidly deteriorates, and patients with this disease are gravely ill after 10 to 15 hours of fever. The patient may find it difficult to produce more than small amounts of sputum in the early hours of illness; however, blood-tinged sputum usually appears within the first 12 hours. Bloody, frothy, liquid sputum typical of plague pneumonia is produced in large quantities late in the disease at a time when the prognosis is uniformly poor.

Laboratory Findings. Peripheral blood leukocytosis with total counts of 12,000 to 15,000 and neutrophilia usually occur in both types of human plague. There is elevation of the erythrocyte sedimentation rate, but other hematologic abnormalities have not been observed. Proteinuria and mild hematuria may accompany the acute febrile phase of plague.

Diagnosis. The clinical diagnosis of plague is confirmed by conventional bacteriologic techniques and inoculation of susceptible laboratory animals. *Y. pestis* may be isolated in pure culture after 48 to 96 hours from bubo aspirates, blood, and sputum, using blood agar and infusion broth. Inoculation of these materials into mice or guinea pigs produces bacteremia and death of the animal in two to five days. A smear of heart's blood of these animals will reveal numerous bipolar staining rods.

In all instances, however, a tentative diagnosis of plague must be made on clinical and epidemiologic grounds, there being dire consequences of a missed diagnosis, especially of plague pneumonia. Careful examination of stained smears of bubo aspirates or sputum will usually reveal the presence of small gram-negative bacilli, and proper isolation precautions and specific therapy must be based on the judgment of this examination. Stained smears from organs of cadavers in cases of sudden death in plague endemic areas should be examined with great diligence to avoid catastrophic spread of this disease.

Patients recovering from plague develop specific antibodies that may be demonstrated in convalescent-phase serum by bacterial agglutination, agglutination of erythrocytes sensitized with capsular antigen, complement-fixation, and mouse protection tests. Antibodies make their appearance early in the second week of disease and continue to rise up to the fourth or fifth week. In all cases, serodiagnosis is retrospective but of value in establishing the presence of infection with *Y. pestis* as well as the immune status of a vaccinated population.

Plague infections in man must be differentiated from tularemia, lymphogranuloma venereum, and other causes of localized lymphadenopathy. The disease is frequently confused with malaria, influenza, enteric fevers, and various causes of acute pneumonia, among them Klebsiella, staphylococcal, tularemic, and viral infections of the lung. In the absence of buboes or pneumonia, bacteremia caused by a variety of gram-negative organisms may resemble acute septicemic plague.

Treatment. *Y. pestis* is readily inhibited in vitro by relatively small concentrations of streptomycin, chloramphenicol, and the tetracyclines. The disease responds readily when antimicrobial therapy is started during the early phase of illness, but it rapidly becomes refractory to specific treatment as it progresses. In view of the ease and uniform success of early therapy, delay in diagnosis and administration of chemotherapy is a grave error in clinical judgment. Pneumonic plague is uniformly fatal, and becomes difficult to treat after the twelfth to fifteenth hour of fever. Bubonic plague is generally less severe, but may progress to death with equal swiftness.

Early studies with sulfonamides revealed that mortality from bubonic plague could be reduced to 5 to 20 per cent by the administration of sulfadiazine or sulfamerazine at the rate of 12 grams daily for four to seven days. These drugs were found to be ineffective in plague pneumonia.

Streptomycin or the broad-spectrum antimicrobials represent the therapy of choice in all plague infections. Streptomycin should be administered parenterally at the rate of 4 grams daily for two days followed by 8 to 10 grams given over a period of five additional days. Chloramphenicol should be administered at the rate of 6 to 8 grams daily for the first 48 hours followed by 3 grams (50 to 75 mg per kilogram) daily for a total dosage of 20 to 25 grams. Chloramphenicol should be given intravenously and orally during the first 48 hours of therapy if the latter route of administration is feasible. Tetracyclines should be administered in a similar manner, large doses (4 to 6 grams daily) being given during the first 48 hours of therapy. Intravenous therapy during the first 24 hours is mandatory in severely ill patients but should be supplemented by oral administration of the drug if this is tolerated by the patient.

When specific therapy is not instituted within the first 15 hours of overt illness in plague pneumonia, antimicrobial therapy usually will not favorably alter the outcome of the disease.

Supportive care includes the use of intravenous fluid therapy, pressor drugs to support failing peripheral circulation, and oxygen therapy when respiratory function has been compromised by widespread pneumonitis. Tracheostomy frequently results in improved pulmonary function and facilitates care of patients severely ill with primary respiratory disease.

Prevention. Prevention of plague is best accomplished by control programs to reduce rodent infections in endemic foci. Improvement in living standards is usually associated with spontaneous disappearance of this disease or at least its confinement to natural foci. However, there are many areas where such an evolution is not likely to occur and natural foci will probably always exist. Under such circumstances, three general approaches to plague control are available. In practice, rodent control has proved to be the least effective method in most endemic regions, primarily because human living standards cannot be sufficiently improved. Rodenticides in common use include sodium fluoroacetate (1080), arsenic trioxide, red squill, alpha-naphthylthiourea (ANTU), and anticoagulants such as warfarin. In economically underdeveloped areas, vector control with insecticides is probably the most effective single control method. The residual effect of 10 per cent DDT dust or 5 per cent spray dispersed around rat habitations and human dwellings is sufficient to reduce sharply the flea populations and thus eliminate large numbers of vectors. However, resistance to DDT has been observed in the most important vector, *X. cheopis,* and local vectors should be tested for susceptibility to various insecticides. In practice, the application of insecticides should always precede any employment of rodenticides. Finally, although millions of human beings have been inoculated with living, attenuated or formalin-killed plague vaccines, the protective effect of these immunoprophylactics has not been assessed adequately. However, there is evidence to support the concept that the production of specific antibodies in man is associated with a significant degree of resistance to plague infection. Protection of human populations against plague is best assured in endemic areas when all available control measures are employed.

Baltazard, M.: Déclin et destin d'une maladie infectieuse: La peste. Bull. W.H.O., 23:247, 1960.

Burkle, F. M.: Plague as seen in South Vietnamese children. Clin. Pediatr., 12:291, 1973.

Butler, T.: A clinical study of bubonic plague. Am. J. Med., 53:268, 1972.

Cavanaugh, D. C., and Steele, J. H.: Trends in research in plague immunization. J. Infect. Dis., 129:S1, 1974 (Supplement, May).

McCrumb, F. R., Jr., Mercier, S., Robic, J., Bouillat, M., Smadel, J. E., Woodward, T. E., and Goodner, K.: Chloramphenicol and Terramycin in the treatment of pneumonic plague. Am. J. Med., 15:284, 1953.

Meyer, K. F.: Effectiveness of live or killed plague vaccines in man. Bull. W.H.O., 42:653, 1970.

Poland, J. D.: *In* Hoeprich, P. D. (ed.): Infectious Diseases. New York, Harper & Row, 1972, p. 1141.

Pollitzer, R.: Plague. W.H.O. Monograph 22, Geneva, 1954.

W.H.O. Expert Committee on Plague. W.H.O. Tech. Rep. Ser. No. 447, 1970.

218. TULAREMIA

Theodore E. Woodward

Definition. Most cases of tularemia are characterized by the formation of a focal ulcer at the site of entry of the causative bacillus, enlargement of regional lymph nodes, and a constitutional reaction of fever, prostration, myalgia, and headache. There may be pneumonia, which is occasionally accompanied by pleurisy or a typhoid-like illness.

Franciscella tularensis, the microbial agent, is

transmitted to humans by insect vectors such as ticks or deer flies, by the handling or ingestion of infected animal tissues, or by inhalation of infected aerosols. The clinical diagnosis is confirmed by demonstration of bacteremia, by isolation of the bacillus from the sputum, tissue exudates, or gastric washings, and by demonstration of serum agglutinins in early convalescence.

Historical Features. The knowledge of the ecology and clinical features of tularemia has been developed in the United States through the pioneering work of Francis and other Public Health Service investigators. McCoy described the disease in 1911 while studying a plaguelike illness in ground squirrels in Tulare County, California. The first clinical description and bacteriologic proof of illness is attributed to Wherry and Lamb in 1914. In a series of studies conducted in Utah and elsewhere, Francis (1928) incriminated rabbits as important animal hosts and established the transmissibility of disease by deer flies.

Etiology, Specific Laboratory Diagnosis, and Epidemiology. Tularemia is of considerable interest because the causative microorganism is a member of the important gram-negative group characterized by intracellular parasitism about which basic information on immunity mechanisms is incomplete. The bacillus is pleomorphic and nonmotile, and propagates best on such artificial media as blood-glucose-cysteine agar or after inoculation of animals with suspensions of infected tissues.

Culture. During the early stages of illness, *F. tularensis* is isolated readily by direct culture in appropriate media or by the subcutaneous or intraperitoneal inoculation of exudate into mice or guinea pigs. Positive cultures are obtained from the local ulcer or regional lymph nodes during the first several weeks in patients with ulceroglandulary type of illness. Regardless of the clinical type of tularemia, viable organisms may be isolated from nasopharyngeal or gastric washings during the active systemic phases of illness. Pleural fluid and bronchial secretions are suitable for cultural purposes. Bacteremia may be demonstrated in all forms, although isolation from the blood by culture on an artificial medium is difficult because of the paucity of organisms present. Organisms have been isolated from cerebrospinal fluid or bone marrow, although such cultural procedures are rarely indicated. Under ideal conditions, if suitable media are inoculated with appropriate material, the organism may be identified within two to four days. Impression smears of splenic tissues often reveal the characteristic coccal or bacillary forms intracellularly after preparation with Giemsa or Wayson's plague stain.

Serologic Diagnosis. The conventional serum agglutination reaction is a very useful diagnostic test, because specific agglutinins appear within eight to ten days from the onset of illness. Maximal titers are reached in about four weeks. Demonstration of a rise in titer through examination of serial specimens is confirmatory evidence of infection, although single titers of 1:160 or more are usually significant. Sera from patients with brucellosis or tularemia may show cross-agglutination, although the titer is usually higher with the homologous antigen.

Cutaneous Test. Foshay described a diagnostic skin test that consists of the intradermal inoculation of a purified antigen consisting of a killed suspension of *F. tularensis.* The reaction is of the delayed tuberculin type, becoming positive in 48 hours. The test is highly specific and becomes positive during the first week of tularemia either prior to or coincident with the development of agglutinins. The test remains positive for years.

Epidemiology. Tularemia has been detected in many countries of the Northern Hemisphere, including Japan, Central Europe, Asiatic and European Russia, and Scandinavia. *F. tularensis* has been found in practically all animal species. In much of North America cottontail rabbits are the most important animal host and were formerly a very common source of the ulceroglandular and typhoidal forms of tularemia. Restricted sale of wild rabbits in metropolitan areas resulted in a sharp decline of the disease.

The clinical infection develops after puncture wounds by bony spicules of infected rabbits or by the ingestion of improperly cooked food. Foxes, squirrels, rats, mice—indeed, all rodents—have been incriminated as sources of infection. Streams are contaminated for variable periods by infected animal carcasses (or by other less well understood routes), so that drinking the water or handling aquatic mammals such as muskrats may be hazardous.

Many cases have their origin from infected arthropods such as ticks, deer flies, or mosquitoes. In North America the ticks *Dermacentor andersoni, Dermacentor variabilis,* and the Lone Star tick are important reservoirs and vectors. Infected female ticks transmit *F. tularensis* transovarially. A primary ulcer often forms at the site of tick attachment.

Tularemia occurs in all seasons: among hunters and trappers in the fall and winter, and during the spring and summer when ticks and deer flies are active. All ages and both sexes are susceptible. Since 1967, fewer than 200 cases have been reported annually in the United States. During a four-week period in the spring of 1968, 47 patients acquired the disease in Vermont after the handling of muskrats.

Mechanism of Infection and Pathology. The disease may present in a variety of forms with two major subdivisions, depending on whether or not the initial site of entry can be visualized. In all forms there is lymph node involvement. In most instances there is a primary ulcer, variable in size, which may be located on the skin (ulceroglandular), in the eye (oculoglandular), or in the nasopharynx with necrotizing lesions. Sometimes the cutaneous lesion may be insignificant, so that the picture is that of "glandular tularemia" without an overt primary lesion. The entry also may be through the intestinal tract (enteric or typhoidal) or via the lungs (pulmonary).

After infection, *F. tularensis* reaches the blood via the lymphatics and nodes; the microbe, although phagocytized, resides intracellularly without loss of viability. Granulomatous lesions develop within the reticuloendothelial system, particularly in lymph nodes, liver, and spleen. These lesions, usually hyperplastic, bear some resemblance to tuberculosis and may caseate or form small local abscesses. The macrophage is the predominant cell type that surrounds an area of caseous necrosis. Langhans' cells are observed occasionally, and the larger lesions are liable to central abscess formation.

Bronchopneumonia is a common development in tularemia, occurring in approximately 30 per cent of patients who acquire the disease, regardless of the type of infection. Histologically, the early lesion is edematous, and consists of fibrin and leukocytes associated with necrosis of alveolar walls. In non-necrotic areas the exudate consists of the large mononuclear type. The gross lesions resemble the bronchopneumonia of tuberculosis, although histologically there is less epithelioid cell transformation. Tubercle-like nodules are more common in lymph nodes than in the lungs. Mediastinal nodes are involved frequently.

Clinical Manifestations. The incubation period of tularemia ranges from two to ten days. Headache, fever, and toxic signs characterize all forms of the illness and are in no way dissimilar to those in other infectious illnesses. The pertinent historic and epidemiologic features are often helpful clues, and in approximately three fourths of all patients there is a primary lesion associated with adenopathy.

Ulceroglandular Tularemia. The initial lesion begins as a reddish papule, which is often undermined and more extensive than the small area of superficial induration indicates. Neighboring and draining lymph nodes are enlarged, tender, and discrete. Fluctuation of these nodes occurs later in the illness, after two or more weeks, when other acute signs may have partially abated. Such diseased nodes may subsequently require incision and drainage. The lymph nodes during the early stages are laden with *F. tularensis* and, if incised, may provoke bacteremia and toxemia. Fluctuant buboes four or more weeks old are usually sterile. Generalized lymphadenopathy occurs. Systemic signs of toxemia may be severe in ulceroglandular tularemia, although most cases are mild or moderate in severity. Pneumonia of all gradations may accompany this type of infection.

Occasionally, tularemia referred to as the glandular type may occur as generalized adenopathy and toxemia but without cutaneous lesions.

Enteric Form of Tularemia (Typhoidal or Cryptogenic). After ingestion of infected animal tissues or water, ulcerative lesions of the buccal mucosa, pharynx, and intestine, and subsequent involvement of cervical, pharyngeal, and mesenteric lymph nodes may occur. The course of illness may be fulminant and fatal unless the disease is recognized and treated properly. Certain of these patients manifest illness that is similar to various forms of gastroenteritis and typhoid fever. These patients may be severely ill with sustained high fever, profound toxicity, stupor, and delirium or coma. This typhoidal systemic reaction may typify any of the clinical varieties of tularemia regardless of the presence of a cutaneous lesion. The term "cryptogenic" has often been used to connote the absence of an obvious portal of entry.

Pulmonary Tularemia. Lung involvement occurs in all forms of tularemia, subsequent to the bacteremia. Available evidence suggests that primary tularemic pneumonia is an entity, particularly in those persons such as laboratory workers who are exposed to infected aerosols. The incubation period varies from two to five days, depending upon the number of viable bacteria inhaled. In addition to headache, fever, malaise, and prostration, there is a nonproductive harassing cough and a sensation of substernal discomfort. Later the sputum may be mucoid or bloody and, in severely ill patients, pleural pain, dyspnea, tachycardia, and cyanosis occur.

In spite of extensive pulmonary involvement, there may be a paucity of physical signs. The early roentgenographic signs, seldom evident before the second to the fourth day of fever, consist of small irregular oval lesions with hilar adenopathy. Later in the illness, the infiltrate may be annular. True abscess formation is rare, although during resolution and convalescence, which in untreated patients or in those treated late may be prolonged, shadows suggesting abscess formation may be noted. Pleuritis with effusion is not uncommon.

Oculoglandular Tularemia. After ocular contamination there may be pain, photophobia, intense congestion, itching, lacrimation, chemosis, and a mucopurulent discharge. Small yellowish granulomatous lesions may appear on the palpebral conjunctivae or cornea and may eventually ulcerate. The preauricular and other regional lymph nodes may enlarge and ultimately suppurate. In untreated patients, serious ocular complications, including corneal perforation or optic atrophy, may ensue.

Other General Manifestations. Initially, in severely ill patients, there is a rigor followed by pyrexia that persists for a month or more. The fever may be continuously high or remittent, and defervescence is usually gradual. Hepatomegaly and splenomegaly with tenderness over the respective organs are relatively common. Toxic signs in all cases include fever, headache, myalgia, and nausea. Rashes are very uncommon; when present, they consist of localized papular lesions along the peripheral lymphatics or maculopapular body eruptions. In untreated patients or in those first given antimicrobial therapy late in the course of illness, convalescence may be prolonged with sporadic episodes of fever, weakness, muscular pains, and chronic respiratory signs.

Nonspecific Laboratory Findings. The erythrocyte sedimentation rate and C-reactive protein are elevated during the active stages. In contrast, the total blood leukocyte count is usually normal or low. Occasionally there may be moderate leukocytosis. Mild albuminuria may occur at the height of illness.

Differential Diagnosis. Ulceroglandular tularemia is recognized readily in endemic areas. Punctate lesions with surrounding erythema at the site of prior arthropod attachment suggest *Rocky Mountain spotted fever,* particularly when associated with fever, headache, and toxic signs. The absence of a rash would favor tularemia, because patients with rickettsial disease develop a characteristic exanthem. *Meningococcemia* is recognized by its fulminant character, the typical exanthem, leukocytosis, and the bacteriologic findings. Fever, toxic signs, pharyngitis, adenitis, hepatomegaly, and splenomegaly are common to tularemia and *infectious mononucleosis.* The hematologic and serologic findings are usually distinctive. *Cat scratch disease* is characterized by peripheral ulceration and regional adenopathy; a history of contact with cats, the cutaneous reaction to specific antigens, and the absence of agglutinins for *F. tularensis* are distinguishing features. *Ecthyma* and *furunculi* are similar in some respects to this form of tularemia, although lymphadenitis and systemic signs are less likely to develop.

The lesions of *sporotrichosis* are multiple, occur along the course of lymphatics, attach themselves firmly to the skin, and are freely movable.

Certain forms of tularemia may present with clinical features similar to those of psittacosis, Q fever, and mycoplasmal pneumonia. Broad-spectrum antimicrobial drugs are effective in each of these conditions. Appropriate serologic tests or viral isolation may be required to define the precise cause. Influenza with associated pneumonia is similar but does not respond to specific drugs, and its clinical course is short. Fungal diseases, such as *histoplasmosis* and *coccidioidomycosis,* may be acute and may simulate pulmonary tularemia. Consideration of the history, the epidemiologic data, and the cutaneous manifestations, as well as the bacteriologic and serologic findings, usually will permit proper identification.

The presence of unexplained pleural effusion, similar to tuberculous fibrinous pleurisy, requires differentiation. The results of cultural and serologic tests will aid in differentiation.

Complications. Pericarditis and meningitis are distinctive but unusual complications of tularemia. Pericardial involvement may develop by direct extension from the pulmonary lesions or lymph nodes, and is characterized by a fibrinous or fibrocaseous exudate. In untreated patients constrictive pericarditis may ensue. Tularemic meningitis is characterized by a lymphocytic pleocytosis in the cerebrospinal fluid, and was usually fatal prior to the availability of specific antimicrobial drugs. Rare instances of tularemic peritonitis, perisplenitis, osteomyelitis, and endocarditis have been reported.

Treatment. *Specific Therapy.* Tularemia is very amenable to treatment with antimicrobial drugs. Streptomycin is preferable, but the broad-spectrum antimicrobials are equally beneficial in ameliorating the active manifestations. They are less effective, however, in eradicating the organism, primarily because of their bacteriostatic mode of action. With the latter drugs, relapses are liable to occur if treatment is initiated within the first week of illness.

STREPTOMYCIN. Streptomycin, when given in doses of 1.0 gram daily to adults for about one week, results in prompt recovery. Most patients are improved within 24 hours, and are afebrile within 48 hours. Relapses are uncommon with streptomycin except when insufficient drug is given during the very early stages of illness. Strains resistant to streptomycin do appear, a fact which is of no clinical significance when infection is acquired naturally.

TETRACYCLINE AND CHLORAMPHENICOL TREATMENT. Broad-spectrum antimicrobials are very effective in rendering the patient afebrile and free from toxicity within 48 to 72 hours. Relapses are uncommon when therapy is initiated 10 to 12 days after the onset of illness, but are frequent if it is given during the first week. *F. tularensis* does not develop resistance to chloramphenicol or tetracycline; hence, retreatment leads to prompt response.

The following dosage schedule is considered optimal: for tetracycline, an initial oral dose of 25 mg per kilogram of body weight; and for chloramphenicol, 50 mg per kilogram of body weight. Subsequent daily doses are calculated on the same basis as the initial loading dose, dividing the requirement equally and giving it at six- to eight-hour intervals. Antimicrobial therapy is continued until the patient is improved and has been afebrile for about five to seven days.

No supplementary chemotherapy is necessary with any of the aforementioned regimens. Tetracycline is preferred solely because reactions to it are potentially less serious.

General Management. An adequate diet with appropriate protein intake is advisable. Oxygen treatment is indicated for all severely ill patients with pneumonia whether or not cyanosis is present. Other supportive measures useful for treating patients with pneumonia, such as frequent turning and the performing of a tracheostomy to provide a proper airway, are indicated. Thoracentesis for removal of fluid will allay respiratory embarrassment. The presence of any superimposed infection is detected by appropriate examination of the sputum, blood, or tissues.

The local ulcer requires no special measures. During the early several weeks of illness, lymph nodes should not be manipulated unduly or incised. Later, fluctuant buboes, which are usually sterile, may require incision and drainage. Recovery ensues rapidly.

Prognosis and Postinfection Immunity. In untreated patients, the case fatality rate in ulceroglandular tularemia was formerly approximately 5 per cent. However, of those patients with typhoidal tularemia or with pulmonary manifestations, about 30 per cent succumbed. With the advent of streptomycin and later the broad-spectrum antimicrobials, death from tularemia has been virtually eliminated and the morbidity shortened drastically to several days after institution of treatment, even among severely ill patients.

Second attacks of tularemia with systemic complications are uncommon, because recovery from the initial episode usually confers immunity. However, it is not unusual for patients to develop primary lesions when reinfected long after the initial systemic infection. Viable *F. tularensis* may be isolated from such recurrent primary ulcers, which resemble a Koch reaction. Under these conditions, systemic manifestations are unusual.

Under test conditions in volunteers, when streptomycin is given soon after intradermal infection (before the onset of clinical illness), an attack may be aborted fully. Immunity does not develop, agglutinins fail to appear, and such subjects are prone to further infection. This phenomenon is of little practical significance, as patients are usually encountered after a week or more of active clinical illness. Partial to complete resistance to infection follows such antigenic stimulation.

Control Measures. *General.* In infected areas those measures designed to repel ticks, mosquitoes, or deer flies should be employed. Gloves should be used for handling all potentially infected animals, particularly rabbits, and animals to be consumed should be cooked thoroughly. Laboratory workers exposed to infected aerosols should exercise care by wearing suitable masks and utilizing other protective devices.

Vaccination. The available killed vaccines afford only partial protection to man against tularemia. Viable attenuated preparations have been used with considerable success in the Soviet Union. The vaccine is administered intradermally and provokes a reaction similar in severity to that which follows smallpox immunization. Significant protection has been demonstrated in volunteers in the United States vaccinated with a similar viable product and who subsequently were exposed to virulent strains of *F. tularensis* by the respiratory or cutaneous routes. In those subjects who have developed clinical illness after immunization, the disease has been mild.

Foshay, L.: Tularemia. Ann. Rev. Microbiol., 4:313, 1950.
McCrumb, F. R.: Aerosol infection of man with *Pasteurella tularensis.* Bact. Rev., 25:262, 1961.
Meyer, K. F.: Pasteurella and franciscella. *In* Dubos, R., and Hirsch, J. G. (eds.): Bacterial and Mycotic Infections of Man. 4th ed. Philadelphia, J. B. Lippincott Company, 1965, Chap. 27, p. 659.
Young, L. S.: Tularemia epidemic, Vermont, 1968. Forty-seven cases linked to contact with muskrats. N. Engl. J. Med., 280:1253, 1969.

DISEASES CAUSED BY MALLEOMYCES

Leighton E. Cluff

219. GLANDERS (Farcy)

Definition. Glanders, or farcy, is an infectious disease of horses, mules, and donkeys caused by *Malleomyces* *mallei.* The infection is occasionally transmitted to man, and is characterized by an acute fulminant febrile illness or a chronic indolent disease with abscesses of the respiratory tract or skin. Farcy refers to the nodular abscesses observed in skin, lymphatics, and subcutaneous tissues.

Etiology. Glanders was described by Aristotle about 330 B.C., and the occurrence of the disease in horses was observed by Apeyrtos about 375 A.D. Royer's (1837) monograph on glanders in man remains the classic description of the disease. The microorganism responsible for glanders was isolated in 1882. It is a gram-negative bacillus culturable aerobically on ordinary nutrient media. It is variously called *Malleomyces mallei, Bacillus mallei,* or *Pfeiferella mallei. M. mallei* is nonmotile. It elaborates a specific antigen (mallein) upon lysis that is used as a skin test material for diagnostic purposes. The bacillus is antigenically separable from *M. pseudomallei,* which causes melioidosis. When grown on potato slices or potato infusion agar, *M. mallei* produces a brown pigment resembling that of *Pseudomonas aeruginosa.* The bacillus produces fatal infection experimentally in guinea pigs and hamsters but will not cause disease in rats, cattle, hogs, or fowl.

Incidence and Prevalence. Glanders has probably never been a common disease in man. It occurs almost exclusively in persons handling horses, and therefore is an occupational disease. It has been reported from all parts of the world. It has been eradicated in the United States and the United Kingdom, but may still occur in Asia and South America.

Epidemiology. Glanders is a communicable disease among horses, and it may occur sporadically in other animal species in contact with horses. In horses, glanders is manifested by nasal symptoms and abscesses and by cutaneous nodules or abscesses (farcy). Glanders is transmitted to man by direct contact with infected horses, the bacillus preferentially invading areas of abraded or injured skin. Experimental infection can be induced in animals by inhalation of the bacillus, and certain laboratory-acquired infections indicate that infection may develop in man after inhalation of the microorganism. *Unlike melioidosis, glanders can be transmitted from person to person.*

Pathology and Pathogenesis. Characteristically glanders is associated with cellulitis, necrosis, abscess, and thromboses with septic embolization. Healing occurs by fibrosis, and, rarely, by calcification.

Clinical Manifestations. Glanders may occur as a fulminant acute febrile disease, as a chronic indolent and relapsing disease, or as a subclinical occult infection detectable incidentally at postmortem examination or by serologic test. The two principal features of glanders are (1) nasal cellulitis and necrosis-producing septal perforation, palatal and pharyngeal ulceration; or (2) cutaneous cellulitis, vesiculation, and ulceration at the site of inoculation of the bacillus into the skin, followed by lymphangitis with nodular abscesses along the lymphatics and lymphadenopathy (farcy).

Pulmonary involvement is common in glanders, producing pneumonia, abscesses, pleural effusion, and empyema. Occasionally, in chronic indolent glanders, small nodular granulomatous lesions may be found in the lungs. Hilar lymph node enlargement is common in pulmonary glanders.

When glanders becomes disseminated, destructive polyarthritis, subcutaneous and muscular abscesses, osteomyelitis, meningitis, and pustular skin lesions, particularly over the joints and face, are seen. Prostration and stupor may develop, and are followed by death in two to three weeks.

Chronic glanders may be punctuated by recurrent acute relapses with bacteremia, often resulting in a fulminant course and death. Amyloidosis may be a complication of chronic glanders.

Fever and chills, headache, and backache are common in acute glanders. Leukopenia or a normal leukocyte count is the rule, but leukocytosis has been observed.

Diagnosis. There are no pathognomonic clinical featues of glanders. The nodules along lymphatics resemble those seen in sporotrichosis. The respiratory lesions may be difficult to distinguish from other ulcerative infections of the nose and mouth. The cutaneous lesion often resembles streptococcal cellulitis. The multiple abscesses mimic many mycotic and staphylococcal infections and are difficult to distinguish from those of melioidosis. The acute fulminant illness may resemble typhoid fever or disseminated tuberculosis. The diagnosis of glanders can be established by combination of a history of exposure to horses, isolation of M. mallei, serologic tests (agglutination, complement-fixation), and skin test with sterile culture filtrate (mallein). Inoculation of infected material into guinea pigs may facilitate identification of the microorganism.

Treatment. There are reports of successful treatment of glanders with sulfonamides. Tetracycline, chloramphenicol, and streptomycin may be useful, but there is little clinical experience with these drugs in glanders. Because of the serious prognosis and the lack of documented experience with drug therapy, it is advisable to administer daily streptomycin (1.0 gram) in association with a sulfonamide or a tetracycline until all evidences of disease have disappeared. Incision, drainage, and excision of abscesses must be done with caution, for the infection may be disseminated by such manipulation.

Prognosis. Although a few patients have been cured with chemotherapy, the effect of treatment on the mortality rate is not known. *More than 90 per cent of patients with glanders will die from the disease if untreated.* However, the frequency of occurrence of occult or subclinical glanders is not known.

Prevention. Infected horses have been identified by skin tests with mallein and by serologic tests. Destruction of infected animals has eliminated glanders as a public health problem in the United States and most other countries.

Eghbal, M., Rafyi, A., Chamey, H. M., and Farvar, B.: Development of bacterial resistance to sulfonamides during therapy of glanders in man. Presse Méd., 61:1535, 1953.

Howe, C., and Miller, W. R.: Human glanders. Report of six cases. Ann. Intern. Med., 26:115, 1947.

Mendelson, R. W.: Glanders. U.S. Armed Forces Med. J., 1:781, 1950.

220. MELIOIDOSIS

Definition. Melioidosis is a rare disease of man caused by *Malleomyces pseudomallei.* It has been observed most frequently in Malaysia, the People's Republic of China, Burma, India, and other parts of the Far East and Southeast Asia, but has only rarely been observed in North and South America. It is a disease of wild rodents and some domesticated animals, and probably is transmitted to man by contact with diseased animals or animal excreta and possibly by contact with contaminated soil. The disease in man appears in a subclinical (only positive serologic tests), pulmonary, septicemic, or extrapulmonary form. The septicemic and pulmonary disease may be acute and fatal. The pulmonary and extrapulmonary infection with abscesses may be chronic and debilitating.

Etiology. Melioidosis was first identified by Whitmore and Krishnaswami (1912) in Rangoon. The disease was recognized as similar to glanders and attributable to a gram-negative bacillus resembling but differing from *Malleomyces mallei.* The microorganism causing melioidosis has been variously called *Malleomyces pseudomallei, Bacillus whitmori,* and *Pfeiferella whitmori.* It is a motile bacillus that grows aerobically on nutrient agar. Culturally it may resemble Klebsiella and *Pseudomonas aeruginosa. M. pseudomallei* is antigenically distinguishable from *M. mallei.* It produces fatal infection in guinea pigs, rabbits, and other laboratory animals.

Epidemiology. *M. pseudomallei* has been found to cause disease sporadically, endemically, and epidemically among a wide variety of animal species, including rats, rabbits, goats, hogs, dogs, cats, and horses. In addition, the bacillus has been found to be harbored by mosquitoes and fleas. Frequently, the initial manifestations of melioidosis in man are cutaneous abscesses, diarrhea, and pneumonia; therefore it is probable that the disease is transmitted by direct contact with infected animals or by ingestion or inhalation of contaminated material. All these routes of inoculation can produce the disease experimentally in animals. It is unlikely that melioidosis is ever transmitted from man to man. Infection has been observed in narcotic addicts, and in infants, or in patients with diabetes mellitus, renal or liver disease, and pregnancy as predisposing factors.

Clinical Manifestations. Melioidosis may appear acutely or insidiously, and most often follows a fulminant course with septicemia or a chronic indolent course with multiple abscess formation. The incubation period of the disease is not known. The acute illness is often associated with fever, chills, cough, production of bloody and purulent sputum, diarrhea, or abdominal pain. Physical examination may reveal signs of pneumonia, empyema, lung abscess, hepatomegaly, jaundice, and splenomegaly. *A subacute or chronic illness may follow the acute disease or may develop in the absence of an acute illness.* In this situation the patient often has osteomyelitis, suppurating lymphadenopathy, subcutaneous abscesses, psoas abscess, lung abscess, pyelonephritis, or liver or spleen abscess. Bronchocutaneous and other types of fistulas may appear. Patients with this chronic illness may survive for many months, and occasionally may recover.

Diagnosis. Melioidosis may resemble typhoid fever, malaria, mycotic infection, and occasionally acute staphylococcal septicemia or staphylococcal pneumonia. The chronic pulmonary disease most resembles tuberculosis. Melioidosis can be differentiated from these diseases only by bacteriologic identification of the bacillus from blood, sputum, urine, or pus. Hemagglutination and complement fixation tests may be useful when acute and convalescent serologic titers are compared. A single positive test may only indicate previous clinical and subclinical infection.

The leukocyte count of the peripheral blood often is normal in melioidosis, but may rise to levels of 20,000 per cubic millimeter. Urinalysis may show pyuria and hematuria.

Treatment and Prevention. There is no available antigen for active immunization against melioidosis. Prevention of the disease is possible by controlled sanitation and improved standards of living. Patients have been successfully treated with chloramphenicol, sulfonamides, or tetracycline, given over long periods of time. The drug susceptibility of *M. pseudomallei,* however, is variable. In adults, 3 grams of tetracycline a day orally for 90 days, or, alternatively, in septicemia, large doses of chloramphenicol are preferred. Surgical drainage of abscesses is essential for proper management.

Buchman, R. J., Kmiecik, J. E., and LaNove, A. M.: Extrapulmonary melioidosis. Am. J. Surg., 125:324, 1973.

Khaira, B. S., Young, W. B., and Hart, P. DeV.: Melioidosis. Br. Med. J., 1:949, 1959.

Prevatt, A. L., and Hunt, J. S.: Chronic systemic melioidosis. Review of literature. Am. J. Med., 23:810, 1957.

Spotnitz, M., Rudnitsky, A., and Rambaud, J. J.: Melioidosis pneumonitis. J.A.M.A., 202:950, 1967.

221. ANTHRAX

Leighton E. Cluff

Definition. Anthrax is an infectious disease of wild and domesticated animals caused by *Bacillus anthracis.* Occasionally it is transmitted to man. A necrotic ulcer of the skin or mucous membranes is the most common feature of the disease, but hemorrhagic mediastinitis and disseminated infection with hemorrhagic meningitis may also develop. Depending upon the most prominent feature of the disease, anthrax has been variously referred to as *malignant pustule, splenic fever, woolsorters' disease, milzbrand,* and *charbon.*

Etiology. *Bacillus anthracis* was identified in 1849 by Davaine, and was further characterized by Koch in 1877. It is a gram-positive, spore-forming, encapsulated, hemolytic, aerobic microorganism. It resembles *B. subtilis* and *B. cereus* but can be differentiated from these organisms by its virulence for laboratory animals such as the mouse and rabbit, by its lack of hemolytic activity on blood agar, and by lysis of *B. anthracis* with specific bacteriophage. In broth, the bacillus elaborates an antigen that can be used for specific immunization ("protective antigen"). The spores of *B. anthracis* are killed by boiling for ten minutes but survive for long periods of time in soil, in animal carcasses, and after aerosolization.

Epidemiology. Anthrax has occurred sporadically and in epidemics throughout the world. Cattle, sheep, goats, horses, and swine are most commonly found to have anthrax; outbreaks of the disease in these animals rarely occur in the United States. Although the disease has been acquired by butchering, skinning, or dissecting infected carcasses, human infection in the United States is observed almost exclusively in persons handling imported contaminated hides, wool, goat hair, or other animal products. There has been a progressive decrease in anthrax in the United States in the past several years (17 cases from 1956 to 1964). The infection may be transmitted to man by direct contact, inhalation, and ingestion of infected material.

Pathology and Pathogenesis. Anthrax is characterized by edema, hemorrhage, necrosis, and various degrees of inflammation. *B. anthracis* possesses a glutamyl polypeptide capsule that interferes with phagocytosis, and this contributes to its pathogenicity. The gelatinous edema of anthrax infection contains large amounts of bacterial capsular material. The serum of many animals has lytic activity against the bacillus, but this anthracidal substance seems to bear little, if any, relationship to natural resistance. It is probable that *B. anthracis* initiates infection in the skin only through abrasions, cuts, or other types of injury. During the course of lethal anthrax infection in laboratory animals a bacterial toxin is produced that is responsible for death. This lethal toxin can be neutralized by specific antitoxin.

Clinical Manifestations. The skin lesion of anthrax usually begins as a small erythematous papule that becomes vesicular, necrotic, and covered with a dark crust or eschar. Intense nonpitting edema, which may not be erythematous, often surrounds and may extend a considerable distance from the eschar. Characteristically the lesion is pruritic but not very tender or hot. The skin lesion is commonly on exposed areas of hands, arms, neck, or face; and there may be mild regional lymph node enlargement. Lymphangitis is not usually observed. Constitutional symptoms and fever are frequently absent unless the skin disease is severe or the infection becomes disseminated, when high fever, prostration, and death may occur.

Infrequently anthrax may develop without a lesion, possibly after inoculation into the skin, but probably more commonly after inhalation of spores of the bacillus in contaminated air. Characteristically, this form of anthrax is severe and is associated with disseminated infection. *Hemorrhagic mediastinitis,* often without pneumonia, and *hemorrhagic meningitis* may occur. Death is common in this form of anthrax; the illness may begin abruptly, be of short duration, and terminate rapidly. Dyspnea and cyanosis are indicative of respiratory or ventilatory insufficiency. Roentgenographic examination of the chest in inhalation anthrax reveals widening of the mediastinum. Leukocytosis is ordinarily not pronounced. Pleural effusion may complicate pulmonary anthrax. Anthrax in man from ingestion of bacilli is rare.

Diagnosis. Anthrax is most readily diagnosed in persons known to have been exposed to animals or animal products potentially contaminated with *B. anthracis.* Cutaneous anthrax can be differentiated from many other bacterial infections of the skin by the insignificance of regional adenopathy, lymphangitis, and cellulitis in relation to the severity of the eschar and edema. Furthermore, pruritus, lack of tenderness, and intense nonpitting edema are characteristic of anthrax. Small skin lesions, however, may be more difficult to recognize. Pulmonary anthrax can be identified by a history of occupational exposure and acute widening of the mediastinum shown by roentgenographic examination. Anthrax meningitis is confused with subarachnoid hemorrhage or cerebrovascular accident, but is usually associated with prominent signs of infection, and gram-positive bacilli can be seen in the cerebrospinal fluid.

In disseminated anthrax infection, blood cultures are often positive. Occasionally, the bacilli may be identified in the centrifugal sediment of blood treated with 3 per cent acetic acid solution and stained with Wright's stain.

In cutaneous anthrax, the bacilli can usually be cultured from the lesions, or typical encapsulated bacilli will be seen when stained with a polychrome eosin-methylene blue stain (Wright or Giemsa). Their direct cultivation on peptone agar should always be attempted. If the specimen has to be shipped, the specimen should be dried on silk threads or on a sterile glass slide. In view of the occurrence of anthrax-like bacilli on the skin, it is imperative that diagnoses be confirmed by animal inoculations, preferably in guinea pigs or mice or by specific bacteriophage lysis. In pulmonary anthrax, the bacillus has been found microscopically in the sputum and in the pleural exudate.

Prognosis. Cutaneous anthrax is often a self-limited disease, but dissemination of the infection and death may occur in 20 per cent of patients. A fatal outcome in cutaneous anthrax can be averted by appropriate treatment, but treatment of disseminated infection is often unsuccessful in preventing death.

Treatment. *B. anthracis* is susceptible to the action of penicillin and the tetracyclines. Penicillin G should be given in total daily doses of at least 1.2 million units, starting as soon as anthrax is diagnosed or seriously suspected. The effectiveness of the tetracyclines is probably not quite so great as that of penicillin; nevertheless, they are effective in cutaneous anthrax and may be administered in a total daily dose of 2.0 grams. Therapy with penicillin or the tetracyclines should be continued for seven days. It should be emphasized that in patients with disseminated anthrax, the progressive course may be so rapid that antimicrobial drugs may not save the patient's life.

Prevention. Anthrax can be prevented in man by control of infected animals or animal products. Sterilization of wool during manufacture is often impracticable, although this is the means employed to prevent infection from clothing and other products, such as shaving brushes, made of potentially infected materials. Vaccination with "protective antigen" is effective in preventing infection in persons likely to be occupationally exposed.

Brachman, P. S.: Human anthrax in the United States. *In* Hobby, G. L. (ed.): Antimicrobial Agents and Chemotherapy. Baltimore, Williams & Wilkins Company, 1965.

Brachman, P. S., Plotkin, S. A., Bumford, F. H., and Atchison, M. M.: An epidemic of inhalation anthrax. II. Epidemiologic investigation. Am. J. Hyg., 72:6, 1960.

Gold, H.: Anthrax: Report of 117 cases. Arch. Intern. Med., 96:387, 1955.

Hughes, M. H.: Anthrax. Br. Med. J., 1:488, 1973.

Plotkin, S. A., Brachman, P. S., Utell, M., Bumford, F. H., and Atchison, M. M.: Epidemic of inhalation anthrax, first in twentieth century. I. Clinical features. Am. J. Med., 29:992, 1960.

Smith, H., and Keppie, J.: Studies on the chemical basis of pathogenicity of *Bacillus anthracis* using organisms grown in vivo. *In* Howie, J. W., and O'Hea, A. J. (eds.): Mechanisms of Microbial Pathogenicity. London, Cambridge University Press, 1955.

222. LISTERIOSIS

Leighton E. Cluff

Definition. Listeriosis is an infectious disease of animals and man with exceptionally protean manifestations, including meningitis, disseminated granulomas, lymphadenopathy, respiratory symptoms, and ill-defined acute febrile illness. It can produce abortion and fetal or neonatal death. The infection is caused by a gram-positive bacillus called *Listeria monocytogenes* and is worldwide in distribution.

Etiology. Infection of the human being with *Listeria monocytogenes* was identified in 1929 by Nyfeldt. The microorganism was first characterized, however, by

Murray, Webb, and Swann in 1926, during an epizootic among rabbits and guinea pigs. Subsequently the microorganism has been identified as a cause of disease in fox, raccoon, goat, lemming, mouse, rat, hamster, pig, horse, cow, dog, domestic fowl and wild birds, and other animals. *L. monocytogenes* is a gram-positive, nonspore-forming, aerobic or microaerophilic, motile bacillus. It ferments a number of sugars, with formation of acid but no gas. It can be grown on nutrient agar or broth, preferably containing 1 per cent glucose, and produces beta hemolysis on blood agar. *L. monocytogenes* resembles *Erysipelothrix rhuziopathiae* and diphtheroids, but can be differentiated from these bacteria by its motility (best at 20 to 30° C), its specific antigenicity, and its animal pathogenicity. Listeria regularly—and Erysipelothrix occasionally—produces purulent keratoconjunctivitis in rabbits after inoculation into the conjunctival space, whereas diphtheroids do not.

Incidence and Prevalence. Listeriosis in man and animals has been observed throughout the world. It has been recognized more frequently in humans in recent years, but its true incidence is not known. Confusion in bacteriologic differentiation accounts largely for inadequate recognition of listeriosis. In addition, the diverse manifestations of the disease render it difficult to identify clinically.

Epidemiology. Listeriosis may develop after inhalation, ingestion, or direct contact with contaminated food or animal products. The disease is most common in persons living in rural areas. Although infection with Listeria occurs in many domesticated and wild animals, there are only rare instances of epizootics or outbreaks in animals other than man. Transmission of infection from person to person probably occurs under some circumstances, notably in nursery outbreaks. Women can carry Listeria in the vagina, and infection may be transmitted venereally. Whether or not man can be an asymptomatic carrier of Listeria under other conditions is not known.

Pathology and Pathogenesis. Human listeriosis is characterized by disseminated granulomas and focal necrosis or suppuration in involved tissues. Lesions may develop in liver, intestinal tract, gallbladder, skin, mucous membranes of the respiratory tract, lung, heart, spleen, lymph nodes, placenta, and brain. The fetus may be infected transplacentally through the umbilical vein, with production of septicemia. Debilitating diseases such as chronic infection and cancer predispose to the occurrence of listeriosis. Pregnancy may increase susceptibility to infection, but the disease in pregnant women may be less severe than in other persons. Administration of adrenal cortical steroids may also increase susceptibility to listeriosis. Infection also occurs in persons with no underlying disease.

Clinical Manifestations. *Meningitis* is the most commonly recognized form of listeriosis in the United States. It is characterized at onset by symptoms of headache, myalgia, fever, chills, nausea, vomiting, and photophobia, followed by the development of stiff neck, stupor, convulsions, somnolence, and, finally, death. The onset may be abrupt or gradual, and the initial symptoms may be those of gastrointestinal or respiratory illness. Examination reveals manifestations of meningitis or encephalitis in varying degrees of severity. There may be pharyngitis, rhinitis, otitis media, neck rigidity, ocular palsy, and signs of depressed cerebral function. Leukocytosis is common, with granulocytosis and, occasionally, monocytosis, in the early phase of the disease. The cerebrospinal fluid, with decreased sugar, elevated protein, and cell counts of 150 to 3000 per cubic millimeter, is indistinguishable from that in many purulent meningitides. Early, the cells in the fluid may be principally granulocytes, but later there may be a predominance of mononuclear cells.

Febrile pharyngitis with cervical and generalized lymphadenopathy can be caused by Listeria, and may be difficult to differentiate from *infectious mononucleosis.* Patients with this type of illness, however, may have an abrupt onset of fever, chills, headache, myalgia, conjunctivitis, macular rash, and sore throat. Lymph nodes in the neck and elsewhere may enlarge, and there may be hepatosplenomegaly. Blood leukocytes occasionally increase in number with a more or less pronounced monocytosis. The absorbed heterophil serologic test for infectious mononucleosis is negative, Listeria can be isolated from blood and pharynx, and there will be a rising serum agglutinin titer for Listeria.

Lymph node enlargement in the neck and elsewhere without respiratory symptoms may also be attributed to listeriosis. In addition, lymph node enlargement associated only with conjunctivitis may occur. Isolated acute upper respiratory illness may be attributable to listeriosis, although for obvious reasons this diagnosis is seldom established. Chronic urethritis in men has been described, and possibly may be responsible for subclinical or occult infection, demonstrable by culture of the bacillus from bone marrow.

Papular skin lesions associated with disseminated listeriosis have been seen in infants, but adults may acquire primary cutaneous infection after direct contact with infected animal tissues.

Disseminated listeriosis in infants has been reported frequently in Europe, but infrequently in the United States. The disease may arise by transplacental infection of the fetus, causing abortion, fetal death, or serious illness within several days after birth. Outbreaks of infection may develop in newborn nurseries, probably by person-to-person transmission. The disease is characterized by disseminated visceral granulomas and abscesses. When it manifests itself in infants a few weeks old, it often begins as a mild febrile illness with cough, coryza, gastrointestinal symptoms, and pneumonia. Granulomas may be formed on the posterior pharyngeal wall. Granulocytosis and occasionally mononucleosis are present. Pleural and pericardial effusions may develop. Listeriosis has been reported as a common cause of neonatal death and fetal damage in Europe.

Listeriosis in pregnancy may be subclinical or may be associated with an acute febrile illness resembling influenza and occasionally pyelonephritis; it is rarely severe. Its occurrence after the fifth month of pregnancy, however, is likely to affect the fetus seriously. A woman may become a vaginal carrier of Listeria and may possibly infect her infant at birth.

Disseminated listeriosis in adults has an abrupt onset with chill and fever. Meningitis can occur, as well as bacterial endocarditis. Blood cultures are usually positive, and there may be a consumptive coagulopathy. This type of listeriosis is observed most often in patients with carcinoma or debilitating disease, and its development may have been facilitated by adrenal steroid therapy.

Diagnosis. There are no pathognomonic clinical features of human listeriosis. The diagnosis rests on isolation of the microorganism or rising agglutinin titers in the serum. It is likely that the recognition of listeriosis has been difficult because of the failure to differentiate Listeria from diphtheroid bacilli in culture. The isolation of microorganisms resembling diphtheroids from infectious material or blood should alert one to the necessity for further bacteriologic characterization.

Listeriosis may resemble influenza, miliary tuberculosis, typhoid fever, mycotic infections, and several bacterial infections with septicemia. *Infectious mononucleosis* is most often confused with listeriosis in adults, for the two diseases may be clinically alike. However, listeriosis is infrequently associated with monocytosis, does not produce a positive absorbed heterophil serologic test, and in systemic disease the bacillus can be isolated from blood, bone marrow, urine, or upper respiratory tract.

Treatment. *Listeria monocytogenes* is susceptible in vitro to sulfonamides, penicillin, tetracycline, chloramphenicol, erythromycin, novobiocin, and occasionally streptomycin. Penicillin is the drug of choice, but the tetracyclines and erythromycin are also effective. Some have recommended use of the aminoglycosides, but most strains of Listeria are susceptible to less toxic antimicrobial drugs, and these are preferred unless in vitro resistance is demonstrated. Treatment should be continued for a period of several days, depending upon the characteristics of the disease.

Prognosis. Listeria meningitis has a fatality rate of 70 per cent in untreated patients. The fatality rate in treated patients has not been defined, but is considerably lower. The prognosis in adults with pharyngitis and lymph node enlargement is good, whether treated or not, but meningitis may supervene. Recovery from meningitis may leave residual symptoms of central nervous system damage. Infection of the newborn is very serious; the fatality rate and the incidence of congenital defects are high. Untreated, disseminated listeriosis is usually a fatal disease.

Prevention. Listeriosis must be regarded as primarily a contagious disease of animals; prevention of human infection would require elimination of animal reservoirs, but this would not prevent person-to-person transmission. Pasteurization prevents transmission of the disease by contaminated milk. Animal products, including meat, should be declared unfit for consumption if the disease is found in slaughtered animals. Better recognition of the disease should clarify its epidemiology and indirectly facilitate control measures. There are no effective agents for immunization.

Gray, M. L., and Killinger, A. H.: *Listeria monocytogenes* and listeric infections. Bact. Rev., 30:309, 1966.

Hoeprich, P. D.: Infections due to *Listeria monocytogenes*. Medicine, 37:143, 1958.

Lowenstein, M. S., Fox, M. D., and Martin, S. M.: Human listeriosis in the U.S. J. Infect. Dis., 123:328, 1971.

Medoff, G., Kunz, L. J., and Weinberg, A. N.: Listeriosis in humans: An evaluation. J. Infect. Dis., 123:247, 1971.

Moore, R. M., and Zehmer, R. B.: Listeriosis in the U.S., 1971. J. Infect. Dis., 127:610, 1973.

223. ERYSIPELOID OF ROSENBACH

Leighton E. Cluff

Erysipeloid of Rosenbach is a specific infectious disease attributable to *Erysipelothrix rhuziopathia.* It occurs in man after contact with infected animals or animal products, particularly swine, cattle, sheep, fish, birds, dogs, horses, reindeer, rabbits, mink, rats, and mice. The disease in man therefore usually arises in abattoir employees, butchers, kitchen workers, those handling fish, those handling animal hides and pelts, and those working with bone or bone meal. Most infections in human beings can be related to skin injury. The causative microorganism is a gram-positive bacillus, nonspore-forming, that can be grown aerobically or anaerobically on nutrient broth containing 1 per cent glucose or upon blood agar. It produces death in laboratory animals, particularly mice, causing focal abscesses in the liver or cutaneous cellulitis. The bacillus is susceptible in vitro to tetracycline, penicillin, and chloramphenicol.

Erysipeloid in man occurs seasonally, usually in summer and early fall, and is worldwide in distribution. Most commonly it is characterized by a nonsuppurative violaceous lesion of the hand or fingers that is swollen, very slightly tender, and has a sharply defined margin rarely extending above the wrist. In contrast to streptococcal cellulitis there are usually burning, tingling, and itching, but little pain in the involved area; rarely does the patient have systemic symptoms of fever, chills, malaise, or headache. Lymphangitis is infrequent, and when it develops it is often attributable to secondary infection with staphylococci or streptococci. The localized disease is self-limited, lasting a few days, and resolution is rapid, associated with brownish discoloration of the involved skin and rarely desquamation. A bacteriologic diagnosis can be made by culture of material aspirated or biopsied from the margin of the lesion, but isolation of the bacillus is not invariable. Ordinarily, the lesion is sufficiently distinctive to permit a clinical diagnosis when the microorganism is not cultured.

Infrequently Erysipelothrix infections may become disseminated, causing a diffuse involvement of skin. Rarely, bacteremia may develop, and bacterial endocarditis can occur.

Erysipeloid continues to occur frequently in exposed persons. The ubiquitousness of the bacillus has made it difficult to eradicate the disease. The ordinarily benign character of the infection, however, has made it an insignificant public health problem. Treatment of erysipeloid with penicillin has been shown to shorten the illness, but relapses of the disease have occurred in persons who are untreated or who receive inadequate treatment.

Ewing, M.: Erysipeloid. Med. J. Aust., 1:449, 1957.

Klauden, J. V.: Erysipeloid as an occupational disease. J.A.M.A., 111:1345, 1938.

Price, J. E. L., and Bennett, W. E. J.: The erysipeloid of Rosenbach. Br. Med. J., 2:1060, 1951.

Sneath, P. H. A., Abbott, J. D., and Cunliffe, A. C.: The bacteriology of erysipeloid. Br. Med. J., 2:1063, 1951.

224. ACTINOMYCOSIS

John P. Utz

Definition. Actinomycosis is a chronic, systemic disease characterized by multiple indurated abscesses and sinus tracts characteristically in the face, neck, chest, and abdomen.

History. Lebert is credited with the first report, in 1857, of actinomycosis in man. Bollinger described the disease in cattle in 1876. In 1877 Harz named the causative organism *Actinomyces bovis*. In 1878 Israel clearly defined the disease in man by a summary of the clinical and pathologic characteristics observed in 38 patients. The same author in collaboration with Wolff in 1891 succeeded in growing the microorganism in anaerobic culture. In 1910 Lord observed *A. bovis* in and about carious teeth and tonsillar crypts in the mouths of otherwise normal persons.

Etiology. Actinomycosis in man is caused by *A. israelii* and in cattle by *A. bovis*, but species characteristics overlap. In the normal mouth *A. israelii* grows as a pleomorphic rod-shaped bacterium and in tissues as a granule. In draining pus, mycelial clumps measuring 1 to 2 mm in diameter and colored white to yellow have been termed "sulfur" granules. Microscopically these are composed of 0.5 to 1.0 μ filaments which stain gram-positive. On agar media under strictly anaerobic conditions, *A. israelii* grows as a white spherical or lobulated colony. Laboratory animals are generally not susceptible to experimental infection. Although long considered to be a fungus, the microbe is now classified under the bacteria, a designation that more closely fits certain of its major characteristics, including susceptibility to penicillin.

Epidemiology. The disease is worldwide in distribution. During the first part of the twentieth century it was viewed as being the most common of the "systemic mycoses," but the incidence has been decreasing of late. Males are affected almost twice as frequently as females, and the illness seems most common among farmers and in rural areas. Disease is produced by direct invasion of contiguous tissues by *A. israelii* commonly present in the mouth or bowel. There is virtually always concurrent infection with other anaerobic bacteria. Disease in the brain, heart valves, or extremities may be exceptional instances of hematogenous dissemination. Disease in cows, dogs, or swine has no contagious relation to that in man.

Pathology. In tissues the characteristic and classic findings are the actinomycotic granules. These are usually found in abscesses and are surrounded by polymorphonuclear leukocytes. Chronic granulomatous reactions are also seen with giant cells, especially about granules.

Clinical Manifestations. *Cervicofacial Form.* The cervicofacial form occurs in less than half of all cases. Infection probably spreads secondarily to trauma or to carious teeth or infected tonsils. The subcutaneous tissues at the angle of the mandible and of the neck have a characteristic "woody" or indurated feeling, and the skin over these areas is reddened and may have single or multiple draining sinus tracts. Pain is seldom prominent even with osteomyelitic or periosteal lesions of bone.

Thoracic Form. This form of disease arises from aspiration into the bronchi of *A. israelii* or in a few instances from extension of disease from the esophagus to mediastinal tissues and secondarily to pleura and lung. Fever and cough are minimal early in the illness. As disease progresses to consolidation, pleurisy, and draining sinuses, prominent symptoms are weight loss, night sweats, and high fever. Rib involvement occurs occasionally, pleural effusion rarely.

Abdominal Form. Actinomycosis of the abdomen generally follows appendicitis, appendiceal abscess, a perforating lesion of the stomach, or a diverticulum of the large bowel. An abdominal mass is usually palpable, and may be extensive; and there may be burrowing sinus tracts, some of which may open to the skin in the inguinal or other regions. Retroperitoneal and thoracic spread through the diaphragm are common.

Other Forms. Approximately 10 per cent of patients have lesions in the brain, heart valves, anorectal area, or subcutaneous tissue of the extremities. Rare instances of actinomycosis of the finger have been attributed to injury to the hand by an adversary's tooth.

Diagnosis. The diagnosis of actinomycosis is supported by the finding in pus of granules that microscopically are composed of gram-positive, branching, often beaded filaments. It should be emphasized that granules may be expressed from otherwise normal tonsils and may not be found in cerebrospinal fluid in cases of central nervous system disease. The diagnosis is confirmed by the isolation of the microorganism in anaerobic culture from a lesion.

Skin test and serologic methods of confirmation are unreliable and unavailable.

Cervicofacial forms of actinomycosis must be distinguished from Ludwig's angina, tuberculosis, osteomyelitis, and malignancy. The thoracic form of disease is suggestive of tuberculosis, other fungal infections, and malignancy. Abdominal actinomycosis is often suspected of being tuberculosis, malignant disease, and, occasionally, amebiasis.

Treatment. Penicillin, first used for actinomycosis in 1944, continues to be the best drug in treating all forms of the disease. Although most strains are inhibited in vitro by levels of 0.1 unit per milliliter, the nature of the pathologic process leads often to treatment failures and necessitates prolonged therapy. Doses of 10 to 20 million units parenterally daily for at least six weeks or until lesions have healed are recommended. In penicillin-allergic patients, alternative agents are tetracycline, clindamycin, or chloramphenicol.

Surgical resection and incision and drainage of chronically infected tissues are important adjunctive therapeutic measures.

Prognosis. Prior to antimicrobial therapy, prognosis for life was poor in all forms. With penicillin therapy, the approximate recovery rates are as follows: cervicofacial, 90 per cent; abdominal, 80 per cent; and thoracic, 40 per cent.

Cope, V. Z.: Actinomycosis. London, Oxford University Press, 1938.
Lerner, P. I.: Susceptibility of pathogenic actinomycetes to antimicrobial compounds. Antimicrob. Agents Chemother., 5:302, 1974.
Peabody, J. W., Jr., and Seabury, J. H.: Actinomycosis and nocardiosis. J. Chronic. Dis., 5:374, 1957.

225. NOCARDIOSIS

John E. Bennett

Definition. Nocardiosis is an uncommon acute or chronic suppurative infection, most often originating in the lung, with a marked tendency to spread to brain and other organs.

History. Eppinger described the first case in 1890 and isolated the etiologic agent.

Etiology. *Nocardia asteroides* is the etiologic agent in most cases of nocardiosis. *Nocardia brasiliensis* causes an occasional case of nocardiosis, but this organism more typically is responsible for mycetoma or, rarely, a lymphocutaneous disease resembling sporotrichosis. Both Nocardia species are aerobic, higher bacteria with branching hyphae 0.5 to 1.0 μ wide. Hyphae are gram-positive and weakly acid fast. Nocardia grow readily at

25 or 37° C on many antibiotic-free culture media. Colonies are initially smooth and white or cream colored, later becoming chalky with an orange or yellow hue. Growth is often apparent in the first week of incubation. Identification of an isolate as *N. asteroides* or *N. brasiliensis* is a complex task, best assigned to a reference laboratory.

Epidemiology. Nocardia organisms are soil saprophytes. Portal of entry is the lung or, rarely, through trauma to the skin or gastrointestinal tract. Man-to-man transmission is unknown. Nocardiosis is infrequent but worldwide. Infection in males is two to three times as common as in females. Disease occurs at any age but is more frequent in older adults. No occupational predisposition is known. Many patients have pre-existing debilitating conditions, such as neoplasia, immunosuppressive therapy, or alveolar proteinosis.

Pathology. The lung lesion is a bronchopneumonia, with a tendency to suppuration, empyema, and abscess formation. Brain lesions are poorly encapsulated abscesses, often multiple. Purulent meningitis may result from rupture of a brain abscess into the cerebrospinal fluid. Neutrophils are the most prominent inflammatory cell in all sites, but lymphocytes and plasma cells also occur. Giant cells or epithelioid cells are unusual. Branching filaments of Nocardia are scattered in the lesion, with no granule formation. Hyphae are best demonstrated histologically by a tissue Gram stain, such as Brown and Brenn. An overstained Gomori methenamine silver procedure can also be used.

Clinical Manifestations. Presenting symptoms usually refer to the lung, brain, or subcutaneous tissue, in that decreasing order of frequency. Pulmonary infection may be acute or of many months' duration. Symptoms include fever, cough, purulent sputum, weight loss, anorexia, fatigue, dyspnea, and chest pain. Radiologic appearance of the lung lesion is variable, but typically there are one or more areas of dense pneumonia. Lesions tend to cavitate with time. Empyema is frequent. Infection sometimes extends from the lung into the chest wall, forming a subcutaneous abscess. The central nervous system is infected in 30 per cent of cases. This may be the initial or sole manifestation of the disease or may be a late complication of pulmonary nocardiosis. Clinically the neurologic disease presents as a brain abscess or purulent meningitis. Skin or subcutaneous abscesses also occur in about 30 per cent of cases, usually in the presence of pulmonary nocardiosis. Dissemination to many other organs may occur, particularly heart, kidney, spleen, and liver.

Diagnosis. A refractory, suppurative pneumonitis should suggest the possibility of nocardiosis, particularly in the presence of chest wall extension, brain abscess, or skin abscesses. Sputum, bronchoscopic washings, pleural fluid, percutaneous lung aspirates, and pus aspirated from other sites should be Gram stained and cultured for Nocardia. Cultures of blood, bone marrow, urine, or cerebrospinal fluid are rarely positive. Branching, gram-positive filaments on smear raise the possibility of actinomycosis or nocardiosis. Nocardia can usually, but not always, be distinguished from Actinomyces on smear by the absence of granules and weak acid-fastness of the former. Acid-fastness is best demonstrated by a modified Ziehl-Neelsen stain or in tissue by a modified Fite-Faraco stain. Use of 1 per cent sulfuric acid during destaining is critical. Diagnosis of nocardiosis by culture alone is fraught with problems. Nocardia organisms are difficult to isolate from heavily contaminated specimens, such as sputum, and accurate culture identification of Nocardia requires both time and expertise.

Nocardia is sometimes isolated from a specimen, usually sputum, but the patient's condition is best explained by other diagnoses. Either the Nocardia is a laboratory contaminant or it is causing a mild, self-limiting disease. Although this situation does occur, it is much more common for subsequent developments to indicate that nocardiosis had been the cause of symptoms incorrectly ascribed to tuberculosis, neoplasm, or another disorder.

Treatment. Treatment of choice is enough sulfadiazine to give serum concentrations of 10 to 15 mg per 100 ml. Six to nine grams per day is usually required for an adult. Copious fluid intake and urine alkalinization with oral sodium bicarbonate are necessary to prevent crystalluria. After about a month, if the patient is improving, sulfadiazine dosage may be reduced to 4 to 6 grams per day, or an equivalent amount of sulfisoxazole or trisulfapyrimidines may be used instead. Therapy is usually continued at this dose for 12 to 18 months. Pus in the brain, pleura, or soft tissues should be drained. Whether or not drugs other than sulfonamides are useful is an open question. Only a few patients not receiving sulfonamides have survived. It is common practice for patients responding poorly to sulfonamides to be given an additional drug, particularly ampicillin, 150 mg per kilogram per day. Cycloserine, erythromycin, and minocycline also have their advocates.

Prognosis. Clinically apparent nocardiosis is usually fatal without treatment. With appropriate therapy, nocardiosis confined to the lung has the best prognosis (50 to 60 per cent survival) and central nervous system infection the worst (13 per cent survival). The occurrence of nocardiosis in the presence of immunosuppressive therapy portends a poor prognosis.

Grossman, C. B., Bragg, D. G., and Armstrong, D.: Roentgen manifestations of pulmonary nocardiosis. Am. J. Roentgenol., 96:325, 1970.

Kurup, P. V., Randhawa, H. S., and Gupta, N. P.: Nocardiosis: A review. Mycopathologia, 40:193, 1970.

Murray, J. F., Finegold, S. M., Froman, S., and Will, D. W.: The changing spectrum of nocardiosis. Am. Rev. Respir. Dis., 83:315, 1961.

Orfanakis, M. G., Wilcox, H. G., and Smith, C. B.: In vitro studies of the combined effect of ampicillin and sulfonamides on *Nocardia asteroides* and results of therapy in four patients. Antimicrob. Agents Chemother., 1:215, 1972.

226. BRUCELLOSIS

(Undulant Fever, Malta Fever)

Vernon Knight

Definition. Brucellosis is an infectious disease caused by microorganisms of the genus Brucella, transmitted to man from lower animals. The disease may be acute, subacute, subclinical, chronic, or relapsing, and infection may localize in various viscera and tissues.

Etiology. Brucellae are small, gram-negative, aerobic, nonmotile, and nonspore-forming coccobacilli. Three species, characterized by their affinity for a particular animal host, account for most human infections: *Brucella abortus* (cattle), *Brucella melitensis* (sheep and goats), and *Brucella suis* (pigs). A newly described species,

Brucella canis, causes abortion in beagles and has, on infrequent occasions, been transmitted to humans in contact with infected dogs.

History. Brucellae were first isolated by Bruce in 1887 from the spleens of British soldiers dying on the island of Malta. This disease, now known to have been caused by infection with *B. melitensis,* was contracted by drinking raw goat's milk. Bang, in 1897 in Denmark, isolated a strain of the species now designated *B. abortus* from cattle with infectious abortion. Traum in 1914 isolated the third species, *B. suis,* from an infected sow.

Epidemiology. In the United States, reported cases of brucellosis in man now number slightly less than 200 per year, representing a low plateau after a steady decrease since 1947, when 6300 cases were reported. The cases occur principally in persons associated with swine- and cattle-slaughtering operations and to a lesser extent among workers involved in producing and marketing livestock. Two thirds of infections result from exposure to swine, and a smaller proportion results from exposure to cattle. In keeping with this, the majority of isolations of Brucella from human cases have been *B. suis,* and less frequently *B. abortus* or *B. melitensis. B. canis,* the cause of disease in dogs, has been isolated from a few human patients. A small number of patients reported exposure to milk or cheese as a possible source of infection. Of interest is the fact that in recent years about two thirds of American cases have occurred in Iowa, California, Virginia, Texas, and Minnesota.

The decrease in human brucellosis in this country is a result of almost uniform pasteurization of milk and milk products and reduction of the infection in cattle. The latter has been accomplished by a State-Federal eradication program whereby movement of infected or exposed animals is restricted and infected animals are slaughtered. In addition, a program of vaccination of calves with live strain 19 Brucella vaccine has contributed to control of the disease. Recently a program to eradicate porcine brucellosis was started.

In Great Britain about 300 cases of brucellosis in man are reported annually. These arise from ingestion of milk and milk products and contact with infected cattle. It is estimated that 300,000 cattle, involving one third of the dairy herds in Britain, are infected. In Britain, brucellosis occurs chiefly in cattle, and infections caused by *B. melitensis* and *B. suis* do not occur except for a small number of cases whose infection was acquired from sources outside Britain. In other countries that use sheep and goats more extensively, these animals may be the principal sources of infection.

Pathogenesis and Pathology. In the case of ingested dairy products, the organism penetrates the gastrointestinal mucosa; with direct contact the organism enters through breaks in the skin or the conjunctiva. It presumably may also be inhaled, because brucellae have been isolated from the air of a slaughterhouse where infected animals were killed, and infection is readily transmitted to laboratory animals by aerosol. Many persons have become infected with the organism in the laboratory, and one laboratory accident involving apparent airborne spread has been described. Brucellae are destroyed in milk and milk products by pasteurization; otherwise, they may remain viable in refrigerated milk for 10 days and in cheese up to 90 days. They may persist in meat for several weeks.

After penetration of skin or mucous membranes, the organisms spread via lymphatics to regional nodes and thence to thoracic duct and the bloodstream. Hematogenous dissemination leads to localization in spleen, bone marrow, liver, kidneys, endocardium, and elsewhere. In cattle, swine, sheep, and goats, organisms also localize in mammary glands, male and female genital organs, and in the pregnant uterus, fetal fluids, and membranes, causing abortion. Correlated with genital, uterine, and fetal infection is the finding in these tissues of a 4-carbon, polyhydric alcohol, erythritol, which promotes the growth of brucellae. Although erythritol is apparently not present in the human testicle, orchitis is paradoxically a complication of human Brucella infection. Erythritol is not present in human placentas, and brucellosis is rarely associated with abortions in humans.

Characteristically, Brucella infections are granulomas consisting of foci of lymphocytes, epithelioid cells, plasma cells, and multinucleated giant cells. In severe cases, necrosis and abscess formation may occur, a finding most characteristic of infection with *B. suis.* Brucella infection causes the development of the usual array of humoral antibodies which can be measured as agglutinins, opsonins, bacteriocidins, and precipitins, and by complement fixation. These apparently participate in the control of acute infection, aided by macrophages which ingest and destroy large numbers of organisms. Despite increased capacity of macrophages from infected animals to destroy brucellae, infection may persist in intracellular foci in macrophages or in other cells at local sites of infection, to become the source of chronic or relapsing infections.

Clinical Manifestations. The incubation period varies from a few days to a few weeks or even months. Onset may be insidious, with nonspecific findings such as low-grade fever, headache, weakness, joint pains, insomnia, sweats, and low back pain. Less commonly, onset may be abrupt, with high fever, chills, and prostration, but with few localizing signs. It is probable that fever and some of the other acute manifestations of infection are an effect, at least in part, of Brucella endotoxin, which resembles endotoxin from other gram-negative bacteria. Some lymphadenopathy occurs in about one half of cases, and splenomegaly occurs in about one third, usually in the more severely ill.

The initial illness, when untreated, may persist a few days to several weeks, and improvement may be followed by one or more relapses. Disability may persist for a year or more. Treatment is usually followed by prompt recovery, but relapse may occur in a small percentage of patients. The accompanying figure illustrates the prompt response to treatment with tetracycline of a patient with acute *B. melitensis* infection. Her disease relapsed a few weeks later but was successfully retreated with the same drug.

Infrequent but severe complications of brucellosis include *meningoencephalitis, spondylitis, endocarditis, orchitis, pancytopenia, nephritis, hepatic and splenic suppuration, cholecystitis, arthritis,* and *uveitis.* When the complication is the presenting complaint, as is sometimes the case, the diagnosis of brucellosis may not be suggested. For that reason the varied involvement possible with this disease should be kept in mind. Suppurative lesions of the liver and spleen often calcify with the passage of time, and calcific densities in roentgenograms of liver or spleen may be a clue to diagnosis. Such cases usually respond to treatment, although recovery is slow, and relapses may occur.

Brucellosis has been diagnosed occasionally in patients with Hodgkin's disease and other forms of reticu-

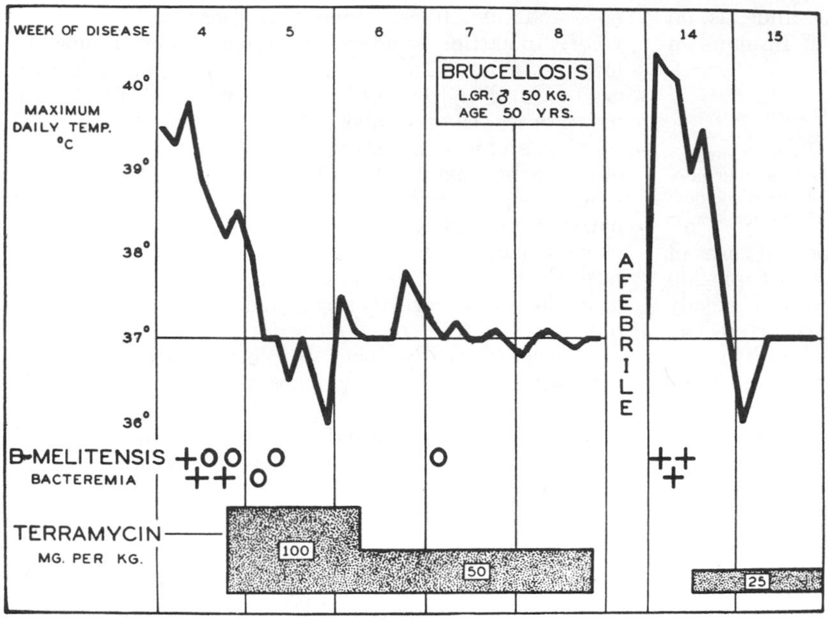

Bacteremic relapse in *B. melitensis* infection and successful retreatment with oxytetracycline. (Case of Dr. F. Ruiz Sanchez, Guadalajara, Mexico; from Knight, V.: Ann. N.Y. Acad. Sci., 53:332, 1950.)

loendothelial neoplasia. Apparently, when such neoplastic processes affect patients with Brucella infection, the neoplasia may interfere with cellular immunity and lead to dissemination of the organism from localized foci of infection.

Subclinical Disease. "CHRONIC BRUCELLOSIS." Occasionally the physician will be consulted by a patient who is chronically ill with something called "chronic brucellosis." Usually such patients have chronic arthralgias, intermittent low fever, lassitude, and a considerable overlying anxiety. Serologic tests for anti-Brucella antibodies may be present, but are of low titer (less than 1:100); the skin reaction to Brucella antigen is positive; but multiple blood cultures are negative for Brucella. Such patients seldom give a history of a well-documented attack of acute brucellosis, although they may well have received anti-Brucella chemotherapy. As a general proposition, it is extremely difficult to establish with certainty that any particular infection is *not* present. With due recognition of this fact, it can be stated that as a practical matter (1) almost certainly these patients do not have brucellosis; (2) the possibility of a Brucella infection should not be accepted as a satisfactory explanation for whatever symptoms they do have; and (3) they should not receive anti-Brucella chemotherapy. There are two sorts of experience in support of these assertions. First, a high proportion of persons occupationally exposed to infection show clean-cut bacteriologic evidence of infection, yet such subclinical infections are an asymptomatic affair. Second, the clinical syndrome of the alleged "chronic brucellosis" does not progress to detectable Brucella disease, nor is it suppressed by anti-Brucella chemotherapy.

SUBCLINICAL INFECTION. Among those occupationally exposed, unless stimulated by further exposure, the titer of antibody declines to normal in a few months to a few years. In the absence of symptoms, in this form of undoubted Brucella infection, antimicrobial treatment is probably not indicated. However, disseminated infection and bacteremia may occur with mild illness. Persons repeatedly exposed maintain high titers of antibody, and may display hypersensitivity to the Brucella organism as evidenced by excessive reaction to accidental exposure to live strain 19 Brucella vaccine or the occurrence of skin rash after handling of Brucella-infected animal tissues. As discussed previously, however, illness in people with Brucella antibody should not be assumed to be brucellosis without other diagnostic studies, in order not to miss infectious mononucleosis and other diseases which mimic brucellosis.

Diagnosis. Definitive diagnosis is best made by isolation of the organism from blood, bone marrow, or local sites of involvement. Cultures should be examined for growth every four to five days, and not be discarded before six weeks of incubation.

The organisms may be isolated in trypticase soy or tryptose phosphate broth; the primary isolation of *B. abortus* requires the presence of 10 per cent carbon dioxide. Virulent organisms possess a capsule and grow as small, glistening translucent colonies on agar. This property is gradually lost by cultivation on artificial media (smooth → rough mutation). *B. abortus* is inhibited by thionine, whereas *B. suis* and *B. melitensis* are inhibited by basic fuchsin and crystal violet. *B. suis* may be distinguished from the other species by production of H_2S. Within species, patterns of metabolic activity and other characteristics permit the definition of several "biotypes," which may be of value in epidemiologic work.

Cross-reacting agglutinating antibodies are formed in response to two principal antigenic determinants common to virulent strains of the three major species. Studies suggest that the antigens are specific, surface polysaccharides. They are designated M and A (M for *melitensis*, which predominates in this species, and A for *abortus*, which predominates in *B. abortus* and *B. suis*). These characteristics permit serologic differentiation of *B. melitensis* from the other two species.

Agglutinating antibody is usually present by the time the patients are first seen. In primary infections a large fraction of the antibody may be IgM, but IgG later becomes the predominant antibody moiety. Titers of 1:80 or greater are indicative of past or present infection. There is considerable variation in the titer of agglutinating antibody in both acute and chronic brucellosis, but a rising titer of antibody suggests the presence of active infection. In some cases, lower dilutions of serologic tests will not show agglutination when higher dilutions are positive (prozone reaction). This reaction is caused by incomplete or blocking antibodies, and can be avoided by using 5 per cent sodium chloride or albumin solution as a diluent instead of physiologic saline. A Coombs-type antiglobulin test will also reveal Brucella antibody obscured in the prozone reaction. A complement-fixing antibody test is also available.

An *intradermal skin test* is available, utilizing several preparations of Brucella antigen. It is of the delayed hypersensitivity type, and has about the same significance as the tuberculin test. As positive skin tests are frequent in endemic areas, the test is of little value in diagnosis of individual cases; moreover, the test may elicit a low titer of circulating Brucella agglutinins.

Differential Diagnosis. Acute febrile brucellosis must be differentiated from diseases whose onset is associated with fever but without localizing signs. These include influenza, other viral respiratory infections, infectious mononucleosis, early stages of infectious hepatitis, malaria, typhoid, primary histoplasmosis, disseminated tuberculosis, and lymphoma. The possibility of other illness in patients with subclinical brucellosis should be kept in mind. *The skin test should not be depended upon for diagnosis of brucellosis.*

Treatment. Tetracycline and its derivatives are usually effective in relieving the acute manifestations of the infection. Tetracycline, 0.5 gram four times daily for a period of 21 days, is recommended for uncomplicated Brucella infection in adults. Some patients in the first few hours of treatment will have a Herxheimer-like reaction characterized by increased fever, weakness, hypotension, and generalized discomfort. These manifestations clear spontaneously and, in the writer's experience, have not been a serious problem. In more severe cases streptomycin, 0.5 gram twice daily, may be given during the first two weeks of tetracycline treatment. Relapses can be retreated by the same regimen used initially.

Trimethoprim and sulfamethoxazole in combination have produced remission in acute brucellosis. Treatment prolonged to six weeks may prevent the occasional relapses seen with shorter periods of treatment. The dose used was 10 mg of trimethoprim and 50 mg of sulfamethoxazole per kilogram per day, equivalent in an average adult to 4 tablets, each containing 80 mg of trimethoprim and 400 mg of sulfamethoxazole.

In patients with the rare but serious complication of pancytopenia, steroids, such as prednisone, 40 to 60 mg per day, should be given for the first seven to ten days of antimicrobial treatment. Steroids may also be beneficial in relieving the prostration of more severely ill patients.

Prognosis. Most acute cases of brucellosis respond to a course of antimicrobial therapy with a prompt and lasting recovery. Relapse may occur one or more times in about 5 per cent of cases treated 21 days or longer, but responds to retreatment. There is some evidence that there may be residual damage in patients with Brucella nephritis. In untreated brucellosis, the mortality is less than 2 per cent, and the majority of the patients make a complete recovery within three to six months. When symptoms are prolonged in brucellosis, it may be due to hypersensitivity to Brucella antigen. The exact mechanism of such reactions is not known, but both cellular and humoral immune responses may be involved.

Prevention. Present programs in the United States to control the disease in cattle and pigs are succeeding, and the disease in man is expected to disappear here in the next few years. Elsewhere control measures are less advanced. The major preventive measure for the general population is to consume only pasteurized dairy products. There is no way to prevent spread of infection to workers from infected animals or animal tissues.

Busch, L. A., and Parker, R. L.: Brucellosis in the United States. J. Infect. Dis., 125:289, 1972.

Hassan, A., Erian, M. M., Farid, Z., Hathout, S. D., and Sorensen, K.: Trimethoprim-sulphamethoxazole in acute brucellosis. Br. Med. J., 3:159, 1971.

Henderson, R. J., and Hill, D. M.: Subclinical Brucella infection in man. Br. Med. J., 3:154, 1972.

Morgan, W. J. B.: Brucellosis in animals: Diagnosis and control. Proc. R. Soc. Med., 62:1050, 1969.

National Brucellosis Committee (subcommittee of Office of Veterinary Public Health Services): Brucellosis in the United States, 1970. Arch. Environ. Health, 25:66, 1972.

Swenson, R. M., Carmichael, L. E., and Cundy, K. R.: Human infection with *Brucella canis*. Ann. Intern. Med., 76:435, 1972.

DISEASES DUE TO MYCOBACTERIA

227. TUBERCULOSIS

Roger Des Prez

GENERAL CONSIDERATIONS

Tuberculosis is a chronic infection, potentially of lifelong duration, caused by two species of mycobacteria, *M. tuberculosis* and, rarely, *M. bovis.* It is almost always initiated by inhalation of infectious material, rarely by ingestion, and more rarely still by cutaneous inoculation (prosector's wart). Early in infection a silent bloodstream spread seeds the lymphatic system and other organs throughout the body, leaving foci which may cause clinical illness after long periods of latency. Tuberculosis must be differentiated on bacteriologic grounds from chronic infections caused by other species of mycobacteria.

Although paleopathologic evidence indicates that humans were infected with tuberculosis in neolithic times, the infection became epidemic with the Industrial Revolution, which produced the crowded living conditions most favorable to its spread. In the mid-nineteenth century, it is said to have accounted for one quarter of adult deaths in Europe. During that century three great strides led to an accurate conception of the disease and its cause. In 1804 Laennec published the opinion that the many different forms of tuberculosis in the lungs and elsewhere, previously regarded as different diseases, were actually different manifestations of one disease. By 1839 the term *tuberculosis* came into use, reflecting the unifying anatomic feature of tubercle formation. In 1865, Villemin established the contagious nature of the process by infecting laboratory animals with diseased tissue. In 1882 Koch reported isolation and culture of the tubercle bacillus and successful production of disease in animals by these isolates.

The sanatorium movement, which began because of emphasis on climate in treatment, received further impetus from the demonstration of the infectious nature of the process. As a result, phthisiology became a distinct and sophisticated medical specialty but one which was separated from the mainstream of medicine. The development of diagnostic radiology led to an appreciation of the pivotal importance of cavity formation. Treatment, other than general supportive measures and bed rest, became directed almost entirely at the goal of cavity closure, utilizing methods such as pneumoperitoneum, therapeutic pneumothorax, and collapse of the chest wall by surgical measures (thoracoplasty).

By 1947 it had become established that streptomycin (SM) was a truly effective antituberculous drug, initiating the chemotherapy era. Soon after, it was shown that combination of SM with para-aminosalicylic acid (PAS) tended to prevent treatment failures associated with development of bacterial resistance to SM, establishing the principle of combined drug therapy. The availability of effective drug treatment also made it possible for the first time to resect diseased tissue, a procedure which had previously frequently resulted in spread of infection. Some form of pulmonary resection became a part of treatment of many if not most cases. This attitude persisted for some 15 years until it became clear that resection added very little to the long-term results of effective and extended drug therapy.

In 1953 isoniazid (INH) was established as an antituberculous drug of a different and higher order than SM, and tuberculosis became a medically curable illness in most cases. Since patients on treatment became rapidly noninfectious and required little bed rest or specialized therapeutic methods aimed at cavity collapse, the need for sanatoriums disappeared, and tuberculosis became, perhaps for the first time, the legitimate province of the general physician and general hospital. Treatment began to be applied not only to patients with demonstrably active cases but also to individuals in whom active disease seemed only reasonably likely to develop (chemoprophylaxis). Finally, the more meticulous bacteriologic techniques required to determine drug susceptibility of infecting strains was, more than anything else, responsible for the recognition and eventual definition of many other pathogenic mycobacteria, all of which are less susceptible to isoniazid.

BACTERIOLOGY

Mycobacteria are acid-fast, nonmotile, nonsporulating, weakly gram-positive rods classified in the order Actinomycetales. Until recently, only *M. tuberculosis,* the human tubercle bacillus, and *M. bovis* were regarded as pathogenic for man. *M. avium,* which causes tuberculosis in poultry and swine, is thought to produce human disease only rarely. Recently other mycobacteria, previously either unrecognized or regarded as saprophytes, have become recognized as human pathogens. The clinical importance of these "atypical" mycobacteria is discussed in Ch. 244.

Such distinguishing characteristics as slow growth rate, resistance to chemical disinfectants, and the ability to survive within phagocytic cells are attributed to the hydrophobic, lipid-rich (60 per cent of dry weight) mycobacterial cell wall. Its relative impermeability accounts for the typical diagnostic staining characteristics. In the Ziehl-Neelsen method, staining with carbolfuchsin is facilitated by steaming the smear. Subsequent treatment with acid-alcohol elutes carbolfuchsin from other bacteria and organic material, but "acid-fast" mycobacteria resist decoloration.

When pulmonary tuberculosis is sufficiently advanced to cause symptoms, most cases will demonstrate a positive sputum smear. Sputum for culture is usually collected over a 24-hour period, but some authorities prefer the first sputum raised in the morning. When sputum is not produced, the respiratory secretions can be obtained by gastric aspiration or by inhalation of heated, hypertonic aerosols (10 per cent saline). The aerosol is inhaled for 15 minutes, and all sputum raised then and for a 15-minute period thereafter is collected.

Differentiation of Clinically Important Mycobacterial Species

Definitive identification of mycobacteria is usually accomplished by reference laboratories, but good species identification can be achieved by a few simple observations. Rate of growth and production of pigment were used by Runyon to classify the so-called "atypical" mycobacteria into four groups; Group I is characterized by formation of yellow colonies after brief exposure to light (photochromogens), Group II by production of yellow or orange colonies without light stimulation (scotochromogens), Group III by nonpigmented colonies, and Group IV by growth within seven days. These characteristics, together with nonsusceptibility to isoniazid, lack of production of niacin, and production of the enzyme catalase, suffice for tentative identification of those mycobacteria known to be of pathogenic importance in man. *M. tuberculosis* usually requires two or three weeks for visible growth. Colonies are rough, and no pigment is produced. It is the only species which produces a positive niacin test. Isoniazid-susceptible strains of *M. tuberculosis* produce catalase, whereas isoniazid-resistant strains are usually catalase negative. *M. bovis* resembles *M. tuberculosis* but does not produce niacin. The *photochromogenic* property of *M. kansasii* (Runyon Group I) is its most distinguishing characteristic. Growth is slow, colonies are either rough or smooth, moderate isoniazid resistance is usual, catalase production is marked, and niacin is not produced. *M. marinum* (Runyon Group I) resembles *M. kansasii* except that growth is poor at 37° C and good at room temperature. *M. avium* and *M. intracellulare* (the Battey bacillus) grow slowly, produce smooth, thin, nonpigmented colonies, are highly resistant to isoniazid, produce catalase, and do not produce niacin. They are serologically closely related and differ only in that *M. avium* grows well at 45° C and *M. intracellulare* does not. They are classified in Runyon's Group III. *Scotochromogenic mycobacteria* (Runyon Group II) produce yellow to orange pigment in the dark, grow slowly, have smooth colonies, are highly resistant to isoniazid, produce catalase, and do not produce niacin. *Rapid growers* (Runyon Group IV) produce colonies within seven days, are catalase positive, niacin negative, and very resistant to isoniazid.

EPIDEMIOLOGY

In much of the world, bovine tuberculosis remains a significant problem and infection by mouth is frequent. In Western nations, however, infection is almost always by inhalation. Most importance is attached to the dried residues of droplets aerosolized by cough, called *droplet nuclei,* which may remain suspended in air for prolonged periods and are sufficiently small to reach terminal air passages where removal is difficult and bacterial multiplication can begin. Well-studied epidemics in certain closed environments such as naval vessels and boarding schools indicate that one person with cavitary disease may "poison" the environment with droplet nuclei and infect virtually all susceptibles in the same environment, even in the temporary absence of the infectious person himself. A tuberculosis ward is probably not a place of great risk when care is taken, because persons receiving chemotherapy become rapidly noninfectious. Infected urine may be contagious, especially for young children using the same toilet facilities, owing to droplet nuclei formed from urine aerosolization. Transmission of tuberculosis by the genital route is rare. Inoculation of abraded skin by contaminated tissues at autopsy examination may produce a primary skin infection in tuberculin-negative individuals (prosector's wart). Fomites are not important in the spread of infection.

Incidence and Prevalence. The decline in tuberculosis mortality which began in the middle of the last century was probably due to improved living conditions and heightened social awareness. In the past 20 years of drug treatment, mortality has declined somewhat more rapidly, but the incidence of new cases has fallen less, suggesting a residue of older individuals infected in earlier years. In the young, it is clear that the new case rate has drastically fallen in urban United States. In 1928, 53 per cent of 16-year-old schoolchildren in Philadelphia were tuberculin positive. By 1968, this had decreased to 1.4 per cent. The incidence of new disease in older groups will eventually also surely decline, but active tuberculosis in the United States is at present most frequently seen in nonwhite older males, presumably infected while young and succumbing to age- and race-dependent factors favoring evolution of infection into disease.

IMMUNOLOGIC RESPONSE AND PATHOLOGIC FEATURES

Tuberculosis is the prototype of infections which require cellular immune responses for control. Infection induces a rich antibody response, but what role, if any, these antibodies play in control of infection is not clear. In the first few weeks after infection, the previously unexposed host has virtually no defense against multiplication of the infectious inoculum either at the initial site or at various metastatic foci established by lymphohematogenous dissemination. During this silent period, lymphocytes genetically coded to react with antigens of the tubercle bacillus proliferate and circulate throughout the lymphatic system. At some interval, usually three to six weeks after infection, the population of specifically reactive lymphocytes usually reaches sufficient size and dissemination to bring the infection under control. The mechanism by which this is accomplished is the elaboration, by reactive lymphocytes in contact with antigen, of a series of lymphocyte products which attract or entrap macrophages at the site of the lymphocyte-antigen interaction, stimulate them to a metabolically more active state in which their mycobactericidal activity is greatly enhanced, and cause some macrophages to differentiate into epithelioid cells and fibroblasts. This sequence of events results in a quite efficient control of infection. However, activated lymphocytes may also elaborate cytotoxic materials which in some instances, particularly when large concentrations of antigen interact with large populations of reactive lymphocytes, may cause cellular necrosis, an event of central importance in the progression of the infection. Although the details of these antigen-lymphocyte-macrophage interactions are by no means clear, *in a general sense tissue hypersensitivity, as manifested by the tuberculin reaction and by cellular necrosis, and cellular immunity, as manifested by successful containment of the infection, are parallel consequences of the appearance of a population of specifically reactive lymphocytes.*

The pathologic response to tuberculous infection is determined in large part by interaction of these two factors, the population of specifically reactive lymphocytes present in the host and the mass of antigen present in the lesion, as modified by structural characteristics of the tissue involved. Small numbers of bacilli in a host with well established lymphocyte reactivity to tuberculosis antigens induce *tubercle formation,* characterized by central multinucleated giant cells surrounded by a cluster of epithelioid cells. More peripherally, lymphocytes are seen admixed with fibroblasts and, in older lesions, fibrosis. Visible bacilli are few or absent. Lesions of this histologic character are termed *productive* and represent successful local containment of infection. When large bacterial concentrations coexist with high levels of lymphocyte reactivity, an exudate rich in fibrin and a nonspecific inflammatory reaction containing polymorphonuclear leukocytes, monocytes, and small numbers of epithelioid and giant cell results; such lesions, termed *exudative,* may progress to *caseous necrosis.* In contrast to many other infections, tissue autolysis in tuberculosis is initially incomplete. The term caseous depicts its cheesy, semisolid, or solid consistency, which appears microscopically as amorphous, homogeneous, eosinophilic material. When specific lymphocyte reactivity has waned because of age or intercurrent illness, and breakdown of a previously quiescent chronic focus leads to extensive bacteremia, the cellular response may be minimal or lacking entirely in the presence of large concentrations of multiplying bacteria in the miliary foci. This histologic picture has been termed *nonreactive tuberculosis.*

Since the histopathologic response is determined in part by local factors, quite different patterns may occur simultaneously in the same individual and even in different parts of the same lesion, some representing progression and some successful containment. In pulmonary caseous foci, for instance, the histologic response at increasing distances from the caseous center (where antigen concentration is greatest) comes more and more to resemble that associated with successful containment of infection, with tubercle formation and fibrosis predominating. It is important to emphasize that these histologic features are not diagnostic of tuberculosis and may be seen in some combination in a wide variety of other conditions.

PATHOGENESIS

The tubercle bacillus requires ready access to oxygen for growth, and even under the most favorable circumstances cell division occurs no more frequently than every day or two, explaining the chronic character of tuberculous disease. In unfavorable circumstances it may become metabolically dormant and persist in necrotic tissue for years. Infection by inhalation requires very few infectious units under favorable circumstances. The initial focus is usually in the mid or lower lung fields where there is greater ventilation. Bacterial multiplication proceeds with little or no reaction, spreads to regional nodes in the hilum of the lung, and thence gains access to the bloodstream. *It is important to emphasize that asymptomatic lymphohematogenous dissemination of the primary infection before the acquisition of tuberculin hypersensitivity probably occurs in all instances; it is this event which sets the stage for the development of chronic pulmonary and extrapulmonary tuberculosis at a later time.* The metastatic bacterial colonies throughout the body also multiply in unimpeded fashion prior to development of tuberculin reactivity. Circulating bacilli are most efficiently cleared from the bloodstream by reticuloendothelial organs, but bacterial multiplication is favored in those areas known to be associated with clinical tuberculosis, notably the apices of the lungs, lymph nodes, kidneys, richly vascularized skeletal areas, and the central nervous system.

As mentioned, the subsequent development of *tuberculin hypersensitivity* and *cellular immunity* greatly alters the balance in favor of the host. Activated macrophages reduce the bacterial population at both initial and metastatic foci, and further bacterial growth is inhibited. It is likely, however, that slowly metabolizing viable bacilli persist at most foci. When antigen concentration at the site of initial infection and in the regional lymph nodes is sufficiently large, cellular necrosis may develop and eventually calcify, producing the so-called *Ghon complex.* This roentgenographic finding, for years considered pathognomonic of tuberculosis, is now known to be also caused by certain fungi, notably histoplasmosis and coccidioidomycosis, and other mycobacteria.

Fate of the Primary Infection. In possibly 99 per cent, the infection remains quiescent after the development of tuberculin hypersensitivity and is of no further clinical significance. In very few, infection may evolve into clinical tuberculosis in a number of ways. In some, particularly the very young, the preallergic bacteremia (early hematogenous dissemination) may progress directly into generalized acute hematogenous tuberculosis. The resemblance of the resulting disseminated tubercles to millet seeds led to the designation, *miliary tuberculosis.* At times it is the strategic location of miliary tubercles rather than progression of the bacteremia which is critical, particularly with respect to development of *tuberculous meningitis,* because subependymal foci in brain or spinal cord may rupture into the subarachnoid space and produce spread of the infection via the subarachnoid fluid. Meningitis may occur in the setting of obvious, progressive bloodstream infection but also may be due to a nonprogressive and otherwise asymptomatic bacteremia.

Local rather than hematogenous events will also determine the outcome. The initial focus may directly evolve into progressive pneumonia (*progressive primary*); rarely cavitation may result. Large hilar nodes may become necrotic, liquefy, discharge into the bronchial tree, and produce tuberculous pneumonia in this fashion, or, particularly in the young, often partially compress the major bronchi, producing bronchial obstruction and collapse of a pulmonary segment or lobe. When the site of the initial infection is subpleural in location, rupture into the pleural space may occur, producing the clinical picture of *serofibrinous pleurisy with effusion.* A hematogenous focus located near the pleural surface can also produce this syndrome.

Numerically, the most frequent serious sequel of the preallergic bacteremia is chronic pulmonary tuberculosis. Pulmonary sequestration of blood-borne bacteria occurs in a distribution proportional to blood flow, but conditions in the superior and posterior aspects of the lungs greatly favor bacterial multiplication. Over the years it has been a matter of controversy whether chronic apical pulmonary tuberculosis of the so-called *reinfection type* results from breakdown of latent residua seeded at the time of the initial infection (*endogenous reinfection*) or from acquisition of new infection from the environment (*exogenous reinfection*). Many authorities assume that both can occur. However, it now seems likely that exogenous reinfection is considerably less important, and that apical pulmonary tuberculosis is almost always a direct consequence of the primary infection, with progression (then or later) in that area caused by local factors favoring bacterial growth, whereas the initial focus in the mid or lower lung fields almost always regresses.

The time at which apical pulmonary tuberculosis appears depends on three factors: first, the period of life in which infection occurs; second, normal, age-dependent factors favoring or inhibiting growth of the apical lesion; and third, non-age-related factors altering resistance to progression of the infection. All mortality curves from urban populations in the early part of this century, in which infection in childhood was the rule, demonstrate a peak in the first three years of life owing to the relative deficiency in cellular immunity which characterizes this period of life. In very young children, progressive hematogenous tuberculosis, particularly miliary and meningeal disease, constituted a large part of the over-all mortality. Older prepubertal children (roughly between 5 and 15), although in no way resistant to *infection*, very seldom manifested progressive *disease*. After puberty a second mortality peak was seen which continued through the second and into the third decade and was more pronounced in females than in males. Thereafter, the death rate continued at a lower level until old age, when a third, less dramatic mortality peak was seen. At present, in countries with low prevalence, clinical tuberculosis is becoming more a disease of the elderly, particularly the older male, presumably caused in part by waning immunologic competence in old age.

As mentioned, persons infected during the disease-resistant period of childhood (roughly 5 to 15) are prone to develop clinical tuberculosis in the postpubertal and early adult period of life, presumably owing to age-dependent host factors favoring evolution of the infection. In contrast, apical pulmonary tuberculosis caused by infection after childhood most often becomes manifest within two years of initial infection. Beyond this period of maximal jeopardy, quiescent foci in the lungs and elsewhere may evolve to produce clinical disease at any time when a combination of local and systemic factors favor reactivation.

The importance of local factors in reactivation of previously quiescent foci is illustrated by development of tuberculous arthritis after injury, activation of pulmonary tuberculosis by destructive lung disease such as lung abscess, and the appearance of late hematogenous dissemination after trauma. Thus any tuberculin-positive individual is at risk to develop any form of tuberculosis, often as a result of a remote and clinically undetectable primary infection. The role of immunologic senescence or other processes altering cellular immunity needs to be emphasized; reactivation of tuberculosis becomes progressively likely as individuals become more aged.

Endobronchial Spread of Chronic Pulmonary Tuberculosis: The Importance of Cavity Formation. In contrast to the earliest stages of tuberculous infection in which lymphohematogenous dissemination is the rule, once chronic pulmonary tuberculosis has become established, further spread occurs for the most part via the bronchial tree. The cavity, which is responsible both for progression of pulmonary disease in the individual and for infection of others, has provided the environment which has nurtured the tubercle bacillus through so many centuries of coexistence with the human species. *Especially in the era prior to the availability of effective drugs, cavity formation was the pivotal event in the course of pulmonary tuberculosis, to the prevention or treatment of which most forms of therapy were directed.*

Late Hematogenous Dissemination. Foci seeded at the time of the preallergic bacteremia may, after prolonged quiescent periods, break down and liberate bacteria into the bloodstream. Chronic pulmonary foci may cause late bacteremia in this manner, but extrapulmonary and often clinically inapparent foci, particularly in lymph nodes, bones, and the urogenital system, cause most instances of miliary and meningeal tuberculosis in older individuals.

THE TUBERCULIN TEST

The tuberculin test is best performed by intracutaneous injection of 0.1 ml of purified protein derivative (PPD of Seibert). Proper introduction will be indicated by a raised white area that persists for some minutes after injection. PPD in solution rapidly adsorbs to glass or plastic with loss of potency. Accordingly, injection should be made promptly after mixing the tablet with the provided diluent; preferably a solution containing an agent preventing adsorption of antigen (Tween-stabilized tuberculin) should be employed. Dosage is expressed in terms of tuberculin units (1 TU is 0.00002 mg, bioequivalent to 1:10,000 Old Tuberculin or OT; 5 TU is 0.0001 mg; 250 TU is 0.001 mg, bioequivalent to 1:100 OT). In children or in persons with coincidence of ocular involvement, the 1 TU dose is used. In adults a 5 TU dose is employed first. *Production of visible and palpable induration over 10 mm in diameter after 48 to 72 hours is considered virtually diagnostic of infection with M. tuberculosis.* A smaller reaction is of uncertain significance, because it may be due to other mycobacterial infections. If this is negative, retesting with 250 TU is carried out. A positive reaction to this larger (second-strength) dosage is also of uncertain significance, because it may reflect cross-reactivity. A negative reaction in a *nonfebrile, relatively well individual* is strong evidence against tuberculosis. However, as many as 15 per cent or more of persons constitutionally ill with proved tuberculosis may fail to react to 250 TU when first tested, becoming reactive again as health returns. Associated illnesses such as Hodgkin's disease, sarcoidosis, less commonly other neoplasias, and acute infections, notably the viral exanthemata, may also cause false negatives. False positives are almost always due to infections with other mycobacterial species.

FACTORS MODIFYING THE COURSE OF TUBERCULOSIS

Nutritional status, mental and physical stress, and exhaustion modify the course of tuberculosis, as is well illustrated by the peak in mortality statistics observed during the major wars in both belligerent and nonbelligerent nations. *Pregnancy, delivery, and the puerperium,* long regarded as risk periods, have probably been overemphasized. Although statistical evidence is lacking, there is little doubt that *prolonged therapy with corticosteroids* predisposes to exacerbation of tuberculosis, as does *therapy with oncolytic or immunosuppressive agents. Diabetes* predisposes to clinical tuberculosis and the disease tends to be more fulminant, particularly in young, poorly controlled diabetics. *Silicosis* or *anthracosilicosis* alters host rcpsonse to tuberculosis in important ways. Instances of infection with the usually nonpathogenic *M. avium* is observed in silicotics. Once established, silicotuberculosis may produce massive conglomerate fibrosis with little potential for resolution and little response to antituberculous drugs. Moreover, conglomerate fibrosis often contains quite small bacterial populations, making bacteriologic diagnosis difficult. In times past, *sarcoidosis* was thought to predispose to the progression of tuberculosis, but this no longer appears to be the case. *Hodgkin's disease, leukemia, and other lymphatic neoplasms* are often confused with tuberculosis and may also be complicated by active tuberculosis caused presumably by the detrimental effects of these diseases on cellular immune mechanisms. *Carcinoma* and *destructive infections* such as histoplasmosis, other mycobacterial infections, and lung abscess may erode an old tuberculous focus, releasing tubercle bacilli which may or may not produce disease. Severe viral illness, notably rubella and influenza, may have detrimental effects on the course of tuberculosis. *Gastric resection,* for unknown reasons, favors the development of pulmonary tuberculosis. *Pulmonary surgery* may also cause progression of quiescent pulmonary foci. The role of various types of trauma in activating latent foci has been mentioned previously.

PREVENTION OF TUBERCULOSIS

Vaccination

BCG (bacille Calmette Guérin) is a strain of *M. bovis* with attenuated virulence for man. Several large studies have produced convincing evidence that vaccination with an effective strain of BCG will result in a significant decrease in the incidence of clinical disease. Also of benefit is the fact that vaccinated persons who do become ill develop less progressive forms of tuberculosis. Miliary and meningeal disease in young children, for instance, is rare after BCG vaccination, a major advantage, considering the gravity of these conditions in the very young. (Disseminated infection with BCG itself is so rare as to be of no importance.) The difficulty with BCG stems from the lack of a satisfactory animal model for testing its immunizing potency, and by no means could all "vaccines" be called effective. This problem with BCG is not unlike that with antityphoid vaccine and, in the case of BCG, has been largely solved by the use of dry frozen vaccine from a batch known to have shown full effectiveness in large-scale field trials.

BCG vaccination programs have been carried out with substantial success in some European countries and the United Kingdom. In the United States the irregular performance of the early vaccines acted against its general use. By the time a generally effective dry frozen vaccine was developed, the falling rates of infection and disease in the United States made employment of the vaccine a procedure of value in only specialized circumstances (see below). One source of reluctance has been the fact that tuberculin positivity is induced by BCG, thus destroying the major indicator of early infection, an important consideration in areas of low prevalence. The success of isoniazid prophylaxis (see below) was another factor that weighed against widespread vaccination. Almost all authorities advise the use of BCG in tuberculin-negative children in areas in which 20 per cent or more of secondary schoolchildren are tuberculin-positive. (Vaccination is, of course, of no use in tuberculin-positive persons.) Vaccination may also be appropriate for missionary or government personnel prior to assignment to areas of known high prevalence, in groups of health professionals with high (over 20 per cent) incidence of infection, and even in some military personnel. Vaccination of infants born to tuberculous mothers or who must live in known high-risk environments is the procedure of choice, but is compromised somewhat by the problem of keeping the infant isolated for the four- to ten-week period required for development of tuberculin hypersensitivity in response to BCG vaccination. A strain of *M. microti* (the vole bacillus), naturally attenuated for man, is of the same order of effectiveness as BCG, but this has not been widely used.

Chemoprophylaxis

The term chemoprophylaxis has been applied to two distinct situations: first, the treatment of tuberculin-negative individuals in the hope of preventing infection in high-risk situations; and second, treatment of tuberculin-positive persons in the hope of preventing evolution of infection into disease. In a practical sense, it means treatment with isoniazid, because of its effectiveness, convenience, low cost, and relatively low toxicity.

Circumstances in which *infection prophylaxis* (primary prophylaxis) is indicated are few. When an infant cannot be isolated from a mother with active tuberculosis long enough to establish tuberculin hypersensitivity with BCG, isoniazid may be administered to the child until and for a few months after the mother achieves a negative sputum under treatment. When the period of risk cannot be defined, such as in households with recalcitrant infectious patients or in geographic pockets of known high risk, it may be useful to continue therapy for two years or more, because the morbidity associated with meningitis is less in older children. Alternatively, it may be reasonable to stop chemoprophylaxis at some point for a period long enough to achieve vaccination and tuberculin conversion and then to resume therapy for another year, assuming that the conversion might be due to either vaccination or infection, and that in either case protection would result. Prophylactic treatment of tuberculin-negative household contacts of newly discovered active cases is advised by many. The decision to do so should take into consideration the hepatotoxicity of isoniazid, particularly as related to the age of the individual and the practical aspects of monitoring for this toxic manifestation (see below).

Certain exposure to highly contaminated material, as in laboratory accidents or in mouth-to-mouth resuscitation of positive patients, may be covered with prophylactic isoniazid for a period of several months. In the latter situation, attention should be given to the possibility of isoniazid resistance if these data are available, and therapy adjusted accordingly. The status of the tuberculin test during and after treatment should be monitored.

In certain conditions, notably sarcoidosis and Hodgkin's disease, cutaneous anergy may make it impossible to determine whether or not infection has occurred. Moreover, both roentgenographic and histologic abnormalities in sarcoidosis and to a lesser degree in Hodgkin's disease may resemble those produced by tuberculosis. Further, both these conditions may require corticosteroid therapy (see below). For these reasons, many persons with sarcoidosis, Hodgkin's disease, and related lymphomas are treated with isoniazid without certain knowledge as to whether or not infection has in fact occurred. Similarly, prolonged corticosteroid therapy in gravely ill individuals is ordinarily accompanied by isoniazid, because all debilitating conditions may produce cutaneous anergy, making it impossible to exclude either old or active tuberculosis.

In contrast, *disease prophylaxis* (secondary prophylaxis) is a frequently employed and well established procedure. Its greatest use is in the recent tuberculin converter, which in point of fact represents treatment of an early and active infection. Treatment of children under five years with a positive reaction to a 5 TU dose of tuberculin is recommended without exception. This may also be the case in older persons in whom tuberculin conversion is known to be a relatively recent (within two years) event. The degree of tuberculin reactivity is important in reaching the decision to treat; most weak tuberculin reactions (requiring large tuberculin doses to be elicited) have entirely different implications and do not require treatment. It seems likely, although not yet established, that the incidence of tuberculosis in later life will be substantially reduced by early treatment of the tuberculin converter.

In addition to treatment of the preclinical infection, as defined above, a number of situations known to be prejudicial to the course of tuberculous infection constitute sufficient reason for chemoprophylaxis in tuberculin-positive individuals. These include silicosis, severe and poorly controlled diabetes, the postgastrectomy state, progressive neoplastic disease of the lung or of the myeloid or lymphatic systems (particularly when treatment with oncolytic agents is employed), and prolonged treatment with corticosteroids. The occurrence of severe viral illness in a tuberculin-positive individual is regarded by some as an indication for chemoprophylaxis. Persons with an undiagnosed pulmonary infiltrate and a positive tuberculin reaction, in whom for one reason or another definitive diagnosis is not indicated, may be given prophylaxis. It is essential in such circumstances, however, to ensure that the period of prophylaxis does not serve to postpone appropriate diagnostic approaches for more serious diseases. Finally, persons with known, presumably arrested tuberculosis never treated with chemotherapy should receive isoniazid. Often, previously stable infiltrates will regress under this therapy, demonstrating that the presumed inactivity was illusory.

Chemoprophylaxis in adults consists of isoniazid in dosage of 300 mg once daily for a period of a year or two, depending on the circumstances. In children, the dose is 6 to 8 mg per kilogram. The indications for the use of isoniazid in these uncertain situations should be balanced against the real risk of hepatotoxicity, particularly in older persons. It must be recalled that transient liver function test abnormalities are observed in 10 per cent of persons receiving isoniazid and clinical jaundice in 1 per cent; in one large study at least, death from severe hepatitis occurred in approximately 0.1 per cent. These figures undoubtedly overestimate the extent of the problem because of the difficulty of sorting out hepatic diseases of other causes. Nevertheless, everyone receiving isoniazid should be told of the symptom complex which might represent drug-induced hepatitis, and ideally should be seen monthly by a knowledgeable medical worker. If careful surveillance of symptoms is maintained, periodic liver function testing is probably not necessary. As mentioned above, the presence of established unrelated liver disease complicates the picture. There is no clear evidence that liver disease predisposes to an increased incidence of isoniazid hepatotoxicity. However, the detection of isoniazid-induced hepatotoxicity is rendered more difficult by the presence of unrelated liver disease. Finally, it is reasonable to assume that the consequences of hepatotoxicity might be more serious in the presence of an already damaged liver. Age appears to be an important factor; toxic reactions are rare in childhood and seem to be particularly severe in postmenopausal women. The histologic picture of isoniazid-induced hepatitis resembles viral hepatitis, including chronic active hepatitis, and prolonged reactions may lead to cirrhosis. These severe and at times fatal reactions have always been associated with continual ingestion of the drug for a week or more, usually for a much longer period, after the appearance of symptoms, emphasizing the need for patient education and continued supervision.

228. PULMONARY TUBERCULOSIS

Robert Goodwin

SYMPTOMATIC PRIMARY INFECTION

The primary infection is most often symptomatic in infants and young children because of an age-related tendency to extensive lymphadenitis and lymphohematogenous spread, and accordingly has traditionally been termed childhood tuberculosis. At the time of tuberculin conversion, fever and lassitude may be briefly present; rarely *erythema nodosum* or symptomatic inflammation of the eye *(phlyctenular keratoconjunctivitis)* will develop. Hilar lymphadenitis may partially compress the major bronchi, producing a brassy cough and occasionally sputum and localized bronchial obstruction. The chest roentgenogram will often reveal hilar adenopathy, usually unilateral, and at times a small parenchymal infiltrate. Diagnosis is based on a positive and usually vigorous tuberculin test. Microscopy of the sputum smear is occasionally positive, and positive cultures can probably be demonstrated in most patients if obtained repeatedly. Symptoms are most often either lacking or evanescent, but syndromes based on hilar adenopathy, pleural effusion, and, rarely, direct progression of the initial pulmonary infiltrate may be seen.

Hilar adenopathy may compress the small and relatively flaccid bronchi in the very young, thus producing partial or complete bronchial obstruction and obstructive pneumonitis. Involvement of the bronchial wall and mucosa by direct extension from contiguous tuberculous lymphadenitis can seed tuberculous foci distally. Prolonged obstruction and endobronchial scarring may result in distal bronchiectasis. Occasionally a node will rupture into a bronchus, producing intense bronchitis and pneumonitis which may go into caseation. (This may also occur in the adult [see below].) *Tuberculous pleurisy and effusion* (see Part XI, Section Nine) is an important and not uncommon complication occurring soon after infection in both children and young adults. Although this syndrome is itself usually self-limited, three fourths of the patients will subsequently develop progressive pulmonary or extrapulmonary tuberculosis; accordingly tuberculin-positive patients should be treated as having active tuberculosis unless another cause of the effusion can be definitely established. The term *progressive primary* connotes direct evolution of the initial infiltrate into a pneumonic, caseous process. It differs from apical chronic pulmonary tuberculosis in that hilar adenopathy is prominent and the process involves the middle or lower lung fields.

Features characteristic of childhood tuberculosis may also be seen in isolated populations into which tuberculous infection has only recently been introduced. In such circumstances, instead of being infected in childhood, the major portion of the population acquires infection in young adulthood.

Treatment. Children are usually given a larger dosage of isoniazid (10 to 15 mg per kilogram) than adults, because the risks of isoniazid toxicity are negligible in the young. An uncomplicated infection is usually treated with isoniazid alone except when drug resistance seems likely on epidemiologic grounds (contact with a patient with a known drug-resistant strain). Symptoms caused by bronchial compression may be benefited by brief corticosteroid treatment (prednisone, 20 to 40 mg daily). Treatment of progressive, caseous pulmonary parenchymal disease requires more than one drug (see below).

CHRONIC PULMONARY TUBERCULOSIS

Pulmonary tuberculosis in adults is predominantly an apical parenchymal process almost always caused by evolution of hematogenous foci seeded during the preallergic phase of the initial infection. This may occur fairly promptly or after long periods of quiescence. Whether or not a latent period intervenes, these metastatic foci gain largest size and are therefore most unstable in the superior areas of the lung in which local factors favor bacterial growth.

Chronic pulmonary tuberculosis begins as a small patch of bronchopneumonia surrounding a growing bacterial colony, most commonly in the posterior or apical segment of an upper lobe or the apical segment of a lower lobe. The inflammatory response in the sensitized host produces fibrin-rich alveolar fluid containing a mixture of inflammatory cells. Intense inflammation may progress to caseous necrosis which, while intact, is an effective mechanism of host defense, causing the death of most organisms. (Invariably, however, a few metabolically dormant organisms persist.) The critical factors which may reverse this favorable trend are the tendency of caseous foci in upper lung zones to liquefy and discharge into the bronchial tree, producing a cavity in open communication with inspired air, from which infectious secretions spread via the bronchi to other areas of the lung and to the outside environment. *Once reactivation occurs, the progressive nature of tuberculosis in the sensitized host is largely due to the combination of these three factors: the tendency of apical caseous foci to liquefy; the access of liquefied infectious material to the bronchial tree; and the aerobic nature of the organisms, resulting in extremely large bacterial populations within open cavities.*

Bronchogenic spread of infectious material is enhanced by coughing, which aerosolizes infectious material and then on inhalation distributes it widely throughout the lung. Sooner or later new foci of disease develop, which then may undergo caseous necrosis and then heal, or liquefy, slough, and produce another cavity. New lesions usually appear first in the segment or lobe initially involved, producing scattered, patchy disease. The apical posterior areas of the contralateral lung are quite apt to become involved. In addition to the exudative response, some associated productive tissue reaction is usually found, characterized by giant cells and epithelioid cells forming tubercles and leading eventually to fibrosis and healing. This is particularly true in the anterior and basal portions of the lung and in areas which respond to continual bronchogenic seeding from apical cavities with granuloma formation, fibrosis, and scarring but very rarely become necrotic or cavitary. Almost all lesions will contain some mixture of exudative and productive tissue responses, with progression in one area and regression in another. Moreover, the pace and tempo of progressive disease is highly variable from one patient to the next and in the same individual at different times. Intercurrent or genetic factors, vigorous hypersensitivity reactions, and large numbers of organisms favor acute and rapidly progressive reactions which may produce confluent pneumonia *(tuberculous pneumonia or phthisis florida)*. At the other end of the spectrum, relatively effective immunity and low bacterial populations favor predominantly productive lesions with a greater tendency to spontaneous healing. Large thick-walled cavities in a shrunken, extensively carnified lobe *(chronic fibroid tuberculosis)* may persist for years without causing symptoms but will nevertheless be highly contagious.

Mechanisms of healing are basically the same whether they occur spontaneously or after drug treatment. Theoretically, the exudative component of the early infiltrate could resolve with preservation of normal lung architecture. More often it is replaced with fibrous tissue. Solid caseous foci may become encapsulated by fibrosis. An open cavity may occasionally become obstructed by granulation tissue at the bronchocavitary junction, and become inspissated and encapsulated, producing a tenuous form of healing. An open cavity probably always remains infectious except after prolonged antimicrobial therapy, which may eliminate all necrotic and infectious tissue and result in a clean fibrotic cavity wall. Regardless of the type and extent of healing, however, it is probable that dormant organisms capable of renewed growth and reactivation of disease persist in all cases.

Symptoms. Small apical infiltrates may persist for months or even years in tenuous balance, undergoing minor extensions and regressions and producing no symptoms. Discovery of such cases by chest roentgenogram is a fortunate event. When the infection reaches a certain size, however, absorption of antigenic substances results in entirely nonspecific *constitutional symptoms* such as anorexia, fatigue, fever, chilliness, night sweats, and wasting. Constitutional symptoms usually begin insidiously and progress slowly. Weight loss and fatigue are more likely to lead to medical attention than is fever, which usually occurs in the afternoon and is often unrecognized. Often the magnitude of the illness becomes apparent to the patient only when viewed in retrospect after drug treatment.

Symptoms caused by local pulmonary inflammation are also variable in degree and in time of onset. *Cough* and *sputum* are the most consistent, both because of bronchial involvement and because of secretions from a cavity. Accordingly, their presence indicates advanced disease. Material from cavities mechanically irritates draining bronchi and, since it is highly infectious, eventually causes superficial mucosal and submucosal tuberculous disease. Depending upon the degree of bronchial reaction, the size of cavities, and the quantity of drainage, cough may vary from mild to severe, and sputum may be scant and mucoid or copious and purulent.

Hemoptysis and *chest pain* are unpredictable symptoms which cause the patient great concern. Hemoptysis may be due to slough of a caseous lesion or bronchial ulceration. It is usually minor in degree but is most often associated with advanced disease. Particularly in late chronic disease, bleeding may be copious and sudden, owing to rupture of an artery within the fibrous wall of a cavity (Rasmussen aneurysm). Exsanguination is unusual, but, particularly in extensive disease, there may be a real threat of drowning, requiring prompt positioning for draining (prone or Trendelenburg) and avoidance of drugs which suppress cough. *Pleural pain* is usually due to extension of inflammation to the pleural surface with involvement of the parietal pleura without production of pleural fluid *(dry pleurisy)*. Much less commonly, pleural pain will be associated with serofibrinous pleurisy with effusion (which usually occurs prior to established apical pulmonary tuberculosis), and rarely tuberculous empyema will be discovered. Hemoptysis and chest pain are the symptoms most likely to lead to a diagnosis of tuberculosis. Rarely, medical attention is not sought until disease occurs in other tissues bathed in highly infectious pulmonary secretions, such as in painful pharyngeal ulcers; hoarseness and dysphagia caused by laryngeal involvement; tuberculous otitis media; or anal pain caused by a tuberculous perirectal abscess. Shortness of breath is common in pneumonic or extensive destructive disease.

Lower and Middle Lobe Tuberculosis in Older Persons. As tuberculosis in young adults becomes less frequent, certain atypical presentations in older persons are being recognized. A progressive infiltrate in the lower or midlung field may rarely be due to a progressive primary infection, presumably because of deficient immune mechanisms in the elderly. Also, tuberculous hilar lymph nodes from a remote infection may rupture into a bronchus, causing tuberculous pneumonia in the associated lobe or segment.

Physical Examination. Although there are no physical findings diagnostic of tuberculosis, examination does provide valuable information regarding the degree of illness, the presence of associated disease, and anatomic and functional pulmonary changes. In patient assessment, information derived from the physical findings must be correlated with the chest roentgenogram. *Neither is adequate without the other.* Physical findings usually underestimate the extent of involvement and may be entirely normal, even with advanced disease. In spite of these inadequacies, physical examination provides some information not obtainable in any other way, such as asymmetry in respiratory excursion, contraction of the hemithorax, and deviation of the trachea. Dullness associated with decreased fremitus may detect pleural thickening or pleural fluid. Auscultation may reveal rales, but very frequently these can be detected only during quick inspiration after a short cough (post-tussic rales). (Interestingly, rales may persist for years after disease has become inactive, presumably owing to permanent distortion of small bronchi.) With large or fortuitously located lesions, tubular breath sounds and whispered pectoriloquy may be heard. Distant, hollow tubular breath sounds heard over cavities are termed amphoric, because they resemble sounds made by blowing across the mouth of a jar (amphora). Forced hyperventilation may detect local stenosis and obstruction of a bronchus. Careful funduscopic examination may reveal choroidal tubercles. In a particular situation any one of these observations from a careful physical examination may be of considerable help in arriving at a correct diagnosis. It can hardly be too strongly emphasized, however, that in the usual course of events, the physical examination of the chest of a patient with tuberculosis can be completely normal. Consequently, the diagnosis of pulmonary tuberculosis must not be excluded on the basis of a normal chest examination.

Roentgenologic Findings. The chest roentgenogram is central to diagnosis, determination of extent, and character of disease, and evaluation of response to treatment. Although not diagnostic, the finding of a patchy infiltrate located in the apical posterior area is highly suggestive of tuberculosis. Cavities can usually be seen on the standard posteroanterior chest roentgenogram, but may be overlooked, and are much more clearly seen with planigrams. Certain histopathologic characteristics of the infiltrates can be estimated from the chest roentgenogram. Exudative lesions tend to have soft indistinct margins. Increased density suggests caseation. Productive lesions tend to be small and nodular with sharply defined margins. Scar tissue produces quite sharp margins and tends to contract. Healing exudative lesions first become smaller and less dense and then, as scarring develops, become more sharply defined. When the roentgenographic changes have stabilized except for slow further contraction, one criterion indicating achievement of quiescent or inactive status is met.

Other Laboratory Findings. A normocytic, normochromic anemia is usual and may be severe. The white blood count is usually normal; a monocytosis of 8 to 15 per cent may be seen. Prolonged and severe infections may cause hyperglobulinemia and hypoalbuminemia. Hematuria or pyuria may disclose coexisting renal tuberculosis; marked albuminuria may indicate amyloidosis. A low serum sodium is sometimes found in extensive chronic pulmonary tuberculosis, more often caused by abnormal retention of water (inappropriate secretion of antidiuretic hormone) than by coexistent Addison's disease. It is important to exclude the presence of diabetes.

Diagnosis. A strong presumptive diagnosis may often be made on the basis of roentgenographic characteristics alone. A sputum smear positive for acid-fast bacteria on microscopy, a usual finding in extensive disease, will, in the proper setting, provide nearly conclusive evidence of pulmonary tuberculosis. It must be remembered, however, that any destructive process in the lung, particularly in the apical posterior area, may erode an inactive focus and cause appearance of acid-fast bacilli in the sputum without development of new, active tuberculosis. This should seldom be a cause of confusion, however, because such excretion of tubercle bacilli is apt to be short lived and, above all, because such a necrotizing pneumonia should be recognizable in other ways (see Ch. 181 to 183 and 195). A positive tuberculin test, although of great use in children, has limited diagnostic significance in older age groups. A negative reaction to 250 TU is strong but not conclusive evidence against active tuberculosis. *Histologic demonstration of granulomatous disease* provides only presumptive evidence of tuberculosis, and even demonstration of acid-fast bacteria is not definitive in that they may represent mycobacteria other than *M. tuberculosis.* Definitive diagnosis requires culture and speciation of the organism.

Differential Diagnosis. Although tuberculosis may be confused with virtually any intrathoracic condition, certain diseases are frequently considered in differential diagnosis. *Fungal disease,* particularly histoplasmosis, and disease caused by other mycobacteria can be indistinguishable from chronic cavitary or fibroid tuberculosis. (Coexistence of histoplasmosis and tuberculosis in the same individual is not rare.) *Bronchiectasis* may present with symptoms suggesting tuberculosis, and bronchiectatic areas surrounded by infiltrate may mimic cavitation roentgenographically. *Cavitary lung abscess* often involves the dorsal segments of the lower lobes and posterior segments of the upper lobes owing to patterns of aspiration during unconsciousness. Typically, lung abscess causes little in the way of physical findings, may have a fluid level, and is not associated with patchy bronchogenic infiltrates. *Acute bacterial pneumonias* may resemble florid tuberculosis in all particulars except for the sputum examination and response to antimicrobial drugs. *Neoplasm* may resemble tuberculosis, as in an isolated coin lesion, an obstructing and inconspicuous endobronchial tumor causing distal chronic inflammation, or a cavitating neoplastic mass. (An irregular cavity wall suggests necrotic neoplasm.) The association between neoplasm and tuberculosis is complex: first, in that cancer may erode into and reactivate a latent tuberculous focus; second, in that saprophytic mycobacteria may be found in association with a destructive neoplasm; and third, in that chronic scarring in a tuberculous focus may induce neoplastic degeneration. New roentgenographic progression of a previously stable, fibrotic tuberculous focus may be due to "scar cancer" rather than to progressive infection.

Classification of Pulmonary Tuberculosis. Previous classifications included the following description of the extent of disease. *Minimal:* The total area of disease, taken in the aggregate, is less than the area from the second chondrocostal junction and the fifth vertebral body to the apex of the lung on one side, and no cavity is demonstrable (planigrams usually required). *Moderately advanced:* The aggregate total area of scattered, small lesions is less than one lung field, or of dense, confluent lesions less than the equivalent of one third of one lung field. The total diameter of cavitation, if present, is less than 4 cm. *Far advanced*: Disease greater in extent than moderately advanced.

The present classification (American Thoracic Society, 1974) is as follows:

Basic Classification

0. *No tuberculosis exposure, not infected* (no history of exposure, negative tuberculin skin test)

I. *Tuberculosis exposure, no evidence of infection* (history of exposure, negative tuberculin skin test)

II. *Tuberculous infection, without disease* (positive tuberculin skin test, negative bacteriologic studies [if done], no roentgenographic findings compatible with tuberculosis, no symptoms due to tuberculosis)
Chemotherapy status (preventive therapy):
- A. None
- B. On chemotherapy since (date)
- C. Chemotherapy terminated (date)
  - 1. Complete (prescribed course of therapy)
  - 2. Incomplete

III. *Tuberculosis: infected, with disease*
The current status of the patient's tuberculosis shall be described by the following characteristics:
- A. *Location of disease*
  - 1. Pulmonary
  - 2. Pleural
  - 3. Lymphatic
  - 4. Bone or joint
  - 5. Genitourinary
  - 6. Miliary
  - 7. Meningeal
  - 8. Peritoneal
  - 9. Other

  The predominant site shall be listed for each patient. Other sites may also be listed if significant. More precise anatomic sites may be specified.
- B. *Bacteriological status*
  - 1. Positive by
    - a. Microscopy only (date)
    - b. Culture only (date)
    - c. Microscopy and culture (date)
  - 2. Negative (date)
  - 3. Pending
  - 4. Not done
- C. *Chemotherapy status*
  - 1. None
  - 2. On chemotherapy since (date)
  - 3. Chemotherapy terminated (date)
    - a. Complete (prescribed course of therapy)
    - b. Incomplete

The following data are necessary in certain circumstances:
- D. *Roentgenogram findings*
  - 1. Normal
  - 2. Abnormal
    - a. Cavitary or noncavitary
    - b. Stable or worsening or improving
- E. *Tuberculin skin test*
  - 1. Positive reaction
  - 2. Doubtful reaction
  - 3. Negative reaction
  - 4. Not done

Tuberculosis suspect: Patients may be so classified until diagnostic procedures are complete. This classification should not be used for more than three months.

TREATMENT OF PULMONARY TUBERCULOSIS

The capacity of the tubercle bacillus to retreat into a metabolically dormant state allows some viable cells to survive all drugs presently available. Therefore, although effective drug therapy may control the active phase of pulmonary tuberculosis, slow drug-independent healing processes are required for permanent control and the disease is chronic, its course measured in many months or years.

Principles of Drug Therapy

Controlled clinical trials have established certain basic principles, but new concepts gradually emerge, many of which have not been fully evaluated and are in some cases controversial (see also Ch. 267 and 268). A textbook presentation must offer a definite and simple plan of approach which in the author's judgment is the most reasonable at the time; it cannot present both sides of all controversial points.

Effective use of drugs now available should provide cure in 95 to 100 per cent of previously untreated cases. In actual practice, results are less satisfactory. In part this may reflect poor medical direction, but much more important is the often carefully obscured failure of the patient to follow his drug regimen.

The Antituberculous Drugs. *Isoniazid* (INH) remains the keystone of original treatment of pulmonary tuberculosis. It is highly effective (bactericidal against actively metabolizing cells, bacteriostatic against metabolically dormant cells), well absorbed, distributed throughout all tissues in effective concentrations, of low toxicity, and inexpensive. Drug resistance may emerge in the presence of very large bacterial populations such as are associated with pulmonary or renal cavities, and one or more companion drugs must be added to prevent this. However, isoniazid, in contrast to all other antituberculosis drugs, may retain some in vivo effectiveness even when in vitro studies indicate resistance, probably caused in part by a slightly decreased pathogenicity of isoniazid-resistant strains. Accordingly, it is advisable to continue administration of isoniazid in spite of development of in vitro resistance, while adding other effective drugs. The incidence of isoniazid-resistant isolates from previously untreated patients has remained for some years at approximately 2 per cent in the United States and England, although in other areas this figure may be higher. Allergic reactions to isoniazid are uncommon. Transient elevations of SGOT occur in 10 per cent of patients, and isoniazid-related hepatitis, reversible in its early stages, occurs in less than 1 per cent below age 35 but up to 2.5 per cent in higher age groups, particularly in subjects using alcohol excessively. Isoniazid depletes body pyridoxine stores and may induce peripheral neuritis, particularly in nutritionally compromised patients such as alcoholics. Pyridoxine (50 mg a day) is often given with isoniazid and is mandatory with doses greater than 300 mg daily and in severe alcoholics. Isoniazid dosage is 5 mg per kilogram of body weight, which in most adults is usually rounded off to 300 mg in a single daily dose. Larger doses (10 to 15 mg per kilogram) may be given at the cost of greater toxicity (pyridoxine always added) in extensive caseous disease and in isoniazid-resistant infections, particularly when supporting drug therapy is weak.

Rifampin (RMP) is a new antituberculous agent of the same order of effectiveness, low incidence of toxicity, and high degree of patient acceptance as INH. Its cost is almost prohibitively high. Its effectiveness (with companion drugs) in INH-resistant treatment failures has radically changed the prognosis in such cases from uncertain at best to favorable in the majority. Its role in initial treatment has yet to be established. Clinical and experimental evidence indicates that RMP plus INH is more effective than any other regimen. However, to date the evidence for increased clinical effectiveness is confined to patients treated for only six months. In these it is clear that INH plus RMP leads to fewer relapses after discontinuation of therapy than is the case with any other regimen administered for this period of time. However, when therapy is continued for 18 months, which is routinely recommended although at times hard to achieve, the advantage of the combined use of these two most potent agents disappears. Further, it seems likely that hepatotoxicity is increased by the use of INH and RMP together in comparison to regimens containing only one or the other. Finally, in contrast to INH, RMP loses all effectiveness when resistant strains emerge. At present it seems justifiable to employ both agents in treatment of cases of extraordinary gravity such as extensive miliary or caseous pulmonary tuberculosis associated with marked debility. At the time of this writing, however, it is the author's practice to reserve RMP for retreatment in the usual case of pulmonary tuberculosis.

Rifampin is excreted by the liver and rarely if ever should be used in the presence of liver disease. Rarely it may cause bilirubinemia, usually with larger than ordinary dosage. Its use combined with INH increases the incidence of liver function abnormalities. Thrombocytopenic purpura and a serum sickness type of reaction have been observed. These allergic phenomena are rare at conventional daily dosage but are not uncommon when larger than usual dosage and intervals greater than 24 hours are employed. The recommended dosage is 450 to 600 mg administered by mouth in a single daily dose given at least an hour before or after meals, because food makes absorption unreliable.

Streptomycin (SM) is the second major commonly used antituberculosis drug. It is often administered for a few months as the third drug in three-drug therapy (INH plus EMB plus SM) of severe disease. In conjunction with INH, it offers a strong two-drug regimen for hospitalized patients. SM is excreted by the kidneys, and toxic levels may develop when renal function is compromised. Eighth nerve toxicity (especially the vestibular branch) is a troublesome complication, more serious in those over 50, in whom the ability to compensate for loss of vestibular function is less effective. Streptomycin is administered intramuscularly in a dose of 1 gram daily in active treatment circumstances but may be reduced to 1 gram two or three times weekly in suppressive usage.

Ethambutol (EMB) is the most useful oral companion drug for INH (replacing para-aminosalicylic acid) in original treatment cases, and, if not previously used, for RMP in retreatment (INH-resistant) cases. A tendency to induce optic neuritis (loss of visual acuity, field constriction, and loss of green color discrimination) limits dosage. An acceptable incidence of 2 per cent allows the use of 25 mg per kilogram of body weight in hospitalized patients, but 15 to 20 mg per kilogram is recommended for outpatient treatment, at which dosage the incidence of optic neuritis is negligible.

Para-aminosalicylic acid (PAS), the principal companion drug to INH for years, has now been replaced by the much less toxic EMB. PAS is difficult to take and is poorly tolerated because of gastric irritation. In addition, it causes serious hypersensitivity reactions more frequently than any other antituberculous drug. PAS is now used mainly as a companion drug in retreatment cases with limited drug options. It is usually administered as the sodium salt in a dose of 5 grams three times daily with meals or 10 grams in a single daily dose given on a full stomach.

Pyrizinamide (PZA) follows SM in antimicrobial effectiveness, but its value is limited by early development of drug resistance (as early as six weeks in an active infection). This may be offset by its use with multiple drugs, with a strong drug, or in an already fairly well controlled infection. SM plus PZA is a good combination. Hepatotoxicity is a limiting factor, with 15 per cent showing altered liver function tests and 3 per cent frank jaundice, and with reported fatal hepatitis in as high as 1 per cent. The usual oral dosage is a total of 2 to 3 grams daily given in two to three divided doses.

Ethionamide (ETH) is moderately effective in retreatment cases as a companion drug with a strong agent or as one of three or more weak drugs. Patient intolerance is moderately high owing to central nervous system mediated nausea. It is administered by mouth in a dose of 500 to 1000 mg daily, most often 250 mg three times daily.

Cycloserine (CS) is a toxic and rather ineffective drug used in retreatment with a strong drug or as a member of a combination of three or more drugs. Its tendency to induce a variety of central nervous system symptoms, including convulsions, limits the dosage to 0.5 to 1.0 gram daily, the lower being of questionable effectiveness and the higher a dose that few tolerate. A regimen of 250 mg three times daily is a reasonable compromise.

Capreomycin (CM) is an aminoglycoside that approaches SM in effectiveness, with similar dosage requirements and toxicity. There is no cross-resistance with SM, and in general it can be substituted for that drug, but it is best to include it in a three-drug regimen.

Viomycin (VM) and *kanamycin* (KM), aminoglycosides that are less effective and more toxic than SM or CM, are used only in retreatment when the drug options have become quite limited. The aminoglycosides have additive toxicities, and only one can be used at a time.

Combined Drug Therapy. Drug resistance may be *primary* (in previously untreated patients) or may emerge during treatment. Although a matter of continuing concern, primary resistance is not yet a major problem in most areas. Continuing surveys in the United States, Great Britain, and elsewhere indicate a rather stable level of 2 to 3 per cent of previously untreated infections primarily resistant to either INH or SM, and less than 1 per cent to both drugs. However, some careful studies have demonstrated a higher incidence of primary drug resistance in children in urban areas of known high prevalence.

Drug resistance emerging during treatment is a major problem recognized ever since earliest drug trials. Canetti's detailed studies provide insight into the mechanisms of this phenomenon. Naturally occurring mutants resistant to INH appear at a predictable rate of 1 per 10^5 or 10^6 bacterial cells. This is true with respect to SM and probably other antituberculous drugs. When INH is administered alone and the bacterial population is large, drug-susceptible cells are killed or suppressed and resistant mutants may in time repopulate the site of infection. This is of little practical importance in closed lesions with a low bacterial population (10^3 to 10^5 cells per gram of tissue), but is extremely important in open lesions associated with very large bacterial populations. Pulmonary cavities usually contain 10^7 to 10^9 but occasionally 10^{10} or more organisms; therefore as many as 10^3 or more INH-resistant bacteria might be present from the outset, providing an ample nidus for establishment of a drug-resistant infection once the larger susceptible population is suppressed. Under these circumstances, significant numbers of resistant organisms may appear in the sputum in a few weeks, and after three to four months the major portion of the bacterial population may be INH resistant. If two effective drugs are used at the same time, and organisms resistant to each are present in a ratio of 1 to 10^5 bacterial cells, then the population of organisms resistant to both would be approximately 1 in 10^{10} bacteria, making emergence of resistance unlikely. This is the basis of the principle of combined therapy in which two or more effective drugs are used, each active against organisms resistant to the other.

Although combined therapy is primarily intended to prevent development of drug resistance, it may also increase drug effectiveness. It is important to accomplish either or both of these aims with minimal drug toxicity. The character and severity of the disease should determine the drug combinations used. Cavities with thick necrotic walls and large areas of caseation provide both the greatest hazard of drug resistance and the severest test of drug therapy. Consequently, two or three drugs, including two of the most potent (INH, SM, RMP), are recommended for severe disease.

Prolonged Therapy. The principle of prolonged therapy was also established early by the occurrence of relapse when treatment was terminated too soon, ordinarily caused by organisms still susceptible to the agents administered. Since the antituberculosis drugs are bacteriostatic for dormant organisms, suppressive therapy must be continued until the slow processes of host healing mechanisms secure control of residual infection. Strangely, there have been few studies designed to determine how long is "prolonged" and what circumstances should modify the duration of suppressive therapy. General experience indicates that for disease without residual cavity or large areas of caseation, two years of overall drug treatment usually secures permanent healing. For years, persistent cavities were resected to diminish risk of relapse. As more prolonged periods of drug therapy came into use, it became clear that the persistent "open negative" thin-walled cavity was not a serious threat and eventually became sterilized. Two to three years of drug therapy is usually indicated when thin-walled cavities persist. Caseous "open negative" thick-walled cavities require longer suppressive therapy, and surgical excision may occasionally be advisable. Some patients with extensive, necrotic disease are treated with indefinite administration of INH.

Stages of Therapy. Drug treatment consists of an *active treatment phase* during which a combination of drugs is administered in the presence of large numbers of organisms, and a *suppressive phase* during which isoniazid, usually as a single agent, is continued when the infection is reduced to a few dormant organisms.

Patient Participation. Drug regimens are always dependent on patient cooperation. Patient failure to take drugs is the most frequent and important cause of treatment failure. There are many reasons such as simple forgetfulness, the illusion of health associated with disappearance of symptoms, and the always underestimated reluctance of almost all individuals to subject themselves to any discipline for prolonged periods. Some discontinue drugs when they feel well. Alcoholics frequently forget or don't care. There are many less obvious reasons, including imagined drug reactions, queer health ideas, and rumors passed on by other patients. There is a strong tendency to cover up lapses. Every physician who treats tuberculosis has often observed relapse in a patient who indignantly maintains that he has taken his drugs faithfully, only to find that the infection is still drug susceptible and that the disease promptly responds to the same drugs given under supervision. It is important that the physician remain constantly aware of this human element.

A Plan of Drug Therapy

Initial Treatment. *Active Phase of Therapy.* Usually treatment is best initiated in a hospital where the patient can be isolated, observed, and kept at reduced activity, and where appropriate roentgenologic laboratory facilities are available. In ideal circumstances, treatment can be initiated in the home. But even under the worst circumstances, reasonably good results may be obtained if only the patient will take the drugs. The first consideration in any event is institution and maintenance of effective drug therapy.

In selecting initial drugs, it is reasonable to assume that the organism is susceptible to all agents (see above, Combined Drug Therapy). The first choice is always INH. The decision concerning companion drugs must be based on the character and severity of the disease, assessed primarily by roentgenologic findings. In *severe cavitary disease,* INH, plus daily SM and EMB, provides maximal drug effectiveness and protection against development of resistance. In *moderate cavitary* or *noncavitary disease,* two drugs are sufficient, usually INH and EMB. The antimicrobial activity of INH suffices, and ethambutol is adequate to prevent emergence of resistant strains. Since this clinical category includes the major portion of pulmonary tuberculosis, INH-EMB is the most frequently employed regimen.

In *minimal, noncavitary disease* with at most a very few organisms in the sputum, it is permissible to use INH alone, but in most cases it is preferable to begin with INH and EMB, continuing the EMB for only two or three months if the sputum becomes promptly noninfectious.

Ordinarily a bacteriologic diagnosis is established at least by smear before institution of drugs. If smears are negative on microscopy, five or six adequate sputum specimens should be cultured before initiating drugs. In severely ill patients, drugs should be started immediately, because a few days of antituberculous drugs will not interfere with demonstration of tubercle bacilli in a sputum smear or culture. Complete roentgenographic studies, including, if possible, planigrams, should be obtained at the outset and during progress on treatment. During the early course of treatment, it is best that the hemogram and urinalysis be repeated at weekly intervals and that liver and renal function be monitored frequently. Throughout the active treatment phase, chest roentgenograms and sputum specimens should be obtained at least monthly. During the early period, it is best to obtain sputum specimens at weekly intervals or clusters of three at fortnightly intervals in order to establish convincingly that tubercle bacilli either have disappeared from the sputum or are now drug resistant. Drug susceptibility studies for the commonly used drugs should be obtained before treatment, again in three or four months if the sputum still contains tubercle bacilli, or at any time of bacteriologic relapse.

The most significant event in the course of the active treatment phase is the disappearance of tubercle bacilli from the sputum. In noncavitary disease or in patients with small thin-walled cavities, this frequently occurs within one or two months. In some patients with extensive cavitary disease, reversal of infectiousness occurs rapidly, i.e., in about two months. This has important prognostic significance, because such patients demonstrate lower relapse rates than those in whom reversal of infectiousness requires four months or longer. The persistence of tubercle bacilli in the sputum after four months is associated with a rapidly rising incidence of drug resistance, and after six months the finding of drug resistance is likely. Between the four- and six-month period, therefore, there is need to consider strengthening the drug regimen in patients who continue to discharge bacilli in the sputum. A more potent companion drug, such as SM, may suffice, particularly if there are few organisms in the sputum. If there are many organisms still present in the sputum, two new drugs are needed. If the original regimen was INH and SM, it is best to continue these drugs and add RMP or EMB, or EMB and ETH, pending drug susceptibility studies. Significant resistance to any of these drugs requires a regimen containing at least two drugs (one major) to which the organisms are susceptible, and three if the new regimen does not contain a major drug. INH is always continued, even with high degrees of in vitro resistance; other drugs to which resistance is demonstrated are usually discontinued.

When discharge of tubercle bacilli in the sputum has been shown to have ceased for three consecutive months, when appropriate roentgenologic improvement has occurred (much less important), and when no cavities or large areas of caseation persist, the active treatment phase may be superseded by the suppressive phase (usually INH alone). If cavities persist ("open negative"), combined therapy should be continued for a longer time. For thin-walled cavities, the total period of combined drug therapy should be at least nine months. Persisting thick-walled cavities require combined drug therapy for at least a year and perhaps a good deal longer. Expert judgment is required in these cases.

The persistence of tubercle bacilli in the sputum after six months of drug therapy ordinarily means either drug resistance or patient noncompliance. Drug susceptibility studies will determine which possibility is present. If the patient's cooperation cannot be relied on, surgical excision may be advisable before all effective drugs are dissipated.

Decisions as to length of hospitalization, isolation, and return to work must be individualized, taking into consideration young children in the patient's environment, his social responsibility (covering cough), reliability in drug taking, history of alcoholism, and similar factors. Under ideal circumstances, in limited infections shedding relatively few organisms, work may be resumed or even continued without interruption after two or three weeks of effective drugs. Individuals with more severe infections may leave the hospital and return to work when control of the infection seems imminent or is accomplished.

Suppressive Phase of Therapy. Once control has been stabilized during the active phase, combined therapy is supplanted by a prolonged period of suppressive treatment. In all but the most severe cases, the patient will have returned to work by this time. Ordinarily, INH alone in a single daily dose of 300 mg is used. In disease without significant residual cavitation (none or thin-walled cavities), therapy is continued until 18 to 24 months after tubercle bacilli have disappeared from the sputum. The presence of thick-walled residual cavitation, persistence of large areas of unsloughed caseation, and slow bacteriologic conversion require longer periods of suppressive therapy. Decisions must be individualized under these circumstances, but total treatment periods of three or even four years may be reasonable, and occasionally therapy is continued indefinitely.

Retreatment. In most retreatment circumstances it is very important that the patient be managed in a hospital experienced with tuberculosis. Expert judgment is particularly important in drug-resistant tuberculosis in order to attain maximal effectiveness from limited drug resources. Even though resistance to INH is demonstrated or suspected, it is important to continue the use of this drug, usually in higher (up to 10 to 15 mg per kilogram) than normal doses (see above).

There is an infinite variety of circumstances attending each retreatment case. The determination of the susceptibility of the organism to all available drugs is critical to proper management. Some circumstances and principles of retreatment are tabulated here: (1) A relapse after prompt reversal of infectiousness almost always indicates that drugs have been stopped too soon, usually by the patient. If drugs were stopped completely, most will harbor drug-susceptible strains and respond again to the initial drug regimen. (2) If lapse in treatment and relapse is followed by irregular drug ingestion, resistant organisms will probably be present. (3) A patient who continues to shed tubercle bacilli in the sputum for more than six months is probably excreting drug-resistant organisms. (4) Under circumstances of suspected or presumed drug resistance, a two- or three-drug combination, including an unused strong drug (INH, RMP, SM) and an unused companion type drug (EMB, PZA, ETH, PAS, CS), may be added to INH while awaiting drug susceptibility studies. (5) CM can replace SM in the aforementioned regimens. VM and KM are less effective and more toxic, and their use is limited to last resort situations. (6) SM, CM, VM, and KM have similar and additive toxicities, and no more than one should be used at the same time.

Other Forms of Treatment. The effectiveness of drug therapy in untreated disease has made most other forms of treatment largely unnecessary. Bed rest and surgery may still have a place in retreatment cases and treatment failures.

Bed Rest. Strict bed rest, long the mainstay of treatment, is insignificant compared to effective antimicrobial drug therapy, and is no longer generally used in any circumstance. Modified bed rest is beneficial during the symptomatic stage of the early treatment period. In treatment failures, with infections resistant to all drugs, modified bed rest and continued use of INH may together in time salvage many apparently hopeless cases. In retreatment cases with tubercle bacilli resistant to all but the weakest drugs, modified bed rest will improve chances of success.

Surgery. Surgery is now rarely used, because effective use of combined and prolonged drug therapy has demonstrated the relative innocuousness of the "open negative" status. Surgery is no longer recommended for the thin-walled cavity when the sputum becomes promptly noninfectious. Surgical resection remains important and is advisable (1) in cases of drug treatment failure, provided there is sufficient pulmonary reserve and sufficient drug coverage available to avoid complications, and (2) in cases with any persistent cavity in which lack of patient cooperation compromises the prospects of prolonged drug therapy. When a drug-resistant strain is present, lobectomy is less apt to lead to complications than is segmental resection.

Adjunctive Therapy with Corticosteroids. Corticosteroids will suppress the hypersensitivity state in tuberculosis, and relatively low doses (30 mg daily of prednisone) will abolish constitutional symptoms. High dosage (60 to 80 mg of prednisone) is required to block the local inflammatory reaction, and the cost in terms of side effects is usually greater than the benefit. Steroid therapy may, however, be of great benefit in extensive disease in which hypersensitivity-induced debility may be fatal before the stores of absorbable antigen are significantly reduced (several weeks after control of bacterial growth by antimicrobial agents); the use of corticosteroids will abolish these constitutional symptoms and may tide the patient over this critical period. Also, in less serious disease in which fever, anorexia, and anemia of infection lead to weeks of serious morbidity, corticosteroids will produce prompt symptomatic recovery and repair of the anemia. In these two circumstances a moderate dose of corticosteroids (approximately 10 mg of prednisone three times daily) will suffice; it is usually possible to taper the dose by 2.5 mg decrements every four or five days. In the rare instance of hypoxia caused by a diffusion defect, usually in severe miliary tuberculosis, a large anti-inflammatory dose of corticosteroids (60 to 80 mg of prednisone daily) may be necessary for a few days before quickly decreasing to 30 mg of prednisone daily and then tapering. The unusual coexistence of Addison's disease and active pulmonary tuberculosis should be borne in mind. The adverse effect of steroids on tuberculous infection can be disregarded in the presence of effective antituberculous therapy.

Hospitalization. The classic reasons for hospitalization (bed rest and isolation) are no longer pertinent. Bed rest is not necessary in initial drug treatment, and effective drug therapy reduces the period of significant infectiousness to a few weeks. However, proper management of pulmonary tuberculosis requires a variety of services, including roentgenographic facilities, a bacteriologic laboratory competent to culture tubercle bacilli and to determine drug resistance, availability of a variety of laboratory studies for evaluation of possible drug susceptibility reactions, diagnostic facilities for evaluation of associated disease, opportunity for frequent patient observation during the early stages of treatment, and, above all, the availability of expert judgment in severe or difficult cases. Home care is entirely adequate if these services are available, but in most circumstances they are best provided through the specialty service of the hospital, either on an ambulatory basis or as an inpatient. Hospitalization is actually more important in retreatment cases, because frequent drug susceptibility studies, the advice and skills of an experienced thoracic surgical service, and expert judgment are critically important when drug resources are limited.

Desensitization. In most instances there will be sufficient alternative therapies to make it unnecessary to resort to desensitizing patients to any of the antituberculous drugs. In the rare incidence in which this might become necessary, the reader is referred to Simpson and Hubaytar (Am. Rev. Respir. Dis., 84:738, 1962), for a simple and effective method of desensitization to SM and INH.

EXTRAPULMONARY TUBERCULOSIS

Roger Des Prez

229. INTRODUCTION

Extrapulmonary tuberculosis falls into two groups on the basis of pathogenesis. The first comprises conditions resulting from *lymphohematogenous dissemination (miliary tuberculosis, tuberculosis of bones and joints, renal tuberculosis,* most cases of *tuberculous lymphadenitis, female genital tuberculosis, peritonitis, pericarditis, meningitis,* and some instances of *pleural effusion).* These illnesses may coexist with tuberculosis elsewhere or *may be isolated clinical manifestations.* The second comprises conditions which complicate pulmonary tuberculosis, caused either by bronchial or gastrointestinal spread of infectious secretions (*intracanalicular spread*) or by direct contiguous invasion (pleura, pericardium, esophagus). Urogenital tuberculosis may represent a combination when a hematogenous renal focus cavitates and seeds the lower urinary tract via the ureters.

230. PRINCIPLES OF DRUG THERAPY

Most extrapulmonary tuberculosis responds more readily to drugs than does advanced pulmonary tuberculosis, because the bacterial populations are small. The exception is cavitary renal tuberculosis which may contain large bacterial populations, requiring combined drug therapy. In the remainder, the likelihood of drug resistance developing on therapy is negligible, and the choice of a drug regimen depends on how life-threatening the illness is judged to be. Those conditions carrying a threat of early mortality (miliary and meningeal tuberculosis, and probably spondylitis and pericarditis) are treated with maximal drug therapy (isoniazid and daily streptomycin, or isoniazid and rifampin) at least until response is established, thus increasing antimicrobial potency and eliminating the small possibility of a primarily isoniazid-resistant infection. Less threatening conditions such as involvement of serous membranes, lymph nodes, the skeletal system (excluding the spine), and genital tuberculosis may be treated with isoniazid alone. Usually response is good, and only prolonged isoniazid therapy is required. When it is not, other drugs may be added without significant loss.

231. TUBERCULOSIS OF THE PLEURA

Substantial subpleural foci established prior to tuberculin hypersensitivity may, when this develops, rupture into the pleural space, evoking a brisk allergic reaction and the clinical syndrome of *primary serofibrinous pleurisy with effusion.* This occurrence, of itself usually self-limiting, is important in identifying rather extensive initial infections which are very likely to result in progressive tuberculosis elsewhere at a later time (see Part XI, Section Nine). Pleural effusion may also result from subpleural hematogenous foci and, uncommonly, as a complication of established chronic pulmonary tuberculosis, which more frequently causes local inflammation and adhesions (dry pleurisy), precluding sudden delivery of large amounts of antigenic material into the pleural cavity. Rarely, rupture of a necrotic chronic focus into the pleural space may produce tuberculous empyema and secondary bronchopleural fistula.

232. ENDOBRONCHIAL TUBERCULOSIS

Cavitary tuberculosis inevitably produces bronchial mucosal infection in the immediate vicinity of the cavity and usually in spotty distribution elsewhere. In the days before drug therapy, such involvement at times obstructed the bronchocavitary junction or even a whole segment or lobe, with subsequent inspissation, fibrosis, and contraction, an important although tenuous healing mechanism. Superficial bronchial lesions respond promptly to chemotherapy, and now usually require little attention. However, partial degrees of bronchial cicatrization may cause nontuberculous complications such as atelectasis and obstructive pneumonitis. Some degree of permanent bronchial distortion probably occurs in all moderately extensive pulmonary tuberculosis. Tuberculosis of the trachea, now rare, is an extension of florid endobronchial tuberculosis. The consequences of bronchial involvement in childhood are discussed in Ch. 228.

233. TUBERCULOSIS OF THE LARYNX

Prior to drug therapy, tuberculosis of the larynx was a dread late complication of extensive pulmonary tuberculosis. The onset of hoarseness, dysphagia, and perhaps pain referred to the ear often initiated downhill course, with extensive bronchogenic spread throughout both lung fields from copious, thin, laryngeal secretions. This is now almost never seen, even in patients with a drug-resistant strain and highly infectious sputum. Rarely, isolated ulcers or nodules with intact mucosa, resembling carcinoma, are diagnosed as tuberculosis either by biopsy or by association with active pulmonary tuberculosis. Hematogenous laryngeal tuberculosis is usually accompanied by hematogenous involvement of the lung as well. Response to drug therapy is excellent, and surgery is usually unnecessary.

234. GASTROINTESTINAL TUBERCULOSIS

Gastrointestinal tuberculosis frequently complicated extensive pulmonary tuberculosis in years past, and was also caused by ingestion of milk containing tubercle bacilli. It is now rare, but occasionally complaints related to a gastrointestinal focus may lead to recognition of pulmonary tuberculosis; even more rarely, gastrointestinal tuberculosis presents without recognizable active pulmonary disease.

Tuberculosis of the tongue and mouth may present as painful ulcers or as a nonhealing tooth socket after dental extraction. Untreated, the process is indolently progressive, but response to chemotherapy is rapid. Extension of oropharyngeal disease via the eustachian tube may produce *tuberculosis of the middle ear and mastoid bone. Tuberculosis of the tonsil and pharyngeal lymphatic tissue* was common when bovine tuberculosis was epidemic; draining regional nodes were termed *scrofula. Tuberculosis of the esophagus* may very rarely result from penetration of an adjacent node, leading to bronchoesophageal fistula or to ulcerative or hyperplastic disease of the esophageal wall. *Tuberculosis of the stomach* may resemble diffuse neoplastic involvement (linitis plastica type) or a nonhealing ulcer, and may, if caused by extension from an adjacent lymph node focus, present as an isolated clinical manifestation. Hyperplastic or ulcerative *duodenal tuberculosis* may resemble peptic or neoplastic obstructive disease. Tuberculosis of the intestine may produce ulceration with bleeding and a tendency to perforation and fistula formation, hyperplasia with obstructive symptoms, or a combination of the two. *Tuberculosis of the small intestine* is more liable to produce perforation than disease elsewhere. *Ileocecal tuberculosis* is the most frequently observed form of bowel involvement, presumably because of cecal pooling of infectious fecal material producing mucosal disease, occult bleeding, obstruction, or fistula formation. *Tuberculosis of the ascending and transverse colon* is much less common, and may present as a concentric, hyperplastic lesion producing obstruction. *Tuberculosis of the sigmoid colon* may resemble carcinoma, atypical ulcerative colitis, or diverticulitis. All these lesions may perforate and produce *tuberculous perirectal and pelvic abscesses* and fistula in ano. Diagnosis is now almost always an unexpected finding at surgery; but if it is established by nonsurgical means, the effects of chemotherapy should be determined, because even advanced lesions may respond satisfactorily.

235. MILIARY TUBERCULOSIS

The term *miliary tuberculosis* was coined to describe the appearance of lungs and other organs from fatal cases of progressive tuberculous bacteremia in which the disseminated small tubercles suggested millet seeds. It is at present applied to any form of persistent or recurrent hematogenous dissemination. The hematogenous phase of the primary infection is especially liable to evolve into miliary tuberculosis in very young children, and, together with the associated meningitis, accounts for most tuberculosis deaths in this age group. In adults miliary tuberculosis may be due to old residua of remote infections which reactivate, undergo necrosis, and seed the circulation. A pulmonary focus may be responsible, but more frequently a previously undetected extrapulmonary focus in the lymphatic, genitourinary, or skeletal system is the cause. Such foci may cause multiple bacteremic episodes, and the process may be protracted, intermittent, and low grade. Host factors such as debility, advanced age, intercurrent therapy with oncolytic agents, immunosuppressives, or corticosteroid hormones, malignant disease, particularly of the lymphatic and hematopoietic systems, and occasionally local injury are frequently associated with activation of latent foci.

Clinical Features and Diagnosis. In the very young, the illness is acute and severe, with high intermittent fevers, night sweats, and occasionally rigors. Complications such as pleurisy, peritonitis, or meningitis occur in as many as two thirds, usually developing several weeks after the onset of constitutional symptoms. A similar acute illness is usual in adults as well. The presenting syndrome is similar to that seen in an acute viral or rickettsial infection or in typhoid fever or brucellosis. The onset, although perhaps not actually abrupt, can nevertheless be dated. The patient is prostrated, frequently has a moderately severe headache, and, although conscious and oriented, usually seems to wish to be left alone. A leukopenia is present, sometimes as low as 3500 to 4000 cells per cubic millimeter, and there is a considerable increase of immature forms. Although meningeal signs may be absent, eventually meningitis appears in about two thirds of patients. In some patients, however, miliary tuberculosis may be covert and subtle, with weeks or months of nonspecific, slowly progressive, constitutional symptoms such as weight loss, weakness, and low-grade or absent fever. This clinical picture, ascribed to small, intermittent bacteremic episodes, has been designated *chronic hematogenous tuberculosis.* As in the more acute form, the presenting complaint may be due to serous membrane involvement, meningitis, or, less commonly, disseminated lymphatic involvement. Choroidal tubercles are often absent. Splenomegaly is uncommon.

Diagnostic studies are usually initiated because of the appearance of a typical miliary infiltration on chest roentgenogram. However, *individuals may succumb to miliary tuberculosis before the miliary pulmonary infiltrate has become roentgenographically detectable.* The tuberculin test is of little help, because as *many as one fourth of proved cases may be initially tuberculin negative,* reactivity returning when treatment results in improvement. Anemia is usual. The white blood count is usually normal or depressed initially (see below). Gastric and urine cultures, although frequently positive for *M. tuberculosis,* are of little immediate diagnostic help. Culture of the cerebrospinal fluid may be positive for tubercle bacilli despite the absence of pleocytosis, protein elevation, or meningeal signs. Evidence of associated tuberculosis is helpful but often lacking. In many, a tentative diagnosis is made when granulomatous lesions are discovered on bone marrow aspiration or liver biopsy. Culture of these tissues may be positive without histologic evidence of disease, and negative findings do not exclude the diagnosis.

Primary Hepatic Tuberculosis. In rare cases the sole clinical manifestations of miliary tuberculosis may be hepatic dysfunction and fever. The hepatic findings may resemble those of neoplastic or nontuberculous granulomatous origin (elevation of serum alkaline phosphatase, less elevation of serum bilirubin, and little indication of hepatocellular damage). At times the presenting findings will resemble those of extrahepatic obstruction with ascending cholangitis. Diagnosis is made by liver biopsy.

Miliary Tuberculosis of the Aged. Miliary tuberculosis in older persons may present simply as a wasting illness with intermittent, low-grade fever or no fever at all, commonly misdiagnosed as neoplasm, and frequently discovered only at autopsy. In such cases, a therapeutic trial of isoniazid will often be diagnostic and may be a conservative alternative to diagnostic laparotomy.

Miliary Tuberculosis and Hematologic Disease. Many hematologic illnesses may be mimicked by miliary tuberculosis (leukemoid reaction, leukopenia, thrombocytopenia, aregenerative anemia, hemolytic anemia, leukemia, myelofibrosis, and even polycythemia). The often associated histologic picture of foci containing myriads of acid-fast organisms but little specific cellular reaction has been termed *nonreactive tuberculosis.* Many such cases are misdiagnosed as leukemia, a confusion compounded by the fact that miliary tuberculosis may complicate true leukemia. Further, the steroid therapy administered for a hematologic illness may reactivate a latent tuberculous focus, leading to secondary miliary tuberculosis. Since steroid therapy is often indicated for serious hematologic disease, awareness of the possibility that the underlying cause may be cryptic miliary tuberculosis is very important.

Electrolyte Abnormalities. A surprising number of patients with miliary tuberculosis, especially but not exclusively those complicated by meningitis, will demonstrate hyponatremia. Although coexistent adrenal insufficiency is always a concern, the syndrome of inappropriate secretion of antidiuretic hormone is a much more frequent cause.

Treatment and Prognosis. Treatment of miliary tuberculosis with regimens including isoniazid should be successful in virtually all patients except those dying within the first few weeks or those with serious underlying disease. The prognosis with concurrent meningitis is less favorable. Maximal drug therapy with isoniazid and rifampin is recommended. When a good response has been established and the infecting strain is known to be isoniazid susceptible, rifampin may be discontinued. Isoniazid should be continued for a total of at least two years. (A good response to isoniazid in a therapeutic trial of unproved disease makes it unnecessary to add another drug.) Response to treatment may be dramatic or require some weeks. Adjunctive therapy with corticosteroids is advisable in severe cases with extensive pulmonary involvement and serious hypoxemia, and also in cases with poor response owing to severe debility. It is, of course, mandatory in the rare instance of coexistent adrenal insufficiency. Other causes for poor response to treatment, such as miliary disease caused by mycobacteria other than *M. tuberculosis* or by isoniazid-resistant *M. tuberculosis,* are rare, presumably owing to the decreased virulence of these organisms.

236. TUBERCULOUS MENINGITIS

Tuberculous meningitis is invariably fatal when untreated and is often associated with incapacitating neurologic damage, particularly in the very young, even with prompt therapy. It was long regarded as primarily a children's disease, but at present one half or more of cases are observed in adults. Meningitis complicates the majority of untreated cases of miliary tuberculosis. The infection reaches the subarachnoid space by direct extension from a subjacent focus, most frequently a small, subependymal tubercle, less frequently a tuberculoma or parameningeal focus in the spine, middle ear, or elsewhere. Since the critical factor is location, extensive bacteremia merely enhances the probability of meningeal involvement, which may also follow a small, transient, otherwise inapparent hematogenous phase. Once infectious material ruptures into the subarachnoid space, an allergic inflammatory response spreads infection via the cerebrospinal fluid, implanting bacilli elsewhere on the meningeal surfaces. Involvement is usually most marked at the base of the brain and may produce a grossly thickened space-occupying exudate, causing pressure injury to adjacent cranial nerves and long tracts. Obstructed basilar foramina may cause hydrocephalus. Vascular thrombosis and ischemic brain damage may also occur.

Clinical Features and Diagnosis. The illness may be abrupt and severe, or subtle and chronic. In some instances defects in mentation or affect may develop, with little to suggest infection. Extrameningeal tuberculosis is clinically apparent in half the patients and the tuberculin test is positive in three fourths, *but the absence of both does not exclude the diagnosis.* A variety of neurologic abnormalities may develop, including cranial nerve palsies, blindness, deafness, long tract signs, subarachnoid block, disorders of consciousness ranging from mild confusion to dementia or coma, and, as mentioned, the syndrome of inappropriate secretion of antidiuretic hormone.

An increase of cells in the cerebrospinal fluid, more than half mononuclear cells, is the rule. Cell counts are rarely over 1000 per cubic millimeter, more frequently in the 50 to 200 range, and may be as low as only a few lymphocytes. In acute severe disease, the cerebrospinal fluid may contain predominantly polymorphonuclear leukocytes, thus resembling pyogenic meningitis. The cerebrospinal fluid protein is almost always elevated and glucose is usually depressed in comparison with simultaneously determined blood glucose. Smears of the cerebrospinal fluid sediment will be positive for acid-fast bacilli in less than 25 per cent; this return may be improved if the pellicle on the top of the fluid specimen is stained and examined. Culture will eventually be positive for *M. tuberculosis* in at least 75 per cent of cases. Of the cerebrospinal fluid abnormalities, only the degree of pressure elevation has prognostic import, higher pressures being associated with a tendency to herniation at the base of the brain. Accordingly, the cerebrospinal fluid should be removed cautiously and slowly.

Treatment and Prognosis. Therapy should always include isoniazid and either rifampin or streptomycin, probably the former. Early in the course, isoniazid should be administered in larger than conventional dosage (8 to 12 mg per kilogram in the adult, and 15 to 20 mg per kilogram in children) with pyridoxine (100 mg per day). If response is favorable, these dosages may be reduced after four weeks or so. Isoniazid may be given by mouth or by intramuscular administration if oral therapy is not possible (equal total dose). Rifampin is administered as described for pulmonary tuberculosis. Intrathecal therapy is not indicated.

Bacteriologic cure should be achieved in three fourths or more of the patients, but permanent neurologic residua (weakness, paralysis, blindness or deafness, other cranial nerve palsies, hydrocephalus, compromised intelligence, and, rarely, symptoms and signs of pituitary or hypothalamic dysfunction such as precocious puberty, obesity, diabetes insipidus, and panhypopituitarism) may result in as many as 25 per cent. These are local complications of the inflammatory response, and accordingly adjunctive anti-inflammatory therapy might be advantageous. Use of *corticosteroid hormones or corticotrophin* has received wide acceptance. Although evidence is conflicting, most studies reveal a slight but definite survival advantage in groups receiving adjunctive corticosteroid therapy, particularly in prevention of brainstem herniation. The response to corticosteroid therapy may be dramatic, with rapid clearing of sensorium, regression of abnormalities in the cerebrospinal fluid, defervescence, and loss of headache. Even if long-term benefits are slight, this symptomatic improvement justifies corticosteroid therapy. Prednisone (60 to 80 mg per day) is recommended in all cases of tuberculous meningitis complicated by altered consciousness, neurologic abnormality, subarachnoid block, or cerebrospinal fluid pressures in excess of 300 mg of water. This will include most cases. The corticosteroid therapy may be tapered rapidly in the second or third week to a level of 30 mg, and then decreased at a slower rate every third or fourth day, using the signs and symptoms of meningeal inflammation as a guide to reduction of dosage. The hormone can usually be discontinued entirely after six to eight weeks.

237. TUBERCULOMAS

Tuberculomas, once the most frequent cause of intracranial mass lesions in children, are now rare. Except in cases in which meningitis develops owing to extension to the subarachnoid space, the symptoms are those of an expanding cerebral or cerebellar mass. Diagnosis is usually made at surgery. Antimicrobial therapy should be administered when the diagnosis is made, both in hope of some resolution and to prevent development of meningitis.

238. TUBERCULOUS PERICARDITIS

The subject of pericarditis is covered in Ch. 571 to 576, and this discussion concerns only aspects unique to tuberculous pericarditis. The pericardium is most often contaminated by an adjacent mediastinal node, less frequently by a pulmonary focus, and rarely via the bloodstream, evoking an allergic effusion which disseminates the infection over the entire pericardial surface. Associated pleural effusion is present in approximately one half of the patients, and peritoneal involvement may also occur, a syndrome termed *tuberculous polyserositis.* Although always associated with other tuberculosis foci, frequently pericarditis is the only clinically apparent manifestation. Prior to the era of chemotherapy, tuberculous pericarditis was fatal in 90 per cent or more of the cases, with deaths caused both by progressive infection and by acute and chronic cardiovascular complications such as tamponade, constriction, restriction, and myocardial and coronary artery involvement.

Features tending to differentiate tuberculosis from other causes of pericarditis are the somewhat chronic course, less prominent pain and rub, and symptoms of chronic systemic infection, although frequently a symptom complex resembling progressive right heart failure leads to diagnosis. Etiologic diagnosis of tuberculous pericarditis, once the anatomic process has been established, is always difficult. The tuberculin test is usually positive (over 90 per cent), but may be negative. *Pericardiocentesis* is often employed for both diagnosis and relief of tamponade. *This procedure is associated with significant morbidity and mortality, and, if done, should always be preceded by unequivocal evidence of pericardial fluid.* It is not only risky; it also provides meager diagnostic information. The character of the fluid will not differentiate tuberculous disease from other causes of pericardial exudate (with the possible exception of pyogenic pericarditis). The fluid is rarely positive for acid-fast bacilli on microscopy, and culture (positive in approximately 40 per cent) requires too much time to be of immediate therapeutic assistance. It is the writer's preference to advise pericardiocentesis only for temporary relief of tamponade or to exclude the possibility of a pyogenic process when associated clinical manifestations (high spiking fever, marked leukocytosis, associated nontuberculous infection) make this uncommon process a serious consideration. Pericardiocentesis is best carried out in association with right heart catheterization and only after arrangements for prompt thoracotomy have been made, should this become necessary. When the presence of documented tuberculous disease elsewhere makes tuberculous pericarditis likely and little hemodynamic compromise is present, therapy may be initiated with isoniazid and rifampin and the course carefully followed. If, because of uncertain diagnosis, unfavorable hemodynamic conditions, or less than prompt improvement, this approach becomes unsatisfactory, and if the general condition of the patient is otherwise fairly good, we advise thoracotomy and anterior pericardial stripping. The advantages of this approach are (1) accurate diagnosis; (2) relief of tamponade and very probably prevention of some instances which would otherwise progress to constrictive or restrictive disease; (3) a favorable surgical technical situation prior to the development of chronic inflammation, scarring, and fibrosis; and (4) relief of right atrial hypertension which favors fluid retention, venous thrombosis, and pulmonary embolization. Our personal experience with patients succumbing to pulmonary embolic disease has led us to this rather prompt and decisive diagnostic and therapeutic approach.

Some authorities advise the use of corticosteroids to favor resolution of the inflammatory process. Although this is acceptable in the presence of a certain diagnosis and the absence of substantial right atrial hypertension, such circumstances rarely obtain in the individual case.

Further, the risk of an infectious process not susceptible to antituberculous drugs, although minor, is always present.

239. TUBERCULOUS PERITONITIS

Tuberculous peritonitis usually results from rupture of an adjacent caseous lymph node, fallopian tube, or subserosal tubercle into the peritoneal cavity, and is often the only clinical manifestation of infection. Peritoneal involvement from a bowel focus is rare. The process may become loculated or may involve the entire peritoneal surface, and the response may vary from copious, thin ascitic fluid with a few inflammatory cells to a hyperplastic reaction with gelatinous exudate tending to fibrosis or caseation. The onset may resemble pyogenic peritonitis, or may be quite subtle, suggesting occult malignancy, fever of unknown origin, bowel obstruction, or unexplained ascites. Fever may be absent and the tuberculin test negative. Recognition of tuberculous peritonitis in cirrhotics may be difficult, because the symptoms may resemble those of uncomplicated cirrhosis with ascites, requiring paracentesis for detection (ascitic fluid in uncomplicated cirrhosis usually contains less than 200 cells).

Diagnosis is usually made at laparotomy or on the basis of response to specific antituberculous chemotherapy. The peritoneal fluid resembles that found in tuberculous pleurisy with effusion, but is indistinguishable from that which may occur in peritoneal carcinomatosis. In acute cases the leukocytosis may be predominantly polymorphonuclear, suggesting a pyogenic process. Acid-fast stain of the fluid sediment is rarely positive and tubercle bacilli can be cultured in less than 20 per cent of cases. Needle biopsy of the parietal peritoneum (Cope or Abrams needle) will be diagnostic in most patients, but has resulted in death from occult intraperitoneal bleeding. Accordingly, if tissue is required, a limited exploratory laparotomy is preferable. When the therapeutic implications of tissue diagnosis are limited to the question of whether or not to treat for tuberculosis, a trial of isoniazid is often an acceptable alternative. Multiple drug therapy is advised by some authorities, but single drug therapy with isoniazid for a period of 24 months has produced completely satisfactory responses in all cases known to the writer.

240. TUBERCULOUS LYMPHADENITIS

Prior to the control of bovine tuberculosis, cervical tuberculous lymphadenitis or *scrofula* was commonplace, owing to local infection of the oropharynx and draining cervical lymphatics. This mode of acquisition of tuberculous cervical lymphadenitis is now extremely rare in areas with no bovine tuberculosis problem. In contrast, cervical granulomatous lymphadenitis in children caused by mycobacteria other than *M. tuberculosis* and *M. bovis* is almost certainly acquired by the oral route (see Ch. 244).

The term tuberculous lymphadenitis is now used to describe superficial lymph node involvement either caused by extensive lymphatic spread from a primary pulmonary focus or as a part of a generalized lymphohematogenous dissemination. The cervical and mediastinal nodes are most frequently involved. Clinical evidence of associated tuberculosis is lacking in more than half of the cases. Painless or, less frequently, painful node enlargement is the usual presenting complaint, but many patients have symptoms of systemic infection. The nodes may become fluctuant and drain.

Drugs should be administered before surgery is resorted to, because often even large, necrotic, chronically draining nodes will resolve completely and resection is rarely needed. Drug therapy should be given for at least a year and probably two. Most recommend use of isoniazid and a companion drug, but isoniazid given as a single agent is adequate therapy in almost all instances. Prolonged rest or hospitalization is not necessary once a favorable response has been established. Careful bacteriologic investigation is particularly important in view of the frequency of granulomatous lymphadenitis caused by other mycobacterial species, which are quite drug resistant and require a different therapeutic approach emphasizing surgical removal.

241. GENITOURINARY TUBERCULOSIS

RENAL TUBERCULOSIS

Renal tuberculosis develops from foci in the cortex seeded via the bloodstream. Although usually unilateral when detected, 50 per cent of the cases will become bilateral in the absence of treatment, presumably because of progression of contralateral hematogenous foci. The bacilli lodge in the cortex, but infection does not become progressive until it reaches the medulla (via the renal tubules) where the environment is much more favorable to progression. Foci in the renal papillae may cause obstruction and retrograde involvement of the obstructed segment, or may undergo necrosis, excavate, and seed the ureteral and vesical mucosa. Papillary obstruction with infection may cause segmental renal destruction; scarring in the renal pelvis and ureters may cause obstructive hydronephrosis; and the contaminated urine may cause bladder irritability, contracture, and scarring, as well as infection of the male genitalia.

Symptoms are usually subtle and are often lacking even with advanced cavitary renal tuberculosis. Sterile pyuria should suggest tuberculosis, especially with frequency and dysuria. Pyuria may be intermittent and low grade (10 white blood cells per high power field). Intermittent hematuria may also be seen. Fever and backache are uncommon and probably late symptoms. Male genital tuberculosis may be the first clue to renal involvement. History of prior tuberculous infection or coexistent extrarenal foci other than in the bladder and genitalia are the exceptions.

Diagnosis is based on the isolation of tubercle bacilli from early morning specimens of urine. Demonstration of acid-fast bacilli by microscopy of concentrated sediment should be regarded with suspicion, but could be caused by smegma bacilli. Intravenous or retrograde pyelography may provide the first evidence of disease and is necessary to assess the degree of involvement. However, unless calcification is present, the findings are nonspecific.

Treatment with a two-drug regimen, including isoniazid, for a period of at least two years will arrest the disease in most instances. Relapse is usually associated with emergence of drug resistance, and retreatment with two drugs to which the infection is susceptible is advised. Intravenous pyelograms should be obtained at three-month intervals to detect and treat ureteral strictures complicating the healing process. Very rarely obstruction with complicating pyogenic infection or pain may require removal of renal tissue, but this is to be avoided if possible.

MALE GENITAL TUBERCULOSIS

Male genital tuberculosis affects the *prostate,* the *seminal vesicles,* the *epididymides,* and more rarely the *testes;* it may be secondary to recent or remote renal tuberculosis or to lymphohematogenous spread. Most instances present as an epididymal lesion, varying from a firm, painless, small nodule to an inflamed and draining mass. Diagnosis is usually made by prostatic or epididymal biopsy. Some instances may be detected because of poor healing and fistula formation complicating prostatic or scrotal surgery; in these, diagnosis may require a therapeutic trial of isoniazid, because culture of the draining material is often unrevealing. Response to drug therapy is excellent in most patients, and surgery is usually not required except for diagnosis. Combined drug therapy is usually recommended; but in the absence of active renal disease, isoniazid is adequate therapy.

FEMALE GENITAL TUBERCULOSIS

Female pelvic tuberculosis begins as a hematogenous endosalpingeal focus. Infection may spread to the ovary, the endometrium, and rarely the cervix, producing an ulcerating granuloma that resembles carcinoma. Local or generalized peritonitis may also develop. The most common symptoms are menstrual disorders and abdominal pain. Most patients are sterile. In a smaller number, pregnancy and delivery appear to activate a previously latent focus. When conception does occur, tubal disease favors ectopic pregnancy. Pelvic inflammatory disease unresponsive to antimicrobial therapy may lead to the recognition of tuberculosis. In the majority, however, local and constitutional symptoms are mild or absent. Diagnosis is made by histologic study and culture of endometrial scraping, by culture of menstrual blood, and often by exploratory laparotomy. Response to a drug regimen containing isoniazid or to isoniazid alone is usually excellent, and surgery is only rarely necessary to remove large tubo-ovarian abscesses.

242. TUBERCULOSIS OF BONES AND JOINTS

Blood-borne tubercle bacilli tend to lodge in the anterior aspects of vertebral bodies and in the metaphyseal areas of long bones. Evolution of foci in bone may produce cystic areas of osteomyelitis without joint involvement but often erode the end plate and involve the nearby joint space. At present, bone and joint tuberculosis is not common in the United States, but several cases are seen each year on most medical services. It remains a major problem in other areas of the world.

TUBERCULOUS SPONDYLITIS

The most grave form of skeletal tuberculosis is *tuberculous spondylitis* or *Pott's disease.* The originating focus is usually in the anterior aspect of the vertebral body near an intervertebral disc. The developing infection may erode the cortex, destroy the intervertebral disc, and involve the adjacent vertebral body. The roentgenographic picture of rarefaction and destruction of adjacent areas of two vertebral bodies, loss of the intervening disc space, and a tendency to anterior wedging or collapse is typical of tuberculous spondylitis, but is also caused by other infectious processes. The anterior foreshortening and angulation of the spine may result in a visible and tender posterior bony prominence or gibbus. Less frequently, the infection may begin in the center or posterior aspect of the vertebral body. The thoracic, thoracolumbar, cervical, and lumbosacral areas are involved in order of decreasing frequency. More than one area may be involved with intervening normal vertebrae. Characteristically, the infection dissects anterolaterally from the vertebral body, producing a paraspinal abscess. In the thoracolumbar area, this may be seen as mediastinal widening or a pear-shaped retrocardiac density on the chest roentgenogram. In the lumbar area, the psoas shadow may be lost. In the cervical area, the abscess may displace anteriorly and obstruct the esophagus and trachea. The firm paraspinal ligamentous structures may result in high pressure in the abscess and produce ischemic paralysis in the subjacent spinal cord. The abscess pressure also may cause it to dissect along ligamentous planes and present as a fluctuant or firm mass in the groin, the gluteal area, or the supraclavicular space.

Clinical Features and Diagnosis. Symptoms are usually insidious and prolonged and may not include fever, although weight loss is common. Local back pain is frequent, and referred pain imitating renal colic or abdominal disorders occurs. Walking may be painful, and the gait may become stilted. Miliary, meningeal, or pulmonary tuberculosis may develop and dominate the picture in the untreated case. Severe anterior angulation of the spine may eventually produce a hunchback deformity. Frequently, however, it is the development of *weakness or paralysis* which leads to medical attention. Paralysis, now the most serious consequence of Pott's disease, may develop owing to pressure from abscess fluid, to generalized inflammatory edema, or to intrusion of a bony sequestrum or granulation tissue on the anterior aspect of the cord. Paralysis caused by angulation and displacement is unusual, because the anatomic abnormality develops slowly, but violent movement may produce cord transection when spine instability is marked.

In prior years most infectious spondylitis was tuberculous. However, it is now clear that entirely similar roentgenographic and clinical pictures can be produced by several other organisms, notably staphylococci, gram-negative enterobacteria, fungi, and rarely mycobacteria other than *M. tuberculosis.* Accordingly, in the absence of strong ancillary evidence for tuberculosis, aspiration or open biopsy of the vertebral body is indicated.

Treatment. Treatment of Pott's disease is based on antimicrobial therapy and immobilization. Usually isoniazid and streptomycin or rifampin for a period of two years or more is recommended. Most orthopedists advise some form of prompt surgical intervention such as debridement of the abscess cavity and spinal fusion, followed by a prolonged period of body casting. Others, particularly in areas in which surgical facilities are limited, have reported comparable results using just drug therapy and a brief period (two or three months) of bed rest without casting. When paralysis develops or fails to improve on therapy, surgery is required, and the procedure, whether abscess evacuation, debridement of granulation tissue, or removal of sequestra, is dictated by the findings at operation. Usually some form of spinal fusion will also be carried out. Although the course of therapy is usually decided by the responsible orthopedist, it is the writer's preference to assess the effects of drug therapy and bed rest while maintaining close surveillance of the neurologic status, because many individuals will achieve stable spines and remission of neurologic symptoms without operative intervention or casting.

TUBERCULOUS ARTHRITIS

Clinical Findings and Diagnosis. Tuberculous arthritis involves the hips, knees, elbows, shoulders, and small joints of the hands and feet in roughly that order. The initial symptoms are pain on motion or weight bearing, usually with some swelling. The process is usually monarticular, chronic, and associated eventually with considerable muscle wasting, pain, and stiffness. A history of trauma to the involved joint can frequently be obtained. In the absence of proved associated tuberculosis, diagnosis requires biopsy, histologic study, and culture. The need for verification by culture has been emphasized by reports of cases of granulomatous arthritis caused by mycobacteria other than *M. tuberculosis* (see Ch. 244).

Treatment. Most authorities recommend isoniazid and daily streptomycin. It is the writer's practice to utilize isoniazid alone. Intra-articular injection of drugs is not recommended. Many and perhaps most instances of tuberculous arthritis will heal with preservation of joint function when treated with mild immobilization, bed rest in the case of weight-bearing joints, and chemotherapy. When progress is not entirely satisfactory, joint exploration and removal of hypertrophied and fragmented synovial granulation tissue may be required. Casting and procedures to effect joint fusion are rarely necessary and are often detrimental.

OTHER FORMS OF SKELETAL TUBERCULOSIS

Cystic tuberculosis of bone (tuberculous caries or *tuberculosa multiplex cystica*) is a rare condition in which osteolytic cystic areas of long and flat bones and occasionally of the tubular bones of the hands or feet are caused by tuberculosis. *Tuberculosis of the costochondral junction* may present as a cold abscess overlying the area of involvement. *Tuberculosis of the tendon sheaths and bursae is* usually secondary to involvement of the adjacent joint. These are responsive to antimycobacterial drug therapy with isoniazid alone or combined with streptomycin.

243. RARE FORMS OF TUBERCULOSIS

Ocular tuberculosis is one of the causes of *granulomatous intraocular infection. Phlyctenular keratoconjunctivitis* is a rare allergic external ocular inflammation observed in children at the time of the primary infection and characterized by small blisters (phlyctenules) at the junction of conjunctiva and cornea. *Choroidal tubercles* often provide a clue to the presence of disseminated tuberculosis. They produce no symptoms and are difficult to differentiate from other retinal exudates.

Cutaneous tuberculosis, once important but now only rarely seen, is usually grouped into two categories. The first, in which organisms are present, includes *lupus vulgaris, tuberculosis verrucosa cutis* (anatomic or prosector's wart), *scrofuloderma* (the skin changes surrounding a draining tuberculous sinus or overlying a tuberculous node), and *tuberculosis orificialis* (nodular and ulcerated lesions around the mouth or other orifice through which highly infectious material passes). These are all very responsive to isoniazid. The second group comprises the *tuberculids* (including *erythema induratum* or Bazin's disease). These reactions are thought to be allergic and comprise a variety of erythematous, papular, and ulcerative forms. Their relationship to tuberculosis is poorly understood. *Tuberculosis cutis miliaris acuta disseminata* is a rare complication of overwhelming miliary tuberculosis, usually in children.

Tuberculosis of the adrenals is important only as a now uncommon cause of adrenal insufficiency. Tuberculosis of the *spleen, thyroid, pancreas,* and *breast* may all occur and mimic other infections or neoplastic change in these organs.

Bentley, G., and Webster, J. H. H.: Gastrointestinal tuberculosis. A 10-year review. Br. J. Surg., 54:90, 1967.

Bobrowitz, I. D.: Ethambutol compared to streptomycin in original treatment of advanced pulmonary tuberculosis. Chest, 60:14, 1971.

Brown, A. B., Gilbert, R. A., and TeLinde, R. W.: Pelvic tuberculosis. Obstet. Gynecol., 2:476, 1953.

Canetti, G.: Present aspects of bacterial resistance in tuberculosis. Am. Rev. Respir. Dis., 92:687, 1965.

Diagnostic Standards and Classification of Tuberculosis. New York, National Tuberculosis and Respiratory Disease Association, 1969.

East African/British Medical Research Councils: Controlled clinical trial of short-course (6-month) regimens of chemotherapy for treatment of pulmonary tuberculosis. Lancet, 1:1079, 1972.

Garibaldi, R. A., Drusin, R. E., Ferebee, S. H., and Gregg, M. B.: Isoniazid-associated hepatitis. Report of an outbreak. Am. Rev. Respir. Dis., 106:357, 1972.

Goyette, E. M.: Treatment of tuberculous pericarditis. Prog. Cardiovasc. Dis., 3:141, 1960.

Kent, D. C.: Tuberculous lymphadenitis: Not a localized disease process. Am. J. Med. Sci., 254:866, 1967.

Konstam, P. G., and Blesovsky, A.: The ambulant treatment of spinal tuberculosis. Br. J. Surg., 50:26, 1962.

Mackaness, G. B.: The immunology of antituberculous immunity. Am. Rev. Respir. Dis., 97:337, 1968.

Moulding, T.: Chemoprophylaxis of tuberculosis: When is the benefit worth the risk and cost? Ann. Intern. Med., 76:761, 1971.

Munt, P. W.: Miliary tuberculosis in the chemotherapy era: With a clinical review in 69 American adults. Medicine, 51:139, 1971.

Newman, R., Doster, B., Murray, F. J., and Ferebee, S.: Rifampin in initial treatment of pulmonary tuberculosis. A U.S. Public Health Service tuberculosis therapy trial. Am. Rev. Respir. Dis., 103:461, 1971.

Proudfoot, A. T., Akhtar, A. J., Douglas, A. C., and Horne, N. W.: Miliary tuberculosis in adults. Br. Med. J., 2:273, 1969.
Rich, A.: The Pathogenesis of Tuberculosis. 2nd ed. Springfield, Ill., Charles C Thomas, 1952.
Smith, D. T.: Diagnostic and prognostic significance of the quantitative tuberculin tests. Ann. Int. Med., 67:919, 1967.
Smith, D. T.: Isoniazid prophylaxis and BCG vaccination in the control of tuberculosis. Arch. Environ. Health, 23:235, 1971.
Sochocky, S.: Tuberculous peritonitis. A review of 100 cases. Amer. Rev. Resp. Dis., 95:398, 1967.
Stead, W. W.: Pathogenesis of a first episode of chronic pulmonary tuberculosis in man: Recrudescence of residuals of the primary infection or exogenous reinfection? Am. Rev. Respir. Dis., 95:729, 1967.
Twomey, J. J., and Leavell, B. S.: Leukemoid reactions to tuberculosis. Arch. Intern. Med., 116:21, 1965.
Vall-Spinosa, A., Lester, W., Moulding, T., Davidson, P. T., and McClatchy, J. K.: Rifampin in the treatment of drug-resistant *Mycobacterium tuberculosis* infections. N. Engl. J. Med., 283:616, 1970.
Youmans, G. P., and Youmans, A. S.: Recent studies on acquired immunity in tuberculosis. Curr. Top. Microbiol. Immunol., 48:129, 1969.

244. DISEASES DUE TO MYCOBACTERIA OTHER THAN M. TUBERCULOSIS AND M. LEPRAE

Robert Goodwin

The term tuberculosis traditionally refers to infection associated with *M. tuberculosis (var. hominis* and *var. bovis).* It has long been known that other mycobacterial species exist in nature, some of which cause disease in animals. For years their role in human disease was unappreciated, owing largely to the overwhelming prevalence of *M. tuberculosis.* When found, their significance was denied because of the notion that mycobacteria were human pathogens only if they produced disease in the guinea pig (these did not). In recent years modern culture methods and drug susceptibility studies stimulated by the chemotherapy era have identified many mycobacterial species other than *M. tuberculosis* in human disease tissue.

Much of the most important bacteriologic work on these "atypical" mycobacteria has been carried out by Runyon, who classified them into four groups primarily on the basis of the presence and type of pigment production and growth rate. (See Bacteriology in Ch. 227). Most recently most of the known human pathogens have received tentative species designations, which will be employed herein. The relationship of these to the Runyon classification is as follows: *M. kansasii* and *M. marinum*—Runyon Group I (photochromogens); *M. scrofulaceum*—Runyon Group II (scotochromogens); *M. intracellulare* (Battey bacillus), *M. avium,* and *M. xenopi*—Runyon Group III (nonpigmented species); *M. fortuitum*—Runyon Group IV (rapid growers).

Human infection with many of these organisms is widespread throughout tropical and subtropical areas of the world. Their epidemiology is obscure. Many of the organisms involved are widespread in nature, being found particularly in the soil and in water. *M. kansasii* has been recovered from milk in Dallas and tapwater in California, but its source in nature is not clear. *M. intracellulare* is readily found in soil and in house dust, and has been demonstrated in throat swabs of normal individuals. *M. avium,* also of widespread distribution, is found in chickens and other birds as well as in household mammals. *M. scrofulaceum* has been isolated from soil and water, and is frequently found in oropharyngeal secretions of healthy men. *There is no evidence of man-to-man transmission of any of these, and no source case has ever been identified in human disease.*

The diseases produced by these organisms have roentgenologic, pathologic, and, to some extent, clinical similarities to tuberculosis, but there are distinct differences in virulence, treatment, and prognosis. The term *mycobacteriosis* has been suggested to differentiate them from tuberculosis. However, species orientation is preferable, because there are differences in organ susceptibility, treatment, and prognosis. It is convenient from a clinical standpoint to group these infections according to organ involvement. Pulmonary disease, mainly in older white men, is the most common clinical manifestation. Lymphadenitis in children and granulomatous skin lesions in all age groups are next in frequency. Injection abscesses are not uncommon. Rarely, disseminated disease, meningitis, renal or skeletal involvement, and penetrating wound infection are reported.

PULMONARY DISEASE

M. kansasii and *M. intracellulare* (Battey bacilli), and less frequently *M. avium,* may produce a tuberculosis-like pulmonary disease in susceptible individuals, as may rarely the less virulent *M. fortuitum, M. xenopi,* and *M. chelonei* (subsp. chelonei) and even more rarely *M. aquae, M. szulgai,* and *M. scrofulaceum.*

Prevalence. In the United States and Europe, 1 to 2 per cent of hospital admissions for tuberculosis are due to infection with either *M. kansasii* or *M. intracellulare.* There are geographical variations, particularly in the United States. The prevalence of *M. intracellulare* infections is relatively high in Georgia and northern Florida, and *M. kansasii* infection is much more frequent in the Dallas and Chicago areas. In some localities the incidence is as high as 7 to 10 per cent of annual hospital admissions for tuberculosis.

Clinical Manifestations. Pulmonary disease caused by *M. kansasii, M. intracellulare,* and *M. avium* primarily affects white males over the age of 45, less frequently, females and blacks. Chronic bronchitis and emphysema are present in some series in 40 per cent of patients with disease caused by *M. kansasii* and in 60 per cent of those with disease caused by *M. intracellulare.* Although virulence is less, disease, once established, tends to become cavitary and progressive. The clinical picture at any given time is indistinguishable from that of chronic pulmonary tuberculosis. Although in general slower in tempo than untreated tuberculosis, these infections may produce relentless destruction of pulmonary tissue and lead to death from respiratory insufficiency. Constitutional symptoms are much less prominent, local symptoms of cough and sputum are similar, and hemoptysis may occur somewhat more frequently than in tuberculosis. Roentgenographic studies usually reveal far-advanced disease at the time of discovery. Cavities are more frequently thin walled and pneumonic lesions less prominent than in tuberculosis, but there is much overlap, and roentgenographic differentiation is not possible in the individual case. Lesions have the apical posterior localization characteristic of tuberculosis. Pleural effusions are uncommon, and pleural changes of any sort are inconspicuous. Pathologic changes cannot be distinguished from those of tuberculosis, although in general the process appears more chronic with more fibrosis and less caseation.

Diagnosis is dependent upon bacteriologic identification of the specific organisms. With the exception of *M.*

kansasii, mycobacteria other than *M. tuberculosis* may be found in oropharyngeal secretions of normal persons, and therefore diagnosis of disease requires repeated demonstration of the organism in significant numbers in the presence of compatible pulmonary disease. A tuberculosis-like disease that does not respond to antimicrobial therapy or the demonstration of a high order of primary drug resistance should suggest the possibility of another mycobacterial species.

Treatment. Mycobacteriosis, excepting to some extent *M. kansasii* infection, differs most strikingly from tuberculosis in conspicuous lack of susceptibility to the antituberculous drugs. Pulmonary disease caused by these less virulent agents is therefore much more difficult to treat than drug-susceptible tuberculosis. *M. kansasii* is partially responsive to antituberculous drugs, and their use is usually recommended. Isoniazid-streptomycin-ethambutol is an effective starting regimen, which should be modified when drug susceptibility reports are available. In vitro and animal studies suggest that rifampin may be highly effective. The addition of this drug to the aforementioned regimen or its substitution for ethambutol in serious infection is reasonable, but a final statement awaits further clinical trials. Surgical excision may be necessary in treatment failures. The use of drugs is generally disappointing in disease caused by *M. intracellulare,* and probably entirely ineffective against *M. avium, M. fortuitum,* and other rare atypical pulmonary mycobacterial infections. There is no established plan for drug management of disease caused by *M. intracellulare* or the other drug-resistant mycobacterial infections. Although some strains are occasionally partially susceptible to some of the drugs, this is quite unpredictable. The most commonly useful drugs are isoniazid, ethambutol, ethionamide, pyrazinamide, and cycloserine. Rifampin should be tried. Multiple drugs increase the chance of success but at greater risk of toxicity. When effective, drugs are usually continued for one year after the sputum is free from bacilli. To the degree that drug therapy is less useful, other methods of treatment become more so. Hospitalization and a fairly confining type of rest therapy are recommended. Most agree that residual cavities should be resected, if possible, whether or not the sputum has been rendered noninfectious. The incidence of surgical complications is remarkably low even without effective drug coverage.

A statement of *prognosis* must be quite broad. The persistence of the bacilli in the sputum despite drug treatment is an unfavorable sign. Sputum free from bacilli for a year with no residual cavity (with or without surgery) indicates a good prognosis with a relapse rate perhaps no greater than 5 to 10 per cent. With vigorous treatment, including the use of surgery when indicated, the best success rates in pulmonary disease caused by *M. kansasii* are in the range of 85 per cent, and in disease caused by *M. intracellulare,* 75 per cent.

LYMPHADENITIS

Infants and young children may respond to a primary infection with certain atypical mycobacteria with the clinical manifestations of scrofula. Reports from the United States, Europe, and Australia in recent years indicate that 75 per cent of granulomatous cervical adenitis suggestive of tuberculosis is actually caused by mycobacteria other than *M. tuberculosis. M. scrofulaceum,* a scotochromogen, *M. avium, M. intracellulare,* and, less commonly, *M. kansasii* are the responsible agents. Each of these may be the predominant cause of adenitis in certain geographical areas and not found at all in others. In the vast majority the adenitis is cervical, occasionally preauricular, and rarely inguinal, axillary, or epitrochlear. Cervical adenitis most commonly occurs in the submaxillary and submandibular areas and is almost always unilateral, in most instances representing a regional component of a primary infection. Submaxillary and submandibular involvement suggests that the buccal mucosa is the portal of entry; involvement of the preauricular node implies conjunctival infection. In the extremities the infection usually follows a puncture wound. The pathology of the lesion is similar to that of tuberculosis, as are the clinical manifestations. Enlarged, firm, and nontender single nodes or groups of nodes may appear and persist unchanged or progress to fluctuation, drainage, and sinus formation, sometimes quite rapidly. Surgical excision is usually employed for both diagnosis and treatment. Infections with *M. kansasii* may be an exception, and a trial of drug treatment is indicated (see Pulmonary Disease, above). Isoniazid treatment of granulomatous cervical adenitis is recommended prior to cultural identification, because the infection may be due to *M. tuberculosis.* If antigens are available, the demonstration of skin hypersensitivity to some other mycobacterial species and a negative or smaller reaction to PPD-S *(M. tuberculosis)* is regarded as diagnostic. PPD-B (Battey) may be used for this purpose. Although recurrence may develop in an adjacent lymph node, surgical excision of grossly involved nodes is usually curative.

SUPERFICIAL SKIN DISEASE

In addition to *M. leprae* (leprosy) and *M. tuberculosis,* two other mycobacteria, *M. marinum* and *M. ulcerans,* occasionally produce skin infections. Both have temperature requirements below 37° C, accounting for limitation of infection to superficial areas of the skin. *M. marinum,* previously referred to as *M. balnei,* is a photochromogenic saprophyte first described in marine fish. It is widely distributed in nature, occurring in soil, water and freshwater fish as well. The temperature for optimal growth is 30 to 32° C. It has been implicated in epidemics of granulomatous skin disease traced to infected swimming pools, beaches of several of the Hawaiian Islands, and more rarely tropical fish aquariums. The granulomas occur at the site of minor abrasions, most commonly on the elbows, but also on the knees, toes, fingers, dorsum of the feet, and bridge of the nose, appearing two to three weeks after exposure as papules or nodules which increase slowly in size and may ulcerate. Spontaneous healing is to be expected after several months. Diagnosis may be established by culturing a biopsy of the lesion at 30° C. Histologically, the tissue usually suggests a tuberculosis-like granuloma, but may appear to be a nonspecific chronic inflammatory reaction. Rifampin may speed spontaneous healing.

Disease caused by *M. ulcerans* is relatively rare in most areas of the world but strangely is quite common in the Buruli district of the upper Nile in Africa. This organism has a limited temperature requirement in the range of 32 to 33° C. Disease begins as a painless nodule, usually on the extremities, which may grow rapidly and ulcerate. The ulcers (Buruli ulcers), seldom less than 5 cm in diameter and often much larger, have characteristic undermined margins. They tend to be persistent and progressively destructive. Surgical excision is curative and is much simpler when the lesion is recognized in the preulcerative stage.

OTHER INFECTIONS

More than 100 cases of *injection abscesses* have been reported, mostly caused by the common saprophyte, *M. fortuitum,* but also by *M. chelonei* (subsp. abscessus). These have occurred mostly in adults and respond to incision and drainage. The same organisms, and more rarely *M. kansasii,* have occasionally caused penetrating wound infections. *M. fortuitum* infection may result in corneal ulceration after trauma.

A dozen or so usually fatal cases of *disseminated* infection have been reported in young children and more rarely in immunologically deficient adults. Many different mycobacteria have been implicated, including *M. kansasii, M. avium, M. intracellulare, M. scrofulaceum,* and *M. fortuitum.* Multiple and single *bone and joint* lesions have been reported, mostly in children. Rare cases of *meningitis* in children and adults are reported with *M. avium* and *M. kansasii.* One case of renal infection caused by *M. kansasii* has been found.

Bates, J. H.: A study of pulmonary disease associated with mycobacteria other than *Mycobacterium tuberculosis:* Clinical characteristics. Am. Rev. Respir. Dis., 96:1151, 1967.
Lincoln, E. M., and Gilbert, L. A.: Disease in children due to mycobacteria other than *Mycobacterium tuberculosis.* Am. Rev. Respir. Dis., 105:683, 1972.
Pfuetze, K. H., and Hubble, R.: Nontuberculous mycobacterial diseases. Disease-a-Month, September 1968.
Schaefer, W. B., and Davis, C. L.: A bacteriologic and histopathologic study of skin granuloma due to *Mycobacterium balnei.* Am. Rev. Respir. Dis., 84:837, 1961.
Selkon, J. B.: 'Atypical' mycobacteria: A review. Tubercle (Suppl.), 50:70, 1969.

245. LEPROSY (Hansen's Disease)

M. F. R. Waters

Definition. Leprosy is a chronic inflammatory disease of man caused by *Mycobacterium leprae,* which displays a wide clinical "spectrum" related to host ability to develop specific cell-mediated immunity (CMI). In high resistant "tuberculoid" leprosy, the localized signs are restricted to skin and nerve. Low resistant "lepromatous" leprosy is a generalized disease involving many systems, with widespread lesions of skin, peripheral nerves, upper respiratory tract, eyes, testes, and the reticuloendothelial system. Common complications include more acute, immunologically mediated, inflammatory episodes ("reactions"), secondary inflammation in the anesthetic areas which result from nerve damage, and deformity of hands, feet, and face.

Etiology and Microbiology. Although Hansen recognized the leprosy bacillus in 1873, as yet *M. leprae* has not been cultured in vitro. There is no known animal reservoir. Past attempts to infect human volunteers were unsatisfactory, and successful experimental transmission was not achieved until 1960, when Shepard reported limited infection in mouse footpads. Since that date, leprosy has been one of the fastest growing points in medical research. In 1967, Rees and his colleagues obtained lepromatous leprosy in thymectomized-irradiated mice. More recently, Kirchheimer and Storrs (1971) have described lepromatous leprosy developing in a proportion of immunologically normal nine-banded armadillos inoculated with leprosy bacilli.

M. leprae is an intracellular, rod-shaped, acid-fast organism, 1 to 7 μ long and 0.25 μ in width; morphologically it resembles *M. tuberculosis.* However, in suspensions prepared from lepromatous tissues, bacilli are frequently arranged in characteristic "cigar-bundle" groups and in larger aggregates or "globi" derived from multinucleate Virchow giant cells. The cytoplasm of many bacilli is fragmented; such bacilli are dead. The percentage of solid-staining, presumed viable bacilli is known as the morphologic index (MI). Dead organisms are only slowly broken down, and may remain in tissues for many months or years.

In normal mice, a footpad inoculum of 5000 or 10,000 bacilli yields 10^6 after about six months, but no subsequent increase occurs. During the log phase of multiplication, the generation time is 12 to 13 days, the longest of any known bacterium. In thymectomized-irradiated mice, yields of 10^9 bacilli per footpad are not uncommon and systemic spread occurs, but the generation time remains unchanged. The footpad technique has been applied to studying the effect of drugs in leprosy, the detection of drug resistance, and the immunology and pathogenesis of the disease.

M. leprae is most easily detected in patients by Wade's "scraped incision" method. After cleansing, the skin is pinched to exclude blood, and a small cut made in the skinfold some 2 to 3 mm deep. One side of the cut is then scraped with the back of the scalpel point. The tissue pulp collected on the blade is spread on a glass slide, dried, fixed, and stained by the Ziehl-Neelsen method, care being taken never to overheat the carbolfuchsin. Leprosy bacilli are very scanty in tuberculoid lesions, and are often not detected by routine methods. They become more numerous as the spectrum is crossed and are present in huge numbers in lepromatous lesions. A lepromatous patient may have more than 10^{12} bacilli in the body. The density of bacilli in smears or tissues is termed the bacterial index (BI).

A standardized, autoclaved suspension of *M. leprae* is used as a prognostic intradermal skin test, the "lepromin test," which gives an accurate assessment of specific CMI in leprosy patients; it is negative in lepromatous and positive in tuberculoid leprosy. However, the test is often positive in nonleprosy patients, including those who have never visited leprosy endemic areas, and shows some cross-reactivity with tuberculin. Therefore it is of no diagnostic or epidemiologic value.

Incidence and Prevalence. Although governmental returns indicate a world total of 11 million leprosy patients, many consider that 15 million is a more accurate estimate, and that 1 million new patients will arise over the next 5 years. The importance of leprosy lies not only in numbers but also in the chronicity of the disease, which frequently disables but now seldom kills. Therefore it makes disproportionate demands on the health services and economies of developing countries.

Leprosy occurs in almost all tropical and warm temperate regions, including Japan and Korea, and is endemic in several states of the United States. It has only recently died out in certain northern European countries and Canada. It seems to be related particularly to overcrowding, so that as living standards rise, the disease becomes less common.

Epidemiology. Because *M. leprae* cannot be cultured, and because there is no simple, specific immunologic test of past or present infection, epidemiologic studies have hitherto been restricted to clinical cases. These have been further hampered by the long incubation period of three or more years. Close (household) contacts of lepromatous patients may show a tenfold higher incidence of leprosy and those of tuberculoid patients a twofold higher incidence than the general population. Lepromatous patients are thought to form the main source of infection in the community.

The lepromatous dermis is full of bacilli, but these are not shed in significant numbers through the intact epidermis. However, leprosy bacilli are excreted freely in lepromatous nasal secretions, so that 24-hour yields are comparable in numbers to those of *M. tuberculosis* coughed up in cavitary pulmonary tuberculosis. Bacilli from dried nasal secretions remain viable after being kept in the dark for at least 24 hours, and thus could be largely responsible for the spread of leprosy. The possibility of insect spread is also being reinvestigated. It has been assumed, without proof, that *M. leprae* gains entry through the skin or the respiratory tract.

Studies in twins and other subjects suggest that lepromatous disease is a host-determined characteristic possessed by a fixed proportion of all people. Godal (1971) has recently developed a specific lymphocyte transformation test (LTT) which may help to clarify the epidemiology of leprosy.

Pathology and Clinical Manifestations. Leprosy has two special features. One is the invasion by *M. leprae* of certain superficial nerves, which may become thickened and firm. The other is the wide range of clinical and histologic manifestations, reflecting the intricacies of the host-parasite relationship. Skin lesions, which are best seen in good oblique light, may occur anywhere, save on the hairy scalp and perineum. Nerves of predilection, which should always be palpated, include the ulnars at and above the medial humeral epicondyle, the superficial radials and medians at the wrist, the great auriculars at the edge of the sternocleidomastoid muscle, and the lateral popliteals (common peroneal) at the neck of the fibula. Appropriate muscle weakness and wasting may occur, resulting in claw hand (ulnar and/or median), foot drop, claw toes, and facial nerve paralysis, the last-named usually incomplete but including lagophthalmos. Wrist drop is comparatively rare.

The spectrum of leprosy has been particularly well defined by Ridley and Jopling, who proposed a five-group system of classification according to certain immunologic features, principally *the cytology* of the host cells of the macrophage-histiocyte series (whether histiocytic or epithelioid), *the bacterial density,* and *the degree of infiltration by lymphocytes.* Their classification enables the majority of patients to be diagnosed accurately from the clinical features, although the intermediate "borderline" (dimorphous) groups are relatively unstable, and tend to move toward lepromatous in the absence of treatment and toward tuberculoid after institution of effective chemotherapy. The five groups are, in order across the spectrum, *tuberculoid* (TT), *borderline-tuberculoid* (BT), *borderline* (BB), *borderline-lepromatous* (BL), and *lepromatous* (LL). Their distinctive clinical manifestations are now described, and these, with their corresponding pathologic, bacteriologic, and immunologic features, are summarized in the accompanying table.

Tuberculoid (TT). The typical tuberculoid lesion is large and annular, with a sharply raised outer edge and a thin erythematous rim which slopes gradually to a hypopigmented, flattened center. In profile, it resembles a saucer the right way up. The surface is dry, hairless, and sometimes scaly, with loss of sweating and marked anesthesia. Sometimes the lesion is a plaque with a dry, pebbly surface, or a macule. The lesion is usually single—at most two or three may be present—and, frequently, running to it may be palpated a thickened cutaneous sensory nerve in which caseation may occur. Sometimes, one of the nerves of predilection in the region of the skin lesion may be enlarged; rarely the only sign is a thickened nerve. Tuberculoid leprosy appears to be related to delay in the development of adequate cell-mediated immunity, and it forms a stable group.

Borderline-Tuberculoid (BT). The skin lesions resemble those of TT leprosy, but are usually multiple, though asymmetrical, and smaller in size, or else small "satellite" lesions may be present near the periphery of larger lesions. Sharp-edged papules may also occur. Enlarged cutaneous sensory nerves are less commonly found, but frequently one or more nerves of predilection are thickened. Therefore BT leprosy is often associated with deformity of one or both hands and/or feet; a patient may present with, or later develop, a plantar ulcer in an anesthetic foot or burns or infection of anesthetic fingers. Lagophthalmos may result in exposure keratitis.

Borderline (BB). The rather numerous, though asymmetrical, skin lesions are erythematous or hyperpigmented, and vary markedly in size. They occur as papules, plaques, and most characteristically as annular lesions with broad rims. The outer edge is often flattish and irregular; it rises to a thick inner edge, and the anesthetic, hypopigmented center is always sharply "punched out." The profile resembles a saucer the wrong way up, except that where the cup should sit is a deep central depression. Satellite lesions are common. Moderate and widespread, though asymmetrical, enlargement of the nerves of predilection may occur with or without associated muscle weakness and wasting.

Borderline-Lepromatous (BL). The skin lesions are numerous, but are not usually bilaterally symmetrical. They consist of erythematous or hyperpigmented papules, nodules, or plaques which appear moist and succulent, and which possess normal sensation or show only mild hypoesthesia. Small, indefinite-edged, hypopigmented macules may also be present. Some nodules may be dimpled, and often one or two lesions, usually the first to appear, have punched-out, hypopigmented, anesthetic centers, indicating progression from BB leprosy. Nerves of predilection close to the latter are often markedly thickened; elsewhere they may be only slightly enlarged. Ear lobes may appear normal, or be asymmetrically (more rarely symmetrically) enlarged. The eyebrows, nasal cartilage, and eyes are unaffected. Although bacilli are very numerous in the lesions, they are often undetected in normal-looking skin.

Lepromatous (LL). Lesions show marked bilateral symmetry. Skin lesions are very numerous, with erythematous, smooth, shiny surfaces, and are neither anes-

Summary of the Clinical, Histological, Bacteriological and Immunological Findings of the Five Groups of the Leprosy Spectrum

	TT	BT	BB	BL	LL
Skin lesions					
Numbers	1 to 3	Very few to moderate	Moderate	Moderate to many	Very many
Symmetry	Very asymmetrical	Asymmetrical	Asymmetrical	Slightly asymmetrical	Symmetrical
Anesthesia	Very marked	Marked	Marked to moderate	Slight to nil	Nil
Nerve enlargement					
Cutaneous sensory	Common	May occur	0	0	0
Peripheral nerves*	0 or one	Common; asymmetrical	Common; asymmetrical	Moderately asymmetrical	Symmetrical
Skin histology					
Granuloma cell	Epithelioid	Epithelioid	Epithelioid	Histiocyte	Foamy histiocyte
Lymphocytes	+++	+++	+	± or ++	±†
Dermal nerves	Destroyed	Mostly destroyed	Some visible	Visible	Easily visible
Bacilli numbers (routine examination)	0	0, + or ++	+, ++ or +++	++++	+++++
Lymph nodes					
Paracortical infiltrate	Nil; immunoblasts	Sarcoid-like	Diffuse epithelioid	Diffuse histiocytes	Massive infiltrate with foamy histiocytes and Virchow cells
Germinal centers	Normal	Normal	Normal	Some hypertrophy	Gross hypertrophy
Lepromin test	+++	++	± or 0	0	0
Reactions					
ENL	0	0	0	Rare	Very common
Lepra	?	Common	Very common	Very common	(Rare)‡

*Nerves of predilection, i.e. ulnar, median, lateral popliteal, facial, great auricular, and posterior tibial.
†In LL leprosy, the peripheral blood shows an absolute decrease in T and an absolute increase in B lymphocytes.
‡Lepra reactions are occasionally seen in treated LL patients who have developed from borderline (BT, BB, or BL) in the absence of treatment.

thetic nor anhidrotic. Early cases may have numerous, small, hypopigmented macules with vague edges and small papules with indefinite edges; nerves may be but slightly thickened at this stage, although significant involvement of the nasal mucosa is frequently detected. With time, plaques and nodules develop, and the skin progressively thickens as lepromatous infiltrate increases; rarely, but especially in Central America, infiltrate alone occurs. The ear lobes enlarge, and the lines of the face coarsen and deepen (leonine facies). The lips often swell, and the eyebrows and eyelashes become scanty and are lost. Iritis and keratitis are common. Nasal blockage occurs, with ulceration and blood-streaked discharge, and in time the nasal cartilage and bones may be gradually destroyed, resulting in saddle-nose deformity. Lepromatous laryngitis may cause hoarseness. Edema of the extremities may occur, lymph nodes often enlarge, and testicular involvement frequently leads to atrophy and occasionally to gynecomastia. Dermal nerve damage leads to a progressive pseudo-"glove-and-stocking" anesthesia; light touch, pain, and temperature sensation are eventually lost over most of the body except scalp and flexures, but position sense is well preserved. Very numerous bacilli are present not only in the skin, in the draining lymph nodes, and in nerves of predilection, but also in the liver, spleen, bone marrow, and blood; there are relatively few in the kidney, and the lungs, heart, and central nervous system are not clinically involved in the infection.

In some peoples, such as the Chinese, many of the lepromatous cases originate as borderline, and a small number of residual BB-type lesions may be found; otherwise the signs are consistent with LL. In treated LL patients whose disease relapses, the new lesions are usually asymmetrical initially, but otherwise retain lepromatous characteristics.

Indeterminate Leprosy. Some child contacts of adult cases develop a single (occasionally two or three) hypopigmented macule, 2 to 5 cm in diameter, which shows hypoesthesia and decreased sweating. Histologically, there is lymphocytic infiltrate around the dermal appendages and neurovascular bundles. If left untreated, about one quarter later develop leprosy which may be of any type on the spectrum.

Reactions. ***Erythema Nodosum Leprosum (ENL)—Lepromatous Lepra Reaction.*** More than 50 per cent of treated LL patients, and the occasional untreated LL or treated BL patient, suffer from episodes of erythema nodosum leprosum. Over the course of a few hours, a crop of painful erythematous papules develops, typically on the exterior surfaces of the limbs and the face, but in severe attacks over much of the body except the scalp. The papules last for two to three days, becoming more purple, and then gradually subside, leaving dark staining of the skin. The episodes are usually associated with fever and general malaise. They may be isolated or may occur continuously over months or years, leading, if untreated, to gross prostration, weakness, and occasionally death. In severe ENL, the papules may form sterile pustules and ulcers. A frequent complication is painful neuritis, usually of the ulnar, median, or lateral popliteal nerves, and muscle weakness may increase. Lymphadenitis, iritis, and orchitis may also occur, and more rarely nephritis and large-joint arthritis. The ENL is due to immune complex formation, resulting in vasculitis and polymorphonuclear infiltrate. The antigen is probably derived from the cytoplasm of dead leprosy bacilli, and serum immunoglobulin levels are markedly elevated in LL leprosy.

Nonlepromatous Lepra Reactions. These occur very frequently in BT, BB, and BL leprosy. The leprous lesions themselves become markedly swollen, erythematous, and often scaly, and new lesions may appear. The reaction lasts for many weeks or months. Systemic upset and fever are uncommon, but neuritis may occur, and ulceration of the friable skin may lead to unsightly scarring. The reaction is often associated with change in specific CMI and therefore of a patient's leprosy classification, so that untreated patients become more lepromatous and treated patients more tuberculoid.

Diagnosis and Differential Diagnosis. It is essential to consider leprosy in all patients with skin or peripheral nerve lesions who have resided in endemic areas. The three most helpful findings are (1) thickening of one or more nerves, either of predilection or cutaneous sensory; nerve enlargement is found in some TT, many BT, and the great majority of BB, BL, and LL patients; (2) anesthetic skin lesions, which are found in almost all TT, BT, and BB patients, in many BL patients, and in those LL patients who have evolved from borderline; and (3) acid-fast bacilli (AFB) in skin smears, which are positive in many BT and in all untreated BB, BL, and LL patients. Smears are usually taken from both ear lobes and up to six typical skin lesions. Leprosy should be suspected when skin or nasal symptoms persist despite routine treatment; in chronic, painless, plantar ulceration; in foot drop unassociated with trauma; or in unusual presentations of arthritis and erythema nodosum. Confirmation should be obtained by skin biopsy or, in neural leprosy without skin lesions, by biopsy of a thickened sensory nerve.

Lack of anesthesia differentiates vitiligo, mycotic infections, lupus erythematosus, and psoriasis from TT and BT leprosy. Nerves are not enlarged in neurologic conditions such as syringomyelia, motor neuron disease, and Friedreich's ataxia; they are enlarged in hereditary sensory neuropathy of Déjérine and Sotta, which can be differentiated by the absence of skin lesions and of AFB and by the familial history. Dermal leishmaniasis, yaws, secondary syphilis, and neurofibromatosis may resemble LL leprosy, but there is no nerve thickening, and smears for AFB are negative.

Treatment. Treatment is made difficult by the excessive prejudice and outdated fear of leprosy persisting in many cultures, and by the extreme chronicity of the infection and slowness of response to treatment which is related in part to the unique generation time of *M. leprae*.

Treatment of the Infection. The drug of choice remains DDS (dapsone, 4-4′diaminodiphenyl sulfone), which is as cheap as aspirin and may be administered by mouth or parenterally. In LL and BL patients, clinical improvement is detected from about three months after starting DDS (often earlier in TT, BT, and BB leprosy), and around this time bacilli from nose and skin will no longer infect mice. The MI reaches zero by six months, but the BI takes many years to become negative. Small numbers of viable bacilli have been shown to persist, possibly in Schwann cells and other special sites, in LL patients treated continuously for at least ten years; such patients may relapse if treatment is stopped. Therefore it is recommended that DDS be given for the following minimum periods:

Intermediate and TT	3 years
BT	5 years
BB	7 years
BL	10 years
LL	20 years or for life

Although the minimal effective dose of DDS is less than 1 mg, the recommended standard adult dose in LL and BL leprosy is 100 mg daily by mouth or 300 to 400 mg twice weekly by injection. This results in an incidence of drug resistance of only 2.5 per cent, whereas the incidence may be many times higher on lower dosage, especially if irregularly taken. DDS resistance has not yet been reported from the other types of leprosy (TT, BT, BB, and indeterminate), in which bacillary loads are so much lower. In these, a dosage of 25 to 50 mg DDS daily is acceptable.

Sulfone resistance has been detected 5 to 25 years after the start of treatment, sometimes long after the patient has become smear negative. New active lesions, usually asymmetrical papules and small plaques with high BI and MI, are found on a background of old, resolving, or resolved lepromatous leprosy. Bacilli from these lesions will grow in the footpads of mice treated with DDS mixed in their diet (Pettit and Rees, 1964). Clinically, resistance must be distinguished from relapse off treatment by a therapeutic trial of DDS, 400 mg given regularly twice weekly by injection. In drug-susceptible relapse, uninterrupted improvement occurs. In resistant patients, some initial improvement may occur if there is a mixed bacterial population of partially and highly resistant organisms, but the MI is unlikely to fall to 0, and further new lesions, with raised MI, will sooner or later appear.

Toxic effects of DDS include dose-related sulfhemoglobinemia and hemolytic anemia, the latter especially in glucose-6-phosphate dehydrogenase–deficient patients. Drug allergy, which occurs in one in several hundred cases, may be serious and even fatal; three to seven weeks after starting DDS the patient develops fever, pruritus, and dermatitis, which may become exfoliative, and jaundice and psychosis sometimes occur. DDS must be stopped immediately and prednisolone given for several weeks.

Alternative treatment is required in sulfone allergy and in proved cases of sulfone resistance. *Clofazimine* (B663, Lamprene), a rimino-phenazine dye, is both antimycobacterial and, in high dosage, anti-inflammatory. It is relatively nontoxic, its chief disadvantage being that it causes a reddish-brown pigmentation of the skin which is objectionable to most light-skinned patients. In a dose of 100 mg daily, it appears clinically and bacteriologically approximately as effective as DDS. Clofazimine resistance has not yet been reported, although the drug has been given for over ten years to sulfone-resistant patients. It is used widely in dark-skinned races, in a dose of 100 mg three or four times a day, to control ENL and lepra reactions, although several weeks elapse before its full anti-inflammatory effect is produced.

Rifampin is bactericidal. It kills leprosy bacilli faster than any other drug tried hitherto, so that patients may be rendered minimal public health risks within a few days; clinical improvement is seen in about three weeks, and the MI falls to zero within six weeks. It has been used for over six years in the treatment of DDS-resistant leprosy, usually in combination with the second-line drug thiambutosine, with excellent results, although the

BI falls no faster than with clofazimine. Dosage is 600 mg daily, and intermittent therapy is under trial. Rifampin combined with DDS may also be of value in the initial therapy of sulfone-sensitive LL leprosy, when a rapid therapeutic effect is especially desirable.

Treatment of Reactions. In mild erythema nodosum leprosum, paracetamol or aspirin may suffice. Somewhat more severe episodes often respond to two or three courses of stibophen, 2 ml daily parenterally for five days. In severe continuous ENL, or in all episodes complicated by significant neuritis or iritis, there are three alternative regimens. Prednisolone, given in addition to DDS, rapidly suppresses ENL, but in the long term severe steroid toxicity is common. Therefore steroids are best reserved for short-term cover for operations, childbirth, and similar situations. The drug thalidomide is equally effective in controlling reactions, but its use is contraindicated in women because of its teratogenic potential. The dosage is initially 200 mg twice daily; subsequently it is progressively lowered to a maintenance dose, usually of 50 to 100 mg nightly, which may be continued for years. DDS must not be discontinued. The third alternative is clofazimine in high dosage. In light-skinned males and postmenopausal females thalidomide is probably the drug of choice; in dark-skinned patients and premenopausal women clofazimine is the safest drug, provided that a rapid action is not required. *Lepra reactions* can often be controlled with paracetamol, with or without stibophen. But whenever neuritis occurs or when there is risk of skin ulceration, the signs of inflammation should be suppressed with prednisolone. Although steroids may be required for some months, toxicity is rare, because the dosage is usually less than for ENL and the total duration of the reaction is shorter. In dark-skinned patients, clofazimine can be commenced with the prednisolone, and the latter drug slowly withdrawn. Thalidomide is useless in this type of reaction.

Other Treatment. Patients must be educated to protect their anesthetic limbs. The healing of plantar ulcers is aided by rest and plaster splints. Reconstructive surgery and physiotherapy are valuable in the rehabilitation of deformed patients. The use of transfer factor in LL and BL leprosy is being assessed.

Prognosis. Even without treatment, patients with TT leprosy and three quarters of those with "indeterminate" disease eventually cure themselves; however, the patients with BL, most BB, and many BT forms of disease tend to lose cell-mediated immunity, and their disease becomes more lepromatous. Widespread nerve damage may develop in the BT and BB groups. Patients with the LL form used to die from uncontrolled leprosy, intercurrent infection, or amyloid nephritis, and blindness was common. With correct treatment, the prognosis now is good. Death from leprosy is rare, although amyloidosis is still seen occasionally, especially in inadequately treated ENL. Patients who fail to care for anesthetic extremities may suffer from repeated trauma or infection, resulting in gradual absorption of digits, or amputation may become necessary for chronic osteomyelitis. Even with careful management, reactional neuritis may sometimes cause increased deformity, and ENL may also, if rarely, result in blindness or significant renal damage.

Prevention. Because *M. leprae* cannot be grown in vitro, there is no specific vaccine. The precise value of BCG in protecting against early leprosy is being further assessed. Prophylactic DDS or acedapsone (diacetyl DDS) may be justified in special local situations. Otherwise prevention rests on early diagnosis of cases, and annual examination of known contacts may be rewarding.

Rees, R. J. W., and Waters, M. F. R.: Recent trends in leprosy research. Br. Med. Bull., 28:16, 1972.
Ridley, D. S., and Jopling, W. H.: Classification of leprosy according to immunity. A five-group system. Int. J. Lepr., 34:255, 1966.

TREPONEMAL DISEASES

Thorstein Guthe

246. SYPHILIS

Definition. Syphilis is a chronic infectious disease caused by *Treponema pallidum.* From the portal of entry—usually the genitals—there is lymphatic invasion and blood-borne spread (treponemia), and the infection is generalized from the beginning. Subsequently the disease becomes localized and dispersed. The early lesions are benign and the late manifestations destructive in character. Several organs of the body may be involved, but late treponemia and establishment of further lesions occur rarely in the acquired disease; this reflects the relative stability of the immunity that develops during the course of the disease. The host response includes specific humoral and cell-mediated immunity. Immune responses can be detected by serologic and other tests. Despite its slow evolution and remarkable immunologic features, syphilis will, if untreated, eventually incapacitate one of five and kill one of ten infected persons.

Treponema Pallidum. *T. pallidum,* discovered by Schaudinn and Hoffman in 1905, is a helical cell about 0.15 μ wide and 6 to 15 μ long. Around its central protoplasmic core is wound a bundle of three to four axial fibrils that provide the "muscle," giving *T. pallidum* a characteristic motility pattern. Treponemes undergo transverse fission. Multiplication time is 30 to 35 hours. *T. pallidum* has not been cultivated in vitro. It can remain viable for many hours on special media, or indefinitely if preserved at extremely low temperatures (carbon dioxide ice, liquid nitrogen).

Transmission. A few treponemes suffice to implant infection (Magnuson et al., 1956). Transmission is facilitated by moist conditions and congenial temperature, and occurs almost exclusively by direct contact with infectious lesions. Injured or inflamed areas will favor implantation. Sexual transmission is the rule. Not infrequently genito-oral, genito-rectal or mouth-to-mouth transmission takes place. The chain of infection sometimes involves both heterosexual and homosexual prac-

The author wishes to acknowledge the valuable advice of his colleague Dr. O. Idsøe, Consultant on Treponematoses, World Health Organization, Geneva, concerning this chapter.

tices. As many as 30 to 40 infected persons have been brought to treatment on the basis of a single index case. "Innocent" transmission by adults or children occasionally occurs. Contact between an infector, the moist object, and the susceptible must be rapid to achieve indirect transmission. Inoculation into the skin or a vein has resulted from an accidental needle prick. An initial lesion does not arise in blood-borne transmission when it occurs in utero of pregnant syphilitic women (prenatal syphilis) or more rarely by blood transfusion from an infected blood donor (syphilis d'emblée). A macerated fetus and the mucocutaneous lesions of early prenatal syphilis are highly contagious. Some infected individuals can pass asymptomatically through the early stages of syphilis, as distinct from those whose early trivial symptoms were misinterpreted or "masked" by treatment of other conditions, e.g., gonorrhea. Physiologic secretions (salivary, vaginal, seminal) may contain treponemes from contagious lesions. Direct intrauterine infection of the egg or the fetus from semen of a syphilitic male cannot arise.

Epidemiology. The health of the public is affected when syphilis spreads within and between countries. Propagation is facilitated by the properties of the agent, by its mode of transmission, and by behavioral, social, and several environmental factors. In recent years the climate of opinion concerning sexual behavior has become overtly permissive among the young. The pattern of promiscuity and of heterosexual and homosexual relations has altered. Industrialization, urbanization, migration, and unprecedented tourism have facilitated human contact and sexual encounters with concomitant risk of acquiring sexually transmitted disease. Paradoxically, medical advancements have contributed in the same direction. Thus fear of infection has been removed by easy and effective antimicrobial therapy and fear of pregnancy by oral contraceptives and intrauterine devices. Generally it has become clear that medical advances have been to some extent outweighed by the complex ecologic forces in a rapidly changing environment. It has been recognized that new ways are needed to promote the mental and physical health of individuals and communities, e.g., health education, recreation, city planning.

The long-term trend of syphilis in the last 100 years has been downward. However, the epidemic outbreak of syphilis (and gonorrhea) during World War II was first followed by a rapidly declining incidence until 1958, since which time there has been a noticeable recrudescence of these conditions. Examples of reported incidence of *early syphilis* per 100,000 population are United States, 3.9 in 1958 and 10.1 in 1971; Poland, 18.6 in 1958 and 51.9 in 1971; and France, 3.3 in 1958 and 8.3 in 1971. It has been shown (United States) that for each reported case of early infectious syphilis three additional cases are diagnosed and treated by private physicians but not reported to the health authorities. A decline in *late* cardiovascular and neurosyphilis and in *congenital syphilis* has been observed since the mid-1940's. This decline has occurred despite the experience that late syphilis can be expected to increase after periods of high incidence of early syphilis. *The prevention of the late forms of syphilis by the penicillin treatment of early syphilis is one of the great achievements of the chemotherapy era.*

Host-Treponeme Relationship. Man is the only natural host of *T. pallidum.* Hormonal and genetic factors may affect susceptibility to infection. The host-treponeme interaction is best portrayed by the rhythm and features in the development of lesions during the course of untreated syphilis.

Natural Course of Syphilis. After implantation and local multiplication of *T. pallidum* and extension of the infection to lymph nodes, treponemes spread rapidly to all body tissues via venous blood, the pulmonary circulation, and the arterial system. Human syphilis therefore ceases rapidly to be a local disease (even incubating infection can cause blood-transfusion syphilis). The agent does not grow in the bloodstream, but on passage through the small vessels, numerous metastatic foci are set up in the body, e.g., in the skin, mucous membranes, and nervous system. After the appearance of the initial lesion, some three weeks after infection, multiplication continues for several weeks in these metastatic foci. Some eight to nine weeks after the original implantation the first generalized mucocutaneous outbreak occurs. The primary lesion heals spontaneously within a few weeks, and the secondary eruption within a few weeks or months. The treponemes in the metastatic foci of internal organs are presumably killed in most instances, but sometimes they become only temporarily inactivated (latent), giving rise to further manifestations. In the untreated disease further secondary episodes occur in 25 per cent of patients within the first four years, mostly within two years. With increasing duration of infection the hematogenous "showers" of treponemes generating these contagious episodes become less frequent and less rich in treponemes. The cutaneous lesions tend to group and localize, or may occur solitarily until the mucocutaneous system no longer responds to treponemes with pathologic changes. The further course of the untreated infection is illustrated by data from the University Clinic, Oslo, where by the turn of the century some 1100 patients with diagnosed early syphilis remained untreated under hospitalized conditions and were subjected to follow-up studies. In the last representative follow-up investigation 50 to 60 years after the original infection (Gjestland), late "benign" syphilis had occurred in 15 per cent, cardiovascular syphilis in 10 per cent, and neurosyphilis in 6.5 per cent of these patients. Ten per cent died as a direct consequence of their disease. In about two thirds, latency continued indefinitely after subsidence of the secondary attacks. They went through life without major physical or mental consequences of their disease.

These features of the host-treponeme relationship in syphilis raise the question of the mechanisms concerned in the pathogenesis of lesions and their nature in both early and late disease, and point to the remarkable role of the defense forces of the host against the invading pathogen during the natural course of the infection.

Immunology. The immune response of the host directed against the pathogen is reflected in the natural course of syphilis as outlined above. The underlying waning treponemia, the decrease in demonstrable treponemes in late lesions, and the presence of presumed resistance to superinfection after the initial phase of the disease are among the signals. Moreover, a varying degree of cross-resistance to syphilis in persons infected with yaws and pinta suggests the broader role of immunity in treponematoses. Knowledge is limited, however, concerning the effector mechanisms in the protective host responses. It is possible to demonstrate humoral immunity by passive transfer of immune serum in laboratory animals (Turner et al.,

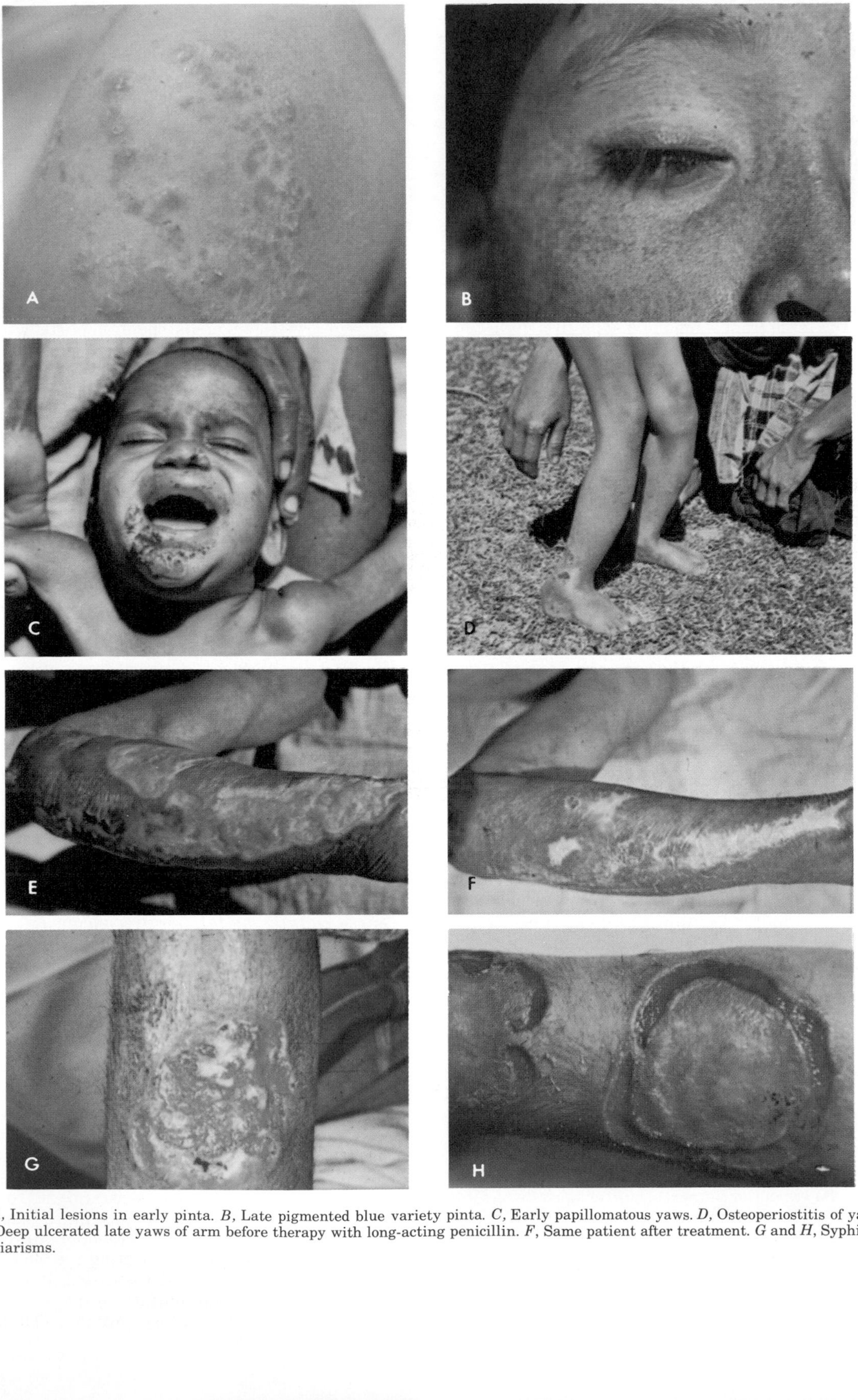

A, Initial lesions in early pinta. *B*, Late pigmented blue variety pinta. *C*, Early papillomatous yaws. *D*, Osteoperiostitis of yaws. *E*, Deep ulcerated late yaws of arm before therapy with long-acting penicillin. *F*, Same patient after treatment. *G* and *H*, Syphilitic tertiarisms.

1973). A cellular immunity response also occurs, but its significance has not been determined (Levene et al., 1971). In animal experimentation successful immunization can reportedly be achieved by the use of gamma-irradiated *T. pallidum* vaccine (Miller, 1973).

The humoral response involves formation of two main antibody types, reagin* and treponemal antibody.

Reagin develops early, four to five weeks after infection, and forms more rapidly than treponemal antibody described below. It declines when the disease moves toward latency, and may fall below detectable levels in late disease. It is affected considerably by therapy in the early phase of syphilis. A rising titer is a precursor of clinical outbreak, and reagin is therefore a useful gauge of disease activity, but of limited value as indicator of immunity. All evidence contradicts a protective role of reagin which is directed against cardiolipin present in the tissues of the antibody-producing host. Reagin is presumably an autoantibody formed in response to tissue destruction during the pathologic process (WHO, 1970; Wright and Doniach, 1971). It is not known if reagin has a pathogenic significance.

Of the *treponemal antibodies* the immobilizin appears to be the more important. Fluorescent and agglutinating treponemal antibodies also appear. Immobilizin is operative in the treponemal antibody immobilization test (TPI). It appears late—two to three months after the infection. It is formed slowly but can persist for life as an indicator of infection. Immobilizin reflects roughly the development of host resistance, although the evidence is equivocal that it has a direct protective role.

In syphilis antibody-producing plasmocytes are characteristically present in early lesions and in lymph nodes. Antibody demonstrated by reagin tests may belong to both IgM and IgG immunoglobulins. IgM is produced early in the infection. IgG exclusively forms the immobilizing antibody when it appears later in the infection. In immunofluorescent tests both IgM and IgG antibodies react with *T. pallidum*. Whether or not formation of antibody continues after treponemes have been eradicated by treatment—as well as the circumstances under which such eradication may take place—is not known (see Persistence of Treponemal Forms, below). IgG antibodies can pass the placenta, in contrast to IgM. The presence of IgM in the serum of newborns suggests local formation of antibodies and therefore prenatal active infection. IgG also passes the blood-brain barrier when the meninges are inflamed. This explains why serodiagnostic tests that mainly identify IgG antibody are preferred in examining the cerebrospinal fluid for syphilis of the nervous system.

Cell-mediated immunity manifests itself as delayed hypersensitivity demonstrable by the response to intradermally injected antigen after 12 to 48 hours. Interaction of antigen with specifically sensitized lymphocytes and cell structures is believed to be the underlying mechanism. Although knowledge is very limited, cell-mediated immunity apparently does not play a major role during the secondary eruptions of syphilis (Levene, 1969). However, it is believed to be operative in gummatous lesions. Moreover, the striking clinical and histopathologic similarity of late destructive skin and bone lesions in venereal syphilis, bejel, and yaws suggests a common cell-mediated or other mechanism of the host response at this stage.

Immunopathologic mechanisms involving tissue damage are very little known in syphilis. Multiple humoral antibodies circulate in all phases of the disease, antigen is present, and antigen-antibody complexes may have pathogenic significance. Nevertheless a direct cytotoxic effect on host cells has not been established. Immunopathologic mechanisms have been suggested in a few and rare manifestations engendered by syphilitic infection, notably biphasic paroxysmatic cold hemaglobulinuria and membranous glomerulonephritis (syphilitic "nephrosis"). The occurrence of cryoglobulins in syphilis has also been reported.

In recent years there have been several important scientific developments in basic immunology concerning humoral and cellular immunity and immunopathology (WHO, 1964 and 1969), which may be expected to be applied also in syphilis and other treponematoses. *At present the clinical and laboratory findings can only illustrate the capacity of immunocompetent cell systems to react to antigenic stimuli in the early phase of syphilis, and to generate protection against further metastatic spread and superinfection with the pathogen. The human host can contain the infection at the time of latency by establishing a notable equilibrium between the pathogenic potential of treponemes and the immune forces, as evidenced by a relatively infrequent disturbance of this equilibrium resulting in occurrence of late injurious manifestations.*

Persistence of Treponemal Forms. Adequate penicillin therapy of early syphilis will usually heal lesions and prevent late manifestations in most instances. Symptomatic manifestations after penicillin therapy of latent syphilis are rare. When occurring, they signal survival of pathogenic treponemes notwithstanding the immune forces and therapy. When not occurring, e.g., late latency, and persistently positive serologic tests have sometimes in the past been considered to be due to persistent antibodies produced by "immunologic memory" rather than to treponemes persisting in the host. However, persistence of treponemal forms (treponeme-like structures) in host tissues has been reported in recent years. Thus in some instances of treated late syphilis treponemal forms were described in lymph nodes and cerebrospinal fluid (Collart et al.), in aqueous humor of the eye (Smith and Israel), and in treated congenital syphilis, as well as in pathologic and nonpathologic ophthalmic situations apparently unrelated to syphilis. Rarely treponemal forms have also been found (lymph nodes) after treatment of early syphilis (Yobs et al.). The treponemal forms that have been demonstrated after treatment of early and late syphilis have only rarely been shown by animal infectivity tests to be viable (Turner). Others may be modified or "dormant" *T. pallidum,* acting as antigenic stimulus for continued treponemal antibody production, whereas others may be saprophytic organisms indigenous to the human host. In some instances these situations may coexist. Persistence of abated forms of microorganisms in the face of normally

*The term *reagin* is used throughout this chapter. It is widely accepted by physicians, clinicians, and epidemiologists to denote antibodies to cardiolipin-type antigens formed in syphilis and other treponematoses. Reagin is often referred to by immunologists and allergists to describe antibodies concerned in the immediate types of skin hypersensitivity and anaphylactic reactions.

effective drugs has already been studied in mycobacteria and corynebacteria, and is a phenomenon apart from true drug resistance (McDermott). There is no evidence that penicillinase-producing, resistant pathogenic treponeme strains have developed. Knowledge concerning immunologic tissue and humoral aspects of persistent treponemal forms is extremely limited, but regardless of the extent to which such forms are viable or modified pathogenic treponemes—or related indigenous organisms—their role may be significant in the immunologic life of the host. *For the physician it is important to realize that studies in this area are very few, that accepted treatment practices need not be reconsidered in early syphilis, and that in late syphilis special considerations continue to pertain.*

Pathology. The early treponemia and the resulting metastatic foci are reflected in the diversity of the body organs involved in the pathology of this chronic inflammation. The macroscopic characteristics of skin manifestations are described later. The histopathology of lesions is basically characterized by endarteritis and periarteritis of the small vessels and capillaries, which show infiltration of lymphocytes and plasmocytes and multiplication of histiocytes. Granulomatous inflammation is typical of the late stages of syphilis as of other chronic infections, e.g., tuberculosis.

In the *early skin lesions* in which many treponemes are present, lymphocytosis and plasmacytosis are particularly marked, although varying in intensity. Acanthosis usually occurs. Many treponemes are present. *Lymph nodes* in the early disease show adenitis with prominent follicles, plasmacytosis, sometimes focal necrosis, fine fibrosis, and presence of treponemes. The histologic picture in lesions and lymph nodes is compatible with antibody production by stimulated cells (WHO, 1970). *Late nodular and gummatous lesions* (usually treponeme-free) are the results of delayed hypersensitivity and show chronic granulomatous tissue with lymphocytes, epithelioid cells, and eventually giant cells in addition to the endovascular changes of early lesions. In *cardiovascular syphilis* there is endarteritis of the vasa vasorum, particularly in the ascending aorta and arch. All layers of the large vessel are involved with destruction of elastic and muscle tissue, weakening the entire structure and predisposing to aneurysm. The aortic ring may also be weakened with shortening and thickening of valve leaflets leading to regurgitation. Coronary ostia may become narrowed, resulting in rare ischemic heart disease. *Central nervous system* syphilis is either meningovascular with inflammation of the pia-arachnoid and its vessels or parenchymatous with the nervous tissue attacked. The leptomeningitis may be acute or chronic. Infiltration of small meningeal vessels may cause thrombosis and local brain damage. The parenchymatous process may engender paresis if the brain is predominantly involved, or tabes dorsalis if the spinal cord is predominantly involved. Tabes begins as extradural leptomeningitis around the dorsal nerve roots, followed by degeneration of axis cylinders and demyelinization of posterior columns of the spinal cord. Optic atrophy may occur from basal meningitis or interstitial neuritis in the nerve or chiasma, or central gummatous lesions may affect the optic nerve directly. Involvement of afferent vessels to the spinal cord may lead to degeneration of pyramidal tracts and a rare condition known as Erb's spastic paraplegia. *Ophthalmic lesions* include uveitis with serofibrinous exudate and synechiae in acquired syphilis, and interstitial keratitis with substantial lymphocytic infiltration in congenital syphilis. Rare membranous *glomerulonephritis* ("nephrosis") in early syphilis shows peculiar vascular or granulomatous tissue changes. Other forms of visceral syphilis, e.g., interstitial nephritis, may occur. In *prenatal syphilis* the placenta is often voluminous, thickened, and pale with enlarged cotyledons and perivascular fibrosis throughout the villi, such as can also be seen in erythroblastosis (Rh-negative mother). Fibrous proliferation and monocellular infiltrates characterize fetal tissues in congenital syphilis; but in addition to the placenta changes, the most characteristic findings are in the lungs (pneumonia alba) and the bones (osteochondritis and periostitis), the latter changes being diagnosable roentgenologically.

Notwithstanding the diversity of the organs affected and the multiformity of the lesions underlying the clinical picture, the elementary pathologic changes in all syphilitic processes are of vascular and inflammatory nature.

Clinical Manifestations and Diagnosis. Untreated acquired syphilis shows a great variety of clinical manifestations, depending inter alia on the duration of the infection and the immunologic state of the host. The accepted classification of syphilis into *early syphilis* of less than four years' duration and *late syphilis* of more than four years' duration is based on these immunologic grounds, as well as on clinical and epidemiologic considerations rather than on definite "stages" of disease that may sometimes merge or overlap. In congenital syphilis, in which there is prenatal hematogenous transmission of *T. pallidum* to the fetus from the syphilitic mother, the disease is usually divided into *early congenital syphilis* in children less than two years old and *late congenital syphilis* in those who are older.

Early Syphilis. The incubation period, initial lesions, secondary manifestations, and early latent period are included in this designation.

THE INITIAL LESION (PRIMARY CHANCRE). Following an incubation of two to six weeks after the original infection, the initial lesion appears at the site of implantation of *T. pallidum:* in males usually on the penile shaft, coronal sulcus, glans, or prepuce, and occasionally intraurethrally; and in females on the external genitalia and cervix. In 5 to 10 per cent of patients the initial lesions are extragenital (lips, tonsils, fingers, within the anus, but also anywhere else). The initial lesion is usually a painless lenticular papule, rapidly eroding and becoming a flat indurated infiltrate, usually with elastic consistency, 3 to 20 mm in diameter, and of round or oval shape. However, lesions are frequently "atypical," modified by size, location, and the nature of underlying tissue, if not by treatment. Solitary chancres are usual. Multiple chancres may appear after manifold simultaneous implantation of *T. pallidum,* especially in women. Regardless of site, initial lesions are accompanied by moderate enlargement of regional lymph nodes, usually recognizable clinically within a week of their appearance. The nodes are firm, freely movable, and painless. The initial lesion heals slowly (two to six weeks), and may or may not leave an atrophic scar. Lymphadenopathy may last for several months. With approaching secondary manifestations metastatic lesions of skin and mucous membrane sometimes go unrecognized while the primary sore is still present. On the other hand, the initial lesion is occasionally absent from the beginning, the secondary lesions nevertheless developing in due course (syphilis d'emblée).

In *diagnosis* of a suspected solitary genital or other lesion, careful general clinical examination of the patient should be undertaken in addition to mandatory dark-field examination for *T. pallidum* in material from the sore and the repeated performance of serologic tests, e.g., VDRL. These may be reactive as early as four weeks after the infection and one week after the appearance of the lesion. If treponemes are not found but seroreactivity has been established, the diagnosis is made in conjunction with clinical and anamnestic data. The most common lesions to suggest, erroneously, syphilitic sores are *chancroid* (which may coexist with chancre) and *granuloma inguinale. Balanoposthitis, erosion and carcinoma of the cervix uteri, and lymphogranuloma venereum* should also be considered. Other conditions include *traumatic sore, herpes progenitalis, condylomata acuminata, lichen planus, scabies, fissura in ano,* and *Vincent's angina.* Differential diagnostic considerations may vary from one country to another, according to the prevalence of the various conditions.

From its earliest phases the incubation period of syphilis is one of considerable biologic activity. When the patient with an initial lesion is first seen by the physician, generalized infection has already occurred as a result of the early treponemia, although generalized symptoms may not as yet have appeared. Unless initial lesions give rise to suspicion of disease, the patient may not seek medical care during the early period of infectiousness. Local genital lesions should therefore always be considered suspect of syphilis until proved otherwise.

SECONDARY MANIFESTATIONS AND EARLY LATENCY. About the sixth week of the infection there is *generalized lymphadenitis* with palpable superficial lymph nodes. Lymph nodes, otherwise seldom swollen, are involved, e.g., the pre- and postauricular, occipital, and supratrochlear lymph nodes. All nodes are firm, freely movable, and painless. *Cutaneous rashes,* notably the macular rash, appear six to eight weeks after the initial lesion, the vestiges of which remain in some patients. The macules are pale red, roundish patches 5 to 10 mm in diameter, neither infiltrated nor scaling, and do not itch. They are usually bilateral, and are distributed to the trunk and proximal parts of extremities. On black skin, macules appear as darker patches. Macular rashes last one to two months. *Papular lesions* often develop before disappearance of macules. The papules are coppery-red, round infiltrates 3 to 10 mm in diameter, sometimes leaving pigmented patches on healing, e.g., "necklace of Venus." The papules are distributed anywhere, and include scalp, soles, and palms. The latter show up as flat, slightly scaly lesions or as a characteristic bluish-red rash covered by normal keratin. The papular rash may last two to four weeks.

In its further development and notably during relapses many varieties of papules may appear in syphilis. Large hypertrophic papules ("condylomata lata") are localized to skin folds, e.g., genitals, anus, axillae, under pendulous breasts, and elsewhere, and are often humid and eroded. Split papules at the oral angles resemble perlèche. On black skin circinate and arciform papules are common around the mouth and on the chin. Seborrheic, psoriasiform, and acneiform papules may occur. Varioliform papules are sometimes encountered in the tropics. They may give the impression of smallpox, but the base of the latter is less infiltrated beneath the pustule which shows umbilical depression and later also characteristic crusts. Follicular and corymbiform grouped papules are late manifestations in secondary syphilis. Patchy loss of hair occurs three to eight months after infection and gives a moth-eaten appearance. It is evident from the above that polymorphism characterizes the early and particularly the subsequent relapsing lesions in secondary syphilis, even in the same person. *Mucous membranes,* notably in the mouth, vulva, and anus, may be involved separately or conjointly with skin manifestations. Erosive superficial mucosal patches are often covered by a thin gray membrane with a red halo. Ulceromembranous tonsillitis and pharyngitis may cause moderate symptoms (hoarseness). Mucous membrane lesions are very contagious. At least 20 per cent of patients with early syphilis will have transient *subacute meningitis* ("meningeal rash"), causing headache and increase of cells and protein in the cerebrospinal fluid. *Ophthalmic conditions* may occur, notably iritis with demonstrable synechiae, but seldom before six months after the infection. *Interstitial nephritis* may give minor or no symptoms. *Periostitis,* particularly of the long bones, is common and shows up as swelling, tenderness, and ostealgia (nocturnal pains).

RELAPSING SYPHILIS. Condylomata lata are likely to recur. The skin manifestations tend to be unilateral, the eruptions more dense, marked, with fewer lesions, and sometimes solitary. They are also more infiltrated and of somewhat longer standing, and have some characteristics that resemble the skin lesions in late syphilis. This reflects the increasing immunity with the duration of the early disease. Neurorecurrences, as well as ophthalmic and other relapsing manifestations, may occur. If the patient has been inadequately treated, relapses may be delayed.

DIAGNOSIS OF SECONDARY SYPHILIS. The diagnosis of secondary syphilis is made on the basis of lymphadenopathy, mucocutaneous lesions, demonstration of *T. pallidum* by dark-field examination of lesion fluid or lymph node aspirate, and seroreactivity in reagin tests. The history may or may not be helpful. In the presence of mucocutaneous manifestations, the necessary serologic tests are usually obtained by the physician. Errors arise from a syphilitic lesion that is misinterpreted as representing some localized body lesion of nonmicrobial origin, e.g., an anal fissure, or from solitary lesions that may be considered "trivial." Close search for clinical manifestations other than the presenting symptom may well reveal lesions on other parts of the skin or simultaneously occurring mucosal eruption, e.g., oral or genital mucous patches, loss of hair, palmar or volar lesions, pointing to the serious systemic nature of the condition.

The most common eruptions that should be considered in differential diagnoses of early generalized secondary syphilitic rashes are *acute microbial disease, exanthemata,* and *drug eruptions.* In the later phase of secondary syphilis when lesions become more localized, the following conditions are of differential diagnostic importance: *pityriasis rosea, perleche, psoriasis,* and *superficial fungus infections.* Also *lichen planus* and sometimes certain forms of *tuberculids, scabies, venereal warts,* and *Reiter's disease* may come into purview. *Aphthous stomatitis* and *Stevens-Johnson* syndrome are among oral cavity manifestations to be considered.

As a whole it is noted that manifestations of secondary syphilis have a very wide range; they involve the skin and other body systems, often extensively, but sometimes in a more limited way and discretely, with corresponding variation of clinical symptomatology in patients who are usually not feeling subjectively ill. *Hardly in any other disease is it of such importance as in suspected syphilis to make a careful and complete examination of the entire skin, mucous membranes, and body systems. Laboratory examination should always be undertaken in suspected cases.*

EARLY ASYMPTOMATIC (LATENT) SYPHILIS. This designation serves to identify seroreactive persons who have no signs and nonreactive cerebrospinal fluid within the first four years of infection. *In view of the tendency of early syphilis to contagious secondary relapses and the potential seriousness of neurosyphilis, which sometimes may develop after two years' duration of the infection, patients in whom a diagnosis of early latent syphilis is established should be treated and kept under surveillance by the physician in the same way as is done for symptomatic secondary syphilis.*

Late Syphilis. In the natural course of syphilis, further infectious mucocutaneous relapses seldom occur after the second, and hardly ever after the fourth year. "Refractory" or premunitory immunity has then been established, and persists for life in two thirds of patients who remain asymptomatic. In the remainder, slow chronic destructive inflammation and fibrosis continue in various affected tissues, giving rise to late manifestations.

LATE ASYMPTOMATIC (LATENT) SYPHILIS. Latent syphilis has reactive serologic tests as its sole evidence. The cerebrospinal fluid is nonreactive, and there is absence of all manifestations at the time of diagnosis four years or more after the original infection. The history, antecedent treatment, and previous serologic tests are important in establishing the diagnosis. Confirmatory treponemal antibody tests (FTA/TPI) are essential to exclude biologically "false" seroreactivity. In addition to careful clinical examination of skin, mucous membranes, and eyes, examination of the cerebrospinal fluid and roentgenologic studies of the heart and aorta are mandatory.

LATE SYMPTOMATIC SYPHILIS. Late symptomatic syphilis may cause inapparent to severe damage of body systems. *Late "benign" syphilis* may show mainly nodular or squamous skin lesions of destructive character, containing few or no treponemes, with tendency to peripheral extension, central healing, and scar formation, a pattern usually not encountered in other skin lesions except lupus vulgaris. Certain forms of *skin tuberculosis, deep mycosis,* and occasionally *cancer* are the main differential diagnostic problems. Serologic examination is obviously important. The typical lesion of late syphilis is the *gumma,* which can involve the skin, mucous membranes, skeletal system, and viscera. Nodular ulcerative lesions spread peripherally, the subcutaneous gumma infiltrating and later perforating the skin, creating a roundish ulcer with cut-out, not undermined, borders in contrast to tuberculous ulcerations. The hard and soft palate can be perforated. In rare instances the total anterior or central part of the palate and nose may be mutilated by gummatous and other involvement of skin and bones, a condition known as rhinopharyngitis mutilans ("gangosa"), which is also encountered in late yaws and bejel. *Skeletal lesions* involve mostly periosteum, more rarely cortex and medulla, and are of a diffuse or localized gummatous nature, particularly affecting the long bones, e.g., tibia, clavicle. Pain, swelling, and roentgenologic findings are diagnostic characteristics. Syphilitic joint lesions are less frequent. Charcot's joints, frequently associated with tabes dorsalis, are considered as a neuroarthropathy. *Nervous system syphilis* includes affliction of cranial nerves from basal syphilitic meningitis, giving symptoms according to the nerve involved, e.g., eighth-nerve deafness, diplopia. Damage to the central nervous system can otherwise give rise to a very wide range of neurologic and other signs and symptoms which characterize meningovascular and parenchymatous neurosyphilis, e.g., general paresis, tabes dorsalis. The latter is frequently associated with primary optic atrophy. *Cardiovascular syphilis* manifests itself primarily as aortitis of the ascending aorta and may lead to aortic insufficiency and aneurysm. Roentgenography is as essential as cerebrospinal fluid examination for the diagnosis of late syphilis. (See Ch. 386 and 587.)

A relatively frequent coexistence of cardiovascular syphilis with neurosyphilis (10 to 15 per cent), neurosyphilis with "benign" late syphilis (13 per cent), and the latter with cardiovascular syphilis (10 per cent) should be kept in mind by the physician. Almost all fatalities in syphilis result from neurosyphilis or syphilis of the heart or aorta. These most serious forms of the disease are discussed elsewhere in Ch. 386 and 587 and in a monograph on venereology (Willcox).

Maternal and Prenatal ("Congenital") Syphilis. The manifestations of maternal syphilis depend on the stage of disease; diagnosis is established on usual anamnestic, clinical, and serologic criteria. Serologic screening may detect pregnant women with no past history of disease. These should be investigated and treated as early latent syphilis. During the first years of infection most pregnancies will terminate in fetal death if the mother is left without treatment. Later in the course of the infection the risk decreases, and untreated syphilitic women may give birth to healthy children. Presumably this is related to the lessening likelihood of the occurrence of treponemia with time. Nevertheless, occasionally an untreated syphilitic woman may deliver a congenitally syphilitic child many years after infection.

EARLY PRENATAL SYPHILIS. Early congenital syphilis is prenatally acquired infection diagnosed in children less than two years old. The fetus is infected after the fourth month of pregnancy. The lesions on delivery depend on the time of infection, and may vary from marasmic to apparently healthy infants. Fibrotic visceral lesions are characteristic. Osteochondritis is diagnosed by roentgenographic examination. The child may be born with "snuffles" from affliction of the nasopharynx with mucous and sometimes hemorrhagic discharge. The cutaneous rash after birth can be impressive papular and bullous eruptions in the palms and soles (exceptional in acquired syphilis), and tend characteristically to affect facial, circumoral, anogenital, and diaper areas, and palms and soles. Such lesions are highly contagious, and *T. pallidum* can easily be demonstrated. Infants without signs of disease, who are suspected of being infected by a seroreactive mother, should be clinically and serologically kept under surveillance for at least six months to establish active infection or passive reaginemia.

LATE PRENATAL SYPHILIS. Late congenital syphilis is a prenatally acquired infection that has persisted and developed in children over two years of age. On discovery the condition is often latent and should be confirmed by FTA/TPI tests. Residual manifestations of early lesions may be present, notably rhagades radiating from the prolabium and frontal bosses and saber tibia from periostitis of the shaft. There may be osseous destruction (saddle nose) and dental deformities, with wedge-shaped, widely spaced, often notched permanent upper central incisors (Hutchinson's teeth). Other "signs" include eighth nerve deafness and syphilitic synovitis in both knee joints (Clutton's joints). The most common affliction is *interstitial keratitis,* usually appearing in late childhood and eventually becoming bilateral. There is photophobia, ground glass appearance of the cornea, and vascularization of adjacent sclera. Other late manifestations resemble those of acquired late adult syphilis of similar duration. Meningovascular syphilis, paresis, and tabes occur, but cardiovascular syphilis is rare.

The profound pathologic processes of prenatal syphilis and the personal and social limitations that they impose are preventable through routine serologic testing of all pregnant women and adequate treatment of those found infected.

Interpretation of Laboratory Findings. In addition to clinical and anamnestic examination, the diagnosis of syphilis depends on laboratory findings. In early syphilis dark-field examination of lesions and serologic tests are indispensable; in late syphilis in addition to serologic tests examination of the cerebrospinal fluid is the most important laboratory procedure.

Dark-Field Examination. *T. pallidum* cannot be readily identified in dried, fixed fluid, or tissue specimens by silver, chromatic, or fluorescent staining. Its presence can best be ascertained in the living state by microscopic dark-field examination which can be done by the trained physician. Material for examination includes tissue fluid from initial and secondary lesions after saline washing and gentle squeezing or an aspirate from an enlarged lymph node. Preferably, specimens should be examined on the spot. They can, however, be collected in a capillary tube, sealed with wax, and mailed to a competent laboratory. Care must be taken in interpreting the findings. *T. pallidum* may resemble spirochetes normally inhabiting genitalia and the oral cavity. The regular corkscrew-like coils, the slow, rotating, forward-backward motions, and graceful sideways bendings help in identification of *T. pallidum. Repeated failures to demonstrate T. pallidum with adequate technique in a suspected lesion may mean that the lesion is healing, that the patient has received topical or systemic treatment, or that the lesion is nonsyphilitic. Before the lesion is diagnosed as nonsyphilitic, an examination of lymph node aspirate should be made.*

Serologic Tests. Serologic tests are indispensable for individual diagnosis of syphilis, for following the effect of therapy, for routine screening of pregnant women, blood donors, and other "risk groups," and for case and contact finding in community, national, and international health programs. It is essential for the physician to utilize laboratories that employ standard reagents and methods and that partake in a proficiency testing program of sensitivity, specificity, and reproducibility in cooperation with a regional or national reference center. Serologic tests detect antibodies formed during the course of the syphilitic infection.

Reagin tests use cardiolipin antigen according to different methods. These may vary from one country to another, but are based on either complement fixation or flocculation techniques, e.g., VDRL.*

The pattern of antibody production has been outlined under Immunology, indicating that treponemal antibody, notably the immobilizin, is specific and reflects roughly the immunity status of the patient, whereas reagin is rather an indicator of disease activity. *The use of quantitative reagin methods† is essential to permit the physician to assess the effect of treatment and compare antibody titers of periodically examined serum specimens in the post-treatment surveillance of the patient.*

Three types of *treponemal antibody tests* are in use: (1) The treponema immobilization test (TPI) uses live *T. pallidum* as antigen, immobilized by antibody in the presence of complement. It is the only test in which the biologic action of serum antibody can be determined directly under the microscope. (2) The fluorescent treponemal antibody test (FTA) uses killed treponemes as antigen. Syphilitic serum is bound to the surface of treponemes fixed onto a slide, and the antibody is made visible by use of fluorescein-tagged antiserum against human globulin. Nonspecific antibodies are removed either by dilution of serum (FTA_{200} test) or "absorbed" (FTA/ABS test). (3) The passive treponemal hemagglutination test (TPHA) uses disrupted *T. pallidum* as antigen, coated onto tannin treated sheep erythrocytes which are agglutinated in the presence of specific antibody.

"False" reaginemia occurs in certain pathologic conditions not caused by syphilis. Transient low-titer seroreactivity may, for example, arise from acute bacterial and viral infections, or after vaccinations, e.g., for smallpox. "False" seroreactivity occurs also from disease of connective tissue, e.g., disseminated lupus erythematosus, leprosy, and malaria; from the continued use of heroin; or from conditions affecting serum globulins, e.g., malnutrition. Moreover, both reagin and treponemal serologic tests for syphilis are also reactive by definition in other treponematoses (yaws, pinta, and bejel). *It should be realized, however, that syphilis remains the most common cause of reagin seroreactivity and that in screening examinations only one of ten VDRL seroreactive persons may be a problem case requiring confirmation with a specific treponemal test.* If TPI or FTA tests, or both, are needed and such tests are not undertaken by a local recognized laboratory, serum specimens can be mailed for examination to a laboratory of repute. If there is doubt about the interpretation of serologic tests, consultation should be arranged with a syphilologist.

Reagin tests may generally confirm a diagnosis of syphilis when a suspected initial lesion is present, although they are usually subordinate to dark-field findings of T. pallidum in the early stage. Reagin tests are reactive in all instances of secondary syphilis; they are im-

---

*Among the reagin tests, flocculation reactions, e.g., VDRL, Kline, Eagle, and complement fixation reactions, e.g., Kolmer, are used. In the present chapter the Venereal Disease Research Laboratory (VDRL) test is referred to as the prototype of reagin tests. It is subjected to national proficiency testing within and between laboratories in several countries and is based on the use of antigens referable to International Standard Preparations for the components used.

†In quantitative serologic tests a series of a progressively higher dilution of serum is made and each dilution is tested separately. The highest dilution that is reactive represents the titer.

portant in the diagnosis of congenital syphilis, offer a clue in latent syphilis, and have supplementary value in late syphilis. Treponemal antibody tests are essential for diagnosis in patients with repeated low or fluctuating reagin titers, in patients without anamnestic and/or clinical evidence, and in acquired and congenital disease, as well as in suspected late manifestations.

Cerebrospinal Fluid Examination. Lumbar puncture* can be undertaken at the physician's office or at a clinic. Examination of the cerebrospinal fluid serves to establish a diagnosis of latent syphilis by exclusion of asymptomatic neurosyphilis, aids in following the effect of therapy once such diagnosis has been made, and generally assures surveillance of patients in different phases of the disease. In syphilitic meningitis there occurs an increase of lymphocytes, proteins, and in some instances antibody. The first sign of asymptomatic neurosyphilis or meningitis arising from latency is pleocytosis of more than four cells per cubic milliliter, closely followed by an increase in protein to 40 mg or more (depending on laboratory method) and reactive antibody tests. When progressing to parenchymatous neurosyphilis, 150 cells or more, marked protein increase (globulin) and strongly reactive antibody tests are encountered. Complement-fixation tests for reagin (Kolmer) and treponemal antibody tests (TPI/FTA) are most suitable in cerebrospinal fluid examinations. When reactive they are pathognomonic of neurosyphilis; flocculation tests are sometimes nonreactive when antibody is present. Successful treatment leads to rapid regression of the cell count. Normalization of protein requires more time. Reversal of serologic tests may take several years.

*In some countries suboccipital puncture is preferred.

Therapy. Mahoney and co-workers (1943) introduced penicillin therapy in syphilis, and this drug has replaced previous metal therapy. Benzyl penicillin G is a more effective antitreponemal agent than the newer penicillins, e.g., ampicillin, methicillin. Injection therapy is preferred, and oral therapy is not recommended. The reproduction time of treponemes is of long duration (30 to 35 hours), and they may lodge in places where they do not multiply. Sustained, uninterrupted treponemicidal blood and tissue levels are therefore held to be more effective than intermittent penicillinemia and also minimize the arising of resistant mutants. Long-acting penicillin preparations such as procaine pencillin G in oil and monostearate (PAM) and benzathine penicillin G (DBED) as well as short-acting aqueous penicillin G preparations are all effective when used in treatment schedules providing adequate time:dose relationships. Aqueous preparations require frequent injections, higher dosages, and more involved patient management. The characteristics of the penicillin preparation used are more important than number, frequency, and total dosages of treatment schedules of undefined preparations. The accompanying table shows generally accepted treatment schedules.

Early Syphilis. Usually *T. pallidum* disappears from initial lesions within 24 hours, somewhat more slowly from secondary lesions. There is rapid involution of the lesion after adequate penicillin therapy, and the long-term outcome is highly satisfactory. A cooperative international study of 688 serononreactive and 494 seroreactive patients with primary syphilis, adequately treated and followed up to 11 years, showed no clinical relapses. Among 499 adequately treated patients with secondary syphilis, also followed up to 11 years, fewer than 5 per cent were retreated for clinical relapse, seroresistance, and—in most cases—reinfection. In 2485 patients with

Penicillin Treatment Practices in Syphilis

Indications for Syphilis Therapy†	Dosage and Administration*		
	N,N-Dibenzylethylenediamine Dipenicillin G (DBED) or Benzathine Penicillin G	*Procaine Penicillin G in Aluminium Stereate Suspension (PAM)*	*Aqueous Benzyl Penicillin G or Procaine Penicillin G*
Primary, secondary, and early latent syphilis with nonreactive cerebrospinal fluid and adequate opportunity for follow-up; epidemiological treatment	Total of 2.4 megaunits; single dose of two injections of 1.2 megaunits in one session	Total of 4.8–6.0 megaunits; first dose of 2.4 megaunits, and 1.2 megaunits at each of subsequent injections 3 days apart (over 9 days)	Total of 6.0 megaunits in doses of 600,000 units daily for 10 consecutive days
Late latent or when cerebrospinal fluid not examined in "latency": asymptomatic neurosyphilis, symptomatic neurosyphilis, cardiovascular syphilis, late benign (cutaneous, osseous, visceral gumma)	Total of 6 to 9 megaunits in doses of 3 megaunits at 7-day intervals, over 14–21 days	Total of 6 to 9 megaunits given in doses of 1.2 megaunits at 3-day intervals, over 15–21 days	Total of 6–9 megaunits in doses of 600,000 units daily, over 15 days
Congenital			
Early			
Up to 2 years of age	Total of 50,000 units per kg in a single or divided dose at one session	Total of 100,000 units per kg given in three divided doses at 2- to 3-day intervals	Total of 100,000 units per kg as 10,000 units per kg per day for 10 consecutive days‡
Late			
2 to 12 years, weight 32 kg (71 lb) or less	Same as early congenital syphilis	Same as early congenital syphilis	Same as early congenital syphilis
Over 12 years, or over 32 kg	Same as adult latent syphilis	Same as adult latent syphilis	Same as adult latent syphilis

*Individual doses can be divided for injection in each buttock to minimize discomfort.
†In *pregnancy*, treatment is dependent on the stage of syphilis.
‡Preferable in very small children.

nonspecified "early syphilis" followed up to 12 years, retreatment in different subseries of patients varied from 1 to 9 per cent with an average of 1.5 per cent retreated for serorelapse, seroresistance, and clinical relapse, the remainder being reinfections (Idsøe et al., 1972). *For the physician it is therefore unnecessary to subject all patients with early syphilis to the intensive treatment required by the few patients who experience seroresistance or relapses after currently accepted therapy schedules. But the need for proper post-treatment observation and surveillance of the patient is obvious. For community health reasons it is essential that a large "epidemiologic dose" of penicillin be administered immediately on diagnosis of infectious syphilis (see table), rendering the patient rapidly noninfectious and providing protection against spread of infection should the patient default from further treatment.*

After adequate penicillin treatment of *early syphilis,* the VDRL titers begin to descend, usually after two months, and a subsequent rapid fall is to be expected in most cases. As a whole, the time to reach seronegativity depends on the duration of infection when treatment was started, although in the majority of cases it is achieved within six months. At the ninth month 5 to 10 per cent may still be seroreactive at a low titer.

A few patients will retain seroreactivity at the end of the second year, mostly those treated in the late secondary and early latent phases. Fluctuations of titers during post-treatment surveillance examinations may occur. Only a persistent rise from nonreactivity or a fourfold titer increase from previous titer level should be considered as *serologic relapse.* Failures occur within one to two years, most of these within three to nine months. Serologic relapse usually precedes or accompanies infectious clinical relapse in which the mucocutaneous lesions are often localized. Cerebrospinal fluid examination is then essential, and retreatment should be provided at once. Occasionally, titers fail to decrease the first six to nine months after therapy. Retreatment is also then indicated. Retreatment should be intensive, usually effected by doubling the previous dosage scheme. The few patients who retain a residual low reagin titer after the second year and who after CSF examination have no evidence of syphilis may safely be followed without further treatment. Both these as well as the reagin nonreactive patients can be considered as "cured" of syphilis when the surveillance scheme has been completed. Whether or not the last treponeme has been eliminated—or will eventually be eliminated by the immunity forces—is another matter. *Long-term practical experience shows no convincing evidence that late clinical manifestations occur after penicillin therapy of early syphilis, providing that it was adequate and that the exceptional early failures were retreated; the assurance that can be given to the patient is thus of a high order.* Distinction between infectious relapse and reinfection is sometimes not possible except on epidemiologic grounds. If the patient is cured of his infection before his immunity defenses have been mobilized, reinfection may occur on renewed exposure to *T. pallidum.*

Late Syphilis. During the course of untreated late syphilis, regression or reaginemia as a rule takes place very slowly and may occasionally reach nondetectable levels by usual reagin tests. Such reagin nonreactivity may be encountered in parenchymatous or cardiovascular syphilis. Treatment does not substantially affect reagin reactivity, or serologic nonreactivity is reached only after many years. Treponemal antibody tests (TPI/FTA) are normally reactive in late syphilis, and despite treatment may remain so throughout life.

The considerable capacity of the immunity in untreated syphilis to prevent progression of late latent infection to symptomatic disease has already been emphasized. This function cannot, however, be accurately measured by serologic tests as distinct from the clinical effect of therapy, although the latter is convincing. It has been estimated by McDermott (1967) that probably less than 2 per cent of diagnosed late latent syphilitics may develop serious manifestations after proper penicillin therapy. Principally, these are older patients with preestablished unrecognizable manifestations, e.g., aortitis, at the time they are treated for their presumed late latent infection. In the treatment of actual late manifestations, the character, location, and extent of the latter dictate the amount of specific therapy; the indications given in the table—mainly based on the generally accepted schedules applied in the United States Public Health Service VD control program—should be considered only as norms in this respect. Functional and other damage caused by the syphilitic processes require supporting therapy and collateral medical care.

As gummatous lesions may coexist with or precede cardiovascular and/or neurosyphilis, routine physical examination, including roentgenologic examination of the cardiovascular system and examination of the crebrospinal fluid, should be made before treatment, which should be adjusted to the findings. Gummas resolve rapidly, but require several months to heal, depending on size and location.

Maternal and Prenatal ("Congenital") Syphilis. The provision of treatment in diagnosed maternal syphilis is often urgent. Even with diagnosis late in pregnancy, a normal infant can be expected after adequate penicillin therapy. Treatment of maternal syphilis depends on the stage of disease as in other infected persons. With solely anamnestic or serologic evidence of syphilis, the need for treatment should be evaluated at each pregnancy. Confirmation of past adequate therapy and subsequent absence of evidence of active syphilis justify withholding treatment unless reinfection occurs. *If doubt exists concerning diagnosis or previous therapy, pregnant women should be retreated adequately, regardless of reagin titer.*

Infants with manifest early congenital syphilis are often seriously ill and require treatment and medical care in hospital. Penicillin is provided by body weight of children and preadolescents. Patients with interstitial keratitis should be hospitalized for intensive treatment (0.3 megaunit of benzyl penicillin G daily for three weeks) and local hydrocortisone application. Treatment of ocular, aural, osseous, and late systemic manifestations requires consultation with specialists.

Prophylactic Treatment. In persons with suspected or known exposure to infectious syphilis lesions, it is fallacious to await development of clinical or serologic symptoms before treatment. If the chain of infection involves a pregnant woman, it is generally accepted that prophylactic treatment should be given immediately. However, prophylactic treatment is increasingly being accepted in other circumstances also, because considerations applicable in previous arsenical therapy (long-treatment courses and toxicity) do not apply to present-day antimicrobial drugs. Syphilis is often acquired from promiscuous heterosexual or homosexual practices. Physicians cannot influence behavioral patterns of contacts. In individual cases, however, the physician can endeavor to elicit contact information comprising the three previous months in primary, six months in secondary, and twelve months in latent syphilis as a basis for epidemiologic action and treatment by a local clinic or health authorities.

When prophylactic treatment is given by the physician, it should be adequate, meaning curative for early syphilis, so as to prevent any hidden or asymptomatic infection from developing, and appropriate clinical and laboratory post-treatment surveillance should be arranged.

Patients Previously Treated. Older patients sometimes confront the physician with information concerning previous injections of arsenicals and/or bismuth or penicillin. Such patients may show low titer reagin tests and TPI/FTA seroreactivity. The physician is justified in treating these patients as newly discovered cases of late latent syphilis after exclusion of systemic involvement when adequate history of disease or therapy cannot be obtained.

Penicillin Side Reactions. An acute systemic febrile reaction—the Herxheimer reaction—with intensification of lesions occurs in about half the patients with early syphilis when treated with antitreponemal drugs, e.g., penicillin. It occurs within 12 to 24 hours, and lasts for 6, seldom for 24 hours after the first injection. Corticosteroid preparations appear to attenuate Herxheimer symptoms. Reaction to subsequent penicillin injections signals intolerance to the antimicrobial drug in late syphilis, e.g, aortitis or paresis. The Herxheimer reaction can be severe, but does not—according to modern authorities—indicate interruption of therapy, gumma of larynx being among particular exceptions.

Penicillin may give rise to drug-induced hypersensitivity based on antigen-antibody reactions. The *immediate* or accelerated type shows urticaria, angioneurotic edema, and anaphylactic shock. It is common practice therefore for the patients to be observed for 20 to 30 minutes after penicillin administration, which should not be used in those with known or suspected penicillin hypersensitivity. Syphilis in allergic, e.g., asthmatic, or atopic patients should be managed with caution during treatment sessions. The physician should always have resuscitation remedies readily available, notably epinephrine (Adrenalin), 0.5 ml subcutaneously, which may be lifesaving, aminophylline, and corticosteroids. The *late* or delayed penicillin hypersensitivity reaction causes dermatitis, various skin eruptions, and exfoliation, and occurs within days or weeks after challenge. The condition is successfully treated with corticosteroids and antihistamines (see Ch. 72).

The true extent of penicillin hypersensitivity is unknown, but reactions appear to be relatively rare. The frequency varies from 0.07 to 10 per cent, depending on degree of selection in patient material studies in different countries. Fatality from anaphylactic shock is 15 to 20 per million treated patients (Idsøe et al.). Most deaths are preventable if resuscitation remedies are used immediately. Objective prediction of adverse reactions is not possible. Immunodiagnosis (skin testing, serohemagglutination) is not yet suitable for general practical use.

Alternatives to Penicillin. In persons with suspected or known penicillin hypersensitivity, other antimicrobial drugs must be used. None are as effective as penicillin in the treatment of syphilis. The experience with cephaloridines, for example, must be regarded as experimental; others have marked side effects. The usefulness of orally administered erythromycin and tetracycline, on the other hand, has been demonstrated. A total dose of 30 to 40 grams over 10 to 15 days (750 mg four times daily) of both erythromycin and tetracycline is given. In pregnant women erythromycin and not tetracycline should be used. The latter in large dosages may cause serious conditions in the mother (pancreatitis, azotemia, fatty liver), and teratogenic effects, e.g., dental deformities, in the offspring. In indicated retreatment of early syphilis and in late manifestations, the total dosage should be doubled or another drug used.

Surveillance. The short period of actual penicillin treatment is in contrast to the relatively long post-treatment surveillance required. The demonstrated persistence in host tissues of treponemal forms after presumably adequate therapy and the continued TPI reactivity that may signal presence of *T. pallidum* in host tissues suggests a prudent attitude to be justified in post-treatment surveillance of syphilis patients.

Early Syphilis. Quantitative reagin tests should be undertaken at 1, 2, 3, 4, 5, 6, 9, 12, 18, and 24 months after treatment, with FTA/TPI tests at 18 and 24 months; in addition to periodic clinical examinations, the cerebrospinal fluid should be examined at 24 months. (1) If all serologic tests are nonreactive and the cerebrospinal fluid normal at 24 months, the patient can be discharged. (2) If reagin titers are persistently low or nonreactive, the cerebrospinal fluid normal, and FTA/TPI tests reactive at 24 months, further six-monthly serologic follow-up examinations are indicated, with renewed cerebrospinal fluid examination four years after original treatment. (3) If the cerebrospinal fluid is reactive in (1) or (2), it is necessary to proceed as in neurosyphilis.

Late Latent Syphilis. Quantitative reagin tests should be undertaken at 3, 6, 9, 12, 18, and 24 months and FTA/TPI tests at 1, 12, and 24 months, with examination of the cerebrospinal fluid and radiologic examination of the heart and aorta *before* treatment. Unless there is roentgenographic or other evidence of cardiovascular syphilis, the patient can be discharged from observation.

Neurosyphilis. In asymptomatic neurosyphilis, clinical examination, quantitative reagin tests, FTA/TPI tests, and cerebrospinal fluid examination should be undertaken every six months for four years. If the cerebrospinal fluid becomes reactive, the patient should be retreated, the cerebrospinal fluid examination repeated six months later, and the subsequent follow-up observations conducted as above. In symptomatic neurosyphilis, quantitative reagin tests, FTA/TPI tests, and cerebrospinal fluid examination should be obtained at six-month intervals for four years. If there is no improvement at six months, the patient should be retreated and the surveillance continued. If two nonreactive cerebrospinal fluid tests are obtained a year apart, no further tests are necessary (see Ch. 386).

Cardiovascular Syphilis. In addition to clinical and roentgenographic surveillance, quantitative reagin tests and FTA/TPI tests should be undertaken every six months for four years, cerebrospinal fluid examination having been made before treatment. In cases of reactive fluid, the patient should be treated as in neurosyphilis (see Ch. 587).

Late "Benign" Syphilis. The follow-up observations for late "benign" syphilis are the same as for late syphilis when cardiovascular and/or neurosyphilis are present.

Maternal and Prenatal ("Congenital") Syphilis. In the first pregnancy, clinical examination and quantitative reagin tests should be undertaken preferably at monthly intervals after treatment until term, and thereafter as appropriate for the stage of disease. In subsequent pregnancies in women with previously adequately treated syphilis, quantitative reagin tests should be undertaken at least on the initial visit and during the last month before delivery. Thereafter they should be obtained whenever appropriate in terms of the stage of disease. In *early prenatal syphilis* when lesions are present, the patient should be treated as in "early syphilis." If no lesions are apparent, quantitative reagin testing of child and mother should be carried out at one, two, three, four, five, and six months to ascertain possible differential titers. If reaginemia of the child is passive and no diagnosis of syphilis appears justified, this decision should be reconfirmed at 12 and 24 months. If disease is "active," the patient should be treated as appropriate for early latent syphilis. In *late prenatal syphilis* (over two years) quantitative reagin tests should be obtained at three-month intervals in the first year, at six-month intervals in the second year, and thereafter at yearly intervals for four years. If the cerebrospinal fluid is reactive or if other late involvement is present, the patient should be treated accordingly.

Aspects of Prevention. Efforts at containment of syphilis and other sexually transmitted diseases through broad social and educational prevention have apparently been outweighed by behavioral and environmental changes in a permissive society. Moreover, sex education—when undertaken in schools—does not always include sufficient information on venereal diseases. Even in enlightened community programs concerning sex and family-life education, the sexually transmitted diseases are often ignored. Although the physician can provide a measure of health education, prevention of disease ultimately depends on individual decisions influenced by knowledge, motivation, and convenience. These decisions concern protection from risk of infection by some (chemoprophylaxis, condoms, postexposure measures), while causing others to report for early treatment should symptoms occur.

The physician should take into account the *psychologic effect* of a diagnosis of syphilis and give the patient sufficient time to alleviate his anxiety, distress, and ignorance; on the other hand, the indispensability for the patient to provide contact information, to complete treatment, and to accept post-treatment surveillance should be emphasized. The physician should put forward a balanced view concerning the communicability of the disease to others, risk of late manifestations, anticipated course of serologic tests, and similar matters. To patients contemplating marriage, interpartner transmission of infection and the chances of having nonsyphilitic children are particularly important. The physician should advise against marriage until the danger of infectious relapse is minimal. Such advice has less meaning if the couple are already living together. Advice concerning pregnancy prevention may then be required, and the physician should specifically inquire as to the need. Late manifestations, e.g., neurosyphilis, should receive consideration similar to other physical handicaps. General paresis is a contraindication for marriage. A dilemma arises when syphilis has been acquired from an extramarital source. The patient must then be urged to arrange for examination of the spouse. Careful surveillance is obviously needed.

The early stages of syphilis and other sexually transmitted diseases are health problems for large numbers of people. The late stages are also chronic social and economic burdens of the individual and the community. To those not seeking the services of the private physician, the community should in its prevention program make available *treatment facilities free of charge* in addition to laboratory, case finding, and social services. In several countries these are provided by state or national public health services. Internationally, the Brussels Agreement administered by the World Health Organization provides these facilities to seafarers in major ports regardless of nationality. *It is important that the private practitioner and specialist diagnosing syphilis in any community take advantage of the epidemiologic facilities of the health authorities so as to have contacts of infectious cases and their associates brought for examination and treatment by him, by a colleague, or at a clinic.*

Collart, P., Borel, L. J., and Durel, E.: Étude de l'action de la pénicilline dans la syphilis tardive: persistance due tréponème pâle après traitement. Première partie: La syphilis tardive expérimentale. Seconde partie: La syphilis tardive humaine. Ann. Inst. Pasteur, 102:596, 692, 1962.

Gjestland, T.: The Oslo Study of untreated syphilis: An epidemiologic investigation of the natural course of the syphilitic infection based upon a re-study of the Boeck-Bruusgaard material. Acta Derm. Venereol. (Stockh.), 35, Suppl. 34, 1955.

Idsøe, O., Guthe, T., and Willcox, R. R.: Penicillin in the treatment of syphilis. The experience of three decades. Bull. WHO (Suppl.), 47:1, 1972.

Levene, G. M., Wright, D. J. M., and Turk, J. L.: Cell-mediated immunity and lymphocyte transformation in syphilis. Proc. R. Soc. Med., 64:426, 1971.

McDermott, W.: Microbial persistence. Yale J. Biol. Med., 30:257, 1957/58.

McDermott, W.: Microbial Persistence. The Harvey Lectures, Series 63. New York, Academic Press, 1969.

Miller, J.: Immunity in experimental syphilis. Successful vaccination of rabbits with *Treponema pallidum,* Nichols strain, attenuated by irradiation. J. Immunol., 110:1206, 1973.

Smith, J. L., and Israel, C. W.: The presence of spirochetes in late seronegative syphilis. J.A.M.A., 199:980, 1967.

Syphilis and other venereal diseases. Med. Clin. North Am., 48:613, 1964.

Turner, T. B., Hardy, P., Newman, B., and Nell, E.: Effect of passive immunization on experimental syphilis in the rabbit. Johns Hopkins Med. J., 133:241, 1972.

United States Department of Health, Education and Welfare: Syphilis: A Synopsis. Public Health Service publication No. 1660. Washington, D.C., U.S. Government Printing Office, 1968.

Willcox, R. R.: A Textbook of Venereal Diseases and Treponematoses. 2nd ed. Springfield, Ill., Charles C Thomas, 1964.

World Health Organization: Cell-mediated immunity responses. Report of a Scientific Group. WHO, Tech. Rep. Ser. 423, 1969.

World Health Organization: Report of a Scientific Group on Treponematoses Research. WHO, Tech. Rep. Ser., 455, 1970.

Wright, D. J. M., and Doniach, R.: Recent advances in the immunology of syphilis. Proc. R. Soc. Med., 64:419, 1971.

Yobs, A., Clark, J. W., Jr., Mothershed, S. E., Bullard, J. C., and Artley, C. W.: Further observations on the persistence of *Treponema pallidum* after treatment in rabbits and humans. Br. J. Vener. Dis., 44:116, 1968.

NONSYPHILITIC TREPONEMATOSES: YAWS, BEJEL, PINTA

247. INTRODUCTION

The course and manifestations of venereal syphilis include many of the features of other nonsyphilitic treponematoses endemic among children and adults in tropical, subtropical, or adjoining regions, where rural populations reside in unhygienic and poor socioeconomic conditions. Clinical features have given distinct names to each of these conditions: yaws, bejel, and pinta. Each is caused by treponemes morphologically indistinguishable from *T. pallidum,* and a scale of pathogenicity can be established based on the degree and type of tissue damage. *T. carateum (pinta)* is the least invasive, affecting only human skin. *T. pertenue (yaws)* affects both the cutaneous and osseous systems. The *treponeme of bejel* affects, in addition, mucous membranes. In contrast to venereal syphilis, there is as a rule no cardiovascular and nervous system involvement or congenital disease in the nonsyphilitic treponematoses.

In addition to the treponemes causing the human infections, the related *T. cuniculi* is responsible for a naturally occurring sexually transmitted spirochetosis of rabbits. The organism is morphologically indistinguishable from pathogenic human treponemes and gives rise to the formation of reagin and treponemal antibodies; the condition responds to antisyphilitic drugs and shows some degree of reciprocal immunity to syphilis and yaws. Finally, cynomolgous monkeys in Africa sometimes have a naturally occurring, apparently asymptomatic treponematosis with significant treponemal serum antibody levels. When isolated and "reactivated" by experimental hamster passages, the treponemes found in lymph nodes are apparently closely related to *T. pertenue* of yaws (Fribourg-Blanc et al.; Sepetjian et al.).

In controlled laboratory experiments, each disease condition usually reproduces itself. However, long-term exposure of infected animals to different environmental conditions may, in some circumstances, modify the biologic characteristics of the particular treponemes. The extent to which this phenomenon occurs in nature has given rise to several speculations concerning the origin and phylogenesis of treponematoses through the ages (Hudson; Willcox; Hackett).

All persons with nonsyphilitic treponematoses develop reagin and treponemal antibodies just as in venereal syphilis; there is a varying degree of cross-immunity between these conditions, and all respond to penicillin and other antisyphilitic drugs. This group of infections—including venereal syphilis—is therefore referred to as treponematoses, notwithstanding individual clinical, biologic, and epidemiologic differences within the group, reflected in problems of diagnosis, treatment, prevention, and community control.

In the past two decades yaws, pinta, and bejel have been subjected to mass penicillin campaigns in the areas of the world where they prevail. Millions of persons with clinical or latent infections or contacts have been treated with long-acting penicillin preparations under the aegis of the World Health Organization, resulting in a remarkable regression of disease and infection, as evidenced in long-term seroepidemiologic postcampaign studies. The application of such methods has become of interest also in the study of "disappearing disease" in relation to the dynamics and theory of epidemic diseases in general (Guthe et al., 1972).

Fribourg-Blanc, A., Niel, G., and Mollaret, H. H.: Note sur quelques aspects immunologiques du cynocéphale Africaine. Bull. Soc. Pathol. Exot., 59:54, 1966.

Guthe, T., Ridet, J., Vorst, J., D'Costa, J., and Grab, B.: Methods of surveillance of endemic treponematoses and sero-immunological investigations of "disappearing" disease. Bull. WHO, 46:1, 1972.

Hackett, C. J.: On the origin of the human treponematoses. Bull. WHO, 29:7, 1963.

Sepetjian, M., Tissot-Guerraz, F., Salussola, D., Thivolet, J. Z., and Mournier, C.: Contribution à l'étude du tréponème isolé du singe par A. Fribourg-Blanc. Bull. WHO, 40:141, 1969.

Willcox, R. R.: Evolutionary cycle of treponematoses. Br. J. Vener. Dis., 36:78, 1960.

248. YAWS
(Frambesia Tropica, Pian, Bouba, Parangi, Patek)

Definition. Yaws is produced by a spirochetal microorganism, *T. pertenue,* which causes a chronic human infection, most often with onset in childhood. An initial cutaneous lesion usually appears, followed by relapsing infectious secondary nondestructive lesions of the skin, periosteum, and bones, frequently interspersed with symptom-free periods. Late manifestations include destructive and deforming lesions of skin, bones, and joints. Hyperkeratosis, notably of the soles, may develop in secondary and late yaws. There is no evidence of cardiac or nervous system involvement or of prenatal manifestations. Infected persons slowly develop relative immunity, and humoral antibodies can be detected by serologic tests reactive also in other treponematoses (syphilis, pinta).

History. Yaws probably existed in Africa from remote times. Early accounts suggest that it was brought to the West Indies with the slave trade in the sixteenth century. By the eighteenth century it had become a serious health problem of the Antilles, Central America, and South America, as well as in areas of Oceania and Southeast Asia. Sauvages (1778) proposed the name frambesia for the disease because of the raspberry-like appearance of its papillomatous secondary lesions. Moseley (1800) observed its clinical course, notably that yaws ends in enlarged nodes and destructive lesions. Maxwell (1839) determined its incubation period to be three to four weeks after inoculation of lesion material into humans. Castellani (1905) identified *T. pertenue* as the causative microorganism of yaws. Lambert (1923) first attempted community-wide treatment with arsenicals in the Pacific Isles. The advent of long-acting penicillin preparations and single injection therapy revolutionized case treatment and made possible important reduction of yaws by mass penicillin campaigns (World Health Organization, 1950–1970) in the tropics.

Etiology. The causative agent, *T. pertenue,* is a helical cell 8 to 12 μ in length and about 0.2 μ in diameter, with several closely set spirals. It resembles *T. pallidum* (syphilis) and *T. carateum* (pinta) morphologically in dark-field illumination and structurally in electron microphotographs. *T. pertenue* has not been grown in vitro, but will survive in special media for several days without multiplication. Strains stored in glycerin remain virulent for many years at −70° C (CO_2 ice) or lower temperatures, e.g., liquid nitrogen or helium. *T. pertenue* is pathogenic for the same animal species as *T. pallidum.* The latter causes subclinical "silent" infection in the hamster, whereas *T. pertenue* causes a specific dermatitis—a procedure sometimes used to differentiate between treponemes in the laboratory (Vaisman, 1969). Pathogenic treponemes closely resembling or identical with *T. pertenue* have been isolated from wild cyno-

The author wishes to acknowledge the valuable advice of his colleague Dr. J. Ridet, Medical Officer, Communicable Diseases Division, World Health Organization, Geneva, concerning this chapter.

molgous African monkeys (Fribourg-Blanc et al.; Sepetjian et al., 1968).

Epidemiology and Pathogenesis. Despite mass penicillin campaigns in recent years, yaws has remained a disease of many rural communities in the intertropical zone in Africa, the Americas, Southeast Asia, and Oceania. Areas of high prevalence of active yaws sometimes lie within a few miles of communities where the disease is rarely observed, depending on the ecologic situation, the evolutionary stage of endemicity, and the number of susceptibles at any given time. There is also a higher frequency of early yaws lesions in the rainy than in the dry season (Harding, 1947). Moreover, skin lesions are less frequent in cooler climates in mountainous tropical communities where they also become less moist and where papillomas tend to erupt in sweaty, mucocutaneous junctions and skin folds rather than involving the flat body surfaces (Ramsey, 1925). Furthermore, the occasional yaws lesions encountered after mass penicillin campaigns appear to be less extensive and less moist. In areas where no further lesions are encountered after such campaigns, continued specific seroreactivity (TPI) in a small proportion of children born after the campaigns could suggest the possibility of asymptomatic infection taking place in the new circumstances.

T. pertenue is incapable of penetrating unbroken skin. It is also unable to pass the placenta and cause congenital yaws. Transmission usually occurs through contact of skin abrasions, cuts, or lesions, e.g., trauma, injury, dermatoses, with infectious yaws lesions of another person. Indirect transmission via contaminated hands is believed to occur among children. Nursing mothers are sometimes infected directly by their infants. In addition to early infectious lesions, untreated latent yaws cases—which are liable to relapse with active lesions—form an important part of the reservoir maintaining the disease in rural communities. Humidity, moisture-holding soil, and mean annual temperatures of 27° C or more are also necessary for the spread of yaws. Moreover, transmission is favored by scant clothing, bare feet, crowded dwellings, and deficient personal hygiene. The gradual improvement of environmental and socioeconomic conditions will reduce the attack rate of yaws (Saxena and Prasad, 1963).

No true vector has been found in which *T. pertenue* actually multiplies, but it has been shown that disease can be transmitted by experimentally infected gnats. In some areas *Hippelates pallipes* may serve as mechanical carriers (Kumm and Turner, 1936). Geographic coexistence of foci of human yaws and natural treponematoses of wild cynomolgous monkeys have been observed in Africa (Baylet et al., 1970).

The age distribution of yaws depends on the rate of transmission and level of endemicity. In hyperendemic communities, e.g., the former Netherlands New Guinea (Kranendonk), the highest incidence of infectious lesions was in the two- to five-year-olds, with a seroprevalence of more than 90 per cent, pointing to an early, almost complete epidemic "saturation" of the community with yaws. In areas of moderate or low endemicity the highest seroprevalence is in older age groups. After mass penicillin campaigns, maximal seroprevalence was in the 45- to 59-year-olds, e.g., Nigeria, signaling regression of a hyperendemic situation many years ago. In the latter instance many more young individuals are susceptible to yaws in the new generation, but there are also more barriers to impede renewed spread of the infection, e.g., education, health consciousness, chemotherapy, and health services. On the other hand, the greater number of serologically nonreactive young people in the new generation have, when reaching puberty, less protective cross-immunity to infection with venereal syphilis. This, in turn, has been reported to be among the reasons for the increased incidence of syphilis noted in tropical countries in the last decade.

Pathology. A main pathologic feature of yaws is the involvement of the skin. In early lesions the epidermis is thickened. There are cell infiltration ("plasmocytoma") of the dermis, hyperplasia, edema, and the presence of many treponemes. The papillae are elongated, often with thickening of the interpapillary pegs. Proliferation of vascular endothelium and obstruction of vessels are less characteristic of yaws than of syphilis. The epithelium may show hyperkeratosis, become superficially eroded, and be covered by dried exudate. The acanthotic epidermis and the papillary proliferation give rise to a fungating, frambesiform, crust-covered lesion. Diffuse periostitis and cortical rarefaction of the long bones are common in early yaws and are more marked than in venereal syphilis. The late lesions of yaws are due to a different tissue response, and endarteritis is observed histopathologically. Late lesions include ulcerating granulomatous nodules and gumma of the skin and bones. The gumma is built of elements similar to syphilitic lesions. Late skeletal affliction is mostly characterized by periosteal proliferation, rarefaction, or destruction of multiple areas of the long bones which can lead to extensive deformities.

Clinical Characteristics. At the site of entry of *T. pertenue* an initial lesion usually develops after an incubation period of three to four weeks. The implantation is facilitated by previous breaks in the skin (abrasion, injury, vaccination). The lesion is a papule situated on the legs in more than half the cases. In babies and toddlers it often appears on the buttocks or in the perineum. The papule grows into a round, broad-based granulomatous lesion ("mother yaw") covered by a serous crust from which *T. pertenue* can be recovered. The regional lymph nodes are frequently enlarged, not "shotty," and do not suppurate. An initial lesion will heal spontaneously within three to six months; ulcerating initial lesions require more time to heal.

As a result of early treponemia a generalized secondary eruption appears before or after the healing of the initial lesion. The most frequent and characteristic eruptions are roundish, raised, rough, granulomatous papules ("yaws" or frambesides), often covered by a brownish crust. These lesions appear anywhere on the skin, but rarely on the scalp. They sometimes show arciform arrangements. Secondary lesions may last for more than six months. A new crop may appear before the preceding lesions heal. Relapsing crops tend increasingly to become localized, e.g., to periaxillary, perianal, or circumoral areas. Sometimes the papilloma may be solitary. Plantar papules appear late, often after the generalized eruption, and are modified by a thick keratotic layer characteristic of barefoot people: a cherry-like granuloma appears in a well of cracked horny layer, frequently giving rise to painful disability ("crab yaws"). On the body, micropapular as well as various forms of macular or desquamative macular ("pian dartre") lesions may also appear. Lesions of mucous membranes are rare, but occur. Desquamatous macules can develop in the palms and notably on the soles, which are sometimes covered by a thick hyperkeratotic layer. In addition to skin eruptions in early yaws, there is superficial lymph node enlargement. In many cases there are pain and tenderness of the tibial shaft and other long bones owing to early periostitis. Such periostitis sometimes leads to saber tibia and polydactylitis. In many cases the general health of the patient appears little affected; in others there are systemic manifestations, with irregular fever, loss of appetite, and weight loss.

The secondary lesions begin to regress after several months, but relapses may occur on and off for four to five years before true latency is reached. The latter can be interrupted by late lesions of several types. (1) *Superficial ulcerations* of the skin with central healing tendency are observed, and *cutaneous and subcutaneous nodules* with ulceration and marginal healing may leave markedly dyspigmented atrophic scars, sometimes with deforming contractures. (2) *Diffuse or more localized hyperkeratosis* of the soles – less frequently of the palms – with fissuring and pitting can result in a characteristic mottled pattern, occasionally complicated by ulceration and sometimes developing more than 15 years after the infection. (3) *Osteal or periosteal gummatous lesions* of the tibia and other long bones may penetrate subcutaneous and cutaneous tissues, resulting in chronic ulcerations. These may also affect tarsal and carpal bones, the scapula, the sternum, and the skull. Affliction of palatonasal structures may lead to gangosa (rhinopharyngitis mutilans), a spectacular condition similar to that in syphilis. The osteitis and periostitis can occur both in association with generalized skin lesions and after these have receded.

Other yaws lesions are less common and include painless subcutaneous fibromatous juxta-articular nodes, paranasal egg-shaped swelling of the superior maxillary bone (goundou), chronic late macular or hyperkeratotic lesions of palmar surfaces, and volar aspects of wrists and insteps of soles, frequently followed by depigmentation.

Diagnosis. Typical early yaws lesions are generally not confused clinically with other conditions. Ulcerated initial leg lesions may sometimes be mistaken for other ulcerations, e.g., tropical ulcer. Also, spirochetes found in tropical ulcers resembling *Borrelia vincentii* may be mistaken for *T. pertenue.* Facial yaws papules may look like crusted impetigo. Individual lesions may resemble those of secondary syphilis or cutaneous leishmaniasis. Demonstration of treponemes by microscopic dark-field examination of exudate from the lesion and seroreactivity in reagin and treponemal antibody tests (VDRL, FTA, TPI, TPHA) serve to distinguish yaws from other conditions except those of the treponematosis group. Reagin tests become positive in serum about a month after the initial lesion (Li and Soebekti, 1955), and TPI titers can be very high (1:2560) in early yaws (WHO, Eastern Nigeria, 1968). Ulcerating contractures and mutilating lesions may present differential diagnostic problems in relation notably to leprosy and tuberculosis. Hyperkeratosis of the soles is often confused with other plantar conditions, mainly keratoma plantare sulcatum, plantar pitting, and tropical hyperkeratotic conditions of unknown origin (Hackett and Lowenthal).

Prognosis. In infected persons the prognosis is favorable when early treatment is provided. Otherwise, periodic infectious recurrences over many years give rise to months of incapacity. An undetermined number of infected persons develop late lesions. Others go on to spontaneous clinical cure; some also become serologically nonreactive ("burnt-out yaws"). Among those developing late chronic lesions, extensive invalidism and deformities often result.

Treatment and Control. The aim of treatment of individual patients is cure of the early disease and prevention of late manifestations. Intramuscular injection of 1.2 megaunits of benzathine penicillin (DBED) or 2.4 megaunits of PAM (procaine penicillin G in oil and 2 per cent monostearate) in adults and half doses for children suffices to cause disappearance of early lesions and prevent relapses. The response is dramatic. The early lesions usually become dark-field-negative within 48 hours, and healing takes place within 1 to 2 weeks. Serologic titers decline, but many retain low-titer reagin seroreactivity, depending on the duration of the infection (D'Mello and Krag, 1955). Penicillin sometimes causes a Herxheimer reaction. The usual safeguards against hypersensitivity reactions to penicillin should be taken (see Ch. 246). Persons with late yaws lesions may require repeated therapy. Oxytetracycline and chlortetracycline are reported to be useful in cases of deforming osteoperiostitis, indolent gummas, or ulcerations. Two grams daily for five to ten days in adults and proportionately less for children are given. Ulcerations of late yaws may also require application of local antiseptic dressings. Deformities caused by chronic osteitis and contractures may necessitate local surgery in addition to drug therapy.

In the efforts to achieve community-wide control of yaws, the previous work of the Jamaica Yaws Commission (1936) was in recent years extended under the auspices of the World Health Organization. Since 1950 some 200 million people in 45 countries were examined, and some 50 million treated with long-acting penicillin in large-scale control programs. The aim was (1) to survey entire area populations so as to control the reservoir of infection, (2) to interrupt the spread of yaws through mass treatment, rendering early cases noncontagious, preventing infectious recurrences, and aborting incubating disease, and (3) to undertake postcampaign yaws surveillance by periodic resurveys to detect and promptly treat overlooked cases or new infections that might arise. Untreated early cases free of clinical symptoms between outbreaks form an important part of the reservoir of infection and contribute to maintain the disease in rural communities. Accordingly, mass treatment criteria in these campaigns were based on a certain association in the population between the occurrence of clinically active lesions and of seroprevalence owing both to such lesions and to clinically symptom-free infections (Hackett and Guthe, 1956). The criteria for mass treatment are as follows: (1) When the prevalence of active yaws cases is 10 per cent or higher (hyperendemic areas), more than 50 per cent of the population is seroreactive, and all members of the community are to be treated. (2) When there are 5 to 10 per cent of active cases (mesoendemic area), all children and their obvious contacts are treated, because most contagious cases occur in the lower age groups. (3) When there are less than 5 per cent active cases (hypoendemic areas), solely case and contact treatment is provided. This wide use of penicillin results in rapid regression of active lesions. The prevalence thus has declined within a few years from more than 20 per cent to less than 1 per cent after mass campaigns in many areas. Examples of reduction in *infectious* yaws are: in N. Nigeria from 4.2 (1954) to 0.1 per cent (1964); in W. Samoa 3 per cent (1955) to nil (1965).

Indifference must be anticipated in rural populations toward long-term surveillance after mass campaigns that resulted in "disappearance" of community-wide diseases. In the case of yaws, seroepidemiologic studies have shown continued low-level transmission with tendency to focal outbreaks ten to fifteen years after mass campaigns (Guthe). Using cardiolipin serology, 40 per cent of children in areas of Indonesia remained seroreactive four to eight years after treatment, and 13 per cent of the seroreactive children still had high seroreactivity titers. A potential for clinical relapses therefore remains. It is really not possible to drive a community disease out of existence by the use of a drug alone even if the population coverage in mass campaigns is nearly complete. Broader measures are needed, notably development of basic health services, into the functions of which the continued surveillance of communicable diseases can be integrated following mass campaigns, e.g., against yaws. (World Health Organization, 1970).

Prophylaxis. Prevention of yaws depends on avoidance of minor injuries to the skin, and of shielding of open wounds and abrasions from contamination by flies. Open infectious lesions should be protected. Health education should aim at improvement of personal hygiene (soap) and community hygiene (water). Children with infectious lesions should be treated and excluded from school until noninfectious. Mass therapy represents an important control measure. No method of artificial immunization is available.

Fluker, J. L., and Hewitt, A. B.: Late yaws. Br. J. Vener. Dis., 46:264, 1970.

Guthe, T.: Clinical, serological and epidemiological features of framboesia tropica (yaws) and its control in rural communities. Acta Dermatovener. (Stockholm) 49:343, 1969.

Hackett, C. J., and Guthe, T.: Some important aspects of yaws eradication. Bull. WHO, 15:869, 1956.

Hackett, C. J., and Lowenthal, L. J. A.: Differential Diagnosis of Yaws. WHO Org. Monograph Series No. 45, Geneva, 1960.

Kantor, I., et al.: Test patterns of yaws antibodies in New Zealand. Arch. Dermatol., 103:226, 1971.

Turner, L. H.: Notes on the Treponematoses with an Illustrated Account of Yaws. Kuala Lumpur, Government Press (Institute for Medical Research, Federation of Malaya, Bulletin No. 9), 1959.

Turner, T. B., and Saunders, G. M.: Yaws in Jamaica: 1. An epidemiological study of two rural communities. Am. J. Hyg., 21:483, 1935.

World Health Organization: Bibliography on yaws 1905–1962. Geneva, 1963.

World Health Organization: Scientific Group of Treponematoses Research. WHO Techn. Rep. Ser., No. 455, 1970.

249. BEJEL
(Endemic Syphilis, Nonvenereal Childhood Syphilis, Belesh, Dichuchwa, Niovera, Skerljevo)

Definition. Bejel is a chronic, inflammatory childhood disease of the treponematosis group. The early disease is characterized by infectious mucocutaneous lesions and osseous manifestations resembling those of secondary syphilis. After disappearance of early lesions and an undetermined latency period, late manifestations may develop. There are skin and bone lesions similar to those of late "benign" venereal syphilis. If they occur at all, cardiovascular, nervous system, and prenatally acquired manifestations are extremely rare.

Etiology. The bejel treponeme is morphologically indistinguishable from *T. pallidum, T. pertenue,* and *T. carateum.* It is present in early lesions or lymph node aspirate. The organism has not been cultivated in vitro. In laboratory animals Turner and Hollander showed consistent differences in clinical reaction as compared with that of yaws and venereal syphilis treponemes. The bejel treponeme is apparently an intermediate between the two (Paris-Hamelin et al., 1968). Like other treponematoses, bejel is accompanied by antibody formation with seroreactivity in reagin, e.g., VDRL, and treponemal antibody (TPI/FTA) tests. Childhood infection with bejel protects against later infection with syphilis.

Epidemiology. Humans are the reservoir of bejel. Treponemes are most likely transmitted directly among children by skin-to-skin contact, or by hands moistened with treponeme-containing saliva, or indirectly via drinking flasks, the spouts of which have been demonstrated to contain treponemes (Grin). Treponeme implantation is generally facilitated by labial and oral fissures, occurring in dry climates, or by small mucosal lesions. Bejel is a household disease. In some instances 60 to 70 per cent of rural community populations have been reported to be infected. Narrow huts, crowded dwellings, unhygienic living conditions, and low socioeconomic standards favor transmission.

There are many scattered endemic centers of bejel in backward rural areas north and south of the tropics. Bejel occurs along the Kalahari and Sahara deserts in Africa, in the countries of the Balkans and the Eastern Mediterranean region, on the Arabian peninsula, in central Asian countries, and in Australia. It prevails in arid areas in contrast to yaws, which is encountered in moist, tropical jungle regions. Bejel was first described as a disease of nomadic people, subsequently to occur in settled rural populations, e.g., among the Dogons of Mali, the Islamic descendants of Bosnia, and the Bakwenas of Botswana. Previously it was widespread in the Middle East and Europe. Bejel has not been observed in the Western Hemisphere, where pinta and yaws are the prevailing childhood treponematoses. Bejel is in regression from its higher prevalence of two to three decades ago as a result of extensive mass penicillin campaigns and some improvement of health services. In certain areas the prevalence of bejel has remained higher than that of yaws because of occurrence in nomadic tribes, on account of geographic inaccessibility of endemic foci, and inadequacy of health services (Basset, 1963). It is likely to recur when mass treatment has been incomplete. Thus in Niger infectious lesions (5 per cent) and seroreactivity (30 to 40 per cent) were found some years after a mass treatment campaign.

Clinical Manifestations and Diagnosis. The experimental incubation period is approximately three weeks. Initial lesions are rarely encountered. The earliest lesions are "mucous patches" of the secondary type localized to the oral and faucial mucosa. "Split papules" occur at the oral angles. Local papular condylomata lata or anal, genital, or other intertriginous skin areas were observed in 25 per cent of infected children in Iraq (Guthe and Luger). Generalized secondary rashes and alopecia are relatively rare. Regional lymphadenopathy is common. Polyadenitis is rare. The early disease is followed by a latency period of undetermined duration, with seroreactivity as the sole sign of infection. Late "benign" manifestations of the skin develop in some patients. They do not differ in character from those in late venereal syphilis. Superficial tuberoulcerative skin lesions and characteristic serpiginous nodular ulcers occur. Nasopharyngeal ulcerations may occur and range from palate perforation to rhinopharyngitis mutilans as in yaws and syphilis (gangosa). Gummatous ulceration of the breast may occur in women previously infected with bejel who are suckling a child with oral lesions, a phenomenon which supports the concept that gumma may be delayed hypersensitivity reactions from repeated exposure (see Ch. 246). Juxta-articular nodes have been described in some geographic areas.

Bone lesions are the most frequent manifestations of late bejel, affecting the clavicle, other long bones, and the frontal bones, giving rise to swelling, tenderness, and pain. There is periosteal and endosteal proliferation, and deformities may result. Isolated cases of cardiovascular and neurologic system involvement have been described in Bosnia (Grin) and Botswana (Murray et al.). Incidental cases of prenatally acquired disease have also been reported. No case of prenatal or systemic disease was observed in several thousand examinations in a WHO project in Syria which included radiologic and cerebrospinal fluid examinations. When observed, the systemic manifestations may be due to the occurrence also of venereal syphilis in the geographic area concerned.

Diagnosis. The diagnosis of early bejel is established on epidemiologic and clinical grounds. It may be confirmed by dark-field demonstration of treponemes in the lesions or in node aspirate and by serologic tests (VDRL), reactive in nearly 100 per cent of cases. Serodiagnostic tests cannot differentiate latent bejel from latent yaws or syphilis. Because late clinical lesions are similar to those of yaws and syphilis, the local epidemiologic situation is an important diagnostic consideration. As distinct from the manifestations of late prenatal syphilis, dental deformities and interstitial keratitis are not observed in bejel.

Treatment and Prevention. Penicillin is as effective against bejel as it is against yaws, syphilis, and pinta. In the control campaigns initiated by the World Health Organization in several countries, one dose of 1.2 megaunits of long-acting penicillin PAM or benzathine penicillin G (DBED) was given intramuscularly in early cases, with two further doses at three- to seven-day intervals to patients with late manifestations. Half doses are used for contacts. The longer acting benzathine penicillin is preferred in contact treatment among nomadic tribes. Rapid healing of early lesions was followed by seroreversal in a large proportion of cases. Late destructive lesions required more time. Healing with scars progressed slowly but definitely and with some reduction in reaginemia, but with little or no effect on treponemal antibody tests (TPI/FTA), as in syphilis.

Seroepidemiologic studies undertaken in Bosnia, Yugoslavia, 20 years after the penicillin mass campaign—which was followed by systematic periodic surveillance over ten years—showed that childhood infection had been reduced to nil, the community seroimmunologic profiles indicating complete interruption of transmission. During this period adequate basic health services were provided, health education promoted, and general socioeconomic development took place. Bosnia remains the only example of eradication of endemic treponematoses. However, eradication of childhood infection has resulted in a population susceptible to venereal syphilis in later life. The absence of protective cross-immunity has thus created a new epidemiologic situation in which sporadic cases of the sexually transmitted treponematosis occurs.

Grin, E. I., and Guthe, T.: Evaluation of previous mass campaigns against endemic syphilis in Bosnia and Herzegovina. Br. J. Vener. Dis., 49:1, 1973.

Guthe, T., and Luger, A.: Epidemiological aspects of non-venereal "endemic" syphilis. Dermatologica, 115:248, 1957.

Hudson, E. H.: Non-venereal Syphilis. Edinburgh and London, E. & S. Livingstone, Ltd., 1958.

Turner, T. B.: Syphilis and the treponematoses. *In* Mudd, S. (ed.): Infectious Agents and Host Reactions. Philadelphia, W. B. Saunders Company, 1969.

Turner, T. B., and Hollander, D. H.: Biology of the Treponematoses. WHO Monograph series no. 35, Geneva, 1957.

250. PINTA
(Mal del Pinto, Carate)

Definition. Pinta is a chronic skin infection caused by *Treponema carateum*, giving rise to an initial lesion and a generalized secondary rash, both containing treponemes. Late skin manifestations comprise extensive dyschromic (treponeme-containing) and achromic (treponeme-free) conspicuous splotches. Antibodies are produced, detectable by serologic tests reactive also in syphilis and yaws. Organ systems are not involved, physical health is not impaired, and prenatal disease is not known.

History. Manifestations of pinta were described in Berochea and by Corona (1811). Frequent seroreactivity (Wassermann complement fixation test) in pinta patients led Menck (1926) to imply association with syphilis and made Herrejon (1927) assume a treponeme to be the causative microorganism. Armenteros and Triana (1938) identified *T. carateum* in Cuban pinta. Leon Blanco (1939) obtained early generalized eruptions by self-inoculation of dark-field-controlled material from lesions. In therapy Corona (1811) showed the usefulness of mercury, Maria Graz (1913) of arsenobenzoles, and Varela (1944) of penicillin.

Etiology. The etiologic agent, *T. carateum*, is a slender helical cell, 8 to 35 μ long and 0.2 to 0.3 μ wide. It has regular spirals, performs characteristic movements in microscopic dark-field examination, and is morphologically indistinguishable from the treponemes causing syphilis and yaws. *T. carateum* has not been cultivated in vitro.

Epidemiology. Pinta is an endemic treponematosis of large rural populations in tropical forest and valley regions of Central and South America. For example, in rural areas of Mexico the prevalence of pinta varied from 1.3 to 9 per cent (1964) of the census population. Pinta cases occasionally reported from Pacific islands, India, Indonesia, and West Africa have not been verified and may have been "pintide" yaws. Unlike yaws, pinta is not a disease of earliest childhood. Community data (Mexico) indicate age-specific prevalences of early pinta lesions to be 2.5 per cent below five years of age, 8.8 per cent between five and ten years, and 12.2 per cent between ten and fifteen years. In late life some early lesions occur also after 40 years of age.

Transmission presumably takes place by person-to-person contact and is facilitated by poor hygiene, low economic standards, and limited health services. Treponemes are present in early lesions as well as in

---

The author wishes to acknowledge the valuable advice of his colleague Dr. S. Christiansen, Scientific Adviser, WHO Reference Centre for Treponematoses, State Serum Institute, Copenhagen, Denmark, concerning this chapter.

extensive late dyschromic lesions, where they can be found up to 40 years after the infection. Pinta does not appear to be very contagious, because an infected spouse with treponeme-containing lesions may sometimes not infect a serologically nonreactive partner or other family members. Scratches and insect bites may provide portals of entry for the agent. Blanco found 63 per cent of 257 initial lesions located on the legs and dorsum of feet. Arthropods (Simuliidae, Hippelates, or Ornithodorus) have not been convincingly demonstrated to be reservoirs of treponemes or biologic vectors, although mechanical transmission cannot be excluded.

Host-Treponeme Relationship. Experimental animal infection has been achieved in the chimpanzee (Kuhn et al., 1968). Man is the only known natural host of *T. carateum.*

As in syphilis, two types of antibody are formed during the human infection: (1) *Reagin,* detectable by cardiolipin antigen tests (VDRL), appears two to six months after the infection. (2) *Treponemal antibody,* identified in treponemal tests (fluorescent [FTA], hemagglutinating [TPHA], and immobilizing [TPI] antibody tests), is produced notably during dyschromic late manifestations but possibly before this stage. In untreated pinta the antibodies persist for many years. Asymptomatic seroreactors in communities affected by pinta are rare or absent. Superinfection can be achieved experimentally during the early generalized erythrosquamous stage of disease, but not after establishment of dyschromic late lesions. Varying degrees of cross-immunity between pinta, syphilis, yaws, and bejel have been reported (Medina, 1965). However, knowledge of humoral and cell-mediated immunity mechanisms is lacking. The same applies to immunologic (immunopathologic) processes possibly concerned in the genesis of lesions. Related aspects are discussed in Ch. 246.

The histopathology of pinta is characterized by a perivascular infiltrate of inflammatory cells composed of lymphocytes, some plasma cells, histiocytes, and macrophages. Swollen endothelial cells show no proliferation, arterioles and capillaries are not obliterated (as is the case in syphilis), and granulomatous tuberculoid structure is not observed. In dyschromic lesions accumulation of melanin-filled chromatophores in the upper corium is characteristic, and is caused by pigment "fallout" from the epidermis. This might be a consequence of the primary process. In achromic lesions the picture is quite different—epidermis is atrophic with flattened rete pegs, melanocytes and melanin are lacking, elastic fibers are destroyed, and there is collagenic sclerosis, which explains the porcelain whiteness of achromic lesions. The pigment changes may result from direct action of *T. carateum* on the epidermal "melanin unit" (a melanocyte with a pool of associated malpighian cells [Duchon et al., 1968]). Pinta lesions are localized to skin areas exposed to sunlight. This is unrelated to the number and distribution of melanocytes. A photosensitization process is therefore unlikely.

Clinical Manifestations and Diagnosis. The incubation period in experimental pinta is 7 to 21 days. In man, the initial manifestation is a small papule developing by extension or by coalescence with satellite lesions into a scaly maculopapular lesion. There is regional lymphadenopathy. A generalized erythrosquamous rash develops three to nine months after infection, and can be of the "wandering" type. Palpable polyadenitis is not a feature of secondary pinta in contrast to secondary syphilis. One to three years after the initial lesion, sizable dyschromic macules develop. These late lesions develop from secondary pintides or independently, and pass from slate blue through violet to brown and white—the final achromic phase of the pathogenic process. The time required to pass through these stages varies for different patches in the same individual, and the coexisting colored and white skin areas present a mottled appearance. Dyschromic lesions are usually located on frontal skin, cheeks, ears, forearms, back of hands, and dorsum of feet, but never the scalp. Blue lesions may be punctate, but most often appear as smudges on the brow, cheeks, and side of nose, and may last for one to two years. Brown lesions last much longer, and white elements are of lifelong duration. The achromic lesions are porcelain white and exhibit a "geographic coast" appearance; the skin is not supple and has no skin lines or lanugo. A different clinical course of pinta has been described in Cuba (Pardo-Castello, 1942), where the early phase is limited to palms and soles, with hyperpigmented spots turning into keratotic elements. The hyperpigmentation extends to the backs of hands and forearms. In Cuba implication of the cardiovascular and nervous systems has also been suggested. Such systemic involvement has not been verified in other pinta-affected areas of Central and South America. For instance Mazotti (1966) found nonreactive treponemal antibody tests (TPI) in the cerebrospinal fluid of a series of advanced pinta patients in Mexico. Neither were abnormalities found in the cerebrospinal fluid of pinta patients in Venezuela (Lawton-Smith and Medina, 1971).

Early pinta may be difficult to differentiate from *neurodermatitis* (dark-field examination is decisive even if there is seroreactivity); *trichophytosis of the glabrous skin* (pinta does not have vesicles or pustules); *pityriasis alba* (early pinta is more infiltrated); *tinea versicolor* (secondary pintides are more sharply delineated and infiltrated); or *psoriasis* (on removal of scales in pinta no bleeding points appear on a smooth surface). In *late pinta* the leukoderma may closely resemble similar lesions in *syphilis* and *yaws* (scarring); *vitiligo* (supple skin in scalp and perianal areas); *chloasma* (pregnancy and disorders of female genitals); *melanosis* (telangiectasis and poikiloderma are not features of pinta); or *incontinentia pigmenti* (urticaria prior to spots in infancy, pattern of splotches different, concomitant retinal and organ disease).

Laboratory Methods. A diagnosis of pinta depends on microscopic dark-field demonstration of *T. carateum* in fluid from early initial and secondary generalized lesions and late dyschromic lesions, as well as on serologic reagin and treponemal antibody tests. Methodologic considerations and interpretations concerning these are related to those in syphilis.

Treatment. The treatment of choice is repository, long-acting penicillin, notably procaine penicillin G in oil with aluminium monostearate (PAM) and benzathine penicillin G (DBED). The considerations regarding time-dose relationship, oral therapy, and alternative antimicrobial drugs in persons hypersensitive to penicillin are the same as are discussed in Ch. 246. Rein et al. (1952) obtained highly satisfactory treatment results with 2.4 to 4.8 megaunits of PAM in early and late pinta. Injections of 2.4 megaunits of the longer-acting benzathine penicillin G can be effectively applied in a single dose or two injections of 1.2 megaunits in each buttock in one session.

Prognosis. Pinta neither endangers life nor gives rise to prenatal disease. It has little appreciable effect on general health of patients. Treatment causes treponemes to disappear rapidly from the lesions, which sometimes regress very slowly, depending on their extent. Achromic patches in which atrophy of the epidermis has occurred do not change. However, the disfigurement from pinta, notably of younger persons, is sometimes associated with psychologic misery and social ostracism. Freedom of choice of habitat, mate, and employment is curtailed.

Prevention. Pinta prevention consists in examination and treatment with long-acting penicillin, of all patients and their contacts, along with improvement of rural health services, hygiene, and economic standards. In the frame of the international treponematoses program of the World Health Organization (WHO) and the Pan-American Health Organization (PAHO) extensive penicillin treatment campaigns have been undertaken in rural endemic pinta areas by several national health administrations in Central and South America during the last two decades. For instance, in Mexico more than 350,000 pinta patients and contacts have been treated since 1959. Prevalence was reduced from 5.9 to 0.4 per cent in five main states.

Chandler, F. W., Kaufmann, A. F., and Kuhn, U. S., III: The histopathology of experimental pinta in the chimpanzee. J. Invest. Dermatol., 58:103, 1972.

Mazotti, L.: Negatividad de la prueba de inmovilizaciom de treponemas (TPI) en el liquido cefalorraquideo de 10 enfermos de pinto (carate). Rev. Inst. Salubr. Enferm. Trop., 22: Nos. 1 and 2, 1962.

Rein, C. R., Kitchen, D. K., Marquez, F. and Varela, G.: Repository penicillin therapy of pinta in the Mexican peasant. J. Invest. Dermatol., 18:137, 1952.

Smith, J. L., et al.: Neuro-ophthalmological study of late yaws and pinta. II. The Caracas project. Br. J. Vener. Dis., 47:226, 1971.

SPIRILLARY AND LEPTOSPIRAL DISEASES

251. RELAPSING FEVERS

(Recurrent Fever, Famine Fever, Tick Fever, Mianeh Fever, Carapate Disease, Kimputu)

Thorstein Guthe

Definition. Human relapsing fevers are acute arthropod-borne infections characterized by toxemia and febrile episodes that subside and recur over a period of weeks. They are caused by spirochetes of the genus Borrelia and occur in an epidemic form usually transmitted through the louse *Pediculus humanis,* and an endemic form transmitted through tick species of the genus Ornithodoros. The ecology and epidemiologic features are not alike. The clinical course and manifestations tend to be similar, although some characteristics are different.

History. Rutty (1739) first described the disease clinically. Henderson (1843) reported an epidemic in Edinburgh, differentiating the disease from typhus. Obermeier (1868) discovered spirochetes in the blood of relapsing fever patients. Munch (1874) and Motchoukoffski (1876) confirmed the etiology of the disease by self-inoculation of blood from relapsing fever patients. Flugge (1891) suggested the body louse to be a vector. Ross and Milne (1904) showed that "tick fever" mentioned by Livingstone in 1857 was caused by spirochetes in the peripheral blood. Dutton and Todd (1905) described the mechanism of infection in *Ornithodoros moubata* and the passing of the infection to its progeny. Koch (1906) confirmed the mechanism of ovarian transmission.

Etiology. Relapsing fever spirochetes are classified in the genus Borrelia. They are delicate helical organisms with length varying from 8 to 30 μ and width from 0.3 to 0.5 μ, with five to ten loosely wound irregular coils. These vary in different strains or in the same strain in varied conditions. The organism divides by transverse fission, is actively motile, and colors readily with usual blood stains.

Among numerous species of relapsing fever spirochetes, *B. recurrentis (B. obermeierei)* is generally accepted as the louse-borne species pathogenic for man. *B. carteri, B. berbera,* and *B. aegypti*—also louse-borne—may be subspecies or possibly only synonyms. Among tick-borne spirochetes *B. persica, B. hispanica, B. duttoni, B. turicatae,* and *B. venezuelensis* are strains with affiliation to natural transmitters of related tick species in different parts of the world. Morphologically the organisms do not differ significantly. They induce essentially the same clinical syndromes in humans. Based on animal experimentation and epidemiologic features, a distinction between louse-borne and tick-borne fevers is generally maintained. Staining methods, antigenic characteristics, serologic, and other methods have not shown consistent differences between strains as a basis for classification. Distinction of the tick-borne strains according to their Ornithodoros species vector has been attempted.

Borreliae cannot withstand desiccation and are susceptible to many chemical agents. They survive in citrated blood for three months at 0 to 2° C. When frozen at −72° C, strains are viable for long periods of time. Present culture methods on artificial media have maintained the organism alive for several months without multiplication. Borreliae multiply abundantly in developing chick embryos. Rodents can also be used for maintenance of strains (rats, hamsters). The long life of ticks *(O. tholazani* can live for 25 years) makes these insects suitable for preservation of tick-borne strains.

Transmission. Under natural conditions relapsing fevers are transmitted by body lice and ticks, although head lice, bedbugs, and fleas have sometimes also been implicated as vectors. (1) When *lice* feed on patients during attacks of relapsing fever, borreliae enter the midgut. Within five to six days the organisms penetrate into the celomic cavity outside the gut, and feces do not contain Borrelia. These do not reach the salivary glands, ovaries, or eggs. Thus borreliae are not injected into humans who are bitten by infected lice. Mutilation or crushing is necessary to transfer infection through abraded skin or by the hand to the conjunctiva, or to the gastrointestinal tract by ingestion. The louse remains infected during its short lifetime (27 to 50 days). Since transovarian transmission is not generally accepted, it is assumed that man is the only host. (2) The many *tick vectors* of relapsing fever—mainly belonging to genus Ornithodoros—attach themselves to the host for a short time, taking up blood. Several methods of infection have been reported, including infected saliva reaching capillaries opened by the bite, gut content being evacuated by the end of the meal and excreta being passed from the malpighian tubules, and infected coxal gland fluid being passed while feeding. Continued transovarian passage of Borrelia to the progeny takes place, and Ornithodoros are invertebrate hosts acting as chronic vectors in the transmission of relapsing fever to man.

Epidemiology. The epidemicity or endemicity of relapsing fevers is dependent on the biology of the vectors.

Louse-Borne Relapsing Fever. Louse-borne relapsing fever is typically epidemic under conditions in which overcrowded poor populations live under unhygienic conditions that facilitate wide dissemination of body lice. Louse-borne fever has been the scourge of armies campaigning in the field, as with typhus, with which it is sometimes confused. Cold spells or climates and heavy clothing favor lousiness and transmission of infection. Louse-borne disease has occurred in sporadic outbreaks, spreading with great rapidity across whole continents, thereafter dying down and disappearing, often for long periods. Epidemics with extensive mortality include those in Russia and Central Europe (1919 to 1923), and in West Africa and French Equatorial Africa (1920 to 1930). More recently a serious epidemic in North Africa (1942 to 1944) spread to the Eastern Mediterranean region and Europe. An estimated one million persons became ill, and some 50,000 died. Since then louse-borne relapsing fever has mainly been reported to occur in the cooler highlands of West, East, and Central Africa, representing possibly a transition from louse- to tick-borne disease. Cases of louse-borne disease have also been reported in the Far East and in several countries in the Americas (Felsenfeld, 1973).

Tick-Borne Relapsing Fever. Tick-borne relapsing fever is endemic with many circumscribed centers in the Eastern and Western Hemispheres, and has been reported from the Far East, Africa, Central America, tropical and temperate South America, the United States (western and central western states), and Canada (British Columbia). Wild rodents and other small animals constitute the vertebrate reservoir for many Borrelia species (rats, foxes, weasels, jackals, chipmunks, squirrels, owls, marmosets, and bats). A variety of tick species of genus Ornithodoros are of ecologic importance. They feed on these animals as well as on man. The frequency of relapsing fever transmission by ticks to man depends on the contact opportunities with humans. Many small animals which are common hosts of ticks bring these into houses and dwellings.

Pathology. Borreliae circulate in the peripheral blood during the pyrexial attacks, disappear prior to the crisis, and are probably present in the internal organs during remissions. In autopsy material their presence can be demonstrated notably in the spleen and brain. The pyrexial attack, the intercalate period, and subsequent relapses probably reflect an immunity pattern in which antibody is first produced against the original Borrelia strain with subsequent formation, persistence, and multiplication of antigenic variants. These in turn give rise to further specific antibody varieties in a cyclical manner. Eventually lysins and immobilizins seem to be the most important antibodies in modifying and eliminating Borrelia from the body of animals and man (Felsenfeld). Knowledge of immunologic aspects is inadequate.

Clinical Characteristics. Variations occur in symptoms of toxemia, severity of clinical manifestations, and recurrence of febrile periods, not only between louse-borne and tick-borne fevers, but also within outbreaks of each of these varieties. Generally, louse-borne fever has a longer incubation (up to 15 days), fewer relapses (usually one or two), longer pyrexial episodes (four to seven days), and longer intercalate periods (seven to ten days) than tick-borne fever. The incubation of the latter has been reported as short as one day *(B. hispanica)*. As many as 14 waning relapses with pyrexial periods of two days' duration have been described *(B. persica)*.

In both types of fever the initial attack is ushered in with chills, nausea, vomiting, joint and muscle pain, photophobia, and fever. The temperature rises rapidly to 40 to 40.5° C, remains elevated during the attack, except for slight morning remissions, and usually falls by crisis. Cough and bronchitis are frequent. An erythematous, evanescent macular or petechial rash develops in some patients, notably in louse-borne fever. The rash involves the neck, shoulders, chest, and abdomen. There are abdominal pain, splenomegaly, hepatomegaly, and sometimes jaundice of varying intensity. Epistaxis, hemoptysis, hematuria, or hematemesis occurs. Uterine hemorrhages and abortion are not infrequent. Headache, delirium, and symptoms of meningeal irritation may occur; pleocytosis and Borrelia in the cerebrospinal fluid have been described. The initial attack ends with crisis. There are profuse sweating, sometimes prostration, and occasionally cardiac weakness or collapse. In the intercalate period there is usually noticeable clinical improvement. The relapse sets in acutely with remanifestation of previous symptoms, although milder with each subsequent attack. The pyrexial attacks become shorter and the intercalate period longer.

In tick-borne fever ophthalmic and neurologic manifestations are special features. Iritis, iridocyclitis, retinitis, choroiditis, and temporary blindness may occur. Cerebral involvement may generate coma, focal hemiplegia, meningitis, aphasia, and cranial nerve palsies. These may appear late and remain as sequelae.

Convalescence in both fevers is protracted. The mortality is reported at from 2 to 8 per cent. It can be much higher in epidemic outbreaks of louse-borne fever.

Diagnosis. Except in epidemic periods, definitive diagnosis of relapsing fever depends on demonstration of borreliae present in the peripheral blood, mostly in the early pyrexial period. Borrelia can sometimes also be found in the lesions of the rash. In wet blood films borreliae can be seen under the light microscope, but preferably by dark-field illumination. The organisms are diagnosed in Wright- or Giemsa-stained films. When these methods fail, intraperitoneal inoculation of infected whole or citrated blood (0.2 to 0.5 ml) into young white mice or rats gives rise to detectable borrelemia within 24 to 48 hours.

From the onset there is a marked polymorphonuclear leukocytosis, 15,000 to 25,000 per cubic millimeter, with increase in immature forms. Blood sedimentation is accelerated. There are secondary anemia and urobilinuria, and sometimes also albuminuria and hematuria.

Agglutinating, complement-fixing, immobilizing and borrelicidal antibodies can readily be demonstrated in the serum of infected persons. IgG hyperglobulinemia occurs initially after infection, followed by a rise in IgM immunoglobulin (Felsenfeld, 1969). Inconstant variations between species and strains and variability of antigen and antibodies, even during the fever attack in the same person, limit the usefulness of serodiagnostic procedures. Reagin tests, e.g., VDRL for syphilis are reactive in 10 to 20 per cent of cases. The Weil-Felix test is reactive in titers of 1:80 or higher. Lice removed from patients can be shown to contain borreliae after grinding, suspension, and inoculation of mice. Demonstration of borreliae in ticks in this way is only presumptive evidence, because some ticks carry the organism but are unable to transmit it to the human host. Chick embryos can be infected, and this is the basis for a method of detecting positive ticks collected in nature (Bairamova).

In the differential diagnosis of relapsing fever, confusion may arise with other acute infectious fevers, notably *malaria, typhus,* and *dengue,* but also *influenza* and *early smallpox.* When jaundice is present, *yellow fever* and *leptospirosis* should be considered. The differences emerge as the attack develops. However, definitive diagnosis depends on detection of Borrelia.

Treatment. The patient with relapsing fever is extremely ill. Bed rest, careful nursing, ample fluid, and careful diet are necessary. Antimicrobial drugs are therapeutically effective. One of the tetracyclines (tetracycline, oxytetracycline, or chlortetracycline) is the treatment of choice (Bryceson et al., 1970). When proper medical and nursing care of individual sporadic cases is possible, intravenous injection is preferred during the later phase of febrile attacks. Oral administration is indicated during afebrile intervals or in older patients, e.g., 0.5 gram every four to six hours for three to five days, and then 1 gram twice daily for another three to five days. In children under ten years of age, half doses are used. Chloramphenicol, streptomycin, and novobiocin are also effective, but for various reasons are not the preferred treatment. In epidemic situations with many cases and when individual nursing care is not possible, repository or other penicillin preparations should be given in large doses to prevent failures. All borrelicidal drugs may give rise to initial exacerbation of symptoms in a Herxheimer type of reaction similar to that observed in treponematoses. A more cautious therapeutic approach and subsidiary treatment of the general and particular symptoms of the patient may then be required (e.g., hydrocortisone prior to drug administration).

Prevention. No effective vaccine has been developed. Antimicrobial drugs, e.g., repository penicillin used prophylactically, have been described to be effective under epidemic conditions. Prevention of louse-borne relapsing fever is through avoiding exposure to body or head lice, notably by personal hygiene, cleanliness, and disinfestation of louse-infested clothing and persons. DDT-resistant louse strains have developed since World War II, and control may depend on the use of other insecticidal powders or residual sprays, e.g., the dimethyldithiophosphate group (Malathion).

Tick-borne relapsing fever is much more difficult to control, because the vectors do not live on the victim. The ticks inhabit cracks of walls and floors of houses, caves, burrows of small animals, and so forth. Some ticks are night feeders and require intensive search to be discovered. Newer insecticides have a high, but not complete, degree of success against ticks, e.g., benzene hexachloride (Lindane), dimethyl dithiophosphate (Malathion), naphthylmethylcarbamate (Carbaryl). In rural endemic relapsing fever areas, avoidance of ticks might mean a change in the domestic environment and habits of residents. Exclusion of animals, maintenance of smooth walls and floors, installation of windows, and upgrading of housing are generally necessary for long-term prevention.

Bairamova, R. A.: Experience in infecting chick embryos with tick spirochetes by means of infected Ornithodoros. Journal Microbial (Moscow), 40:83, 1963 (English summary).

Bryceson, A. D. M., Parry, E. H. O., Perrine, P. L., Warrell, D. A., Virkotich, D., and Leithead, C. S.: Louse-borne relapsing fever. Quart. J. Med., 39:130, 1970.

Coffey, E., and Eveland, W. C.: Experimental relapsing fever initiated by *B. hermsi.* J. Infect. Dis., 117:23, 28, 29, 1967.

Correa, P., Baylet, R. J., and Brougein, P.: À propos d'un cas de fièvre recurrent chez un nouveau-né ou l'infection par voie transplacentaire parait peu contestable. Bull. Soc. Med. Afr. Noire Lang. Fr., 9:215, 1964.

Felsenfeld, O.: Borrelia. Strains, Vectors, Human and Animal Borreliosis. St. Louis, W. H. Green, 1971.

Felsenfeld, O.: Borrelia. *In* Burrows, W. (ed.): Textbook of Microbiology. 20th ed. Philadelphia, W. B. Saunders Company, 1973.

Gefel, A., Anzarut, A., and Pruzanski, J.: Clinical picture and therapy of tickborne relapsing fever. Israel Med. J., 23:211, 1964.

World Health Organization: Louseborne relapsing fever. Wkl. Epid. Rec., 44:425, 1969.

252. PHAGEDENIC TROPICAL ULCER

Thorstein Guthe

Ulcerative skin processes are often encountered in outpatient clinics and hospital practice in the intertropical zone. In addition to clinical types recognizable etiologically, as in treponematoses, leprosy, blastomycosis, and leishmaniasis, the phagedenic ulcer is sufficiently common and characteristic to be considered as a distinct entity. It prevails in tropical Africa, the West Indies, Central and South America, Asia, and Oceania.

Repeated experimental ulcer production in human volunteers (Panja, 1951) supports attributing an *etiologic role* to spirochetes resembling *Borrelia vincentii* and/or fusiform bacilli which are present in sloughs and deep tissues of phagedenic tropical ulcers. Proteus, staphylococci, and hemolytic streptococci are invaders of ulcers of one week's duration. Hot, humid climate furthers the occurrence – sometimes epidemic – of phagedenic ulcers in the intertropical zone, notably in jungle-forest regions. Trauma is a precipitating factor, whether by excoriation, insect bite, or wound. They provide portals of entry for the infective agents on unprotected skin, usually of young males with an active occupation, rarely in females. Forest and plantation workers, labor gangs, campaigning soldiers, and similar workers, as well as individuals of all races, are attacked. Some 90 to 95 per cent of lesions occur on the lower third of the limbs. Deficiency of protein, vitamin A, and other nutrients may favor the occurrence of ulcers, if not their chronicity. The latter is also ascribed to impaired local circulation, anoxemia, and formation of arteriovenous shunts, as in varicose ulcers.

The *course* of phagedenic ulcers is characterized by an acute phase of one to ten days' duration. A papule rapidly develops into an angry hemorrhagic bulla with surrounding inflammation and necrotization, which leads to a round, cup-shaped, fetid, painful ulcer, 3 to 6 cm in diameter, with ragged edges and a sloughing debris-covered base. The ulcer is usually single. In serious cases it may extend and affect deeper tissues, exposing muscle tendons and periosteum. Regional lymphadenopathy is usually absent; fever is moderate and inconsistent. In the later indolent phase the pain subsides and the ulcer base becomes cleaner, with hypertrophic edges owing to epithelial hyperplasia and dermal sclerosis. Ulcers may recur in the same or other areas in 8 to 10 per cent of the cases, suggesting absence of immunity. Prior to penicillin therapy, ulcers sometimes required hospitalization and local treatment for many months. Acute complications are rare (septicemia, gangrene). Chronic complications include carcinomatous changes in ulcers of long duration (Serafino and Menye).

Diagnosis is established on the basis of anamnestic information and the characteristics of the lesion. Demonstration of fusospirochetal organisms is of relative value. Histopathologic characteristics are nonspecific unless malignant changes occur. Among early differential diagnostic considerations are ecthyma, boils, and gangrene, and later the ulcerations of leprosy and treponematoses (notably yaws), leishmaniasis ("oriental sore"), and septic sore ("desert sore"). Phagedenic ulcers may become papillomatous when *T. pertenue* of yaws is implanted. Varicose ulcers are rare in indigenous populations in the intertropical zones. Sickle cell anemia is a not uncommon cause of ulceration, and the presence of sickling should be excluded by appropriate hematologic examinations.

Treatment in the acute stage includes bed rest and local application of mild antiseptic dressings. Intramuscular injections of long-acting benzathine penicillin G (DBED), 1.2 megaunits a week apart with half doses for children (Basset), usually control infection within a few days. Reinforcement of dietary proteins and vitamins has been recommended. In old chronic cases skin grafting is required.

Prevention of phagedenic ulcers is aided by improvement of rural sanitation, development of local health services, and health education. The latter is directed toward bodily cleanliness, protective clothing and footwear, prompt disinfection when injuries occur, and correction of dietary deficiencies.

Basset, A.: Tropical phagedenic ulcer. *In* Simons, P., and Marshall, J. (eds.): Essays on Tropical Dermatology. Amsterdam, Excerpta Medica Foundation, 1969, pp. 25–33.

Castellani, A.: The common ulcers of the leg, cosmopolitan and tropical. J. Trop. Med. Hyg., 60:55, 91, 1957.

Panja, G.: Tropical phagedenic ulcer (Vincent's ulcer.). *In* Gradwohl, R. B. H., Soto, L. B., and Felsenfeld, O. (eds.): Clinical Tropical Medicine. St. Louis, C. V. Mosby Company, 1951, pp. 641–646.

Serafino, X., and Menye, P. A.: Les ulcères phagédéniques cancérisés de jambe. Bull. Cancer (Paris), 55:353, 1968.

253. THE RAT-BITE FEVERS
(Sodoku, Haverhill Fever)

Thorstein Guthe

Definition. Rats are sometimes infected with two independent agents, *Spirillum minus* and *Streptobacillus moniliformis,* also called *Actinobacillus muris.* Rat-bite fever in humans is a clinical syndrome characterized by local lesion, irregular septicemia, metastatic rash, and febrile episodes that commonly follow bites by infected rats, infrequently bites by some other rodents, and rarely bites by carnivores or other animal sources of infection. In humans both the spirillary fever (Sodoku) and streptobacillary fever (Haverhill fever) have similar clinical courses with certain differential characteristics. An etiologic diagnosis can best be established by laboratory means.

Etiology. *S. minus* is a short, thick spirillum 2 to 5 μ long and 0.2 μ wide with three to four regular coils and pointed extremities with tufts of flagella. It exhibits rapid, darting motions in the dark-field microscope. Cultivation in vitro has not been achieved. *Str. moniliformis* is a pleomorphic, nonmotile, gram-negative bacillus 2 to 15 μ long and 0.1 to 0.4 μ wide. It grows in liquid media showing single rods, chains, or long filamentous forms. On solid media symbiont microscopic colonies appear adjacent to or beneath other colonies, and are made up of pleuropneumonia-like stable L-form organisms. Serologic evidence suggests that *Str. moniliformis* may be an intermediate between Corynebacterium and its own L-form (Peace).

Epidemiology. The distribution of both rat-bite fevers is worldwide and coincidental with reservoirs of infected rats where these live in close association with man. Although the rat is the principal natural host, both agents may also inhabit other rodents, e.g., mice, squirrels, ferrets, weasels, and some higher species such as cats, dogs, and pigs. By bites or ingestion of infected cadavers animals infect each other and in turn infect humans. Infection with *S. minus* is usually inapparent in its natural hosts. The agent is mainly in the blood and lacrimal secretion in rodents transmitting infection. Traumatic bleeding of gums and mucosal lesions of the oral cavity may explain nasopharyngeal presence of the agent. Reported prevalence of *S. minus* in rats varies greatly, i.e., 25 per cent in London, 2 to 22 per cent in India, 6 to 14 per cent in Japan, and nil in Atlanta (Brown and Nunemaker). *Str. moniliformis* is found in the saliva and nasopharynx of rodents with inapparent infection. The agent has also been reported to be associated etiologically with epizootics of septicemic infections of wild and laboratory rodents. Apart from bites, streptobacillary fever in humans can also occur by ingestion of food containing infected excreta. Epidemics caused by contaminated raw milk were reported in Haverhill, Massachusetts, and "Haverhill fever" became synonymous with streptobacillary rat-bite fever in the literature (Place and Sutton). Sporadic cases, sometimes in the late stages, continue to be reported (Osimani et al., 1962; McCormack et al., 1967).

Pathology. In spirillary rat-bite fever at the bite site there are intense cellular infiltration, edema, and degeneration leading to necrosis. Degenerative changes occur in the liver and kidneys. Hyperemia of cerebral cortex has been noted. *S. minus* is present at the bite site, in regional lymph nodes, and sometimes in the blood, whereas *Str. moniliformis* can invariably be recovered from the blood as well as from local tissues. The morbid anatomy and histopathology of the rat-bite fevers have not been thoroughly studied. This also applies to the possible role of humoral or cell-mediated immunity in the pathogenesis of the disease. Spirillolytic substances appear in the serum. Cardiolipin antigen tests for treponematoses can be reactive in spirillary infection. In the streptobacillary infection serum agglutinates antigens of the bacillus.

Clinical Manifestations. The clinical features are similar but not identical in both fevers. The incubation periods described vary with averages of two to three weeks in spirillary fever and three days to a week in streptobacillary fever. The modes of presentation of septicemias are diverse, although the onset of symptoms is usually ushered in by chills, nausea, and fever. There is activation of the quiescent bite lesion in spirillary fever, with pain, swelling, edema, and sometimes ulceration of the site of the infecting bite. Regional lymph nodes are also swollen, firm, and nonadherent (Gilbert et al., 1971). This is not a prominent feature in streptobacillary fever. General symptoms include muscle pain, tenderness, and prostration. With each of several episodes of spirillary fever, pain returns with exacerbation of local symptoms. In the streptobacillary variety there may be few fever episodes, even a single one. Migrating arthralgias are encountered in *S. minus* infections, whereas polyarthritis with fibrinous synovial fluid characterizes streptobacillary fever. In spirillary fever the temperature may rise to 40° C and last for two to three days with abrupt fall. All symptoms fade and temperature returns to normal between pyrexial periods. There can be six to eight attacks separated by three to seven days. The attacks then get less frequent, shorter, and milder. The rash may develop with the first or a subsequent fever attack. It is macular or maculopapular in both fevers, and in the spirillary variety sometimes petechial. In spirillary fever the color is notably of a deep purplish shade. The rash is distributed to the trunk and extremities and is not associated with itch. It fades and disappears with the fall of the temperature. It reappears in periods of remission. Endocarditis is reported as a late complication in both fevers; pericarditis has also been described in streptobacillary fever (Carbeck et al., 1967). Sometimes motor and sensory disturbances occur. Urticaria is occasionally observed. The fatality rate in the spirillary fever previously reported at 2 to 10 per cent is greatly reduced by antimicrobial therapy. Most untreated cases subside spontaneously, but others may go on indefinitely.

Diagnosis. A history of rat or other animal bite, infiltration at the bite site, the pattern of the fever, and the rash will in many instances justify a presumptive diagnosis by the physician. Differentiation from other relapsing or trench fevers may be difficult. Malaria may coexist. Weil's disease is rarely transmitted by actual rat bite. The rash may be confused with secondary syphilis or yaws.

Dark-field examination of exudate from the bite site, serous fluid from rash, or aspirate from lymph nodes may confirm a diagnosis of suspected spirillary fever. It is difficult to demonstrate *S. minus* in thick blood drop preparations even at the height of fever attacks. The serum agglutinates spirillum in low dilutions. Reagin tests for treponematoses may be reactive in individuals known not to have had syphilis, yaws, pinta, or bejel. Diagnosis is best confirmed by inoculation of blood, lymph, or excised bite site into the scrotal skin of guinea pigs or intraperitoneally in mice. In streptobacillary fever the microorganism can readily be recovered by culture from the blood, wound serum, or synovial fluid. High serum agglutination titers after three to four weeks are considered of diagnostic value. Reagin tests for treponematoses are usually nonreactive.

Treatment. Lourie and Collier (1943) demonstrated the *spirillocidal* effect of penicillin. This drug is also effective against *Str. moniliformis,* although possibly less so. Time-dose relationship studies in rat-bite fevers concerning choice of short-acting or long-acting penicillin have not been published. Benzyl penicillin G structured preparations are preferable. The extensive appraisal of therapy in rat-bite fevers by Roughgarden emphasizes that intramuscular dosages of penicillin should (in both fevers) be no less than 0.4 to 0.6 megaunit daily for seven days in the early disease, and that the dosages should be doubled if little or no effect is observed. In endocarditis the dosages should be as in similar conditions of streptococcal origin: 10 to 15 megaunits daily for three to four weeks. Streptomycin, 0.5 gram twice daily for three to four days and half dose for children, and oxytetracycline 0.5 gram initially and half-maintenance doses for several days, have been shown to be effective. These drugs are in reserve for use in penicillin-hypersensitive persons and in patients with streptobacillary infection attributed to persistence of penicillin-resistant L-forms of the organism.

Prevention. Prevention rests on rat destruction. Antiplague measures to extinguish rats also affect the distribution of rat-bite fever, as shown in Manila. Rat-bite wound in children and adults should be treated promptly with antiseptic dressing and a prophylactic dose of penicillin or other effective antimicrobial drug.

Brown, T. M., and Nunemaker, J. C.: Rat-bite fever: A review of the American cases with re-evaluation of etiology; report of cases. Bull. Hopkins Hosp., 70:201, 1942.
Gilbert, G. L., Cassidy, J. F., and Bennet, N. M.: Rat-bite fever. Med. J. Aust., 2:1131, 1971.
McCormack, R. C., Kaye, D., and Hook, E. W.: Endocarditis due to streptobacillus moniliformis. J.A.M.A., 200:77, 1967.
Mollaret, P.: Infektionen nach Katzen- oder Rattenbisse. Münch. Med. Wschr., 111:13, 1969.
Peace, P.: Evidence that *Streptobacillus moniliformis* is an intermediate stage between a corynebacterium and its L-form or derived PPLO. J. Gen. Microbiol., 29:91, 1962.
Roughgarden, J. W.: Antimicrobial therapy of rat-bite fever. Arch. Intern. Med., 116:39, 1965.
Tiriba, A. da C.: Rat bites: Clinical and epidemiological considerations on subsequent infections. Med. Bras., 17:127, 1971.

254. LEPTOSPIROSIS

Jay P. Sanford

Definition. Leptospirosis is an inclusive term applied to disease caused by all leptospires regardless of specific serotype. Correlation of clinical syndromes with infection by differing serotypes indicates that a single serotype of Leptospira may be responsible for a variety of clinical features; likewise, a single syndrome, e.g., aseptic meningitis, may be caused by multiple serotypes of leptospires. Hence, the general term leptospirosis is preferred rather than the synonyms such as Weil's disease, Canicola fever, etc.

Etiology. The genus Leptospira contains only one species, *L. interrogans,* which may be subdivided into two complexes, interrogans and biflexa. The interrogans complex includes most of the pathogenic strains, whereas the biflexa complex includes mainly saprophytic strains with no recognized hosts. Within each complex the organisms show antigenic heterogeneity which is stable and allows classification into serotypes. Certain serotypes with common antigens are arranged into serogroups. Despite contrary common usage, an example of the correct designation of leptospira is as follows: pomona serogroup of *L. interrogans,* not *L. pomona.* The interrogans complex now contains about 130 serotypes arranged in 16 serogroups (the number in parentheses refers to number of serotypes within the serogroup): Icterohemorrhagiae (13), Hebdomadis (28), Autumnalis (13), Canicola (11), Australis (10), Tarassovi or Hyos (10), Pyrogenes (9), Bataviae (8), Javanica (6), Pomona (6), Ballum (3), Cynopteri (3), Celledoni (2), Grippotyphosa (2), Panama (2), and Shermani (1). At least 22 serotypes of Leptospira occur naturally in the United States.

Prevalence. Leptospirosis, although not a common disease, has been reported from all regions of the United States. Between 1960 and 1973, about 75 cases have been reported annually. Occasional upswings in the number of cases have been the result of common source outbreaks.

Epidemiology. Infection in man is incidental and is not essential to the maintenance of leptospirosis. The infection occurs in a wide range of domestic and wild animal hosts. In many species, such as opossums, skunks, raccoons, and foxes, infectivity ratios in the range of 10 to 50 per cent are not unusual. Interspecies spread of specific serotypes of leptospires between animal hosts is frequent, e.g., *pomona*, a serotype principally associated with livestock, has been demonstrated in dogs. The infection in animals may vary from inapparent illness to severe fatal disease. The carrier state may develop in many animals wherein the host may shed leptospires in its urine for months to years.

It has not been established that pathogenic leptospires are capable of multiplication outside a host. Survival in nature is governed by factors including pH of the urine, soil, or water into which they are shed and ambient temperature. Acid urine permits only limited survival; however, if the urine is neutral or alkaline and is shed into a similar moist environment which has low salinity and is not badly polluted with microorganisms or detergents, and with a temperature above 22° C, leptospires may survive for several weeks. Human infections can occur either directly by contact with urine or tissue of an infected animal or indirectly through contaminated water, soil, or vegetation. The usual portals of entry are abraded skin, particularly about the feet, and exposed mucous membranes, conjunctival, nasal, and oral. The concept that organisms can penetrate intact skin has been questioned. Although leptospires have been isolated from ticks, they appear to be unimportant in transmission.

With the ubiquitous infection of animals, leptospirosis in man can occur in all age groups, at all seasons, and in both sexes. However, it is primarily a disease of teenage children and young adults (at least 50 per cent of patients are between ages 10 and 39 years), occurs predominantly in males (75 per cent), and develops most frequently in hot weather (in the United States two thirds of infections occur from June to October). The wide spectrum of animal hosts results in both urban and rural human disease. Leptospirosis has been considered an occupational disease; however, improved methods of rat control and better standards of hygiene have reduced the incidence among occupational groups such as coal miners and sewermen. Currently less than 20 per cent of patients in the United States have direct contact with animals, i.e., farmers, abattoir workers, or veterinarians. The majority of patients have incidental exposure, two thirds being children, students, or housewives. Swimming or partial immersion in contaminated water has been implicated in one fifth of patients and has accounted for most of the recognized common source outbreaks.

Pathology. In patients who have died with hepatic involvement (Weil's syndrome), renal involvement, or both, the significant gross changes include hemorrhages and bile-staining of tissues. The hemorrhages, which vary from petechial to ecchymotic, are widespread but are most prominent in skeletal muscle, kidneys, adrenals, liver, stomach, spleen, and lungs.

In skeletal muscle, focal necrotic and necrobiotic changes thought to be rather typical of leptospirosis occur. Biopsies early in the illness demonstrate swelling, vacuolation, and subsequently hyalinization. Leptospiral antigen has been demonstrated in these lesions by the fluorescent antibody technique. Healing ensues by the formation of new myofibrils with minimal fibrosis.

The renal lesion in the acute phase involves the tubules predominantly and varies from simple dilatation of distal convoluted tubules to degeneration, necrosis, and basement membrane rupture. Interstitial edema and cellular infiltrates, consisting of lymphocytes, neutrophilic leukocytes, histiocytes, and plasma cells, are uniformly present. Glomerular lesions either are absent or consist of mesangial hyperplasia and focal foot process fusion, which are interpreted as representing nonspecific changes associated with acute inflammation and protein filtration. Microscopic alterations in the liver are not diagnostic, and correlate poorly with the degree of function impairment. The changes include frequent double nuclei and cloudy swelling of hepatocytes, disruption of liver cords, enlargement of Kupffer cells, and bile stasis in biliary canaliculi. The changes in the brain and meninges are also minimal and are not diagnostic. Thickening of the meninges with a polymorphonuclear leukocytic infiltration has been observed. Microscopic evidence of myocarditis, including focal hemorrhages, interstitial edema, and focal infiltration with lymphocytes and plasma cells, has been recorded. Pulmonary findings consist of a patchy, localized hemorrhagic pneumonitis. Special staining techniques utilizing silver impregnation methods have demonstrated organisms in the lumina of renal tubules but rarely in other organs.

Clinical Manifestations. *General Features.* The incubation period after immersion or accidental laboratory exposure has shown extremes of 2 to 26 days, the usual range being 7 to 13 days and the average, 10 days.

Leptospirosis is typically a biphasic illness. *The leptospiremic or first phase* is characterized by the presence of leptospires in the blood and cerebrospinal fluid. The onset is typically abrupt (75 to 100 per cent of patients). Initial symptoms include headache, which is usually frontal, less often retro-orbital, but occasionally may be bitemporal or occipital. Severe muscle aching occurs in most patients, the muscles of the thighs and lumbar areas being most prominently involved and often accompanied by pain on palpation. The myalgia may be accompanied by extreme cutaneous hyperesthesia. Chills followed by high fever are prominent. The leptospiremic phase typically lasts four to nine days. Features during this interval include recurrent chills, high spiking temperatures (usually 39° C or greater), headache, and continued severe myalgia. Anorexia, nausea, vomiting, and abdominal pain are encountered in about one half of patients. Occasional patients have diarrhea (7 to 29 per cent). Pulmonary manifestations, usually either cough or chest pain, have varied in frequency of occurrence from less than 25 to 86 per cent. Hemoptysis occurs but is rare. Examination during this phase reveals an acutely ill febrile patient. A relative bradycardia may be noted. The blood pressure is usually normal, although European authors comment on early hypotension. Disturbances in sensorium may be encountered in up to 25 per cent of patients. The most characteristic sign is conjunctival suffusion which usually appears on the third or fourth day. It may be lacking in some patients, but more often it is overlooked because of its benign nature. This may be associated with photophobia, but serous or purulent secretion is unusual. Less common findings (in 10 to 50 per cent of patients) may include pharyngeal injection, nuchal rigidity, lymphadenopathy, cutaneous hemorrhages, and skin rashes that are usually macular, maculopapular, or urticarial, and usually occur on the trunk. Uncommon findings (usually less than 10 per cent) are splenomegaly, hepatomegaly, or jaundice. Defervescence and improvement in symptoms coincide with the disappearance of leptospires from the blood and cerebrospinal fluid.

The second phase has been characterized as the "immune" phase and correlates with the appearance of circulating antibodies which have been characterized as predominantly IgM class antibodies. The clinical manifestations of this phase exhibit greater variability than those during the first phase. After a relatively asymptomatic period of one to three days, the fever and earlier symptoms recur and meningismus may develop. The fever rarely exceeds 39°C and is usually of one to three days' duration. It is not uncommon for fever to be absent or quite transient. Even when symptoms or signs of meningeal irritation are absent, routine examination of cerebrospinal fluid after the seventh day has revealed pleocytosis in 50 to 90 per cent of patients. Less common features include iridocyclitis, optic neuritis, and other nervous system manifestations, including encephalitis, myelitis, and peripheral neuropathy.

Some clinicians recognize a third or convalescent phase, usually between the second and fourth weeks, when fever and aching may recur. The pathogenesis of this stage is poorly understood.

Leptospirosis during pregnancy may be associated with an increased risk of fetal loss.

Specific Features. WEIL'S SYNDROME. Weil's syndrome, which may be due to serotypes other than *icterohemorrhagiae*, is defined as severe leptospirosis with jaundice, usually accompanied by azotemia, hemorrhages, anemia, disturbances in consciousness, and continued fever. There is uncertainty as to the pathogenesis of the syndrome, i.e., whether it represents direct toxic damage caused by leptospires or whether it is the consequence of immune response to leptospiral antigens. The consensus favors toxic damage.

The onset and first stage are identical with the less severe forms. The distinctive features of Weil's syndrome appear from the third to the sixth day but may not reach their peak until well into the second stage. As in the other forms of leptospirosis, there is a tendency for the fever to lyse about the seventh day; however, with its recurrence it is marked and may persist for several weeks. Either renal or hepatic manifestations may predominate. Hepatic disturbances include tenderness in the right upper quadrant and hepatic enlargement, both of which are common when jaundice is present. SGOT values are rarely increased more than two- to threefold regardless of the degree of hyperbilirubinemia, which is predominantly conjugated (direct); e.g., serum bilirubin 39 mg per 100 ml, SGOT 105 Sigma Frenkel units. The mechanism of hyperbilirubinemia appears to be an intracellular block to bilirubin excretion.

Renal manifestations consist primarily of proteinuria, pyuria, hematuria, and azotemia. Dysuria is rare. The maximal level of blood urea nitrogen is usually reached on the fifth to seventh day. Serious renal damage usually occurs in the form of acute tubular necrosis associated with oliguria. Hemorrhagic manifestations include epistaxis, hemoptysis, gastrointestinal bleeding, hemorrhage into the adrenal glands, hemorrhagic pneumonitis, and subarachnoid hemorrhage. These have been explained on the basis of capillary injury. In addition, in some patients hypoprothrombinemia and thrombocytopenia have been observed.

ASEPTIC MENINGITIS. A leptospiral cause has been incriminated in 5 to 13 per cent of patients with aseptic meningitis. The pleocytosis is not present before the immune phase, when it develops rapidly. There are usually tens to hundreds of cells, occasionally 1000 per cubic millimeter, which may be neutrophils or mononuclear cells. The cerebrospinal fluid glucose level is almost always normal, i.e., greater than 60 per cent of the concomitant blood glucose, but occasional instances of lowered glucose levels have been recorded. In contrast to the observations with many viral causes of aseptic meningitis, with leptospirosis the cerebrospinal fluid protein may exceed 100 mg per 100 ml early in the course. Xanthochromic cerebrospinal fluid has been observed in the presence of jaundice. Each of the serotypes of leptospires that are pathogenic for man is probably capable of association with this syndrome. The most prevalent serotypes have been *Canicola, Icterohemorrhagiae,* and *Pomona.*

PRETIBIAL (FORT BRAGG) FEVER. An illness was observed in the summer of 1942 that had an onset identical with that of the first phase of leptospirosis. The most distinctive feature was the development of a rash on about the fourth day, characterized by 2 to 5 cm slightly raised erythematous lesions that were usually symmetrically distributed over the pretibial areas. In contrast to other leptospiral syndromes, splenomegaly occurred in 95 per cent of these patients. This outbreak, which related to exposure while swimming, was caused by the Autumnalis serogroup. Subsequently Pomona has been observed in association with rashes, which are usually truncal in distribution but have also been pretibial in location.

MYOCARDITIS. Cardiac arrhythmias, including paroxysmal atrial fibrillation, atrial flutter, ventricular tachycardia, and premature ventricular contractions, have been described, but are usually of little clinical significance. However, on rare occasions definite cardiac dilatation with acute left ventricular failure has been observed. Associated manifestations have included jaundice, pulmonary infiltrates, arthritis, and skin rashes. The serogroups thus far incriminated have included Icterohemorrhagiae and Pomona.

Laboratory Features. Leukocyte counts vary from leukopenic levels to mild elevations in the anicteric patients. In patients with jaundice, leukocytosis as high as 70,000 per cubic millimeter may be present. However, regardless of the total leukocyte count, neutrophilia of greater than 70 per cent is very frequently encountered during the first stage.

Hemolytic substances have been demonstrated in cultures of pathogenic leptospires. In contrast to many hemolysins of bacterial origin, which are not hemolytic in vivo, the leptospiral hemolysins appear active in vivo. In patients with jaundice, anemia may be severe and is most characteristically due to intravascular hemolysis. Anemia owing to leptospirosis is unusual in anicteric patients.

Rarely thrombocytopenia sufficient in magnitude to be associated with bleeding is encountered. The erythrocyte sedimentation rate is elevated in more than one half of patients but is usually less than 50 mm per hour.

Urinalyses during the leptospiremic phase reveal a high frequency of abnormalities, including mild proteinuria, casts, and an increase in cellular elements. In anicteric infections, these abnormalities rapidly disappear after the beginning of illness. Proteinuria and abnormalities in urine sediment are usually not associated with elevations in blood urea nitrogen values. Since the anicteric form of the disease has often gone undiagnosed, estimates of the frequency of azotemia and jaundice are probably high. Azotemia has been reported in approximately one fourth of patients. In three fourths of these patients the blood urea nitrogen is less than 100 mg per 100 ml. Azotemia is usually associated with the occurrence of jaundice. The serum bilirubin levels may reach 65 mg per 100 ml; however, in two thirds of patients the levels are less than 20 mg per 100 ml.

Diagnosis. Diagnosis is based upon either cultural or serologic studies. The most common initial diagnostic impressions in patients with leptospirosis are meningitis, hepatitis, nephritis, "FUO," and influenza. Leptospires may be isolated quite readily during the first phase from blood and cerebrospinal fluid or during the second phase from the urine. Leptospires may be excreted in the urine for up to 11 months after the onset of illness. Whole blood should be inoculated immediately into tubes containing semisolid medium, such as Fletcher's. If culture medium is not available, leptospires reportedly will remain viable up to 11 days in blood anticoagulated with sodium oxalate. Animal inoculation (preferably of either suckling hamsters or guinea pigs) may also be used and is of particular value if specimens, e.g., urine, are contaminated. Direct examination of blood or urine by dark field methods so frequently results in failure or misdiagnosis that it should not be employed as the only diagnostic test. Antibodies appear from the sixth to the twelfth day of illness. Four serologic tests are available: the macroscopic plate agglutination test (the easiest to perform but a relatively insensitive technique), hemolytic test (complex in performance but requiring only a single antigen), microscopic agglutination test (complex in performance but most specific), and complement-fixation test. Serologic criteria for diagnosis include a fourfold or greater rise in titer during the course. Cross-agglutination reactions between various serotypes commonly occur so that the infecting serotype often cannot be determined with certainty without isolation of leptospires.

Prognosis and Sequelae. Between 1965 and 1968, there were 10 deaths (4 per cent) in 277 patients reported in the United States. Age is the most significant host factor related to increased mortality. In a representative series, the mortality rose from 10 per cent in men less than 50 years of age to 56 per cent in those over 51 years of age. The virulence of the infecting leptospires correlates best with the development of jaundice. In anicteric patients, mortality is essentially unknown. With the occurrence of jaundice, mortality in various series has ranged from 15 to 40 per cent. The long-term prognosis after the acute renal lesion of leptospirosis is good. However, a few patients exhibit residual tubular dysfunction, e.g., a defect in renal concentrating ability, and a patient with permanent renal damage has been recorded.

Therapy and Management. A variety of antimicrobial drugs, including penicillin, streptomycin, the tetracycline congeners, erythromycin, and oleandomycin, have been effective in vitro and against experimental leptospiral infections. The data obtained from controlled observations in man are conflicting as to over-all efficacy. If antimicrobial drugs have any beneficial effect, they must be administered within four days, and preferably within two days, of the onset of illness. The agents most studied have been penicillin G and the various tetracycline congeners. Turner states that large doses of penicillin G or tetracycline are indeed advantageous. Within four to six hours after initiation of penicillin G therapy, a Jarisch-Herxheimer type reaction may occur, which suggests antileptospiral activity. There is general agreement that antimicrobials administered after the fifth day have no beneficial effect. Since diagnosis within the first five days requires a very high index of suspicion, management is primarily supportive. The clinical impression exists that early bed rest may minimize the subsequent morbidity. The presence of azotemia and jaundice requires meticulous attention to fluid and electrolyte therapy.

Alston, J. M., and Broom, J. C.: Leptospirosis in man and animals. Edinburgh and London, E. S. Livingstone, Ltd., 1958.

Berman, S. J., Tsia, C. C., Holmes, K., Fresh, J. W., and Watten, R. H.: Sporadic anicteric leptospirosis in South Vietnam. Ann. Intern. Med., 79:167, 1973.

Edwards, G. A., and Domm, B. M.: Human leptospirosis. Medicine, 39:117, 1960.

Heath, C. W., Jr., Alexander, A. D., and Galton, M. M.: Leptospirosis in the United States. Analysis of 483 cases in man, 1949–1961. N. Engl. J. Med., 273:857, 915, 1965.

Nelson, K. E., Ager, E. A., Galton, M. M., Gillespie, R. W. H., and Sulzer, C. R.: An outbreak of leptospirosis in Washington State. Am. J. Epidemiol., 98:336, 1973.

Ooi, B. S., Chen, B. T. M., Tan, K. K., and Khoo, O. T.: Human renal leptospirosis. Am. J. Trop. Med. Hyg., 21:336, 1972.

Turner, L. H.: Leptospirosis. Br. Med. J., 1:537, 1973.

Section Five. THE MYCOSES

255. INTRODUCTION

John P. Utz

Recent developments in epidemiology and histopathologic techniques and the development of amphotericin B as an effective antifungal drug have led to a great increase in awareness of the medical problem of systemic fungal disease. The fact that infection occurs with fungi that are free-living forms in soil, decaying vegetation, and bird excreta poses a difficult problem of control. The deliberate impairment of immune response, e.g., to decrease host versus graft reactions in patients with organ transplants, has created still another setting for infection by "opportunistic" fungi. It is a safe speculation that systemic mycotic infection will continue to be an increasing cause of human disease.

Although the chapters that follow are devoted to the mycoses per se, it should be pointed out that fungi have other pathways through which they can produce disease. P. K. C. Austwick has well summarized these phenomena:

Fungi cause three main types of animal and human disease:

Mycoses: diseases resulting from the invasion of living tissues by the fungus.

Allergies: diseases resulting from the development of hypersensitivity to fungal antigens.

Toxicoses: consisting of the *mycotoxicoses* resulting from the ingestion of toxic fungal metabolites formed in food, and the *mycetisms* resulting from the ingestion of toxic fungal fruiting bodies.

There are also three indirect ways in which fungi can be involved in pathogenic processes in animals, viz., by inducing the formation of toxic substances (including estrogens) by a host plant which is then eaten by an animal; by so degrading a foodstuff that macro-nutrient deficiencies appear in animals feeding on it; and by forming substances such as enzymes, which, although not acting directly on metabolic processes themselves, affect the availability of growth substances to the animal, e.g., vitamins, which may lead to micro-nutrient deficiency.

Fungal pathogenicity thus covers a much wider range of activity than that seen in other pathogenic microorganisms, and its height of complexity may be realized when it is possible for all three types of disease to be present in one individual animal, each caused by the same species of fungus playing three different roles at one and the same time. After all, infection and allergy together due to *Aspergillus fumigatus* are not uncommon in man.

Further complications arise in the existence of two types of fungal thallus morphology in vivo. Firstly, apical hyphal growth leads to spherical or disc-like colonies whose spread is by peripheral extension and by fragmentation, a process compensating for its slowness of dissemination by the provision of relatively large inocula for its extension, and so of more certainty of success. Secondly, the self-replication of single cells either as yeast cells or endosporulating spherules can more readily play a leading role in the dissemination of infection in the body, but for this the fungus is generally dependent upon phagocytosis. It may be said that, in the first instance, the fungus is essentially active, making its own way through the tissues and, in the second, passive and dependent on the bloodstream or blood cells for transport. The latter type of growth is also directly comparable to that in many bacterial and viral infections, being frequently accompanied by acute pyrexial symptoms, while the former is generally associated with a chronic inflammatory process extending sometimes over many years.

Failure to understand this fundamental difference in the behavior in vivo of fungi has led to much confusion in the classification of fungal disease, and it still remains a major problem when trying to generalize on the pathogenesis of the mycoses. The ability of fungi to adopt a wide range of vegetative morphology according to their environment is being increasingly observed, and a number of filamentous saprophytic fungi are now known to be capable of budding as yeast cells under defined experimental conditions, e.g., *Mucor rouxii* and *Aspergillus parasiticus* (Bartnicki-Garcia and Nickerson, 1962; Detroy and Ciegler, 1971). The possession of hyphae or of a unicellular state therefore bears no relationship to the classification or to the potential pathogenicity of the species.*

The systemic mycoses have important properties in common in addition to this point of origin in nature. With few exceptions, they are not contagious from animal to man or man to man, and epidemics or outbreaks arise from a common source. Infection is acquired by inhalation or, in a few instances, by traumatic implantation. The primary focus is usually the lung, and infection spreads hematogenously or, less commonly, by direct extension. The gross and microscopic appearance of infected tissue is that of a granulomatous process. The immunologic response is generally effective (reinfection is rare), and cellular and serologically mediated immune mechanisms have been demonstrated (see Ch. 60 to 70).

256. HISTOPLASMOSIS

John P. Utz

Definition. Histoplasmosis is a systemic fungal disease, respiratory in origin, that spreads to the pulmonary lymphatics and by the blood to the mediastinal lymph nodes, spleen, liver, adrenals, gastrointestinal tract, kidneys, skin, central nervous system, heart, and other organs. It may be asymptomatic, acute, and benign, or progressive and eventually fatal.

History. Darling in Panama in 1905 reported three fatal cases of disseminated disease, which he considered to be due to a *"plasmodium"* with a rigid wall or *"capsule,"* in *histiocytes* which he termed *Histoplasma capsulatum.* In a study of tissue section, da Rocha Lima concluded in 1913 that the agent was a fungus. In 1934 De Monbreun correctly identified the fungus in cultural and in laboratory animal studies. Ten years later Christie and Peterson recognized the benign form of human disease with pulmonary calcification and associated skin hypersensitivity to histoplasmin. Subsequently, Palmer

---

*From Austwick, P. K. C.: The pathogenicity of fungi. *In* Microbial Pathogenicity in Man and Animals. Twenty-second Symposium of the Society for General Microbiology, Imperial College, London. Cambridge, England, Cambridge University Press, 1972.

showed widely varying rates of hypersensitivity according to geographic areas in this country.

Etiology. *H. capsulatum* has two morphologic forms, *yeast* and *hyphal*, dependent upon a variety of environmental factors. The yeast form seen in tissues measures 2 to 3 by 3 to 4 μ and has a clear area resulting from shrinkage of cytoplasm from the rigid cell wall. In artificial media or natural substrate the yeast form is converted readily at room temperatures to the hyphal form with the production on Sabouraud's glucose medium of a white to brown cottony mold. On microscopic examination this is composed of branched hyphae, characteristic spherical forms with spiny projections (tuberculate macroconidia) 8 to 14 μ in diameter, and smaller forms (microconidia) measuring 2 to 5 μ. Conversion of the hyphal to the yeast form occurs characteristically after inoculation into animals or less readily on enriched media at 37° C. Skin hypersensitivity, complement-fixing, and other antigens have been demonstrated. Mice and guinea pigs are susceptible to experimental infection.

Epidemiology. Histoplasmosis occurs with highest frequency in infancy and old age and equally in the sexes except more often in the male in old age. It has been reported in more than 30 countries in both temperate and tropical zones. Skin hypersensitivity rates are as high as 80 to 90 per cent in some parts of the eastern and midwestern United States. Rates of skin reactivity increase rapidly with age to young adulthood and then more slowly thereafter. Man and animals are infected by inhalation of the fungus in dust. Soil from chicken houses or from areas contaminated or composted by bat or bird dung is especially rich in organisms. Massive exposure through such activities as destruction of chicken houses, exploration of caves, or community "clean-up" activities has resulted in outbreaks. Fifty per cent of dogs and cats in some areas and many species of wild animals are known to be infected. *Histoplasma duboisii*, a closely related fungus, produces in African patients a disease marked by lymphadenopathy and bone, joint, and skin involvement.

Pathology. The tissue reaction is characteristically engulfment of yeast forms by histiocytes or macrophages derived from organs of the reticuloendothelial system. Epithelioid or histiocytic granulomas are formed, with tubercle-like nodules, caseation necrosis, and calcification in the lung, lymph nodes, liver, spleen, adrenals, and other organs. The organism can best be identified in tissues by culture or by use of special stains (periodic acid–Schiff, Gridley, or Gomori methenamine silver methods). However, fungal cells may be few, crowded, and not differentiated with certainty from those of *H. duboisii, Blastomyces dermatitidis, Torulopsis glabrata,* or *Candida albicans.*

Clinical Manifestations. On the basis of delayed cutaneous hypersensitivity studies, it appears that primary infection with *H. capsulatum* is usually asymptomatic or produces a respiratory illness that is not distinctive.

Primary Acute Form. The primary acute form is characterized by respiratory symptoms of cough, shortness of breath, pleuritic chest pain, hoarseness, hemoptysis, and cyanosis in that order. Associated generalized symptoms are commonly fever, chills, myalgia, malaise, and weight loss. In focal outbreaks where there is exposure to large numbers of spores, sudden onset and pleuritic pain are common. Pleural effusion, however, is rare. The chest film may show bilateral disease with the characteristic diffuse miliary type of lesion, or, more commonly, localized infiltrations, especially in the lower lobes. There may be hilar and peritracheal lymphadenopathy unaccompanied by other lesions. That infection is not localized to lungs alone is attested to by the frequent splenic calcification seen later and the occasional isolation of *H. capsulatum* from urine during the acute illness. In many patients lesions resolve completely, but in others calcification or fibrotic scarring persists. Calcified peribronchial nodes may compress the bronchus leading to bronchiectasis or may erode and result in broncholithiasis. A distinctive residue of primary infection is the solitary nodule of the lung, located just beneath the pleura, appearing roentgenographically as a "coin lesion."

Progressive Disseminated Form. Rarely the disease progresses and resembles that form originally described by Darling. Pulmonary findings are often not prominent; illness is characterized instead by fever, enlargement of the liver and spleen, generalized lymphadenopathy, weight loss, anemia, and leukopenia. One particular feature may predominate, and illness then appears as endocarditis, pericarditis, meningitis, adrenal insufficiency, or multiple ulcerations of mouth, pharynx, larynx, stomach, or small or large bowel. Granulomatous uveitis has been considered, but not yet proved, to be due to *H. capsulatum.*

Chronic Cavitary Form. In older adult males especially, a chronic, cavitary pulmonary disease occurs that closely simulates and is often labeled tuberculosis. This form is characterized by cough, weight loss, dyspnea, low-grade fever, chest pain, and hemoptysis. This form is most likely a reactivation of a previously quiescent primary infection.

Diagnosis. The isolation in culture and microscopic identification of the fungus establish the diagnosis. In suspected cases of acute primary disease both sputum and urine should be cultured. In the widely disseminated forms, blood, bone marrow, cerebrospinal fluid, ulcer swabs, urine, sputum, lymph nodes, and material from liver biopsy may yield the fungus on culture. Conversion of a skin test from negative to positive and a titer of the complement-fixing antibodies that rises and falls or is in excess of 1:32 only support the clinical impression. A single positive histoplasmin skin test indicates only recent or remote exposure to this or related antigen. Frequently, both skin and complement-fixation tests will be negative in a patient with severe or early disease. Careful microscopic study of properly stained tissue sections may reveal characteristic fungal forms, providing additional supporting evidence for the clinical diagnosis (see Pathology).

Acute primary histoplasmosis should be considered in the differential diagnosis of any persistent febrile respiratory disease, especially those occurring after exposure to chicken or other bird excreta and in any pneumonia without appropriate bacteria in sputum. Hepatosplenomegaly, lymphadenopathy, anemia, and leukopenia of the severe disseminated form may closely simulate Hodgkin's disease and leukemia. Mucosal alterations so closely resemble cancer that repeated biopsies for tissue study have been performed, all with negative results, before cultures were done. As a general rule, histoplasmosis should be suspected in any patient with findings suggestive of tuberculosis but without supporting laboratory data.

Treatment. Amphotericin B is the most active of the

presently available antifungal drugs for the treatment of the disease in man. The drug is customarily given intravenously; a dose of 1.0 mg dissolved in 500 ml of a 5 per cent glucose solution is recommended as the first dose. Dosage should be increased daily by increments of 5 to 10 mg. At present there are many recommendations and no consensus as to optimal daily dosage (from 0.5 to 1.0 mg per kilogram), duration of therapy (from 6 to 14 weeks), or total dosage (from irrelevant to at least 2 grams). Each infusion should be administered over at least a two-hour period. Such undesired side effects as local thrombophlebitis, fever, chills, nausea, vomiting, anorexia, rise in serum urea nitrogen, hypokalemia, and anemia may occur in approximately 80 per cent of patients but should not require abandonment of the therapy. After treatment is stopped, most indices of renal function return toward normal, but in about 80 per cent of patients on higher drug doses values are never again the same as before treatment. Salicylates, antihistamines, and corticoids reduce the severity or frequency of such side effects of treatment as nausea, chills, and fever.

A few patients with localized disease in the lungs have been helped by surgical excision of lesions.

Sulfonamides have a measurable benefit in infections in laboratory animals and a reported activity in disease in children.

Prognosis. Except in localized outbreaks with inhalation of large numbers of fungi, acute primary histoplasmosis is almost always a benign illness from which the patient recovers rapidly. Therapy usually has not been administered.

Since progressive disseminated disease is fatal in 80 to 90 per cent, and the chronic cavitary form in 30 per cent of cases, chemotherapy is indicated. Approximately 80 to 90 per cent of patients with severe disease have recovered with amphotericin B treatment.

Corticoid treatment has been associated with deleterious effects in experimental infections of animals and with relapse after amphotericin B therapy in man.

Austwick, P. K. C.: The pathogenicity of fungi. *In* Microbial Pathogenicity in Man and Animals. Twenty-second Symposium of the Society for General Microbiology, Imperial College, London, April 1972. Cambridge, England, Cambridge University Press, 1972.

Butler, W. T.: Pharmacology, toxicity and therapeutic usefulness of amphotericin B. J.A.M.A., 195:371, 1966.

Drutz, D. J., Spickard, A., Rodgers, D. E., and Koenig, M. G.: Treatment of disseminated mycotic infections: A new approach to amphotericin B treatment. Am. J. Med., 45:406, 1968.

Furcolow, M. L., Doto, I. L., Tosh, F. E., and Lynch, H. J., Jr.: Course and prognosis of untreated histoplasmosis. J.A.M.A., 177:292, 1961.

Vanek, J., and Schwarz, J.: The gamut of histoplasmosis. Am. J. Med., 50:89, 1971.

257. COCCIDIOIDOMYCOSIS (Valley Fever)

Demosthenes Pappagianis

Definition. Coccidioidomycosis is a fungal infection usually acquired by the respiratory route. In most cases it is arrested in the lungs, but it may spread to virtually all organs or tissues. Chronic persistent infection may ensue. Infrequently the infection is fatal.

History. The disease we recognize as coccidioidomycosis was first described in 1892 by Alejandro Posadas in an Argentinian man in Buenos Aires. In the infected tissues a cystlike organism thought to be a protozoan was observed. The second case was reported in 1894 by Rixford in California, the place of origin of the succeeding several hundred recognized cases, and resemblance of the organism to the protozoan Coccidia led to the name Coccidioides. Ophuls and Moffitt in 1900 recognized the causative organism to be a cultivable mold in vitro. Most early recognized cases of coccidioidal infection were severe, often with widespread cutaneous and visceral lesions, and frequently fatal, but Gifford and Dickson in the early 1930's established that San Joaquin or valley fever was a mild infection caused by *Coccidioides immitis*. Introduction of amphotericin B in 1956 led to successful therapy in coccidioidal infections with an otherwise dismal outlook.

Etiology. In the infected host, *C. immitis* exists as a spherule (sporangium), 20 to 100 μ in diameter, and reproduces by formation of few to several hundred endospores. These endospores are released and in turn enlarge to mature spherules. The filamentous septate *mycelial* form usually found in cultures and in nature produces chains of *arthrospores*. These arthrospores (about 2×5 μ) are readily airborne and constitute the inhaled infectious form of the organism. Confirmation of the identity of *C. immitis* requires demonstration of the spherule form of the organism in the patient or by animal inoculation, and constitutes the single best diagnostic procedure.

Epidemiology. Coccidioidomycosis is usually encountered in the southwestern United States (California, Arizona, New Mexico, Texas, southern portions of Nevada and Utah), Mexico, Central America, Argentina, Paraguay, Venezuela, and Colombia. These areas correspond to location of *C. immitis* in the soil. Travelers may acquire the infection during brief visits to these areas. Rarely exportation of the fungus on some product of the endemic region can lead to infection elsewhere. The true *incidence* is likely greater than the 300 to 400 cases reported per year in California, or the more than 500 per year in Arizona. Some 50 deaths per year caused by coccidioidomycosis are reported in the United States. It has been estimated that 25,000 to 35,000 new infections occur per year in California. About a fifth of those so affected will have symptomatic infections that bring them to a physician. The *prevalence* of coccidioidomycosis increases during the dry, dusty summer and fall. An occupational risk of infection exists in agricultural or other disturbers of the soil. In some endemic areas the proportion of the population which has been infected increases with time of residence and may exceed 85 per cent. *C. immitis* survives for months at -20 to $42°$ C and a pH of 4 to 9. It can be found in rodent burrows and elsewhere, persisting for years in the soil. Rodents, dogs, cattle, sheep, and other animals are also infected by inhalation of arthrospores. The infection is not spread from animals to man or from man to man (although one case of in utero infection has been reported).

Humans from a few weeks to 85 years of age have been infected. In general, infection may be milder in children. In adults, about 60 per cent of infections are asymptomatic. Of the 40 per cent with symptomatic infections, most will recover. Approximately 1 in 100 adult white males with symptoms will develop disseminated coccidioidomycosis. Filipinos and blacks have higher rates of dissemination. Adult white females less frequently develop disseminated coccidioidomycosis, perhaps because of their greater tendency to develop the prognostically favorable erythema nodosum.

Pathogenesis and Pathology. The nature of the response to infection with *C. immitis* appears related to the morphologic states of the organism and to the development of delayed hypersensitivity. Endospores appear to induce a granulocytic response, spherules a macrophagic response. Lesions may resemble closely the granulomatous lesion of tuberculosis or sarcoid, but frequently there is juxtaposed suppuration. The mixed inflammatory reaction may yield amorphous necrosis, hyalinization, fibrosis, and calcification. The contribution of delayed hypersensitivity to pathogenesis is not clear, but anergy to coccidioidin is prognostically unfavorable.

Primary infection usually presents as a pneumonitis. (Fewer than 20 cases of primary cutaneous coccidioidomycosis have been reported.) The infection is usually arrested in the pulmonary parenchyma and regional nodes. Occasionally the organisms spread lymphogenously and hematogenously to virtually any tissue (the gastrointestinal mucosa has not been involved, and the brain and the endocardium only rarely). Such dissemination usually ensues early after the primary infection, but occasionally the pulmonary lesion has cleared by the time dissemination is apparent. In about 5 to 10 per cent of patients with primary pulmonary coccidioidomycosis, a chronic cavity or granuloma will develop. Viable *C. immitis* may persist for years in such lesions, although the patient's clinical status remains favorable. Pulmonary cavities occur and recur more frequently in patients with diabetes mellitus.

Clinical Manifestations. Clinically apparent primary pulmonary coccidioidomycosis will develop in 7 to 28 days (average, 10 to 16 days) after inhalation of the spores, presenting with fever, malaise, pleuritic pain, dry cough, night sweats, anorexia, headache, and weight loss. Chest pain is common and may be severe. Early after onset of symptoms, a macular, urticarial, scarlatiniform or morbilliform rash may develop transiently. It may be seen particularly in the inguinal areas and on the palms and soles, and often before coccidioidin sensitivity develops. Such a rash is seen more frequently in children.

Along with the respiratory component, "valley fever" classically includes erythema nodosum of the anterior tibia or erythema multiforme of the extensor aspects of the upper extremities, palms, and upper thorax and neck. This may be seen in about 40 per cent of adult white females and 5 per cent of adult white males who have symptomatic infections, and is accompanied by arthralgia and swelling of ankles and knees. Erythema nodosum indicates marked sensitivity to coccidioidin and is not likely to be coccidioidal in cause if the skin test is negative. Initially primary coccidioidomycosis may be bronchial or peribronchial. The chest x-ray may reveal pneumonitis resembling acute bacterial, mycoplasmal, viral, or other fungal pneumonias with lobar, lobular, or scattered patches of infiltrate. Hilar densities (parenchymal and adenopathy) and pleural effusion are common. Infrequently there is pericardial effusion. A transient cavity occasionally develops during the acute phase. Primary infection of the skin yields an ulcerative lesion and regional adenopathy. Resolution of primary pulmonary coccidioidomycosis usually occurs within several weeks, although asthenia and easy fatigability may last for several months. There may be persistent and unexplained chest pain despite recovery from the acute infection.

Dissemination of the infection to metapulmonary tissues usually occurs during the early weeks or months of infection. However, meningitis or other forms of dissemination may also be recognized only after the primary pulmonary lesion has faded. The progression is sometimes difficult to discern clinically until an overt lesion of bone, skin, lymph node, or meninges is detected. It may be suspected from deterioration of the patient with persistent fever, weight loss, marked bronchomediastinal adenopathy, or mental deterioration (in meningitis), or from labratory parameters to be discussed below.

Chronic cavities, coccidioidomas, or *bronchiectasis* may remain after apparent clearing of the primary pneumonitis, or they may be detected on routine roentgenograms years after the primary infection. Hemoptysis may be the first indication of a pulmonary cavity.

Diagnosis. Awareness of the extreme variability of clinical patterns offered by coccidioidomycosis is essential. It may resemble influenza; bacterial, mycoplasmal, or other mycotic pneumonia; acute or chronic tuberculosis or histoplasmosis; or neoplasms. The hilar or bronchomediastinal adenopathy may resemble that of sarcoid or lymphomas. The chronic pulmonary cavity is characteristically thin-walled on x-ray, but may resemble a pulmonary abscess or be partially filled with fluid. Coccidioidal fibrosis or bronchiectasis may resemble that of other causes. Lesions of bones or soft tissues may resemble those of blastomycosis, tuberculosis, or other bacterial infections. The erythrocyte sedimentation rate is elevated, and there is often a moderate leukocytosis, sometimes with eosinophilia. Sustained eosinophilia is unfavorable.

Coccidioidal meningitis may resemble tuberculosis or other mycotic meningitis. Decrease in the cerebrospinal fluid (CSF) glucose is often an early significant change. Occasionally in the early stages there may be a polymorphonuclear pleocytosis, but the onset is usually more insidious and the CSF changes in cell and protein are suggestive of chronic or "aseptic" meningitis. A "paretic" colloidal gold curve often accompanies these changes.

Coccidioidomycosis is confirmed by direct demonstration of endosporulating spherules in biopsied tissue or exudates utilizing special fungal stains. *Cultures* from lesions or sputum also yield a diagnosis, provided that animal inoculation is used to confirm the production of spherules. The CSF should be cultured but often fails to yield *C. immitis.*

The time involved and hazard of working with *C. immitis* cultures require that appropriate skin test and serologic studies be carried out. The coccidioidin (mycelial phase antigen) skin test may become positive in three days to three weeks after onset of symptoms. A positive coccidioidin skin test means past or present infection. A negative test does not exclude a coccidioidal cause, for the test is often negative in disseminated infections or with old pulmonary lesions (cavities or coccidioidomas). The skin test should be repeated in following the course of the illness, for anergy is unfavorable. The skin test does not interfere with coccidioidal serologic studies. A newly developed skin test antigen derived from spherules may be more sensitive in detecting sensitivity. Precipitins (IgM) are produced early and assist in diagnosis of primary infections. These are detected by a tube test and by a latex particle agglutination test. They fade within the first few weeks but may persist in severe infections and may reappear, e.g., with a bronchopleural fistula or in reinfection via ventriculoperitoneal or ventriculoatrial shunt. Complement-fixing (CF) antibodies (IgG) appear later and may persist for many months or years after recovery. They are readily detected by immunodiffusion. The CF antibody titer rises proportional to severity (extent of involvement). Thus metapulmonary dissemination is usually reflected in an elevated titer (usually above 1:16, but this level may vary between laboratories), and declining titer indicates improvement. Pleural, joint, and cerebrospinal fluids may contain CF antibody, although usually at lower titer than in the serum. Indeed in coccidioidal meningitis the CSF is occasionally seronegative but the serum positive. The basilar meningitis may yield CF-positive cisternal and lumbar fluids even though the ventricular fluid is negative. Complement fixing by the CSF is usually diagnostic of coccidioidal meningitis, although an extradural (paravertebral) abscess can yield CF antibody in the CSF. In this instance the CSF protein is up, with glucose and cells normal.

The CF test is positive in about 60 per cent of cases with chronic coccidioidal cavities, but is often negative in patients with asymptomatic coccidioidomas. Thus diagnosis of the latter is often not assisted by serologic tests. Cross-reactions occur between *C. immitis, Histoplasma capsulatum*, and *Blastomyces dermatitidis* in serologic and skin tests. Primary coccidioidal infections are sometimes accompanied by higher CF titers with Histoplasma and Blastomyces antigens. Sequential sera should yield higher homologous titers.

Treatment. Symptomatic therapy is indicated for primary coccidioidomycosis. Amphotericin B is the only useful antifungal agent in coccidioidomycosis and should be applied in most cases of disseminated disease. Occasionally, as with a small single cutaneous lesion, excision may be curative. In the absence of overt evidence of dissemination, systemic amphotericin may be administered for severe primary coccidioidal infection or when the clinical or laboratory picture indicates likelihood of dissemination. Amphotericin may be administered intravenously on alternate days, with the dose gradually raised to 1.0 mg per kilogram of body weight or according to the sensitivity of the strain of *C. immitis.* Prolonged therapy is often needed in coccidioidomycosis, increasing the risk of nephropathy, hypokalemia, anemia, phlebitis, and other side effects. Meningitis can be treated preferably by intracisternal administration of up to 1.0 mg, usually three times a week. Arachnoiditis has frequently complicated lumbar administration; however, recent experience with amphotericin given with 10 per cent (hyperbaric) glucose had less of this complication. Under some circumstances amphotericin may be given by the intraventricular route via the Ommaya reservoir and catheter. The total dose required must be determined by the progress of the patient. Therapy of meningitis should be continued for at least three months after the CSF becomes normal, but continued vigilance for years is required because of the possibility of relapse.

Excisional therapy may also be needed for osseous, articular, or soft tissue lesions. Pulmonary cavities, although generally benign, may be resected if complicated by progressive enlargement, rupture into the pleural space, hemorrhage, or secondary infection. Pre- and postoperative therapy with amphotericin is advisable, although some thoracic surgeons have had few complications without such coverage. The usually benign solitary pulmonary nodule may have to be resected for differentiation from other lesions.

Immunotherapy with Lawrence's leukocyte transfer factor from coccidioidin-sensitive donors has had limited trials. This may provide an important additional therapeutic modality, particularly in anergic patients who have not responded to amphotericin or who may be at risk of recurrence of cavities, e.g., diabetics.

Prognosis. Prior to amphotericin therapy, more than half the patients with disseminated infections and all with coccidioidal meningitis died. With amphotericin therapy, patients with coccidioidal meningitis have survived for 10 to 15 years, some apparently cured. Nonmeningeal disseminated infections have also been successfully treated, although infections involving joints may be recurrent despite treatment with amphotericin B. Recovery from infection leads to resistance to reinfection (exogenous reinfection has occurred only in a very few laboratory workers). Immunosuppressive therapy of intercurrent disease such as Hodgkin's disease with accompanying cytotoxic therapy may reactivate old arrested coccidioidomycosis.

Prevention. A vaccine prepared from killed spherules has provided good protection of laboratory animals and has appeared safe in humans. However, it has not had a field trial in humans exposed to infection. Avoidance of exposure to the arthrospores would prevent infection, but the widespread distribution of the organism and impracticality of eradicating if from the soil make avoidance difficult in those who are occupationally tied to the soil. The use of lightweight masks or other measures to reduce inhalation of spores during overt dusty exposures is justified.

Ajello, L. (ed.): Coccidioidomycosis. Tucson, University of Arizona Press, 1967.

Einstein, H.: Coccidioidomycosis, *In* Buechner, H. A. (ed.): Management of Fungus Diseases of the Lungs. Springfield, Ill., Charles C Thomas, 1971, Chap. 4.

Fiese, M. J.: Coccidioidomycosis. Springfield, Ill., Charles C Thomas, 1958.

Huntington, R. W., Jr.: Coccidioidomycosis. *In* Baker, R. D. (ed.): Human Infection with Fungi, Actinomycetes and Algae. New York, Springer-Verlag, 1971, Chap. 6.

Smith, C. W., Saito, M. T., and Simons, S. A.: Pattern of 39,500 serologic tests in coccidioidomycosis. J.A.M.A., 160:546, 1956.

258. BLASTOMYCOSIS (North American)

John P. Utz

Definition. Blastomycosis is a chronic systemic fungal disease, respiratory in origin, which, classically, disseminates to the skin and occasionally to subcutaneous tissue, bone, and other organs.

History. In 1894 Gilchrist and in 1898 Gilchrist and Stokes reported the first two cases and named the responsible fungus *Blastomyces dermatitidis*.

Etiology. *B. dermatitidis* is a dimorphic fungus existing in tissue as a yeastlike form (8 to 15 μ, rarely 30 μ), with a characteristic thick wall (0.5 to 0.75 μ). The yeast form reproduces by budding, and the typical bud is characterized by its large size and attachment to the parent cell by a persistent wall and a wide pore. On Sabouraud's glucose medium *B. dermatitidis* grows as a white mycelium composed of slender hyphae to which are attached, either directly or by lateral slender stalks (conidiophores), smooth spherical 2 to 10 μ forms (conidia). Skin hypersensitivity, complement-fixing, and other antigens have been demonstrated. Mice and other laboratory animals are susceptible to experimental infection.

Epidemiology. Blastomycosis was at first exclusively American in distribution: Canada, Mexico, Central

America, northern Latin America, and, in 98 per cent of reported cases, the United States. Recently, however, cases have been reported from widely separated sites in Africa. The disease affects all ages, but there is a slightly higher frequency in the third and fourth decades. Males are affected six to nine times more frequently than females. Man is usually infected by inhalation of conidia, but the saprophytic source of the fungus in nature is not known. In one reported instance genital infection was acquired conjugally. Benign, subclinical cases have been reported, but skin test studies do not support a high incidence of infection in certain areas similar to that of histoplasmosis and coccidioidomycosis. Multiple cases in one small town have been reported.

Pathology. The characteristic tissue response to *B. dermatitidis* is a combination of suppuration and epithelioid and giant cell granulomas. In the lung the disease may be localized or may spread as a bronchopneumonia. Cavitation and circumscribed, calcific nodules are rarely encountered. The skin lesions reveal characteristically pseudoepitheliomatous hyperplasia and microabscesses in which *B. dermatitidis* may be seen. In bone, subcutaneous tissue, meninges, prostate, epididymis, and other organs the histologic appearance is again a combination of suppuration and granulomas.

Clinical Manifestations. *Primary Pulmonary Form.* Primary pulmonary blastomycosis begins usually as a mild respiratory infection (rarely as a fulminant pneumonia) with cough, pleuritic chest pain, and, occasionally, hemoptysis. As the disease progresses, generalized symptoms of fever, night sweats, anorexia, and weight loss appear. Physical signs may not be prominent. However, there may be dullness, bronchial breath sounds, and rales characteristic of consolidation. Roentgenographically, manifestations vary from those of a consolidated lobar pneumonia to multiple infiltrations. Hilar adenopathy is common, localized nodules are less so, and cavitation is rare. Although pleural disease is common, effusion is characteristically extremely rare.

Cutaneous Form. Although cutaneous blastomycosis represents spread from a primary pulmonary infection, the presenting complaint of many patients is a cutaneous lesion, either solitary or multiple. The initial papule or pustule progresses within weeks or months into an ulcerated or warty lesion. The advancing border of this lesion is serpiginous, dusky red, or violaceous, elevated 1 to 3 mm, and has an outer edge that slopes abruptly. The base of the lesion contains small abscesses, from which characteristic budding yeast cells can be demonstrated. The central area may become crusted or, in older lesions, may be healing with a thin atrophic scar. In contrast to the skin lesion that follows accidental laboratory implantation, regional lymphadenopathy does not occur.

Other Systemic Forms. A subcutaneous form of the disease consists of single or more often multiple soft to firm nodules, palpable deep beneath the skin. These may enlarge to become bulging abscesses, but in various stages contain pus. The skin over the nodules may have a slightly reddish hue.

Osteomyelitis or periostitis of long bones or spine occurs frequently. The first manifestation of disease may be a psoas abscess. A septic arthritis may occur either alone or by extension from bone.

Genitourinary blastomycosis is frequently seen in men and is manifested by pain and swelling of the epididymis, prostate, or seminal vesicles.

There may also be involvement of the central nervous system, eye, adrenals, thyroid, and larynx. In contrast to paracoccidioidomycosis, the gastrointestinal tract is almost never involved.

Diagnosis. Although skin lesions may be strongly suggestive, the diagnosis of blastomycosis is confirmed by the finding of typical budding yeast cells in direct preparations or by the culture and identification of *B. dermatitidis* from pus or lesions. When appropriate, sputum, urine, cerebrospinal fluid, bone marrow, or other biopsy and autopsy tissue should also be cultured. Skin tests are almost always negative and, especially in earlier stages of the disease, serologic procedures may show a higher titer or a positive reaction only to *Histoplasma capsulatum.*

The pulmonary form of the disease is rarely diagnosed clinically or roentgenographically and is usually thought to be tuberculosis or, less frequently, sarcoidosis, acute bacterial pneumonia, malignancy, or other fungal infections more common in the geographic area. Skin lesions are suggestive of basal cell carcinoma, tuberculosis, nodulo-ulcerative syphilid, pyoderma, or other fungal infections. Other systemic manifestations mimic those of tuberculosis or other chronic bacterial infection.

Treatment. Amphotericin B has been used extensively for all forms of blastomycosis. Details of administration are given in Ch. 256. Rather less drug is necessary, however, and for involvement of organs and tissues other than bones, 1 to 2 grams is usually sufficient.

2-Hydroxystilbamidine, administered intravenously, is probably less toxic than amphotericin B. It is a satisfactory alternative only in nonprogressive cutaneous disease. The usual dosage has been 225 mg per day and 8.0 grams per course of therapy.

Surgical drainage of abscesses is frequently indicated. Chemotherapy before and after surgery is advisable.

Prognosis. Pulmonary infection of an inapparent or benign form occurs only rarely. Blastomycosis is, if untreated, a chronic and usually progressive disease. Cutaneous and other disseminated disease is eventually fatal in 10 to 30 per cent of cases.

Except with moribund patients chemotherapy usually effects a prompt recovery. Relapse requiring additional therapy has occurred, however, in at least 10 to 15 per cent of patients.

Lockwood, W. R., Allison, F. L., Batson, B. E., and Busey, J. F.: The treatment of North American blastomycosis: Ten years' experience. Am. Rev. Respir. Dis., 100:314, 1969.

Witorsch, P., and Utz, J. P.: North American blastomycosis. A study of 40 patients. Medicine, 47:169, 1969.

259. PARACOCCIDIOIDOMYCOSIS
(South American Blastomycosis)

John P. Utz

Definition. Paracoccidioidomycosis is a chronic systemic fungal disease, probably respiratory or gastrointestinal in origin, with dissemination to the lymph nodes, skin, lung, and other organs.

History. Lutz in 1908 first described the disease and the organism observed in tissues of a Brazilian patient. In 1909 and 1912, Splendore described more fully the characteristics of the disease and the fungus.

Etiology. The disease is caused by a dimorphic fungus, *Paracoccidioides brasiliensis,* which appears in tissues and exudates as a multiple-budding yeast 2 to 60 μ in diameter. The bud is characterized by a thin wall (0.2 to 1.0 μ) and narrow pore. At temperatures less than 30° C on Sabouraud's glucose medium, a white (later brown) membranous or wrinkled mycelium appears that microscopically is composed of branching hyphae and oval forms (conidia). Delayed cutaneous hypersensitivity and complement-fixing antigens have been demonstrated. Guinea pigs and mice can be experimentally infected.

Epidemiology. Except for reports of occasional patients in North America, the disease occurs exclusively in residents of Central and South America and is especially prevalent in Brazil. It is approximately ten times more frequent in males, and is slightly more frequent in persons 40 to 50 years of age. Manual laborers and farmers seem especially susceptible. Infection is probably acquired by the respiratory route, but a saprophytic, environmental source of fungi is not known. Disease in animals and animal-to-man or man-to-man spread are unknown. Widespread infection of a benign form has been suggested by skin test surveys.

Pathology. The histopathologic reaction to *P. brasiliensis* may be suppurative with abscess formation; in other sites it may be granulomatous with fibroblasts, macrophages, lymphocytes, caseation, and giant cells containing organisms. Lesions are seen in the mucosa of the gastrointestinal tract, lymph nodes, spleen, lungs, and liver.

Clinical Forms. *Primary.* The primary lesion is commonly on the oral or nasal mucosa. Rarely, the conjunctival or anorectal mucosa may be involved. The earliest lesion is a papule that ulcerates and spreads to adjacent tissue.

Cutaneous Form. A variety of skin lesions may be seen, most of which progress to an ulcerative, crusted form suggestive of blastomycosis. In contrast, however, regional lymphadenopathy frequently accompanies skin lesions only in paracoccidioidomycosis. A keloidal form (Lobo's disease) of milder nature, without lymphadenopathy and caused by a different species (*P. loboi*), may be another type of paracoccidioidomycosis.

Lymphangitic Form. In this form there are lymphangitis and enlargement of regional lymph nodes, which suppurate and drain. Cervical and submandibular nodes are most commonly affected.

Visceral Form. The gastrointestinal tract is frequently involved as a primary site of infection. The spleen, adrenals, lungs, and liver may be affected by hematogenous spread. Bone, myocardium, and central nervous system involvement are less frequently seen.

Diagnosis. The diagnosis is established by the culture and identification of *P. brasiliensis* and is only supported by positive skin and complement-fixation tests.

The disease must be differentiated from syphilis, tuberculous adenitis and skin disease, yaws, leishmaniasis, and other fungal infections.

Treatment. Amphotericin B (see Ch. 256) is the drug of choice. In the past, continuous sulfonamide therapy resulted in remission but not cure.

Prognosis. All forms of the disease are fatal if untreated. Over 90 per cent of cases are cured by amphotericin B.

Furtado, T. A., Wilson, J. W., and Plunkett, O. A.: South American blastomycosis or paracoccidioidomycosis. Arch. Dermatol., 70:166, 1954.
Hildick-Smith, G., Blank, H., and Sarkany, I.: Fungus Diseases and Their Treatment. Boston, Little, Brown & Company, 1964.
Kroll, J. J., and Walzer, R. A.: Paracoccidioidomycosis in the United States. Arch. Dermatol., 106:543, 1972.

260. MADUROMYCOSIS (Mycetoma, Madura Foot)

John P. Utz

Definition. Maduromycosis is a chronic systemic fungal disease that follows traumatic or imperceptible implantation of the skin. It is characterized by swelling, induration, suppuration, and draining sinuses of the skin, subcutaneous tissue, and bone, typically of the foot.

History. The disease was first recognized and described in 1712 by Kaempfer in India, and was called Madura foot, after the city of that name. It has been suggested, however, that Madura foot was described by Sophocles in the hero of *Philoctetes.*

Etiology. Many species of ten genera have been reported as etiologic agents; the most common of these have been *Madurella mycetomi, Nocardia brasiliensis,* and, in the United States, *Allescheria boydii.* In tissues or pus these fungi, except for Nocardia (see Ch. 225), are characterized by the appearance of "grains" of oval or irregular shape measuring 0.5 to 2.0 mm, and of white, red, black, or yellow color. Microscopically they are composed of 2 to 4 μ segmented, branched hyphae or round encysted forms (chlamydospores).

A. boydii grows rapidly on Sabouraud's glucose medium, forming a white (later gray or brown) cottony, aerial mycelium, which microscopically consists of thin hyphae to which are attached short or long stalks (conidiophores) bearing a single 8 to 10 by 5 to 7 μ pyriform or ovoid form (conidium). Large (50 to 200 μ) flask-shaped vessels containing asci and spores (4 to 7 μ) can be seen when material from the surface of agar is crushed and examined.

When inoculated intraperitoneally into mice, *A. boydii* is pathogenic, but progressive disease similar to that in humans has not been produced.

Epidemiology. Although occasionally reported from temperate areas, the disease is seen most often in those tropical zones where few people wear shoes. The disease occurs chiefly in adults and more often in males. Most causative organisms are saprophytes of soil or plants. The disease has been reported in the dog, cow, and horse, but animal-to-man or man-to-man spread has not been reported.

Pathology. The typical swollen foot has numerous draining sinuses communicating with abscesses of the skin, subcutaneous tissue, or bone. Drainage sites have characteristic collars of fibrous or epithelial tissues. Suppuration with epithelioid, plasma, and giant cells is intermingled with areas of fibrosis, and one or the other reaction may predominate. With Gram, hematoxylin and eosin, or periodic acid–Schiff stains, fungal cells may be seen either in pus or within macrophages or giant cells.

Clinical Forms. Although lesions have been reported on the leg, torso, hand, and face, the characteristic site of disease is the foot. The first manifestation consists of a papule, small nodule, indurated area with a vesicle, or an abscess that ruptures with sinus tract formation. Infection spreads and new nodules appear, leading to generalized swelling and distortion of the toes. Pain is infrequent, and there are few generalized symptoms. Roentgenographic examination may show lytic lesions with reaction and proliferation of the bone.

Diagnosis. Diagnosis is confirmed by the demonstration of granules in draining material, but the specific cause is dependent on isolation of the fungus in culture. Serologic and skin tests have not been developed for most of the responsible fungi. Maduromycosis must be distinguished from other fungal infections and from tuberculosis, yaws, neoplasms, and elephantiasis.

Treatment. With the variety of antimicrobial agents available, each with specific activity, it is essential that definitive mycologic studies be done prior to treatment to determine the identity and, if feasible, the drug susceptibility of the causative fungus. The failure to do so in many past reports is undoubtedly a factor in the generally pessimistic attitude toward treatment and the early resort to amputation.

The drug of choice for infections caused by *Nocardia brasiliensis* is a sulfonamide (see Ch. 225), whereas for those caused by Aspergillus, amphotericin B is indicated (see Ch. 265). Tetracycline and diaminodiphenylsulfone have been reported to be successful in a few cases of *M. mycetomi* infections. Amphotericin B has been reported ineffective in two cases of *A. boydii* infection. Recently, there have been intriguing reports of benefit in this latter infection related to experimental or clinical use of estrogens.

Prognosis. The disease is usually progressive and rarely self-limited.

Butz, W. C., and Ajello, L.: Black grain mycetoma. Arch. Dermatol., 104:197, 1971.

Carrion, A. L., Hutner, M. S., Nadal, H. M., and Belaval, M. F.: Maduromycosis: An unusual case with a description of the causative fungus. Arch. Dermatol., 82:371, 1960.

Mohr, J. A., and Muchmore, H. G.: Maduromycosis due to *Allescheria boydii*. J.A.M.A., 204:335, 1968.

Zeisler, E. B.: A case from Sophocles. Arch. Dermatol., 84:136, 1961.

261. CHROMOMYCOSIS

John P. Utz

Definition. Chromomycosis is a chronic systemic fungal disease, acquired in the cutaneous form by traumatic or imperceptible implantation, and characterized by wartlike, ulcerated, crusted lesions of the skin and subcutaneous tissues.

History. Although rare in this country, chromomycosis was first reported from Boston in 1915, separately by Lane and Medlar, and the organism responsible was named *Phialophora verrucosa* by Thaxter. Subsequently, cases caused by other genera of fungi were described by Brumpt and Carrion.

Etiology. A number of fungi have been incriminated, but chiefly *Phialophora verrucosa, P. pedrosoi, P. compactum,* and *Cladosporium carrioni.* In tissues these fungi resemble each other and appear as single or clustered, round, thick-walled, 6 to 12 μ budding cells of a striking brown color, from which the disease draws its name. On culture, mycelia are produced that vary according to genus and species. Skin hypersensitivity and complement-fixing antigens have been demonstrated in some fungal species. Laboratory animals are susceptible to experimental infection, but the equivalent of natural disease in man is not produced.

Epidemiology. The disease is seen more often in adult males in the rural areas of the tropics, especially in Brazil, Puerto Rico, and Cuba. The responsible fungi are saprophytes of soil, but are found more often in decaying wood and vegetation. Infection in animals has not been reported, and animal-to-man or man-to-man spread is unknown.

Pathology. Varying degrees of hyperkeratoses, acanthosis, and pseudoepitheliomatous hyperplasia are seen. In the cutis the reaction may be granulomatous with mononuclear, epithelioid, and Langhans' giant cells. Fungal cells are seen readily with hematoxylin and eosin stains.

Clinical Forms. Chromomycosis is a disease of the skin and subcutaneous tissue.

The first patient reported had lesions of the buttock. The most common site is the lower extremity. The disease appears also, in descending order of frequency, on the hand, forearm, arm, neck, and shoulders. The earliest lesion is a nodule or pustule that, over a period of weeks to months, ulcerates, drains, enlarges, dries, and becomes violaceous and wartlike. There is rarely pain, but itching is common. Lesions do not spread generally, but scratching results in autoinoculation and satellite or secondary distal lesions.

Diagnosis. Although older typical skin lesions may be clinically and histologically suggestive, the diagnosis is confirmed by the culture and identification of the causative fungus.

Early lesions may be confused with blastomycosis, tuberculosis, leprosy, yaws, and syphilis.

Treatment. Surgical resection of early skin lesions has been the most common and efficacious therapy. Amputation has been required in a small number of cases. Most of the fungi causing chromomycosis are resistant to amphotericin B, but successful treatment has been reported in two cases when the drug was injected locally into the skin. This drug needs further trial in this disease.

Prognosis. The cutaneous form of chromomycosis is chronic and compatible with long life (in one case, 40 years).

Costello, M. J., De Feo, C. P., Jr., and Littman, M. L.: Chromoblastomycosis treated with local infiltration of amphotericin B solution. Arch. Dermatol., 79:184, 1959.

Vanbreuseghem, R.: Mycoses of Man and Animals. London, Sir Isaac Pitman & Sons, 1958.

262. CRYPTOCOCCOSIS (European Blastomycosis, Torulosis)

John E. Bennett

Definition. Cryptococcosis is a systemic fungal infection, its most common and most lethal manifestation being meningoencephalitis.

History. Busse, who reported the first case in 1894, observed the fungus in tissue and isolated the causative agent. That same year Sanfelice isolated from peach juice the same fungus, naming it *Saccharomyces hominis*. The fungus received no less than 37 additional names until 1952, when Lodder and Kreger-Van Rij's monumental taxonomic study of yeast gave the fungus its current name, *Cryptococcus neoformans*. The fungus was rarely isolated from natural sources until 1955, when Emmons demonstrated that *C. neoformans* was a frequent saprophyte in weathered pigeon droppings. This lent support to the emerging concept that the disease was acquired by inhalation of fungus-laden dust. The discovery of amphotericin B, reported by Gold and co-workers in 1956, was to provide the first successful chemotherapy of cryptococcosis.

Etiology. Cryptococcosis is caused by *Cryptococcus neoformans,* a round or oval yeastlike fungus measuring 4 to 7 μ in diameter. It reproduces by budding. This fungus is unique among systemic mycoses of man in that it is highly encapsulated in tissue. The polysaccharide capsule releases into the host the soluble antigen which provides a means of serologic diagnosis. The fungus can be isolated as a smooth, creamy white colony on a variety of common laboratory media. Culture identification is by gross and microscopic appearance, biochemical reactions, and growth at 37° C.

Epidemiology. The disease is sporadic throughout the world, with no clear focal outbreaks in man or sharply defined areas of high endemicity. Disease occurs occasionally in warm-blooded feral and domestic animals, excluding birds. Cryptococcal mastitis may spread through dairy herds, probably by way of milking machines, and contaminate unpasteurized milk. No spread of infection from animal to man or man to man has been reported. Reservoir of infection is probably saprophytic sources in nature, such as weathered pigeon droppings. Presumed portal of entry is the lung, although this site is often clinically inapparent. The fungus is not a part of the normal flora of man or animals, although occasionally it appears to colonize a patient's damaged bronchial tree. No occupational group is known to be predisposed to cryptococcosis. Infection is uncommon before puberty and is more frequent in males. Predisposing factors include Hodgkin's disease, lymphoma, leukemia, sarcoidosis, and supraphysiologic doses of adrenal corticosteroids.

Pathology. The most frequent and characteristic abnormality on gross examination occurs in the brain, which shows basilar arachnoiditis and focal collections of small, glistening, gelatinous cysts, particularly in the cortical gray matter and basal ganglia. Microscopic examination reveals the cysts to be clumps of cryptococci, with little surrounding inflammation. A dense inflammatory response to the fungus may be noted in meninges or brain but is more characteristic of extraneural lesions. Cellular response consists of macrophages, giant cells, and lymphocytes. Necrosis is seen occasionally at the center of a dense inflammatory response, particularly in the lung. Features notable for their infrequency include polymorphonuclear leukocytes, calcification, extensive scarring, and hemorrhage.

Clinical Manifestations. *Meningoencephalitis.* Symptoms begin with the insidious onset of headache, followed by nausea, vomiting, blurred vision, or decreased mental acuity. Less frequent symptoms include photophobia, diplopia, and gait ataxia. Gradually the patient becomes lethargic and prefers to remain undisturbed. Somnolence or irritability may appear. Fever is low grade or absent. Although no one physical finding is highly frequent or characteristic, examination may disclose papilledema, mild to moderate nuchal rigidity, cranial nerve palsies, or extensor plantar response.

Extraneural Cryptococcosis. Pulmonary cryptococcosis is the second most common clinical manifestation. Even patients with no clinically apparent pneumonitis but with cryptococcosis elsewhere in the body are often found to have a pulmonary focus on careful postmortem examination or sometimes on sputum culture. Chest symptoms and radiologic findings, when present, commonly mimic primary or metastatic carcinoma in the lung. Pleural effusions, cavitation, and hilar adenopathy are not common. Skin lesions occur in 10 per cent of patients with cryptococcosis, and bone lesions occur in about 5 per cent. Either may be the sole clinical manifestation of the infection or may be associated with disease in other organs. Skin lesions begin as asymptomatic papules, pustules, or soft subcutaneous nodules. They tend to become painful as they slowly enlarge, ulcerate, and drain glary pus. Osteolytic lesions may appear in almost any bone and present as a cold abscess. Rare clinical manifestations include prostatitis, hepatitis, endocarditis, pericarditis, renal abscess, and endophthalmitis.

Diagnosis. Lumbar puncture in patients with symptomatic cryptococcal meningoencephalitis usually reveals one or more of the following abnormalities: elevated opening pressure, pleocytosis predominantly composed of mononuclear cells, increased protein concentration, and hypoglycorrhachia. A smear of cerebrospinal fluid sediment, mixed with India ink, reveals encapsulated yeast in about half the cases. The smear may be difficult to interpret and provides only a tentative, albeit useful, diagnosis. Another rapid diagnostic aid is serologic detection of cryptococcal antigen in serum and cerebrospinal fluid. With current techniques, about 70 to 80 per cent of patients with cryptococcal meningitis have detectable antigen if both sites are tested. Extraneural cryptococcosis may result in serum antigen if infection is extensive. A falling antigen titer during recovery is a favorable prognostic sign.

Final diagnosis depends upon culture or biopsy. Several milliliters of cerebrospinal fluid should be cultured for cryptococci in cases of indolent meningoencephalitis and also in every case of documented extraneural cryptococcosis, in order to detect subclinical extension to the central nervous system. The frequency of subclinical renal infection in disseminated cryptococcosis makes urine culture useful. Sputum, blood, prostatic fluid, and pus from cutaneous lesions may also yield the fungus. Biopsy may be required to diagnose cryptococcosis in the lung, skin, or bone. Histologic diagnosis can usually be made with accuracy by those experienced in this area.

Therapy. Intravenous amphotericin B is the treatment of choice for cryptococcosis of the central nervous system. Treatment should be continued for at least four weeks after all weekly cultures become negative. 5-Fluorocytosine should rarely if ever be used alone, but studies currently in progress with combinations of 5-fluorocytosine and amphotericin B appear promising. Intrathecal amphotericin B may be a useful adjunct in patients failing an adequate trial of intravenous therapy or with such poor renal function that reduced doses of intravenous amphotericin B are obligatory. Development of communicating or noncommunicating hydrocephalus may require neurosurgical intervention.

Intravenous amphotericin B is the usual treatment of choice for extraneural cryptococcosis. A probable exception is the patient without either hematologic malignancy or immunosuppressive therapy who, on thorough study, has infection confined to one focus in lung, skin, or bone. Surgical excision of skin or lung lesions, curettage of bone lesions, or simply prolonged observation may be warranted if the lesion is not extensive and is stable or regressing.

Prognosis. Cryptococcal meningoencephalitis is invariably fatal unless treated. With currently available therapy, the case fatality rate is about 25 per cent. Patients with Hodgkin's disease, lymphoma, or leukemia or who require continued immunosuppressive therapy fare less well. Death usually results from the sequelae of coma or from brainstem compression. Despite successful therapy, patients may be left with optic atrophy, hydrocephalus, personality changes, or decreased mental acuity.

Fetter, B. F., Klintworth, G. K., and Hendry, W. S.: Mycoses of the Central Nervous System. Baltimore, Williams & Wilkins Company, 1967.
Littman, M. L., and Zimmerman, L. E.: Cryptococcosis. New York, Grune & Stratton, 1956.
Salfelder, K.: Cryptococcosis. *In* Baker, R. D. (ed.): Human Infections with Fungi, Actinomycetes and Algae. New York, Springer-Verlag, 1971, pp. 383–464.

263. SPOROTRICHOSIS

John P. Utz

Definition. Sporotrichosis is a chronic systemic fungal disease, acquired usually by traumatic implantation and localized to cutaneous lymphatic tissues, or rarely by the respiratory route with dissemination throughout the body.

History. From a patient at Johns Hopkins Hospital, in 1896 Schenck isolated a fungus that was identified by E. F. Smith as Sporotrichum; it was called *Sporotrichum schenckii* by Hektoen and Perkins in 1900. A great number of cases were seen subsequently in France, and more than 2800 cases in a single epidemic in the gold mines of South Africa.

Etiology. *Sporothrix schenckii,* a dimorphic fungus, is occasionally observed in tissues as round to cigar-shaped yeast- or bacteria-like forms. On Sabouraud's glucose medium at room temperature, a white, cottony, aerial mycelium appears that in three to seven days becomes wrinkled and changes in color from cream to black. Microscopically, branching, septate hyphae are seen, 2 μ in width, bearing directly or on lateral branches ovoid to spherical bodies (conidia) measuring 2 to 4 by 2 to 6 μ in diameter. Mice are susceptible to experimental infection. Delayed cutaneous hypersensitivity and agglutinogen antigens have been demonstrated.

Epidemiology. The disease is worldwide in distribution; it has appeared epidemically in South Africa and in localized outbreaks in Mexico and Florida. It is more common in the male. It frequently affects laborers, farmers, and florists and is considered a true occupational disease. The fungus exists in its saprophytic form in soil, peat moss, and decaying vegetation and on thorns. In the cutaneous lymphatic forms, infection results from accidental implantation into the skin. In disseminated forms, the mode of entry is probably respiratory. Spontaneous sporotrichosis has been reported in dogs, horses, mules, cats, and other animals, and human disease has resulted from animal contact. Direct transfer from man to man is not known to occur.

Pathology. The histopathologic reaction to *S. schenckii* is varied, frequently acute and suppurative, but also subacute or chronic. In some instances granulomas are seen with epithelioid and giant cells either diffusely distributed or localized in a typical tubercle. Fungi may be seen more readily after staining with a modified Schiff-MacManus technique.

Clinical Forms. *Cutaneous Lymphatic Form.* The earliest lesion is a pustule, papule, or nodule of the skin appearing characteristically on a finger and at a site where the patient may recall an earlier, seemingly insignificant scratch or prick. The nodule enlarges, becomes red to violaceous, and is followed by a chain of subcutaneous nodules along regional lymphatics. These at first freely movable nodules may become attached to the skin, and may ulcerate and drain a thin gray to yellow pus. Streaking and pain characteristic of acute lymphangitis are not present. Generalized symptoms are rare.

Other Forms. Other forms may appear secondary to the cutaneous lymphatic lesion either by direct extension to contiguous, subcutaneous tissue, bone, and joint or by hematogenous spread to distant sites. Sometimes the original site of infection is inapparent, and the disease presents as a septic arthritis or osteomyelitis. Less frequently, there may be involvement of the eye, lungs, gastrointestinal tract, central nervous system, or skin. In disseminated disease, systemic symptoms of fever, weight loss, inanition, malaise, pain at sites of lesion, anemia, and leukocytosis are commonly present. Disease limited to the lungs or localized there suggests that there is a respiratory form acquired by inhalation of the fungus. Too few cases have thus far been reported to characterize this form at present.

Diagnosis. Although the diagnosis may seem readily apparent in the cutaneous lymphatic form of disease, the clinical impression is confirmed by the culture and identification of the fungus. Agglutination or complement-fixation serologic and skin tests may be helpful, but are not generally available.

Cutaneous lymphatic sporotrichosis must be distinguished from tularemia, pyoderma of bacterial origin, and other fungal infections. Disseminated disease resembles tuberculosis, staphylococcal osteomyelitis, or neoplastic disease.

Treatment. The cutaneous lymphatic form of disease responds slowly but progressively to the oral administration of iodides in the form of a saturated solution (1 gram per milliliter) of potassium iodide given in dosage of 2 ml four times daily. Treatment should be prolonged one to two months beyond the time of apparent healing.

Disseminated disease, especially of bone and joints, is frequently resistant to iodide therapy. Dramatic improvement has been seen in a few patients treated with amphotericin B, and for this form of disease this drug is recommended.

Prognosis. Untreated cutaneous lymphatic sporotrichosis may persist for many months to years. Treated lesions respond slowly but completely. Disseminated disease is progressive and usually fatal unless treated.

Baum, G. L., Donnerberg, R. L., Stewart, D., Mulligan, W. J., and Putnam, L. R.: Pulmonary sporotrichosis. N. Engl. J. Med., 280:410, 1969.
Gladstone, J. L., and Littman, M. L.: Osseous sporotrichosis. Am. J. Med., 51:121, 1971.
Wilson, D. E., Mann, J. J., Bennett, J. E., and Utz, J. P.: Clinical features of extracutaneous sporotrichosis. Medicine, 46:265, 1967.

264. MUCORMYCOSIS

John E. Bennett

Definition. Mucormycosis is an acute, often fatal infection caused by fungi of the order Mucorales. Phycomycosis is a term which encompasses mucormycosis and several other mycoses.

History. Two cases of pulmonary mucormycosis reported by Fürbringer in 1876 were probably the first cases described with enough clarity to permit any confidence in the diagnosis. It was not until 1943 that Gregory described mucormycosis originating in nose and paranasal sinuses.

Etiology. Rhizopus and Mucor species are the principal pathogens of mucormycosis. These fungi appear in tissue as hyphae 6 to 50 μ wide, rarely septate, irregular in contour, and tending to branch at nearly right angles. Hyphae may be demonstrated histologically by staining with hematoxylin and eosin, Gomori methenamine silver, or periodic acid–Schiff. Growth at 25 or 37° C is profuse and rapidly spreading on most media. Identification of the culture is based largely on microscopic appearance. Only very specialized laboratories are competent to pursue identification beyond a tentative designation of genus.

Epidemiology. Mucormycosis is uncommon and sporadic around the world, usually afflicting patients with serious pre-existing disease. *Cranial mucormycosis occurs predominantly in patients with poorly controlled diabetes mellitus.* Pulmonary and disseminated mucormycosis occurs occasionally in diabetics but is most prevalent in immunosuppressed patients, particularly treated leukemics. Among the varied underlying disorders present in patients with gastrointestinal mucormycosis, uremia, severe malnutrition, and diarrheal diseases seem prominent. Mucormycosis occurs at any age, with no strong predilection for race or sex. It does not spread from man to man. Disease is probably acquired by inhalation of fungal spores. Mucorales are ubiquitous in the environment, growing on decaying vegetation, dung, and foods of high sugar content.

Pathology. Necrosis is the predominant gross and microscopic finding. This is accounted for in part by the propensity of hyphae to proliferate within small and medium-sized arteries, producing thrombosis. Infarcted areas may be ischemic or hemorrhagic. Neutrophils predominate in the inflammatory response.

Clinical Manifestations. Mucormycosis originating in the nose and paranasal sinuses produces a characteristic clinical entity. Initial symptoms mimic bacterial sinusitis, with low-grade fever and sinus pain. However, nasal discharge is not purulent but is thin and sometimes blood streaked. Over the next few days, infection spreads to contiguous structures. Invasion of the orbit may lead to reduced range of ocular motion, proptosis, chemosis, or blurred vision. Direct invasion of the globe or thrombosis of the ophthalmic artery may occur. Nasal turbinates or hard palate develop areas which are black, friable, and bloodless. Frontal or temporal lobes of the brain may be infected by direct extension, producing headache and deepening stupor. Invasion of the carotid artery within the cavernous sinus may cause embolization, mycotic aneurysm, or thrombosis. Without treatment, the patient usually dies in coma a few days to a few weeks from onset.

Pulmonary mucormycosis presents as a rapidly progressive dense bronchopneumonia, accompanied by high fever, toxicity, and tachypnea, but with little cough or sputum. The necrotic central portion of a lesion is sometimes expectorated, producing hyphae in sputum and a cavity on chest x-ray. Gastrointestinal lesions of mucormycosis begin as one or more shallow ulcerations in esophagus, stomach, or intestine. The ulcer tends to enlarge, deepen, and perforate the viscus. Disseminated mucormycosis may originate in nasal area, lung, or gastrointestinal tract. Sometimes no portal is evident. Hematogenous spread may involve brain or other organs. Pulmonary and disseminated mucormycosis are clinically indistinguishable from invasive aspergillosis.

Diagnosis. *Cranial mucormycosis* is easily mistaken for bacterial sinusitis with cavernous sinus thrombosis. The diagnosis requires biopsy of infected mucosa in the nose or sinus. Hyphae are often abundant on histologic section or wet smear of crushed tissue. Hyphae seen in cross-section may be mistaken for yeast. Occasionally hyphae are confused with capillaries, or vice versa.

Pulmonary and disseminated infections caused by Mucorales, Aspergillus, and *Pseudomonas aeruginosa* have many similarities. Diagnosis of mucormycosis, like aspergillosis, requires biopsy. In the proper clinical setting, demonstration of broad, nonseptate hyphae in bronchial brush specimens or sputum would be strongly suggestive. Culture of biopsy specimens is certainly of interest, but isolation of a ubiquitous organism like Mucorales must be interpreted with caution. Blood cultures are very rarely positive for the fungus.

Treatment. Mucormycosis originating in the nose and paranasal areas should be treated by optimal regulation of diabetes mellitus, extensive surgical debridement, and intravenous amphotericin B. After debridement, sinus cavities can be irrigated daily with amphotericin B, 1 mg per milliliter. Although good guidelines for dose and duration of intravenous amphotericin B are not available, it has been customary to treat vigorously at least until disease progression halts. Treatment should probably continue for another month beyond that. Tomograms of the orbit and sinuses can be very helpful in evaluating disease progression. Carotid arteriogram may demonstrate extension to the ophthalmic artery or carotid siphon. Electroencephalogram and lumbar puncture provide late evidence of intracranial extension.

Intravenous amphotericin B is probably useful in other forms of mucormycosis, but too few patients have been treated for this question to be answered.

Prognosis. A substantial number of cures have been reported recently in mucormycosis of the nose, sinus, and orbit. Prognosis is poor once central nervous system signs appear. Other forms of mucormycosis have largely been diagnosed post mortem.

Baker, R. D.: Mucormycosis. *In* Human Infection with Fungi, Actinomycetes and Algae, New York, Springer-Verlag, 1971, pp. 832–918.

Bartrum, R. J., Watnick, M., and Herman, P. G.: Roentgenographic findings in pulmonary mucormycosis. Am. J. Roentgenol., 117:810, 1973.

Battock, D. J., Grausz, H., Bobrowsky, M., and Littman, M. L.: Alternate-day amphotericin B therapy in the treatment of rhinocerebral phycomycosis (mucormycosis). Ann. Intern. Med., 68:122, 1968.

Meyer, R. D., Rosen, P., and Armstrong, D.: Phycomycosis complicating leukemia and lymphoma. Ann. Intern. Med., 77:871, 1972.

Price, D. L., Wolpow, E. R., and Richardson, E. P.: Intracranial phycomycosis: A clinicopathological and radiologic study. J. Neurol. Sci., 14:359, 1971.

265. ASPERGILLOSIS

John E. Bennett

Definition. The term aspergillosis embraces a variety of diseases which have in common growth of the fungus Aspergillus in tissue or within air-containing spaces of the body, such as bronchus or pulmonary cavity.

History. Micheli first described the genus Aspergillus in 1729. The first case of aspergillosis in man was probably observed by Sluyter in 1847, although disease in birds had been reported before then. In 1856 Virchow reviewed the literature and reported four autopsied cases. Renon's classic paper of 1897 attracted attention to the disease.

Etiology. The etiologic agent Aspergillus is a fungus largely composed of septate hyphae about 4 μ in diameter. Sporulating structures, called conidial heads, may be seen when the fungus is growing in nature, on artificial medium, or within air-containing spaces of the body. The most frequent pathogen for man is *Aspergillus fumigatus.* However, many other species can clearly cause either invasive or noninvasive disease in man, particularly *Aspergillus flavus.* Aspergilli grow rapidly on many routine laboratory media and, because of their ubiquity, are encountered in the laboratory as airborne contaminants. Identification is by gross and microscopic appearance.

Epidemiology. Aspergilli are often found growing on decaying vegetation. Under proper conditions millions of spores, about 2 to 4 μ in diameter, may be released into the air. Inhalation of these spores must be a common event, but disease is infrequent. Both insects and animals may acquire aspergillosis. The disease is an economically important cause of mycotic abortion in cattle and horses. In man the disease is sporadic and worldwide, with no clear occupational predisposition. Transmission from animal to man or man to man has not been encountered.

Pathology. The fungus is capable of eliciting a wide variety of tissue responses, depending upon site and host. A ball of hyphae may be situated within an ectatic bronchus or epithelialized lung cavity and provoke little or no histologic response. During invasion of tissue in a markedly immunosuppressed host, blood vessel invasion by hyphae, thrombosis, necrosis, and hemorrhagic infarction are prominent features. In invasion of more normal tissue, a pyogenic necrotic reaction is common, but epithelioid granulomas with giant cells may be observed instead. Chronic, fibrosing, non-necrotizing granulomatous inflammation has typically been seen in the paranasal sinus and orbit.

Inhalation of Aspergillus spores may provoke an allergic response without invasion of the body, but this condition will not be considered here. Certain aspergilli, given proper growth conditions, produce proteolytic enzymes or toxins. As far as is known, these substances play no important role in aspergillosis.

Clinical Manifestations. *Pulmonary Aspergillosis.* Aspergillus can colonize ectatic bronchi, cysts, or cavities in the lung. Colonization is usually a sequel of a chronic inflammatory process, such as tuberculosis, bronchiectasis, histoplasmosis, or sarcoidosis. A ball of hyphae may form within an air-containing space, particularly in the upper lobes, and is termed an aspergilloma. The fungus rarely invades the wall of the cavity, cyst, or bronchus in such patients. During bacterial pneumonia, lung abscess, or empyema in a colonized patient, Aspergillus may appear in the inflammatory process, although its role is uncertain. In most patients it is difficult to determine clinically whether specific symptoms or signs of disease progression are due to the underlying condition or to some allergic, inflammatory, or obstructive process caused by Aspergillus. The most common symptoms are chronic productive cough and hemoptysis. Uncommonly, Aspergillus appears to be the sole cause of chronic pulmonary inflammation. In a few instances, acute bilateral bronchopneumonia has occurred in normal persons, usually after a presumed massive inhalation of spores. However, the majority of patients with invasive aspergillosis now being encountered are markedly neutropenic or are receiving corticosteroid therapy, or both. A patch of bronchopneumonia appears and steadily becomes larger and denser. The lesion may remain focal or, at any time, may spread hematogenously to one or more sites in the lung, brain, or other organs. The lung lesion may also erode directly through the diaphragm or pericardium.

Lesions of Extrapulmonary Origin. Necrotizing lesions originating in the palate, paranasal sinuses, epiglottis, or gastrointestinal tract may occur in the immunosuppressed patient. Aspergillus may infect intracardiac or intravascular prostheses. Chronic granulomatous inflammation may originate in the paranasal sinuses and spread to orbit or brain. Progressive mycotic keratitis caused by Aspergillus may follow corneal trauma. Growth of Aspergillus on cerumen and detritus within the external auditory canal is termed otomycosis.

Diagnosis. Culture of Aspergillus from sputum usually has no clinical significance. Repeated isolation of Aspergillus from sputum or demonstration of hyphae on sputum smear suggests endobronchial colonization. Precipitins to Aspergillus antigens are often demonstrable in the sera of such colonized patients. Radiologic appearance of an aspergilloma is distinctive. In the severely immunosuppressed patient, isolation of Aspergillus from even a single sputum should raise suspicion of possible invasive infection. Biopsy is usually required to diagnose invasive aspergillosis in lung, paranasal sinus, orbit, or brain. Histology may provide evidence of tissue invasion and permit a presumptive diagnosis of aspergillosis. For absolute confirmation and determination of species, the biopsy should be cultured. Neither serologic tests nor cultures of blood, cerebrospinal fluid, or urine are helpful in most forms of invasive aspergillosis.

Treatment. Surgical excision may be helpful in fungus ball of the lung or in aspergillosis of the paranasal sinus and orbit. Measures to improve bronchopulmonary drainage may assist the patient with endobronchial colonization. Intravenous amphotericin B is not helpful in endobronchial or endocavitary aspergillosis, but in invasive pulmonary aspergillosis a prolonged course of treatment will occasionally arrest progression. Ultimate cure of invasive pulmonary aspergillosis requires not only intravenous amphotericin B but also significant restoration of the host's defense mechanisms.

Prognosis. Endobronchial or endocavitary aspergillosis rarely becomes invasive or disseminated. Although the condition is not usually the sole cause of death, it may contribute problems to an already damaged lung. Cure is infrequent in invasive aspergillosis of the lung, heart, paranasal sinus, orbit, or brain.

Green, W. R., Font, R. L., and Zimmerman, L. E.: Aspergillosis of the orbit. Arch. Ophthalmol., 82:302, 1969.

Kilman, J. W., Ahn, C., Andrews, N. C., and Klassen, K.: Surgery for pulmonary aspergillosis. J. Thorac. Cardiovasc. Surg., 57:642, 1969.
Young, R. C., Bennett, J. E., Vogel, C., Carbone, P. P., and DeVita, V. T.: Aspergillosis. Spectrum of the disease in 98 patients. Medicine, 49:147, 1970.

266. CANDIDIASIS (Candidosis, Moniliasis, Thrush)

John E. Bennett

Definition. Candidiasis is an infection of the skin, mucous membranes, or viscera caused by species of Candida, a yeastlike fungus. Thrush refers to candidiasis of mucous membranes, as in the mouth or vagina.

History. Thrush as a clinical entity has been appreciated for centuries, but its relationship to fungi was unknown until Langenbeck isolated the pathogen from a patient's throat in 1839. Among the many names applied to this fungus, the most significant have been *Oidium albicans* (given by Robin in 1853), *Monilia albicans* (Zopf, 1890) and *Candida albicans* (Berkhout, 1923).

Etiology. *Candida albicans* is the usual cause of candidiasis. A substantial number of cases of disseminated candidiasis have been caused by other species of Candida, particularly *C. tropicalis* and *C. parapsilosis.* The size and shape of Candida cells are variable, but most commonly the cells are oval and 4 to 6 μ in their longest axis. Growth usually appears within a few days of incubation at 25 or 37° C. Deep inoculation into certain media, such as corn meal Tween 80 agar, causes Candida to grow as long tubules called pseudohyphae. Individual species of Candida are distinguished by their ability to utilize or ferment certain sugars. For routine laboratory purposes, *C. albicans* can be identified by its ability to form chlamydospores or, in the presence of serum, to form germ tubes. Candida species look very similar in infected tissue, but usually can be distinguished from other fungi. Candida generally, but not always, grows in tissue as both budding yeast and pseudohyphae. Both tissue forms are well demonstrated by Gomori methenamine silver, periodic acid–Schiff, or tissue Gram stains.

Epidemiology. *C. albicans* is a frequent commensal in the human mouth, gastrointestinal tract, and vagina. Candida is also commonly isolated from the gut of animals. Isolation of this fungus from the environment is unusual, and most of the exceptions could have represented contamination by animals or man. This leads to the presumption that the fungus is spread from man to man and animal to animal. It is usually impossible to trace this spread, because colonization is asymptomatic. A probable exception is the newborn infant, in whom colonization usually leads to oral thrush. Later in life, disease seems to occur when a previously colonized patient becomes more vulnerable to tissue invasion. A wide variety of conditions predispose to candidiasis, particularly diabetes mellitus and therapy with either broad-spectrum antimicrobials or adrenal corticosteroids. Chronic maceration predisposes to cutaneous candidiasis, as in paronychia of bartenders and housewives, intertrigo of obese patients, or diaper rash. Women in the later months of pregnancy are particularly susceptible to vulvovaginal candidiasis. Patients with acute leukemia are prone to gastrointestinal and systemic candidiasis. An important route for acquiring systemic candidiasis is through unsterile intravenous injections of narcotics or through use of plastic intravenous catheters. When the infusion through the catheter is designed to meet the patient's total caloric requirement, the risk of systemic candidiasis goes even higher.

Pathology. In mucocutaneous candidiasis, pseudohyphae and yeast tend to be confined to the epithelium. Leukocytes infiltrate the epithelium as well as the submucosa or corium. Parakeratosis is usual. Ulceration and hyphal invasion of the submucosa is a more frequent characteristic of gastrointestinal candidiasis. In systemic candidiasis, abscesses may be found in almost any organ, but kidney, lung, spleen, heart, and liver are frequent sites. Such abscesses on gross inspection may appear as small, white, firm, cheesy nodules. Histologically these foci show necrosis, leukocytes, pseudohyphae, and yeast. Giant cells are seen occasionally. In the immunosuppressed patient, inflammatory cells may be scanty or absent. Patients with plastic intravenous catheters may develop at the catheter tip an endovenous fibrin sleeve containing Candida. Presumably, this can continue to seed the bloodstream for several days after withdrawal of the catheter.

Clinical Manifestations. The mouth is the most common site of candidiasis. *Oral thrush* is usually an acute, self-limiting disease which presents as discrete and confluent white plaques on the oral and pharyngeal mucosa. The plaque is a pseudomembrane which can be scraped off with difficulty, exposing a red base. *Candida denture stomatitis* is characterized by well-circumscribed areas of erythema and edema in the mucosa under the upper dentures. Candida also appears to cause chronic hyperplastic oral lesions resembling leukoplakia. All the aforementioned oral lesions tend to be asymptomatic. *Cutaneous candidiasis* can present as diaper rash, red macerated areas in large skin folds, fissuring and desquamation in interdigital areas, angular cheilitis, paronychia, balanitis, or pruritus ani. *Chronic mucocutaneous candidiasis,* also called *Candida granuloma,* is an uncommon disease, usually beginning in early childhood, in which hyperkeratotic lesions wax and wane in the skin and mucous membranes for many years. The most severe skin lesions occur on the face, scalp, and hands. Involvement of mouth, vagina, and nails is usual. Children with this disorder frequently seem to have defective function of thymus-derived lymphocytes and tend to develop hypofunction of the parathyroid, thyroid, or adrenal glands.

The most common symptom of *Candida vaginitis* is pruritus. Other frequent symptoms include discharge and burning pain, the latter being worse on urination or intercourse. Speculum examination reveals an inflamed vaginal mucosa and a thin exudate, sometimes with white curds. Within the gastrointestinal tract, the *esophagus* is the most common site of candidiasis and the only site likely to be symptomatic. Substernal burning and either pain or a sense of obstruction on swallowing may occur. Blood-borne *Candida abscesses* are usually manifest only as fever and toxicity. Hematogenous dissemination to the choroid is detected on funduscopic examination as fluffy white retinal exudates. The abscesses gradually enlarge and extend into the vitreous humor, which becomes increasingly hazy. Cells and flare may also appear in the anterior chamber. The most common symptoms are orbital or retro-orbital pain, blurring, scotoma, and opacities floating across the visual field. *Candidiasis of the endocardium* or around the edges of an intracardiac prosthesis resembles bacterial infections in these sites. *Candida meningitis* clinically mimics cryptococcosis. *Pulmonary and renal candidiasis* are usually hematogenous in origin and cause no focal symptoms. Extensive renal cortical abscesses may cause azotemia. *Candidiasis in the lining of the bladder or renal pelvis* usually appears in a diabetic patient with chronic or recurrent bacterial urinary tract infections or after instrumentation or surgery on the urinary tract. Dysuria, pyuria, and passage of pseudohyphae in the urine are frequent findings. Rarely, pseudohyphae will be found packed in a necrotic renal papilla. A sloughed papilla, largely then a ball of fungus, may obstruct a ureter.

Diagnosis. Demonstration of pseudohyphae on smear with confirmation by culture is the procedure of choice for diagnosing candidiasis of epithelial surfaces. Scrapings for this purpose may be made of skin, oral mucosa, vagina, or nails. Cerebrospinal fluid and joint fluid cultures are helpful in diagnosing Candida meningitis or arthritis. Progression of funduscopic findings usually permits an operational diagnosis of Candida endophthalmitis. Esophagram and esophagoscopy can aid the diagnosis of Candida esophagitis. Biopsy is required to diagnose candidiasis of lung or liver. Blood cultures are very useful in diagnosing Candida endocarditis but are less commonly positive in other forms of systemic candidiasis. The fungus can be isolated from blood, using the same routine media employed for bacteria, but one to three weeks of incubation are often required. Rarely, Candida is seen on blood smear. Skin tests with Candida antigens are so commonly positive in normal people that they are not useful in diagnosing candidiasis. Diagnostic interpretation of serologic tests for candidiasis remains controversial.

Treatment. Oral thrush is best treated by rinsing the mouth with and then swallowing nystatin suspension, 100,000 units four times daily. Painting the lesions with 1 per cent aqueous gentian violet is a messy but effective alternative. Vaginal thrush usually responds to deep insertion of a nystatin vaginal suppository once or twice daily for two weeks. Cutaneous candidiasis of macerated areas requires measures to keep the skin dry plus topical nystatin or amphotericin B. Mild symptoms of Candida esophagitis may respond to the patient's sucking on a nystatin suppository three or four times daily. With pronounced esophageal symptoms, a short course of intravenous amphotericin B is more beneficial. Bladder thrush may be eradicated by bladder irrigation with amphotericin B, 50 μg per milliliter. If a Foley catheter is not in place, oral 5-fluorocytosine is an alternative. Isolation of Candida from blood may or may not indicate the need for intravenous amphotericin B. If the patient is febrile and severely immunosuppressed, a single positive blood culture for Candida is generally an indication for prompt chemotherapy. All too often the patient dies before additional blood cultures are reported positive. In the patient who is not immunosuppressed, significance of candidemia depends upon the number of positive cultures and the presence or absence of a plastic intravenous catheter. Multiple positive blood cultures in the absence of such a catheter indicate the need for chemotherapy. In the presence of such a catheter, discovery of candidemia should prompt removal of the catheter and culturing of its tip. If the patient is not seriously ill and is improving, treatment may be postponed to await clinical progress and the results of subsequent blood cultures. The species of Candida isolated is irrelevant to the decision about therapy. Temporization is inappropriate when endocarditis, endophthalmitis, arthritis, or other hematogenous lesions are detected. Systemic candidiasis is treated with the same daily doses of intravenous amphotericin B as are used with other systemic mycoses. Adequate guidelines for judging duration of therapy are not known. There is also inadequate information to judge whether 5-fluorocytosine has a role in the treatment of systemic candidiasis.

Prognosis. Most forms of mucocutaneous candidiasis are benign and respond to local treatment, although relapse is not rare. Chronic mucocutaneous candidiasis of children responds to intravenous amphotericin B, but relapse is virtually inevitable. For some reason these children rarely develop systemic candidiasis. The ability of treatment to prevent death from most forms of systemic candidiasis and to eradicate candidiasis of the urinary and gastrointestinal mucosa depends largely on the severity of the underlying condition. Candidiasis of the endocardium or around an intracardiac prosthesis is usually fatal despite treatment.

Eras, P., Goldstein, M. J., and Sherlock, P.: Candida infection of the gastrointestinal tract. Medicine, 51:367, 1972.

Fishman, L. S., Griffin, J. R., Sapico, F. L., and Hecht, R.: Hematogenous Candida endophthalmitis—a complication of candidemia. N. Engl. J. Med., 286:675, 1972.

Kirkpatrick, C. H., Rich, R. R., and Bennett, J. E.: Chronic mucocutaneous candidiasis. Ann. Intern. Med., 74:955, 1971.

Winner, H. I., and Hurley, R.: Candida Albicans. Boston, Little, Brown & Company, 1964.

Section Six. CHEMOTHERAPY OF MICROBIAL DISEASE

267. DRUGS AND MICROBES

Walsh McDermott

In choosing the initial therapy for a patient with a presumed microbial disease, the physician is confronted with a formidable dilemma. On the one hand, if therapy is to be maximally effective, the correct drug or drug-pairing must be chosen quickly so that it may be administered before significant tissue damage or irreversible physiologic changes have occurred. On the other hand, if the choice is to be made quickly, it is difficult to make it exactly; for there are still only a few techniques by which the cause of an infection can be positively identified during the early hours of acute illness. Thus the physician is in the uncomfortable position of knowing that if he is to obtain the greatest advantages of antimicrobial therapy for his patient, he must make the correct choice of drugs one to five days before solid evidence of the identity of the infection will be forthcoming.

An obvious way out of the dilemma would be by the introduction of rapid diagnostic methods illustrated by techniques such as the use of fluorescent-tagged antibody to swiftly identify organisms. However, surprisingly little effort has been devoted to developing a better, more rapid diagnostic technology. Given this situation, the physician has to rely on his *clinical* acumen and a full knowledge of all the microbial diseases that might reasonably be expected to institute threats to his patients. In actuality, to make this choice of the initial drug regimen from evidence obtained at the bedside is not as difficult as it sounds once the physician realizes what it is that he should be trying to do. While doing it, he can also be comforted by the thought that the expert consultant must go through exactly the same exercise; for he, too, seldom has any secret diagnostic weapons, and is equally hampered by the slowness of the available diagnostic tests. Attempts should be made to differentiate, on clinical grounds, those situations or syndromes that require immediate and intensive action from those that properly may be left to unfold until precise identification becomes possible. Moreover, when a choice of therapy is made, it should be made on the basis of careful consideration of the most serious threats to the patient that are likely. The drug or drugs chosen should be the ones that do most to protect the patient overnight or for a somewhat longer interval against the reasonably likely threats, while at the same time do the least to mask the identity of other infections that might conceivably be present. Above all, once the identity of the infecting microbe *is* established, the physician should be quick to discontinue all but the scientifically relevant therapy.

An example of the exercise involved is as follows:

A young man was first seen with a high fever, a cough, and obviously excruciating pleural pain. His systolic blood pressure was 90 mm of mercury; his leukocyte count was 4000 per cubic millimeter, with a marked increase in immature neutrophils. Less than four hours previously, he had been enjoying himself at the theater, although he had had a mild respiratory infection for the preceding five or six days.

It was apparent that he had an infection, that it was progressing rapidly, and that it involved lung and pleura. What reasonable inferences could be drawn concerning the identity of the infection and hence both its relative threat to him and the appropriate choice of therapy?

At least four microbial species, Pneumococcus, Streptococcus, *S. aureus*, and Klebsiella (Friedländer's bacillus), are capable of producing this particular situation, and faced with the individual case there is absolutely no way of differentiating one from another at the bedside. Nevertheless, the clinician knows that this syndrome occurs in such a severe fulminating form in less than 5 per cent of pneumococcal pneumonias, whereas such severity is the characteristic picture of the rapidly necrotizing pneumonias caused by staphylococci, streptococci, or klebsiellae. He also knows that primary staphylococcal pneumonia is extremely rare in the absence of viral influenza, but that as a complication of viral influenza it is by no means uncommon. Here his day-to-day "community epidemiologic knowledge" can stand him in good stead, for he should know whether viral influenza "is around" or has not been seen for some time; in this case, it has been "around." He likewise is aware that staphylococci acquired from hospitalized patients are more apt to be penicillinase-producers than staphylococci acquired in the world at large, so to speak, and he knows that his patient is a medical student. He knows that primary streptococcal pneumonia of this severe type is a rarer phenomenon than primary staphylococcal pneumonia except in the middle of an outbreak of viral influenza. By contrast, Klebsiella pneumonia, although a not unlikely possibility in such a severe pneumonia syndrome, characteristically occurs in middle-aged weakened hosts and would be a most unlikely happening in an otherwise healthy young man.

In this situation as described, the amount of immediately useful knowledge that was produced is considerable. Armed with this knowledge, the physician who knows that he must start drug therapy right away actually has a pretty good idea of the nature of the problem. Indeed, the assembled information made it seem most likely that the patient had a primary staphylococcal pneumonia. Be that as it may, the physician knows the drug regimen he chooses must provide maximal protection against pneumococcus and Streptococcus (penicillin); maximal protection against Klebsiella (streptomycin or gentamicin); and maximal protection against Staphylococcus, including penicillinase producers (oxacillin or a similar drug, along with streptomycin or gentamicin). Eighteen to 24 hours later when the identity of the infection presumably would become known, the therapy could be modified appropriately. It so happened that the cause of the illness was discovered to be a penicillinase-producing strain of *S. aureus* which was well controlled by the therapy. It should be stressed that once the microbe is identified, the physician's responsibility to modify the therapy is great. Almost invariably the patient has been receiving one or more drugs that are now known to be unnecessary, and the risks of their toxicities should be terminated promptly.

The body of knowledge from which selectivity of the sort described can be obtained is presented in the various chapters on bacterial and mycotic diseases. There are other sorts of knowledge also necessary to the clinician – knowledge about antimicrobial therapy and the drugs themselves (see Ch. 268) and information about some of the microbial mechanisms whereby the impact of drug therapy could be withstood and the microbe survive. One form of survival, viewing the microbial world as a whole, is the "new diseases" that emerge as *endogenous microbial diseases* (see Ch. 178). These "new diseases" are a form of microbial survival of drug challenge, because they ensure that *some* microbes will endure. To ensure the survival of a particular microbial species and hence a particular disease, however, there are two other and quite different survival patterns, *microbial persistence* and *microbial drug resistance*. The latter phenomenon, under the name "drug-fastness," had been recognized since the early days of this century. Microbial persistence, on the other hand, was not recognized – indeed could not be recognized – until the development of penicillin, because it was only then that a powerful antimicrobial drug could be given in virtually any dosage and thus permit exclusion of the obvious possibility that the microbial survival was only a consequence of underdosage.

Microbial Persistence. Microbial persistence can be defined as the phenomenon whereby a microbial strain that is susceptible to a drug in the test tube is nevertheless capable of surviving long-term exposure to that drug in the body. Persistence is thus sharply distinguished from drug resistance, which is a heritable property of a microbial strain and is demonstrable in the test tube as well as in the body. In numerical terms, microbial persistence is of the greater importance, because it is the phenomenon that is responsible for most instances of post-treatment relapse, that interferes with the effectiveness of chemoprophylaxis, and that balks attempts to use drugs for the "eradication" of microbes (see Ch. 268). Once recognized and studied, it became clear that microbial persistence – the drug-related phenomenon – was only one aspect of the larger phenomenon of latent microbial infection with its potentiality for evocation as endogenous microbial disease. As our knowledge accumulates, it is likewise beginning to appear as if microbial persistence and genotypic drug resistance are veering toward each other, and may eventually come to overlap. Persistence thus serves as a link between the other two phenomena, and indeed all three may ultimately be seen to shade into each other. However, we are not yet at that point. Recognition of the present clearly visible difference among the three has been most valuable in that it has made it possible for each to be recognized, reasonably well defined, and isolated for study. For more detailed consideration of these phenomena, the reader is referred to the references at the end of this chapter. Certain aspects of microbial persistence and heritable drug resistance deserve mention at this point.

Until microbial persistence was recognized in the 1940's, the conceptual base of antimicrobial therapy was *therapia sterilisans magna* as originally conceived by Ehrlich; namely, the goal was to effect a total eradication of the infecting microbes from the host. With penicillin and the subsequently introduced drugs, it was discovered that such total eradication did not occur uniformly and predictably. In a significant number of cases of virtually any bacterial disease, drug-susceptible cells of the infecting strain could be isolated well after completion of drug therapy. At times these persisters would increase and produce clinical relapse, which was then easily treatable by the appropriate drug. At other times they would persist in the carrier state or might ultimately disappear either into latency or presumably by leaving the host altogether. Evidence was obtained that this microbial survival could not be explained by failure of drug delivery, namely, that the microbes were located in some sanctuary such as a body compartment or the center of a necrotic area where they could not be reached by the molecules of drug in the extracellular fluid; nor could the phenomenon be explained on the basis that the drug molecules were deviated from making contact with the microbes because the inflammatory-necrotic lesion either chemically degraded the drug or wholly bound it in some way. On the contrary, convincing evidence exists that the capacity to persist is a nonheritable property of a minority of the microbial population, and it is mediated by the ability to assume a metabolic state that has been termed "drug indifference" or "physiologic" spore formation. To what extent bacterial pleomorphism, including such forms as protoplasts, plays a role in persistence is not known. Whatever may be the mechanism or mechanisms, it is also clear that even though an infecting microbial population may be wholly drug susceptible in the conventional sense, actual therapy with that drug will not be uniformly or predictably *eradicative.* This is the case irrespective of whether the drug is classified as "bacteriostatic" or "bactericidal." It is this capacity of drug-susceptible bacteria to survive and outlast periods of drug administration that is responsible for most clinical relapse, failures to eliminate the carrier state, and certain failures of chemoprophylaxis. It is not generally known that Ehrlich in his late years came to perceive that *magna sterilisans* conceived as eradication was untenable. He then subtly changed the *concept* of the "sterilisans" without changing the *word,* and offered the idea that the bacteria in the tissues were in effect rendered sterile, i.e., incapable of having progeny. In the last analysis all that is added to this "latter-day Ehrlich" by the present concept of microbial persistence is the point that the sterile state is reversible.

Drug Resistance. Strictly speaking, any microbial strain that is unaffected by appropriate concentrations of a drug in vitro could be called drug resistant. In actual practice, however, the designation is reserved for the drug-resistant representatives of bacterial species that are customarily susceptible to the drug in question. *Primary resistance* refers to situations in which the infecting bacterial strain is already drug resistant at the time it initiates the infection. *Emergent resistance* refers to the emergence to predominance of a drug-resistant population during the treatment of a microbial disease that was drug susceptible when treatment was started.

All drug-susceptible bacterial species possess the capability to show emergent resistance—that is to say, to escape during therapy—to *some* drug or drugs. But *all drugs* are not associated with emergent resistance. Specifically, no instance of emergent resistance to penicillin has been observed,* and all penicillin resistance is primary. Whether drug resistance can emerge or not thus *depends not on the bacterial species but on the drug.* This clearly indicates that there exists a type of drug action on a microbe wherein the emergence to predominance of drug-resistant forms is not to be feared. The existence of this type of drug action is of obvious importance in considerations of the possible mechanisms involved in multiple drug regimens, as discussed below.

Four Different Forms of Drug Resistance. The pluralistic nature of the broad phenomenon called "drug resistance" can readily be seen by examining different drugs or drug-microbe pairings. At least four distinct forms are identifiable. There is the *sulfonamide-streptomycin form,* in which the resistant bacteria maintain full pathogenic potential and are otherwise altered little, if at all, except for their loss of susceptibility to the drug. There is the *major isoniazid form,* in which certain enzymes have been lost (catalase and peroxidase), and the pathogenicity for laboratory animals, including primates, has been significantly reduced. (There is another, much less frequently encountered form of isoniazid resistance in which full pathogenicity is maintained.) There is a form characterized by *episomal or plasmid transfer,* exemplified by enteric bacteria but also by staphylococci. There is also a form seen most clearly with penicillin and staphylococci in which the critical element in producing the resistance is the *presence of a beta-lactamase,* so-called penicillinase. In some strains of staphylococci the enzyme is inducible; in other strains and species it can be constitutive. Combinations of these various forms of phenomena occur. For example, some strains of isoniazid-resistant tubercle bacilli are of the sulfonamide-streptomycin form, although these are rare; the genetic capability of staphylococci to elaborate penicillinase can be passed from one cell to another by episomal transfer, and the actual enzymatic process of synthesizing penicillinase is induced by exposure to the substrate penicillin.

Episomal transfer is an example of nonchromosomal inheritance, for bacteria not only have chromosomal genes, they also have what are in effect free-floating genes that can pass from one cell to another as if they were a virus. The particles are of two sorts: *the episomes* and *the plasmid.* The difference between them is that the plasmid does not attach itself to the chromosome at any time, whereas the episome can either exist freely in the cytoplasm or at times attach itself to the chromosome. Synergism between an episomal gene and a chromosomal gene can occur. In one such experiment, two genes, one present in the episomal factor and the other in the chromosomal, each of which singly conferred resistance to streptomycin concentrations of 25 mg per milliliter, *co-operated* to yield organisms to 1000 mg per milliliter. It is believed that the synergism was acquired as a direct result of genetic recombination between the chromosome and the episomal factor. The "infection" of the strain of *E. coli* in the form of the episomal factor could be removed by treatment with an acridine dye—in effect, a form of drug therapy in vitro. The last-named observation is of considerable theoretic significance when one attempts to analyze the ways in which two-drug therapy

*The penicillin-resistant pneumococci reported from Australia (Hausman et al., 1971) were not isolated in a situation of *emergent* resistance. This also appears to have been the case with the strains isolated by Tempest et al. (1974) at the Navajo Medical Center.

can be more effective than the more powerful drug used alone.

Aid to the Clinician. In what way is the clinician benefited by acquaintance with this expanding body of knowledge on the multiple forms of what can only loosely be called "drug resistance"? The principal gain—and it is by no means a minor one—is that he is able to perceive that *the results of testing a microbial strain for drug susceptibility in vitro represent only one bit of information, and one that is not always relevant to the therapeutic problem presented by his patient.* The identity of the microbial species, its probable source, e.g., whether acquired in hospital or acquired from a drug-treated household contact, and the *history* of drugs received earlier in the illness and their observed effects usually represent a body of evidence of greater reliability and predictive value than drug-susceptibility tests as they are frequently performed. For example, the highly successful streptomycin-penicillin treatment of enterococcal endocarditis would never have been instituted had the results of the streptomycin-susceptibility tests been the controlling factor. Likewise, a patient's pulmonary tuberculosis may respond well to isoniazid despite isoniazid resistance of the patient's strain when subjected to conventional drug-susceptibility tests. But this is not always the case, which merely reflects that there is obviously more than one form of isoniazid resistance. What is clear is that the clinician should be very wary of abandoning a particular drug therapy that appears to be working satisfactorily and introducing a substitute *solely* on the basis of drug-susceptibility tests. Like many ancillary laboratory procedures, drug-susceptibility tests have a role, but it is usually more a confirming one than a determining one.

Drug Pairings. Consideration of the mechanisms of drug resistance leads to scrutiny of the use of two antimicrobial drugs together. One of the avowed goals of such multidrug therapy is to postpone or prevent drug resistance of the emergent type; the other is to obtain greater antimicrobial effectiveness per unit of time. Conceivably the same process could be responsible for both effects, although this is not the customary way of looking at the matter. With respect to drug resistance, the orthodox explanation dates from Ehrlich's day and is based on the notion that emergent resistance is prevented or postponed because drug A is effective against those bacterial mutants that are resistant to drug B, and vice versa. By this concept it would be possible for a two-drug regimen to affect emergent resistance without exerting an enhanced antimicrobial effectiveness per unit of time. The enhanced effectiveness phenomenon, which is seen, for example, in the penicillin-streptomycin treatment of enterococcal endocarditis, presumably would have to be explained on some other basis. The issue here is not whether, in appropriate circumstances, two-drug therapy can affect emergent resistance or increase total antimicrobial effectiveness. The question is *how* these phenomena are brought about. If the combined drug action is exerted independently, with drug A acting on cells resistant to drug B, virtually any two-drug regimen would be expected to be effective. Contrariwise, if the respective drug actions are dependent, it would presumably represent a highly specialized phenomenon. To settle this issue would thus be a matter of considerable practical importance. Unfortunately, a reasonably complete and authoritative answer cannot be given at this time.

It can be said from the relatively few sets of observations available that enhancement of antimicrobial effectiveness by concurrent administration of two drugs appears to be a *dependent* phenomenon, *with both drugs generally acting on the same microbial cell.* The phenomenon seems to have considerable specificity in terms of drugs and microbial species involved; hence superior drug pairings are relatively rare, and are not to be expected with just any pairing and any drug-susceptible parasite. Whether the "dependent" mechanism is also the major way by which two-drug regimens influence emergent resistance is less clear. In the writer's judgment, there is considerable reason to believe that this is indeed the case and that *when a drug pairing does exert an influence on emergent resistance, it does so by the action of both drugs on the microbes susceptible to both drugs.* Hence in large measure the action would consist of both drugs acting on the same microbial cell. As in the situation with enhancement, such effective drug pairings would represent highly specialized sets of circumstances.

The indication that drug pairings superior to the more powerful drug alone are special affairs is in agreement with the rarity with which multiple drug regimens are of demonstrated value in clinical medicine. Indeed to all intents and purposes, the examples are largely limited to infections with enterococci, tubercle bacilli, and viridans streptococci. Conceivably with further experience it might be possible to add to the list the gentamicin/carbenicillin treatment of Pseudomonas infections. It is important for the physician to keep reminding himself that, except for these few microbial diseases, the justification for the use of more than one antimicrobial drug at a time is largely limited to situations in which an etiologic diagnosis has not yet (or never) been established. Usually, as discussed above, this occurs only during the early hours of treatment, and the physician should be quick to change to single drug therapy as the situation is clarified.

Need for Selectivity. The day has gone by when the physician could prescribe all two or three of the available antimicrobial drugs to an acutely febrile patient and relax with the comforting thought that all that modern science could do was being done. With today's multiplicity of drugs, the emergence of "new" microbial diseases, and our considerably expanded knowledge about mechanisms of microbial survival, the physician must be highly selective in his drug choices, and hence must have mastery of a considerably greater body of clinical and laboratory-derived knowledge than was needed even a few decades ago. The physician's "comforting thought" today is of quite a different sort. It consists of the knowledge that, however difficult modern science is making things for *him* in the management of infections, it is making things ever so much better for his patients.

Davis, B. D., Dulbecco, R., Eisen, H. N., Ginsberg, H. S., Wood, W. B., Jr., and McCarty, M. (eds.): Microbiology. 2nd ed. New York, Harper & Row, 1973.

Dubos, R. J.: Man Adapting. New Haven, Yale University Press, 1965.

McDermott, W.: Microbial Persistence. Harvey Lecture Series No. 63, 1969, pp. 1–31.

McDermott, W.: Microbial drug resistance. Barnwell Lecture. Am. Rev. Respir. Dis., 102:855, 1970.

268. ANTIMICROBIAL THERAPY

Richard B. Roberts

The announcement of the first sulfonamide in 1935 ushered in the modern era of antimicrobial therapy, an era characterized by the dramatic reduction in incidence, morbidity, and mortality of many infectious diseases. The most outstanding examples include the reduction in disease incidence or death caused by pneumococcal pneumonia, microbial endocarditis, and tuberculosis. The impact by this class of agents on medical, public health, and economic factors related to disease states has been unparalleled in the history of drug therapy.

The abuse of these therapeutic agents, however, is alarming. In the United States, production of antimicrobial agents and the use of these drugs by physicians has steadily increased in the past decade, i.e., a 60 per cent increase in use over this period of time. Antimicrobial agents are a commonly prescribed medication in office practice (about 15 per cent of all drugs), and approximately one third of hospitalized patients receive such drugs. Surveys have suggested that two thirds of these patients receive the incorrect agent or an inappropriate dose. Indiscriminate use of these drugs may be accompanied by such complications as adverse reactions (allergic or dose related), superinfection, emergence of resistant organisms, and delay in identifying the causative organism.

Since many clinical situations dictate that antimicrobial therapy be instituted prior to identification of the specific etiologic microbe, intelligent use of these drugs requires a thorough knowledge of the suspected infectious process as well as of the changing patterns of microbial resistance. In addition, an understanding of the physical and chemical properties of antimicrobial agents is important, because these properties determine adequate drug levels and toxicity, depending on absorption, distribution, and excretion of these drugs.

SELECTION OF ANTIMICROBIAL AGENTS

Host Determinants

Age and Weight. The dose of an antimicrobial drug is usually calculated on the basis of body weight and, less commonly, body surface (Table 1). The route of administration, dosage, and the incidence of adverse reactions may also vary, depending on the age of the patient. For example, in the neonate and aged patient, renal function may be compromised, and the dosage of drugs excreted by the kidney should be adjusted accordingly. *Tetracycline* should not be used in pregnant women, infants, or young children, because this drug may cause enamel hypoplasia, tooth discoloration, and disturbance in bone growth. *Sulfonamides* should not be given to newborns because of possible elevated serum levels owing to abnormalities in acetylation or kernicterus owing to displacement of bilirubin from serum albumin. Similarly, the liver of premature and newborn babies produces only small amounts of glucuronyl transferase, the enzyme necessary to inactivate *chloramphenicol.* High levels of the biologically active drug may cause the "gray baby syndrome," characterized by abdominal distention, progressive pallor and cyanosis, vasomotor collapse, and death.

Site of Infection. The anatomic location of an infectious process often determines the choice of the antimicrobial and the route of its administration. Clinical studies have shown that adequate levels of most antimicrobial agents except the polymyxins are achieved in inflamed joints, making intra-articular instillation unnecessary. Antimicrobial drugs also penetrate inflamed pleura. Aminoglycosides should not be instilled into a body cavity (i.e., pleural or peritoneal), because neuromuscular blockade and respiratory paralysis may occur. Adequate drainage in addition to effective drug levels in the blood are necessary in infections associated with obstruction in the respiratory, biliary, or urinary tracts. Adequate levels of an antimicrobial agent in the cerebrospinal fluid are determined in part by the pharmacologic properties of the drug and meningeal inflammation. The penicillins, because of their low toxicity, can be given in sufficient dosage parenterally to achieve adequate levels in the cerebrospinal fluid. Chloramphenicol and sulfonamides cross the blood-brain barrier and are effective in bacterial meningitis. However, therapeutic levels of cephalothin and clindamycin in the cerebrospinal fluid are not achieved in the presence of normal or inflamed meninges, and these drugs should not be used in bacterial meningitis. Gentamicin and polymyxin B cross the blood-brain barrier poorly and should be given intrathecally as well as parenterally to patients with gram-negative bacillary meningitis.

Underlying Disease. Serious and life-threatening infections in the compromised host present as one of the most difficult diagnostic and therapeutic challenges in medicine. A variety of microbes, including bacteria, viruses, fungi, and protozoa, infect patients who have malignant disorders or who receive immunosuppressive and cytotoxic therapy for cancer, rheumatic diseases, and renal transplantation. These patients often require antimicrobial therapy before the etiologic agent or agents are identified. Since infections in the compromised host are usually severe and are caused by a number of diverse microorganisms, an aggressive diagnostic approach, often culminating in invasive biopsy procedures, may be necessary. Initial antibacterial therapy should include a penicillinase-resistant penicillin or a cephalosporin and gentamicin. Carbenicillin is added if the clinical or laboratory findings are consistent with Pseudomonas bacteremia. Clindamycin should be given if anaerobic organisms, especially *Bacteroides fragilis,* are suspected. These drugs should be given in maximal doses parenterally. If the initial bacterial cultures are negative after three to five days, the patient should be re-evaluated. If diagnostic studies are negative, the drug therapy should be discontinued, because superinfection with resistant gram-negative bacilli and fungi may occur. Even with appropriate therapy, clinical response may be delayed and may ultimately depend on remission of the underlying disease or reduction of immunosuppressive therapy.

Function of the liver and kidneys may be affected by many underlying diseases. Since these are the major excretory organs for antimicrobial drugs, either many antimicrobial drugs should not be used or their dosage should be modified in the face of compromised hepatic or renal function. These precautions are discussed subsequently under the heading Excretion.

Genetic Factors. The genetic background of patients

TABLE 1. Antimicrobial Agents for Bacterial, Fungal, and Viral Infections

	Adult Daily Dosage (Time Interval of Divided Doses)	Route	Mechanism of Action
Amantadine hydrochloride	200 mg/day	PO	Unknown
Aminosalicylic acid	12 grams/day (t.i.d.)	PO	Replacement of para-aminobenzoic acid
Amphotericin B	1.0 mg/kg/day or every other day (total dose: 2–3 grams) or 15–50 mg/day × 10 weeks	IV	Interaction with sterols of cell membrane
Bacitracin	t.i.d.	Local	Inhibition of cell wall synthesis
Capreomycin	1 gram/day	IM	Unknown
Cephalosporins			Inhibition of cell wall synthesis
Cephalothin	4–12 grams/day (q. 4–6 hours)	IV	
Cephapirin	4–12 grams/day (q. 4–6 hours)	IM, IV	
Cephaloridine	2–4 grams/day (q. 6 hours)	IM	
Cefazolin	2–6 grams/day (q. 6–8 hours)	IM, IV	
Cephaloglycin	1–2 grams/day (q.i.d.)	PO	
Cephalexin	1–4 grams/day (q.i.d.)	PO	
Chloramphenicol	1–4 grams/day (q. 6 hours)	IV	Inhibition of protein synthesis (50S ribosomal binding)
	1–4 grams/day (q.i.d.)	PO	
Clindamycin	0.6–4.5 grams/day (q. 6–8 hours)	IM, IV	Inhibition of protein synthesis
	0.4–1.2 grams/day (q.i.d.)	PO	
Cycloserine	500–750 mg/day (q. 12 hours)	PO	Inhibition of cell wall synthesis
Cytarabine	10–100 mg/square meter/day	IV	Inhibition of nucleoprotein synthesis
Erythromycins			Inhibition of protein synthesis (50S ribosomal binding)
Erythromycin ethylsuccinate	1–4 grams/day (q. 6 hours)	PO	
	400 mg/day (q. 6 hours)	IM	
Erythromycin stearate	1–4 grams/day (q. 6 hours)	PO	
Erythromycin gluceptate	1–4 grams/day (q. 6 hours)	IV	
Erythromycin lactobionate	1–4 grams/day (q. 6 hours)	IV	
Ethambutol	25 mg/kg/day × 6 weeks, then 15 mg/kg/day	PO	Unknown
Ethionamide	500–750 mg/day (q. 12 hours)	PO	Unknown
Flucytosine	150 mg/kg/day × 6 weeks (q. 6 hours)	PO	Inhibition of nucleoprotein synthesis (competition with cytosine)
Gentamicin	3–5 mg/kg/day (q. 8 hours)	IV, IM	Inhibition of protein synthesis (30S ribosomal binding)
	4–5 mg/day	IT	
Idoxuridine	100 mg/kg/day	IV	Inhibition of nucleoprotein synthesis (competition with thymidylic acid)
		Local	
Isoniazid	300 mg/day	PO	Inhibition of enzymes requiring pyridoxal as cofactor
Kanamycin	15 mg/kg/day (q. 8–12 hours)	IV, IM	Inhibition of protein synthesis (30S ribosomal binding)
	4–8 grams/day (q. 4–6 hours)	PO	
Lincomycin	2–8 grams/day (q. 6 hours)	IV, IM	Inhibition of protein synthesis (50S ribosomal binding)
	2 grams/day (q.i.d.)	PO	
Methenamine mandelate	4–12 grams/day (q.i.d.)	PO	Unknown
Methisazone	1.5 grams/day × 8 days	PO	Inhibition of nucleoprotein synthesis
Nalidixic acid	2–4 grams/day (q.i.d.)	PO	Unknown
Neomycin	4–8 grams/day (q. 6 hours)	PO	Inhibition of protein synthesis (30S ribosomal binding)
	t.i.d.	Local	
Nitrofurans			Unknown
Nitrofurantoin	5–10 mg/kg/day (q.i.d.)	PO	
Novobiocin	2–4 grams/day (q. 6 hours)	PO	Unknown
	1–2 grams/day (q. 6 hours)	IV	

may play a determinant part in the use of some antimicrobial agents. Although there may be other examples as yet unrecognized, the following known phenomena are important in determining, in part, the response to therapy as well as the risk of adverse reactions.

The rate at which isoniazid and sulfapyridine are conjugated and biologically inactivated in the liver is genetically determined. These drugs are inactivated in the liver by acetylation. Studies have shown that certain groups of patients receiving a sulfonamide or isoniazid acetylate the drug rapidly and others slowly. The rate of acetylation determines the concentration and duration of biologically active drug in the serum. Although sulfapyridine is not commonly used, salicylazosulfapyridine, which is often administered to patients with mild ulcerative colitis, is metabolized by the microbial flora of the colon to sulfapyridine and 5-aminosalicylic acid. The former metabolite is rapidly absorbed into the systemic circulation and is responsible for the adverse reactions that accompany the use of salicylazosulfapyridine.

Acute hemolytic anemia is associated with the administration of certain antimicrobial agents in patients with glucose-6-phosphate dehydrogenase deficiency. This enzyme abnormality is transmitted as a sex-linked partially dominant characteristic with full expression in homozygous males. Affected females are usually heterozygous. The antimicrobial agents that may precipitate acute hemolysis in these patients are chloramphenicol, niridazole, nitrofurantoin, primaquine, and sulfonamides. Sulfonamides may also be responsible for acute hemolysis in patients with certain hemoglobinopathies.

Drug Susceptibility. One of the most important determinants in the selection of an antimicrobial agent is the susceptibility of the causative organism. It is imperative that appropriate stains and cultures of blood, secretions, cavity fluids, and the like be obtained prior to the institution of antimicrobial therapy. Once the organism has been isolated, drug-susceptibility determinations may be performed by either one of two methods: the disc (agar) *diffusion* technique, or the tube (broth) or plate (agar)

TABLE 1. Antimicrobial Agents for Bacterial, Fungal, and Viral Infections (*Continued*)

	Adult Daily Dosage (Time Interval of Divided Doses)	Route	Mechanism of Action
Nystatin	1.5–3 million units (t.i.d.)	PO	Interaction with sterols of cell membrane
Penicillins, penicillinase-sensitive			Inhibition of cell wall synthesis
Aqueous crystalline penicillin G	0.6–20 million units/day (q. 2–6 hours)	IV, IM	
Procaine penicillin G	600,000–4.8 million units/day (q. 6–12 hours)	IM	
Benzathine penicillin G	600,000–2.4 million units (q. 4 weeks)	IM	
Phenoxymethyl penicillin	1–4 grams/day (q.i.d.)	PO	
Penicillins with gram-negative bacillary activity			Inhibition of cell wall synthesis
Amoxicillin	0.75–1.5 grams/day (q. 8 hours)	PO	
Ampicillin	4–12 grams/day (q. 4–6 hours)	IV, IM	
	1–4 grams/day (q. 6 hours)	PO	
Carbenicillin	2–40 grams/day (q. 4 hours)	IV, IM	
	2–4 grams/day (q.i.d.)	PO	
Penicillins, penicillinase-resistant			Inhibition of cell wall synthesis
Cloxacillin	2–4 grams/day (q. 6 hours)	PO	
Dicloxacillin	1–2 grams/day (q. 6 hours)	PO	
Methicillin	6–12 grams/day (q. 4–6 hours)	IV, IM	
Nafcillin	4–8 grams/day (q. 4–6 hours)	IV, IM	
Oxacillin	4–8 grams/day (q. 6 hours)	IV, IM	
	2–4 grams/day (q. 4–6 hours)	PO	
Polymyxins			Disruption of cell wall–membrane complex
Polymyxin B	2.5 mg/kg/day (q. 8 hours)	IV, IM	
	5.0 mg/day	IT	
Polymyxin E			
Colistimethate sodium	5.0 mg/kg/day (q. 6 hours)	IV, IM	
Colistin sulfate	5.0 mg/kg/day (q. 6 hours)	PO	
Pyrazinamide	40–50 mg/kg/day (q. 8–12 hours)	PO	Unknown
Rifampin	600 mg/day	PO	Inhibition of DNA-dependent RNA polymerase
Spectinomycin	2.0 or 4.0 grams/day	IM	Inhibition of protein synthesis (30S ribosomal binding)
Streptomycin	1–2 grams/day (q. 12–24 hours)	IM	Inhibition of protein synthesis (30S ribosomal binding)
Sulfonamides			Competition with para-aminobenzoic acid
Sulfisoxazole	4–6 grams/day (q. 6 hours)	PO, IV	
Salicylazosulfapyridine	4–8 grams/day (q. 3–6 hours)	PO	
Tetracyclines			Inhibition of protein synthesis
Tetracycline HCl	IV: 0.5–1.0 gram/day (q. 12 hours)	IV, PO	
Chlortetracycline		IV, PO	
Oxytetracycline	PO: 1–2 grams/day (q. 6 hours)	IV, PO	
Demethylchlortetracycline	0.6–1.2 grams/day (q. 6 hours)	PO	
Methacycline	0.6–0.9 gram/day (q. 6–12 hours)	PO	
Doxycycline	0.2–0.4 gram/day (q. 12 hours)	PO	
Minocycline	0.1–0.4 gram/day (q. 12 hours)	PO	
Trimethoprim/sulfamethoxazole	4 tablets/day (q. 12 hours) (1 tablet = T80 mg/S400 mg)	PO	Sequential inhibition of folic acid reduction
Vancomycin	2 grams/day (q. 6 hours)	IV	Inhibition of cell wall synthesis
Viomycin	1 gram twice weekly	IM	Inhibition of protein synthesis

dilution technique. The former method is routinely used in most clinical laboratories. Because of the many factors which may influence drug-susceptibility determinations, standardization of this method must take into account the growth of the organism, the inoculum size, the type and quantity of media employed, the size and concentration of drug-impregnated discs, and the duration and environmental conditions of incubation. If these conditions are adhered to, the diameter of the area of growth inhibition about the impregnated disc distinguishes resistant from susceptible strains. In addition, precautions concerning specific bacteria or drugs must also be taken into consideration. Resistance of *Staphylococcus aureus* to methicillin is reliable only if the zones are measured within 20 hours of incubation, because methicillin deteriorates rapidly at incubating temperatures. Fastidious and slow-growing organisms such as Bacteroides and certain streptococci may not produce visible colonies within 24 hours, and reports of susceptibility may not be reliable. Disc susceptibility tests performed in anaerobic jars may give misleading results. Colistin and polymyxin B diffuse poorly in agar, and the drug-susceptibility results may be inaccurate. The standardized disc test is not recommended for gonococci or for *Mycobacterium tuberculosis.*

In certain clinical settings, namely patients with endocarditis and osteomyelitis, a more precise method for determining the susceptibility of an organism may be indicated. The *dilution method*—that is, twofold dilutions of the drug in broth or agar containing a standardized inoculum of the infecting organism—is the technique commonly employed in many laboratories. Results are expressed as the minimal inhibitory concentration or MIC, which is the smallest amount of drug that will inhibit growth after 18 to 24 hours of incubation.

The serum antibacterial activity may also be determined. At a specified time after the drug is given (usually one hour after parenteral administration), serum is collected and serially diluted in a medium inoculated with the organism. A serum dilution of 1:8 or greater that inhibits the growth of the test organism is indicative of an adequate blood level for serious and life-threatening infections. Accurate serum concentrations can be determined by impregnating discs with known concentrations of a drug and other discs with serum dilutions from the patient. These discs are placed on agar previously inoculated with the organism, and zones of growth inhibition are compared after incubation.

Knowledge of the drug-susceptibility patterns of bacteria is important for the intelligent use of antimicrobial agents. For example, despite the common use of penicillin G, group A streptococci, pneumococci, and meningococci have remained susceptible to it. Methicillin-resistant *Staphylococcus aureus* strains, however, have been reported especially from Denmark and less commonly from England and the United States. These strains are also resistant to the cephalosporins. Patterns of susceptibility and resistance of gram-negative bacilli vary from hospital to hospital as well as temporally within the same institution. This phenomenon is principally due to the widespread use of antimicrobial agents active against gram-negative bacilli and the development of emergent resistance. Because of the changing patterns of susceptibility and resistance of bacteria, continuous laboratory surveillance of the incidence and susceptibility of isolates by hospital epidemiologists and clinical laboratories is extremely important. The antimicrobial susceptibilities of various microbes are discussed later in this chapter.

Bactericidal and Bacteriostatic Drugs. Bactericidal agents are drugs that kill organisms at or near the minimal inhibitory concentration. Examples of bactericidal agents include the penicillins, cephalosporins, vancomycin, aminoglycosides, and polymyxins. In general, patients with severe infections should receive bactericidal drugs. This is especially true in patients with abnormal host defense mechanisms involving antibody function, phagocyte function, or cellular immunity. Bacteriostatic drugs inhibit the growth of organisms and include erythromycin, lincomycin, clindamycin, chloramphenicol, tetracycline, and the sulfonamides. Erythromycin, lincomycin, and clindamycin may have bactericidal activity at high concentrations against certain organisms. An intact immunologic system is an important determinant in the response of patients receiving bacteriostatic drugs. In many clinical situations, such as upper respiratory tract infections, anaerobic infections, and uncomplicated urinary tract infections, bacteriostatic drugs are as effective clinically as bactericidal agents.

Combination Therapy. The administration of more than one antimicrobial agent at the same time is indicated for (1) initial therapy in a critically ill patient when the causative organism is not known, (2) polymicrobial infection in which the organisms are not susceptible to one antimicrobial agent, (3) reducing or postponing the emergence of resistance to one or both agents, such as in the therapy for tuberculosis, and (4) synergism. Synergism is best exemplified by the penicillins, the cephalosporins, vancomycin, and the aminoglycosides. In vitro studies suggest that this enhanced antimicrobial effect by bactericidal agents may be due to the inhibition of cell wall synthesis by the penicillins or vancomycin resulting in increased permeability and penetration of the aminoglycosides. The combination of penicillin or vancomycin with streptomycin or gentamicin should be used in patients with enterococcal endocarditis. Limited clinical studies suggest that carbenicillin and gentamicin may be more effective than either drug alone in severe *Pseudomonas aeruginosa* infections. (For additional discussion of multiple drug therapy, see Ch. 267.)

Antagonism between two antimicrobial agents can be demonstrated in vitro. Since bactericidal drugs such as penicillin inhibit cell wall synthesis of rapidly multiplying bacteria, the simultaneous use of a bacteriostatic drug may interfere with bactericidal activity. It is uncommon, however, to detect adverse effects clinically with combined bactericidal and bacteriostatic therapy.

Absorption and Distribution

Pharmacologic properties differ markedly between classes of antimicrobial agents and between agents within the same class. Knowledge of these properties is important for the intelligent use of these drugs. Antimicrobial drugs may be administered by various routes, including topical, oral, and parenteral (intramuscular and intravenous). *Topical administration* should be restricted to special circumstances whenever possible because of possible absorption into the systemic circulation, allergic reactions, and the development of microbial resistance. Examples of appropriate local administration include severe burns, intravenous catheter sites, and purulent conjunctivitis. The *oral route* is used chiefly in initial therapy for mild to moderately severe infections and for the completion of therapy in patients with severe infections. Because of the variable absorption of antimicrobial agents in the presence of gastric acidity, oral medications should be given in the fasting state, i.e., 1 to 2 hours before or after meals. *Parenteral administration* of antimicrobial drugs is indicated for severe infections that require high and sustained blood levels. Many drugs cannot be administered intramuscularly because of severe pain. These include cephalothin, vancomycin, erythromycin, chloramphenicol, and tetracycline. *Intravenous administration* is indicated in patients with severe infections or hypotension, or when appropriate levels cannot be achieved by the intramuscular route. Intravenous appliances must be changed every 24 to 48 hours to avoid thrombophlebitis and local infection with or without bacteremia. In general, medications should be diluted in 50 to 100 ml of solution and allowed to run in over a period of 15 to 30 minutes. Adverse reactions, especially associated with the aminoglycosides and polymyxins, may occur with rapid intravenous administration. Intrathecal and intra-articular therapy may be necessary in gram-negative infections. Complications associated with intrathecal administration include arachnoiditis with severe pain, paresthesias, and transient to permanent paralysis. The intrapleural or intraperitoneal administration of antimicrobial drugs is not recommended.

The distribution of a drug is a complex phenomenon and depends on many factors, including (1) molecular size, (2) electrical charge at pH 7.4, (3) lipid solubility, (4) plasma protein binding, and (5) presence of inflammation. If adequate blood levels are present, most antimicrobial agents will enter infected synovial and serous fluids. However, even in the presence of inflamed meninges, therapeutic levels of cephalothin, clindamycin, polymyxin, or gentamicin may not be achieved.

Excretion

The liver and the kidneys are the two principal excretory organs for antimicrobial agents. Renal clearance, by either glomerular filtration or tubular secretion, or both, is a major determinant of serum levels. Probenecid increases and prolongs the serum level of those antimicrobials excreted by tubular secretion (i.e., the penicillins and cephalosporins). Repeated evaluation of hepatic and renal function must be performed when antimicrobial agents are given in high doses for a prolonged period of time. Ampicillin, nafcillin, erythromycin, tetracycline, chloramphenicol, lincomycin, clindamycin, and novobiocin should be used with caution in patients with liver disease. In the face of impaired renal function, the following agents should be administered with caution, and the dosage reduced accordingly: amphotericin B, cephaloridine, colistimethate, flucytosine, gentamicin, kanamycin, methenamine mandelate, neomycin, nitrofurantoin, penicillins, polymyxin B, streptomycin, sulfonamides, tetracycline, and vancomycin. Many of these agents not only are excreted largely by the kidney but also are nephrotoxic. Although the initial loading dose is the same, subsequent doses are reduced or the duration between doses is prolonged. Formulas for drug dose and interval between doses have been derived based on renal function, i.e., serum creatinine or creatinine clearance. These guidelines are useful but cannot be relied upon alone. Adjustments are best guided by repeated determinations of the serum concentration of the drug. In addition, knowledge of the dialyzability of antimicrobial agents with hemodialysis and peritoneal dialysis is necessary for the management of patients with acute and chronic renal failure.

Adverse Reactions

The administration of antimicrobial agents may be associated with toxic or allergic reactions. Adverse reactions are widely variable, as shown by the following examples: (1) local irritation at the site of administration; (2) hypersensitivity reactions; (3) dose related hepatic, renal, and bone marrow toxicity; and (4) adverse reactions caused by the composition of the drug preparation (i.e., hyperkalemia with potassium penicillin G, fluid retention with disodium carbenicillin). The adverse reactions associated with specific antimicrobial agents are discussed below.

SPECIFIC ANTIMICROBIAL AGENTS

Antimicrobial agents may be classified as to their chemical structure, mechanism of action, antimicrobial spectrum of activity, and bactericidal versus bacteriostatic properties. Table 1 lists the common antibacterial agents with their route of administration, dosage, and mechanism of action. More detailed descriptions of the indications for each drug are included in the chapters dealing with specific organisms or infectious diseases. The antituberculous drugs (isoniazid, rifampin, streptomycin, para-aminosalicylic acid, pyrazinamide, capreomycin, cycloserine, ethambutol, ethionamide, and viomycin), the antiviral drugs (amantadine hydrochloride, cytarabine, idoxuridine, and methisazone), and the antifungal agents (amphotericin B, flucytosine, and nystatin) are included in Table 1 and are discussed in detail in the chapters dealing with the respective diseases for which they are used. Table 2 lists the antiprotozoan and antimetazoan drugs with their clinical indications, dose, route of administration, and toxicity. The following antiparasitic drugs are not approved by the Food and Drug Administration for general use in the United States: antimony sodium gluconate, bithional, melarsoprol, niclosamide, niridazole, pentamidine, and suramin. These agents, however, may be easily obtained for therapy of the indicated diseases by calling the Parasitic Diseases Branch of the Center for Disease Control at 404–633–3311.

Penicillins. *Penicillinase-Sensitive Penicillins.* The penicillins that are susceptible to penicillinase are penicillin G (benzyl penicillin), phenoxymethyl penicillin, ampicillin, and carbenicillin. Penicillin G has three intramuscular forms which differ in the rate of absorption, thus affecting the concentration and duration of drug in serum. *Aqueous crystalline penicillin G* is well absorbed but is painful and is therefore usually given intravenously. *Procaine penicillin G* is well tolerated intramuscularly and is slowly absorbed so that injections are only necessary every six to twelve hours. *Benzathine penicillin G* is also given intramuscularly and is slowly released from the site of injection over three to four weeks. Procaine penicillin G and benzathine penicillin should not be administered intravenously. Penicillin G is unstable in the presence of gastric acid. *Phenoxymethyl penicillin,* although ten times less active than benzyl penicillin, is acid stable and is preferred for oral therapy. Renal clearance of the penicillins is by glomerular filtration and tubular secretion, and the simultaneous administration of probenecid will increase and prolong serum levels. However, probenecid may cause such adverse reactions as nausea, vomiting, hypersensitivity reactions (rash and fever), and rarely the nephrotic syndrome, hepatocellular injury, and aplastic anemia. Acute gout as well as the development of uric acid stones may be precipitated by probenecid. Penicillin G is active against streptococci of groups A, B, C and G, viridans streptococci, pneumococci, nonpenicillinase-producing staphylococci, *Corynebacterium diphtheriae, Listeria monocytogenes,* anaerobic streptococci, Fusobacterium, Clostridia, treponemes, Leptospira species, Neisseria, Pasteurella multocida, and Actinomyces.

Penicillins with gram-negative bacillary activity include ampicillin and carbenicillin. *Ampicillin* differs from penicillin G only in the presence of an amino group on the side chain. This minor alteration is responsible for the difference in antimicrobial activity. Ampicillin is active against enterococci, *Hemophilus influenzae,* Shigella, Salmonella, *Escherichia coli,* and *Proteus mirabilis.* Indole-positive Proteus species (i.e., *P. rettgeri, P. morgani, P. vulgaris*) and Pseudomonas species are resistant. Ampicillin may be given either parenterally or orally, and the serum half-life is twice as long as that of penicillin G. *Amoxicillin,* an analogue of ampicillin, is available for general use and has several pharmacologic advantages over ampicillin. It is more stable in the presence of gastric acid and thus better absorbed. Serum levels are higher and more prolonged than those of ampicillin. Both drugs have the same spectrum of antibacterial activity.

Carbenicillin is also similar in structure to penicillin G except for a carboxyl group on the side chain. It is active in vitro against *E. coli,* Pseudomonas species, Pro-

TABLE 2. Antimicrobial Agents for Protozoan and Metazoan Infections

Protozoan Infections	Infecting Organism	Antimicrobial Agent	Adult Dose	Route	Adverse Reactions (Most Frequent Are *Italicized*)
Amebiasis	*Entamoeba histolytica*				
Asymptomatic cyst		Diiodohydroxyquin	650 mg t.i.d. × 3 weeks	PO	*Iodine toxicoderma,* rash, slight thyroid enlargement, nausea
Intestinal disease		Metronidazole	750 mg t.i.d. × 5–10 days	PO	*Nausea,* vomiting, diarrhea; *headache,* vertigo, insomnia, ataxia
Hepatic disease		Metronidazole	750 mg t.i.d. × 10 days	PO	See above
Giardiasis	*G. lamblia*	Metronidazole or	250 mg t.i.d. × 10 days	PO	See above
		Quinacrine	100 mg t.i.d. × 5 days	PO	*Vomiting, vertigo, headache;* psychosis, blood dyscrasia, ocular damage, rash, hepatic necrosis
Leishmaniasis					
Visceral	*L. donovani*	Antimony Na gluconate	600 mg q.d. × 10 days	IM	Similar to antimony potassium tartrate but less severe
Cutaneous	*L. tropica*	Antimony Na gluconate	600 mg q.d. × 10 days	IM	See above
Mucocutaneous	*L. brasiliensis*	Antimony Na gluconate	600 mg q.d. × 10 days	IM	See above
Toxoplasmosis	*T. gondii*				
Moderate–severe illness		Pyrimethamine and	75 mg first day, then 25 mg q.d. × 4 weeks	PO	*Folic acid deficiency,* blood dyscrasia, rash, vomiting, convulsions, shock
Immunosuppressed host		Sulfadiazine plus	1 gram q.i.d. × 4 weeks	PO	*Rash,* photosensitivity, hepatic and renal toxicity, blood dyscrasia, vasculitis
		Folinic acid	6 mg q. 2 days	IM	
Malaria	*Plasmodium vivax, malariae, ovale*	Chloroquine followed by	1 gram, then 500 mg in 6 hours, then 500 mg q.d. × 2 days	PO	*Vomiting, headache, pruritus,* ocular damage, convulsions, psychosis, rash; hair, nail, and mucous membrane discoloration
		Primaquine	26.3 mg q.d. × 14 days	PO	*Hemolytic anemia* in G-6-PD deficient patients, neutropenia, nausea, hypertension
	P. falciparum				
	Chloroquine-susceptible	Chloroquine	1 gram, then 500 mg in 6 hours, then 500 mg q.d. × 2 days	PO	See above
	Chloroquine-resistant	Quinine and	650 mg t.i.d. × 14 days	PO	*Cinchonism, hypotension, arrhythmias,* blood dyscrasias, photosensitivity, blindness
		Pyrimethamine plus	25 mg b.i.d. × 3 days	PO	See above
		Sulfadiazine	500 mg q.i.d. × 5 days		See above
	Comatose patient	Quinine	600 mg/300 ml saline q. 8 hours until PO tolerated	IV	See above
Trichomoniasis	*T. vaginalis*	Metronidazole	250 mg t.i.d. × 10 days	PO	See above
Trypanosomiasis	*T. gambiense*	Pentamidine	4 mg/kg/day × 10 days	IM	*Nausea, vomiting,* hypoglycemia, hypotension, blood dyscrasias, renal and hepatic toxicity
	T. rhodesiense	Suramin followed by	1 gram on days, 1, 3, 7, 14, and 21 after 100 mg test dose	IV	*Rash, pruritus, paresthesias, vomiting,* peripheral neuropathy, shock
		Melarsoprol	2.0–3.6 mg/kg q.d. for 3 days; repeat after 1 week and, if necessary, after an additional 10–21 days	IV	*Encephalopathy,* vomiting, neuropathy, rash, myocarditis, hypertension
Pneumocystosis	*P. carinii*	Pentamidine	4 mg/kg/day q.d. × 12–14 days	IM	See above

Metazoan Infections	Infecting Organism	Antimicrobial Agent	Adult Dose	Route	Adverse Reactions (Most Frequent Are *Italicized*)
Intestinal nematodes	*Ascaris lumbricoides* (roundworm)	Pyrantel pamoate	11 mg/kg (maximum 1 gram), single dose	PO	*GI disturbance,* headache, dizziness, rash, fever
	Enterobius vermicularis (pinworm)	Pyrantel pamoate	11 mg/kg, single dose; repeat after 2 weeks	PO	
	Necator americanus (hookworm)	Pyrantel pamoate	11 mg/kg, single dose	PO	
	Ancylostoma duodenale (hookworm)	Pyrantel pamoate	11 mg/kg, single dose	PO	
	Trichuris trichiura (whipworm)	Thiabendazole	25 mg/kg b.i.d. × 2 days	PO	*Nausea, vomiting, vertigo, rash,* leukopenia, color vision disturbance, tinnitus, shock
	Strongyloides stercoralis	Thiabendazole	25 mg/kg b.i.d. × 2 days	PO	
Tissue nematodes					
Filariasis	*Wuchereria bancrofti*	Diethylcarbamazine	2 mg/kg t.i.d. × 14 days	PO	*Allergic and febrile reactions* due to worm disintegration; encephalopathy
	Loa loa	Diethylcarbamazine	2 mg/kg t.i.d. × 14 days	PO	See above
River blindness	*Onchocerca volvulus*	Diethylcarbamazine plus	2 mg/kg t.i.d. × 14 days	PO	See above
		Suramin	1 gram per week × 5 weeks	IV	See above
Trichinosis	*Trichinella spiralis*	Thiabendazole and/or	25 mg/kg q.d. until symptoms subside	PO	See above
		Corticosteroids	40 mg q.d. for 3–5 days	PO	
Cestodes (tapeworms)	*Taenia saginata* (beef tapeworm)	Niclosamide	2 grams in a single dose	PO	Nausea, abdominal pain
	Diphyllobothrium latum (fish tapeworm)	Niclosamide	2 grams in a single dose	PO	
	Taenia solium (pork tapeworm)	Niclosamide	2 grams in a single dose	PO	
Trematodes (flukes)					
Schistosomiasis	*S. mansoni*	Stibophen	4 ml q.o.d. to 100 ml	IM	Similar to antimony potassium tartrate but less severe
	S. haematobium	Niridazole	25 mg/kg q.d. × 5–7 days	PO	*Vomiting, diarrhea, dizziness, headache,* EKG changes, rash, insomnia, paresthesias, convulsions, psychosis, hemolysis
	S. japonicum	Antimony potassium tartrate	q.o.d. 8, 12, 16, 20, 24 ml, then 28 ml q.o.d. × 10 doses	IV	*Bradycardia, vomiting, cough,* myalgias with rapid administration, rash, pruritus, colic, diarrhea, hemolytic anemia, hepatic and renal toxicity, shock
Paragonimiasis	*P. westermani*	Bithionol	50 mg/kg q.o.d. × 15 doses	PO	*Photosensitivity, urticaria, abdominal pain, vomiting,* and *diarrhea*

teus species, and some strains of Enterobacter. The minimal inhibitory concentrations for Pseudomonas are very high when compared to other drug susceptibilities (i.e., 75 to 100 μg per milliliter). However, carbenicillin is a relatively nontoxic agent which can be given in doses of 30 to 40 grams per day intravenously with serum levels of 200 to 400 μg per milliliter. One half this dose is usually adequate for *E. coli,* Proteus, and Enterobacter infections. Carbenicillin is principally excreted by the kidneys, and very high urine levels are present after 0.5 or 1.0 gram is given parenterally (1000 μg per milliliter of urine or more). Thus a dose of 4 to 6 grams per day is adequate for uncomplicated urinary tract infections. Since *Pseudomonas aeruginosa* may develop resistance during therapy, especially if the drug is given in suboptimal doses, carbenicillin should not be used alone in patients with severe infections, cystic fibrosis, or chronic urinary tract obstruction when prolonged therapy may be indicated. In addition, superinfection, especially with Klebsiella species and Serratia species, is not uncommon. An oral form of carbenicillin, the indanyl salt of the sodium ester, is indicated only in uncomplicated urinary tract infections caused by susceptible organisms. Whereas serum levels are low after 0.5 to 1.0 gram orally, urine levels are in excess of the minimal inhibitory concentration of susceptible gram-negative bacilli.

Penicillinase-Resistant Penicillins. The semisynthetic penicillins that resist penicillinase are methicillin, nafcillin, oxacillin, cloxacillin, and dicloxacillin. The principal indication for using these penicillins are infections caused by *Staphylococcus aureus* which produce penicillinase. These drugs are also active against group A streptococci and pneumococci. Cloxacillin and dicloxacillin are acid stable and are the preferred agents for oral therapy. Nafcillin is the only penicillinase-resistant penicillin excreted primarily by the liver, and the dose need not be significantly altered in patients with renal failure.

Adverse Reactions to the Penicillins. In general, severe adverse reactions to the penicillins are uncommon, and a wide range exists between therapeutic and toxic serum levels. Hypersensitivity reactions occur in 2 to 5 per cent of patients. These reactions may take two clinical forms: (1) immediate reactions, including anaphylaxis, accelerated urticaria, and angioneurotic edema; and (2) delayed reactions, which are more common and include delayed urticaria, morbilliform eruption, and serum sickness. Hypersensitivity reactions have been reported with all the penicillin derivatives. Patients allergic to one penicillin are allergic to all congeners. Drug fever is not uncommon. Coombs-positive hemolytic anemia may result from the formation of antibody to penicillin-coated red cells. This is most likely to occur when large parenteral doses are given over a long period of time. Central nervous system toxicity, characterized by myoclonus and generalized seizures, may be seen when high doses of parenteral penicillins are administered to patients especially with renal insufficiency. Hyperkalemia may be seen in patients with renal insufficiency, because the potassium salt of penicillin G has 1.6 mEq of K^+ per million units. Diarrhea is common in patients receiving oral ampicillin. Skin rashes have been reported to be more common in patients with infectious mononucleosis who receive oral ampicillin. Carbenicillin must be used with caution in patients in whom sodium restriction is important, because 1 gram of carbenicillin contains 4.7 mEq of sodium. Carbenicillin may cause elevated hepatic enzymes, neutropenia, and increased clotting and prothrombin times with bleeding in patients with renal insufficiency. Methicillin and, less commonly, penicillin G have been reported to cause interstitial nephritis and reversible azotemia. Bone marrow depression with anemia and leukopenia has also been associated with methicillin therapy.

Cephalosporins. Six cephalosporins are currently marketed in the United States: cephalothin, cephapirin, cefazolin, cephaloridine, cephaloglycin, and cephalexin. The cephalosporins are active against most organisms susceptible to the penicillins, i.e., group A streptococci, viridans streptococci, pneumococci, *Staphylococcus aureus,* and *C. diphtheriae.* Susceptible gram-negative bacilli include *Escherichia coli,* Klebsiella, and *Proteus mirabilis.* Enterobacter species, indole-positive Proteus strains and Pseudomonas species are resistant to the cephalosporins. Cephalothin, cephapirin, cefazolin, and cephaloridine are used parenterally, cephaloglycin and cephalexin, orally. *Cephalothin* is usually given intravenously, because intramuscular injections of greater than 0.5 gram are painful. Renal clearance is rapid, and the drug should be given every four hours. *Cephapirin* has antibacterial spectra and pharmacologic properties similar to cephalothin. *Cefazolin* has several pharmacologic advantages over cephalothin. Because of its low renal clearance and longer half-life, serum levels are two to three times higher and more sustained. Cefazolin may produce less thrombophlebitis than cephalothin and may be given intramuscularly. *Cephaloridine* should be given only by the parenteral route and must be avoided in patients with renal insufficiency. *Cephaloglycin,* the first available oral cephalosporin, is poorly absorbed and is indicated only for urinary tract infections when cephalexin is not available. *Cephalexin* is acid stable and well absorbed. Urine levels are within the therapeutic range after a 0.5 to 1.0 gram oral dose. Since the excretion of the cephalosporins is by tubular secretion, serum levels may be increased and prolonged with the simultaneous administration of probenecid. Since the cephalosporins do not achieve therapeutic levels in the cerebrospinal fluid, these agents should not be used in patients with bacterial meningitis.

Adverse reactions to the cephalosporins are relatively uncommon. The question of cross-allergenicity between the penicillins and the cephalosporins remains controversial. The incidence of cross-sensitization must be low, because cephalosporin compounds have been given successfully to many patients with prior penicillin reactions. However, the cephalosporins should probably not be administered to patients with a documented history of an immediate hypersensitivity reaction to penicillin. Thrombophlebitis is commonly seen with the intravenous use of large doses of cephalothin and cephapirin, and frequent changes of the intravenous site are necessary if these drugs have to be given over an extended period of time. A positive Coombs test without hemolysis may occur with large doses of cephalothin; leukopenia is rare and usually responds to discontinuing the drug. Cephaloridine is nephrotoxic, especially if the dose is greater than 4 grams per day or if patients are receiving ethacrynic acid or furosemide. Acute tubular necrosis has also been reported in patients receiving cephalothin and gentamicin. The specific role of either drug or the combination in this complication is unknown. Nausea and vomiting may accompany the administration of the oral cephalosporins. The presence of cephalexin in the urine may give a false positive test for glucose with Benedict's solution or Clinitest tablets.

Vancomycin. Vancomycin is active against penicillinase-producing *Staphylococcus aureus* and *S. epidermidis,* viridans streptococci, and enterococci. It is an important alternative drug in patients allergic to the penicillins and the cephalosporins who have severe staphylococcal infections or endocarditis caused by penicillin-resistant viridans streptococci and enterococci. Methicillin-resistant *Staphylococcus aureus* strains are usually resistant to the cephalosporins but sensitive to vancomycin. All gram-negative bacilli are resistant to this antimicrobial. Vancomycin can only be administered intravenously. Pain at the site of injection is frequent and thrombophlebitis common. Chills, fever, and urticaria may also accompany its administration. The more severe adverse reactions include reversible nephrotoxicity with albuminuria, casts, and azotemia, and ototoxicity with deafness when very high blood levels are achieved.

Erythromycin, Lincomycin, and Clindamycin. *Erythromycin* is one of two macrolide antimicrobials. It should be classified with lincomycin and clindamycin, because all three drugs have the same mechanism of action (inhibition of protein synthesis by binding the 50S ribosomal unit). The spectrum of activity of these drugs, with a few exceptions, is similar. Erythromycin is active against group A streptococci, pneumococci, and *Staphylococcus aureus. Mycoplasma pneumoniae* and *T. pallidum* are also susceptible to it. Erythromycin may be used in patients allergic to penicillin who have respiratory tract or soft tissue infections caused by pneumococci and group A streptococci, respectively. It may be used as the primary drug in *M. pneumoniae* infections. Erythromycin should not be used for serious *Staphylococcus aureus* infections. Local irritation at the site of parenteral administration is common, and gastrointestinal disturbance may be associated with oral therapy. Erythromycin estolate may produce reversible cholestatic hepatitis, and other preparations of erythromycin should be used. Hypersensitivity reactions, such as rash and eosinophilia, and drug fever are uncommon.

Triacetyloleandomycin is also a macrolide antimicrobial, but it is used infrequently because of adverse reactions.

Lincomycin and clindamycin (a chloro-derivative of lincomycin) are also active against group A streptococci, pneumococci, and penicillinase-producing staphylococci. Enterococci, gram-negative bacilli, and *Mycoplasma pneumoniae* are resistant. Many strains of *Staphylococcus aureus* resistant to erythromycin are also resistant to lincomycin and clindamycin. Staphylococci resistant to erythromycin but susceptible to lincomycin or clindamycin may rapidly develop resistance to the latter drugs during lincomycin-clindamycin therapy (dissociated cross-resistance). Clindamycin is well absorbed from the gastrointestinal tract and produces higher serum levels than oral lincomycin. Clindamycin is also more active against many anaerobes, especially *Bacteroides fragilis,* and has become the drug of choice in the initial therapy of severe anaerobic infections. Erythromycin crosses the blood-brain barrier, but lincomycin and clindamycin do not, and therefore the latter agents should not be used in bacterial meningitis. Gastrointestinal disturbances such as nausea, vomiting, abdominal cramps, and diarrhea occur with clindamycin and lincomycin. Pseudomembranous colitis has been observed with both drugs. Rapid intravenous administration may be associated with cardiopulmonary arrest. Reversible hepatocellular toxicity and bone marrow depression (leukopenia) have been reported after clindamycin therapy. Hypersensitivity reactions such as rash and generalized pruritus are rare.

Novobiocin. The antibacterial spectrum of novobiocin is similar to that of penicillin G and erythromycin; *Staphylococcus aureus* and pneumococci are susceptible to this antimicrobial. It is well absorbed from the gastrointestinal tract and may also be given intravenously. However, the high incidence of adverse reactions precludes the routine use of this drug, and it is rarely prescribed at present. Toxic reactions include gastrointestinal disturbances (nausea, vomiting, diarrhea, and bleeding), bone marrow depression (pancytopenia), hypersensitivity reactions (eosinophilia, rash, fever, angioedema, exudative erythema multiforme), alopecia, and yellow discoloration of the skin and sclera caused by a degradation product of the drug.

Bacitracin. Bacitracin is a polypeptide antimicrobial agent for topical use only. *Staphylococcus aureus, Staphylococcus epidermidis,* enterococci, viridans streptococci, and group A streptococci are susceptible to it. Gram-negative bacilli are resistant to bacitracin. The antibiotic is stable in ointments only when it is incorporated in petrolatum. Bacitracin is indicated in open superficial skin infections such as eczema, dermal ulcers, and minor wounds infected with drug-susceptible bacteria. Purulent conjunctivitis and infected corneal ulcers may also respond to topical bacitracin when caused by similar organisms. Furunculosis, impetigo, pyoderma, and subcutaneous abscesses should not be treated with topical bacitracin alone. Adverse reactions are rarely seen with this topical antibiotic.

Aminoglycosides. The four drugs that belong to this class of antimicrobial agents are streptomycin, neomycin, kanamycin, and gentamicin. *Streptomycin,* one of the first aminoglycosides available for parenteral administration, was widely used in the 1940's and 1950's, because *Mycobacterium tuberculosis* and gram-negative bacilli, especially *Escherichia coli,* Klebsiella-Enterobacter species, and Proteus strains were susceptible. However, with the development of other drugs for these infections and because adverse reactions, notably vestibular toxicity, are a risk, the use of intramuscular streptomycin is now limited to a few specific diseases. Most strains of enterococci are resistant to streptomycin in vitro. Nevertheless, streptomycin in combination with penicillin or vancomycin is the therapy of choice in patients with penicillin-resistant viridans streptococcal and enterococcal endocarditis. These drug combinations should also be used for prophylaxis against enterococcal bacteremia in patients with underlying congenital or valvular heart disease who have urogenital or gastrointestinal manipulation. Streptomycin has substantial activity against *M. tuberculosis,* and the indications for its use in this disease are discussed in Ch. 228. Streptomycin may also be used in the therapy of plague, tularemia, and brucellosis. *Neomycin,* also discovered in the 1940's, has limited clinical application because of nephrotoxicity and neurotoxicity. The drug is poorly absorbed from the gastrointestinal tract and is therefore useful in patients with severe hepatic disease with impending or frank coma, inhibiting bacterial growth in the intestinal tract and reducing absorption of nitrogenous compounds. Unfortunately, neomycin is widely used in topical antimicrobial preparations, many of which are available without a prescription. There is no evidence from controlled studies that neomycin is effective in healing or preventing skin infections. Indeed, topical neomycin frequently causes contact dermatitis. Injudicious use of neomycin in patients with extensive wounds or burns or instillation into body cavities may result in absorption of the drug and life-threatening adverse reactions.

Kanamycin is closely related to neomycin but is less toxic. It is active against most gram-negative bacilli, including *E. coli,* Klebsiella-Enterobacter species, and Proteus species. The antibiotic is also active in vitro against Shigella, *Staphylococcus aureus,* and *M. tuberculosis,* but is not indicated for clinical use in these infections, because less toxic agents are available. *Pseudomonas aeruginosa* strains are universally resistant to kanamycin. Ampicillin plus kanamycin has been the initial therapy of choice in suspected neonatal sepsis. However, if it is known that kanamycin-resistant gram-negative organisms have been isolated from the nursery, ampicillin plus gentamicin is recommended.

Gentamicin is widely used for serious gram-negative bacillary infections. It is active against Pseudomonas species as well as *E. coli,* Klebsiella-Enterobacter species, and Proteus species. *Staphylococcus aureus* strains are also susceptible to gentamicin; however, less toxic antistaphylococcal agents are available, and gentamicin should not be used for this purpose. Gentamicin may be given by either the intramuscular or the intravenous route. Therapeutic levels in the cerebrospinal fluid are usually not achieved with parenteral administration, and intrathecal injections are indicated in patients with gram-negative bacillary meningitis. In patients with urinary tract infections, the urine should be alkaline for maximal antimicrobial activity. Carbenicillin when mixed with gentamicin in the same solution will inactivate the latter drug over a prolonged period of time.

Adverse reactions are commonly seen with administration of the aminoglycosides. These agents are excreted principally by the kidneys and should be avoided or the dose adjusted in patients with compromised renal function. Furthermore, the therapeutic serum level often approximates the toxic level, and adverse reactions may be unavoidable in patients with life-threatening infections. Since gentamicin has such a wide spectrum of activity against aerobic gram-negative bacilli, it is often used in conjunction with a penicillinase-resistant penicillin or a cephalosporin for the initial therapy in patients with malignancies or who are on immunosuppressive or cytotoxic agents. If the infecting organism proves to be susceptible to a less toxic drug, gentamicin should be discontinued and that agent instituted for the remainder of the patient's therapy. The aminoglycosides should never be injected into body cavities or given rapidly by vein, because neuromuscular blockade with respiratory arrest may ensue. This curare-like effect may be reversed with neostigmine or calcium gluconate. All the aminoglycosides are nephrotoxic and neurotoxic. Neomycin and kanamycin cause auditory toxicity with deafness. Deafness is more commonly seen in patients with renal insufficiency or in patients receiving ethacrynic acid or furosemide. Streptomycin and gentamicin usually cause vestibular damage which may be irreversible. Occasionally deafness may also occur. During long-term therapy, patients must be closely followed with daily tandem-walking and weekly caloric reactions and audiograms. Paresthesias, peripheral neuropathy, and optic neuritis are rarely observed. Hypersensitivity reactions have been reported with each of the aminoglycosides.

Polymyxins. Polymyxin B and polymyxin E are polypeptide antimicrobials that are active against *E. coli,* Klebsiella-Enterobacter species, and Pseudomonas species. Proteus species are resistant to these drugs. Polymyxin B is given parenterally and may also be administered intrathecally. The polymyxins do not cross the blood-brain barrier and must be given both parenterally and intrathecally in patients with gram-negative bacillary meningitis. Polymyxin E has two forms, parenteral colistimethate sodium and oral colistin sulfate, a nonabsorbable antimicrobial. Although active in vitro against many species of gram-negative bacilli, polymyxin is most useful in the therapy of *Pseudomonas aeruginosa* infections. Since the polymyxins are excreted by the kidneys, caution must be used when these agents are given to patients with renal insufficiency. Serious adverse reactions are dose related. Neurotoxic reactions include circumoral or fingertip paresthesias that are usually reversible. Ataxia, slurred speech, and blurred vision are uncommon. Respiratory paralysis may occur with rapid intravenous administration or in patients receiving succinylcholine and may be reversed by intravenous calcium gluconate but not neostigmine. Azotemia and impaired renal function are seen with high doses. Hypersensitivity reactions have been reported and include eosinophilia and rash.

Spectinomycin. Spectinomycin is active against *Neisseria gonorrhoeae* and has been approved only for use in uncomplicated gonorrhea. The drug does not have treponemicidal activity. It should be considered for use in patients with gonococcal urethritis and cervicitis who are allergic to penicillin, because it can be given as a single dose intramuscularly. There is no cross-resistance between spectinomycin and penicillin. Although spectinomycin inhibits protein synthesis by binding 30S ribosomal subunits (similar to the aminoglycosides), adverse reactions, except for fever and urticaria, have been uncommon to date.

Chloramphenicol. Chloramphenicol has a broad spectrum of activity against the rickettsiae, gram-positive bacteria, gram-negative bacteria, including Salmonella and Shigella, and anaerobic bacteria. The drug is well absorbed from the gastrointestinal tract. It is metabolized by the liver and can therefore be used in patients with renal insufficiency. Adequate levels in the cerebrospinal fluid are present after intravenous injection. Chloramphenicol causes bone marrow aplasia and fatal pancytopenia in 1 of every 40,000 or more courses of therapy or 1 of 25,000 to 50,000 people exposed. This severe toxic reaction is a form of hypersensitivity or idiosyncratic reaction which cannot be predicted before therapy. For this reason, chloramphenicol should be used only for certain specific, severe infections. These indications include (1) typhoid fever or other Salmonella infections, (2) as an alternative drug for ampicillin in *Hemophilus influenzae,* pneumococcal, and meningococcal meningitis, (3) severe anaerobic infections for which clindamycin is not effective, (4) gram-negative bacillary infections that do not respond to other antimicrobial agents, and (5) severe rickettsial infections when tetracycline is not effective.

Anemia which is dose related and not a hypersensitivity reaction may occur with prolonged use. This form of bone marrow depression is reversible and is characterized by interference with iron metabolism, with increased serum iron and saturation of iron-binding globulin, decreased reticulocyte count, and vacuolization of red cell precursors. Patients receiving chloramphenicol must have repeated complete blood counts and serum iron and saturation determinations. This type of anemia is most commonly seen in patients with liver disease or renal insufficiency and in those receiving high doses. Fatal toxicity may develop in neonates ("gray baby syndrome"). Optic neuritis and peripheral neuropathy are rarely seen with prolonged therapy. Hypersensitivity reactions have been reported.

Tetracyclines. The tetracyclines have a broad spectrum of activity. Rickettsia, Chlamydia, *Mycoplasma pneumoniae,* gram-positive and gram-negative bacteria, certain anaerobic organisms, and *T. pallidum* are susceptible to the tetracyclines. At present, 25 to 50 per cent of group A streptococci, 5 to 10 per cent of pneumococci, and most *Staphylococcus aureus* isolates are resistant. In addition, many aerobic gram-negative bacilli and Bacteroides species are also resistant. These changing susceptibility patterns since the introduction of tetracycline in the 1940s have made it necessary to restrict the use of these drugs to the following indications: (1) Rickettsia infections; (2) *M. pneumoniae* infections; (3) Chlamydia infections, including psittacosis, trachoma, lymphogranuloma venereum, and nongonococcal urethritis; (4) granuloma inguinale and chancroid; (5) alternative therapy for gonorrhea and syphilis; and (6) urinary tract infections caused by susceptible gram-negative bacilli.

Tetracycline has replaced *chlortetracycline* and *oxytetracycline* as the agent of choice. It may be given orally or intravenously, although thrombophlebitis often accompanies the latter route of administration. Tetracycline should be avoided in patients with renal insufficiency. Four long-acting tetracyclines are available: *demethylchlortetracycline, methacycline, doxycycline,* and *minocycline.* The rate of renal excretion of these agents is less and oral absorption greater than those of tetracycline, resulting in prolonged serum levels. Minor variations in the degree of antibacterial activity exist among the four preparations which are reflected in the amount of drug recommended per dose. Doxycycline does not accumulate in the serum of patients with renal insufficiency and may be advantageous when the status of renal function is unknown. However, because of the low renal clearance of both doxycycline and minocycline, their usefulness in urinary tract infections may be limited by low urinary concentrations. Unlike the other tetracyclines, minocycline decreases nasopharyngeal carriage of meningococci and may therefore be indicated in prophylaxis of infection caused by sulfadiazine-resistant meningococci. With few exceptions all the tetracycline compounds produce the same adverse reactions. These include gastrointestinal disturbances such as nausea, vomiting, and diarrhea, thrombophlebitis with intravenous administration, staining and hypoplasia of dental enamel and disturbed bone growth in neonates and young children, pseudotumor cerebri with bulging fontanelles and increased cerebrospinal fluid pressure in infants, and acute fatty degeneration of the liver in pregnant women and patients with renal insufficiency. Photosensitivity reactions are not infrequently seen with the long-acting tetracyclines. A variant of the Fanconi syndrome caused by toxic products may occur with administration of outdated tetracycline preparations. Superinfections with resistant gram-negative bacilli, *Staphylococcus aureus,* and Candida may occur with prolonged therapy.

Sulfonamides. For four decades, sulfonamides have been widely prescribed for a variety of clinical infections. However, their present use is limited because of resistance of gram-positive and gram-negative organisms, the availability of more active antimicrobial agents, and adverse reactions. The major indications are (1) nocardiosis; (2) suppressive therapy for paracoccidioidomycosis; (3) prophylaxis in sulfadiazine-sensitive meningococcal infections; (4) alternative prophylaxis for acute rheumatic fever in patients allergic to penicillin; (5) uncomplicated urinary tract infections caused by susceptible organisms, especially *E. coli;* (6) salicylazosulfapyridine therapy in patients with mild ulcerative colitis; (7) certain protozoal infections (toxoplasmosis, *Pneumocystis carinii,* and chloroquine-resistant P. falciparum malaria); and (8) when administered in combination with antifolate compounds, chronic urinary tract infections and possibly also typhoid fever.

Sulfisoxazole is well absorbed from the gastrointestinal tract and may also be administered parenterally if necessary. The drug is chiefly excreted by glomerular filtration and thus is not affected by probenecid. *Sulfamethoxazole* is a congener of sulfisoxazole, but is absorbed less and the renal excretion is delayed. The more potent *sulfadiazine,* once widely used, is less soluble and tends to cause crystalluria. The incidence of crystalluria is decreased by increasing fluid intake and maintaining an alkaline urine. Long-acting sulfonamides, such as *sulfamethoxypyridazine* and *sulfadimethoxine,* although widely used in the past, have no place in clinical antimicrobial therapy because of their toxic effects. The poorly absorbed sulfonamides, *succinylsulfathiazole* and *phthalylsulfathiazole,* are principally used to decrease bacterial counts in the intestine prior to surgery. These agents are of doubtful value. *Salicylazosulfapyridine* may decrease the severity of disease in patients with mild ulcerative colitis. This effect may be due to the antibacterial action of sulfapyridine or the anti-inflammatory effect of 5-aminosalicylic acid.

Adverse reactions caused by the sulfonamides include the following: hypersensitivity reactions with fever, rash, photosensitivity, and rarely vasculitis; nephrotoxicity with crystalluria and renal tubular necrosis; kernicterus in the newborn; hepatitis (occasionally with noncaseating granuloma); agranulocytosis and aplastic anemia; and acute hemolytic anemia in patients with G-6-PD deficiency. Long-acting sulfonamides may cause Stevens-Johnson syndrome and myocarditis.

Trimethoprim-Sulfamethoxazole. This drug combination sequentially inhibits the utilization of para-aminobenzoic acid by bacteria in the synthesis of folic acid. A double sequential blockage is thus produced, and relatively low concentrations of each drug are required for antimicrobial activity. At present, the drug combination (trimethoprim, 80 mg; sulfamethoxazole, 400 mg), has been approved in the United States only for chronic urinary tract infections. Clinical trials suggest that it may be useful in patients with bronchitis, gonorrhea, and possibly typhoid fever resistant to both chloramphenicol and ampicillin. Adverse reactions are the same as those described for the sulfonamides, including the Stevens-Johnson syndrome, and trimethoprim, including nausea, vomiting, skin rashes, and macrocytic anemia caused by folic acid deficiency. Serious nephrotoxicity has been reported in patients with diminished renal function.

Nitrofurantoin. Nitrofurantoin is an oral antibacterial agent that is excreted in the urine by both glomerular filtration and tubular secretion. The drug is most active against *E. coli,* Klebsiella-Enterobacter species, and some strains of enterococci. The susceptibility of Proteus strains is variable, and Pseudomonas species are resistant. Nitrofurantoin should be used only for uncomplicated urinary tract infections or suppressive therapy in patients with chronic urinary tract infections. The drug is most active in the presence of an acid urine, and emergent resistance has not been noted. It should not be prescribed in pregnant women, because it crosses the placenta, or in patients with renal insufficiency. Adverse reactions include nausea and vomiting, hypersensitivity reactions (fever, rash, allergic pneumonitis), paresthesias which may progress to severe polyneuropathy if the drug is not discontinued, acute hemolytic anemia in patients with G-6-PD deficiency, and cholestatic hepatitis.

Nalidixic Acid. Nalidixic acid is also an oral antimicrobial agent used in the therapy of uncomplicated urinary tract infections. The drug is active against strains of *E. coli,* Klebsiella-Enterobacter species, and Proteus species; Pseudomonas species are resistant. Gram-negative bacilli may rapidly develop resistance to this agent, and repeated urine cultures with drug-susceptibility determinations should be performed during therapy. Adverse reactions include nausea, vomiting, hypersensitivity reactions (rash, eosinophilia, photosensitivity), and rarely cholestatic jaundice, blood dyscrasias, visual disturbances, toxic psychosis, and convulsive seizures. Severe headache associated with papilledema has been observed in children.

Methenamine Mandelate and Hippurate. These antimicrobial compounds are the salts of methenamine and mandelic acid and hippuric acid, respectively. They are well absorbed from the gastrointestinal tract and rapidly excreted in the urine. They are bactericidal in acidic urine (pH less than 5.5). An acidifying agent is necessary if the infecting organism forms ammonia. Methenamine mandelate or hippurate may be used for chronic suppression of urinary tract infections. *Escherichia coli* is susceptible to these drugs. Proteus species and Pseudomonas species are usually resistant. Adverse reactions are uncommon and include epigastric pain, dysuria, crystalluria, and metabolic acidosis, especially in patients with renal insufficiency.

FAILURE OF ANTIMICROBIAL THERAPY

The failure of a patient to respond to antimicrobial therapy may be due to factors related to the host and the nature of the disease or to an error in the choice, dosage, or route of administration of the drug. The following causes are most common: (1) incorrect diagnosis; (2) impaired host defense mechanisms; (3) inadequate dose, route of administration, or distribution of drug; (4) closed space infection; (5) presence of a foreign body; (6) superinfection; and (7) microbial drug resistance.

Resistance of microorganisms to antimicrobial agents may be classified as primary (natural) or emergent (acquired) (see Ch. 267). Microorganisms acquire resistance by either mutation or episomal transfer. Mutation patterns may be multi-step, involving a number of genes, or large-step, involving one gene. The efficiency of mutation is increased in the presence of low-dose antimicrobial drug administration. Both gram-positive and gram-negative bacteria develop resistance by mutation. Recognition of episomal transfer of resistance is presently restricted to gram-negative bacilli and *Staphylococcus aureus.* The transfer of cytoplasmic DNA (R factor) requires cell-to-cell contact and is termed conjugation. The transfer of resistance may be single or multiple, and occurs most commonly in the gastrointestinal tract. It is often designated infectious drug resistance.

CHEMOPROPHYLAXIS

Antimicrobial agents are often administered to individuals who are believed to be at some increased risk of acquiring a bacterial infection.

Prophylaxis is usually successful only when a single drug is given for a specific organism. The antimicrobial drugs and their clinical indications which are considered to be of value are summarized in Table 3. Antimicrobial prophylaxis is not effective in viral respiratory diseases, viral exanthems, clean abdominal surgery, and congestive heart failure. Unlike the therapeutic situation in which the identity of the offending microbe might be in doubt and there is urgency in selecting therapy, with chemoprophylaxis there is usually no urgency, and the microbe in question is known. Consequently, the use of antimicrobial drugs in chemoprophylaxis should be more rational than in therapy. Unfortunately, this is not always the case, and in many instances the prophylactic use of antimicrobial agents is unwarranted, ineffective, and often dangerous because of toxic reactions, superinfection, and emergent resistance. The matter of drug toxicity requires comment. Selection of a drug is a matter of

TABLE 3. Recommendations for Antimicrobial Prophylaxis

Disease or Clinical Setting	Etiologic Agent	Antimicrobial Drug
Acute rheumatic fever (recurrent)	Group A streptococcus	Penicillin, erythromycin, sulfonamide
Meningococcal infections	*Neisseria meningitidis*	
	Sulfonamide-susceptible	Sulfisoxazole
	Sulfonamide-resistant	Minocycline
Microbial endocarditis		
Oral cavity instrumentation	Viridans streptococcus	Penicillin, cephalosporin
Urogenital and gastrointestinal instrumentation	Enterococcus	Penicillin or vancomycin plus streptomycin
Open heart surgery	*Staphylococcus aureus* and *epidermidis*	Penicillinase-resistant penicillin, cephalosporin
Newborn nursery epidemics	Enteropathic *E. coli*	Neomycin, Colistin
	Staphylococcus aureus	Penicillinase-resistant penicillin
	Group A streptococci	Penicillin
Tuberculin reactors of certain sorts	*Mycobacterium tuberculosis*	Isoniazid
Malaria	Plasmodia	
	Chloroquine-susceptible	Chloroquine followed by primaquine
	Chloroquine-resistant (*P. falciparum*)	Chloroguanide and sulfone
Ophthalmia neonatorum	*Neisseria gonorrhoeae*	Silver nitrate, penicillin
Burns		Silver sulfadiazine, silver nitrate
Bronchitis (chronic)	Pneumococcus or *Hemophilus influenzae*	Ampicillin, tetracycline

weighing offsetting risks. It is easy to forget that a degree of drug toxicity that is acceptable when weighed against an instance of a particular disease may be unacceptable when weighed against the chance that someone *might* acquire that disease. Finally, although one must emphasize the need for caution in chemoprophylaxis, it is fitting to remember that in terms of the number of people benefited, the use of the drugs in this way represents one of the greatest achievements of modern biomedical science and technology.

Gavin, T. L., et al.: Antimicrobial Susceptibility Testing. American Society of Clinical Pathologists, 1971.
Goodman, L. S., and Gilman, A.: The Pharmacological Basis of Therapeutics. 4th ed. New York, Macmillan, 1970.
Handbook of Antimicrobial Therapy. The Medical Letter on Drugs and Therapeutics (revised ed.), 1974.
Kunin, C. M., et al.: Use of antibiotics. A brief exposition of the problem and some tentative solutions. Ann. Intern. Med., 79:555, 1973.
Pratt, W. B.: Fundamentals of Chemotherapy. New York, Oxford University Press, 1973.
Weinstein, L., and Dalton, A. C.: Host determinants of response to antimicrobial agents. N. Engl. J. Med., 279:467, 1968.

Part IX
PROTOZOAN AND HELMINTHIC DISEASES

269. INTRODUCTION

Philip D. Marsden

With rapid air travel, so-called parasitic infections are becoming more important in temperate climes. They have always been important in the tropics.

Parasitic disease is usually taken to imply infections caused by protozoa and helminths, although, in their relationship to the host, bacteria, viruses, and rickettsiae equally fulfill the general criteria used to describe an organism as parasitic. The reason for this nomenclature is historic; because they are bigger organisms, helminths and protozoa were discovered relatively early by medical investigators. Ascaris and tapeworms are dramatic enough to have been recognized in ancient times, and protozoa were seen with the first crude microscopes.

For the correct diagnosis of parasitic disease the physician must be as competent at the microscope and in using the laboratory procedures to find parasites as he is at defining the clinical presentation at the bedside and interpreting it. As with other infectious diseases, a firm diagnosis rests on finding the infectious agent. Recently serologic tests have been used much more to aid diagnosis, and, interpreted wisely, they are valuable. Broadly speaking, they mean that a patient has developed antibodies of a certain type to a parasitic antigen. Rarely do they give any confirmation about the status of the parasite in the body of man in terms of numbers present or whether they are multiplying. Positive serologic findings should often be an indication for redoubling one's efforts to find the parasite.

Whether a complement fixation test, hemagglutination test, fluorescent antibody test, or gel diffusion test is positive at a significant titer must be decided in the light of known facts about the specificity of the tests.

Many of the drugs used are toxic to man but more toxic to the parasites. We know little of the mechanism of drug action in many cases, e.g., Pentostam in leishmaniasis. With some drugs such as heavy metal containing compounds and emetine the toxic dose for man is near the therapeutic dose. Physicians should be especially careful to check their prescriptions of these drugs, especially if they are not used to prescribing them often.

The National Communicable Disease Center, Atlanta, Georgia, offers unique services to the physician in the United States for the management of parasitic disease. Not only is there a laboratory for diagnostic serology, but recently a number of rare drugs previously not available in the United States and mentioned in this book have become available through the Parasitic Disease Drug Service in the Epidemiology Program. These include drugs for the treatment of both types of human trypanosomiasis, leishmaniasis, amebiasis, pneumocystis infection, and schistosomiasis.

With regard to diagnostic serology, Dr. Irving G. Kagan has kindly provided the accompanying table of serologic tests available for parasitic diseases in the United States.

Immunodiagnostic Tests for Parasitic Infections

	Complement Fixation	Precipitin	Particle Agglutination Tests: *Bentonite Flocculation*	*Hemagglutination*	*Latex Agglutination*	*Cholesterol Flocculation*	Fluorescent Antibody	Methylene Blue Dye
Trichinosis	+	+	+*	±*	+*	+*	+*	
Echinococcosis	+	+	+*	+*	+*		+	
Schistosomiasis	+*		±*	±*		+*	+*	
Ascariasis/toxocariasis			+*	+*			0	
Filariasis	±		+*	+*	0		0	
Cysticercosis	+	0		+*			0	
Chagas' disease	+*	±	0	+*	0		0*	
Leishmaniasis	+			+*			0	
Toxoplasmosis	+*			+*	0		+*	+*
Amebiasis	+*	+	±*	+*	±		±*	
Malaria				±*			+*	

* = Tests available in the U.S.
0 = Under experimental investigation.
± = Used for diagnosis, but requires further evaluation for routine use.
+ = Generally accepted useful routine diagnostic test.
Adapted from data supplied by Dr. Irving Kagan, Center for Disease Control.

Section One. PROTOZOAN DISEASES

270. INTRODUCTION

Philip D. Marsden

Malaria remains the greatest challenge in parasitic disease both in terms of prevalence (over 500 million people still live in malarious areas) and in the amount of morbidity and mortality it causes. In many tropical countries, notably Africa, malaria has a profound influence on the pattern of clinical medicine.

Trypanosomiasis is a good example of geographically restricted disease. *Trypanosoma brucei* infections are restricted to Africa because tsetse flies (Glossina species) are not found elsewhere. African sleeping sickness demands attention because human infections once established are so frequently fatal. Also, this same group of trypanosomes are responsible for widespread fatal disease in cattle, profoundly influencing animal husbandry. South American trypanosomiasis (Chagas' disease) is restricted to the Americas because again the great majority of reduviid bugs occur in this location. The significance of this infection as a public health problem is a matter of current concern. One estimate suggests that 7 million people are infected and 30 million exposed to the risk of infection. Permanent cardiac damage often ensues, and at the time of writing there is no cure.

Also in the family Trypanosomatidae, the genus *Leishmania* is responsible for considerable human suffering. Visceral leishmaniasis is a debilitating infection, and without treatment the terminal event is usually a secondary bacterial infection, often a pneumonia. Cutaneous and mucocutaneous leishmaniasis can be disfiguring infections. Therapy is far from satisfactory.

Amebiasis ranks fourth in this consideration, because, although bowel infections are widely prevalent, invasive disease is less common. Then come a miscellany of rarer protozoal disease entities.

The reader will appreciate that the first three groups of diseases caused by protozoa all have arthropod vectors: Anopheles for malaria, Glossina and Reduviidae for trypanosomiasis, and Phlebotomus for leishmaniasis. It is relevant and important for medical men to have some knowledge of these vectors. A few examples of why this is so will suffice. At the time of writing there have been a few cases of indigenous vivax malaria recognized in the United States. Epidemiologic work has revealed vector Anopheles in the area. Xenodiagnosis using clean Reduviidae is the best way of finding *Trypanosoma cruzi* parasites in a patient with a chronic infection, and because of this these insects are most important, as they are used in diagnostic medicine. Phlebotomus remains very susceptible to DDT, and spraying of this insect's habitats will result in the control of human leishmaniasis.

Another medical consideration worth emphasizing is that blood protozoa can be transmitted by blood transfusion. Particularly important in this respect are malaria and *Trypanosoma cruzi* infections. Suitable selection of donors in temperate countries is necessary to avoid this complication in nonimmune persons exposed to the risk of malaria parasites in transfused blood. *Trypanosoma cruzi* infections transmitted by blood transfusion are said to be particularly acute. It is of interest that recent advances in immunology enable us to screen blood donors for malaria with the indirect fluorescent antibody test, whereas for *Trypanosoma cruzi* the valuable complement-fixation test or an indirect fluorescent antibody test is available.

Belding, D. L.: Textbook of Parasitology. 3rd ed. New York, Appleton-Century-Crofts, Inc., 1965.

Faust, E. C., and Russell, P. F.: Clinical Parasitology. 8th ed. Philadelphia, Lea & Febiger, 1970.

Hunter, G. W., Frye, W. W., and Swartzwelder, J. C.: A Manual of Tropical Medicine. 4th ed. Philadelphia, W. B. Saunders Company, 1966.

Wilcocks, C., and Manson-Bahr, P. E. C.: Manson's Tropical Diseases. 17th ed. Baltimore, Williams & Wilkins Company, 1972.

271. MALARIA

Thomas C. Jones

General Considerations. Malaria is characterized by shaking chills, relapsing fever, prostration, splenomegaly, and anemia. After the initial illness, the disease may follow a chronic or relapsing course. It is caused by four species of the genus Plasmodium (*P. vivax, P. falciparum, P. malariae,* and *P. ovale*). The infection is maintained in nature by the feeding habits of female mosquitoes of the genus Anopheles, in which sporogony occurs, feeding on blood of humans, in which schizogony and gametocytogony occur. Malaria remains a common cause of morbidity and mortality in the world. Delay in diagnosis or inappropriate therapy may lead to severe complications which include coma, acute renal failure, severe anemia, pulmonary edema, or shock. Recognition of the association between malaria and hemoglobinopathies, persistent hypergammaglobulinemia, Burkitt's lymphoma, and the tropical splenomegaly syndrome has emphasized the often subtle but significant influence of malaria on populations living in endemic areas.

History. The term malaria originated in the seventeenth century in Italy where the death of patients after intermittent or so-called Roman fevers was attributed to the bad air (mal'aria) of the marsh and swamp lands. These fevers were recognized in ancient times in China, India, and Mesopotamia, but the earliest record of quotidian, tertian, and quartan fevers was that of Hippocrates in the fifth century B.C. The Greeks and Romans were aware of the association of these fevers with marsh lands and conducted one of the earliest public health campaigns by draining the stagnant water. Cinchona bark was recognized as being effective against fevers in 1600 in Peru, after which it was widely used in Europe. Torti, in 1712, clearly distinguished the fevers that responded to cinchona from those that did not.

The protozoan was first described in the blood of a patient by Charles Laveran in 1880, who observed the parasite in an unstained smear of fresh blood. In 1891 Romanowsky developed a technique for staining blood smears for accurate study of the erythrocytic stage of malaria. In 1897, William MacCallum observed penetration and fertilization of the female gamete, documenting that a sexual cycle occurred in malaria. The role of the mosquito as a vector in malaria was postulated by Sir Patrick Manson after he documented that filaria could develop in the mosquito. Theobald Smith showed a few years later that an insect vector (the tick) could actually transmit disease among cattle. The careful studies of Sir Ronald Ross in 1898 documented that in avian malaria the protozoan developed in the stomach of infected mosquitoes and migrated to the salivary glands, from which it could infect healthy birds. Several months later Bignami, Bastianelli, and Grassi documented the transmission of malaria to man by Anopheles mosquitoes. Our present knowledge of the malaria cycle was completed in 1948 when Shortt, Garnham, Bray, and others confirmed the presence of the pre-erythrocytic stage in man.

A decrease in the prevalence of malaria during this century has resulted from campaigns to control mosquitoes and the widespread use of drug therapy directed against malaria. The systematic approach to mosquito control organized by Col. William Gorgas in the Canal Zone in 1906 was one of the outstanding achievements in preventive medical sciences. Effective insecticides were first introduced in 1939, and a number of synthetic antimalarial drugs were developed. The global program of malaria eradication was instituted during the 1950's with impressive results. It has become clear recently that various technical and socioeconomic problems in some countries have required that careful methods of malaria control be substituted for attempts at eradication of the disease.

Epidemiology. Malaria is an endemic disease in parts of Africa, Asia, and Central and South America, where environmental factors, including temperature, humidity, and standing water, support the breeding of mosquitoes and where there is close contact between the mosquitoes and man. The disease in these areas contributes to a high infant mortality and syndromes of chronic malaria. The prevalence of malaria in endemic areas is usually determined by documenting the proportion of people with large spleens (spleen rate) or the proportion of people with blood smears positive for malaria parasites (parasite rate). It has been estimated that 100 million cases of malaria occur each year. Approximately 1 per cent of these patients die of the disease, although this figure can vary from less than 1 per cent to over 10 per cent, depending on the species of Plasmodium most prevalent, the level of immunity of the host, and the availability of prompt medical care.

Acute disease caused by malaria often occurs when nonimmune persons enter endemic areas. Through the centuries the most impressive effects of malaria have been recorded during time of war when large numbers of nonimmunes are placed in malarious areas. This has certainly been the major factor contributing to the incidence of malaria in American citizens in the past 35 years. The number of cases of malaria in the United States rose from less than 100 in 1960 to 4000 in 1970 as a direct result of the exposure of nonimmune military personnel to the disease in Vietnam.

Epidemics of malaria may occur when the parasite is introduced into a region with a large nonimmune population. This occurred in the Soviet Union after World War I when more than 5 million cases were reported in 1923; and in Ethiopia in 1958 when 3 million cases and 150,000 deaths caused by malaria were reported. Such epidemics are reminders of the potential threat to localities where effective malaria eradication has created a large nonimmune population but where mosquito vectors persist in large numbers. Vectors for transmission of plasmodia, primarily *A. quadrimaculatus* and *A. freeborni,* persist in parts of the United States. Since 1963, 14 cases of malaria have been documented in which infection occurred within the United States.

Falciparum and vivax malaria are widely spread throughout the tropics and subtropics, particularly in hot, humid regions. Malariae malaria is also widespread, but it is of lower prevalence, and it tends to be less evenly distributed. Ovale malaria is primarily seen in West Africa.

During the past decade malaria has been found to be associated geographically with several other conditions, including various erythrocyte abnormalities and Burkitt's lymphoma. Patients with sickle hemoglobin have been shown to acquire falciparum malaria as frequently as those with normal hemoglobin, but their disease is less severe. The malaria parasite appears less able to divide in these abnormal erythrocytes. Other hemoglobinopathies and inherited enzyme defects, including hemoglobin C, D, E, K, O, b-thalassemia, and glucose-6-phosphate dehydrogenase deficiency, have also been shown to occur more commonly in areas endemic for malaria. These defects appear to provide some selective advantage for survival in malarious areas, and their high frequency is a good example of the concept in population genetics of balanced polymorphism. Correlation of the prevalence of Burkitt's lymphoma with prevalence of malaria has led to suggestions that chronic malaria suppresses mechanisms for immunologic surveillance, leading to expression of this tumor. Some work in laboratory animals chronically infected with malaria supports this view, but the relationship needs further clarification.

The epidemiology of malaria is inseparable from the epidemiology of its mosquito vectors. Entomologists must document different and changing characteristics of the numerous species of anopheline mosquitoes, including their flying and resting habits, feeding habits, and degree of resistance to insecticides. For example, a recent change in mosquito living habits from domestic to sylvatic in Central America has rendered the usual technique of household DDT residual spraying less effective. Several instances have been recorded in which mosquito feeding habits changed from cattle to man, resulting in epidemic malaria.

Although the mosquito is the primary vector for malaria, direct transfer of infected erythrocytes from one individual to another by blood transfusion or syringe usage in common by addicts will cause malaria. In these cases the sexual cycle in the mosquito and the pre-erythrocytic stages of malaria in man are bypassed. In the past 15 years 45 cases of malaria transmitted by transfusions were reported in the United States. The American Association of Blood Banks has recommended that blood not be taken from anyone who has emigrated from an endemic area or had malaria during the preceding three years, or who has visited a malarious area during which antimalarial prophylaxis was taken in the preceding two years. Travelers to malarial areas who remained symptom free and who did not take antimalarials may donate blood after six months. An epidemic of vivax malaria (which affected 47 persons) was reported from California after the sharing of heroin injection equipment by drug addicts. One of the members of the group had just returned from Vietnam. In the past, malaria was transmitted intentionally by physicians as a method of causing fever in patients for treatment of neurosyphilis and other diseases. Congenitally acquired malaria has rarely been reported. Transmission of malaria of monkeys, *P. knowlesi* and *P. cynomolgi,* from monkey to man has been demonstrated in the laboratory and rarely documented in nature.

The major thrust against malaria has been the worldwide cooperative program of malaria eradication begun approximately 20 years ago. The program was a unified approach divided into four carefully defined phases: preparatory, attack, consolidation, and maintenance. The techniques included concentrated spraying with residual insecticides, use of antimalarial drugs, and case-detection surveys. Recently, a number of problems have challenged the completion of malaria eradication using these techniques: inadequate finances in some regions; social disorganization during war and natural disaster; resistance of mosquitoes to insecticides; resistance of plasmodia to antimalarial drugs; and the demonstration that the malaria of monkeys can be transmitted to man.

Realization of these limitations has led to programs concentrating on malaria control rather than eradication. Perhaps related to this, there has been an increased interest in malaria immunity, both to define mechanisms of natural or acquired resistance and to develop potentially useful vaccines.

The Protozoan. Over 100 different species of Plasmodium are capable of infecting the red blood cells of mammals, birds, and reptiles. There are several hundred species of Anopheles mosquitoes which can be infected by the protozoan and therefore transmit the disease. Male anopheline mosquitoes feed on nectar and therefore do not transmit the infection. The female requires products of a blood meal for egg production. Female mosquitoes vary in their feeding habits so that only 50 species participate in transmission of human malaria. During the process of feeding, the mosquito injects fluid from the salivary glands. Sporozoites may be released with the salivary fluid if the mosquito ate a blood meal two to four weeks previously which contained male and female malaria gametocytes (Fig. 1).

The sporozoites enter the circulation immediately, and a transient parasitemia occurs which lasts less than one hour. During this period the sporozoites enter hepatic parenchymal cells, initiating the *pre-erythrocytic* stage of plasmodium infection by forming a primary hepatic schizont. The duration of this pre-erythrocytic stage is usually short in *P. falciparum* (5.5 to 7 days) and *P. vivax* (6 to 8 days) but somewhat longer in *P. ovale* (9 days) and *P. malariae* (13 to 16 days). Merozoites are then released from the hepatic cells and enter circulating erythrocytes. Occasionally, when the number of sporozoites inoculated is very low, the period from infection to onset of erythrocyte infection lasts for months or even years. In falciparum malaria the tissue phase terminates at the beginning of the *erythrocyte cycle;* in other Plasmodium species, the hepatic forms persist.* This species variation necessitates different therapeutic approaches in treating malaria. The species also differ in the number of merozoites released after primary hepatic schizogony: *P. falciparum* – about 40,000 from each infected cell; *P. ovale* – 15,000; *P. vivax* – 10,000; and *P. malariae* – 2000. The large number of merozoites released into the circulation in *P. falciparum* may contribute to the high levels of parasitemia seen in this infection and perhaps to the increased frequency with which erythrocytes are observed to contain multiple organisms.

The merozoite enters the red blood cell by inducing erythrocyte endocytosis, and the organism begins to develop within a vacuole in the erythrocyte. Using Giemsa or Wright stains, the parasite is first identified with light microscopy as a characteristic "ring-form," an early *trophozoite* (Figs. 2*A* and 2*B*). The organism increases in size, partially filling the red blood cell; this is termed the late *trophozoite.* Later the nuclear material is segregated by schizogony, and the red cell becomes partially filled with the cytoplasm and the multiple nuclei of the *schizont* (Fig. 2*C*). The erythrocyte cycle is completed when the red blood cells rupture, releasing the merozoites formed from the schizont, which then invade other erythrocytes. This cycle takes 48 hours in *P. falciparum, P. vivax,* and *P. ovale* malaria, and 72 hours in *P. malariae* infection. Symptoms of fever and chills coincide with the release of merozoites; hence the clinical descriptions of tertian malaria (fevers on days one and three) and quartan malaria (fevers on days one and four). The number of merozoites formed during erythrocyte schizogony is helpful in species diagnosis. Examination of a mature schizont of *P. malariae* will reveal 6 to 12 developing merozoites, *P. ovale* 6 to 16, and *P. vivax* 12 to 24.

By mechanisms which remain completely unknown, some merozoites do not continue the cycle of schizogony but develop into female and male gametocytes (Fig. 1). These first appear in the peripheral blood several days after the onset of the erythrocytic cycle, and they may

*The exoerythrocytic state is described in this chapter as "persistent" rather than cyclic, based on the arguments presented by Coatney et al. in the first cited reference. It is recognized that not all malariologists agree with this recent change in terms or the implied change in the nature of tissue schizogony and the mechanism of relapse.

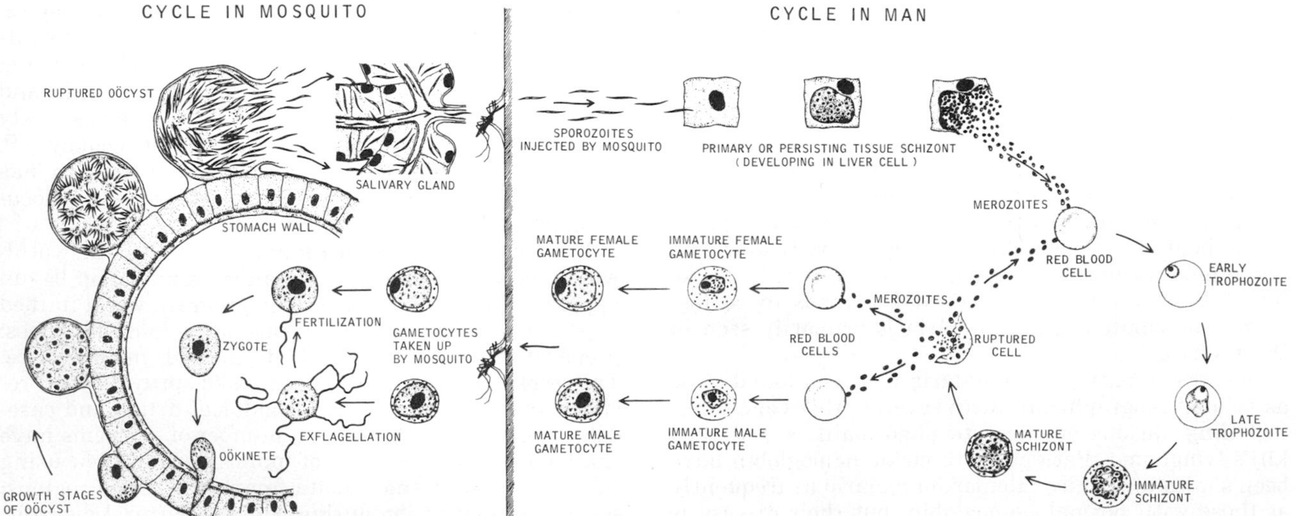

Figure 1. Life cycle of Plasmodium in mosquito and man. (Adapted from Alvarado, C. A., and Bruce-Chwatt, L. J.: Scientific American, Vol. 206, May, 1962.)

persist for weeks after schizogony has been suppressed. During the blood meal of an Anopheles mosquito, the gametocytes are ingested. Conditions exist in the stomach of the mosquito for the male gametocyte to form motile male gametes (exflagellation) which then fertilize the female gamete. After fertilization, the *zygote* becomes a motile *öokinete,* penetrates the stomach wall, and multiplies in an enlarging *öocyst.* Rupture of this cyst allows release of sporozoites which are distributed throughout the mosquito and accumulate in the salivary gland. The formation of sporozoites completes the process of *sporogony,* the sexual or mosquito cycle of malaria.

Pathogenesis and Immunity. There has been no documentation of generalized or significant host injury or response during the periods of sporozoitemia or hepatic schizogony, although antisporozoite antibodies have been demonstrated. After release of merozoites from the hepatic cells into the circulation, however, marked changes occur. Parasitized and nonparasitized red blood cells undergo alterations. In *P. falciparum* infection the erythrocytes develop electron-dense knoblike projections, take unusual shapes, and become less deformable. They also become more adhesive to vascular endothelium and more permeable to sodium, and demonstrate increased osmotic fragility. During the erythrocyte cycle, red blood cells are damaged at the time merozoites are released, leading to intravascular hemolysis and progressive anemia. Damage to vascular endothelium also occurs. B lymphocytes begin to produce IgM and IgG antibodies directed against the merozoites, and excess antibody is seen in the plasma in several days. These antibodies coat merozoites, after which they do not enter uninfected red cells, and they are removed from the circulation by phagocytic cells in the bone marrow, spleen, and liver. T lymphocytes release materials which stimulate increased metabolic and phagocytic activity of macrophages. This series of events produces the clinical and pathologic changes observed in acute and chronic malaria.

In acute falciparum malaria a number of complications result from alteration of the red blood cells and the vascular endothelium. The severe anemia and the adherence of red cells to capillary endothelium decrease oxygen supply to the tissues. The anoxia causes serious functional impairment of the brain and kidneys, less commonly of the liver, myocardium, and bone marrow. In fatal cases of falciparum malaria the brain is edematous, and blood vessels are occluded by parasitized erythrocytes, and surrounded by areas of hemorrhage and necrosis. The kidney may show ischemia of the renal cortex and diffuse glomerulitis, as well as tubular necrosis. The liver may show centrilobular degeneration and necrosis. These changes in the kidney and liver are believed related more to ischemia secondary to severe anemia and hypovolemia than to vascular obstruction by erythrocytes. In patients who die in pulmonary edema unrelated to fluid overload, the cardiac and pulmonary vessels are filled with parasitized red cells. Impaired bone marrow function in man is manifested by thrombocytopenia, absence of reticulocytes, and varying degrees of leukopenia.

Accelerated intravascular coagulation is occasionally documented in patients with malaria; that is, factors V, VII, VIII, X, fibrinogen, and platelets are decreased, prothrombin and partial thromboplastin times are prolonged, and fibrin degradation products are increased. However, disseminated intravascular coagulation is not a prominent feature at autopsy of patients who die of malaria.

During the acute attack of falciparum malaria, most patients develop vasodilation, just as in some other acute febrile diseases. This results in decreased effective circulating blood volume and orthostatic hypotension. Changes secondary to this include increased aldosterone levels, increased plasma volume, hyponatremia, and reversal of the urinary sodium to potassium ratio.

Some of the clinical and pathologic features of malaria are related to the host immune response. Patients occasionally have a Coombs-positive hemolytic anemia. This may partially explain the rapid intravascular hemolysis which exceeds that attributable to the level of parasitemia alone. "Blackwater fever," the complication of falciparum malaria characterized by rapid hemolysis and acute renal failure, occurs both in patients who have received quinine and in patients who have a history of previous exposure to the Plasmodium who have not received quinine. Antibody damage to red cells has been postulated in both situations. The pathologic changes seen in blackwater fever include renal ischemia and tubular necrosis. Recent evidence has suggested that the glomerulitis seen in some patients with falciparum malaria may be induced by immune complexes.

The pathologic picture in malaria of long duration is in large part that due to the immune response. Marked elevation of the serum immunoglobulins (IgG and IgM) is seen, and the liver and spleen are enlarged consistent with continued stimulation to the reticuloendothelial system. Anemia is common. A number of patients in an area hyperendemic for malaria develop marked splenomegaly (tropical splenomegaly syndrome). Parasites may not be demonstrable in peripheral blood smears, but elevated fluorescent antimalarial antibody titers are present, and the patients respond to prolonged therapy with antimalarials. Liver biopsy frequently shows hepatic sinusoidal lymphocytosis. In *P. malariae* infection of long duration, nephrotic syndrome is not uncommon. There is good evidence that this is related to immune complex injury to the glomerulus. Preliminary evidence has suggested that patients with chronic malaria have depressed cellular immune responses.

Host Resistance. Resistance to malaria involves numerous complex metabolic and immunologic factors. As mentioned previously, certain hemoglobinopathies and enzyme defects of the erythrocytes render patients less vulnerable to the severe complications of malaria. For unknown reasons, blacks appear less susceptible to *P. vivax* infection than whites. *Acquired immunity* to malaria requires both humoral and cellular defense mechanisms. Circulating antibodies are of primary importance in control of the acute infection, documented by studies in which antimalaria IgG was transferred to infected hosts and found to be protective. This protection was species specific. The role of antibody has been shown by the transfer of immunity from mother to fetus, with protection of the neonate during the period in which maternal IgG persists. Whether decreases in immunoglobulin levels contribute to relapse of malaria has not been clearly shown. The importance of cellular defense mechanisms has been assumed because of the intense phagocytic activity of cells of the reticuloendothelial system during malaria infection.

Clinical Manifestations. The patient with malaria experiences chills and fever, often associated with frontal

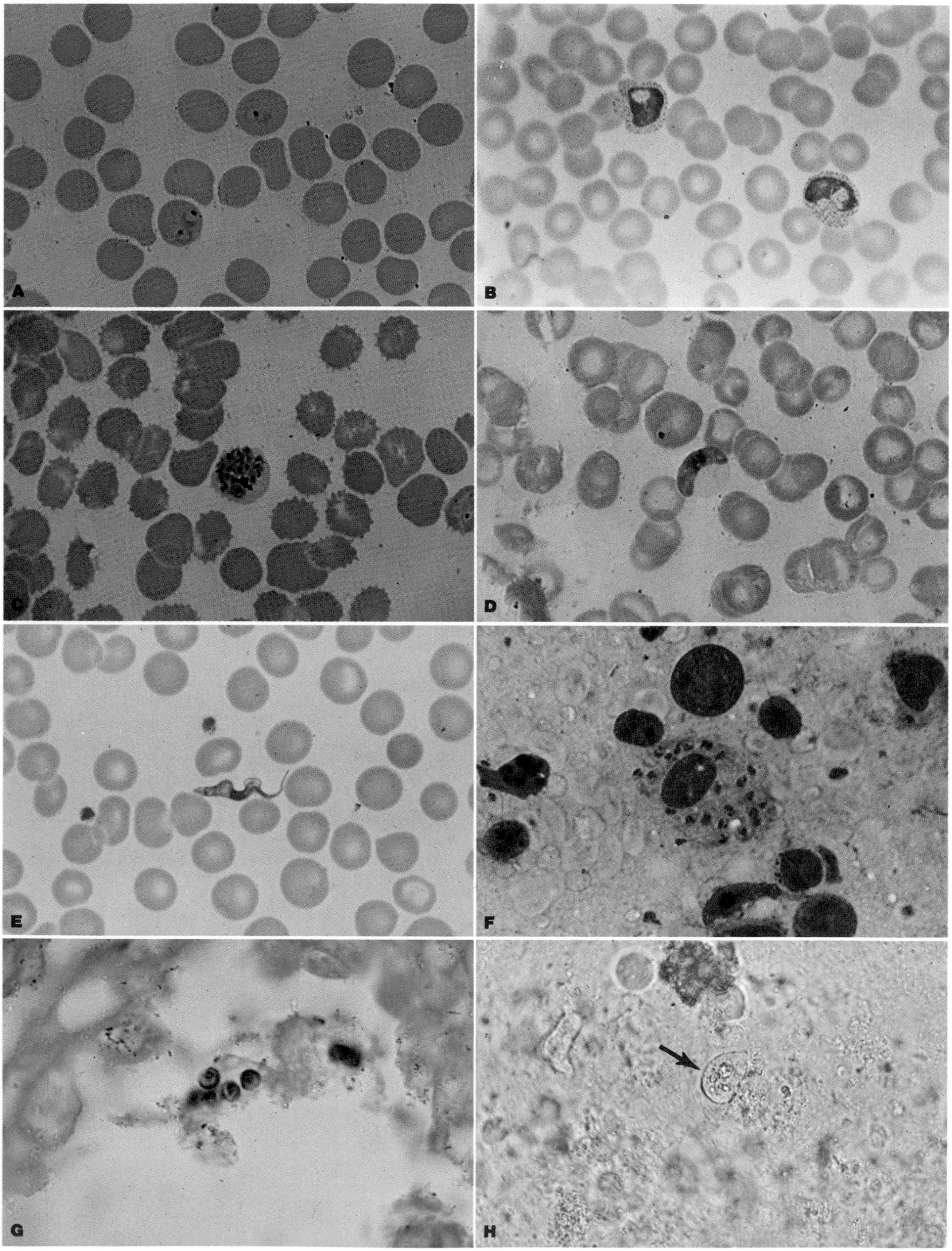

Figure 2. *See opposite page for legend.*

headache and myalgias. In the early period of the illness the fever may be persistent for several days before developing into a synchronous periodicity, the hallmark of tertian or quartan malaria. When the typical pattern has been established, the patient has a chill, a rise in temperature to 40 to 41° C, headache, and myalgias. This is followed in several hours by diffuse sweating and a fall in temperature. In vivax and ovale malaria these paroxysms occur every 48 hours (benign tertian malaria) and in malariae malaria every 72 hours (quartan malaria). In falciparum malaria the temperature is usually persistently elevated, but it may occasionally progress to a 48-hour cycle (malignant tertian malaria). Between the paroxysms of chills and fever, the patient often feels well except for some weakness or fatigue.

The illness may begin with nonspecific symptoms such as *sore throat, dry cough,* and *abdominal pain.* Most patients have *nausea* and *anorexia; vomiting* is less common. These symptoms may mislead the physician into making a diagnosis of pharyngitis, influenza, or gastroenteritis. Occasionally, the only sign of malaria is fever. In the postoperative surgical patient, fever caused by malaria is frequently confused with that caused by drug allergy. Rarely fever may be absent.

Physical examination reveals a tachycardia, and the skin is warm and flushed. *Jaundice* is not common, but occasionally it can be a prominent feature of the illness. *Hepatomegaly* is commonly found, and the liver may be moderately tender. The spleen is often palpable in acute malaria and is usually quite soft and occasionally tender. Attempts to palpate the spleen should be made carefully in view of the relative ease with which splenic rupture can occur. *Splenomegaly* is more commonly found in the early stage of vivax and ovale malaria than in falciparum malaria. Orthostatic hypotension can be documented in falciparum malaria. Lesions of herpes simplex virus may be seen.

Examination of peripheral blood after several days of illness reveals a normochromic, normocytic anemia which is usually mild, but it may be severe in prolonged infections or in those presenting with high parasitemia or acute hemolysis. The number of reticulocytes is usually normal until several days after therapy is begun; then reticulocytosis is seen. The white blood cell count is normal or low. Monocytosis may be present, but eosinophilia is not a feature of malaria. Thrombocytopenia of a moderate degree is usually present. Serum $\alpha 1$ glycoproteins are increased, whereas $\alpha 2$ glycoproteins (containing haptoglobin) are decreased. A false positive VDRL may occur. The serum transaminases are almost always elevated to moderate degrees and total bilirubin is often elevated. This is predominantly indirect bilirubin, but occasionally increased conjugated bilirubin is seen. Severe cases of malaria may be associated with sufficient liver dysfunction to be misdiagnosed as infectious hepatitis. Tests for determining intestinal absorption have been shown to be abnormal in some malaria patients. Urinalysis reveals trace amounts of albumin and bilirubin in uncomplicated cases, and rarely marked proteinuria has been documented. In falciparum malaria hyponatremia, reversal of the urinary sodium/potassium ratio, and transient increases in serum creatinine and blood urea nitrogen can frequently be recorded.

Fever and related symptoms gradually subside over several weeks in untreated vivax, ovale, and malariae malaria. However, relapse of vivax or ovale infection may occur months or even years later. The illness at the time of relapse is usually milder and of shorter duration than the initial illness. Death caused by infection with these organisms is very uncommon.

Complications. In falciparum malaria high levels of parasitemia and serious complications may develop rapidly. The most important of these complications are *coma, severe hemolytic anemia, acute renal failure,* and *acute pulmonary edema.* The patient may first demonstrate confusion with increasing lethargy, and within a few hours be unconscious. Focal neurologic signs are uncommon, but hyperreflexia and Babinski signs may be seen. Examination of the cerebrospinal fluid will reveal increased pressure and increased protein, without pleocytosis. *Massive intravascular hemolysis* may result from high levels of parasitemia, quinine therapy, drug administration to patients with glucose-6-phosphate dehydrogenase deficiency, or hypersensitivity after previous malaria infections. Hemoglobinuria, acute tubular necrosis, and renal failure may result. *Hemolysis, hemoglobinuria,* and *renal failure* make up the striking clinical picture of severe malaria known as "blackwater fever." Acute renal failure may occur in the absence of signs of intravascular hemolysis and can be detected early only

---

Figure 2. *A* to *D* show various erythrocyte forms of falciparum or vivax malaria (× 1500).
A, "Ring forms" of *Plasmodium falciparum.* Note the delicate rings and an erythrocyte containing two organisms.
B, Trophozoite of *Plasmodium vivax.* The red cell is enlarged, Schüffner's dots are seen, and the parasite is large and ameboid.
C, Schizont of *Plasmodium vivax* with at least 18 merozoite nuclei.
D, Gametocyte of *Plasmodium falciparum.* The crescent or banana shape is characteristic.
E, Trypanosoma rhodesiense in the peripheral blood. It has a nucleus, posterior kinetoplast, an undulating membrane, and flagellum (× 1500).
F, Spleen smear showing a cell filled with *Leishmania donovani.* The rod-shaped kinetoplast and large round nucleus appear as two adjacent red dots.
G, Methenamine silver nitrate stain of clump of Pneumocystis cysts. They appear as black circles against the blue background (× 800).
H, Stool sample observed by light microscopy, showing a motile *Entamoeba histolytica* moving in a straight line across the field. The ameba contains lucent vacuoles and shows a pseudopod directed to the upper right (× 500).
(*A, C, D,* and *F* are photographs taken by T. C. Jones from the Cornell Parasitology teaching slides; *B* is from the collection of H. Zaiman, originally photographed by M. Wittner; *E* and *G* were provided by R. B. Roberts; *H* is a photograph of fresh material provided by T. C. Jones.)

by careful monitoring of the urine volume and serum creatinine or urea nitrogen levels. Acute pulmonary edema is an uncommon complication, but it may develop rapidly and be particularly refractile to therapy. Pulmonary edema may be due to excessive fluid administration, but a number of cases have been reported in which intravascular volume was normal. Patients may present with signs and symptoms of vascular collapse—so-called algid malaria. A rare complication of malaria is splenic rupture, the only complication which is probably more common in vivax than falciparum malaria. Patients who survive untreated falciparum malaria may have recurrences of symptoms for a number of months, but thereafter they remain asymptomatic.

Syndromes Associated with Chronic Malaria. Syndromes associated with chronic malaria are most likely the result of repeated exposure of immune patients to Plasmodium and occur predominantly in hyperendemic areas of malaria. The patients may be asymptomatic, but they have intermittently detectable parasitemia, hypergammaglobulinemia, elevated antimalaria antibody titers, anemia, and splenic enlargement. Some patients develop marked splenomegaly—the tropical splenomegaly syndrome. Patients infected with *P. malariae* may develop nephrotic syndrome (quartan nephrosis). This is most common in children. It is associated with a poor prognosis and does not respond well to corticosteroid administration.

Diagnosis. The diagnosis of malaria must be suspected in every patient with fever, coma, or shock who has lived or traveled in a malarious area, has received a blood transfusion, or may be a drug addict. The only technique for confirming the clinical suspicion of malaria is the identification of plasmodia in fixed, stained blood smears. The diagnosis may be made by an alert technician during examination of a differential white count. However, it is usually only when a high suspicion of the possibility of malaria exists that the proper smears will be done and the necessary time taken to make the diagnosis.

Thin blood smears are made by placing a drop of blood on the end of a glass slide, touching the drop with another slide, and rapidly moving the edge of the second slide along the surface of the first. A thick blood smear is made by placing a drop of blood on a slide, then spreading it to fill a diameter of about 1 cm. The slides are allowed to dry. The thin blood smear is fixed in methanol and stained with Giemsa, or fixed and stained with Wright's. The thick blood smear is first dipped in water to lyse the red blood cells, then fixed and similarly stained. For the inexperienced observer the thin smear is easiest to examine and most likely to yield the diagnosis in the nonimmune patient with malaria. Careful examination of several thousand red blood cells on a properly stained smear will usually reveal the protozoan. When malaria is suspected but smears do not reveal the orgainism, smears should be repeated several times a day. The highest level of parasitemia is said to be demonstrable several hours *after* a chill. A thick smear can be particularly helpful for finding the characteristic gametocyte of falciparum malaria (Fig. 2*D*), but it may also reveal organisms when they are too infrequent to be easily identified on a thin smear.

The correct diagnosis of the species of plasmodium is critical in determining therapy and prognosis in malaria. The following brief description and the photomicrographs in Figure 2 were selected to aid in differentiating *P. vivax* and *P. falciparum* in peripheral blood.

Differentiation of P. vivax and P. falciparum in Blood Smears. The following characteristics can be used to identify *P. falciparum.* Only the ring forms are usually seen in the peripheral blood; they are small and delicate, often with two chromatin dots (Fig. 2*A*). The erythrocytes containing these protozoa are not conspicuously enlarged, and red dots (Schüffner's dots) are not present. The level of parasitemia may be high (more than 5 to 10 per cent of the erythrocytes infected), and some erythrocytes may contain several parasites. Organisms may appear to be on the surface of the erythrocyte (appliqué forms). *P. vivax* ring forms are often larger than falciparum rings and in later stages appear quite pleomorphic (Fig. 2*B*). The infected erythrocytes are usually larger than normal, and if properly stained, Schüffner's dots can be identified. By examining blood films at various times, the maturation of *P. vivax* in the peripheral blood can be documented. The mature schizont (Fig. 2*C*) contains 12 to 24 chromatin dots, and the parasite cytoplasm almost fills the red blood cell. The gametocyte of *P. falciparum* is very characteristic (Fig. 2*D*) and should be looked for carefully since it substantiates the diagnosis. It has a crescent or banana shape, whereas the shape of *P. vivax* gametocytes is globular.

Mixed Infection. Even after one species of malaria is identified, it must be kept in mind that the patient could have a mixed infection (1 to 2 per cent of cases). Mixed infection can best be diagnosed by careful review of several thin blood films. Repeated blood films for one to two days after the start of treatment should show decreasing levels of parasitemia. If a *P. vivax* infection is diagnosed and treated with chloroquine but parasitemia is seen to be increasing, a mixed infection with chloroquine-resistant *P. falciparum* should be suspected. At present, *P. falciparum* infection acquired in Southeast Asia and some parts of South America is resistant to chloroquine (see below). All patients diagnosed as having *P. falciparum* should have repeated smears during therapy to ensure that the parasitemia is decreasing.

Chloroquine Susceptibility Test. A technique for documenting whether *P. falciparum* is susceptible or resistant has been developed. At the time of initial diagnosis and before therapy is instituted, a sample of the patient's blood is defibrinated and added to vials (1 ml each) containing varying concentrations of chloroquine and 5 mg of glucose per 100 ml. During 24 hours of incubation, *P. falciparum* will mature to the schizont stage in the vials containing insufficient levels of chloroquine. Chloroquine susceptibility can be calculated from these data.

Antibody Tests. Antibody tests for malaria are not useful in the diagnosis of the acute illness. The indirect fluorescent antibody and hemagglutination tests are of value in testing populations to determine the prevalence of malaria and in screening blood donors when tracing cases of transfusion-induced malaria.

Differential Diagnosis. The differential diagnosis of malaria is lengthy and varies, depending upon the area of the world, the dominant malaria species, and whether the disease is acute or chronic. The fever of malaria must be separated from fever caused by dengue and other arboviruses, typhus, amebiasis, typhoid, relapsing fever, heat stroke, drug allergy, influenza, bacterial pneumonias, and wound infections. Intermittent chills secondary to antipyretics may simulate the chills and fever of malaria in all these conditions. Cerebral malaria must be distinguished from viral encephalitides, drug overdose, and other causes of coma. The jaundice of malaria must be distinguished from viral hepatitis and leptospirosis. In more chronic malaria infection in which splenomegaly and anemia are prominent, one must also consider bacterial endocarditis, schistosomiasis, visceral leishmaniasis, and lymphoma.

Therapy. *Elimination of Parasitemia.* The initial therapeutic goal in the treatment of malaria is to eliminate the erythrocytic stage of the infection, because all the acute symptoms are due to this hematogenous process. Chloroquine, a 4-aminoquinoline, is the drug of choice to accomplish this purpose. It can be given orally, or parenterally if the patient is vomiting. Chloroquine diphosphate is given orally as follows: 1 gram initially (600 mg of base), followed by 500 mg (300 mg of base) at 6 hours, 24 hours, and 48 hours after the initial dose (total dose 2.5 grams; 1.5 grams of base). Children should receive a loading dose of 17 mg per kilogram, followed by 8.5 mg per kilogram at 6, 24, and 48 hours. Chloroquine hydrochloride is available for intramuscular or intravenous injection. It is important to note that the hydrochloride salt contains a different quantity of chloroquine base than the diphosphate salt. Chloroquine base, 300 mg, is given intramuscularly every six hours for three doses (total of 900 mg base). On the second and third days therapy may be changed to oral medication, or single intramuscular injections can be continued until a total dose of 1.5 grams chloroquine base is reached. Intravenous medication with chloroquine is seldom indicated, because the patient in shock or coma will usually be given quinine realizing the possibility of a drug-resistant infection (see below). If intravenous chloroquine is considered necessary, 300 mg of base is diluted in 300 ml of saline and given over 30 to 60 minutes. It can be given every six to eight hours, but not in excess of a total daily dose of 1000 mg of base.

The exact mechanism of action of chloroquine remains unknown. It interrupts the vacuolar digestive mechanisms of protozoa, and it binds strongly to nucleic acids. Higher concentrations of the drug are found in infected erythrocytes than in uninfected cells or plasma. This enhanced uptake of chloroquine by parasitized cells may be very important, as suggested by the observation that chloroquine-resistant strains do not enhance the concentration of chloroquine by erythrocytes. In spite of the fact that chloroquine is also concentrated in the liver, it is ineffective in inhibiting tissue schizogony. Chloroquine is absorbed rapidly from the gastrointestinal tract. Fifty per cent becomes bound to plasma proteins, and only about 10 per cent of the active compound is excreted in the urine. Most of the drug is concentrated in tissue, and degradation probably occurs in the liver. It disappears from tissue over a period of several weeks after the drug is stopped. Chloroquine is usually well tolerated, but it can cause transient headache, visual disturbances, nausea, and vomiting. At toxic levels it can cause delirium, psychotic reactions, and convulsions. Its use is not contraindicated during pregnancy for treatment of malaria. When given for prolonged periods in doses higher than that used in malaria chemoprophylaxis, punctate keratitis and retinitis have been recorded. Amodiaquine is as effective as chloroquine for treating malaria.

Drug-Resistant Plasmodia. When falciparum malaria is diagnosed, a careful history must include the country where the infection was acquired. If the illness was acquired in South America, Central America, or the Philippines and the level of parasitemia is greater than 2 per cent of erythrocytes, or if it was acquired in Vietnam, Laos, Thailand, Malaysia, Cambodia, or Burma, regardless of the level of parasitemia, or if the source of the infection is unknown (such as in transfusion malaria) and parasitemia is high, then quinine sulfate should be used instead of chloroquine. *P. falciparum* acquired in the areas cited has been documented to show varying degrees of resistance to chloroquine.

Resistance of plasmodia to antimalarial drugs has been recognized for many years. Shortly after pyrimethamine and proguanil were introduced, strains resistant to these drugs were identified. This was not unexpected, because protozoa have been known to rapidly develop resistance to inhibitors of folate metabolism. Strains of *P. falciparum* which required higher than standard doses of quinine to be eradicated were recorded many years ago. Only in the past decade, however, has the problem of drug resistance been brought to particular attention by appearance of resistance of *P. falciparum* to previously accepted therapeutic levels of chloroquine. Resistant strains appeared in several parts of the world at about the same time, unrelated to whether chloroquine had been commonly used in the area or not.

Resistance of *P. falciparum* to chloroquine has been divided, based on response in level of parasitemia after initiation of therapy: no reduction (termed RIII level of resistance), and partial reduction (termed RII). The first level of chloroquine resistance (RI), to be considered in more detail below, is one in which *patent* parasitemia is eradicated, but parasitemia and clinical symptoms recur in a few days to several weeks; i.e., recrudescent malaria. At present, quinine is effective in removing patent parasitemia in these cases; however, a number of other drugs are necessary to prevent recrudescence. Careful attention to the diagnosis of chloroquine-resistant malaria is now an integral part of the management of patients with malaria (see Diagnosis).

To eradicate parasitemia in cases suspected to be caused by chloroquine-resistant strains, quinine is given orally, 650 mg every eight hours for seven to ten days. Quinine dihydrochloride is used intravenously in patients unable to take the drug orally. Quinine, 600 mg, is dissolved in 100 to 200 ml of 5 per cent glucose and water and administered over 30 minutes. This is repeated every eight hours. The mechanism of action of quinine against the malaria parasite is unknown. It has been shown to block protein synthetic and glycolytic pathways. It is absorbed readily from the gastrointestinal tract, and over 70 per cent is bound to plasma proteins. Like chloroquine, it is concentrated in tissues, including erythrocytes. Only 5 per cent of administered quinine is excreted unchanged in the urine. The most common side effects of quinine are tinnitus, vertigo, nausea, and vomiting. Although these symptoms are annoying, they are not indications to discontinue medication. A Coombs-positive hemolytic anemia is a rare complication of quinine therapy.

Prevention of Recrudescent Falciparum Malaria. Recrudescence of falciparum malaria occurs frequently in patients whose infection was acquired in Southeast Asia, Central America, or South America. Recrudescence is due to persistence during an asymptomatic period of erythrocytic stages of *P. falciparum* at undetectable levels, followed by increased parasitemia and symptoms several days to six weeks after apparently successful control of the illness by chloroquine or quinine. This is the first level of chloroquine resistance (RI). To prevent this, several drugs have been added to the initial therapeutic program for treatment of falciparum malaria acquired in the areas previously mentioned. Most commonly, pyrimethamine is given, 50 mg orally per day for three days in combination with dapsone, 25 mg orally per day for one month. If dapsone is unavailable, sulfadiazine, 1 gram every six hours for three days, is given concomitant with pyrimethamine. These drugs act by blocking folate metabolism at the paraminobenzoic acid and the dehydrofolate reductase steps. They can cause bone marrow suppression and allergic reactions. Difference of opinion exists over whether these drugs should be started on the first day of chloroquine or quinine therapy or several days later. We recommend that the drugs be started at the end of chloroquine treatment or on the fourth day of quinine therapy. This reduces the possibility of complicating the clinical picture by potential side effects of the drugs. Recently clindamycin or tetracycline has been found effective in combination with quinine against recrudescence of falciparum malaria. In cases in which recrudescence has occurred repeatedly, intravenous quinine has been used in place of oral quinine in combination with these drugs.

Gametocytes usually disappear from the peripheral blood within a few days after schizogony is interrupted, and no specific therapy is needed. Primaquine is an effective gametocidal drug and can be used in the rare patient with prolonged asymptomatic gametocytemia.

Prevention of Relapse Due to Persistent Hepatic Schizonts. Relapse of *P. vivax* and *P. ovale* malaria is caused by the persistence of hepatic schizogony.* Primaquine, an 8-aminoquinoline, is usually effective in preventing relapse (approximately 90 per cent of patients are cured). Since relapse is common in these infections, chloroquine therapy should always be followed by a course of primaquine. The adult dose is 15 mg of base daily for 14 days. Children should be given 0.25 mg per kilogram of body weight per day for 14 days. If relapse occurs after a full course of primaquine, the dose of primaquine should be doubled during a second 14-day period of therapy. The mechanism of action of primaquine is unknown, but it does appear to block glycolysis.

Primaquine can induce hemolysis in patients whose erythrocytes are deficient in glucose-6-phosphate dehydrogenase. Therefore patients should be tested for this deficiency before therapy is started, and if glucose-6-phosphate dehydrogenase deficiency is documented, red blood cell counts should be monitored carefully during treatment.

Supportive Therapy. Treatment of malaria is often accomplished with ease even in cases of falciparum malaria. However, since the course of falciparum malaria is unpredictable and complications may develop rapidly, all cases should be approached as medical emergencies. The management of a patient with malaria includes complete bed rest during the period of orthostatic hypotension. In the occasional patient with very high fever, this should be controlled by continuous antipyretic administration, sponging, and cooling. Frequent determinations of hematocrit, electrolytes, creatinine, urine volume, bilirubin, and transaminases are necessary. The level of consciousness should be carefully monitored.

The patient with falciparum malaria should receive transfusions with packed erythrocytes if severe anemia develops. The vascular volume and cardiac function should be monitored carefully by following the blood pressure, and in severe cases monitoring the central venous pressure may be necessary. Intravenous fluids should be given judiciously with full knowledge of the vascular volume, renal function, and serum electrolytes.

If cerebral malaria develops, the patient should be managed according to procedures used in the care of any comatose patient (see Ch. 319). Corticosteroids have been advocated in these cases to reduce cerebral edema. Heparin therapy should be used in the rare cases documented to have disseminated intravascular coagulation.

If the patient develops oliguria, a trial of furosemide or mannitol may be given. However, when acute renal failure is present, judicious administration of fluids associated with hemodialysis or peritoneal dialysis is indicated (see Ch. 604). The dose of quinine should be reduced to half in patients with renal failure, but maintained at therapeutic levels once hemo- or peritoneal dialysis is instituted.

If signs of pulmonary edema develop, standard therapeutic approaches are indicated, including digitalis preparations and methods to reduce the central venous pressure (see Ch. 520). This complication, however, has been quite refractory to treatment.

Prevention. An individual entering an area where malaria remains endemic must avoid contact with mosquitoes and systematically take drug prophylaxis. Use of mosquito netting, screens, insecticides, and mosquito repellents are the main mechanisms for avoiding contact with mosquitoes. The best repellent available at present is N,N-diethyltoluamide. It remains effective for up to 18 hours, a considerable advance over the odor repellents which are of value for only two or four hours.

The best means of malaria prevention is chemoprophylaxis. This is a cumbersome method, requiring intelligence, compulsiveness, and often willingness to tolerate the mild side effects of the medication. Travelers should check with medical officials in the area they visit for up-to-date advice on malaria chemoprophylaxis. The primary drug recommended for prophylaxis for travelers from the United States is chloroquine diphosphate or sulfate. Five hundred milligrams (300 mg of chloroquine base) is taken once a week. Children of ages 8 to 12 should receive 250 mg; ages 4 to 7, 200 mg; and ages 1 to 3, 125 mg; infants should receive 75 mg weekly. Where malaria is hyperendemic, 500 mg twice weekly has been recommended. Chloroquine should be started one to two weeks before entering the malarious area and continued for six weeks after departure from the area. Chloroquine does not prevent the hepatic infection, but simply suppresses the erythrocytic stage; *therefore the period of prophylaxis after leaving the malarious area is very important.* It is this period which travelers most often ignore and which leads to their illness several weeks after leaving the endemic area. After chloroquine prophylaxis, primaquine (15 mg of base per day) should be given for 14 days to eradicate the hepatic stages of plasmodia infections.

A single tablet containing 300 mg of chloroquine base and 45 mg of primaquine base was used for chemoprophylaxis by the U.S. military during the Vietnam war. This tablet is not recommended for use in preference to chloroquine alone. However, if primaquine is unavailable, this drug combination may be used after the traveler leaves the endemic area; it will prevent chloroquine-sensitive falciparum malaria and relapsing malaria. One table is taken per week for eight weeks. It is important that this combination *not* be used in the *treatment* of malaria, because the dose of primaquine base is at toxic levels when 1.5 grams of chloroquine base is given.

Prophylaxis When Cloroquine Resistance Is Present. Chloroquine prophylaxis may be ineffective in areas

*See footnote, page 474.

such as Southeast Asia and parts of Central and South America where chloroquine-resistant falciparum malaria is encountered. Travelers to these areas must balance their likely level of exposure to infected mosquitoes with the dangers of more vigorous chemoprophylaxis. The Communicable Disease Center has recommended that travelers to these countries take chloroquine in the dose usually recommended for other areas of the world (500 mg once weekly). Chloroguanide hydrochloride (100 to 200 mg per day) is probably an effective alternative to chloroquine chemoprophylaxis. The traveler must be told that these drugs may not be effective, and they should seek medical care promptly if fever occurs. A drug combination which at present is completely effective in preventing chloroquine-resistant falciparum malaria is pyrimethamine, 25 mg, plus sulfadoxine, 500 mg, taken once a week. This combination is not available in the United States, but it can be obtained in many other countries. Another effective drug combination is chloroguanide hydrochloride, 100 mg per day, plus dapsone, 25 mg daily. However, an increased risk of agranulocytosis caused by dapsone makes it less desirable as chemoprophylaxis for civilian travelers unless heavy exposure to infected mosquitoes is anticipated. Further testing will be needed to determine if tetracycline, long-acting sulfonamides, or repository drugs have a place in the chemoprophylaxis of malaria.

Prevention in a Community. Prevention of malaria in communities in endemic areas requires a coordinated effort directed at reducing the number of Anopheles mosquitoes and identifying and treating human cases of malaria. Anopheles are reduced in the environment by draining or filling breeding areas and by the use of larvicides. Effective campaigns against adult mosquitoes usually include spraying of all buildings with residual insecticides twice a year. DDT has been particularly effective for this purpose in the past; however, because of mosquito resistance and potential unacceptable side effects of DDT, other drugs such as hexachlorocyclohexane, dieldrin, malathion, and carbamates are now being used.

In areas endemic for malaria, use of chemoprophylactic drugs is usually reserved for children or pregnant women (to prevent congenital transmission of malaria). In some areas entire populations are treated by including the drug in the salt distribution for daily use. These approaches are used to reduce morbidity and mortality before adequate immunity is acquired. Hopefully, some form of active immunization could replace this method in the future.

Coatney, G. R., Collins, W. E., Warren, M., and Contacos, P. G.: The Primate Malarias. U.S. Department of Health, Education, and Welfare, National Institutes of Health. Washington, D.C., U.S. Government Printing Office, 1971.

Inter-American Malaria Research Symposium. Am. J. Trop. Med. Hyg., 21:613, 1972.

Maegraith, B., and Fletcher, A.: The pathogenesis of mammalian malaria. Adv. Parasitol., 10:49, 1972.

Miller, L. H.: Malaria. *In* Hoeprich, P. D. (ed.): Infectious Diseases. Hagerstown, Md., Harper & Row, 1972, p. 1113.

Neva, F. A., Sheagren, J. N., Shulman, N. R., and Canfield, C. J.: Malaria: Host-defense mechanisms and complications. Ann. Intern. Med., 73:295, 1970.

Powell, R. D., and McNamara, J. V.: Infection with chloroquine-resistant *Plasmodium falciparum* in man. Ann. N.Y. Acad. Sci., 174:1027, 1970.

Russell, P. F., West, L. S., Manwell, R. D., and MacDonald, G.: Practical Malariology. 2nd ed. London, Oxford University Press, 1963.

World Health Organization: Chemotherapy of Malaria and Resistance to Antimalarials. WHO Tech. Rep. Series No. 529, 1973.

TRYPANOSOMIASES

272. AFRICAN TRYPANOSOMIASIS (African Sleeping Sickness, Maladie du Sommeil, Schlafkrankheit)

W. E. Ormerod

Definition and Etiology. African trypanosomiasis (sleeping sickness) is a meningoencephalitis caused by the protozoan *Trypanosoma brucei* (Plimmer and Bradford, 1899), discovered by Sir David Bruce to be the cause of nagana of cattle in Zululand. The disease occurs in several clinicoepidemiologic patterns. The two principal patterns of disease in man are Gambian sleeping sickness, which is chronic, and Rhodesian sleeping sickness, which is relatively acute. Another form, Zambezi sleeping sickness, although chronic, is more like the acute (Rhodesian) form in its epidemiologic behavior. The terms "Rhodesian" and "Gambian" are used today without geographic implication.

There is no clear-cut difference between the strains of organisms causing Gambian and Rhodesian forms of the disease, but there are strains previously regarded as *T. brucei (sensu stricto)* which, although identical in every other respect, will not infect man. This has given rise to difficulty, because they could not be identified with even moderate precision without experimental infection of man, a procedure which was seldom justifiable. A new test devised by Rickman and Robson and improved by Hawking, which subjects the trypanosome to trypanocidal substances in human serum, is now helping to classify isolates in terms of whether they are likely or not to be infective for man.

Other African species of trypanosomes, *T. congolense* and *T. vivax*, are important causes of disease in domestic livestock, but as they do not infect man they are of no medical interest. Trypanosomiasis can cause serious losses in domestic cattle and, where good husbandry is practiced, can reduce the food supply. By contrast, in Africa where husbandry is usually bad, and the yields are negligible, the existence of cattle trypanosomiasis acts as an important restraint on overgrazing and consequent soil erosion.

T. brucei gives a cyclical infection in the mammalian host but, unlike malaria, the cycles usually overlap, giving a variety of different stages in the blood at any one time. Ormerod and Venkatesan ascribe this cycle to the liberation of "long-thin" blood forms from a visceral stage in the leptomeninges. The blood forms divide until their division is inhibited by the uptake of lipids from the serum with consequent activation of trypanosomal lysosomes. Lysosomal action inhibits some forms completely; they contract into the "short-stumpy" forms which are removed by lysis and phagocytosis. A few, however, partially inhibited, develop multiple nuclei and flagella and, as giant forms, are filtered out of the circulation by mesodermal capillaries to renew the visceral phase.

Epidemiology. ***Prevalence.*** Although animal strains of *T. brucei* occur throughout the tsetse belt of Africa, that is to say, south of the Sahara and north of the Limpopo River and the Kalahari, human strains are not so widespread. The chronic (Gambian) form is to be found in West Africa from the Gambia to the Congo, penetrating inland to Lakes Chad, Victoria, and Tanganyika. The chronic (Zambezi) form with similar pathology is also to be found in Botswana, Rhodesia, Zambia, and Portuguese East Africa, but, as mentioned above, in its epidemiology it resembles the more acute (Rhodesian) form now found in Tanzania, Uganda, Kenya, and (most recently) Ethiopia. Distinction among these forms is not always useful to the clinician, because today the treatment of all forms is the same. Nevertheless, there is some difference in the prognosis of the different forms, and to the epidemiologist the differences are of great importance.

Transmission. *T. brucei* is transmitted by several species of the tsetse fly Glossina. When the fly bites an infected host, if its feeding is interrupted it can pass the infection to a second host by regurgitating part of the first feed. This mode of infection may occur at the height of an epidemic when other biting flies such as Stomoxys or tabanid (horse) flies may also be involved. Usually, however, the trypanosomes develop in the tsetse into noninfective forms, and this process continues for about 20 days until infective trypanosomes are formed; these remain in the salivary gland of the fly until it dies from other causes. The duration of the developmental cycle in the fly varies with temperature and does not continue below 18° C.

Rhodesian Sleeping Sickness. The Rhodesian strains of *T. brucei* are transmitted mainly by *G. morsitans*. This fly is associated with the edge of Brachistegia woodland (the miombo of Tanzania) and with the woodland that fringes watercourses in which, during the dry season, its habitat resembles that of *G. pallidipes*, also a transmitting agent. Although these flies feed on the blood of a wide range of species of game animals, there is evidence that the only important wild animal reservoir of Rhodesian sleeping sickness is the bushbuck *Tragelaphus scriptus*. This small antelope differs from other game in that it can live in close proximity to man, runs only a short distance when disturbed, and returns to its original "stand" in a thicket where it shares the same population of Glossina with man if he happens to be present. Sporadic Rhodesian disease is spread by this means, but epidemic Rhodesian strains are spread by *G. morsitans*, ranging widely in or between scattered thickets at the edge of the miombo, and under these conditions direct "man-fly-man" transmission occurs. Domestic cattle may also act as a reservoir.

Epidemic Rhodesian sleeping sickness occurred in Tanzania in the 1930's and large areas remain depopulated, because the disease has become "enzootic" and is still liable to break out again and cause acute disease in man. To the north of Lake Victoria, where epidemics have occurred more recently, the disease is spread mainly by *G. pallidipes* which ranges widely in the lakeside thickets. In Kenya a recent epidemic has been attributed to *G. fuscipes*, a fly related to *G. palpalis*, which has otherwise always been associated with Gambian sleeping sickness. This serves to emphasize the unstable and fluctuating epidemiology of the disease in this area, in contrast to the more stable epidemiology of the disease in the more southerly part of its range.

Zambezi Sleeping Sickness. Zambezi sleeping sickness is similar to Rhodesian sleeping sickness in its epidemiology. It is also transmitted by *G. pallidipes* and *G. morsitans*, especially when the fly is concentrated into "fringing forest" during the dry season: the bushbuck is also the most important, if not the only, reservoir. The disease is very sporadic and few of the indigenous population at risk contract it: some present as "healthy carriers"; others develop chronic wasting disease, but outsiders may suffer a very acute infection. Blair et al. point out that the epidemiologic pattern in Rhodesia has remained unchanged for the past 60 years.

Gambian Sleeping Sickness. Gambian sleeping sickness is transmitted mainly by *G. palpalis*. This fly obtains its blood meal from reptiles, birds, and man; it is a shade- and moisture-loving fly, and consequently transmission occurs most readily when a population of flies becomes isolated by unfavorable climate around a small woodland area. Frequently in West African savannah country such woodlands contain the water supply of a village. Here interchange of trypanosomes between fly and man takes place, and a focus of infection is built up. *G. tachinoides*, a fly associated with river thickets of West Africa, also transmits Gambian strains. This fly feeds on the blood of mammals other than man; consequently, it cannot be stated with confidence that there are not other animal reservoirs of Gambian sleeping sickness. Indeed, the dog and the domestic pig have been shown to harbor strains, but there is no evidence that these are of more than occasional epidemiologic importance.

Pathology. The extent of pathologic lesions depends on the duration of the disease. The most acute cases, those in which death occurs within two months, show little effect other than that associated with infectious disease generally. There are general wasting, hemorrhages into lung and bone marrow, and cellular proliferation in lymph nodes and in the malpighian bodies of the spleen. Acute myocarditis is believed to be the cause of death in some cases, but is rarely observed post mortem. Most cases of acute disease show some small round-cell infiltration of the meninges, but the brain appears normal. After about six months, the lymph nodes and malpighian bodies lose much of their cellularity, and fibrosis occurs in lymph nodes and vessels. At this stage the red bone marrow decreases, and a normocytic anemia and a leukopenia with a relative increase in lymphocytes occur. There is slight infiltration of the brain substance with small round cells, but heavy infiltration of the leptomeninges. Where the leptomeninges extend into the Aschoff-Robin space that surrounds meningeal vessels as they penetrate into the brain substance, the lesion known as *perivascular cuffing* is produced; this may vary from a single layer of infiltrating cells surrounding the vessel, in cases lasting for about six months, to a depth of about 20 cells when the disease has continued for two or more years. The nature of the cellular reaction has not been studied in detail, but there is one type of cell, the large *morular cell* (Mott's cells) with loculated eosinophilic cytoplasm, that is present in the leptomeninges or the cuffing (rarely in the brain substance). The presence of this cell is considered pathognomonic of advanced sleeping sickness. Thrombosis is liable to occur in the cuffed vessels and gives rise to the cerebral degeneration that causes the progressive mental deterioration and coma from which the disease is named.

Pathogenesis. The tsetse fly feeds by rupturing small vessels and sucking from the subcutaneous pool that is formed. It may inject trypanosomes either into the bloodstream or into the pool where they lodge and grow to form a *chancre*, a hard painful nodule that contains trypanosomes. Initial growth of the trypanosomes is in the blood and, in man, seldom reaches a level greater than one organism per cubic millimeter. With each wave of the infection the organism appears with a different surface antigen, and over 20 have been observed with a single strain. The host responds by production of immunoglobulins in amounts sufficient to produce very high erythrocyte sedimentation rates; these globulins are in the IgM (19S) rather than in the IgG (7S) range, which is normally associated with infectious disease. It is doubtful whether much of the globulins are "protective" or even "specific," and it is likely that the main immunologic action lies in a cell-mediated response against the visceral phase of the organism.

Clinical Manifestations. The clinical diagnosis of sleeping sickness is usually difficult, for there are few reliable physical signs of the disease. A history of exposure to tsetse bite is essential. A chancre may develop at the site of the bite of the infected tsetse fly, although more frequently this passes unobserved or may be confused with the reaction to a normal tsetse bite, which can occasionally be severe. The occurrence, site, and appearance of the chancre vary greatly between different areas and individual patients.

With typical *Rhodesian disease* the bite will have occurred about two weeks before the first symptoms. With *Gambian* and *Zambezi disease*, however, the symptoms may be delayed for several years; the history of, or the scar from, a chancre may be useful in diagnosing the disease in a European.

Irrespective of the demonstration of a previous bite, the most important early symptom of sleeping sickness is the *severe headache*. This is associated with loss of nocturnal sleep and a *feeling of oppression* that African patients will often recognize, causing them to trek many miles to a sleeping sickness clinic. Wasting, mental disturbance, and drowsiness occur only when the disease is established in the central nervous system.

Physical signs in the early stages include fever, which may be high and fluctuating, especially in the Rhodesian and Zambezi disease. A fleeting circinate erythematous rash occurs on the chest and shoulders of some European patients, but is not seen in Africans. Enlarged lymph nodes are associated with Gambian disease and are found characteristically in the posterior triangle of the neck. Periosteal tenderness is described as a diagnostic sign but is neither frequent nor specific; similarly, swelling of the dorsum of the foot is easily confused with famine edema, which may coexist in the type of population at greatest risk of acquiring trypanosomiasis.

Diagnosis. Because there is nothing conclusive about the clinical manifestations of trypanosomiasis, the diagnosis depends entirely on demonstration of the presence of the organism. In the *Rhodesian disease* it is usually made by microscopic examination of a thick (unfixed) blood film stained with Giemsa, a tedious but fairly reliable procedure in the hands of a well-trained microscopist. Injection of blood into rats or mice is of value in doubtful cases. Zambezi strains are more difficult to diagnose by microscopy but are very easily isolated in rats and mice.

Gambian disease cannot with certainty be diagnosed by microscopic examination of the blood or by injection of laboratory animals. Microscopic examination of the fluid obtained by puncture of swollen lymph nodes is the best method in early cases. In later cases microscopy of cerebrospinal fluid is preferable, although concentration of the trypanosomes by centrifugation is often necessary. Culture of the organism as a method of diagnosis is difficult and uncertain as compared with culture of *T. cruzi*. Immunologic methods are not usually successful in the diagnosis of sleeping sickness, except for the fluorescent antibody test which shows promise as a specific diagnostic method. A method of selecting cases for further study is based on the formation of precipitin bands by the patient's serum or cerebrospinal fluid in a gel containing antiserum against IgM, β_2 macroglobulins. Immunodiffusion plates prepared for this purpose can be obtained commercially.

It is impossible at present to distinguish sleeping sickness from other febrile and wasting diseases without demonstrating trypanosomes. These organisms must be sought with care in any patient who has been exposed to tsetse bites in an area in which sleeping sickness has ever been known to occur.

Treatment. The two essential drugs for treatment of sleeping sickness are *suramin* (Bayer 205) and *melarsoprol* (Mel B). Suramin can be used in the early febrile stage of the disease; but because it is a large molecule unable to pass the blood-brain barrier, it becomes ineffective once the central nervous system has been invaded; consequently examination of the cerebrospinal fluid is of importance in deciding which drug to use. If the cerebrospinal fluid is normal, suramin alone may be used, but if trypanosomes, lymphocytes, or a raised protein is found, melarsoprol becomes the drug of choice, preferably after a preliminary course of suramin. Suramin is given intravenously in a course of five doses of 1.0 gram every second day, and this may be repeated after a week. Suramin produces some toxicity to the kidney, with the appearance of casts and albumin in the urine. It causes fetal abnormality in rats, but this has not been noted in man. In Nigeria, 1 in 2000 patients has a dangerous sensitivity to suramin; this can be detected by giving a preliminary dose of 0.2 gram.

Melarsoprol is very dangerous and is contraindicated if suramin can be used, but it is effective in all stages of the disease and is active against most strains of *T. brucei,* including some that are tryparsamide resistant. Doses are given intravenously as the 3.6 per cent solution; three doses of 0.5, 1.0 and 1.5 ml are given at daily intervals, and after a week three more doses of 1.5, 2.0 and 2.5 are given, and so on until a total of 35 ml has been given. Thomson gives slightly higher dosage together with promethazine hydrochloride, 25 mg twice daily throughout the course, and he treats patients showing signs of encephalopathy with BAL, 2 ml every four hours. It must be emphasized, however, that this very high dosage should be reached only if the patient shows no signs of toxicity, notably of arsenic encephalopathy. Sudden death with encephalopathy may occur in the early stages of melarsoprol therapy; this may be due to sensitivity to arsenic or to the rapid liberation of trypanosomal antigen. It is therefore wise to begin therapy of the Rhodesian form with suramin to reduce the number of parasites before continuing with melarsoprol. The effect of melarsoprol therapy can be assessed by following the reduction of protein levels in the cerebrospinal fluid, but it can only be a rough guide because melarsoprol will of itself raise the level of protein for periods up to six months after injection. Melarsonyl potassium (Mel W) may be given intramuscularly, but less experience has been acquired concerning its curative effect. Nitrofurazone, which can be given by mouth (0.5 gram three times a day for 15 days) is even more toxic, but it may be the drug of choice in cases in which the patient is known to be sensitive—or his trypanosomes resistant—to arsenic. It is likely to cause polyneuritis and cardiac arrhythmia, and in patients with hereditary glucose-6-phosphate dehydrogenase deficiency it can cause severe hemolytic anemia (a property which it shares with melarsoprol). Tryparsamide is also used in combination with suramin for mass therapy of Gambian disease; it is not suitable for patients treated individually and is ineffective in the Rhodesian disease. It can produce toxic ambylopia leading to optic atrophy in some patients. The treatment of the trypanosomiasis should always be accompanied by an antimicrobial drug, because sleeping sickness leads to an increased susceptibility to bacterial infection.

Prognosis. Relapse may follow treatment, especially after suramin, when the central nervous system had been already involved at the time chemotherapy was started. Relapse may also occur because of drug resistance. Recovery after treatment is usually complete when the disease is treated at an early stage. If treatment is first given late in the disease, the survivors are often mentally sluggish and sometimes obese. A patient from whom trypanosomes have been isolated will sooner or later be killed by the disease unless it is treated. With Rhodesian disease the patient dies fairly soon, but with both Zambezi and Gambian disease the patient may survive for several years. It is suggested that some patients may be able to overcome the infection by natural means. If this in fact occurs, it is so exceptional that adequate treatment of diagnosed cases should always be performed. The neglect of an outbreak of sleeping sickness may result in extermination of the human population of the locality.

Prevention. African sleeping sickness can be prevented by measures aimed at destroying the habitat of the vector, the shade trees, and the other vegetation upon which the tsetse flies rest. As individual communities become larger, and especially when water sources are provided inside the villages, the risk to the inhabitants is reduced. The use of insecticides may also supplement this process. Elimination of the blood meal of the fly by game destruction programs has no effect on human sleeping sickness; neither has the liberation of sterile male tsetse met with much success.

Probably the most effective measures against the Rhodesian disease involve the isolation of human populations from areas known to harbor infective game and systematic search for and treatment of all infected humans. Search for and treatment of cases are even more important in Gambian disease, because man himself is the reservoir of infection.

Pentamidine, administered intramuscularly, is the

only suitable drug for *chemoprophylaxis,* and is of established effectiveness only against the Gambian disease. Its use is limited to the protection of a controlled population, such as a labor force, exposed to the Gambian disease. Pentamidine should not be used for therapy of individual cases of the disease, because, like suramin, it is not active within the nervous system. A single injection of 4 mg per kilogram is believed to provide a preventive effect in the Gambian disease for at least six months.

Blair, D. M., Burnett Smith, E., and Gelfand, M.: Human trypanosomiasis in Rhodesia. Cent. Afr. J. Med., 14 (Suppl.):1–12, 1968.

Hawking, F.: The differentiation of *Trypanosoma rhodesiense* from *T. brucei* by means of human serum. Trans. R. Soc. Trop. Med. Hyg., 67:517, 1973.

Mulligan, H. W., and Potts, W. H. (eds.): The African Trypanosomiases. London, Allen and Unwin, 1970.

Ormerod, W. E., and Venkatesan, S.: The occult visceral phase of mammalian trypanosomes with special reference to the life cycle of *Trypanosoma (Trypanozoon) brucei.* Trans. R. Soc. Trop. Med. Hyg., 65:722, 1971.

Robertson, D. H. H.: Chemotherapy of African trypanosomiasis. Practitioner, 188:80, 1962.

Thomson, K. D. B.: Melarsoprol tolerance in sleeping sickness patients of the Benue endemic zone. *In* Proceedings of 1st Medical Research Seminar, Yaba, Lagos, 1972, p. 242.

273. CHAGAS' DISEASE

Heonir Rocha

Definition. Chagas' disease is caused by an infection with a protozoan, *Trypanosoma cruzi.* It has a self-limited acute phase, detected only in a minority of infected persons. The disease usually presents as a chronic process, characterized by cardiac and digestive manifestations. In most cases there is no clinical evidence of the infection. In an endemic area, however, Chagas' disease is an important cause of morbidity and mortality.

Etiology. In the blood, *T. cruzi* is a spindle-shaped trypanosome showing a scanty undulating membrane and a large kinetoplast. Following penetration of tissue cells the parasite changes into Leishmania forms, which are round or ovoid bodies containing a large nucleus and a rodlike kinetoplast. Multiplication is cyclical and takes place intracellularly by binary fission. Within tissues there is production of intermediate forms, from which the circulating trypanosomes are derived. There are strains of *T. cruzi* with widely different virulence for mice; also, great differences in tissue tropism and antigenic structure have been documented. These variations have been considered of possible significance in clinical infections, and they could explain some of the diversity of the clinical picture of this disease in different geographic areas.

Epidemiology. Men and probably domestic animals (chiefly dogs and cats) infected with *T. cruzi* are the main reservoirs for contamination of the insect vectors. These vectors are winged but capable of only short flights, and are strictly hematophagous. They belong to the family Reduviidae, subfamily Triatominae, of which several dozen species have been found to be infected. However, only three species, *Triatoma infestans, Panstrongilus megistus,* and *Rhodnius prolixus,* well adapted to human dwellings, are major transmitters of the infection in large areas of South and Central America.

The insect vectors live in cracks and holes in walls and roofs, behind objects hanging on the walls, and in the thatch of primitive adobe houses. Their habits are very much like those of bedbugs; they feed at night or in the dark and seek shelter by day. The flagellate forms of *T. cruzi* are ingested with the blood meal by the insect, and after a series of changes and multiplications in the digestive tract of the vector, the metacyclic trypanosome forms are produced in large numbers and are discharged in the feces. The transmission of the disease usually results from contamination of mucous membranes or broken skin with feces containing the infective trypanosomes (so-called posterior-station transmission).

Occasionally man can be infected by blood transfusion or accidental laboratory contamination. Infection of the newborn via the placenta has also been documented. Transmission via breast milk and by eating infected meat has been reported.

Chagas' disease has been detected in a large area in the Western Hemisphere extending from the southern United States (Texas) to Argentina.

In the United States several species of wild rats, opossums, armadillos, and house mice have been found to be infected; also, several species of triatomid bugs have been found to have *T. cruzi.* However, the disease in humans is practically nonexistent in the United States. The major feature of the epidemiology of Chagas' disease is the association of infection in man and domestic animals with the presence of species of the insect vector in the domestic habitat. This intimate contact of man and vector is apparently lacking in the United States.

The incidence of Chagas' disease has been shown to be greatly variable, depending on the existence of favorable conditions for endemicity. Well-conducted epidemiologic studies are certainly needed to give a better picture of its geographic distribution. So far the disease has been reported only in the Americas, where it has been estimated that at least 7 million people are infected and 30 million are exposed to the risk of infection.

Pathogenesis and Pathology. The invading organism, after penetration through mucous membranes or skin, multiplies within cells of surrounding tissues or regional lymph nodes as Leishmania forms. These forms produce pseudocysts that eventually rupture, causing an inflammatory and lymphatic reaction. The liberated bodies either again penetrate adjacent tissue cells or invade the blood.

The lesions and clinical manifestations of the *acute stage* of the disease are mainly related to the destruction of cells by growth and multiplication of the parasite and the resulting inflammatory reaction. Practically every organ of the body may be invaded, but the reticuloendothelial system, muscle fibers (especially cardiac), and neuroglial cells of the central nervous system are more likely to be involved.

Inflammation is seen mainly around ruptured pseudocysts containing Leishmania, particularly in muscles. In the cardiac muscle there is diffuse interstitial mononuclear cell infiltration and interfibrillar edema, with many pseudocysts of Leishmania in the cardiac fibers; various degrees of muscle degeneration are also seen, waxy and fatty degeneration predominating. In the brain and meninges there is frequently a mild mononuclear infiltration.

Parasitemia may persist for 4 to 12 weeks, after which the parasite remains quiescent in tissues as Leishmania forms with occasional transient blood invasion.

In the *chronic stage,* the main pathologic lesions are observed in the heart and digestive tract. The heart is dilated and hypertrophied, with no valvular or specific vascular lesions. There are frequent mural thrombi, particularly in the right atrium and at the apex of the left ventricle with thinning of this region. Although this thinning may be extreme, leading to aneurysm of the apex, it does not seem to lead to rupture of the ventricle. The myocardium shows a variable degree of mononuclear inflammatory reaction, degenerative changes, and a predominant diffuse interstitial fibrosis. Quantitative studies of the intrinsic nervous system of the heart have shown a pronounced reduction in the number of parasympathetic ganglion cells. The presence of Leishmania within muscle fibers is detected in only about 30 per cent of chronic cases (Fig. 1). Embolic infarcts resulting from intramural thrombi are frequently found in the lungs, spleen, kidneys, and, occasionally, in the brain of patients dying from this disease.

Frequently the patients with digestive tract involvement have megaesophagus and/or megacolon with only minor inflammatory reaction in the myocardium; occasionally there also is severe diffuse myocarditis. In the esophagus and colon there is a marked decrease in the number of cells of the autonomic nervous system, and there are focal inflammatory lesions in the muscular layer. It is thought that megaesophagus and megacolon are the result of destruction of the intramural nervous system, probably related to the parasitic infection and to the secondary inflammatory and vascular lesions.

The detection of widespread inflammation in the myocardium, not associated with the presence of the parasite, the production of similar tissue lesions in mice injected with just an extract of *T. cruzi,* the continuous destruction of muscle fibers, and the necrotizing arteriolar lesions described in muscular layers of the esophagus have suggested an immune allergic mechanism for lesions of the acute phase and particularly of the chronic phase of this disease. Furthermore, the reduction of the intrinsic nervous control of the heart and digestive tract has been taken as an important pathogenic mechanism in this parasitic infection.

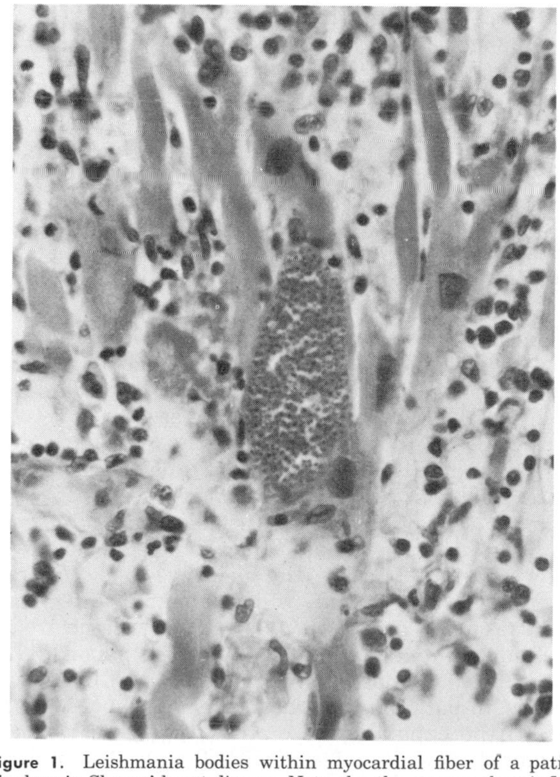

Figure 1. Leishmania bodies within myocardial fiber of a patient with chronic Chagas' heart disease. Note also the mononuclear inflammatory reaction and edema.

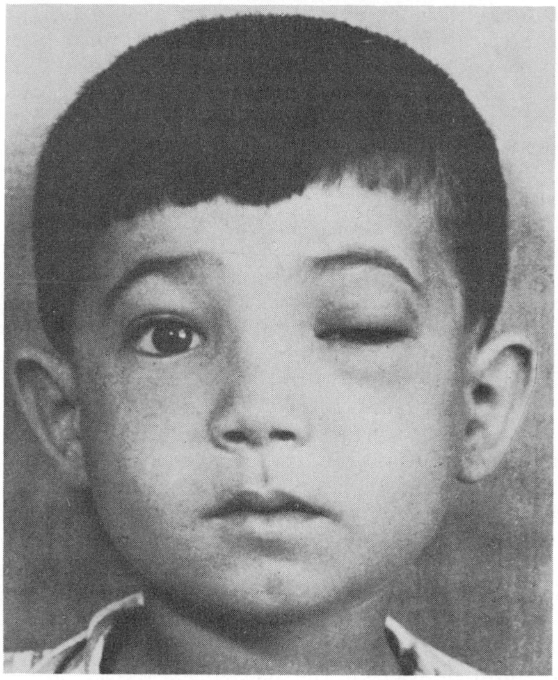

Figure 2. Romaña's sign in acute Chagas' disease. Note unilateral periorbital edema. (Courtesy of Professor Aluizio Prata, Salvador, Bahia, Brazil.)

Clinical Manifestations. In the course of Chagas' disease there are distinct phases with peculiar clinical features.

Acute Form. In an endemic area, the acute manifestations of Chagas' disease usually occur in the first decade of life, and are recognized in only a small minority of infected cases. The local signs at the portal of entry frequently call the attention of the physician to the condition. Characteristically there is *unilateral* painless periorbital edema with mild conjunctival reaction, a bluish or darkish discoloration of the skin, and satellite lymphadenopathy usually with enlarged preauricular lymph nodes. These physical findings are referred to as Romaña's sign (Fig. 2). The subsidence of the palpebral edema usually takes four to eight weeks.

In a minority of cases, the initial lesion occurs in other exposed areas of the skin. It is usually a lesion resembling a furuncle that increases to become a purplish indurated papule, 4 to 6 cm in diameter, with regional adenopathy, leaving a pigmented scar when it subsides.

Concomitantly with the local signs the patient develops a variable clinical picture usually characterized by malaise, anorexia, remittent or continuous fever, mild generalized nontender lymphadenopathy, moderate hepatosplenomegaly, and, in some instances, peripheral edema or a generalized edema of varying degrees which supervenes later on in the course. In a few cases a morbilliform or maculopapular erythematous skin rash is present. The pulse is usually fast (even when fever is absent) and regular. In severe cases there may be marked cardiac dilatation, gallop rhythm, and signs of heart failure. Myocarditis of variable degree probably occurs in all cases, but it is severe only in a very small percentage. Laboratory findings include a moderate leukocytosis with lymphocytosis, increased sedimentation rate, increase in alpha-2 and gamma globulins, and decrease in serum albumin. The serum glutamic oxaloacetic transaminase (SGOT) has been found elevated in severe cases. Electrocardiographic (EKG) abnormalities are present in about 50 per cent of patients, commonly showing prolongation of P-R interval, low voltage of QRS, and primary T wave changes. These are more pronounced in the most severe cases. The presence of intraventricular block is a very ominous sign.

The disease subsides within two or three months in 90 to 95 per cent of cases. The 5 to 10 per cent fatality rate is usually related to severe myocarditis, acute meningoencephalitis (occurring in the newborn or in the very young), or complicating bronchopneumonia. *In the great majority of patients with the chronic form of Chagas' disease there is no history of an acute phase.* It is thought that probably only 1 per cent of infected subjects have noticeable clinical signs following the initial contamination.

Indeterminate or Latent Phase. Patients who had acute manifestations of the disease, as well as those with inapparent infection, may remain asymptomatic for periods of 10 to 30 years, or for their whole lives. Those patients show only serologic evidence of the disease by complement-fixation (positive Machado-Guerreiro reaction), and occasionally the parasite can be recovered from their blood. This is actually the most common situation in an endemic area. Yet, there are few clinical and anatomic data available concerning this particular stage of the disease.

Chronic Form. The chronic manifestations of *T. cruzi* infection are primarily due to cardiac and digestive involvement.

CARDIAC MANIFESTATIONS. Approximately 20 to 40 per cent of patients with chronic *T. cruzi* infection in an endemic area exhibit evidence of heart damage. This is the most important finding in the chronic phase of this disease. Symptoms and signs are the result of a progressive diffuse chronic myocarditis.

In the early stages the patient may have no symptoms, and the diagnosis of heart disease rests on the electrocardiographic changes.

With the advanced disease the patient may present a clinical picture of heart failure of gradual onset, with serious systemic congestion. Signs of right-sided heart failure usually predominate over those of left ventricular failure. The pulse is weak and irregular because of ventricular premature contractions. The heart is greatly enlarged, the heart sounds are muffled, and there is a systolic murmur of functional mitral insufficiency and sometimes one of tricuspid regurgitation. A widely split second pulmonic sound and an apical third heart sound are commonly heard. The heart shadow roentgenographically shows marked global enlargement, with clear pulmonary fields (Fig. 3). The course of these patients is usually complicated by pulmonary or systemic embolism arising from the frequently occurring mural thrombi. Occasionally, the episode of heart failure begins abruptly, without apparent precipitating cause, usually running a short fatal course; on other occasions it is brought on by pregnancy or delivery, severe pulmonary infection, or an associated severe chronic anemia.

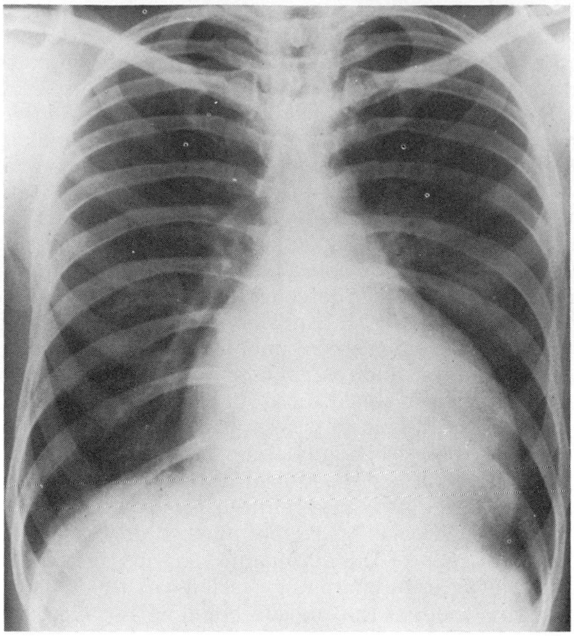

Figure 3. Chest film in a case of chronic Chagas' heart disease. Marked global enlargement of cardiac shadow, with clear pulmonary fields.

In some instances the patient may complain only of palpitation or syncopal attacks resulting from disturbances in cardiac rhythm (ventricular premature contractions or atrioventricular block, Adams-Stokes attacks). In cases of complete atrioventricular block the patient may present with Adams-Stokes syndrome. Rarely, the first manifestation of chronic Chagas' disease is a cerebral embolism owing to dislodgement of a thrombus located in the left ventricle.

A great variety of EKG abnormalities are detected in chronic Chagas' heart disease. Complete right bundle branch block is the most frequent conduction disturbance, occurring in about 50 per cent of cases; similarly, ventricular premature contractions (usually multifocal) are present in half the patients; also frequent are negative symmetric T waves. Atrioventricular block of variable degree occurs in one third of cases, but complete A-V block is detected in only about 10 per cent. Atrial fibrillation or flutter is relatively uncommon (about 10 per cent), and left bundle branch block is rare.

DIGESTIVE MANIFESTATIONS. Megaesophagus and megacolon are important manifestations of chronic *T. cruzi* infection. The evidence for the etiologic role of the parasite in these conditions is (1) the high incidence of these abnormalities in endemic areas of Chagas' disease; (2) the finding of a positive Machado-Guerreiro reaction in 85 per cent of patients with megacolon or megaesophagus in endemic areas. When xenodiagnosis is also performed in these cases, the incidence of *T. cruzi* infection rises to 95 per cent, which is significantly higher than that in the general population of the same area; (3) the frequent detection of EKG changes (about 50 per cent), similar to those described in chronic Chagas' myocarditis, in patients with megacolon or megaesophagus; and (4) the capability of reproducing these lesions in animals chronically infected with *T. cruzi.* This infection in animals and humans produces a marked decrease in the number of cells of the autonomic nervous system in esophagus and colon with disturbance in motility, even in the absence of anatomic changes of these organs. Conversely, fibrosis and degeneration of autonomic ganglia have been demonstrated in the heart of individuals with megaesophagus.

Patients with megaesophagus complain of longstanding progressive dysphagia, regurgitation, retrosternal discomfort, and sometimes paroxysmal attacks of night cough. They may get repeated respiratory infections as a result of aspirations of esophageal contents. The esophagus becomes enormously dilated, and in some cases it can be seen in a plain chest film as a right paramediastinal shadow.

Megacolon is characterized by persistent severe constipation of many years' duration. The incidence of fecal impaction and volvulus with intestinal obstruction is high in endemic areas of Chagas' disease.

The concomitance of megaesophagus, megacolon, and heart failure is not common. Most frequently, patients with digestive involvement present only EKG abnormalities or a moderate enlargement of the heart.

Prenatal Chagas' Disease. Prenatal transmission of *T. cruzi* infection has been verified by clinical and experimental observations. The mother may be in the latent or indeterminate phase of the disease.

The infected newborn may present generalized edema, enlargement of liver and spleen, petechiae or purpuric manifestations, sometimes jaundice, and a picture of meningoencephalitis. The pathologic findings are those of acute Chagas' disease. A microscopic picture of placentitis occurs in those instances. The characteristic feature is the finding of Leishmania within histiocytes of the inflammatory reaction. It has been shown that this infection may be responsible for premature birth or fetal death. The possibility exists of evolution to chronicity of a prenatally transmitted *T. cruzi* infection, but conclusive demonstration in humans is needed.

Diagnosis. In the acute stage, the diagnosis lies mainly in the demonstration of the parasite in the blood of the patient. *T. cruzi* may be seen in a fresh blood smear, in a thick-drop preparation of blood, or in a buffy coat smear up to three months after the onset of the disease. As the parasitemia decreases, or if blood preparations are negative, xenodiagnosis or animal inoculation of freshly drawn blood or blood culture can be used. Xenodiagnosis is a method of having laboratory-bred triatomid bugs feed on patients and examining the insects 40 days later for the presence of *T. cruzi* in the intestinal tract. The method is practical and is very sensitive in the detection of this stage of Chagas' disease. Blood culture in NNN media and inoculation of blood in young mice or guinea pigs require special laboratory facilities, but can be helpful particularly when xenodiagnosis is not available. A precipitin reaction using antigen obtained from *T. cruzi* culture gives positive results in almost every acute case.

The clinical diagnosis of chronic Chagas' heart disease is based on the following: (1) epidemiologic evidence (patient from endemic area, usually of poor socioeconomic group); (2) clinical picture of primary myocardial disease (enlarged heart, with no signs of valvular, coronary artery, or any other cause of heart disease); (3) EKG changes of the types (previously mentioned) usually seen in Chagas' disease; and (4) serologic evidence of infection or isolation of *T. cruzi.*

The most valuable procedure in diagnosing chronic Chagas' disease is the complement-fixation test (Machado-Guerreiro reaction), which is positive in about 95 per cent of cases. Xenodiagnosis is positive in only about 20 per cent of chronic cases.

Differential diagnosis may include rheumatic heart disease, particularly when there is a loud systolic murmur simulating organic valvular disease, in patients under 30 years of age. Coronary heart disease may be another difficult problem in patients over 40. It is often impossible on clinical grounds to dissociate chronic myocarditis owing to Chagas' disease from certain cardiomyopathies of unknown cause. Besides the great help derived from careful evaluation of clinical and epidemiologic data, the Machado-Guerreiro reaction and xenodiagnosis are of major importance in making a definite diagnosis of Chagas' disease.

Clinical Course and Prognosis. Acute Chagas' disease is relatively benign, with subsidence of symptoms in 90 to 95 per cent of cases. The chronic form usually has a slowly progressive course. It is clear that by no means all of those infected ultimately develop the serious forms of the disease, but the exact proportion that do so is not known. This important question could be settled only by a large-scale, long-term prospective epidemiologic study; the need for such a study is great.

Sudden and unexpected death is common in Chagas' disease. Complete A-V block, multifocal premature ventricular contractions, ventricular tachycardia, and marked enlargement of the heart with signs of heart failure are severe prognostic signs. Pulmonary embolism is a frequent terminal complication in patients with heart failure.

Treatment. There is no satisfactory treatment for *T. cruzi* infection. Several chemotherapeutic agents have been tried without success, including primaquine, pyrimethamine, nitrofurans (levofuraltadone), aminopterin, intravenous gentian violet, amphotericin B, and puromycin, among others. These agents may cause transient disappearance of parasitemia, but follow-up studies usually show a relapse. This is probably related to the ineffectiveness of all those agents against the tissue forms of the parasite. Some of them (nitrofurans) may demonstrate great potency against *T. cruzi* in tissue cultures, and also in experimental infection in mice. However, despite extensive killing of intracellular parasites, some intact leishmanial bodies can always be found in the tissues of the laboratory animal. None of the drugs commonly employed in the treatment of African trypanosomiasis have shown value in Chagas' disease (see Ch. 272). Several new drugs are under trial, Bayer 2502 ("Lampit") being one of them. Unfortunately the results have not been uniformly promising.

After a certain degree of tissue damage has occurred, even the eradication of the parasite may not prevent the progression of the disease. In chronic cases, therapy is only symptomatic, comprising the usual measures for heart failure, Adams-Stokes syndrome, megaesophagus, megacolon, or one of its complications. Digitalis preparations should be managed with great care because of the unusual degree of sensitivity to toxic effects.

Prevention. Controlling the transmission of the disease is the most important preventive measure. This requires housing of satisfactory quality; moreover, it requires the repeated systematic application of residual insecticides (benzene hexachloride) effective against the triatomid bugs. For individual short-term protection, fine-mesh bed nets are useful.

Blood transfusion is a potential hazard in endemic

areas. The incidence of positive Machado-Guerreiro reactions among blood donors may be as high as 15 per cent. To prevent infection from transfusions, the addition of gentian or crystal violet to the blood has been used. Persons having a positive complement-fixation test should not be accepted as potential blood donors.

The production of a vaccine to prevent human infection is, certainly, another possible approach. Mice can be protected against a fatal *T. cruzi* challenge by prior inoculation with a strain of mild pathogenicity. However, as it is impossible to predict the potential virulence to man of a *T. cruzi* strain of low pathogenicity to lower animals, only vaccines of killed parasites should be tried at present, and so far they have failed to be protective.

Anselmi, A., and Moleiro, F.: Physiopathology of Chagas' heart disease: Correlations between clinical and experimental findings. Bull. WHO, 44:659, 1971.

Köberle, F.: Chagas' heart disease (pathology). Cardiologia (Basel), 52:82, 1969.

Laranja, F. S., Dias, E., Nobrega, G., and Miranda, A.: Chagas' disease. A clinical, epidemiologic and pathologic study. Circulation, 14:1035, 1956.

Prata, A., Köberle, F., and Puigbo, J. J.: Chagas' heart disease. Cardiologia, 52:79, 1968.

Resenbaum, M. B.: Chagasic myocardiopathy. Prog. Cardiovasc. Dis., 7:199, 1964.

Woody, N. C., and Woody, H. B.: American trypanosomiasis. I. Clinical and epidemiological background of Chagas' disease in the United States. J. Pediatr., 58:568, 1961.

World Health Organization: Chagas' Disease, Report of a Study Group. Technical Report Series No. 202, 1960.

274. PNEUMOCYSTOSIS

Thomas C. Jones

Pneumocystosis is an acute pulmonary disease characterized by fever, tachypnea, dyspnea, and cyanosis which occurs in immunodeficient patients and malnourished or premature infants. It is caused by species of the genus Pneumocystis, organisms of uncertain classification, but probably protozoa. The organisms cause asymptomatic infection in healthy mammalian hosts and are seen extracellularly in cysts in the pulmonary alveoli.

History. In 1909 Carlos Chagas described what he thought was a stage of sporogony of *Trypanosoma cruzi* occurring in the lungs of experimentally infected guinea pigs. The next year Carini observed the same forms in rats infected with *T. lewisi*. In 1912 Delanoe and Delanoe recognized that the "cyst of Carini" was not part of the life cycle of trypanosomes, but was a different organism. The first reports of such an organism in humans appeared in 1938 when Ammich and Beneke independently described them in the lungs of infants dying during the first year of life. Epidemics of the disease in institutionalized children were subsequently described throughout Europe. In 1953 Vanek, Jirovec, and Lukes recognized the relationship between Pneumocystis and the pathologic entity interstitial plasma cell pneumonia. Reports of pneumocystosis have increased since that time, associated with the increased use of corticosteroids and antimetabolites as therapy in malignant disease or in patients undergoing organ transplantation, and with the increased life span of patients with congenital immunodeficient syndromes.

Organism. The life cycle of Pneumocystis is unknown. At present, one can only postulate that the life cycle in lungs of infected mammals includes an extracystic body or trophozoite which changes to a cyst followed by the development of oval bodies within the cyst. These are then released to initiate another cycle. A trophozoite-to-trophozoite cycle may also occur. The cyst stage of the organism is found in exudate within the alveoli. It is 5 to 6 μ in diameter, and its outer wall stains well with methenamine silver nitrate (see Fig. 2*G*, Ch. 271), Gram-Weigert stains or periodic acid–Schiff reagents. Using Giemsa stain, the oval bodies (1 to 2 μ in diameter) can be recognized within the cyst and are usually eight in number. Under the electron microscope these oval bodies are seen to have a nuclear mass, endoplasmic reticulum, ribosomes, and mitochondria. The oval bodies are released from the cyst, after which they are termed trophozoites or extracystic bodies; they move freely about the alveoli, and become the nidus for new cysts to form.

Epidemiology. Pneumocystis species are widely distributed, affecting rodents, rabbits, sheep, dogs, and other mammals, in addition to humans. It is unlikely that animals serve as a reservoir for infection of humans, since organisms of different mammals appear to be host specific. For the same reason, the species name *P. carinii* should not be used to name the organism seen in humans, but should be reserved for the organism identified in rodents. Evidence at present best supports the thesis that infection is transmitted by the respiratory route by droplet spray. In a few cases congenital infection has been considered the most likely route of infection.

Epidemiologic data suggest that the organism is highly infectious, that infection is usually asymptomatic, and that apparently healthy, infected individuals can transmit the disease to immunodeficient patients. This is supported by observations in animals that healthy rats and rabbits when caged communally acquire the infection, and when the animals are rendered immunodeficient by corticosteroid administration, disease may be manifest. It is supported in humans by the high prevalence (4 per cent) of the organism in routine autopsy studies, the increased prevalence of antibodies to Pneumocystis in personnel working in medical institutions (7 to 15 per cent), the epidemics of disease in the institutionalized patients, and the sporadic clusters of cases in hospitalized immunodeficient patients.

Disease that follows recent infection or is associated with latent infection has been seen most commonly in patients with hypogammaglobulinemia of immunoglobulins G or M, in patients in the second to fourth months of life (when passively transferred maternal antibodies first reach low levels), or in patients receiving corticosteroids or antimetabolites. A few patients not on immunosuppressive drugs and with normal immunoglobulin levels and a few patients with isolated defects in cellular immunity have acquired the disease. Organisms reach high numbers in the lungs of infected persons showing clinical disease, and it is likely that these patients can more readily spread the disease than asymptomatic carriers.

Pathology and Pathogenesis. When conditions exist in the alveoli for the multiplication of Pneumocystis, an inflammatory response is elicited which includes transudation of fluid into the alveoli and thickening of alveolar interstitial spaces. The alveoli become filled with foamy, proteinaceous material in which trophozoite nuclei are found along with clumps of the Pneumocystis cysts. The interstitial spaces have been noted to contain predominantly plasma cells and alveolar epithelial cells when pathologic material was studied in malnourished or premature infants; hence the origin of the pathologic description, interstitial plasma cell pneumonia. However, in the immunodeficient child or adult, this pattern is not seen. The inflammatory response in these patients has been described as primarily lymphocytes, macrophages, and occasionally eosinophils. Polymorphonuclear leukocytes are not seen. The lung is usually diffusely involved with this process, although localized disease has occasionally been described. The lung is firm and rubbery in consistency. Other organisms, such as cytomegalovirus or bacteria, are frequently found in association with Pneumocystis. Less commonly, Pneumocystis is found in lungs which also contain mycobacteria, fungi, or toxoplasma. Rarely, pneumocystis may become generalized, involving lymph nodes, spleen, and bone marrow.

Clinical Manifestations. The major symptoms of pneumocystosis are tachypnea and a nonproductive cough. These symptoms often develop insidiously over a period of several weeks and may be associated with fever, dyspnea, and cyanosis. It has been noted that these symptoms may first appear during the period when corticosteroids are being withdrawn. The disease may also present with an abrupt onset (over two to three days) of high, spiking fever, cough, dyspnea, and cyanosis, with the patient reaching a moribund state within a few days. Most of the patients presenting with this rapid course have been on continuous high doses of corticosteroids. In the United States at present the disease which presents with an abrupt onset may be more common than the more insidious onset characteristic of the illness seen in institutionalized infants in Europe. After renal transplantation, pneumocystosis has been recorded as responsible for 10 per cent of pulmonary infections and usually occurs three to four months after transplantation.

On physical examination the patient shows signs of respiratory distress (tachypnea and dyspnea) associated with fever and cyanosis. Auscultation of the lungs may reveal no abnormalities, although scattered rales and rhonchi may be heard.

There are no diagnostic laboratory tests. *The white blood cell count* may reflect the underlying disease of the patient or other complications, but leukocytosis may be seen. Significant eosinophilia has occasionally been reported, particularly in children with humoral immune deficiency. *The blood gases* will usually indicate hyperventilation and decreased oxygen saturation even while the patient is on continuous oxygen, consistent with an alveolar capillary block syndrome. Some have reported associated mild respiratory acidosis. *The chest radiograph* usually shows diffuse mixed alveolar and interstitial pneumonitis. This appears as a granular haziness beginning in the hilar region. A few cases of more localized disease have been seen, giving a segmental distribution. An air bronchogram is often seen. Pleural effusion does not occur.

Course. In immunodeficient patients the course of pneumocystosis will usually be one of progressive deterioration unless improvement occurs in the underlying immune defect. Increasing pulmonary consolidation, cyanosis, and death are the natural history of the disease. After institution of specific therapy against pneumocystis, improvement begins in five to ten days. The roentgenographic findings may become transiently worse after institution of therapy, but will then show gradual improvement over one to three weeks. Some have suggested that pneumocystosis of long duration may lead to interstitial fibrosis or emphysema. This has been difficult to document in view of the many factors leading to pulmonary changes in these patients.

Diagnosis. Once the suspicion of pneumocystis is raised by the clinical setting of immune deficiency and progressive pulmonary symptoms, the patient should be considered for lung biopsy or "brush" biopsy. Most centers now recommend open lung biopsy rather than needle biopsy because the latter provides no visualization of the lung, a smaller sample, and a greater risk of lung collapse or bleeding. Biopsy is required to distinguish pneumocystosis from drug-induced interstitial fibrosis, cytomegalovirus infection, aspergillus or other fungi, unusual forms of bacterial bronchopneumonia, toxoplasmosis, or leukemic infiltration. Impression smears of the biopsy specimen at the time of surgery can be fixed in methanol and stained with Giemsa, methenamine silver, or Gram-Weigert stains and carefully examined for the presence of Pneumocystis cysts. Specimens are also preserved for bacterial and fungal cultures. If the biopsy must be delayed, or if surgery is believed to be contraindicated for other reasons, then a therapeutic trial with specific drugs against Pneumocystis should be instituted. Recently, use of bronchoscopy with a "brush" biopsy has been considered. This may show Pneumocystis; however, the sampling error and absence of tissue for histologic examination make it less valuable than open lung biopsy. Examination of sputum for cysts should be attempted, although in the immunodeficient patient this has usually not been revealing. Increased use of appropriate fixing and staining techniques on sputum and more careful sputum examination may improve the value of this simple test. Immunofluorescent antibody tests are now being evaluated. However, they show significantly elevated titers in only about 30 per cent of cases of pneumocystosis. Although measurement of antibody response using fluorescent antibody techniques is relatively insensitive, it appears to be specific. Thus a change in titer from negative to positive adds support to the diagnosis, whereas the absence of such a change does not exclude it.

Treatment. Therapy for pneumocystosis if started early in the disease has proved to be quite successful. During the past decade pentamidine isethionate has been used. This has reduced mortality from Pneumocystis infection from near 100 per cent to 10 to 50 per cent. The drug is made rapidly available by calling the Parasitic Disease Drug Service, U.S. Public Health Service (404-633-3311). The patient is given 4 mg per kilogram per day intramuscularly for 12 to 14 days. The mechanism of action of the drug remains unknown, but it does cause megaloblastic cell changes, inhibits incorporation of nucleotides into DNA and RNA, and inhibits oxidative phosphorylation. Folinic acid therapy can be used in patients who develop signs of folate deficiency without interfering with action of the drug against the organism. Pentamidine may also cause hypoglycemia, hyperglycemia, and nephrotoxicity. When given intravenously, hypotension can occur. The possibility that pentamidine causes pulmonary interstitial fibrosis has been raised by studies in animals. Because of these observed and potential toxic effects, another drug combination, pyrimethamine and sulfadiazine, has been tested for treatment of pneumocystis. Although there have been fewer patients treated with this combination than with pentamidine, it appears to be effective. These drugs interfere with the synthesis of folinic acid. For treatment of adults, pyrimethamine is given, 25 mg per day, and sulfadiazine, 1 gram four times daily. Folinic acid, 6 mg daily intramuscularly, will prevent significant bone marrow toxicity.

Because of the relationship between the occurrence of

pneumocystis and hypogammaglobulinemia, gamma globulin administration has been recommended. However, commercially available gamma globulin has proved to be of little value when given alone for treatment of pneumocystis. In general, attempts should be made to reduce the dose of corticosteroids when signs of pneumocystosis appear; however, in some patients whose respiratory symptoms developed during tapering of corticosteroids, a transient *increase* in the dose of these drugs while pneumocystosis therapy is started should be considered. Supportive measures such as oxygen therapy, assisted ventilation, and careful fluid and electrolyte balance are important parts of the management.

Prevention. In order to interrupt spread of pneumocystis infection, a great deal must be learned about its life cycle. Since the diseased patient may be able to spread the organism to other patients, healthy personnel, and relatives, appropriate respiratory precautions should be considered when the diagnosis is suspected. Attention to preventing contact between susceptible patients and diseased patients in open wards and in clinics may reduce the spread of the disease. The disease will be controlled only when the relationships between certain types of immune deficiency or corticosteroids and rapid proliferation of the organism are better understood.

Burke, B. A., and Good, R. A.: *Pneumocystis carinii* infection. Medicine, 52:23, 1973.

Norman, L., and Kagan, I. G.: Some observations on the serology of *Pneumocystis carinii* infections in the United States. Infect. Immun., 8:317, 1973.

Robbins, J. B.: *Pneumocystis carinii* pneumonitis. A review. Pediatr. Res., 1:131, 1967.

Rosen, P., Armstrong, D., and Ramos, C.: *Pneumocystis carinii* pneumonia. A clinicopathologic study of twenty patients with neoplastic diseases. Am. J. Med., 53:428, 1972.

Vogel, C. L., Cohen, M. H., Powell, R. D., Jr., and DeVita, V. T.: *Pneumocystis carinii* pneumonia. Ann. Intern. Med., 68:97, 1968.

LEISHMANIASIS

Anthony D. M. Bryceson

275. INTRODUCTION

Definition. Leishmaniasis is an infection with parasites of the genus Leishmania. It is usually a zoonosis transmitted by phlebotomine sandflies between wild or peridomestic animals, especially rodents or canines. Man is infected when he interrupts the natural cycle.

In man the infection is either visceral or cutaneous. Visceral leishmaniasis is a severe chronic infection of the reticuloendothelial system, characterized by fever, chills, weight loss, splenomegaly, leukopenia, anemia, and a high natural mortality. It is caused by *L. donovani.* Cutaneous leishmaniasis is characterized by single or several chronic sores which usually heal spontaneously. In parts of South and Central America, severely mutilating metastatic lesions of the mouth and nose are seen. Cutaneous leishmaniasis is caused by *L. tropica* in the Old World, and by members of the *L. mexicana* and *L. braziliensis* groups in the New World.

Etiology. Leishmania exist in two forms, one in the vertebrate host, including man, and the other in the sandfly and in artificial culture. In the vertebrate host the parasite is in the amastigote (Leishman-Donovan body) stage, so called because it has no flagellum. It is a round or oval body 2 to 3 μ across, containing a nucleus and a smaller kinetoplast which stain respectively red and purple with Geimsa, Wright's, or Leishman's stain, and stand out against the pale blue cytoplasm. Leishmania are strict intracellular parasites and are found in macrophages in which they multiply by binary fission. Heavily parasitized host cells rupture, and fresh cells are invaded. Sandflies become infected when they feed on an infected person or animal and take up parasites from blood or skin. In the sandfly the parasite is in the promastigote (leptomonad) stage, so called because of the anterior origin of its flagellum. Promastigotes are supple, highly motile, spindle-shaped organisms, 15 to 25 μ long and 1.5 to 3.5 μ broad. Promastigotes are found in the midgut of the sandfly, where they divide and whence they migrate forward into the pharynx and buccal cavity, rendering the sandfly infective. The cycle of development in the sandfly takes about seven days. Once inoculated into man, the promastigote rapidly penetrates macrophages, flagellum first, and transforms into an amastigote.

Immunology. The patterns of disease in man are partly determined by the species of parasite (trophism for skin or viscera, differences in immunogenicity and allergenicity) and partly by man's response to the parasite. Resistance to Leishmania depends upon the development of specific cell-mediated immunity. The capacity of individuals to mount such a response varies, and consequently leishmaniasis presents a spectrum of disease in the same way that leprosy does. At one end of the spectrum lie visceral leishmaniasis and diffuse cutaneous leishmaniasis, characterized by abundance of parasites, absence of lymphocytes in lesions, insensitivity to leishmanin, and poor prognosis. At the other end lie the self-healing sores, with relatively scanty parasites, marked lymphocytic infiltration, and leishmanin sensitivity. Accompanying cell-mediated immunity is delayed hypersensitivity to numerous parasite antigens, which causes the destructive pathology of leishmanial ulcers, especially in the chronic conditions of espundia (see below) and leishmaniasis recidiva (see below) in which the normal balance between immunity and hypersensitivity has been lost. The mechanisms underlying these abnormal immune responses are not understood.

Antibody, which is produced in large quantities in visceral leishmaniasis, is not protective, and it has been suggested that it may even contribute to the pathogenesis of hemolytic anemia, nephritis, and amyloidosis. Healing is usually accompanied by long-lasting immunity to the particular species of Leishmania involved, but not to other species.

Leishmanin (Montenegro) Test. Leishmanin is a suspension of 10^6 promastigotes in 1 ml of 0.5 per cent phenol saline. The test is performed by injecting 0.1 ml intradermally into the volar surface of the forearm. A palpable nodule, 5 mm or more in diameter after 48 to 72 hours, is considered positive. The test is an index of delayed hypersensitivity, but not necessarily of immunity to Leishmania. It is not species specific. It is used to map out the extent of past infection in a community and may be of help in diagnosis in individual patients.

276. VISCERAL LEISHMANIASIS (Kala-Azar, Ponos)

Epidemiology. It has been suggested that the zoonotic origin of *L. donovani* was among jackals in the steppes of Central Asia, where sporadic cases of visceral leishmaniasis are still sometimes seen among nomads and in settlers in the outskirts of rapidly expanding towns. From here the disease spread and developed three distinct epidemiologic patterns.

Visceral Leishmaniasis with a Canine Reservoir. This is the pattern in a belt which stretches from Portugal to Peking between latitudes 30 and 48 degrees North, the most important areas being the Mediterranean littoral, including North Africa, the shores of the Caspian Sea, central Soviet Asia, and northeast China. The main vectors are *Phlebotomus perniciosus* in Western Europe, *P. major* in Eastern Europe, *P. papatasii* in the Middle East, and *P. chinensis* in China. In the Mediterranean and Chinese foci, the host-parasite relationship is relatively stable, and the disease is most common among children between one and four years of age. For this reason the parasite is sometimes called *L. infantum,* although adults in areas into which the disease has newly been introduced or visitors of any age are highly susceptible. Domestic dogs and foxes are the reservoir.

Portuguese and Spanish settlers probably introduced *L. donovani,* also called *L. chagasi,* into the New World and initiated a zoonosis among foxes and dogs, although man may still be important as a reservoir. The likely vector is *P. longipalpis*. Visceral leishmaniasis is epidemic in northeast Brazil and sporadic in Amazonia, northern Argentina, and Paraguay and extends up through Venezuela and Colombia as far as Guatemala and Mexico. In Brazil male children are most commonly affected.

Visceral Leishmaniasis with a Rodent Vector. This is the pattern in Africa south of the Sahara from Lake Chad in the west to Somalia in the east, sparing the highlands of Ethiopia. The apparent absence of the disease in West Africa and south of the equator is unexplained. In the Sudan the zoonosis is between the Nile rat (*Arvicanthus niloticus*) and *P. orientalis* on the flood plains of the Nile and its tributaries. Visceral leishmaniasis is found among nomads who occupy temporary villages in riverine acacia woodland and migrant workers from adjoining countries.

In Kenya the disease is associated with termite hills where the vector *P. martini* rests and around which village men gather in the evenings. The reservoir is probably the gerbil *Tatara vicina*. The disease is usually sporadic, but epidemics have occurred. Males are affected four times as often as females, and the disease is most common in teenagers.

Visceral Leishmaniasis with a Human Reservoir. This is true epidemic kala-azar and is the pattern of the disease in northeast India, Bangladesh, Assam, and Burma. Classically the disease spreads along the Brahmaputra valley every 20 years or so. Transmission is by the highly anthroposophilic, domestic sandfly *P. argentipes*. Often, many cases are found to have originated from one house. The age and sex pattern is the same as in Africa. Man is the only reservoir, and *P. argentipes* is readily infected from blood or from the lesions of post-kala-azar dermal leishmaniasis. The disease virtually disappeared over large areas as a result of DDT spraying for malaria control, but could spread again now that spraying has stopped.

Factors Affecting Transmission. Opportunities for contact with infected sandflies largely determine the pattern of disease in a given area. This is modified by the level of immunity of the population or individual. An attack of visceral leishmaniasis confers lifelong immunity, which determines the periodicity of epidemics. Subclinical infections with *L. donovani* or possibly even lizard and rodent species of Leishmania affect the pattern of spread in Africa.

Pathology. The organs most severely affected are the spleen, liver, bone marrow, lymph nodes, intestines, and skin. The patient suffers from hyperplasia within and damage to these organs and from effects secondary to splenomegaly, reticuloendothelial blockage, and chronic parasitemia. Histologically the disease is characterized by massive proliferation of parasitized macrophages with little or no lymphocytic response. In Africa and Central Asia a cutaneous nodule or leishmanioma commonly develops at the site of parasite inoculation. Parasites multiply within histiocytes which may become the focus of a tuberculoid granuloma that heals spontaneously, and the infection proceeds no further. In the majority of cases, however, after a period of months, the infection disseminates.

The spleen is grossly enlarged, smooth, and firm and the capsule thick. The pulp is friable and infarcts are usual. There is massive hyperplasia of reticuloendothelial cells which are heavily parasitized. In the liver, Kupffer cells are hyperplastic and contain parasites. Occasionally parenchymal cells are parasitized. In chronic untreated cases there is parenchymal cell degeneration which may be followed after several years by fibrosis and even cirrhosis with clinical and biochemical evidence of hepatic dysfunction.

The bone marrow is heavily infiltrated with parasitized macrophages. Erythropoiesis and granulopoiesis are normal in the early stages of the disease, but may be depressed later. The peripheral blood shows anemia and leukopenia. The anemia is probably due to increased plasma volume, sequestration of erythrocytes in the spleen, and hemolysis. Leukopenia is said to predispose the patient to secondary infections. Lymph nodes and lymphoid tissue of the nasopharynx and gut are enlarged and contain many parasitized cells.

Kidneys may show cloudy swelling of tubular cells. In fatal cases hyaline thickening of the glomerular mesangium has been found, and in chronic cases amyloidosis can develop. The skin, although normal in appearance, contains many intracellular parasites. In *post-kala-azar dermal leishmaniasis* there is variable infiltration with lymphocytes, histiocytes, and parasites.

In visceral leishmaniasis there is an enormous overproduction of IgG, only a small fraction of which is specific antibody. Some of it is autoantibody.

Clinical Features. The incubation period is normally two to six months, but may be as short as ten days or as long as nine years. The onset is usually insidious, especially in indigenous peoples who may feel well and have a good appetite despite daily bouts of fever; however, in those who are poorly nourished and have several underlying parasitic infections, the disease may then progress rapidly. In Africa a primary cutaneous nodule may be noticed for a few months before there are any systemic symptoms. The earliest symptom is fever. This is usually gradual in onset and accompanied by sweats, often without preceding chills. Alternatively, the onset is sudden with high fever and chills. This is common in Americans and Europeans who have contracted the disease while visiting an endemic area. Associated with fever there may be dizziness, weakness, and weight loss. Other common early symptoms include cough, diarrhea, pain, or discomfort in the left hypochondrium and symptoms of complicating secondary infections.

The important physical findings are fever, splenomegaly, lymphadenopathy, and skin changes. Fever at first is often inconstant, with apyrexial periods of several days or weeks. In over 80 per cent of cases, however, the fever eventually develops a characteristic pattern with twice daily elevations reaching 38 to 40° C (100 to 104° F), and may then undulate as in brucellosis. In the most acute cases fever and toxemia may be the only signs. Splenic enlargement is not necessarily rapidly progressive, nor does the size of the spleen correlate with the duration of the disease. In many instances, however, it reaches the right iliac fossa. It is firm and not tender unless there has been a recent subcapsular infarct. The liver enlarges more slowly and becomes palpable in about 20 per cent of cases and is likewise firm and not tender. Generalized lymphadenopathy is common in patients from Mediterranean countries, Africa, or China. Various changes have been reported in the skin. Classically there is hyperpigmentation of hands, feet, and abdomen. This may be missed in black Africans; in lighter-skinned Indians it looks gray or black (kala-azar means black sickness). In Africans warty eruptions or ulcers of the skin and oronasal lesions are occasionally seen.

Course and Complications. As the disease progresses,

anemia becomes clinically apparent. There may be bleeding from the nose or gums. In longstanding cases jaundice and signs of hypoalbuminemia may develop, namely, brittle hair, opaque nails, subcutaneous edema and ascites. Finally, after a course which may run for a few months or for five years, the patient becomes emaciated and exhausted. Intercurrent infections are the cause of death in 90 per cent of fatal cases. The most common are cancrum oris, pneumonia, pulmonary tuberculosis, bacillary dysentery, amebic dysentery, and, in Africa, brucellosis. Massive gastrointestinal hemorrhage accounts for another 1 to 2 per cent.

Post-Kala-Azar Dermal Leishmaniasis. About 20 per cent of Indian patients develop a rash one to two years after treatment or spontaneous recovery. The lesions develop slowly and may last for several, even 20, years. In Africa the rash develops in 2 per cent of cases, usually during treatment, and does not persist. It commonly starts as hypopigmented or erythematous macules on the face and sometimes on the arms, legs, and trunk. On the face the rash gradually becomes papular or nodular, especially on the forehead, cheeks, and earlobes, and closely resembles lepromatous leprosy. In 25 per cent of cases the lesions resolve spontaneously.

Diagnosis and Laboratory Findings. The diagnosis must be suspected in any person living in, or having visited, an endemic area who has a prolonged fever. The diagnosis is likely in the presence of splenomegaly, granulocytopenia, anemia, and hyperglobulinemia and is made by isolation of the parasite or by characteristic immunologic changes.

Isolation of Parasite. This is best done by needle aspiration of bone marrow, spleen, liver, or lymph nodes. Material obtained is:

1. Used to make a thin film on a glass microscope slide, stained, and examined under oil immersion for amastigotes, which must be distinguished from platelets. Parasitized macrophages usually rupture on smearing and free parasites must be looked for (see Fig. 2*F*, Ch. 271). Bone marrow aspiration is the procedure of choice. However, splenic puncture is safe so long as the tip of the spleen is well below the costal margin and the prothrombin and bleeding times are normal. A hypodermic needle on a syringe is inserted into the spleen, allowed to rest a moment, and withdrawn without suction. Organisms are seen in about 90 per cent of splenic aspirates and rather less often from other tissues. Buffy coat preparations show parasites in over 90 per cent of cases in India, but in only about 1 per cent in Africa.
2. Inoculated onto NNN (Novy-MacNeal-Nicolle) medium overlaid with balanced salt solution, containing streptomycin and penicillin (but not amphotericin). Cultures are kept in the dark at 22 to 25° C (not at 37°C), and every three to four days a drop of fluid is taken and examined wet for promastigotes. If after four weeks no parasites are seen, the fluid overlay is reinoculated onto a fresh NNN slope. Culture greatly improves the chances of making a diagnosis.
3. Inoculated intraperitoneally into hamsters, which are susceptible to a single amastigote. Though sensitive, this method is slow and seldom valuable.

Immunologic Tests. Antileishmanial antibodies can be demonstrated by indirect immunofluorescence of promastigotes in 100 per cent of cases and by precipitation in gel in 95 per cent. Cross reactions with *Trypanosoma cruzi* antibodies can be absorbed out. Complement fixation is positive in 65 per cent, but if the older antigen made from Kedrowsky's bacillins is used, reactions may be expected in some patients with mycobacterial disease. Serum obtained by eluting blood dried onto filter paper in the field can be used satisfactorily in all these techniques. The leishmanin test is *negative* in cases of active visceral leishmaniasis, but becomes positive after recovery, being most intense after one to two years, after which it fades slowly.

Total serum proteins are raised up to and over 10 grams per 100 ml. This increase is due almost entirely to the IgG fraction of gamma globulin. On immunoelectrophoresis the IgG pattern is characteristically skewed. In some cases IgM is also slightly increased, but this is said to be transient and to revert rapidly to normal on treatment. In advanced cases serum albumin levels fall. This disturbed globulin pattern underlies the older diagnostic aldehyde test which is also positive in other diseases with a grossly disturbed globulin pattern.

Laboratory Findings. The principal laboratory findings have to do with the blood and with the plasma proteins.

Blood Changes. Leukopenia is the most characteristic finding. The total count is below 2000 cells per cubic millimeter in 75 per cent of cases. There are an absolute neutropenia and eosinopenia and a relative lymphocytosis and monocytosis. Agranulocytosis occasionally develops. Anemia is slower in onset but becomes severe. It is normocytic and normochromic unless complicated by bleeding or deficiency states. There is often a mild reticulocytosis, and erythrocyte half-life is reduced. Thrombocytopenia is usual and progresses with the disease. Early on, tests of clotting are normal but later the prothrombin, partial thromboplastin, bleeding, and clotting times are prolonged. There are no characteristic findings in the urine.

Differential Diagnosis. In Europeans, Americans, and others who are not immune, malaria must be exluded by examination of thick and thin blood films. In immunes, malarial parasites in the blood film are of no diagnostic significance. In many parts of the tropics where malaria and schistosomiasis are endemic, a palpable spleen is commonplace and is usually unrelated to a recent febrile illness. Diseases which can be confused with visceral leishmaniasis include aleukemic leukemia and lymphomas, tropical splenomegaly syndrome (serum IgM, liver biopsy), cirrhosis of the liver with portal hypertension and hypersplenism, miliary tuberculosis, histoplasmosis, acute schistosomiasis, brucellosis, typhoid, and other septicemias, including bacterial endocarditis.

Prognosis. Untreated, 75 to 90 per cent of patients die. Treated, in all early cases, patients should recover. The mortality of late or severe disease in malnourished patients treated under difficult conditions can be over 25 per cent. Bad prognostic signs include extreme emaciation and toxemia, agranulocytosis, and the absence of the lymphocytosis which usually appears during treatment.

Treatment. *Chemotherapy.* Pentavalent antimony is the drug of choice, and, of the available preparations, sodium stibogluconate (Pentostam, Solustibostam) is probably the best. This is marketed as a solution containing 100 mg per milliliter. The dose is 0.2 ml per kilogram of body weight daily by intravenous or intramuscular injection, not exceeding 10 ml per dose. In India six injections are usually adequate, but elsewhere 30 are considered necessary. Alternative preparations include the following: (1) Meglumine antimoniate (Glucantime, 30 mg per ml), 0.4 ml per kilogram of body weight daily for 14 days. (2) Ethyl stibamine (Neostibosan) which must be freshly prepared as a 5 per cent solution. The adult dose is 0.1 ml the first day, 0.2 ml the second day, and 0.3 ml daily thereafter for 8 to 16 doses by intravenous injection. (3) Urea stibamine, 100 to 200 mg intravenously on alternate days for 15 doses. Side effects of pentavalent antimony are cumulative but rare. They are nausea, vomiting, urticaria, bradycardia, and electrocardiographic changes. In 5 to 10 per cent of patients, less in India, more in Africa, the response to antimony is unsatisfactory. The choice then lies between two toxic drugs, pentamidine isethionate (Lomidine, 40 mg per milliliter) and amphotericin B (Fungizone). The dose of pentamidine is 0.1 ml per kilogram of body weight by intramuscular injection every three to four days for ten doses, or less frequently if side effects develop. If the drug is accidentally injected intravenously, the patient will collapse, but recovers quickly if the feet are raised. Cumulative side effects include fatigue, anorexia, nausea, abdominal pain and, in 2 per cent of cases, prolonged hypoglycemia. Ten per cent of patients develop diabetes whose onset is not related to the duration of treatment. If this drug has to be used, a glucose tolerance test should be performed weekly. Amphotericin B is given by slow intravenous infusion in 5 per cent dextrose in a dose of 1 mg per kilogram of body weight on alternate days to a total of 2 grams for an adult. Side effects include rigors, thrombophlebitis, nausea, vomiting, fatigue, anemia, and uremia. This drug is more difficult to administer than pentamidine but is preferable.

Supportive Treatment. Bed rest, good nursing care, oral hygiene, an adequate fluid intake and sufficient food are all desirable. Complicating infections must be sought and treated. Anemia responds as the patient recovers, but if severe, and especially if there is bleeding, blood transfusion should be given. Deficiencies of iron, folate, and other vitamins need treating.

Response to Treatment. Little improvement may be seen until the course of treatment is nearly over. The patient then continues to improve steadily. There are lymphocytosis and reticulocytosis. No criterion of cure has been established. The patient should be seen monthly for six months and at a year. At each visit blood is cultured for Leishmania, spleen size is measured, and hemoglobin and serum IgG estimated. Complement-fixing antibody should not be detectable after six months. The spleen does not always become impalpable, and may indicate cirrhosis.

Relapses and Post-Kala-Azar Dermal Leishmaniasis. These usually respond to a further course or courses of antimony. If not, one of the other drugs may be used. One month should elapse before repeating a course. Rarely, if repeated courses of drugs fail to eliminate the parasite, the spleen remains huge, and the patient suffers from hypersplenism, splenectomy may be indicated. It must be followed by a course of chemotherapy, and in malarial areas by antimalarial prophylaxis for life.

Prevention. On a mass scale the detailed epidemiology of the local disease must be known. This will enable reservoir control (destruction of stray dogs, early detection, and treatment of cases) and vector control (insecticide spraying in the right places) to be carried out, and people may be able to avoid contact with infected flies, e.g., Kenyan termite hills. Personal prophylaxis depends on wearing protective clothing in the evenings, the use of insect repellants, and sleeping under fine mesh netting.

277. CUTANEOUS LEISHMANIASIS OF THE OLD WORLD (Oriental Sore)

Epidemiology. The innumerable names of this disease (Delhi or Bagdad boil, Biskra button, Aleppo evil, bouton de Crete, little sister) testify to its extent and familiarity throughout the Mediterranean basin, the Near and Middle East, and parts of India. Four epidemiologic situations are recognized.

"Rural" leishmaniasis throughout these areas is caused by the subspecies *L. tropica major.* The disease is a zoonosis among the desert gerbils *(Rhomobomys opimus)* and is transmitted to man by *Phlebotomus papatasii.* Where village settlements are close to gerbil colonies, up to 100 per cent of the population become infected, usually in early childhood. Travelers, hunters, and soldiers also get the disease. In "urban" leishmaniasis, the parasite *L. tropica minor* is adapted to dogs and to man, either of whom can act as reservoirs. *P. sergenti* is the main vector. This disease was the scourge of Middle Eastern cities; every adult inhabitant bore the scar, and few visitors were spared.

In Africa two distinct zoonoses exist. In West Africa the situation is "rural." Human cases are uncommon and sporadic. The vector and reservoir are not definitely established, but rodents and dogs are probably involved. In Ethiopia the disease is confined to the highlands, where the reservoir is the rock Hyrax (Procavia). The vector is *P. longipes,* which bites villagers at night in their houses.

Pathology. At the site of inoculation there is a massive infiltration with monocytes and histiocytes which take up the parasites and support their growth. The lesion then becomes surrounded by or mixed with lymphocytes and a few plasma cells. Macrophages develop into epithelioid cells, and parasites diminish. In later cases loose tubercles composed of loosely packed cells may develop. The overlying dermis ulcerates. The epidermis shows hyperkeratosis, acanthosis, pseudoepitheliomatous hyperplasia, intraepidermal necrosis, and ulceration. Healing is accompanied by fibrosis and is followed by lifelong immunity. Second infections are seen in only about 2 per 1000 cases, and then often in association with a generalized depression of immunity.

If cell-mediated immunity fails to develop, the patient gets diffuse cutaneous leishmaniasis, the disease spreading to other parts of the skin. Histologic study shows masses of heavily parasitized macrophages with little or no lymphocytic infiltration or epidermal change. The leishmanin test is negative.

In leishmaniasis recidiva, failure to heal is associated with exquisite delayed hypersensitivity, extreme chronicity, a tuberculoid histology with epithelioid giant cells but without caseation, and scanty or undetectable parasites.

Clinical Manifestations. The earliest lesion is a small erythematous papule, appearing two to eight weeks after the sandfly bite. It may itch slightly. The typical "urban" sore grows slowly into a nodule 1 to 2 cm across, and after a period of weeks or months forms a central crust under which is a shallow ulcer. The edge of the lesion is characteristically studded with small satellite papules. The sore usually remains in this state for a few more months and then heals gradually, leaving a depressed mottled scar. The whole process takes from three months to two years. The most common site is the face, followed by the arms and legs. There may be one or several sores. About 1 per cent of urban sores develop *leishmaniasis recidiva (lupoid leishmaniasis).* The ulcer fails to heal completely, scarring centrally but spreading peripherally, or heals and recrudesces at the edge of the scar. The lesion lasts for many years and resembles cutaneous tuberculosis.

There are many variants of the typical pattern of Oriental sore. "Rural" sores are commonly multiple, rapid in evolution, more florid, and produce more scarring. Ethiopian lesions are solitary, facial, milder, and slower in evolution, although lesions affecting the mucocutaneous border of the nose are extremely chronic and disfiguring.

Ethiopia is the only Old World country where *diffuse cutaneous leishmaniasis* is found. It is a rare condition,

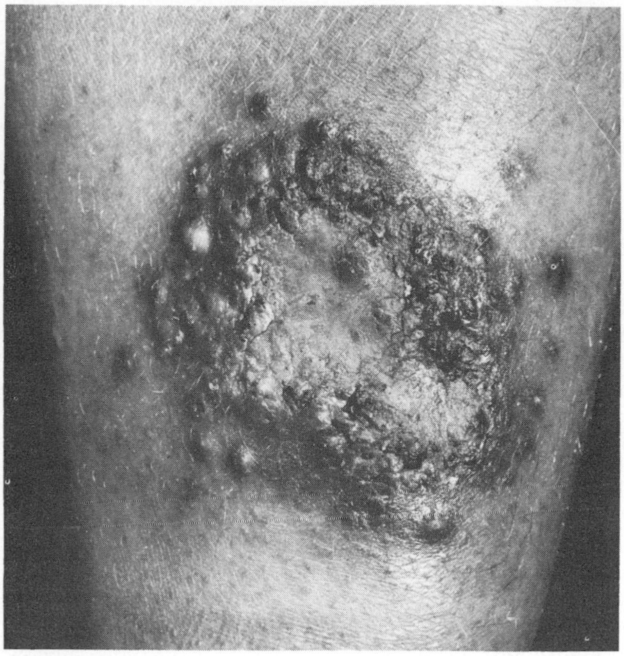

Figure 1. Cutaneous leishmaniasis—"Oriental sore."

occurring in perhaps 1 in 100,000 cases. The primary nodule does not ulcerate, but after a period of months or years starts to spread locally, and the disease disseminates to other parts of the skin, notably on the face and

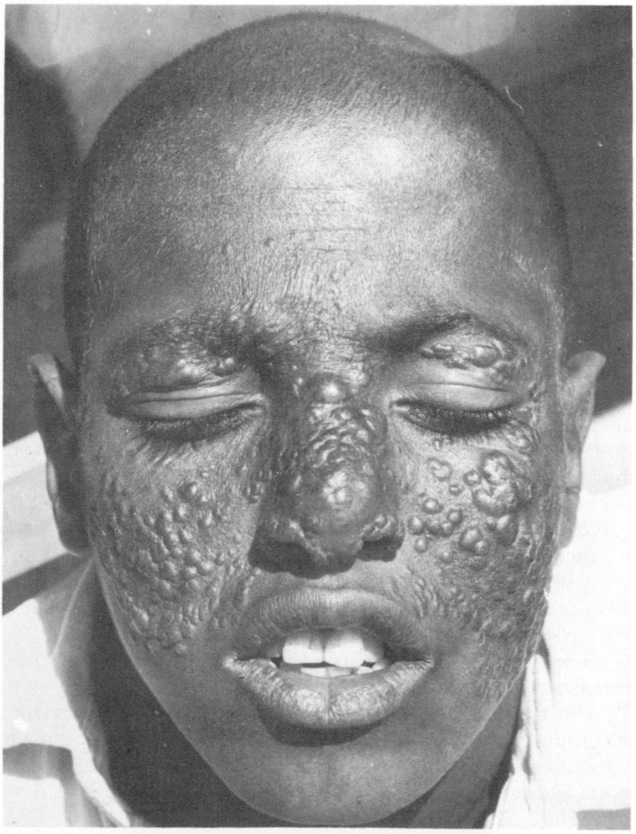

Figure 2. Early diffuse cutaneous leishmaniasis in an Ethiopian. Post-kala-azar dermal leishmaniasis may also look like this.

the extensor surfaces of the limbs, producing infiltrative and nodular lesions which may resemble lepromatous leprosy and do not heal spontaneously. The viscera are not involved, and the patient feels well.

Diagnosis. Leishmaniasis must be suspected as the cause of any chronic nodule or ulcer in a person living in or having recently visited an endemic area. Typical sores are diagnosable on sight. Diagnosis is confirmed by finding parasites in stained slit skin smears taken from a nonulcerated part of the lesion. The slit must reach the dermis, and the smears must contain tissue juice, not blood or pus. If unsuccessful, the crust is removed, the ulcer cleaned of all debris, and smears made of tissue scraped from the base of the ulcer. These methods are simpler and more likely to show parasites than is histology. In healing lesions and lupoid leishmaniasis, parasites are scanty and culture of juice or biopsy tissue may be necessary.

The leishmanin test becomes positive as the lesion ulcerates and is of diagnostic value in patients who do not live in endemic areas; it also may help to distinguish lupoid leishmaniasis from cutaneous tuberculosis, late syphilis, and fungal granulomas, which may be histologically similar.

There are no characteristic blood changes, and antibodies are difficult to demonstrate by usual techniques.

Treatment. Treatment remains unsatisfactory, but, as almost all cases heal spontaneously, the systemic use of toxic drugs is seldom justified. Fortunately most cases respond to a course of pentavalent antimony or to local infiltration with 0.5 ml 2 per cent berberine sulfate or 15 per cent mepacrine. Indolent sores may respond to heating to 50° C by coned infrared rays, to curettage and skin grafting, or to intralesional injections of corticosteroids combined with a course of antimony. Secondary infection is treated with the customary antimicrobial drugs.

Prevention. Detailed epidemiologic knowledge has permitted attacks on the reservoir in Central Asia and in Middle Eastern cities, where demolition of mud buildings and antimalarial spraying have reduced the number of sandflies. Immunization with live, virulent organisms is practiced on a mass scale in Russia and traditionally in the Middle East (see R. A. Neal, 1968).

278. CUTANEOUS LEISHMANIASIS OF THE NEW WORLD

(Including American Mucocutaneous Leishmaniasis or Espundia)

Epidemiology and Parasitology. Cutaneous leishmaniasis is endemic in Central and South America as far south as the Parana Estuary in the east and the Peruvian Andes in the west. In this extensive and varied terrain many different zoonoses exist, each associated with its own reservoirs and vectors and a particular pattern of human disease. Two main groups of parasites are now distinguished, those of *L. mexicana* and of *L. braziliensis.* The former, which grows easily in NNN medium and in the hamster, is responsible for most of the cutaneous leishmaniasis in Central America and a little in Brazil. The latter, which grows poorly in NNN medium and in the hamster, is responsible for most of the disease in

Cutaneous Leishmaniasis of the New World: Epidemiology

Parasite	Vector to Man	Reservoir	Geography	Human Disease
L. mexicana mexicana	*Lutzomyia olmeca*	Numerous rodents	Yucatan, Central America	"Chicle ulcer, bay sore" in forest workers; single skin lesions, healing in six months; diffuse cutaneous leishmaniasis
L. mexicana amazonensis	*Lutzomyia flaviscutellata*	Numerous rodents	Brazil, Trinidad; ? = *L. pifanoi,* Venezuela	Rare, single skin lesions; diffuse cutaneous leishmaniasis
L. braziliensis braziliensis	*Lutzomyia ssp, Psychodopygus ssp.*	Uncertain	All Amazon forests, esp. Brazil	"Espundia"; single or few large persistent destructive skin ulcers; oronasal metastases common
L. braziliensis guyanensis	*? Lutzomyia anduzei*	Unknown	Guyanas, into Brazil, Venezuela	"Forest yaws, pianbois"; multiple, widespread, deep skin ulcers, with nodular lymphatic metastases; ? oronasal metastases
L. braziliensis panamensis	*? Lutzomyia trapidoi*	Rodents, ? sloths	Panama	Single or few deep skin ulcers with nodular lymphatic metastases; ? oronasal metastases
L. peruviana	*? Lutzomyia peruensis*	Dogs	Peru, west slopes of Andes to 3000 meters	"Uta"; single or few skin lesions, healing in one year

South America, including espundia. Epidemiologic details are summarized in the accompanying table.

Cutaneous leishmaniasis presents a formidable obstacle to the development of the Central and South American forests, in large areas of which transmission of the infection is extremely high. This is particularly true in Brazil, where almost all workers on the trans-Amazonian highway become infected and run the risk of developing mutilating oronasal metastatic lesions. Amerindians, on the other hand, very rarely get leishmaniasis, although by the age of 40 years up to 100 per cent are sensitive to leishmanin.

Pathology. The pathology of cutaneous lesions is similar to that of Oriental sore. Metastatic lesions of espundia arise in the mucosa of the nose and mouth and show at first a typical leishmanial granuloma with numerous parasites, which later become scanty, and can be seen also in cells in cartilage, which is rapidly invaded and destroyed. There is vasculitis with edema, necrosis, and fibrosis.

Clinical Manifestations. Cutaneous lesions develop and heal in the same way as Oriental sores, but tend to be less nodular and more ulcerative and destructive. Lesions of the pinna are very chronic. Regional variations are given in the table.

In espundia, from 2 per cent (Panama) to 80 per cent (Paraguay) of primary cutaneous sores are followed after a period ranging from a few days to five years by metastatic lesions of the nose or mouth, most commonly on the mucocutaneous borders, but sometimes on the palate or larynx. These lesions may arise long after the primary lesion has healed. At first there is crusting or polyp formation, and then ulceration and perforation of the septum. Alternatively, large protruding granulomas of the nose and lips develop. The lesion heals slowly, if at all, after many years. Scarring may constrict the nose or mouth, producing gross deformity and making eating difficult. Secondary sepsis is common and increases the patient's debility.

Diffuse cutaneous leishmaniasis is a rare disease found mainly in Venezuela. Its clinical features are the same as in Ethiopia.

Diagnosis. The approach to diagnosis is set forth in Ch. 276 and 277. In late cases of espundia it may be impossible to isolate the parasite, but geographic history, clinical pattern, and leishmanin sensitivity make the diagnosis likely. Antibodies are detectable by immunofluorescence in over 90 per cent of patients with cutaneous or oronasal lesions, and disappear when the disease has been successfully treated. Blastomycosis is added to the list of differential diagnoses.

Treatment. The milder varieties of solitary sores seldom need treatment, unless they are disfiguring. Cycloguanil pamoate, 5 mg per kilogram of body weight as a single (painful) repository injection, is said to speed the healing of lesions of *L. mexicana.* If there is any suspicion that a sore has been caused by *L. braziliensis,* it must be treated by a course of pentavalent antimony (see Ch. 276). Established oronasal lesions frequently do not respond to antimony, or are liable to relapse. Amphotericin B (see Ch. 276) is then the drug of choice. Diffuse cutaneous leishmaniasis responds initially to antimony, but becomes resistant in relapse. Amphotericin B should then be tried.

Prevention. Prevention in South America is difficult. Intensity of transmission in the forest and lack of detailed epidemiologic information make mass prophylaxis a hopeless approach at the moment. People who are obliged to enter the forest could attempt to follow a regimen of the application of insect repellents every few hours and of sleeping under a fine mesh netting, but admittedly both of these procedures can produce considerable discomfort.

Lainson, R., and Shaw, J. J.: Leishmaniasis of the New World: Taxonomic problems. Br. Med. Bull, 28:44, 1972.

Manson-Bahr, P. E. C., and Winslow, D. J.: Cutaneous leishmaniasis. *In* Marcial-Rojas, R. A. (ed.): Pathology of Rickettsial and Helminthic Diseases. Baltimore, Williams & Wilkins Company, 1971, p. 97.

Most, H., and Lavietes, R. H.: Kala-azar in American military personnel. Medicine, 26:221, 1947.

Symposium on leishmaniasis. Bull. W.H.O., 44:477, 1971.

Turk, J. L., and Bryceson, A. D. M.: Immunological phenomena in leprosy and related diseases. Adv. Immunol., 13:209, 1971.

Walton, B. C., Brooks, W. H., and Arjona, I.: Serodiagnosis of American leishmaniasis by indirect fluorescent antibody test. Am. J. Trop. Med. Hyg., 21:296, 1972.

Wilcocks, C., and Manson-Bahr, P. E. C. (eds.): Manson's Tropical Diseases. 17th ed. Baltimore, Williams and Wilkins Company, 1972.

Winslow, D. J.: Visceral leishmaniasis. *In* Marcial-Rojas, R. A. (ed.): Pathology of Rickettsial and Helminthic Diseases. Baltimore, Williams & Wilkins Company, 1971, p. 86.

279. AMEBIASIS

Richard Knight

Definition. Amebiasis is caused by infection with *Entamoeba histolytica.* This species normally lives as a commensal within the large bowel lumen, where it may persist for several years. Symptoms of the disease may be produced by bowel invasion which may lead to submucosal ulcerations or which may allow spread of the organisms to the liver and other organs.

Etiology. Four species of Entamoeba infect man, but only *E. histolytica* has pathogenic potential. Noninvasive trophozoites of *E. histolytica* within the bowel of an infected host may round up and eliminate their cytoplasmic inclusions to form a precystic ameba. These organisms each secrete a substance which envelops them to become uninucleate spherical cysts (10 to 16 μ in diameter); immature cysts contain a large glycogen vacuole. The cysts mature either within the bowel lumen or outside the body. Most mature cysts have four nuclei resulting from two nuclear divisions; they contain a number of cigar-shaped chromatoid bars that constitute a ribosome store. When these mature cysts are ingested, they undergo one additional nuclear division. The cyst wall is destroyed in the small intestine, releasing eight motile uninucleate amebae or trophozoites. A population of trophozoites can thus become established in the proximal colon and cecum where they live adjacent to the mucosa and multiply by binary fission about every eight hours. These noninvasive forms measure 10 to 20 μ in diameter and feed upon bacteria and exfoliated epithelial cells.

Invasive *E. histolytica* are larger than noninvasive forms, up to 50 μ, and move much more actively by unidirectional pseudopodial movement. They contain ingested erythrocytes – hence the term hematophagous – and few or no bacteria.

Freshly isolated strains of *E. histolytica* behave differently when inoculated intracecally into weanling rats, those from patients with dysentery often being the most pathogenic. In culture, this virulence tends to decrease, although it may usually be restored by animal passage. A few strains have been isolated that differ from *E. histolytica* antigenically and by their ability to grow at room temperature and in hypotonic media. These *E. histolytica* – like amebae are probably never pathogenic; all other strains of *E. histolytica* are potentially virulent.

E. hartmanni is closely related to *E. histolytica* but is smaller, the peripheral nuclear chromatin is more clumped, and the quadrinucleate cysts are less than 10 μ in diameter (mean, 8 μ). *E. hartmanni,* formerly called "small race" *E. histolytica,* is not pathogenic. *E. coli* is another common commensal, whose sluggish trophozoites (20 to 30 μ) have coarse granular endoplasm. The karyosome is eccentric and the peripheral chromatin coarser than that of *E. histolytica.* Mature cysts (12 to 20 μ) have eight nuclei and thin pointed chromatoids. *E. polecki* is primarily a pig parasite and is rare in man except in parts of New Guinea where pigs and man live in close association. The mature cyst has only one nucleus and resembles an immature *E. histolytica* cyst.

Epidemiology. About 10 per cent of the world's population harbor *E. histolytica.* In the United States the prevalence is 2 to 5 per cent, in some tropical countries over 40 per cent. Poverty and poor sanitation encourage infection. Cysts may survive a month in water but are killed by drying. Rats, dogs, and certain monkeys are sometimes infected, but almost all human infections are from cysts passed by human carriers. *Encystment does not occur outside the body,* so patients passing only trophozoites in their stools are not infectious. Food is the most common vehicle of transmission; it may be contaminated by infected food handlers or flies. Direct contamination with human feces used as fertilizer is most common with uncooked fruit and salad vegetables. Direct fecal spread is important among children or the mentally handicapped in institutions, where infection rates may be very high.

Water-borne infection occurs, sometimes in epidemic form, as in the famous Chicago epidemic in which there were 1400 known cases and more than 100 deaths. Epidemics are probably not often recognized because the incubation period is so variable and many infections asymptomatic. Cysts may appear in the stool as early as four days after infection. The rate of spontaneous loss of infection is perhaps 15 per cent per year, so returning Americans infected in the tropics may remain infected for five years or more. In countries where there is continuous transmission, prevalence rates remain stable from year to year. In certain parts of the world, such as Mexico, parts of South America, the West Coast of Africa, Natal, and Southeast Asia, invasive disease is especially common. The incidence of disease does not necessarily correlate with the prevalence of infection.

Pathogenesis and Pathology. Commensal trophozoites thrive adjacent to the colonic mucosa where the oxygen tension is moderately low and the pH between 6.0 and 6.5. Host tissues appear to be damaged only by direct contact with amebae; lysosomal enzymes are released, possibly by activating a contact-sensitive surface organelle. The relatively anoxic and acid conditions of cell necrosis favor further penetration of amebae into the tissues. Although some amebic bowel lesions are secondarily infected, the role of intestinal bacteria in pathogenesis is still uncertain. They may act mainly by creating a milieu suitable for amebic growth.

Amebic ulceration is most common in the cecum and rectosigmoid, but may affect any part of the large bowel, appendix, and terminal ileum. The initial lesions are small, discrete superficial mucosal erosions which may then extend more deeply through the muscularis mucosae and spread laterally, producing ulcers that are flask-shaped in cross section. Lesions may coalesce, causing extensive mucosal loss. Blood vessel involvement usually results in local thrombosis. Penetration may extend through the muscle coats, causing *peritonitis,* the most dangerous complication of intestinal amebiasis. Microscopically, tissue necrosis is the main change; amebae occur throughout the lesion, but particularly at the advancing edge, and even beyond into healthy tissue. In tissue sections, amebae may appear shrunken and be surrounded by a clear space. They stain rather indistinctly with ordinary hematoxylin and eosin but stand out clearly as bright red bodies with periodic acid–Schiff stain; iron hematoxylin staining is necessary to show the nuclear structure clearly. The lymphocytic inflammatory response is slight or moderate; some neutrophils are also present, especially if there is secondary bacterial infection.

Ulcers heal rapidly after treatment, and persistent scarring is uncommon. Sometimes localized bowel lesions show a more vigorous host response, with edema and a marked inflammatory reaction producing an amebic granuloma or ameboma. These are most common in the cecum and rectosigmoid and may be multiple.

Although strain virulence may influence the probability of tissue invasion, host factors are also important.

Women in late pregnancy and the puerperium are especially susceptible, as are patients on cytotoxic or corticosteroid therapy. Colonic cancers may be secondarily invaded by *E. histolytica. Trichuris trichiura* infections and intestinal schistosomiasis may also encourage invasion. The high carbohydrate low-protein diets of developing countries perhaps enhance host susceptibility.

Hepatic Involvement. In many patients with invasive intestinal disease, amebae probably reach the liver via the portal vein, but most are destroyed. Hepatomegaly is not unusual in acute amebic dysentery because of products of colonic tissue destruction or bacteria reaching the liver. Established amebic infection of the liver usually causes progressive cytolytic lesions that extend in all directions, with trophozoites proliferating near the advancing edge. Perhaps these lesions begin at the sites of venous embolism or thrombosis. Secondary bacterial infection is rare, and the content of such a "liver abscess" is necrotic liquefied liver tissue. The abscess is sharply demarcated from surrounding liver, which shows edema, hyperemia, and a narrow zone of lymphocytic and polymorphonuclear infiltration; a fibroblastic reaction occurs in longstanding lesions. Most liver abscesses are solitary and occur long after any clinically evident bowel ulceration; but both solitary and the rarer multiple abscesses may develop during or shortly after a bout of dysentery. The term *amebic hepatitis* has been used by clinicians, but there is no pathologic basis for a diffuse lesion of this kind. In adults, 80 to 90 per cent of amebic liver abscesses occur in men, but before puberty both sexes are similarly affected. No other host factors have been definitely identified, although pre-existing liver disease and alcoholism may be relevant. Most complications of liver abscess are due to direct spread to adjacent structures.

Antibody Response. Tissue invasion provokes a humoral antibody response, mainly IgG, and a skin sensitivity to injected amebic antigen. It is not known whether this response has any protective function. Using sensitive techniques, antibodies can be detected in 25 per cent or more of apparently healthy carriers, suggesting that mild self-limiting bowel invasion is more common than has been supposed.

Clinical Manifestations. *Intestinal Amebiasis.* Most persons with *E. histolytica* in the stool have no symptoms, and many will remain symptomless carriers for the whole duration of their infection. Invasive bowel disease begins most commonly between one and six months after infection but sometimes much later, especially in an immunologically compromised host.

Involvement of the colon without diarrhea is the most common form of bowel disease; the ulceration is localized and not severe enough to produce dysentery. The patient complains of colicky pains in the right or left iliac fossa, flatulence, and an altered bowel habit, often with some diarrhea. A little blood or mucus may be noted in the stool; there is little constitutional upset. The cecum or sigmoid colon may be tender or feel abnormal on palpation. Symptoms may persist intermittently for months thereafter, and spontaneous cure is not uncommon.

Widespread colonic or rectosigmoid ulceration produces amebic dysentery with frequent bloody stools. Dysentery may begin abruptly, but often follows a varied period of the milder colonic symptoms noted above. Initially, many patients remain ambulant, but later, fever, colicky abdominal pains, and tenesmus appear. The illness is usually less acute than bacillary dysentery and dehydration less evident. There may be colonic tenderness and some hepatomegaly. The stool is often offensive and contains some fecal matter; much of the blood present is altered unless there is rectal ulceration. In the rare fulminating form of the disease, toxic megacolon occurs with progressive abdominal distention, vomiting, dehydration, and electrolyte loss; some very ill patients have relatively few bowel actions. Sigmoidoscopy and barium enema examination should not be carried out in patients with severe dysentery; when the diagnosis is in doubt, a limited endoscopy may be justified.

Amebomas may present as a tender abdominal mass, sometimes with fever and constitutional upset. Partial bowel obstruction may occur, especially when the lesion is annular. The appendix may be affected primarily, or secondarily by a cecal lesion. This may resemble simple appendicitis, except that pain begins in the right iliac fossa, and guarding and rigidity are slight unless perforation has occurred.

COMPLICATIONS. A grossly diseased and atonic large bowel may perforate at several points. Absent bowel sounds with relatively little pain, rigidity, or tenderness should suggest this very dangerous possibility. Free gas in the peritoneum confirms it. Less commonly, when perforation is localized, classic signs of peritonitis are produced. Local perforation can also lead to pericolic abscess or retroperitoneal fecal cellulitis. *Fibrous strictures* of the colon rarely follow amebic dysentery or amebomas, but may require surgical relief. Serious hemorrhage is uncommon, but can be life threatening. Amebic ulceration or an ameboma may rarely initiate a cecocolic intussusception. Irritable bowel syndrome may follow amebic colitis and persist for several months. Much rarer is the syndrome of postdysenteric colitis which can continue for several years despite eradication of the amebic infection. It is distinct from simple ulcerative colitis and is associated with very high amebic antibody titers; endoscopy shows reddened edematous mucosa, sometimes with superficial erosions. Barium enema examination will exclude the rare possibility of internal fistulas.

Cutaneous amebiasis takes the form of deep, painful, and rapidly spreading ulceration. The most common sites are the perianal area, perineum, laparotomy incisions, and colostomy stomas. Rarely, the uterine cervix is affected, giving lesions that may resemble carcinoma. Penile lesions may follow anal coitus.

Hepatic Amebiasis. About half of all patients with liver abscess have a history suggestive of amebic dysentery between a week and many years previously. Solitary lesions are most common in the upper part of the right lobe; multiple lesions are often associated with coexistent dysentery. The illness begins insidiously with fever, sweating, and pain in the liver region. If the diaphragm is involved, there may be right pleuritic or shoulder pain. Most patients present within a few weeks of onset; as the disease progresses, there are weight loss and anemia. *Those developing the condition in temperate countries after returning from the tropics rarely have bowel symptoms.* Hepatomegaly is always present, but if enlargement is mainly upward, it may not be very evident on abdominal palpation. Left lobe lesions are palpable as an epigastric mass. Liver tenderness is mainly localized to the site of the lesion, and, in suspected cases, all the lower right intercostal spaces should be carefully palpated. Pain on heavy percussion or compression of the liver is not a very specific sign, because many types of liver and chest disease will be painful with these procedures. Crepitations and signs of lung consolidation or pleural fluid in the lower right chest are quite common. Jaundice occurs only when lesions are very large or numerous. The blood sedimentation rate is raised, and normally there are a polymorphonuclear leukocytosis and some normocytic normochromic anemia. Levels of serum transaminase and alkaline phosphatase are variable and of little diagnostic value. *The most suggestive roentgenographic finding* is an immobile, raised, or bulging right hemidiaphragm; lung or pleural involvement may also be visible. Radioisotope liver scans help considerably to show the site, size, and number of lesions present. *Diagnostic needle aspiration* with the finding of relatively odorless brownish or pink material with no bacteria on Gram staining is almost pathognomonic. An 8 cm pleural aspiration needle 1.5 to 2.0 mm in diameter connected to a large syringe via a three-way tap is normally used. When there is no definite clinical evidence as to the site of the lesion, the eighth or ninth right intercostal space should be explored in the midaxillary line.

COMPLICATIONS. Rupture through the diaphragm can produce amebic lung abscess or empyema and sometimes a bronchohepatic fistula so that the patient coughs up amebic pus. Extension to the body surface may lead to sinus formation and cutaneous lesions. Amebic peritonitis follows rupture into the peritoneum, and the primary source may be evident only at laparotomy. The gut, stomach, vena cava, spleen, and right kidney can also be involved by direct spread. A dangerous complication of left lobe lesions is *amebic pericarditis;* urgent aspiration may be necessary to relieve tamponade, and fibrous constrictive pericarditis is a rare late sequel. More than 100 cases of *amebic brain abscess* have been reported. All have been associated with liver abscess and, so far, all patients have died. This condition should not be confused with primary amebic meningoencephalitis caused by free-living amebae (Naegleria and Hartmanella). Hematogenous lesions also occasionally occur in the lung and perhaps elsewhere.

Differential Diagnosis. *Intestinal Amebiasis.* Amebic dysentery may resemble bacillary dysentery, nonspecific ulcerative colitis, intestinal salmonellosis, and, more rarely, heavy infection with intestinal schistosomiasis or *Trichuris trichiura.* Patients with nondysenteric colitis are often suspected of having irritable bowel syndrome, and blood in the stool may be attributed to hemorrhoids. Diverticulitis, carcinoma, and Crohn's disease of the colon may require exclusion by barium enema and sigmoidoscopy. *The finding of* E. histolytica *should not delay the search for another disease, especially because amebic ulceration may be superimposed upon a carcinoma.* Amebomas may mimic neoplastic, infective, and granulomatous conditions of the large bowel, including lymphogranuloma venereum when the rectum is involved. The interpretation of therapeutic trials with tissue amebicides may be difficult, and the delay can make a tumor inoperable.

Hepatic Amebiasis. In the differential diagnosis of hepatic amebiasis, it is necessary to exclude primary and secondary neoplasms of the liver, abscesses caused by migrating Ascaris worms, and purulent subphrenic or intrahepatic disease. Other conditions to be considered are hydatid cyst, the painful or tender hepatomegaly of viral or alcoholic hepatitis, and various pleural or lung lesions of the right lower chest. Radioisotope hepatoscans are particularly useful in the detection and localization of space-occupying lesions.

Laboratory Diagnosis. *Microscopy and Culture.* Diagnosis is based upon the finding of hematophagous trophozoites in stool specimens or fresh material obtained during endoscopy. Although sigmoidoscopic appearances are not pathognomonic, this procedure is valuable for initial assessment and follow-up. The disease spectrum is wide, and the clinical picture depends upon the severity and extent of bowel involvement.

Hematophagous trophozoites should be sought in temporary wet mounts of dysenteric stools, bowel wall scrapings, material from suspected skin lesions, and in the last portion of pus obtained at liver aspiration. If necessary, the material should be diluted with buffered saline (ideally, pH 6.8). In nondysenteric stools, flecks of mucus or pus should be looked for and examined. Trophozoites remain active and recognizable for about 30 minutes above 18° C (see Fig. 2, Ch. 271). If delay will inevitably be longer than this, the specimen should be kept cool as activity is restored, even after several hours at 4° C. If necessary, amebae may be preserved in polyvinyl alcohol and identified after staining with Heidenhain's iron hematoxylin or Gomori's trichrome stain; alternatively, a smear may be fixed in Schaudinn's fixative and stained later. In wet mounts, the definitive identification of nonhematophagous *E. histolytica* is not possible, and even in stained preparations, it is not easy; for this reason, purged stool specimens are of no help unless hematophagous amebae are obtained. On the other hand, *E. histolytica* cysts can be readily recognized in wet mounts, using dilute Lugol's iodine to define nuclear and chromatoid morphology. Cyst concentration techniques using formol ether sedimentation or zinc sulfate flotation give a diagnostic sensitivity of about 70 per cent per specimen compared with 30 per cent without concentration. Examination of concentrates from stools obtained on three separate days is normally sufficient to exclude an intraluminal amebic infection. Cysts in stool may be preserved in 10 per cent formalin, but this reduces the effectiveness of concentration procedures.

Cultivation of *E. histolytica* from fresh stool is not difficult with appropriate media, and is sometimes helpful in confirming the diagnosis. Stained preparations of isolates must be made for accurate identification. If amebic liver pus is to be cultured, the medium should be preconditioned with *Escherichia coli.*

Serologic Tests. Amebic antibodies may be detected by several techniques; in order of decreasing sensitivity, the most used are indirect hemagglutination, indirect fluorescent antibody, complement fixation, and gel diffusion precipitation. Over 90 per cent of patients with liver abscess normally have positive serologic tests, compared with 60 to 80 per cent of those with invasive intestinal disease. Results must be interpreted with caution; as antibody may persist for several years and in endemic areas, some asymptomatic carriers and noninfected persons will have positive reactions. However, negative serologic tests are quite strong evidence against a diagnosis of liver abscess. Serologic tests are also valuable in suspected amebomas and other localized colonic lesions beyond the reach of sigmoidoscopy.

Treatment. *Clinical Pharmacology.* TISSUE AMEBICIDES. Intramuscular emetine hydrochloride and the synthetic compound, dehydroemetine dihydrochloride, are the most rapidly acting tissue amebicides, but both are toxic and cumulative. Emetine is given in a dose of 1 mg per kilogram of body weight daily (maximum, 65 mg daily) for up to ten days. *Serious cardiotoxicity* is suggested by hypotension, dyspnea, precordial pain, tachycardia, and palpitations, but is unusual until at least six doses have been given. Electrocardiographic changes include T wave inversion, prolongation of PR interval, widening of the QRS complex, and arrhythmias. Less serious side effects are weakness, nausea and vomiting, local myositis at the site of injection, and, rarely, a more generalized myositis. A course of treatment should not exceed ten days and should not be repeated without an interval of at least two weeks. Complete bed rest is essential. The drug should not be given to patients with cardiovascular disease, and is not generally recommended for pregnant women or children. Dehydroemetine is excreted more rapidly in the urine than emetine, and a daily dose of 1.25 mg per kilogram of body weight (maximum, 90 mg daily) is necessary; it is probably less cardiotoxic.

Metronidazole (Flagyl) is a potent and safe amebicide that can only be given by mouth; it is rapidly absorbed from the small bowel to reach all tissues. This compound is also useful in the treatment of intraluminal infections, because some is excreted in the bile in modified form and some directly into the colon. A five- or eight-day course of 750 or 800 mg thrice daily is effective in all forms of invasive amebiasis. Paradoxically, higher doses are required to eliminate a bowel infection than to destroy all tissue-invading amebae. Side effects very rarely necessitate stopping treatment; they include dizziness, nausea, abdominal pain, a metallic taste in the mouth, brownish discoloration of the urine, and a confusional state if alcohol is taken. The effectiveness of metronidazole has greatly simplified the chemotherapy of amebiasis, but its action is slightly less rapid than that of emetine, and there is no parenteral preparation.

The main indication for chloroquine is hepatic amebiasis, because the drug is concentrated by, and accumulates within, the liver. The usual regimen consists of 150 mg base twice daily for three weeks. Some toxicity may occur with this regimen, including T wave changes on the electrocardiogram. *Patients being treated for invasive intestinal amebiasis with drugs other than emetine or metronidazole should be given a two-week course of chloroquine to prevent the development of hepatic lesions.*

LUMINAL AMEBICIDES. Tetracycline can be very useful in some patients with invasive intestinal disease; it acts mainly upon bacteria within the lesions, but also alters the bacterial flora of the gut, and has some direct amebicidal activity. Tetracycline is used especially in children, in situations when a parenteral drug is needed, and when metronidazole or emetine is contraindicated or not available. If the drug is used alone, parasitic cure is uncommon, and there may be clinical relapse. For adults, the dosage is 250 or 500 mg every six hours for five to ten days.

Numerous substances have been used to eliminate the bowel infection in symptomless carriers and in patients with invasive disease who are not given metronidazole. The most effective are diiodohydroxyquin (Diodoquin), diloxanide furoate (Furamide), and paromomycin (Humatin). The only adverse effects of Diodoquin are mild diarrhea, pruritus ani, rashes, and rarely iodism. The related compound clioquinol (iodochlorohydroxyquin) has been incriminated as a rare cause of myelo-optic neuropathy.

Management. INTESTINAL AMEBIASIS. Amebic dysentery and nondysenteric colitis should be treated with emetine, metronidazole, or tetracycline, depending upon drug availability and contraindications. If emetine is given, only a three- to six-day course is normally required to control the acute phase of the disease. It should be combined with or followed by metronidazole or tetracycline with chloroquine. Tetracycline should probably be given to all patients with severe dysentery. Amebic peritonitis should be treated medically with gastric suction and intravenous fluid and electrolytes, together with emetine and parenteral tetracycline. If the diagnosis is made at laparotomy, surgical repair is usually not possible because the bowel wall is so friable. Amebomas may be successfully treated with a full course of metronidazole or a ten-day course of emetine. In all forms of intestinal disease, if metronidazole is not used, a luminally active drug must also be given to eradicate the infection.

In countries where transmission rates are low, such as the United States and Western Europe, it is generally recommended that all detected symptomless infections should be treated to prevent later invasive disease or transmission to others. Suitable regimens for adults are Diodoquin, 650 mg thrice daily for 21 days; entamide furoate, 500 mg thrice daily for 10 days; or paromomycin, 500 mg thrice daily for seven days. Alternatively, a full course of metronidazole can be given, particularly if there is suspicion of tissue invasion or concurrent infection with *Giardia intestinalis.*

HEPATIC AMEBIASIS. Liver abscess may be successfully treated with a ten-day course of emetine plus chloroquine for three weeks and a luminal amebicide. Alternatively, a five- or eight-day course of metronidazole may be used; 400 or 500 mg thrice daily will cure the liver lesion, but 750 or 800 mg should be given to eliminate the coexistent gut infection which must be assumed to be present.

Aspiration of the liver is sometimes necessary for therapeutic purposes as well as for diagnosis. The principal indications are as follows: (1) very large lesions and those in the left lobe, especially when there is clinical or radiologic evidence that rupture is imminent; (2) after rupture, if this has occurred into the pleural cavity or pericardium (these also must be aspirated); and (3) poor clinical response after five days of medical treatment. Sometimes the procedure may have to be repeated two or three times. The principal complications are hemorrhage and introduction of bacterial infection; the latter is suggested if the aspirate changes color, becomes very liquid or offensive, or contains gas. Bleeding is less common than might be expected because in liver abscess the right hemidiaphragm rarely moves with respiration.

Occasionally therapeutic drainage by an elective laparotomy is necessary. The indications are as follows: (1) when aspiration is strongly indicated on clinical grounds, but attempts by percutaneous route have failed to locate or adequately drain the lesion; (2) when the lesion continues to refill despite chemotherapy and several percutaneous aspirations; and (3) in the presence of left lobe lesions when not superficial or when the diagnosis is uncertain. An indwelling soft rubber drain is rarely required after surgical drainage, but if used it must be connected to a sterile underwater seal and removed early.

Amebic lung lesions will respond to treatment given for the associated liver lesion. Cutaneous lesions respond to either emetine or metronidazole.

Prognosis. Despite a normally rapid response to treatment, invasive intestinal disease may relapse if the infection is not eliminated. Host factors may be relevant in some persons, including perhaps those with mild nonspecific colitis. If symptoms recur, care must be taken to exclude other colonic disease. There is so far no evidence of drug resistance by any strain of *E. histolytica.* Amebic peritonitis, especially when there are multiple gut perforations, carries a grave prognosis; but permanent sequelae after any form of amebic colitis are rare. Hepatic scanning suggests that filling defects normally disappear within two or four months after treatment of liver abscess. Failure to aspirate large lesions adequately may lead to clinical relapse or much slower resolution. Healing occurs with little scar formation, but if the lesion was secondarily infected, bizarre hepatic calcification may be seen years afterward. Published reports of unselected patients suggest that a 10 per cent mortality is not unusual in liver abscess, but the prognosis can be much better with early diagnosis and adequate treatment.

After successful treatment for amebiasis, there is no reason why a person from a temperate country should not return to the tropics.

Prevention. Chlorination of water supplies does not destroy *E. histolytica* cysts, but proper filtration is effective. A weak solution of iodine is a more potent cysticide than chlorine. Salads and vegetables may be soaked in vinegar or potassium permanganate solution; these are procedures of doubtful benefit, and for some they render the food inedible. A solution of sodium hypochlorite has been found useful. Visitors to the tropics should avoid purchasing food from street vendors and from premises where flies are evident. Fruit that can be skinned should be safe. Boiling water for five minutes kills cysts. Members of domestic staffs involved in food handling should have their stools examined.

Intermittent mass chemotherapy with entamide furoate and metronidazole has been successfully attempted in Mexico and elsewhere where invasive disease is common; it may also be useful in mental institutions in temperate countries. *Personal chemoprophylaxis* by visitors to the tropics is not recommended, and it is better for such persons to avoid eating uncooked foods and to have their stools examined on return.

Amoebiasis: Report of a WHO Expert Committee. WHO Technical Report Series No. 421, 1–52, 1969.

Biagi, F. F., and Beltran, H. F.: The challenge of amoebiasis: Understanding pathogenic mechanisms. Int. Rev. Trop. Med., 3:219, 1969.

Elsdon-Dew, R.: The epidemiology of amoebiasis. Adv. Parasitol., 6:1, 1968.

Powell, S. J.: New developments in the therapy of amoebiasis. Gut, 11:967, 1970.

Wilmot, A. J. Clinical Amoebiasis. Oxford, Blackwell, 1962.

OTHER PROTOZOAN DISEASES

280. INTRODUCTION

Philip D. Marsden

Apart from *Entamoeba histolytica,* at least four genera and seven species of amebae have been established as living in man. Common stool amebae are *Entamoeba coli, Endolimax nana,* and *Iodamoeba buetschlii.* They are nonpathogenic, but such protozoa have a double importance. First, they must be distinguished from the pathogenic *E. histolytica* by the available clear morphologic criteria. Second, they provide an index of fecal contamination. If any stool protozoan is encountered, it is wise to examine a further specimen, for, because of the variable appearance of protozoa in the stool, the second specimen may reveal a pathogen. *Dientamoeba fragilis* is a delicate ameba without a cystic stage. Some clinicians believe it is a cause of mild diarrhea, but the evidence is not convincing.

Several flagellates are also found in the stool, among them the nonpathogenic *Trichomonas hominis* and *Chilomastix mesnili.* Information on the differential diagnosis of these intestinal protozoa can be found in texts of parasitology. Here we will consider briefly the clinical significance of five pathogenic protozoa: *Giardia lamblia* and *Trichomonas vaginalis* (both flagellates), *Balantidium coli* (a ciliate), *Isospora belli* (a coccidium), and *Naegleria gruberi* (an ameba).

Knight, R., Schultz, M. G., Hoskins, D. W., and Marsden, P. D.: Intestinal Parasites. Gut, 14:145, 1973.

281. GIARDIASIS

Philip D. Marsden

Abdominal pain, distention and flatulence, and recurrent diarrhea may be associated with *Giardia lamblia* infection, especially in children. Inhabiting the duodenum and upper jejunum, the parasite is a pear-shaped flagellate, anteriorly broad and rounded and tapering to a point not unlike a tennis racket. It is convex dorsally with a ventral attachment disc. There are sets of identical structures on either side of the median line. When stained, there are two nuclei, four pairs of flagella, and a parabasal body. In fresh stool this trophozoite is actively motile with an irregular characteristic progression. It reproduces by longitudinal binary fission.

The thick-walled cysts are 10 to 14 μ by 6 to 10 μ and have two to four nuclei with curved rods or axostyles. In some infections several million cysts per gram of feces may be passed. Only in patients with very rapid bowel transit times do trophozoites appear in the stool, although they may be found in duodenal aspirate. Cultivation of Giardia in vitro has recently been achieved.

The infective cysts are transmitted in food and drink, and the infection is cosmopolitan. The great majority of patients are asymptomatic, but there is no doubt that heavy infections are associated with symptoms. Diarrhea is the most common symptom, and the stools are pale and contain mucus. Giardia is in fact a cause of steatorrhea, and patients have abnormal fat balances and D-xylose tests which return to normal after successful treatment. The hypothesis that this malabsorption is the result of a mechanical barrier produced by large numbers of parasites attached to the microvillar surface is attractive, but effects on digestive enzyme activity and microvillar function are possible. Villous flattening with inflammatory infiltration has been demonstrated in one study.

Diarrhea may alternate with constipation, and apart from these symptoms epigastric pain resembling a peptic ulcer may be a disabling symptom. Anorexia, meat intolerance, and loss of weight may occur. Although Giardia may be found in the gallbladder, the evidence that it is responsible for cholecystitis is unsatisfactory. Giardiasis must be distinguished from other causes of malabsorption and peptic ulcer.

Giardiasis, symptomatic or not, should always be treated. Two drugs are equally effective. Quinacrine hydrochloride (Atabrine), in a dose of 100 mg three times a day after food for seven days, is an established therapy, but the drug has a bitter taste, and nausea and vomiting may result. It may also stain the skin yellow, but psychosis does not occur at this dosage level. Metronidazole (Flagyl), 200 mg three times a day after food for ten days, is equally effective with few side effects. Both drugs have about an 80 per cent cure rate, and in the event of failure of one drug the other can be tried. The follow-up procedures are similar to those in amebiasis.

Hoskins, L. C., Winawer, S. J., Broitman, S. A., Gottlieb, L. S., and Zamchek, N.: Clinical giardiasis and intestinal malabsorption. Gastroenterology, 53:265, 1967.

Yardley, J. H., Takano, J., and Hendrix, T. B.: Epithelial and other mucosal lesions of the jejunum in giardiasis: Jejunal biopsy studies. Bull. Hopkins Hosp., 115:389, 1964.

282. TRICHOMONIASIS

Thomas C. Jones

Another group of lumen-dwelling protozoa with flagella are the trichomonads. Three species of the genus Trichomonas frequently inhabit man: *Trichomonas hominis, Trichomonas tenax,* and *Trichomonas vaginalis.* Only the last-named is considered pathogenic and is a common cause of infection and disease in the genital tract.

T. vaginalis is a pear-shaped, colorless, single-celled organism 10 to 20 μ in size with two pairs of anterior flagella, an eccentrically located nucleus, an undulating membrane, and a structure termed an axostyle leading to a posterior flagellum. The flagella and undulating membrane move the organisms rapidly through exudative material in a jerky, rotating manner. Vaginal pH may determine its survival since it loses activity at a pH below 5.

The organism can persist in endocervical or urethral glands without causing symptoms, or under appropriate conditions it can induce inflammation on the mucosal surfaces of the vagina, urethra, urinary bladder, or prostate. The inflamed area takes on a characteristic "strawberry-like" appearance owing to vasodilation. Exudate filled with polymorphonuclear leukocytes and mononuclear cells covers the surface. Phagocytosis of the protozoan has been recorded. Trichomonas infection can make interpretation of cervical Papanicolaou smears more difficult for the cytologist. There is no evidence that chronic *T. vaginalis* infection contributes to carcinoma of the cervix.

Patients usually present with symptoms of vaginal itching or burning, and a yellow blood-tinged discharge. These symptoms are more commonly associated with menstruation. If the urethra is involved, symptoms of dysuria and a mild urethral discharge are seen. Approximately 20 per cent of females with documented Trichomonas infection are asymptomatic.

Diagnosis is made by observing the motile organisms in fresh specimens of vaginal discharge. A drop of warm saline is mixed with the exudate and examined immediately, using low-power microscopy. *T. vaginalis* can also be cultured. Metronidazole is effective therapy when given in doses of 250 mg three times daily for ten days. Females should also receive 500 mg vaginal suppositories for ten days. Both male and female partners should be treated at the same time. Failure to do this results in reinfection, so-called "Ping-Pong" vaginitis. The infection is usually acquired by sexual intercourse. It can be transmitted to infants at the time of birth, and may survive on nonmucosal surfaces for a sufficient time to be spread in places such as mental institutions where personal hygiene is poor.

283. BALANTIDIASIS

Philip D. Marsden

Balantidium coli is the largest protozoan of man, measuring 50 to 70 μ in length by 30 to 60 μ in width. It infects the colon of man and may produce diarrhea and dysentery. When viewed under the low power of the microscope in a saline smear of stool, the grayish-green trophozoite can be seen gliding across the field powered by spiral longitudinal rows of cilia. There is a large oral macronucleus and a smaller micronucleus. A cytostome or mouth ingests organic matter that circulates as food vacuoles. Erythrophagocytosis has been observed. Reproduction is by binary fission or conjugation. A resistant cyst form is passed in formed stools, and this is the infective form. *Cosmopolitan in distribution, it is a rare infection of man although common in pigs.* When man and pig share shelter, human infections are common, and this accounts for the high incidence of human infection in parts of New Guinea (20 per cent) and Peru. *B. coli* of man can be transmitted to monkeys, cats, guinea pigs, and rats, but the importance of these animals as reservoirs is minor. Handling pigs in slaughterhouses may be an occupational risk.

This ciliate can be a tissue invader, and similar factors to those mentioned for *E. histolytica* may well determine this behavior. Proteolytic secretions produce necrosis and ulceration of the mucosa. Columns of balantidia may be seen lying in the submucosa. Secondary infection with bacteria results in an accompanying inflammatory reaction. The ulcers are often quite large and deep, with a broad, indurated base. A liver abscess with *B. coli* in situ has been described, and balantidia have been found in the lung and heart in isolated cases.

Less than one fifth of infected persons have symptoms. Severe infections are associated with diarrhea and the passage of blood and mucus in the stools. Constitutional symptoms of fever, nausea, vomiting, and asthenia are described. Examination of fresh stools reveals the trophozoite or cyst. Culture of the stools on media similar to those used for amebiasis may reveal an infection when conventional microscopy has failed; in symptomatic patients this is usually not necessary. Balantidiasis must be differentiated from amebic dysentery and ulcerative colitis. Although arsenical preparations have been used in the past, oxytetracycline is probably the drug of choice in an adult dose of 500 mg three times a day for ten days. Paromomycin (Humatin) is also effective. Spontaneous recovery has been noted. The infection may be fatal if bowel perforation occurs.

Arean, V. M., and Koppisch, E.: Balantidiasis: A review and report of cases. Am. J. Path., 32:1089, 1956.

Van der Hoeven, J. A., and Rijpstra, A. C.: Intestinal parasites in the central mountain district of Netherlands, New Guinea. An important focus of *Balantidium coli*. Docum. Med. Geog. Trop., 9:225, 1957.

284. COCCIDIOSIS

Philip D. Marsden

Coccidia have alternate asexual and sexual generation in the same host, and the nature of the cycle is not dissimilar to plasmodia in the forms produced. There is probably only one human species, *Isospora belli*, which parasitizes the small intestinal epithelium. The cycles of schizogony and gametogony have now been described in small bowel mucosal biopsies from symptomatic patients, and it has been suggested that this organism causes a malabsorption syndrome. Until recently the case for the pathogenicity of Isospora rested mainly on laboratory infections that resulted in diarrhea lasting about three weeks, accompanied by the passage of the diagnostic form of the parasite in the stool. This is a thick-walled oocyst 25 to 35 $\mu \times 12$ to 16 μ in size. Both ends are rounded, and one is contracted to form a neck. This stage is the zygote. Further development in two to four days results in the formation of two sporoblasts, which mature into oval sporocysts. Each sporocyst ultimately contains four sporozoites. These oocysts are very resistant to physical and chemical insult and will readily sporulate in potassium dichromate. Many instances of spurious parasitemia have been reported in man when oocysts of various animals and fish coccidia have passed unchanged through the bowel to appear in the stool and pose a diagnostic problem. The mild persistent diarrhea during the active phase of the infection is usually accompanied only by nausea and abdominal discomfort. In the recent report cited below, the patients had severe diarrhea and steatorrhea unresponsive to therapy, and three died.

Brandborg, L. L., Goldberg, S. B., and Breidenbach, W. C.: Human coccidiosis—a possible cause of malabsorption. The life cycle in small bowel mucosal biopsies as a diagnostic feature. N. Engl. J. Med., 283:1306, 1970.

Smitskamp, H., and Oey-Muller, E.: Geographical distribution and clinical significance of human coccidiosis. Trop. Geogr. Med., 18:133, 1966.

285. PRIMARY AMEBIC MENINGOENCEPHALITIS

Philip D. Marsden

Recently it has been realized that *free-living amebae* are capable of producing severe brain lesions in man. Several species are implicated, but *Naegleria gruberi* has been the species usually identified when cultures are made. They can be cultured on plain agar plates with *Aerobacter aerogenes* as a nutrient source, but we need to know more about their cultural requirements. The Naegleria amebae possess the capacity to transform in culture from ameboid trophozoites to highly mobile flagellates. Another organism, *Acanthamoeba castellani*, was among the first to be recognized. An ameba 6 to 8 μ long, with foamy cytoplasm, a nucleus of 2 μ, and a 1 μ darkly staining central karyosome, it is present as a commensal in human mouths and throats and was shown to be pathogenic for mice and monkeys before the first cases were reported in man. An initial report from Australia in 1965 described a rapidly progressive meningitis that proved fatal. Early symptoms in the first two days or so are fever, severe frontal headache, defects of olfactory sense, lethargy, sore throat, and obstructed nostrils. By the third day vomiting and impaired consciousness may be present, progressing to deepening coma and death on the fourth day. At postmortem, destruction of the inferior surface of the frontal lobes and olfactory bulbs was seen, associated with a purulent exudate. Histologic examination revealed columns of amebae extending into the brain substance, especially via the perivascular spaces.

This clinical entity has now been reported from several parts of the United States (Florida, Virginia, Texas), Great Britain, and Czechoslovakia. It is usually found in children and young people, and is invariably fatal. It appears to be acquired by swimming, diving, or water skiing in lakes known to contain large numbers of free-living amebae. Pressure changes under water probably force the amebae through the cribriform plate. Naegleria has repeatedly been found in the cerebrospinal fluid of man. The CSF also shows an increased protein level, decreased sugar, neutrophils, and red cells, but is bacteriologically sterile. Most of the patients to date have died, usually because the diagnosis has been missed.

Emetine, arsenicals, sulfonamides, tetracyclines, and metronidazole have been used without success. Amphotericin B therapy has resulted in recovery of a patient in whom Naegleria organisms were recovered from the CSF, and in vitro studies show that therapeutic concentrations are amebicidal. In one recent fatal case *Naegleria gruberi* was recovered from the lungs, liver, spleen, and heart blood, as well as from the central nervous system. Since such free-living amebae are ubiquitous, doubtless reports from other countries will appear in the future.

Culbertson, C. G.: Pathogenic acanthamoeba (Hartmannella). Am. J. Clin. Path., 35:195, 1961.

Duma, R. J., Rosenblum, W. I., McGehee, R. F., Jones, M. M., and Clifford, N. E.: Primary amoebic meningoencephalitis caused by Naegleria. Ann. Intern. Med., 74:923, 1971.

Fowler, M., and Carter, R. F.: Acute pyogenic meningitis probably due to Acanthamoeba sp.: A preliminary report. Br. Med. J., 2:740, 1965.

286. TOXOPLASMOSIS

Thomas C. Jones

General Considerations. Toxoplasmosis is a common infection of mammals and birds which occasionally results in protean disease. It is caused by the protozoan *Toxoplasma gondii*. In man, tissue parasitism during the proliferative phase may occur without signs or symptoms; it may lead to a transient illness characterized by lymphadenopathy, fever, and fatigue; or it may cause extensive damage to the brain, eyes, muscle, heart, liver, or lungs. Severe manifestations of the disease most commonly occur when a fetus is infected (congenital toxoplasmosis) or when infection occurs in patients with impaired immunity. Chronic infection may lead to a recurrent inflammatory process usually recognized by progressive ocular damage. When members of the cat family ingest Toxoplasma organisms, infection of epithelial cells in the intestinal tract results in production of oocysts which, when excreted, provide an important means by which the infection is transmitted in nature. Viable organisms within cysts in muscles and brain of infected animals provide a continued source of infection to carnivores.

History. In 1907 *Toxoplasma gondii* was recognized as a distinct protozoan and named by Nicolle and Manceaux. The first human case of congenital infection was recorded in 1923 by Janku in Prague, and in 1938 Wolf, Cowen, and Paige described the first cases from which the parasite was isolated. Toxoplasmosis in adults was first described by Pinkerton and Henderson in 1941. Eye damage caused by Toxoplasma in adults was first suggested by Frenkel and confirmed after observations made by Wilder in 1952. The present realization that 500 million humans are infected with the protozoan evolved from the extensive epidemiologic studies of Feldman, Desmonts, Thalhammer, and Jacobs, and from the recognition by Siim and others of the varied, often mild clinical patterns of acquired infection. In 1967, Hutchison first suggested that the cat played a role in the life cycle of *Toxoplasma gondii*, a cycle which was subsequently delineated in 1970.

The Protozoan. When mammals or birds ingest either infective oocysts or cysts in muscle or brain of other animals, an *intermediate* or asexual cycle of Toxoplasma infection is initiated. This consists of an obligate intracellular *proliferative* stage and a *cyst* stage. In the proliferative stage, *trophozoites*, which are ovoid or arc shaped, 3 to 4 μ in diameter, 6 to 7 μ in length, enter host cells by endocytosis and then divide by endodyogeny; two daughter cells are formed within each parent. Division continues until the host cell ruptures, releasing organisms which in turn infect adjacent cells. As the host develops immunity, parasite proliferation gradually slows, and a firm wall (cyst) forms around the organism allowing the Toxoplasma to persist for years in this cyst stage.

When *cats* ingest cysts or oocysts of *Toxoplasma gondii*, however, an addition process can occur, i.e., the *definitive* or sexual cycle initiated within the cat's intestinal epithelial cells. Parasites released from cysts or oocysts penetrate the epithelial cells where they first enter a proliferative stage and then mature by gametogony into *macro-* or *microgametocytes*. A *zygote*, formed by union of the gametocytes, matures in one to four days into an infective *oocyst*. The mature infective oocyst is oblong, 9 μ by 13 μ, and it contains two *sporocysts*, each of which contains four *sporozoites*. Oocysts are excreted by the cat for one to three weeks, beginning three to five days after ingestion of the Toxoplasma containing tissue. Cats generally also acquire a systemic infection (intermediate cycle) at the time of first exposure to Toxoplasma, just as other mammals do. They occasionally repeat the sexual cycle after reinfection, although the period of oocyst shedding may be shorter.

Epidemiology. *Toxoplasma gondii* infects almost all mammals and birds. The usual life cycle in nature is among cats, small mammals, and birds, but man has intruded on this cycle with his taste for uncooked meats and his close association with cats. In some areas, such as Tahiti and the Easter Islands, the prevalence of Toxoplasma infection is near 100 per cent. In most parts of the world the prevalence ranges between 20 and 60 per cent of the population. Only in very dry areas, such as Arizona, and in very cold areas, such as northern Alaska, are low prevalence rates found. A few small islands in the Pacific, where cats have never been introduced, have remained free of toxoplasmosis.

The means by which the parasite is transmitted varies from one area to another: in one, oocyst ingestion seems more likely; in another, cyst ingestion. For instance, the very high rates in certain parts of the tropics are believed to be due to close contact with cat feces. In these areas infection is often acquired in childhood. The oocysts are resistant to drying and to a wide range of temperatures, and may remain infectious in moist soil for a year. Ingestion of oocysts is made more likely by the demonstration that cockroaches and flies can disseminate them to various exposed foods. In the United States the population appears to acquire the infection more commonly by ingesting uncooked infected meat. The infection is acquired at a rate of 1 per cent of the population per year of life from age 15 to age 50. Mutton and pork have been found to be more frequently infected than beef. Rarely, transmission of infection has followed accidental inoculation of trophozoites by laboratory workers, organ transplantation, and leukocyte transfusion from immunosuppressed donors. Blood transfusions from healthy donors have not been shown to be a means of transmitting toxoplasmosis.

Transplacental Transmission. Transplacental transmission in humans occurs only at the time of parasitemia, during the acute infection. The frequency of this secondary form of transmission therefore follows the frequency of acquisition of infection during child-bearing years. In the United States and Europe 0.5 to 1.0 per cent of women have been demonstrated to have rising or very high antibody titers to Toxoplasma during pregnancy. Forty per cent of these adult infections are transmitted to the fetus. This may result in abortion or stillbirth, or an infant with clinical signs of toxoplasmosis (one third to one half of infected infants). Alternatively, infected infants may be completely asymptomatic but may show an antibody response to Toxoplasma antigens as evidence of transplacental infection. These infected asymptomatic infants are believed to make up a population which later in life may show signs of recurrent retinochoroiditis. There is no significant relationship in humans between chronic Toxoplasma infection and either recurrent abortion or prematurity.

Pathogenesis and Immunity. Multiplication of Toxoplasma organisms within cells causes little obvious disturbance to host cell function until the dividing parasites cause the cell to rupture. Adjacent cells are then infected, resulting in progressive tissue necrosis and an acute inflammatory response (edema and infiltration with mononuclear cells and a few polymorphonuclear leukocytes). Organisms are disseminated hematogenously throughout the body. New sites of necrosis and inflammation are initiated, particularly in myocardium and skeletal muscle. In those patients who develop severe generalized toxoplasmosis significant encephalitis, myocarditis, myositis, pneumonitis, hepatitis, and skin rash have been documented.

Generalized lymph node enlargement, along with other signs of systemic infection such as fever and malaise, develops one to two weeks after ingestion of infectious tissue. These lymph nodes show histocytic hyperplasia rather than follicular hyperplasia, giving the hematoxylin-eosin stained section a rather typical appearance of containing predominantly eosin reactive cells. The architecture of the lymph node is preserved. Necrosis and giant cells are not seen, and only rarely can groups of Toxoplasma organisms be identified. Occasionally, even in relatively mild infections, myositis or myocarditis can be demonstrated.

Associated with the development of marked lymphoreticular activity, both humoral and cellular immunity can be demonstrated. Antibodies against various Toxoplasma antigens can be demonstrated in the peripheral blood. Later Toxoplasma antigen induces lymphocyte proliferation and lymphokine production, and mononuclear cells no longer support division of intracellular Toxoplasma. The acute infection resolves, but Toxoplasma organisms remain viable within cysts in the infected tissue for the lifetime of the host.

Congenital Infection; Immunologic Deficiency. Although the healthy adult usually deals effectively with the Toxoplasma infection, the immunologically deficient patient does not. The best example of this is the pathologic changes of congenital toxoplasmosis. The infected placenta may show areas of necrosis, inflammatory cells, and parasites, more frequently on the fetal than on the maternal side of the placenta. The fetal brain shows necrosis, glial cell proliferation, and perivascular lymphocytic infiltration. Toxoplasma can be identified in these lesions. High ventricular fluid protein, aqueductal obstruction, and hydrocephalus are often seen. If the infant survives several months, calcification of these areas occurs. Necrotic lesions in the retina are also seen. Organisms can be isolated from numerous organs of the body, but extensive inflammation is most often identified as pneumonitis, myocarditis, hepatitis, and splenitis.

About half the infections which occur in utero are caused by a sufficiently low number of organisms or are of low enough virulence that infection is manifest only by the appearance of humoral and cellular immune responses. Cysts develop and persist in brain, retina, and cardiac and skeletal muscle. Rupture of these cysts, many years later, can lead to transient episodes of inflammatory response and scarring. These inflammatory lesions are usually well localized, but in the retina they lead to significant organ impairment. The enucleated eye may show areas of necrosis in the retina often associated with proliferating Toxoplasma organisms, as well as a granulomatous inflammation of the choroid and sclera. The eye damage is the result of proliferation of organisms released at the time of cyst rupture which invade other cells, combined with damage caused by the vigorous hypersensitivity reaction.

In the patients with abnormal or suppressed immune responses, primary infection or cyst rupture may lead to symptomatic myositis, myocarditis, retinochoroiditis, or encephalitis.

Clinical Manifestations. Manifestations of toxoplasmosis can be divided into four clinical patterns: acquired disease in otherwise healthy individuals, congenital infection, retinochoroiditis, and disease in the altered host.

Acquired Toxoplasmosis. Patients with acquired toxoplasmosis usually present with lymphadenopathy (90 per cent), fever (40 per cent), or malaise (40 per cent). Lymph node enlargement may be the only sign, and since cervical lymph node enlargement is particularly common, the patient may seek medical attention only because of concern about a neck mass. The nodes are usually nontender and rubbery in consistency. Generalized lymphadenopathy occurs in over half the cases, and transient splenomegaly has been recorded in approximately one third. The fever is usually low grade, but occasionally it may be high and of prolonged duration. Fatigue is often rather marked and may be associated with generalized muscle discomfort. Less commonly recorded signs or symptoms have included sore throat, headache, and a maculopapular rash. The pharynx is usually hyperemic; exudative pharyngitis is not seen. Specific organ involvement in this form of the disease includes myocardium (rarely pericardium), skeletal muscle, rarely liver, skin, and brain. When such organ involvement occurs, the abnormalities in organ function may dominate the clinical picture. Retinochoroiditis in association with the acute acquired disease is very unusual.

The course of the illness is quite variable. Occasionally fever, malaise, and specific organ involvement are marked and the illness prolonged. More commonly, fever lasts only a few days or weeks, although fatigue and lymphadenopathy may persist for several months. Lymph nodes will occasionally fluctuate in size during the recovery period.

Laboratory tests usually reveal a normal total leukocyte count with a slight monocytosis or lymphocytosis. Atypical lymphocytes may be described, but they are usually not present in large numbers. Hematocrit and hemoglobin are usually normal; however, a Coombs-negative hemolytic anemia has occasionally been reported. Serum transaminases are usually normal, but early in the illness they may be slightly elevated (less than 100 U). The Paul-Bunnell test for heterophil antibodies is negative. The electrocardiogram may show ST and T wave abnormalities in cases in which myocarditis is prominent. The chest film is usually normal; hilar adenopathy is very rare. Lymph node biopsy shows histocytic hyperplasia. Antibodies against Toxoplasma antigens are present in high or rising titers.

Congenital Toxoplasmosis. Cases of congenital toxoplasmosis may be manifested as microophthalmia, microcephaly, seizures, retardation, hepatosplenomegaly, pneumonitis, rash, and fever. If aqueduct of Sylvius obstruction has occurred, hydrocephalus will be prominent. Occasionally, signs may not be obvious at birth, but they may progress during the first months of life. Cerebral calcification may be seen after several months. The infant will show progressive signs of failure to thrive, followed by death. Cases of congenital toxoplasmosis may be mild, demonstrating only mental retardation, a seizure disorder, or retinochoroiditis. Laboratory tests reflect the severity of the specific organ involved. Toxoplasma antibody titers are elevated and will show a persistent or rising titer as maternal antibody disappears.

Toxoplasmic Retinochoroiditis. This form of toxoplasmosis is almost always a late sequela of otherwise asymptomatic congenital infection. Symptoms are usually first noted in the second or third decade of life. Patients have recurrent episodes of ocular pain and decreased vision associated with progressive loss of vision. The lesion is retinal, with an associated posterior uveitis. Toxoplasma infection probably does not cause an isolated anterior uveitis. Systemic signs of Toxoplasma infection are not usually present. Toxoplasma antibody titers are frequently low and tend not to change.

Toxoplasmosis in the Altered Host. Toxoplasmosis may present as a disseminated disease in patients with neoplasms of the lymphatic system, particularly Hodgkin's disease, or in patients being treated with immunosuppressive drugs. The clinical manifestations of the systemic disease are variable. Fever, encephalitis, myositis, hepatosplenomegaly, or myocarditis may occur. Pneumonitis has been described rarely in this setting. Lymphadenopathy may or may not be present. The primary difficulty is in separating the numerous other causes of these signs or symptoms from those caused by toxoplasmosis. At present one clinical pattern seems dominant, that is, progressive signs of encephalitis (confusion, headache, coma). In a patient with altered cellular immunity, these signs should lead to a consideration of and probably treatment for toxoplasmosis. If untreated, this illness is almost always progressive and fatal. Toxoplasma antibody titers are usually elevated.

Diagnosis. The diagnosis of toxoplasmosis rests on the presence of changing or elevated titers of antitoxoplasma antibodies and on isolation of the parasite from infected tissue. The antibody tests available include the indirect fluorescent antibody test (IFA), the Sabin-Feldman dye test, and a complement fixation test. The IFA and dye test show high antitoxoplasma antibody titers usually from the time of earliest symptoms (one to two weeks after infection). A titer of 1:1024 or higher, or evidence of a rising titer, is suggestive of active infection. The high titers will decrease during the subsequent months and after two to four years reach low levels (1:16 to 1:256) for the lifetime of the individual. There has been no cross-reactivity between dye test antibodies and other antigens; thus the test is very specific. An indirect hemagglutination test is also available. However, many feel that the rise in antibody titer is too slow to be as helpful clinically as the Sabin-Feldman dye test.

The complement fixation test becomes positive later than the dye test, three to six weeks after infection, when symptoms are often present. Thus one is often able to see a changing titer over several weeks by using this test in a patient whose dye test is elevated. A significant complement fixation test is a titer of 1:8 or greater or a fourfold increase in titer. This test usually becomes negative within a few years after infection. In conjunction with the dye test it can help separate those patients with persistently high dye test antibody titers from those with recent infection. This may help in deciding if symptoms which began weeks or a few months previously are due to recent Toxoplasma infection or, in an asymptomatic pregnant female, whether the infection was recently acquired. Treatment may transiently decrease complement fixing antibody titers.

In congenital toxoplasmosis the contribution of transferred maternal IgG antitoxoplasma antibody must be excluded. This is done by performing several tests over the first few months; if positive titers are due to maternal antibody, the titer will fall about 50 per cent per month over four to six months. If the infant had been infected, the titer would remain stable, dip transiently, or increase. One may also test for IgM antitoxoplasma antibodies by using an IFA test to determine if the observed antibodies are fetal or maternal in origin. Since IgM antibodies do not cross the placenta, their presence indicates fetal antibody synthesis. In some infected infants this test may be falsely negative.

The diagnosis of Toxoplasma retinochoroiditis by serologic means is difficult. Since the infection is chronic, dye test and IFA titers are usually positive in low titer, and complement fixing antibodies are absent. The diagnosis of toxoplasmic retinochoroiditis may be suggested by finding higher antibody titers in the anterior chamber fluid than in the serum, or by isolating the organism at the time of enucleation. A negative dye test or IFA excludes Toxoplasma as the cause of retinochoroiditis.

The use of serologic tests in the immunodeficient patient to determine "activity" of the infection has also been difficult. Some patients with repeatedly low antibody titers have demonstrated a sudden rise in titer associated with a moribund state and death; however, at autopsy, disseminated toxoplasmosis could not be implicated as a factor contributing to death. Investigators are now examining whether changes in lymphocyte response to Toxoplasma antigen may be of more predictive value. At present, elevated antibody titers, plus progressive encephalitis, should be sufficient to warrant antitoxoplasma therapy in an immunodeficient patient. Evidence of the organism on biopsy of organs such as muscle, kidney, lung, and liver should also be an indication for therapy in these patients.

The diagnosis of toxoplasmosis can be substantiated by isolation of the organism. Biopsy material (particularly lymph node or muscle), tissue at the time of autopsy, or blood, sputum, or cerebrospinal fluid can be inoculated intraperitoneally into Toxoplasma-free laboratory animals. Smears of peritoneal fluid can be made at seven to ten days, stained by Giemsa technique, and examined for the protozoa. If the smear is negative, the peritoneal fluid should be injected intraperitoneally into another animal. If the infected animals survive for three weeks, they are sacrificed and their brains examined for Toxoplasma cysts and their serum for Toxoplasma antibody. Isolation of Toxoplasma organisms from human tissue should be correlated with histopathology of the tissue and antibody titers.

The differential diagnosis in a patient with lymphadenopathy and fever usually rests between lymphoma and infectious mononucleosis, although numerous infections, such as tuberculosis, brucellosis, tularemia, cat scratch disease, and certain systemic viral and rickettsial illnesses, must be considered. Toxoplasmosis can be distinguished from infectious mononucleosis by absence of marked atypical lymphocytosis and heterophil antibodies and normal or nearly normal hepatic transaminases; and from lymphoma by absence of anemia, hilar adenopathy, and a lymph node biopsy which shows histocytic hyperplasia rather than neoplastic cells. The other numerous causes of lymphadenopathy and fever must be excluded by appropriate serologic and skin tests, biopsy, and cultures.

Congenital toxoplasmosis must be distinguished from cytomegalovirus infection. Microcephaly is more common in cytomegalovirus infection than in toxoplasmosis. Ventricular fluid protein content is often higher in toxoplasmosis than in cytomegalovirus infection. Bacterial and fungal meningoencephalitis must be excluded by appropriate cultures. Viral encephalitis, particularly the rubella syndrome, must be considered. Congenital malformations are unusual in toxoplasmosis.

Toxoplasmic retinochoroiditis must be distinguished from cytomegalovirus, herpes, tuberculosis, histoplasmosis, and sarcoidosis by appearance of the retinal lesion and appropriate serologic and skin tests.

Treatment. A combination of pyrimethamine (Daraprim) and sulfadiazine has been shown to be effective in controlling Toxoplasma during the proliferative stage. There is no known therapy for eradicating organisms in the cyst stage. Pyrimethamine is given orally, 75 mg the first day, followed by 25 mg per day for one month. Infants are given 1 mg per kilogram per day for the first three days, and then 0.5 mg per kilogram per day thereafter. An intramuscular preparation is not commercially available. Sulfadiazine is given orally, 4 grams daily in divided doses for one month. Infants can be given 100 mg per kilogram per day. Recently, sulfalene and trimethoprim, a similar drug combination, has been found effective. Other sulfonamides such as the triple sulfonamides can be substituted for sulfadiazine; however, sulfisoxazole (Gantrisin) has been found ineffective. Other drugs such as spiramycin, tetracyclines, and sulfones are less effective than the aforementioned drugs. Since pyrimethamine and sulfonamide inhibit folate synthesis, folinic acid (leucovorin), 6 mg per day, should be used in conjunction with the aforementioned therapy to prevent potential bone marrow toxicity. Platelet counts and white blood cell counts should be performed twice weekly during therapy.

Study of the effectiveness of these drugs in acquired human toxoplasmosis has been limited by the marked variability and spontaneous improvement without therapy. However, in some cases there has been evidence that this treatment shortens the period of fever and malaise, although lymphadenopathy may persist. It has therefore been recommended that only patients with fever, myalgias, or malaise be considered for therapy. Asymptomatic adults should be considered for treatment (1) after accidental laboratory infection and (2) when a pregnant female demonstrates serologic evidence of recent infection, only after appropriate consultations and considerations have led to a rejection of therapeutic abortion and have weighed potential fetal damage from the drugs. There is no adequate evidence to recommend treating dye-test-positive women who wish to become pregnant or who abort habitually, or in treating asymptomatic women after delivery of a congenitally damaged infant.

Congenital toxoplasmosis should be treated whether asymptomatic or symptomatic, because the proliferative stage may continue for several months before adequate cellular immunity has developed to control the infection. Treatment will not be effective when given late in the course of the disease or when severe central nervous system damage has already occurred.

In toxoplasmic retinochoroiditis, the primary therapy should be directed at controlling the hypersensitivity response with corticosteroids. Pyrimethamine and sulfadiazine should be used in conjunction with this therapy to prevent dissemination of infection and to limit local damage caused by proliferating organisms.

In patients with altered immunity and toxoplasmosis, good therapeutic response to this drug combination has been recorded. Fever has been controlled, and evidence of progressive encephalitis has been reversed. In these patients long-term therapy has to be considered because appropriate immunologic responses do not occur, making relapse of the disease likely.

Prevention. Toxoplasmosis is commonly transmitted by consumption of undercooked meat or Toxoplasma oocysts. Thus, dye-test-negative pregnant women or patients with depressed cellular immunity should avoid both these sources of infection. Meat should be cooked at a temperature in excess of 60° C (140° F) for at least 15 minutes. Susceptible individuals should avoid soil or sand boxes where cats may defecate, because oocysts may survive in these places for months. If cats are kept in the house, they should not be fed raw meat or allowed access to wild rodents or birds.

Since infection-immunity in human adults prevents congenital toxoplasmosis, it is reasonable that an appropriate vaccine might be developed in the future. Laboratory workers should take precautions to avoid accidental needle puncture. Baseline antibody testing should be done in patients who are to receive immunosuppressive drugs, who have lymphatic malignancies, or who are to act as organ or leukocyte donors.

Beverley, J. K. A.: Toxoplasmosis. Br. Med. J., 2:475, 1973.

Carey, R. M., Kimball, A. C., Armstrong, D., and Lieberman, P. H.: Toxoplasmosis: Clinical experiences in a cancer hospital. Am. J. Med., 54:30, 1973.

Feldman, H. A.: Toxoplasmosis. N. Engl. J. Med., 279:1370, 1431, 1968.

Frenkel, J. K.: Toxoplasma in and around us. Bio. Science, 26:343, 1973.

Frenkel, J. K.: Toxoplasmosis. *In* Marcial-Rojas, R. D. (ed.): Pathology of Protozoal and Helminthic Diseases. Baltimore, Williams & Wilkins Company, 1971, p. 254.

Kean, B. H.: Clinical toxoplasmosis – 50 years. Trans. R. Soc. Trop. Med. Hyg., 66:549, 1972.

Remington, J. S.: Toxoplasmosis – recent developments. Ann. Rev. Med., 21:201, 1970.

Wallace, G. D.: The role of the cat in the natural history of *Toxoplasma gondii*. Am. J. Trop. Med. Hyg., 22:313, 1973.

Section Two. HELMINTHIC DISEASES

287. INTRODUCTION

Philip D. Marsden

Compared to protozoans, helminths are very large organisms with a complex cellular structure. As they feed on host tissue, their metabolism results in various protein secretions and excretions; and because they themselves largely consist of complex protein, it is not surprising that invasion of the body by worms is frequently associated with an eosinophilic response. Thus, in the invasive stage of schistosomes, hookworm, ascaris, and similar parasites, an eosinophilia is usual. Yet when these worms have matured and settled at their site of election, eosinophilia often is not found. It might be argued in the case of intestinal nematodes that this is because they are in the gut and in a strict sense outside the body, but because the phenomenon also occurs with schistosomiasis and tissue filariae this is too facile an explanation. At present the mechanisms and course of eosinophilia produced in a host in response to a foreign protein are not clearly understood.

With regard to immunology, understandably, complex helminths produce complex crude antigens of low specificity. At the moment, with a few exceptions, group-specific reactions with antigens for schistosomes, hermaphroditic flukes, nematodes, and cestodes are all that are available using tests such as complement fixation or indirect hemagglutination. Skin tests on the whole are much less satisfactory than those based on serology. Many of these helminths are recognized by the presence of characteristic progeny in the form of either eggs in the stools, sputum, or urine, or larvae in the tissues.

The concept of the over-all population or load of worms is important in human disease, as *the parasitic load* is one of the factors determining the extent of pathology (another would be the host response). Today many helminthic infections can be quantitated, and these methods will be mentioned under diagnosis. Another important aspect of worm infections is their relatively long life. Many flukes live for decades after the infection has

TABLE 1. Prevalence of Common Helminth Infections in Man*

Parasite	Source of Infection	Approximate Locality	Estimated Incidence in U.S. and Canada	Estimated World Incidence
Trematodes (flukes):				
Schistosoma japonicum	Water through skin	Far East	–	46,000,000
Schistosoma haematobium	Water through skin	Africa, Middle East	–	39,200,000
Schistosoma mansoni	Water through skin	Africa, South America, Caribbean	–	29,200,000
Clonorchis sinensis	Fish	Far East	In Chinese immigrants	19,000,000
Opisthorchis felineus	Fish	Far East	–	1,100,000
Paragonimus westermani	Crabs, crayfish	Africa, South America	–	3,200,000
Fasciolopsis buski	Water nuts	Far East	–	10,000,000
Cestodes (tapeworms):				
Diphyllobothrium latum	Fish	Around Arctic Circle, N. Europe, Russia, America	†	10,400,000
Taenia saginata	Beef	Cosmopolitan	10,000	38,900,000
Taenia solium	Pork	Cosmopolitan	†	2,500,000
Echinococcus granulosus	Dog feces	Cosmopolitan	†	†
Nematodes (roundworms):				
Intestinal nematodes				
Strongyloides stercoralis	Human feces	Cosmopolitan	400,000	34,900,000
Hookworm	Human feces	Cosmopolitan	1,800,000	456,800,000
Ascaris lumbricoides	Human feces	Cosmopolitan	3,000,000	644,400,000
Trichuris trichuria	Human feces	Cosmopolitan	400,000	355,100,000
Enterobius vermicularis	Human feces	Cosmopolitan	18,000,000	208,800,000
Tissue nematodes				
Trichinella spiralis	Pork	Cosmopolitan	21,100,000	27,800,000
Wuchereria bancrofti and *Brugia malayi*	Mosquitoes	Africa, South America, South Asia	–	189,000,000
Loa loa	Chrysops	Equatorial Africa	–	13,000,000
Dipetalonema perstans	Culicoides	Africa, South America	–	27,000,000
Mansonella ozzardi	Culicoides	South America	–	7,000,000
Onchocerca volvulus	Simulium	Equatorial Africa, Central America	–	19,800,000
Dracunculus medinensis	Cyclops	Middle East, India, Africa	–	48,300,000

*Based on data calculated by N. R. Stoll (J. Parasit., 33:1, 1947). Since the world population has increased by more than 50 per cent, all the figures given can be regarded as extremely conservative. For instance, it is said that 180 million people in the world are infected with one of the three species of schistosome that infect humans.

†Represents less than 100,000 infections.

been acquired, and similarly many filarial species are long lived. This illustrates the importance of obtaining a very detailed history of the patient's movements around the world because a visit to an endemic area 20 years ago may be connected with a current clinical problem.

It must be remembered that there are a large number of helminths that rarely infect man, and many cannot be included in this book. For information on these a standard textbook on parasitology (see references in Ch. 270) should be consulted. An important topical point is that we are now beginning to realize that for every worm adapted to man there are many others which gain access to man's tissues but fail to mature because they are natural parasites of other mammals or birds. These may cause very puzzling clinical problems. An increasing proportion of unexplained eosinophilia encountered in clinical practice is being explained on a basis of invasion of the body by a worm that will not mature in man because he is not the definitive host.

By a simple classification, worms may be separated into trematodes or flukes, cestodes or tapeworms, and nematodes or roundworms. A check list adapted from H. W. Brown's table in the twelfth edition of this text is given here in Table 1, together with information on the source of infection and the main areas of occurrence in the world. The most important helminthic infections in terms of disease in man and incidence are schistosomiasis, hookworm, and filariasis.

THE CESTODES
(Tapeworms)

Philip D. Marsden

288. INTRODUCTION

The cestodes are endoparasitic flatworms, the hermaphroditic adults of which are flat and ribbonlike and inhabit the intestinal tract of vertebrates. The larval forms may require more than one intermediate host and develop in the tissues of vertebrates, and in some instances invertebrates. Most adult tapeworms consist of a scolex or head equipped for attachment with suckers, hooks, or grooves and a strobila or tapelike chain of progressively developing segments or proglottides. The neck is the site of segment generation, and mature segments are complete hermaphroditic units with both sets of sex organs. There is no digestive system, food being absorbed directly through the cuticle. There are

TABLE 2. Common Important Tapeworms

Official Name	Intermediate Host(s)	Stage in Man
Diphyllobothrium latum	Water fleas, freshwater fish	Adult worm
Taenia saginata	Cattle (beef)	Adult worm
Taenia solium	Pigs (pork)	Adult worm and larval stage
Hymenolepis nana	Man	Adult worm and larval stage
Echinococcus granulosus	Man, sheep, cattle	Larval stage
Echinococcus multilocularis	Man, sheep, cattle	Larval stage

longitudinal primitive excretory systems and a nervous system. In gravid segments the uterus is loaded with eggs, and these pass out of the bowel either in the segment or free in the stool. The delicate outer membrane of the eggs is often lost, but the thick-walled inner membrane contains a form infective for the intermediate host.

When eggs are ingested by the appropriate intermediate host, larvae (termed onchospheres) are released which are capable of penetrating the intestinal mucosa. The method by which the larvae develop into encysted forms differs among the cestodes and leads to different clinical patterns. Onchospheres in *Taenia solium* each develop into a small (0.5 to 1.0 cm) fluid-filled structure containing a single inverted "head." These are called *cysticerci,* or bladder worms, and many such larvae distributed in various organs cause the disease cysticercosis. The oncospheres in *Hymenolepis nana* penetrate only into the intestinal mucosa. They develop similarly to those just described; however, fluid is usually not present in the larva, and hence it is termed a *cysticercoid.* In the case of *Echinococcus granulosus,* usually only one onchosphere is able to develop (unilocular) within the intermediate host. However, this larva develops an internal germinating membrane capable of producing an entire population of daughter and granddaughter cysts within the primary cyst. This cyst is called an *echinococcal* or *hydatid* cyst. It continues to enlarge as the population of scolices within increases and will commonly reach a diameter of 20 to 30 cm after many years.

The clinical pattern of disease reflects these various methods of development; the cysticercoid of *H. nana* presents as intestinal irritation; the cysticercus of *T. solium* leads to multiple small lesions, often in the brain, causing seizure disorders; the Echinococcus produces a single large space-occupying lesion which often because of its size interferes with liver, lung, or cardiac function.

In the following chapters, we will deal with only the six most common of the 30 or more species of tapeworm which have been found in man. These are listed in Table 2. They will be discussed in the order cited in the table: first those in which man is the definitive host, then those in which he serves as both definitive and intermediate host, and finally those in which only the larval stage can develop in man.

289. DIPHYLLOBOTHRIUM LATUM (The Fish Tapeworm)

Infection with the fish tapeworm is most common in temperate areas such as Scandinavia and around the Baltic Sea. It also occurs in Canada and in the northern United States, notably Alaska. Central Europe is an endemic focus. In the tropics relatively few reports have appeared from the Philippines, Madagascar, Botswana, Uganda, and Chile. A human parasite, *Diphyllobothrium pacificum,* has been described from Peru. The adult is the largest tapeworm of man, reaching 10 meters and having 4000 segments. (The spatulate head has two deep sucking grooves for attachment to the wall of the ileum.) The gravid segment disintegrates, and operculated ova are passed in the feces.

From the egg a ciliated embryo is eaten by a freshwater flea (Cyclops or Diaptomus species) in which it develops to a *procercoid.* When the infected flea is swallowed by freshwater fish, e.g., salmon, pike, further development takes place in the muscles of the fish to the *plerocercoid,* the form infective to man. The plerocercoid on being liberated into the small intestine grows to an adult in three to six weeks. Although the adult worm causes no pathologic lesion, there is a very important complication to this infection, namely a megaloblastic anemia. This appears to be due to the avidity of the worm for vitamin B_{12}, as 44 per cent of a single dose of Co^{60} labeled vitamin B_{12} was absorbed by the worm, the radioactivity being concentrated in the proximal growing part. Also the nearer the worm is to the jejunum, the greater the chance of developing megaloblastic anemia. It is not clear why the worm needs so much vitamin B_{12}. The worm also appears to require folic acid in the same way. The full range of neurologic symptoms of subacute combined degeneration of the cord may appear, particularly in severe cases of multiple parasitism. Peripheral neuritis appears very early in the parasitism, and recently optic atrophy has been reported.

The *diagnosis* is made by direct examination of the stools, because the eggs are present in very large numbers. Yellowish-brown and operculated, they have to be distinguished from fluke eggs such as Paragonimus, but the large number in the stool favors the diagnosis of fish tapeworm even to the uninitiated. The operculum is actually less conspicuous in Diphyllobothrium, and there is a small knob at the anopercular end (mean size 70 by 45 μ). Because the treatment for the tapeworms of this group and of the Taenia genus is the same, they are considered together later.

Prophylaxis is readily accomplished by thoroughly cooking fish before consumption. Freezing of fish for 48 hours at $-10°$ C will also prevent infection. The infection is not uncommon in New York among Jewish housewives who make their own gefilte fish and sample it in the process.

SPARGANOSIS

This condition requires mention here, because it is the name of an infection caused by the migrating larvae or spargana of several species of tapeworm related to *D. latum* but requiring final hosts other than man. It presents as a migrating subcutaneous painful swelling suggesting a cellulitis. Marked eosinophilia is usually present. The eye may be involved with orbital swelling or even actual penetration of the globe. In China this results from applying infected frogs on poultices to the eye. Biopsy reveals inflammatory tissue reactions and an immature cestode, many of which are quite impossible to identify. *Diphyllobothrium mansonoides (Spirometra mansonoides)* is a common offender. So-called *Sparganum proliferum* is unknown in the adult stage, but may distribute thousands of larvae throughout the body, and in contrast to other forms carries a poorer prognosis. This type of infection is rare, but occurs in many tropical countries, diagnosis being made by finding the plerocercoid larvae in tissues.

290. TAENIA SAGINATA (The Beef Tapeworm)

The beef tapeworm has a cosmopolitan distribution, being particularly common in the Middle East, Kenya, and Ethiopia. In the last-named country people habitually take a monthly purge of herbs to get rid of an impressive length of worm, but rarely get rid of the head. Beef tapeworm is also common in parts of South America, Mexico, and Russia. In all these countries it is acquired by eating undercooked or raw beef—a delicacy in Ethiopia. In one series in the United Kingdom, fashion models seemed commonly infected because rare steaks were fashionable at the time. In spite of the harmless nature of the parasitism, a fastidious fashion model with a beef tapeworm can be a real problem in medical management. It is doubtful whether *T. saginata* causes any symptoms, although epigastric pain, appetite disturbances, and general malaise have been ascribed to the presence of the worm. It is possible that multiple worms may be associated with symptoms. Very rarely the worm may block the pancreatic or cystic duct or appendix, producing acute inflammation (16 such cases have been reported). The 5- to 10-meter adult worm has four suckers on the head to attach it to the wall of the small intestine. The gravid segments are usually recognized in the stool, but, being muscular, they can traverse the anal sphincter and appear in the underclothing. They contain more than 12 uterine branches, which distinguish them from *T. solium,* although recently some doubt has been cast on the reliability of this criterion. Characteristic Taenia eggs may be found in the stool or on the anal margin. When the eggs are swallowed by cattle, llamas, or buffaloes, the hatched embryos gain the skeletal muscles by the bloodstream after bowel penetration and develop into the encysted bladder-like larval forms or cysticerci which are infective for man.

Man is the only definitive host in which the adult worm can develop. The larval cysticercus form has been reported only three times in man, so host specificity seems to be strict. Treatment will be discussed later; prevention consists in not ingesting beef containing cysticerci.

291. TAENIA SOLIUM (The Pork Tapeworm Causing Human Cysticercosis Due to Cysticercus Cellulosae)

In contrast to *T. saginata,* both larval and adult forms of this species can develop in man. Again this worm is cosmopolitan in distribution although relatively rare in North America and western Europe; cysticercosis is the most common identifiable cause of epilepsy in the Durban African population and is a serious disease because of the frequency of brain involvement. Man, again the only definitive host of importance, acquires the infection by eating undercooked measly pork containing cysticerci. Pigs and wild boars are the usual intermediate hosts.

The adult worm usually causes no symptoms in the small intestine. For attachment the head has four suckers and two rows of hooklets on a prominent rostellum. It is smaller than *T. saginata* (2 to 4 meters). Its segments are more delicate than *T. saginata* and there are usually less than twelve branches to the uterus in the gravid segment. The eggs are indistinguishable from *T. saginata,* both being approximately 35 μ, thick-walled, brown, and containing an embryonic oncosphere with six hooklets. In *T. solium* infection, however, these eggs are infective to man, but must pass through the stomach and undergo tryptic digestion before hatching occurs. The usual way in which man is infected with eggs is by external autoinfection, transferring eggs from the anus to the mouth or to food fecally contaminated by a carrier of the worm. Internal autoinfection by regurgitating segments of the worm into the stomach is a theoretic possibility, but has not been recorded.

Once free from the egg in the intestine, the oncosphere penetrates the intestinal wall with its hooklets and, as in the pig, settles in the body tissues. The invaded organs in order of frequency are subcutaneous tissue, brain, eye, muscles, heart, liver, lung, and peritoneum. The cysticercus matures in four months to an ellipsoidal translucent cyst, 10 to 20 by 5 to 10 mm, with an opaque invaginated scolex with suckers and hooks. It is gradually surrounded by a thick fibrous capsule and may live for years. Death is frequently associated with calcification.

The invasive phase may be associated with fever, headache, muscle pains, and high eosinophilia. Usually years after this stage more serious symptoms occur owing to brain involvement, with the onset of epilepsy, personality changes, signs of raised intercranial pressure, or long tract signs. In every patient with epilepsy of late onset coming from an endemic area this possibility should be excluded by (1) taking a detailed history, especially in relation to a past history of tapeworm infection; the stool should be examined for Taenia eggs and segments, because rarely the worm may still be in situ; (2) having a full physical examination, especially for subcutaneous nodules containing cysticerci; biopsy will establish the diagnosis; (3) taking roentgenograms of the skull, buttocks, and thighs for calcified cysticerci which have a characteristic size and shape; and (4) performing either a complement-fixation test or an indirect hemagglutination test, using antigen from lyophilized pig cysticerci.

More rarely the globe of the eye is involved, as well as the heart and skeletal muscle. A cysticercus may be visible on the tongue. Sometimes the cysticerci become secondarily infected. In the brain, inflammation around them may produce internal hydrocephalus. Although the adult worm can be eradicated easily, there is no medical treatment for *Cysticercus cellulosae* save palliative anticonvulsants. Rarely surgical intervention may be necessary in cases of raised intracranial pressure. Again prophylaxis rests on avoiding opportunities of eating infected meat and the inspection and thorough cooking of pork.

292. TREATMENT OF INFECTIONS WITH ADULTS OF THE FISH, BEEF, AND PORK TAPEWORM

Quinacrine hydrochloride (Atabrine, Mepacrine) is an effective drug for treatment of all three species of adult worm. The rationale is that a single comparatively large dose of this drug causes the worm to release its hold and it can then be voided. The most successful technique for adults is as follows: Admit the patient to hospital and give only fluids for 36 to 48 hours. Then pass a tube into the duodenum and, with the patient resting quietly, inject 1 gram of quinacrine hydrochloride down the tube in 40 ml of water, using a 20-ml syringe. Half an hour later a saline purge is injected down the tube, and all feces saved for the next 24 hours. Long lengths of the worm stained yellow with the drug are passed, and the head should be identified. If the head is not dislodged, the worm will regenerate in two to three months, and segments will reappear in the stools. The duodenal tube reduces the chances of vomiting the drug, which is a particular hazard with *T. solium* infections. (Obviously, in many endemic areas it will not be possible to get every patient into hospital.) If the head of the worm is found, one can usually reassure the patient that the worm is eliminated unless it is a rare case of multiple infection.

Niclosamide (hydroxychlorobenzamide) is a relatively new drug that may well replace Atabrine, as it is said to be safe, effective, and easy to administer. When the patient wakes in the morning, two tablets of 0.5 gram each are chewed thoroughly and swallowed with a little water. The same procedure is repeated one hour later. No fasting or purgation is necessary, and children receive a proportionately smaller dose. The worm disintegrates so that unfortunately the head cannot be sought as proof of cure. For this reason follow-up at six months is desirable. Although no report has appeared, some authorities believe that this drug should not be used in *T. solium* infection because worm disintegration may be followed by cysticercosis. It must be remembered that feces from patients harboring *T. solium* are an infectious risk. The patient should scrub his hands after defecation and pass his feces into disinfectant.

293. HYMENOLEPIS NANA (Dwarf Tapeworm)

H. nana is less important as a cause of symptomatic disease than the other tapeworms described here. However, since it is spread directly by contact with contaminated stool, the infection can reach epidemic proportions in institutions where fecal-oral exposure is difficult to control, such as in mental hospitals or schools for young children. In a recent study, almost 8 per cent of the children at Willowbrook State School were found to be infected.

Clinical manifestations of this infection include anorexia, diarrhea, and abdominal pain secondary to irritation of the intestinal mucosa. In addition, systemic signs and symptoms such as headache, dizziness, and occasionally seizures are not infrequent. The treatment of choice is hydroxychlorobenzamide (niclosamide), 2 grams daily for three days, followed a week later by a second course of therapy. This treatment schedule has been developed because relapse occurred when shorter courses of therapy were used. Relapse is thought to occur for two reasons: first, the chlorobenzamide is only effective against the adult; and second, the cysticercoid stage may persist in the mucosa for several weeks before developing into an adult.

294. ECHINOCOCCOSIS (Hydatid Disease)

There are two species of the genus Echinococcus which infect man, *Echinococcus granulosus* and *Echinococcus multilocularis.* They are the most important cestodes producing serious disease in man because of the size and location of their larval form, the hydatid cyst. Man is only one of a number of intermediate hosts, other important ones being sheep, cattle, and deer. The definitive hosts for these very small adult tapeworms are canines such as dogs, wolves, jackals, and foxes.

Hydatid disease is cosmopolitan because infected stock have been distributed all over the world for breeding purposes. The incidence of human infection is low in many countries, but where the triad of man, dog, and sheep or cattle is common, hydatid disease is relatively frequent. Examples are countries such as Australia, Argentina, Chile, Kenya, New Zealand, and Wales. It has been reported from 15 states in the United States. Canada and Alaska seem to enjoy a distinct variant, *E. granulosus var. canadensis.*

Human infection follows ingestion of the eggs excreted by infected dogs. The adult tapeworm measures only 2.5 to 9.2 mm and has a head with hooklets and suckers, a growing neck, and only three segments: immature, sexually mature, and gravid. Heavy infections of dogs are common, but the worm lives for only about six months in the upper jejunum. The eggs produced are indistinguishable from Taenia eggs and like them produce an oncosphere with six hooklets. On reaching the intestine of the intermediate host such as man, they pass through the intestinal wall and circulate in the blood and can develop in any body tissue. It may take 20 to 30 years before the slowly growing hydatid cyst causes symptoms. Often they remain small (less than 10 cm), but they may grow as large as the human head. The host parasite factors determining growth are not clearly understood, but growth is variable from 0.25 to 1 cm a year. The structure of a developed hydatid cyst is complex. Briefly, it really consists of a whole colony of infective larval forms, for inside the laminated, defined cyst wall is a germinal layer that is constantly budding off new infective individuals. The cyst is filled with fluid, and second and third generation cysts containing thousands of infective forms or scolices are suspended in this fluid. There is little wonder that when a dog eats an infected sheep's liver he acquires many adult Echinococcus organisms.

When the infective embryo or oncosphere passes into the portal circulation of man, it is first held up in the liver where more than half (59 per cent) of those that survive develop. Many are destroyed by phagocytic cells. The next tissue filter is the lungs, where 27 per cent lodge. Finally, 15 per cent escape into the general circulation to involve the abdominal cavity, muscle, kidney, spleen, bone, heart, and brain.

ECHINOCOCCUS GRANULOSUS

Echinococcus granulosus is the common species; there are several types of cysts, as follows: (1) The classic unilocular cyst is usually fertile and surrounded by a false capsule of host tissue fibrosis. Rupture of such a cyst will cause dissemination of daughter cysts with secondary hydatids. (2) Alveolar hydatids have a reticulated irregular outline and resemble those of *E. multilocularis,* but there is no metastatic growth. Owing to irregular growth of the germinal membrane, this cyst usually occurs in the liver and is difficult to remove. It is often sterile, and its contents degenerate. (3) Osseous hydatid. The nature of bone does not permit a host or parasite capsule to form. Daughter cysts form in the bone medulla, erode the cortex, and produce a pathologic fracture. If they escape from the bone, the cysts grow in their normal spherical shape with the usual capsules in the extraosseous tissues.

Clinically, the hydatid cysts may produce signs of a space-occupying lesion in relation to the organ in which it occurs. In the liver abdominal pain and vomiting may be presenting symptoms, a mass being visible or palpable. Usually the cysts are too tense to show fluctuation. In the lung they are usually detected on routine chest films as spherical, well-defined shadows. They are more common in the right lung, and rarely are associated with cough and hemoptysis. Those of the brain are indistinguishable from a cerebral tumor. In the kidney, hematuria or loin pain may be the first sign, whereas hydatid cyst of bone may present as a pathologic fracture.

The *complications* of hydatid disease are important. The most serious is rupture and dissemination of further infective larvae. Patients with suspected hydatid disease should always be gently palpated – a leaking cyst may present as anaphylactic shock with an urticarial rash and high eosinophilia. The cyst may become secondarily infected with bacteria and present similarly to a liver or lung abscess.

A suggestive tumor in a patient from an endemic area demands the following investigations. An eosinophilia may be present. Plain roentgenograms may show calcification in the cyst wall, although this does not mean that the cyst is not infective. An isotope scan of the liver reveals the extent of the tumor, but gives no clue as to its nature. In the chest film the round, uniformly dense shadow is suggestive. A fluid level with air in the cyst means communication with a bronchus and possibly secondary infection. A skin test using cyst fluid is positive in the majority of patients, but it has been shown that the reaction depends on the concentration (nitrogen content) of protein in the fluid injected. A cross-reaction occurs in patients with schistosomiasis. Until there is universal acceptance of a standard skin test antigen, a negative result is meaningless. Hydatid complement-fixation tests, hemagglutination tests, and bentonite flocculation tests are all practicable and are helpful. A scolex antigen is probably the best (Bull. WHO). Rarely cyst fragments, such as scolices, may be found in the sputum or urine. It must be recalled that one in five patients has multiple cysts, so that if a cyst is located in one site, especially if it is not the liver, there may be others. A liver scan should be done in every patient with an extrahepatic cyst. *Diagnostic aspiration is never indicated because of the risk of rupture.* In the liver and lung, carcinoma and abscess are often difficult differential diagnoses.

It should be emphasized that many hydatid cysts never get very large (5 to 10 cm) and never cause symptoms. There is no medical treatment. Surgery is only indicated in cysts that are enlarging, producing pressure symptoms, or developing complications. The physician should consult a surgeon who has experience with this problem. If possible the cyst should be removed entirely. To prevent spillage and dissemination, the cyst is usually aspirated at operation after packing off the site; 20 ml of fluid is withdrawn, and an equal quantity of 2 per cent formalin, 1 per cent iodine, or 30 per cent sodium chloride is introduced to kill the scolices. Injection of a 1 per cent aqueous solution of iodine in a volume amounting to one twentieth of the whole cyst volume is lethal to scolices within one minute. It is said to produce fewer complications than formalin. Anaphylactic reactions owing to spillage during operation may require corticosteroids.

E. granulosus var. canadensis is common in Alaska and Canada where it has a sylvatic cycle in deer and wolves. It produces smaller and more delicate cysts in man than the classic *E. granulosus;* the latter are more frequent in the lung, usually asymptomatic, and almost never cause serious complications so that the distinction is important.

ECHINOCOCCUS MULTILOCULARIS

The medical importance of distinguishing between these two species is that *Echinococcus multilocularis* does not produce large single cysts with endogenous growth and well-defined fibrous tissue encapsulation but rather an aggregate of innumerable small cysts that multiply by exogenous budding to produce the so-called alveolar or malignant hydatid. More than 90 per cent occur in liver, which is progressively honeycombed by a multitude of small cysts. They may become confluent and even metastasize like a malignancy. Intrahepatic or portal hypertension develops with splenomegaly, and biliary obstruction may produce icterus. The hepatic infection may be difficult to differentiate from a malignancy. This species of cestode occurs in south central Europe, Russia, and Alaska. Rarely cases have occurred in Australasia, England, and Argentina.

Prevention of infection with both these species entails elimination of the infection from dogs by worming with arecoline hydrobromide regularly and preventing their eating infected offal. Contamination of the hands, food, and drink with dog feces should be avoided.

295. OTHER TAPEWORMS

Two other species of adult tapeworms that parasitize the human intestine are usually mentioned, but in comparison with those discussed above they are of little importance in human disease. The rat tapeworm *Hymenolepis diminuta* is acquired by swallowing infected insects carrying the Taenia eggs from rats. *Dipylidium caninum* is the common tapeworm of cats and dogs throughout the world, and is transmitted by their fleas to children handling their pets. The gravid proglottids are shaped like melon seeds and may be seen in the stool. For these parasites niclosamide is usually used, although recently paromomycin has given high cure rates in most of the human intestinal cestodes.

Coenurus infections of man, like hydatid, take the form of cystlike larvae in the tissue; 64 cases have been recorded to date. Infection in temperate regions is probably due to the larval cyst *Multiceps multiceps* (a dog tapeworm) and usually occurs in the central nervous system. Similar cysts are found in the brain of sheep, producing a fatal disease known as gid, which is characterized by somnolence, loss of weight, visual disturbance, and ataxia. In Africa *Taenia brauni* seems to be responsible for similar "hydatid-like" cysts in the subcutaneous tissues of man.

Araña Iniguez, R.: Hydatid echinococcosis of the nervous system. *In* Spillane, J. D. (ed.): Tropical Neurology. New York, Oxford University Press, 1973, p. 408.

Bjorkenheim, G.: Neurological changes in pernicious tapeworm anaemia. Acta Med. Scand., 140 (Supplement):260, 1961.

Dew, H. R.: Hydatid Disease. Sydney, Australian Publishing Co., Ltd., 1928.

Echinococcosis. Bull. WHO, 39, No. 1, 1968.

Jalayer, T., and Askavi, I.: A study of the effect of aqueous iodine on hydatid cysts in vitro and in vivo. Ann. Trop. Med. Parasitol. 60:169, 1966.

Katz, A. M., and Pan, C.: Echinococcus disease in the United States. Am. J. Med., 25:759, 1958.

Keeling, J. E. D.: The chemotherapy of cestode infections. *In* Goldin, A., Hawking, F., and Schnitzer, R. J. (eds.) Advances in Chemotherapy. London and New York, Academic Press, 1968, Vol. 3, pp. 109–152.

Pawlowski, Z., and Schultz, M. G.: Taeniasis and cysticercosis (*Taenia Saginata*). Adv. Parasitol., 10:269, 1972.

Powell, S. J., Procter, E. M., Wilmot, A. J., and McLeod, I. N.: Cysticercosis and epilepsy in Africans: A clinical and serological study. Ann. Trop. Med. Parasitol., 60:152, 1966.

Swartzwelder, J. C., Beaver, P. C., and Hood, M. W.: Sparganosis in the southern United States. Amer. J. Trop. Med. Hyg., 13:43, 1964.

Templeton, A. C.: Anatomical and geographical location of human Coenurus infection. Trop. Geogr. Med., 23:105, 1971.

Vik, R.: The genus Diphyllobothrium. Exp. Parasitol., 15:361, 1964.

Wilson, J. F., Diddams, A. C., and Rausch, R. L.: Cystic hydatid disease in Alaska: A review of 101 cases of *Echinococcus granulosus* infection. Am. Rev. Respir. Dis., 98:1, 1967.

Yoeli, M., Most, H., Hammond, J., and Scheinesson, G. P.: Parasitic infections in a closed community. Results of a 10-year survey in Willowbrook State School. Trans. R. Soc. Trop. Med. Hyg., 66:764, 1972.

DISEASES CAUSED BY TREMATODES (Flukes)

296. SCHISTOSOMIASIS (Bilharziasis)

Kenneth S. Warren

Definition. Schistosomiasis, a chronic infection of more than 200,000,000 people in Asia, Africa, the Caribbean, and South America, is caused by three different worm species, *Schistosoma mansoni, S. japonicum,* and *S. haematobium.* Infection occurs during immersion in fresh water containing schistosome cercariae. These larval forms penetrate the skin and migrate via the lungs and liver to the final habitat of the half-inch-long adult worms: the veins of the intestines and urinary bladder. The worms themselves do not multiply within man, but produce large numbers of eggs, many of which remain in the body, damaging primarily the intestines, liver, and urinary tract. Eggs that are excreted in the urine and feces and that reach fresh water hatch into ciliated miracidia. These organisms penetrate into snails, multiply, and develop into cercariae, the infective form for man.

Etiology. Although the cercariae of many different schistosome species penetrate human skin, there are three major species that complete their life cycles in man and are thus capable of causing systemic disease: *Schistosoma mansoni, japonicum,* and *haematobium.* The life cycles of these schistosomes are essentially similar, all being digenetic trematodes alternating a sexual phase of reproduction in man (definitive host) with an asexual reproductive phase in snails (intermediate host). Nevertheless, at each phase of the life cycle there are differences among the species that play crucial roles in the epidemiology, pathogenesis, and clinical picture of the disease.

The adult worms or schistosomes are members of the class Trematoda of the phylum Platyhelminthes or flatworms. The male worms (10 to 20 $\times$ 0.5 to 1 mm) have cleft bodies within which the longer and thinner females reside, *S. japonicum* being the largest of the three species. The worms may live in man for as long as 30 years, but recent evidence suggests that their mean life span is five to ten years. The habitats of the adult *S. mansoni, japonicum,* and *haematobium* worms are, respectively, the veins of the large intestine, small intestine, and urinary bladder.

The worms absorb metabolites through both their intestines and integument. Their energy processes depend on anaerobic catabolism of carbohydrates; the schistosomes utilize an amount of glucose equivalent to one fifth of their dry body weight each hour and convert 80 per cent of it to lactic acid. In addition, the ingestion of red blood cells appears to be of nutritional significance, as the worms contain a proteolytic enzyme that breaks down globin; the remaining insoluble hematin-like pigment is regurgitated, because the schistosome intestine terminates blindly. The rapid metabolic rate of these worms may in part be related to their continual output of large numbers of eggs, estimated at 1400 to 3000 per day for *S. japonicum* and one tenth that number for *S. mansoni.* The eggs of the last-named species are released singly, whereas those of the other two species are deposited in clutches of as many as ten. They embryonate over a period of six days and increase in size, reaching a mean of 66 × 155 μ for *S. mansoni,* 60 × 143 μ for *S. haematobium,* and 67 × 89 μ for *S. japonicum.* The shape of the eggs is distinctive, *S. mansoni* being ellipsoidal and having a lateral spine; *S. haematobium,* also ellipsoidal but with a terminal spine; and *S. japonicum,* spheroidal with a tiny knob. The eggs remain viable for approximately 21 days after laying, during which time they must pass out of the body if their life cycle is to be completed. Passage from the blood vessels through the tissues and into the lumen of the excretory organs is apparently facilitated by enzymatic secretions of the eggs plus muscular movements of the gut or bladder. A large proportion of the eggs, however, either remain in the intestinal and vesical tissues or break free in the bloodstream and are carried into the liver and lungs.

The eggs that pass out of the body in feces or urine and reach fresh water hatch rapidly into free-swimming ciliated miracidia. The miracidia of *S. mansoni* are negatively geotropic and positively phototropic, although those of *S. haematobium* appear to be the opposite. Their average life span is about six hours. If during this time a snail is encountered, the organisms may penetrate it, and if it is of the genus Biomphalaria for *S. mansoni,* Bulinus for *S. haematobium,* or Oncomelania for *S. japonicum,* the organism can complete its life cycle. The former two snail genera are aquatic, the latter amphibious. The miracidium remains close to the site of penetration, developing into a mother sporocyst. After about ten days daughter sporocysts begin to migrate into the digestive gland of the snail, and at about five weeks from the inception of the process cercariae produced from the daughter sporocysts begin to be shed by the snail. Maximal stimulus for shedding of *S. mansoni* and *haematobium* cercariae is provided by light, but darkness seems to favor the output of *S. japonicum* cercariae. The average daily output of *S. mansoni* and *S. haematobium* cercariae is about 700, but that of *S. japonicum* cercariae is only about two. These organisms may live for two to three days under ideal conditions, but their infectivity begins to decrease by 24 hours. The fork-tailed schistosome cercariae are about 125 to 200 μ in length by 50 to 75 μ in width. *S. mansoni* and *haematobium* cercariae alternate periods of rest, during which they sink slowly, with periods of movement, during which they rise toward the surface of the water. In contrast, *S. japonicum* cercariae attach themselves to the surface film where they tend to remain at rest. When cercariae encounter mammalian skin, they attach themselves with suckers, and by mechanical means, aided by enzymatic secretions, the head penetrates, leaving the tail behind. This process occurs during immersion in water or while the skin remains moist (drying kills the organism), and takes four to ten minutes for *S. mansoni,* but only a few seconds to three minutes for *S. japonicum.*

As the worms do not multiply in the mammalian host, each cercaria that penetrates the skin can develop into only one worm. Many cercariae die in the skin, however, and in the best of experimental hosts only about 60 per cent of the *S. mansoni* organisms reach maturity. Within a few hours to days the schistosomula (the cercariae are completely changed both biochemically and physiologically immediately after penetration) migrate to the lungs by either the blood stream or lymphatics. After a few days in the pulmonary vessels the schistosomula migrate to the liver, either directly through the lungs and diaphragm or by the bloodstream. This phase takes ten to twelve days for *S. mansoni,* a somewhat shorter period for *S. japonicum,* and a longer one for *S. haematobium.* Once in the intrahepatic portal venules the worms rapidly reach maturity, mate, and move against the blood flow to their final habitats. Egg output is detectable at five to six weeks for *S. japonicum*, seven to eight weeks for *S. mansoni*, and ten to twelve weeks for *S. haematobium.*

Epidemiology. *Incidence and Prevalence.* Initial infection in schistosomiasis usually occurs in childhood, and reinfection may continue as long as there is contact with fresh water. It must be remembered that the worms do not multiply in the human body, that complete immunity apparently does not occur, and that the worms may live for decades. Under these circumstances the incidence of schistosomiasis in endemic areas is low and occurs principally in children, but the prevalence of the disease may build up to massive proportions.

The worldwide prevalence of schistosomiasis is now estimated at over 200,000,000 cases. It is known to be endemic in 71 countries that have a total population of 1,362,635,000.

In Africa, *S. haematobium* and *S. mansoni* are widespread. Only the former species occurs in Tunisia, Algeria, Morocco, Mauritania, Portuguese Guinea, Niger, the Congo Republic (Brazzaville), Somalia, and the island of Mauritius. Both species are found in all other countries, including the Malagasy Republic. Sixty per cent of Africans live in areas where exposure to schistosomes is possible, and 40 per cent of these (about 75,000,000 people) are infected.

In Southwest Asia, *S. haematobium* is endemic in Aden, Saudi Arabia, Yemen, Israel, Iraq, Iran, Syria, Turkey, and Lebanon. *S. mansoni* occurs in the first four of these countries, and is particularly prevalent in Yemen, where half the 3,500,000 population are thought to be infected. The highest prevalence rate for *S. haematobium* occurs in Iraq, where 20 per cent of the exposed population of 5,000,000 are infected. Of the 87,003,000 population of Southwest Asia an estimated 10,745,000 are exposed to infection.

In the Orient, *S. japonicum* occurs in China, Japan, the Philippines, and the Celebes. The prevalence in China was estimated at 32,000,000, but it is reported that this number has been substantially reduced by a recent massive control campaign. Schistosomiasis is under control in Japan, but seems to be spreading in the Philippines. Small foci of schistosomiasis japonica have recently been discovered in Thailand and Laos. Of the 868,531,000 population of Southeast Asia, 337,051,500 are estimated to be exposed. A small focus of *S. haema-*

tobium infection was found in India, in Maharashtra State, but it is now believed that transmission there has ceased.

In endemic areas of the New World (population 98,339,000) where only *S. mansoni* is found, 18,199,750 people are estimated to be exposed. Brazil has the largest number of cases, estimated at 8,000,000, and the infection seems to be spreading. Schistosomiasis also occurs in Venezuela, where it is apparently on the wane, and in Surinam. It is endemic in the following Caribbean islands: Puerto Rico, Vieques, Dominican Republic, Antigua, Guadeloupe, Martinique, and St. Lucia. The parasite has not been found in any of the Central American countries.

The one tiny focus of schistosomiasis in Europe, *S. haematobium* in southern Portugal, has now been eliminated.

The life cycle of schistosomiasis will become established only in areas where there is a susceptible snail species. Thus the infection is prevalent on the West Indian island of St. Lucia, although St. Vincent, 30 miles away, is completely free of the parasite. There are 1,450,000 Puerto Ricans now living on the mainland of the United States, and 100,000 immigrants from other areas endemic for schistosomiasis entering this country each year, but the presence of susceptible snails in the continental United States has not been established. Prevalence rates within endemic areas may be exceedingly variable, ranging from close to 100 per cent in some localities to almost none in others. This is governed by the interaction of multiple local ecologic factors relating to both the snail and human populations. Another important factor in the epidemiology of schistosomiasis is the variation in geographic strains of the species; for example, *S. japonicum* on Formosa is highly infective to domestic and wild animals but not to man, and *S. mansoni* in Africa south of the Sahara appears to be relatively avirulent.

Animal reservoirs are undoubtedly of significance in maintaining the life cycle of *S. japonicum*—in particular, cows and dogs. Natural *S. mansoni* infections have been found in rodents, baboons, insectivores, and dogs in Africa, but it is generally believed that animal reservoirs do not play a significant role in the life cycle of this species. *S. haematobium* is rarely encountered in animals.

Although *transmission patterns* differ among the three species of schistosomes, *there is little question that for each species agricultural development, particularly irrigation, may lead to a marked increase in the prevalence of schistosomiasis.* A major epidemic occurred in Egypt after the construction of the low Aswan dam, and in Rhodesia after development of large scale irrigation schemes.

In regard to morbidity and mortality, precise demographic figures are not available, particularly because schistosomiasis is such an insidious disease. The few investigations of morbidity now available show little or no effect of schistosomiasis on educational attainment or work capacity. Most studies suggest, however, that disease and death in schistosomiasis are correlated with intensity of infection. As the worms do not multiply in man, the number of parasites in a given individual is related to the degree of water contact and perhaps the occurrence of partial immunity. Under these conditions, schistosomes have an overdispersed distribution in which most members of the host population bear low worm burdens. As far as has been determined, little or no morbidity occurs in the large majority of the population carrying infections of low intensity. Though the proportion of heavily infected individuals is small, when this figure is multiplied against the vast number of people with schistosomiasis, it becomes obvious that this helminthic infection constitutes a major medical problem. In addition, there is no question that in all its forms schistosomiasis is potentially lethal—Katayama fever in *S. japonicum* infections, portal hypertension with hematemesis in both schistosomiasis japonica and mansoni, uremia in *S. haematobium* infection, and cor pulmonale in all three. Schistosomiasis may also potentiate the development of other diseases such as hepatitis, hepatoma, cirrhosis, and cancer of the urinary bladder.

Pathogenesis and Clinical Manifestations. Basic to an understanding of the disease processes in schistosomiasis are these facts: the schistosomes do not multiply in man; complete immunity does not follow initial infection; repeated infections usually occur; the worms are relatively long lived; most individuals have low worm burdens, but large numbers of worms may accumulate; and a large proportion of schistosome eggs are not excreted but remain within the body. Disease is correlated with the intensity of infection and is related not only to the presence of the various stages of the schistosomes in the body tissues and their secretions and excretions, but to the inflammatory responses of the host as well.

Clinically, three distinct syndromes occur at different stages of schistosome infection. Within one day of cercarial penetration, swimmer's itch, a pruritic papular rash, may appear. Several weeks later Katayama fever, a self-limited but possibly fatal illness resembling serum sickness, may develop. Finally, after many years, during which the infection may be either asymptomatic or associated with relatively mild intestinal or urinary tract symptoms, fibrosis of the liver may result in the signs and symptoms of portal hypertension in schistosomiasis mansoni and japonica; fibrosis of the ureters and bladder in schistosomiasis haematobia may result in changes associated with urinary tract obstruction.

Schistosome Dermatitis. Schistosomiasis begins with penetration of the skin by cercariae. These organisms are not discriminating and will penetrate the skin of most animals whether they are susceptible or insusceptible, living or dead. When nonhuman schistosomes, those that complete their life cycle in animals or birds, enter the skin of man, they die. Even in highly susceptible experimental hosts many *S. mansoni* cercariae die in the skin and perhaps in the lung; in the hamster almost 40 per cent are lost in this manner. In the highest primate thus far studied, the chimpanzee, 4 to 8 per cent of *S. mansoni* cercariae, 14 to 40 per cent of *S. haematobium* cercariae, and 1 to 48 per cent of *S. japonicum* cercariae were recovered as adult schistosomes. In most laboratory animals the recovery rate for *S. japonicum* is higher than that for the other two species.

The death of cercariae in the skin leads to the development of a pruritic papular rash known as *swimmer's itch.* This syndrome occurs in its most severe form after exposure to animal schistosomes, and has been shown to be a sensitization phenomenon, rarely occurring on primary exposure. Papules appear in sensitized persons at 5 to 15 hours, and there is massive round cell invasion of the dermis and epidermis, suggesting a delayed hypersensitivity response. Swimmer's itch has been demonstrated in infected patients experimentally re-exposed to

S. mansoni and *S. haematobium* cercariae. A mild form of swimmer's itch appears to occur in patients exposed to *S. japonicum* cercariae, but the rice paddy dermatitis of the Far East is caused mainly by avian schistosomes.

Katayama Fever. The next clinical phase of schistosomiasis begins 20 to 60 days after exposure and has been known in Japan as Katayama fever since the mid-nineteenth century. This syndrome occurs most frequently and is most severe in *S. japonicum* infections; in schistosomiasis mansoni it is usually found only in patients with very heavy initial infection; it is rarely if ever seen in schistosomiasis haematobia. In addition to fever, the patient suffers from chills, sweating, anorexia, headache, diarrhea, and cough. Hepatosplenomegaly is frequent, and generalized lymphadenopathy and urticaria are often seen. Eosinophilia occurs in most cases, averaging about 40 per cent. The fever may last for several weeks; when it subsides the other signs and symptoms also disappear. Death may occur in the Katayama fever stage of schistosomiasis japonica, but rarely does so in *S. mansoni* infection. At autopsy, massive infection is almost invariably found, with large numbers of eggs in the liver and intestines; 1608 worm pairs were demonstrated at autopsy in a Brazilian child. Katayama fever, which usually appears on initial infection, begins at about the time of onset of egg-laying by the worms; thus large amounts of antigen are suddenly added to moderate levels of cross-reacting antibody formed in response to the developing worms. It is possible, therefore, that this serum sickness–like syndrome may be a form of immune-complex disease.

Chronic Schistosomiasis. A correlation between the number of worms and the development and extent of chronic disease (except for patients with advanced liver fibrosis) was recently demonstrated by techniques quantitating human worm burdens at surgery and at autopsy. Heavy worm burdens were apparently a prerequisite for the development of severe disease, whereas light infections appeared to be of little consequence pathologically. *Thus, patients with few worms may never show any signs or symptoms related to schistosome infection.*

It is said that patients with chronic schistosomiasis mansoni or japonica may complain of fatigue, abdominal pain, and intermittent diarrhea or dysentery. Although this may be true in selected hospital populations, recent controlled field studies have revealed few such signs and symptoms, even in heavily infected individuals. On sigmoidoscopy, particularly in Egypt, granulomatous nodules or polyps may be observed. In *S. haematobium* infection, terminal hematuria, and, occasionally, dysuria and frequency are found. Mild chronic blood loss has been measured by radioisotope labeling in both *S. mansoni* and *S. haematobium* infections, but anemia is not usually seen in areas where there is normal iron intake. All the aforementioned signs and symptoms are related to the passage of eggs through the mucosa of the intestine and the urinary bladder.

Many eggs do not, however, leave the body; in laboratory animals less than half of them are excreted. Over a period of 20 years, for each *S. mansoni* worm pair producing eggs at a rate of 300 per day, at least 1,000,000 eggs will remain in the body. This figure can be multiplied by 10 for each *S. japonicum* worm pair.

In *S. mansoni* and *S. japonicum* infections, some of the eggs remain in the intestinal walls, but many of them enter the circulation and are carried into the liver. In schistosomiasis haematobia many eggs remain in the tissues of the bladder and adjacent organs, but some (usually too few to cause significant disease) enter the lungs via the inferior vena cava as well as the liver via the portal system. Granulomatous inflammation develops around the eggs trapped in the tissues; in the case of *S. mansoni* this has been demonstrated to be an immunologic response of the delayed hypersensitivity type. Both the eggs and the reactions to them are being constantly resorbed, but if large numbers of eggs gather together, the fibrosis subsequent to inflammation may remain. In schistosomiasis mansoni and japonica this leads to hepatic portal fibrosis, and in schistosomiasis haematobia, to fibrosis of the ureters and bladder.

Hepatosplenic Schistosomiasis. As the liver parenchyma is relatively unharmed by the pathologic processes involved in hepatic schistosomiasis japonica and mansoni, the clinical consequences of the disease relate primarily to granulomatous inflammation and portal fibrosis. Pathophysiologically this results in an intrahepatic block to portal blood flow and the development of portal hypertension and portal-systemic collateral circulation. The lesion is presinusoidal; thus intrasplenic and portal pressures are markedly elevated, whereas wedged hepatic vein pressure is normal. Total liver blood flow tends to remain within normal limits owing to a compensatory increase in arterial flow.

Clinically, the earliest sign of significant liver involvement is hepatomegaly. With progression, the spleen enlarges and becomes firm in consistency. Eventually it may extend to well below the umbilicus. At this point the patient tends to be in good general health, but may consult a physician because of a dragging feeling in the left upper abdominal quadrant.

The other major factor bringing the patient to the physician is a sudden hematemesis because of bleeding esophageal varices. Such an episode may not reappear for many years or may recur at fairly frequent intervals. The consequences of hematemesis in schistosomiasis are very different from those in cirrhosis of the liver: the blood ammonia concentration tends to remain normal, hepatic coma rarely occurs, and mortality is very low, being primarily due to exsanguination. This is consistent with relatively normal liver function. Jaundice is almost never seen in uncomplicated schistosomiasis, and the levels of both conjugated and unconjugated bilirubin are usually normal. Serum albumin concentration is normal or only slightly decreased, and globulin is somewhat elevated. As a consequence, ascites and edema are rarely encountered. Even sulfobromophthalein retention is often normal in these patients. Stigmata of chronic liver disease such as palmar erythema, spider angiomas, altered hair distribution, and gynecomastia are rare. Patients may suffer multiple severe hematemeses, but aside from temporary changes, liver function tends to remain relatively normal.

In spite of moderate chronic and occasional severe acute intestinal blood loss, a significant degree of anemia rarely occurs in uncomplicated schistosomiasis. The white blood count is usually within normal limits, but there is a moderate eosinophilia. Splenomegaly, however, may result in hypersplenism, the patient developing leukopenia, thrombocytopenia, and anemia with decreased red blood cell life span.

Patients with decompensated hepatic disease characterized by liver parenchymal malfunction and all the physical stigmata of this state, including jaundice and ascites, are seen in localities in which schistosomiasis is endemic. This is particularly common in the case of schistosomiasis japonica, and may, perhaps, be related to overwhelming embolization of the liver with the large numbers of eggs produced by this parasite. Pathologists have stated, however, that *it has not been possible to prove the transformation of advanced schistosomal fibrosis into true cirrhosis.* In Egypt it has been suggested that patients with schistosomiasis might concomitantly have other forms of liver disease. Finally, it must be recognized that all those infected with *S. mansoni* and *S. japonicum* perforce have some degree of liver involvement, and that the effect of malnutrition, hepatotoxins, and hepatitis may be potentiated; such interrelationships have been demonstrated in laboratory animals.

Pulmonary Schistosomiasis. Pulmonary schistosomiasis, which in its most severe state is characterized by signs and symptoms of cor pulmonale, is a complication of hepatosplenic schistosomiasis. Portal-systemic collateral circulation enables the eggs to bypass the liver, and they are trapped in the pulmonary capillary bed. Arteritis with angiomatoid formation occurs, and there is obstruction to pulmonary blood flow. Pulmonary hypertension is found in every case, but cardiac output usually remains within the normal range. Arterial oxygen saturation is usually normal, and cyanosis is rare. The lungs are often involved in schistosomiasis haematobia because of the passage of eggs from the vesical plexuses into the inferior vena cava, but egg embolization appears to be relatively light, and significant disease is uncommon.

Urinary Tract Schistosomiasis. Severe urinary tract disease may occur in both the early and late phases of *S. haematobium* infection. Initially there may be ureteral obstruction owing to florid granulomatous inflammatory reactions to the eggs in both the ureters and the bladder; these lesions appear to be highly reversible after antischistosomal therapy. Later in the course of the disease irreversible fibrosis may supervene. Bladder fibrosis and calcification lead to frequency and dysuria. On cystoscopy, so-called sandy patches may be seen on the bladder walls; these are made up of large numbers of schistosome eggs. The disease may progress through hydronephrosis, secondary infection, and finally uremia. An association between cancer of the bladder and urinary schistosomiasis has been demonstrated.

In the past decade there has been a growing impression among Brazilian clinicians and pathologists that there is an increased frequency of renal disease in patients with schistosomiasis mansoni. Initially proteinuria was noted in patients with hepatosplenic schistosomiasis, and then, at autopsy, the renal glomeruli of similar patients were found to have pathologic changes. This was followed by ultrastructural and immunocytochemical studies which revealed electron-dense deposits in the glomerular basement membranes which contained immunoglobulins. Similar deposits have been observed in laboratory animals. It should be pointed out, however, that specific schistosomal antigen has not been demonstrated as yet, and comparable lesions have been found in the kidneys of patients with cirrhosis of the liver.

Central Nervous System Schistosomiasis. Schistosomiasis of the central nervous system, although relatively rare, is an important complication of the infection. *S. japonicum* usually involves the brain, whereas *S. mansoni* and *S. haematobium* tend to affect the spinal cord. Schistosomiasis japonica is reputed to be one of the important causes of focal epilepsy in the Far East. The disease may also present as a space-occupying lesion or occasionally as a generalized encephalitis. Cerebral schistosomiasis japonica may appear at any time in the course of infection from the first three weeks on. At autopsy the lesions almost always consist of large collections of eggs in the venous circulatory system, suggesting the presence of adult worms, although they have never been found. *S. mansoni* and *S. haematobium* in the spinal cord may be associated with a transverse myelitis-like syndrome; at surgery or autopsy large granulomas made up of eggs are usually found.

The development of chronic salmonellosis has been described in schistosomiasis in both man and laboratory animals. In the latter, schistosomiasis has also been associated with increased severity of viral hepatitis and intestinal amebiasis.

Diagnosis. When schistosomiasis is considered as a diagnosis in nonendemic areas, the first question that should be asked is: "Where have you been?" It must then be determined whether there was contact with fresh water, whether transient pruritus was observed soon thereafter, and if there was a febrile episode several weeks later. For schistosomiasis mansoni and japonica, abdominal symptoms and signs might be considered, and for *S. haematobium* infection, terminal hematuria, dysuria, and frequency are important. The presence of eosinophilia is a useful sign of schistosome infection. A wide variety of serologic tests (e.g., complement-fixation, flocculation, fluorescent antibody, and circumoval precipitin) and a skin test of the immediate type are available. *These immunologic methods, which are all based on detection of circulating antibody, essentially have no place in the diagnosis of the individual case,* as cross-reactions with other parasitic infections providing false positive results are relatively common; false negative reactions also occur.

Definitive diagnosis can be made only by finding schistosome eggs in the excreta (feces or urine) or in a biopsy specimen – usually rectal. Eggs may not be present in the early stages of acute schistosomiasis. Schistosome eggs are relatively large, and are easy to identify because of their distinctive shape. Direct fecal smear is too insensitive, but techniques which provide both concentration and quantitation of eggs in the feces have been developed. This is important, because correlations between egg output and intensity of infection have been made. The Kato thick smear technique is a simple and highly effective method for fecal egg counting. A small portion of stool (schistosome eggs are distributed randomly in feces) is passed through 105-mesh stainless steel bolting cloth (W. S. Tyler Co., Cleveland, Ohio) and 50 mg is added to a tared glass slide and covered with a cellophane cover slip (no. 124PD, E.I. DuPont de Nemours, Inc., Film Department, Wilmington, Delaware) impregnated with 50 per cent glycerin. The slides are inverted and pressed onto a bed of filter paper, turned face up, and left for a period of at least 48 hours during which the fecal matter clears. Although the embryo within the egg also clears, the characteristic shape of the egg shell can be easily seen. After counting all the eggs in the sample, multiplication by 20 provides the number of eggs per gram of feces.

Rectal biopsy is a highly efficient method for the diagnosis of *S. mansoni* and *japonicum* infection, and will often help detect *S. haematobium* eggs. Through a proctoscope, snips are taken from the valves of Houston (8 to 10 cm from the anus), pressed between glass slides, and examined immediately under a microscope. Sometimes only opaque dead eggs are observed, suggesting a burnt-out or successfully treated infection. Liver biopsy has been suggested as a means of diagnosis, but will only rarely detect an infection not revealed by the aforementioned methods.

For the diagnosis of schistosomiasis haematobia, urine is collected at midday, because a diurnal variation in egg output has been demonstrated. The urine specimen is centrifuged and the sediment examined. For quantitative data the Bell technique is effective; this involves sieving a 10 ml aliquot of urine collected between 1100 and 1300 hours onto filter paper, staining with ninhydrin and counting the eggs. *S. mansoni* eggs are occasionally found in urine.

For determining the severity of intestinal disease, sigmoidoscopy and barium enema are of value. The extent of liver disease may be estimated by liver biopsy, barium swallow, esophagoscopy, and especially splenoportography with measurement of intrasplenic pressure. In schistosomiasis haematobia, cystoscopy and intravenous pyelography are useful techniques.

Treatment. Antischistosomal treatment should never be instituted without proof of infection by the demonstration of living eggs in excreta or biopsy specimens, except in the rare case of suspected schistosomiasis of the central nervous system. A positive serologic or skin test does not provide a definitive diagnosis. Complete cure is not necessary and indeed is not always desirable in schistosomiasis (particularly in endemic areas where reinfection may occur), because disease is related to intensity of infection, surviving worms do not multiply, and immunity may be premunitive, i.e., dependent on the presence of living organisms. The recent use of quantitative egg counts has shown that in cases in which cure is not achieved by the full course of treatment with an established drug, egg output is usually reduced by over 90 per cent. Thus striving for cure by increasing the drug dosage or repeating the course of treatment is rarely necessary and, because of the toxicity of the antischistosomal drugs, may actually be harmful.

None of the drugs now available for human use have any effect on the schistosomes during their early migratory phases in the body (the first three to six weeks), thus rendering it difficult to treat Katayama fever; steroids have been used to suppress the clinical manifestations during this stage of the infection. The three schistosome species vary considerably in their response to drugs, *S. haematobium* being the most susceptible and *S. japonicum* the most resistant. Under these circumstances it is generally stated that it is still necessary to treat schistosomiasis japonica with the highly toxic antimony potassium tartrate (tartar emetic). In a recent report (1972) of a World Health Organization consultant group, however, it was noted that the cure rates in *S. japonicum* infections with tartar emetic, stibocaptate (Astiban), and niridazole (Ambilhar), respectively, ranged between 40 to 75, 40 to 75, and 40 to 70 per cent. Thus it can be recommended that those infected with any of the three species of human schistosomes be treated with niridazole or stibocaptate, the latter when there are signs or symptoms of liver or cerebral disease. Both these drugs may be obtained from the Parasitic Disease Drug Service of the Center for Disease Control, Atlanta, Georgia 30333. Particularly in the case of *S. mansoni* infections, it would not be unreasonable to withhold treatment with these drugs in asymptomatic individuals with very low egg counts.

Niridazole is administered orally in two divided daily doses totaling 25 mg per kilogram of body weight for a period of five to seven days. Vomiting, diarrhea, cramps, and dizziness may occur. Side effects are greatly exacerbated in patients with signs and symptoms of liver or cerebral disease. Under these circumstances stibocaptate can be substituted; this antimony compound is administered intramuscularly in a dose of 8 mg per kilogram once per week for five weeks. Antimony compounds are cardiotoxic; stibocaptate is also associated with anorexia, vomiting, abdominal pain, headache, and pain at the site of injection.

Utilizing a combination of surgery and a single dose of an antischistosomal drug, many of the worms can be sieved out of the bloodstream. Although such extracorporeal hemofiltration is a valuable research tool, it should be used as a form of treatment only under special circumstances.

In general, the surgical treatment of schistosomiasis should be approached with caution. Many of the apparently irreversible lesions of urinary tract schistosomiasis will resolve completely after antischistosomal treatment, particularly in young patients. Cerebral schistosomiasis japonica is frequently cured or markedly ameliorated by drug therapy. Finally, prophylactic portacaval shunts should never be performed in hepatosplenic schistosomiasis, because hematemesis is not invariable and is unpredictable in onset, and, when it occurs, mortality is low. If the creation of shunt by surgery is necessitated by repeated bleeding episodes, splenorenal anastomosis is preferable to portacaval shunt because of a much lower incidence of chronic portal systemic encephalopathy. Prior to shunting, however, antischistosomal therapy is necessary to prevent prolonged passage of eggs into the lungs which may lead to the development of cor pulmonale.

Prognosis. The prognosis is usually good. Many patients with schistosomiasis never have symptoms or signs of disease, or have only relatively mild ones. Epidemiologically, both the infection and the disease reach their peak in early adult life and decline with age. Disregarding the factor of death among heavily infected patients, this may be due to decreased exposure to infection, gradual death of the worms, slow development of immunity, and diminution in the inflammatory response to the parasite and its products.

The early stages of hepatic or urinary tract disease appear to be reversible after antischistosomal therapy. Although late disease seems relatively irreversible, progression may be halted and gradual improvement may follow drug therapy. In hepatosplenic schistosomiasis the prognosis in patients suffering a hematemesis is far better than in those with cirrhosis, because the former do not tend to go into hepatic coma. Patients with cerebral schistosomiasis japonica may show remarkable improvement after antischistosome therapy.

Prevention. On the individual level, schistosomiasis may be prevented by avoidance of contaminated waters. If this is not possible, boots should be worn; if contaminated water reaches the skin, rapid drying or rubbing with alcohol will prevent infection. Storage of water for several days will ensure the death of cercariae, as will the boiling of drinking water. Sea water is safe for swimming, although the mouths of rivers and streams should be avoided; chlorination of swimming pools will prevent infection. Repellents are of no great value, and vaccines or prophylactic drugs are not available.

There are three approaches to the control of schistosomiasis on a mass basis: (1) destruction of the snail intermediate host, (2) prevention of snail infection by the treatment of human infection and the construction of privies, and (3) elimination of contact with contaminated water by the provision of safe water supplies. Destruction of the snail is primarily based on the use of molluscicides such as the various copper salts, sodium pentachlorophenate, Bayluscide, and n-trityl-morpholone. Molluscicides, however, are quickly inactivated by sunlight and adsorption to mud and organic matter; they pass rapidly through running water or are diluted in vast bodies of still water, and they often destroy other aquatic fauna and flora. Also, although molluscicides may appear to be highly effective, only a few surviving snails can rapidly repopulate an area. Many biologic control measures have been advocated, including the use of nonsusceptible snail species which may compete for miracidia, food, and space; snail-eating fish and ducks; and snail pathogens. None of these measures has shown outstanding promise. The snails that transmit *S. japonicum* are amphibious and are frequently found along the banks of water courses; their eradication can necessitate the use of earth-moving equipment and flame throwers. When the snails are "buried" in this way, as in the campaigns in the People's Republic of China, it appears to reduce the infectivity of the environment.

An attempt to break the life cycle at the stage of transmission from man to the snail has been hampered by the lack of practical mass therapy. The recent development of effective oral drugs and of a single-dose intramuscular drug offers great promise for the future. An important adjunct to this approach is the construction of privies. Breaking the cycle at the stage of transmission from the snail to man can be accomplished by the provision of safe water supplies for washing and recreational purposes.

Control measures based on the destruction of snails are an end in themselves, and in addition may be inimical to the environment. In contrast, mass antischistosomal treatment coupled with the construction of privies or the provision of safe water supplies should contribute greatly to the general health of the population.

Cheever, A. W.: A quantitative postmortem study of schistosomiasis mansoni in man. Am. J. Trop. Med. Hyg., 17:38, 1968.

Clark, W. D., Cox, P. M., Jr., Ratner, L. H., and Correa-Coronas, R.: Acute schistosomiasis mansoni in 10 boys. An outbreak in Caguas, Puerto Rico. Ann. Intern. Med., 73:379, 1970.

Lehman, J. S., Jr., Farid, Z., Smith, J. H., Bassily, S., and El-Masry, N. A.: Urinary schistosomiasis in Egypt: Clinical, radiological, bacteriological and parasitological correlations. Trans. R. Soc. Trop. Med. Hyg., 67:384, 1973.

von Lichtenberg, F., Edington, G. M., Nwabuebo, I., Taylor, J. R., and Smith, J. H.: Pathologic effects of schistosomiasis in Ibadan, western State of Nigeria. II. Pathogenesis of lesions of the bladder and ureters. Am. J. Trop. Med. Hyg., 20:244, 1971.

Warren, K. S.: The immunopathogenesis of schistosomiasis: A multidisciplinary approach. Trans. R. Soc. Trop. Med. Hyg., 66:417, 1972.

Warren, K. S.: Regulation of the prevalence and intensity of schistosomiasis in man: Immunology or ecology? J. Infect. Dis., 127:595, 1973.

Warren, K. S., Reboucas, G., and Baptista, A. G.: Ammonia metabolism and hepatic coma in hepatosplenic schistosomiasis. Patients studied before and after portacaval shunt. Ann. Intern. Med., 62:1113, 1965.

WHO Reports on Schistosomicidal Drugs. II. Report of a WHO consultant group on the comparative evaluation of new schistosomicidal drugs for use in treatment campaigns. Bol. Of. Sanit. Panam. (English), 6:89, 1972.

HERMAPHRODITIC FLUKES

Philip D. Marsden

297. INTRODUCTION

The hermaphroditic flukes, unlike Schistosoma flukes, have both sets of sex organs in the same worm, and frequently self-fertilization occurs. These flukes are flat leaflike worms with oral and ventral suckers. They have a complex life cycle. The egg hatches to produce a motile ciliated *miracidium,* which penetrates the soft tissue of a snail and undergoes a cycle of development similar to that in schistosomiasis. *Cercariae* are produced by the snail after a few weeks, but unlike schistosomes these cercariae encyst in a second intermediate host, either fish, crab, or plant. These encysted cercariae or *metacercariae* are a relatively resistant form which can survive adverse conditions. If the metacercaria is then ingested by man, it hatches to produce an immature fluke which migrates through the body tissues to gain its site of final development. This varies with the species concerned, being the liver for Clonorchis and Fasciola, the lung for Paragonimus, and the intestine for *Fasciolopsis buski.*

Initial invasion is often accompanied by eosinophilia, but it takes a month or longer before the characteristic eggs are produced. All the eggs have an operculum or lid through which the miracidia escape, unlike Schistosoma eggs. Some of these flukes live for a long time, producing progressive damage in the tissues of the host. When searching for the ova of trematodes in the biliary tree, duodenal aspiration may be more rewarding than stool examination. Therapy, especially in the hepatic hermaphroditic trematodes, is unsatisfactory.

298. HEPATIC HERMAPHRODITIC FLUKES

Clonorchiasis (Clonorchis sinensis). Man is infected by eating the flesh of undercooked or raw freshwater fish in which the metacercariae are encysted. More than 40 species of fish, mainly of the carp and salmon (cyprinoid) group, have been found to harbor metacercariae. The natural definitive hosts other than man are fish-eating mammals, including cats, dogs, mink, and rats. Widespread in the Far East, the main endemic areas of human infection are Japan, Korea, China, and Vietnam. As the flukes live for decades (20 to 30 years) in the biliary tree, immigrants from Asia have been found infected in many countries. A proportion of the Chinese in New York and San Francisco are infected. Infections recorded in Hawaiians are attributed to imports of infected frozen, dried, or pickled fish from Japan.

It appears that most of the larval flukes ascend the biliary tree directly from the duodenum, but some may pass via the portal circulation to the liver. They mature in the bile ducts, and the grayish-brown adults, measuring 10 to 20 mm by 2 to 4 mm, move sluggishly around by means of their suckers in the distal biliary passages. They feed on secretions from the mucosa of the bile duct and possibly also on cellular elements. Occasionally they gain access to the gallbladder and pancreatic ducts. In effect they cause a chronic cholangitis with inflammation of the biliary tree, proliferation of the biliary epithelium, and progressive portal fibrosis. The severity of these changes depends upon the load of flukes.

After ingesting the metacercariae, the patient may present with epigastric pain, malaise, and tender hepatomegaly. An eosinophilia is usually present in the early stages, but no eggs can be found until about one month has passed and the flukes have matured. Light infections are often asymptomatic, but a firm liver edge is often discovered within the costal margin on routine examination. In an Asian, this finding should prompt a careful search for ova in the stool. In heavy infections (10,000 to 20,000 flukes), more serious sequelae occur. The marked portal fibrosis may be associated with signs of portal hypertension. Extension of the fibrosis into the liver parenchyma may be associated with liver cell death and fatty change. Jaundice is more likely to be associated with biliary obstruction owing to a mass of flukes or stone formation. Cholangiocarcinoma is a late complication of severe clonorchiasis, a metaplastic change occurring in the irritated biliary epithelium. In Hong Kong there is a high incidence in males after the fourth decade, the adenocarcinomas showing varying degrees of differentiation. Suppurative cholangitis caused by superimposed bacterial infection may present as hypoglycemic coma. Chronic pancreatitis is a rare complication.

The diagnosis is made by finding the eggs in the stool. Unfortunately they are not characteristic and can be easily confused with a number of other trematodes producing small, similar eggs (Heterophyes, Opisthorcis, Metagonimus). The eggs average 29 by 16 μ; they are light brown and ovoid. There is a definite shoulder in a shell wall near the operculum and a boss at the anopercular end.

The invasive stage must be distinguished from that of other fluke infections, *visceral larval migrans,* and *hepatic amebiasis.* The last-named condition is not associated with eosinophilia. The late stages may resemble cirrhosis and uncomplicated cholecystitis. Hypoglycemic coma can also be a manifestation of a hepatocellular carcinoma. In the elderly, repeated nonparasitic cholangitis is sometimes a difficult diagnosis to establish in patients with pyrexia of unknown origin.

Treatment and Prevention. Most investigators agree that the drugs available for treating this infection are often ineffective and disappointing. Prolonged chloroquine therapy is chiefly suppressive; however, it is still the drug of choice. Chloroquine diphosphate in a dose of 300 mg base (two 250 mg tablets) three times a day for three to six weeks is a standard course. Some workers have increased this dose or used it for periods of up to a year. Various percentages of cures are claimed, but it depends on the criteria used and especially on what stool concentration technique is employed and how frequently. At the higher dosage levels the more severe side effects of chloroquine toxicity may be seen, namely, corneal deposits and retinopathy, central nervous system changes (a parkinsonian-like syndrome), dyspigmentation, cardiac arrhythmias, and peripheral myopathy and neuropathy. A new compound, hexachloroparaxylol, proved effective, but alarming toxicity tests in recent animal studies have resulted in its withdrawal. Biliary obstruction may require surgical relief, and at surgery as many flukes as possible should be removed from the biliary tree. Prevention of this infection relates to the competent cooking of freshwater fish.

Opisthorchiasis (Opisthorchis viverrini and felineus). *Opisthorchis felineus* is prevalent in the Philippines, India, Japan, and Vietnam, as well as in the USSR and parts of Eastern Europe, whereas *Opisthorchis viverrini* is common in north Thailand and Laos. The life cycles of these flukes are similar to that of *Clonorchis sinensis* and are completed in about four months under favorable conditions. Snails are infected by fecal contaminants of water from infected persons or animal reservoirs, e.g., cats. In northeast Thailand 90 per cent of people more than ten years of age are infected with *O. viverrini,* and 3.5 million in the whole country. With all infections of this type, as might be expected, the incidence rises with age. The source of infection is a popular dish of raw fish, rice, vegetables, and spices.

The pathologic findings are similar to those in *Clonorchis sinensis,* although stone formation is said to be unusual. Cholangiocarcinoma has also been reported to be associated with this infection. The eggs are indistinguishable from Clonorchis. This emphasizes the importance of a geographic history, for the only other way of distinguishing the parasite would be by examination of the adult flukes. Percutaneous transhepatic cholangiography may reveal radiologic changes such as a single cystic cavity or mulberry-like dilatation of the intrahepatic bile ducts.

Dicrocoeliasis. *Dicrocoelium dendriticum* is acquired by eating ants in which the metacercariae have developed following ingestion by the ant of slime balls containing cercariae secreted by the snail. Infections are generally uncommon, but occur in Europe and Asia and around the Mediterranean basin. Being light infections, their main importance is for the physician to recognize the small, fully embryonated thick-shelled eggs ($40\ \mu \times 25\ \mu$) for what they are. Spurious parasitism, in which nonhuman species ingested in liver pass through the bowel unchanged, is well documented.

Fascioliasis (Fasciola hepatica). This is also a biliary fluke, but it is less well adapted to man than is *Clonorchis sinensis.* It is a common parasite of sheep, producing marked liver damage. Worldwide in distribution in sheep, it is prevalent in low wet pastures where suitable species of snails are indigenous. The metacercariae encyst on plants, and man is infected mainly as a result of eating wild watercress and other plants gathered in these pastures. Human infections are more common where such salad is favored, e.g., Europe, Cuba, and Chile. In England outbreaks are associated with particularly wet summers.

The adult fluke is large, 2 to 3 cm in length by 0.8 to 1.3 cm in breadth, and may occlude the *common bile duct.* Indeed, many human infections have been first recognized at surgery for biliary obstruction. Again an invasive stage of fever, eosinophilia, and hepatomegaly is associated with larval flukes moving through the liver substance to gain the biliary tract, for the larval flukes produced from the metacercariae in the jejunum pass across the peritoneal cavity to pierce Glisson's capsule and move through the liver substance. Far fewer flukes than Clonorchis are found in man, but again hyperplasia, necrosis, and cystic dilation of the biliary tract, accompanied by leukocytic infiltration and eventually periportal fibrosis, can ensue if the load of flukes is heavy enough. The differential diagnosis is similar to that of clonorchiasis.

The *diagnosis* depends on finding large yellowish operculate eggs 130 to 150 μ in length in the feces or aspirated bile. Liver should be excluded from the patient's diet in areas where raw liver is eaten, because eggs in such livers will pass through the intestinal tract unchanged. A complement-fixation test using an extract of the adult fluke as antigen is a useful diagnostic aid, especially in infections in which the flukes are ectopic. A hemagglutination test has also been developed.

Unlike the other hepatic hermaphroditic flukes, *Fasciola hepatica* and the closely allied *Fasciola gigantica* are occasionally found in sites other than the liver. This could be related to man's being a relatively poor host species. Thus a migrating subcutaneous swelling associated with intense eosinophilia may contain such an immature fluke, and there are records of occurrences in many sites, including the brain.

A further oddity associated with *Fasciola hepatica* infection is the parasitization of the pharynx by young post-metacercarial flukes which are acquired by eating raw liver in which the young flukes are actively migrating. This occurs in Lebanon, where such raw sheep and goat livers are eaten; the patient complains of intense inflammation of the back of the throat. This syndrome of parasitic pharyngitis, known as halzoun, can also be produced by a leech or a pentosomid (a wormlike arthropod).

Emetine hydrochloride is still considered by many the most effective therapy in a dose of 65 mg intramuscularly daily for ten days, but cure is rarely achieved. (For side effects see Ch. 279. It may be replaced by the less toxic dehydroemetine.) Some physicians give chloroquine concurrently, 300 mg of base three times a day for a longer period, although chloroquine alone fails to cure. Bithionol has been shown to be effective in a dose of 50 mg per kilogram on alternate days for 10 to 15 doses, and, being less toxic, may be used as an alternative. Ectopic flukes are removed surgically.

Clonorchiasis

Hou, P. C.: The relationship between primary carcinoma of the liver and infestation with *Clonorchis sinensis*. J. Pathol., 72:239, 1956.

Komiya, L.: Clonorchis and clonorchiasis. *In* Dawes, B. (ed.): Advances in Parasitology. London, Academic Press, 1966, Vol. 4, pp. 53–106.

Viranuvatti, V., and Stitnimankam, T.: Liver fluke infection and infestation in South East Asia. *In* Popper, H., and Schaffner, F. (eds.): Progress in Liver Disease, Vol. 4. New York, Grune & Stratton, 1972, pp. 537–547.

Weng, H. C., Chung, H. L., Ho, L. Y., and Hou, T. C.: Studies in *Clonorchis sinensis* in the past 10 years. Chin. Med. J. (Peking), 80:441, 1960.

Opisthorchiasis

Harinasuta, C.: Opisthorchiasis in Thailand: A review. *In* Harmasuta, C. (ed.): Proceedings of the Fourth Southeast Asian Seminar on Parasitology and Tropical Medicine: Schistosomiasis and Other Snail-Transmitted Helminthiases. Manila, 1969, pp. 177–199.

Fascioliasis

Hardman, E. W., Jones, R. L. H., and Davies, A. H.: Fascioliasis—a large outbreak. Br. Med. J., 3:502, 1970.

Khalil, G. M., and Schacher, J. F.: *Linguatula serrata* in relation to halzoun and the Marrara syndrome. Am. J. Trop. Med., 14:736, 1965.

Neghume, A., and Ossandan, M.: Ectopic and hepatic fascioliasis. Am. J. Trop. Med., 23:545, 1943.

Pantelouris, E. M.: The Common Liver Fluke. Oxford, Pergamon Press, 1964.

299. LUNG HERMAPHRODITIC FLUKES (Paragonimiasis)

Although *Paragonimus westermani* is the most common species of this group infecting man, recently a number of other human pathogens have been recognized in the genus Paragonimus, which to date numbers more than 31 species. These include *P. africanus* found in Nigeria, the Cameroons, and the Congo, and two new Chinese flukes, *P. skrjabini* and *P. heterotremus*. *P. westermani* is widely distributed in the Far East, occurring as an important human infection in China, Japan, Vietnam, Korea, Formosa, the Philippines, and Thailand. Species also occur in South America in Peru, Colombia, Ecuador, and Venezuela.

Paragonimiasis is a chronic lung infection of man caused by this group of flukes, the adults living in cystic spaces in the lung. Reddish-brown plump oval flukes, they resemble in size a coffee bean (0.8 to 1.6 cm long by 0.4 to 0.8 cm wide). They are covered with little spines and live singly or in pairs in the lung parenchyma, feeding on host exudates. They live five to six years usually. Oval yellowish-brown operculated ova (85 μ by 35 μ) are coughed up in thick, blood-stained sputum. These hatch to produce a miracidium which invades specific snails. The cercariae subsequently produced by these snails encyst as metacercariae in the muscles and viscera of freshwater crabs. Man acquires the infection by eating the crabs raw or partly cooked. The larval flukes released from the metacercariae usually migrate to the lung via the peritoneal cavity, penetrating the diaphragm, but may mature in the abdomen or brain.

For many species man is not the definitive host, felines being preferred. For instance, other hosts apart from man for *P. westermani* are cats, tigers, leopards, mink, badgers, dogs, lions, and rats. *P. westermani* was discovered by Westerman in 1877 in a tiger in the Amsterdam zoo.

Pathogenesis and Pathology. The larval fluke tunnels into the lung at the periphery. There is an inflammatory reaction around it with many eosinophils. Later it forms a cystic space with a fibrous tissue wall. These cysts usually communicate with a bronchus and often become secondarily infected with abscess formation. Death of the fluke is often followed by calcification. Ova may be reaspirated, with an eosinophilic inflammatory response and the formation of small lung granulomas.

Although the target organ for Paragonimus is the lung, it must be realized that often adults go astray, and if the invading species is one less adapted to man, this is more liable to happen. Thus a characteristic feature of *P. skrjabini* infection is migrating subcutaneous nodules that contain active flukes. Such granulomas in the subcutaneous tissue may require excision as in fascioliasis.

In the brain the temporal and occipital lobes are occasionally the site of an eosinophilic granuloma containing flukes and, in a few cases, ova. A transverse myelitis is known. Flukes in the peritoneal cavity produce adhesions and abscesses, and ulceration of the intestine occurs with ova in the stool. Adult and mature flukes have been found in many other organs, including intestine, spermatic cord, testis and scrotum, vagina, and muscles.

Clinical Manifestations. Lung infections are encountered with symptoms of persistent hemoptysis, breathlessness on exertion, pleural pain, and recurrent pulmonary infections. The condition is known as endemic hemoptysis. Clubbing of the fingers is common, and persistent rales may be heard over the affected lung segments as in nonparasitic bronchiectasis. A lung abscess may be present. Pneumothorax, pleural effusion, and empyema are rarer complications. Chest films early in the disease show infiltrations, but later dense nodular opacities or ring shadows indicate the site of the cysts. Pleural adhesions and calcification are late signs. Coexistent pulmonary tuberculosis occurs in some patients. There are rarely more than 20 parasites in the lungs.

It has been estimated that there were 5000 cases of cerebral paragonimiasis in South Korea in January 1968. Cerebral paragonimiasis may present signs of a space-occupying lesion with epilepsy and paresis of varying degrees. Ophthalmic signs are optic atrophy associated with papilledema or direct involvement with the inflammatory process. The cerebrospinal fluid shows a raised protein, and eosinophils are present. There may be calcifications present on skull roentgenograms; pneumoencephalography may show the site of a pseudotumor. Abdominal paragonimiasis is a difficult condition to diagnose, but an abdominal mass in a patient with lung disease should raise this suspicion.

Diagnosis. This rests mainly on finding ova in the sputum. One third of patients also have ova in the stools because of swallowed sputum or a coincidental intestinal lesion. Complement-fixation tests are useful, and positive results correlate closely with an active infection. Yokogawa has treated patients on this basis alone. The intradermal test remains positive for a long while after active infection and is not a reliable guide. Work goes on defining the antigenic structure of the parasite. The extent to which the Paragonimus antigen cross-reacts with other flukes is not clear.

Pulmonary paragonimiasis may resemble bronchiectasis, lung abscess, bronchial carcinoma, or—most important of all—pulmonary tuberculosis. Cerebral paragonimiasis mimics other space-occupying lesions but especially other helminths in the brain. These include Fasciola, *Schistosoma japonicum, Angiostrongylus cantonensis*, and hydatid.

Prognosis. Fatalities are rare, and lung lesions resolve spontaneously in five to ten years. Cerebral involvement may be associated with persistent epilepsy. Two per cent of lung paragonimiasis is complicated by pulmonary tuberculosis.

Treatment. Bithionol (Actamer, Biton) is 2,2′-thiobis(4,6-dichlorophenol) and is given orally in a dose of 30 mg per kilogram of body weight on alternate days for 20 days. Skin reactions and gastrointestinal irritation are rarely severe enough to interrupt treatment. Results are far superior to those obtained with chloroquine or emetine drugs used in the past. Granulomas containing Paragonimus adults and ova may require surgical removal from the skin, testis, abdominal organs, or brain.

Prevention. It might be thought that it would be a simple matter to dissuade people from eating raw, fresh salted, pickled, or imperfectly cooked crabs and crayfish, but such local delicacies are not easily relinquished. Drunken crab, a favorite dish, involves immersing live crabs in alcohol prior to consumption. In Korea and West Africa, fresh crab juice is used as a home remedy in the treatment of measles.

Chang, H. T., Wang, C. W., Yü, C. F., Hsü, C. F., and Fang, J. C.: Paragonimiasis, a clinical study of 200 adult cases. Chin. Med. J., 77:3, 1958.
Grados, O. B., Cuba, C. C., Morales, F. N., and Mazabel, T. C.: Epidemiologia de la paragonimiasis en el Peru. Arch. Peruanos Pat. Clin., 26:33, 1972.
Miyazaki, I.: Lung Flukes in the Western Hemisphere. Tokyo, Overseas Technical Cooperation Agency, 1972.
Nwokolo, C.: Endemic paragonimiasis in Eastern Nigeria. Clinical features and epidemiology of the recent outbreak following the Nigerian Civil War. Trop. Geogr. Med., 24:138, 1972.
Yokogawa, M.: Paragonimus and paragonimiasis. *In* Dawes, B. (ed.): Advances in Parasitology. London, Academic Press, 1969, Vol. 7, pp. 375–387.
Yokogawa, S., Cort, W. W., and Yokogawa, M.: Paragonimus and paragonimiasis. Exp. Parasitol., 10:81, 139, 1960.
Yokogawa, M., Okawa, T., Tsuji, M., Iwasaki, M., and Shigeyasu, M.: Chemotherapy of paragonimiasis with bithionol. III. The follow-up studies for 1 year after treatment with bithionol. Jap. J. Parasit., 11:103, 1962.

300. INTESTINAL HERMAPHRODITIC FLUKES

FASCIOLOPSIASIS
(Fasciolopsis buski)

Fasciolopsis buski is a large fleshy fluke, 3 cm long and 1.2 cm wide. It is found mainly in China but also in India, Indonesia, Thailand, Malaya, and Taiwan, normally as an intestinal parasite of pigs. The eggs are passed in the feces, and miracidium is released to penetrate a snail. The cercariae subsequently produced encyst as metacercariae on edible water plants called water caltrop or water chestnuts. The tubers and fruits of these plants are eaten fresh and raw from July to September and as they are peeled with the teeth, people are easily infected. The ponds are often fertilized with night soil or contaminated by pigs.

Most infections are asymptomatic, but foci of inflammation may occur at the site of attachment of the worms in the small intestine. In heavy infections abdominal pain may simulate a peptic ulcer, and there may be alternating diarrhea and constipation. A recent investigation does not suggest that malabsorption occurs. Intestinal stasis, ulceration, and even obstruction have occurred. Several thousand worms may be harbored by the patient, and in severe cases, especially in children, edema of the face and trunk has been described. The mechanism of this edema may be complex, as anemia and hypoproteinemia from blood loss in the bowel are possible. Definite allergic edemas do not appear to be reported in the literature, but there is a variable eosinophilia with heavy loads. Brown, in a previous edition of this textbook, suggested that an absorption of toxic metabolites may be responsible for this edema. Ascites and death from exhaustion are rare.

Diagnosis. Diagnosis depends on finding the characteristic eggs in the stool. These are large, 130 to 140 μ by 80 to 85 μ, yellowish, and rather similar to Fasciola but with a smaller operculum. Occasionally an adult fluke may be vomited or passed in the stool. Facial edema may raise the question of differentiating fasciolopsiasis from trichinosis or the nephrotic syndrome.

Therapy. Tetrachloroethylene is effective (see Treatment in Ch. 304). Some advocate hexylresorcinol in an adult dose of 1 gram. Either drug should be given on an empty stomach. Not all the flukes may be eradicated, but the therapy can be repeated after a few days. Prevention entails cooking the offending plants, eradicating snails with molluscocides, and preventing fecal contamination of ponds.

OTHER INTESTINAL HERMAPHRODITIC FLUKES

Two very small intestinal flukes—*Heterophyes heterophyes* and *Metagonimus yokogawai*—deserve mention. The former is found in Egypt, Tunisia, South China, India, and the Philippines, and the latter occurs in the Far East and Indonesia. Both are acquired by eating raw or inadequately cooked fish that contain the respective metacercariae. The adult flukes, 2 to 3 mm long, are attached to the mucosa of the small intestine and are alleged to produce superficial inflammation and ulceration. Usually they are not present in sufficient numbers to produce symptoms. Very rarely eggs may gain access to the circulation and be found in internal organs. Usually they are passed in the stool and closely resemble Clonorchis eggs, which is perhaps their main importance. Both species can be treated with tetrachloroethylene as used for hookworm. Many species of the genus Echinostoma can also infect man in the Far East, but again rarely produce symptoms. Their eggs resemble those of Fasciola but are smaller. *Gastrodiscoides hominis* is a fascinating fluke with a large ventral sucker. Like the others, it can produce diarrhea. It occurs in Assam, Indochina, India, and Malaysia. In Canada the eggs of *Metorchis conjunctus* are occasionally found in the stools of man.

Barlow, C. H.: The life cycle of the human intestinal fluke *Fasciolopsis buski* (Lankester). Amer. J. Hyg., Monograph 4, 1925.
Cross, J. H.: Fasciolopsiasis in South East Asia and the Far East: A review. *In* Harmasuta, C. (ed.): Proceedings of the Fourth Southeast Asian Seminar on Parasitology and Tropical Medicine: Schistosomiasis and Other Snail-Transmitted Helminthiases. Manila, 1969, pp. 177–199.
Plaut, A. G., Kampanort-Sanyakorn, C., and Manning, G. S.: A clinical study of *Fasciolopsis buski* in Thailand. Trans. Roy. Soc. Trop. Med. Hyg., 63:470, 1969.

THE NEMATODES (ROUNDWORMS)

Philip D. Marsden

301. INTRODUCTION

Roundworms have an intestinal tract and a large body cavity bordered by a complex cuticle and containing the reproductive, nervous, and excretory systems. They have elongated, cylindrical, bilaterally symmetrical, smooth, nonsegmented, translucent, flesh-colored bodies, often filiform, with a pointed posterior and rounded anterior end. The Nematoda constitute the second largest class in the Animal Kingdom, with 500,000 species. Many are free living. They are unisexual, and the female is usually bigger than the male. There is a great variation in size among the common human species. For example, in the intestinal nematodes a female Ascaris may reach 18 cm whereas a female Strongyloides is smaller than 1 mm. Their bodies are muscular and require high carbohydrate reserves.

The common human nematodes can be roughly divided into the *intestinal nematodes*, of which the common ones in order of importance are hookworms, Ascaris, Strongyloides, Trichuris, and Oxyuris, and the *tissue nematodes*. The latter group includes Trichinella and the various filarial worms. Heyneman has suggested that the life cycles of the intestinal nematodes of man can be shown to demonstrate an increasing dependence upon the host and a decrease in the proportion of metabolically active time in the free-living stages if they are arranged in a certain sequence. This sequence reflects different degrees of adaption by the parasite to the host and is presented in Table 1.

Rhabditis, a free-living nematode which rarely infects man, is but one step away from the relatively common *Strongyloides stercoralis*. Strongyloides represent the first stage in parasitic adaption. Hookworms are obligate parasites with no free-living stage. Both these nematodes and Ascaris have a phase of lung migration by immature larvae in the host, the explanation of which is not known. Ascaris, Trichuris, and Enterobius have progressively shorter oval maturation times. *Trichinella spiralis* is viviparous; the intestinal phase is transient, and the larvae persist in the host muscle.

Although the adult Trichinella organisms are intestinal nematodes, from a clinical viewpoint trichinosis can be considered as a tissue parasitic infection, as it is the larvae that produce the disease syndrome. The final break from the free-living state is illustrated by the filariae, in which the adult worms live in the host tissue, specific arthropods serving as the intermediate hosts. Whether filariae evolved from insect parasites or arose by adaption of intestinal parasites to insects after ingestion of eggs by coprophagic insects is a matter for speculation.

As in schistosomiasis, the number of worms present in the host determines the clinical manifestations, and many mild infections are asymptomatic. Quantitative

TABLE 1. Sequence for Common Human Intestinal Nematodes (Heyneman)

Species	Details of Life Cycle
Strongyloides stercoralis	Most primitive since parasitism is irregular and exists in free-living adult stage in soil
Necator americanus	Regular parasitism; no free-living adults, only larvae in soil
Ancylostoma duodenale	
Ascaris lumbricoides	All hatched larval stages as well as adults in host; only eggs in soil
Trichuris trichiura	Similar to Ascaris, but newly hatched larvae do not migrate through host's body; all development confined to the intestine
Enterobius vermicularis	Eggs infective shortly after being laid; soil phase for eggs rarely involved
Trichinella spiralis	No eggs laid; larvae hatch within female, are deposited in mucosa, which they penetrate, and migrate via blood stream to encyst in tissues

techniques to determine adult worm load are commonly used in some nematode infections. Among the intestinal nematodes, Strongyloides and Oxyuris infections cannot be quantitated owing to the variability in excretion of progeny. Ascaris produces so many eggs that quantitative techniques are usually not worthwhile, but hookworms and Trichuris eggs can be quantitated by a stool-dilution technique. For example, in Stoll's method 3 grams of stool is emulsified in 42 ml of water in a special flask. Tenth normal sodium hydroxide may be used to soften hard feces. Glass beads and shaking after standing produces a uniform fine emulsion; 0.15 ml volume of this is pipetted onto a glass slide, and all the eggs counted in this volume are equivalent to 0.01 gram of feces. Knowing the number of eggs per gram of stool, the total volume of stool, the egg output per female worm, and the usual sex ratio of the species population, it is possible to calculate the approximate worm load. Tissue helminths can also be quantitated in terms of larval output by expressing results in *Trichinella spiralis* infections as the number of larvae per gram of skeletal muscle or the number of microfilariae per milliliter of blood at a certain time of day. Onchocerca infections are likewise expressed as number of microfilariae per milligram of skin.

Another important feature of nematode infections is the frequency with which infections with nonhuman parasites are encountered as abortive infections, with larvae only rarely maturing to adults, thus suggesting helminths in a process of adaption into man. A number of such parasites will be mentioned in the text that follows, including the genera Oesophagostomum, Toxocara, Anasakis, Angiostrongylus, Dirofilaria, and others of clinical importance.

Heyneman's sequence is followed in the present discussion of the nematodes, although it is important to point out that, in terms of human suffering, hookworm and Bancroftian filariasis are by far the most serious infections.

Beaver, P. C.: Wandering nematodes as a cause of disability and disease. Am. J. Trop. Med., 6:433, 1957.

Beaver, P. C.: The nature of visceral larva migrans. J. Parasitol., 55:3, 1969.

Heyneman, D.: The life cycle of the nematodes parasitic in man: An evolutionary sequence. Med. J. Malaya, 20:249, 1966.

Knight, R., Schultz, M. G., Hoskins, D. W., and Marsden, P. D.: Intestinal parasites, a progress report. Gut, 14:145, 1973.

Marsden, P. D., and Schultz, M. G.: Intestinal parasites, a progress report. Gastroenterology, 57:724, 1969.

INTESTINAL NEMATODES

302. STRONGYLOIDIASIS (Cochin-China Diarrhea)

Definition. Strongyloidiasis is an infection of the small intestine with the invasive small nematode *Strongyloides stercoralis.* Most infections are asymptomatic, but a few can be life threatening; because of this, treatment is always necessary.

Etiology and Transmission. The parasitic female worm is small (2.2 mm long) and lives in the mucosa of the intestinal villi. The parasitic male has rarely been observed, and experimental work suggests that parthenogenesis is the rule. The eggs produced by the female hatch rapidly, producing larvae in the small intestine, and these may reinvade the bowel mucosa before being voided in the feces (internal autoinfection). On the other hand, they may invade immediately after voiding via the perianal skin (external autoinfection). Other larvae become infective within hours of contact with the soil, and invasion of a fresh host occurs via the skin. Alternatively, voided larvae may develop into *free-living adults in the soil.* These adults produce further generations of infective larvae in the soil. These alternative cycles make the life history of Strongyloides the most difficult one to grasp.

After skin penetration, the infective larvae undergo the same curious migration as hookworms via the venous system to the lungs (in 24 to 48 hours). Autoinfective forms may take a peritoneal or lymphatic route to the same site. From the lungs the developing larvae ascend the trachea, drop down into the stomach, and mature in the small intestine. Because of the frequency of autoinfection this nematode is self-perpetuating, and infections can last for 30 to 40 years. Man is the only common host, although primates and dogs can be experimentally infected.

Distribution. The parasite is cosmopolitan, but it is more frequent in the tropics. Local habitats where warmth, moisture, and lack of sanitation favor the free-living existence are endemic sites. Curiously enough, in nearly all populations, however, the infection seems to be sporadic and an incidence comparable with that seen in hookworm infection is not encountered. Conceivably, however, this may be due to diagnostic difficulties, as mentioned below. This infection, like all intestinal parasitic infections, has been reported in high incidence from some mental institutions. Resistance to reinfection has been suggested by animal studies.

Pathology and Pathogenesis. The adult female worms burrow through the intestinal submucosa above the muscularis mucosae, depositing eggs as they go. They cause a chronic inflammatory cell infiltrate with many eosinophils. The rapidly hatching larvae are responsible for most of the pathologic findings, and their powers of penetration are such they can be distributed widely throughout the body. For reasons not clearly understood, the whole process may be accelerated (the so-called hyperinfective syndrome). Debility on the part of the host, malnutrition, or corticoid administration favors the development of this syndrome. Obviously prolonged bowel transit time would increase the possibility of internal autoinfection. Inflammation of the small bowel may be so intense as to cause malabsorption, thickening, and edema visible roentgenographically. The mesenteric lymph nodes enlarge, and ulceration and necrosis of the mucosa may occur. The lungs and liver may also show abscess formation, and fatty changes in the liver may indicate primary or secondary malnutrition. In recent years several series of fatal cases have been described from the West Indies, Brazil, and Africa. Acute small bowel obstruction has been described, as well as *E. coli* bacteremia with meningitis, the latter perhaps arising from bacteria being introduced from the bowel on migrating larvae. The gut may be invaded at any level by larvae, and gastric and colonic involvement are well documented. Rarely larvae are found in other abdominal organs. Involvement of the kidney, heart, and endocrine glands is described.

Clinical Manifestations. Dermal invasion, either as a result of primary exposure or by external autoinfection, may be characterized by linear, erythematous, urticarial wheals, which are the sites of migrating larvae. Particularly common around the buttocks, they may occur anywhere, and are often recognized for what they are, as they are relatively fast moving. It is a form of cutaneous larva migrans (see Ch. 305). Lung invasion may be associated with signs of bronchospasm or bronchopneumonia. These may be short-lived or recurrent if several waves of larvae arrive in the lung. Hemoptysis is not uncommon as the larvae burst through the pulmonary alveoli. They may be found in the sputum, and there is usually a marked eosinophilia. Bowel involvement may give rise to a variety of clinical manifestations, but again it must be stressed that many light infections are asymptomatic. The most common gastrointestinal symptom is epigastric pain, which is often to the right of the midline, constant, and of a dull, aching character, mimicking peptic ulcer. Tenderness may be present on abdominal palpation over the duodenum. In heavy infections diarrhea is common; it may not be just the result of inflammation but may also reflect the coexistent malabsorption. Upper abdominal pain and vomiting from the involved upper gut are frequent, but intestinal obstruction is rare. Marked large bowel involvement may resemble ulcerative colitis. In the hyperinfective syndrome death may result from disseminated inflammatory lesions, often with superimposed bacterial infection.

Diagnosis. Strongyloidiasis must always be thought of in patients with unexplained eosinophilia. The high eosinophilia is probably associated with recurrent larval invasion. The diagnosis is made by finding the larvae in the stool, preferably by using a concentration technique. Unfortunately there are a number of difficulties. In warm climates fresh stool should be examined, as hookworm larvae hatch quickly from the eggs; they can be differentiated, but only by an expert. The excretion of larvae in strongyloidiasis is intermittent, and multiple stool specimens should be examined. The Baermann funnel technique and filter paper culture technique have facilitated diagnosis. Sometimes larvae are demonstrated in the duodenal aspirate or sputum when other techniques have failed. Jejunal biopsy may show larvae and adult parasites in section in the mucosa. The filarial complement-fixation test is invariably positive and of diagnostic help in difficult cases. Barium studies may show thickening and deformities of the small bowel owing to inflammatory edema.

Treatment. As so little is known about the conditions governing development of serious infections, all patients should be treated with thiabendazole, 25 mg per kilogram twice daily for two days. Given orally, this drug is effective, with few side effects. The tablets should be chewed; they have an orange taste. Assessment of parasitologic cure requires repeated stool examinations using special techniques. The eosinophilia should fall within eight weeks. The prognosis is good in otherwise healthy subjects, but may be poor in the exceptional circumstances described above. Prophylaxis involves avoiding unsanitary conditions when infection is likely. Strongyloides of nutria and raccoons have caused transient creeping eruptions (cutaneous larva migrans) in Louisiana trappers.

Bras, G., Richards, R. C., Irvine, R. A., Milner, P. F. A., and Ragbeer, M. M. S.: Infection with *Strongyloides stercoralis* in Jamaica. Lancet, 2:1257, 1964.

Kanani, S. R., and Rees, P. H.: The diagnosis of strongyloidiasis with special reference to the value of the filarial complement fixation test as a screening test. Trans. R. Soc. Trop. Med. Hyg., 64:246, 1970.

Stemmerman, G. N.: Strongyloidiasis in migrants. Pathological and clinical considerations. Gastroenterology, 53:59, 1967.

Tanaka, H.: Experimental and epidemiological strongyloidiasis of Amaini Oshima Island. Jap. J. Exp. Med., 28:159, 1958.

303. CAPILLARIASIS

Until recently the genus Capillaria appeared to infect man so rarely that it would not have merited inclusion in a general work of this kind. The most common form, *Capillaria hepatica* (less than 20 cases reported), was recognized by finding Trichuris-like eggs encapsulated in the liver. Species of the genus had also been reported in the lungs and skin of man.

Recently, however, a new parasite of man *Capillaria philippinensis,* has been described from the northern Philippines, where more than 1000 cases and 100 deaths have been confirmed to date. Patients with intestinal capillariasis have colicky abdominal pain, chronic diarrhea, muscle wasting, and edema, which may lead to debility and death in four months. Clinical studies have shown the presence of a severe protein-losing enteropathy in these patients with malabsorption of fats and sugars.

A tiny nematode (3 to 4 mm by 0.03 to 0.04 mm), *C. philippinensis* is confined to the small intestine, particularly the jejunum. The eggs detected in the stool are similar to *Trichuris trichiura* (to which the Capillaria are closely related) but are smaller, are more oval, and have less prominent bipolar plugs. There is evidence that hatching may occur in the small intestine, and tissue invasion of the bowel similar to strongyloidiasis has been noted at postmortem examination. The mode of transmission of the disease is not fully worked out, but three species of fish have been found to contain infective larvae. It is still uncertain whether interhuman transmission occurs.

Apart from intravenous feeding in severe cases, success in eliminating this parasite has been reported by using high doses of thiabendazole.

Cross, J. H., Banzon, T., Clarke, M. D., Basaca Servilla, V., Watten, R. H., and Dizon, J. J.: Studies on the experimental transmission of *Capillaria philippinensis* in monkeys. Trans. R. Soc. Trop. Med. Hyg., 66:819, 1972.

Detels, R., Gutman, L., Jaramillo, J., Zerrudo, E., Banzon, T., Valera, J., Murrell, K. D., Cross, J., and Dizon, J. J.: An epidemic of intestinal capillariasis in man. Am. J. Trop. Med., 18:676, 1969.

Whalen, G. E., Rosenberg, E. B., Strickland, G. T., Gutman, R. A., Cross, J. H., Watten, R. H., Uylangco, C., Dizon, J. J.: Intestinal capillariasis, a new disease in man. Lancet, 1:13, 1969.

304. HOOKWORM DISEASE (Ancylostomiasis, Miner's Anemia)

Definition. The two common hookworms of man, *Ancylostoma duodenale* and *Necator americanus,* attach themselves to the small bowel by their buccal capsules and suck blood, thereby causing chronic blood loss. Depending on their number and the iron stores of the host, a variable degree of anemia often results. A distinction is made between hookworm infection when the load is too light to produce symptoms and hookworm disease.

Pathogenic Chain. *Etiology.* The human hookworms measure about 1 cm in length, the female being slightly longer than the male, which is recognizable by an expanded posterior end, the copulating bursa. *A. duodenale* is larger than *Necator americanus,* and the two species are differentiated most easily by the fact that *A. duodenale* has two pairs of teeth in its buccal capsule, whereas *N. americanus* has a pair of cutting plates only. The eggs of the two species are indistinguishable and are passed in the feces. In warm moist soil the larva hatches within 48 hours. The rhabditiform larva has a free-living cycle in the soil, feeding on bacteria, during which time it molts twice. The filariform larvae resulting from the second molt are the infective stage for man and can survive several months in favorable conditions. They tend to migrate up grass stems or gain any elevation up to 3 feet, and on coming into contact with the skin of man, quickly penetrate it, enter the bloodstream, and are transported to the lungs. Like Strongyloides, there they leave the vascular system and emerge into the alveoli, migrate up the bronchi and trachea, and down the esophagus to reach the small intestine where maturity is attained. Eggs appear in the stool five or more weeks after invasion, and the adults live one to nine years.

Epidemiology. Over 400 million people have hookworm infections, but in the majority the worm load is small. *Ancylostoma duodenale* is the Old World hookworm, being prevalent in Europe, North Africa, and the Middle and Far East. *Necator americanus* is found more in the New World and tropical Africa. During the past 30 years both parasites have become widely distributed, and rigid geographic demarcations are not possible.

The survival of larvae is favored by a damp sandy soil, high in humus content at a temperature of 24 to 32° C. Promiscuous defecation and the absence of shoes are the chief factors responsible for infections. Such conditions occur in mines as well as on the surface of the ground. Urban people tend to have less hookworm than agricultural rural workers at locations where night soil is often used as fertilizer. Infection can be acquired by ingesting or handling contaminated vegetables. Coffee, banana, sugar cane, rice, and sweet potato fields are ideal for the growth and development of larvae. Often one locality is used as a communal latrine in the area, and people reinfect themselves by visiting these sites again and again. *The distinction between hookworm infection and hookworm disease is important.* Methods of estimating the intensity of the infection show that in endemic areas most patients have few worms and no significant anemia. Those who have hookworm anemia have more worms, and these heavy infections could be the result of repeated exposure or a failure of immunity on the part of the host. With canine hookworm, small repeated infections give almost complete immunity. Antibodies have been demonstrated in sera of infected patients.

Pathology and Pathogenesis. Inflammatory cell infiltration is seen at the site of penetration of the hookworm larvae, and in the lungs small hemorrhages occur with eosinophilic and leukocytic infiltration. An eosinophilia is present during the invasive phase. The main feature of the established disease is the active sucking of blood by the worms. They create a negative pressure in the buccal capsule and suck in a piece of mucosa which acts as both an anchorage and a source of blood. It is still not clear what hookworms abstract from the blood. Vital preparations in vitro show red cells being vigorously expelled from the posterior end. Ancylostoma sucks between 0.16 and 0.34 ml of blood per day and Necator, 0.03 to 0.05. The development of anemia depends upon three factors: the iron content of the diet, the state of the iron reserves, and the intensity and duration of infection.

When iron intake is high, a heavy worm load is needed to produce a significant anemia. Up to 60 per cent of the iron from the hemoglobin extracted by the hookworm is reabsorbed in the intestine. At open operation small punctate hemorrhagic spots are encountered at the site of attachment. In addition to anemia, hypoalbuminemia occurs owing to a combination of blood loss and a low rate of albumin synthesis, possibly associated with anoxia affecting liver cell function. Malabsorption is said to occur in a few cases with partial villous atrophy and chronic inflammatory cell infiltration of the lamina propria.

Clinical Manifestations. The site of skin penetration by the larvae is associated with pruritus and the development of an erythematous papular eruption (ground itch) which may last several days or even longer, depending on the host's immune response. Within a week after penetration the patient may have a transient asthmatic attack, but this is not as commonly seen as in invasive ascariasis.

Established hookworm disease is associated with general symptoms of anemia, weakness, fatigue, dyspnea, palpitation, and mental and physical retardation. Pica may be noted. On examination the skin and mucus membrane are pale. Peripheral edema is due possibly to a variety of factors, namely, hypoalbuminemia, a rise of capillary venous pressure, and tissue anoxia. In severe cases there is evidence of congestive cardiac failure. The pulse is rapid with a high pulse pressure. On auscultation of the enlarged heart, a third heart sound and an ejection type of systolic murmur are commonly heard; regurgitant systolic and even diastolic murmurs may occur and disappear when the anemia is corrected. For this reason it is very unwise to diagnose a valvular lesion clinically in such anemic patients until that anemia has been corrected. The hemoglobin may be very low (2 grams per 100 ml) and the patient still ambulant. The patient may complain of upper abdominal pain, and radiologic changes suggestive of a duodenitis have been reported.

Diagnosis and Differential Diagnosis. Stool microscopy, either by a direct smear or by a concentration technique, reveals hookworm ova. Quantitation of the egg excretion enables the physician to decide whether the patient has a significant worm load. This is done by diluting a known volume of stool and counting a sample (Stoll technique). Hookworm ova are 60 to 70 μ long by 35 to 40 μ wide and have a characteristic morphology with a clear shell and developing embryo inside. They must be distinguished, however, from both Trichostrongylus and *Ternidens deminutus,* both of which have larger eggs. Test tube cultivation of ova and differentiation of the resultant larvae are of value in doubtful cases. A skin test using an extract of *Necator americanus* larvae of standard nitrogen content has proved useful in screening a hookworm-infected population. Fluorescent antibody, complement-fixation, and hemagglutination tests have been developed but have little clinical application.

The anemia of hookworm disease is a classic iron deficiency anemia with a low hemoglobin, mean corpuscular hemoglobin concentration and serum iron, and a high iron-binding capacity. On the film the red cells are microcytic and hypochromic. Folic acid deficiency may sometimes be superimposed on macrocytosis. The serum albumin is low, and liver function tests may be abnormal. In the edematous patient there may be confusion with kwashiorkor, wet beriberi, or the nephrotic syndrome. The anemia has to be differentiated from other iron deficiency anemias.

Treatment. Tetrachloroethylene in a dose of 0.1 mg per kilogram of body weight is effective (maximum of 5 ml in a single dose). It is usually dispensed in 1-ml gelatin capsules or in a liquid that should be kept in the refrigerator in a dark bottle. It is given in the morning on an empty stomach; all food should be withheld for six hours and any fatty foods withheld for the rest of the day. Repeated treatments may be necessary. Vertigo, vomiting, and dizziness may follow therapy. Bephenium hydroxynaphthoate (Alcopar) is more expensive but is being increasingly used. The standard dose for an adult is 5 grams containing 2.5 grams of bephenium base; it is taken as granules in a glass of water on an empty stomach. Three daily doses may achieve total eradication. Loose stools, nausea, and vomiting have followed treatment. Both drugs will remove a large number of worms at the first dose, but to get rid of the last 5 to 10 per cent is often very difficult. In many areas total eradication may not be desirable or necessary. In general, tetrachloroethylene is said to be more effective in *Necator americanus* infections. If Ascaris are also present, Alcopar is preferred, or both Ascaris and hookworm will respond to thiabendazole. Tetrachloroethylene irritates Ascaris and may cause migration.

The anemia responds well to ferrous sulfate, 200 or 400 mg three times daily. Occasionally the hemoglobin is so low, or there is an associated acute infection, that the patient presents in extremis owing to heart failure. Pregnancy may also precipitate acute heart failure. Intraperitoneal blood transfusion or exchange transfusions have been life-saving. The prognosis is good in most cases. It is wise to delay treating the hookworm infection until the hemoglobin is above 50 per cent after oral iron. Without treatment of the worm infection, the anemia will relapse when iron therapy is discontinued. *Prevention* involves the sanitary disposal of human excreta and the prevention of soil pollution. The wearing of shoes cuts down the opportunities for infection.

Gilles, H. M., Williams, E. J. W., and Ball, P. A. J.: Hookworm infection and anemia. Quart. J. Med., 33:1, 1964.
Roche, M., and Layrisse, M.: Nature and causes of hookworm anemia. Am. J. Trop. Med., 15:1031, 1966.
Stoll, N. R.: On endemic hookworm, where do we stand to-day? Exp. Parasitol., 12:241, 1962.
Stoll, N. R.: For hookworm diagnosis is finding one egg enough? Ann. N.Y. Acad. Sci., 98:712, 1962.

305. CUTANEOUS LARVA MIGRANS (Creeping Eruption)

Cutaneous larva migrans is considered at this point because its most common cause is *Ancylostoma braziliense,* although it may be produced by a variety of other helminths. It is characterized by an erythematous, serpiginous, intracutaneous track or burrow, the anterior end of which is observed to migrate at the rate of 1 to 2 cm per day. There is often intense irritation, and secondary infection may result from scratching. This migration is due to the infective larva of *A. braziliense* (the cat and dog hookworm), which does not visceralize in man but wanders around in the skin. This migration may last for 2 to 50 weeks before the larva dies. Rarely some larvae reach the lungs, causing high eosinophilia and patchy pulmonary infiltration.

Patients are often infected by lying on beaches contaminated by dog or cat feces. The feet, legs, and hands are the most common sites, and the appearance of the lesion is usually diagnostic. It is virtually impossible to remove the larva from the skin.

Anyclostoma braziliense is found in the southern United States, Central America, and tropical South America, as well as in tropical Africa and parts of the Far East, especially the Malay peninsula. There have been several reports of the worm maturing in the gut of man and eggs appearing in the feces, so there is not an absolute host specificity. Two other dog hookworms, *Uncinaria stenocephala* and *Ancylostoma caninum,* can produce similar lesions. Occasionally the ground itch of the two common human hookworms may persist and resemble creeping eruption in immune subjects.

The larva migrans track of *Strongyloides stercoralis* tends to be a short line, erythematous and rapidly moving (larva currens). Rodent Strongyloides may produce similar lesions but no mature worms. A form of myiasis with the horse bot fly maggot (Gasterophilus) can produce a larger deeper migrating form of cutaneous larva migrans.

Treatment. Thiabendazole by mouth, 25 mg per kilogram per day for two days, is usually effective. If not, the dose can be doubled and repeated. Alternatively, the advancing end of the burrow can be treated with topical thiabendazole sprinkled on elastoplast or in a cream containing 15 per cent thiabendazole powder in a hydrosoluble base. This drug has completely superseded the other, more unsatisfactory treatments such as ethyl chloride spray and Hetrazan.

Battistini, F.: Treatment of creeping eruption with topical thiabendazole. Tex. Rep. Biol. Med., 27 (Supplement 2):645, 1969.
Beaver, P. C.: Larva migrans. Exp. Parasitol., 5:587, 1956.
Stone, O. J.: Systemic and topical thiabendazole for creeping eruption. Tex. Rep. Biol. Med., 27 (Supplement 2):659, 1969.

306. TRICHOSTRONGYLIASIS

The adult worms of the genus Trichostrongylus are much smaller than hookworms, being under 100 mm long. They lie embedded in the mucosa of the duodenum and jejunum, where they suck a small quantity of blood. Eight species have been reported in man. Infections are most frequent in the Far East, especially in Japan, Korea, and Indonesia. High infection rates have been reported in Iran. South and Western Asia, Chile, and Brazil are areas where human infections also occur. Worm loads in man are usually light and asymptomatic. Infection is acquired by ingesting salad contaminated with infective third-stage larvae. The importance of Trichostrongylus lies in the fact that the egg is frequently mistaken for hookworm, and this group is not very susceptible to antihelminthics used in the treatment of hookworm (e.g., Tetrachlorethylene). These "hookworm eggs" appear to persist after therapy and are termed drug resistant. Frequently, these so-called drug-resistant hookworms turn out to be Trichostrongylus. The eggs of Trichostrongylus are larger and more sharply pointed at one end and have more advanced embryonation than hookworm ova. They are from 73 to

94 μ in length and 40 to 50 μ in width. Larvae recovered from fecal culture of the ova can also be distinguished from hookworm. Treatment is seldom needed, but thiabendazole is probably effective in the majority of cases.

Ghadirian, E., and Arfaa, F.: Trichostrongyliasis, a prevalent zoonotic infection in Iran. *In* Abstracts of Invited Papers, Ninth International Congress on Tropical Medicine and Malaria, Athens, 1973, p. 156.

Marcial Rojas, R. A.: Trichostrongyliasis. *In* Marcial Rojas, R. A. (ed.): Pathology of Protozoal and Helminthic Disease with Clinical Correlation. Baltimore, Williams & Wilkins Company, 1971, p. 753.

307. GNATHOSTOMIASIS

Although Gnathostoma species are more closely related to Ascaris, this group is mentioned at this point because it also presents as *creeping eruptions* or, more commonly, as *migratory swelling in the subcutaneous tissues.* More than 100 human infections with the immature stages of *Gnathostoma spinigerum* have been reported from the Far East, particularly Thailand. Normally a parasite of wild felines, dogs, and foxes, Gnathostoma infects man when he eats the larvae in undercooked fish (fermented fish is a Thai delicacy). The larva causes a migratory swelling, often in the subcutaneous tissues, associated with an intense eosinophilia. Occasionally the larva comes to the skin surface and resembles cutaneous larva migrans, but the area of involvement is larger. Sometimes the larva burrows deep into the internal tissues and may lodge in the gut wall or elsewhere and produce an abscess. Indeed, secondary infection frequently occurs. Brain involvement in fatal cases with eosinophilic meningitis has been reported. Eye involvement with iritis and orbital cellulitis is also described. If the worm does not reach the body surface, the symptoms can persist for months. Some recommend extraction of the worm, but Hetrazan has been said to be useful. There is insufficient experience with thiabendazole thus far to permit a definite statement of its value, but its trial seems reasonable.

Miyazaki, I.: On the genus Gnathostoma and human gnathostomiasis with special reference to Japan. Exp. Parasitol., 9:338, 1960.

308. OESOPHAGOSTOMIASIS

Oesophagostomiasis is more closely related to hookworm and Strongyloides than to Gnathostoma, but like Gnathostoma it may rarely form a tumor in the human gut wall. Again, man is not the definitive host. The infection is often carried by pet monkeys, and the clinical picture is usually one of intestinal obstruction. Bacterial infection of the tumor nodule is common. Surgical excision of the tumor shows it to contain worms of Oesophagostomum species.

Anthony, P. P., and McAdam, I. W. J.: Helminthic pseudotumours of the bowel: Thirty-four cases of helminthoma. Gut, 13:8, 1972.

309. ASCARIASIS

Definition. Ascariasis is infection with *Ascaris lumbricoides,* the large roundworm of man. The adults mature in the small intestine and can produce disease by intestinal obstruction or migration. The passage of larvae through the lungs may result in pneumonitis.

Etiology. Ascariasis is a large whitish nematode; the female (20 to 35 cm) is larger than the male (15 to 30 cm), which often has a curly tail. The vulva of the female is situated ventrally at the junction of the anterior and middle thirds of the worm. Frequent copulation is necessary to ensure the continuous production of fertile eggs. A female worm has a reproductive capacity of 26 to 27 million eggs and a daily output of 200,000. The life span of the adult worms is relatively short (12 to 24 months). They are not attached to the wall of the jejunum, but bridge themselves across the lumen and by their muscle tone maintain themselves against the fecal stream. In a largely anaerobic environment they obtain nourishment from the semidigested food of the host and possibly from epithelial cells of the intestinal mucosa. The high protein and vitamin content of the parasite suggests that they deprive the host of nutrients.

The brownish eggs with a thick shell and albuminous coat become infective ten days after being passed in the stool. Fertile and infertile eggs have a different morphology. On ingestion of infective eggs by man, the larvae hatch in the small intestine, and, penetrating its wall, are carried by the blood and lymphatic system to the lungs. It has been suggested that this migration is necessitated by the need for oxygen, which is not available in the intestine, at this stage of the life cycle. Here, like hookworm and Strongyloides, the larvae migrate up the respiratory passages to the epiglottis and down to the esophagus. A new generation of eggs appears in the feces approximately two months after the ingestion of embryonated eggs.

Epidemiology. Although cosmopolitan, this worm is most abundant in the tropics, where sanitation is poor. One in every four people in the world is infected with *Ascaris lumbricoides.* The eggs are killed by direct sunlight and temperatures above 45° C; nevertheless, under optimal conditions they may remain viable for ten years. The eggs pass unchanged through the intestine of animals with the possible exception of the pig. The pig Ascaris, *Ascaris suum,* is morphologically identical to the human Ascaris, and there is some evidence that cross-infections can occur. The susceptibility to infection is greatest in childhood, reaching a peak at puberty, and transmission is by fecal contamination of food and drink. Circulating antibodies appear to play some role in host immunity.

Pathology and Clinical Manifestations. Light infections of a dozen or so worms often pass unnoticed, especially in adults. During the phase of larval migration, especially if many eggs have been ingested, respiratory symptoms may appear 4 to 16 days after infection. The pulmonary migration of larvae is associated with fever, cough, occasionally hemoptysis, and either crepitations or more rarely the signs of consolidation on auscultation of the chest. The sputum contains larvae and eosinophils, and there is a high blood eosinophilia. Sections of the lungs at this stage would show larvae in the bronchioles with patchy infiltration of alveoli with polymorphs and eosinophil leukocytes. Aberrant larvae may lodge in the liver, producing granulomatous lesions and hepatomegaly. More rarely such larvae, which fail to re-enter the circulation, are found in other abdominal organs.

When adult worms are present in the intestine, the established infection is often associated with occasional colicky abdominal pain and some abdominal distention.

These adults may produce complications by mechanical effects within the gastrointestinal tract, or by wandering outside it, or more rarely by producing allergic manifestations in a sensitized host.

Heavy loads of worms may particularly be associated with intestinal obstruction, intussusception, volvulus, appendicitis, and hernial strangulation. A bolus of Ascaris may be a common cause of intestinal obstruction in childhood in an endemic area. Before undertaking bowel surgery, an Ascaris infection should always be excluded, because these worms are difficult to control once the bowel is opened, and considerable peritoneal soiling may result. Migration of adult worms may occur spontaneously or as a result of some stimulus such as fever or tetrachloroethylene. The Ascaris adults may perforate a suture line or cause a bile or pancreatic duct obstruction. Occasionally they migrate into the stomach and are vomited up, or pass down into the large bowel and out with the stool. Adult worms have been described issuing from umbilical fistulas, and even from the nose or ear. Obstruction of the bile duct is associated with cholangitis, and eggs may be deposited in the liver. *A. lumbricoides* has been said by some to be second only to *E. histolytica* in producing liver abscesses. Blockage of the pancreatic duct results in acute pancreatitis. Once the adult worm has left the bowel, it often dies, releasing foreign protein that may produce a reaction in a sensitized host. These reactions range from facial edema and giant urticaria to acute local necrosis and anaphylaxis. Laboratory personnel who work with Ascaris invariably become sensitized to the worms. Young pigs infected with Ascaris do not gain weight normally, and it is possible that heavy loads of human Ascaris may affect children similarly, as the worms will consume much food in the actively growing phase.

Diagnosis. Examination of the feces reveals the characteristic ova. Usually in view of the number of ova produced, they can be found in ordinary direct smear. Although fertilized eggs are easy to recognize, unfertilized eggs assume bizarre shapes and may be mistaken for debris. Rarely one encounters infections of immature worms or only male worms. Sometimes an infection is diagnosed in barium meal examination, as the barium can be seen in the Ascaris gut. Although many serologic tests have been developed for Ascaris, including complement-fixation, hemagglutination, and gel diffusion, they are seldom used for diagnostic purposes.

Treatment. Piperazine citrate is the drug of choice in the treatment of Ascaris infestations. The piperazine salts are simple, safe, and efficient. They act by blocking the neuromuscular junctions of the worm. The paralyzed worm can no longer bridge itself across the intestinal lumen and is carried along in the fecal stream and passed in the stool. Piperazine citrate is given in a dose of 75 mg per kilogram to a maximal single dose of 4 grams. This will clear 75 per cent of patients of their worms, but the dose can be repeated the following day with safety. No special preparation or purgation is necessary. Neurotoxic effects from piperazine have been reported in patients with renal failure who cannot excrete the drug.

Thiabendazole in the same dose as for strongyloidiasis and Alcopar in the same dose as for hookworm are both effective in ascariasis as well. In the presence of Ascaris plus one or another of these intestinal parasites, single drug therapy may be preferred. However, neither of these drugs is as effective in ascariasis as piperazine. In multiple intestinal helminthic infections, Ascaris should always be treated first.

When examining stools for ova after therapy, it must be remembered that eggs may be passed in the stool for up to a week after the worms have been eradicated owing to the delay in the colonic circulation of feces.

The following regimen is suggested to deal with *intestinal obstruction* owing to Ascaris. Initially conservative treatment with nasogastric suction, intravenous fluids, and piperazine therapy should be tried for 48 hours. If no improvement follows, at laparotomy it is often possible to manipulate the bolus of worms into the large bowel through the terminal ileum. Only if this is not possible should enterotomy and worm extraction be performed.

Prevention. This consists of disposal of human excreta in sanitary privies and toilets. Children must be taught to use these facilities and avoid contamination of food with ova.

Chang, C. C., and Han, C. T.: Biliary ascariasis in childhood. A clinical analysis of 788 cases. Chin. Med. J. (Peking), 85:167, 1966.

Gelpi, A. P., and Mustafa, A.: Seasonal pneumonitis with eosinophilia: A study of larval ascariasis in Saudi Arabia. Am. J. Trop. Med. Hyg., 16:646, 1967.

Lejkina, E. S.: Research in Ascaris immunity and immunodiagnosis. Bull. WHO, 32:699, 1965.

Otto, G. F., and Cort, W. W.: The distribution and epidemiology of human ascariasis in the United States. Am. J. Hyg., 16:657, 1934.

Piggott, J., Hansbarger, E. A., and Neafie, R. G.: Human ascariasis. Am. J. Clin. Path., 53:223, 1970.

The Control of Ascariasis. World Health Organization Technical Report, Series No. 379, 1967.

310. TOXOCARIASIS (Visceral Larva Migrans)

Toxocariasis is an accidental human infection with the cat and dog Ascaris (*Toxocara cati* and *Toxocara canis*). The eggs of these species are infective two to three weeks after being passed, and if ingested by man the second stage larvae emerge. These penetrate the intestinal wall and reach the liver. The majority remain in the liver but others migrate to other organs, particularly the brain and the eye. Rarely they complete their cycle of development in man and produce adult worms in the bowel. Children are particularly susceptible because of more frequent soiling of the fingers and habits of playing with puppies, in which the incidence of infection is very high. Initially reported from the southern United States, these parasites are common in dogs and cats in many parts of the world. Although many reports have come from North America and Europe, it is likely that this syndrome also occurs in other parts of the world.

The migrating larvae produce "eosinophilic trails" and tissue inflammation in the affected organ. Usually a granuloma forms with epithelial cells, fibroblasts, lymphocytes, plasma cells, and occasional giant cells. A fibrous capsule eventually encloses the larva, which may remain alive for months. The granulomas can be seen macroscopically as small grayish-white spots. Such granulomas have been found in the lungs, eyes, brain, heart, kidney, and striated muscle.

The most common clinical form is that of a patient with a mild fever and tender hepatomegaly. Routine investigation reveals a marked eosinophilia (50 to 60 per cent), and further questioning often brings to light a history of contact with dogs. These signs and symptoms may persist for 18 months. The serum globulins may be elevated and anti-τ globulins are found. Another clinical form is as an *endophthalmitis* with a space-occupying granuloma visibly distorting the contour of the retina on funduscopy. In the past such granulomas were often mistaken for retinoblastomas, and the eye was removed. Several such series of "retinoblastomas" have been examined, and many of the tumors were found to consist of granulomas containing Toxocara larvae. Many mild infections are asymptomatic.

The syndrome of tender hepatomegaly and eosinophilia must be distinguished from invasive schistosomiasis or fascioliasis. A variety of nematodes can produce visceral larva migrans in special circumstances, among them *Ascaris lumbricoides, Necator americanus,* and *Strongyloides stercoralis.* Other nonhuman nematodes such as Gnathostoma, Capillaria, Hepaticola, and Dirofilaria may be involved in granuloma formation in the liver. Sarcoidosis and periarteritis nodosa may mimic this disease. Blind liver biopsy is seldom helpful, but where facilities exist, direct visualization of surface granulomas of the liver with a peritoneoscope may enable biopsy of a granuloma to be made. A definitive diagnosis can often be made by examination of this granuloma. A diagnosis of second-stage rhabdoid Toxocara larva can be made on a section at mid-gut level, showing a maximal width of 12 to 20 μ and lateral alae. A variety of serologic tests are available but lack specificity, as they cross-react with other helminthic infections. However, in areas where such infections are rarely encountered, a fluorescent antibody test or an indirect hemagglutination test may be helpful.

Treatment. Diethylcarbamazine (see Bancroftian Filariasis in Ch. 316) has been used and does kill some larvae in the tissues of infected mice. A resolution of symptoms has followed the use of thiabendazole in one case in a dose of 25 mg per kilogram twice daily for seven days. The prognosis is good if the source of infection is removed by treating the dog with piperazine. Care must be taken to worm pets regularly, especially puppies, if they are in contact with children.

Huntley, C. C., Costas, M. C., Williams, R. C., Lyerly, A. D., and Watson, R. G.: Anti-γ-globulin factors in visceral larva migrans. J.A.M.A., 197:552, 1966.
Kagan, I. G.: The serological diagnosis of visceral larva migrans. Clin. Pediatr. (Phila.), 7:508, 1968.
Mok, C. H.: Visceral larva migrans: A discussion based on a review of the literature. Clin. Pediatr. (Phila.), 7:565, 1968.
Nelson, J. D., McConnell, T. H., and Moore, D. V.: Thiabendazole therapy of visceral larva migrans: A case report. Am. J. Trop. Med. Hyg., 15:903, 1966.
Woodruff, A. W.: Toxocariasis. Br. Med. J., 3:663, 1970.

311. ANISAKIASIS

Although the full life cycle is still unknown, it appears that man is occasionally infected by the ascarid *Anisakis marina,* which has its larval stages in herrings. The adult worms develop in marine mammals such as seals, dolphins, porpoises, and whales. Man is infected by eating raw or undercooked herrings, and infection has occurred where such food is considered a delicacy, namely, northeastern Europe (Denmark particularly) and Japan. The larvae appear to burrow into the wall of the stomach or small bowel to produce an eosinophilic granulomatous mass that may be mistaken for a malignancy. Perforation of the bowel wall has been reported, as has stenosis following granuloma formation. Usually the correct diagnosis is not made until the specimen is examined after surgical resection.

Van Thiel, P. H.: The final hosts of the herring worm *Anisakis marina.* Trop. Geogr. Med., 18:310, 1966.
Yokogawa, M., and Yoshimura, H.: Clinicopathologic studies on larval anisakiasis in Japan. Am. J. Trop. Med. Hyg., 16:723, 1967.

312. TRICHURIASIS (Whipworm Infection, Trichocephaliasis)

In trichuriasis, the adult worms are shaped like a whip. The long anterior threadlike portion of the worm consists of a cellular esophagus buried deep into the submucosa of the colon, making it difficult to dislodge. These adults are pinkish-gray and are 30 to 50 mm long. The male is distinguished from the female by its coiled caudal extremity. The female produces 5000 to 10,000 eggs per day. The eggs are 50 to 55 μ long, golden brown with prominent characteristic bipolar plugs. Under favorable conditions they become infective in three to five weeks, and when ingested by man the first stage larva hatches in the small intestine and spends three to ten days in the intestinal villi. Then it passes down to the large bowel where it matures in 30 to 90 days. The adult worms live for years.

Of worldwide distribution, trichuriasis is most frequently encountered in the tropics. Often in a particular endemic locality, the infestation has a patchy distribution because of dense shade, heavy rainfall, and the clay soils that hold water as well as fecal pollution, thus facilitating transmission. In the United States, whipworm infection is found in the southern Appalachians and southwestern Louisiana; it is not infrequent in Puerto Rico.

The great majority of infections are asymptomatic; only heavy loads of worms cause clinical illness. The worms are distributed throughout the colon and rectum, and heavy infections may be associated with colic and diarrhea with blood. *Trichuris trichiura* abstracts 0.005 ml of blood per worm from the host each day. In children in precarious iron balance a load of over 800 worms may be associated with an iron deficiency anemia. Up to 5000 worms have been recovered from heavily infected children. In such infections rectal prolapse may complicate the diarrhea, and the appearance of the congested mucosa associated with the whitish bodies of the worms has been described as the "coconut cake" rectum. Early infections may be associated with a mild blood eosinophilia. Trichuris has been implicated as a predisposing factor to acute amebic dysentery by causing an initial breach of the mucosa, this suggestion being based on finding a higher incidence of Trichuris in patients with acute bowel amebiasis than is normal for the area. Trichuris is often associated with other helminthic and protozoal infections. Appendicitis and peritonitis with the presence of worms in the peritoneal cavity have been described.

Diagnosis is made by finding the eggs in the feces, either on direct smear or by concentration methods. In the rare Trichuris dysentery the eggs may appear in aggregates in the mucoid stools, together with eosinophils and Charcot-Leyden crystals. Egg counts below 10,000 per gram are unlikely to be associated with symptoms.

Treatment is not very satisfactory. Dithiazanine iodide was formerly used, but it has caused nine deaths, and has been withdrawn from the market. Treatment should be confined to heavily infected individuals presenting with symptoms and to those employed as food handlers, nurses, and so forth. Thiabendazole in a similar dose to that used in Strongyloides (25 mg per kilogram of body weight twice daily for two days) eradicates the infection in one third of cases, and the course can be repeated after one week. Mebendazole, a new broad-spectrum anthelmintic, appears to be effective. An oral dose of 100 mg twice a day for three days gave a cure rate of 64.3 per cent in one trial. It is well tolerated and has a direct ovicidal effect.

Boon, W. H., and Hoh, K. K.: Severe whipworm infection in children. Singapore Med. J., 2:34, 1966.

Franz, K. H., Schneider, W. J., and Pohlman, M. H.: Clinical trials with triabendazole against intestinal nematodes infecting humans. Am. J. Trop. Med. Hyg., 14:383, 1965.

Jung, R. C., and Jelliffe, D. B.: The clinical picture and treatment of whipworm infection. West Afr. Med. J., 1:11, 1952.

Layrisse, M., Apariedo, L., Martinez Torres, C., and Roche, M.: Blood loss due to infection with *Trichuris trichiura*. Am. J. Trop. Med. Hyg., 16:613, 1967.

Sargent, R. G., Savoury, A. M., Mina, A., and Lee, P. R.: A clinical evaluation of mebendazole in the treatment of trichuriasis. Am. J. Trop. Med. Hyg., 23:375, 1974.

Wagner, E. D., and Chavarria, A. P.: In vivo effects of a new anthelmintic, mebendazole (R 17,635), on the eggs of *Trichuris trichiura* and hookworm. Am. J. Trop. Med. Hyg., 23:151, 1974.

313. ENTEROBIASIS (Oxyuriasis, Pinworm or Seatworm Infection)

Infestation with the pinworm, *Enterobius vermicularis,* is not limited to rural communities and the poor as with many intestinal nematodes, but occurs also in urban communities. Reportedly worldwide in distribution, it appears to be much rarer in the tropics. Children are more commonly infected than adults.

The adult female worm is 8 to 13 mm long, and the male, which is rarely seen, 2 to 5 mm. Both live in the cecum and adjacent large and small bowel. The females migrate at night to the anal orifice, where they deposit their eggs. Within a few hours larvae develop in the eggs, which are then infectious and on ingestion hatch in the duodenum and migrate to the large bowel where they mature in 15 to 28 days. The ova can be transferred from the anal margin to the mouth by contamination of the hands, and ova lodge under the nails after scratching of the anal margin. The eggs also become widely disseminated in the environment, notable in bedclothes and dust samples. It has been suggested that hatching of larvae on the anal margin may result in the colon's being colonized from below as a form of autoinfection. Fortunately the eggs are relatively susceptible to drying, and in a warm dry environment survive only a few days.

Usually pinworm infestation is harmless and is often asymptomatic. Pruritus ani is the chief complaint caused by the migrating female worms. Numerous other symptoms have been described, including enuresis, irritability, and insomnia, which may result from the pruritus. Less convincing reported manifestations are abdominal pain, teeth grinding, nausea, and weight loss.

Rarely the female worm may penetrate into the mucosa of the bowel, where it has been a primary cause of appendicitis. Occasionally female worms migrate into the vagina, causing an intense vulvitis. Prostatitis is a rare complication in the male, and secondary ischiorectal abscesses may follow perianal eczema. Granulomas may form around worms that enter tissues, and such granulomas have been described in the uterus, fallopian tubes, and peritoneum, presumably associated with migration of worms up the female genital tract. A rare case not reported in the literature occurred in a mentally deficient child who developed pulmonary eosinophilic granulomas owing to massive inhalation of Enterobius eggs present in the dust of the mental institution.

The best method for finding Enterobius eggs is by means of the sealing tape (Scotch tape) swab. A piece of Scotch tape 2 inches long is folded, sticky side out, over the end of a wooden tongue depressor and pressed firmly against the perianal region. The tape is then stuck to the slide, acting as a coverslip, and the specimen is scanned for the typical eggs, which are 50 to 60 μ in length, are flattened on one side, and contain a developing embryo. The patient can be given six such swabs, and he does the examination every morning for six mornings on rising and before taking a bath. All can then be examined at the laboratory. Adult worms are rarely observed in feces or on the perianal skin, or seen with the sigmoidoscope. All members of the family should be examined in view of the frequency with which whole families are infected. The eosinophil count is rarely elevated in this infection.

Treatment with piperazine citrate, 65 mg per kilogram (maximal daily dose 2.5 grams) daily for eight days, is usually effective. Single-dose treatment is becoming more fashionable with either pyrvinium pamoate, 5 mg per kilogram (maximum, 250 mg), which can be repeated after two weeks, or thiabendazole, 25 mg per kilogram twice daily for one day, repeated seven days later. Pyrvinium pamoate (Povan) turns the stool red, and may occasionally be associated with vomiting, diarrhea, and skin rashes. The methods of transmission should be explained to the patient, and care of personal hygiene (short nails, frequent baths, and clean underclothes) instituted before treatment. Follow-up tape swabs are necessary. There is a tendency for some patients to become overanxious about this infection, occasionally with the development of a "worm neurosis." They should be strongly reassured.

Cram, E. B.: Studies on oxyuriasis, xxviii. Summary and conclusions. Am. J. Dis. Child., 65:46, 1943.

Deruiter, H., Rijpstra, A. C., and Swellengrebel, N. H.: Ectopic *Enterobius vermicularis;* variations on its pattern. Trop. Geogr. Med., 14:375, 1962.

Most, H., Gellin, G. A., Yager, R., Aron, B., Friedlander, M., and Quarfordt, S.: Enterobius (pinworm infection): A study of 951 Puerto Rican and 315 non-Puerto Rican children in New York City. Am. J. Trop. Med. Hyg., 12:65, 1963.

TISSUE NEMATODES

314. TRICHINOSIS* (Trichiniasis, Trichinellosis)

Definition and Etiology. Trichinosis is a self-limited infection of the intestine (by the adult parasite) and of the striated muscle (by the larvae) produced by a small nematode, *Trichinella spiralis.* The same animal host

*The present chapter is based on the article on trichinosis prepared by Dr. Harold W. Brown for the twelfth edition of this book. Little new clinical information has developed in the interval; what has appeared has been incorporated in the basic article. P.D.M.

thus acts as both the final and the intermediate host, harboring the adults temporarily and the encysted larvae for long periods. When infected meat containing larvae is ingested, these larvae are released into the upper small intestine by the action of digestive juices. They become adult in five to seven days, the males and females mate, and the fertile female begins to deposit larvae into the mucosa. These larvae pass into the circulation through the hepatic and pulmonary filters, and are carried to all parts of the body. They burrow into the muscles and encyst and complete their development in striated muscle. In other tissues such as the myocardium, brain, and eye, the larvae disintegrate and are absorbed. Among the muscles heavily parasitized are the diaphragmatic, masseteric, intercostal, laryngeal, extraocular, nuchal, pectoral, deltoid, gluteus, biceps, and gastrocnemius. A total of 1500 larvae are liberated by each female worm, usually in four to eight weeks but up to 16 weeks, after which the females die.

Larvae attain a size of 0.4 by 0.025 mm in a cyst in the muscle by the thirty-fifth day. The capsule is complete in three months, and calcification occurs within six months to two years. Recent evidence suggests that there may be strain differences in relation to host susceptibility. The parasite is chiefly found in man, hogs, rats, bears, foxes, walruses, dogs, and cats, but any carnivorous or omnivorous animal may be infected.

Epidemiology. Generally of worldwide distribution, the parasite has not been reported from the islands of the Pacific or Australia. It occurs more frequently in the Northern Hemisphere than in the tropics. It is common in Europe and the United States. Fatal cases have recently been described from Kenya and Chile. It is rare east of the Suez Canal. In the United States there has been a marked reduction in the incidence of the infection, owing to laws requiring the cooking of garbage fed to hogs, storage of meat at low temperature, and education of the public resulting in thorough cooking of pork.

Until quite recently, trichinosis was relatively common in New York City, as pork was being obtained from garbage-fed hogs in New Jersey. However, hog-rearing in this way has substantially declined. Pigs become infected by eating infected meat and occasionally infected rats. Rats are infected in the same way. One of the main methods of transmission is in sausages, wursts, or hamburgers in which the beef is diluted (or actually contaminated in mechanical grinders) with a little pork. Infections from bear and walrus meat have been reported. The low incidence in the tropics is probably due to the fact that meat of any kind is a luxury to many people. Hindus, Jews, and Moslems eschew pork, and the Chinese cook it very well.

Pathology and Pathogenesis. Three to four days after invasion of the muscle, the fiber becomes edematous, loses its cross striations, and undergoes basophilic degeneration. The nuclei increase in number and size, and there is interstitial inflammation around the muscle with a chronic inflammatory cell infiltrate. The severity of the disease depends on the adult worm load, the age of the patient, and the degree of host resistance as well as the numbers of organs involved.

In the heart a focal interstitial myocarditis may occur. Acute nonsuppurative meningitis may be associated with larvae in the cerebrospinal fluid. Larvae may cause lesions in the choroid and retina. Catarrhal enteritis, pulmonary edema, and bronchopneumonia may occur in the early stages of the disease.

Clinical Manifestations. The cardinal features of trichinosis are fever, orbital edema, myalgia, and eosinophilia. Only a small percentage of infected patients have sufficient parasites, however, to produce such clinically recognizable disease. The clinical picture can be divided into distinct stages in a symptomatic infection. First, there is the stage of adult maturation during the first weeks after infection associated with transient gastrointestinal symptoms. From the seventh to the fourteenth day larviposition begins, and muscle penetration commences. This is usually associated with an irregular persistent fever (37.8 to 40.5° C), urticarial rash, and occasionally respiratory symptoms in the form of cough and bronchospasm. Muscle pains become prominent and unusual, but the characteristic physical signs are bilateral orbital edema and subungual and subconjunctival hemorrhages. A severe infection may result in death four to eight weeks after infection from toxemia, secondary pneumonia, myocardial failure, or trichinous encephalitis. Severe muscle involvement may render breathing, masticating, swallowing, or locomotion painful. An eosinophilia beginning seven days after the infection may rise to very high levels (70 per cent) and persist for months. Serum transaminases are also elevated in the invasive stage.

Diagnosis and Differential Diagnosis. Although the rising eosinophilia together with a suggestive clinical picture leads one to suspect this diagnosis, it is proved by finding the larvae in a muscle biopsy. This should be done in the fourth week of infection when a small piece of muscle is removed from the deltoid or gastrocnemius. Crushed between two microscope slides and examined under the low-power objective of the microscope, the living coiled larvae can be seen. In light infections when the direct examination is negative, the biopsy specimen can be incubated overnight in an acid-pepsin mixture and the centrifuged deposit examined for larvae.

Calcified cyst and calcified larvae represent older infections, as calcification usually takes 18 months, but the larva may live inside the calcified cyst for many years. Calcified cysts appear as tiny white spots in fresh muscle, but are too small to be detected radiologically.

A variety of serologic tests are available. The bentonite flocculation test is as sensitive as the complement-fixation test and much easier to perform. It is usually positive four weeks after infection, but may be present earlier. A change from a negative to a positive test during the illness is significant. The indirect fluorescent antibody test detects some infections at an earlier stage. Few other parasitic infections are associated with such persistent fever or generalized muscular aches and tender muscles. Polymyositis of nonparasitic cause may present like this and be associated with eosinophilia. Periarteritis nodosa may also mimic trichinosis.

Treatment. Patients with symptomatic trichinosis should be confined to bed and given a smooth high-calorie, high-protein diet. Congestive cardiac failure should be searched for and, if present, should be treated. Mild analgesics can be given for the muscle pain. Anti-inflammatory steroids (prednisolone, 5 mg three times daily) relieve fever, edema, and muscle pain in severe acute cases but are said not to affect the adult worms' fecundity or the number of larvae settling in the muscle. In patients with central nervous system involvement this effect of steroids is dramatic.

Thiabendazole, in a dose of 25 mg per kilogram of body weight for five to seven days, has also produced a marked resolution of the symptoms of fever and muscle pain, but living larvae have still been recovered on muscle biopsy after much larger courses of the drug. In severe infections the use of corticosteroids and thiabendazole may be lifesaving, but when the parasite load is not considerable, the prognosis is good even without treatment.

Prevention. The ultimate prevention of trichinosis is dependent on its elimination in hogs, and the incidence in these animals can be greatly reduced by heat-sterilizing garbage. Freezing meat at −32° C for a few hours (or at 15 to 30° C for several weeks) kills larvae, as does gamma radiation of the meat. Pigs fed on a diet containing 0.1 per cent thiabendazole fail to incubate *T. spiralis* on challenge. Routine meat inspection does not detect the infection, and serologic and skin tests on pigs have not been helpful in detecting infected animals. The chief safeguard at present is the thorough cooking of pork at 60° C for 30 minutes for each pound of meat.

Gould, S. E.: Trichinosis. Springfield, Ill., Charles C Thomas, 1945.
Hennekeuser, M. H., Pabst, K., Poeplau, W., and Gerok, W.: Thiabendazole for the treatment of trichinosis in humans. Tex. Rep. Biol. Med., 27 (Supplement 2):581, 1969.
Maynard, J. E., and Kagan, I. G.: Trichinosis (serology). Practitioner, 191:622, 1963.
Moser, R. H.: Trichinosis from Bismarck to polar bears. J.A.M.A., 228: 735, 1974.
Proceedings of the International Commission in Trichinellosis: No. VI. Wiad. Parazyt., 14:127, 1968.
Zimmerman, W. J., Steele, J. H., and Kagan, I. G.: The changing status of trichiniasis in the U.S. population. Public Health Rep., 83:957, 1968.

315. ANGIOSTRONGYLIASIS

Angiostrongylus Cantonensis. Eosinophilic meningoencephalitis, a syndrome caused by *Angiostrongylus cantonensis* (the rat lung worm), was first recognized in New Caledonia in 1950, and has since been reported from Hawaii, Tahiti, other Pacific Islands, Indonesia, and Thailand. The human disease has only been reported from the Far East and the Pacific to date, although infected rats have been found in Madagascar, Mauritius, Ceylon, and Sarawak.

The life cycle was described by workers in Australia in 1955 before the importance of the worm as a human pathogen was known. A delicate filiform nematode, 17 to 25 mm in length, the adult lives in the lungs of rats, and the eggs are coughed up, swallowed, and pass out in the feces as first-stage larvae. Further development occurs in slugs and snails to the third-stage infective larvae. These larvae are ingested by man either while in this intermediate host or after they have been shed by it onto some other article of food, e.g., lettuce. Crabs and freshwater prawns have also been found to be infected with these metastrongyloid larvae, but probably act as paratenic hosts. The dispersal of the giant African land snail *Achatina fulica* may have assisted the spread of the infection. When infective larvae are ingested by the rat, they migrate to the brain and reach young adulthood in four weeks. They then migrate to the pulmonary arteries and after two more weeks start laying eggs. Unfortunately if man accidentally ingests these infective larvae, they migrate to the brain (as in the rat), and there produce the clinical picture of a meningoencephalitis associated with fever, signs of cerebral irritation, mental deficit, and varying degrees of loss of consciousness. Mild blood eosinophilia is present, and lumbar puncture reveals a fluid under increased pressure with increased protein and many eosinophils (from 100 to 3000 per cubic millimeter). Occasionally patients present with a facial nerve lesion or complaints of diplopia and parasthesia. A complement-fixation test using an extract of adult worms as antigen has been developed. The illness usually persists for some weeks or months and then the patient recovers spontaneously.

Young adult worms have been found in the brain and cerebrospinal fluid of man, and experimental infection of monkeys produces a similar syndrome. The pathology of the brain in fatal cases is one of focal areas of softening, the meninges and subarachnoid space being infiltrated with plasma cells, lymphocytes, eosinophils, and neutrophils. There is perivascular cuffing with chronic inflammatory cells in the brain substance. Careful sectioning of the brain is necessary to find the 0.16 to 8 mm nematodes.

This condition must be differentiated from a variety of other parasitic infections involving the central nervous system. In Thailand cerebral gnathostomiasis and Angiostrongylus infections occur. Cerebral paragonimiasis could be an important differential diagnosis in parts of the Far East. In other situations the syndrome of eosinophilic meningitis could be produced by cysticercosis, hydatid, schistosomiasis, fascioliasis, trichinosis, and possibly strongyloidiasis. Refinements of serologic diagnostic techniques will help in this sometimes difficult clinical problem.

The author has been able to trace no references to treatment with thiabendazole, although this would seem to be the drug to try. Prevention entails education regarding dangerous foods such as raw crabs and prawns and undercooked snails, and making sure that lettuce is free of slugs and snails. Freezing of crustaceans and molluscs at −15° C for 12 hours has been found to be effective in destroying the infective larvae of *A. cantonensis.*

Angiostrongylus Costaricensis. Human disease caused by this parasite has recently been described from Costa Rica where 130 cases have been studied. The worm also occurs in Honduras and Panama. Patients, usually children, present with right iliac fossa pain, fever, and blood eosinophilia, and often an abdominal mass is palpable. At operation an eosinophilic granulomatous cecal pseudotumor is found to contain adult worms and eggs.

The intermediate host is a slug, *Vaginulus (Sarasinula) plebius,* and the definitive hosts are at least five species of rodents, including *Rattus rattus.* Infected slugs contaminate lettuce leaves with infective third-stage larvae, and man acquires the disease by ingesting the slug itself on contaminated salad. In the rodent host—and probably in man—the cycle occurs in the abdominal cavity. The third and fourth larval molts occur in lymph vessels. After three months the young adults move to radicles of the mesenteric arteries, mate, mature, and oviposit. Arteritis and thrombosis may be followed by macro- or microinfarcts of the gut, with ulceration and necrosis of the gut wall. Fistulization or generalized peritonitis may ensue. Neither larvae nor eggs are usually detected in the stools of man.

In *Angiostrongylus costaricensis* infection of man, sexually mature adult worms develop, and as such this species is better adapted to man than *Angiostrongylus cantonensis.*

Alicata, J. E.: Present status of *Angiostrongylus cantonensis* infection in man and animals in the tropics. J. Trop. Med. Hyg., 72:53, 1969.
Mackerras, M. T., and Sanders, D. F.: The life history of the rat lungworm *Angiostrongylus cantonensis* (Chen) (Nematoda; Metastrongylidae). Aust. J. Zool., 3:1, 1955.

Morera, P.: Life cycle and redescription of *Angiostrongylus costaricensis* (Morera and Cespedes 1971). Am. J. Trop. Med. Hyg., 22:613, 1973.
Schollhaminer, G., Aubry, P., and Rigaud, J. L.: Quelques réflexions sur la méningite à éosinophiles a Tahiti. Étude clinique et biologique de 165 observations, à propos d'un cas atypique. Bull. Soc. Pathol. Exot., 59:341, 1966.

316. FILARIASIS

GENERAL CONSIDERATIONS

To talk of filariasis as such is to use a general term like anemia, for there are seven types of nematodes found in man belonging to the superfamily Filarioidea, as well as one member of the superfamily Dracunculoidea (the guinea worm), which is usually included in a consideration of this group. Of these Filarioidea, the embryos or microfilariae are found in the blood in five and in the subcutaneous tissues in two species. The adults are viviparous, and the blood microfilariae demonstrate a periodicity in the peripheral blood, depending on the species. They may remain ensheathed in their elongated egg shell or have no sheath. These microfilariae are distinguished on their criteria as well on as the pattern of distribution of nuclei seen in stained specimens in their tails. Giemsa stain can be used, but better results of sheath staining are obtained with Delafield's hematoxylin or Mayer's acid hemalum.

In Table 2 the various species are listed and the characteristics of their microfilariae are shown. The adult worms live for many years, whereas blood microfilariae have a life of three to six months. After being bitten by an infected arthropod it may take 1 year to 18 months before microfilariae are present in the peripheral blood, a long prepatent period. The controlling mechanism for periodicity has never been satisfactorily explained for many of these human species. However, Hawking's recent work suggests that at least two circadian rhythms are involved, one mechanism within the microfilariae themselves, and the other some physiological tide in the host (body temperature for certain animal species). This periodicity fits the habits of the insect vector; for instance, the Loa insect vector flies by day, but most bancrofti infections are transmitted nocturnally. The geographic distribution of these species is of particular importance, because in some it is markedly restricted. For instance *Loa loa* is a filarid of Equatorial Africa, and *Mansonella ozzardi* is only found in South America.

Not all the species listed are significantly pathogenic. Few symptoms have been ascribed to *Mansonella ozzardi* infections, and the case for the pathogenicity of *D. perstans* is very shaky. Two of these filarial infections are notable in terms of their importance in man. These are the *Wuchereria-Brugia complex,* which produces bancroftian filariasis with lymphatic obstruction and elephantiasis, and *onchocerciasis,* which is a common cause of blindness in endemic areas. Multiple infections occur, in endemic areas, for instance, in parts of West Africa a patient may be seen infected with *Loa loa,* bancrofti, perstans, and onchocerciasis.

This final group of the most modified nematodes will be considered in the order in which they are listed in Table 2, except that the guinea worm will be considered first. Dirofilariasis and pulmonary tropical eosinophilia will then be reviewed.

Hawking, F.: Advances in filariasis. Trans. R. Soc. Trop. Med. Hyg., 59:9, 1965.
Hawking, F., Moore, P., Gammage, K., and Worms, M. J.: Periodicity of microfiliae. XII. The effect of variations in host body temperature on the cycle of *Loa loa, Monnigofilaria setariosa. Durofilaria immitis,* and other filariae. Trans. R. Soc. Trop. Med. Hyg., 61:674, 1967.

DRACONTIASIS
(Guinea Worm)

Infection with the guinea worm (*Dracunculus medinensis*) usually presents as a skin ulceration at the site of emergence of the female adult worm. Man is probably the only reservoir, although monkeys and dogs can be experimentally infected. Human infections are widespread in the tropics, occurring in local distribution in West Africa and the Nile Valley, the Middle East, India and Pakistan, the Caribbean Islands, Guyana, and Brazil. Infection occurs on ingesting infected water fleas (Cyclops) present in drinking water from shallow wells or ponds. The infective larvae in the Cyclops penetrate the intestinal walls and mature in the loose connective tissue under the skin, especially that of legs and feet. The male worm is small and dies after copulation. The female requires a year to become gravid, and then measures up to a meter long and is 2 mm in diameter. When ready to discharge larvae, she approaches the skin surface, and a blister is produced by secretion of a toxic substance from the anterior end of the worm. The blister breaks down to form an ulcer a few centimeters across, and the anterior end of the worm protrudes into this ulcer. On contact with water the head of the worm ruptures, and the uterus periodically discharges the tightly coiled larvae infective to the water flea. Secondary infec-

TABLE 2. Common Filarioidea of Man as Distinguished by Characteristics of Microfilariae

	Periodicity of Microfilariae	Sheathed or Unsheathed	Tail Morphology
Microfilariae in blood:			
Wuchereria bancrofti	Majority nocturnal	Sheathed	Nuclei not to tip of tail
Brugia malayi	Majority nocturnal	Sheathed	Two distinct nuclei in tail tip
Loa loa	Diurnal	Sheathed	Nuclei to tip of tail
Mansonella ozzardi	Nonperiodic	Not sheathed	Nuclei not to tip of tail
Dipetalonema perstans	Nocturnally subperiodic	Not sheathed	Nuclei to tip of tail
Microfilariae in subcutaneous tissues:			
Onchocerca volvulus	Nonperiodic	Not sheathed	Nuclei not to tip of tail
Dipetalonema streptocerca	Nonperiodic	Not sheathed	Nuclei to tip of tail, which is crooked

tion of the ulcer with resultant cellulitis is common. Generalized allergic symptoms may occur prior to the blister formation or when surgical removal of the worm is attempted. Multiple infections are common. The lesion is usually on the lower leg, but may occur on the genitalia, buttocks, or upper limbs. In water carriers lesions have been observed on the back, suggesting that the worm is positively hydrotropic. Alternatively, the mature female may never reach the surface of the body and may be absorbed or calcify in the tissue. The radiologic appearance is pathognomonic because the worm is so large. If a gravid worm dies in situ or is broken during extraction, cellulitis and secondary infection often occur. This may give rise to contractures. Also *Clostridium tetani* may contaminate the wound and tetanus may result. Rarely the adult worm involves serous cavities, the extradural space, or joints. Guinea worm arthritis appears to be due to the presence of the adult worm or larvae in the joint. A microscopic diagnosis can be made by finding embryos in the exudate from the guinea worm ulcer after exposure to a few drops of water.

Gradually winding the worm out of the ulcer by turning it on a stick a few centimeters a day is still common practice. Surgical extraction is also practiced. Recently niridazole (Ambilhar) has been reported to be lethal to the adult worm, which can readily be withdrawn after a course of 25 mg per kilogram of body weight for seven days. Thiabendazole is also effective. Prevention involves contructing water sources that cannot be contaminated and killing cyclops by chlorination or boiling water to be used for drinking.

Muller, R.: Dracunculus and dracunculiasis. *In* Dawes, B. (ed.): Advances in Parasitology, Vol. 9, New York, Academic Press, 1973, p. 73.
Raffier, G.: Efficacy of thiabendazole in the treatment of dracunculiasis. Texas Rep. Biol. Med., 27(Supplement 2):601, 1969.

BANCROFTIAN FILARIASIS

Etiology. Bancroftian filariasis is caused by the filarial worm *Wuchereria bancrofti.* The adult worms reside in the lymphatic system and produce recurrent lymphangitis with fibrosis and obstruction. The infection is transmitted by culicine and anopheline mosquitoes.

The threadlike adult worms are 4 to 10 cm long and live for decades. The female worm is viviparous, producing microfilariae 130 to 320 μ long which are found in the peripheral blood; in some forms this occurs only at night, whereas during the day the microfilariae are in the lungs. If ingested by a suitable mosquito, these microfilariae develop in the thoracic muscles of the insect and are present in the mouth parts after two weeks. They enter the skin through the puncture wound when the mosquito next feeds, and, finding their way to the lymphatics of the host, the males and females mate and mature. More than a year after infection microfilariae appear in the peripheral blood.

Epidemiology. Man is the only definitive host of this common type of filariasis. Periodic bancroftian filariasis is found throughout tropical Africa and North Africa, as well as in the tropical coastal borders of Asia and Queensland. It is endemic in the West Indies and the northern countries of South America. In the northern Pacific bancroftian filariasis exhibits nocturnal periodicity, but in the Pacific Islands east of 160 degrees of longitude (including New Caledonia, Fiji, Samoa, the Ellis and Cook Islands, Society Islands, and the Marquesas) the microfilariae are nonperiodic, being present in the peripheral blood throughout the 24-hour period. The term *W. bancrofti var. pacifica* has been applied to this strain.

Pathology. The severity of the lesions probably depends on the adult worm load and their site of development and the susceptibility of the host. Light infections are often asymptomatic, and microfilariae are detected on incidental blood examinations. Maturing adults in the lymphatics are associated with endothelial thickening, fibrin deposition, and infiltration with eosinophils, histiocytes, and lymphocytes. Giant cells occur. Fibrotic and inflammatory changes tend to obstruct the lymphatics, and this process is exacerbated by death of the worms, which may calcify. There is reactive hyperplasia in the lymph nodes, and small granulomas are seen. An eosinophilic endophlebitis of the small veins is present in the lymph nodes. The testicles and epididymis often show similar changes with evidence of chronic inflammation. Worms may not be present at the site of inflammation. Secretions of the worm, especially after molting, are thought to be responsible for some of these changes. As lymphatic obstruction becomes more extensive, chronic edema develops in the infected areas. Recently lymphedema has been produced in laboratory animals with longstanding bancrofti infections.

Clinical Manifestations. Attacks of fever, headache, and lymphadenopathy sometimes associated with urticarial rashes are known as filarial fever and occur in the acute phase of the disease. Often, however, no history of this early phase can be obtained. Epididymitis may occur as a lone lesion. Lymphatics most affected are those of the inguinal region, upper arms, and spermatic cord. Chronic lymphadenopathy is often the only sign of infection for years. Retrograde lymphangitis may be noted. In a small proportion of infected individuals, with increasing lymphatic obstruction over the years, all degrees of chronic edema occur, affecting especially the lower limbs and scrotum. Initially the edema is pitting, but as organization of collagen occurs in the edematous subcutaneous tissues, it becomes nonpitting. Eventually the giant limbs of elephantiasis are produced. The skin over the affected part, at first smooth, later becomes scaly and is fissured at the points where the fascia is attached to the skin. Hyperkeratosis produces warts and nodules. Varicose nodes in the groin are the result of lymphatic dilatation and may lead to scrotal lymphedema. Infection may supervene in any of these lesions with formation of a chronic discharging sinus. Chronic inflammatory disease of the testicle and epididymis with or without hydrocele occurs.

Chyluria may be renal or vesical in origin, depending on the level at which the lymph varix communicates with the urinary tract. Cystoscopy and intravenous or retrograde pyelography help to establish the site of communication.

Diagnosis. In the early stages and when lymphadenopathy only is present, microfilariae are usually present in night blood films. Although the motile microfilariae are easily seen in fresh films, staining is necessary for identification. Microfilariae may be absent in the late stage; thus only 4 per cent of patients with elephantiasis and 30 per cent of patients with hydrocele had microfilariae in one series. Concentration techniques are available for microfilariae, and they may be found in the chylous urine or hydrocele fluid. Eosinophilia is not a constant finding. The filarial complement-fixation test and skin test, although only group specific, are useful in suggesting a filarial cause for a lymphedema. Lymphangiograms reveal the extent of the lymphatic obstruction and may be a useful preoperative measure. It is rarely justified to remove an enlarged lymph node to find the adults because this still further prejudices the lymphatic circulation. In an endemic area surgeons frequently encounter adult worms when operating on the groin.

The differential diagnosis depends on the type of clinical syndrome. Lymphadenopathy caused by other infections and neoplasms must be considered. Elephantiasis may be associated with congenital defects of the lymphatic drainage as well as tuberculous inguinal lymphadenitis. Tuberculosis, *Schistosoma haematobium,* and gonorrhea produce epididymitis, and relatively few hydroceles are filarial. Lymphatic obstruction caused by many other agents may produce lymphedema and chyluria.

Treatment. Diethylcarbamazine (Banocide, Hetrazan) is believed to kill a large proportion of adults as well as microfilariae. A dose of 3 mg per kilogram of body weight is given, rising to a maximum of 12 mg per kilogram over four days. This dose is then given daily for 14 days. Reactions are mild in comparison with those seen in onchocerciasis, but fever, nausea and vomiting, and skin rashes may occur as with any drug. The arsenical Mel W and the antimonial Astiban (sodium dimercaptosuccinate) kill adult filariae, but are too toxic for general use. All patients with microfilaremia should receive an adequate course of treatment.

The management of lymphedema depends on its severity. Mild degrees are best treated with elevation of the foot of the bed and an elastic stocking. Careful instructions regarding foot care should be given, as ascending streptocccal cellulitis is common in the edematous tissues and further prejudices the lymphatic circulation. Some workers believe the Streptococcus to be more important in producing lymphangitis than the worms themselves. Any foot sepsis requires early and vigorous treatment with antimicrobial drugs. Tinea infections should be eradicated. Banocide therapy is often given in elephantiasis on the ground that it may prevent further lymphatic damage, but clinical improvement is seldom observed.

A variety of surgical operations have been devised to remove the edematous subcutaneous tissue from the leg, scrotum, and breasts. Success depends on the type of operation and the skill of the surgeon. In scrotal elephantiasis care must be taken to preserve the testicles. Hydroceles can be treated by the injection of sclerosing agents. Chyluria of bladder origin can be terminated by fulgurating the leaking bladder lymphatics. Renal chyluria is best left alone, although in the past kidneys have been wrapped in cellophane with the subsequent production of renal hypertension.

Prevention. Diethylcarbamazine, 3 mg per kilogram per month for 12 to 18 months, has been effective in mass treatment for preventive purposes. Residual DDT or dieldrin is effective against many of the mosquito vectors, and systematic destruction of mosquito-breeding sites has also met with success. Biologic control of mosquito vectors is receiving intensive field trials, but thus far they have not resulted in methods for mass application.

MALAYAN FILARIASIS

A disease similar to bancroftian filariasis is produced by a closely related filarial worm, *Brugia malayi.* The sheathed microfilariae of this species have two distinct caudal nuclei. Transmitted by mansonoides mosquitoes, it is the only filarial infection of man in Malaya and Borneo, whereas in India, Ceylon, and tropical China it coexists with *W. bancrofti. Brugia malayi* is responsible for only mild lymphedema in man, usually below the knee, with enlargement of the popliteal and femoral nodes. In contrast to bancroftian filariasis, the microfilaremia rates in the Malayan form are quite high in children younger than five years. In this infection, also, there are two types of organisms, one with nocturnal periodicity, and another subperiodic form. The latter is found in many animals (primates, carnivores, and rodents) and is a true zoonosis.

Galindo, L., Von Lichtenberg, F., and Baldison, C.: Bancroftian filariasis in Puerto Rico: Infection pattern and tissue lesions. Am. J. Trop. Med., 11:739, 1962.

Nelson, G. S.: The pathology of filarial infections. Helminth. Abst., 35:Pt. 4, 311, 1966.

Schacher, J. F., and Sahyoun, P. F.: A chronological study of the histopathology of filarial disease in cats and dogs caused by *Brugia phangi* (Buckley and Edeson, 1956). Trans. R. Soc. Trop. Med. Hyg., 61:234, 1967.

Turner, L. H.: Studies on filariasis in Malaya: the clinical features of filariasis due to *Wuchereria malayi.* Trans. R. Soc. Trop. Med. Hyg., 53:154, 1959.

Wilson, T.: Filariasis in Malaya—A general review. Trans. R. Soc. Trop. Med. Hyg., 55:107, 1961.

LOIASIS

Loa loa infection is characterized by the appearance of transient swellings mainly on the limbs; these are thought to be the site of the migrating adult worms in the subcutaneous tissue. Occasionally a worm will traverse the conjunctiva of the eye.

The male adult worm is 30 mm long and the female 70 mm. They live for many years, and gain access to the body through the proboscis of biting flies (deer flies of the genus Chrysops). These worms appear to be in a state of continuous migration in the subcutaneous tissues of the body. It is not clearly understood how the sexes locate each other, but they meet and mate, and the female produces microfilariae that appear in the blood during the day and are infective to the insect vector.

Man is the only reservoir host, with the possible exception of monkeys. Human loiasis is restricted to Africa, mainly the West Coast. It occurs from Sierra Leone to the Cameroons and extends into the heart of Africa in the region of the Congo basin.

Clinical Manifestations. The main clinical manifestation is the repeated occurrence of hot erythematous swellings (5 to 10 cm or more) called Calabar swellings after the endemic area of Calabar. These occur in the upper limbs particularly, are painful, and subside in a few days. They are associated with the presence of an adult worm. A similar swelling occurs around the eye when the adult worm crosses the eye beneath the conjunctivae. The patient notices the worm in his line of vision ("like a submarine, doctor") and it is worth inquiring for such a history. Calabar swellings seem to occur more frequently in the extremities. Why this is so is not known. Routine roentgenography in endemic areas often reveals calcified dead worms lying between the metacarpals. Rarely, neurologic symptoms may be associated with the infection if the Calabar swelling involves a peripheral nerve. Also the parasite has been found in the cerebrospinal fluid associated with a meningoencephalitis.

Diagnosis. The initial diagnosis is usually based on a history of Calabar swellings in a patient coming from an endemic area. Examination of the daytime blood reveals sheathed microfilariae with a characteristic distribution of caudal nuclei. In early loiasis, microfilariae may not be detected even by concentration techniques. Very high eosinophil counts are encountered at this stage (50 to 70 per cent). A positive filarial complement-fixation test is usually present. Occasionally the adult worm can be extracted as it crosses the eye. It has been suggested that another human filarid, *Acanthocheilonema perstans*, may cause Calabar swellings.

Treatment. Diethylcarbamazine (Hetrazan) kills both adults and microfilariae. One course of 12 mg per kilogram of body weight for 14 days is all that is necessary. Reactions are rare.

Woodruff, A. W.: Loiasis. *In* Fairley, N. H., Woodruff, A. W., and Walters, J. H. (eds.): Recent Advances in Tropical Medicine. London, J. & A. Churchill, Ltd., 1961, pp. 178–194.

MANSONELLA OZZARDI

Mansonella ozzardi is found only in the New World, occurring in South America and certain foci in the Caribbean. The adult worms are embedded in visceral adipose tissue. Although they are usually regarded as nonpathogenic, fever, headache, lymphadenitis, and erythematous irritant skin rashes have been reported in association with their presence. Cold extremities, the result of peripheral vasoconstriction caused by a postulated filarial toxin, have been reported. The microfilariae show no particular periodicity and are about twice the size of perstans and have a different caudal morphology. *Simulium amazonicum* has been implicated as the vector, and midges of the genus Culicoides have also been suggested. A recent survey, cited below, showed that of 810 Colombian Indians, 96.2 per cent harbored microfilariae of *Mansonella ozzardi.*

Marinkelle, C. J., and German, E.: Mansonelliasis in the Comisaría del Vaupes of Colombia. Trop. Geog. Med., 22:101, 1970.
Undiano, C.: Importance and present-day concepts of the pathogenicity of Mansonella infections. Fev. Fac. Cienc. Med. Univ. Cordoba, 24:183, 1966.

DIPETALONEMA PERSTANS

Filariasis caused by *Dipetalonema perstans* has an extensive distribution in Equatorial Africa, the Caribbean, and South America, where it sometimes overlaps with *Mansonella ozzardi.* The adult worms are found in association with the serous cavities of the body, usually behind the limiting membrane. They may be seen at postmortem examination moving behind the peritoneum or pleura. The small (100 μ) unsheathed microfilariae are found in the blood throughout the 24 hours, but there is a peak in the peripheral blood population at night. A Culicoides species, a small black midge, is responsible for transmission.

The vast majority of patients exhibiting microfilaremia have no symptoms, but there have been recent reports of clinical symptoms associated with this infection. These reports include fever, Calabar swellings, arthritis, and upper abdominal pain associated with hepatomegaly. A high eosinophilia is often present in cases with scanty embryos, and such a finding in a patient from an endemic area should prompt a careful search for these. Diethylcarbamazine (Hetrazan) has little effect on the adults or on the microfilariae.

Wiseman, R. A.: *Acanthocheilonema perstans:* A cause of significant eosinophilia in the tropics. Comments on its pathogenicity. Trans. R. Soc. Trop. Med. Hyg., 61:667, 1967.

ONCHOCERCIASIS
(River Blindness)

River blindness is a form of cutaneous filariasis caused by infection with *Onchocerca volvulus* and is characterized by skin irritation, corneal opacities, and skin nodules.

Etiology. The threadlike adult worms lie tangled together in fibrous nodules in the subcutaneous tissues or fascial planes. Microfilariae produced by the females become widely distributed in the surrounding skin. Female black flies (buffalo gnats) of the genus Simulium ingest these larvae while taking a blood meal. After development in the fly for one week, the larvae are infective for man and are deposited when the fly next bites. They take more than a year to mature, mate, and produce microfilariae. Adult worms live 7 to 15 years.

Epidemiology. Human onchocerciasis is found on the West Coast of Africa from Sierra Leone to the Congo and in the east from the Sudan to Nyasaland. It also occurs in Guatemala, Mexico, Eastern Venezuela, Northern Brazil, and Surinam. Simulium larvae and pupae are usually found in rapidly running highly oxygenated water. Small insects (3 mm long), the flies bite low on the legs in Africa, but more around the head in Central America, which may account for the high incidence of nodules on the head in the latter locality. In East Africa *Simulium naevi* larvae and pupae evaded detection for many years until they were found on the shells of freshwater crabs.

Pathogenesis and Pathology. An initial inflammatory reaction around the adult worm is followed by a foreign body granulomatous reaction and fibrous capsule formation. The nodules are literally the graveyards of the adult worms, for these eventually die and degenerate, sometimes with secondary abscess formation. The microfilariae in the surrounding subcutaneous tissues produce a low-grade inflammatory reaction with lymphocytes, plasma cells, and eosinophils. Thickening of the epidermis and dermis owing to fibrosis eventually occurs, with destruction of elastic fibers and sometimes reduction in pigmentation.

Microfilariae migrate into the tissues of the eye to produce important inflammatory lesions which may result in blindness. Punctate keratitis is associated with death of microfilariae in the cornea, and such multiple corneal opacities may result in permanent corneal scarring. A low-grade iritis and iridocyclitis result in pupillary distortion and even occlusion. Choroidoretinitis also occurs.

Clinical Manifestations. Any patient who has a persistent irritating skin rash or visual disturbances and has been in one of the endemic areas may have onchocerciasis. More rarely, the presenting complaint takes the form of deep-seated muscular pains. The early skin lesions consist of an erythematous papular irritant rash. In heavy infections definite thickening and hyperkeratosis of the skin occurs (craw-craw or crocodile skin). Rarer late complications are depigmentation and pendulous bags in the groins containing sclerosed lymph nodes.

Nodules vary much in size from a few centimeters to as big as a tennis ball. They are frequently detected over bony prominences such as the greater trochanter, the iliac crest, the olecranons, ribs, and occiput. Often the adult worms are located deep in the fascial planes, and no nodules are palpable. To detect the small milky dots of punctate keratitis near the limbus the eyes should be examined with a strong pencil torch, the beam directed obliquely across the cornea. Signs of iritis may be present. With a slit lamp, microfilariae may be visible in the aqueous humor. Funduscopic examination may reveal the much rarer posterior segment lesion.

Diagnosis. Skin shavings are used to demonstrate microfilariae. Thin sections of the superficial skin are removed with a razor blade, mounted in saline, teased out, and examined. Many motile microfilariae emerge from those snips within an hour after they have been made. Blood contamination can be avoided if the shavings are superficial, and this is important if there is a coexistent blood microfilaremia. If there is a definite site of skin irritation, shavings should be taken from this area. In lightly infected patients multiple shavings may be necessary to detect microfilariae, and quite often they are not found. The reaction to a test dose of 50 mg of diethylcarbamazine (Mazzotti's test) in the form of an exacerbation of the itching rash is suggestive, as are an eosinophilia and a positive filarial complement-fixation test. In up to 35 per cent of cases microfilariae can be found in the urine.

Scabies and superficial mycoses are the most common irritant skin rashes of the tropics and are important differential diagnoses. Streptocerciasis caused by infection with the rare, closely related filarid *Acanthocheilonema streptocerca* also presents as an irritating rash and requires only mention. Although an infection with no mortality, the recurrent irritation of onchocerciasis can be most distressing. Severe ocular lesions may induce total blindness, and this is the blinding filarid.

Treatment. When practicable, all nodules should be excised; this simple measure will reduce the load of adult worms. Suramin is effective in killing adult worms. The side effects and method of administration of this drug are mentioned under African Trypanosomiasis (Ch. 272). A suitable course for onchocerciasis is 1 gram weekly for six weeks. As the drug is nephrotoxic, treatment should be stopped if more than 30 mg per 100 ml of protein appears in the urine.

Diethylcarbamazine is effective in killing microfilariae but does not kill the adult worms. In sensitized individuals, reactions occur when the microfilariae die in the tissues. Skin irritation becomes more intense, and there may be edema of the skin with fever, headache, and malaise. More serious is acute inflammation of the eye which may prejudice sight. As these reactions are dose related, it is usual to start therapy with a small dose of the drug (0.5 mg per kilogram) and increase gradually to the doses recommended in the previous article. Eye reactions can be controlled with 1 per cent cortisone acetate eye drops and the general reactions controlled with antihistamines and, in severe cases, with systemic steroids.

Prevention. Simulium larvae and pupae are very sensitive to small concentrations of DDT in the river water (less than 1 part per million), and this has been the most effective form of control of the insect vector. Personal prophylaxis is possible to a limited extent by avoiding places where biting Simulium are numerous.

Buck, A. A. (ed.): Onchocerciasis. Symptomatology, Pathology, and Diagnosis. Geneva, World Health Organization, 1974.
Duke, B. O. L.: Onchocerciasis. Br. Med. J., 4:301, 1968.
Nelson, D. S.: Onchocerciasis. *In* Dawes, B. (ed.): Advances in Parasitology. Volume 8. New York, Academic Press, 1970, p. 173.
WHO Expert Committee on Onchocerciasis. World Health Organization Technical Report Series No. 335, 1–92, 1966.
Woodruff, A. W., Choyce, D. P., Muci-Mendoza, F., Hills, M., and Pettitt, L. E.: Onchocerciasis in Guatemala: a clinical parasitological study with comparison between the disease there and in East Africa. Trans. R. Soc. Trop. Med. Hyg., 60:695, 1966.

STREPTOCERCIASIS

Dipetalonema streptocerca is carried by midges of the genus Culicoides. It occurs in Central Africa, particularly in the Congo and neighboring countries. The adult worms are found in the region of the shoulder girdle, and the microfilariae produced in the skin cause a reddish brown irritant rash which may be associated with some degree of edema. Skin shavings reveal the unsheathed microfilariae with the crooked tails and the nuclei going down to the tip. Treatment with diethylcarbamazine is effective.

Meyers, W. M., Connor, D. H., Harman, L. E., Fleshman, K., Moris, R. and Neafie, R. G.: Human streptocerciasis: A clinicopathologic study of 40 Africans (Zairans), including identification of the adult filaria. Am. J. Trop. Med. Hyg., 21:528, 1972.

DIROFILARIASIS

Several Dirofilariae have been reported to occasionally cause symptoms in man, particularly in the United States. Such infections have also been reported from the Mediterranean basin, South America, and Africa. In Louisiana and Texas a subcutaneous filarid of raccoons *(Dirofilaria tenuis)* occasionally invades man, but does not mature. It produces a painful subcutaneous nodule, consisting of an eosinophilic inflammatory reaction around the worm; this may be a granuloma or may be located in a lymph node. The diagnosis is usually made after biopsy. Mosquitoes transmit the infection.

Other species found in man include *D. conjunctivae, D. repens,* and *D. immitis.* Adult worms have been detected in the heart and great vessels and in the eye. They have also caused infarcts in the lung and "coin" lesions at the hila which may be mistaken for a bronchial carcinoma and excised before the nature is known. In sections the worm is seen in cross section in the center of an infarcted area infiltrated with eosinophils.

Beaver, P. C., and Orihel, T. C.: Human infection with filariae of animals in the United States. Am. J. Trop. Med. Hyg., 14:1010, 1965.
Beskin, C. A., Colvin, S. H., Jr., and Beaver, P. C.: Pulmonary dirofilariasis, cause of a pulmonary nodular disease. J.A.M.A., 198:665, 1966.

POSSIBLE HUMAN MENINGONEMIASIS

Recently Orihel has pointed out that microfilariae recovered from patients with neurologic disorders in

Rhodesia and thought to be *Dipetalonema perstans* more closely resemble *Meningonema peruzzii*. The adults of this species inhabit the leptomeninges of the brainstem in African monkeys.

Orihel, T. C.: Cerebral filariasis in Rhodesia—a zoonotic infection. Am. J. Trop. Med. Hyg., 22:596, 1973.

PULMONARY TROPICAL EOSINOPHILIA
(Eosinophilic Lung, Weingarten's Syndrome)

Since the early part of this century Indian physicians have recognized a syndrome of paroxysmal cough and nocturnal bronchospasm associated with high eosinophilia, and have called it pulmonary tropical eosinophilia. Low fever, dyspnea, and malaise may be accompanying symptoms. The absolute eosinophil count is above 3000 per cubic millimeter, and may reach very high levels. Chest films may show increased reticulation, prominence of bronchovascular markings, or diffuse miliary mottling of the lung fields. In Ball's series of 1000 cases the great majority were Indian; the condition is much more common among Indians in Singapore. It is now generally accepted that this syndrome is caused by occult filarial infections. The evidence that this is so can be listed as follows: (1) Patients have a consistently high titer of filarial complement-fixing antibodies in the absence of evidence of microfilariae in the blood. (2) There is a clinical, hematologic, and serologic response to therapy with the antifilarial drug diethylcarbamazine. (3) The syndrome has been produced in a volunteer by inoculation of *Brugia malayi* infective larvae and *Brugia pahangi* (a feline filaria). (4) Microfilariae have been demonstrated in lung granulomas in such cases by several groups of workers.

It is possible that eosinophilic lung results from an alteration in host immunity to the filarial parasite, giving rise to allergic phenomena manifested by persistent hypereosinophilia and pulmonary symptoms. What is not yet settled is the precise identification of the parasite. It is likely that several species of filaria of the genera Wuchereria and Brugia, some human, some animal, may be involved, depending on the locality in which the syndrome occurs. The high incidence in Indians is noteworthy and may suggest a genetic predisposition in certain racial groups. The course of diethylcarbamazide recommended is similar to that for bancroftian filariasis. Often the symptoms get temporarily worse after starting the drug, but invariably they resolve, and a second course of the drug or the use of carbarsone as an alternative is seldom necessary.

The question of occult filariasis has recently been reviewed, and it has been pointed out that in many instances it has not been possible to identify the helminth responsible because of the difficulty of interpreting the microfilariae in tissue sections even if they are found. Quite apart from the well defined clinical entity of pulmonary tropical eosinophilia there are patients presenting with signs of reticuloendothelial activation (enlarged lymph nodes, hepatosplenomegaly) and eosinophilia for which it is difficult to find a cause.

Ball, J. D.: Tropical pulmonary eosinophilia. Trans. R. Soc. Trop. Med. Hyg., 44:237, 1950.
Donohugh, D. L.: Tropical eosinophilia, an etiologic enquiry. N. Engl. J. Med., 269:1357, 1963.
Danaraj, T. J., Pacheco, G., Shanmugaratnam, K., and Beaver, P. C.: The etiology and pathology of eosinophilic lung (tropical eosinophilia). Am. J. Trop. Med. Hyg., 15:183, 1966.
Islam, N.: Tropical eosinophilia. East Pakistan, Islam A. Chittagong, 1964.
Lie Kian, J., and Shandosham, A. A.: The pathology of clinical filariasis due to *Wuchereria bancroft* and *Brugia malayi* and a discussion of occult filariasis. *In* Sandosham, A. A., and Zaman, V. (eds.): Proceedings of Seminar on Filariasis and Immunology of Parasitic Infections, and Laboratory Meeting. Kuala Lumpur, Malaysia, Rajiv Printers, 1969, p. 125.

TROPICAL PYOMYOSITIS

Philip D. Marsden

This is a condition of a large deep-seated abscess, single or multiple, occurring in any voluntary muscle. Strange lumps for diagnosis in the tropics sometimes turn out to be deep-seated abscesses. By far the most frequent organism isolated is *Staphylococcus aureus*, and in Uganda 60 per cent of such organisms are phage gpII. Histologically there are areas of focal muscle necrosis with inflammatory cell infiltration. The regional lymph nodes are rarely affected, and there may be no fever or leukocytosis in the peripheral blood. The cause is unknown. Subcutaneous helminthic infection, particularly filaria, and sickle cell disease have been suggested as predisposing conditions, but as yet there is no convincing evidence to this effect. Treatment consists of antimicrobial therapy (initially with penicillin) and surgical drainage.

Elebute, E. A.: Pyomyositis. *In* Schwartz, S. I., Adesola, A. O., Elebute, E. A., and Rob, C. G. (eds.): Tropical Surgery, New York, McGraw-Hill Book Company, 1971.
Marcus, R. T., and Foster, W. D.: Observations on the clinical features, aetiology and geographical distribution of pyomyositis in East Africa. East Afr. Med. J., 45:167, 1968.

EOSINOPHILIA IN RELATION TO HELMINTHIC INFECTIONS

Philip D. Marsden

Hypereosinophilic states are considered elsewhere in this book, and conditions such as periarteritis nodosa, eosinophilic leukemia, and allergic diseases are discussed in the appropriate chapters. However, the author believes that a number of the cases of unexplained eosinophilia seen today in diagnostic units will in time be explained on the basis of helminthic infections, and it is worthwhile making one or two general points in relation to such infections.

As can be seen from the preceding chapters, almost all

helminthic infections in contrast to protozoal infections are at some time or other associated with eosinophilia. In terms of the parasites for which man is the definitive host, the eosinophilia often coincides with the invasive phase of a trematode, cestode, or nematode infection, and the diagnosis may not be apparent until several weeks or months later when the adults begin to produce progeny. For this reason obscure eosinophilia should always be kept under observation, and stool or tissue specimens re-examined. Some parasites are notorious in presenting a problem of eosinophilia for diagnosis, notably Strongyloides and Trichinella infections. After effective treatment of helminthic infections, particularly those in close contact with body tissues, there is often a pronounced rise in circulating eosinophils.

Perhaps more interesting is the clinical situation in which a patient has a significant human helminth load and yet little or no expected eosinophilia in the absence of cortisone therapy. Recent work suggesting that sensitized lymphocytes play an important role in the genesis of eosinophilia may throw some light on this problem.

Eosinophilia is a prominent feature of infections with nonhuman helminths, e.g., Angiostrongylus, and situations in which there is an abnormal host response, e.g., pulmonary tropical eosinophilia. It appears that a small number of nonhuman helminths passing through man's tissues may engender marked eosinophilia and even hypergammaglobulinemia, e.g., toxocariasis, gnathostomiasis. To find the helminths responsible is impossible in many patients, and when found they may be very difficult to identify. Our elucidation of this clinical problem appears to rest on the elaboration of more specific and sensitive serologic tests, and the techniques of indirect hemagglutination, gel diffusion, fluorescent antibody tests, and similar procedures are useful here to detect host response to helminthic antigens. However, much difficult work will be needed to characterize these complex antigens.

Finally, in a clinical consideration of this problem, common things occur commonly. A survey of a series of patients with occult eosinophilia in a large teaching hospital in New York City revealed a few cases of strongyloidiasis, but eosinophilia was most frequently one of the signs of a reaction to drug therapy.

Part X

DISORDERS OF THE NERVOUS SYSTEM AND BEHAVIOR

317. INTRODUCTION

Fred Plum

Almost all diseases use the nervous system to express themselves and it is this fact that often makes neurology seem complex and difficult to the physician. Pain, sensory loss, weakness, disturbed thinking, and impaired mood or alertness are not specific indicators of specific diseases. To be sure, in many instances, they are symptoms of primary disease of the nervous system. Even more often, however, they reflect disease in some other system or organ of the body. Finally, and perhaps most frequently, these symptoms derive from man's faulty adjustment to his environment. Symptoms are error signals, and the nervous system is as sensitive to symbolic threats as it is to physical ones.

Based on the aforementioned concepts, the goals of the chapters that follow are to present neurologic disease as a problem to be approached logically and for which certain principles repeatedly provide the key for diagnosis and treatment. These principles are based on our current knowledge of how the brain functions as an adaptive organ, adjusting man to his external as well as to his internal environment.

Part X is organized in two main categories. In the first, the more general functions of the nervous system are considered: how it is organized, how it handles certain normal activities, and how it expresses psychologic and somatic symptoms in response to both real and symbolic threat or injury. In the second, the more traditional approach is taken, and neurologic diseases are discussed according to anatomic and causative categories. Heavy emphasis is placed on the biochemistry of disease and the specific physiology of signs and symptoms. It must be recognized, however, that this century's revolution in biologic science is just beginning to attack effectively the problems involved in understanding brain function, behavior, and neurologic disease. Thus these pages often expose our ignorance as much as they do our knowledge.

A word about treatment. Man's brain is his uniquely human organ. Damage it and life loses its meaning in direct proportion, no matter what other physiologic benefits may accrue in the process. The brain cannot be regenerated, repaired, or homotransplanted. It accumulates no metabolic debts and, unless supplied continuously by an effective circulation carrying large amounts of oxygen and glucose, it digests itself irreparably. This means that one cannot "let the brain go" while solving other medical problems. For example, if an elderly man with severe anemia suffers an ischemic stroke while awaiting accurate blood studies, there is no satisfaction later in a correct hematologic diagnosis. If an adolescent girl suffers permanent dementia from hypoglycemia while having her diabetes regulated, the perfect control of glycosuria seems hardly worth it. The integrity of the nervous system must be the first goal in therapeutics.

Section One. CONSCIOUSNESS AND ITS DISTURBANCES

318. INTRODUCTION

Fred Plum

William James remarked that everyone knows what consciousness is until he tries to define it. Full consciousness is generally taken to imply not only wakefulness but the total complement of human mental faculties: complete awareness of self and environment. In clinical medicine, when one speaks of consciousness as opposed to unconsciousness or coma, a less encompassing state is usually meant, consisting of behavioral wakefulness plus the capacity to respond appropriately to at least a limited number of external stimuli. *Dementia, apathy, amnesia,* or *aphasia* may impair the content of consciousness, but as long as enough appropriate responses remain in other behavioral functions, consciousness is considered to be preserved. *Obtundation* and *drowsiness* describe states of dull behavior with blunted alertness in which part of the content of consciousness is lost, often with an excessive tendency to sleep. *Stupor* is a state wherein subjects respond when vigorously stimulated, but immediately sink back again as soon as external stimuli are withdrawn. *Coma* is complete unresponsiveness. In light coma, semi-appropriate movements occur in response to noxious stimuli, but in deep coma, subjects retain only primitive reflexes or no response at all.

The present physiologic concept of consciousness is that it depends upon close interaction between the intact cerebral hemispheres and the central gray matter of the upper brainstem. The hemispheres contribute most of the specific components of consciousness, including language, memory, intellect, and learned responses to sensory stimuli. But in order for the cerebrum to function, the organism must be aroused or activated by more caudally placed mechanisms that reside in the thalamus, hypothalamus, midbrain, and upper pons. An important component of this arousal mechanism is located within what Magoun and his colleagues called the ascending reticular activating system; other brainstem systems also influence cerebral cortical activity and the state of consciousness.

The relation of the cerebral cortex to consciousness is more quantitative than qualitative: All hemispheric lesions undoubtedly reduce, at least to some degree, the content of man's consciousness, and the total loss of the cortex causes at least several weeks of coma even if the brainstem is intact. Between the extremes of an injury so small that it is clinically almost undetectable and so large that it causes coma lies a continuum along which the size of the lesion and the impairment of mind, memory, wit, and personality are roughly proportional.

319. THE PATHOGENESIS OF STUPOR AND COMA

Fred Plum

The preceding paragraphs have described how stupor or coma results when a disease process either diffusely and bilaterally blots out the function of the cerebral hemispheres or blocks brainstem-activating structures so that the cortex cannot be aroused. A potentially bewildering series of individual maladies can have one or both of these effects, as may be seen in the accompanying table. However, if one examines the mechanisms by which neurologic diseases cause coma, all these maladies fall into three categories that can be distinguished by their signs and symptoms: (1) supratentorial mass lesions, (2) subtentorial compressive or destructive lesions, and (3) metabolic brain diseases.

SUPRATENTORIAL MASS LESIONS

Supratentorial masses are rarely so large that they produce coma by directly destroying or replacing the cerebral hemispheres. Rather, they interfere with consciousness because they shift and squeeze the contents of the supratentorial compartment and, in so doing, compress the diencephalon. The expanding process can originate anywhere in the hemisphere and ultimately produce this reaction because the fibrous tentorium and the bones of the base of the skull resist movement except toward the tentorial opening. As a result, when supratentorial masses demand room for expansion, the diencephalic tectum and adjacent midbrain are particularly likely to be compressed, and sometimes the diencephalon is even displaced downward through the tentorial notch (transtentorial herniation).

How do supratentorial masses progress so that these reactions occur? The brain has certain common responses to injury, including edema, vascular dilatation, and the invasion of leukocytes and proliferation of glial cells. The intensity, tempo, and exact contribution of each of these responses varies according to the nature of the original lesion and the rate at which it appears, but each shares in the brain's defenses against neoplasms, infections, infarcts, and irritants. Thus the original lesion gradually enlarges and tends to impair structures ever more remote from itself in the inexpansible intracranial cavity. The remote effects are due partly to edema spreading away from the edges of the primary lesion and partly to an actual shift of the brain within the skull, compressing normal tissues and blood vessels against rigid structures such as the falx cerebri and the tentorium. At this stage, clinical signs of increased intracranial pressure are common and imply that an intracranial lesion is already exerting generalized deleterious effects.

The clinical picture of supratentorial mass lesions producing stupor or coma has several distinctive features. If a history is available, localizing symptoms such as frontal headache, focal seizures, or other changes consistent with hemispheric disease will usually be found to have preceded unconsciousness. Physically, most patients demonstrate a combination of *focal* hemispheral signs, e.g., sensorimotor defect, aphasia, and visual field defect, reflecting the site of the original pathologic process, plus *diffuse* signs of supratentorial dysfunction, indicating that the lesion is exerting remote effects on the opposite hemisphere and the deep diencephalon. An important negative finding is that, unless the patient is in the terminal stages of illness, no evidence of direct subtentorial brainstem dysfunction can be found: pupillary and oculovestibular reflexes remain intact. If a patient with a supratentorial lesion progresses in his illness, the neurologic signs and symptoms evolve in a characteristic, orderly, rostral-caudal pattern. The more rostrally located neurologic functions first disappear, followed by more caudal impairment, first in the diencephalon and then down the brainstem almost as if the structures were being progressively transected from above downward, each plane of function being removed almost completely before the next is impaired.

The aforementioned description needs amplification to be complete. Some supratentorial masses begin and enlarge in neurologically silent areas such as the frontal lobes or the subdural space and lack a focal signature. Lesions of this type may be revealed only when the patient develops signs of diffuse forebrain dysfunction plus, perhaps, headache and evidence of increased intracranial pressure.

Stupor or coma with supratentorial lesions is ominous

The Common Causes of Stupor and Coma

Supratentorial lesions (causing upper brainstem dysfunction)
- Cerebral hemorrhage
- Large cerebral infarction
- Subdural hematoma
- Epidural hematoma
- Brain tumor
- Brain abscess (rare)

Subtentorial lesions (compressing or destroying the reticular formation)
- Pontine or cerebellar hemorrhage
- Infarction
- Tumor
- Cerebellar abscess

Metabolic and diffuse lesions (see also Table 1 in Ch. 320)
- Anoxia or ischemia
- Hypoglycemia
- Nutritional deficiency
- Endogenous organ failure or deficiency
- Ionic and electrolyte disorders
- Exogenous poison
- Infections
  - Meningitis
  - Encephalitis
- Concussion and postictal states

because it implies that the deeply located upper brainstem is already compressed or distorted and that the much more serious complication of herniation of the forebrain downward into the tentorial notch is about to occur. Such herniation begins either with direct downward displacement of the diencephalon (central herniation) or with the uncus of the temporal lobe squeezing into the tentorial notch and against the midbrain (uncal herniation). Either way, if the hernia develops fully, it usually impacts the midbrain and nearly always results in permanent brain damage or death. A characteristic constellation of symptoms heralds each of these patterns of transtentorial herniation. With impending *central* herniation, stupor becomes gradually deeper, and the subjects sigh, yawn, or develop periodic respirations. The pupils shrink to as little as 1 to 2 mm in diameter, but retain their light reflexes. Oculovestibular reflexes are brisk, and the extremities stiffen into bilateral rigidity or spasticity, combined with extensor plantar responses. With *uncal* herniation, signs are in many ways similar to the above except that as the uncus slides over the tentorial edge, it often compresses the third nerve ahead of it, even before the diencephalon is squeezed. The result is that the pupil on the side of the herniation begins to dilate more than its fellow. Eventually, the pupil dilates widely and becomes light-fixed, and the patient becomes stuporous. Shortly afterward, oculomotor functions of the third nerve are usually impaired, and the involved eye turns outward. If the herniating process continues, the opposite third nerve becomes involved as well, and then the brainstem. To initiate effective treatment one must recognize the process before this advanced stage and halt it with osmotic decompressing agents or surgical treatment. Otherwise, when conditions progress this far, few subjects recover without substantial, permanent neurologic injury.

SUBTENTORIAL MASS OR DESTRUCTIVE LESIONS

These conditions cause stupor or coma if they destroy or compress the centrally located activating systems in the brainstem anywhere above approximately the midpons. Expanding lesions of the posterior fossa have the same effect if they compress the midbrain upward. Compression against the medulla oblongata with an ensuing cerebellar pressure cone produces stiff neck, along with respiratory and cardiac irregularities, but does not directly cause loss of consciousness.

The characteristic clinical feature of subtentorial destruction or compression causing coma is the presence of restricted and usually asymmetrical signs of focal brainstem dysfunction, which frequently can be anatomically pinpointed to a single locus by the clinical findings. Seldom do the signs indicate complete brainstem transection. This restricted, discrete localization is unlike metabolic lesions causing coma in which the signs commonly indicate incomplete dysfunction at several different levels of the brain, and also is unlike the secondary brainstem dysfunction and coma that follow supratentorial herniation, in which *all* function at any given level tends to be lost as the process progresses from rostral to caudal along the neuraxis.

Purely compressive lesions of the posterior fossa rarely cause coma until late in their course when the patient is near death. The pathologic process is usually a hemorrhage, abscess, or tumor of the cerebellum or fourth ventricle, and occipital headache, nystagmus, diplopia, nausea, vomiting, cranial nerve signs, and ataxia usually precede unconsciousness. Important points in distinguishing both destructive and compressive posterior fossa lesions from metabolic depression of the brainstem are that in metabolic depression oculovestibular responses are generally preserved until the advanced stages, and pupillary light reflexes are nearly always preserved. By contrast, structural brainstem lesions causing coma always disrupt the oculovestibular responses, and those involving the midbrain also interrupt the pupillary reflexes.

METABOLIC DEPRESSION OF THE BRAIN CAUSING COMA

Primary metabolic encephalopathies are intrinsic to the neuron, the glial cell, or the white matter, respectively. They often produce dementia, but rarely cause coma except terminally. *Secondary* metabolic encephalopathies are those in which brain function is disrupted either because the brain is not supplied with a required substance, e.g., thiamine, oxygen, or glucose, or because it is poisoned by an ingested or endogenous toxin, e.g., depressant drugs or the products of uremia. The secondary metabolic encephalopathies are frequent causes of delirium as well as of stupor and coma; their relationship to the normal metabolism of the brain is discussed in detail in Ch. 320.

Experimental evidence conflicts as to whether most metabolic agents causing coma depress mainly the brainstem reticular formation or the cerebral cortex. Clinically, most patients with metabolic encephalopathy appear to suffer depression of the forebrain more than of the brainstem. However, the striking finding with most metabolic agents is that they selectively depress certain susceptible functions at several different brain levels, but at the same time spare other functions that emanate from identical levels. For example, most metabolic poisons depress the reticular and motor functions of the midbrain, yet nearly all of them spare the pupillary light reflex so that reactive pupils persist into the deepest stages of metabolic coma until asphyxia intervenes. (Poisoning with glutethimide or parasympathomimetics provides the only exception to this rule, both drugs blocking the light reflex in large, coma-causing doses.) Most of the metabolic encephalopathies cause delirium before stupor or coma, and many of them are accompanied in their early stages by asterixis, a flapping irregular tremor of the outstretched hands, or by random myoclonic muscle twitches. Although the metabolic encephalopathies occasionally produce asymmetrical motor signs, they more characteristically impair body movement symmetrically, and they never impair central sensory pathways except as an accompaniment to the over-all depression of the sensorium.

To epitomize, diseases causing stupor or coma fall into three categories:

1. Supratentorial mass lesions, which present with asymmetrical neurologic signs of hemispheral dysfunction combined with evidence of intact subtentorial brainstem function. As supratentorial lesions evolve, the signs indicate progressive rostral-caudal neurologic deterioration, almost as if the brain were being serially sectioned from top to bottom.

2. Subtentorial compressive and destructive lesions, which present from the outset with either cranial nerve abnormalities or other focal brainstem signs, including pupillary and oculovestibular reflex abnormalities. Long tract motor signs are usually present and asymmetrical.

3. Metabolic brain diseases, which present a picture of either diffuse cortical depression or, more often, of impaired function in both the hemispheres and the brainstem accompanied by retained pupillary light reflexes. The multifocal distribution of metabolic encephalopathy is usually symmetrical and not accompanied by sensory impairments.

APPROACH TO THE PATIENT IN STUPOR OR COMA

The physician must ensure that the brain and other vital organs receive no further injury while he obtains whatever history, examinations, and laboratory data are required. Before anything else he must provide a free and open airway and determine that the subject is breathing deeply enough to oxygenate his lungs and eliminate carbon dioxide. Next, the heart and blood pressure should be examined, and possible sources of bleeding checked to be certain that cardiac output and blood volume are sufficient to supply the metabolic needs of the brain and kidney. In all patients in coma an intravenous infusion should be started, using a large-bore needle. Blood samples for typing and cross-matching, as well as for other appropriate laboratory determinations, can be obtained at this time. Whenever the cause of coma is doubtful, and particularly when the clinical signs suggest a metabolic disorder, blood should be taken for sugar determination, and then 50 ml of 50 per cent glucose given intravenously. Hypoglycemic encephalopathy can take many forms, some of which mimic other diseases. If glucose is given promptly, no further cerebral damage occurs while the doctor awaits definitive laboratory diagnosis. Intravenous sugar harms nothing if the coma has another cause.

Beyond these immediate, lifesaving measures, it requires considerable restraint to approach a patient in a coma methodically, for the urge to act without delay is understandably strong, but potentially dangerous. Inquiry into both the past medical history and the circumstances under which the patient lost consciousness generally discloses more of diagnostic value than any other maneuver. Is there any suggestion that head trauma could have occurred recently? Has there been renal, hepatic, or myocardial disease? Could a seizure have preceded the present unconsciousness? Has the subject been taking insulin? Have there been recent changes in mood, behavior, or neurologic function to suggest an evolving intracranial process? Was the subject "blue," depressed, or moody, and did he have access to depressant drugs? Is he a "spree" drinker? These and other questions must be covered comprehensively with relatives, past physicians, friends, police, or ambulance personnel.

One must perform both a meticulous neurologic examination and a thoughtful physical review of every body system, because disease in remote organs often causes or accentuates dysfunction in the brain.

Fever implies infection, or, less often, lymphomatous neoplasm. On the other hand, hypothermia (30 to 36° C [86 to 96.8° F]) in a patient not severely exposed to cold suggests depressant drug poisoning, hypoglycemia, or severe lower brainstem injury, as by infarction. Hypertension may be the cause of hypertensive encephalopathy or the underlying cause of cerebral hemorrhage. Conversely, an elevated blood pressure can be a symptom of subarachnoid hemorrhage in a subject not previously hypertensive. Hypotension in a supine patient implies low blood volume (hemorrhagic or traumatic shock; severe nutritional and fluid depletion), low cardiac output (myocardial infarction), or low peripheral resistance (depressant drug poisoning). Tachycardia (over 160 per minute) can mean that unconsciousness is the result of lowered cardiac output from a supraventricular cardiac arrhythmia. Bradycardia suggests heart block and the Adams-Stokes syndrome or a myocardial infarct.

The pattern and depth of respiration are often informative in evaluating both neurologic function and acid-base balance, so much so that the evaluation of breathing is discussed more fully in Ch. 320.

The skin should be searched for petechiae (thrombocytopenic or nonthrombocytopenic purpura, meningococcemia, and bacterial endocarditis), bruises, evidence of nutritional deficiency, icterus, angiomatous spiders, and the bright pinkness of carbon monoxide poisoning. Fleshy or clubbed fingertips suggest carcinoma of the lung, or, less often, lung abscess or congenital heart disease (with brain embolism or abscess). A meticulous examination of the optic fundi is imperative but should be completed without cycloplegics, the use of which destroys the potential diagnostic value of pupillary reactions in coma. In the fundus oculi, the pathologic changes of many diseases causing coma can be viewed directly: increased intracranial pressure, hypertensive vascular disease, diabetes, blood dyscrasia, tuberculosis, sarcoidosis, bacterial endocarditis, cryptococcosis, collagen vascular disease, and even subarachnoid hemorrhage producing subhyaloid bleeding.

Chest examination has two potentially rewarding findings: cardiac murmurs suggest bacterial endocarditis with consequent focal, embolic encephalitis; the wheezes and obstructive sounds of the pulmonary cripple suggest CO_2 retention causing narcosis. In the abdominal examination, the presence of masses suggesting polycystic kidneys increases the chances that subarachnoid hemorrhage has occurred, whereas liver enlargement (hepatic coma is common with hepatomas) or splenic enlargement (both blood dyscrasias and infectious mononucleosis can cause encephalitis-like illnesses) can provide valuable leads.

During the neurologic examination, certain potentially informative steps are sometimes overlooked. The skull should always be palpated and inspected meticulously. Edema of the scalp commonly overlies fresh fracture lines, and basal skull fractures predispose to blood pigment stains behind the ear (Battle's sign) and about the orbit (raccoon eyes). Blood also may escape from basal fractures into the ear canals, the middle ears, or the nostrils. The skull should be percussed, because focal or unilateral skull tenderness, manifested by grimacing or withdrawal in a stuporous subject, often overlies an intracranial mass lesion. The neck should be tested carefully: stiff neck can reflect meningitis, cerebellar tonsillar herniation, or, occasionally, simply skeletal muscle spasticity. The stiff neck of acute bacterial meningitis is rarely equivocal; that of impending herniation is commonly less severe and lacks accompanying signs of infection or a prominent Kernig sign. It usually requires several hours or a day or more for stiff neck to develop after subarachnoid bleeding.

It is useful to watch the unconscious patient for a time, observing whether or not the extremities move equally and whether tremor, myoclonus, or single or repetitive seizures involve any part of the body. Status epilepticus with focal continuous epilepsy is not uncommon, but is often overlooked.

Laboratory Examination of the Patient in Coma

Patients should be subjected to a skull roentgenogram (looking for fracture lines, densities, and pineal shifts), a blood count and smear, and a urinalysis. When the clinical findings are consistent with metabolic encephalopathy but the cause is uncertain, the blood glucose and serum sodium, potassium, and bicarbonate should be obtained promptly. Knowledge of the arterial pH often can be almost diagnostic of the cause of metabolic coma (see Table 3 in Ch. 320).

When to do a lumbar puncture is always a serious question. All physicians are aware that in patients with increased intracranial pressure the procedure sometimes induces fatal herniation of the brain through the tentorium or foramen magnum. For this reason, lumbar puncture is best avoided if the physician strongly suspects his patient of having an expanding intracranial mass, particularly in the posterior fossa. However, there are certain treatable diseases such as meningitis that can be diagnosed only by lumbar puncture, and many others in which the procedure yields valuable preliminary diagnostic information. When the advice of neurologic specialists is unavailable, the doctor has no choice but to proceed with lumbar puncture if the diagnosis is in doubt and he believes the procedure has a reasonable chance of offering valuable information. Certain steps minimize the risk. One is to use a small (No. 20), sharp needle. Another is to fill the manometer with saline and attach it to the needle before releasing fluid, a technique that prevents sudden subarachnoid pressure shifts. Finally, jugular manometrics should *never* be performed, for they offer little useful data and increase the risk of impacting potential intracranial herniations.

Magoun, H. W.: The Waking Brain. 2nd ed. Springfield, Ill., Charles C Thomas, 1963.
Petito, F., and Plum, F.: The lumbar puncture (editorial). N. Engl. J. Med., 200:225, 1974.
Plum, F., and Posner, J. B.: The Diagnosis of Stupor and Coma. 2nd ed. Philadelphia, F. A. Davis Company, 1972.

320. DELIRIUM AND EXOGENOUS METABOLIC BRAIN DISEASE

Jerome B. Posner

INTRODUCTION

There are few situations in clinical medicine that confuse and upset the physician so much as when he confronts a patient whose state of consciousness is rapidly changing. The physician's task in such a situation is both enormous and exacting. First he must decide which of three major categories of disease is responsible for the patient's condition: (1) structural brain disease (e.g., brain tumors, subdural hematomas, cerebral infarctions); (2) "functional" brain disease (e.g., schizophrenia, manic-depressive psychosis); or (3) metabolic brain disease or delirium (see definitions below). If the patient's disorder falls into one of the first two categories (discussed elsewhere in this book), the physician can obtain help from highly skilled specialists in those areas (neurologists, neurosurgeons, or psychiatrists). If the patient's behavioral change is due to metabolic encephalopathy, the general physician must then determine himself which of a bewildering variety of metabolic defects is responsible (Table 1) and must rapidly begin treatment to assure that the metabolic defect does not produce irreversible brain damage. While he is carrying out these exacting tasks, he is often impeded by the fact that the patient is noisy, obstreperous, and uncooperative, and by his own knowledge that appropriate treatment is essential and inappropriate treatment (e.g., injudicious use of sedative drugs) potentially deleterious or even fatal. To deal with metabolic brain disease, the physician must understand some pathophysiologic aspects of cerebral metabolism and must undertake a systematic and thorough physical and laboratory examination of the patient.

DEFINITIONS

Metabolic encephalopathy is a term applied to the behavioral changes which result from diffuse or widespread multifocal failure of cerebral metabolism. When the cerebral disorder arises from an intrinsic failure of neuronal or glial metabolism, it is referred to as *primary or endogenous metabolic encephalopathy*. The primary disorders usually begin insidiously, progress inexorably, and produce a clinical picture of dementia, as discussed in Ch. 326 to 331. When the encephalopathy results from interference with brain metabolism by extracerebral disease, it is called *secondary or exogenous metabolic encephalopathy*. The secondary encephalopathies usually begin acutely or subacutely and often subside with time and treatment. They produce a clinical picture in which confusion, thinking errors, behavioral abnormalities, disorders of consciousness, and abnormal motor activity predominate. The causes of secondary metabolic encephalopathy are as many and varied as the illnesses that disturb body chemistry. Some examples of metabolic encephalopathy are listed in Table 1.

Metabolic brain disease is common and often misdiagnosed. When mild, it produces intellectual dullness, social indifference, and vague perplexity easily mistaken by observers for psychogenic depression or simply low intelligence. More severe encephalopathy elicits either a florid picture of tremulous agitation, rich and frightening hallucinations, and periods of seemingly complete loss of contact with the environment, or a more quiet, withdrawn, akinetic state which may fade into stupor or coma. The former, often called *delirium* or *toxic psychosis,* may be confused with a functional psychosis, and the latter, often called *acute* or *subacute confusional state,* is likely to be mistaken for structural brain disease. Although certain specific systemic disorders characteristically cause one or another of the aforementioned

TABLE 1. Causes of Metabolic Brain Disease

I. Deprivation of oxygen, substrate, or metabolic cofactors
*A. Hypoxia (interference with oxygen supply to the entire brain—cerebral blood flow normal)
1. Decreased oxygen tension and content of blood
Pulmonary disease
Alveolar hypoventilation
Decreased atmospheric oxygen tension
2. Decreased oxygen content of blood—normal tension
Anemia
Carbon monoxide poisoning
Methemoglobinemia
*B. Ischemia (diffuse or widespread multifocal interference with blood supply to brain)
1. Decreased cerebral blood flow resulting from decreased cardiac output
Stokes-Adams syndrome, cardiac arrest, cardiac arrhythmias
Myocardial infarction
Congestive heart failure
Aortic stenosis
Pulmonary embolus
2. Decreased cerebral blood flow resulting from decreased peripheral resistance in systemic circulation
Syncope: orthostatic, vasovagal
Carotid sinus hypersensitivity
Low blood volume
3. Decreased cerebral blood flow due to generalized increase in cerebrovascular resistance
Hypertensive encephalopathy
Hyperventilation syndrome
Increased blood viscosity (polycythemia), cryo- and macroglobinemia
4. Decreased local cerebral blood flow due to widespread small vessel occlusion
Disseminated intravascular coagulation
Systemic lupus erythematosus
Subacute bacterial endocarditis
Cardiopulmonary bypass
*C. Hypoglycemia
Resulting from exogenous insulin
Spontaneous (endogenous insulin, liver disease, etc.)
D. Cofactor deficiency
Thiamin (Wernicke's encephalopathy)
Niacin
Pyridoxine
B_{12}
Folate

II. Diseases of organs other than brain
*A. Diseases of nonendocrine organs
Liver (hepatic coma)
Kidney (uremic coma)
Lung (CO_2 narcosis)
*B. Hyper- and/or hypofunction of endocrine organs
Pituitary
Thyroid (myxedema-thyrotoxicosis)
Parathyroid (hyper- and hypoparathyroidism)
Adrenal (Addison's disease, Cushing's disease, pheochromocytoma)
Pancreas (diabetes, hypoglycemia)
C. Other systemic diseases
Diabetes
Cancer
Porphyria
Sepsis
Fever

III. Exogenous poisons
*A. Sedative drugs
B. Acid poisons or poisons with acidic breakdown products
Paraldehyde
Methyl alcohol
Ethylene glycol
C. Other enzyme inhibitors
Heavy metals
Organic phosphates
Cyanide
Salicylates
D. Psychotropic drugs
Tricyclic antidepressants and anticholinergic drugs
Amphetamines
Lithium
Phenothiazines
LSD-mescaline
Monoamine oxidase inhibitors
E. Others
Penicillin
Anticonvulsants
Steroids
Cardiac glycosides

IV. Diseases producing toxins or enzyme inhibition in CNS
A. Meningitis
B. Encephalitis
C. Subarachnoid hemorrhage

V. Abnormalities of fluid, ionic or acid-base environment of CNS
A. Water and sodium (hyper- and hyponatremia) (hypo- and hyperosmolality)
B. Acidosis (metabolic and respiratory)
C. Alkalosis (metabolic and respiratory)
D. Potassium (hypokalemia)
E. Magnesium (hyper- and hypomagnesemia)
F. Calcium (hyper- and hypocalcemia)

VI. Miscellaneous diseases of unknown cause
A. Seizures and postictal states
*B. "Postoperative" delirium
C. Concussion
*D. "Sensory deprivation"

*Alone or in combination, the most common causes of delirium seen on medical or surgical wards.

syndromes, each can occur with any of the metabolic brain diseases; thus the terms "delirium," "toxic psychosis," and "confusional state" are used interchangeably in this chapter to describe the wakeful stage of metabolic encephalopathy. A patient who is drowsy but can be coaxed to respond to verbal stimuli is *obtunded.* When he no longer responds to verbal stimuli but responds appropriately to noxious cutaneous stimuli, he is *stuporous.* If he does not respond appropriately to noxious stimuli, he is *comatose.* The term *dementia* is used operationally to describe an irreversible loss of memory and cognitive functions, usually insidious in onset and due to intrinsic disease of the brain. It is the irreversibility of dementia which clearly distinguishes it from delirium. An insidiously developing, quiet delirium may be clinically indistinguishable from the early stages of dementia.

SOME PATHOPHYSIOLOGIC ASPECTS OF METABOLIC BRAIN DISEASE

Pathologic changes in metabolic brain disease depend upon the nature and severity of the illness. The brains of some patients delirious during life are entirely normal at postmortem examination. In most cases, however, at least microscopic pathologic changes can be identified if the process causing delirium has lasted for some hours or days prior to death. The pathologic changes are bilateral, symmetrical, and usually diffusely distributed in the cerebral hemispheres. Lesions may be present in the neurons, the glial cells, or the white matter, depending on the nature of the primary illness.

Perhaps the most common pathologic cerebral changes are observed after anoxia, ischemia, or hypoglycemia.

The mildest abnormalities are visible only microscopically and consist of "microvacuoles" in neuronal cytoplasm of neocortex and hippocampus. The microvacuoles are swollen mitochondria, and this change is probably reversible. With more severe insults there is dissolution of the Nissl granules (particles of ribonucleic acid) and generalized pallor of staining. Finally, the nuclei shrink and become hyperchromatic, and irregular basophilic rings and granules appear in the swollen cytoplasm. These changes are not reversible. After severe and prolonged insults, all neurons in the cerebral cortex may disappear, and the third layer of the cortex may completely degenerate so that the naked eye detects a thin line of spongy necrosis (laminar necrosis). Anoxic changes also affect the basal ganglia to cause grossly visible focal necrosis of the globus pallidus. Occasionally, there may be diffuse demyelination of the subcortical white matter. Characteristically, the brainstem and spinal cord are spared unless the process has been overwhelmingly severe.

A nonspecific but common pathologic change in patients who have died with uremia, hyponatremia, diabetic coma, or CO_2 narcosis is cerebral swelling, recognized grossly by flattened gyri, obliterated sulci, and small ventricles. The cut brain may appear either "wet" or "dry," but, microscopically, large perivascular and perineuronal spaces attest to the presence of edema.

Unusual glial cells with ballooned, lobulated nuclei are found in the cortex and basal ganglia of patients who die in hepatic coma, and are relatively specific for this disorder. Widespread perivascular "cuffs" of lymphocytes or polymorphonuclear leukocytes indicate an inflammatory lesion of the brain and meninges from viral or bacterial invasion.

In all cases of metabolic brain disease, the cerebral oxygen uptake declines in rough proportion to the degree of brain dysfunction observed clinically. So far, we understand in only a few instances how systemic illnesses interfere with cerebral metabolism, but these few serve as models to suggest the possible mechanisms for the others. The following material outlines some of our knowledge of normal and abnormal cerebral metabolism.

Glucose. Glucose is the brain's only substrate under physiologic conditions, and is transferred across the blood-brain barrier by facilitated transport. Other substances can serve as substrates of brain in extraordinary circumstances (e.g., ketone bodies during starvation). Under normal circumstances, each 100 grams of brain utilizes about 5.5 mg of glucose per minute, which represents almost the body's entire basal glucose consumption. Eighty-five per cent of brain glucose uptake reacts with oxygen to form CO_2, water, and energy; the remainder is probably accounted for by lactic acid production even in the presence of ample oxygen supplies. Under anaerobic conditions, lactic acid is the end product of glucose metabolism, but the energy so produced is insufficient to maintain neuronal function. There are about 2 grams of reserve glucose (as such and as glycogen) in the brain, an amount that allows the brain of a hypoglycemic patient to survive (although not to function at a normal metabolic rate) for about 90 minutes without suffering irreversible damage. The blood glucose concentration at which cerebral metabolism fails and clinical symptoms develop is variable from patient to patient, but, in general, levels below 30 mg per 100 ml cause confusion, and below 10 to 15 mg per 100 ml, coma.

Oxygen. Oxygen, the other substance vital for normal cerebral function, is not stored by the brain, and a few seconds of anoxia is sufficient to cause coma. After a variable period of time, usually minutes, both hypoxia and ischemia cause irreversible neuronal damage. The normal brain consumes about 3.5 ml of oxygen per 100 grams per minute and produces an equal amount of carbon dioxide (R.Q. = 1). Cerebral oxygen consumption represents 15 to 20 per cent of the total body oxygen consumption at rest and is remarkably constant in normal man, whether awake or sleeping. However, significant deviations in oxygen consumption occur with brain dysfunction. Clinically, delirium usually accompanies oxygen uptakes below 2.5 ml and when the uptake falls below 2.0 ml per 100 grams per minute, most patients are unconscious. The degree of hypoxia necessary to cause clinical symptoms depends not only on the blood oxygen tension but also on hemoglobin concentration, cerebral blood flow, and serum pH. In general, Pa_{O_2} values below 50 mm Hg cause delirium, and below 25 mm Hg, coma.

Blood brings both glucose and oxygen to the brain. Under resting conditions, the brain receives 55 ml of blood each minute, about 15 per cent of the cardiac output. If the flow falls, the brain compensates by extracting more oxygen and more glucose from the blood it receives. Increased extraction of oxygen maintains normal metabolism in the face of a decreased cerebral blood flow up to the point where so much oxygen has been extracted that the oxygen tension of the brain's venous blood falls to about 20 mm of mercury (a level at which hemoglobin is about 35 per cent saturated). At this point, which is reached when cerebral blood flow falls to about half of normal, the oxygen tension is too low to maintain normal metabolism, and the patient loses consciousness. With hemoglobin concentrations below about 8 grams per 100 ml, cerebral blood flow must increase to assure an adequate oxygen supply. Profound anemia thus becomes a potential contributor to cerebral hypoxia.

Other Substances. In addition to glucose and oxygen, the brain requires other substances (e.g., enzymes, vitamins, amino acids, electrolytes) to maintain metabolism, synthesize transmitter substances, preserve cellular structure, and maintain membrane potentials. Abnormalities of any of these essential substances lead to metabolic brain disease. The unique function of nervous tissue is to transmit electrical impulses, both within cells and by synaptic transmission across cells. The integrity of intracellular transmission depends not only on energy from oxidative metabolism (to maintain the sodium pump) but also on finely controlled intra- and extracellular electrolyte balance. Thus, for example, alterations of extracellular sodium, an ion necessary for propagation of the action potential, produce behavioral changes and delirium. Lithium, a cation with properties similar to both sodium and potassium, changes behavior in manic patients and, in overdose, can lead to severe delirium and coma, perhaps by interfering with normal electrolyte function. The integrity of intercellular transmission is regulated by the synthesis, release, re-uptake, and breakdown of transmitter substances and by maintenance of postsynaptic transmitter receptor sites. Several substances have been identified as putative transmitters in the nervous system, including norepinephrine, dopamine, serotonin, acetylcholine, and amino acids, especially glycine, gamma-aminobutyric acid, and glutamic acid. Most psychotropic drugs are believed to exert their behavioral effects by altering the activity of biogenic amines in the central nervous system, and in overdose most of these drugs produce delirium and sometimes coma. By the same token, severe alterations in amino acid metabolism lead to delirium. Interference with transmitter function may occur when the synthesis, breakdown, or release of the transmitter is inhibited, or when a foreign substance having a structure similar to the transmitter competes for sites on the postsynaptic receptor. Such a "false transmitter" may be the mechanism by which hallucinogenic drugs act, and may also be responsible for the production of "hepatic coma." However, despite these considerations, in no instance is the exact mechanism of delirium in either electrolyte or putative transmitter abnormalities clearly understood.

The biochemical common denominator of metabolic brain disease is decreased oxygen uptake: Is there an anatomic common denominator? Two concepts have arisen delineating a principal locus of metabolic brain disease. One is that the neurons of the cerebral cortex are affected first and, as the process becomes more severe, subcortical structures are affected from the rostral end downward, the phylogenetically oldest and most caudal structures resisting most strongly. This view is supported by the pathologic distribution of cerebral anoxic and hypoglycemic changes and by physiologic studies of hypoglycemic animals in which abnormal electrical activity was recorded from the cortex before it appeared in the hypothalamus.

The second concept is that the neurons of the brainstem reticular formation are the most susceptible to metabolic change and, at least at first, the cortical neurons cease to function only because they lose their reticular stimulation. This concept is supported by physiologic experiments on animals, demonstrating that moderate degrees of hypoxia, hypoglycemia, anesthesia, and cyanide poisoning all block electrical conduction through the reticular formation before they block the ability of cortical neurons to receive messages via other afferent pathways (the lemniscal system).

Neither of these experimental concepts fully explains the several human disease states in which metabolic lesions clinically affect several different levels of the neuraxis simultaneously, with the major locus of early dysfunction differing not only from patient to patient but sometimes from one attack to the next in the same patient. This phenomenon is exemplified by the varied picture of hypoglycemia: Some patients first suffer loss of consciousness and have bilaterally synchronous slow waves in the EEG, suggesting an initial reticular involvement. Others first experience restricted cerebral motor or sensory signs unaccompanied by either EEG abnormalities or impaired consciousness. Still other patients convulse with one attack of hypoglycemia but suffer only quiet coma in the next. It appears that in the clinical situation, regional cerebral factors such as blood flow and energy requirements must vary from moment to moment to predispose first one part of the brain and then another to metabolic insult.

CLINICAL FEATURES OF METABOLIC BRAIN DISEASE

The purpose of the physical and laboratory examination in a patient with suspected metabolic brain disease is twofold: first, to establish if the patient is delirious as opposed to suffering behavioral changes from structural brain or psychiatric disease; and second, to determine exactly the type of metabolic defect causing the delirium. In general, examination of the state of consciousness, motor activity, and autonomic activity, as detailed below, helps to answer the first question, whereas the general physical examination, examination of ventilation, and laboratory examination (the latter two detailed below) help to answer the second question. It cannot, however, be overemphasized that, despite the difficulties of examining a delirious patient, a thorough and systematic general physical, neurologic, and laboratory examination *must* be undertaken if a definitive diagnosis is to be established and definitive treatment to be applied. Some principles of the examination are outlined in Table 2.

TABLE 2. Physical Examination of Patients with Suspected Metabolic Brain Disease

History (from relatives or friends)
- Previous medical illnesses (diabetes, uremia, heart disease)
- Previous psychiatric history
- Access to drugs (sedative, psychotropic drugs)
- Recent complaints (headache, depression)

General physical examination
- Evidence of trauma
- Evidence of chronic or acute systemic illness
- Ventilation (see Table 3)

Neurologic examination
- Mental status
  - Affect (agitated, depressed, apathetic)
  - Alertness (delirium, obtundation, stupor, coma)
  - Orientation (time, place, person)
  - Perceptual abnormalities (illusions, delusions, hallucinations)
  - Psychomotor activity
- Motor examination
  - Focal weakness
  - Tremor
  - Asterixis
  - Myoclonus
  - Seizures
- Autonomic examination
  - Pupillary size and responses
  - Temperature
  - Heart rate and rhythm
  - Diaphoresis

State of Consciousness and Mental Content. Mental changes are the earliest and most subtle sign of metabolic brain disease. Restlessness or lethargy, emotional lability, insomnia or drowsiness, and vivid nightmares may appear before other mental changes. Patients often appear fearful and anxious, or depressed. They may express the fear that they are "going crazy." Patients may lie quietly or sleep when left alone, and they rarely read or tend to the world around them. Alternately, they may be restless, irritable, and easily distracted. With more severe metabolic disturbances, patients become drowsy and finally stuporous or comatose. The particular affect that prevails in patients with metabolic encephalopathy depends partly on the nature of the illness and partly on the rapidity of its development; previous personality often has surprisingly little influence. Thus, barbiturate- or alcohol-withdrawal syndromes, acute liver necrosis, and porphyria often cause an agitated delirium, whereas uremia, pulmonary encephalopathy, and anoxia usually produce a more quiet illness. Rapidly occurring metabolic processes are more likely to produce agitated delirium than those that develop slowly.

Disturbances in cognition appear along with altered alertness and awareness and are characterized by difficulties with immediate recall and the ability to abstract. Normal subjects readily recall and repeat 6 or 7 digits forward and 5 or 6 backward and can identify the common denominator between such pairs as an apple and an orange or a fly and a tree, but delirious patients cannot. However, innate intelligence and education also determine cognitive abilities and, unless the physician has examined the patient previously, it is difficult to attribute mild disturbances to a metabolic defect. An early sign of delirium, although usually not as early a sign as altered alertness and cognition, is impairment of memory and orientation. Loss of memory for recent events with relative preservation of remote memory is a hallmark of metabolic and other organic brain disease and is tested by asking the patient about the names of his doctors, some important current events, and his recent activities. Orientation to place and time should be specifically tested by asking the date and year, the day of the week, and the present location. Orientation for time, particularly the year, is lost early in patients with delirium and orientation for place a little later.

Perceptual errors, e.g., mistaking the physician for an old friend or family member, illusions, and hallucinations are common accompaniments of delirium. They frighten and agitate some patients, but are quietly tolerated by others. The nature of the illusions and hallucinations seems to be a property of the individual's personality, and often the same hallucinations accompany separate episodes of delirium. A quiet, withdrawn patient must be specifically asked about hallucinations, because he often fails either to volunteer the information or to behave as if he were hallucinating. Hallucinations of metabolic origin are usually visual by contrast with those of schizophrenia, which are usually auditory.

Fluctuations of the mental status are a hallmark of metabolic encephalopathy. Patients may be totally out of contact one moment and lucid the next. Lucid intervals appear unpredictably and last for minutes or hours. Some of the fluctuation is environmentally related. Thus delirious patients characteristically become more disoriented at night, in unfamiliar surroundings, and in situations in which restraints and background noise and unfamiliar activity decrease familiar sensory stimuli. One study demonstrated a significantly higher incidence of postoperative delirium in patients treated in a windowless intensive care unit than in those treated in a similar one with windows.

Motor Activity. Tremor, asterixis, and multifocal myoclonus are characteristic of metabolic brain disease, and the specificity of the latter two makes them the most important physical signs that distinguish metabolic encephalopathy from psychiatric illness or from structural brain disease.

The *tremor* of delirious patients is coarse and irregular at a rate of about eight to ten per second. It is usually absent at complete rest. It is best seen in the fingers of the outstretched hands. It is less specific than asterixis and multifocal myoclonus, and may be seen in patients with psychiatric disease as well as systemic illness not associated with delirium.

Asterixis is an abnormal, involuntary jerking movement elicited in the hands by asking patients to dorsiflex the wrist and spread the extended fingers. In its mildest form there are irregular random lateral jerking movements of the fingers at the metacarpal phalangeal joints. With fully developed asterixis there is sudden palmar flexion of the fingers at the metacarpal phalangeal joint and of the wrist. The movements are asynchronous in the two hands, occur every 2 to 30 seconds, recover quickly, and cannot be controlled by the patient, even when he is aware of their presence. Asterixis may also involve the feet and tongue. In the lightly unconscious patient the same movement can sometimes be evoked by passively dorsiflexing the wrist or the ankles. Bilateral asterixis almost universally accompanies metabolic encephalopathy at some stage of the illness. It is absent in patients with psychiatric disorders unless they are taking large amounts of drugs, and is encountered extremely rarely, and then unilaterally, in patients with gross structural brain disease such as decompensating subdural hematomas or deep hemispheral infarcts encroaching on the diencephalon.

Multifocal myoclonus consists of sudden nonrhythmic, nonpatterned gross muscle contractions in a resting person. The movements are most common in the face and shoulders but occur anywhere in the body. Multifocal myoclonus can often be elicited, if not present at rest, by passive movements of the shoulder and upper arm. It occurs in a later and more severe stage of metabolic illness than does asterixis, and may physiologically represent a more intense and widespread manifestation of that abnormal movement. Multifocal myoclonus makes its most frequent appearance in uremia, hypercarbic-anoxic encephalopathy, and penicillin overdose, but can occur in virtually all metabolic encephalopathies.

Psychomotor activity ranges from extreme hyperactivity to total immobility. Delirious patients may be unwilling or unable to stay in bed, pacing the halls, in constant movement, with outbursts of aggressiveness which may culminate in attacks on others. With more severe delirium, there may be groping movements, picking at the bedclothes, and constant tossing and turning. Such patients may fall out of bed and injure themselves. Increased psychomotor activity is typically observed in acute deliria such as delirium tremens and drug withdrawal states. More commonly, delirium is manifested by reduced activity, with the patient lethargic, drowsy, and generally bradykinetic. The same patient may run the gamut from psychomotor overactivity to reduced activity during the course of the same delirium. *Speech* is often abnormal. Patients with increased psychomotor behavior often speak rapidly, with a muttering or slurred speech which, because of its speed, is incomprehensible. Patients with reduced psychomotor activity may speak slowly, monotonously, and so softly as not to be clearly heard.

Seizures, weakness, and *hyperactive stretch reflexes* frequently accompany severe metabolic brain disease. The seizures are usually generalized, and the motor abnormalities are usually symmetrical. Focal paresis and focal seizures are by no means rare, however, especially with anoxia or hypoglycemia. Signs of focal disturbance make it more difficult to distinguish between metabolic and structural brain disease. However, in metabolic brain disease the focal signs are usually less severe and more fleeting, and they are accompanied by more widespread neurologic dysfunction than in gross structural disease.

Autonomic Activity. Pupillary light reactions are always preserved in metabolic coma with the few exceptions to be mentioned, and absence of the pupillary light reaction strongly suggests a structural lesion. The exceptions are glutethimide intoxication, which may produce mid-position or slightly dilated fixed pupils; anticholinergic drug administration, which produces fixed, dilated pupils; and exposure to severe anoxia, or asphyxia, which produces fixed dilated pupils and, if sustained, probably implies irreversible brain damage.

Hypothermia is common in delirious patients with myxedema, hypoglycemia, and barbiturate intoxication. Hyperthermia with profuse perspiration and tachycardia accompanies most agitated deliria and is especially common with delirium tremens. Hyperthermia without perspiration suggests anticholinergic drug ingestion or infection. Hyperthermia also marks salicylate and occasionally phenothiazine overdosage.

Ventilation. The clinical features of delirium that have been described are common to many metabolic disorders and aid little in the differential diagnosis of specific types of metabolic coma. Ventilation is an exception. A rapid evaluation of the patient's ventilatory status, coupled with an estimate of blood acid-base balance, frequently narrows the range of possible causes of metabolic coma. Some causes of metabolic brain disease associated with ventilatory abnormalities are listed in Table 3. A careful clinical examination of the respiratory rate and depth usually allows the physician to estimate whether his patient is hyperventilating, eupneic, or hypoventilating. Caution must be exercised in evaluating patients with severe emphysema whose respiratory effort is increased and who may be tachypneic but nevertheless hypoventilating because of ineffective lungs. Caution must also be used in evaluating patients poisoned with depressant drugs who appear to be hypoventilating but are actually eupneic because their metabolic needs are so low. Unexplained abnormalities in the respiratory pattern demand rapid determination of blood gas and acid-base status. As may be seen in Table 3, a delirious and clinically *hyperventilating* adult with a low serum pH probably has diabetic ketosis, uremia, lactic

TABLE 3. A Differential Analysis of Hyperventilation and Hypoventilation in Delirious Patients

Clinical and Laboratory Findings	Probable Diagnosis
I. Hyperventilation:	
A. Metabolic acidosis	
(arterial pH <7.30, Pco_2 <35, HCO_3^- <10 mEq per liter)	
1. BUN > 60 mg per 100 ml	Uremic encephalopathy
2. Hyperglycemia (blood sugar > 250 mg per 100 ml)	Diabetic coma
a. 4+ Serum acetone	Diabetic ketoacidosis
b. No acetonemia	Diabetic lactic acidosis
3. Cyanosis (Po_2 <50 mm Hg) – shock	Anoxic lactic acidosis
4. History: diarrhea; hyperchloremia, ±hypokalemia	Diarrheal acidosis
5. Hyponatremia, hyperkalemia, ±hypoglycemia	Addison's disease
6. BUN, sugar, oxygen, blood pressure – normal	Exogenous poisoning
a. Paraldehyde odor on breath	Acidosis secondary to paraldehyde ingestion
b. Hyperemic optic discs, dilated sluggish pupils	Methyl alcohol poisoning
c. Oxalate crystals in urine	Ethylene glycol poisoning
7. None of the abnormal findings above	Spontaneous lactic acidosis
B. Respiratory alkalosis	
(arterial pH >7.45, Pco_2 <35, HCO_3^- >15 mEq per liter)	
1. Po_2 >50, hepatomegaly, serum NH_3 elevated	Hepatic encephalopathy
2. Po_2 <50, cyanosis	Cardiopulmonary disease
a. Rales, elevated venous pressure, cardiomegaly	Pulmonary edema
b. No heart disease	Pneumonia, alveolar-capillary block, pulmonary emboli
3. Absent pupillary and oculovestibular responses, decerebrate rigidity	Central neurogenic hyperventilation
4. Nystagmus on caloric testing, normal examination	Psychogenic hyperventilation
C. Mixed respiratory alkalosis and metabolic acidosis	
(arterial pH >7.35, Pco_2 <35, HCO_3^- <15 mEq per liter)	
1. Fever, tachycardia, hypotension	Gram-negative sepsis
2. Hyperthermia, positive urine $FeCl_3$ test	Salicylate poisoning
3. Abnormal liver function tests	Hepatic encephalopathy
II. Hypoventilation:	
A. Respiratory acidosis	
(arterial pH <7.30, Pco_2 >45, HCO_3^- >20 mEq per liter)	
1. Serum HCO_3^- >20 mEq per liter but <30 mEq per liter	
a. Normal lungs	Depressant drug poisoning
b. Rales, emphysema, Po_2 <40 mm Hg	Chronic pulmonary disease with acute CO_2 retention
2. Serum HCO_3^- >35 mEq per liter	
a. Normal lungs	
(1) Obesity	Pickwickian syndrome
(2) Not obese	"Central alveolar hypoventilation"
b. Rales, emphysema, Po_2 <40 mm Hg	Chronic pulmonary disease with slowly developing CO_2 retention
B. Metabolic alkalosis	
(arterial pH >7.45, Pco_2 <55, HCO_3^- >35 mEq per liter)	
a. Alkali ingestion	
History of peptic ulcer	$NaHCO_3$ ingestion alkalosis
b. Gastric acid losses	
Vomiting, hypotension, hypovolemia	Gastric HCl depletion
c. Renal acid losses	
(1) Edema, heart disease	Diuretic therapy
(2) Hypokalemia, moon face, truncal obesity	Cushing's syndrome secondary to adrenal hyperfunction, steroid therapy, hormone-secreting lung neoplasms
(3) Hypertension, hypokalemia	Primary hyperaldosteronism

acidosis, or poisoning with an acidic product. Severe metabolic acidosis, if not treated, is rapidly lethal. Uremia, diabetes, and Addison's disease can be treated specifically (see Ch. 603, 806, and 846), and the others often respond to prompt and urgent treatment of the acidosis by infusion of bicarbonate. If, however, the serum pH is elevated in the delirious and hyperventilating adult, pulmonary disease, cardiac disease, hepatic coma, or neurogenic hyperventilation are the possible causes. Pneumonia is probably the most common cause of mild respiratory alkalosis in unconscious patients; the others can be evaluated by appropriate laboratory tests. When the serum pH is elevated and the bicarbonate is between 10 and 15 mEq per liter (mixed respiratory alkalosis and metabolic acidosis), sepsis, especially with gram-negative organisms, salicylism (which causes acidosis in children, alkalosis in adults), and severe hepatic coma are the probable causes.

A similar analysis can be applied to *hypoventilating* patients. In these, the severe problems are depressant drug poisoning, which produces a low serum pH with a normal bicarbonate, and chronic pulmonary failure, which produces a low serum pH and usually a high serum bicarbonate. (The serum bicarbonate level indicates the duration of hypoventilation.) Both situations demand ventilatory support.

Electroencephalogram (EEG). The EEG is useful in evaluating patients with metabolic brain disease because it is slower than in normal subjects and because it is symmetrical. The slowing indicates that there is neural dysfunction, and the bilateral symmetry suggests a diffuse process. The degree of slowing roughly parallels the severity of the encephalopathy. The normal EEG has a basic frequency of 8 to 13 per second. In metabolic disease, bilateral, synchronous, paroxysmal bursts of 1 to 3 per second activity are frequently superimposed upon a background of mildly slow 5 to 7 cps activity. A normal EEG is incompatible with severe delirium, and an EEG with focal or unilateral slow activity strongly suggests a structural and not a metabolic brain disorder.

Other Laboratory Tests. The causes of metabolic coma are legion, and a final diagnosis usually depends on extensive laboratory tests. The tests which should be performed immediately to establish the presence of life-threatening metabolic defects are listed in Table 4, along with those whose results are not available immediately but should be done as soon as possible if the diagnosis is unclear.

TABLE 4. Laboratory Evaluation of Metabolic Brain Disease

Test	Reason for Test
Immediate:	
Glucose	Hypoglycemia, hyperosmolar coma
Na^+	Osmolar abnormalities
Ca^{++}	Hyper- or hypocalcemia
BUN	Uremia
pH, Pco_2	Acidosis, alkalosis
Po_2	Hypoxia
Lumbar puncture	Infection, hemorrhage
Later:	
Liver function tests	Hepatic coma
Sedative drug levels	Overdose
Blood and CSF culture	Sepsis, encephalitis, meningitis
Full electrolytes, including Mg^{++}	Electrolyte imbalance
EEG	

DIAGNOSIS OF METABOLIC ENCEPHALOPATHY

The physician should consider metabolic encephalopathy as the possible diagnosis for every patient whose thinking, behavior, or state of consciousness has recently become disordered. The diagnosis requires, first, that one establish that metabolic encephalopathy rather than psychiatric disease or a structural brain lesion is causing the abnormal behavior and, second, that one identify the specific metabolic illness responsible.

Psychiatric disease is distinguished in the awake patient by examination of the mental status and the motor function. Patients with psychogenic amnesia who are disoriented claim to be confused about who they are as well as to the place and time; patients with metabolic brain disorders always know who they are. Hallucinations in psychiatric illness are usually auditory; in metabolic illness they are usually visual. Recent memory and cognitive abilities are generally preserved in psychiatric patients but are lost early in patients with metabolic illness. Tremor plagues anxious patients, and occasionally generalized seizures wrack those with catatonic schizophrenia, but asterixis and multifocal myoclonus are never present in psychiatric disease. Asterixis, if carefully searched for, is present in most patients with metabolic brain disease. Rarely, a patient with "hysterical coma" will present a diagnostic problem. Such patients are quietly unresponsive, and all their limbs are flaccid, but they often strongly resist passive eye opening. If the diagnosis is doubtful, irrigating the tympanum with 50 ml of cold water is informative; this procedure produces physiologic nystagmus in the patient with "hysterical coma," but only tonic eye deviation in the comatose patient with metabolic disease. The EEG in "hysterical coma" shows a normal awake record; it is always abnormal in metabolic coma.

Supratentorial mass lesions that encroach on the diencephalon produce diffuse brain dysfunction (see Ch. 319). However, supratentorial lesions produce focal motor and/or sensory signs early in the illness, often before mental changes, and these focal signs either persist or grow worse. Hemiparesis or hemisensory defects, although occasionally present in metabolic disease, are usually mild, often fleeting, and generally appear only after consciousness is lost. Late in the course of mass lesions, when transtentorial herniation has impaired midbrain function, bilateral decorticate or decerebrate rigidity usually replaces unilateral motor signs. These motor signs of midbrain dysfunction may also be present in metabolic coma, but in metabolic coma the pupillary light reflexes are retained, thereby ruling out a structural lesion. The EEG of a patient with a supratentorial mass lesion is usually slow either focally in one area or laterally over one hemisphere; that of a patient with metabolic brain disease, even when focal neurologic abnormalities are present, is symmetrically slow. Skull roentgenograms of patients with structural lesions reveal shift of the pineal gland (if calcified) away from the side of the mass, but the pineal is midline in metabolic disease. If doubt still persists, brain scanning or angiography outlines structural lesions causing coma but is unremarkable in metabolic disorders.

Subtentorial structural lesions are distinguished from metabolic brain disease by the presence in the former of signs of cranial nerve and focal brainstem dysfunction. In patients with subtentorial lesions causing changes in consciousness, the pupils are almost always abnormal, either because pontine and medullary sympathetic pathways are involved or because the third nerve nuclei or fibers are destroyed. Both pupillary light reflexes and the ciliospinal reflex (pupillary dilatation to noxious cutaneous stimuli) are preserved in metabolic disease. Dysconjugate eye movements are common with subtentorial lesions, rare with metabolic disease. Unilateral facial weakness involving both the brow and lower face, unilateral facial anesthesia, absent caloric responses to one side, or eye deviation toward a paralyzed arm and leg all suggest a subtentorial lesion and are against the diagnosis of metabolic disease.

Dementia is the expression of irreversible metabolic brain disease in which the primary metabolic error usually resides in the brain rather than affects the brain secondarily. For this reason, the incipient signs of dementia can resemble delirium, and distinction may sometimes be difficult. In general, dementia begins gradually, whereas delirium begins either acutely or subacutely. Recent memory loss, cognitive difficulties, and disorientation to place occur early in dementia and precede any change in consciousness, whereas lethargy, apathy, decreased awareness, and disorientation in time are early marks of delirium. Tremor, asterixis, and myoclonus are rare in dementia (except myoclonus in Creutzfeldt-Jakob disease). Mild or moderate dementia reduces the brain's defenses against metabolic insults, and thus it is common for a fully reversible delirium to complicate mild systemic illnesses in demented patients. In these cases only treatment of the systemic disorders will separate the delirious component from the dementia (see Ch. 326 to 331).

Differential Diagnosis. Delirium means that a metabolic illness is so advanced that it not only threatens brain function but may threaten life itself unless promptly diagnosed and reversed by treatment. Since the neurologic manifestations of the various metabolic encephalopathies are often similar, specific diagnosis by physical examination is often impossible, so some systematic approach to the problem is needed.

In Table 1 are listed all of the common and many of the less frequent causes of metabolic brain disease. Those marked with an asterisk either alone or in combination account for most of the delirium encountered on general medical wards. The table is designed as a checklist; the specific symptoms, signs, and management of each of the systemic disorders causing delirium can be found elsewhere in this book.

When the cause of delirium is unclear, the first conditions to consider are *hypoxia, hypoglycemia,* and *metabolic acidosis.* Unless promptly treated, all three are potentially rapidly lethal, and the first two very quickly damage the brain irreversibly.

Certain physical signs, such as respiratory abnormalities, convulsions, and fever, suggest specific diagnoses. The examination of respiration aids in the diagnosis of pulmonary encephalopathy, sedative drug poisoning, gram-negative sepsis, and hepatic coma (Table 3). Often an early clue to the diagnosis of hepatic coma is the presence of respiratory alkalosis, which then prompts liver function tests or a blood ammonia determination to support the diagnosis. *Generalized convulsions* occur in many metabolic brain disorders, especially with hypoxia and hypoglycemia. Repeated seizures are dangerous since they create the risk of brain damage and should be treated even before their cause is clear. If hypoxia and hypoglycemia are not the cause, repeated seizures suggest sedative drug withdrawal, uremia, hyponatremia, hypocalcemia, or penicillin encephalopathy.

Agitated delirium accompanied by fever prompts immediate consideration of intracranial infection. Often the patient with meningitis is so combative that nuchal rigidity cannot be adequately assessed, and only lumbar puncture confirms the diagnosis. A lumbar puncture should be performed on any patient who is delirious without obvious cause and who lacks evidence of sustained increased intracranial pressure. Encephalitis and subarachnoid hemorrhage often present initially with delirium accompanied by little or no fever and no nuchal rigidity, and may not be diagnosed unless the cerebrospinal fluid is examined. In any delirious patient with nystagmus or ocular palsies, thiamin deficiency encephalopathy (see Ch. 404 to 406) should be immediately considered, because if this condition is untreated, cardiovascular collapse and death may follow.

Once the dangerous and potentially lethal illnesses detailed above are excluded, there is time to consider the many other causes of metabolic brain disease and to make the tests appropriate to their diagnosis. In most cases, a single cause for delirium is not found. Instead, the patient has multiple metabolic defects, no one of which is sufficient to produce delirium, but the sum total of which in a susceptible patient is responsible. A common example is an *elderly* patient with mild *congestive heart failure, anemia,* and *hypoxia* being given *sedative drugs* for agitation and diuretics which have caused an electrolyte imbalance. The dismay caused by the multiplicity of diagnostic possibilities is partially offset when the physician makes the happy therapeutic discovery that treatment of any one of the metabolic disorders may substantially improve his patient's delirium.

PROGNOSIS AND TREATMENT OF METABOLIC BRAIN DISEASE

Metabolic brain disease can be definitively treated only by correcting the systemic disorder responsible for the delirium, and the effectiveness of this correction, in turn, determines the prognosis of the delirium. With the exception of severe hypoxia, hypoglycemia, or thiamin deficiency, all of which can cause neuronal death, delirium clears as the systemic disorder causing it improves. Often, however, the encephalopathy improves much more slowly than the systemic illness so that severe encephalopathy may persist four to five days or more after the systemic disorder has been fully reversed. Such a delay need not portend an unfavorable outcome, and vigorous efforts to prevent infections and other complications of delirium and coma are indicated during this period, for full recovery of cerebral function still is possible.

Certain general therapeutic measures apply to all delirious patients (Table 5). An adequate *airway* and *oxygenation* of the blood must be assured. For stuporous or comatose patients, this may require an endotracheal tube or tracheostomy. *Blood volume, cardiac output,* and *blood pressure* must be maintained at near normal levels to assure adequate cerebral blood flow. If the cause of coma is not known, a blood glucose should be obtained; but even before the results are reported, intravenous glucose (50 ml of 50 per cent solution) should be given to assure that hypoglycemia will not cause irreversible brain damage. Abnormalities of *acid-base balance* and of

TABLE 5. Immediate Treatment of Metabolic Brain Disease

1. Assure oxygenation
2. Maintain circulation
3. Give glucose
4. Restore acid-base balance
5. Treat infection
6. Control body temperature
7. Stop seizures

electrolyte balance should be corrected. Correction should be carried out over several hours, because too rapid correction often leads to other metabolic abnormalities. Infection should be treated and fever lowered.

The awake, delirious patient should be kept in a quiet room, away from the unfamiliar noises and bustle of the general ward. The room should be well lighted, and a light kept burning at night, because darkness accentuates disorientation and hallucinations. Physicians and nurses can reassure the patient by introducing themselves at each contact and quietly apprising him of his whereabouts. All procedures must be carefully and often repetitively explained before they are done. Drugs not essential for treatment of the patient's systemic illness should be withdrawn. This applies particularly to sedatives, narcotics, and tranquilizers, all of which commonly cause or accentuate delirium; it also applies to extensive use of diuretics, antihypertensive drugs, anticonvulsants, and even digitalis, medications that are less widely recognized to cause or accentuate delirium. If the patient is agitated and hyperactive, small doses of diazepam, starting with 5 mg orally or intramuscularly, and increasing as necessary, can be given to quiet him but not to render him unresponsive.

Careful attention is required to other systemic disorders that, although not of themselves sufficiently severe to cause delirium, may increase an already present encephalopathy. Oxygen should be given to mildly hypoxic patients, and transfusions should be administered to those with significant anemia. Mild electrolyte disorders such as hypokalemia and hyponatremia are diagnosed by periodic serum electrolyte determinations and are corrected by appropriate fluid control. Such measures often improve a patient's delirium considerably, even if the primary cause cannot be treated. Fluid losses should be routinely measured and replaced parenterally if the patient is not eating. Vital signs and the state of consciousness must be checked frequently to ensure that sudden worsening does not go undetected.

Lipowski, Z. J.: Delirium, clouding of consciousness and confusion. J. Nerv. Ment. Dis., 145:227, 1967.

Plum, F., and Posner, J. B.: The Diagnosis of Stupor and Coma. 2nd ed. Philadelphia, F. A. Davis Company, 1972.

Sokoloff, L.: Circulation and energy metabolism of the brain. *In* Albers, R. W., Siegel, G. J., Katzman, R., and Agranoff, B. W. (eds.): Basic Neurochemistry. Boston, Little, Brown & Company, 1972, Chap. 15, pp. 299–326.

321. SLEEP AND ITS DISORDERS

Fred Plum

DEFINITION

Adult man spends one third of each day asleep. Yet why he sleeps and what "rest" does for his tissues are questions which thus far defy satisfactory answers.

Sleep is a recurrent state of relative inactivity of mind and body movement, readily interrupted by external stimuli but largely preventing any awareness of self or environment while it exists. The mere physiologic ability to cycle between sleep and wakefulness requires relatively little brain, although the amount of brain present modifies the cyclic pattern. Newborn babies, in whom the cerebral hemispheres are still little developed, sleep two thirds of each 24 hours in a series of relatively short sleep-wake cycles; anencephalic infants, whose brain stops at the midbrain, tend to do the same, as do adults who have suffered extensive injury to the cerebral hemispheres. Paralleling the evolving functional development of the hemispheres in older children, periods of continuous wakefulness become longer and longer until at about the age of six the adult diurnal pattern of sleep is established. Children up to about the age of 13 sleep more than adults, and women sleep more than men. Data reviewed by Kleitman indicate a mean duration of sleep in healthy adults of about eight hours, with little difference among subjects of different ethnic groups, occupations, or intelligence.

THE PHYSIOLOGY OF SLEEP

Knowledge about the fundamental physiology of underlying states of sleep and wakefulness has accumulated rapidly during the past two decades. These have disclosed that sleep is an active state composed of several identifiable stages regulated by the relations between distinct nuclear areas in the lower brainstem reticular formation and their connections with both more rostral and more caudal neural structures. Sleep is thus a very primitive vegetative function in the organization of the mammalian nervous system. Furthermore, different stages of sleep and wakefulness appear to depend on activity in anatomic pathways employing distinct neurotransmitter agents, lending hope that pharmacologic approaches may lead to better future methods of treating disordered sleep in patients.

The anatomy of sleep, like that of its antithesis, wakefulness, depends upon projections from centers located mainly in the caudal pontine reticular nucleus, the locus caeruleus, the vestibular nuclei, and the oculomotor control centers. Very little brain above the level of the midbrain is required for sleeping and waking to occur, because sleep-wake cycles exist in the most primitive vertebrates as well as in humans born with little or no brain tissue above the midbrain level. Sleep has at least two different forms, one characterized by low voltage fast activity on the EEG and accompanied by skeletal muscle atonia and rapid eye movements (thus the term REM sleep), and the other by increasingly slower waves on the EEG (SW sleep) as sleep becomes deeper. Most dreaming occurs during REM sleep. All evidence indicates that in the healthy state a balance occurs between REM and SW sleep in which REM occupies about one-quarter of the total time and recurs in episodes about every 100 minutes. Drugs which alter sleep affect these different stages in different ways, and there is evidence that human beings have a specific biologic need for a certain minimum of REM sleep as well as of total sleep.

Although few symptoms are more distressing than insomnia, it is not clear just why one needs sleep or what function the state serves. Over-all cerebral metabolism does not change during sleep. However, both Pappenheimer and Monnier have extracted from the cerebrospinal fluid or cerebral blood of sleep-deprived animals a factor that induces sleep when infused into wakeful recipients. Recent studies suggest that the induction and maintenance of the stages of sleep and waking are controlled at least in part by local concentrations in the brainstem of the biogenic amines serotonin and norepinephrine. Furthermore, these amines may serve as transmitters in specific brainstem pathways involved in sleep functions. However, the experimental evidence in the field still has inconsistencies, and it is not yet possible to describe a pharmacologic-physiologic model which fits all the observed requirements. The following references supply the most recent information in this fast-developing field.

Koella, W. P., and Levin, P. (eds.): Sleep. Proc. 1st European Congress of Sleep Research. Basel, Karger, 1973.

Pappenheimer, J. R., Fencl, V., Karnovsky, M. K., and Koski, G.: Peptides in cerebrospinal fluid and their relation to sleep and activity. *In* Plum, F. (ed.): Brain Dysfunction in Metabolic Disorders. Res. Publ. Assoc. Res. Nerv. Ment. Dis., 53:201, 1974.

Williams, H. L.: The new biology of sleep. J. Psychiatr. Res., 8:445, 1971.

DISORDERS OF THE QUALITY OF SLEEP

Too little sleep is known as *insomnia* and too much as *hypersomnia.* Insomnia most frequently results from functional disorders, whereas hypersomnia is often, but not invariably, a sign of organic neurologic disease.

Insomnia. Insomnia has three patterns: difficulty in falling asleep after retiring, intermittent waking throughout the period of attempted sleep, and early awakening. Direct observations on patients suffering from insomnia almost always reveal that they are less wakeful than they think, and there is little evidence that chronic insomnia takes any physical toll. Nevertheless, even brief difficulties in falling or staying asleep cause great subjective distress and lead to a large annual consumption of sedatives.

Physical causes of insomnia are comparatively few. Patients with chronic pain often suffer more at night, which keeps them awake. Those with unrecognized orthopnea resulting from heart disease sometimes translate their difficulties into a primary complaint of sleeplessness; the same is true of patients with marginal pulmonary insufficiency, in whom inability to sleep may be the first sign of respiratory decompensation. Insomnia can be an early symptom of acute infectious illness and is common in Sydenham's chorea and in bulbar poliomyelitis. Aside from these occasional associations with physical illness, difficulty in sleeping reflects mainly anxiety, worry, or depression. Whether insomnia occurs on going to bed or with early awakening helps relatively little in estimating its seriousness as a symptom.

To treat insomnia requires understanding, patience, a close attention to its accompaniments, and a willingness to discuss psychologic issues. Patients with difficulty in sleeping should be advised to eat light evening meals and to avoid stimulants such as coffee or tea after midday. Early morning awakening in the elderly most frequently reflects a declining need for sleep, and is best met by having the subject plan his day better and avoid afternoon naps. All patients are reassured by knowing that sleeplessness will not harm their bodies, and many regain the ability to sleep after a sympathetic physician has taken the time to discuss with them the issues that keep them awake. Patients with insomnia should always be asked sympathetically but directly if they are depressed and particularly if they have considered suicide. Drugs to treat insomnia should be used sparingly. All sedatives are potentially addicting, and most subjects with severe insomnia rapidly develop tolerance to sedation. Alcoholic nightcaps are inadvisable; the sedative effect is moderate and the temptation to "drown" anxiety is great. The most widely used sedatives and their recommended starting dose in grams are chloral hydrate, 1.0; secobarbital sodium, 0.1; pentobarbital sodium, 0.1; and glutethimide, 0.5. Any of these agents are also satisfactory for sedating patients in hospital, and the dosage can be repeated safely at least once or even twice in that setting. When insomnia is associated with depression, amitriptyline, 25 to 100 mg, is useful; the entire dose should be given at bedtime, starting at the lower dose and increasing. Insomnia coupled with more severe symptoms of depression demands close supervision and skilled psychologic management.

Hypersomnia. Hypersomnia occasionally signifies nothing more serious than boredom and mild depression, particularly among adolescents and young adults. Young women sometimes develop transient hypersomnia during menstruation. Occasionally one encounters hysterical hypersomnia, with which patients may claim to sleep for days at a time, then awaken fully. More often, however, excessive sleepiness signifies either narcolepsy or structural nervous system disease; among patients with the latter, the dividing line between prolonged hypersomnia and coma may be difficult to establish. Many neurologic conditions prolong or excessively deepen sleep. These include increased intracranial pressure, neoplasms around the third ventricle or in the posterior fossa, head trauma, encephalitis, and many metabolic disorders, including carbon dioxide retention, hepatic encephalopathy, uremia, pituitary insufficiency, and the surreptitious taking of drugs. With so many potential causes, the approach to hypersomnia of unknown cause resembles that employed to evaluate undiagnosed coma.

A rare condition of recurrent hypersomnia combined with excessive eating is sometimes observed in adolescent males, and is known as the *Kleine-Levin syndrome.* The cause is unknown, but the attacks last several days to a week or more, during which the patient eats voraciously and often develops disturbed behavior. Intervals of months to years of normal behavior separate the attacks. There is no treatment, and the attacks tend to disappear as the patient reaches adulthood.

Narcolepsy. *Definition and Etiology.* Narcolepsy is a chronic disorder characterized by recurrent and excessive drowsiness or sleepiness from which subjects are readily awakened. It is frequently accompanied by cataplexy, sleep paralysis, and, less often, hypnagogic hallucinations. As with most illnesses of unknown origin, many causes have been suggested. Some observers postulate a defect in the reticular formation of the brainstem, particularly since the REM stage tends to appear at the onset of narcoleptic sleep rather than approximately 90 minutes later, as with normal sleep. Other workers have been struck with the high incidence of psychologic disturbances (about 10 per cent of narcoleptics develop schizophrenic reactions), and have tended to regard this as the cause rather than an associated symptom of the illness. A high familial incidence of narcolepsy has been invoked as indirect evidence that the syndrome has a constitutional basis.

Clinical Findings. Narcolepsy is uncommon but not rare. Both men and women are affected, and there appears to be no ethnic predilection. The onset is usually insidious during adolescence or young adulthood. Once the predisposition to excessive sleepiness starts, it is likely to last a lifetime if not treated. The symptoms range from mild drowsiness, which intrudes upon lecture hours, social events, or after-dinner conversations, to severe sleepiness in which subjects spend nearly the entire day drifting in and out of sleep, unable to work, play, or supervise the home. The sensation is reported as ordinary, uncontrollable drowsiness, perhaps with diplopia, but indistinguishable from that which normally follows severe fatigue. As witnessed by others, the sleep looks natural and is readily interrupted by stimuli. The naps refresh, but only briefly, and somnolence quickly recurs.

Cataplexy is a phenomenon of acute, brief, episodic, generalized muscular weakness, precipitated by feelings of emotion. It affects about three quarters of narcoleptic patients. In general, the stronger the emotion, the greater the muscular paresis, and patients relate that laughter, anger, or surprise "turns them to jelly" and induces brief collapse or aphonia without impaired consciousness. *Sleep paralysis* is a sensation of being unable to move while drifting into sleep or, less often, just upon awakening. Usually, brief contact with another person or strong effort interrupts the sensation, which lasts only a few seconds anyway. *Hypnagogic hallucinations* principally coincide with the early drifting phase of sleep when sleep paralysis occurs. Their intensity, the completeness of the visual or auditory recollections, and the time of onset distinguish them from dreams.

Physical abnormalities are lacking in primary narcolepsy. Laboratory studies are similarly normal. Neither hypothyroidism, hypoglycemia, nor any other endocrine abnormality has been substantiated in these patients, although the basal metabolic rate is low in many, reflecting their tendency to sleep through the test. The blood gases, and particularly the arterial carbon dioxide tension, are normal if obtained while the subject is awake, and no higher than in sleeping normal persons if drawn during drowsiness. The EEG contains normal patterns but a high percentage of sleep frequencies.

Differential Diagnosis. Narcolepsy must be distinguished from psychogenic hypersomnia on the one hand, and occult central nervous system lesions on the other. Narcoleptic-cataplectic symptoms are intensifications of experiences known in a minor way to nearly everybody, and the exact point where excessive drowsiness, weakness during emotion, and sleep paralysis become a syndrome rather than a psychologic reaction to the environment can be difficult to decide in mild cases. Narcolepsy is favored if the symptoms date back to adolescence or have been present for several years, or if the drowsiness appears as a primary complaint interfering with other activities. Hypersomnia caused by toxins or central nervous system lesions usually resembles narcolepsy very little. Its onset is generally recent and fairly sharply identified in time. Also, the sleep is commonly deep, arousal is difficult, and the patients are slow and apathetic when awake in contrast to narcoleptic patients, who are alert as long as stimulated into wakefulness. Brain lesions causing hypersomnia often produce dementia and headache, neither of which complicates primary narcolepsy. Finally, structural brain lesions causing hypersomnia usually either are large or are situated near the deep midline structures of the third ventricle, and in both cases almost always result in physical signs of oculomotor, skeletal motor, or sensory dysfunction on the neurologic examination. In doubtful cases, lumbar puncture should be obtained as well as an electroencephalogram, which is almost always abnormal when a structural lesion produces hypersomnia.

Treatment. The treatment of narcolepsy is largely symptomatic. General measures include drinking coffee or tea with meals and otherwise increasing everyday stimuli to a maximum. Most patients can continue to drive automobiles, for enough warning is experienced for them to pull off the road to sleep. Narcolepsy has no relation to epilepsy, and anticonvulsants have no place in treatment. Many individual stimulants have been tried, dextroamphetamine (Dexedrine) and methylphenidate (Ritalin) being most successful. Dextroamphetamine is usually initiated with doses of 10 mg three times daily. If patients require much larger doses, slow-release capsules yield sustained effects. Methylphenidate is the present stimulant of choice and is initiated in doses of 5 to 10 mg three times daily, then gradually increased until it either relieves drowsiness or produces unwanted nervousness and irritability. In addition, the tricyclic antidepressant imipramine in doses of 25 mg three times daily is quite effective in relieving cataplexy and should be combined with methylphenidate. Monoamine oxidase inhibitors have also been used to treat narcolepsy, but produce so many undesirable side effects that their use is not recommended. All stimulant drugs cause anorexia, and subjects must prevent weight loss by making conscious efforts to eat. Serious blood dyscrasias have not been reported. Occasionally the drugs produce excessive excitement or disturbed behavior, and must be discontinued.

Critchley, M.: Periodic hypersomnia and megaphagia in adolescent males. Brain, 62:627, 1962.

Guilleminault, C., Carskadon, M., and Dement, W.: On the treatment of rapid eye movement narcolepsy. Arch. Neurol., 30:90, 1974.

Kety, S. S., Evarts, E. V., and Williams, H. L. (eds.): Sleep and Altered States of Consciousness. Res. Publ. Ass. Res. Nerv. Ment. Dis., Vol. 45, 1967.

Kleitman, N.: Sleep and Wakefulness (revised and enlarged edition). Chicago, University of Chicago Press, 1963.

Zarcone, V.: Narcolepsy. N. Engl. J. Med., 288:1156, 1973.

Section Two. FOCAL DISTURBANCES OF HIGHER NERVOUS FUNCTION

Norman Geschwind

322. LANGUAGE, APHASIA, AND RELATED DISORDERS

Language is one of the most striking biologic attributes of man. Recent evidence suggesting that some potential for language exists in chimpanzees may open up new possibilities for investigation of the neurologic foundations of linguistic behavior. At present, however, nearly all our knowledge of the neural substrate of language is based on man. Detailed postmortem studies of well-described patients have provided the majority of the information, but useful data have been accumulated from patients with other types of disorders and from studies of the effects of stimulation of the brain during operations.

A striking feature of the human brain is dominance, i.e., the superiority of one hemisphere in the performance of certain functions. Dominance is not known to exist in any mammal other than man. About 93 per cent of people are right-handed, and at least 99 per cent of right handers have left hemisphere dominance for speech.

The situation is more complex and less well defined in the non-right-handed, i.e., the left handers and those with varying degrees of ambidexterity. Such a patient becomes aphasic as a result of lesion in *either* hemisphere, although left hemisphere lesions generally produce more lasting disability. A third group, *pathologic left handers,* who have suffered early childhood injury to the left hemisphere, are usually right-brained for speech.

The cause of dominance was in dispute for many years. We now know that the temporal speech region on the left is generally larger than the corresponding area on the right. The nondominant side is, however, endowed genetically with the capacity to develop language. Thus if the dominant hemisphere is damaged before age 10 or 12, there is nearly always excellent recovery of language, although the over-all degree of mental development is slowed. Spontaneous recovery from aphasia can also occur in later life, but much less frequently. Dominance in the intact human can be studied by two recently developed techniques. The Wada test consists of the injection of sodium amytal into the internal carotid artery. This causes a hemiplegia on the side opposite the injection, but aphasia results only from injection on the dominant side. This test is especially useful to neurosurgeons to ascertain the dominant side, especially in non-right-handed patients. Another technique, the *Kimura test,* is that of dichotic listening, in which different words are simultaneously presented to the two ears. Normal individuals tend to report the words presented to the ear opposite the dominant hemisphere.

323. APHASIA

The aphasias may be defined as disorders of language secondary to lesions of the brain. In most cases there is disorder of the output of speech. In the experience of the author, aphasia in spoken speech is invariably accompanied by similar abnormalities in writing. Aphasia in spoken language is of two major types: (1) Nonfluent aphasia, in which few words are produced slowly and with great effort, and sounds are incorrectly articulated. Production of grammatical words is relatively more affected so that sentences tend to be ungrammatical, e.g., "Weather sunny." (2) Fluent aphasia, in the more extreme forms of which the patient produces runs of well-articulated speech, which has the rhythm and melody of normal language and a basically normal grammatical structure, but which tends to convey little information, e.g., "I was at the other one and then I was at this one," a fluent aphasic's circumlocutory manner of explaining that he was in another hospital previously. The speech of these patients usually contains many incorrect words, called *paraphasias. Literal* (or phonemic) *paraphasias* are substitutions of well-articulated but incorrect sounds, e.g., "spoot" for "spoon," and *verbal paraphasias* are incorrect usages of words, e.g., "knife" for "fork," or "department" for "hospital."

In differential diagnosis, one must be wary of describing *mutism* as aphasia, because even severe aphasics are usually not mute. Causes of mutism are (1) uncooperativeness, (2) psychiatric disorders, e.g., severe depression or schizophrenia, (3) widespread disorders of brain, such as trauma, subarachnoid hemorrhage, or metabolic disorders, (4) lesions of mesencephalic and pontine tegmentum, and (5) bilateral lesions of the cranial nerves serving the speech organs, their nuclei, or their supranuclear pathways.

Dysarthria should not be confused with aphasia. Dysarthric speech is incorrectly articulated, but, if transcribed, shows correct grammar and word usage. A helpful clue is that if a patient who is mute or has completely unintelligible speech can produce fully normal language (not just his own name) in writing or on a typewriter, he is almost certainly not aphasic.

A common error is to misdiagnose a fluent aphasia as schizophrenic word-salad. Several clues help to make the differential diagnosis. Fluent aphasia is much more common than schizophrenic word-salad. The schizophrenic speech disorder usually develops in chronic "back ward" schizophrenics. By contrast fluent aphasia may come on abruptly as the result of a stroke in a previously well person. Finally, fluent aphasia from vascular disease usually occurs in older people, whereas schizophrenia almost always is manifest before the age of 30.

Aphasic Syndromes and Their Localizations. *Broca's aphasia* is the result of a lesion of Broca's area, i.e., the portion of the frontal lobe just anterior to the face, lip, tongue, and mouth area of the motor cortex. This produces a nonfluent aphasia, and writing is also involved. Comprehension of language is intact. There is nearly always a right hemiplegia. *Wernicke's aphasia* results from a lesion of Wernicke's area, the posterior portion of the superior temporal gyrus. The aphasia is typically fluent. Written language is equally impaired. Comprehension of spoken and written language is severely impaired. Repetition of spoken language is poor. There is usually no hemiplegia, and other elementary neurologic signs are usually lacking. *Conduction aphasia* results from a lesion of the parietal operculum, i.e., the region lying above the sylvian fissure. There is fluent aphasia involving speech and writing, with severely impaired repetition but intact comprehension. Elementary neurologic signs are usually absent, with the occasional exception of cortical sensory loss on the opposite side. *Anomic aphasia* is characterized by fluent aphasia in speech and impairment of written language, but with intact comprehension and repetition. The components of the Gerstmann syndrome (discussed subsequently) are often present. In this syndrome the lesion, if focal, is at the region of the parietotemporal junction, but a similar syndrome is produced in nonfocal widespread disease of the brain, such as is caused by metabolic disease or by large tumors with raised intracranial pressure.

These four syndromes are the most common, and although overlapping forms are common, relatively pure forms are not rare. Certain other syndromes are much less common.

In *isolation of the speech area* there is a large lesion involving the cortex and underlying white matter in a C-shaped configuration that spares Broca's area, Wernicke's area, and their interconnections, but destroys the cortex and underlying white matter that surround the speech region. These patients either may show little spontaneous speech or may have fluent abnormal speech. The most striking characteristic of this disorder is that despite an almost total lack of comprehension, the patient can repeat well without dysarthria. This lesion is usually the result of anoxia or of carotid insufficiency. *Alexia without agraphia* is a syndrome in which the patient speaks and writes normally but cannot comprehend written language. The lesion, almost always the result of infarction in the distribution of the left posterior cerebral artery, consists of destruction of the left visual cortex and the splenium, i.e., the posterior portion, of the corpus callosum. In *alexia with agraphia* the patient can neither write nor comprehend written language, but other language functions are normal. Other components of the Gerstmann syndrome (see below) may be present. The lesion involves a portion of the left angular gyrus. A right visual field defect may occur if the lesion extends deeply into the white matter but is often absent. *Pure word-deafness* describes a syndrome in which there is dense incomprehension of language in the presence of intact hearing, although other language functions are intact. Two types of lesion produce this: either a single lesion lying subcortically in the posterior temporal lobe or bilateral lesions of the middle portion of the first temporal gyrus. *Pure agraphia* is extremely rare as the result of any focal lesion, but is common in patients with confusional states of toxic, metabolic, or traumatic origin.

324. OTHER DISORDERS OF THE HIGHER FUNCTIONS

Apraxia. Apraxia is the inability to perform a learned act in response to a stimulus which would normally elicit it, and which cannot be accounted for by weakness, incoordination, reflex change, sensory loss, incomprehension, inattention, or uncooperativeness. Three lesions may produce apraxia. With lesions of the corpus callosum there will be apraxia of the left side of the body, but not of the right or of the face. Patients with Broca's aphasia (who usually have a right hemiplegia) will show apraxia that is usually most marked in the face and is also often present in the left limbs. With lesions in the left parietal operculum, producing a conduction aphasia, there is usually apraxia in the face (where it is most marked) and in the limbs of both sides of the body. In all forms of apraxia whole-body movements, e.g., "stand up," "sit down," "turn around," and movements of eye-closing and eye-opening are best preserved. In all forms of apraxia the defect is most marked to verbal command (although the patient comprehends), usually somewhat less marked on imitation of the examiner, and least marked in the handling of objects, although in some patients even this latter category is impaired.

Agnosia. Agnosia is a failure of recognition of complex stimuli in the face of preserved elementary perception. The most common form is visual agnosia, in which there are usually bilateral posterior occipital lobe lesions. The agnosias are less well understood than the aphasias or apraxias.

Callosal Syndromes. These were first brilliantly described by Hugo Liepmann in the early 1900's, but have been rediscovered only in recent years. In some cases of anterior cerebral artery occlusion there is infarction of the anterior four fifths of the corpus callosum. The patient will carry out verbal commands with the right hand but not the left. He will name objects held (concealed from vision) in the right hand but not the left. He can, however, with the left hand draw or select from a group of objects the one previously held in the left hand. He manifests, in brief, inability to transfer information between the two hemispheres. Involvement of the splenium of the corpus callosum plays a role in alexia without agraphia (see Ch. 323).

Gerstmann's Syndrome. This consists of agraphia, right-left disorientation, acalculia (difficulty in carrying out calculations), and finger agnosia (inability to name fingers or to identify them). The patient almost invariably also shows constructional disorder, i.e., a difficulty in drawing or copying designs, especially three-dimensional ones. When all the components of this syndrome are present, the lesion almost invariably lies in the left posterior parietal region. It should, however, be kept in mind that a single component has little localizing value. Thus constructional difficulty without the other components may result from lesions in many locations.

Right Hemisphere Syndrome. Lesions of the right parietal region produce constructional difficulty that is more severe on the average than that produced from any other site. Patients with lesions in this location may also show a dressing disorder manifested by great difficulty in putting on clothes. Milder degrees of the difficulty may be brought out by such maneuvers as putting one sleeve of the bathrobe inside out; the patient may be unable to get the bathrobe on properly.

A striking feature of acute lesions of the right hemisphere is *anosognosia,* i.e., a tendency to deny or neglect disability, or when admitting its presence, to be unconcerned with it. It is a common experience that the patient with an acute left hemiplegia will show this type of behavior, although by contrast the patient with an acute right hemiplegia will, even if aphasic, show appropriate awareness of disability and will be depressed. These disorders in right hemisphere lesions are always accompanied by a curious mental state, in which the patient shows apathy, poor attention, and often jocularity. These states (and the accompanying unconcern with illness) are usually transient, but are sometimes permanent in cases of large right parietal lesions. Patients with transient cases, however, do not necessarily have parietal lesions.

It should be noted that not all patients who deny illness suffer from right hemisphere disease. Weinstein has shown that a patient with any disability may deny illness if he is sufficiently obtunded. Thus a patient may deny blindness resulting even from disease of the eyes if he develops a confusional state from metabolic disorder or drugs.

325. MEMORY

Memory describes the processes by which past experience is stored and retrieved. Disorders of memory include *anterograde amnesia,* i.e., the failure to store new memories, or *retrograde amnesia,* i.e., disorders of storage or retrieval of memories laid down in the past.

Certain separable stages in memory storage have become clear from clinical observation. There is a stage of *immediate* memory, which is the ability to retain material presented as long as attention is not distracted. This is examined by such tests as digit span, i.e., the ability to repeat a series of digits spoken by the examiner. Most normal persons can immediately repeat a series of seven such digits. The next step is *transfer* to the long-term memory store. The first step in this is *intermediate memory* storage, and the later step is called *remote memory.* The reasons for separating these steps will become clear when we discuss the clinical syndromes.

ANATOMY OF MEMORY

Memories are probably held in short-term store simply by continuation of nervous activity. The transfer to the long-term store probably involves some molecular change either in nerve membrane or in intracellular organelles. The neural structures most involved appear to lie in the limbic system, especially the hippocampal region, mammillary bodies, and, according to some authors, the dorsomedial nuclei of the thalamus (Victor et al.). The intactness of these structures appears to be important, in some as yet undefined way, in the transfer of memories from the intermediate to the long-term stores. The memories are probably not laid down in these limbic structures, because their destruction does not lead to loss of remote memories. They must therefore act on the structures which are the sites of storage. The limbic structures are also important, as will be seen below, in retrieval from the intermediate store.

CLINICAL DISORDERS OF MEMORY

Memory disorder may be evident in widespread disorder of the brain such as may be produced by drugs or metabolic disorders. On the other hand, memory may be relatively or dramatically spared in many of the dementias. Thus memory is much less impaired than such functions as calculation and abstraction in general paresis. By contrast, in Alzheimer's disease, in which involvement of hippocampus is prominent, memory disorder is a salient feature of the initial stages.

Disease processes predominantly affecting the hippocampal-mammillary system will produce significant memory disorder with little or no effect on other intellectual functions. This clinical state is called *Korsakoff's syndrome.* When caused by thiamin deficiency, the most striking lesions are in the mammillary bodies. The hippocampus may be involved in Alzheimer's disease, head injury, or tumors. Disease of the posterior cerebral artery may cause infarction of the hippocampus. Herpes simplex encephalitis has a predilection for all the structures of the limbic system. Occasional cases of severe memory loss have been reported after bilateral removal of the medial temporal structures surgically.

In order to produce a permanent memory deficit, bilateral lesions of the mammillo-hippocampal system are required. However, a unilateral lesion of the *left* hippocampus will produce a transient memory disorder, which may last as long as three months (Geschwind and Fusillo).

The memory disorder that sometimes follows head injury illustrates well the different states of the memory process outlined above. A patient who shows this disorder, let us say a week after the episode, may exhibit the following picture. He will be alert, awake, and cooperative and may, on a standard IQ test, score in a normal or even superior range. In addition his immediate memory, as shown, for example, by digit span, will be normal. By contrast he shows an anterograde amnesia, i.e., an inability to learn new material. He also shows a retrograde amnesia extending back from 3 to 20 years. More remote memories, in particular most of what was learned before the age of 12, are much better preserved. Over the next two or three months the condition improves. The ability to learn new material reappears (but the patient will have a permanent gap in his memory for the period in which he lacked this ability). The retrograde amnesia gradually shrinks until it reaches its permanent form, with a duration of seconds to minutes. The long retrograde amnesia must therefore have been a disorder of retrieval, rather than storage. It thus appears that the integrity of the limbic structures is necessary for the retrieval from intermediate, but not remote memory. In cases of persistent Korsakoff's syndrome, such as occur frequently with other forms of disorders that produce permanent bilateral limbic system damage, the retrograde amnesia does not improve significantly.

A prominent feature of many but not all cases of Korsakoff's syndrome, especially in the early stages, is confabulation, i.e., the tendency of the patient to invent fanciful replies to questions whose answers he doesn't know.

Functional amnesia occurs in hysteria (usually young women) or in older patients who are depressed. A similar clinical picture seen in malingerers is usually easy to recognize. The patient may show either a highly selective memory disorder, e.g., denying that he is married, although all other recent and remote facts are preserved, or a global disorder, e.g., professing total amnesia for all events of his life. Failure of a patient without aphasia to state his own name is invariably not organic in origin.

Another common syndrome is the fugue state in which the patient denies any memory of his activities for a period of time ranging from hours to weeks, during which his external activities appeared normal or during which he disappeared and traveled extensively. Although some short-lasting fugue states may occasionally be the result of temporal lobe epilepsy, the author's experience has been that these are nearly all functional in origin.

Benign memory disorder, a common complaint with onset in the forties or even the late thirties, is the appearance of difficulty in recalling proper names or other specific features which are, however, usually recognized promptly. This problem often arouses great anxiety, but studies indicate that although this delimited difficulty may continue to progress over many years, it is usually not a forerunner of serious intellectual deterioration, and is often compatible with the highest levels of professional activity. It is called "benign" memory disorder to distinguish it from the rapidly progressive and disabling malignant forms in which even in the early stages the memory difficulty involves recollection of the over-all significance of many situations, rather than just isolated facts.

Geschwind, N.: Disconnexion syndromes in animals and man. Brain, 88:237, 585, 1965.
Geschwind, N.: The organization of language and the brain. Science, 170:940, 1970.
Geschwind, N., and Fusillo, M.: Color-naming defects in association with alexia. Arch. Neurol., 15:137, 1966.
Victor, M., Adams, R. D., and Collins, G. H.: The Wernicke-Korsakoff Syndrome. Philadelphia, F. A. Davis, 1971.
Zangwill, O. L.: Cerebral Dominance and Its Relation to Psychological Function. Springfield, Ill., Charles C Thomas, 1960.

Section Three. DEMENTIA

Paul R. McHugh

326. INTRODUCTION

General Considerations. Dementia means deterioration in intellectual capacity. The condition is distinguished from mental retardation, in which subnormal intellectual ability has been lifelong and may or may not be caused by brain injury; and from aphasia and Korsakoff's psychosis, in which specific intellectual skills (language and memory, respectively) have deteriorated without a proportional disturbance in other cognitive functions.

Dementia is a clinical entity. Any pathologic process affecting the cerebral hemispheres can lead to an impairment in intellectual capacity. The extent of the brain injury and not the location of injury or the nature of the neuropathology determines its severity. The diagnostic task is twofold: first, the physician must recognize the symptoms of dementia; then, he must identify the cerebral pathology producing it. The first aspect of diagnosis requires skill in testing mental function; the second, knowledge of the mode of onset of different pathologic conditions and of their particular neurologic features and diagnostic laboratory data.

Clinical Manifestations. The earliest symptoms of dementia can pass almost unrecognized. They appear as disturbances in the patient's capacities for problem solving, grasp of situation, and agility of thought. He may carry out his daily routines at home and at work adequately, but he becomes inefficient in them and may fail in the tasks that are demanding or require his special skills. Thus a physician with dementia manages his familiar patients but is less able to diagnose or prescribe for new ones. A lawyer maintains his office but misses opportunities that depend on judgment and brisk decisions. A teacher spends unusual effort for a routine lesson and is puzzled by questions from his students that go beyond the prepared material. These changes are hard to distinguish from fatigue or boredom. The appreciation of their importance will depend on how well the examiner knows the patient and on how much the patient's livelihood depends upon mental capacity. Thus relatives and fellow workers usually notice a change before doctors can be sure of it; and professional, managerial, or skilled workers are more quickly brought for help than are individuals with unskilled occupations.

As a dementia progresses, however, the disability will be obvious to all because its symptoms are defects in basic mental functions. Memory failure is often the first definite symptom. The patient becomes forgetful particularly of the events of the day, overlooks appointments, fails to remember conversations, or forgets the purpose of his errands.

Other symptoms reflect the patient's bewilderment in the face of complexity. He becomes lost in attempting to find his way in the city. He fails to understand a conversation, particularly if several people are involved, as at a meeting. He cannot follow directions that involve a series of steps.

Language presents special difficulties. He is unable to use words with facility and pertinence, but depends on clichés and habitual forms of expression. His conversation becomes rambling and repetitious, his letters long and vague, his directions to others involved and obscure. Defining a word or a proverb for his examining physician is very difficult because he is unable to call up the meaning of abstract words and concepts.

At this stage in a dementing illness, habit sustains the patient's social behavior. Yet this façade of customary manners and speech cannot hide his deficits in mental capacity if examination is carried beyond casual interchange to test his memory, his orientation, or his grasp of situations and concepts.

The dementing patient often suffers from emotional disturbances. Sudden outbursts of emotion, taking the form of anger, tears, or aggressiveness may occur when the patient is attempting a task that is beyond his present mental skill. These *catastrophic reactions* are usually of short duration, but their repeated appearance may be a prominent feature of the illness almost from its onset. They can appear under circumstances in daily life such as during a difficult decision at work or during the mental status examination if a challenging problem is presented. Any such outburst will usually last until the extra demands on the patient are relieved, and during such an outburst the patient will be unable to solve problems that are within his capacity when he is in emotional control.

More sustained and chronic emotional disorders, such as depression and anxiety, are also seen in dementing illness for reasons that are not immediately obvious. They may represent a response of the patient comprehending his growing difficulties but may also represent an injury to central nervous system mechanisms mediating emotional expression.

A symptom seen in some patients and easily confused with depression is a progressive apathy or mental inertia. This may at first be just a loss of sparkle or liveliness of character, but progresses to involve initiative and the physical energy of the patient. Such apathy can result in much poorer performance in daily affairs than can be explained at first by the cognitive disabilities, but worsens as the dementia progresses and can reach such a state of unresponsiveness that the patient is inaccessible to examination.

Finally, if the dementing disorder is relentlessly progressive, the patient will lose all his mental powers. He will be unable to care for himself or appreciate any of his surroundings. He loses his remote memories, now failing to recognize his closest relatives. He cannot care for any of his physical needs and becomes bedridden and totally unaware of his situation. At this point his life is dependent on nursing care and usually is lost to intercurrent infection or malnutrition.

Dementia is thus a decline in all intellectual functions, reflected in every aspect of behavior.

Diagnosis. It is not difficult to recognize intellectual impairment in individuals late in the course of a cerebral disease. The more taxing problem is the recognition of the intellectual impairment when it is slight and potentially reversible. The tests of cognitive function that are part of the neurologic examination of every patient are intended to accomplish this. But they must be interpreted with care.

It is customary to test (1) orientation to time, place, and person; (2) language skills, by naming common objects and comprehending commands; (3) fund of knowledge, such as the names of some capital cities and of presidents; (4) recent memory, by setting three objects to be remembered for 5, 10, and 30 minutes; (5) attention span, by asking for a serial subtraction of 7 from 100 or any other arithmetic task that requires "carrying over"; (6) abstract reasoning power, by asking for definitions of proverbs or the similarity of words such as apple-orange, ear-eye, poem-statue; and (7) constructional capacity, by asking the patient to draw simple objects such as a clock or to copy an abstract design.

The results of these tests must be interpreted in the light of other knowledge about the patient. If the patient was a gifted professional person whose family has noted a decline in his judgment and an increasing forgetfulness, the discovery that he cannot hold three words in mind for five minutes and that he interprets proverbs clumsily provides some evidence that he is suffering from a disturbance to his intellectual power. On the other hand, if the patient was not a person with intellectual achievements in the past and has received a poor education, difficulties in proverb interpretation or fund of knowledge are less likely to represent brain disease. Although it is possible to find all the intellectual functions disturbed in dementia, the tests for recent memory, for attention, and for constructional capacity are most useful. Deficiencies here are easy to document; these functions are affected early in the course of many brain diseases and they are little dependent on education. Also, tests for recent memory are useful in differentiating a patient with mental retardation from an individual of limited intelligence who is developing a brain disease, since memory function is intact in the mildly retarded individual.

It is important to differentiate Korsakoff's syndrome and aphasia. The patient with Korsakoff's syndrome will fail the tests of recent memory. He will be disoriented to time and place, but he will be able to name objects, obey commands, and accomplish tasks of abstract reasoning and drawing if he can hold the question in mind. His disorder is in memory. The rest of his intellectual function is relatively spared. The aphasic patient will have severe problems in naming objects and comprehending words. But if this difficulty can be surmounted, it will be evident that it is language specifically that is disturbed, and other mental functions such as memory, orientation, and the capacity to draw are relatively intact.

It is often useful to supplement the bedside tests of mental function with standardized examination of intellectual skills. The Wechsler Adult Intelligence Scale (WAIS) is most often employed. Nothing about this psychologic examination is different in concept from the bedside tests. It measures the intellectual performance of a patient by asking him to attempt problems in several different areas. Since a mathematical score is given, an objective comparison of his performance with that of others is possible. Although the WAIS includes problems similar to those given at the bedside, it adds several "performance" tests which are actually unfamiliar tasks, such as recognition of errors in pictures, design of patterns from colored blocks, and assembly of parts of puzzles. These tests most specifically examine the ability of a patient to put his mind to an unfamiliar situation and solve it. They are less dependent on learning and decline early in a dementia, producing a discrepancy between these "performance scores" and the "verbal scores" which tend to remain intact for a longer period.

Diagnostic Issues in Dementia. As mentioned previously, the symptoms of dementia appear with an injury to the cerebral hemispheres, and are not specific for a particular pathology. It is the course of their development, the associated neurologic signs, and the laboratory findings that permit diagnosis of the pathologic entities producing the dementia.

Since the same symptoms can be produced by curable, reversible pathology as by incurable and progressive disorders, the first diagnostic consideration should reflect a search for the treatable pathologic entities. Each of the following conditions should be considered in every patient with the symptoms of dementia: general paresis, myxedema, neoplasms and other chronic intracerebral lesions, hepatolenticular degeneration (Wilson's disease), avitaminosis B_{12}, and occult hydrocephalus. Many of these conditions can be diagnosed by evidence derived from the clinical examination; others demand clinical laboratory studies. Thus the Argyll Robertson pupil of cerebral syphilis, lateralized motor-sensory signs of neoplasm, the Kayser-Fleischer ring of Wilson's disease, and a gait disorder caused by a spastic weakness of legs in hydrocephalus should all be sought in the physical examination of the demented patient. A group of laboratory tests are required in the diagnostic evaluation. As a routine, all patients should have a lumbar puncture to measure intracerebral pressure and to obtain a sample of cerebrospinal fluid for analysis. Cell count, protein content, and a test for the syphilitic precipitants will be needed in cerebrospinal fluid. Blood serologic examination, analysis for protein-bound iodine and serum B_{12} analysis are also indicated. An electroencephalogram is useful, as it may reveal a local lesion or a severe generalized slowing of the rhythms characteristic of delirium. Skull roentgenograms can also reveal a local lesion. In many patients it is necessary to proceed to a pneumoencephalogram in order to exclude some of the rarer but curable forms of dementia such as occult hydrocephalus.

The onset and course of a dementing disorder must be carefully analyzed when considering the likely pathologic entities. Was the onset abrupt or insidious, was the subsequent course a gradual and relentless loss of mental faculties, or was it a series of sudden losses producing a steplike decline in the mental faculties? Did it require months or only a few weeks to develop? Different pathologic entities produce different clinical histories in these respects. Thus the dementia associated with vascular disease of the brain will have a sudden onset and increase in an intermittent and variable fashion. The dementia of general paresis tends to be subacute and steadily progressive; that of degenerative disease is more insidious in onset and slow in development.

The characteristics of four known cerebral degenerations will be reviewed as they exemplify some of these general statements about dementia. These conditions are Alzheimer's disease, Pick's disease, Creutzfeldt-Jakob disease, and Huntington's chorea.

327. ALZHEIMER'S DISEASE

Alzheimer's disease is a progressive degenerative process of the brain that produces a dementia in middle to late life.

The brain in Alzheimer's disease gradually atrophies, nerve cells disappearing from the cortex. The major brunt of the atrophic process appears to be in the frontal and occipital regions of the brain, but microscopic examinations will demonstrate pathologic changes throughout the cortex. Many of the neurons that remain show a peculiar alteration of their neurofibrils, which are thickened and twisted into distinctive "neurofibrillary tangles." Within the atrophic cortex there are many "senile plaques." These are microscopic collections of granular argyrophilic particles which tend to form in a halo around an indefinite center containing sudanophilic fat or an amyloid-like substance. Exactly what these plaques are is uncertain, but they appear to represent collections of degenerating brain substance.

The dementia that accompanies Alzheimer's disease has few distinctive characteristics. All the symptoms of dementia enumerated above eventually appear. Onset is insidious and progress slow. A disturbance in recent memory is usually the first symptom. Affective disturbances such as depression or anxiety and disorientation in time and place appear soon after. Often there is a considerable emotional unrest in these patients, prompted in some 30 to 40 per cent by delusionary false beliefs. A sizable fraction of patients also have auditory and visual hallucinations during illness. Focal neurologic signs are rare early in the course of the disease, but with progression of the illness, focal cortical symptoms of aphasia, apraxia, and agnosia often become prominent. Seizures, both focal and generalized, are common only in far-advanced instances. With these intellectual and emotional disturbances there is the development of a disorder of gait. This takes the form of difficulty in starting the rhythmical movements of walking. A synchronous activation of agonist and antagonist muscles results in a locking of the legs and a hesitant shuffle.

The progress of all these symptoms is much the same in all patients. It is slow, but usually within five to eight years of the onset of symptoms the patient reaches a terminal stage. Here there is a profound dementia and a decerebrate physical state with flexion contractures of all limbs. Death comes from an intercurrent infection or some other complication of the bedfast condition.

The age of onset varies. Because this disorder was first recognized among relatively young people, the term "presenile dementia" has been applied to Alzheimer's disease. This implies a distinction in kind between this condition and "senile dementia" that appears when many other changes of aging are evident. But the cerebral pathology and the clinical course of patients who develop symptoms before or after age 65 are the same. Alzheimer's disease, defined as it is by the cerebral pathology of atrophy with senile plaques and neurofibrillary tangles, is a disorder appearing with increasing frequency as people age.

Alzheimer's disease is not an uncommon disorder, but it is more common in females than in males. Autopsy diagnoses vary from 1 to 10 per cent in mental hospitals, the particular figure depending on whether the observers make a distinction between Alzheimer's disease and senile dementia.

The cause of Alzheimer's disease is unknown. Most examples occur sporadically, but a few patients have a family history of dementia. It is not even certain whether Alzheimer's disease is a specific response to one noxious biologic process or whether it is a more general response of the brain to injurious processes. The latter possibility is suggested by the occasional appearance of Alzheimer pathology in such different situations as the punchdrunk syndrome of boxers, Down's syndrome (trisomy 21), and postencephalitic parkinsonism.

The diagnosis of Alzheimer's disease is made most often by exclusion. An individual who has a slowly progressive dementia without prominent neurologic signs and without any of the clinical and laboratory findings of the treatable conditions mentioned, as well as a pneumoencephalogram demonstrating a moderate dilation of the cerebral ventricles with some atrophy of cortex, is most likely to be suffering from Alzheimer's disease. Only by cerebral biopsy can more conclusive evidence for diagnosis be found, and this cannot be recommended in the usual clinical situation.

328. PICK'S DISEASE

Pick's disease is also a degenerative disorder of the cerebral cortex that produces dementia in middle and late life. It is distinguished from Alzheimer's disease by its morbid anatomy.

In contrast to Alzheimer's disease, in which the cerebral atrophy is diffuse, in Pick's disease the atrophy is relatively circumscribed and confined to the frontal and temporal lobes, where the atrophy is severe. The microscopic pathology is also distinctive in Pick's disease; a particularly degenerating neuron characterized by the accumulation close to the nucleus of a globular argyrophilic mass that distends the neuron into a swollen ballooned form is seen in the disorder. This is the *Pick cell* and it is usually found widespread in the atrophying areas of cortex. There are usually neurofibrillary tangles and senile plaques as well in the atrophic parts of brain.

It is difficult to distinguish an example of Pick's disease from Alzheimer's disease on clinical grounds. Patients with Pick's disease may have less difficulty in gait than patients with Alzheimer's disease. Otherwise, the conditions seem clinically identical. Pick's disease is considerably less common than Alzheimer's disease, but, as in that condition, no definite cause has been identified. Some examples of Pick's disease appear to be transmitted by a dominant gene in a family, but many examples are without a family history.

329. CREUTZFELDT-JAKOB DISEASE

The dementia in Creutzfeldt-Jakob disease is rapidly progressive, advancing noticeably day by day from its onset to a fatal termination, usually within a year. The dementia is accompanied by a variety of neurologic symptoms such as ataxia, aphasia, paralysis, and visual disturbances and by prominent myoclonic jerking of the limbs and body at some stage in the disorder. The EEG is abnormal early in the disturbance, its normal rhythms lost and replaced with a distinctive mixture of slow and sharp waves useful for diagnosis. The condition is the result of a degeneration of cerebral cortex thought to be caused by a transmissible agent of the latent or slow virus variety. It is more thoroughly discussed in Ch. 400.

330. HUNTINGTON'S CHOREA

Huntington's chorea is a distinctive disease entity in which a dementia associated with chorea appears usually in the fourth or fifth decade of life. Its neuropathology is characteristic, and the disease is transmitted as an autosomal dominant.

The dementia of Huntington's chorea appears insidiously but is relentlessly progressive over the 12 to 15 years from onset to fatal termination of the illness. Although most of the cognitive disabilities of these patients are similar to those with other brain diseases, patients with Huntington's chorea can suffer from a profound mental apathy as the illness advances. This apathy can lead to unresponsiveness and mutism late in the course. The absence of aphasia at any stage of the disorder is a noteworthy distinction of this dementia from that in Alzheimer's disease.

Mood changes resembling manic-depressive illness are common in Huntington's chorea. Patients can have discrete periods of severe depression accompanied by psychomotor retardation and delusions of guilt that may prompt suicide attempts. The high incidence of suicide in Huntington's chorea (7 to 10 per cent is reported) is due in most part to these periods of delusional depression. Electroconvulsive treatment combined with antidepressant medication (imipramine, 150 to 250 mg per day) has proved efficacious in the treatment of these depressions. Periods of manic excitement with overactivity and delusions of wealth, strength, and worldly importance can alternate with the depressive periods. The manic symptoms respond to phenothiazine treatment (chlorpromazine, 300 to 500 mg per day).

In some patients symptoms of dementia or mood disorder may appear prior to the onset of choreic movements, and therefore these patients can present diagnostic difficulties. The correct diagnosis is made when the family history is discovered or chorea appears. Of particular interest is the possibility that the degenerative changes in Huntington's chorea may be affecting a particular neurochemical system that might provide a model for the appreciation of biologic mechanisms in both manic-depressive disorder and dementia.

Other characteristics of this disorder are given in Ch. 370.

331. TREATMENT OF THE DEMENTED PATIENT

With the obvious exception of the specific treatments for curable diseases, the issue of treatment for the demented patient is most often that of management of particular symptoms rather than reversal of a pathologic process. Often, a treatment based on some research finding is proposed for the degenerative disorders only to prove of little value when employed in a clinical trial. Thus the discovery that cerebral oxygen consumption is reduced in Alzheimer's disease led to treatments with both oxygen inhalation and hyperbaric chambers. But these treatments failed to produce significant improvement, almost certainly because the observed reduction in oxygen consumption is due to a reduction in the number of viable neurons rather than to an inadequate oxygen supply. Any treatment that is proposed for these distressing conditions is liable to be uncritically acclaimed, with eventual disappointment. The importance of the clinical trial with double-blind technique in assessing these treatments cannot be exaggerated.

Some general principles of management of the demented patient can be emphasized. First, complicating medical conditions such as congestive heart failure, dehydration, iron deficiency anemia, infections, and electrolyte imbalance can, even if not severe in themselves, make the mental condition of a patient with degenerative brain disease much worse. A meticulous correction of all medical complications will do much to aid the patient. Second, much of the emotional unrest in demented patients is due to fear produced by their disorientation, misidentifications, and misinterpretations and to *catastrophic reactions*. Great relief of these symptoms can come from a willingness of nurses and doctors to explain repeatedly to the patient his situation and the proper interpretation of what is happening. Changes in surroundings and in nursing personnel should be minimized; well lighted rooms, preferably with familiar possessions, serve best, and an attitude toward the patient that is accepting and supportive will do much to assist him. Any obligations that require effort beyond his capacity and so produce *catastrophic* reactions must be eliminated. Third, considerable help for individual symptoms can be gained by the use of pharmacologic measures. Sleep disturbances in demented patients are best treated with chloral hydrate, up to 1.0 to 1.5 grams at night. Acute confusional aggression or agitation can be relieved by phenothiazine medication, and thioridazine in doses of 50 to 100 mg three or four times daily has been effective. Depressive symptoms can respond to antidepressant medication (imipramine, 50 mg three times to four times per day).

All these drugs should be used sparingly, as the patient with cerebral degeneration may demonstrate toxic signs at much lower doses than normal patients. Drug toxicity can worsen the condition severely.

In general, the management of the demented patient rests on an appreciation of the nature of his psychologic disabilities and the application of psychosocial medical and nursing principles. The response to this management is often gratifying.

Corsellis, J. A. N.: Mental Illness and the Ageing Brain. London, Oxford University Press, 1962.

McHugh, P. R., and Folstein, M. F.: Psychiatric syndromes of Huntington's chorea. Semin. Psychiat., 1974.

Post, F.: Clinical Psychiatry of Late Life. New York, Pergamon Press, 1965.

Sjogren, T., Sjogren, H., and Lindgren, A. G. H.: Morbus Alzheimer and morbus Pick: A genetic, clinical and pathological study. Acta Psychiat. Scand. (Suppl. 82), 1952.

Strachan, R. W., and Henderson, J. G.: Psychiatric syndromes due to avitaminosis B_{12} with normal blood and marrow. Quart. J. Med., 34:303, 1965.

Wolstenholme, G. E. W., and O'Connor, M. (eds.): Alzheimer's Disease and Related Conditions. Ciba Foundation Symposium. London, Churchill, 1970.

Section Four. PSYCHOLOGIC ILLNESS IN MEDICAL PRACTICE

Paul R. McHugh

332. THE CONCEPT OF DISEASE IN PSYCHIATRY

Any general hospital can provide an experience in psychiatry, because an example of every psychologic disorder will eventually appear among patients admitted to its services. However, many skilled physicians feel unsure of their ability to manage these disorders. They are apt to contrast their knowledge of somatic illness founded firmly in morbid anatomy and pathophysiology with their understanding of psychologic medicine in which classifications seem based on confusing mixtures of symptomatology and speculative theories, and the most effective treatments are empirical. Such physicians will continue uncertain until they grasp how the basic concept of disease can bring order to psychiatry as it does in all of medicine. This they must accomplish before they can profit from a review of the clinical facts of particular psychiatric conditions; hence this chapter.

The term "disease" is difficult to define, because it is a concept and not something concrete or given in nature. It is intended to convey the idea that among all the morbid changes in physical and mental health it is possible to recognize groups of abnormalities as distinct entities or syndromes separable from one another and from the normal and that these separations will prove to have some biologic explanation when the entities have been thoroughly investigated.

All abnormalities can logically be viewed as quantitative changes merging imperceptibly into one another and into the normal, and can then be explained as consequences of disturbed interactions of a few vital processes. The Galenic concept of "humors" is just such a view. In fact the concept of disease based on qualitatively distinct syndromes is a convention proposed first by Sydenham, and remains but a convention today. However, this has been the most useful convention in the natural sciences. It has become so indispensable in medical thinking that it is taken for granted in most discussions. Neglect of this convention explains much of the difficulty faced by students in psychiatry. Its logic thus needs review here.

The concept of any given disease passes through several stages as knowledge increases. At each stage attention focuses on certain features of the condition which are the "defining characteristics." At the first stage a "clinical disease entity" is recognized and defined as a constellation of symptoms and physical signs running a more or less predictable course or natural history. Dropsy, hemophilia, and epilepsy are typical clinical disease entities. But these entities are not pure species. Each can be the expression of any one of several different pathologic conditions. Dropsy, for example, is found with different pathologic conditions: glomerulonephritis, congestive heart failure, constrictive pericarditis. Thus the second stage is the division of the clinical disease entity into several "pathologic disease entities." When a disease can be conceived as a pathologic entity, the defining characteristics on which concept and diagnosis rest are results of laboratory tests that reveal pathologic function or morbid anatomy. Again, by way of example, the demonstration of an elevated blood urea nitrogen and albumin and casts in the urine of a patient with dropsy leads to a presumptive opinion that the pathologic disease entity responsible for his condition is glomerulonephritis. This presumptive diagnosis is confirmed by studying the histopathology of the kidney. The third and final stage in the concept of a disease is the recognition of a particular etiologic agency. This recognition can derive from any aspect of biologic knowledge:

Genetics, microbiology, and biochemistry have all made their contributions. For glomerulonephritis the etiologic agency is the phenomenon of autoimmunity, and it will be from investigations of this phenomenon that physicians can expect to gain a complete understanding of glomerulonephritis as well as a treatment that can prevent and cure it.

For many medical diseases the mark of the twentieth century has been the discovery of etiologic agencies and their action. Not so for psychiatry. For most psychiatric disorders knowledge has not passed the first stage on the traditional path, and for many even the hold on this stage is insecure. This insecurity arises in part from the difficulty of the subject matter, but also from a neglect of the standards of observation and history-taking that are required in defining a clinical disease entity.

This neglect has been defended by a common opinion in psychiatry that all psychologic disturbances are to be viewed as emotional reactions to some form of environmental distress, and thus are quantitative abnormalities differing from normal in a continuous and smooth fashion rather than grouping into qualitatively distinct entities with separable pathologies and etiologies.

One objection to this view has to be the practical one that it discards for no obvious advantage a convention that has ordered other abnormalities successfully. Another is that it oversimplifies mental disturbances to make them all expressions of a few psychologic mechanisms. A consideration of the forms of disorder for which psychiatry assumes responsibility will demonstrate the utility found in the concept of disease for some of them.

Three groups of disturbances fall into manageable psychiatric categories. *The first holds all those disturbances in mind and behavior that are a result of observable brain pathology.* Represented here are the clinical disease entities of delirium, dementia, and mental retardation. The conceptual and investigative approach to these conditions is indistinguishable from that for other somatic diseases. Such pathologic disease entities as Alzheimer's disease and such etiologic agencies as perinatal hypoxia, infections, and metabolic changes have been discerned.

The second group holds the two functional psychoses in which no obvious brain pathology is evident; schizophrenia and manic-depressive disorder. That these conditions are not unlike somatic disorders and should be conceived as clinical disease entities defined by symptoms and course is impossible to prove at this time. But this view was first prompted by the alien character of the symptoms that seemed unaccountable from an empathic understanding of the patient's temperament and his recent life experiences. It has been strengthened by the discovery of pharmacologic treatments specific to each entity and by the recognition of a few morbid conditions of the central nervous system leading to identical clinical conditions – temporal lobe epilepsy, amphetamine toxicity leading to a schizophrenia-like disorder, and the reserpine reaction that mimics a depressive disorder. It is now more conceivable that we are on the threshold of discoveries that will provide pathologic disease entities and etiologic agencies for these conditions than that they will be explained as quantitative exaggerations of emotional reactions.

The third group of disturbances in mind and behavior are the personality disorders and neurotic symptoms. The concept of disease does not fit these conditions. They seem to be quantitative rather than qualitative abnormalities in psychologic functions. It is difficult to say for these where normal leaves off and abnormal begins since they do seem to be extremes of normal variation. Personality disorders seem no more diseases than are shortness of stature, plainness of face, and dullness of wit. Neurotic symptoms such as anxiety or depression, like any symptoms of disturbance, can be evoked by many causes, including somatic or psychiatric diseases, but they most commonly appear as understandable reactions of an individual with a disordered personality faced with an environment that strikes at his special vulnerability.

Thus the concept of disease does provide in psychiatry a means for organizing clinical material that is similar to that used in general medicine. In the following chapters its application in the detailed consideration of the separate conditions will be attempted.

Jaspers, K.: General Psychopathology. Translated by J. Hoenig and M. Hamilton. Manchester, Manchester University Press, 1963.
Scadding, J. G.: Diagnosis: The clinician and the computer. Lancet, 2:877, 1967.
Taylor, F. K.: Psychopathology. Its Causes and Symptoms. London, Butterworth and Co., Ltd., 1966.
Wightman, W. P. D.: The Emergence of Scientific Medicine. Edinburgh, Oliver and Boyd, 1971.

FUNCTIONAL PSYCHOSES

333. INTRODUCTION

The psychoses form a loose category that gathers together several different clinical entities. To be placed within the category an entity must produce disturbances in thinking and perception that are inexplicable solely as responses to experience and are severe enough to distort the patient's appreciation of the real world and the relationship of events within it. The category psychosis has no uniform foundation as in somatic pathology nor any more objective aspects of psychopathology to mark its distinction from other collections of psychiatric symptoms. It is thus a term difficult to use with precision. Sometimes psychosis is used as a euphemism for insanity, sometimes as a synonym for schizophrenia, one of the entities within the category, and sometimes to draw an elusive and dubious distinction as between neurotic and psychotic depression.

The unmodified term can be qualified by a differentiation into organic psychoses and functional psychoses. Here the term psychosis means only severe mental illness. The organic psychoses, delirium, dementia, and Korsakoff's syndrome, are produced by a variety of cerebral pathologies. The functional psychoses, schizophrenia and manic-depressive disorder, lack a recognizable neuropathology.

This differentiation is practical. It draws a distinction in kind that affects treatment and prognosis, and it indicates the character of the clinical problem. For the organic psychoses the central problem is the cause of the pathologic changes. For the functional psychoses the central problem is consistent diagnosis.

Schizophrenia and manic-depressive disorder are clinical disease entities. The criteria for their diagnosis are their symptoms alone. There are no objective tests verifying a diagnosis. Only the natural history or response to empirically discovered treatments can confirm a diagnostic opinion. Since they lack a recognized neuropathology and are by definition inexplicable as responses to experience, there are no comprehensive etiologic explanations for these disorders. Treatment therefore is symptomatic rather than fundamental. Both prevention and radical cure await a chance discovery or a major scientific advance in understanding the biologic foundations of human behavior.

334. SCHIZOPHRENIA

Schizophrenia is a most devastating mental illness. It is a disturbance of mind and personality appearing in clear consciousness and characterized by several distinctive alterations in mental experiences, modes of thinking, and mood that are seldom completely resolved. The most characteristic features occur during the active phases of the disturbance, and take the form of hallucinations, delusions, and altered behavior toward others. Specific intellectual and affective disabilities varying from minimal to severe can develop insidiously or remain after an attack. A crucial element of the definition is that all these symptoms occur in a patient free of any relevant and discernible pathologic change in his nervous system.

Clinical Manifestations. The symptoms of schizophrenia can begin at almost any stage in life, but most commonly occur during adolescence and early adulthood and then either insidiously or as an acute attack followed by a series of attacks, each leaving behind personality defects of increasing severity.

In some patients it is possible to recognize a particular premorbid personality. They may have seemed more timid or seclusive than others. They may have been bookish, unsociable, and preoccupied with philosophic and religious ideas to the exclusion of friendships and community experiences. But this so-called *schizoid personality* is not found in most patients who develop schizophrenia. At least half of schizophrenic patients had premorbid personalities indistinguishable from normal.

Among the mental changes that mark the onset of a schizophrenic illness, only some are specific to this disorder. Emotional unrest, uncertainty, perplexity, and confusion can be found in many disorders other than schizophrenia, and therefore a diagnosis of schizophrenia cannot rest on them. There are, however, a number of mental changes that are more or less diagnostic. These can be usefully divided into abnormal mental experiences and disturbed modes of expression. The abnormal mental experiences are somewhat more reliable evidence of the illness simply because they are easier to elicit with confidence and less dependent upon interpretation than disturbances in expression.

Hallucinations and delusions are the outstanding schizophrenic mental experiences. Although hallucinations can occur in many disorders such as delirium, dementia, and occasionally manic-depressive disorder, certain forms of hallucinations are more specific for schizophrenia. Thus auditory hallucinations are the most common hallucinations in schizophrenia, and certain kinds of auditory hallucinations are almost diagnostic. Thus hearing one's thoughts aloud or hearing voices commenting about one's every action or several voices engaged in a conversation in which derogatory and praising remarks are passed with the patient discussed in the third person are the most typical schizophrenic hallucinations.

Although delusions, i.e., false beliefs that are incorrigible, idiosyncratic, and preoccupying, can be found in many disorders other than schizophrenia, in this illness delusional experiences are dramatic and well developed. They can begin as vague, fearful interpretations and "half-beliefs" and develop into firm incorrigible convictions. A delusion coming on suddenly, not prompted by any hallucination or previous delusion, nor related in any obvious way to the patient's mood, is called a "primary delusion" and is highly suggestive of schizophrenia. Many other schizophrenic experiences are of delusional form, but have such individual characteristics that they have been named for themselves.

Commonly schizophrenics have delusions about bodily control, the so-called passivity experiences. The patient feels as though he were under the control of some outside force or power making him behave as an automaton without a will of his own. He may feel hypnotized and feel forced to make particular movements, speak with a special voice, or walk to certain areas. The patient may believe these feelings come to him as penetrating waves from electronic or telephonic equipment.

The schizophrenic patient may experience changes in his thinking. Particularly he may feel that his thoughts are disrupted by some outside agency, that his thoughts are withdrawn from his mind, or that other thoughts are inserted into it. He may believe that people can hear his thoughts, which are leaving his mind as waves broadcast to others.

In contrast to these abnormalities of experience are the disturbances in the patient's mode of expression. Particularly noticeable is his abnormal language. Characteristically, he is difficult to understand. His thinking is expressed in a vague and awkward fashion with words poorly chosen and ideas poorly related to one another. Strikingly, the patient makes no effort to correct the vagueness of his thinking or to improve the clarity of his talk. Often, asking a question of the patient, the examiner receives a reply that is off the point and that goes into unnecessary details. Although the questions of the interview seem to start the patient toward a particular answer, it is never reached, but the patient takes up abstract and unnecessary ideas and must be redirected toward his goal. The examiner, laying the responsibility for the confusion on himself, may work to express himself more clearly, and only after considerable effort recognize that the difficulty in communication rests with the odd replies from the patient.

Another prominent disturbance is emotional expression of these patients. They seem distant, unresponsive, and cold. On some occasions the patient's emotional attitude seems incongruous, particularly for the thoughts he is expressing. Thus he may laugh while saying that he is in mortal danger. This cold or incongruous attitude and manner give the schizophrenic patient his most striking features, and even when at their mildest can be baffling and distressing symptoms to his family.

Other abnormal modes of expression of the schizophrenic patient are disturbances in stance and mobility called catatonic symptoms. Gestures may seem stiff, slow, and mannered. Some schizophrenic patients make repetitive movements or facial grimaces. Others may become totally immobile and mute. Still others may assume unnatural postures and hold them for long periods.

During the active phases of the schizophrenic illness the flamboyant subjective experiences are most prominent. During the chronic phase of schizophrenic illness expressive disturbances in thought and emotion are more evident, varying from mild to severe. Although at times some patients seem free of residual symptoms, usually a careful examination will reveal mild disturbances in thinking and emotional responsiveness.

Diagnosis. The diagnosis of schizophrenia rests on recognition of the distinctive clinical symptoms of this disorder and the exclusion of other conditions which may produce similar symptoms.

Many disorders of brain function can imitate schizophrenic symptoms; but with the exception of the three schizophrenia-like disorders to be discussed, patients with the other brain disturbances also manifest disturbed consciousness, disorientation, and disruption of cognitive abilities, particularly recent memory function, that are not found in schizophrenia.

Mania or depression can be confused with schizophrenia (to the considerable embarrassment of the diagnostician when the patient recovers completely on receiving treatment appropriate for these conditions). A source of difficulty is the occurrence of delusions, which are common enough in mania and depression but usually spring directly from the attitudes of self-confidence or self-blame that are so prominent in those disorders.

In schizophrenia disturbances in experience, including the auditory hallucinations and delusions just described, form the most secure basis for diagnosis. Thus, in a person free of brain disease or drug intoxication, recognition of formed auditory hallucinations, primary delusional experiences, passivity experiences, or disturbances in "thought control" permit the diagnosis of schizophrenia to be made with some confidence.

If these symptoms cannot be found, then diagnosis must rest upon recognition of manifest disturbances in thought and emotional expression. It should be pointed out, however, that opinion holding a person's thought to be illogical and vague, or his affective responses to be inadequate or incongruous, is an evaluative judgment and must be held with somewhat less confidence, if the difficulties are minimal or inconstant, than opinion resting on recognition of delusions and hallucinations.

Catatonic symptoms of immobility, posturing, and grimacing, along with the disturbances in behavior described as negativism or reluctance to cooperate, must be carefully interpreted. Only in those patients in whom no evidence of a prominent mood change can be found should a diagnosis of schizophrenia be made. Motility changes in the direction of psychomotor retardation are prominent features of depressive disorder, a condition as common as schizophrenia and more common than the catatonic variety of schizophrenia, and excitement with hyperactivity can appear in mania.

Symptoms of emotional unrest, anxiety, withdrawal, and hostility can be found in schizophrenic patients, but these are common to many other psychiatric disorders, and therefore can never form the basis for a secure diagnosis of schizophrenia. However, that diagnosis is rendered more likely if it can be established that the patient was developing normally without an apparently vulnerable personality, and if these symptoms appeared without a change in the patient's mood or the pattern of his life. Since these more general symptoms can be found in both schizophrenia and many other psychiatric disturbances, it is important to search carefully for the more basic symptoms of hallucinations and delusions from which emotional unrest and unpredictable behavior may stem. Often repeated efforts are required to gain cooperation of the patient so that he will divulge the existence of those basic symptoms that make a diagnosis of schizophrenia certain.

Etiology. There is no neuropathology or consistent pathophysiology that can be observed to develop with progression of the disorder and that might give some hint of causation. An approach to a consideration of etiology has to be more circuitous and the opinions derived held with somewhat less assurance than is true of other clinical entities. Two aspects of etiology can be conveniently separated for the purpose of organizing the information we have. One aspect is "cause," that is, any prerequisite element needed to set in motion a train of events leading to the entity. The other is "mechanism," that is, the particular nature of the train of events, be they psychologic, neurologic, or biochemical, that produce the symptoms. For schizophrenia there is some information relating to "cause" and also to "mechanism," but it is far from conclusive.

"Cause" or Prerequisite Elements in Schizophrenia. The genetic constitution has been decisively demonstrated to be one of the "causes" of schizophrenia. The risk of schizophrenia increases with the closeness of blood relationship to a schizophrenic patient. Thus only 1 per cent of very distant relatives of a schizophrenic patient will themselves suffer from the disorder. This is no higher than the risk in the general population. But 5 to 6 per cent of siblings and 40 to 50 per cent of monozygotic twins of schizophrenic patients will have schizophrenia.

The possible objection that these data merely reflect the increasingly common environment of progressively closer relatives has been refuted by observations on monozygotic twins brought up apart who continue to show an identical high risk. Heston made the same point in a different fashion by studying a group of offspring of schizophrenic mothers. These particular children were raised from earliest infancy in foster homes by normal, nonschizophrenic mothers and fathers. The incidence of schizophrenia in these children was exactly the same as that reported for children raised by a schizophrenic parent. They thus resembled their biologic mother although reared apart from her.

It has nevertheless been impossible to fit schizophrenia into a clear mendelian pattern of dominant or recessive inheritance. Some students of the disease would describe the hereditary contribution to schizophrenia as polygenic, i.e., the sum of a number of contributions from the genes no one of which is solely responsible. The polygenic concept might permit environmental factors to play a larger role in causation. Thus a mild genetic vulnerability might express itself in a schizophrenic phenotype only in those who face stressful environments, whereas those carrying a more severe genetic vulnerability might show the disorder in any environment. It is difficult at the moment to propose a test that would exclude the polygenic hypothesis as a possibility.

Some studies that have established a genetic contribution to the etiology of schizophrenia have also given evidence of the inadequacy of genetics as a sufficient cause for the disorder. That 50 per cent of monozygotic twins of schizophrenic patients are free of this illness means one of the following: (1) Although the genetic constitution is necessary and sufficient to produce schizophrenia, the symptoms employed to define a case fail to provide an adequate means of recognizing all examples of the disorder, and 50 per cent are mistakenly called normal. (2) The defining symptoms encompass a mixed group of disorders, and in only 50 per cent of these disorders are genetic features necessary and sufficient causes for the symptoms. (3) A genetic vulnerability for schizophrenia is necessary but not sufficient. It must be combined with certain life experiences that need not be common for genetically identical individuals.

The present inadequacy of the genetic hypothesis to provide a complete description of the "cause" for schizophrenia reinforces a search for environmental and experiential causes. It has proved just as difficult to determine an environmental contribution as to define the genetic contribution. Thus the experiences of being raised by a cold and distant mother, or of receiving insistent, simultaneous, but incompatible directions from the parents, or of simply living in a disharmonious family incapable of providing a healthy environment for psychologic growth have all been considered causes of schizophrenia.

Such disturbed experiences have been found in the lives of some schizophrenic patients when viewed retrospectively after the onset of the illness. But none has proved to be a common experience in all schizophrenic people. Nor has it been possible to predict an increased incidence of schizophrenia among individuals living in comparably disturbed situations. Presently the most economical view of the role of life experiences in the "cause" of schizophrenia holds that *any* adversity, be it a psychologic shock, abnormality in critical relationships, or physical injury (particularly brain injury) may provide a partial contribution in causing schizophrenia, but that most of these adversities are exerting their causal effects upon a genetically vulnerable individual.

"Mechanism" of the Schizophrenic Syndrome. This is the other aspect of etiology. Given that some combination of genetic and environmental attributes is probably prerequisite for the illness, by what derangements are the symptoms produced? Are they produced by some change in a psychologic function that might have been learned or developed through experience, or are they produced by some morbid change in the nervous system that alters the normal capacity to perceive, integrate, and respond? There have been proposals for each of these "mechanisms."

Many distinguished psychiatric studies have proposed that the mechanism of the disturbance has been through the production of a particular psychologic change fundamental to the whole syndrome and from which all the symptoms can be explained. Thus Federn has proposed a "loosening of ego boundaries" as the essential feature mediating this illness, whereas Bleuler proposed a basic disturbance in associational thinking. A crisis of identity has been proposed by exponents of existential psychiatry. These views have a ring of plausibility perhaps derived from their resemblance to experiences common to all men, part of which can seem to be reflected in the behavior of schizophrenic patients. But they depend on concepts that are difficult to define except in terms of what they purport to explain.

Other studies have attempted to demonstrate the possibility that the mechanism is a change in the central nervous system. No such change has been demonstrated in schizophrenia as yet, so supporters of this possibility have had to reason by analogy.

Three well documented conditions affecting the brain can give rise to a mental disturbance resembling schizophrenia. The most familiar is the syndrome found with *amphetamine intoxication.* In this condition the patient is alert and oriented but preoccupied by auditory hallucinations and delusional ideas indistinguishable from those seen in schizophrenia. The disturbance may last from several days to a few weeks, but disappears eventually after the withdrawal of the stimulant.

Slater, Beard, and Glithero have demonstrated that among patients suffering from *psychomotor epilepsy,* caused by an irritative lesion in the limbic portions of the temporal lobe, a certain number develop a paranoid schizophrenia-like syndrome after 10 to 15 years of epilepsy. This condition displays all the classic delusional and hallucinatory symptoms of schizophrenia, but there is less tendency toward deterioration of thinking and personality.

Finally, certain patients, *withdrawing from excessive alcohol ingestion,* suffer from a period of auditory hallucinations. Although in most of these patients the hallucinatory experience clears within 24 to 48 hours, in a small proportion a chronic condition of persisting auditory hallucinations associated with delusional beliefs, incongruous affect, and disturbed thought develops. This chronic condition may be indistinguishable from the schizophrenic syndrome, and may persist for many years.

For all these schizophrenia-like conditions the possibility exists that the pertinent features might be the expression of a latent predisposition for schizophrenia in the affected individuals. But there is no evidence of a predisposition. The relatives of these patients do not have an increased incidence of schizophrenia, and the patients themselves do not have schizoid traits in their premorbid personalities.

The existence of these conditions demonstrates that the symptoms of schizophrenia are capacities of the damaged human brain. Yet we are ignorant of any common pathologic feature of these brain disorders that could by implication be the fundamental mechanism for schizophrenia. One possibility is that each of these disorders represents an extraexcitatory arousal of the brain, particularly of the reticular formation and limbic system, either directly via amphetamine or epileptic discharge or in rebound from long-continuing action of the depressant ethanol. It may be that the condition of schizophrenia itself is thus produced by some stimulatory action on these same regions evoked by the genetic-environmental "causes" discussed above.

Another proposed mechanism for producing schizophrenia is through some change in body metabolism or chemistry that could itself alter cerebral and psychologic functions. Many students have been prompted to consider this alternative because of the remarkable growth in biochemical methodology. In fact the difficulties in establishing a role for biochemistry in the etiology of schizophrenia rest not with the chemical methodology but with such issues as defining the group being studied, avoiding chemical artifacts related to dietary habits or medications given chronically hospitalized people, and deciding what biochemical change to look for with little knowledge of what kinds of change might produce symptoms. The papers of Kety should be consulted for a more thorough discussion of these difficulties. A rare condition, periodic catatonia, has been documented by Gjessing to be associated with a phasic change in nitrogen balance, but no relationship between this disorder and schizophrenia in general has been found.

Thus our knowledge of "mechanism," as much as our knowledge of "cause," is still fragmentary and provisional. But on the bits of evidence at hand, the view that most examples of schizophrenia will prove to be due to some deranged neural mechanism that itself is produced by an anomaly of the genetic constitution seems easiest to defend.

Treatment. The treatment for any schizophrenic patient is complex and should not be attempted by the inexperienced. A period of hospitalization will usually be required. There a program to include drug therapy, psychologic treatment, and social evaluation can be planned.

The sheet anchor of treatment now for schizophrenia is the *phenothiazine* drugs, discovered in the 1950's almost by accident. To date there is no good explanation for their effectiveness. Clearly they are not simply acting by virtue of their sedative effect, since their remarkable action is not mimicked by other sedatives. They can remove the symptoms of schizophrenia, including the delusions, hallucinations, and disordered thought, and are not restricted to relieving excitement or anxiety as the term tranquilizer might imply.

The most versatile phenothiazine preparation is the original: chlorpromazine. The dose required to treat acute symptoms varies widely from patient to patient, and amounts from 200 to 2000 mg per day may be necessary. Maintenance dosage is similarly an individual matter, but 200 to 300 mg per day is usually an effective range. Since cessation of treatment results in the reappearance of symptoms in 60 to 70 per cent of patients within six months, drug therapy is often given over years. This practice, however, is being re-evaluated in light of a movement disorder (tardive dyskinesia) that may appear with prolonged use of phenothiazines.

The *psychotherapy* suitable for the schizophrenic patient has been a subject of intense controversy. The more radical approaches based on psychologic and particularly psychoanalytic views of the genesis of schizophrenia have not achieved their optimistic goals of curing the patient by relieving some basic psychologic conflict. More modest psychotherapy is indispensable when it is intended to help the patient in his everyday affairs, taking advantage of those personal assets that persist despite his illness, and establishing a relationship of friendly rapport in order to guide him in his management of personal and social issues, which, if mishandled, can lead to distress and further illness. A particularly pressing issue for the schizophrenic patient is the social situation into which he is placed after hospitalization. His psychiatrist, usually at first with the help of a psychiatric social worker, must strive to find a job that is regular and well within the patient's power but not excessively challenging, a domestic arrangement that is calm and supportive but not too emotionally demanding, and a daily routine that combats the tendency to withdraw from all social contacts into an isolated and perhaps fantasy-ridden existence. To accomplish these goals is one of the most challenging exercises in medical treatment. The growth of "halfway houses" as residences for previously hospitalized schizophrenic patients has been prompted by recognition of the need for stable and structured social environments for schizophrenic patients once they have improved enough to leave the hospital.

Prognosis. Prognosis for any patient diagnosed as schizophrenic is always guarded. Certain features carry a good prognosis: high intelligence, a normal premorbid personality, an acute onset, catatonic features in the illness, and a family history of affective disorder. Other features carry a poor prognosis: low intelligence, schizoid premorbid personality, insidious onset of the illness, symptoms of thought disorder, affective blunting in the illness, and a family history of schizophrenia.

The use of phenothiazines has considerably improved the prognosis of schizophrenia, 30 to 50 per cent of patients having complete remissions on follow-up over five years. Another 30 to 40 per cent show some residual symptoms but are able to live in the community, and only 10 to 20 per cent require further hospitalization if phenothiazine treatment is begun and maintained after their first attack of the illness.

Connell, P. H.: Amphetamine Psychosis. Maudsley Monographs, No. 5. London, Chapman and Hall, Ltd., 1958.

Fish, F. J.: Schizophrenia, Bristol, John Wright & Sons, 1962.

Heston, L. L.: Psychiatric disorders in foster home reared children of schizophrenic mothers. Br. J. Psychiatry, 112:819, 1966.

Kety, S. S.: Biochemical theories of schizophrenia, I and II. Science, 129:1528, 1590, 1959, 1969.

Klein, D. F., and Davis, J. M.: Diagnosis and Drug Treatment of Psychiatric Disorders. Baltimore, Williams and Wilkins Company, 1969.

Schneider, K.: Clinical Psychopathology. Translated by M. W. Hamilton. New York, Grune & Stratton, Inc., 1959.

Shields, J.: The Genetics of schizophrenia in historical context. *In* Coppen, A. J., and Walk, A. (eds.): Recent Developments in Schizophrenia. Brit. J. Psychiat., Special Publication No. 1, pp. 25–41, Ashford Kent, 1968.

Slater, E., Beard, A. W., and Glithero, E.: The schizophrenia-like psychoses of epilepsy. Br. J. Psychiatry, 109:95, 1963.

Victor, M., and Hope, J. M.: The phenomenon of auditory hallucinations in chronic alcoholism. J. Nerv. Ment. Dis., 126:451, 1958.

335. MANIC-DEPRESSIVE PSYCHOSIS

The essential feature of this psychosis is an excessive disturbance of mood and self-appraisal from which its other mental symptoms seem to arise. This disturbance can be in the direction of elation and self-confidence or sadness and self-blame. The course tends to be episodic, even periodic, with attacks of elation (mania) or sadness (depression) interspersed with periods of apparent mental health varying in length from weeks to years. Individual patients may suffer attacks of only one kind throughout their lifetime. Single or repetitive attacks of depression seem to be the most common manifestation, but attacks alternately manic and then depressive or even repetitively manic are not unusual.

Clinical Manifestations. *Depression.* During an attack of depression the patient complains of feeling miserable and uncertain of himself. He may give evidence of his sadness by a dejected appearance and by restlessness and distractibility. Some patients are slowed in their activity, and this can progress to a psychomotor retardation of such severity that the patient seems totally unresponsive.

Mental examination of the depressed patient usually brings to light not only his feelings of sadness or misery but also a lowered self-esteem that can vary in intensity from feelings of inadequacy and incompetence to convictions of personal worthlessness, blameworthiness, and evil. This combination of depressed mood with self-blame is the diagnostic sign of this condition. It will also explain most of the other symptoms, modes of behavior, and dangers faced by the depressed patient.

Other symptoms include delusional extrapolations of the attitudes of self-blame. These can increase to a belief that the patient's guilt is notorious, that he is to be arrested, and that he will be condemned to die or to suffer some extraordinary punishment either in this world or the next. Suspiciousness and fear of mistreatment based on these delusional beliefs may be difficult to distinguish from similar attitudes in the paranoid schizophrenic patient. A useful if not cast-iron distinction is the depressive's belief that the suspected ill treatment comes as a justified punishment and not, as with the schizophrenic, as an undeserved persecution.

In some severely depressed patients delusional ideas can become bizarre and even grandiose in concept. Thus they come to believe that they have been the cause of cosmic disasters, that the sun is darkened by them, that whole cities have been deserted because of their presence, or that they and their progeny are accursed in the sight of the Divinity. Delusions of bodily change may take the form that their brains are rotting, their bowels totally blocked, or their bones fractured and dislocated.

Delusional ideas may concern the relationship of the patient to the world and to others. He may believe that he has lost all his money, that he has become a burden to others, that he is universally despised, or even that he gives off such a bad odor that people cannot stand his presence. Again, these beliefs are usually reflective of the patient's inner attitude of self-blame, self-contempt, and hopelessness.

The point about these opinions is that they are delusional and not just false. They are unshakable opinions held in the face of all contrary evidence. Only treatment of the depressive disorder will remove them.

The most worrisome symptom of the depressed patient is *inclination to suicide.* It is easily appreciated that attitudes of such hopelessness and despair as have been described could prompt self-destruction. But it is not necessary to have such exaggerated delusions for suicide to be a distinct risk. Vigilance for suicidal intentions must be maintained throughout the course of the depressive disturbance. There is nothing to prevent a physician's asking any depressed patient about thoughts of self-injury. Often this simple action will reveal both the severity of the mood disturbance and the need to bring the patient into hospital for his own protection.

Homicide is also a possibility for the depressed patient, and is particularly likely in those who harbor beliefs that their family shares in their guilt and accursed characteristics. Any suggestions by the patient that he might prefer death should be most seriously believed.

Along with these psychologic symptoms the depressed patient will often suffer from disturbances in his sleep, particularly waking early in the morning and being unable to return to sleep. Other physical disturbances include bodily aches and pains, loss of appetite, constipation, and weight loss. These features may combine with the retardation to give the appearance of chronic physical ill health. In fact, many depressed patients will first consult internists complaining of such physical symptoms. Helpful to the differentiation of the patient whose somatic symptoms are part of a depressive illness is a discovery of the features of depressed mood, and attitudes of self-blame or hopelessness when these features are combined with complaints of poorly localized pains, with loss of appetite or weight loss, or even with preoccupations about the state of the inner organs.

Mania. Symptoms that are almost the exact opposite of those seen during an attack of depression appear during an attack of mania. Now the patient says that he is in excellent spirits, that he feels well, and in fact has never felt better. He is active and restless, and appears energetic, confident, and quick-witted. These characteristics tend to worsen, and it is in their more extreme form that they become recognized as symptoms. The restlessness and energy become overactivity, with the patient moving constantly and planning progressively less plausible projects. His speech becomes incessant, rapid, and disjointed, one idea following another with little connection between them. His attitude of confidence is that of grandiose self-satisfaction. He may be overbearing and pompous. He often will be irritated by his surroundings, easy to anger, and perhaps suspicious that the efforts being made to control him are unjust.

Although a manic patient can usually be recognized by his overactivity, ebullience, and great self-confidence, he can develop as well ideas of resentment and feelings that he is being in some way unfairly noticed or persecuted. These ideas, on investigation, are found to derive from his own delusional opinion that he is so important that he must be under scrutiny by forces such as foreign powers. Occasionally, these persecutory ideas are so prominent that a diagnosis of schizophrenia is entertained. It is, however, the direct connection of these ideas to the attitude of self-confidence that allows a diagnosis of mania to be made.

With the mental changes manic patients exhibit disturbed social behavior. They may have increased sexual interest and may become promiscuous. They tend to overspend and be reckless with money. They may insult their employers and so be fired from their jobs. In the first attack of mania and before the severe restlessness and disorganization of thought appear, these activities may not be recognized as the products of mental illness, but may be construed as actions for which the patient can be held accountable. Thus the patient can be subjected to severe losses, to legal actions, or to moral criticism that can hamper his life long after his manic attack is over. To protect him from these consequences hospitalization of the manic patient may be required.

Etiology. *"Cause" or Prerequisite Elements in Manic-Depressive Disorder.* As with schizophrenia, an important genetic contribution to the etiology of the manic-depressive disorder seems certain. There is a progressive frequency of incidence with increasing blood relatedness so that with monozygotic twins the concordance rate is over 50 per cent. It is likely that genetic constitution is a necessary but not sufficient cause for this disorder. Certain other features of the illness require consideration. First, the illness does appear in attacks interspersed with periods in which the person appears to be normal. Second, the attacks are somewhat seasonal, appearing more frequently in the spring and fall than in summer and winter. Third, although many attacks occur spontaneously, many seem to be precipitated by some disturbing event. Presumably some other elements must combine with the genetic vulnerability to explain these features. Again, the most easily defended position would hold that a necessary cause for manic-depressive disorder is the genetic constitution of the patient, but that any of a large number of environmental disturbances can bring out the disorder.

Mechanism in Manic-Depressive Disorder. As with schizophrenia, a pharmacologically induced disorder has enhanced confidence that, whatever the "cause," the mechanism for affective disorder is a neural one. Treatment with reserpine for hypertension produced depression in up to one of four patients, and this depression was accompanied by the typical delusional attitudes of the manic-depressive psychosis. The discovery that reserpine depleted brain neurons of biogenic amines, particularly norepinephrine and serotonin, has prompted a variety of hypotheses that propose some lack of norepinephrine, serotonin, or other biogenic amines at synaptic sites in the brain for emotional control. That many effective antidepressant agents also influence these same amines has been a further support to these hypotheses.

Treatment. The first rule in managing either manic or depressed patients is that most of them should be in hospital. Their conditions can bring catastrophe to themselves and their families in the form of financial mismanagement in mania and suicide in depression. If these diagnoses are strongly suspected, then psychiatric opinion should be immediately sought so as to determine whether hospitalization should be imposed. It is critical to have expert help, because the patient can often hide the severity of the disorder in a mass of explanations which may appear quite plausible.

It is crucial to diagnose these patients and separate them from those with other conditions, because new drug treatments have proved effective for them and are specific to the affective disorders. Two classes of pharmacologic agents are effective in *depression.* Seemingly more effective are the so-called *tricyclic antidepressants,* the prototype of which is imipramine. This drug, given in doses of from 75 to 300 mg per day, will relieve a depressive attack in 50 per cent of patients. Maintenance therapy of 100 to 150 mg per day should be continued in such patients for six to eight months after their recovery. If it is ineffective, the logical practice should be to switch to the other class, which includes the drugs that have as their primary action the capacity to inhibit the enzyme monoamine oxidase. These drugs, in doses of 45 to 75 mg per day, have also proved useful in depression.

If *monoamine oxidase inhibitors* are used, the patient must be warned to avoid foodstuffs such as cheese, broad beans, and some yeast extracts, which have pressor amines of the phenyl-ethyl-amine group that includes tyramine. If absorbed by patients whose monoamine oxidase enzyme is depleted, they can cause sudden elevation of blood pressure with headache, blurred vision, and even cerebrovascular hemorrhage.

The mainstay of treatment for severe depression is *electroconvulsive treatment* (ECT). In contrast to the drugs which relieve the symptoms of depression, ECT will terminate an attack of depression usually in four to eight treatments. This treatment can produce the most dramatic and quick recovery from the depths of a life-threatening depression, and should not be withheld from a delusional patient or any seriously depressed patient who has failed to respond to drug treatment after three to four weeks. Maintenance with imipramine, 100 to 150 mg per day for six months, is recommended after ECT for the avoidance of relapse shortly after successful treatment.

The *treatment of mania* is often very difficult, particularly if the patient is suspicious about medicines. Haloperidol in doses of 2 to 10 mg thrice daily taken orally has proved effective. This compound is liable to produce severe extrapyramidal side effects which can be combated with antiparkinsonian drugs and with Benadryl. Chlorpromazine in doses of 300 to 1000 mg per day can also be tried.

A recent and effective measure for controlling mania has been the use of lithium ion in the form of lithium carbonate. This compound is available in 300 mg tablets, and daily intake of 900 to 2400 mg per day can relieve manic excitement. It is, however, essential to follow plasma lithium concentration in these patients, because toxic signs of disorientation, tremor, anorexia, and diarrhea can appear if plasma lithium concentration rises above 2 mEq per liter. The therapeutic level and the toxic level of lithium are close, and therefore the medication must be started when the patient can be carefully supervised in a hospital. Maintenance lithium treatment can be recommended, because there is fair clinical evidence that in this fashion some further attacks of mania may be avoided.

Prognosis. The prognosis for a single attack of mania or depression is excellent. Even without treatment patients tend to recover completely within six months. With antidepressant treatment the medication can be withdrawn after six to eight months with fair assurance that symptoms will not recur at this time.

The longer-range prognosis is not so favorable. Eighty per cent of people who have suffered one attack of affective disturbance will have another at some time in their lives, but this may not be for many years. Some patients, however, will have recurrent attacks of mania or depression interrupted by only brief intervals of normal behavior. A role for lithium in improving their prognosis is presently under study but cannot as yet be considered established.

The best advice to give patients who have suffered from their first affective attack is that they will very likely be quite well for years, but that they and their family should be aware that their mood changes are to be considered seriously, and they should seek psychiatric attention promptly if such a mood change tends to persist or worsen.

Astrup, C., Fossum, A., and Holmboe, R.: A follow-up study of 270 patients with acute affective psychoses. Acta Psychiatr. Scand. (Suppl. 135), 1959.

Lewis, A.: Melancholia. J. Ment. Sci., 80:277, 1934.

Schildkraut, J. J.: The catecholamine hypothesis of affective disorders: A review of supporting evidence. Am. J. Psychiatry, 122:509, 1965.

336. PERSONALITY DISORDERS AND NEUROTIC SYMPTOMS

General Considerations. The concept of disease entities that supports our understanding of the functional psychoses does not suit all psychologic disturbances and particularly those that are described as personality disorders or neurotic symptoms. There is uncertainty both in terms and in concept here. For example, the designation neurosis is ambiguous in that it seems a name for a clinical entity with some sharp distinction from normal, but a cardinal symptom of one neurosis, *anxiety,* is an experience of all people at some time and is an appropriate mood in certain circumstances. What then is abnormal in *anxiety neurosis?* Is this abnormality of a quantative or a qualitative nature? To what kind of patient can the term anxiety neurosis be applied? Should we use it only for patients in the emotional "state" of anxiety, or is it suitable regardless of the present state if a patient has "traits" that make him prone to this emotion?

The term *personality* and particularly its extension, *personality disorder,* can be just as troublesome. Personality seems a word similar to such terms as character or temperament, words intended to describe aspects of human psychologic variation distributed in a smoothly graded fashion in the population. But if that is true, then the distinction personality disorder can seem an arbitrary, socially contrived, or judgmental decision, since no sharp dividing line is to be expected in smoothly graded characteristics. In this chapter an attempt is made to dispel some of these ambiguities while considering several emotional disturbances often called neurotic that occur in a general medical setting.

Although many mental changes and emotional disturbances in patients can be ascribed to known or presumed pathologic changes in brain function, certain varieties of human psychologic constitution and certain life experiences can themselves provoke emotional disturbance and disrupted behavior. The terms personality disorder and neurotic symptoms are intended to describe the disturbances that result from variation in human constitution and experience by invoking the concepts of potential and response. Personality always means *potential.* It encompasses and describes the abiding and distinctive traits or tendencies of an individual to react to circumstances in a particular fashion. Thus by "optimistic personality" is meant an individual who can be expected to respond with cheerfulness and optimism in situations in which others are less likely to do so. An individual's personality is the sum of numerous traits, and a comparison with others is implicit in the description of each trait. Thus every trait can be conceived as a dimension of variation along which people can be dispersed in a fashion similar to their dispersal along the dimensions of height, weight, or intelligence. Any definition of an individual's personality is an attempt to place him in relationship to others in respect to one or more traits. An individual can be said to have a disorder of personality if he deviates to such an extreme along the range of variation for some trait that either he or others complain of its effects.

Whereas personality and personality disorder indicate potential, the neurotic symptoms are emotional *responses* displayed when the individual is troubled by circumstances. For anyone certain environments and life events are conducive to anxiety, others to depression, and still others to suspiciousness. People with a disorder of personality have an increased potential for these responses and are provoked to them by less extreme circumstances and less specific stimuli. Thus paranoid personality disorder is a term used to describe an individual who tends to show attitudes of suspiciousness and feelings of persecution (the neurotic symptoms) in settings so minimally threatening that they will seldom provoke such attitudes in others. If, however, his life is relatively free of threatening features, these feelings will be diminished and, despite his personality traits, symptoms may be avoided.

Before such concepts can be used in the evaluation and management of a particular patient, that patient must be well known to the doctor, and the possibility of other conditions that could produce similar symptoms must be excluded. For this a detailed psychiatric history, mental status, and physical examination are needed. The latter two can be obtained during the first interview, but historical information about the patient's family background, developmental milestones, sexual adjustment, scholastic and occupational achievement, habits, and medical problems may require several hours of examination. Observations from his relatives improve the accuracy of such information, and their descriptions of his personality are indispensable. All these data, combined with the knowledge of the patient's present condition, form the basis for diagnosis, treatment, and prognosis, and to embark on such matters without this information is to commit a capital error. The result is often failure of treatment, because the patient has been misunderstood and emphasis given to minor rather than major features of his problem.

As it becomes clear that a given patient's disturbance is the outcome of the kind of person he is and the situations that he faces, the data of the psychiatric history and the mental status examination can usually be divided into three categories which, although closely related, are usefully distinguished: (1) the predisposing factors for the disturbance, including personality traits and formative life experiences; (2) the precipitating factors; and (3) the symptoms themselves and their effect on the patient.

Predisposing Factors. Predisposing factors are those features special to an individual that make him vulnerable to emotional disturbance. The most critical factor is personality, the traits of which are distinguished in the patient's temperament, attitudes, and predictable responses. But personality is the outcome of genetic constitution, intellectual endowment, and lifetime experiences, and each of these is a predisposing factor in itself. As intriguing examples of studies in these issues, the work of O'Connor on the role of intellectual subnormality in emotional instability and the study of Granville-Grossman on the relationship of parental loss to depression in adulthood can be recommended. Predisposing factors often overlooked are the patient's social status and cultural situation. The scholarly study of Dr. Beatrice Berle, *80 Puerto Rican Families in New York City,* and the recent work of the Dohrenwends in social psychiatry are excellent examples of empirical work in these areas.

Finally, the state of health is an important predisposing feature, because physical illness, through the distress it produces or by direct effects on the central nervous system, interferes with a person's capacity to cope with circumstances and thus leads to psychologic symptoms.

Precipitating Factors. The precipitating factors are events or experiences that have disrupted emotional equilibrium and bear a close temporal relationship to the disturbance for which the patient seeks help. The common-sense expectations that personal illness, or conflict produced by changes in family or occupational circumstances, could precipitate psychologic distress have been confirmed in studies such as those of Brown and Birley. Holmes has attempted to grade life events in a hierarchy of emotional stressfulness, and many workers have found his scale useful for estimating the relative distress different patients have endured. Some psychologic precipitants are more recondite, because they depend on a special meaning an individual gives events, perhaps a symbolic meaning derived from the particular patient's early life experiences. Before emphasizing these more abstruse precipitants of a unique character, it is usually wise to consider the more immediate and obvious ones that may be present.

Symptoms. In this chapter, the symptoms of anxiety,

depression, and hysterical reaction are discussed, because they are common in the general practice of medicine.

All these neurotic symptoms emerge as complaints either of the patient himself or of others who must deal with him. They are symptoms in the sense that they disturb the patient's sense of well-being or they interfere with his behavior and his adaptability to circumstances. They can vary from mild to severe, and they can be acute or chronic.

In the assessment of these symptoms the patient should be encouraged to describe how he feels, how the symptoms developed, what seems to make them worse or better, what they are like when compared to previous emotional reactions, and how they disturb him now. *The aim is to come to appreciate these symptoms as understandable responses of this particular person to his particular circumstances.* The over-all principle is that we are considering here not classes of patients suffering from distinct disease entities, but individuals troubled by their special life circumstances and needing assistance tailored to their particular personal nature and situation. The specific symptoms, their characteristic predisposing and precipitating factors, their effects on behavior, and modes of treatment will be considered in the balance of this chapter.

ANXIETY

Definition. Anxiety is an unpleasant mood of tension and apprehension. It is fear's first cousin and, like fear, has prominent autonomic effects when severe. But fear is an emotion sharply focused on immediate dangers, whereas anxiety is usually imposed by the anticipation of future danger, distress, or difficulties. As an emotional response common to all men, anxiety is useful. Activities that arouse it are avoided and those that diminish it are sustained. Although anxiety may spur people to perform difficult tasks skillfully and admirably, when excessive it is a hindrance, as some well prepared students demonstrate when facing a critical examination. *Anxiety is a medical problem when it is excessive, inappropriate, or without obvious cause.*

Predisposing and Precipitating Factors. Anxiety is the psychologic response to anticipated troubles, real or imagined, dimly or accurately perceived. But men and troubles vary. Some persons, the timid, the inexperienced, the excessively conscientious, are frequently anxious in situations that seem not to affect others. Most people are at least mildly anxious whenever they seek medical advice, and when threatening dangers are intense or prolonged, as in chronic painful illness or in battle, even the most resistant individuals can develop incapacitating anxiety.

Resistance to anxiety varies with physical condition, and when tired, sick, or injured, people are more easily threatened. Also, they are more vulnerable to anxiety when their powers of analysis and discrimination are failing or underdeveloped. Thus, because of inadequate comprehension or imprecise perception, the immature, the elderly, or the person with brain damage may become anxious in situations in which a person with a healthy, mature brain is comfortable. In fact, one of the first indications of a dementia can be an attack of severe anxiety without obvious provocation.

Common precipitants of anxiety in daily life are circumstances of conflict in which an action is demanded but the correct action may be difficult to discern. Thus a person may be anxious over difficult decisions on which rest his economic and social success or because the decisions produce an unpredictable response in an inconsistent superior. Laboratory models for this kind of situation and its effects on the emotional state have been easy to produce. Pavlov trained dogs to respond to the picture of a circle by rewarding such responses with food. He did not reward responses to an ellipse. Then, by simply compressing the ellipse so that it gradually approached a circle in shape, he made the discrimination progressively more difficult. The emotional response of these dogs was remarkable. They became ferocious and violent when put into harness for the experiment. They tore at their restraints, barked uncontrollably, and refused to attempt the discrimination. In this state, not only did they make many mistakes, but they became unable to make discriminations that had previously been easy. It is not difficult to see analogies in both situation and behavior between Pavlov's dogs and men with emotional conflicts.

An emotional state of anxiety can be produced in other ways than as an understandable response to anticipated difficulties. An intractable anxiety state can follow a head injury as one of the symptoms of the so-called *postconcussional syndrome.* Similarly, a mood of tension and agitation with tremulousness can occur in the delirious states, such as those that follow withdrawal of alcohol or barbiturates and are sometimes produced by the hallucinogenic drugs such as LSD-25. In these situations, it may be disturbed perceptions and misinterpretations that arouse anxiety, but often the anxiety is independent of anything that the patient definitely experiences or understands. Roth describes a peculiar and chronic anxiety state that can follow a calamitous emotional experience. This condition, referred to as the *phobic anxiety syndrome,* occurs in mildly obsessional persons after a severe fright. The disturbance can last for many months. These patients are in a state of considerable anxiety, mostly unformulated, and, associated with this, they have an unwillingness to leave their homes because of vague fears. The peculiar psychologic response of *depersonalization,* which is a change in the awareness of self such that the person feels unreal, is present in many of these patients. In the phobic anxiety syndrome the mood of anxiety follows rather than precedes difficulty, demonstrating that anxiety, normally an anticipatory psychologic response, may take on a self-sustained activity after certain experiences such as severe frights or sudden disasters.

The role of learning and of conditioning has too often been neglected in considerations of anxiety. This probably derived from attempts to explain all anxiety in terms of basic instinctive drives. That a fear-provoking situation could train an individual to experience symptoms of anxiety in circumstances that resembled these situations is very likely, and is indicated by research on emotion in animals. The capacity to develop anxiety via conditioning mechanisms seems the probable explanation for certain cases of phobic anxiety focused on specific objects.

Manifestations of Anxiety. The manifestations of anxiety are divisible into three groups. *First* are the inner feelings of tension, apprehension, and dread that form the anxious mood itself. *Second* are disturbances of the intellectual power of the anxious patient. He is unable to think clearly, to use proper judgment, to learn efficiently, or to remember accurately. *Third* are the autonomic, visceral, and endocrine changes that have been analyzed by Walter B. Cannon and his followers as the companions of emotional excitement and particularly of anxiety or fear. These include tremor, tachycardia, hypertension, increased perspiration, dilated pupils, and reduced salivation and gastric secretion. Increased activity of the sympathetic nervous system and of the adrenal medulla mediates the majority of these visceral responses to anxiety.

A model anxiety state is to be seen among front-line soldiers. The infantryman is a prepared subject for anxiety. He is always threatened with death or mutilation. He must go without sleep, remain exposed to the weather, and often be hungry. He is usually unable to understand what is happening around him. He is repeatedly frightened by gun fire and distressed by the death of comrades. If he is exposed long enough, he develops a severe and persisting anxiety state sometimes called "battle fatigue." He becomes tense and easily startled. His judgment is poor, and he cannot efficiently sustain a complex offensive action. Among other physical complaints, he suffers from headache, anorexia, and diarrhea. He is usually convinced that death is imminent. Almost all men develop this condition if exposed to battle long enough. Wolff reports that the average man in the army of the United States reached this point after 85 days of combat; 75 per cent could be expected to break down by combat day 140, and 90 per cent by combat day 210. These figures vary little among nations, although few are willing to publish them. They make the point that, in his resistance to crippling anxiety, even the bravest man has a "breaking point." On reaching it, he does not betray his group or run from the enemy, but rather he becomes less efficient in protecting himself and runs a high risk of death.

The symptoms of anxiety that physicians see in patients are not different. The patients all have the same three groups of symptoms, but, depending in part on the cause, these symptoms can appear as a relatively brief attack or as a more prolonged, chronic disturbance of mood.

Anxiety attacks may be single episodes or may be periods of exacerbation in a chronic state of tension. They are short periods of tension, varying in severity from mild apprehension to severe panic. An anxiety attack can occur at any time. A favored time is when the patient is traveling in a plane, bus, or train. Most commonly, though, an attack develops at night when, with the disappearance of daytime distractions, a patient begins to ruminate on his troubles. The apprehensions grow to preoccupy his thoughts, and he develops visceral responses of fear. Clear thinking becomes impossible, as does sleep. The heart pounds. A common complaint in an anxiety attack is the sensation of tightness in the chest as though the lungs could not be adequately filled. The patient responds to this sensation by deep and sighing respirations. Sometimes he may produce in this way a respiratory alkalosis with feelings of giddiness and vertigo, tingling of his fingertips, and even tetany with carpopedal spasm. This is the *hyperventilation syndrome,* and the resulting symptoms may add to anxiety.

Full-blown anxiety attacks have an hysterical flavor and may, in part, depend on personal tendencies to self-dramatization and suggestibility. But they also can be the results of a psychic chain reaction, the initial apprehensions and anxiety stirring up cardiac and respiratory changes that are themselves frightening. Granville-Grossman and Turner have provided more evidence that visceral responses to anxiety can increase the subjective symptoms of anxiety by demonstrating that these latter symptoms are improved when an anxious patient is treated with propranolol, a drug that blocks the adrenergic beta-receptors of the sympathetic nervous system and slows the heart rate.

Chronic anxiety may be punctuated by or may begin with an acute attack, but it may be just a steady and distressingly prolonged disturbance of mood. The symptoms are less intense although not different in quality from those of acute anxiety. The patient is tense and "on edge." He may also report some feelings of sadness or hopelessness along with his anxiety. It can be difficult to differentiate his condition from an agitated depression. His intellectual powers are diminished, and he has considerable difficulty in concentration and in thinking. He will score poorly on intelligence tests, particularly on the performance subtests, just as does a patient with dementia. He will have a number of somatic complaints: frontal or occipital headache, anorexia, diarrhea, and weight loss, among other things. On examination, he may have the physical signs of tension, a fine tremor of the extended arms and brisk tendon reflexes, rapid heart beat, increased blood pressure, and pupillary dilatation. More extensive laboratory studies may reveal other visceral and endocrine disturbances, such as reduced gastric acid secretion or increased adrenocortical activity.

Diagnosis. Usually diagnosis is not difficult. In both acute and chronic anxiety, the patient's major complaint is the distressing emotional state. Associated disturbances in thinking and autonomic function serve to confirm the diagnostic impression. For these patients, the major issue is not the diagnosis of anxiety, but rather the question of why they have become anxious now. This question must be answered from knowledge of the circumstances and personality of the patient.

An occasional patient focuses his complaints on his physical symptoms, such as irregularities in the beat of his heart, the change in bowel habits, weight loss, anorexia, or easy fatigability. From these symptoms a more severe illness such as a hidden malignancy, a chronic infection, or some endocrine disorder like hyperthyroidism or Addison's disease may be suspected. Although these conditions are usually seen to be only remote possibilities, laboratory studies may be required to exclude them. As with all psychologically disturbed patients, laboratory studies should not be delayed or protracted but should be decided upon, and this phase of the examination should be finished as promptly as possible.

Treatment. Treatment will vary with the cause and severity of anxiety. Many mildly anxious patients can be helped by a physician who is willing to listen carefully to their difficulties and offer some support and occasional advice. Most patients with anxiety have this mild type. Their disturbances are transient and are based on some particular problem or self-doubt that has developed acutely and is eventually resolved.

Those with more severe anxiety can be aided by a combination of pharmacologic treatment and repeated compassionate discussions of their troubles. Barbiturates have been the preferred agents for relief of anxiety in the past. However, barbiturates can be addictive, and there is the ever-present danger that they may be used in a suicide attempt by an anxious patient who is also depressed. In several double-blind clinical trials, chlordiazepoxide (Librium) has been found as effective as barbiturates for treating anxiety, and can be recommended. Dosage of 10 mg three to four times a day is usually effective. Up to 20 to 25 mg three times daily can be given to severely disturbed patients.

Patients with persisting anxiety can be referred with some confidence to specialists in psychotherapy. The effectiveness of psychotherapy seems to depend on the comfort provided by frequent sympathetic discussions and an increased recognition by the patient of the irrational aspects of his anxiety. The particular school of psychotherapeutic theory subscribed to by the therapist seems less important.

Only the most severely anxious patients need hospitalization and then usually only for an acute attack of anxiety. They are treated best with sedation; chlordiazepoxide in doses of 25 to 30 mg three times daily can be used. The somatic symptoms from the respiratory alkalosis of the hyperventilation syndrome can be treated by placing a bag over the nose and mouth that will retain the expired CO_2 for rebreathing.

Careful consideration should be given to any evidence that the anxious patient may be depressed. Agitated depression can be easily confused with simple anxiety. If depression is thought to be the diagnosis, then antidepressant medication, such as imipramine, 25 to 50 mg three to four times a day, should be given rather than sedatives.

For those individuals with restricted anxieties prompted by particular stimuli, i.e., phobias, there is growing evidence that deconditioning techniques based on learning theory may have an important place in therapy. Certainly some impressive controlled trials have been published indicating a faster response to this mode of management than to interpretive therapy for individuals suffering from a single phobia. This treatment, like any other, should not be attempted without experience and guidance.

DEPRESSION

Definition. Depression is a term for a mood of sadness and gloom. It can be a symptom of manic-depressive psychosis, and Ch. 335 should be consulted for a complete consideration of the subject. Here we are dealing with depression that occurs as a response to troubled life circumstances. Such depression can usually be given a more specific name, such as discouragement, demoralization, or grief—terms that carry specifically the connotation of an emotional reaction.

The troubled mood is usually not hard to recognize. The patient appears miserable, his face expressive of sadness and perhaps tension. He may move without confidence or purpose and report that his energy is decreased and his thinking slow and difficult. Appetite is usually lessened, often with weight loss, and sleep is restless and diminished. Sexual interest will be greatly reduced. The patient may also say that he is irritable and fearful. Depending on the severity of his depression, the patient will seem socially disorganized, proving inefficient in work, failing in duties, and neglectful of appearance. His acknowledged inadequacies in these respects may add to his sense of misery and may prompt thoughts of resigning from work, leaving his family, or even committing suicide.

Although various troubles can provoke depression, there is a specific response that illustrates features common to many depressive reactions. That response is *grief*, well studied recently by Dr. C. M. Parkes.

Grief is an experience in almost every lifetime and is the response that follows the loss, usually by death, of some relative or friend. The severity of the reaction and its duration depend upon many factors, but the most important is the closeness of the relationship and degree of dependence of the mourner on the lost individual.

Grief is a state that follows a pattern of development in which certain stages can be recognized even though the transition from one to the next is not possible to define exactly and features from one can persist in the others. *The first stage,* which lasts several days, begins upon learning of the death. The mourner feels stunned and appears bewildered, does not seem to grasp his loss fully or to relate its implications to his feelings coherently. He may appear irritable, tearful, or anxious, but can also seem calm and capable. Although his emotions and behavior may be unpredictable, they are often culturally modified as he carries out such customs as funeral rituals. He himself will usually report afterward that his emotions were blunted and his thinking uncertain, and that his depressed mood was not fully experienced. Parkes refers to this period as the stage of numbness, blunting, or shock.

This stage ends gradually but usually within one week of the bereavement, when there is an increase in the emotion of sadness and the appearance of an intense sense of loss that comes in waves, called pangs of yearning or pining by Parkes. In this *second stage,* between these surges of distressing feelings, which are so frequent at first as to be almost continuous, the patient is usually irritable and sad, with sleep and appetite diminished. Activity, which often takes the form of aimless moving about rather than productive work, may be increased, particularly so during a depressive surge, a point Parkes uses to support his analogy of this stage of grief to the searching behavior of animals separated from their mates. It is the phenomenon of *surges of misery,* however, that is most characteristic of grief and usually aids in its recognition. With time these occur less often, but it is common experience to have such a wave of depressive feelings sweep over a person following a reminder of the loss years after the bereavement.

The third period of grief appears with a diminution in the attacks of yearning and the anxious restlessness. This phase, usually entered into within several weeks of bereavement, customarily lasts the longest. It is a stage of depressed feelings with apathy and a disinclination to find purpose or interest in work. The patient is no longer restless, sleepless, or without appetite, but his emotional state is one of gloom and discouragement and his capacity for enjoyment or for physical or intellectual work is greatly reduced. Parkes refers to this as the stage of *disorganization,* when the patient seems withdrawn, may complain of ill health, and fails to plan ahead. This state may last over a year and only gradually be replaced with more customary feelings. Recovery may be brought about in part by the natural but chance occurrence of new integrative activities and friendships, and can be facilitated by efforts of the mourner to expose himself to the opportunities for these restorative experiences.

Depressions that are responses to difficulties in life other than bereavement are very similar to this third stage. Symptoms like those in the first two stages of grief can appear briefly in distressing situations that have a sudden onset, such as being informed of an unexpected personal misfortune. But these are usually transient features and are soon replaced by a mood of sadness and discouragement very like that of the third stage.

Precipitating Factors. In this form of depression it is usually not difficult to recognize the change as a response to some difficulty, for the patient is often preoccupied with the trouble itself and is ready to draw the link between it and his present mood. Precipitating situations can be of many kinds. They can be sudden and specific events in which something is lost, such as a relationship or a job. Other provocations are situations chronically thwarting to the sense of achievement and self-esteem, as in an education program in which students are confronted with their errors but given little effective teaching to overcome them. Moving away from home can provoke the very unpleasant depressive reaction, homesickness, especially in persons who depend a great deal on the support of friends and family. In general, circumstances that disturb a person's sense of stability, security, effectiveness, or worth provoke depressive responses.

The more such a precipitant is prolonged or accompanied by a growing realization of his difficulties, the more likely the person is to show a depressive response. A paradigm of these features for a precipitant is found in debilitating physical illnesses such as cancer. Here the protracted and continually worsening clinical situation provides constant reminders of losses suffered and brings more each day. That depression is a universal occurrence in such circumstances has been demonstrated by Hinton in his study of the dying.

For reasons not fully understood, there are some physiologic states and physical illnesses that commonly provoke depressive moods. Patients with hepatitis or influenza are particularly prone to report a depressive mood and to find reasons for it in trifles that did not trouble them when they were well. Endocrine alterations such as the postpartum state, Cushing's disease, or Addison's disease are also precipitants of depressive feelings that can be very distressing to the patient and of such profound degree as to occasionally promote a suicidal action. Certain brain diseases, particularly stroke, may also precipitate a prolonged and distressing depressive state. In all these circumstances the mood of depression may rest on some disturbed physiologic mechanism in the central nervous system as yet unknown. Their possible relationship to manic-depressive disorder is discussed in Ch. 335.

Predisposing Factors. Given that situations of difficulty can lead to depression, there are features of personality that can make an individual more vulnerable to this response, perhaps by making him assess losses and difficulties more acutely and by inhibiting his power to resolve them. Especially vulnerable are those insecure and sensitive individuals who perceive criticism when none is intended and find a source of depressive feelings in their self-doubting.

Another depressive predisposition is that of the self-dramatizing and emotionally unstable and immature individual who tends to amplify emotional reactions of all sorts. When such an individual finds himself in situations of discomfort in which his feelings may be neglected, he seems more prone than others to develop a sense of dissatisfaction, distress, and depression. Slavney and McHugh present empirical evidence of this predisposition in their report of depressive symptoms in 80 per cent of patients hospitalized with the diagnosis of hysterical personality.

Finally, individuals limited in their capacity to cope with difficulties are predisposed to depressive responses. Particularly vulnerable for this reason are the mentally retarded. Even modest impairment in intellectual endowment will interfere with the person's ability to find solutions to situations that present him problems, and his failure and uncertainty tend to provoke a depressive mood. Borderline mental retardation is often overlooked in the search for predisposing factors, and a history of poor occupational and scholastic performance in a depressed patient warrants formal intelligence testing.

Differential Diagnosis. The differential diagnosis of depressive states can be difficult, particularly if it is not carried out methodically. The most important distinction to draw is that between depression as a response to troubled circumstances and depression as a symptom of manic-depressive disorder. This important discrimination rests on clinical grounds and cannot be made with certainty in all situations. Thus, although the depressions of the widow, the homesick, and the patient with a fatal illness can all be recognized as responses, the trap is in making this understandable connection with every depression and explaining it always as being due to some recent difficulty. If the family of the patient says he is more depressed than they would expect him to be under the circumstances, the diagnosis of a depressive response might be questioned. Also, the presence in the patient of remarkable changes in self-attitude such as the appearance of beliefs that he is a criminal or deserves punishment for minor transgressions, or that he is infectious and filled with physical corruption, are not seen in the usual depressive response and should lead to the consideration of manic-depressive psychosis. Finally, a previous history of mania or of depression, or a family history of affective disorder should influence the interpretation of depression and sway the diagnosis away from the depressive response (see Ch. 335).

Treatment. Although the depressive response is characteristic enough to be recognized easily again and again, the particular predispositions, precipitants, and interactions are never the same from one patient to another. Treatment is based on these particulars and is thus unique to some extent on each occasion. It is therefore hard to describe the treatment of depression without some sense of dissatisfaction because, although the principles are simple, no list of them applies to every patient.

An important early decision in treatment is the need for hospitalization. This is usually determined by how severely the mood disturbance interferes with self-care, by the availability of a supportive and protective environment at home, and particularly by the presence of suicidal features. To assess the last, the patient must be asked if he has been considering self-injury. Although judgment is required in evaluating his answers, a sequence of questions probing for suicidal thoughts should be routine for every patient with depression. A proportion of the patients will deny all thought of self-injury and can be assumed to be of lesser suicidal risk. Those who admit to such thoughts should be asked if they have any means in mind. To that question still more patients will reassure the doctor that their thoughts on suicide have not reached so severe an intensity. Those patients, however, who admit to having considered a means (pills, gas, shooting) must be considered of higher risk, and thought must be given to protecting them, perhaps by hospitalization or by guaranteeing that they are under the supervision of friends or relatives. Finally, the patients should be asked if they have acquired any means or done anything to try them out. Again a proportion of patients will say that they have not been that despondent, but those who say that they have done such things are at very high risk and should in most cases be hospitalized.

Once a decision is made about the site of treatment, in a hospital or on an outpatient basis, the act of reaching a secure diagnosis of a depressive reaction in a patient is the first step in its treatment, because this judgment requires that the doctor has come to understand the patient and his predicament. To gain this understanding the doctor's first meetings should be devoted to listening to the patient's description of his circumstances, of his emotional changes, and of the connections he draws between his experiences and his depressive mood. If appropriate, other informants such as relatives can amplify on the patient's statements and give details of his past modes of coping with trouble. All these efforts are intended to bring the doctor an appreciation of this particular individual and the circumstances that he faces.

Such knowledge, combined with the relationships of trust, respect, and empathy that develop naturally in its acquisition, provides the resources for treatment.

The therapeutic efforts from this foundation are directed toward re-engaging the patient in life experiences in which success can be found, replacements for losses enjoyed, and a sense of integrity and control regained. Usually the first need of the patient is some help in simple tactics for the management of his current troubles and for the avoidance of their repetition in the future.

At this stage a sense of helplessness often prompts the patient to abandon many of his activities and efforts, but if at all possible he must be encouraged not to give in to these promptings, because doing so tends to perpetuate the disturbed mood by holding him from opportunities to reassess his situation and to try out solutions. His daily work, even when less efficiently performed, is often helpful in directing his attention to matters other than his troubles.

With assistance in simple matters of personal management, the patient can be helped to some success in his circumstances, bringing him encouragement and promoting a willingness to maintain his efforts and to plan for the future. Educating the patient in how certain circumstances strike his particular vulnerabilities and so provoke depressive responses can be helpful.

The most useful ingredient of the treatment is the support and interest of the doctor. This encourages the patient to express his feelings and discuss his circumstances. In this way not only is the physician provided with more information about assets and vulnerabilities of the patient, but often there is spontaneous recognition by the patient of causal features for his difficulties that brings both relief to his mood and self-perceived tactics for their resolution. If this supportive relationship can be maintained and developed, improvement of depression can be expected. For the occasional patient with whom such a relationship fails or who succumbs frequently to depressive reactions because of some intractable predisposition, more prolonged treatment by specialists in psychotherapy can be recommended.

Finally, treatment with pharmaceutical agents may help. Chlordiazepoxide, 10 mg three times daily, may relieve agitation somewhat in the bereaved or otherwise relatively depressed. A sleeping medication, flurazepam hydrochloride (Dalmane), is helpful for the sleeplessness. *The antidepressant medications,* although most useful in the manic-depressive psychoses, can be tried in some patients with a prolonged depressive response. Imipramine in a dose of 150 to 250 mg a day or the monoamine oxidase inhibitor phenelzine, 15 mg three times daily, has helped individual patients, but this symptomatic relief should be considered a minor part of the treatment plan in patients with this form of depression.

HYSTERIA

Definition. Hysteria is a disturbance of behavior in which symptoms and signs of physical ill health are imitated more or less unconsciously for some personal advantage. As the phrase "more or less unconsciously" implies, hysteria may be hard to distinguish from "malingering," in which the imitation of illness is a well-appreciated fraud. Frank malingering is rare, though, because the power of human self-deception is usually adequate to persuade a person of the validity of his own symptoms. The only ones who can be called malingerers with any confidence are some self-mutilating patients and the remarkable pathologic liars, picturesquely called examples of the *Munchausen syndrome,* who travel from hospital to hospital gaining admission by means of dramatic acts of illness.

Predisposing and Precipitating Factors. Hysterical symptoms are to be seen as responses to distressing experiences. They can occur in almost any person facing danger or difficulty, especially if, as with soldiers in battle or prisoners, the distress is intense and prolonged and physical symptoms can provide a viable escape. Dull-witted or immature persons with inadequate powers of introspection and self-control may produce transparently hysterical symptoms in response to milder distress, such as school difficulties or family problems. Some of the exaggerations and elaborations of medical symptoms common in hospitalized patients may be similarly interpreted as responses to the distress of illness by persons whose capacity for self-control has been weakened by somatic illness. Hysterical symptoms can be the first manifestations of a dementing illness or of a depressive or schizophrenic psychosis, and these disorders must be considered when a previously well balanced adult develops a suspiciously hysterical symptom.

Commonly, though, hysteria is a disturbance in the behavior of a person predisposed by an attention-seeking, emotionally unstable, and egocentric personality. In fact, these characteristics form what has become known as the "hysterical personality" even though hysteria can occur in other types of people, and these characteristics do not invariably produce hysterical symptoms. Most easily recognized in such people is their flair for the dramatic. They show this tendency in flamboyant dress and in exaggerated, even melodramatic, responses to questions about their symptoms. They are never so happy as when they are the center of attention. Karl Jaspers characterized the hysterical personalities as those who "crave to appear, both to themselves and others, as more than they are and to experience more than they are ever capable of." The zeal of these patients for exaggeration and drama renders them more liable to hysterical symptoms. But other kinds of people can have these symptoms. In all of them usually a discouraged, depressive mood has been prompted by difficulties in life, and the hysterical symptoms then emerge from this mood state.

Symptoms and Signs. Many of the phenomena of somatic illness can be imitated by hysteria. The accuracy of the imitation depends on the medical sophistication of the patient. A doctor or nurse is more likely to produce a convincing imitation than is an unqualified person.

Common hysterical symptoms are vague subjective disorders, such as generalized weakness, dizziness, indigestion, or pain. Hysterical pain can occur in any part of the body, but the head and neck, the region over the heart, and the low back are particularly favored. Hysterical pain can be of any character, from dull aching to sharp and stabbing pain, but it is often described by the patient in vivid similes such as "like a bullet," "like a bolt of lightning," "aches like an abscessed tooth," or "sore as a hot boil." Usually, hysterical pain is not confined to a local area as around a pathologic lesion, nor is it referred into the distribution of a particular nerve or dermatome. Rather, hysterical pain is felt in a general region of the body and spreads, sometimes in bizarre ways, into contiguous areas without regard to neuroanatomic boundaries. Thus pain beginning in the face may spread along the side of the head and into the back, crossing from the region of the trigeminal nerve into the upper cervical nerve regions. Hysterical pain often varies in its character, intensity, and distribution, changing considerably with attention or suggestion. Occasionally it can be remarkably improved by a small amount of intravenous amobarbital sodium when analgesics do not help.

Although vague symptoms of a subjective kind such as pain or dizziness are the present vogue in hysteria, crude and gross symptoms are still seen. These may be psychologic, such as the amnesia or fugue states, in which memory is partially lost, often in situations in which the patient is depressed or anxious. Other psychologic symptoms shown occasionally include auditory and visual hallucinations and even flamboyant delusions. These must be carefully judged, but appear most commonly in young people who have read popular books on psychology and psychiatry and are apparently suggested into these symptoms by their reading at a time when they are distressed over other matters.

Motor disturbances in the form of abnormal movement, disturbed gaits, seizures, or paralyses are occasionally hysterical symptoms. Hysterical seizures can usually be distinguished from epileptic ones. The patients only rarely injure themselves, bite their tongues, or lose their urine. They do not have the typical tonic and then clonic phases of a seizure, but tend to show a dramatic flailing of the limbs. Consciousness is partially retained, and seizures hardly ever occur when the patient is alone. The EEG is normal.

Sensory disturbances are particularly favored hysterical symptoms. Thus, *blindness* or *deafness* is common, often developing dramatically at a time of emotional distress. Loss of sensation over one side of the body to pin prick or light touch is frequently found after a susceptible patient has been examined by a neurologist.

Diagnosis. Diagnosis of hysteria is seldom easy and never popular. Ideally, it should rest on three supports: first, the *form* of the hysterical manifestation; second, the *personality* of the patient; and third, the *setting* in which the symptoms developed. Often it is not possible to find all three supports to a diagnosis, but all should be sought.

Commonly, hysterical symptoms are vague and variable. In fact, the more definite and consistent a patient's description of the onset, location, nature, and duration of his symptoms, the less likely the symptoms are to be hysterical. Hysterical symptoms and signs are also usually incompatible with what is known of anatomy and physiology. Thus sensory losses do not conform to patterns of nerve distribution; reflexes remain intact and unchanged in the palsies of arm and leg; seizures of the entire body do not disturb consciousness; total blindness appears without a disturbance of pupillary reflex or of opticokinetic nystagmus. The hysterically mute person can phonate on coughing. The hysterically deaf person speaks louder to be heard over increased ambient noises. Many other hysterical symptoms have been analyzed for such inconsistencies by Head.

Knowledge of the personality and past history of the patient is helpful to a diagnosis of hysteria. The recognition that the symptoms are occurring in an hysterical personality should prompt an observer to look very closely at the symptoms before embarking on extensive laboratory tests or upon surgery. Similarly, knowledge of a previous vague and poorly understood medical disturbance can lend weight to an opinion that a new symptom that has eluded diagnosis is occurring in an individual prone to hysteria. Conversely, hysteria can usually be eliminated as an explanation for symptoms in an emotionally stable, middle-aged person. People who have passed through adolescence and young adulthood without resorting to hysterical behavior are unlikely to employ it when older.

The setting in which the symptoms develop should be carefully scrutinized, and a search made for a distressing event that may have provoked an hysterical reaction or for any purpose that the hysterical symptoms may serve. Occasionally, a clear association between the symptoms chosen and a particular recent disturbance in the life of the subject can be found, such as an amnesia developing in a person who has done something shameful or criminal, or weakness and pain persisting in a person who is seeking financial compensation for an injury. Often, though, motivations behind hysterical symptoms are vague and uncertain. It is usual to find that the patient is unhappy or anxious about some aspect of his life circumstances and that the hysterical symptoms serve to call attention to his distress. Also, it may be possible to demonstrate that the development of particular symptoms has been prompted by suggestion: weakness of legs, for example, developing in a nurse caring for a paraplegic patient, or peculiar falling attacks after the patient has witnessed an epileptic seizure.

A careful study of the symptoms, the personality, and the life setting of a patient usually allows a reasonably certain differentiation of hysterical symptoms from those of a medical illness. There are, however, certain medical problems that are notoriously easily confused with hysteria. These are the diseases that produce vague and changing symptoms that seem to vary with the patient's motivation and, at least in their early phases, lack convincing physical signs. If such an illness occurs in a patient who has features of the hysterical personality and who will therefore describe the symptoms in a dramatic and flamboyant fashion, physicians may be even more persuaded to believe that the illness is only deceptively physical. Examples of diseases frequently confused with hysteria because of their subtle clinical features are the first attack of multiple sclerosis, particularly if sensory changes alone are produced; the weakness of arms and legs seen early in acute idiopathic polyneuritis of the Guillain-Barré type; the difficulty in swallowing of bulbar myasthenia gravis; the attacks of muscular weakness in periodic paralysis; the tonic posturings and oculogyric crises of postencephalitic parkinsonism; the pain of a cauda equina tumor; and the abdominal pain of acute intermittent porphyria.

Management of Hysteria. The management of hysterical patients is difficult. No one method can be recommended unqualifiedly. But there are certain principles that can be followed. To help hysterical patients it is essential to have sympathy for them. Many doctors find these patients irritating. It is just as possible to see them as individuals displaying an intriguing aspect of human behavior that has profound implications in their lives. It is pointless to argue with these patients about the validity of their symptoms. A useful approach is to agree that they have had an illness producing their symptoms, but that they are now improving even though total recovery has not arrived.

It is important to diagnose hysteria promptly. Hesitation in diagnosis leading to several hospital admissions for extensive laboratory investigations is a good way to solidify hysterical symptoms in a patient. Among other things, the uncertainty of doctors helps persuade a patient that the symptoms are real. Repeated examinations increase the consistency with which symptoms are reported. Long hospitalization, mounting bills, and the inconvenience caused to others make it difficult for a patient to abandon symptoms without embarrassment. The gratifying attention given to the patient in the hospital, perhaps as an example of an intriguing diagnostic problem, can feed the self-dramatizing tendencies and so encourage the behavior.

There is always risk of error in any diagnosis, because diagnosis is only a weighing of probabilities. The diagnosis of hysteria, though, depends purely on a physician's judgment and, before relief of symptoms is accomplished, can be confirmed in the laboratory only by evidence of health. Physicians, for obvious reasons, fear more the error of calling a physically sick patient hysterical than the error of mishandling hysteria. They often prefer to exclude, by laboratory examination, progressively more unlikely diseases than to study carefully the symptoms and the individual who has produced them, even though this would lead more directly to a definite diagnosis as well as an understanding of the response. It may be unwise to counsel too strongly against this behavior because medical diagnosis is never easy. A compromise can be found in the admonition to perform immediately the laboratory tests that seem necessary for a patient, but when hysteria is suspected, to bring the period of investigation as quickly as possible to a close so that management of the specific symptom can be begun.

Treatment of the specific symptoms rests basically upon persuasion. The doctor is persuading the patient to perform the functions that the patient claims are disabled. Intravenous amobarbital sodium given to the point where the patient is mildly intoxicated and his speech slurred is particularly helpful in making and establishing a persuasion. Usually, some ingenuity is required for success. The hysterically blind person can, for example, be persuaded first that he can distinguish light from dark and then gradually to distinguish forms, to read large print, and, finally, small newsprint. The person who claims he cannot walk can be encouraged first to move his legs in bed, and then to stand, to make a few tentative shuffles, and finally to stride out. The hysterically deaf person can be persuaded to hear through a stethoscope and then gradually that he can hear without it. A dramatic show of some kind is often helpful in removing these symptoms. If a physician has success in partially removing hysterical symptoms, he should persist in his treatment without interruption in order to bring about as much improvement as possible and even to restore full function. When there is recovery of function, the patient should perform his recovered skills in public—before his family, other patients and several doctors—to prevent his relapsing immediately into his former state.

The fear that sudden removal of hysterical symptoms will result in a disastrous psychologic collapse is exaggerated. Rarely, a depressed patient with hysterical symptoms has an increase in depression, but it is clear that in those situations a depression was overlooked and the more secondary hysterical symptoms were emphasized.

Some hysterical disorders are refractory to treatment. Among these are the disorders assumed for some material gain, such as compensation. They usually are not improved until some settlement is made. Episodic disorders such as hysterical seizures can be hard to control. Sometimes, however, a statement to the patient that they will not recur, given with full authority by a physician whom the patient trusts and respects, may eliminate these symptoms. The longer the patient has hysterical symptoms, the harder they are to remove. This is a corollary to the aforementioned observation that hysterical symptoms produced for transparent reasons and bordering on malingering are more difficult to eliminate than are the ones produced by an attention-seeking personality in some emotional distress. Symptoms held for a long time cannot be easily abandoned without embarrassing the patient.

Simultaneously with treatment of the specific symptoms, the emotional state and present life of the patient should be studied to discover any distress that may have precipitated the hysterical symptoms. Then advice, social assistance, or guidance can be offered to aid the patient in resolving these difficulties. This aspect of their psychologic treatment depends on developing a relationship of friendship and mutual respect identical to that found necessary in treating an anxious or depressed person.

Long-term management of hysterical patients is much more difficult than treatment of individual symptoms. It is not wise to have the average hysterical patient embark on depth psychotherapy, because he tends to produce more symptoms and to recount involved sexual and other fantasies in order to maintain the interest of his doctor. If possible, these patients should be followed by one physician who understands them and the behavior that they are liable to produce and is also competent to recognize physical illness should it arise. This physician can save these patients from needless surgery and long hospitalization. He can remove hysterical symptoms promptly by being alert to the diagnosis and providing help for the difficulties that precipitate them.

Berle, B. B.: 80 Puerto Rican Families in New York City. New York, Columbia University Press, 1958.

Brown, G. W., and Birley, J. L. T.: Social precipitants of severe psychiatric disorders. *In* Hare, E. H., and Wing, J. K. (eds.): Psychiatric Epidemiology. New York, Oxford University Press, 1970.

Dohrenwend, B. P., and Dohrenwend, B. S.: Social Status and Psychological Disorder. A Causal Inquiry. New York, John Wiley & Sons, Inc., 1969.

Granville-Grossman, K. L.: The early environment in affective disorder. *In* Coppen, A., and Walk, A. (eds.): Recent Developments in Affective Disorder. Br. J. Psychiatry, Special Publication No. 2, 1968.

Granville-Grossman, K. L., and Turner, P.: The effect of propranolol on anxiety. Lancet, 1:788, 1966.

Head, H.: The diagnosis of hysteria. Br. Med. J., 1:827, 1922.

Hinton, J. M.: Physical and mental distress of the dying. Quart. J. Med., 32:1, 1963.

Homes, T. H., and Rahe, R. H.: The social readjustment score. J. Psychosom. Res., 11:213, 1967.

Jaspers, K.: General Psychopathology. Manchester, Manchester University Press, 1962.

O'Connor, N.: Psychology and intelligence. *In* Shepherd, M., and Davies, D. L. (eds.): Studies in Psychiatry. New York, Oxford University Press, 1968.

Parkes, C. M.: The first year of bereavement. Psychiatry, 33:444, 1970.

Roth, M.: The phobic anxiety-depersonalization syndrome and some general aetological problems in psychiatry. J. Neuropsychiatry, 1:293, 1960.

Slavney, P. R., and McHugh, P. R.: The hysterical personality: A controlled study. Arch. Gen. Psychiatry, 30:325, 1974.

Walters, A.: Psychogenic regional pain, alias hysterical pain. Brain, 84:1, 1961.

Wolff, H. G.: Every man has his "breaking point." Milit. Med., 125:85, 1960.

Section Five. PSYCHOLOGIC TESTING IN CLINICAL MEDICINE

Paul R. McHugh

337. INTRODUCTION

The intent of this section is to describe some methods of psychologic testing that have proved helpful in clinical settings. The goal is to provide some capacity to evaluate critically any psychologic test instrument, whether presently in use or likely to be devised in the foreseeable future.

Psychologic tests are intended to assist clinical evaluation of behavioral disorders by bringing accurate measurement to the mental examination. Physicians are familiar with instruments that bring accurate measurement to observations in the physical examination; the clinical thermometer and sphygmomanometer give information in numerical form about body temperature and blood pressure that cannot be collected with such accuracy without their assistance. They are so easy to employ that knowledge of the normal readings in the human population and implications of deviations from normal have been established. Although psychologic tests are aimed at more abstract phenomena such as intelligence or personality, they similarly attempt to bring precision through numerical or graphic measurements and provide a means by which an individual can be compared in these features with others.

The mere provision of a numerical expression does not prove a test useful, as the numbers may not be meaningful. Often in our fascination with a new test and its intriguingly plausible scales for measurement, we overlook its failure to satisfy the criteria of *reliability* and *validity*.

The reliability of a measuring instrument, whether it be for a physical or a psychologic function, is an expression of the accuracy and reproducibility of its findings. No instrument is perfectly reliable, but the range within which it is unreliable must be a small fraction of the potential range of measurement if it is to be capable of detecting a genuine deviation in the variable under study.

The validity of a measuring instrument is an expression of its capacity to measure what it claims to measure. The clinical thermometer does measure body temperature. How can we be sure that psychologic tests are actually measuring the psychologic variables that they claim to measure? How can we be sure that intelligence tests, for example, measure intelligence? The only proof that a psychologic test is valid is the demonstration that scores on it predict behavior in life thought to be the expression of the trait it claims to measure. For example, results on a valid intelligence test should correlate to some extent with scholastic performance.

The issues of reliability and validity can perhaps be made clearer with a homely example. The common ruler is an instrument designed to measure distances. It is a reliable instrument in that repeated measurements of the same object, say a cube one foot to a side, will give the same results. It is also a valid instrument for the measurement of the cube's dimensions. It is not, however, a valid instrument for measuring the cube's weight. This is determined by the material of the cube, and no number of repeated measurements with the reliable ruler will make it give a valid measure of weight.

338. INTELLIGENCE

The quantitative measurement of the mental attribute, intelligence, was first attempted by Binet at the turn of the century. His success and the Stanford-Binet battery of tests developed from his work brought such predictive power to the study of intelligence that they provide an impetus to the development of tests to examine other mental functions. But the tests of intelligence have through their revisions, particularly the *Wechsler Bellevue Intelligence Scale* published in 1939 and the *Wechsler Adult Intelligence Scale (WAIS)* of 1955, remained the most secure and useful tests of mental function.

Intelligence is difficult to define. It is the abstract concept used to explain the observation that individuals vary in their mental capacities and in the effectiveness with which they employ them. Intelligence is more easily defined in practice by pointing to instances of its action. This way is in fact used in our daily life. We judge a man's intelligence by observing his bearing, his speech, his apparent grasp of situations, his judgments, and his emotional control. Then in the light of our past experience of watching other men, we call an individual bright or dull. We are doing nothing conceptually different when we estimate intelligence at the bedside or by means of psychologic tests. We organize the testing so that a series of observations can be made within a reasonable period of time. We add scope to our examination by asking for performance in several different kinds of mental activity. We bring accuracy to the observations by scoring the performance.

The questions on orientation, memory, attention and concentration, fund of knowledge, and capacity to reason abstractly that constitute the tests of cognition routinely carried out at the bedside in the course of the physical and mental examination provide a doctor an estimate of his patient's intellectual functioning. In the light of knowledge of the patient's past life and demonstrated abilities, the doctor makes a judgment whether there has been damage to intellectual functioning. Psychologic tests are able to give a more accurate estimate of the intelligence of a patient at the moment of testing than do these bedside examinations, because these tests have proved both reliable and valid.

All these approaches, from the casual observations to the most refined test, are applications of a fundamentally identical method: an assessment of a performance thought on practical grounds to be a reflection of intelligence. However, any performance will be influenced by other factors, particularly the factors of education and experience. *Since these factors derive from opportunities and social heritage of the subject, every one of these assessments must be qualified and interpreted in the light of the subject's cultural and educational background.*

Subcultural differences that are obvious on bedside examination, being recognized as modifications in expression and in experience, *are allowed for almost automatically in that assessment but are sometimes forgotten when formal intelligence test scores are displayed.* Just as there is no culture-pure bedside examination, there is no culture-pure intelligence test. Test scores must be interpreted in relationship to all that is known about the patient. Particular care in the interpretation is demanded if he is a member of a subculture different from the standard criterion group employed in the development of the formal tests: urban, school-educated whites. The greater his divergence in this respect, the greater the allowance needed in interpreting the scores of his tests. Emotional disturbances or other preoccupations that interfere with the patient's concentration or cooperation will also obviously affect these performances. Allowances must be made for any of these features in assessing test scores, just as allowance is made for these features on bedside examination.

The *Wechsler Adult Intelligence Scale* is the most reliable and valid instrument we have for measuring the intellectual function of the adult. Its reliability has been demonstrated by the close correlation of test scores given on separate occasions to the same individuals and by the similarity of scores when one half of a test is compared with another half (split-half method). Its validity has been demonstrated by its correlation with life performances of individuals it scores as intelligent or dull.

In its present form the WAIS consists of 11 subtests of mental skill. Six of these subtests are "verbal tests." In these the patient is requested to define words, to recognize similarities between words, to do arithmetic, to remember numbers forward and backward, to answer questions on his fund of knowledge, and to judge and interpret proverbs. These tests are followed by five "performance tests," in which a patient is asked to work with rather unfamiliar material and solve problems set to him by that material. Tests here include the putting together of puzzles, work with symbols, the setting out of logical stories from pictures disorganized for the test, construction of patterns from multicolored blocks, and the recognition of things missing from drawings. The performance tests seem somewhat less related to the education of a person than are the verbal tests. All the subtests that have been chosen for the WAIS have a long history of investigation. They are combined together to produce a thorough and accurate instrument.

The scoring of the WAIS is in the form of the *Intelligence Quotient (I.Q.).* In fact, the WAIS derives a verbal I.Q. from the verbal tests and a performance I.Q. from the performance tests. A full-scale I.Q. is derived from the combination of all 11 subtests.

The I.Q. compares an individual with others. Historically it was developed for children. I.Q. then was the ratio of mental age over chronologic age times 100 when mental age was defined in terms of a child's ability to succeed on tests which the average child of a given age could do. Thus a child solving problems which the average nine-year-old could solve had a mental age of nine. If he, himself, was nine years old at the time of the test, he had an average ability and an I.Q. of $9/9 \times 100$, or 100; if his chronologic age was six, he would be an advanced child with an I.Q. of $9/6 \times 100$, or 150. Terman demonstrated the constancy of I.Q. in the growing child.

But a ratio of mental to chronologic age is unlikely to be useful in adults because tested intelligence does not increase after the late teens. The WAIS and many other tests for adult intelligence continue to use the term I.Q. This is possible because of the fact that tests of intelligence appear to distribute individuals in a "normal" or gaussian fashion. This curve has a mean at I.Q. 100 and a standard deviation of ±15 I.Q. points. It is possible to divide the curve into percentiles of the population. The WAIS score of any person places him in the percentile of the population with similar scores, and his I.Q. can be extrapolated from percentile by means of the distribution curve. Thus an individual whose performance on the WAIS is equal to 50 per cent of the population is said to have an I.Q. of 100, whereas individuals whose test performances exceeded 98 per cent of the population will be said to have an I.Q. of 135 or above.

The WAIS has found its greatest clinical utility in the study of patients with brain disease. Any damage to the cerebral hemispheres will injure intellectual ability and disturb the scores on the WAIS. An intriguing observation is that early in the course of brain disease performance tests are disturbed before the verbal test scores change. This may indicate that verbal tests measure more what an individual has learned and practiced, whereas performance tests measure his capacity to meet new problems. The verbal and performance scores of normal individuals are usually comparable. The verbal I.Q. can be considered a fair estimate of the original intellectual endowment of an individual suffering from a brain injury. The decline of the performance I.Q. is a useful measure of the degree of injury to the cerebral tissue the patient has endured. With an advancing brain disease verbal I.Q. will fall eventually, but a patient will usually continue to demonstrate higher verbal than performance scores.

Emotional unrest such as anxiety or depression will also interfere with WAIS scores. Here, as with cerebral disease, the performance I.Q. will fall below the verbal I.Q., demonstrating that the capacity to work with unfamiliar material is disturbed more than tests of what has been well learned. But because these findings are identical to those in persons with brain disease, the differentiation of an emotional disturbance from dementia cannot come from WAIS results. It must rest on other information such as is derived from the history, physical examination, and mental status.

The WAIS is useful not only in demonstrating deterioration of intellectual function but also when done serially can document recovery of function with treatment. Since it is so simple to employ, its increasing utility in clinical research is assured.

339. PERSONALITY

By personality is meant all the abiding traits of character that constitute an individual's potential to respond in particular ways to circumstances. All physicians are aware of how much information they must acquire through several interviews with the patient and from independent sources before they can have much confidence in their diagnostic opinion on personality. Tests that could elucidate personality more accurately and more rapidly would be useful. Two alternative approaches have been developed, "projective" tests and questionnaires, and each approach has raised particular problems.

In the so-called projective tests of personality ambiguous situations are set before the patient, and his responses are recorded. Thus he is presented with sentences to complete, a picture to interpret, or, in the most well known projective test, the Rorschach test, he is presented with a standardized set of ink blots and asked to describe the forms that he can recognize within them. Since there is nothing in the situations themselves that force any particular response, the responses of the patient are thought to derive from his personal predilections and inner needs, drives, and conflicts. This seems logical. But logic is not the essential criterion for a test intended to aid the clinical examination. It must be demonstrated that the responses on projective tests provide measurements that are reliable and valid. This remains to be done.

Certain features of a patient can be expected to be seen in any set of his responses. For instance, overly conscientious persons will tend to be fixed on details, the schizophrenic patient with his disordered thought will demonstrate this feature in distorted expression, and the depressed patient will speak of unhappy themes as he discusses any matter. These features will appear whether the patient is being examined by his doctor or doing a projective test. Until the reliability and validity of projective tests can be demonstrated, it cannot be known whether they are superior to the clinical examination, and if they are not superior to the clinical examination, they are of doubtful utility to the physician. The question of their value is shrouded in controversy.

The other approach to personality measurement is the questionnaire. This was developed from the clinical examination. Since questions are used there to gain information from the patient, it seemed logical that a questionnaire including these and many other questions would improve on the clinical examination. It came as a surprise when tests developed in this fashion proved to be unreliable and invalid. This was demonstrated when different questionnaires intended to probe similar features of personality, such as introversion, did not correlate well with one another, and in fact could give quite opposite impressions of the same person. Questionnaires developed in this fashion proved so misleading that the method fell into disrepute. It was, however, eventually recognized that these early tests gratuitously assumed that questions would be accurately answered by patients. Consider the question, Do you lack self-confidence, yes or no? To presume that a person will understand this question exactly the same way as the examiner intends and that his criterion for a yes or no answer is the same as that of all other people is to presume too much. Also these early tests failed to consider that many individuals might attempt to show themselves in some more favorable light and therefore not answer questions truthfully.

The most intriguing conceptual advance in the study of personality was the recognition that an objectively truthful answer to questions was not needed for a valid, useful test. In fact, more information can be obtained from observing the patient's replies to questions than from any belief that the statements they agree to or reject are in themselves accurate descriptions of their personality. The task of building questionnaires changed from finding questions that would display the inner feelings of people to finding questions that would be answered differently by different personality types.

To build such a questionnaire the first step was to gather together specific groups of people for study: normal people, anxious patients, hysterical patients, depressed patients, for as many groups as could be differentiated. These patients, the criterion groups, were asked a large number of questions, and the replies were compared from group to group. The questions which differentiated the groups best were then collected for the questionnaire. This questionnaire then given to an individual was interpreted not from the content of questions rejected or affirmed but from the number of questions replied to in the same fashion as in one or more of the criterion groups.

The most useful questionnaire that has been developed is the *Minnesota Multiphasic Personality Inventory (MMPI)*. The questions in that test have been carefully studied and chosen so that they differentiate the groups to the greatest degree possible with it. Because of the complexity of issues of personality, the numbers of questions needed to derive a profile with this test is 550. It was possible in the MMPI to fit in many questions that give an indication of the tendency of the patient to lie, exaggerate, or misunderstand questions.

The results of the MMPI are expressed as a series of ten scales or dimensions along each of which an individual is placed by means of his responses that correspond to responses of nine criterion groups. These scales were originally derived from clinical groups and given clinical names, i.e., hypochondriasis, depression, hysteria, psychopathic, masculine-feminine dimension, paranoid, psychaesthenic, schizophrenic, manic, and social introversion. Three so-called reliability scales are also scored for each test.

The MMPI is a reliable instrument, the accuracy and reproducibility of its readings having been demonstrated in repeated testing of individuals over many years. The validity of its scales varies. Some of the scales measure the personality characteristics for which they are titled. Scores on the psychopathic and manic scales do correlate with the clinical features intended by these terms. Scores on the schizophrenic and hysterical scales do not correlate well with these clinical disorders but with aspects of bizarreness and self-dramatization, respectively, features not specific to schizophrenia or hysteria. In an effort to avoid these invalid implications, the MMPI scales are no longer referred to by clinical titles, but by numbers or letters derived from the original names.

The tendency to look at specific scales for diagnostic impressions has been replaced by consideration of the "profile," or pattern of the several scales together, hoping to derive in this way a more global view of personality structure. This approach emphasizes the multidimensional character of personality. It takes advantage of the features of reliability found in this test. But, once again, the establishment of validity for these profiles must be accomplished. This is being attempted by matching the life course of individuals with predictions from the profiles, but work is still in progress.

Current practice is to find the MMPI useful as a screening and probing instrument that often suggests aspects of personality difficulty that might well be more carefully studied. However, its validity for the differentiation of clinical psychiatric entities or specific personality types is uncertain, and thus it must not be regarded as the arbiter in differential diagnosis.

Butcher, H. J.: Human Intelligence, Its Nature and Assessment. London, Methuen & Co., Ltd., 1968.
Penrose, L. S.: The Biology of Mental Defect. London, Sidgwick and Jackson, Ltd., 1963.
Terman, L. M., and Oden, M.: The Gifted Group at Mid-Life. Genetic Studies of Genius, Vol. V. Stanford, California, Stanford University Press, 1959.
Welsh, G. S., and Dahlstrom, W. G.: Basic Readings on the MMPI. Minneapolis, University of Minnesota Press, 1956.
Williams, M.: Mental Testing in Clinical Practice. London, Pergamon Press, 1965.

Section Six. MEDICAL ASPECTS OF SEXUALITY

Harold I. Lief

THE PHYSICIAN'S ROLE

Once almost completely neglected in medical education, sex counseling is now included in the curriculum of approximately 90 medical schools in the United States. Physicians now recognize the frequency and importance of sexual problems in medical practice. About 40 per cent of the emotional problems for which patients ask their doctors for help are related to marriage, and the most frequent marital difficulties, as perceived by a representative sample of physicians surveyed by Herndon and Nash, are problems of sexual adjustment. In the Marriage Council of Philadelphia clinic, about 75 per cent of couples report some sexual maladjustment, including 15 per cent for whom a sexual problem is a major problem and a primary cause of marital difficulty.

The frequency with which sexual problems arise in practice varies with three factors: the specialty, whether the physician routinely asks about sex problems, and the comfort of the physician in discussing sex with the patient. The highest frequencies, according to Burnap and Golden, are found in the practice of psychiatry, obstetrics-gynecology, urology, and in general practice. If the physician routinely asks about sex problems, the average frequency of patients with sexual problems is 14 per cent, whereas it drops to 7.9 per cent among the physicians who inquire about sexual matters "only when indicated." Among the group of physicians who might be thought to display discomfort with sexuality, the frequency of sexual problems reported in their practices was only 2.7 per cent, as compared with an average of 15 per cent among those physicians who were reasonably comfortable.

The importance of taking a sexual history is emphasized by the results of a study by Pauley and Goldstein, who found that most physicians who routinely take a sexual history from their patients identify significant sexual problems in at least half of them. On the other hand, the great majority of physicians who do not actively inquire about sex activity estimate that less than 10 per cent of their patients have sexual problems.

Most sexual problems presented to physicians are in the context of a marital relationship, as either primary causes of marital dysfunction or as consequences of other areas of marital discord, but which, nevertheless, augment and maintain marital unhappiness. It seems reasonable, then, to make sex and marriage counseling a "package" in the training of the physician and in the delivery of medical care. Even in the case of the pediatrician, it is still logical, for he soon comes to recognize the direct connection between the marital relationship of the parents and the sexual problems of the child.

The busy physician or the physician who shies away from marital therapy may have to treat the couple by dealing with one patient only. And many situations can be handled adequately in this fashion, e.g., the urologist who cures male dyspareunia by clearing up the patient's prostatitis, the internist who helps restore his patient's potency by reassuring him that sexual activity will not give him another coronary occlusion, the gynecologist who reassures his patient that she will suffer no loss of sexual drive after hysterectomy. Yet, sexual behavior involves a relationship, and hence, in most instances, therapy should also be directed toward the relationship.

Not only are marital and sexual problems in medical practice frequent, but they are often overlooked or avoided—either because of the physician's lack of training and his feeling of incompetence in this area or because these problems impinge on his own marital and sexual conflicts or values and make him uncomfortable. Even if he consciously or unconsciously ducks the issue by failing to follow cues, changing the subject by responding with a trite and stereotyped form of reassurance, e.g., "this is just a phase—your problem will disappear in time," he is carrying out counseling of sorts. Vincent has stated it well:

> The theoretical position that the physician cannot or should not engage in any marriage or sexual counseling becomes meaningless when the patients expect this role of their physician and when their illnesses have sexual and marital implications—if not origins. The majority of physicians literally have no choice; even to do and say nothing in response to the patient's questions and/or presentation of symptoms in the sexual and marital areas is, by default, one form of counseling.

In dealing with sexual and marital problems, the physician has an unequaled opportunity to practice preventive as well as therapeutic medicine. By aiding patients to obtain greater sexual satisfaction, he may prevent the escalation of marital discord and consequent family disorganization through emotional conflict with or without divorce. Anything that seems to strengthen family life has positive repercussions on the next generation as well. Early intervention can occur in a number of clinical situations, e.g., premarital counseling, family planning services, during pregnancy, postpartum care, early marriage, as well as through family life education for teenagers and young adults. The pediatrician and obstetrician have especially significant points of entrance into the system of health care, enabling these specialists to practice effective prevention.

To be competent in handling the therapeutic and preventive aspects of the sexual, marital, and family problems he sees almost daily in his practice, the physician must not only have a store of *information,* but must also develop a set of *skills* and *attitudes* that facilitate his making optimal use of his information. Surely the key factor in competent sex and marital counseling is the degree of comfort of the counselor. His skill in interviewing, in eliciting salient data about the most intimate, personal dimension of patients' lives, will depend directly on his capacity to react, not with anxiety, anger, or self-righteousness, but with openness, ease, and a clear desire to achieve an atmosphere of genuine communication—of feelings as well as thoughts. In the absence of these skills and attitudes, his quantity of information, even if vast, is of little use.

SEXUALITY

Sexuality refers to the totality of one's sexual being, of which physical sex is only a part. In this sense, our sexuality is what we "are" rather than what we "do." One's sense of being male and masculine, female and feminine, and the various roles these self-perceptions engender or affect are important ingredients of sexuality. Cognitive, emotional, and physical sex all contribute to the totality.

Sexuality may be described in terms of a system analogous to the circulatory or respiratory system. The components of the sexual system are set forth in the accompanying table.

Abnormalities in biologic sex may be minor or major. Major abnormalities create problems of intersexuality, which may, if not corrected early in life, lead to conflicts in sexual or gender identity. The sex assigned is, with rare exceptions, more important in determining gender identity than is biologic sex, and sex change procedures are usually unwise after the age of 18 months. Some of these patients and some without evident biologic defect have grave difficulties in developing a core gender identity of the same biologic sex. These are transsexuals, mostly biologic males who think of themselves as "a female trapped in a male body."

With these relatively rare exceptions, development of sexuality leads to a secure sense of maleness or femaleness, which is generally complete by the age of three. However, in our culture, doubts and conflicts about masculinity and femininity are ubiquitous. Serious disturbances lead to such sex deviations as transvestitism, fetishism, voyeurism, and exhibitionism.

Homosexuality. Homosexuality is a special variant of gender identity. Although homosexuals do not question their maleness or femaleness (sexual identity), many, if not most, of them question their masculinity or femininity, at least in cultures which promote heterosexuality and marriage as much as does ours in the United States. (By the time they are ten years old, 90 per cent of girls and 80 per cent of boys already are fantasizing about marriage.)

The physician should not automatically come to the conclusion that every homosexual who consults him for any medical problem wants to "go straight," i.e., to become heterosexual. In fact, most homosexuals prefer their sexual adaptation, and only those who are in great distress about their homosexual behavior should be considered for psychotherapeutic intervention, and then only after a thorough evaluation of their motivation for change. Family pressure for change is insufficient reason to undertake intervention.

Sexual System and Personality. Far more commonly, the physician is called upon to deal with less overt conflicts about gender identity that create significant marital problems with sexual connotations, examples of which are the Don Juan who has to prove his masculinity by sexual conquests; the promiscuous housewife who tries to prove to herself her femininity by finding the elusive orgasm, or by demonstrating her attractiveness; the woman who cannot respond sexually because she is afraid of being completely dominated or possessed by a male; and the husband who cannot have sexual intercourse with his wife on top, because it seems unmanly. The "battle of the sexes" is carried out not only in bed, but in every area of marital interaction, generally by people who are uncertain of their masculinity or femininity and who fight to gain self-respect by derogating the partner. Several generations ago, these sexually related social roles were handed down or "assigned" by tradition; today, roles are negotiable, and problems become serious when negotiation is impossible to attain because of faulty communication, or when it breaks down because of disturbed perception or the fear of compromise.

The sexual system develops as such an integral part of personality development that sexuality and personality are inseparably interwoven. The physician who wishes to be an effective sex counselor, therefore, must deal with sexual relations in the context of human, especially marital, relations.

Sexual System (Sexuality)

1. Biological sex—chromosomes, hormones, primary and secondary sex characteristics
2. Sexual identity (sometimes called core gender identity)—sense of maleness and femaleness
3. Gender identity—sense of masculinity and femininity
4. Sexual role behavior: (1) sex behavior—behavior motivated by desire for sexual pleasure, ultimately orgasm (physical sex); (2) gender behavior—behavior with masculine and feminine connotations.

PROBLEM AREAS

Sexual disturbances in marriage may be the result of (1) sufficient psychopathology on the part of one or both spouses, (2) a poor relationship or "fit" between the spouses, or (3) relative ignorance of one or both partners. An example of the first category is the wife whose life experience taught her that sex is nasty and sinful and who cannot experience sexual pleasure, for the pleasure would increase her guilt inordinately. Patients in this category with longstanding sexual dysfunction are generally referred to psychiatrists. Patients whose difficulties stem largely from a poor marital relationship may be seen by the nonpsychiatric physician, who, unless he has had special training in sex and marriage counseling, must be mindful of his own capacities and limitations.

The physician who is comfortable in dealing with sexual problems and whose values do not push him to impose his own standards on his patients can clear up many sexual concerns by giving appropriate information. Sexual misunderstanding and misinformation are extensive; only a few examples are given here: the adolescent boy who thinks his penis is too small, or the teenage girl who thinks she is abnormal because of her sexual urges; the idea that the person who desires sex frequently is a "sex maniac"; the notion that oral-genital sex is a perverse activity; the frequent concept that coital orgasm is the only form of orgasm that is normal; that masturbation leads to mental illness (1650 out of 11,000 medical students who took the Sex Knowledge and Attitude Test, or SKAT, expressed this belief!); that direct clitoral stimulation must be continued until penetration occurs; that waxing and waning of sexual excitement is abnormal; that sexual activity during pregnancy or weeks after recovery from a coronary occlusion is dangerous; or that after the age of 50 or 60 or 70 a person is sexually "over the hill."

In evaluating any sexual problem it is necessary to determine how much weight to attach to the three factors contributing to the problem. Often, all three are represented. The woman who has the concept of sex as a sinful activity and who inhibits her responsivity may have only a hazy idea of what pattern of stimulation (called by Masters and Johnson "sensate focus") is best suited to increase her sexual excitement, and may make all sorts of excuses to her husband ("I'm tired"; "I have a headache"; "It's my period") to avoid sex, or she may grant or withhold sex as a weapon to punish her husband or in bargaining for something she wants.

Although the sexual problems that arise in marriage constitute the most frequent and most important need for professional intervention, additional characteristic sexual problems arise during the life cycle. Including marital sexual problems, some of the more frequent problem areas are the following:

1. Helping children and their parents deal with problems of sexual development. This includes concern about masturbation, sex play among children, menstruation, wet dreams, sexual fantasies, and possible coital activity among teenagers. "How do I, as a parent, talk to my children about sex?" is a question often asked of physicians.

2. Concerns of teenagers about masturbation, penis size, "how far to go during petting," the relation of sex to the relationships between sexes (how does sex relate to love?), erotic arousal for members of the same sex, contraception, and sexual performance. Unwanted pregnancy creates a need for abortion or "problem pregnancy" counseling. Venereal disease may occur at any age level, but it is increasing rapidly among teenagers.

3. Among young adults contemplating marriage, concerns about sexual performance and compatibility, as well as about family planning.

4. During marriage (or other intimate relationships), concerns about sexual interest, frequency, responsivity, coital positions, aspects of noncoital sex such as oral-genital sex, extramarital sex, contraception, abortion, and infertility. Of increasing concern to young people are conflicts about sex-role behavior (what is appropriate for men and women in their relations with each other). Life cycle events such as pregnancy, childbirth, moving to another locality, change of jobs, death, or chronic illness often have important effects on sexual feelings and behavior. Bodily complaints and physical symptoms may mask sexual and marital problems.

5. Other illnesses—psychic, such as depression, or physical, such as heart, lung, metabolic, or neurologic disease—may create special sexual concerns and inhibitions of function, as does ablative surgery.

6. Separation such as occurs with divorce or death in the middle-aged or elderly creates very special sexual problems. The loss of companionship and affection may be even more important than the decrease in sexual opportunities, although the interest in sex itself among the elderly is characteristically unrecognized or minimized by the physician.

Although childhood sex play and masturbation are now recognized as part of normal psychosexual development, parents are frequently concerned enough to ask their physicians about these behaviors. In most instances reassurance is all that is needed. If the sexual activity is "excessive" (and this is often subject to varying interpretation), it indicates a narrowing of the range of healthy social activities of the child, rather than the abnormality of the sexual behavior per se. Parents who ask how to talk about sex with their children can be referred to a number of books on this topic. A list of recommended reading can be obtained from the Sex Information and Education Council of the United States (SIECUS), 1855 Broadway, New York, N.Y. 10023. Similarly, a list of excellent books for teenagers to read can be obtained from the same source. The physician should read any recommended text so that he can answer questions in a more informed manner. The basic points in talking to children or teenagers is to be as comfortable as possible, and to be brief, concise, and factual once the real concerns are elicited by gently encouraging the child to talk, and above all, to avoid lecturing in a pontifical fashion. The physician is more apt to be "heard" if he discusses the pros and cons of sexual decision-making, rather than expressing his own value-position in a forceful manner.

The problem of premarital coitus is characteristically presented by the unmarried girl who asks her physician for the "pill." If freedom of the physician is not restricted by his own set of values, this provides him with an opportunity to discuss with the young patient her feelings and expectations about her relationship with her actual or intended partner. Physicians are often concerned that prescribing contraception for the unmarried girl will be a license for sexual activity. Actually, the young girl asks *after,* rather than before, the initial coital experience. A study of over 500 unwed never-pregnant teenagers aged 13 to 17, who for the first time sought professional help to obtain contraception, shows that 96 per cent of those teenagers who asked for contraception were previously sexually active; most of them had been having intercourse for more than a year; few were using any contraceptives, and still fewer were using one of the most effective methods. It should be clear that if a minor requests contraception, she needs it. This study and others suggest that contraceptive information and educational programs directed at minors will not be a significant factor in their decision to become sexually active.

A special area of increasing concern to physicians is called *"problem pregnancy" counseling.* This is not restricted to teenagers, as the majority of abortions are performed on married women. The unmarried pregnant teenager, however, is in a highly vulnerable position, because pregnancy and childbearing may seriously interfere with her educational and economic status, let alone the negative social sanctions that still persist despite the Supreme Court's decision legalizing abortion. The various options, i.e., continuing with the pregnancy and giving up the baby for adoption, or bringing the baby home, whether to marry or not, or whether to terminate pregnancy, have to be discussed thoroughly, and outside pressures for decision-making separated from internal conflict. The availability of legal abortion has eased the situation greatly, but the decision for abortion should never be made lightly, because the physician should be fairly certain that the patient will not be in the small minority who suffer from depression or remorse after the abortion. This applies to married women as well as to the unmarried. Most patients (who are not harmed by the abortion procedure per se) would derive special benefits by more intensive contraceptive, sex, and family counseling than is ordinarily provided to women seeking abortion.

Family-planning counseling gives the physician an unparalleled opportunity for exploring the connections between sexual attitudes and behavior and contraceptive concerns. The choice of the appropriate method of contraception is influenced by the frequency of coitus, attitudes toward responsibility and decision-making, fears of bodily damage, and desires for greater sexual spontaneity, as well as religious and moral values. Contraceptive failures are related to risk-taking, to the failure to learn how or under what conditions conception occurs, or to the individual's being under stress so that "contraceptive vigilance" is reduced. Adequate communication with the partner about contraceptive planning is an important consequence of appropriate counseling.

Family planning is much more than the prescription of a contraceptive method. It includes the timing of marriage, timing of the first child, child-spacing, the total number of children desired, and sex and marriage counseling, as well as contraception, problem-pregnancy, and sterilization counseling. Genetic counseling may also be a significant dimension of family planning. In this sense, family-planning counseling is an essential feature of premarital counseling, but is of course applicable throughout the child-bearing years.

Patients frequently misperceive the spouse's desired frequency of intercourse; most often the wife overestimates her husband's desired frequency. In one sixth of the cases studied, there was a gross underestimation of the wife's desires. The *perception* of the problem is usually more significant than the *reality*. The physician can often help by asking each spouse separately how often he wants intercourse and his perception of his spouse's desires. Better communication is the first step toward relieving this problem, and in many instances may be all that is required. The physician also has to bear in mind that the sex drive in the male is at a peak between the ages of 15 and 25, whereas in the female it peaks a decade later.

Inadequate responsivity in the female is due either to faulty preparation or to the inhibiting influence of emergency emotions – fear, anger, and guilt. Faulty preparation may be due to ignorance or unconcern of the husband or the inability of the wife to communicate her needs and preferences to her husband. The physician should try to clear away areas of ignorance before tackling the more difficult problems of inhibition caused by emotions designed for emergency "survival" rather than for pleasure. The long-range goal of therapy is to substitute the welfare emotions – love, pride, hope, and joy – for the emergency emotions. Newer techniques of sexual education and re-education, increasing the couple's awareness of the "sensate focus" and increasing each spouse's positive regard for his own body, have been developed by Masters and Johnson.

Premature ejaculation is again due either to a faulty perception of the bodily cues signaling impending ejaculation or to the influence of emergency emotions. Unless the patient is diabetic, impotence is generally related to a fear of failing in penetration, superimposed on emergency emotions related to his feelings about his partner. The vast majority of men with this disorder can be helped by removing the fear of performance, as John Hunter discovered two hundred years ago. He counseled his patients to avoid coitus "in six consecutive amatory experiences" and reported signal success.

Extramarital intercourse is sometimes dealt with more easily by marital partners than one might think. If, however, it threatens to have a destructive effect on the marriage, referral to an experienced marriage counselor is appropriate.

The astute physician has to be on the lookout for the presence of sexual or marital problems that lie behind a host of physical symptoms – headache, backache, fatigue, menstrual irregularities, or dysmenorrhea. Osler said of syphilis that it was "the great imitator" of other disease states. It may be said more accurately that sexual dissatisfaction plays that role today.

Chronic illness often has sexual connotations. Most physicians do not even discuss sex with their postcoronary patients, and when they do they may offer vague and uncertain advice, such as "take it easy." Patients who have chronic illness, or who have had organ ablation such as hysterectomy *are* concerned about their sexual function: How often? Under what circumstances? Am I still virile or attractive? are questions many patients are too embarrassed to ask.

DOCTOR-PATIENT RELATIONSHIP

Many patients are in doubt about what constitutes normal sexual behavior. These include questions about masturbation, oral-genital sex, sexual positions, coital frequency, sex during menstruation, pregnancy, or in the postpartum period, and sex in mid-life or later. The well-informed physician will be able to deal effectively with these concerns if he takes the trouble to inquire about the patient's sex life or is alert to cues that the patient wishes to discuss this area. History taking should utilize open-ended questions that preclude a yes or no answer and that go from less sensitive areas to ones of greater potential discomfort to the patient, e.g., from a discussion of marital relations to sex, or from menarche to petting to coitus, or from frequency to foreplay to coital positions.

If the physician is interested in this area, if he is reasonably comfortable and tactful, and has an appreciation of the role his own feelings and attitudes play in his interviewing and management of his patients' sexual problems, he will be able to establish a feeling of confidence and hope in his patient. This emphatic relationship coupled with the physician's growing fund of information and skills in interviewing makes possible the competent management of marital and sexual problems that heretofore have been either neglected or mishandled. In no other area of his practice can the physician derive greater reward and satisfaction from his efforts.

American Medical Association, Committee on Human Sexuality: Human Sexuality. Chicago, A.M.A., 1973.

Burnap, D. N., and Golden, J. S.: Sexual problems in medical practice. J. Med. Educ., 42:673, 1967.

Calderone, M. S.: Manual of Family Planning and Contraceptive Practice. 2nd ed. Baltimore, Williams & Wilkins Company, 1970.
Group for the Advancement of Psychiatry, Committee on Medical Education: Assessment of Sexual Function: A Guide to Interviewing. Vol. 8, Report No. 88, November 1973.
Herndon, C. N., and Nash, E. M.: Premarriage and marriage counseling: A study of North Carolina physicians. J.A.M.A., 180:395, 1962.
Katchadourian, H. A., and Lunde, D. T.: Fundamentals of Human Sexuality. New York, Holt, Rinehart & Winston, 1972.
Kinsey, A. C., Pomeroy, W. B., and Martin, C. E.: Sexual Behavior in the Human Male. Philadelphia, W. B. Saunders Company, 1948.
Kinsey, A. C., Pomeroy, W. B., Martin, C. E., and Gebhard, P. H.: Sexual Behavior in the Human Female. Philadelphia, W. B. Saunders Company, 1953.
Klemer, R. H.: Counseling in Marital and Sexual Problems: A Physician's Handbook. Baltimore, Williams & Wilkins Company, 1965.
Lief, H. I.: Preparing the physician to become a sex counselor and educator. Pediatr. Clin. North Am., 16:44, 1969.
Lief, H. I.: New developments in the sex education of the physician. J.A.M.A., 212:1864, 1970.
Masters, W. H., and Johnson, V. E.: Human Sexual Response. Boston, Little, Brown & Co., 1966.
Masters, W. H., and Johnson, V. E.: Human Sexual Inadequacy. Boston, Little, Brown & Co., 1970.
McCary, J. L.: Human Sexuality. New York, Van Nostrand, 1973.
Money, J., and Ehrhardt, A. A.: Man and Woman, Boy and Girl. Baltimore, Johns Hopkins University Press, 1972.
Nash, E. M., Jessner, I., and Abse, D. W.: Marriage Counseling in Medical Practice. Chapel Hill, University of North Carolina Press, 1964.
Pauley, I. B., and Goldstein, S. F.: Physicians' perception of their education in human sexuality. J. Med. Educ., 45:745, 1970.
Settlage, D. S. F., Baroff, S., and Cooper, D.: Sexual experience of younger teenage girls seeking contraceptive assistance for the first time. Fam. Plann. Perspect., 5:223, 1973.
Sex Information and Education Council of the United States (SIECUS): Sexuality and Man. New York, Charles Scribner's Sons, 1970.
Sorenson, R. C.: Adolescent Sexuality in Contemporary America. New York, World, 1973.
Trainer, J. B.: Physiologic Foundation for Marriage Counseling. St. Louis, C. V. Mosby Company, 1965.
Vincent, C. E.: Human Sexuality in Medical Education and Practice. Springfield, Ill., Charles C Thomas, 1968.
Vincent, C. E.: Sexual and Marital Health: The Physician as Consultant. New York, McGraw-Hill Book Company, 1973.
Zubin, J., and Money, J. (eds.): Contemporary Sexual Behavior: Critical Issues in the 1970's. Baltimore, Johns Hopkins University Press, 1973.

Section Seven. DRUG ABUSE, ADDICTION, AND INTOXICATION

340. INTRODUCTION

Robert B. Millman

Drug abuse is behavior that results from the complex interaction of an individual, his social and cultural environment, and the pharmacology and availability of particular drugs. There is frequently no sharp line that distinguishes appropriate use from misuse of any drug. Drug abuse may therefore be defined as the use of any substance in a manner that deviates from the accepted medical, social, or legal patterns within a given society. This section will consider the abuse of drugs that are primarily used to induce alterations in mood, perception, and behavior. These may be grouped into six major classes: (1) opiates; (2) central nervous system depressants, including alcohol, hypnotics, and tranquilizers; (3) central nervous system stimulants, including the amphetamine group and cocaine; (4) cannabis; (5) psychedelics; and (6) miscellaneous inhalants.

Abuse of some drugs may be intermittent and lead to little physical, psychologic, or social deterioration. In other cases, the user may become dependent on the drug in order to function at what he perceives to be a satisfactory level. This *psychologic dependence,* or habituation, varies in intensity and may culminate in *compulsive drug abuse,* in which the supply and use of particular drugs become primary concerns of living. In addition, certain drugs have the capacity to produce *physical dependence.* This is an altered physiologic state induced by the repeated administration of a drug that requires the continued administration of the drug to prevent the appearance of a syndrome characteristic for each drug, the *withdrawal,* or *abstinence, syndrome.* The term *"addiction"* has been used in the literature to refer to either behavioral or pharmacologic events. As used herein, it refers to a pattern of compulsive drug use that includes both physical dependence and an overwhelming involvement with the supply and use of a drug. Neither a diabetic who is on insulin nor a well-adjusted patient in methadone maintenance treatment is an addict in this sense of the term, although both are physically dependent on their medication.

Etiology. No single factor is the basis of all drug-taking experience, and no person's drug taking has a single cause. Drugs are taken to reduce pain, to influence mood, to change activity levels, to reduce tension and anxiety, to decrease fatigue and boredom, to facilitate social interaction, to heighten sensation and awareness, to satisfy curiosity, and for many other reasons. If caffeine, nicotine, alcohol, and prescription and over-the-counter depressants and stimulants are included, few people in the United States would be found who take no psychoactive drugs. Some people experiment with drugs that are considered dangerous from a medical or legal point of view and do not repeat the experience. Others persist in drug-abuse behavior patterns for a variety of reasons.

Sociologic Factors. Social and cultural factors determine which drug-abuse patterns are acceptable for a given group; and in some cases, groups derive their identity from particular drug-using behavior. The use of alcohol is condoned and even encouraged in many segments of society. Cannabis and psychedelic use are an integral part of membership in some white middle-class groups. Heroin use, until recently, was an involving, exciting pursuit in inner-city ghetto areas. Given the limited opportunities to experience pleasure, satisfaction, or pride in certain underprivileged groups, moreover, the aggressive, goal-oriented life of a heroin addict may appear attractive to a young boy or girl. Social factors also determine the availability of particular drugs. Heroin is easily available in the inner city, whereas the suburban dweller may have to travel long distances to obtain the drug. Patterns of abuse change rapidly in response to a variety of social and cultural factors. Currently (1974), the incidence of heroin addiction may be decreasing in New York City and some other urban areas, whereas the extent of multiple-drug use, including alcohol and hypnotics, may be increasing.

Psychobiologic Factors. Personality characteristics, in part, determine the psychoactive effects that drugs elicit in individual users and influence the choice of drugs and patterns of abuse. Amphetamines may produce tranquility in some people. Alcohol and barbiturates impair behavior control in others and may permit more aggressive personality types to "act out" in a hostile and violent manner.

Controversy exists whether drug abuse implies a personality disturbance that antedates drug use and that can be classified in distinct groups according to the drug and pattern of abuse. Most authorities agree that the experimental or intermittent abuse of drugs is not necessarily an indication of psychopathology. Compulsive drug use is frequently associated with serious psychopathology. Some workers describe addictive or alcoholic personality types, characterized by a mixture of neurotic traits and character disorders. Narcotic addicts have been described as passive individuals who experience intolerable anxiety related to physical pain, sexuality, hunger, and aggression. Opiates relieve this anxiety and permit the addict to withdraw from these inner tensions.

Evidence is accumulating to suggest that personality characteristics in drug-abusing populations vary considerably and that psychologic factors play a markedly variable role in the etiology of drug abuse. It is well known that some seriously disturbed people have experimented with alcohol, opiates, and other drugs and have not become compulsive users. *Moreover, no predictive test or system has been developed that will determine whether or not a person will become a compulsive user, nor which people will use which drugs.* Although premorbid personality disturbances are crucial in the etiology of some cases of compulsive drug use, the psychopathology noted in other cases may be a reaction to the behavioral patterns of compulsive abuse in a society that condemns the drug-dependent life.

Learning influences the nature of the drug experience and patterns of abuse. Conditioned factors have been implicated in the drug-craving and abstinence symptoms that occur when an abstinent ex-addict returns to a site of former drug use.

Various disease states are treated with psychoactive drugs for prolonged periods. The drug use of a small percentage of patients may come to exceed medically recommended dosages or indications and eventuate in addiction in some cases. Psychologic and sociologic factors should be considered in the etiology of these behavior patterns in addition to the physical and pharmacologic determinants. Genetic and physical factors may also influence the response to drugs in some individuals.

Pharmacologic Factors. The nature of the psychic and physical effects of particular drugs is a determinant of their initial abuse potential. Considerations of physical dependence and tolerance influence the pattern of abuse. *Tolerance* refers to the decreased effect obtained from repeated administration of a given dose of a drug or to the need for increased amounts to obtain the effects that occurred from the first dose. Tolerance may be either *drug disposition* (metabolic) in type, in which there is more rapid inactivation or excretion of a drug, or *pharmacodynamic* (cellular), in which cells in the nervous system adapt to drug concentrations. Both may occur with the same drug. The physical dependence that develops concurrently with tolerance to opiates, barbiturates, and alcohol is poorly understood and may be related to pharmacodynamic tolerance mechanisms. *Cross-dependence* refers to the ability of one drug to suppress abstinence symptoms produced by withdrawal of another. Cross-dependence may be complete or partial, as with alcohol and the barbiturates.

Diagnosis. Diagnosis of specific patterns of drug abuse and dependence requires careful history taking, when possible, and a complete physical examination. Drug abusers are often poor historians and may minimize or exaggerate the extent of their drug use, depending on their perception of the situation, their needs, and the attitudes of the examiner. The nature and degree of drug-induced psychoactive effects and any abstinence symptoms and signs should be assessed. Adverse effects of particular drugs should be sought.

Evaluation of the mode of administration of the drugs of abuse is important in establishing a diagnosis. Signs of repeated intravenous injections ("tracks") suggest heroin, amphetamine, or cocaine abuse. These drugs are also "sniffed," whereby the material is inhaled and absorbed through the mucous membranes of the nasopharynx and respiratory tract. Chronic sinusitis or perforation of the nasal septum may suggest this mode of administration. Personal hygiene and patterns of behavior and dress may further define the clinical picture.

Routine qualitative procedures for the detection in urine of morphine (the major metabolite of heroin), methadone, amphetamines, cocaine, and the most frequently abused general depressants are currently available in many laboratories. Results will generally be positive if a dose sufficient to produce pharmacologic effects has been taken within 24 hours prior to the urine sample. Since results are not immediately available ordinarily, and since false positives occur, these tests should be used to confirm the clinical impression. They are most useful as an adjunct to the long-term evaluation of patients already in treatment. In emergency situations, blood levels of suspected drugs may usually be obtained immediately.

Treatment and Prevention. Treatment procedures should vary according to the individual and his social set, the pattern and extent of abuse, and the pharmacology of the abused drugs, as well as the goals of treatment. As distinct from most other patients, drug abusers frequently know more about the behavior and disability incident to drug taking than do their physicians. Serving to further complicate therapeutic efforts, drug abusers are often faced with prejudice and hostility on the part of treatment personnel, e.g., "they did it to themselves." Since many of their personality characteristics and behavior patterns occur in response to the attitudes of society, an inquiring, compassionate attitude is crucial in the treatment of this group of patients.

Drug-abuse prevention programs have focused on educational efforts in which the risks of drug abuse are publicized, and on increased legal stringency. Both approaches have serious deficiencies. Perhaps more important than either of these would be the provision of reasonable, attractive vocational, recreational, and educational alternatives to drug abuse in those most at risk, namely, the young and socially disadvantaged. Finally, physicians must be extremely prudent in their prescribing practices with respect to potentially abusable drugs.

341. THE OPIATES

Robert B. Millman

Opiates or narcotic analgesics refer to natural or synthetic drugs that have pharmacologic actions similar to the derivatives of opium. Opium is obtained from the poppy plant *Papaver somniferum* and contains more than 20 alkaloids, of which morphine and codeine are relevant to this discussion. Heroin, the principal opiate of abuse in the United States, is converted from morphine by the addition of two acetyl groups (diacetyl-morphine). Demerol and methadone are synthetic narcotic analgesics. Pentazocine is a synthetic analgesic compound that has actions similar to both the opiates and the narcotic antagonists.

Incidence. People have used opium for medical, religious, or recreational purposes since ancient times. Marked changes have occurred in the characteristics of the opiate-abusing population in the United States during the past 100 years. The use of patent medicines containing opiates was widespread in the middle class during the period from 1850 to 1906, when the labeling requirements of the Pure-Food and Drugs Act caused many preparations to be withdrawn. The Harrison Narcotics Act of 1914 and Supreme Court decisions in the 1920's made possession of narcotics without a prescription a crime and created a climate in which addicts were considered to be criminals and in which physicians could not prescribe narcotics to addicts. The number of oral opiate users declined, and the primary remaining group were those who injected heroin or morphine. Illegal dealers became the only source of opiates. Prices rose precipitously, and addicts frequently resorted to criminal activity to finance their addiction. The addict population from the 1930's to the second world war included predominantly white individuals involved in criminal activity or the entertainment professions who used intravenous heroin as well as morphine, cocaine, and other drugs. The growth of urban black ghettos and the development of efficient production and delivery systems ushered in the present era of extensive heroin use associated with a pervasive street culture that supports the heroin-dependent life. Surveys completed in 1971, estimated between 200,000 and 300,000 heroin addicts in the United States. The majority of these were members of ethnic minority groups and lived in urban areas. Males predominated over females, and the population was quite young. In New York City in 1971, heroin addiction was the major cause of death in males aged 15 to 35. Large numbers of affluent white suburban youths were also becoming addicted. At present, evidence suggests that the incidence of heroin addiction may be decreasing in many urban areas owing to a multiplicity of factors, including changing social and cultural styles, the proliferation of effective treatment programs, and decreased availability of heroin. A recent phenomenon is the oral methadone abuse that is occurring as a result of its increased availability.

Patterns of Abuse. People initially experiment with heroin for many reasons, including a search for pleasure, curiosity, anxiety, immaturity, sexual problems, psychopathology, and peer pressure. In some urban ghetto areas, given the lack of attractive alternatives, using and selling heroin appears to be a rewarding, involving "career" that carries with it the illusion of wealth and significance. Users are generally introduced to the drug by a friend or acquaintance already using the drug. The role of the nonaddicted drug dealer ("profiteer") is minimal in exposing new users to the drug. Street heroin ("smack," "scag," "junk," "dope") is adulterated ("cut") with quinine, lactose, maltose, and other sugars as it passes from the importer to the street user. The final amount of heroin in a street package costing from two to ten dollars may vary from 3 to 30 mg.

Initial street use is generally by "sniffing," in which the material is absorbed through the mucous membranes of the nasopharynx and respiratory tract. A user's first experience with the drug is often characterized as somewhat unpleasant because of nausea, vomiting, and anxiety; these symptoms abate with subsequent use. Effects may then be perceived as a sense of relaxation and peace with relief of worry and tension, a euphoric state in which all things are as they should be. At the outset, use may be intermittent and separated by weeks or months. It is not known how many people experiment with the drug and do not continue its use. Those who do continue to use heroin develop tolerance to its euphoric effects. In an attempt to maximize the euphoric effects of a given street amount, users will begin to inject the drug subcutaneously ("skin-popping") and eventually intravenously ("mainlining"). Intravenous injection produces a warm flushing of the skin and pleasurable sensations in the entire body, described as similar to sexual orgasm and called a "rush" or "kick." Many years of intravenous use of opiates and other drugs may result in obliteration of patent, available veins, necessitating a return to the subcutaneous mode of injection.

As tolerance increases and the awareness of physical dependence becomes manifest, more drug must be used more often. The urban street addict, with little access to legitimate sources of money or drug, must devote all of his time and energy to the acquisition of heroin to support his addiction ("habit"). Involvement in the "junkie" subculture, with its own language and behavioral systems, ensures his supply of drug and provides for the transmission of skills, information, and ideology that makes it possible to live as an addict. Any source of money is acceptable; males frequently engage in theft and forgery, whereas females will be prostitutes and shoplifters. Every user is a potential "dealer" of drugs, since this is the most efficient way of making money. Food, clothing, sexual desires, and dignity may become subordinate to the ever-present need for opiates. An unknown number of heroin addicts, particularly those in the entertainment professions, are able to maintain their employment and their families and do not become immersed in the behavior patterns of the street "junkie."

If heroin is not available or is in poor supply, addicts will use other opiates, particularly methadone because of its long duration of action, to allay their withdrawal symptoms. Few cases of primary methadone addiction have been noted, since it is usually available in oral form only and the intensity of its euphoric properties is less than that of heroin. Barbiturates, other hypnotics, and alcohol may also be used in this regard. Mixed addictions in this group are frequently seen. An integral part of the natural history of this disease consists of repeated arrests, hospitalizations for the complications of addiction, attempts at self-imposed abstinence, periods when drug is not available ("panic"), and failures in treatment programs. These abstinent episodes may serve to lower an addict's tolerance and so decrease the expense and hardship of his "habit."

The patterns of abuse noted in addicted medical personnel or in those few "medical" addicts, who obtain their drugs through licit channels, are quite different from those of the street "junkie." Meperidine, morphine, and pentazocine are generally the drugs of choice in this group. There is little of the social and physical degradation seen in the general addict population. They are frequently able to maintain their employment and the other elements of their lives.

Opiate addicts are a heterogeneous group. The incidence of premorbid psychopathology is probably quite low in the street addict population. This may be due to the high degree of personality integration and resourcefulness required for survival. There may be a higher incidence of pre-existing personality disturbances in the middle-class addict, whose behavior is more deviant for his social situation. Personality characteristics and behavior patterns frequently result from the interaction of the addict and the drug in the sociocultural environment of addiction.

A small number of people are able to function effectively as street addicts but decompensate acutely when the heroin is withdrawn or when methadone is substituted. The relief of anxiety afforded by the opiates may be important in ensuring continued function in these patients with borderline psychologic adjustments. The very structured existence of street heroin addiction may also be useful.

Pharmacology. Opiates are absorbed from the gastrointestinal tract or the nasal mucosa, and after subcutaneous, intramuscular, or intravenous injection. Morphine and heroin lose much of their analgesic potency when taken orally, whereas codeine and meperidine remain quite active and methadone retains most of its analgesic efficacy after oral administration. Heroin is hydrolyzed to morphine in the body, and except for its greater potency and more rapid onset of action, has pharmacologic properties similar to those of morphine. Morphine is concentrated in parenchymatous tissues, skeletal muscle, and, to a lesser extent, brain. It is conjugated with glucuronic acid and excreted primarily in the urine and secondarily in the feces. Traces of morphine can be found in urine for 48 hours, although 90 per cent or more is excreted within the first 24 hours.

Administered subcutaneously, methadone and morphine exert approximately equal analgesic effects; heroin is three times stronger, whereas meperidine and codeine are approximately one tenth as potent. Morphine or heroin taken intravenously is effective almost immediately; duration of action varies from three to six hours. Oral administration prolongs the action of all the opiates, particularly that of methadone, in which the onset of effect occurs within 30 minutes and the duration of action in nontolerant individuals is four to ten hours.

Morphine or heroin administered to a nontolerant individual induces analgesia through a reduction in the anxiety and tension that result from the perception of pain. Somnolence characterized by an inability to concentrate, sleepiness, or "nodding," also occurs. Opiates cause pupillary constriction, depression of respiration by decreasing the responsiveness of the brainstem to carbon dioxide, depression of body temperature, and stimulation of central nervous system centers to produce nausea and vomiting. Other acute effects include decreased motility of the stomach, diminished pancreatic and biliary secretions, decreased propulsive contractions of the small and large intestine, and increased tone of the anal sphincter, leading to constipation. Increased tone of the detrusor muscle leads to a sensation of urgency accompanied by increased tone of the vesical sphincter, resulting in urinary retention. An acute release of antidiuretic hormone is effected, as well as inhibition of release of ACTH, corticotrophin-releasing factor, and gonadotrophin. Peripheral vasodilatation occurs, resulting in pruritus and possibly causing the observed increase in perspiration. Histamine release occurs, frequently resulting in a wheal-and-flare reaction, or "hive," at the site of injection and in a "pins-and-needles" sensation.

Addiction and Withdrawal Processes. Repeated use of narcotic analgesics produces tolerance to most of the acute narcotic effects, and the lethal dose is markedly increased. Whereas a 10-mg dose of morphine may produce euphoria in a nontolerant individual, the daily use of 5 grams has been reported in addicts. The rate at which this tolerance develops depends on the frequency and magnitude of use. Street addicts may spend from $20 to $200 or more daily on heroin and may inject themselves every three to six hours. Tolerance to all the opiate effects does not occur equally, since highly tolerant users will continue to demonstrate pupillary constriction and constipation. Cross-tolerance occurs with all narcotic analgesics. Tolerance to narcotics is primarily due to some form of cellular adaptation to the drug's action, with increased metabolism of lesser importance.

Physical dependence develops concurrently with tolerance and has been demonstrated after only a few exposures on succeeding days. It is marked by the development of an acute abstinence syndrome upon withdrawal of opiates, the "cold-turkey" process. This syndrome is quite variable in severity and characteristics and depends upon the particular drug, the dose, the interval between doses, and the duration of narcotic use, as well as on the personality and immediate environment of the narcotic addict. With heroin, the first withdrawal signs are generally seen shortly before the next scheduled dose. They are purposive in nature and include feelings of anxiety, restlessness, irritability, and drug craving. Lacrimation, rhinorrhea, yawning, and perspiration become apparent 8 to 12 hours after the last dose of narcotic. A restless sleep may intervene, the so-called "yen sleep," from which the addict awakens with more severe withdrawal symptoms and signs, including dilated pupils, sneezing, coryza, anorexia, nausea, vomiting, diarrhea, abdominal cramps, bone pains, myalgias, tremors, weakness, insomnia, goose flesh, and, very rarely, convulsions or cardiovascular collapse. With morphine and heroin, withdrawal symptoms peak at 48 to 72 hours, and most observable symptoms disappear in seven to ten days. With methadone, the onset of withdrawal symptoms is more gradual, the peak is less pronounced and later, and the duration may be more than two or three weeks. The abstinence syndrome may be precipitated within minutes in opiate-dependent persons by administration of a narcotic antagonist such as nalorphine, levallorphan, or naloxone, although there are no medical indications for this diagnostic procedure.

Pentazocine (Talwin), a drug with weak opiate-antagonist effects and moderate opiate-agonist effects, elicits morphine-like subjective effects in nontolerant individuals. Higher doses produce dysphoric effects, including nervousness, anxiety, and, infrequently, bizarre alterations in perception and behavior. Tolerance and physical dependence occur, and cases of addiction to this drug are reported. Abrupt withdrawal of the drug from persons taking 200 to 700 mg daily results in an abstinence syndrome marked by irritability, abdominal cramps, nausea, vomiting, hyperthermia, lacrimation, and drug-seeking behavior. When pentazocine is administered to opiate-dependent patients, its antagonistic actions may precipitate withdrawal symptoms.

Subsequent to the termination of abstinence symptoms or after a course of detoxification with decreasing doses of opiates, most addicts experience recurrent urges for narcotics and generally resume their use of these drugs. The traditional psychologic theory of relapse presumes that, after withdrawal, the physiologic causes of drug taking have been removed, but that addicts have an "addictive personality" disorder that causes them to return to opiate addiction to escape reality. Psychologic factors play a role, although no predictive test has been developed to distinguish future addicts from future nonaddicts, nor are addicts able to be distinguished from nonaddicts by psychologic evaluation when they are observed under the same abstinent conditions. Evidence is accumulating that metabolic and neurophysiologic changes persist long after the detoxification process is completed, as does some tolerance. Protracted abstinence signs, as indicated by alterations in blood pressure, pulse rate, body temperature, respiratory rate, and pupillary size, have been documented and may relate to the chronic drug craving reported and the high incidence of relapse. The conditioned associations abstinent ex-addicts experience when they are exposed to their old neighborhoods and friends are also involved in the persistence of drug craving. Narcotic addiction with its implicit relapses after periods of abstinence should be viewed as a disease of complex etiology in which a persistent neurochemical disturbance as well as profound psychologic and social factors contributes to the dominance of drug-seeking behavior.

Medical Complications. When a known dose of an opiate is administered under aseptic conditions, either occasionally or chronically, medical complications are almost unknown. There are well-documented cases of long-term opiate addiction in physicians and others in whom no adverse physical effects were found. The patterns of use, including life style, unknown and markedly variable opiate dose, lack of hygienic administration techniques, and the variety of adulterants used to dilute the opiate, are responsible for the extensive morbidity and mortality (estimated to be about 1 to 2 per cent per year) associated with opiate abuse and dependence.

Acute heroin reactions secondary to intravenous use of street drug are responsible for more than three quarters of all fatalities from narcotics. Formerly thought of as true pharmacologic overdoses with respiratory depression, these reactions may be due to opiate-induced cardiac arrhythmias or hypoxia by unexplained mechanisms. Acute reactions to adulterants, including quinine, allergic reactions, and synergistic effects from multiple-drug use, may also be implicated. The syndrome is marked clinically by the rapid development of cyanosis, pulmonary edema, respiratory distress, and coma. Increased intracranial pressure and occasionally convulsive seizures are seen. The pathologic picture includes pulmonary congestion and edema and frequently cerebral edema.

Skin abscesses, cellulitis, and *thrombophlebitis* are the most frequent complications of heroin addiction. Skin manifestations are particularly noted after the subcutaneous injection of heroin and its adulterants. Septicemia and acute and subacute bacterial endocarditis with involvement of either or both sides of the heart are seen. *Staphylococcus aureus* is frequently the causative organism in right-sided lesions. Peripheral and pulmonary embolic phenomena occur. Osteomyelitis occurs infrequently. Malaria was a frequent complication in the 1930's. The introduction of quinine as an adulterant and the eradication of malaria in this country have decreased the incidence of this complication. Syringe-transmitted syphilis occurs infrequently.

Viral hepatitis transmitted by the communal use of contaminated needles is a frequent complication of intravenous drug use. Abnormal liver function tests, hypergammaglobulinemia, and increased serum immunoglobulins that persist for long periods of time after the acute episodes and that occur in addicts with no history of hepatitis are due in some cases to variants of chronic hepatitis, but may also be due to effects produced by alcohol, malnutrition, allergic phenomena, adulterants, and recurrent or chronic infections. False positive serologic tests are due to these factors. The nephrotic syndrome has been seen in association with street heroin use as well.

Pulmonary complications include pneumonia, abscess, infarction, and tuberculosis. Disseminated extrapulmonary tuberculosis has been reported. Angiothrombotic pulmonary hypertension and granulomatosis result from the intravenous injection of foreign bodies, including talc or cotton. Vascular lesions include local arterial occlusion, phlebitis, mycotic aneurysm, and necrotizing angiitis.

Neurologic complications of street heroin use include transverse myelitis, peripheral nerve lesions, and muscle disorders, including acute rhabdomyolysis with myoglobinuria and a fibrosing chronic myopathy. Septic states may lead to bacterial meningitis and brain, subdural, and epidural abscesses. In this country, intravenous narcotism is a leading cause of tetanus.

Menstrual irregularities in addicted women have been described, although it is unknown whether these can be ascribed to narcotic-induced suppression of adrenocorticotrophic hormone and gonadotrophic release or to malnutrition, frequent infections, and the general life style of female addicts. There is a high incidence of toxemia and of prematurity in infants born to addicted mothers, probably because of these life-style factors and the lack of prenatal care. Withdrawal symptoms are noted in a variable percentage of these newborn.

Treatment. Methods of treatment of narcotic dependence vary considerably, depending on the treatment goals, the factors that are thought to be most significant in the etiology of a patient's addiction, and the characteristics of individual patients. The magnitude of the addict's desire to stop using opiates is an important factor in the selection of the appropriate treatment modality as well as in the outcome. These motivational factors are difficult to assess, since most addicts want to terminate their addiction within one or two years after its onset. Nevertheless, many continue the compulsive use of heroin for many years and suffer repeated treatment failures. Approaches are primarily psychosocial, pharmacologic, or combinations of these. Since addiction has physical, psychologic, and social determinants, treatment is best provided by a well-organized team approach rather than by individual practitioners.

Withdrawal Techniques. Withdrawal of narcotics is most effectively accomplished by inpatient or outpatient substitution of oral methadone for any of the natural or synthetic narcotic analgesics (detoxification). Doses ranging from 20 to 40 mg daily are instituted, followed by a gradual reduction of dosage over the course of 10 to 14 days or more. Optimally, psychologic, legal, and vocational supportive services should be provided the patient throughout the process and continuing into the drug-free period. In some cases, patients are withdrawn in a drug-free environment without opiate substitution, although this has proved less justifiable on medical and moral grounds. The chronic nature of this disease necessitates continuing treatment after the withdrawal process is completed.

METHADONE MAINTENANCE

In this country, methadone maintenance has been the most successful and most widely used approach in the treatment of opiate dependence. This mode of therapy emphasizes social and emotional rehabilitation rather than abstinence. The treatment is based on the two major properties that distinguish methadone from other narcotics: good oral efficacy and long duration of action. After oral ingestion in tolerant individuals, the duration of action of methadone is extended to 24 to 36 hours owing to a reservoir of drug in tissues. Initially, oral methadone is administered daily in doses that will allay symptoms of abstinence. The dose is gradually increased until a stabilization level is reached at which patients will be tolerant to the euphoric effects of the drug and will experience no persistent craving for opiates. If the stabilization level is high enough (80 to 120 mg), there is a good degree of cross-tolerance to the effects of other narcotics, such that the effects of even large doses of intravenous opiates will not be felt (narcotic blockade). Approximately 75 per cent of patients in well-run programs remain in treatment. Improvement has been noted in the work and school records of patients retained in the program, and the incidence of their criminal activity has declined markedly. Long-term methadone maintenance has been shown to be medically safe, with minimal side effects and no toxicity when properly administered. Performance and learning are normal in methadone-maintained subjects. Medication should be dispensed in a clinic situation that provides medical care and extensive rehabilitative services so as to facilitate satisfactory reentry into nondrug-dominated ("straight") society. Since methadone is subject to abuse and is potentially lethal in nontolerant individuals, adequate provisions must be made to prevent its illicit dispersal.

Programs utilizing methadone maintenance for varying periods of time followed by a slow-detoxification process have shown promise. Research is presently under way with levomethadyl acetate hydrochloride, a synthetic congener of methadone that extends opiate effects for 72 hours. Various programs that would provide heroin under supervision are also being considered (heroin maintenance). The short-acting nature of the drug, coupled with the necessity for injecting it, renders this form of treatment less potentially useful.

NARCOTIC ANTAGONISTS

Narcotic antagonists such as cyclazocine and naltrexane are being evaluated for the treatment of detoxified addicts. These agents block or attenuate the euphoriant effects of narcotics and prevent the development of physical dependence in patients who continue to use narcotics. Drug-seeking behavior might be extinguished insofar as it depends on conditioned associations to euphoric drug effects or abstinence symptoms. Prevention of the development of physical dependence might also minimize the continuation of narcotic use after a spree, and increase periods of abstinence. These drugs do not relieve the chronic opiate-drug hunger, and patients are prone to omit their dose of antagonist and relapse to heroin. A major advance would be the discovery of a medicine that relieves all symptoms of physical dependence, blocks the opiate-induced euphoria, does not itself produce physical dependence, and is not subject to abuse.

PSYCHOSOCIAL APPROACHES—ABSTINENCE PROGRAMS

A diverse array of programs exist that emphasize abstinence from opiates and other drugs as a primary component of treatment. These take the form of either voluntary groups or supervised institutionalization.

Voluntary groups are generally communities that are self-regulatory in nature and staffed predominantly by former drug users. The individual remains in the closed, drug-free environment for variable periods of time, frequently one to two years, and is encouraged to develop a new set of social and living skills that will enable him to remain drug free upon completion of the program. Outpatient programs are also under way. Intensive therapeutic techniques are utilized to eliminate the social and personality deficiencies of residents that led them to drug use. These facilities serve to reduce the sense of isolation felt by many drug users, and attempt to provide role models for responsible behavior. Some of the well-known groups are Synanon, Daytop Village, Phoenix House, and Sera. Although sharing many common methods and doctrines, these communities vary considerably in the nature of the therapeutic milieu created and in the complex system of rewards and punishments provided residents. Therapeutic communities are valuable for many people, although only a small percentage of heroin addicts are motivated to enter a community, and follow-up studies of individuals who have returned to society are not presently available.

An alternative approach is programs which involve the nonpunitive incarceration of an addict for the purposes of rehabilitation (civil commitment). These programs generally include a period of enforced abstinence in a prison, hospital, or other locked facility, followed by careful supervision of the individual in the community. If renewed drug abuse or other antisocial behavior is noted, the addict is reinstitutionalized. To date, these programs have met with meager success. If adequate rehabilitative services and facilities are made available in the future, the efficacy of these programs might be increased.

Results of traditional psychotherapeutic techniques have been disappointing for the majority of compulsive opiate abusers. Specialized forms of group psychotherapy may be useful for some patients. After variable and sometimes prolonged periods of addiction, an unknown number of addicts spontaneously cease opiate use. This "maturing-out" process may be related to advanced age and the difficulty of obtaining drugs, a decline of internal psychologic conflicts, and the cumulative effect of various treatment programs.

342. CENTRAL NERVOUS SYSTEM DEPRESSANTS

Robert B. Millman

All central nervous system depressants are subject to abuse. The most frequently abused drugs in this category are the short-acting barbiturates, particularly pentobarbital (Nembutal) and secobarbital (Seconal), and assorted other hypnotics such as glutethimide (Doriden), methyprylon (Noludar), and methaqualone (Quāālude). Tranquilizers, including meprobamate (Miltown), chlordiazepoxide (Librium), and diazepam (Valium), are implicated in abuse patterns less often. Bromide abuse has become rare. Since many of the characteristics of these drugs are similar, this discussion will center on the barbiturates, with other agents considered when relevant.

Incidence and Patterns of Abuse. There is a continuum of depressant use that extends from appropriate use to compulsive abuse and addiction. Massive quantities of depressants are produced yearly in the United States (over 1 million pounds of barbituric acid derivatives alone). These are prescribed by physicians for hypnosis or sedation in a variety of conditions, including insomnia, depressive and anxiety states, and convulsive disorders. The source of drug for one major category of abuser is physicians' prescriptions. The pattern of use may begin as intermittent use at night to decrease anxiety and ensure sleep, progress to nightly use with increased doses, and culminate in prolonged daily use to maintain an adequate level of functioning. An individual may obtain drugs from several physicians at one time, none of whom are aware of the magnitude of their patient's depressant use. In this group there may be no illicit drug use, although alcohol is frequently used in association with the depressants.

Barbiturate and other hypnotic use is also prevalent in urban drug subcultures. Heroin addicts use hypnotics ("downs") to supplement the poor quality of heroin available. Alcoholics will also use hypnotics when they are available, since the quality of the intoxications are similar. Although some people abuse barbiturates preferentially, concurrent physical dependence on alcohol or opiates is more common than pure barbiturate dependence in these groups. Illicit sources of drugs are most often employed, and a wealth of street names have evolved for the most popular hypnotics, including "reds" (secobarbital), "yellows" (pentobarbital), and "double trouble" (amobarbital and secobarbital). Most use is oral, although some individuals inject the drugs intravenously or intramuscularly. The amounts taken vary markedly, but some individuals have ingested as much as 30 hypnotic doses of the short-acting barbiturates daily over many months.

Recently, a marked increase in the use of illicitly obtained hypnotics has been noted in some adolescent and preadolescent populations. Patterns and extent of use vary markedly, but generally multiple-drug use occurs and is considered appropriate behavior within these groups. Intermittent users may take several times the therapeutic dose, possibly in addition to marijuana, alcohol, and amphetamines if they are available, to get "high" enough to enjoy a concert or party.

The "high" that obtains from abuse of depressant drugs has been characterized as the sense of tranquility or peace that occurs just prior to sleep in normal individuals. The world is seen as limited to the immediate. Inhibitions and anxiety are blunted, and there may be a feeling of aggressiveness, freedom, and pleasant numbness. Sexual pleasure and ability are said to be enhanced at low doses of these drugs; higher doses lead to a decreased ability to perform sexually. Violent and antisocial behavior occurs, frequently serving to isolate depressant abusers ("down heads") from other groups of drug abusers.

There appears to be a high incidence of serious psychopathology in compulsive abusers of the depressant drugs. Users may be seeking obtundation in attempts to cope with anxiety arising from a variety of sources.

Pharmacology. Barbiturates and related hypnotics are rapidly absorbed after oral administration and are distributed throughout the body. They are general depressants of nerves and of skeletal, smooth, and cardiac muscles, although at low doses the central nervous system is primarily affected. Central nervous system effects vary from mild sedation to coma, depending on the particular drug, the dose, the route of administration, the degree of excitability of the nervous system, and tolerance. In some individuals under certain circumstances, small doses produce an initial stimulation not unlike that produced by alcohol. Barbiturate-induced sleep is similar to physiologic sleep except for a reduction in the proportion of rapid eye movement (REM) sleeping time. Duration of action varies with the particular barbiturate. After effects, including drowsiness, depression, impairment of judgment and performance, and occasionally hyperexcitability, may persist for many hours.

Both drug-disposition and pharmacodynamic tolerance to the barbiturates and related hypnotics develop rapidly with repeated administration. Drug-disposition tolerance in the short-acting barbiturates and some other depressants results from the activation of drug-metabolizing liver-enzyme systems and is characterized by the more rapid degradation of the drug and a decrease in sleeping time. The range of tolerance is narrow, and individuals tolerant to the sedating and intoxicating effects of 1 gram of pentobarbital may become intoxicated for prolonged periods upon the addition of 0.1 gram. Although the lethal dose of barbiturates varies in individuals, in distinction to the opiates, tolerance does not increase this dose significantly from that of nontolerant individuals. Severe poisoning is likely to occur when more than ten times the hypnotic dose is ingested at one time. Acute barbiturate poisoning may thus be superimposed on chronic intoxication at any time. The combination of sublethal doses of depressants with opiates or alcohol may also result in acute poisoning. Cross-tolerance develops to all barbiturates as well as to paraldehyde, meprobamate, and chlordiazepoxide. Partial cross-tolerance between alcohol and the depressants occurs.

Clinical Manifestations. Acute depressant poisoning may occur either accidentally or incident to a suicide attempt. Accidental overdoses may be due in some cases to "drug automation"; an individual may fail to fall asleep after several hypnotic doses, become confused, and ingest an overdose. Upon recovery, there may be no memory of the excessive drug ingestion. The clinical manifestations and treatment of poisoning are discussed in Ch. 348. The acute and chronic signs and symptoms of mild hypnotic intoxication resemble those of intoxication with alcohol. The individual shows general sluggishness, difficulty in thinking, slowness of speech and comprehension, poor memory, faulty judgment, emotional lability, and narrowed attention span. Neurologic signs of barbiturate intoxication include thick, slurred speech, nystagmus, diplopia, strabismus, vertigo, ataxic gait, positive Romberg sign, hypotonia, dysmetria, and decreased superficial reflexes. Sensation, deep tendon reflexes, and pupillary responses are unaltered. Skin rashes have been reported. Unexplained seizures in adults should always prompt one to consider chronic depressant drug abuse.

With compulsive users, clothing may be unkempt and nutrition poor; needle marks and abscesses from intramuscular or intravenous use may be present. Adverse effects of chronic barbiturate use are poorly documented, but may be similar to those of alcohol on organ systems and the brain.

Abstinence Syndrome. Physical dependence, as indicated by abstinence signs and symptoms, develops to all the central nervous system general depressants. A characteristic *general depressant withdrawal syndrome* occurs and is similar to the symptoms of withdrawal from alcohol. It varies in severity, depending on the drug, dose, and frequency of use. *In contrast to the opiate withdrawal syndrome, that from depressants may be life-threatening.* The first manifestation of this syndrome might be considered the rebound increase in nightly rapid eye movement sleep, associated with nightmares and a sense of having slept badly, that occurs after discontinuation of use of only therapeutic doses of barbiturates for several nights. After a daily dose of 0.4 gram of pentobarbital for three months, abrupt withdrawal produces paroxysmal EEG changes without other significant symptoms. After 0.6 gram per day for one to two months, 50 per cent of patients experience insomnia, tremors, anorexia, and irritability, and 10 per cent may have a seizure. After continuous intoxication with doses of 0.9 to 2.2 grams per day for one month or less, 75 per cent may have seizures, and 66 per cent delirium; all experience insomnia, tremors, and anorexia. In general, the time required to produce physical dependence is shorter with the short-acting barbiturates and the withdrawal symptoms are more abrupt in onset and more severe than with the longer-acting sedatives.

When short-acting hypnotics are abruptly withdrawn, signs and symptoms of the intoxication clear over the initial 12 to 16 hours, and the patient appears to improve. Increases in restlessness, anxiety, tremulousness, and weakness then occur, which may be accompanied by cramps, nausea, vomiting, and orthostatic hypotension. These symptoms progress, and coarse hand tremors, muscle twitching, hyperactive deep reflexes, and increased blink reflex appear within 24 hours. Symptoms generally attain their peak during the second and third days, and convulsions may occur then or before. Some patients who have seizures may begin to show improvement, but 50 per cent develop a delirium that is marked by sensorial clouding, visual and auditory hallucinations, and disorientation to time and place. During the delirium, which usually occurs between the fourth and seventh days, hyperthermia, tachycardia, and agitation can lead to exhaustion and sometimes to fatal cardiovascular collapse. The abstinence syndrome generally clears by about the eighth day, and there is usually no residual physical damage. Clearing is frequently preceded by a period of prolonged sleep. With longer-acting barbiturates and chlordiazepoxide, seizures may not occur until the seventh or eighth day. Hallucinations sometimes persist for many months, but these may be a manifestation of an underlying psychosis.

Treatment. Treatment procedures include withdrawal and rehabilitative phases. Compulsive abusers of depressants are often considered more difficult to treat than any other class of drug abusers. Outreach and educational programs aimed at intermittent abusers of depressants before they become addicted may be important in this regard. The pattern of use and extent of physical dependence should be evaluated by means of a careful history and physical examination. Depressant abusers frequently distort or are unaware of the magnitude of their use, particularly those with a concurrent addiction to heroin.

If physical dependence is suspected, close observation or hospitalization is indicated. When the diagnosis is established, a suitable general depressant should be administered after the intoxication clears but before major withdrawal symptoms have begun. Pentobarbital orally is a suitable substitute for most of the general depressants, although phenobarbital and secobarbital may also be used. If the patient will not tolerate the oral administration of pentobarbital, intramuscular injections of the same doses may be used. Patients may usually be switched to oral drugs after a few intramuscular injections. Sufficient pentobarbital should be given to produce a mild but manageable level of intoxication, marked by inconstant slow nystagmus on lateral gaze, slight dysarthria, and ataxia. Most patients require from 0.2 to 0.4 gram every six hours, but some may need up to 2.5 grams over a 24-hour period. This "stabilization dose" should be carefully controlled to prevent signs of increased intoxication, such as dysarthria, emotional lability, constant nystagmus, or gross ataxia. Patients should be maintained on this dose for 24 to 48 hours, after which the dose of pentobarbital should be reduced by 0.1 gram or less daily. The patient should be observed carefully for signs of insomnia, tremulousness, and orthostatic hypotension, at which time the withdrawal of pentobarbital should be suspended for one to two days. If symptoms are severe, the patient should be given 0.2 gram intramuscularly immediately, which will usually suppress them. Delirium, convulsions, or fever should be treated as emergencies, with hourly doses until the patient is able to sleep for 8 to 12 hours, after which the stabilization dose is determined, as described above. Once a withdrawal delirium develops, increased doses of pentobarbital may fail to restore equilibrium; agitation and disorientation may persist for several days.

Fluid and electrolyte losses must be replaced, and complicating medical and surgical conditions treated. Increasing fever without evidence of infection necessitates additional sedation, antipyretics, sponging, or cooling blankets. Phenothiazines, butyrophenones, and diphenylhydantoin are not indicated.

In general, the use of the pentobarbital substitution technique may take from ten days to three weeks. It should not be hurried. Patients who are taking large amounts of lesser-known sedatives should probably be withdrawn from the original drug of abuse, if it is known, without substitution therapy. This withdrawal regimen may be carried out concurrently with that for opiates.

After withdrawal is completed, provisions must be made for high-frequency supportive counseling. Patients are frequently withdrawn and depressed, and the danger of relapse or suicide is great. The inclusion of patients in a therapeutic program, either as an inpatient or on an ambulatory basis, should be assured.

Physicians must be cautious when prescribing depressants for the relief of anxiety and insomnia. Attempts should be made to diagnose and treat the source of these symptoms. Whenever possible, tranquilizers such as chlordiazepoxide and diazepam, with a lower abuse potential, should be used in lieu of the short-acting hypnotics to induce sleep.

Bromides. Chronic bromide intoxication (bromism) has become rare, because bromide has been supplanted in modern medicine with more effective and less toxic sedative and analgesic compounds. The bromide ion is very slowly excreted by the kidney, with a half-life in the blood of about 12 days. Consequently, the daily ingestion of small doses will result in an accumulation of the drug to toxic levels over a period of weeks. Central nervous system symptoms and signs are the most common features and include drowsiness, impaired thought and memory, dizziness, and irritability, leading in more severe cases to delirium, hallucinations, lethargy, and coma. High plasma levels are associated with an EEG pattern of diffuse slow waves. Neurologic disturbances include tremors, thick speech, motor incoordination, and decreased superficial reflexes. A characteristic acneiform rash and other skin lesions occur in 20 per cent of cases. Gastrointestinal disturbances include anorexia, foul breath, and constipation. The diagnosis of chronic bromide intoxication is established by serum bromide levels above 9 mEq per liter in association with the aforementioned clinical picture.

Treatment consists of the daily administration of 200 mEq of either sodium or ammonium chloride, together with sufficient fluids to ensure a large urine output. This reduces the half-life of bromide to three or four days. Diuresis with chloruretic drugs may be useful if more rapid displacement of bromide is indicated. Hemodialysis rapidly clears bromides and may be indicated in treating comatose patients.

343. CENTRAL NERVOUS SYSTEM STIMULANTS

Robert B. Millman

Central nervous system stimulants or sympathomimetics that are subject to abuse include the *amphetamines, cocaine, methylphenidate* (Ritalin), *phenmetrazine* (Preludin), and *diethylpropion* (Tepanil). This discussion will consider the amphetamine group primarily, including amphetamine, dextroamphetamine, and methamphetamine, which are synthetic derivatives of ephedrine, and cocaine, an alkaloid of the coca plant which grows in the Andes in South America.

Incidence and Patterns of Abuse. Amphetamine abuse is widespread in industrial societies, particularly in Japan, Sweden, Great Britain, and North America. Patterns of use vary markedly. Until the recent federal and state regulations severely limiting physicians' prescribing practices with respect to the amphetamines and related drugs, enormous quantities were prescribed for the treatment of a variety of conditions, including obesity, depressive syndromes, behavior disorders, narcolepsy, and the reduction of fatigue. Many patients, frequently middle-class women, became dependent on these drugs when they found that they had to continue to ingest the drug to prevent depression and to perform optimally. The advent of tolerance necessitated increased doses, occasionally five to ten times the original 5- or 10-mg amount prescribed. Amphetamine abuse by students, athletes, truck drivers, and others who want to increase their efficiency or productivity is common. In both these patterns, oral preparations are used. Hypnotics are often used by this group to ensure sleep, and concurrent dependence on both classes of drugs is not unusual.

Another category of amphetamine abuser is composed of multidrug users, primarily young, who use these drugs for their mood-elevating properties. Any amphetamine may be used, although methamphetamine ("speed," "crystal," or "meth") is preferred, because it has more pronounced central effects and less peripheral ones. The drugs are taken orally on occasion, although "sniffing" or intravenous use is common in drug-dominated groups. Most methamphetamine is manufactured in illegal laboratories, but commercially available oral preparations are also dissolved for intravenous use.

Upon "sniffing," or particularly after intravenous use, the user experiences a "flash" or "rush" that is described as a sense of increased mental capacity and physical strength, with little need for food or sleep, and a feeling of power and intensity that is quite distinct from the feeling of satiation induced by the opiates. Increased activity, planning, and talking occur. Dissipation of the drug effects after three to six hours is experienced as an unpleasant sense of fatigue and depression ("crashing"). Use may be intermittent and limited to special occasions such as a party or journey, or may be more regular. Rarely, chronic amphetamine abusers report that the daily, controlled use of these drugs decreases the anxiety and tension they experience normally, and enhances their ability to eat, sleep, and generally function.

Some individuals use the drug continuously, to maintain the "high" or stave off the "crash" for several days or even longer (a "run"). As tolerance develops, the dose is increased and the drug taken more frequently, such that 1 gram may be injected every two to four hours. As this stage, the compulsive user, or "speed freak," is usually nervous, irritable, and suspicious. There may be intense involvement in complicated and often unnecessary tasks such as disassembling a television set or reorganizing a room. When the supply of drug is depleted or the user becomes too disorganized or debilitated to continue, the "run" ends. Cessation of amphetamine use is usually followed by a prolonged deep sleep. Hypnotics or alcohol are often used to minimize the duration of the "crashing" phase and facilitate the induction of sleep. Upon awakening, although much of the paranoid ideation may be gone, a feeling of lassitude, apathy, and depression may be present. Intravenous users frequently inject other drugs alone or in combination with amphetamines. The combination of amphetamines or cocaine and heroin is known as a "speed ball."

Most of the psychoactive effects of cocaine are similar to those of the amphetamines with regard to elevation of mood, decreased need for food or sleep, and hyperactivity. Supply is always through illicit channels; it is more expensive than the amphetamines or heroin, and it is much shorter acting. After intravenous administration, the primary mode in this country until recently, effects last 5 to 15 minutes. Intravenous use is generally seen in the same population that abuses heroin. It is often used in "runs" of varying duration, such that 1 to 10 grams may be used during the course of a day via frequent injections. Psychologic dependence and compulsive use occur, but less frequently than with the amphetamine group. Recently there has been a marked increase in abuse of this drug by affluent and middle-class people in urban areas. Use in this group, by sniffing the much-adulterated white powder, is generally intermittent; and marijuana, alcohol, and hypnotics may be used concomitantly.

Pharmacology. Peripheral sympathomimetic effects of amphetamines and cocaine are minor compared with their potent central nervous system activity. Peripheral effects include increased cardiac contraction, increased blood pressure with reflex slowing of the heart rate, relaxation of the bronchial musculature, increased contractility of the urinary bladder sphincter, increased venous pressure, pulmonary arterial pressure, and renal blood flow. Central effects include stimulation of the cerebrospinal axis and the medullary respiratory center. In low doses these drugs increase alertness and physical and cognitive ability, particularly when performance has been compromised by lack of sleep. The significant appetite depression seen is probably due to a combination of factors, including an inhibitory effect on the feeding center in the lateral hypothalamus as well as the improvement in mood that occurs.

Tolerance develops to both the peripheral and central effects of the amphetamines. Tolerance to cocaine is not thought to occur; there may be some degree of psychologic tolerance to the euphoric effects of this drug, although it apparently dissipates rapidly. Cross-tolerance exists between the amphetamines, but no cross-tolerance has been demonstrated between the amphetamines and cocaine.

Cessation of amphetamine or cocaine use does not produce major physiologic symptoms. The depression, increased appetite, lassitude, and prolonged sleep that ensue might be considered an abstinence syndrome and evidence of some physical dependence. Moreover, during this sleep, a characteristic electroencephalographic pattern is produced that shows a marked increase in the percentage of REM sleep, and nightmares may occur.

Adverse Effects. Adverse physical effects in intermittent users of amphetamines or cocaine by the sniffing route may be limited to irritation of the nasal mucosa or perforation of the nasal septum. Chronic users may be markedly debilitated and subject to numerous infections as a result of lack of sleep and poor nutrition. A sensation of something crawling under the skin is described ("cocaine bugs"), such that chronic users will frequently have excoriations and open sores from constant scratching and pinching. The intravenous use of these drugs is fraught with the numerous complications that result from nonsterile conditions, which are detailed in Ch. 341. Reports of necrotizing angiitis and hepatitis resulting from the direct toxic effect of methamphetamine require further clarification. Severe overdose reactions or death from either amphetamines or cocaine are quite rare. Amphetamine toxicity is marked by extensions of the sympathomimetic effects, culminating in cerebrovascular accidents, convulsions, and coma. Cocaine toxicity is characterized by initial sympathomimetic effects followed by cortical depression and anesthetization of the midbrain and medulla, leading to respiratory failure and cardiovascular collapse. Large intravenous dosages of cocaine may cause cardiac arrhythmias by direct action of the drug on cardiac tissue. The lethal dosage of amphetamines is variable, depending on the extent of tolerance; that of cocaine is estimated to be about 1.2 grams.

There is a high incidence of psychopathology in compulsive amphetamine and cocaine abusers. The most frequent complications of amphetamine and cocaine abuse are paranoid ideation and stereotyped compulsive behavior. Chronic users are frequently aware of these characteristics of the drugs and will not act on ideas of persecution. Antisocial or violent behavior may occur when this insight is lacking. Continued use frequently leads to a well-described *amphetamine or cocaine psychosis* that is often indistinguishable from acute paranoid schizophrenia. These reactions appear to be inevitable if the dose and frequency of use of amphetamines and cocaine are continually increased or high doses maintained. Psychotic episodes have also been precipitated in some individuals after only one small dose. The syndrome is marked by paranoid ideation; stereotyped compulsive behavior; visual, auditory, and tactile hallucinations; and loosening of associations occurring in a setting of clear consciousness and correct orientation. The etiology of these disorders may be related to actions of amphetamines and cocaine in inhibiting the re-uptake inactivation of the catecholamines, dopamine, and norepinephrine, thus potentiating their synaptic effects. The psychotic episodes invariably appear while the patients are under the influence of the drug, and generally abate within a few days to several weeks after cessation of drug use. Prolonged psychotic episodes occur and may relate to the premorbid personality of the user.

Treatment. Amphetamine and cocaine abusers are a heterogeneous group who demonstrate markedly diverse patterns of drug use. Accordingly treatment must be flexible. Treatment of the physical complications of abuse are considered in the appropriate chapters of this textbook. Treatment of paranoid ideation or the overt psychotic episodes must ensure cessation of amphetamine or cocaine use and may necessitate short-term hospitalization or, if possible, confinement in a safe, supportive atmosphere. Phenothiazine drugs or other tranquilizers are frequently benefical in the acute situation.

After recovery, depressive symptoms should be sought and the possibility of suicide must be considered. The compulsive abuser may require long-term supportive care under close supervision, with provision for psychiatric and social rehabilitation.

Physicians would do well to prescribe this class of drugs with great caution. Some authorities suggest that the childhood hyperkinetic disorders and narcolepsy are the only indications for their use.

344. CANNABIS (Marijuana and Hashish)

Robert B. Millman

Marijuana and hashish are derived from *Cannabis sativa,* the hemp plant, an herbaceous annual which grows readily in many parts of the world and reaches maturation in four to five months. All parts of both the male and female plants contain varying amounts of the major psychoactive principle, delta-9-tetrahydrocannibinol; its active isomer, delta-8-THC; and numerous other cannabinoids. The concentration of delta-9-THC in the flowering tops of these plants is a function of genetic and environmental factors and varies from less than 0.2 per cent in the fiber-type plants to more than 4 per cent in those plants grown for drug content. In the United States, marijuana refers to the dried mixture of crushed leaves and flowering tops with or without the inclusion of stems and seeds. The flowering tops of the plants secrete a clear, varnish-like resin, which when collected and compressed is called hashish and is thought to be four to eight times more potent than marijuana. Cannabis or its products are also called *kif, bhang, ganja, charas,* and *dagga* in various parts of the world.

Incidence and Patterns of Abuse. Cannabis has been used extensively in many societies since antiquity as a form of folk medicine, as a work adjunct, in association with religious practices, and for recreational purposes. The prevalence of cannabis use has increased explosively in the United States and Western Europe during the past 15 years in association with the changing styles of youth culture. Several recent surveys suggest that the number of people in the United States who have ever used cannabis is 15 to 25 million. Users fall heavily into the teenage and young adult group, although increased use is being noted in older age groups as well. Whereas geographic, social, and cultural considerations are determinants of whether a person will use cannabis, personality characteristics are important in determining the frequency and pattern of use. Many people experiment with the drug and do not continue its use; over half are estimated to use the drug one or more times per month; about one in four who use it that often do so three times or more a week.

The drug is peripheral to the life of the occasional user, and frequently there is no other drug use. Others demonstrate a compulsive abuse pattern, in which their lives are dominated by the acquisition and use of cannabis and other drugs. Occasional users generally smoke in groups, where the ritual of preparation and sharing of the cigarette is an integral part of social interaction. Chronic smokers will also frequently smoke alone.

Marijuana is usually smoked in homemade cigarettes ("joints"). Hashish is smoked in a wide variety of small pipes. Both preparations may be ingested in combination with food or drink, although this is less common. The weight of a marijuana cigarette on the street may vary from 0.5 to 1 gram. In imported material, the delta-9-THC content, although generally less than 1 per cent, may be much more potent.

Pharmacology. Cannabis preparations are three to four times more potent when smoked than when taken orally. After inhalation, effects begin within minutes, peak within one hour, and are dissipated within three hours. After ingestion, effects begin in 30 minutes to two hours, peak at three hours, and persist for four to six hours. The effects of cannabis correlate with the appearance in plasma of active polar metabolites of delta-9-THC, principally the 11-hydroxy-delta-9-THC compounds. Nonpsychoactive polar metabolites are slowly eliminated from the body over a period of more than 1 week.

The acute physiologic effects of cannabis are dose related and include an increase in heart rate, conjunctival vascular congestion, decreased intraocular pressure, bronchodilatation, increased airway conductance, and peripheral vasodilatation. Dryness of mouth and throat, fine tremors of fingers, ataxia, nystagmus, nausea, and vomiting have been noted. Orthostatic hypotension and loss of consciousness occur infrequently. Sleep patterns may be altered.

Psychoactive effects are highly variable and depend on the dose, the route of administration, the personality of the user, his prior experience with the drug, his personal expectations, and the environmental and social setting in which the drug is used. Enhanced perception of colors, sounds, patterns, textures, and taste is common. Mood changes are complex; a sense of increased well-being is frequently experienced, although anxiety and depression may be increased by the drug, as well. Drowsiness or hyperactivity and hilarity may occur. Ideas may seem disconnected, rapid-flowing, and associated with altered importance. Time seems to pass slowly, and short-term memory may be impaired. Motor performance is variably impaired, as is reaction time. Although attention can be maintained in certain situations, it is probable that alterations in attention are responsible for some of the reported decrements in performance and cognitive function.

Inexperienced users of cannabis report fewer subjective effects, but demonstrate more decrement in perceptual and psychomotor performance than experienced users. A learning process may be involved in the initial perception of psychoactive effects, although enzymatic induction with more rapid conversion of delta-9-THC to active metabolites is also possible. A varying degree of tolerance develops to some of the psychologic and physiologic effects of the drug. Physical dependence on cannabis does not occur in man.

Adverse Effects. There are no documented reports of human fatalities caused by an overdose of cannabis in any form. Decreased pulmonary function has been reported in chronic users, with an increased incidence of bronchitis, sinusitis, and nose and throat inflammations. Chromosome breakage, in vitro inhibition of cell-mediated immunity, and cerebral atrophy have been reported but not confirmed.

Adverse reactions are generally psychologic in nature, infrequent, and dependent on dose, the personality of the user, and the setting. The most common adverse effects are simple depression, acute panic reactions, and paranoid ideation. These symptoms usually abate in several hours. An acute toxic psychosis, transient in nature, with confusion, auditory and visual hallucinations, and depersonalization, has been reported as occurring infrequently though unpredictably. There is disagreement as to whether cannabis may precipitate a psychotic episode in a stable, well-structured personality. It is agreed that the drug may trigger a prolonged psychotic episode in people with borderline psychologic adjustments. Larger doses are associated with an increase in these reactions, though in a nonlinear way. "Flashback" phenomena similar to those seen with psychedelic use occur rarely.

An amotivational syndrome has been described, in which chronic, heavy users who are psychologically dependent on cannabis demonstrate apathy, diminished goal-directed activity, inability to master new problems, poor social and work adjustment, poor judgment, magical thinking, and multiple drug use. In addition to possible drug effects, sociologic and psychologic characteristics of users may be implicated in this syndrome.

There is no evidence that cannabis use leads to criminal activity. Socially or psychologically predisposed individuals may experiment with other drugs as a result of positive experiences with cannabis.

Treatment. Treatment of the frequently seen depressive and panic reactions should be personal, supportive, and reassuring. The patient must be continually reminded of the drug-induced nature of his difficulty. Tranquilizers are sometimes indicated in violent or aggressive states. Psychotherapy and hospitalization may be indicated in more severe or chronic disorders. The chronic use of marijuana is frequently associated with a subculture that rejects conventional mores and orientation. To be effective, treatment efforts should be sensitive to these value systems.

345. PSYCHEDELICS

Robert B. Millman

The distinguishing characteristics of this class of substances is their ability to reliably produce characteristic alterations in perception, thought, feeling, and behavior. They are among the oldest known psychoactive drugs, often having been used as an adjunct to religious practices in some societies. They are sometimes classified as hallucinogens, psychotogens, or psychotomimetics. In this country, the most frequently abused drugs in this category are related either to the indolealkylamines such as the synthetic *lysergic acid diethylamide* (*LSD*, "acid"), *psilocybin* ("magic mushrooms"), *psilocin, dimethyltryptamine (DMT),* and *diethyltryptamine (DET),* or to the phenylethylamines such as *mescaline,* which is derived from the peyote cactus, and the substituted amphetamines such as 2,5-dimethoxy-4-methylamphetamine *(DOM, "STP"). Phencyclidine ("angel dust"),* a drug with anesthetic properties, has been abused for its psychedelic effects. Since the pattern of physiologic and psychologic effects produced by other agents is similar to that seen with LSD, this discussion will center on LSD. By virtue of their ability to produce bizarre alterations in behavior, some anticholinergic compounds will be considered in this chapter. Their psychoactive effects are distinct from the other psychedelics, and they might better be classified as deliriants.

Incidence and Patterns of Abuse. LSD became available through illicit channels in 1960, and use apparently peaked in the 1967–1968 period, when the new styles of youth culture and its leaders were being popularized by the mass media. Estimates vary from 500,000 to one million users at that time, and have been lower since then. The incidence of other psychedelic drug use parallels that of LSD. The decline may be due to the real and potential dangers of the drug, increasingly severe legal penalties, and changing social patterns.

Use has been primarily among middle-class, white, educated youth in this country who are seeking an enriching, ecstatic, mystical, or transcendental experience. A complex set of metaphysical and religious beliefs and social styles further distinguish the user.

Use is generally intermittent, frequently less than one "trip" monthly, separated by periods in which marijuana is used. Rarely, individuals may take the drug more often ("acid heads"), and some remain in intoxicated states for prolonged periods. Opiate and excessive alcohol use are not often seen in this population, although intermittent amphetamine and hypnotic use are not unusual in the intervening periods. The drug is generally taken in groups so that support is available in the event of a "bad trip." A naive user will frequently be attended by a guide who has previously had the psychedelic experience. As in the case of cannabis, a supportive, safe environment is sought for the experience to minimize the effects of unpleasant reactions.

LSD is generally synthesized in illegal laboratories and made available in a variety of forms, including impregnated paper or sugar cubes, capsules, and tablets. Users are often unaware of the dose they ingest or of whether the preparation is actually LSD or another of the psychedelics.

Pharmacology. LSD is the most potent psychedelic known. It is more than 100 times more potent than psilocybin and 4000 times more potent than mescaline in producing psychologic effects. The usual illicit street dose is probably around 200 μg, but doses as low as 20 μg produce psychologic effects in susceptible individuals. It is generally taken orally, although it has been injected on occasion. Central sympathomimetic stimulation occurs within 20 minutes after ingestion, characterized by mydriasis, hyperthermia, tachycardia, elevated blood pressure, piloerection, increased alertness, and facilitation of monosynaptic reflexes. Nausea and occasionally vomiting occur.

Psychoactive effects are fully evident within one to two hours; these are quite variable from subject to subject and in the same subject under different conditions of dose, mood, expectation, setting, and time. Perceptions are heightened and may become overwhelming. Afterimages are prolonged and overlap with ongoing perceptions. Objects may seem to move in a wavelike fashion or melt. Illusions and synesthesias, the overflow of one sense modality to another, are common. There may be a sense of unusual clarity, and one's thoughts may assume extraordinary importance. Time may seem to pass very slowly, and body distortions are commonly perceived. True hallucinations with loss of insight may occur in susceptible individuals. Mood is highly variable and labile, and may range from expansive reactions characterized by euphoria and self-confidence to a constricted reaction marked by depression and panic.

The syndrome begins to clear after 10 to 12 hours, and fatigue and tension may persist for an additional 24 hours. The biologic half-life of LSD in man is three hours.

The duration of action of mescaline is about 12 hours, that of psilocybin is four to six hours, that of DOM is six to eight hours, and that of phencyclidine is two to four hours. DMT must be injected or sniffed, and effects last less than two hours.

Tolerance to LSD develops rapidly, repeated daily doses becoming ineffective in three to four days. Recovery is equally rapid, so weekly use of the same dose is possible. Cross-tolerance has been demonstrated between LSD, mescaline, psilocybin, and the amphetamine-based psychedelics, but not between LSD and amphetamine. Physical dependence does not occur with LSD or any of the psychedelic drugs.

Mechanisms of action of LSD are unknown, but may depend on a complex interaction of serotonin and norepinephrine systems in the central nervous system. LSD lowers the threshold for reticular arousal via sensory input and may influence the processes concerned with the filtration and integration of sensory information.

Adverse Effects. Acute physiologic toxicity of the psychedelic drugs is low at doses that produce marked psychologic effects. In man, no deaths directly attributable to the use of these drugs have been reported. Controversy exists as to whether the illicit use of LSD increases the rate of chromosome breakage in users and leads to an increased incidence of congenital defects in children born to parents who had taken this drug. Evidence suggests that pregnant women exposed to illicit LSD had an elevated rate of spontaneous abortions. LSD may inhibit antibody formation and disrupt the body's immune system. Additional study of these adverse effects are necessary, because illicit users of LSD frequently take other drugs and may be malnourished and debilitated.

The acute panic reaction ("bad trip," "freak-out") is the most frequent complication of psychedelic use. These vary in intensity and have led to suicide attempts and accidents on rare occasions. Fear of death or insanity and sensations of breathlessness or paralysis are commonly reported. In most cases, this acute reaction subsides as drug effects are dissipated. Other complications include prolonged psychotic disorders, acute and chronic paranoid reactions, and depressive states. "Flashback" phenomena, the recurrence of some aspect of the drug experience when the individual is not under the influence of the drug, have been reported. The intensity, frequency, and duration of these episodes are quite variable. Adverse psychologic reactions are most frequent in emotionally disturbed individuals in crisis situations or insecure environments, who take the drug in unsupervised settings. High doses of psychedelic drugs lead to an increased incidence of these complications. Whether the psychedelics cause prolonged adverse reactions in emotionally stable people is not clear.

Anticholinergic Compounds. Ingestion of the alkaloids *atropine, hyoscyamine,* and *scopolamine* as they occur in their natural plant forms is reported in other parts of the world, but does not occur in the United States. Use in this country is rare and generally incident to the accidental or voluntary ingestion of these compounds when they are available in pharmaceutical preparations. Excessive use of *antihistaminic* compounds with anticholinergic effects also occurs. Symptoms of the potent peripheral effects of intoxication with these drugs include dilated, fixed pupils, dry skin and mouth, flushing, hyperthermia, and tachycardia. Psychoactive effects are those of an acute toxic psychosis, with clouding of consciousness, delirium, and loss of memory for the period of intoxication. Vivid sensory phenomena are not prominent, although hallucinations may occur.

Treatment. Treatment of the acute panic reaction may usually be accomplished by ensuring a warm, supportive environment with someone in constant attendance and with a minimum of other external stimuli. The user should be reminded continually that the effects he is experiencing are due to the drug and will pass in time. In particularly agitated patients, phenothiazines or diazepam orally or intramuscularly may be used. In the event of precipitation of prolonged psychosis, hospitalization with supportive care may be required. Flashbacks are treated with reassurance and/or psychotherapy when these are severe. In general, the duration and severity of these decrease with time if psychedelic drug use ceases.

Treatment of anticholinergic poisoning is symptomatic and consists of protecting the patient from self-injury, providing fluids, and reducing the fever. Administration of cholinesterase inhibitors is not indicated.

346. MISCELLANEOUS INHALANTS

Robert B. Millman

Nitrous Oxide. Recreational inhalation of nitrous oxide alone or in combination with oxygen is a rarely reported phenomenon that occurs in some youthful populations. Psychoactive effects occur in 15 to 30 seconds and persist for less than five minutes. The experience is described as one of intoxication, euphoria, and hilarity. Adverse effects have not been reported.

Organic Solvents. The inhalation of a wide range of organic solvents, particularly the toluene in glue, has received a good deal of attention from the mass media and law-enforcement agencies. It is likely that this publicity has contributed significantly to the incidence of this practice in the adolescent and preadolescent population. The material is usually squeezed into a plastic bag and the vapors inhaled. Prolonged exposure, as in the case of industrial workers, may have serious adverse effects on a variety of organ systems. As used recreationally, these solvents produce intoxication and dizziness not unlike that experienced with alcohol. Few side effects have been reported, although suffocation caused by the plastic bag has apparently occurred. The inhalation of aerosol sprays containing fluorocarbon propellants has recently been reported. Acute toxicity has not yet been adequately evaluated, although cardiac arrhythmias are considered to be a potentially serious complication.

Amyl Nitrite. Amyl nitrite ("amies," "poppers") inhalation has been reported in the youthful drug-abusing population. Use is intermittent and characterized by an instantaneous feeling ("rush") of dizziness, hilarity, and activity. Effects persist for minutes. Adverse effects include palpitations, postural hypotension occasionally proceeding to loss of consciousness, and headache. Chronic use is extremely rare, and more severe adverse effects have not been reported.

Brecher, E. M., and the Editors of Consumer Reports: Licit and Illicit Drugs. The Consumers Union Report on Narcotics, Stimulants, Depressants, Inhalants, Hallucinogens, and Marijuana, Including Caffeine, Nicotine and Alcohol. Mount Vernon, New York, Consumers Union, 1972.

Cherubin, C. E.: A review of the medical complications of narcotic addiction. Int. J. Addict, 3:167, 1968.

Dishotsky, N. I., Loughman, W. D., Mogar, R. E., and Lipscomb, W. R.: LSD and genetic damage. Science, 172:431, 1971.

Dole, V. P.: Narcotic addiction, physical dependence and relapse. N. Engl. J. Med., 206:988, 1972.

Dole, V. P., and Nyswander, M.: A medical treatment for diacetylmorphine (heroin) addiction. J.A.M.A., 193:646, 1965.

Isbell, H., Altschul, S., Kornetsky, C. H., et al.: Chronic barbiturate intoxication. An experimental study. Arch. Neurol. Psychiat., 64:1, 1950.

Jaffe, J.: Narcotic analgesics and drug addiction and drug abuse. *In* Goodman, L. S., and Gilman, A. (eds.): The Pharmacological Basis of Therapeutics, Fourth Edition. New York, The Macmillan Company, 1970, p. 237.

Kalant, H., LeBlanc, A. E., and Gibbins, R. J.: Tolerance to, and dependence on, some nonopiate psychotropic drugs. Pharmacol. Rev., 23:135, 1971.

Kreek, M. J.: Medical safety and side effects of methadone in tolerant individuals. J.A.M.A., 223:665, 1973.

Oakley, S. R.: Drugs, Society and Human Behavior. St. Louis, Mo., C. V. Mosby Company, 1972.

Snyder, S. H.: Catecholamines in the brain as mediators of amphetamine psychosis. Arch. Gen. Psychiatry, 27:169, 1972.

347. ALCOHOL ABUSE AND ALCOHOL-RELATED ILLNESS

Jack H. Mendelson

Definition. The most widely accepted operational definition of alcohol abuse is excessive drinking which adversely affects an individual's health, impairs social function, or both. Although it is not difficult to assess the impact of alcohol abuse on biologic function, it is often impossible to quantify alcohol-related social impairment. Experts disagree about both the type and the severity of problem drinking which cause social dysfunction because of wide variations in societal norms for characterizing deviant drinking behavior. Attempts to establish criteria for normative drinking behavior based upon volume and consumption frequency indices have not been satisfactory because of conflicting social, cultural, religious, and even political perceptions of how individuals in various societies may consume alcohol.

The frequently used term "alcoholism" is ambiguous. "Alcoholism" is often not synonymous with alcohol abuse, but denotes a series of problems ranging from deviant drinking behavior (as defined by the society in which it occurs) to alcohol addiction. Some of the phenomena which are reported to occur during the progression of *alcohol abuse* to *alcohol addiction* include excessive drinking in normal social situations; drinking in isolation; drinking to reduce anxiety, apprehension, or anger; drinking to facilitate the induction of sleep during conditions of insomnia; early morning drinking; and alterations in memory function (blackout) during heavy episodic alcohol intake. All or none of these phenomena may be reported by individuals who demonstrate evidence of addiction to alcohol, and no specific pattern of events is pathognomonic of behavior attributes for transition of alcohol abuse to alcohol addiction.

Addiction to alcohol is characterized by both tolerance and physical dependence. Tolerance occurs when an individual consumes progressively larger quantities of alcohol over a period of time in order to induce changes in feeling states or behavior which previously were induced by smaller doses of alcohol. Physical dependence occurs when an individual develops subjective discomfort and/or overt withdrawal signs after partial or complete cessation of drinking. It is important to emphasize that withdrawal signs and symptoms may occur in alcohol addicts when they reduce drinking but do not completely cease all alcohol intake. Relatively small decrements in sustained high blood alcohol levels may be associated with precipitation of the withdrawal syndrome.

As with most behavior disorders, it is often impossible to establish a precise definition of clinical status, e.g., alcohol abuse versus alcohol addiction. The physician must make a judgment about the presence and severity of an alcohol-related problem on the basis of careful determination of physical and mental status, occupational performance, social interaction, and—not least important—the patient's own perception of how alcohol consumption enhances or compromises his or her health and well-being.

Etiology. No specific biologic, psychologic, or social variable has been shown to have high predictive value for determining which individuals are at high risk to develop and sustain problem drinking behavior. There are no known psychologic tests which can reliably differentiate alcohol abusers from normal drinkers. Many theories have purported to explain the causation of alcoholism in terms of psychodynamic factors, personality profiles, psychosocial developmental and growth characteristics, nutritional idiosyncrasies, allergic disorders, and specific and nonspecific metabolic derangements. To date, none of these theories of the causation of alcohol abuse or alcohol addiction have significant support from well-controlled laboratory and clinical investigations.

The contribution of specific genetic and environmental factors which may enhance the risk for development of alcohol-related problems has not been clarified. Many patients who develop alcohol-related problems have no family history of alcohol abuse or alcohol addiction. But it is also known that individuals with a family history of alcohol abuse, particularly those who report that both parents had alcohol problems, may be at very great risk for developing alcohol abuse themselves. It is likely that this enhanced risk occurs, in part, as a function of growing up in an environment where excessive drinking is employed for coping with or modifying social stress. Moreover, there are recent data which indicate that a genetic component may be associated with the causation of alcohol problems. Studies of adoptees in Denmark have demonstrated that these individuals are more likely to develop alcohol problems if their biologic parents were alcohol abusers than if the adopted parent had abused alcohol. Thus at present it appears reasonable to conclude that both genetic and developmental factors may contribute to the genesis of alcohol-related illness.

Incidence and Prevalence. Surveys of American drinking practices reveal that approximately two thirds of the adult population of the United States use alcohol at least occasionally. It is estimated that about 12 per cent of the American population are heavy drinkers, i.e., individuals who drink almost daily or who once a week consume five or more drinks per occasion. It is obvious that this definition of heavy drinking may be associated with a number of ambiguities, and it is difficult to rate relative degree of drinking (heavy versus light) from self-written reports about the volume and frequency of alcohol consumed. Thus, individuals may consume the same quantity of alcohol during a given interval of time, but variations in the spacing or the concentrating of the drinking may indicate vastly different drinking patterns. For example, alcohol addicts who are spree drinkers may consume enormous amounts of alcohol in a two- or three-day interval during a month and remain relatively abstinent the remainder of the time.

A recent survey of American drinking practices and problems revealed that the largest population of problem drinkers were city-dwellers of low socioeconomic status. The highest rates of alcohol-related problems were found in young (under 25) urban men; the number of heavy drinkers among white and black males was similar (22 and 19 per cent, respectively). However, black women reported a significantly higher rate of drinking (11 per cent) than white women (4 per cent). American Indians and Eskimos have high reported rates of alcohol abuse and addiction.

Repeated surveys have shown that alcohol problems can be found in anyone who drinks alcohol to excess and that individual variations obliterate the significance of any group, ethnic, or cultural qualities. Case finding in alcoholism is difficult because of the stigma associated with the disorder. However, most agree that alcoholism represents the major drug problem in America today. It has been estimated that about 5 million adults in the United States have significant alcohol-related problems. It is also estimated that an additional 4 million abuse alcohol to the extent that they are at high risk for the development of alcohol addiction. These figures imply that 7 per cent of the adult population have a significant alcohol-related problem.

Pharmacologic Aspects. After the consumption of alcohol, absorption occurs primarily from the small intestine, but gastric emptying and the rate of absorption from the intestine are influenced by a number of factors. The rate of absorption is accelerated with increasing concentrations of alcohol up to a maximum of 40 per cent. Concentrations of ingested alcohol above 40 per cent may be absorbed more slowly as a consequence of delayed gastric emptying. Similarly, high concentrations of congeners in beverage alcohol delay absorption because they impede gastric emptying by inducing pyloric spasm. The ingestion of food along with beverage alcohol also reduces the speed of absorption by delaying the emptying time of the stomach.

After absorption, ethanol is distributed to all portions of the body and achieves equilibrium with body water compartments. Since ethanol is more soluble in lipid fractions, ethanol concentration in body tissues is greatest in those organs and cells containing high concentrations of lipids. No impermeable or semipermeable membranes impede the diffusion of alcohol into any body organ or tissue.

Alcohol is removed from the body primarily by metabolism in the liver, and only 2 to 10 per cent is excreted directly by the kidneys and the lungs. Alcohol is catabolized in the liver by well-known enzymatic mechanisms involving the enzyme alcohol dehydrogenase and the cofactor NAD. The rate of alcohol metabolism in normal drinkers and in abstinent alcohol addicts is not significantly different. However, the rate of ethanol metabolism may increase in alcohol addicts during the course of spree drinking, and it is believed that this increase is due to an ethanol-induced increase in rate of hepatic metabolism.

There are no known pharmacologic agents which may be utilized in clinical practice to enhance the rate of ethanol catabolism in man. Although it has been shown that high dosage administration of fructose may accelerate rates of ethanol metabolism, the clinical use of this is impractical.

Blood alcohol levels depend upon the amount of alcohol ingested and the weight of the individual. For the average man, it has been estimated that the consumption of 180 ml of distilled spirits on an empty stomach will produce a blood alcohol level of approximately 100 mg per 100 ml. Values around 180 mg per 100 ml have been established by most jurisdictions as the legal limit of sobriety for operating a motor vehicle. Blood alcohol levels achieved in usual social drinking situations average about 50 to 75 mg per 100 ml. At this blood level a subjective state of pleasant tranquility and a mild degree of sedation may occur. Overt signs of intoxication usually occur in social (nontolerant) drinkers between 100 and 200 mg per 100 ml. Severe intoxication is observed in social drinkers at levels above 200 mg per 100 ml, but alcohol addicts who are tolerant to the effects of ethanol may appear relatively intact and nonintoxicated with such blood alcohol levels. Regardless of the degree of tolerance, blood alcohol levels above 400 mg per 100 ml produce stupor and/or coma, and concentrations above 500 mg per 100 ml are frequently fatal.

Alcohol and Behavior. *Acute Intoxication.* Although the concomitants of acute intoxication are well known and easily recognized (dysarthria, ataxia, and emotional lability), there is no simple correlation between the volume of alcohol consumed and an individual's ability to carry out cognitive and motor tasks successfully. Indeed, some individuals actually show improved performance on perceptual and psychomotor tasks with low to moderate doses of alcohol. This paradox obtains because small to moderate doses of ethanol may act in a manner similar to a minor tranquilizer, i.e., to reduce anxiety which may affect skill and performance. Individuals who demonstrate little impairment in performance of cognitive and motor tasks with high blood ethanol concentrations (150 to 200 mg per 100 ml) have probably developed tolerance for alcohol as a consequence of recurrent heavy drinking.

Moderate dosage of alcohol usually impairs visual-motor coordination in most social drinkers. In particular, brightness discrimination and visual adaptation after exposure to bright lights is often markedly reduced. Auditory and tactile sensation are usually unchanged. The integration and evaluation of sensory information, rather than the impairment of sensory input itself, are most severely compromised during acute intoxication. An individual's ability to initiate or maintain sustained attention to stimuli and to judge the qualities of stimuli is usually significantly diminished after moderate alcohol intake. Individuals under such conditions tend to underestimate the speed and distance of objects as well as to show impairment in making judgments regarding the passage of time.

Impairments of behavior associated with acute intoxication are also determined by factors related to the setting. If a person consumes alcohol in a situation in which drunkenness is both expected and tolerated, this anticipation may influence his behavior more than the dosage of alcohol ingested. Similarly, individuals who fear the consequences of intoxicated behavior may successfully mask the manifestations of acute inebriation even though they consume relatively large amounts of alcohol.

Alcohol, Aggression, and Accidents. Although it is well known that alcohol ingestion and acute intoxication are significant factors in accidents, the causal significance of alcohol ingestion per se is not a simple one. Alcohol intoxication may effect a number of patterns of behavior which combine to produce enhanced risk for an accident. These include compromised judgment, enhanced emotional lability, and inability to suppress expression of aggression. Acute alcohol intoxication also contributes to situations which result in death and injury as a function of violence and aggressive behavior. Homicide, armed robbery with aggravated assault, and other crimes of violence are frequent in perpetrators or victims who are acutely intoxicated.

Acute alcohol intoxication has been frequently implicated in fatal accidents. For example, over half of the nonhighway accident fatalities involve alcohol addicts or abusers. A recent survey carried out in a general hospital emergency room in which blood alcohol values were determined in accident victims showed that 30 per cent of the individuals involved in highway accidents, 22 per cent involved in home accidents, and 16 per cent involved in occupational accidents had elevated blood ethanol levels.

Alcohol abuse is a significant contributing factor to over 50 per cent of motor vehicle fatalities, and it has been estimated that 28,000 highway deaths during a recent 12-month period were associated with alcohol intoxication. There is increasing evidence, however, that alcohol-related automobile fatalities may not be simply associated with episodic acute intoxication in social drinkers, but rather are phenomena related to chronic intoxication and alcohol addiction. Statistics obtained from studies of blood alcohol levels in individuals involved in single vehicle fatalities indicate that a majority had blood ethanol values above 150 mg per 100 ml. Such high blood levels suggest that the accident victims were not social drinkers but alcohol addicts. Thus it is possible that the preponderance of motor vehicle accidents and deaths in which alcohol is implicated is associated with addiction to alcohol, as defined in pharmacologic terms, and is not a consequence of occasional intemperate drinking.

Alcohol and Sexual Function. The effect of acute intoxication on sexual behavior and function is poorly understood. The classic reference is Shakespeare's perception that intoxication increases desire but impairs sexual performance. Although the effects of acute alcohol intoxication on sexual behavior in moderate drinkers may be quite idiosyncratic, by contrast, sexual function and behavior are often markedly impaired in alcohol addicts. Male alcohol addicts often report sexual impotence and diminished heterosexual desire. A tendency to initiate or increase alcohol intake has been reported by female alcoholics during premenstrual periods. Gynecomastia and testicular atrophy have been reported in male alcohol addicts, particularly those who also show evidence of alcohol-related liver disease. Recent studies have demonstrated that alcohol administration to alcohol addicts is associated with suppression of plasma testosterone levels.

The "Hangover." A well-known consequence of acute alcohol intoxication is a syndrome of generalized somatic discomfort, headache, nausea, agitation, and mild tremulousness which has been termed the "hangover." The physiologic mechanisms related to the hangover have not been determined. Current evidence indicates that the hangover may be the equivalent of a mild withdrawal syndrome. There is no evidence that any specific characteristic of beverage alcohol, such as its congener content, or any unique pattern of drinking, such as mixing different beverages, is the causal basis for the hangover. No specific form of pharmacotherapy is available for treatment of the problem, and there is little evidence that the plethora of popular remedies have any efficacy.

Addiction to Alcohol. Addiction to alcohol is characterized by the presence of both tolerance and physical dependence. Although many individuals may frequently abuse alcohol, not all become physically dependent. Moreover, it is difficult to predict addiction liability on the basis of dosage of alcohol and frequency of consumption alone. There is no question, however, that physical dependence on alcohol is analogous to physical dependence induced by a number of other centrally acting drugs and is not caused by intercurrent illness, vitamin, or nutritional disorders. Withdrawal signs and symptoms have been observed in otherwise healthy alcohol addicts exclusively as a concomitant of cessation of drinking. Physical dependence has also been induced in a number of species of laboratory animals without producing derangements in nutritional or metabolic function.

Tolerance appears to develop more rapidly than physical dependence for alcohol and other drugs which affect the central nervous system (i.e., narcotics, barbiturates, and psychotropic drugs). Three forms of tolerance may be observed in the alcohol addict: behavioral tolerance, pharmacologic tolerance, and cross-tolerance to certain other drugs which have their primary effect on central nervous function.

Behavioral tolerance is manifest when the alcohol addict can consume relatively large amounts of ethanol without impairment in social behavior or psychomotor coordination. It has been observed clinically and demonstrated in research ward studies that some alcohol addicts can consume as much as 1 quart of beverage alcohol per day without evidence of gross intoxication. It has also been shown that many alcohol addicts can perform relatively complex tasks without error when their blood alcohol levels are twice the legal limit of intoxication for many state jurisdictions.

Pharmacologic tolerance reflects a metabolic adaptive change in the alcohol addict as a consequence of long-term drinking. Evidence of pharmacologic tolerance was originally inferred from the finding of low blood alcohol levels in alcohol addicts who had consumed large amounts of alcohol (up to 1 quart of bourbon per day for 20 consecutive days). Subsequent studies demonstrated an enhanced rate of ethanol metabolism in alcohol addicts during protracted episodes of drinking. The pharmacokinetics of alcohol-induced enhancement of ethanol metabolism have not been clarified, but they appear not to persist after long periods of sobriety. Pharmacologic tolerance may contribute to some small aspect of behavioral tolerance, but adaptive processes in the central nervous system are probably far more important for behavioral tolerance than alcohol-induced enhancement in rates of ethanol metabolism.

Clinical reports have stressed that alcohol addicts may show reduced sensitivity and responsivity to a number of other drugs: *cross-tolerance*. There are reports that alcohol addicts require significantly higher doses of both the barbiturate and volatile anesthetics for induction and maintenance of appropriate levels of surgical anesthesia. Alcohol addicts frequently show cross-tolerance for barbiturates, hypnotics, and psychotropic agents such as the minor tranquilizers. However, cross-tolerance and cross-dependence have not been demonstrated between alcohol and the opiates. It is important to point out that cross-tolerance occurs in alcohol addicts when they are temporarily abstaining from drinking. When alcohol addicts are intoxicated, both synergism and potentiation with narcotics, opiates and analgesics, barbiturates, and a variety of other psychotropic agents may occur. In fact, there is some evidence which indicates that the consumption of drugs such as barbiturates during heavy alcohol intake is associated with a decreased catabolic degradation of both agents.

Although tolerance for ethanol may appear to be very great for some alcohol addicts, the degree of tolerance which can be developed for ethanol is much smaller than that which can potentially occur in opiate or barbiturate addiction. Barbiturate addicts may ingest as much as 2 grams of secobarbital or pentobarbital daily without gross impairments of behavior. Heroin addicts may eventually employ a dosage 50 times larger than their initial intake. On the other hand, blood alcohol levels exceeding 450 mg per 100 ml for any drinker, social or addicted, are rarely observed, because this level is almost invariably associated with a comatose state. Moreover, the lethal level of 500 to 600 mg per 100 ml is no different for alcohol addicts as opposed to normal drinkers, because such blood alcohol levels cause severe and often irreversible respiratory depression.

Physical dependence upon alcohol is characterized by the appearance of withdrawal signs and symptoms after cessation of drinking. Tremulousness, delirium, and seizure disorders were first reported by Hippocrates to accompany alcohol abuse, and detailed descriptions of the abstinence syndrome are reported in the medical literature of the late eighteenth century. Systematic studies by Victor and Adams in 1953 are the basis for the classification of the withdrawal syndromes currently identified in clinical practice. Three types of withdrawal states have been differentiated: tremulous states, seizure disorders, and delirium tremens.

Tremulousness is the most frequent and benign type of abstinence syndrome. Although the onset of tremulousness usually occurs 12 to 48 hours after reduction of alcohol intake or initiation of abstinence, this sign may be observed as early as six hours after cessation of drinking. Tremor is usually mild with involvement of the hands, but in some instances it may be generalized with involvement of all extremities as well as the tongue and trunk. Tremor may be increased when the patient extends the arms with the palms upright and the fingers separated. Tremulousness usually remits or is significantly diminished by 72 hours after cessation of drinking, but in rare instances it may persist for five days.

Hallucinosis may be associated with a tremulous state or may occur independent of tremor. Hallucinations also may occur in alcohol addicts during conditions of severe intoxication as well as during conditions of complete or partial cessation of drinking.

Seizure disorders usually occur 12 to 24 hours after cessation of drinking. Seizures may be associated with tremulousness, but may be present without any other evidence of withdrawal signs. The seizure disorder is of the grand mal type, usually not preceded by auras but almost always followed by a postictal state. Seizures may be observed in patients who have no overt evidence of a neurologic disorder and who have no abnormalities of the electroencephalogram. Victor and Adams have emphasized that approximately one third of all patients who have seizure disorders after cessation of drinking progress to develop delirium tremens.

Delirium tremens is the rarest form of the alcohol withdrawal syndrome. Delirium tremens is characterized by confusion, disorientation, delusions, hallucinations, psychomotor agitation, and autonomic dysfunction. The peak incidence of this syndrome is 72 to 96 hours after cessation of drinking. The severe confusional states and delirium which are the hallmark of delirium tremens are rarely observed in the more frequent instances of tremulousness after cessation of drinking. Patients who develop delirium tremens also often have profuse sweating, tachycardia, hypertension, and fever. Delirium tremens is a potentially lethal illness which requires hospitalization and intensive medical care.

Although the basic mechanisms underlying the alcohol withdrawal syndrome remain to be determined, a number of associated disorders affect the severity of the disorder. Significant disturbances in acid-base, water, and electrolyte homeostasis may be associated with the abstinence syndrome. After cessation of alcohol intake, many alcohol addicts develop episodic hyperventilation which may produce respiratory alkalosis and elevations in blood pH. This condition is usually associated with hypomagnesemia. The low serum magnesium levels observed in alcohol addicts during the withdrawal syndrome are probably caused both by poor dietary intake of magnesium during heavy drinking and by magnesium shifts from the intravascular to the intracellular fluid compartments associated with the pH shift of respiratory alkalosis. It is also important to remember that alcohol addicts who develop withdrawal syndromes may be not dehydrated, but in fact, overhydrated.

Intercurrent Illness and Associated Disorders. Alcohol addicts are at high risk for developing a number of disorders which are observed frequently in general medical practice. These are discussed individually in other chapters of this text, but a few merit mention here.

Alcohol-related hepatic disease is a leading cause of morbidity and mortality in adult males. It has been demonstrated that alcohol intake alone without concomitant nutritional deficiency may induce hepatic disorders such as fatty metamorphosis, alcoholic hepatitis, and Laennec's cirrhosis (see Ch. 709). However, since many people consume large quantities of alcohol without developing these disorders, the crucial determinants of the interrelationships between heavy alcohol consumption and hepatic disease remain to be determined. Gastritis and pancreatitis (see Ch. 640 and Ch. 645 and 646) are also frequently in those who abuse alcohol. A variety of malabsorption syndromes may be associated with heavy alcohol intake (see Part XIV, Section Three).

The most severe neurologic disorders seen in alcohol

addicts are peripheral neuropathies (see Ch. 456 to 474) which are characterized by motor and sensory impairments in the upper and lower extremities. Pain, paresthesia, motor weakness, and paralysis may occur as a consequence of poor dietary intake in conjunction with heavy ethanol intake.

Diseases of the central nervous system may also be associated with chronic alcohol abuse. Wernicke's disease and Korsakoff's psychosis (see Ch. 406) are characterized by derangements of memory function and disorders of thought processes. The genesis of many "organic brain diseases," which at present constitute the majority of first admissions to state mental hospitals, may be related to nutritional and metabolic derangements associated with alcohol abuse.

There is accumulating evidence that alcohol abuse may be a factor in the development of coronary artery disease. Individuals who have a familial Type IV hyperlipidemia (see Ch. 817) are at high risk for developing elevations in blood triglyceride levels with even moderate alcohol intake. A number of cardiomyopathies have been found in alcohol addicts. Finally, it has been shown that chronic alcohol abuse may cause derangements in hematopoiesis, produce muscle wasting, and suppress immune mechanisms with consequence of higher risk for infection.

Affective Disorders and Psychosis. Some individuals with neurotic and psychotic affective disorders drink excessively, but many others with severe depression never abuse alcohol. In manic-depressive illness patients are more prone to drink excessively during the manic phase of their disorder than when they are depressed. There is also evidence to indicate that chronic alcohol abuse enhances rather than reduces feelings of depression.

Approximately 25 per cent of all suicide victims have detectable amounts of alcohol in body fluids on necropsy examination. It is estimated that one third of all suicides are associated with chronic alcohol abuse, but these findings may relate mainly to white middle-aged males. Suicide rates for black males over 35 are low, even though drinking problems may be high.

Treatment and Prevention. Although there are occasional reports of children who die of respiratory failure associated with ethanol overdosage, death from *acute ethanol poisoning* is rare. Rapid ingestion of large amounts of ethanol ususally induces vomiting. Those who consume large amounts of ethanol slowly usually become stuporous before they can ingest a dose necessary to produce significant respiratory depression. The rate of ethanol catabolism in man ranges from 15 to 22 mg per 100 ml per hour, and there are no clinically useful or efficacious methods for rapidly decreasing blood alcohol levels.

Acute ethanol intoxication may be complicated by concurrent intoxication with other centrally acting drugs. There appears to be an increasing degree of polydrug abuse in the United States, particularly drugs which act synergistically with or potentiate the actions of ethanol. Alcohol abusers also frequently abuse barbiturates and minor tranquilizers. The most commonly reported form of drug abuse in narcotic addicts maintained on methadone is with alcohol. In hospital practice it is advisable to obtain blood determinations for other possible central nervous system depressants when a severe depression of consciousness is noted in patients who appear only to be intoxicated with ethanol.

Many persons who seek a physician's aid during conditions of acute ethanol intoxication have other medical disorders. These patients should receive the most careful physical examination and diagnostic workup. Most states have adopted legislation requiring that patients with alcohol-related illness, including acute intoxication, should not be denied admission to hospitals and medical facilities. In addition, the American Medical Association and the American Hospital Association have endorsed resolutions against discriminatory policies for patients with alcohol-related problems who seek admission to general medical facilities. Some patients may request hospital treatment for detoxification after chronic alcohol intake when there is no evidence of any significant intercurrent illness. If the patient's motivation for receiving medical assistance appears good, the physician should attempt to provide the best available hospital care. However, involuntary commitment of patients with alcohol problems is not legal in most jurisdictions if hospitalization is initiated only on the basis of a diagnosis of alcoholism without evidence of a serious psychotic disorder.

Treatment of the *alcohol withdrawal syndrome* has improved significantly during the past decade. Less than 15 years ago many hospitals reported a 15 per cent mortality in patients with delirium tremens. The current mortality rate associated with delirium tremens is less than 1 per cent. The major factor affecting reduction in both mortality and morbidity is the application of good general medical care. Patients requiring treatment for the withdrawal syndrome should have the following procedures carried out on a systematic basis: (1) a careful physicial and roentgenologic examination to identify any traumatic injuries (especially trauma to the skull); (2) a search for infection of the pulmonary and genitourinary systems; (3) a search for hepatic, gastrointestinal, and cardiac disorders; and (4) an evaluation of the state of hydration, electrolyte, and acid-base status, with appropriate measures instituted to correct any derangements. It should not be assumed that patients exhibiting the withdrawal syndrome are dehydrated or have any particular derangement in electrolyte or acid-base balance status unless demonstrated by appropriate clinical and laboratory examinations.

Chlordiazepoxide is the best drug for reducing psychomotor agitation in patients who have withdrawal syndromes, provided the agent is used judiciously. In general, the dosage employed should permit reduction of tremor and anxiety without compromising the patient's ability to tolerate fluid and foods orally. Patients exhibiting the withdrawal syndrome should not be sedated deeply simply to produce long periods of sleep. Whenever possible, medication should be given orally, although at the initial stages of the withdrawal syndrome it may be necessary to use the intramuscular route. The routine use of corticosteroids is contraindicated, and the efficacy of diphenylhydantoin (Dilantin) in controlling seizure disorders is questionable. Administration of multivitamins orally or intravenously should be based upon judgment of the patient's nutritional status.

The *treatment of chronic alcohol abuse* is often difficult because most patients with alcohol-related problems tend to deny the severity of their illness and to avoid or reject assistance by physicians and other health care professionals. It has been postulated that the patient's acceptance of treatment can be greatly improved if initial contacts with the physician and the hospital are sympathetic and positive. The point has often been made that treatment for the alcohol abuser and alcohol addict should have limited goals and that alcohol-related illness should be considered as a chronic disease analogous, in some ways, to chronic pulmonary and cardiac conditions. For the most part, physicians treating such illnesses strive to alleviate suffering and to induce compensation rather than achieve absolute cure. A reasonable treatment goal is to restore physical and behavioral status after decompensation in alcohol abusers, even if recidivism is expected. Multimodality therapy suited to the needs of the individual and his resources should be offered. However, the question of which treatment will maximally benefit the patient with alcohol problems remains unanswered.

At present there is no uniformly effective, specific treatment for alcohol abuse. A number of treatment techniques have been employed singly or in combinations which have proved effective for some patients. These include individual and group psychotherapy, Antabuse therapy, referral to self-help groups such as Alcoholics Anonymous, and a number of behavioral modification techniques. It is discouraging that the few relatively well controlled therapy evaluation studies have demonstrated a low rate of alcohol abstinence after therapy. But since these evaluations were carried out in specialized clinic treatment settings, it remains likely that the individual counseling and relationship offered by the family physician will offer a greater degree of success.

The spontaneous recovery rate for alcohol abusers has been estimated to be about 20 per cent over a three-year period. Thus physicians should not assume that alcohol-related disorders are intractable. Since all variants of alcohol abuse are multiply determined, alcohol problems present the treatment challenge of any complex behavioral disorder. Although there is no evidence to indicate that alcohol abuse is invariably associated with a predisposing psychiatric illness, the development of problem drinking rarely occurs in isolation from emotional, interpersonal, and job-related problems.

The physician should employ a multifaceted program of treatment which can be best determined from assessing the patient's motivation, resources, and ability to sustain treatment relationships. For some individuals, self-help groups such as Alcoholics Anonymous may be useful, but one must first explore whether any given patient can effectively utilize this form of assistance. The physician should familiarize himself with all available resources which exist in the patient's community for assistance with alcohol-related problems. It is often essential that the physician involve other members of the family in cooperating with some form of treatment program.

Adequate techniques for *prevention of alcohol-related disorders* have yet to be devised. Although significant emphasis has been placed upon public education and information concerning the responsible use of alcohol, the impact of such programs is difficult to evaluate. Since there are relatively poor incidence and prevalence data for alcohol abuse, it is impossible to argue that public education programs or attempts to shape attitudes have had any impact on alcohol abuse and alcohol addiction. Increased programs of public education and information may appear logical, but it should be remembered that problem drinking usually occurs in situations in which behavior is not determined by logical thinking but rather by internal and external stresses which are not highly amenable to rational persuasion.

Cahalan, D.: Problem Drinkers. San Francisco, Jossey-Bass, Inc., 1970.
Kalant, H.: Absorption, diffusion, distribution and elimination of ethanol: Effects on biological membranes. *In* Kissin, B., and Begleiter, H. (eds.): The Biology of Alcoholism, Vol. 1. New York, Plenum Press, 1971.
Mello, N. K.: Behavioral studies of alcoholism. *In* Kissin, B., and Begleiter, H. (eds.): The Biology of Alcoholism, Vol. 2. New York, Plenum Press, 1972.
Mendelson, J. H., and Mello, N. K.: Alcohol, aggression and androgens. Proc. Assn. Res. Nerv. Ment. Dis., 1974, in press.
Wolfe, S., and Victor, M.: The physiological basis of the alcohol withdrawal syndrome. *In* Mello, N. K., and Mendelson, J. H. (eds.): Recent Advances in Studies of Alcoholism. Washington, D. C., U. S. Government Printing Office, Publ. No. (HSM) 71-9045, 1971.

348. ACUTE DRUG POISONING

Fred Plum

Accidental or intentional drug overdose has become a common medical problem which almost any physician may be called upon to treat. Suicide ranks high as a cause of death among all age groups beyond early adolescence, and its incidence climbs steadily with age in single white males. Furthermore, psychologically engendered drug abuse plagues many countries, with fatal or near-fatal "accidents" often affecting youngsters of secondary school age as well as adults. No social stratum enjoys immunity. The physician's job is made harder by the fact that the mentally unbalanced or those just seeking new sensations have an ever-expanding roster of pharmaceutical or industrial chemicals to draw from. Nevertheless, changing fashions affect the minority, and the most frequent agents causing drug poisonings will undoubtedly continue to resemble those listed in Table 1.

Table 2 lists the most common drug poisonings presently encountered in the United States, gives their principal signs of toxicity, and outlines their treatment. Clinical appraisal still must be used to diagnose the agent causing several of these reaction patterns, specific chemical tests being either unavailable or impractical. Blood levels or size of the dose are generally unreliable guides to the potential danger with almost any of the drugs listed because tolerance develops to their chronic ingestion, making individuals react differently to similar doses. Also, the mixing of drugs with each other and with alcohol adds to the unreliability of blood levels as a guide to treatment or prognosis of the drugs listed in Table 2. Only the opiates and the sedatives create any appreciable risk of death. Opiate poisoning is discussed in more detail in Ch. 348. The rest of this chapter gives details of the management of sedative drug overdose. For the diagnosis and treatment of suspected drug or chemical poisonings not covered in these pages, physicians should consult the *Physicians' Desk Reference* or the Poison Control Center of a large city.

TABLE 1. Drugs Used, in Order of Frequency, Among Severe Overdose Subjects, New York Hospital, 1969–1973

Alcohol	Lithium
Barbiturates, glutethimide	Salicylates
Heroin or methadone	Phenothiazines
Methaqualone	Diphenylhydantoin
Meprobamate	Bishydroxycoumarin, Coumadin
Scopolamine	Tolbutamide, phenformin
Amphetamine	Insulin
Imipramine	

TABLE 2. Common Drug Poisonings, Signs of Toxicity, and Treatment

Drug	Mild Toxic Signs	Tissue for Diagnosis	Treatment	Severe Overdose Signs	Treatment
Opiates:					
Heroin Morphine Demerol Methadone	"Nodding" drowsiness, small pupils, urinary retention, slow and shallow breathing; skin scars and subcutaneous abscesses; duration 4–6 hrs; with methadone, duration to 24 hrs	Urine	Levallorphan 1 mg iv, nalorphine 10 mg iv, naloxine 0.4 mg iv or im; repeat at 15-min intervals not more than twice; repeat in 3 hrs if necessary	Coma; pinpoint pupils, slow irregular respiration or apnea, hypotension, hypothermia, pulmonary edema	Levallorphan, nalorphine, naloxine; if no response by second dose, suspect another cause; treat shock; find and detect infection
Depressants:					
Alcohol Barbiturates Glutethimide (Doriden) Meprobamate (Equanil)	Confusion, rousable drowsiness, delirium, ataxia, nystagmus, dysarthria, analgesia to stimuli	Blood, urine, breath Blood Blood Blood	Alcohol excitement: diazepam or chlorpromazine None needed for acute toxicity; withdraw drug under supervision if patient is a chronic user	Stupor to coma; pupils reactive, usually constricted; oculovestibular response absent; motor tonus initially briefly hyperactive, then flaccid; respiration and blood pressure depressed; hypothermia; with glutethimide, pupils moderately dilated, can be fixed; with meprobamate, withdrawal seizures common; with methaqualone, coma, occasional convulsions, tachycardia, cardiac failure, bleeding tendency	Intubate, ventilate, gavage; drainage position; antimicrobials; keep mean blood pressure above 90 mm Hg and urine output 300 ml/hr; avoid analeptics; hemodialyze severe phenobarbital poisoning
Methaqualone (Quaalude, Sopor, Mandrax)	Hallucinations, agitation, motor hyperactivity, myoclonus, tonic spasms	Blood			As above; diuresis of little help
Chlordiazepoxide (Librium) Diazepam (Valium)	Usually taken with another sedative if poisoning the attempt	Blood			
Stimulants:					
Amphetamines Methylphenidate	Hyperactive, aggressive, sometimes paranoid, repetitive behavior; dilated pupils, tremor, hyperactive reflexes; hyperthermia, tachycardia, arrhythmia Acute torsion dystonia	Blood	Reassurance if mild Chlorpromazine if intense Chlorpromazine	Agitated, assaultive and paranoid excitement; ocsionally convulsions; hypothermia; circulatory collapse	Chlorpromazine
Cocaine	Similar but less prominent than above; less paranoid, often euphoric	None: clinical appraisal only	Reassure	Twitching, irregular breathing, tachycardia	Sedation
Psychedelics (LSD, mescaline, psilocybin, STP)	Confused, disoriented, perceptual distortions, distractable, withdrawn or eruptive, leading to accidents or violence; wide-eyed, dilated pupils; restless, hyperreflexic; less often, hypertension or tachycardia		Reassure; "talk down"; do not leave alone	Panic	Reassure; diazepam satisfactory; avoid phenothiazines
Atropine-scopolamine (Sominex)	Agitated or confused, visual hallucinations, dilated pupils, flushed and dry skin		Reassure	Toxic disoriented delirium, visual hallucination; later, amnesia, fever, dilated fixed pupils, hot flushed dry skin, urinary retention	Reassure; sedate lightly; (1) avoid phenothiazines; (2) do not leave alone
Antidepressants:					
Imipramine (Tofranil), amitriptyline (Elavil)	Restlessness, drowsiness, tachycardia, ataxia, sweating	Clinical		Agitation, vomiting, hyperpyrexia, sweating, muscle dystonia, convulsions, tachycardia or arrhythmia	Symptomatic; gastric lavage
MAO inhibitors: tranylcypromine (Parnate), phenelzine (Nardil), pargyline (Eutonyl)	Hypertensive crises, agitation, drowsiness, ataxia	Clinical	Withdrawal	Hypotension; headache; chest pain; agitation; coma, seizures and shock	Symptomatic; gastric lavage
Phenothiazines	Acute dystonia, somnolence, hypotension	Clinical	Benadryl 0.50; withdrawal	Coma; convulsions (rare); arrhythmias; hypotension	Symptomatic; gastric lavage

SEDATIVE OVERDOSE

Pathogenesis. All the sedative drugs depress the central nervous system, although not equally on a gram-molecular weight basis, and not to the same degree so far as different central structures are concerned. The duration of action varies widely and depends largely on how the particular drug is detoxified or eliminated. The short-acting barbiturates, pentobarbital, secobarbital, and amobarbital, are detoxified by the liver, as is methaqualone. They exert their maximal effects promptly after being absorbed and, even in huge doses, seldom cause neurologic depression lasting longer than three to five days. Barbital and phenobarbital are partially detoxified by the liver and partially excreted in the urine. Severe poisoning with the latter agent can cause coma lasting 10 to 14 days. Glutethimide has a short duration of action comparable to that of secobarbital, but it is poorly absorbed from the gut. This can prolong the effect of an ingested dose. Meprobamate has an intermediate duration of effect lasting for days. Bromide rarely causes full coma, but, once it reaches high levels, it displaces chloride in the blood and tissues, and persists for weeks to cause symptoms without further ingestion.

Although the sedatives have few important effects outside the nervous system, glutethimide and meprobamate in toxic doses tend to produce hypotension. Also, glutethimide possesses unique anticholinergic properties and is the only sedative that predictably produces light-fixed pupils in toxic doses.

A withdrawal syndrome consisting of tremulousness, agitation, and sometimes delirium and convulsions can develop when any of the hypnotic sedatives are stopped after prolonged use. Quantitative information is lacking, but convulsions seem to be a particular problem after withdrawal from meprobamate and methaqualone.

Clinical Manifestations. Stupor or coma caused by depressant drug poisoning presents the characteristic picture of severe metabolic brain disease. The depression of the central nervous system tends to be bilateral and symmetrical, and the drug affects simultaneously many levels, including the spinal cord. Respiratory and circulatory controlling mechanisms in the lower brainstem are affected only with very high doses or not at all, and, except with glutethimide, the pupillary light reflexes are preserved. Early in the course of poisoning, patients can demonstrate muscular hypertonus or even spasticity as the result of uneven depression of different neurologic levels. Within a short time, usually an hour or less, flaccidity supervenes, and the stretch reflexes tend to disappear. Even moderate degrees of drug depression depress or block the oculovestibular reflexes.

Four grades of coma have been described in order to aid in estimating the severity of poisoning and the effects of treatment. *Grade I* is light coma in which vigorous noxious stimulation evokes withdrawal or groaning. *Grade II* is deep coma in which only minimal grimacing or reflex responsiveness can be evoked by a noxious stimulus. In *grade III* subjects fail to respond in any way to a noxious stimulus. In *grade IV* unresponsive patients remain in deep coma for over 36 hours and, in addition, have serious respiratory or circulatory depression. As mentioned above, a relationship between the blood level of a sedative drug and the depth of coma is only approximate. Generally speaking, however, blood levels of short-acting barbiturates of more than 2.5 mg per 100 ml and phenobarbital blood levels of more than 12 mg per 100 ml are associated with grades III and IV coma.

Diagnosis. The combination of unresponsiveness, preserved or sluggish pupillary reactions, absent oculovestibular reactions, motor areflexia, hypothermia, and depression of respiration and circulation is clinically diagnostic of sedative-anesthetic drug poisoning. Only pontine infarction resembles this clinical state, and with lesions of the pons the pupils are usually small or pinpoint, the stretch reflexes are generally preserved or hyperactive, and the plantar responses are extensor. Specific chemical tests will detect barbiturates, glutethimide, meprobamate, methaqualone, and bromides in blood or urine, and are readily done as emergency measures.

Management of Coma. There are no specific antidotes for the sedative drugs. Treatment consists of physiologic support and preventing complications until the drug is detoxified and is excreted. Proper management saves all but a very few patients if they survive to reach the hospital. Among the writer's series of 356 consecutive patients in coma, 11 or 3.1 per cent died, all but three of whom were older than 45 years. To achieve this low rate required meticulous attention to the airway and ventilation, to the circulation, and to the potential complications of the comatose state. In laboratory animals, the fatal dose of barbiturates is seven times that required to produce apnea and almost twice that which first produces circulatory shock. Similar actions by the drugs in man guide the treatment of poisoning.

Airway and Ventilation. Several mechanisms threaten to obstruct the airway of patients in coma from sedative drugs. If the subject lies on his back, the tongue and pooled secretions occlude the hypopharynx, with the result that secretions are aspirated into the lungs. The cough reflex and the ciliary action of the tracheobronchial mucosa are depressed. Many subjects aspirate stomach contents into the lungs, particularly if gastric lavage is attempted before tracheal intubation.

Because of these potentially fatal complications, the first step is to secure the airway. An oropharyngeal airway is sufficient to manage patients in light coma who cough when the larynx is stimulated. A cuffed endotracheal tube should be placed in more deeply anesthetized patients who lack a cough reflex. It is wise to precede intubation with atropine, 0.0008 gram intravenously, to reduce the danger of cardiac arrest. How long to leave the endotracheal tube in place in an unresponsive subject is often a difficult question. One practice is to deflate the cuff hourly for 5 minutes, to replace the tube at 24 hours, and to perform a tracheostomy at somewhere between 36 and 48 hours if the cough reflex has not returned or if no other signs indicate a lessening of coma.

To drain the lungs, patients should be placed in the prone position, as illustrated in the accompanying figure, and suctioned gently through the endotracheal tube

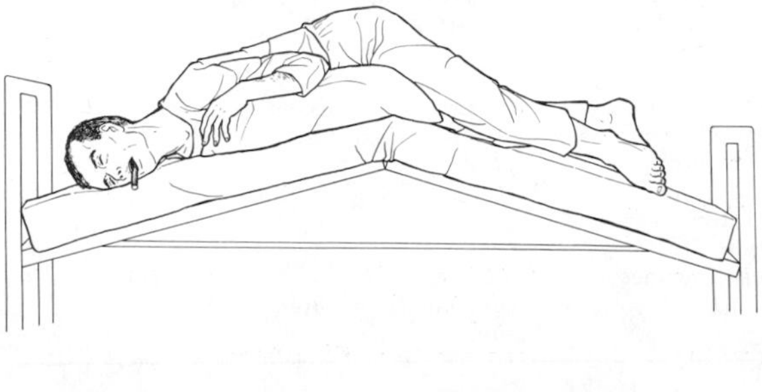

every half hour, or more often if pulmonary secretions accumulate. It is desirable to administer low concentrations (25 per cent) of moistened oxygen, but not to occlude the tube with a large catheter. Tubes are removed when active coughing or bucking returns.

Hypoventilation should be treated with artificial respiration. Shallow breathing in a deeply comatose patient frequently reflects no more than the subject's depressed metabolism, but if the rate falls below 12 per minute or if the physician entertains serious doubts as to the adequacy of ventilation, artificial respiration is indicated. Ideally, arterial blood gases should be measured in deeply comatose patients and artificial respiration initiated if the arterial Pco_2 climbs above 45 mm of mercury. High concentration (>30 per cent) oxygen therapy should be avoided for patients not receiving artificial respiration, for its use increases the risk of hypoventilation and CO_2 retention.

Circulation. Severe shock is rare with depressant drug poisoning unless the patient has been asphyxiated. However, moderate hypotension is common and significantly reduces glomerular filtration and renal clearance of the barbiturates. Fluids should be given liberally to restore blood volume and promote urine flow, and pressor agents, such as metaraminol or levarterenol, are indicated to keep the diastolic blood pressure above 60 mm of mercury and the systolic above 90 mm of mercury. Digitalis or similar compounds are useful only in patients with heart disease. Corticosteroids are unnecessary.

Prevention of Complications. As long as he remains unconscious, the patient should be kept semiprone in the drainage position and changed from side to side in the semiprone position, but never placed on his back. Since the duration of unconsciousness is to be measured in days, the emergence of drug-resistant bacteria is of less concern than is pneumonia caused by already aspirated material. Thus it is useful to administer penicillin or tetracycline.

The blood pressure, pulse, and respiration should be recorded each half hour, and any abnormalities should be met appropriately. Body temperature elevations imply an infection if stimulants have not been given. Hypothermia above 32° C requires no special treatment. To evaluate the rate of urine flow, most physicians prefer to insert an indwelling catheter.

Other Measures. Gastric lavage is desirable for any patient who has ingested depressant drugs within the preceding few hours. The procedure carries the risk of producing pulmonary aspiration, and is best preceded by tracheal intubation with a cuffed tube in deeply comatose subjects. Subjects too lightly anesthetized to tolerate intubation should be turned prone before being lavaged. Care is required to avoid misplacing the tube and irrigating the lungs.

Forced diuresis and alkalinization of the urine have been recommended as adjuncts in treating barbiturate poisoning. Forced diuresis increases the renal clearance of both short- and long-acting barbiturates, and the quantity cleared increases proportionately to the volume of urine. Phenobarbital has a relatively high pK value, and raising the urine pH appears to increase its dissociation and excretion. Several programs have been employed to achieve diuresis. The first step is to assure an adequate blood pressure; the second, to infuse a hypotonic electrolyte solution. The infusions are given at hourly rates up to 600 ml, depending upon urine flow. Close attention must be given to hour-by-hour fluid balance and 12-hour electrolyte balance. If urine flow does not match the infusion rate by the second or third hour, infusions should be slowed and more attention given to raising the blood pressure. Chemical and osmotic diuretics are contraindicated. Hypokalemia is a greater risk than hyperkalemia.

For treating bromide intoxication, diuresis should be combined with a high intake of sodium chloride to displace bromide from blood and tissues.

Hemodialysis is not necessary to treat poisoning with the short-acting hypnotics. However, hemodialysis is indicated for patients who have ingested large amounts of long-acting barbiturates such as barbital or phenobarbital as well as for patients who have severe bromide poisoning. In these instances, dialysis can shorten into a day or less a period of coma or stupor that otherwise would last a week or more.

Analeptics and pharmacologic stimulants are contraindicated for coma caused by depressant drug poisoning. Most carry the risk of overstimulating or producing convulsions in lightly poisoned patients.

Recovery and Prognosis. Patients recovering from coma require close medical supervision. Severe pneumonitis can develop as late as three to four days after recovery. If antimicrobial drugs were started during coma, they are best continued for at least 48 hours thereafter. Permanent physical sequelae to coma are extremely rare. Among 356 cases, residual brain injury was observed only once (in a patient who suffered an acute cardiac arrest). Peripheral nerve injuries from pressure developed in 6 subjects, and 14 subjects had pressure skin lesions leaving scars. There were no other residua.

Later management varies according to the patient's underlying psychiatric disorder and his attitudes upon recovery. Serious suicide attempts are never accidents, and reports of near-fatal ingestion caused by misunderstanding the dose or forgetting previous doses carry little validity. The expert opinion of a psychiatrist should be sought before deciding whether to release a patient or to institutionalize him. The immediate prognosis is good, but long-term results are less encouraging, and there is a high incidence of recurrent attempts at self-destruction over the years.

Driesbach, R. H.: Handbook of Poisoning. Diagnosis and Treatment. Los Angeles, Lange Medical Publications, 1971.

Physicians' Desk Reference to Pharmaceutical Specialties and Biologicals. Published annually by Medical Economics Co., Oradell, N.J.

Section Eight. PROMINENT NEUROLOGIC SYMPTOMS AND THEIR MANAGEMENT

349. PAIN

Jerome B. Posner

INTRODUCTION

Pain is the symptom for which most patients seek medical assistance. Since only the sufferer and not the observer perceives pain, it can have no precise definition. Sir Thomas Lewis described the situation exactly when he said that pain is "known to us by experience and described by illustration." Webster defines pain as the "sensation one feels when hurt mentally or physically; especially distress, suffering great anxiety, anguish, grief, etc., as opposed to pleasure—or, a sensation of hurting or strong discomfort in some part of the body caused by an injury, disease, or functional disorder and transmitted through the nervous system." Webster's definition suggests that there are two aspects to the perception of pain: the first is an emotionally neutral perception of a stimulus which is usually sufficiently strong to produce tissue damage; the second is an affective response to the perception of that stimulus. Pain implies damage to the organism, either physical or psychologic, and chronic pain, if untreated, will itself damage the organism. It is the physician's twofold therapeutic task to discover and treat the *cause* of pain and also to treat the pain itself, whether or not the underlying cause is treatable. To meet this task, the physician must know something of the anatomy and physiology of pain pathways.

ANATOMY AND PHYSIOLOGY OF PAIN

Three theories have been advanced to explain the physiology of pain. The first, the Doctrine of Specific Nerve Energies, by Müller in 1838, envisioned a specific system of receptors and fibers which respond to pain and to pain only, and are different from other receptors and fibers which respond to other specific sensory modalities. A second theory, the Pattern Theory, by Naff in 1927, suggested that any given fiber and pathway could subserve any modality and that perception of pain depends on the temporal and spatial pattern of the impulses which the stimulus produced. A third concept, the Duplex Theory, by Henry Head in 1920, suggested two interacting sensory systems, one composed of slowly conducting small fibers which subserve pain and the extremes of temperature, and another of large, more rapidly conducting fibers which subserve light touch, localization, and temperature discrimination. Head called these two systems protopathic and epicritic. Clinical and experimental evidence has been presented to support and to refute all three theories, and it is likely that some combination of the three explains the physiology of pain. Whatever the correct hypothesis, certain underlying anatomic and physiologic concepts seem incontrovertible. It is generally accepted that so-called "free" nerve endings are the primary receptors for the pain stimulus. Pain receptors are either nociceptors stimulated by tissue injury or chemoreceptors stimulated by chemical substances. There may be several classes of both types of pain receptors. Several chemicals produce pain when appropriately presented to nerve endings. These include acetylcholine, 5-hydroxytryptophan, hypertonic solutions, strong acids or bases, histamine, and potassium ions. Plasma kinins (e.g., bradykinin and kallidin) are potent producers of pain when injected intradermally or applied to the base of a blister. In the clinical situation, pain probably results when tissue injury, not necessarily structural, releases a substance (probably a proteolytic enzyme) which breaks down cellular proteins into pain-producing polypeptides such as kinins, which in turn stimulate pain receptors.

In the peripheral nerves, the stimulus that leads to pain is carried by two types of small fibers. Fast pain, a sensation of short latency and short duration, usually perceived as pricking or sharp, is mediated by delta fibers (the smallest myelinated fibers) which are 1 to 6 μ in diameter. Slow pain, with a longer latency and duration, is perceived as a poorly localized, burning, exceedingly unpleasant sensation and is mediated by small unmyelinated C fibers which are 0.4 to 1.2 μ in diameter. Both sets of fibers have their cell bodies in the dorsal root ganglia and enter the spinal cord through the dorsal roots into Lissauer's tract. They synapse in the substantia gelatinosa or in the posterior horn of the spinal cord. After synapsing, the delta fibers pass through the anterior white commissure to reach the lateral spinothalamic (neospinothalamic) tract contralaterally and ascend to the thalamus. Postsynaptic C fibers also cross the spinal cord in the anterior white commissure to reach the anterior spinothalamic (paleospinothalamic) tract. These neurons also ascend to the thalamus, but along the way give rise to a large number of collaterals to the reticular formation of the brainstem and hypothalamus. The neospinothalamic tract terminates in the ventrobasal complex of the thalamus, and the paleospinothalamic tract in the intralaminar and perifascicular nuclei of the thalamus. The ventrobasal thalamus also receives fibers from the dorsal column–medial lemniscal system (subserving the modalities of touch, position, and vibratory sensation) and projects to two areas of the cerebral cortex: somatosensory area 1 (which in man is part of the sensorimotor cortex surrounding the Rolandic fissure), and somatosensory area 2 in the parietal operculum. The thalamic intralaminar and parafascicular nuclei (paleospinothalamic tract) project diffusely to the cortex and are considered to be part of the reticular activating system of the brainstem. These anatomic facts, combined with clinical and physiologic observations, have led to the hypothesis that the discretely localized neospinothalamic tract carries rather neutral information about pain localization and intensity, whereas the more diffusely projecting paleospinothalamic tract is responsible for the affective component of pain.

The fast conducting dorsal column–medial lemniscal pathway and the slower conducting spinothalamic pathway interact at several levels of the neuraxis, and it is this interaction which has led to the "gate control theory of pain." According to this speculation, sensory fibers have two functions: to carry patterned information, depending on the specialized properties of each unit, and to modulate the effectiveness of synaptic transmission between peripheral nerve and ascending spinal fibers. The first site of the putative modulating action is in the substantia gelatinosa of the spinal cord where large fibers are presumed to activate an inhibitory system and small fibers stimulate an activating system. If large fiber stimulation is sufficient, synaptic transmission is inhibited, and small pain fiber activity which arrives later is less effective in exciting ascending spinal pathways. If the large fiber stimulus is insufficient or absent, small fibers excite the action system and carry pain messages to higher centers. This hypothesis lacks proof, and some recent contrary evidence has been presented. Similar "gates" in the brainstem reticular formation and in the thalamus which add to the modulation of incoming pain impulses have been proposed to circumvent the objections.

Much of the evidence supporting the aforementioned anatomic concepts has come from clinical and experimental studies in man: There are no known primary diseases of the pain receptors, but pain can be produced either by stimuli which damage tissues (e.g., heat greater than 45° C) or intradermal, intra-arterial, or iontophoretic application of the several chemical substances noted above. In man, the same C fiber ending responds to light needle pressure, pinching, radiant heat, and histamine application. Low concentrations of procaine injected into the peripheral nerve selectively anesthetize small fibers; pain is abolished when light touch, position, and vibration sense—modalities conducted by larger fibers—remain intact. Conversely, ischemia produced by a blood pressure cuff over the nerve blocks conduction in larger fibers so that pain remains after the perception of other modalities is abolished; bright, pricking, or fast pain disappears before the slower, burning, unlocalized pain. Peripheral neuropathies (e.g., diabetic neuropathy, postherpetic neuralgia) which selectively involve large, myelinated fibers often lead to a chronic, burning, spontaneous pain exacerbated by touching the denervated area.

The pathogenesis of pain produced by nerve compression is less well understood. Both herniated intervertebral discs and tumors which compress nerves or nerve roots can produce chronic and severe pain, but when normal nerve roots are compressed or manipulated at surgery, pain is not experienced. It is likely that the compressive lesions cause edema and inflammation which make the nerve susceptible to pain. Evidence adduced at surgical operation suggests that nerve roots which had previously been compressed are painful when manipulated, whereas those not previously compressed are not. Central nervous system lesions are sometimes the cause of chronic pain; direct electrical stimulation of the anterolateral columns in man has shown that approximately 50 per cent of the fibers carry nociceptive information, whereas the remainder are divided between warmth and cold. Although lesions made in these tracts usually relieve chronic pain, stimulation or occasionally even lesions of this area produce chronic, burning, dysesthetic sensations. Spontaneous lesions of the spinothalamic pathways in the spinal cord or midbrain generally produce loss of pain and temperature sensation but occasionally are associated with pain. In the thalamus, a lesion of the ventral-basal complex characteristically produces sensory loss, followed in four to six weeks by a spontaneous burning sensation in that part of the body subserved by the damaged area of the thalamus (thalamic syndrome). Lesions rostral to the thalamus are rarely responsible for the production of pain.

DIAGNOSIS OF PAINFUL DISORDERS

A thorough history, general physical examination, and careful neurologic examination are imperative in any patient complaining of pain. Often the description of the nature and distribution of the pain is so characteristic (e.g., trigeminal neuralgia or tabetic lightning pains) (see below) that it allows no other diagnosis. At times the history is so vague and bizarre and the distribution of pain so unanatomic as to suggest that the pain is a somatic delusion and not due to structural or even physiologic abnormality. Inquiry should be made concerning (1) the temporal pattern of pain, (2) its distribution, (3) exacerbating factors, and (4) relieving factors.

For example, headache beginning early in the morning before arising suggests increased intracranial pressure, whereas headache occurring late in the day is more suggestive of tension. Back pain and sciatica made worse by sitting or walking suggest disc disease, whereas back pain and sciatica which are worse while in bed suggest intraspinal tumor. Pain limited to a specific area is usually due to organ disease, whereas pain distributed in the distribution of a peripheral nerve or nerve root suggests that the nerve itself is diseased. Back pain and sciatica exacerbated by cough or sneeze suggest intraspinal disease, whereas similar pain not exacerbated by cough or sneeze suggests disease in the pelvis. Pain in the back or legs exacerbated by straight leg raising suggests disease of the nervous system, whereas a similar pain exacerbated by rotating the hips suggests pelvic or hip disease. Most pain caused by structural disease is relieved at least to some degree by analgesic drugs, whereas psychogenic pain often is not. Skeletal muscle relaxants or local heat may relieve pain of musculoskeletal origin. Both psychogenic and organic pain are relieved to some extent by distraction and a pleasurable environment. Both are exacerbated by anxiety or stress.

A careful general physical examination must be performed. Both the physical and laboratory examination should begin with the assumption that the site of pathologic change is at the site of pain. The painful areas should be examined for swelling and redness as well as for any obvious deformity. (The pain of herpes zoster usually precedes the rash, and occasionally on examination one may note only the faintest reddening of the skin in a dermatomal distribution.) The areas reported as painful should be palpated, the temperature estimated, and points of tenderness sought. (If the site of pain is in a soft tissue, bone, or joint, it should be tender to palpation as well as spontaneously painful.) Joints should be taken through a full range of motion and the effect of movement on the pain assessed. Nerve trunks going to the extremities should be palpated and stretched by movement of that extremity (e.g., straight leg raising, abduction, and extension of the arm). Inflamed and compressed nerve roots and nerve plexuses are more painful when stretched. A careful neurologic examination must also be performed. If there are neurologic abnormalities (e.g., weakness, sensory loss, reflex changes) in the painful part, one can infer that nervous system disease is responsible for the pain. The absence of specific neurologic abnormalities on first examination does not guarantee, however, that the nervous system is free of disease, because the process may simply not have advanced beyond the stage of selectively involving pain pathways.

Finally, laboratory examinations are performed. If the site of disease appears to be in bones or joints, x-rays of those structures or radioisotope scans may localize it. First attention should be paid to the local site of pain, but the physician should acquaint himself with the common referred patterns of pain (e.g., hip disease commonly causes knee pain, cardiac pain is frequently referred to the ulnar aspect of the arm and forearm, the pain of renal colic may be felt primarily in the groin and testicle, and pain resulting from disease of the throat may be referred to the ear).

Referred pain is pain perceived at a site remote from the source of the disturbance. Usually, referred pain is cutaneous and evoked by disease of deep structures innervated by the same dermatome. Referred pain may be associated with cutaneous hyperalgesia and even relieved by procaine injection into the area of referral. When pain is referred to the same dermatome or myotome as innervates the diseased structure (e.g., pain down the medial aspect of the arm [T1-T2] produced by myocardial infarction or angina pectoris), it is often helpful in diagnosis. However, pain is sometimes referred at a great distance from the primary site to segments not similarly innervated, and there the mechanism is perplexing (e.g., anginal pain referred to the jaw). Various theories have been suggested to account for referred pain. Such theories as division of the same nerve into deep and superficial branches, release of chemical mediators in the nervous system, and convergence of cutaneous and visceral nerves into common synaptic pools at the spinal cord all explain the dermatomal referral of pain but fail to explain pain at remote sites. Knowledge of common sites of referred pain often helps in establishing diagnosis of diseased internal organs.

MANAGEMENT OF CHRONIC PAIN

In some patients, pain is best managed by treating the underlying disorder (e.g., steroids for giant cell arteritis relieve headache and muscle pain promptly; radiation therapy for bone pain caused by cancer is often helpful). In others, a particular kind of pain has a particular treatment (see Specific Pain Syndromes, below), but in many patients the pain is chronic and the physician is able neither to treat the underlying disturbances nor to offer specific therapy for that type of pain. In treating this type of chronic and severe pain, certain general principles should be followed:

1. The pain should be treated by the simplest means which will relieve it, but all efforts should be made to relieve it. Chronic pain is both physically debilitating and psychologically demoralizing. It should be treated by the physician as a serious symptom and all efforts made to relieve it to the extent that the patient is comfortable.
2. Pain should be treated early. There is both clinical and experimental evidence that if chronic pain goes untreated for an extended period of time, abnormal self-excitatory states arise in the central nervous system so that treatment directed toward peripheral structures which initially would have relieved the pain are no longer effective. In general, the earlier one undertakes to treat chronic pain, the more successful one is.
3. Pain should be treated promptly. Clinical evidence suggests that if analgesic drug doses are spaced so far apart that severe pain recurs, the analgesic becomes less effective. Thus patients should be encouraged to take analgesic agents when the pain first reappears rather than wait until it becomes unbearable.
4. Various treatments of pain are additive and should be used together rather than separately.

5. Narcotic drugs should be used sparingly but should not be withheld if there is no alternative effective therapy. Experiments in laboratory animals indicate that enough narcotic given long enough produces physical dependence in every individual. However, the percentage of patients who become addicted to narcotics given for pain is unclear. Many physicians are impressed that narcotic addiction is unusual in patients treated for pain if the pain is later relieved by other means. If a patient has severe pain caused by organic disease and does not respond to non-narcotic drugs or to treatment directed at the underlying disease, narcotics should be used to the degree necessary to relieve pain. In patients with terminal cancer, one need not worry about addicting the patient, and in patients with more chronic disease, judicious use of narcotics, although running the risk of addiction, may restore a debilitated and bedridden individual into a comfortable, working, and useful citizen. Methadone maintenance programs have proved that patients can take narcotics in large doses over long times and continue to function usefully in society.

6. Psychogenic factors always play a role in chronic pain—the pain is more severe when the patient is anxious and stressed and less severe when he is relaxed. The physician must assess the psychologic factors in any patient with pain. If these factors are overwhelming, the chemical and physical methods described below are not likely to be very useful and psychotherapy should be undertaken. However, no patient should be diagnosed as having psychogenic pain until an exhaustive examination has ruled out structural disease.

7. Placebo effects are important. In most clinical studies, about one third of patients report relief of pain when given a placebo, although the extent of relief is rarely equal to that achieved by analgesic drugs. The physician can utilize a patient's desire to be free of pain by approaching the therapy in an enthusiastic and reassuring manner. It is less important whether it is the placebo or the drug which was effective than that the patient be relieved of his pain.

8. Multidisciplinary pain clinics which diagnose and treat intractable pain exist in many centers and should be utilized for severe problems.

Analgesic Agents

Analgesics (or analgetics) are drugs which decrease pain without causing loss of consciousness. Analgesics (Table 1) can be divided for clinical purposes into those which are suitable for mild pain, generally non-narcotic agents; those suitable for moderate pain, usually narcotics or narcotic antagonists with low addiction potential; and those which are suitable for severe pain, generally narcotic agents except for methotrimeprazine. The mild analgesics appear to act peripherally by blocking the pain chemoreceptors and perhaps by relieving inflammation. There is also evidence for a central effect of some of these drugs as well. Aspirin has been shown to be a potent inhibitor of prostaglandin formation, and this may be its mechanism of action peripherally.

The physician's strategy in treating chronic pain should begin with the mildest agents possible and add stronger agents or analgesic adjuvants only when mild agents fail to work. Drugs should always be given in sufficient amounts and at sufficiently short intervals to achieve relief of pain. Treatment should begin with aspirin or acetaminophen, 600 mg every three to four hours. If the pain is due to musculoskeletal spasm or if anxiety is prominent, one of the mild tranquilizers (diazepam or meprobamate) can be added. If the pain fails to respond to this mild regimen, one adds drugs used for the treatment of moderate pain (e.g., codeine or pentazocine). If the pain is still unrelieved and the physician satisfies himself that psychogenic factors are not responsible, the agents used for moderate pain should be discontinued, and agents used for severe pain should be added to the mild analgesic. Levorphanol, 2 mg, or methadone, 10 mg, every three to four hours is probably the agent of choice if oral drugs are to be used, and morphine, 10 mg every three to four hours, if a subcutaneous or intramuscular agent is necessary. Other narcotic drugs may be substituted for these, and often several must be tried to find that which relieves the patient's pain but causes fewest side effects. If the pain continues as a chronic and unremitting problem not relieved by these drugs, or if anxiety and depression appear to be a major contributor to the pain, a major tranquilizer (phenothiazine) or antidepressant agent, or both, may be added to the mild analgesics and narcotic agents. At times a satisfactory resolution of an intractable problem may be achieved by the combined use of a narcotic and non-narcotic analgesic and a tranquilizer or an antidepressant. The physician must be careful to adjust the doses of each so as to produce maximal pain relief with minimal sedation and unpleasant side effects. The physician should be prepared to increase the dose of those particular drugs to which tolerance develops as is necessary to control pain. No tolerance develops to non-narcotic analgesics. The more potent analgesics, including codeine but excepting the phenothiazines, are potentially addicting drugs to which tolerance develops and thus no fixed dose can be defined. These drugs act centrally, probably at synapses.

Non-narcotic Mild Analgesics. Aspirin and acetaminophen (Tylenol, Tempra) are the most useful of the mild analgesics. Either aspirin or acetaminophen may be given in doses of 600 mg every three to four hours, either alone for relief of mild pain or in conjunction with more potent drugs for relief of severe pain. The degree of pain relief is linearly related to the logarithm of the dose of the drug, higher doses being not significantly more effective until doses are reached which produce unpleasant side effects. The side effects of aspirin (clotting disorders, dyspepsia, and gastrointestinal bleeding) make acetaminophen, which has almost no such side effects, a safer drug and probably the drug of choice. There is no evidence that aspirin and acetaminophen together are more effective than either one alone, but either aspirin or acetaminophen plus codeine is more effective than codeine alone. There is no evidence that the other mild, non-narcotic analgesics are superior in any way to the two most commonly used drugs.

Narcotic Analgesics. All these drugs are potentially addicting, and tolerance develops to all. Thus there is no set dose of the drug, and with long, continued usage the dose must increase. *The physician is wise to learn to handle two or three of these drugs and use those consistently rather than using all the drugs occasionally.* He must be prepared to use more than one, because some patients find that side effects of the drugs make one preferable to another. Morphine, 10 mg intramuscularly, is the standard by which other narcotic analgesics are judged.

TABLE 1. Analgesic Agents

Type	Generic Name (Proprietary)	Usual Dose* Oral (mg)	Usual Dose* Subcutaneous or Intramuscular	Comment
Some agents used for mild to moderate pain	Aspirin	600 q 3–4 h		Side effects of dyspepsia and GI bleeding
	Acetaminophen (Tylenol)	650 q 3–4 h		Equal to aspirin but without GI side effects; less anti-inflammatory effect
	Phenacetin (aceto-phenetidin)	600 q 3–4 h		Probable renal toxicity with chronic use
	Dextropropoxyphene (Darvon)	65 q 3–4 h		Weak narcotic related to methadone, probably not superior to aspirin
	Phenylbutazone (Butazolidin)	100 qid		Anti-inflammatory agents, probably useful only for pain associated with inflammation (e.g., arthritis) – may cause agranulocytosis
	Indomethicin (Indocin)	25 qid		Useful only for pain associated with inflammation, probably not superior to aspirin
Some agents used for moderate to severe pain	Codeine	30–60 q 4–6 h	120 q 4–6 h	Narcotic with low addiction potential; additive effect if used with mild analgesics
	Oxycodone (with aspirin, phenacetin and caffeine = Percodan)	5 q 4–6 h		No advantages over codeine
	Pentazocine (Talwin)	30–50 q 4–6 h	60 q 4 h	Narcotic antagonist (produces withdrawal in patients physically dependent on narcotics); low addiction potential; hallucinations and dysphoria in doses >80 mg IM or 200 mg po
Some agents used for severe pain: narcotics and antagonists	Levorphanol (Levo-Dromoran)	2 q 3–4 h	2 q 3–4 h	Superior to morphine for postoperative patients in some studies
	Morphine		10 q 3–4 h	The standard narcotic agent for treatment of pain
	Meperidine (Demerol)	50–100 q 3–4 h	75–100 q 2–4 h	More rapid onset and shorter duration of action than morphine; possibly less spasmogenic and better for pain of biliary tree
	Methadone (Dolophine)	10–20 q 4 h	10–15 q 3–4 h	Possibly less sedative effect than morphine
	Fentanyl (Sublimaze)		0.1–0.2	Rapid onset, short duration, used in anesthesia
Non-narcotic	Methotrimeprazine (Levoprome)		20 q 4–6 h	Phenothiazine; no addiction; produces sedation and postural hypotension
Some agents used as analgesic adjuvants (probably little or no analgesic properties per se but used to relieve anxiety and/or depression)	Minor tranquilizers – muscle relaxants:			
	Diazepam (Valium)		5 qid	Useful with mild analgesics for acute or subacute pain associated with muscle spasm and/or anxiety
	Meprobamate (Miltown)		200–400 qid	
	Antidepressants:			
	Amitriptyline (Elavil)		75–100 hs	Reported useful in pain associated with depressive symptoms (esp. atypical facial pain); may be useful when combined with analgesic agents for chronic pain of many kinds; may cause oversedation or anticholinergic symptoms
	Phenelzine (Nardil)		15 tid	
	Imipramine (Tofranil)		25 qid	
	Phenothiazines:			
	Chlorpromazine (Thorazine)		25–50 qid	Reported useful in pain associated with anxiety or depression and in some specific pain syndromes (e.g., thalamic pain, postherpetic pain); these drugs may have analgesic properties or potentiate analgesics; fluphenazine and amitriptyline have been reported to relieve postherpetic pain; may cause oversedation, depression, Parkinson-like syndrome, hypotension, or urinary retention
	Promazine (Sparine)		50–100 qid	
	Promethazine (Phenergan)		25–50 hs	
	Fluphenazine (Prolixin)		1–3 qd	

*Intramuscular dose of narcotics is equivalent to 10 mg of morphine. Since tolerance develops to these drugs, doses must be increased with continued use. Oral doses are not equivalent to intramuscular doses but represent usual starting doses.

Intramuscular morphine has its maximal effect in 60 to 90 minutes and lasts somewhere between three and six hours. It requires 60 mg or more of morphine orally to give the same analgesic effect as 10 mg intramuscularly. Levorphanol has a relatively high oral/parenteral ratio for analgesia; 2 mg given intramuscularly is equal to 10 mg of morphine intrasmuscularly, and 4 mg given orally is equal in total effect to 10 mg of morphine given intramuscularly. Methadone also has a relatively high oral/intramuscular potency ratio; 10 mg intramuscularly or 20 mg orally equals 10 mg of morphine intramuscularly. Codeine and dihydrocodeine are also effective orally and are generally used in doses of 50 to 60 mg as a mild analgesic. They often cannot be used to relieve severe pain, because side effects preclude high doses, but by the same token they are rarely addicting. Pentazocine can be used as a mild analgesic when given in doses of 30 mg and is equal to morphine if given in intramuscular doses of 60 mg. It is a weak narcotic antagonist with a high analgesic potential and has a dependence potential substantially less than that of morphine or meperidine (Demerol). Pentazocine is not included in the Federal Controlled Substances Act. However, hallucinatory effects and toxic psychoses have been noted in its users, and like the other narcotics it can produce respiratory depression. Dextropropoxyphene (Darvon) is structurally related to methadone and is a prescription drug not subject to the Controlled Substances Act of 1970. It is a weak narcotic with low addiction liability and a low analgesic potential.

Other Agents. The phenothiazine methotrimeprazine (Levoprome) is a potent analgesic agent. Given intramuscularly in doses of 15 to 20 mg, it is equivalent to 10 mg of morphine intramuscularly. The drug is not addicting, is an effective antiemetic, and does not suppress cough or respiration but does produce sedation and postural hypotension, making it useful only for hospitalized patients.

Sedative and anticonvulsant drugs as well as other phenothiazines have been utilized by some physicians in the treatment of chronic pain, particularly that associated with depression or other psychologic symptoms. The antidepressant amitriptyline (Elavil), given orally in a single dose of 75 mg at night (when it helps counter insomnia) or orally in divided doses of 25 mg three to four times a day, has been effective in relieving some chronic pain or in decreasing the narcotic dose required. In conjunction with the phenothiazine, fluphenazine, the drug has been reported useful in the treatment of postherpetic neuralgia (see below).

Physical Methods of Pain Relief

There are a bewildering array of physical methods designed to relieve pain (Table 2). These vary from simply rubbing a partially denervated area with a soft towel to placing radiofrequency lesions stereotactically in the thalamic and hypothalamic reticular formations. The simpler procedures can be carried out by the general physician or even by the patient; the more complicated ones, depending on their nature, demand the services of a skilled anesthesiologist or neurosurgeon.

The physician's approach to the use of physical methods for intractable pain should embody certain general principles:

1. Nondestructive procedures should be tried first. Cutaneous stimulation, either by hand or by battery-driven electrodes, or local anesthetic blocks in conjunction with analgesic drugs may be effective in relieving pain. If these simple procedures fail, the services of an anesthesiologist or neurosurgeon should be procured and a treatment plan embodying the use of analgesics and physical procedures outlined.

2. The least destructive procedure which will relieve pain should be tried first. In general, the procedure should be directed first at the peripheral nervous system, and, only if this fails, at the spinal cord, brainstem, or cerebrum. Quantitative data on the incidence of pain relief and its duration are sketchy for most of these procedures and seem to vary from center to center, depending on the skill and enthusiasm of the investigator reporting.

3. Thus the choice of a particular procedure often depends not only on the nature of the patient's disease but on the particular skills, experience, and bias of the physician.

4. If and only if a full trial of analgesic drugs has failed should destructive procedures for relieving pain be tried. These destructive procedures can and should be used in conjunction with analgesic drugs, because, even if the drugs have failed to relieve pain on their own, they may act synergistically with physical methods. Nerve blocks and surgical procedures often yield only temporary relief in patients with chronic pain. Thus many of the enthusiastic reports in the literature refer to patients followed for only a short period of time. When the patients are followed over months or years, the pain which was relieved shortly after the procedure often returns and is as bad as or worse than it was prior to the operation. For this reason, patients with cancer who are not expected to live a long time are often better candidates for surgical destructive procedures than are patients with pain originating from more benign conditions.

5. Patients with chronic pain being considered for destructive procedures must be thoroughly evaluated psychiatrically. If psychogenic factors play a major role in the genesis of pain, surgical procedures will not help, and often the pain will be exacerbated after surgical intervention.

Cutaneous Stimulation. Cutaneous stimulation of a painful area, particularly one which has been partly denervated, is often effective in relieving pain. This procedure, which probably has its greatest use in the treatment of postherpetic neuralgia, consists of rubbing the painful area with a soft cloth or terrycloth towel, almost constantly while awake at first but then with gradually lengthening intervals of rest between rubbing periods. Often a period of rubbing will yield relief which long outlasts the stimulus, and continued intermittent rubbings may totally relieve the pain. The "gate theory" offers an explanation of the rubbing phenomenon, i.e., rubbing stimulates large fiber afferents which may close the gate against incoming pain fibers. Whatever the explanation, the procedure is often useful in the treatment of painful phantom limbs and in chronic cutaneous or extremity pain after surgery. Recently, battery-powered electrical stimulators which give one control over the frequency and intensity of the cutaneous stimulation have become available. The electrodes of the stimulator may be placed over the painful area or over the peripheral nerve supplying the painful area, and stimulation using an intensity and frequency which produces a vibratory sensation is applied.

Acupuncture Analgesia. Acupuncture analgesia has become increasingly popular in the past few years, but no carefully controlled studies have reported on its usefulness. A needle is placed under the skin, often in a place remote from the painful site but at times into the painful site, and the area is stimulated either by twirling the needle or by electrically vibrating it. Several investigators have proposed a "multigate" theory as an explanation for the purported effectiveness of acupuncture, but its mechanism and usefulness in Western medicine for analgesia are still not clear.

Nerve Blocks. Direct block of peripheral nerves, using either anesthetic agents (lidocaine) or neurolytic agents (4 per cent phenol), has been popular in the treatment of thoracic and abdominal pain, particularly that pain which follows surgery. Blocks may be dangerous if used in the extremities, because they may paralyze as well as anesthetize, but in areas where they can be used relief of pain sometimes long outlasts the period of anesthesia. The procedure is a simple one when performed by a skilled anesthesiologist.

Subarachnoid injection of anesthetics or neurolytics directed at nerve roots has been utilized in patients with widespread and intractable pain. Barbotage of nerve roots via lumbar puncture, using either cerebrospinal

TABLE 2. Physical Methods of Pain Relief

I. Directed at end-organs or receptors	
A. Local anesthesia	
Ethyl chloride spray	Often useful for pain due to acute muscle spasm or musculoskeletal tension
Lidocaine injection of painful area	
B. Local stimulation	
Rubbing painful area (with soft towel)	Local stimulation often relieves pain due to partial denervation (e.g., postherpetic neuralgia, postamputation pain, post-thoracotomy pain, causalgia)
Cutaneous electrical or mechanical stimulation (vibrator or battery-powered electrode)	
Acupuncture?	
C. Local destruction	
Surgical undercutting of skin	Rarely successful for intractable postherpetic pain
II. Directed at peripheral nerves and roots	
A. Pharmacologic blockade	
Anesthetic block to nerves, plexus, roots	Repeated anesthetic block to nerves which do not have major motor function may relieve pain for prolonged periods; block should always be tried before surgery is considered; subarachnoid drugs or barbotage often give temporary relief of pain, but motor or autonomic dysfunction may complicate the procedure
Subarachnoid block of sensory roots	
Anesthetics	
Neurolytic drugs (phenol, alcohol)	
Mechanical blocks (CSF barbotage)	
Sympathetic block	For causalgia-like syndromes
B. Peripheral nerve stimulation	Electrical stimulator placed cutaneously over peripheral nerves is reported to successfully relieve some intractable pain
C. Surgical procedures	
Peripheral nerve section	Most useful for thoracic and lumbar pain; good initial results, but long-term results poor; trigeminal rhizotomy effective for tic douloureaux
Dorsal rhizotomy	
Dorsal root ganglionectomy	
Sympathectomy	For causalgia
III. Directed at spinal cord and brainstem	
A. Destructive procedures	
Spinothalamic tractotomy (percutaneous or open)	Most reliable surgical method for pain relief, best for thoracic or lower pain
Myelotomy	For intractable facial pain, high incidence of paralytic complications
Trigeminal tractotomy	
Mesencephalic tractotomy	Lesions in spinothalamic tract above cord for head and neck pain
B. Stimulators	
Dorsal column stimulator	Electrodes placed surgically in dorsal columns and stimulated through the skin reported successful in several kinds of severe pain
IV. Directed at the diencephalon	
A. Destructive lesions (stereotaxic surgery)	
Ventral-basal complex	Not effective for chronic pain; lesions may produce "thalamic" pain
Centre-médian	Appears effective for pain due to malignancy but not phantom pain; probably best for head and neck tumors
Pulvinar	Often a delay of two to three weeks before pain is relieved
Hypothalamus	Only sketchy data available on usefulness or complications
V. Directed at cerebral hemisphere	
A. Destructive lesions	
Cingulomotomy	Designed to relieve "suffering"; only rarely effective; better results if combined with thalamic lesions
Sensorimotor cortex gyrectomy	Occasional relief of phantom pain or facial pain reported
Hippocampus	Not fully evaluated; bilateral lesions required; marked personality change
Frontal lobotomy	Rarely used because of behavioral changes
B. Other	
Hypnotism	All designed to relieve anxiety about pain and perhaps to promote cortical inhibition of pain pathways
Acupuncture?	
Psychotherapy	
Psychotropic drugs	

fluid, hypertonic saline, or iced saline, appears to destroy enough nerve fibers to relieve chronic pain in the lower extremities, at least for a time. The procedure is sufficiently painful that it must be done under anesthesia. Bladder and bowel dysfunction are occasional complications, and the relief of pain is often transient. Phenol, 4 per cent, can likewise be injected into the subarachnoid space and directed at particular nerve roots by positioning the patient. The mechanism of action is destruction of nerve fibers; if material spills into the cauda equina, bladder and bowel dysfunction are common. The relief of pain is usually longer than that achieved with barbotage but may also be transient.

Each nonsurgical procedure directed at the *peripheral nervous system* has its surgical counterpart. In patients with chronic pain such as that which follows herpes zoster, the skin has been undercut in an attempt to totally denervate it. Postoperative infection is a complication at times and the pain relief is only transient, thus contraindicating this procedure. Peripheral nerves can be cut, particularly in the thorax and abdomen, but this should not be done unless prior nerve blocks have indicated that it will be effective and sustained. The peripheral nerves regenerate after a time, and often the pain returns. Dorsal root ganglia in the thorax and abdomen can be removed for chronic pain or the dorsal roots themselves cut. This procedure also should not be done unless nerve blocks have indicated that it will be effective. Several roots must be cut on either side of the painful area if one is to achieve long-term pain relief.

Surgery of the Central Nervous System. There are three kinds of surgical procedures directed at the central nervous system for the relief of pain. The first, a direct outgrowth of the gate theory, involves the placement of electrodes on the dorsal columns with the power source being led under the skin. The patient then uses a transmitter to deliver a stimulus of known frequency and intensity to the dorsal columns. This increases large fiber input to the spinal cord, causes a mild tingling sensation, and often relieves pain for a prolonged period of time. Enthusiastic reports of this nondestructive surgical procedure have come from several centers, but it has not been performed long enough to fully evaluate its usefulness.

The second kind of procedure involves destruction of pain pathways in the spinal cord, brainstem, or brain. Spinothalamic tracts can be destroyed either surgically, after a laminectomy (open cordotomy), or by the placement of a radiofrequency lesion through a needle (percutaneous cordotomy). These procedures are particularly effective in relieving pain in the lower extremities and have the advantage that, although pain and temperature sensations are lost, cutaneous sensation and motor power remain intact. At times the level of anesthesia approaches within one or two cord segments of the level at which the destructive lesion is placed, but often there is a drop to about five segments below the placement of the lesion. Thus the lesion must be placed considerably higher than the site of pain. If the lesion is placed unilaterally, pain often appears in the other side of the body, necessitating another lesion. Bilateral lesions considerably enhance the risk of motor weakness and bladder and bowel dysfunction, but in skilled hands these risks are low. Occasional patients with bilateral percutaneous lesions in cervical cord suffer loss of automatic respiratory function (Ondine's curse). Percutaneous spinothalamic tract cordotomy, when done by a skilled technician, produces satisfactory pain relief in 70 to 90 per cent of patients, with a small mortality (1 to 5 per cent) and morbidity. The procedure is particularly useful in patients with terminal cancer, because the pain relief is usually sustained until death and the procedure does not require a major operation. An analogous lesion in the low brainstem placed in the descending tract of the trigeminal nerve has been reported useful in relieving facial pain. Pain and temperature sensation are lost, but cutaneous sensation remains intact. Lesions have been placed in the spinothalamic tract of the midbrain, so-called mesencephalic tractotomies. The dangers of this lesion are considerably greater than those of spinal cord lesions, and most centers have abandoned the procedure. Several neurosurgeons have placed lesions in the thalamus, both in the ventral-basal complex and in the interlaminar nuclei. Although good results are occasionally reported for both, the ventral-basal lesions appear only to produce transient relief of pain, whereas those placed in the interlaminar nuclei at the end-point of the paleospinothalamic tract appear to be more successful. There are rare reports of removal of sensory portions of the parietal lobe in relieving chronic pain, but the rarity of the reports implies the ineffectiveness of the treatment.

The third surgical method directed at pain relief is to place lesions in the frontal lobe, particularly the limbic projection to the frontal areas, in an attempt to alter the patient's psychologic response to pain rather than alter the pain pathways themselves. Several different surgical procedures, including frontal lobotomy, frontal leukotomy, and cingulotomy, have been tried with varied success. These procedures, which alter the patient's personality as well as his suffering, probably deserve trial only when all other procedures have failed.

Good statistical data comparing the various surgical procedures for pain are difficult to come by. The best extant data indicate that initial relief of pain occurs with almost all procedures in 50 to 80 per cent of patients, with spinothalamic tract cordotomies yielding the best results. Longer-term follow-up suggests that considerably less than 50 per cent of patients achieve lasting relief, in many series the figure being as low as 20 per cent. Patients with malignant disease seem to have greater pain relief even initially than those with more benign conditions, probably because selection of patients with benign conditions often includes many with psychogenic pain.

SOME SPECIFIC PAIN SYNDROMES

Trigeminal Neuralgia. Trigeminal neuralgia (tic douloureux) is a disease characterized by sudden, lightning-like paroxysms of pain in the distribution of one or more divisions of the trigeminal nerve. The pain is usually unassociated with identifiable structural disease of the nervous system (idiopathic trigeminal neuralgia) but occasionally may be a symptom of a gasserian ganglion tumor, of multiple sclerosis, or of a brainstem infarct involving the descending root of the trigeminal nerve (symptomatic trigeminal neuralgia).

The history is diagnostic. The pain occurs as brief, lightning-like stabs, frequently precipitated by touching a trigger zone around the lips or the buccal cavity. At times, talking, eating, or brushing the teeth serves as a trigger. The pains rarely last longer than seconds, and each burst is followed by a refractory period of several seconds to a minute in which no further pain can be precipitated. The pains, however, often occur in clusters so that the patient first may report each pain as lasting for hours. The pain is limited to the distribution of the trigeminal nerve, usually affecting the second and third division or both, and only occasionally affecting the first division. Spontaneous remissions and exacerbations are common, the exacerbations tending to occur in spring and fall seasons. Between paroxysms of pain, the patient is asymptomatic. Tic pain rarely occurs at night. In idiopathic trigeminal neuralgia, the neurologic examination is entirely normal. In symptomatic trigeminal neuralgia, there may be sensory changes in the distribution of the trigeminal nerve, and such a finding should prompt a careful search for structural disease of the nervous system.

Carbamazepine is the drug of choice for the treatment of trigeminal neuralgia. This anticonvulsant drug is given in doses varying from 400 to 800 mg a day, but because of its sedative properties the initial dose is 100 mg twice daily, gradually increased to the required maintenance dose. No more than 1200 mg should be taken daily. The drug is not an analgesic and is only effective for specific kinds of pain such as trigeminal neuralgia, glossopharyngeal neuralgia, and the lightning pains of tabes dorsalis. Occasional cases of aplastic anemia have been reported, and complete blood counts are procured prior to the initiation of therapy and at frequent intervals thereafter. Other side effects include dizziness and sedation. Diphenylhydantoin in doses of 400 mg a day is also effective in trigeminal neuralgia but less so than carbamazepine. There is no evidence that the two drugs are synergistic. If medical treatment fails, section of the nerve root proximal to the ganglion affords permanent relief. Local anesthesia of the ganglion or the peripheral branches of the nerve at some time prior to surgery is desirable, because some patients find the anesthesia produced by nerve section less tolerable than the pain itself.

Glossopharyngeal Neuralgia. Glossopharyngeal neuralgia is characterized by pain similar to that of trigeminal neuralgia but in the distribution of the glossopharyngeal and vagus nerves. The trigger zone is usually in the tonsil or posterior pharynx, and the pain spreads toward the angle of the jaw and the ear. Occasional patients suffer cardiac slowing or arrest during these attacks as a result of the intense afferent discharge over the glossopharyngeal nerve. Carbamazepine is often effective, but if it fails, glossopharyngeal nerve roots are sectioned in the posterior fossa. Symptomatic glossopharyngeal neuralgia is occasionally the presenting complaint in a patient with a tonsillar tumor, and careful examination of the pharynx and tonsillar fossa for mass lesions must be carried out.

Lightning Pains of Tabes. The lightning pains of tabes are acute, short-lived pains in the trunk or lower extremities which occur with structural lesions of the dorsal roots and particularly with tabes dorsalis. Lightning pains are analogous to trigeminal and glossopharyngeal neuralgia. Like those two disorders, the pain usually responds to carbamazepine. There is no surgical therapy.

"Reflex Sympathetic Dystrophies." This is a term which applies to pain, hyperalgesia, hyperesthesia, and autonomic changes, usually after injury to an extremity. If the injury has involved a peripheral nerve, particularly the sciatic or median nerve, the syndrome is called *causalgia* (hot pain). If the injury has not involved a peripheral nerve, such terms as post-traumatic painful osteoporosis, Sudeck's atrophy, post-traumatic spreading neuralgia, minor causalgia, shoulder-hand syndrome, and reflex dystrophy have been applied, the particular term depending on the outstanding symptom. Whatever the term, the pathophysiology of all these disorders appears to be the same, as do their clinical manifestations and response to therapy.

The disorder may follow either a major or minor injury to an extremity, after which severe pain, usually of a burning quality, develops in the extremity. The pain is continuous but exacerbated by emotional stress and is associated with severe hyperpathia, so that moving or touching the limb is often intolerable. At first the pain is localized to the site of the injury or the distribution of the nerve injured, but with time it spreads, often to involve the entire extremity. Along with the pain there are vasomotor changes, first of vasodilatation (warm and dry skin) but later a change to vasoconstriction (edema, cyanosis, cool skin). Other autonomic disturbances include either hyperhidrosis or hypohidrosis; trophic changes in the skin, subcutaneous tissue, and muscles; and osteoporosis. The entire symptom complex is rarely present in any one patient, and one sign or symptom usually predominates. Untreated, severe reflex sympathetic dystrophy leads to muscle atrophy, fixation of joints, osteoporosis, and a useless extremity. The exact mechanism of the pain and sympathetic changes is not understood. The various hypotheses include a reverberating "central excitatory state," "artificial synapses" between partially demyelinated nerves, and a central biasing of the spinal cord "gate."

Treatment should be undertaken as early as possible, because there is evidence that the earlier the treatment, the more effective it will be. Treatment begins with local anesthetic infiltration of the painful site, using 2 to 5 ml of 0.5 per cent lidocaine, repeated frequently enough to maintain relief of pain. When local measures fail, most patients are relieved by sympathetic block with lidocaine. This procedure often gives permanent relief, but if repeated local anesthetics produce only transient benefit, surgical sympathectomy should be performed.

Postherpetic Neuralgia. Postherpetic neuralgia refers to severe and prolonged burning pain with occasional lightning-like stabs in the involved dermatome after an attack of herpes zoster. Severe postherpetic neuralgia is usually a disease of elderly patients and, like most chronic pain, is exacerbated by emotional upset and relieved to some degree by distraction. Touching the involved area usually exacerbates the pain. Treatment of postherpetic neuralgia is not entirely satisfactory, but the initial treatment should be directed toward stimulating the painful area. Brisk rubbing for many hours a day with a terrycloth towel or stimulation of the dermatome with a cutaneous electrical stimulator often brings relief which long outlasts the stimulus. Initially, when therapy is undertaken, the hyperpathia may be so severe that the patient is unwilling to have the area stimulated. One can then spray the area with a local anesthetic (e.g., ethyl chloride) before stimulation is undertaken. During the first 48 to 72 hours, stimulation should be done as often as possible while the patient is awake and then decreased gradually. Care must be taken to keep the rubbing light so as not to excoriate friable skin. Relief of pain may take several weeks. Analgesic drugs are sometimes beneficial, and psychotropic drugs (amitriptyline, 75 mg daily, and fluphenazine, 1 to 3 mg daily) have been reported to be useful. If the pain does not respond to conservative treatment, surgical therapy may be considered as a last resort, but the results are usually poor. In many patients the disease runs its course, and after a year or two the pain disappears spontaneously. Thus mutilating surgical procedures are probably not indicated.

Phantom Limb Pain. Phantom limb pain is a chronic and severe pain appearing to be localized in an amputated or totally denervated limb. All patients suffer phantom sensations after amputation, but in only about 10 per cent is it painful, usually when there has been severe pain prior to operation. The pain is frequently similar to that suffered before amputation, or at times it may resemble muscle pain with the phantom seeming to be in a cramped or uncomfortable position. In most instances, the pain lessens and disappears with time, but in occasional patients it is a chronic and severe problem. Therapy is difficult. A search should be made for painful neuromas, but these are an uncommon cause of phantom pain, and even if small neuromas are found and removed, the pain is not usually relieved. Surgical procedures directed at the central nervous system are often not helpful. The pain may be triggered by touching the amputation stump, but over the passage of time healthy areas of the body when touched may also trigger pain in the phantom. Phantom pain is sometimes permanently abolished by cutaneous stimulation, either rubbing or electrical stimulation, or by repeated anesthetic blocks of peripheral nerves proximal to the stump. Narcotic analgesics may be helpful; other analgesic agents are usually not helpful. Sympathetic blocks have been reported to relieve pain in some patients for prolonged periods, but sympathectomy rarely produces relief as lasting as with causalgia. The mechanism of phantom pain is unknown.

Myofascial Pain Syndromes. Pain arising from skeletal muscle is common. Unaccustomed exercise causes soreness and tenderness in the involved muscles but is rarely a source of patient complaint. Prolonged tonic contraction of skeletal muscles, however, has an underlying pathogenesis of psychologic tension, resentment, and anxiety, and may produce pain in which the cause is not immediately apparent to the patient. Examples are tension headache arising from chronic contraction of paraspinous muscles at the base of the skull, anterior chest pain from contraction of pectoralis major, posterior thoracic or lumbar pain from paraspinous muscle contraction, and abdominal pain from rectus muscle retraction. The pain is initially localized over the area of muscle contraction but may spread widely into a distribution characteristic for the muscles involved. The muscles are usually tender to palpation, and there is often a particular tender area somewhere in the muscle, called a trigger area, which, when palpated, reproduces the entire distribution of the spontaneous pain. When the pain is acute, it may be treated with rest, local heat, and mild analgesic drugs, along with muscle relaxant drugs such as diazepam or meprobamate. When the pain is chronic or severe, particularly when a trigger area is found, local anesthesia with ethyl chloride spray or local injection of 0.5 per cent lidocaine sometimes affords relief. At times, a single injection breaks the pain–muscle tension–pain cycle and permanent relief is achieved. At other times, repetitive injections with the addition of analgesic agents and muscle relaxants are required.

Bonica, J. J.: Management of Pain. 2nd ed. Philadelphia, Lea & Febiger, 1974.
Bonica, J. J. (ed.): Symposium Issue: Management of pain. Postgrad. Med., 53:56, 1973.
Jannetta, P. J., et al.: The neurosurgical approach to the relief of pain. *In* Current Problems in Surgery. Chicago, Year Book Medical Publishers, 1973.
Payne, J. P., and Burt, R. A. P. (eds.): Pain: Basic Principles–Pharmacology–Therapy. Baltimore, Williams & Wilkins Company, 1972.

350. HEADACHE

Fred Plum

INTRODUCTION

Headache is man's most common pain, and in one form or another it affects some 90 per cent of the population. In any consideration of headache, two major points stand out: one is that *most* headaches come from structures *outside* the skull, and the other is that increased intracranial pressure, as such, does not necessarily cause headache. The following is an outline of the principal types:

A. Extracranial headache:

1. Vascular headaches of the migraine type are recurrent and vary widely in intensity, duration, and frequency. The following subtypes are recognized:

a. *Classic migraine,* with sharply defined, transient visual, other sensory and/or motor prodromes.

b. *Hemiplegic or ophthalmoplegic migraine,* featured by sensory and motor phenomena that persist during and after the headache.

c. *Common migraine,* without striking prodromes and less often unilateral than (a) and (d). Synonyms are "atypical migraine" and "sick headache."

d. *Cluster headache,* predominantly unilateral, associated with flushing, sweating, rhinorrhea, increased lacrimation and, often, Horner's syndrome. The headaches are usually brief in duration and occur in close-packed groups separated by long remissions.

e. *Lower half headache,* of possible vascular mechanism, centered primarily in the lower face. In this group are some instances of atypical facial neuralgia, sphenopalatine ganglion neuralgia (Sluder), and vidian neuralgia (Vail).

2. Muscle contraction headaches are occipitofrontal pains or sensations of tightness, pressure, or constriction associated with sustained skeletal muscle contraction and no permanent structural change. The ambiguous and unsatisfactory terms "tension," "psychogenic," and "nervous" headache refer largely to this group.

3. Combination of vascular headache of the migraine type and muscle contraction headache.

4. Anterior headache and nasal discomfort (nasal obstruction, rhinorrhea, tightness, or burning) can result from congestion, edema, and inflammation of nasal and paranasal mucous membranes. This is "sinus" headache.

5. Nonmigrainous vascular headaches associated with generally nonrecurrent dilatation of intracranial arteries.

6. Ocular headache due to spread of effects of noxious stimulation, as by increased intraocular pressure, excessive contraction of ocular muscles, trauma, new growth, or inflammation.

7. Aural headache due to spread of effects of noxious stimulation, as by trauma, new growth, or inflammation.

8. Dental headache.

9. Headache due to spread of pain from noxious stimulation of other structures of the cranium and neck (periosteum, joints, ligaments, and muscles or cervical nerve roots).

10. Cranial neuritides (caused by trauma, new growth, or infection).

11. Extracranial arteritis.

B. Intracranial headache:

1. Traction headache. Headache resulting from traction on intracranial structures, mainly vascular, by masses:

a. Primary or metastatic tumors of meninges, vessels, or brain.
b. Hematomas (epidural, subdural, or parenchymal).
c. Abscesses (epidural, subdural, or parenchymal).
d. Headache following puncture ("leakage" headache).
e. Pseudotumor cerebri and various causes of brain swelling.

2. Headache due to overt inflammation of cranial structures resulting from usually nonrecurrent inflammation, sterile or infectious.

Intracranial disorders: infectious, chemical, or allergic meningitis, subarachnoid hemorrhage, postpneumoencephalographic reaction, arteritis, and phlebitis.

C. Cranial neuralgias: trigeminal (tic douloureux) and glossopharyngeal (see Ch. 349). Trigeminal neuralgia must be distinguished in particular from the brief vascular headache of A 1 c, with which it is often confused.

D. Headaches of a delusional or conversion reaction are those in which a somatic pain mechanism is nonexistent. The diagnosis is rare and must be made cautiously. Closely allied are hypochondriacal and depressive reactions in which tissue abnormalities relevant to headache are minimal.

Pathogenesis of Headache. Wolff and his colleagues identified the principal pain-sensitive structures of the head as (1) *extracranial:* all the tissues, especially the arteries; and (2) *intracranial:* a very limited group of tissues, including the great venous sinuses and their venous tributaries from the surface of the brain, parts of the dura at the base, the dural arteries and the cerebral arteries at the base of the brain, the fifth, seventh, ninth, and tenth cranial nerves, and the upper three cervical nerves.

The cranium (including the diploic and emissary veins), the parenchyma of the brain, most of the dura, most of the pia-arachnoid, and the ependymal lining of the ventricles and the choroid plexuses are not sensitive to pain.

The fifth cranial nerve contains the pathways for pain from sensitive intracranial structures located on or above the superior surface of the tentorium cerebelli.

Pain from these structures is experienced in various regions in front of a line drawn coronally joining the ears across the top of the head.

The ninth and tenth cranial nerves and the upper two or possibly three cervical nerves contain the pathways for pain from pain-sensitive structures on or below the inferior surface of the tentorium cerebelli. Pain from these structures is experienced in various parieto-occipital and upper cervical regions behind the line just described.

HEADACHE FROM INTRACRANIAL SOURCES

Six basic mechanisms of headache from intracranial sources have been formulated: (1) traction on and displacement of the great venous sinuses or of the veins that pass to them from the surface of the brain; (2) traction on and displacement of the middle meningeal arteries; (3) traction on and displacement of the large arteries at the base of the brain and their main branches; (4) dilatation and distention of intracranial arteries; (5) inflammation in or about any of the pain-sensitive structures of the head and portions of the pia and dura at the base of the skull; and (6) direct pressure by tumors on pain-sensitive cranial and cervical nerves. Intracranial diseases commonly cause headaches through more than one mechanism and may also cause secondary extracranial muscle-contraction headache, usually at the occiput, but often elsewhere.

The head pain associated with fever, bacteremia, sepsis, nitrite and foreign protein administration, carbon monoxide inhalation, hypoxia, and asphyxia is due principally to dilatation and distention of intracranial arterial structures. A similar vascular mechanism is the probable basis for the headaches that follow epileptic seizures (with or without convulsions) and certain "hangover headaches," and is a component of many migraine headaches and those associated with arterial hypertension and Meniere's disease. Painful distention of intracranial arteries is likewise responsible for the headaches that accompany sudden brisk rises in the arterial blood pressure, such as occurs with distention of the rectum or urinary bladder in paraplegics, rapid intravenous infusion of epinephrine, and the hypertensive crises occurring with pheochromocytoma.

The headache of meningitis is primarily related to the lowered pain threshold of inflamed tissues. The inflammatory changes are usually most noticeable in the basal dura and pia and in adjacent blood vessels and nerves at the base of the brain. Under these circumstances, even the slight, usually painless arterial dilatation and distention during each cardiac systole become painful; hence, the characteristic throbbing headache.

Lumbar Puncture Headache

Dull, usually pulsating occipital headache develops in about one fifth of patients having lumbar puncture, particularly for the first time. The headache usually begins 12 to 24 hours after the puncture, comes on in the erect position, and subsides if the subject lies flat. The headache usually disappears spontaneously in a day or so, and in most patients is made tolerable by routine analgesics. Occasionally, patients develop more prostrating symptoms that sometimes last as long as 10 to 14 days, accompanied by secondary muscle-contraction headache as well as nausea and vomiting. Vigorous reassurance and sedatives added to the analgesics may help shorten the course.

The cause of postlumbar puncture headache is probably leakage of cerebrospinal fluid through the torn dural sac. The consequent loss of buoyance results in downward traction on unsupported, pain-sensitive posterior fossa tissues, particularly the veins. The headaches can often be avoided by accurate punctures, using No. 20 caliber sharp spinal needles, which minimize drainage through the dural needle wound.

Headache With Brain Tumor: With or Without Increased Intracranial Pressure

The headache with space-occupying lesions is deep, aching, steady, dull, and seldom rhythmic or throbbing. The pain is continuous in one tenth of the patients and is generally more intense in the morning. Aspirin, 0.3 gram, and local application of cold packs usually diminish the pain, and coughing or straining at stool may aggravate it. Some patients prefer the recumbent to the erect position. The headache is rarely as intense as that associated with migraine, ruptured cerebral aneurysm, or meningitis, and seldom interferes with sleep. Even when the tumor directly compresses and displaces pain-sensitive cranial nerves, headache may be absent or slight, and rarely is it as intense as the pain of tic douloureux, unless the tumor intermittently obstructs the cerebral ventricular system. In this instance, pain is excruciating and generalized, and may last 30 seconds to a half hour and then disappear as quickly as it commenced. During such an attack the sudden increases of intracranial pressure can be fatal.

Severe brain tumor headache is associated with nausea and vomiting. However, vomiting caused by new growth may occur with neither nausea nor headache, and is then usually the result of medullary compression. Being unexpected, such vomiting may be projectile.

When the headache is occipital or suboccipital, it is often associated with "stiffness" or aching of the muscles of the neck and tilting of the head toward the side of the lesion.

Pathogenesis. Increased intracranial pressure, per se, is not necessarily associated with headache. The headache with brain tumor results from traction-displacement of intracranial pain-sensitive structures, chiefly the large arteries, veins, venous sinuses, and the cranial and somatic nerves mentioned.

Local traction and direct pressure may be exerted by the tumor upon adjacent pain-sensitive structures. Extensive displacement of the brain evokes pain from structures remote from, as well as adjacent to, the tumor.

Localizing Value. When the site of the headache is interpreted in terms of the following principles of intracranial pain production and pain reference, it may aid significantly in localization of a brain tumor:

(1) About one third of all headaches approximately overlie the tumor. (2) In the absence of increased intracranial pressure, two thirds of headaches are near or immediately over the tumor, and when unilateral are on the same side. (3) Occipital headache is almost always present and is the first symptom of posterior fossa tumors, except cerebellopontine angle tumors. When headache occurs with cerebellopontine angle tumors, it is frequently and sometimes solely postauricular. (4) Frontal headache is a first symptom in about one third of supratentorial tumors. Occipital headache rarely occurs with such growths unless associated with increased intracranial pressure or early tonsillar herniation. (5) A generalized headache with brain tumor signifies extensive displacement of the brain, usually with increased intracranial pressure, and has little localizing value.

Management. The headache itself rarely determines the management. Nevertheless, the most effective treatment for brain tumor headache is surgical removal of the mass. Transient decompression can be achieved by the intravenous infusion of either 500 ml of a 20 per cent sodium mannitol solution or 250 ml of a solution containing 30 per cent urea in 10 per cent invert sugar. Adrenal corticosteroids in high doses can also be employed to reduce brain edema and transiently decompress the mass. Lumbar drainage is contraindicated, nor does it predictably reduce headache of meningitis or subarachnoid hemorrhage.

If an inoperable tumor causes headache, ventricular drainage or shunting is sometimes employed.

Sometimes x-radiation or surgical procedures are justified in attempts to reduce headache caused by clearly defined metastatic disease. Headache resulting from craniopharyngioma or pituitary tumors does not in itself constitute an indication for surgical procedures, because removal provides no assurance that headache will be diminished or eliminated.

HEADACHES FROM EXTRACRANIAL STRUCTURES

Six main categories of head and face pain from extracranial tissues and related structures can be distinguished: (1) headaches due to painful dilatation and distention of cranial arteries; (2) headaches due to sustained contraction of skeletal muscle about the face, scalp, and neck; (3) headache from disease of the nose, paranasal spaces, eyes, ears, and teeth; (4) craniofacial pain of the major neuralgias and the postinfectious neuralgias and postinfectious neuritides; (5) headache due to nonspecific inflammation of cranial arteries ("cranial arteritis," "temporal arteritis"); and (6) head pain due to trauma, infection, or new growth involving extracranial tissues.

More than 90 per cent of all headaches are in the first two of these categories and occur in a life setting that engenders frustration, resentment, anxiety, emotional tension, and fatigue.

Vascular Headaches

Vascular headaches are principally due to painful dilatation and distention of one or more of the extracranial and, probably, intracranial, i.e., dural, branches of the external carotid artery, with associated edema of adjacent tissues. The most common site of vascular headaches of the migraine type is the temple or the forehead, and one or both frontal, supraorbital, and superficial temporal arteries are most frequently involved. Many headaches at the back of the head and neck are associated with painful dilatation and distention of the postauricular and/or occipital arteries, and comprise one type of "occipital neuralgia."

Finally, the lower half of the head and face and the upper jaw in the vicinity of the back teeth may all be the site of pain of vascular origin, with spread to the neck and even the shoulder. Such headaches may be accompanied by the awareness of unusually forceful throbbing in the neck. "Atypical facial neuralgia" is but one of the many designations applied to such headaches, which very probably result in good part from dilatation and distention of the extracranial portion of the middle meningeal artery, of the internal maxillary artery, and of the other branches and the trunks of the external and the common carotid arteries.

Migraine Syndrome

Clinical Features. The migraine syndrome is a pattern of dysfunction integrated within the central nervous system and manifested as widespread bodily disturbances, both nonpainful and painful. The outstanding feature is periodic headache, usually unilateral in onset but at times becoming bilateral or generalized. The attacks may vary in duration from a few minutes to several days and, in severity, from trifling symptoms to prolonged disabling illness. The headaches are associated with "irritability," nausea, and often photophobia, vomiting, constipation, or diarrhea. Although most common in the temple, headaches may be experienced anywhere in the head, face, and neck. The syndrome runs in families.

For a period of several hours to several days preceding the headache, the cranial arteries undergo a variable contractile state indicated by a facial flushing or pallor and by other transient cranial vasomotor phenomena such as vertigo. In the hour preceding the headache, a variety of visual and other neurologic abnormalities caused by transient local constriction of cerebral or retinal arteries occur in about 10 to 15 per cent of the instances. These prodromes may take the form of scintillating scotomas, visual field defects such as unilateral or homonymous hemianopsia, and, occasionally, hemiplegia. More sustained neurologic defects and even cerebral infarction have rarely occurred. As the vasoconstrictor phenomena recede, vasodilator headache commences, sometimes overlapping, sometimes beginning after a short symptom-free interval. The pain is throbbing and aching, is appreciably reduced by pressure on the common carotid and the affected superficial artery, and is characteristically eliminated or reduced by vasoconstrictor agents, particularly ergotamine tartrate. The walls of the dilated cranial arteries and the adjacent tissues become edematous and tender. With sustained vasodilatation for several hours, the easily compressible arteries become rigid and relatively noncompressible, and the pulsatile pain becomes a steady ache. Redness and swelling of the eye with excessive tearing, and redness and swelling of the nasal mucosa with or without epistaxis, may occur along with the headache. A secondary muscle contraction component of the headache may outlast the vascular pain and will not be modified by vasoconstrictor agents.

One variety of headache closely related to migraine syndrome is the *cluster headache,* sometimes called histamine headache. This head pain is almost always unilateral, affects men much more than women, and usually begins between the third and sixth decades. Attacks come on abruptly with intense throbbing pain arising high in the nostril and spreading to involve the region behind the homolateral eye and sometimes the forehead as well. During the attacks, which last up to two hours, seldom more, the nose and eye water. The skin reddens and a homolateral Horner's syndrome with pupillary constriction and ptosis may develop. The attacks tend to occur from once to several times daily, in clusters lasting weeks or, less often, months. Without apparent reason, the cluster subsides as suddenly as it began, and the patient commonly remains free of headache for weeks or months until another cluster begins. During a cluster period, but not between, alcohol is likely to induce attacks. When headaches recur in close succession, the Horner's syndrome may outlast the headache.

Pathogenesis. Before the onset of migraine headache a generalized accumulation of fluid may occur as part of a nonspecific disturbance in fluid and electrolytes that is found in many persons with and without the migraine syndrome during periods of stress. There is evidence of a general abnormality of vascular behavior in many migraine subjects, and the extracranial vessels of such subjects show more variability in their contractile patterns than those of normal subjects even during headache-free periods. Sympathetic nerve stimulation or section has little effect on these vessels or on the migraine attack, and humoral agents have long been sought as the basis of the migraine syndrome. Local fluid collected from sites of swelling at the point of maximal headache and tenderness during an attack contains a vasodilator polypeptide of the bradykinin type that lowers pain thresholds and may be a factor in a local sterile inflammation. However, neither kinins, histamine, nor substances such as acetylcholine satisfactorily explain the generalized manifestations of the disorder. Several lines of evidence suggest that abnormalities in the metabolism of serotonin may play a role in the migraine syndrome. Reserpine, which induces a drop in serum serotonin levels, will often induce a migraine attack, and serum levels of serotonin have been found to drop spontaneously just before migraine attacks. During migraine attacks, an increased quantity of serotonin metabolites has been found in the urine. Methysergide, a powerful serotonin antagonist, prevents or reduces the frequency of migraine attacks in most subjects.

Management. Headaches of low intensity are usually eliminated by 0.3 to 0.6 gram of aspirin, but sometimes require 60 mg of codeine phosphate as well.

For severe vascular headache, the restoration of the painfully dilated vessels to a nonpainful constricted state and the restoration of pain threshold to normal are accomplished best by the prompt intramuscular administration of 0.25 to 0.5 mg of ergotamine tartrate, not to exceed 0.5 mg in any one week. If the agent is administered in amounts of 1.0 to 2.0 mg by suppository, the side effects of nausea, vomiting, and elevated blood pressure are diminished. Ergotamine tartrate may also be given by mouth in 3.0 mg amounts, to be swallowed or absorbed sublingually. This first dose may be repeated in 30 minutes, and a third given in another 30 minutes if the headache persists. Ergotamine tartrate, 1 mg, can also be given in tablets in combination with caffeine, 100 mg, up to 8 tablets for any single headache attack. The amount of ergotamine so administered should not exceed 10 mg in any one week. Administration by mouth or by suppository is less predictably effective than intramuscular administration

Propranolol, 20 mg four times daily, occasionally adds to the benefit received from ergotamine tartrate or ergotamine-caffeine combinations. Short courses of corticosteroids interrupt periods of cluster headache in about half the affected patients. Methysergide is similarly effective in cluster headache.

Prevention. Of utmost importance is a consideration of the personal problems of the patients. Patients with migraine headaches are generally striving, order-loving persons who, during periods of threat or conflict, become progressively more tense, resentful, and fatigued. Although the disease undoubtedly depends on a constitutional background, feelings of anger, depression, or emotional fatigue often form the backdrop for a recurrence of headache. Treatment is best if it allows the patient free and repeated expression of his conflicts, resentments, and dissatisfactions; enables him to recognize the nature of his dilemma and its relationship to the physiologic basis of his pain; and guides him toward a more flexible attitude and personal adjustment. About two of three patients can be appreciably helped by such aid.

For patients in whom attention to psychologic attitudes and adjustment of life situations fail to bring significant relief, two forms of long-term pharmacotherapy have been useful. One is the monoamine oxidase inhibitor phenelzine sulfate, 45 mg daily, which induces a significant reduction in headache frequency in most patients with migraine, and can be given indefinitely. The other is the serotonin antagonist methysergide, which in doses of 2 mg three to four times daily is effective in about two of three cases in preventing headache of the migraine type. However, methysergide must be used with great caution. Both ergotamine tartrate and methysergide possess the ability to induce profound vasoconstriction and are contraindicated in pregnancy, peripheral vascular disturbance, severe hypertension, coronary artery disease, thrombophlebitis, and renal disease. Serious and unexpected vasospastic and psychic reactions have occasionally occurred with methysergide. Retroperitoneal fibrosis producing back pain and ureteral obstruction has been reported. Any of these serious complications necessitate prompt discontinuance of methysergide, and any single course of the drug should not outlast three to six months.

Muscle-Contraction Headaches

The pain of a muscle-contracting headache is a steady, nonpulsatile ache, unilateral or bilateral, in the temporal, occipital, parietal, or frontal regions. Additional descriptive terms include tightness bitemporally or at the occiput, bandlike sensations about the head, which may become caplike in distribution, viselike ache, weight, pressure, drawing, or soreness. Cramplike head pains and "feeling as if the neck and upper back were in a cast" are described by some patients. Pain may be fleeting, with frequent changes in the site and intensity of recurrences, or localized in one region. The headache may last for weeks, months, or even years.

Pathogenesis. Muscle contraction headaches are due to long-sustained contraction of skeletal muscle about the face, scalp, and neck. Concurrent vasodilatation of the associated cranial arteries frequently contributes to the irritability of the involved muscles and to the headaches.

With prolonged sustained contraction, the muscles of the head, jaws, neck, and upper back become tender, causing the patient to limit their motion. Palpation may reveal sharply localized painful areas or nodules. Commonly, it hurts to comb or brush the hair or to don a hat. Exposure to cold, with shivering, may precipitate or aggravate the headache. Pressure on the contracted, tender muscles may augment the intensity and may elicit tinnitus, dizziness, and lacrimation – features that also occur spontaneously.

Sustained muscle contraction giving rise to headache is often secondary to noxious stimuli from other cranial tissues and structures, e.g., from distended arteries in vascular headache, inflammation or other disease in the eye, ear, nose, paranasal spaces, teeth, or scalp, and from brain tumor. Painful, sustained muscle contraction is also the primary source of many headaches associated with emotional tension states, especially in the adverse life situation of tense, aggressive, frustrated, anxious, or depressed persons.

Management. Reassurance, massage, manipulation, and manual stretching of the nuchal and occipital muscles, aspirin, and phenobarbital (30 mg three times a day) reduce or eliminate most such headaches. Bed rest, local heat, warm baths, and the passage of time are important adjuvants. Removal of the primary source of noxious stimuli may eliminate the headaches secondary to disease of the eye, ear, nose, and sinuses or teeth.

Headaches caused by sustained muscle contraction associated with life stress and emotional tension are only temporarily modified by sedatives or analgesics. Treatment should be directed at improving the patient's adjustment, as outlined under the management and prevention of migraine headache. Particularly among patients susceptible to recurrent headache of this type, the antidepressant amitriptyline in doses of 25 to 75 mg daily may bring considerable relief.

Other Types of Extracranial Headache

Recurrent ("Chronic") Post-traumatic Headache. Head injury may rarely be followed by headaches that stem from intracranial sources such as subdural hematomas or subarachnoid hemorrhages. However, post-traumatic headaches more frequently stem from nonintracranial sources, four types being most common: (1) pain or tenderness resulting from local tissue damage in a scar or at a site of impact, (2) muscle-contraction headache, (3) attacks of throbbing and aching vascular headache, and (4) infrequently, delusional headaches for which no tissue abnormality exists. The first two varieties are most common and are sometimes accompanied by fleeting vertigo with sudden movement or rotation of the head, nausea, irritability, and insomnia.

Many injured patients harbor resentment related to the circumstances of their accident or fear that they have sustained permanent brain injury. These reactions and attitudes are intimately related to the pathophysiology and "chronicity" of post-traumatic headaches, and the headache often fails to subside completely as long as compensation claims remain unsettled.

Headaches Associated with Arterial Hypertension. When otherwise symptom-free and in the absence of hypertensive encephalopathy or pheochromocytoma, about 10 per cent of persons with arterial hypertension may experience severe, even disabling, headaches, particularly during the morning hours. Recent studies show that these are principally vascular and muscle-contraction headaches. Fluctuations in blood pressure correlate only poorly with the headaches, nor is the extent of the elevation directly related to the severity of the attacks. However, headache attacks tend to be less frequent when the blood pressure is least elevated.

The headache associated with arterial hypertension resembles the vascular headaches of migraine and muscle tension and often regresses spontaneously with reassurance, bed rest, sedative medication, and the passage of time, especially when the patient is hospitalized. Ergotamine tartrate and methysergide are contraindicated.

Nasal and Paranasal Structures as Sources of Headache. Sinus headache is predominantly a short-lived problem, always associated with objective evidence of acute sinusitis. Most of the discomfort comes from the ostia, which are many times more sensitive than the relatively insensitive walls of the sinuses. Typically, "sinus" headache commences in the morning (frontal) or early afternoon (maxillary) and subsides in the early or late evening. The pain is dull and aching, is made worse by changing head position, and is seldom associated with nausea and vomiting. It is due to mucosal inflammation, and engorged turbinates, ostia, nasofrontal ducts and superior nasal spaces should be visible. Most patients have sinus tenderness. Headache not associated with turbinate engorgement and inflammation is probably not due to sinus or nose disease. Sinus headache is best treated with decongestants and analgesics. Persistent purulent discharges should be cultured and appropriate antimicrobial drugs employed. Chronic suppurative disease in the frontal, ethmoid, and sphenoid sinuses, or in the mastoid air cells, may result in osteomyelitis and inflammation of adjacent cranial tissues. Headache persisting after surgical drainage of the diseased sinus is evidence for extradural and possibly subdural infection.

Head Pain and Disease of the Teeth. Noxious stimuli in a tooth usually evoke local toothache, but pain can be referred to tissues remote from a diseased tooth. Afferent fibers for sensation in the teeth are contained in the second and third divisions of the fifth cranial nerve. Headache in the areas supplied by the latter is, in rare instances, associated with prolonged, intense toothache, or follows a tooth extraction. More commonly, in association with toothache, tooth extraction or a tender, diseased tooth, distant tissues exhibit surface hyperalgesia, tenderness, and vasomotor reactions, such as tender eyeballs, reddening of the conjunctivae, and tenderness of the auricular and temporal tissues. Because of secondary muscle contraction, other sites of tenderness and pain may be noted behind the ears, behind the lower border of the mastoid process, and in the muscles of the occiput, neck, and shoulders.

The teeth in the upper jaws are frequently the site of tenderness and pain in association with disease of the nasal and paranasal structures. Occasionally, in coronary insufficiency, pain is experienced in the lower jaw because of the close approximation of the fifth cranial and upper cervical neural segments in the cord. The teeth rarely cause craniofacial pains or "neuralgias" in the absence of toothache. Headache may not be attributed to a diseased tooth unless the injection of procaine into the tissues about the suspected tooth greatly reduces the intensity of, or eliminates, such headache.

Head Pain and Disease of the Ear. The fifth, seventh, ninth, and tenth cranial nerves contribute to the sensory innervation of the ear, and branches from the upper cervical roots supply the immediately adjacent scalp and muscles. Severe pain in the vicinity of the ear can be caused by disease of the teeth, acute tonsillitis, inflammatory and neoplastic disease of the larynx and nasopharynx, temporomandibular joint disorders, tumors, and inflammation in the posterior fossa and disease of the cervical spine and its soft tissues. Pain in the ear is also associated with vascular headaches and atypical facial neuralgias as well as herpes zoster of the fifth and seventh cranial nerves and, rarely, the glossopharyngeal nerve. True glossopharyngeal neuralgia causes severe pain radiating from the tonsil into the ear. It has the usual timing feature of "tic."

Primary ear disease is relatively infrequent—but important—as a source of headache, because it almost always indicates inflammation or destructive disease. Acute otitis media (purulent or nonpurulent), furunculosis of the ear canal, traumatic rupture of the tympanum, and fracture of the anterior wall of the bony canal all cause pain in the ear associated with sustained tender contraction of adjacent skeletal muscles. Osteomyelitis of the mastoid bone may be associated with inflammation of the nearby periosteum as well as dura and adjacent tissues (epidural abscess)—both sources of pain in or behind the ear. Pain in this region also accompanies tumors of the acoustic nerve and inflammation and thrombosis of the lateral sinus.

The Eye as a Source of Headache. Errors of refraction (hypermetropia, astigmatism, anomalies of accommodation), disturbances of ocular muscle equilibrium, and glaucoma are universally described as causing headache. Refractive errors are also said to give origin to such other symptoms as aching of the eyes, "sandy" feeling in the eyes, pulling sensations in and about the orbit, and conjunctival congestion. Headache usually starts around and over the eyes and subsequently radiates to the occiput and back of the head.

The pain of increased intraocular pressure at first remains localized in the eyeball, then extends along the rim of the orbit and, finally, throughout most of the area supplied by the ophthalmic division of the trigeminal nerve. Nausea and vomiting sometimes accompany such headaches.

Headache accompanying various ocular disturbances is regarded as secondary to (1) sustained contraction of the intraocular muscles, which is associated with excessive accommodation effort, or (2) sustained contraction of the extraocular muscles, resulting from the effort to produce distinct retinal images, and single binocular vision with fusion. Simple myopia, per se, in contrast to the aforementioned ocular defects, does not evoke headache because the myope, in attempting to improve his vision by the contraction of his eye muscles, actually makes his vision worse and soon abandons the attempt.

With inflammation of the iris and ciliary body, light may cause intense pain in the eye and adjacent areas when the light stimulus is accompanied by movement of the inflamed iris. When the iris is immobilized, pain is allayed.

Anthony, M., Hinterberger, H., and Lance, J. W.: The possible relationship of serotonin to the migraine syndrome. Res. Clin. Stud. Headache, 2:29, 1968.

Anthony, M., and Lance, J. W.: Monoamine oxidase inhibition in the treatment of migraine. Arch. Neurol., 21:263, 1969.

Dalessio, D. J.: Wolff's Headache and Other Head Pain. 3rd ed. New York, Oxford University Press, 1972.

Vinken, P. J., and Bruyn, G. W. (eds.): Headaches and Cranial Neuralgias. Vol. 5. Handbook of Clinical Neurology. Amsterdam, North-Holland, 1968.

351. HEARING LOSS

J. R. Nelson

Approximately 3 per cent of the population suffer from hearing loss sufficiently severe to impair the understanding of speech. A new era of treatment of conductive hearing losses has recently begun with excellent surgical results from use of the operating microscope and new microsurgical techniques. Considerable help is available even to those with hereditary or congenital sensorineural losses through improved audiometric detection methods and rehabilitation programs.

Definition. The two major types of hearing loss are *conductive* losses, usually resulting from involvement of the mechanical sound transmission apparatus in the middle ear, and *sensorineural* losses, in which the cochlea, the cochlear nerve, or more central pathways are affected.

Conductive losses gradually narrow the loudness between air-conducted sounds and those produced by direct vibration of the skull (bone conduction). Discrimination of test words presented above threshold is not disturbed. The proper timing and phase relationships of various sound wave frequencies are maintained even though the mechanical oscillations from ear drum to oval window are dampened by disease processes. Simple tests for conductive hearing loss include the *Rinne test,* in which a 512 cps fork is first held against the mastoid process until the sound fades and then is placed 1 inch from the ear. With 20 to 25 db or more of conductive loss, bone conduction is superior to air conduction. A more sensitive test is the *Bing test,* in which a finger is placed in the ear just as the sound from a fork on the mastoid bone fades away. If the sound then reappears, a normal conductive mechanism is likely. The Bing phenomenon may be absent with as little as 5 db of conductive impairment. The *Weber test* involves the lateralization of sound to the diseased ear when a fork is held at midforehead or on a central incisor.

Sensorineural deafness can be due to either cochlear or retrocochlear pathology. With cochlear pathology there is a paradoxically increased response to successive increments of sound intensity. One test of this is the *recruitment* phenomenon, in which the poorest hearing ear is first determined with a low intensity tone. If a second, higher intensity sound is presented to each ear quickly and the previously poorer ear now appreciates sound best, an abnormal loudness-to-intensity gradient has been demonstrated. A similar phenomenon underlies the short increment sensitivity index test (SISI), in which, in normal hearing, small 1 db pips of sound added to a steady tone 20 db above threshold are not heard, but with cochlear damage a near-perfect reception score of such small increments is found. The illusion that a sound is of a different frequency (diplacusis) is also common. With auditory nerve (retrocochlear) lesions, nerve fatigue occurs whereby a steady tone gradually seems to fade in loudness. More than 20 to 30 db of such "tone decay" is suggestive of a retrocochlear type of sensorineural loss. The *Békésy test* involves presentation of continuous tones and interrupted tones at various frequencies. Because of tone decay, with nerve lesions the audiometric graph for continuous tones will show a greater loss than with interrupted tones when the nerve recovers between stimuli. Such recordings are rated type III or IV in contrast to the normal type I or type II response that occurs in cochlear lesions and in some normal ears. The Rinne test is normal with sensorineural loss, and the Weber test lateralizes toward the normal ear, contrasting with conductive losses.

A battery of simple audiometric tests now can differentiate the various types of deafness. Sensorineural losses can be subcategorized into cochlear and retrocochlear types with about 70 per cent or more accuracy. The

Types of Hearing Loss

	Conductive	Cochlear	Nerve	Pontine
Air > bone conduction	Reversed*	Normal	Normal	Normal
Recruitment	Absent	Present	Absent	Often present
SISI Score†	0–20%	80–100%	0–20%	0–20%
Tone decay	None	None	Present	Present
Bekesy (type)	I	I, II	III, IV	III, IV
Speech discrimination	Normal	Fair to good	Poor	Fair

*Except early, then use Bing test.
†SISI – short increment sensitivity index test (% of pips heard).

idealized findings with various sites of pathology are shown in the accompanying table.

The impedance of the middle ear can also be measured now with a relatively simple device to define abnormal patterns with drum, middle ear, and eustachian tube dysfunction. Another exciting new form of testing involves direct recording of cochlear nerve action potentials from the ear drum to evaluate the integrity of the cochlea and nerve directly.

Etiology and Clinical Manifestations. *Hereditary deafness* accounts for up to half of childhood cases and up to a third of adult cases. It is usually of a sensorineural type with either dominant (10 per cent) or recessive inheritance (90 per cent). Onset is usually in childhood with bilateral involvement, but families with adult onset, mostly unilateral findings, or frequency-specific bands of loss are described. Such entities suggest selective abiotrophy ("early aging") of the cochlear neurons. In many cases there are other metabolic defects or malformations of the ear, eye, integument, skeleton, or nervous system (Konigsmark).

Nonfamilial *congenital deafness* syndromes with varying degrees of hypoplasia of the inner ear include complete failure of development of the inner ear (Michel), cochleosaccular dysgenesis (Scheibe), the most common type, and subtotal development of either the membranous labyrinth (Alexander) or the entire osseous and membranous labyrinth (Mondini), both of which may show incomplete hearing loss. These deformities may show characteristic changes on temporal bone laminagrams.

Neurotropic Infections. Both viral and bacterial infections may seriously threaten hearing from embryonic life to adulthood. Maternal German measles (rubella) accounts for at least 20 per cent of congenital deafness and produces a severe bilateral sensorineural impairment in addition to its other teratogenic effects. Reduction of this cause should follow the wide use of the vaccine now available. Only slightly less prevalent are cases of severe postmeningitic hearing loss. The incidence has decreased since the antimicrobial era, but unfortunately it is still all too common in infants and young children. Prematurity probably predisposes to this cause and is an important, poorly understood cause of deafness itself.

Certain cases of sudden, unilateral sensorineural hearing loss are associated with viral upper respiratory infections and produce "cochleitis" with a profound loss, which may be due to direct inflammation or vascular involvement. Some otologists advocate emergency treatment with intravenous histamine for vasodilatation and low molecular weight dextran to reduce blood viscosity. The rate of recovery may be enhanced, but controlled studies are still needed to clarify this point. Mumps is a well recognized cause of unilateral sensorineural deafness, and vestibular involvement may also occur. Other common childhood viral illnesses may occasionally produce hearing loss. Herpes zoster may simultaneously affect the eighth nerve and geniculate ganglion to produce deafness, vertigo, and facial palsy (Ramsay Hunt syndrome) in addition to ear or throat pain and vesicles. The syndrome of sudden unilateral deafness may also be caused by rupture of the round or oval window membranes with coughing, straining, or other unusual pressure gradients between inner and middle ear. Such perilymph fistulas also cause dizziness, and explorations of the ear may reveal a surgically repairable leak (Goodhill).

Otologic syphilis deserves special mention, because a young adult who may have been sucessfully treated for congenital syphilis may still develop late inflammatory changes of recurrent interstitial keratitis, joint effusion (Clutton's joints), and fluctuating progressive sensorineural hearing loss and vertigo. Eventual total deafness is the rule. A low-tone hearing loss is common early, as with Meniere's disease, but explosive total deafness in one ear suggestive of internal auditory artery occlusion may occur. Such inner ear manifestations may appear even in the absence of a positive VDRL in the blood or serum, and more sensitive tests such as the FTA-ABS test may be required. Some authorities believe that all cases of "bilateral Meniere's" should be considered syphilitic until proved otherwise. Softening of the capsular bone about the oval window occurs so that the stapes moves excessively, but only in an outward direction. This provides the basis for *Hennebert's sign,* which is a positive fistula test (vertigo with middle-ear pressure changes) that occurs only with negative suction applied with a pneumatic otoscope. These cases raise the possibility that treatment failure rather than autoimmune responses or late fibrotic reactions accounts for the late-life damage to the ear. Recent evidence suggests that long-term cortisone treatment may partially reverse or halt the progression of deafness and vertigo. Some authorities also recommend intensive retreatment with oral ampicillin, 1.5 grams, and probenecid, 0.5 gram, four times per day for up to four to five weeks.

Otosclerosis. Otosclerosis is a very common cause of hearing loss in Caucasian adults, and is usually inherited as a dominant trait with up to 40 per cent penetrance. Pathologically, the process consists of an overgrowth of labyrinthine capsular bone around the oval window which leads to progressive fixation of the stapes. Hearing loss begins insidiously in early adult life, with slow progression. Pregnancy may accelerate the condition in females. The audiometric findings in far-advanced cases may be misleading with poor reliability about the amount of sensorineural loss. Careful correlation with tuning fork results is essential. Some patients with no measurable hearing loss by audiometry may still have partial recovery after surgery to the point that use of an aid allows serviceable hearing. The surgical treatment of otosclerosis has developed rapidly in the past 25 years with successive adoption of horizontal canal fenestration, stapes mobilization by fracture, and finally stapedectomy with replacement by Teflon plugs, steel pistons, or wire prostheses that bridge the gap between the incus and a new membrane on the oval window that forms over a fascia or Gelfoam graft. Good to excellent long-lasting results occur in over 90 per cent of cases. Some evidence suggests that administration of 25 to 60 mg of sodium fluoride per day for a year may halt the progression of otosclerosis.

A poorly understood sensorineural component often is seen in longstanding cases, probably owing to involvement of the otic capsule of the cochlea.

Middle Ear Infections. Antimicrobial drugs have not entirely eliminated suppurative otitis media, particularly chronic forms, although acute attacks usually respond to the drugs and to myringotomy. Once chronic drainage and infection have been arrested, several reconstructive surgical procedures are possible even though extensive destruction of middle ear structures has occurred. Modified radical mastoidectomy with tympanoplasty may improve function of the middle ear conductive mechanism. Numerous grafting and artificial prosthetic replacement techniques are available. Recurrent cholesteatoma formation represents a special challenge, as these imbedded epithelial fragments may grow to cause extensive destruction of the middle ear and temporal bone.

Chronic serous otitis media is the most common cause of chronic conductive hearing loss in children. A predisposing factor may be poor eustachian tube function from edema secondary to allergy, inflammation, large lymphoid follicles, large adenoids, or a congenitally small lumen. Insertion of a polyethylene tube in the tympanic membrane for several weeks may allow external drainage, equalize the middle ear pressure, and restore hearing while the eustachian tube hopefully regains its patency.

Traumatic Hearing Loss. There are two major types of temporal bone fractures that may be associated with hearing loss. With a longitudinal fracture along the axis of the petrous pyramid, damage to the inner ear is usually slight, but bleeding from the ear and disruption of the middle ear bones are common and may require surgical repair at a later date. In contrast, transverse fractures perpendicular to the petrous pyramid may cause severe inner ear damage and facial palsy. If facial paralysis is immediate, surgical exploration is mandatory.

Noise-induced acoustic trauma is an important cause of hearing loss in industrial settings, but exposure to gun blasts, airplane engines, and even rock and roll music may cause progressive high tone sensorineural hearing loss. Certain individuals are much more sensitive to acoustic trauma and must be protected with ear molds or protective ear covers if it is necessary to work in high noise levels. The magnitude of this problem is great, and has been often neglected in spite of advances in prevention.

Meniere's Disease. Although the episodic attacks of vertigo are more disabling, a fluctuating low-tone "cochlear" hearing loss with eventual involvement of other frequencies is common. This condition and acoustic neuroma, which also produces unilateral tinnitus, deafness, and vertigo, are more fully discussed in Ch. 352.

Ototoxic Drugs. Many antimicrobials, mostly when administered by injection, may cause severe cochlear damage. Dihydrostreptomycin fortunately has been removed from use; streptomycin causes semicircular canal and utricular damage with relative sparing of the cochlea and saccule. Other drugs which may cause deafness when blood concentration is high because of large dosage or renal failure are neomycin, kanamycin, vancomycin, gentamicin, ristocetin, ethacrynic acid, furosemide, and quinine. Use of such drugs should be carefully considered, particularly in patients with renal failure.

Central Causes of Deafness. In order to markedly raise the threshold for hearing with central involvement, bilateral damage of the pontine projections or higher centers is required. Other signs of cranial nerve involvement and sensory and motor pathway damage should be sought. Lesions at the cortical level produce complex aphasic impairments, and are beyond the scope of this chapter.

Rehabilitation of the Hard of Hearing. The education of the deaf child and the assistance needed by all hard of hearing persons is a task requiring skilled efforts by the physician, audiologist, and teacher. Selection of hearing aids must not be made before a full professional evaluation reveals the exact cause of the hearing problem.

Davis, H., and Silverman, S. R. (eds.): Hearing and Deafness. 3rd ed. New York, Holt, Rinehart and Winston, 1970.
Goodhill, V., et al.: Sudden deafness and labyrinthine window ruptures. Ann. Otol., 82:2, 1973.
Hardy, D. B.: Fetal consequences of maternal viral infections in pregnancy. Arch. Otolaryngol., 98:218, 1973.
Jerger, J.: Review of diagnostic audiometry. Ann. Otol., 77:1042, 1968.
Jerger, J.: Clinical experience with impedance audiometry. Arch. Otolaryngol., 92:34, 1970.
Konigsmark, B. W.: Hereditary deafness in man. N. Engl. J. Med., 281:713, 1969.
Patterson, M. E.: Congenital luetic hearing impairment. Arch. Otolaryngol., 87:70, 1968.
Pulec, J. L. (ed.): Meniere's Disease. Philadelphia, W. B. Saunders Company, 1968.
Saunders, W. H.: Sudden deafness and its several treatments. Laryngoscope, 72:1206, 1972.
Shambaugh, G. E., Jr.: The diagnosis and treatment of active cochlear otosclerosis. J. Laryngol. Otol., 85:301, 1971.
Sheehy, J. L., Gardner, G., Jr., and Hambley, W. M.: Tuning fork tests in modern otology. Arch. Otolaryngol., 94:132, 1971.

352. DIZZINESS AND VERTIGO

David A. Drachman

THE COMPLAINT OF DIZZINESS

As a *complaint* rather than a *disease*, the term "dizziness" appropriately includes almost any sensation that a patient chooses to call by that name. By usage the term is applied to a number of uncommon sensations that are *not* part of daily experience. It is the thread of unfamiliar spatial disorientation that appears to bind these complaints together. When one listens carefully to a large number of "dizzy" patients, it is possible to sort their complaints into four types: a *rotational sensation, impending faint, dysequilibrium,* and *vague lightheadedness.*

Type I dizziness is a *definite rotational sensation* (vertigo) in which the patient feels that either he or the environment is spinning. Violent vertigo is often accompanied by nausea, vomiting, and a staggering gait. Oscillopsia—a visual hallucination of to-and-fro movement of the environment—may occur. The onset of vertigo is often instantaneous, and patients sometimes describe a sensation of being hurled to the ground. Although full-blown vertigo is unmistakable, with milder forms the patient may describe only a rocking sensation or vague lightheadedness. Recognition of mild vertiginous episodes is often aided by testing with the dizziness simulation battery described below.

Whenever the patient's dizziness is exclusively rotational, it is due to a disorder of the vestibular system: either the peripheral labyrinth or its central connections. Because of this close relationship, it is important to separate definite rotational vertigo accurately from other types of dizziness.

Type II dizziness is a *sensation of impending faint or loss of consciousness.* Pallor, dimness of vision, roaring in the ears, and diaphoresis, with recovery upon assuming the recumbent position, are common. Type II dizziness of cardiovascular origin is of abrupt onset and short duration. When faintness is gradual in onset or of longer duration, the relationship of the episodes to hypoglycemia should be sought.

The complaint of impending faint usually implies an inadequate supply of blood or nutrients to the entire brain, such as occurs in postural hypotension. It is not a feature of *focal* cerebral ischemia, although this mistaken impression is widely subscribed to by physicians.

Type III dizziness is *dysequilibrium:* the loss of balance *without* an abnormal sensation in the head. This experience occurs only when the patient is walking; it disappears as soon as he sits down. It is due to a disorder of motor system control.

Type IV dizziness is *vague lightheadedness* other than vertigo, faintness, or dysequilibrium. This designation includes dizziness that cannot be identified with certainty as any of the other types. When patients complain of lightheadedness, *fractional* or *poorly described* symptoms of vertigo, faintness, or dysequilibrium must first be looked for, e.g., a rocking sensation instead of spinning. Evidence of *hyperventilation* symptoms should next be sought, as well as symptoms pointing to a *psychiatric disorder,* particularly depression or anxiety. Finally, the evidence for *multiple sensory impairment* should be examined, especially a history of peripheral neuropathy, cervical spondylosis, or cataract surgery in an elderly or diabetic patient.

EVALUATING THE DIZZY PATIENT

The *history* must explore four major questions that critically distinguish the disorders producing dizziness: (1) the type of dizziness (I to IV) experienced by the patient; (2) the *abruptness* of attacks or *continuity* of symptoms; (3) the relation or independence of dizziness to *position or motion* (standing/sitting/lying; sudden change in position; walking); and (4) the *age* of the patient. The relation of these data to differential diagnosis will be discussed with specific entities.

A neurologic examination allows the distinction between central and peripheral causes of dizziness, and may reveal certain *patterns* of involvement that point to the diagnosis: e.g., brainstem syndrome (hemiplegia alternans), cerebellopontine angle syndrome, multiple sensory impairment.

The dizziness simulation battery is a series of eight bedside maneuvers that have proved valuable in distinguishing the various types of dizziness. Some produce dizziness in all patients, whereas others induce it only in patients with underlying disorders. After each maneuver the patient is questioned as to the similarity of the test-evoked sensation to his own dizziness. Identification of a provoked sensation as identical to the patient's dizziness is often more reliable than a verbal description, particularly if a single maneuver exclusively reproduces his symptoms.

1. *Orthostatic hypotension:* Blood pressure is measured supine, immediately on standing, and after three minutes.
2. *Potentiated Valsalva maneuver:* The patient squats for 30 seconds, then stands and blows into a mercury sphygmomanometer, raising the column to 40 mm Hg for 15 seconds.
3. *Carotid sinus stimulation:* The carotid sinus is unilaterally massaged for 15 seconds without continuous compression of the artery. ECG monitoring is required in the elderly, and the test should be omitted in patients with known cardiac disease.
4. *Neck-twist:* The patient rotates his head in each direction for 15 seconds as if watching an airplane fly past. Dizziness may result from "kinking" of a vertebral artery, cervicogenic dizziness, or a vestibular disorder.
5. *Walking and turning:* The patient walks in one direction and then quickly turns, reversing direction. This test reproduces dizziness occurring with multisensory deficits, gait apraxia, and disorders of balance.
6. *Hyperventilation:* The patient breathes deeply for three minutes.
7. *Nylen-Bárány maneuver:* The examiner carries the patient's head backward from a seated position, so that it is hanging 45 degrees below the horizontal and turned 45 degrees to one side. Vertigo *accompanied by nystagmus* indicates positional vertigo. The characteristics distinguishing a "benign" from a "malignant" form of this condition are listed in Table 1.
8. *Bárány rotation:* The patient is seated in a rotating chair, head tilted 30 degrees forward from the vertical. The examiner spins the patient in one direction ten times within 20 seconds, then abruptly stops the rotation.

Laboratory Tests (Table 2). *Caloric testing* can identify disorders of the labyrinth, vestibular nerve, and central vestibular connections. The patient is positioned so that the horizontal semicircular canals are exactly vertical, and each ear is irrigated with cool (30° C) and warm (44° C) water to produce convection flow of endolymph, which mimics rotational stimulation of each canal. Observations of the amplitude, speed, and duration of the ocular deviation and nystagmus generated by this test provide information on the function of the vestibular apparatus.

Audiometric studies are used to evaluate lesions of the middle ear, labyrinth, and cochlear nerve, particularly in Meniere's disorder and cerebellopontine angle tumors. Routine pure tone audiometry indicates the presence or absence of a hearing loss and may also distinguish banal causes (acoustic trauma, aging, otosclerosis) from specific cochlear and nerve disorders. More elaborate testing, including the short increment sensitivity index

TABLE 1. Positional Vertigo

Benign	Central or Malignant
1. Latency of onset of vertigo and nystagmus	1. Immediate onset of vertigo and nystagmus
2. Adaptation and fatigue of vertigo and nystagmus	2. Persistence of nystagmus
3. Direction-fixed nystagmus	3. Direction-changing nystagmus
4. Severe vertigo and systemic symptoms	4. Mild vertigo; few systemic symptoms

TABLE 2. Laboratory Tests in Dizziness

1. Caloric testing with electronystagmography (ENG)	6. Electrocardiogram with rhythm strip
2. Audiometry	7. Serum protein electrophoresis
3. Psychometric testing (MMPI)	8. Thyroid function studies
4. Skull x-rays with Stenvers' views	9. Electroencephalography
	10. Five-hour glucose tolerance test
5. Cervical spine x-rays	*Optional:* Petrous polytomography
	24-hour cardiac monitoring

(SISI), speech discrimination, Békésy, and threshold tone decay tests, improves the accuracy of diagnosis.

SPECIFIC CONDITIONS PRODUCING DIZZINESS

It is not always simple to assemble the clinical and laboratory findings obtained from a dizzy patient into a specific diagnostic entity. A classification is provided here of the causes of dizziness, designed to parallel the four major complaints described earlier.

Vertigo and Other Vestibular Disorders

Vertigo accounts for only about a third of complaints of dizzy patients. When patients present with vestibular disorders, it is most important to distinguish between *peripheral* (labyrinthine) abnormalities and those involving *central* vestibular connections. The key to this distinction is the evidence for or against involvement of neighboring brainstem structures.

Peripheral Causes of Vertigo. *Benign Positional Vertigo.* Benign positional vertigo is probably the most frequent cause of vertigo, accounting for about 25 per cent of patients with this complaint. The patient experiences a sensation of spinning when he rolls over in bed or makes other sudden head movements. Symptoms are greatest when he lies on his side with the affected ear underneath. The vertigo, sometimes accompanied by nausea and vomiting, lasts for less than five minutes, and between episodes the patient is free of symptoms. This condition, brought about *only* on change of position, differs from other vestibular disorders in which vertigo is increased by head motion but is present at other times as well. Benign positional vertigo occurs at any time during adult years; the cause is usually obscure, although it occasionally follows head trauma. The diagnosis is based on the typical history and on finding the "benign" type of vertigo and nystagmus on performing the Nylen-Bárány maneuver (Table 1). Caloric testing reveals depressed labyrinthine function in one ear in about half the patients. In the majority of cases symptoms persist for several weeks, although bouts may recur over a span of years with prolonged symptom-free intervals. This condition must be distinguished from "malignant positional vertigo" (Table 1), which occurs with lesions (tumors, infarcts) involving posterior fossa structures; benign positional vertigo is only rarely associated with such conditions.

Acute Peripheral Vestibulopathy ("Acute Labyrinthitis"; "Vestibular Neuronitis"). This condition is defined as a single bout of spontaneous vertigo, lasting for hours or days. Attacks occasionally follow a trivial respiratory or other infection, but the relation is not clear. Symptoms of vertigo, nausea, and vomiting usually improve within 48 hours, but may persist for 7 to 14 days. On examination the patient appears acutely ill, often pale and diaphoretic, resisting motion of the head. Nystagmus invariably accompanies the vertigo. As the patient recovers, he may feel "off balance" for weeks or months owing to unilateral impairment of vestibular function, present in about 50 per cent of patients. Hearing is not impaired in this condition.

Acute and Recurrent Peripheral Vestibulopathy. Acute and recurrent peripheral vestibulopathy is clinically similar to the entity described above, but consists of *repeated* bouts of vertigo occurring over a period of months or years. This condition occurs in an older age group than acute peripheral vestibulopathy, and is associated with *less* severe vestibular impairment on caloric testing. Approximately half the patients presenting with a single attack of peripheral vestibulopathy experience a recurrence, linking this with the previous condition. The absence of auditory impairment distinguishes this condition from Meniere's disorder.

Meniere's Disorder. Meniere's disorder is widely considered to be one of the most frequent causes of dizziness, but it actually accounts for only about 5 per cent of all dizziness and 10 to 15 per cent of vertigo. It usually occurs in adults and consists of recurring bouts of vertigo associated with *hearing loss* and *tinnitus* which may precede or follow the first bout of vertigo. Patients often complain of "fullness" in the ears, and are sometimes aware of *recruitment* as a sensation of auditory discomfort produced by loud noises. Bouts of vertigo last from hours to days, recurring as often as every week or as infrequently as every ten years. Hearing loss is unilateral in 80 to 90 per cent of patients, with a severe deficit in half the patients. Most patients develop chronic impairment of vestibular function, resulting in the syndrome of vestibular imbalance. In many patients the recurrent episodes of vertigo may "burn out" over the years.

Diagnosis depends on the characteristic history and the audiometric findings (low frequency pure tone impairment, poor speech discrimination comparable to the pure tone hearing loss, and recruitment). Caloric testing demonstrates abnormal vestibular function in 80 per cent of patients.

Pathologic studies have identified distention of the membranous labyrinth with endolymph as the immediate cause of this condition, but the explanation for the excess of endolymph remains obscure.

Toxic Damage to the Labyrinths. Drugs of the aminoglycoside group (e.g., streptomycin) may produce toxic damage to the labyrinths and possibly the eighth nerve. Although toxicity is generally dose related, some patients develop labyrinthine damage after brief treatment with ordinary doses of these drugs, particularly if renal function is impaired. Tinnitus, hearing loss, or vertigo may be the presenting symptom, along with severe impairment of balance, nausea, and vomiting. Vertigo continues for days or weeks. If the ototoxic drug is immediately discontinued, damage to the labyrinth is usually arrested. A characteristic loss of balance follows the acute stage of vertigo and may include blurring of vision on motion owing to loss of the vestibulo-ocular reflexes. With the loss of vestibular sensation, these patients are dependent on visual cues and are unable to walk in the dark. After several months, adaptation to the loss of vestibular sensation develops, and many can lead fairly normal lives.

Diagnosis is based on the history of treatment with one of the ototoxic drugs, followed by the sequence described above. On examination the Romberg test is abnormal. Caloric tests demonstrate bilateral severe hypoactivity of the labyrinths. Bárány rotation may fail to elicit vertigo or nystagmus.

Other Peripheral Causes of Vertigo. Head trauma may be followed by persistent or positional vertigo. Dislocation of the otoliths from the macula of the utricle has been proposed as a cause of this condition. When vertigo immediately follows trauma, the etiologic relationship is clear, but in cases with medicolegal implications vertigo (and other forms of dizziness) may follow head trauma after a lengthy delay. It is often stated that the termination of pending litigation resolves such cases. *Cervicogenic vertigo,* although not vestibular in origin, may present with similar manifestations. Since the articulations and musculature of the cervical region provide extensive input to the brainstem vestibular system, cervical spondylosis or even painful muscular contraction may result in vertigo, nausea, and vomiting. *Dysproteinemias, hypothyroidism,* and *otitis media* are other occasional causes of vertigo.

Treatment. Management of vertigo resulting from most peripheral vestibular disorders is similar. When vertigo is severely disabling, the patient should be placed at bed rest or, in persistent cases, hospitalized. Meclizine, 25 mg four times daily, is of value in suppressing labyrinthine hyperactivity. Atropine tablets, 0.4 mg sublingually at the onset of attacks of vertigo, may abort the development of symptoms. Nausea and vomiting are controlled by trimethobenzamide hydrochloride (Tigan) suppositories, 200 mg every six hours, or in resistant cases by parenteral phenothiazines such as chlorpromazine (Thorazine), 25 mg every six hours. Mild tranquilizers such as diazepam (Valium), 5 mg orally, help control the anxiety that often accompanies vertigo.

Patients with benign positional vertigo may benefit from a soft foam rubber collar that limits cervical motion, thus preventing the stimulus for attacks.

Many patients with peripheral vestibular disorders have residual labyrinthine deficits after the acute vertiginous phase, and benefit from measures to improve their balance. A foam rubber collar is useful to limit neck motion, and methylphenidate (Ritalin) may enable them to react more quickly to the remaining sensory modalities. Balancing exercises help patients to adapt to ambulation in the absence of normal vestibular function.

The treatment of acute attacks of Meniere's disorder is similar to that for other vestibular disorders. A variety of medical and surgical treatments to prevent recurrences of vertigo and/or deterioration of hearing have been proposed; a discussion of their application and merits is beyond the scope of this chapter.

Central Causes of Vertigo. *Cerebrovascular Disease.* Cerebrovascular disease produces vertigo when basilar-vertebral artery ischemia damages the vestibular nuclei or their connections. In virtually all cases injury to adjacent brainstem structures occurs, and vertigo is unlikely to be due to a stroke when other neurologic symptoms or signs are absent. As with other patterns of cerebrovascular disease, elderly hypertensive patients with diabetes, heart disease, or hyperlipidemia are the most likely candidates. Caloric testing may help in the diagnosis by providing evidence of central vestibular involvement.

Transient ischemic attacks may be particularly difficult to diagnose, because at the time of examination the patient may have recovered completely. A reliable history of additional brainstem symptoms is necessary to establish the diagnosis.

The treatment of cerebrovascular disease is discussed in detail elsewhere. Transient ischemia in the basilar-vertebral distribution is a recognized indication for anticoagulation. The role of aspirin, dipyridamole (Persantine) and other agents that affect platelet function is not yet firmly established, but a trial of these relatively safe agents may be justified in those patients in whom differentiation of brainstem ischemia from peripheral vestibulopathy is uncertain.

Multiple Sclerosis. Multiple sclerosis may produce vertigo in young patients, although this condition accounts for no more than 5 to 10 per cent of acute vertigo in those below age 40. Further, although multiple sclerosis may begin with vertigo, this is far less common than onset with optic neuritis or paresthesias. The diagnosis is discussed elsewhere; one must be aware that vertigo associated with ocular motor disorders that cannot be caused by purely peripheral vestibular disease (e.g., persistent diplopia, median longitudinal fasciculus syndrome, ophthalmoplegia) is strongly suggestive of this condition.

Treatment of the vertigo is similar to that for peripheral vestibulopathies; meclizine, atropine, and Tigan are of value in controlling the vertigo and its associated nausea and vomiting.

Cerebellopontine Angle Tumors. Cerebellopontine angle tumors are a *rare* cause of vertigo, but must not be overlooked early in their growth when they are readily removable. The large majority are benign acoustic neuromas arising in the internal auditory meatus. These tumors develop in middle-aged patients who experience vague unsteadiness that progresses over a period of years. Vertigo when present may be of the "malignant" positional type (Table 1), and only rarely does acute spontaneous vertigo occur. Hearing loss, tinnitus, facial numbness or weakness, cerebellar ataxia, and occasional dementia complete the picture. Unilateral or bilateral acoustic neuromas are especially common in von Recklinghausen's disease (neurofibromatosis).

On caloric testing there is a markedly diminished response on the affected side. Audiometry demonstrates the findings of a "retrocochlear" lesion, including rapid tone decay and a Type III or IV curve on Békésy audiometry. Roentgenograms of the petrous bones are diagnostic and show erosion of the affected internal auditory meatus, a finding that is seen even earlier on polycyclic tomography.

Vertiginous Migraine. Vertiginous migraine may occur preceding the headache, during the headache phase, or as a "migraine equivalent" in place of the headache. Since both migraine and vertigo are common conditions, the occurrence of vertigo without a constant time relation to headache may represent only a coincidence in some unfortunate patients. Treatment is directed at prevention of the migraine attacks and control of the symptoms of vertigo, nausea, and vomiting as outlined above.

Viral Infections. Viral infections rarely cause vertigo except when herpes zoster affects the eighth nerve, often in conjunction with the Ramsay Hunt syndrome or geniculate herpes. Facial paralysis, vertigo, and hearing loss occur with herpetic vesicular lesions in the external auditory canal. Lymphocytes and polymorphonuclear leukocytes may be found in the cerebrospinal fluid. The diagnosis is established by demonstrating a rise of antibody titers to herpes zoster. Pathologically, lymphocytic infiltration of the sensory ganglia and nerve roots is seen. Treatment consists of the use of prednisone during the acute phase of the illness and the management of the vertigo, nausea, and vomiting as outlined above.

Vestibular Disorders Not Producing Vertigo. In some patients *hypoactivity* of the labyrinths may occur without antecedent episodes of vertigo. These patients describe lightheadedness on walking, turning, or changing position. The exact cause of the conditions producing these disorders is obscure. With *hyperactive* labyrinths, most often seen in anxious patients, instantaneous vertigo or loss of balance occurs on rapid turning. Caloric testing confirms the abnormal responsiveness of the labyrinths in either case. Patients with hypoactive or asymmetrical labyrinthine function benefit from methylphenidate (Ritalin), head restraint with a foam rubber collar, and a course of balancing exercises. Patients with hyperactive labyrinths are treated with meclizine, 25 mg three times daily.

Faintness: Syncopal and Seizure Disorders

Syncopal Disorders (see also Ch. 353). ***Orthostatic Hypotension.*** In orthostatic hypotension the patient experiences faintness upon standing, resulting from a fall in blood pressure (at least 25/15 mm Hg). Acquired and idiopathic varieties are described. In the closely related Shy-Drager syndrome (see Ch. 377), manifestations of parkinsonism, peripheral neuropathy, dementia, and cerebellar abnormalities contribute to a multifactorial problem of dizziness.

Cardiac Arrhythmias. Patients with brief dizziness caused by episodic cardiac arrhythmias are often unaware of palpitations and complain only of faintness. When the arrhythmia is constantly present, it is easily recognized by auscultation or electrocardiography. With infrequent runs of abnormal heart rhythm, the use of 12- or 24-hour ambulatory electrocardiographic monitoring is necessary.

Carotid Sinus Hypersensitivity. Carotid sinus hypersensitivity resulting in bradycardia or temporary asystole may also present with Type II dizziness. The dizziness occurs abruptly and disappears rapidly, lasting no more than 15 seconds. The diagnosis is established by reproduction of symptoms with cautious carotid massage.

Vasovagal Syncope. Vasovagal syncope causes confusion with other forms of dizziness when the patient experiences faintness rather than actual loss of consciousness. The tendency to occur in young adults, the relation to precipitating emotional factors, the appearance of pallor at the onset, and the short duration are characteristic.

Cough, Micturition Syncope. Some patients experience faintness upon coughing or, with males, upon micturating while standing. The exact temporal relationship of faintness (or loss of consciousness) to these acts is diagnostic; the reproduction of symptoms by a potentiated Valsalva maneuver confirms the mechanism.

Seizure Disorders. Patients with temporal lobe seizures may describe feelings of "remoteness," "unreality," or, rarely, vertigo. When these events precede a typical psychomotor or generalized seizure, the cause is clearly *epileptic dizziness.* When the dizziness occurs as an isolated seizure phenomenon, it presents a diagnostic problem. Such patients *rarely* complain primarily of dizziness, however, because the epileptic phenomena dominate the picture.

Very rarely labyrinthine-induced vertigo may trigger "vestibulogenic epilepsy," a form of reflex seizure akin to reading epilepsy. If caloric testing is carried out while an electroencephalogram is taken, the observation of induced seizure activity establishes the diagnosis.

The reader is cautioned against diagnosing seizure disorders in patients whose dizziness is accompanied by mild abnormalities on electroencephalography without the other criteria mentioned.

Dysequilibrium: Impaired Balance

Bruns' Apraxia of Gait. This is a little-recognized but common disorder of the elderly. The patient walks with a broad-based gait, taking short steps and placing his feet flat on the ground, suggesting a person walking on ice. A tendency to retropulsion increases the danger of falling. On examination, motor power, coordination, and sensation are normal in the legs, although the gait is impaired and hopping on one foot is impossible. The finding of "frontal lobe" deficits, including dementia, grasp and suck reflexes is confirmatory. Most cases of Bruns' apraxia result from a degenerative process similar to Alzheimer's disease. Other causes include such conditions as subdural hematomas, tumors, normal pressure hydrocephalus, or a lacunar state.

When a specific disorder (e.g., a subdural hematoma) is found, treatment is directed toward that condition. In the more common degenerative conditions treatment must be symptomatic. In some patients surprisingly good improvement may result from small doses of L-dopa (1.5 to 3.0 grams per day in divided doses). Mild stimulants (methylphenidate), balancing exercises, and a cane are of benefit, and patients should be encouraged to walk some distance *every day* to avoid lapsing into total dependence.

Parkinsonism. It is not uncommon for patients with parkinsonism and a balance disturbance to complain of dysequilibrium. When tremor is minimal and impaired balance is prominent, it is difficult to distinguish between parkinsonism and gait apraxia. These patients often have a pronounced increase in axial tone, as well as frontal lobe signs and dementia. Treatment is described in Ch. 365.

Cerebellar Lesions. Impairment of balance without other cerebellar signs may be seen in certain cerebellar lesions such as alcoholic cerebellar degeneration or tumors of the vermis. In addition some patients may develop "malignant" positional vertigo. Since a staggering gait and nystagmus are seen in peripheral vestibular disorders, the clinical distinction presents difficulties. Neurodiagnostic studies (radioisotope scan, computerized axial tomography, angiography) may be required to establish the diagnosis.

Astasia-Abasia. Astasia-abasia is impairment of stance and gait on a purely psychiatric basis. In some patients the gait is quite bizarre, but in others it may resemble Bruns' apraxia. The distinction depends on the absence of other frontal lobe signs and on the ability of the patient to walk *normally* under some circumstances, such as only indoors. Other evidence of a phobic or conversion reaction is often present.

Lightheadedness

Vague "lightheadedness" accounts for over 50 per cent of patients' complaints, and includes the largest spectrum of disorders.

Inevitably, some patients provide a *poor description of other types of dizziness* which more introspective or articulate patients would recognize as vertigo, faintness, or dysequilibrium. In addition, *fractional forms of other types of dizziness* are often described as "lightheadedness" even by observant patients. Almost half the patients who initially experience vertigo later complain of lightheadedness as their symptoms subside. The dizziness simulation battery helps to *identify* a sensation which the patient cannot easily *describe* verbally.

Hyperventilation. This is the second most common cause of dizziness after vestibular disorders, and the most common under the age of 40. The disorder is discussed in detail in Ch. 354. In the acute form, young, anxious patients present with brief episodes of shortness of breath, lightheadedness, paresthesias in the fingers and around the mouth, and feelings of panic. More difficult to identify is chronic hyperventilation, seen in patients who periodically sigh deeply. Both forms are recognized by the precise reproduction of symptoms during intentional hyperventilation, but no other maneuver in the dizziness simulation battery reproduces the complaint.

The mechanism of hyperventilation-induced dizziness is presumed to be hypocapnia with secondary cerebral arterial constriction and diminished cerebral blood flow. Treatment of acute attacks with diazepam (Valium), 5 to 10 mg intramuscularly, is often effective.

Multisensory Dizziness. When several sensory modalities are impaired, perception of the environment becomes inadequate to maintain orientation, and the patient experiences dizziness when attempting to walk. The most common combinations of sensory impairment are peripheral neuropathy (with diminished touch, pressure, and proprioceptive sensation), visual loss from cataracts, and cervical spondylosis (with distortion of proprioception from cervical joints). Impaired vestibular and auditory function often add to the sensory disorientation. The aged and diabetic are especially prone to this condition. Patients with multisensory dizziness adopt a broad-based tentative gait, which may superficially resemble Bruns' apraxia of gait, but the "frontal lobe" features are absent. Examination reveals the underlying neurosensory deficit—peripheral neuropathy, visual impairment, cervical arthritis, and hearing loss. Caloric testing may provide evidence of additional sensory impairment. When all five sensory modalities are severely impaired, patients may be unable to walk without assistance.

An important example of this condition is seen in the post-cataract-extraction patient who complains of disabling dizziness despite perfect restoration of visual acuity. Dizziness results from the distortion produced by the corrective lenses used after surgery. Patients who have no other sensory deficits are able to compensate for the visual distortions, but those with peripheral neuropathy cannot. Contact lenses eliminate these distortions, but unfortunately many elderly patients cannot manage them.

Treatment of multisensory dizziness includes balancing exercises and use of a foam rubber collar to eliminate extraneous head motion. A light cane should be used for balance. Methylphenidate (Ritalin) improves the speed of the patient's response to his perceived environment.

Psychiatric Disorders. In addition to patients with astasia-abasia or hyperventilation, some patients experience subjective dizziness on the basis of purely psychiatric disease. Some indicate that their dizziness consists of "difficulty concentrating"; others experience panic states when in crowded places; whereas some frankly psychotic patients describe the bizarre confusion of their perceived environments as "dizziness" for lack of a more explicit term.

In these patients, the diagnosis hinges on elimination of other causes of dizziness combined with evidence of significant psychiatric disease on interview or psychometric testing. It is often useful to demonstrate to such patients the negative findings on extensive tests for organic causes of dizziness, and to assure them that no cause has been overlooked.

Drachman, D. A.: Episodic vertigo. *In* Conn, H. (ed.): Current Therapy 1974. Philadelphia, W. B. Saunders Company, 1974, p. 684.

Drachman, D. A., and Hart, C. W.: An approach to the dizzy patient. Neurology, 22:323, 1972.

Fisher, C. M.: Vertigo in cerebrovascular disease. Arch. Otolaryngol., 85:529, 1967.

Harrison, M. S., and Ozsahinoglu, C.: Positional vertigo: Aetiology and clinical significance. Brain, 95:369, 1972.

Hart, C. W.: The evaluation of vestibular function in health and disease. *In* Otolaryngology. Vol. 1, Chap. 10. Hagerstown, Md., Harper & Row, 1972.

Pulec, J. (ed.): Meniere's Disease. Philadelphia, W. B. Saunders Company, 1968.

353. SYNCOPE

Albert Heyman

Definition. Syncope is the cutting off or transient loss of consciousness. Although the term is usually applied to unconsciousness caused by a temporary decrease in cerebral blood flow, in this discussion a broader definition is employed that includes the brief disturbances in consciousness caused by changes in the chemical composition of the blood as in hyperventilation or hypoglycemia. Syncope is extremely common; in fact, it has been found to occur in as many as 25 to 30 per cent of young, healthy adult males. It should be carefully differentiated from such disorders as epilepsy, vertigo, cataplexy, and strokes, all of which may produce transient disturbances in consciousness, generalized weakness, or inability to stand erect. The loss of consciousness in syncope may not be complete, but may consist of varying degrees of impaired sensorium with transient blurring of vision, weakness, and loss of postural tone. Such attacks may be described by the patient as dizziness, faintness, lightheadedness, or a "drunk feeling." These partial manifestations have the rapid onset, brief duration, and complete recovery characteristic of the fully developed faint.

Pathogenesis. Syncope is most frequently caused by a reduction in cerebral blood flow below a critical level and is usually associated with a sharp fall in blood pressure. This, in turn, is the result of either a loss of peripheral resistance, as seen in vasodepressor faint and in orthostatic hypotension, or a decrease in cardiac output, as in Adams-Stokes attacks. In many patients, however, loss of consciousness is not caused by reduction of blood pressure but by a decrease in such essential blood components as glucose, carbon dioxide, or oxygen. In other instances, as in micturition syncope and cough syncope, the faint seems to result from cerebral ischemia caused by extracardiac disturbances.

There are several features common to almost all types of syncope. Electroencephalographic changes usually appear, and consist of high voltage, 2- to 4-cycle per second slow waves that promptly return to normal after consciousness is regained. Convulsive movements, such as tonic or clonic contractions of the arms or turning of the head, can occur in all types of fainting, depending on the degree and duration of the cerebral ischemia. Fully developed seizures with tongue biting and urinary incontinence, however, are unusual. Recovery is usually hastened in the recumbent posture, which helps restore the normal cerebral circulation. The critical level of cerebral blood flow necessary to maintain consciousness has been estimated to be about 30 ml per 100 grams of brain per minute (normal value is 50 to 55 ml). The duration of asystole or the degree of hypotension necessary to produce critical levels of cerebral ischemia varies, depending upon the posture of the patient, the ability of the cerebral vessels to dilate, and other factors. In normal subjects in the erect posture, a mean arterial blood pressure as low as 20 to 30 mm of mercury or an asystole of four or five seconds' duration is necessary to produce syncope. In the recumbent position, longer periods of asystole may occur before loss of consciousness develops.

Clinical Manifestations. *Orthostatic Hypotension.* Chronic orthostatic hypotension is a disorder of the autonomic nervous system in which syncope occurs when the patient assumes the upright posture. The condition is sometimes seen in diabetic neuropathy and in tabes dorsalis, but in many patients the site of the neurologic lesion is unknown. These people have an abnormality in the baroreceptor reflexes that ordinarily compensates for the pooling of blood in the lower extremities and viscera. When an attempt is made to stand upright, there is an inadequate degree of reflex arteriolar constriction, with a subsequent reduction in venous return. This is associated with an immediate and sharp fall in arterial blood pressure, followed by syncope. The pulse rate remains unchanged during the episode, and there are none of the usual prodromal symptoms of pallor, sweating, and nausea seen in vasodepressor faint. These patients have subnormal values for urinary catecholamines and may have other evidence of autonomic insufficiency such as impotence, bladder disturbances, and loss of sweating in the lower trunk. Orthostatic hypotension has also been associated with a Parkinson-like disorder sometimes referred to as the Shy-Drager syndrome (see Ch. 377).

A new syndrome of orthostatic hypotension known as hyperbradykininism has been reported, in which standing produces a fall in systolic blood pressure, an increase in diastolic pressure and heart rate, and purplish discoloration and ecchymoses over the legs. The disorder is characterized by high plasma levels of bradykinin, which may account for dilatation of the cutaneous venules and capillaries in the legs and reduction in venous return.

Failure of postural adaptation may appear after surgical sympathectomy for hypertension or the administration of vasodilating agents and antihypertensive drugs, especially the sodium-depleting diuretics and ganglionic blocking agents. Syncope has also been noted in patients treated with L-dopa for Parkinson's disease. Patients recovering from chronic wasting illnesses associated with prolonged bed rest may experience syncope when they attempt to assume the upright position. Shorter periods of bed rest, particularly when associated with dehydration or electrolyte deficits, may also be associated with orthostatic hypotension.

Vasodepressor Syncope (the Common Faint). Vasodepressor syncope is by far the most frequent cause of transient loss of consciousness. The condition is characterized by a fall in blood pressure associated with the development of a variety of autonomic manifestations. In the early presyncopal period, there may be pallor, nausea, and sweating; in later stages pupillary dilatation, yawning, hyperpnea, and bradycardia appear. When the mean arterial pressure falls below critical levels, loss of consciousness and characteristic electroencephalographic changes occur. Bradycardia is often severe at the onset of unconsciousness, and pulse rates of 50 to 60 per minute may be observed even after recovery. The duration of syncope is brief, ranging from a few seconds to several minutes. In the postsyncopal period the patient may complain of headaches, weakness, nervousness, and slight confusion. Vasodepressor faint is most often evoked by sudden emotional stress associated with fear, anxiety, or pain. Hypodermic injections, trauma, minor surgery, and the sight of or withdrawal of blood are common precipitating events. Attacks usually occur in the standing or upright posture, and consciousness returns quickly once the patient is recumbent.

The initial event in this complex vascular and neurogenic reaction is dilatation of the vascular bed throughout the body, particularly in peripheral muscles. Vasodilatation in the limb muscles is a normal response to emotional stimuli, and is thought to represent preparation for "fight or flight." The absence of immediate muscle activity, however, and the fall in peripheral resistance are not compensated for by an increase in cardiac output, and as a result there is a reduction in cerebral blood flow.

Adams-Stokes Syndrome. In the early nineteenth century Morgagni, Adams, and Stokes separately observed and described fainting associated with a persistently slow pulse in the range of 40 per minute. Patients with this syndrome usually have a disordered atrioventricular conduction system, secondary to coronary atherosclerosis. In most instances, the loss of consciousness occurs during the changes in rhythm when there may be asystole, ventricular fibrillation, or tachycardia, or a combination of these arrhythmias. Occasionally sudden death results from cardiac standstill. A rare form of syncope caused by ventricular fibrillation has been reported in children with hereditary prolongation of QT interval in the electrocardiogram, sometimes associated with congenital deafness. The clinical picture of syncope caused by cardiac arrhythmias is often characteristic. Loss of consciousness is abrupt; prodromal signs are not usually present. On regaining consciousness, the patient usually shows little confusion or postsyncopal residua. The attacks may occur several times a day and have no relation to posture or activity. Only a brief period of asystole of four or five seconds' duration will produce loss of consciousness in the erect position, but longer periods of asystole are not uncommon. In such instances, neurologic manifestations such as convulsive movements, pupillary dilatation, and prolonged confusion may be observed. The use of radiotelemetered electrocardiographic tape systems has led to more accurate diagnosis of syncope caused by Adams-Stokes attacks. Such monitoring systems, recorded over periods of 10 to 20 hours, give the frequency and nature of the cardiac arrhythmia during the patient's full activity and provide a firm basis for definitive treatment such as implantation of an intracardiac pacemaker.

Reflex Cardiac Standstill. Syncopal attacks may result from cessation of cardiac action in persons without heart disease. In such individuals, the mechanism for cardiac standstill arises from vagal reflex activity. In a few authenticated cases, swallowing or experimental distention of the esophagus with a balloon has induced complete atrioventricular block and syncope. The alterations in consciousness and electrocardiographic changes disappear when the pressure within the esophagus is relieved or after administration of atropine. The syncopal episode occasionally seen during digital prostatic examination, thoracentesis, or bronchoscopic examination may also be due to such a reflex mechanism. Syncope caused by cardiac arrest has been observed in patients with paroxysmal pain in the throat caused by glossopharyngeal neuralgia.

Carotid Sinus Syncope. In relatively few patients this is the mechanism of syncope. Many persons, particularly those more than 60 years of age, show reflex slowing of the heart and fall of blood pressure during massage of one or both carotid sinuses. Such responses are also seen frequently in patients with cardiac disorders, hypertension, or diseases of the carotid vessels such as atherosclerotic thrombosis or stenosis. The most common response to carotid sinus massage is either sinus bradycardia or sinoatrial block, both of which may be abolished by administration of atropine. Much less frequently, there may be a pure vasodepressor response without slowing of the heart. In a third but rare type of carotid response, fainting may appear in a few seconds without significant changes in either blood pressure or pulse; such instances probably occur only with vigorous pressure and when the opposite carotid is already thrombosed. Carotid sinus syncope is not accompanied by the prodromal symptoms seen in the common faint (nausea, sweating, pallor). It is more frequent in men, and usually occurs in the erect posture. It sometimes follows sudden head turning or pressure of a tight collar.

Only very few of the patients who exhibit bradycardia or a reduction in blood pressure on carotid massage experience loss of consciousness caused by these factors. In eliciting carotid sinus responses, care should be taken to avoid obstructing blood flow to the brain by compression of the carotid vessels. Cerebral infarction and even death have been reported after carotid compression and massage. Massage of both carotid sinuses simultaneously may be hazardous.

Organic Heart Disease. Patients with myocardial infarction or valvular lesions may also have transient periods of unconsciousness. The mechanism of syncope in these disorders is not altogether clear, but may be related to a reduction in cardiac output with inadequate cerebral blood flow. In acute myocardial infarction, fainting probably results from decrease in stroke volume owing to a weakened myocardium. Transient arrhythmias, such as ventricular tachycardia, fibrillation, or heart block, may contribute to the syncopal reaction. Transient loss of consciousness may occur during attacks of angina pectoris, and is probably caused by ventricular fibrillation or various types of heart block associated with temporary periods of myocardial ischemia. Syncope also appears during paroxysmal tachycardia even in the absence of structural heart disease. In such cases the loss of consciousness usually occurs at the onset or at the end of the attack, at which time there may be a brief period of cardiac standstill.

Patients with aortic valvular or subvalvular stenosis often have syncope associated with physical exertion (effort syncope). The loss of consciousness in the early phases of such syncopal episodes may be due to shunting of blood to the peripheral muscles, but the later phases have been shown to be associated with transient ventricular asystole, tachycardia, or fibrillation, presumably caused by diminished coronary arterial blood flow. Sudden death may occur during these attacks. Effort syncope is also seen in patients with congenital heart disease such as patent ductus arteriosus or tetralogy of Fallot, as well as in those with pulmonary hypertension or atrial myxoma.

Cough Syncope. Cough syncope usually follows a paroxysm of explosive and vigorous coughing. It is commonly observed in men but rarely in women. In adults, the condition is often associated with chronic lung disease or bronchitis; in children, it may occur during severe pertussis. The syncope is brief, and there are no postsyncopal residua. The condition has also been described following hearty laughter. The loss of consciousness has been attributed to an increase in the intrathoracic and intra-abdominal pressure caused by vigorous coughing. This, in turn, is thought to produce a sudden sharp elevation in cerebrospinal fluid pressure, thereby "squeezing" blood from the intracranial and cerebral vessels. Other theories maintain that the condition is due to a Valsalva effect with reduction in cardiac output or to cerebral "concussive effect" caused by rapid rise in the cerebrospinal fluid pressure. There is clinical evidence to suggest that the presence of an intracerebral lesion such as brain tumor or stenosis of a major cerebral artery may produce increased susceptibility to syncope after paroxysms of cough. Such cases may have focal neurologic symptoms such as paresthesias or clonic movements of one limb prior to loss of consciousness.

Micturition Syncope. This form of syncope is most often seen during or immediately after micturition in men who rise in the middle of the night to urinate. The loss of consciousness is brief and there is no postsyncopal confusion or weakness. Many such people give a history of drinking large quantities of beer before retiring, and considerable bladder deflation may take place during micturition. A similar fainting may be observed after drainage of a distended bladder in urinary retention or after removal of a large quantity of ascitic fluid by abdominal paracentesis. It has been suggested that the loss of consciousness may be due to a reflex vasodilatation of the peripheral vascular system, a situation thought to be the converse of the paroxysmal hypertension seen in paraplegics during bladder distention. It is not likely to be due to a Valsalva maneuver during micturition but may be related to peripheral vasodilation associated with a warm bed and perhaps the recent consumption of alcohol.

Hysterical Fainting. Hysterical fainting is seen almost entirely in young women with emotional illness. It differs from the vasodepressor faint and the hyperventilation syndrome in that the patient is relatively free of anxiety and shows little concern regarding the fainting episodes. The attack usually occurs in the presence of others. The patient generally slumps to the floor gracefully, sometimes dramatically, without injury or awkwardness. It thus resembles the mid-Victorian drawing-room swoon. In earlier decades, hysterical fainting often occurred in groups of young women during mass excitement, particularly that caused by the presence of screen or television idols. Although unusual behavior is now often observed among young women attending "rock" concerts, swooning is seldom seen.

During the attack the patient may be motionless or may show bizarre resisting movements. The attack may last from several minutes to as long as an hour or more, with fluctuations of responsiveness. There are no abnormalities in pulse, blood pressure, or skin color. The electroencephalogram is normal during the attack, indicating that there may be no actual loss of consciousness. The diagnosis can usually be made without difficulty on the basis of the setting of the episode, the patient's underlying emotional disturbance, and the absence of physical abnormalities.

Cerebral Arterial Occlusive Disease. Patients with generalized atherosclerosis may have frequent episodes of loss of consciousness over a period of days or weeks. In most instances the attack is accompanied by signs of focal neurologic deficits such as motor weakness, sensory loss, or cranial nerve disorders. In such cases the diagnosis can be made without difficulty. Occasionally, however, the patient has no localizing symptoms, and complains of vague dizziness, weakness, and visual disturbances. Many such patients are in the older age group and have evidence of hypertensive disease with coronary or cerebrovascular involvement. These cases of "blind staggers" are difficult to categorize, and a definite diagnosis often cannot be made. The symptoms are probably related to postural disturbance associated with vascular or labyrinthine disease.

Hypoglycemia. Low levels of blood sugar often produce symptoms of weakness, trembling, sweating, tachycardia, hunger sensation, and confused behavior. Syncope is not a common occurrence, but prolonged hypoglycemia may result in seizures, coma, and serious brain damage. The majority of patients with these symptoms have anxiety reaction rather than hypoglycemia. The diagnosis of hypoglycemia must therefore be based on documented low levels of blood sugar at the time of the clinical manifestations which, in turn, can be relieved by ingestion of food or sugar. It is also important that the type of hypoglycemia be established. Reactive hypoglycemia is the most common type and may appear in thin, emotionally tense persons a few hours after ingestion of a high carbohydrate meal. It sometimes follows extensive gastric resection in association with the dumping syndrome and occurs in some people with mild diabetes. Hypoglycemia may also be due to islet cell adenoma of the pancreas. In this condition, nervousness, weakness, trembling, and sometimes convulsions occur after fasting and exercise. The fasting morning blood sugar level may be low, in contrast to that of patients with reactive hypoglycemia, in whom this determination is usually normal. Other conditions such as pituitary insufficiency, Addison's disease, hepatic failure, and large sarcomas may also produce hypoglycemia.

Diagnosis. The diagnosis of syncope depends almost entirely upon a careful history of the attack and the setting in which it occurs. Differentiation of syncope from an akinetic epileptic seizure, such as a petit mal or psychomotor attack, may be difficult. Careful evaluation of the electroencephalographic findings, the onset and duration of the attack, and the postsyncopal manifestations can usually distinguish these conditions. These factors are also helpful in differentiating the various types of syncope. In vasodepressor faint, the patient usually has prodromal signs of autonomic hyperactivity such as pallor, sweating, salivation, and bradycardia. In cardiac arrest, orthostatic hypotension, and carotid sinus syncope, loss of consciousness occurs abruptly, and prodromal symptoms are not usually present. Postsyncopal confusion, headache, and weakness often follow vasodepressor faint and the hyperventilation syndrome. In chronic orthostatic hypotension and Adams-Stokes attacks, recovery of consciousness is rapid and complete without postsyncopal symptoms. Most types of fainting occur in the erect or upright position, but in cardiac arrest, syncope may appear while the patient is recumbent. The duration of syncope is brief in postural hypotension but prolonged in hyperventilation and hypoglycemia. Most of these differentiating manifestations can be determined by careful history, but special methods of examination may be necessary. These consist of voluntary hyperventilation for approximately two minutes, massage of the carotid sinuses, and observations of pulse and blood pressure during change in posture from recumbency to erect position. An electroencephalogram is indicated whenever convulsive movements develop during the syncopal episode or when focal neurologic symptoms are noted before or after loss of consciousness. An electrocardiogram and blood sugar levels may also be necessary to arrive at a correct diagnosis.

Treatment. Therapy in syncope consists primarily of treatment of the underlying disorder. In all types of fainting, recovery is usually aided by maintaining the patient in a recumbent position with elevation of the lower extremities. Application of cold water to the face and head and inhalation of spirits of ammonia or other pungent aromatics are time-honored and certainly do no harm.

Ad Hoc Committee on Hypoglycemia: Statement on hypoglycemia. Arch. Intern. Med., 131:591, 1973.
Ebert, R. V.: Syncope. Circulation, 27:1148, 1963.
Engel, G. L.: Fainting. 2nd ed. Springfield, Ill., Charles C Thomas, 1962.
Hedeland, H., Dymling, J.-F., and Hokfelt, B.: Catecholamines, renin and aldosterone in postural hypotension. Acta Endocrinol. (Kbh.), 62:399, 1969.
Pedersen, A., Sandoe, E., Hvidberg, E., and Schwartz, M.: Studies on the mechanism of tussive syncope. Acta Med. Scand., 179:653, 1966.
Thomas, J. E.: Hyperactive carotid sinus reflex and carotid sinus syncope. Mayo Clin. Proc., 44:127, 1969.
Weissler, A. M., and Warren, J. V.: Vasodepressor syncope. Am. Heart J., 57:786, 1959.

354. HYPERVENTILATION

Albert Heyman

Hyperventilation Syndrome. The hyperventilation syndrome is one of the most frequent causes of impaired consciousness, usually producing "faintness" and "lightheadedness" without actual syncope. It is almost always a manifestation of acute anxiety. At the onset of an attack, the patient may complain of tightness of the chest and a feeling of suffocation. He may not be aware of overbreathing but usually recalls excessive deep sighing. Later, a sense of unreality develops, accompanied by feelings of apprehension and sometimes panic. Symptoms related to the heart and gastrointestinal tract often appear. These consist of palpitations or pounding of the heart, precordial oppression, fullness in the throat, and epigastric discomfort. The syndrome may last for as long as a half hour or more and may recur several times a day. Sensations of "numbness" and "coldness" of the hands, feet, and perioral areas often develop, and in prolonged attacks tetany with carpopedal spasm may be noted.

The pathogenesis of the individual symptoms of this disorder is not altogether clear. With normal subjects, hyperventilation in the recumbent posture for as long as an hour will not produce loss of consciousness. They may, however, have sensations of decreased awareness, lightheadedness, and blurring of vision, but do not have the trembling, sweating, palpitations, or precordial distress frequently seen in patients with spontaneous overventilation. The high voltage slow wave activity in the electroencephalogram produced by hyperventilation can be prevented by hyperbaric oxygenation, suggesting that these EEG changes, and probably the alterations in consciousness as well, are due to cerebral hypoxia. The serum calcium level remains normal, but there is often a decrease in serum phosphate within 15 minutes after hyperventilation begins. The hypocapnia caused by overventilation results in cerebral vasoconstriction and sometimes a fall in blood pressure owing to muscle vasodilatation. These factors alone are usually insufficient to produce syncope, and the occasional loss of consciousness with this syndrome is probably due to vasodepressor mechanisms as in the common faint.

The hyperventilation syndrome is often precipitated by acute emotional stress and is most common in nervous, anxious women who have other functional disturbances related to tension. The syndrome can often be reproduced by having the patient hyperventilate voluntarily for two or three minutes. Although the patient is often reassured by the fact that he can control the attack somewhat by breath-holding or breathing in a paper bag, therapy directed at the underlying emotional disturbance is usually necessary.

Hyperventilation Combined with Valsalva Maneuver. The physiologic alterations produced by a combination of hyperventilation and increased intrathoracic pressure (secondary to variants of the Valsalva maneuver) account for several unique types of syncope. The "mess trick," a prank often indulged in by schoolboys, consists of sudden manual compression of the chest of the victim after he has been hyperventilating for about a minute. Loss of consciousness may also occur in the "fainting lark," in which the victim is instructed to hyperventilate in the squatting position, stand quickly, and immediately perform the Valsalva maneuver. The loss of consciousness observed in athletes lifting weights ("weight-lifter's blackout") is due to similar mechanisms. During competition, these individuals often hyperventilate vigorously and then squat before grasping the weight. Lifting of the weight produces high levels of intrathoracic pressure which reduces venous return and causes decrease in cardiac output, stroke volume, and pulse pressure. These alterations, combined with the peripheral vasodilation caused by squatting and cerebral vasoconstriction caused by hyperventilation, result in a reduction in cerebral blood flow and loss of consciousness. Voluntary syncope has also been observed in muscular teenage boys who can maintain a prolonged Valsalva maneuver by vigorous stretching of the trunk and back muscles. Such instances of "stretch syncope" are often self-induced to provide a curiously satisfying experience.

Brown, E. B.: Physiological effects of hyperventilation. Physiol. Rev., 33:445, 1953.
Klein, L. J., Saltzman, H., and Heyman, A.: Syncope induced by the Valsalva maneuver: A study of the effects of arterial blood gas tensions, glucose concentration and blood pressure. Am. J. Med., 37:263, 1964.
Saltzman, H. A., Heyman, A., and Sieker, H. O.: Correlations of clinical and physiologic manifestations of sustained hyperventilation. N. Engl. J. Med., 268:1431, 1963.

Section Nine. NEUROLOGIC DIAGNOSTIC PROCEDURES

Richard P. Schmidt

355. INTRODUCTION

Many special tests and procedures are used to supplement the clinical examination in the establishment of a neurologic diagnosis. These may add precision to the localization and characterization of a disease process, or may record functional alterations as reflected in electrical activity of brain, nerve, or muscle. Their value is related directly to the judgment with which they are used and to the skill with which they are performed and interpreted. Some of the tests outlined below are relatively simple procedures which cause little discomfort, whereas others may be dangerous and must be used only by physicians skilled in the techniques and with full knowledge of potential complications and their treatment. The number of available tests is expanding rapidly, and it has become increasingly important for these to be selectively used and individualized. Those least dangerous and causing the least discomfort are to be used first. Careful clinical examinations may obviate the need for a battery of expensive and time-consuming procedures.

In this section brief descriptions of the useful diagnostic procedures are given. Details of techniques and of interpretations may be found in definitive and specialized monographs.

356. ROENTGENOLOGIC EXAMINATIONS

Roentgenograms of the skull or spine may demonstrate evidence of disease by deformation or involvement of bony structures, by displacement of normal radiopaque structures such as the pineal body, or by abnormal calcification such as may be seen in tumors, vascular malformations, infectious granulomas, or hematomas. Maximal information should always be obtained from plain roentgenograms prior to the institution of more complex studies. Such studies not only may permit a more satisfactory choice, but may also obviate the need for contrast studies such as arteriography or pneumoencephalography. Brain shift may be evident by displacement of a normally calcified pineal body. Increased intracranial pressure over a long period of time characteristically causes demineralization of the dorsum sellae by pressure from an expanded third ventricle or a beaten silver appearance to the inner table of the skull from pressure of the gyri of the cerebral cortex. Diagnosis of some diseases can be confirmed without further examination. For example, pituitary tumors usually cause enlargement of the sella turcica. Meningiomas are often associated with thickening of bone at the site from which they arise. Abnormalities are observed in plain skull films of about half the patients with brain tumor.

Patterns of calcification as seen roentgenographically may be highly specific in diagnosis of disease. Examples include arcuate densities in the wall of an aneurysm or the veins of an arteriovenous malformation, calcification in the pattern of the cerebral cortex in Sturge-Weber syndrome, and diffuse nodular calcification in congenital toxoplasmosis. Amorphous calcification with or without erosion of the pituitary fossa is typical in craniopharyngioma, and the basal ganglia may be calcified symmetrically in hypoparathyroidism.

Lesions of the skull or spine occur frequently in neoplastic diseases. In some instances the appearance is quite characteristic, as in the "punched-out" rarefactions of multiple myeloma. Special attention may be directed to the foramina at the base of the skull through which nasopharyngeal cancer may invade and cause cranial nerve paralysis. Axial projections of the base of the skull may reveal enlargement of these foramina with special advantage. Acoustic neurinoma characteristically enlarges the internal auditory meatus as shown in special projection.

Diagnosis of congenital malformations of the skull and spine can usually be made without contrast material. In basilar impression there is flattening of the basal angle, frequently associated with malformation of the foramen magnum and cervical spine and with hydrocephalus. Injury to the brain in early life may be associated with asymmetric skull growth. Premature closure of the sutures results in microcephaly or in asymmetric growth in the direction of those sutures which remain open.

In examination of the spine special attention should be given to alignment, integrity of the intervertebral disc space, bony excrescences, and evidences of bone destruction. Intraspinal neoplasms commonly erode and cause separation of the vertebral pedicles. Characteristic patterns are seen in such diseases as tuberculosis of the spine, osteoporosis, metastatic carcinoma, and vertebral hemangioma. Oblique views are especially useful for demonstrating intervertebral foramina, which may be enlarged in tumors such as neurofibromas or compromised by osteophytic spurs causing radicular syndromes.

Body section roentgenography may be used for visualization of abnormalities of skull or spine which are otherwise obscure. This procedure has special value in demonstrating changes near the midline or base of the skull, and may also be used to advantage in intraspinal lesions.

Further stages of neuroradiologic diagnosis depend upon making visible structures not seen in plain films by use of radiopaque substances injected into arteries or the subarachnoid space, or by gas (usually air or oxygen) to provide radiolucency in cerebrospinal fluid–containing compartments. With increasing sophistication of instrumentation, the techniques of performing such studies are evolving rapidly, demanding high degrees of skill for their performance and interpretation.

Myelography is used when mass impingement upon spinal or posterior fossa neural structures or nerve roots is suspected, and usually when surgical treatment appears to be required. It is usually done using iodized oil, which is heavier than the cerebrospinal fluid, injected into the subarachnoid space at a reasonable distance from the suspected lesion in the lumbar region or, for special purposes, into the cisterna magna. Oil is manipulated up and down by tilting the patient on a table under fluoroscopic control. Introduction of oil into the cranial cavity is usually avoided, and the oil is removed after completion of the procedure. Adequate myelography with fluoroscopy and spot films at various angles is usually satisfactory for demonstrating mass lesions within or impinging upon the spinal subarachnoid space. It has its greatest usefulness in outlining neoplasms, herniations of the nucleus pulposus, or impingements by spondylotic lesions. At times manipulation of fluid pressure may cause acute exacerbation of the patient's symptoms; if a tumor is present, this may call for urgent surgical intervention. *The test is to be avoided unless there is strong and sufficient reason to suspect a mass lesion.* There may, for example, be exacerbation of multiple sclerosis by the procedure. Iodized oil is a foreign substance to the subarachnoid space, and may initiate a sterile meningeal reaction or, rarely, a progressive adhesive arachnoiditis. For these reasons, in some countries myelography is performed using air-contrast or, less commonly, absorbable water-soluble radiopaque material. When more satisfactory, less irritating agents are found, they will probably replace oil.

In *pneumoencephalography,* oxygen or air is introduced in increments into the lumbar subarachnoid space, from which it ascends into the basal cisterns and enters the ventricular cavities. By proper positioning, the entire ventricular system can be visualized, as can the basal cisterns and subarachnoid spaces over the cerebral cortex. Ventriculography may be used in the presence of increased intracranial pressure or when a tumor is suspected, because of lessened danger of initiating herniation as compared with pneumoencephalography. It is performed by introducing gas directly into the lateral ventricle by a needle introduced through a trephine opening in the skull. Pantopaque may be used for special purposes. It has the disadvantage of limiting the examination to the ventricular system because of failure to fill the subarachnoid spaces. In these tests, atrophic processes or obstructions of fluid paths are reflected by enlargement of the ventricles. In the former, there may be concomitant enlargement of the basal cisterns and of the sulci over the convexity of the brain. Space-taking lesions such as neoplasms may obstruct with "upstream" dilatation appropriate to the site or, as is characteristic, may deform and shift the ventricles.

When appropriately used, pneumoencephalography is a safe procedure; however, it is usually distressing to the patient, and may cause severe headache.

The uses of *angiography* are increasing rapidly. By the injection of appropriate root arteries, positioning of the patient, and timing of serial films, it is now possible to demonstrate practically all the intracranial arterial and venous systems and also to study parent vessels from the aorta upward. Techniques for performance vary, but increasing proportions of these examinations are being done by selective catheterization through the femoral arteries, and fewer by direct puncture of carotid or vertebral arteries in the neck. Special radiologic techniques of magnification, subtraction, and stereoscopic visualization are used to increase diagnostic and localizing capabilities. Special angiographic procedures may be used for lesions of the orbit or spinal cord or for visualizing lesions supplied by the external carotid system such as meningiomas.

Cerebral angiography has certain advantages over gas contrast studies. Pathologic processes of blood vessels such as aneurysms or malformations may be demonstrated. Complete or partial occlusions at any site from the level of the aortic arch to the intracranial vascular tree may be visualized. If surgery for occlusive disease is contemplated, all major vessels must be studied. Angiography is the procedure of choice in delineating neoplasms or other space-occupying lesions. Masses may be localized by displacement of arteries or veins from normal positions and by the filling of abnormal vessels within a neoplasm (tumor stain). It is sometimes possible to predict the histologic type of a tumor from its blood supply and vascular pattern. Subdural hematoma is demonstrated to particular advantage by displacement of superficial blood vessels away from the inner surface of the skull, and is seen best on anteroposterior and oblique projections. Angiography may have an added advantage for patients with increased intracranial pressure in that it is less likely to cause herniation and brain shift than is pneumoencephalography. Patients tolerate the procedure well, and do not have the headache, nausea, and vomiting associated with gas insufflation. Complications may occur, however, especially in children, older patients, and those with vascular and systemic diseases. The complications range from transient dysfunction such as hemiparesis or confusion to more unusual permanent neurologic injuries or even death. Puncture of an artery can cause intraluminal rupture of an intimal atherosclerotic plaque or subintimal dissection. Embolization or thrombosis may occur from the site of puncture.

357. RADIOISOTOPE PROCEDURES

Isotope brain scanning depends upon the ability of certain radioactive substances to localize selectively in neoplasms or in injured tissues (such as infarctions) which damage the normally impermeable blood-brain barrier. Isotopes of short half-life, such as technetium^{99m} pertechnetate are now preferred because they permit a higher level of radioactivity and a much shorter elapsed time to the completion of the procedure. The scan may be recorded with multiple crystals in a scintillation camera or by more conventional scintillation scanners moving across the head and recording the scanning image instrumentally on paper or film. Several projections are used to "view" the head from different directions. With the scintillation camera, dynamic scans may be obtained, giving some evidence of blood circulation or demonstrating large vascular anomalies. Scans are of special worth for locating lesions relatively near the surface, and may be confusing or "negative" with deep or midline lesions. Artifacts may be produced by bruises of the scalp or by such simple processes as contamination by saliva in which the isotope has been secreted. Scans are excellent as screening procedures because of safety and lack of discomfort or serious inconvenience.

358. ELECTRODIAGNOSTIC EXAMINATIONS

Functions of the brain, nerves and neuromuscular apparatus may be examined by appropriate measurements of electrical activity.

The *electroencephalogram* (EEG) is the recording of amplified potentials generated by the brain by means of electrodes applied to the scalp. Recordings directly from the surface or from the depths of the brain may have application in selected instances such as the surgical treatment of foci generating epileptic partial seizures. An adequate routine examination includes the application of 18 or more electrodes on the scalp and observation of the EEG under conditions of nonattentive wakefulness, in response to overbreathing, and during the course of natural sleep. The instruments now used consist of eight or more matched channels for simultaneous recordings, and by convention the record is written in ink on paper moving beneath galvanometer pens. Variation in rhythm occurs with respect to normal processes such as sleep, and there are marked differences between the EEG of the child and the adult. Although the processes that generate the brain waves are largely unknown, normal or usual patterns and deviation from normal are well recognized and may be highly useful in clinical diagnosis. Deviation from normal may be termed a dysrhythmia, and the type of dysrhythmia and its distribution or localization may correlate with the type of the underlying disease. Highly typical patterns are observed in some of the epilepsies, especially the spike-wave pattern associated with petit mal or localized spikes over the temporal lobe in patients with complex partial seizures (psychomotor). A normal EEG does not preclude the presence of serious disease. Mild deviations from normal may be observed in persons with no evidence of cerebral disease. Intelligence cannot be measured and psychologic diagnoses cannot be made by the EEG. The EEG can be properly interpreted only in concert with the clinical data, and it cannot provide precise diagnosis in and of itself.

The EEG may provide evidence for diagnosis and localization of structural lesions such as neoplasms, infarcts, hematomas, and infections. The tool has the great advantage of relative simplicity of application and harmlessness to the patient. If the brain is infarcted, compressed, or disrupted by neoplasms or hemorrhage, slower than normal (delta) waves are observed and may be localized to areas overlying the pathologic processes. Serial or sequential examinations reflect changes of improvement or worsening in the pathologic process, and thus help to delineate the nature of the underlying disorder. Metabolic abnormalities affecting the brain may be followed by the EEG to ascertain the direction of improvement or worsening.

The *electromyogram* (EMG) records the electrical activity in muscle. Detailed diagnostic examination requires use of needle electrodes inserted into the muscles under study. Instrumentation is analogous to that used for the EEG, except that a cathode ray oscilloscope is necessary because of more rapid potential change. Permanent records may be made on photographic film or magnetic tape. Records are obtained during rest, needle insertion, and voluntary contraction, and in response to physical or electrical stimulation. Auditory monitoring with a loudspeaker is customary in many laboratories. The EMG is most helpful in the diagnosis of disease of the motor unit, which includes the ventral horn cell, ventral nerve root, motor nerve, myoneural junction, and muscle. Neuropathic disorders, such as amyotrophic lateral sclerosis or poliomyelitis, produce signs of muscle denervation, including increased insertion activity, fibrillation potentials at rest, and reduced, altered, or absent normal muscle action potentials. Primary muscle disease (myopathy) frequently reduces the amplitude and duration of the muscle action potentials and increases the complexity of their wave form, although the number of potentials is little changed. Myotonia produces a highly characteristic repetitive pattern. Segmental investigation of muscle innervation may be of use in localization and diagnosis of spinal root compression, such as that caused by intervertebral disc protrusion.

Estimates of motor nerve conduction velocity are made by electrically stimulating the nerve, recording electromyographically from the muscle that it innervates, and measuring the latency. Slowing of conduction is observed in a wide variety of peripheral neuropathies and in many instances of neurologically asymptomatic diabetes mellitus. The site of local nerve compression or conduction block can be demonstrated, an example being the local block of median nerve conduction that is found in the carpal tunnel syndrome. Sensory nerve conduction velocity may be measured by recording nerve action potentials after digital nerve stimulation. Sensory neuropathy may produce slowing of conduction or inability to record the nerve potential.

359. ECHOENCEPHALOGRAPHY

High frequency (ultrasonic) sound pulses produced by an electrically activated crystal and conducted in a fluid or solid medium reflect or echo at physical interfaces, and their reflection can, in turn, be detected and recorded. This phenomenon may detect shifts or alterations of structures within the cranial cavity. Present application makes it possible to obtain a rapid, painless, and harmless estimate of the position of midline structures (third ventricle) in the intact cranium. Pulses of ultrasound are delivered to the head through a probe held firmly to the scalp and with liquid or jelly at the interface. A detector may be physically located in the same probe. Proper amplification and display with a cathode ray oscilloscope permit recognition of reflected pulse from skin, ventricle, skull, and other structures. By calibrating the sweep speed of the oscilloscope beam, the distance from the probe to the reflecting surface can be measured in millimeters. Measurement of the position of the midline third ventricle is particularly reliable. This is useful as a screening test for hemispheric mass lesions causing brain shift, and is well adapted to use in emergency hospital services for appraising patients with suspected subdural or epidural hemorrhage. Echoencephalography may also be used to estimate ventricular size and at times to demonstrate abnormal structures such as tumors.

360. NEW AND DEVELOPING TECHNOLOGIES

Improvements in instrument technology and manufacture have greatly expanded the ability to identify and delineate lesions of the central nervous system. Of the recently devised instruments, the EMI-Scanner, developed by EMI Limited in England is achieving acceptance rapidly and is being installed in major centers for neurology and neurosurgery. This instrument uses the principle of differential density absorption of x-rays by lesions and normal structures within the cranial vault. It is composed, in essence, of a rotating x-ray tube and recording device, a small computer, a digital read-out system, and an oscilloscope with its accompanying Polaroid camera. The patient is given no medication before the examination so that it represents a truly noninvasive study. The patient's head is placed in the device, and multiple x-ray pictures are taken by the moving x-ray tube as it courses over the head. These electronic pictures are analyzed by the computer and recorded. Over-all accuracy with the EMI-Scanner appears to be great, and it has the great advantage of being safe and rapid.

Toole, J. F. (ed.): Contemporary Neurology Series, Vol. 3. Special Techniques in Neurologic Diagnosis. Philadelphia, F. A. Davis Company, 1969.

Section Ten. THE EXTRAPYRAMIDAL DISORDERS

361. INTRODUCTION

Melvin D. Yahr

The basal ganglia or extrapyramidal diseases comprise a complex group of clinical disorders characterized by abnormal involuntary movements (dyskinesias), alterations in muscle tone, and disturbances in bodily posture. The major clinical states included under this title are parkinsonism, chorea, athetosis, dystonia, and hemiballism. These terms not only are used to denote particular disease entities, but in a descriptive sense refer to a constellation of symptoms that may occur in a variety of central nervous system disorders involving the basal ganglia and/or their connections. They are recognizable, one from the other, by the degree, form, and combination of the triad of symptoms noted above and are distinguishable as disease entities by the age and mode of onset, the identification of particular etiologic and genetic factors, and the rate and manner of progression of symptoms. Although much is known about the clinical aspects of extrapyramidal disorders, our information is deficient in regard to their fundamental anatomic, physiologic, and pathogenic bases.

The conventional anatomic concept of the basal ganglia as a group of nuclear masses in the forebrain has not proved adequate in explaining the clinical manifestations or what is known about the physiologic or pathologic aspects of these conditions. In consequence, neurologists have devised a functional anatomic approach that includes not only the basal ganglia nuclei, but also related structures in the brainstem as well as a neural network of connections with other parts of the nervous system. The structures of importance in this system are the caudate nucleus and putamen, which, because of their similarities in appearance, cellular structure, and phylogenetic development, are collectively known as the striatum; the globus pallidus or pallidum, an older structure but one in which many nonpyramidal pathways converge; the thalamus, another important way station and integrative region; and the subthalamic nucleus, red nucleus and substantia nigra, all brainstem centers with important connections to the basal ganglia. These nuclear masses, along with their connections with each other and with certain parts of the reticular formation, cerebellum, and cerebrum, make up an anatomic-physiologic unit that collectively has been termed "the extrapyramidal system." The role of this system in maintaining normal motor activity in man is not definitely known, and has only been inferred from studies of animals, in which it is more highly developed and not dominated by the cerebral cortex. In submammalian forms in which motor activities are sterotyped and resemble patterned reflexes, this system appears essential for maintaining normal locomotion, feeding, etc. In higher animals, except man, its integrity is necessary for the production of automatic movements and postural adjustments. Some believe that this same function is carried over to man and that coarse, gross automatic movements are mediated by the extrapyramidal system. Others have implied a more secondary role in which this system is incapable of initiating movements but provides a reinforcing and modulating influence on movements of cortical origin. The latter thesis seems more in keeping with our present knowledge of the integrative function of the nervous system; hence it is best to view the pyramidal and extrapyramidal systems as operating in unison and constant balance. Movements having their origin in the cerebral cortex are mediated through the pyramidal tract but are influenced by reflex regulating mechanisms from various components of the extrapyramidal system. In this context, the prime role of the extrapyramidal system is automatic sensorimotor integration, which can be explained in terms of inhibition and facilitation of motor responses to appropriate stimuli. Hence dysfunction within this system results in motor responses that are delayed, slow, and incomplete and especially affect automatic or involuntary movements.

The manifestations of basal ganglia disorders previously noted fall into two general categories: those of a *positive* nature, such as abnormal movements, tremor, and chorea, and those of a *negative* nature, such as postural changes and loss of associated movements. The positive disturbances arise from an excess of neural activity, and as such cannot derive from destruction of neural elements but must represent the function of surviving structures. They are often termed release phenomena, in that a lesion in one structure removes the controlling or regulating influence on another, with the result that the latter becomes overactive. The negative symptoms, on the other hand, are considered to result from the direct loss or destruction of neural elements. Unfortunately, because of the nature of the disease processes affecting this region it has not been possible to correlate intimately the clinical symptoms with structural changes. Further, there are no naturally occurring animal counterparts to the disturbances of upright posture and of movements that occur in human diseases of the extrapyramidal system. Pathologic studies of most of these diseases show widespread neuropathologic changes throughout the cerebrum, although the basal ganglia and brainstem nuclei suffer the brunt of the damage. In some instances, however, the functional impairment is far more than that expected from the changes found on routine autopsy examination. There is a growing body of information that suggests that the abnormalities in such cases may be chemical rather than morphologic. The content of monoamines, such as dopamine and serotonin, is particularly high in structures such as the caudate nucleus, putamen, and substantia nigra. In at least one disease affecting this system, parkinsonism, the level of dopamine has been shown to be markedly decreased. Experimental lesions in the region of the substantia nigra and the pallidum produce similar effects. Since in many instances the chemical abnormalities do not follow the presumed anatomic connections, a neurochemical network is postulated for this system. In such a neural system chemical transmitter substances, such as dopamine, may be stored in nerve endings of axons whose somata or cell bodies are located in distant areas. The observed chemical changes may reflect injury or damage to a specific chemical system in these instances (a dopaminergic neuronal system) and may be similar regardless of the pathologic process. Extrapyramidal structures have other unique biochemical characteristics as indicated by high levels of acetylcholine as well as the enzymes responsible for its synthesis and degradation. All these findings suggest that better understanding of the extrapyramidal system and its diseases may be derived from intensive study of its chemical topography.

In the clinical evaluation of extrapyramidal disorders it is essential to have a clear understanding of the many and varied symptoms encountered. Those of major significance are abnormal involuntary movements, alterations in muscle tone, and disturbances in bodily posture.

Abnormal Involuntary Movements. *Tremor* is a rhythmic involuntary alternating contraction of opposing muscle groups, fairly uniform in frequency and amplitude. It may involve a limited segment such as fingers or lips, or may be widespread. Characteristically, tremor of extrapyramidal origin is augmented when the part is at rest and diminished or abolished during voluntary movements and sleep. It differs from that of anxiety, thyrotoxicosis, and those due to intoxications by being slower, of greater amplitude, and more rhythmic. Its occurrence at rest and suppression during voluntary movements and sleep distinguishes it from the so-called "action" tremor of cerebellar involvement. The anatomic and physiologic substrate of this type of tremor has not been defined with certainty. In Parkinson's disease in which such tremor is prominent, the substantia nigra invariably undergoes degeneration. However, not all such patients have tremor, and it remains a controversial issue whether the pathologic changes are entirely limited to this structure. Certain thalamic nuclei, particularly the nucleus lateralis posterior, have been implicated, because discharges synchronous with the tremor have been recorded. These findings suggest derangement of a rather complex sensorimotor mechanism with possible multiple pathologic sites.

Athetosis denotes an involuntary movement that results from instability of posture combined with voluntary movement. The result is a slow, writhing, wormlike movement usually most prominent in the fingers and hand, but the face, neck, and feet may also be involved. Multiple areas of the extrapyramidal system, particularly the globus pallidus and striatum as well as the cerebral cortex, have shown pathologic changes when this type of dyskinesia is encountered.

Chorea refers to brief, distal, rapid, explosive movements which at first glance appear to be purposeful and coordinated but on closer inspection are aimless and uncoordinated. They involve upper and lower limbs, face, trunk, and head, and may occur with such rapidity that the individual appears in constant motion. Choreiform movements are accentuated by movement and environmental stimulation, and interfere with normal voluntary function. They are differentiated from tics by being unpatterned, unpredictable, and nonreproducible. Athetosis and chorea may coexist in such a pattern that they are indistinguishable from one another. Pathologic changes accompanying chorea have been found in many areas of the nervous system but especially in the striatum.

Dystonia is a term applied to an abnormally maintained posture resulting from a twisting, turning movement that usually involves the limbs, neck, or trunk. Although there is no specific pattern or posture that describes this disorder, the usual appearance is one of marked distortion of the affected part. The movements appear readily induced by ordinary stimuli, such as walking, talking, or light touch to the skin. The involved muscles appear to be alternately in a state of increased and decreased tone and, usually as the movement starts, the muscles involved appear to gradually build up tone. Patients with this type of movement cannot inhibit, modify, or terminate the posture, and voluntary movements become seriously impaired. In some instances the movements clear, but the abnormal postures become fixed with resultant torticollis, tortipelvis, and deformities of the limbs. Neither the pathologic nor physiologic substrate for this movement disorder has been fully defined. Some have considered it akin to athetosis but different because of the inherent peculiarities of the axial and appendicular musculature that is primarily affected.

Ballism is a violent dyskinesia consisting of forceful, flinging movements of the limbs. The muscles involved are in the shoulder and pelvic girdle, and usually only one side of the body or even one limb is affected. Of all the abnormal movements ballism is the one that appears to be due to a discrete lesion, usually in the subthalamic nucleus of Luys or its immediate connections.

Alterations in Muscle Tone. A wide range of degrees of tension in muscles is to be found in these disorders. Although it is common to associate heightened muscle tonus (rigidity) with extrapyramidal disorders, some, such as chorea and athetosis, may show normal tone or hypotonus of the musculature. Rigidity, which is most commonly encountered in parkinsonism, must be differentiated from spasticity. The former is identifiable by passively flexing and extending the muscles of an extremity or rotating the hand on the wrist. The movement obtained is one of a series of interrupted jerks at regular intervals, the so called cog-wheel effect. Terms such as "plastic" or "lead pipe" are utilized to describe the homogeneous degree of rigidity. Rigidity may be limited to groups of muscles and may be evident only at some joints, or it may be generalized, affecting the entire musculature. The mechanism underlying the rigidity appears to be impairment of reciprocal inhibition of agonist and antagonistic muscle groups. Electromyographic analysis of these muscles shows continuing activity in both groups throughout a movement such as flexion of the forearm. Rigidity reduces muscle power and velocity of movement to some degree, and also contributes to the production of deformities.

Disturbances in Bodily Posture. Patients with extrapyramidal disease in general, and those with parkinsonism in particular, have difficulty in preserving their equilibrium in the erect as well as the sitting position. They also have difficulty in changing from the horizontal to the upright position or in rolling over from back to front. The most profound difficulties are noted in walking, when tendencies to propulsive or retropulsive gait are evident as well as shuffling and festination. Careful analysis of these defects has indicated that the subjects have loss of control of their center of gravity in both sagittal and coronal planes. There are also tendencies to assume abnormal posture such as a flexion of the trunk on standing. There is a notable lack of normal and appropriate use of defense mechanisms, such as putting out the arms when falling. These abnormalities are thought to be due to disturbances in righting reflexes, impairment of vestibular reflexes, and release of proprioceptor mechanisms subsequent to degeneration in the pallidum. They form a distressing and disabling group of symptoms that to date have not been thoroughly investigated.

Denny-Brown, D.: The Cerebral Control of Movement. Springfield, Ill., Charles C Thomas, 1966.
Duvoisin, R.: Clinical diagnosis of the dyskinesias. Med. Clin. North Am., 56:1321, 1972.
Watkins, E. S.: The basal ganglia. *In* Scientific Foundations of Neurology. London, Heinemann, 1972, pp. 75–83.
Yahr, M. D.: Involuntary movements. *In* Scientific Foundations of Neurology. London, Heinemann, 1972, pp. 83–88.
Yahr, M. D., and Purpura, D. P. (eds.): Neurophysiological Basis of Normal and Abnormal Motor Activities. Hewlett, N.Y., Raven Press, 1967.

THE PARKINSONIAN SYNDROME (Paralysis Agitans, Shaking Palsy)

Melvin D. Yahr

362. INTRODUCTION

James Parkinson first described the major manifestations of this syndrome, which is characterized by tremor, muscular rigidity, and loss of postural reflexes. Not only is it one of the most frequently encountered of all the basal ganglia disorders, but parkinsonism is a prominent cause of disability resulting from diseases of all types. Its prevalence has been placed at close to one million patients in the United States, with the addition of 50,000 new cases each year. As a symptom complex its occurrence has been noted in a number of disease processes either as the sole manifestation or in association with other symptoms. However, in the vast majority of cases no definable cause has as yet been found; since the latter seem to have many features in common, particularly in regard to evolution, they have been designated as Parkinson's disease, paralysis agitans, or primary parkinsonism. The cases in which definable processes are found are best classified as secondary or symptomatic parkinsonism. This separation into clinical groups cannot be construed as indicative of a difference in pathophysiology or even pathogenic mechanisms for the production of symptoms, for all parkinsonism may well have a common origin. Indeed, from the standpoint of what is presently known about its chemical pathology, a deficiency of striatal dopamine is common to all types of parkinsonism. In some instances of parkinsonism, regardless of cause, cell loss is consistently found in the substantia nigra in association with other changes diffusely distributed in the corpus striatum and cortex.

363. PARALYSIS AGITANS (Parkinson's Disease)

The largest number of cases of parkinsonism fall into this category. The disease most frequently makes its onset between the ages of 50 and 65 years. A rarely encountered juvenile form has been described. The disease affects both sexes and all races, and there is no evidence to indicate a hereditary factor, although a familial incidence is claimed by some authorities.

The disease begins insidiously with any of its three cardinal manifestations either alone or in combination. Tremor usually in one or sometimes in both hands, involving the fingers in a pill-rolling motion, is the most common initial symptom. This is often followed by stiffness in the limbs, general slowing of movements and inability to carry out normal and routine daily functions with ease. As the disease progresses the face becomes "masklike," with a loss of eye blinking and failure to express emotional feeling; the body becomes stooped, and the gait becomes shuffling with loss of arm swing; and the patient is unable to readily gain and maintain an erect posture. Speech becomes slow and monotonous. There is a tendency to drool. The skin takes on an oily quality, and there is a tendency to seborrheic dermatitis. Although paralysis agitans is invariably progressive, the rate at which symptoms develop and disability ensues is extremely variable. On only rare occasions is the disease so rapidly progressive that the patient becomes disabled within five years of onset. In the majority, intervals of 10 to 20 years elapse before symptoms cause incapacity.

The major neurologic findings are as follows: (1) *Lack of facial expression,* with diminished eye blinking but ready induction of blepharospasm when the frontalis muscle is tapped (Myerson's sign). (2) *Tremor* of the distal segments of the limbs at rest, accentuated by suspension but decreased during active movements and eliminated in sleep. The tremor is rhythmical, alternately affecting flexor and extensor muscles, and may involve upper or lower limbs, mouth, or head. (3) *Muscular rigidity* is readily evident on passive movement of a joint, and is manifested by a series of interrupted jerks (cog-wheel phenomenon) rather than a smooth flowing, easy motion. (4) *Akinesia* is the tendency to slowness in the initiation of movement and sudden unexpected arrests of volitional movements while carrying out purposeful acts. The parkinsonian patient appears disinclined to move, and in the midst of performing a routine function suddenly finds himself "frozen" and unable to move through the sequence of motion necessary to complete the action. This is especially evident in writing or feeding and can be striking when, in attempting to walk, the patient finds that his feet are suddenly "frozen to the ground." (5) *Postural abnormalities* are most evident in the erect and sitting positions. The patient has a tendency to let his head fall forward on the trunk, and his body tends to fall forward or backward when seated on a stool unless supported; when pushed either from in front or behind in the erect position he falls, making no effort to catch himself with either a step or by movement of his arms. There is a tendency to deformities of the trunk, hands, and feet. Kyphotic deformity of the spine, causing a stooped posture, is a hallmark. There are ulnar deviation of the hand, flexion contractures of the fingers, and an equinovarus posture of the foot.

364. SECONDARY OR SYMPTOMATIC PARKINSONISM

In a long list of diseases and conditions of the nervous system parkinsonism has occurred as the predominant manifestation. These include poisoning with carbon monoxide, manganese, or other metals; brain tumors in the region of the basal ganglia; cerebral trauma; degenerative diseases; intoxication with neuroleptic agents, particularly the phenothiazine group of drugs; and infectious processes, such as encephalitis. Cerebral arteriosclerosis has been implicated by some authorities who have even designated a special form of arteriosclerotic parkinsonism. However, it is exceedingly doubtful that such a disorder exists, and pathologic studies to date have not confirmed a vascular basis for the Parkinson syndrome. In most instances of secondary parkinsonism, neurologic abnormalities involving other areas of the nervous system are found, and the parkinsonism itself may show variations from the usual picture. Of all the conditions noted, only two are frequently encountered: postencephalitic and drug-induced parkinsonism.

POSTENCEPHALITIC PARKINSONISM

One of the most prominent sequelae of the epidemic of encephalitis lethargica (von Economo's disease) that occurred between 1919 and 1926 was the parkinsonian syndrome. The syndrome developed after mild as well as severe encephalitis lethargica, and, although in most instances they immediately followed the acute infectious process, in some patients prominent symptoms were not evident for intervals of up to ten years. The causative agent of encephalitis lethargica was never established. However, recent studies suggest that it was produced by a virus of the influenza A variety. Parkinsonism appears to have been a unique sequela of this form of encephalitis because it has rarely followed any other known viral encephalitides. There are still a significant number of survivors of encephalitis lethargica, and the evolution and consequences of this form of parkinsonism differ from others, so its clinical recognition is of importance.

Postencephalitic parkinsonism has a number of distinctive or unique features, including the following: (1) A history of encephalitis lethargica during the epidemic period 1918–1919. Since the pandemic of influenza occurred concurrently with encephalitis, it is essential that careful documentation be undertaken in differentiating these two infectious processes. (2) In addition to any or all of the parkinsonian symptoms indicated above, one or more of the following neurologic deficits may be found: hemiplegia, bulbar or ocular palsies, dystonic phenomena, tics, or behavioral disorders. (3) The parkinsonism itself is as a rule incompletely developed and has been static or slowly progressive over a period of years. (4) Episodes that have been termed oculogyric crises. These consist of attacks in which spasms of conjugate eye muscles occur so that the eyes are deviated upward, downward, or to one side for minutes or hours at a time.

DRUG-INDUCED PARKINSONISM

The use of neuroleptics as psychotherapeutic or antiemetic agents has resulted in the occurrence of a number of extrapyramidal syndromes. Parkinsonism indistinguishable from that previously described, dystonic movements involving the tongue and face, and akathisia, a restless fidgety state with a desire to be in constant motion, are those frequently encountered. Adults are more likely to develop parkinsonism and akathisia, whereas dystonic movements predominate in children. In some instances these reactions are dose-dependent; in others they are related to individual susceptibility. The symptoms usually disappear within a few days when the drugs are withdrawn, but occasionally persist for months. In some subjects permanent remnants of parkinsonian symptoms have been found years after elimination of the drugs. Paradoxically, involuntary movements may make their initial appearance after withdrawal of neuroleptic agents. This condition, termed *tardive dyskinesia,* tends to occur in older patients who have been on phenothiazine drugs for extended periods of time, during which they have shown signs of parkinsonism. Stereotyped, repetitious movements of lips, tongue, and mouth and choreiform movements of limbs and trunk characterize this disorder. It may diminish in intensity or disappear spontaneously after weeks or months, but in some patients it has persisted indefinitely. In most instances the occurrence of basal ganglia symptoms, particularly parkinsonism, can be minimized by the simultaneous administration of one of the centrally active anticholinergic agents, such as Cogentin or Artane. Cautious use of neuroleptics, employing restricted doses and drug holidays in those requiring long-term treatment, may be the best preventive measure.

365. MANAGEMENT OF THE PARKINSONIAN SYNDROME

General Principles. Until the etiology and pathogenesis of parkinsonism are defined, its treatment must be considered as symptomatic, supportive, and palliative. It is only in the exceptional case of symptomatic parkinsonism resulting from the use of drugs or occurring in association with specific disease processes that treatment of the causative factor may result in eradication of symptoms. The more frequently encountered patient will require lifelong treatment, consisting of the administration of specific medications, supportive psychotherapeutic measures, physical therapy, and, in rare instances, surgical intervention. Judiciously employed treatment may control the symptoms of parkinsonism in a large proportion of patients for extended periods of time. In most it allows relatively normal activities of living during most phases of this disorder. The introduction of new therapeutic approaches holds promise of forestalling or preventing the progressive disabling nature of this disorder.

Supportive Psychotherapy. The major symptoms of parkinsonism are markedly influenced by psychic factors, and a patient's outlook and motivation will affect the extent to which he can overcome disability. It is important for the physician to provide reassurance, encouragement, and sympathetic understanding to the patient and family so that they may meet the numerous difficulties to be encountered at various stages of the illness. To allay anxieties both should be counseled regarding the meaning of various symptoms, the nature of the disease in terms of its long and variable course, and the potential that most patients can lead active and productive lives for long periods after symptoms begin.

Physical Therapy. Simple measures such as heat and massage will alleviate painful muscle cramps and the muscle contraction headache that often accompanies pronounced rigidity of the cervical musculature. Exercises help in preventing flexion contractures. Gait training, walking exercises, and minor rehabilitative measures may enable the patient to maintain his independence with regard to personal hygiene and daily living activities for many more years than his disabilities might otherwise allow. Physical therapy in parkinsonism need not be elaborate, but when indicated should be done frequently and for an indefinite period. The patient should be instructed in simple home exercises and encouraged to develop a program of physical activity. Most patients in the earlier stages like to take long walks and should be encouraged to continue this habit as long as reasonably possible. Every effort should be made to keep them gainfully employed and to adjust their occupations as indicated by their symptoms.

Drug Therapy. The drugs now employed in the treatment of parkinsonism are those theoretically capable of restoring normal activity to the striatum. Thus any agent that crosses the blood-brain barrier and enhances the brain's dopaminergic function or that reduces cholinergic activity may be expected to influence parkinsonism favorably. As a general rule a combination of agents with such properties works best.

The dopaminergic system may be functionally enhanced by agents that increase the synthesis of dopamine (this is presumably the modus operandi of levodopa), delay the catabolism of dopamine (monoamine oxidase inhibitors), stimulate its release or its action at receptor sites (amphetamine and its analogues), and block the reuptake of monoamines at the synaptic cleft (anticholinergics). Of the numerous means for improving dopaminergic function that have been tried to date, the most effective thus far has been the administration of levodopa (3,4-dihydroxyphenyl-L-alanine). Given alone or in combination with a peripheral dopa decarboxylase inhibitor (benserazide, carbidopa), it is appreciably more effective and less toxic than any therapeutic agent previously available for the treatment of Parkinson's disease.

In the selection of patients for treatment with levodopa, the over-all severity of parkinsonism and the degree of functional impairment, as well as the existence of concomitant diseases of other organs, must be carefully considered. As previously stated, patients with minimal signs and symptoms who are able to meet the demands of daily living need not involve themselves in a treatment program that may be rigorous and demanding and carries an implicit risk. The presence of occlusive vascular disease involving the heart or brain warrants careful assessment. Severe angina pectoris or transient cerebral ischemic attacks contraindicate the use of levodopa. A history of episodic cardiac arrhythmia presents an additional hazard. When the arrhythmia is associated with myocardial disease, the use of levodopa must be undertaken with extreme caution. Evidence of prior mental illness, particularly affective disorders or major "psychotic breaks," contravenes the use of levodopa. Although requiring careful monitoring, levodopa has been administered without adverse effects to patients with hepatic, renal, gastrointestinal, and hematopoietic disorders. However, the presence of hemolytic anemia and glucose-6-phosphate dehydrogenase (G-6-PD) deficiency contraindicates its use.

Clinical experience with levodopa suggests two phases of treatment with which the physician and patient must be familiar. The first or "introduction phase" extends over a period of weeks or months in which the dosage is slowly built up to the therapeutic range. During this phase, tolerance develops to many of the side effects of levodopa; and although improvement of symptoms occurs in most patients, the optimal therapeutic response may not be evident. A "maintenance phase" follows, in which the full benefits of treatment most often occur, and careful patient monitoring with readjustment of dosage and ancillary therapeutic measures may be required to maintain a stable therapeutic response. Each of these phases requires cooperation on the part of the patient and careful management by the physician to achieve the best therapeutic response.

Levodopa is an aromatic amino acid that is a relatively inert compound by itself, but several of its metabolites have profound pharmacologic effects. These vary, depending on the route of administration, the dosage, and the interval. At present, levodopa has only been validated for oral use in parkinsonism and is available in tablets or capsules of 100, 250, and 500 mg. Treatment may conveniently be initiated with 250 mg given three or four times daily by mouth after meals. If the initial doses are well tolerated, each dose may be increased to 500 mg. Subsequent increments of 125 to 250 mg may be made every two to three days in hospitalized patients or at intervals of one to two weeks in outpatients. It is preferable that no single dose exceed 1.5 to 2.0 grams; hence many patients will be required to take multiple doses throughout a 24-hour period. The dose is gradually increased until either a satisfactory response or a dose-limiting side effect is encountered. The average optimal dose in patients with Parkinson's disease is 5 to 6 grams daily. As a general rule it is often best to settle for a total daily dose that, although failing to control all the symptoms, gives an acceptable degree of improvement and a tolerable level of side reactions. Attempts to eradicate every vestige of the disorder may require doses at which an undue frequency and severity of reactions occur.

It is unusual for patients to enjoy the benefits of levodopa without experiencing some side effects. In most, these effects can be modified to tolerable levels by the judicious use of the drug as well as by ancillary measures. Early on in treatment, the major side effects encountered are nausea, vomiting, and anorexia, requiring reduction of dosage and deferral of further increments until such effects subside. Heightened nervous tension and feelings of anxiety necessitate reduction of dosage and a slower build-up to optimal levels. Acute psychotic episodes with delusions, hallucinations, hypomania, or depression are reactions that make it necessary to withdraw the drug. Cardiac dysrhythmia and/or hypotension with syncope is a combination that rarely permits continued use of levodopa. However, patients with orthostatic hypotension may continue treatment, employing commonly used means for its control. Adventitious involuntary movements develop in most patients on long-term levodopa therapy. When they are mild, treatment may be continued at full dosage. In instances in which the movements are excessive or interfere with function, a reduction in dosage is indicated with an attempt to find a level which compromises between a tolerable level of such movements and some degree of parkinsonian symptoms. Variability in therapeutic response develops in some patients after extended periods of levodopa administration. This apparent loss of "dopa effect" may last for hours or days. Its cause is unknown, and few effective means for relieving it have been found. Occasional transitory alterations in blood chemistry, including elevations of serum glutamic oxaloacetic transaminase (SGOT), alkaline phosphatase, and blood urea nitrogen (BUN), as well as depression of white blood cell count and development of a positive Coombs test, have occurred. To date, these have not been associated with symptoms of dysfunction in organ systems, nor has autopsy material shown structural alterations.

The large daily dose of levodopa required, the delayed onset of therapeutic benefits, and some of its side effects can be avoided by the simultaneous administration of a dopa decarboxylase inhibitor. The use of such a combination prevents the peripheral utilization of levodopa, making it more readily and rapidly available for brain metabolism to dopamine. Hence the beneficial effects make their appearance within a matter of days, and side effects such as nausea, vomiting, and anorexia are virtually eliminated. Those side effects originating in the central nervous system, however, are unaffected. A number of such agents have been developed, but at the time of this writing not all have been validated for general use in all countries. In the United States and some European and South American countries, Sinemet, as tablets containing carbidopa, 10 or 25 mg, plus levodopa, 100 or 250 mg, is marketed. In general, patients will require carbidopa, 100 mg, and levodopa, 1000 mg a day, divided into four equal doses. Available only in some European countries as Madopar is a combination of benserazide, 25 or 50 mg, and levodopa, 100 or 200 mg. The average required daily dose of this combination is benserazide, 200 mg, and levodopa, 800 mg, in four equally divided doses. Aldomet (methyl dopa) in doses of 500 mg (125 mg four times a day) has been used in combination with levodopa, 2 to 4 grams, with some effectiveness, but not to the extent of the previously mentioned compounds. A number of other antiparkinsonian agents are useful as adjunctive drugs with levodopa; they are also indicated for those in whom levodopa is contraindicated and are preferred for patients with very mild symptoms in the very early stages of the disorder. Some are also the drug of choice in drug-induced parkinsonism. Most of these compounds possess central nervous system anticholinergic properties or augment striatal dopaminergic activity. Those most frequently used are trihexyphenidyl (Artane), available in 2 and 5 mg tablets; benztropine (Cogentin), as 1 and 2 mg tablets; cycrimine (Pagitane), as 1.25 and 2.5 mg tablets; and procyclidine (Kemadrin), 2 and 5 mg tablets. All are virtually identical in their therapeutic effectiveness, with little reason except personal preference for choosing one over the other. Treatment should be initiated with small doses such as trihexyphenidyl, 2 mg three times daily, gradually increased until further increases yield no additional benefit or side effects reach an unacceptable degree of severity.

To obtain optimal results with anticholinergic drugs, careful titration of dosage against side effects is required. The goal is to find the dose that yields an optimal compromise between the limited symptomatic improvement of the parkinsonism and the disagreeable symptoms of cholinergic blockade of the central and peripheral nervous systems. Among the latter are blurring of vision, dryness of mouth and throat, anhidrosis, constipation, and urinary urgency or, sometimes, retention. The major symptoms of central anticholinergic intoxication are ataxia, dysarthria, hyperthermia, and a characteristic pattern of mental disturbances, including impairment of recent memory, confusion, delusional thinking, hallucinations, somnolence, and rarely coma.

A number of other agents, not primarily anticholinergics but with mild central anticholinergic properties, are useful. Diphenhydramine (Benadryl), orphenadrine (Disipal), and chlorphenoxamine (Phenoxene) are all similar in pharmacologic action, and there is no reason except personal preference or individual tolerance in choosing one over the other. In general, diphenhydramine has enjoyed the widest use and can be given in divided dosage up to 150 mg a day. It is particularly useful as an adjunct to levodopa, for in addition to benefiting symptoms of parkinsonism, it allays anxiety and tempers insomnia.

The antidepressants imipramine (Tofranil) and amitriptyline (Elavil) are minimally effective when used alone, but in combination with anticholinergic agents or levodopa they may be beneficial. With administration in limited dosage, one may avoid their adverse effects, which may resemble parkinsonism. Not only are they helpful in improving akinesia and rigidity, but depressive symptoms when present are relieved. Imipramine or amitriptyline, 10 to 25 mg given four times a day, can be safely administered for extended periods.

Introduced as an antiviral agent, amantadine HCl (Symmetrel) was accidentally found to have activity against parkinsonism. Its mechanism of action in this regard is unknown, but it has been postulated that it may augment striatal dopaminergic activity or block cholinergic action. When used alone in doses of 100 mg twice a day, its therapeutic effects are evident within 48 to 72 hours, consisting of a mild reversal of symptoms of parkinsonism. More effective action can be achieved when it is added to an existing regimen of treatment consisting of anticholinergic agents or levodopa (or both). On occasion amantadine has proved useful during the induction phase of levodopa therapy. Its effects are short lived, tending to diminish after a month and rarely lasting for more than three months. Many of its side effects are similar to those of the anticholinergic agents, particularly the induction of confusional and delusional states. In some patients after long-term use, edema and a form of livedo reticularis develop over the limbs.

Surgical Measures Surgical attempts to alleviate parkinsonism are primarily directed to the interruption of one or more neural pathways, the integrity of which appears essential for the production of symptoms, and at a site where normal sensory and motor functions will not be affected. Lesions produced by electrocoagulation or freezing in the ventrolateral nucleus of the thalamus have relieved contralateral tremor and rigidity in the limbs. However, akinesia and disturbances in gait, posture, and voice are not appreciably improved, and multiple lesions are necessary to relieve cervical, truncal, and bilateral limb symptoms. Since in most cases tremor and rigidity are bilateral, a good result on one side often encourages an attempt to do the same for the other. Most surgeons prefer to wait six months to one year before operating on the second side to minimize the complications that are apt to occur with bilateral procedures. Even so, the bilateral procedure frequently produces adverse effects on speech and, though recovery usually occurs, the patient may retain some degree of dysarthria and hypophonia. Since in most cases the manifestations become bilateral within a year or two of the onset, and disability is eventually due not so much to tremor or rigidity but to akinesia and postural abnormalities, stereotactic surgery benefits only a limited number of patients. The best candidate for surgery is the patient whose chief manifestation is unilateral tremor and rigidity, preferably in the upper extremity, and whose disease seems to progress slowly. These characteristics represent an early stage of the disease, and usually the patient is not yet seriously disabled. Thus, proponents of stereotactic surgery urge that thalamotomy be considered early in the course of Parkinson's disease, although its critics have pointed out that surgery does not benefit the more advanced patients who most need help, nor does it prevent progression of the disease. The introduction of more effective pharmacologic therapy with its potential of completely controlling parkinsonian symptoms has diminished the enthusiasm for surgical intervention. A balanced judgment would be that thalamotomy be reversed for cases resistant to other forms of therapy and in which relief of upper limb tremor is desired.

Costa, E., Cote, L., and Yahr, M. D. (eds): Biochemistry and Pharmacology of the Basal Ganglia. Hewlett, N.Y., Raven Press, 1966.

Cotzias, G. C., Papavasiliou, P. S., and Gellene, R.: Modification of parkinsonisim: Chronic treatment with L-dopa. N. Engl. J. Med., 280:337, 1969.

Crane, G. E.: Persistence of neurological symptoms due to neuroleptic drugs. Am. J. Psychiatry, 127:1407, 1971.

Crane, G. E.: Tardive dyskinesia in patients treated with major neuroleptics: A review of the literature. Am. J. Psychiatry, 124:40, 1968.

Duvoisin, R. C., and Yahr, M. D.: Encephalitis and parkinsonism. Arch. Neurol. 12:227, 1965.

Hoehn, M. M., and Yahr, M. D.: Parkinsonism: Onset, progression and mortality. Neurology, 17:427, 1967.

Markham, C. H., Brown, W. J., and Rand, R. W.: Stereotaxic lesions in Parkinson's disease. Arch. Neurol., 15:480, 1966.

Yahr, M. D.: The treatment of parkinsonism: Current concepts. Med. Clin. North Am., 56:1377, 1972.

366. ESSENTIAL TREMOR (Familial Tremor)

Melvin D. Yahr

This is a monosymptomatic condition in which tremor involves the hands and/or head and face. The tremor is usually more rapid than that encountered in parkinsonism, is accentuated by emotional factors, may be worsened by volitional movement, and is usually suppressed by the use of alcohol. The age of onset is variable, but in most cases the disorder begins prior to the age of 25 years and tends to persist throughout life. Some progression of the intensity of tremor and spread to other bodily parts usually occur over the years, which may result in significant physical and social disability. There is a strong familial incidence, with occurrence in several successive generations and members of the same family, but the genetic pattern of inheritance has not been determined. Some have suggested its transmission as an autosomal dominant trait. To date no specific pathologic lesion has been reported in the nervous system of people with this condition. It has been suggested that the condition is an abortive form of parkinsonism, but this concept does not appear justifiable at present. There is no specific effective therapy for controlling the tremor, although beta-adrenergic blocking agents such as propranolol in dosage of 120 to 140 mg a day divided equally into three or four doses are occasionally effective. Sedatives such as phenobarbital, in dosage of 15 mg three times a day, may reduce the intensity of the tremor. It is of utmost importance to differentiate essential tremor from parkinsonism. By and large, the distinguishing characteristics are earlier age of onset; lack of severe progression, akinesia, rigidity, or postural abnormalities; and the strong family history of tremor.

Baughman, F. A., Jr., Higgins, J. V., and Mann, J. D.: Sex chromosome anomalies and essential tremor. Neurology, 23:623, 1973.

Critchley, M.: Observations on essential (heredofamilial) tremor. Brain, 22:113, 1949.

Marshal, J.: Observations on essential tremor. J. Neurol. Neurosurg. Psychiatry, 25:122, 1962.

Scopa, J., Longley, B. P., and Foster, J. B.: Beta-adrenergic blockers in benign essential tremor. Curr. Ther. Res., 15:48, 1973.

367. SENILE TREMOR

Melvin D. Yahr

Tremor is a frequent finding in the elderly, most often involving the upper limbs and head. It differs from parkinsonian tremor in that it is finer and more rapid and at first occurs only with voluntary movements. As time goes on it becomes more constant and is also present while the limbs are at rest. There is no associated weakness or alteration in muscle tone. These features differentiate this form of tremor from parkinsonism. The cause is unknown. Since senile tremor has both cerebellar and extrapyramidal features, in that it occurs at rest and with movement, the assumption is that some critical pathway linking these systems has undergone degeneration. There is no effective treatment, although mild benefit may be derived from sedatives or the use of diphenhydramine (Benadryl) given in 25 mg doses three times a day. Most patients accept it as another of the many changes that come with advancing years. Occasional patients have to be reassured that they do not have parkinsonism or some other progressive neurologic disorder.

THE CHOREAS

Melvin D. Yahr

368. INTRODUCTION

There are a number of disease entities that, though wholly unrelated etiologically, have choreiform movements as their major manifestation. In some, intimate relationships with infectious processes have been found, whereas in others familial tendencies have pointed to a strong genetic component. In the light of newer concepts of inheritance, a common pathogenesis for all may be found. Although controversy exists as to the exact anatomic site from which movements of this type may derive, pathologic changes are commonly found in the striatum, particularly in the small cell components of the caudate nucleus and putamen. The classification of chorea into separate entities is at present somewhat arbitrary and is based on age of onset, association with identifiable disease processes or familial tendency, and occurrence of other neurologic abnormalities.

369. ACUTE CHOREA (Sydenham's or Infectious Chorea, St. Vitus' Dance)

Acute chorea is a movement disorder encountered primarily during childhood and having its greatest incidence between the ages of 5 and 15 years. Occurrence beyond this age is uncommon, and then is usually in association with pregnancy or in persons who have had symptoms earlier in life. Females manifest these symptoms at least twice as often as males. Acute chorea has been reported in people of all races.

Considered as a symptom complex rather than as a specific disease entity, acute choreiform movements have been encountered as initial manifestations of a variety of conditions. They have been reported in epidemic encephalitis, in the encephalopathies occurring with exanthema, with pertussis and diphtheria, in idiopathic hypocalcemia, hyperthyroidism, systemic lupus erythematosus, carbon monoxide poisoning, vascular disease, tumors, and degenerative processes of the basal ganglia. These instances, however, account for only a small percentage of cases. The closest relationship appears to be with rheumatic fever. In more than half of the cases, rheumatic manifestations consisting of carditis, valvular heart disease, or arthritis occur prior to, coincident with, or following an attack of chorea.

There are no specific pathologic changes or anatomic sites of involvement that can be correlated with acute chorea. In fact, because acute uncomplicated chorea is rarely fatal, there has been a paucity of detailed pathologic studies. Cases that have come to autopsy have shown scattered changes in the cortex, basal ganglia, cerebellum, and brainstem. These have consisted of varying degrees of arteritis combined with cellular degeneration.

The outstanding clinical features of chorea are involuntary movements, incoordination, muscle weakness, and emotional lability. Although the onset of symptoms may be abrupt and obvious, it is more often insidious and subtle. The most frequent initial complaints include clumsiness of the limbs, evidenced by dropping objects from the hands or an awkward gait, particularly during emotionally tense situations. When these are coupled with irritability, poor performance in school, and generally fidgety behavior, frequently a hasty conclusion is reached, blaming the child or implying a psychiatric disorder. The typical choreatic movements may be noted in any part of the body, limbs, face, hands, tongue, or trunk. They may at first appear to be a part of the natural pattern of coordinated movements but are soon noted to be completely random, jerking, aimless, and purposeless. They occur at rest, are accentuated by any attempt at volitional movement, and disappear in sleep. They may be very mild and may minimally affect normal function or may be so forceful and frequent as to be totally disabling. Facial grimacing and difficulty in speech, chewing, and swallowing occur when the muscles subserving these functions are involved. Interruption of voluntary movements by involuntary ones leads to incoordination so that the person drops objects, walks in an awkward, ungainly fashion and, in general, appears uncoordinated. Attempts to maintain forceful muscular contraction are similarly interrupted, and the resultant "waxing and waning" of motor power results in a relative degree of motor weakness. Although actual paralysis is rare, there is a disinclination to use a part of the body that is severely affected by involuntary movements of this type. Generalized reduction of muscle tone is an invariable feature of chorea and is readily demonstrable by hyperextensibility at finger, wrist, and ankle joints. In almost all choreatic children some degree of emotional lability is evident. It varies from total apathy to irritability, restlessness, and, infrequently, wild, inappropriate behavior.

Certain cardinal features can be found in almost all patients. These include (1) pronation of the forearm when the upper limbs are raised and extended; (2) inability to sustain muscle contraction when the examiner grasps the patient's hand or when the patient protrudes his tongue so that it darts rapidly in and out of the mouth; and (3) abnormal posturing of hands in which the wrist is noted to be sharply flexed and the fingers hyperextended at the metacarpal pharyngeal joints.

There are no specific laboratory tests for chorea. The cerebrospinal fluid is normal. The electroencephalogram may or may not show diffuse abnormalities correlated with the severity of the disease. Unless there are associated disease processes that manifest themselves in abnormalities of blood count, chemistry, or sedimentation rate, these studies are normal.

The age of onset and the distinctive involuntary movements readily differentiate acute chorea from other disorders of the basal ganglia. Tics and habit spasms may be confused with mild cases, but their movements are quite different, being stereotyped repetitive patterns localized to a single group of muscles. Huntington's chorea rarely begins in childhood and, in addition, there is a strong familial tendency with associated dementia. Movement disorders associated with cerebral palsy occur in infancy but have an athetoid element. The use of phenothiazines may induce abnormal movements, but the history of drug ingestion will differentiate these.

Acute chorea is a self-limited disease, recovery occurring in two to six months. Recurrence, with as many as two or three attacks over a period of years, appears in almost one third of the cases. There is no specific therapy. Bed rest and reduction of external stimuli to a minimum, combined with sedative drugs such as phenobarbital or chloral hydrate, are beneficial in controlling the severity of the movements. Paradoxically, the phenothiazines, such as thorazine and chlorpromazine, as well as reserpine in doses commensurate with individual tolerance, although capable of inducing chorea, have also been shown to be effective in its control. Because of the high incidence of rheumatic valvular heart disease complicating acute chorea, prophylaxis with antimicrobial drugs over a long interval of time similar to that utilized in acute rheumatic fever is now recommended. If emotional symptoms are intense, psychotherapy may be in order. When specific abnormalities of calcium metabolism or thyroid dysfunction are found, their correction may completely ameliorate the symptoms. With recovery most patients show few, if any, neurologic sequelae.

Aron, A., Freeman, J., and Carter, S.: The natural history of Sydenham's chorea. Am. J. Med., 38:83, 1965.

Schwartzman, J.: Chorea minor. Review of 175 cases with reference to etiology, treatment and sequelae. Rheumatism, 6:89, 1950.

370. HEREDITARY CHOREA (Chronic Progressive Chorea, Huntington's Chorea)

Hereditary chorea is a progressive degenerative disease of the basal ganglia and cerebral cortex, beginning in adult life and characterized by choreiform movements and mental deterioration. The inheritance of the disease is based on a single dominant autosomal gene. It may be transmitted by either sex, and both sexes are affected in equal numbers. The trait is transmitted from affected individual to affected individual so that those who escape rarely transmit the disease. Only about 50 per cent of the offspring are affected. The disease is relatively rare, although its incidence may be high in geographic regions where affected families have resided for many generations.

Pathologically, widespread degenerative changes with cell loss and reactive gliosis are found, primarily in the cerebral cortex and caudate nucleus. Recently it has been demonstrated that glutamic acid decarboxylase and choline acetylase activity are reduced in the basal ganglia of patients with Huntington's chorea. This results in a deficiency of γ-aminobutyric acid, an inhibitory transmitter substance in brain, as well as depressed function of the excitatory transmitter acetylcholine. Disruption of the homeostatic relationship of these agents may underlie the choreatic manifestations of this disorder.

The clinical manifestations consist of choreatic movements, emotional disturbance, and intellectual deterioration in varying degrees, rate of appearance, and progression. The disease usually makes its appearance between the ages of 35 and 50 years, rather insidiously with any of the aforementioned symptoms, but as a rule with abnormal movements. The movements, though similar to acute chorea, are usually more jerky though less lightning-like and primarily involve the trunk and shoulder girdle and more often the lower limbs than the upper. This pattern of involvement tends to produce a dancing sort of gait, which is a prominent feature of the disease. In rare instances a Parkinson-like rigidity is encountered as the major manifestation rather than involuntary movements. The mental deterioration is similar to that of any organic dementia, with progressive impairment of memory and of intellectual capacity, and inattention to personal hygiene. Emotional disturbances include heightened irritability, bouts of depression, and fits of violent behavior.

With the typical triad of choreiform movements, dementia in adult life, and documentation of similar symptoms in family members, the diagnosis is readily evident. However, there is a tendency for families to deny the existence of mental disease, and it is sometimes difficult to obtain corroborative data even when the diagnosis is strongly suspected. Little difficulty occurs in differentiating hereditary chorea from acute chorea, but senile chorea may raise a problem. The latter, which comes on late in life, involves few mental changes, if any, lacks a familial history, and is usually benign in comparison. Other diseases such as the presenile psychoses, Alzheimer's and Pick's, because of their dementia and similarity in age of onset, may offer some difficulty, especially in instances in which choreiform movements are inconspicuous. Pneumoencephalography demonstrating selective atrophy of the caudate nucleus may help to establish the correct diagnosis in such instances. There is a tendency to overdiagnose hereditary chorea, applying it to diverse neurologic disorders such as cerebellar degenerations and familial tremors. The dire implications of this form of chorea require strict adherence to the diagnostic criteria.

There is no effective therapy. Theoretically, drugs which are capable of elevating brain γ-aminobutyric acid or enhancing its cholinergic activity should be helpful. Although some, such as phenelzine and dimethyl aminoethanol, are undergoing trial, inadequate reports are available at present to comment on their use. Huntington's chorea is relentlessly progressive, leading to total incapacity and inevitably death, usually within 15 years of onset. In the early stages the patient can be managed at home with supervision and the use of phenothiazines or reserpine to reduce the intensity of the movements and to control the behavior to some extent. As the disease advances, confinement to a psychiatric facility becomes necessary.

Chandler, J. H., Reed, T. E., and DeJong, R. N.: Huntington's chorea in Michigan. Neurology, 10:148, 1960.
Lyon, R. L.: Huntington's chorea. Br. Med. J., 1:1306, 1962.
Perry, T. L., Hansen, S., and Kloster, M.: Huntington's chorea: Deficiency of γ-aminobutyric acid in brain. N. Engl. J. Med., 288:337, 1973.

371. SENILE CHOREA

Infrequently, choreiform movements are encountered as an isolated symptom in persons above 60 years of age. As a rule, the movements are mild and may involve the limbs on one side of the body or bilaterally. Involuntary complex movements of the face, mouth, and tongue may occur, in association with limb movements or as the only manifestation of this disorder. No associated mental disturbance occurs in such patients, and no family history indicative of Huntington's chorea can be obtained. In many instances the symptoms come on abruptly, are unilateral, and show little, if any, progression. This has suggested an underlying vascular lesion, which may be found in an exceptional case. More often than not the pathologic findings are similar to those of Huntington's chorea insofar as involvement of the caudate nucleus is concerned, but the cerebral cortex is spared. This has led to the contrary consideration that these cases are a variant of Huntington's chorea occurring sporadically. Probably this form of chorea has several causes. As a rule, the symptoms are mild and the course benign so that therapeutic considerations are unimportant.

Martin, J. P.: Hemichorea resulting from local lesions of the brain. Brain, 50:637, 1927.
Weiner, W. J., and Klawans, H. L., Jr.: Lingual-facial-buccal movements in the elderly. II. Pathogenesis and relationship to senile chorea. J. Am. Geriat. Soc., 21:318, 1973.

372. TICS (Habit Spasms)

Melvin D. Yahr

A tic is a sudden, abrupt, rapid, purposeless, involuntary contraction of a muscle or group of functionally related muscles. Usually an irregular sequence of such contractions occurs that may result in eye blinking, head shaking, shrugging of the shoulder, or any sudden gesture of limbs or face. Tics may be voluntarily controlled for brief intervals, but such a conscious effort is usually followed by more intense and frequent contractions. Many persons experience minor transitory tic phenomena under periods of stress that are of no consequence. More persistent, sustained, and gross movements may be related to particular personality disturbances, and may be amenable to psychotherapy. In some instances tics have occurred during the acute phase of encephalitis; these are thought to be an expression of extrapyramidal dysfunction. Tics in younger patients must be differentiated from chorea. Their patterned, predictable, and stereotyped character makes this distinction.

An unusual form of generalized tic (*maladie des tics, Gilles de la Tourette's disease*) involving facial twitching, continuous gestures associated with echolalia, foul language, and obsessional ideas is occasionally encountered in childhood. The disorder is progressive, and sometimes associated with marked personality changes. Recently, however, a number of reports have appeared suggesting that haloperidol (Haldol) in divided dosage of 6 to 20 mg a day may be effective both in reducing the movement disorder and in overcoming the unfortunate verbal outbursts.

Hansen, M., and Eisler, R. M.: Behavioral approaches to study and treatment of psychogenic tics. Genet. Psychol. Monogr., 87:289, 1973.

Shapiro, A. K., Shapiro, E., and Wayne, H.: Treatment of Tourette's syndrome with haloperidol, review of 34 cases. Arch. Gen. Psychiatry, 28:92, 1973.

373. ATHETOSIS (Mobile Spasms)

Melvin D. Yahr

This involuntary movement disorder is most frequently encountered in early infancy. Although in some respects it resembles chorea and although there are, in fact, transitional forms (so-called choreo-athetosis), the athetotic movements are distinguishable by being slower, coarser, and more writhing. They occur when pathologic conditions involve the basal ganglia, primarily the pallidum, as well as additional motor pathways such as the corticospinal tract. Athetosis is most often found in the heterogeneous group of conditions now lumped together under the term "cerebral palsy" (CP). More often than not, patients with cerebral palsy have marked alteration in muscle tone consisting of a combination of spasticity and rigidity. Their extrapyramidal movements may be widespread or limited and encompass a wide variety of dyskinetic phenomena. Congenital defects, anoxia or trauma at birth, and other degenerative conditions have all been implicated. Some attempt has been made to identify specific entities based on clinicopathologic correlations. One such is athetosis simplex or status marmoratus. Cases of this disorder, which exemplifies all of the features of athetosis, show at autopsy a distinctive marbled appearance of the basal ganglia, the result of an abnormal overgrowth of myelin sheaths and increased numbers of glial cells. The cause of this morphologic abnormality is unknown. Other cases have been grouped together in which the prime pathologic change is cell loss and failure of myelin sheath formation in the region of the basal ganglia—so-called status dysmyelination. Still other cases have been encountered in which abnormal deposits of pigments occur or one of the the lipoidoses or other storage diseases is found with the predominant clinical picture of athetotic movements. Athetosis is infrequently encountered in adult life, but when it is, tumors, vascular insufficiency, or malformations and the effects of toxic agents have been found in the region of the basal ganglia.

Typical athetosis possesses the following features in varying degrees. One or both sides of the body are involved. The movements involve the upper limbs to a greater extent than the lower and primarily in their distal segments. The muscles innervated by the cranial nerves are invariably involved so that facial grimacing, writhing movements of the tongue, and disturbances in articulation and swallowing are encountered. Abnormal postures of the limbs are assumed. In the upper extremities, these consist of adduction and internal rotation at the shoulder, semiflexion at the elbow, flexion of wrist and metacarpal phalangeal joints, and extension at interphalangeal joints. In the lower limbs the foot is maintained in internal rotation and plantar flexion with dorsiflexion of the toes. Superimposed on these abnormal postures are the athetotic movements described above. Muscle tone is increased during movement but is hypotonic during relaxation, and some degree of weakness is usually found. The reflexes may be hyperactive, with abnormal toe responses. In many instances some degree of intellectual impairment may be found.

The abnormal movements and postural abnormalities are distinctive enough to make this condition readily recognizable. The age at onset, the admixture of other neurologic abnormalities, and the manner in which the symptoms progress identify the disease. Since most instances of athetosis appear in early infancy, before one year of age, diseases of the perinatal period are considered primarily. Athetosis occurring in later childhood or adult life may be a part of other extrapyramidal disorders, such as dystonia, chorea, or hepatolenticular degeneration. Less frequently athetosis is a manifestation of a wide spectrum of neurologic disorders already mentioned in which the pallidum is coincidentally involved.

There is no specific therapy for the relief of athetosis. The use of anticholinergic agents as previously indicated under the treatment of parkinsonism may decrease the intensity of the movements. Thalamotomy has on occasion afforded some degree of relief, but one is hesitant to advocate this surgical procedure on a nervous system already extensively damaged by a variety of pathologic processes.

Courville, C. B.: Structural basis of athetosis in cerebral palsied children. Arch. Pediat., 78:461, 1961.

Mettler, F. A., and Stern, G.: On the patho-physiology of athetosis. J. Nerv. Ment. Dis., 135:138, 1962.

Narabayashi, H., and Nakamura, R.,: Clinical picture of cerebral palsy in neurological understanding. Confin. Neurol., 34:7, 1972.

374. DYSTONIA MUSCULORUM DEFORMANS (Torsion Dystonia)

Melvin D. Yahr

The torsion dystonias comprise a group of movement disorders characterized by intense, irregular, sustained torsion spasms of the musculature, with resultant marked abnormalities of bodily posture. The dystonic movements may involve any or all of the musculature, but have a predilection for the trunk and shoulder and pelvic girdles. The cause and morbid anatomy of this condition are unknown.

Three forms can be recognized, based on genetic, clinical, and presumed causative factors. These consist of autosomal recessive, autosomal dominant, and acquired or symptomatic types. Symptomatic dystonic movements occur with hepatolenticular degeneration, postencephalitic parkinsonism, and tumors or other diseases involving the basal ganglia; dystonia musculorum deformans is a distinct clinical entity. Glial scarring in the basal ganglia, thalamus, and cortex has been described in some cases, and some have been associated with status marmoratus and dysmyelination, as indicated in Ch. 373.

The autosomal recessive form is found most often in Ashkenazic Jews, beginning between the ages of 5 and 15 years. Its onset is variable but most frequently begins with intermittent spasmodic inversion of the foot, so that on walking the child finds difficulty in placing the heel on the ground. Bizarre stepping or a bowing gait may be noted when the dystonic movements affect the more proximal muscles of the leg or the spine. As the movements become more intense and the proximal musculature is more prominently involved, lordosis and tortipelvis appear. If the muscles of the neck and shoulder girdle are involved, torticollis is an early finding. Facial grimacing and difficulties in speech become evident as the muscles subserving these functions become involved. The continuous spasms over a period of time result in marked distortions of the body of a degree rarely seen in any other disease process. Although muscle tone and power appear to be normal, the involuntary movements interfere with function to such a degree as to make them useless. No changes in the deep tendon reflexes occur, and mentation remains normal.

The autosomal dominant form has its onset in early adult life and generally involves the axial musculature, with torticollis a frequent presenting symptom. In contrast to the recessive form, it remains more restricted in the regions of the body involved and is more slowly progressive. Recently it has been demonstrated that plasma dopamine beta hydroxylase activity is markedly elevated in the dominant form. This finding is strictly empiric, and although it is helpful in classification of the disease, neither the physiologic nor the biochemical significance of this finding has been elucidated.

In its early stages dystonia musculorum deformans must be differentiated from other movement disorders in which dystonic phenomena may occur. The history and physical findings exclude hepatolenticular degeneration and epidemic encephalitis. The age at onset and the involvement of proximal musculature in the movements are enough to differentiate it from athetosis. Chorea is characterized by movements more rapid and of shorter duration than those of dystonia. Hysteria is often a consideration; if it is not positively established by the personality characteristics of the patient, the course of the disease will soon suggest the correct diagnosis.

There is extreme variability in the rate of progression and eventual disability of both forms of the genetically determined disorder. In their early phases there may be complete remission of symptoms or lack of progression of initial symptoms for intervals of up to five years. Because the natural history is subject to wide variations, evaluation of the effects of treatment is difficult. Dystonic movements have been effectively controlled for varying periods of time by both drugs and surgical intervention. The medicines effective are anticholinergic agents such as those indicated for the treatment of parkinsonism, combined with sedative agents such as phenobarbital. In mild cases a combination of these drugs with some general supportive psychotherapy may be enough to control the patient's symptoms for years. On occasion, carbamazepine (Tegretol) in daily dosage of 800 to 1200 mg a day divided equally in four or five doses has proved effective. Levodopa has been reported as being effective in selected cases. In general a lower daily dose (3 grams per day) than that used in parkinsonism has been required. In more serious cases thalamotomy has produced encouraging results. However, because rather extensive lesions must be placed in the thalamic nuclei, multiple operative procedures are required to produce the desired effect. Although the operations are well tolerated by most patients, they do carry an element of risk and are indicated only in selected cases.

Denny-Brown, D. E.: The nature of dystonia. Bull. N.Y. Acad. Med., 41:858, 1965.

Eldridge, R.: The torsion dystonias: Literature review and genetic and clinical studies. Neurology, 20:1, 1970.

375. SPASMODIC TORTICOLLIS

Melvin D. Yahr

The restriction of dyskinetic movements to neck muscles so that abnormal postures of the head result is the distinguishing characteristic of this symptom complex. Involuntary activity involves the sternocleidomastoids, trapezius, and scalenus muscles in sustained contractions that result in slow, twisting, turning movements of the head (torticollis) or less often forward flexion (anterocollis) or forceful extension (retrocollis). In most instances there is bilateral involvement, and the resultant postural deformity is maintained for varying lengths of time. The muscles of the neck appear under tension, and the continual muscular activity may lead to some degree of hypertrophy, especially evident in the sternocleidomastoid. Similar activity may spread to facial and brachial musculature. The amount of active motion or static postural deformity is extremely variable.

Spasmodic torticollis has variably been described as a psychogenic disorder, a fragment of dystonia musculorum deformans, or a compensatory postural defect in persons with congenital ocular muscle imbalance or defects of the cervical spine or musculature. In some instances it has occurred as part of a wide spectrum of extrapyramidal disorders that follow encephalitis lethargica. There is no information at present regarding either its pathophysiology or pathology.

The disorder has been encountered at all ages, but most frequently makes its appearance during the third to sixth decades of life. The course is extremely variable, being transitory and remitting after a few months in some patients and relentlessly progressive and leading to incapacity in others. Some cases reach a static phase in which movements cease or are minimal, and a minor postural deformity of the head persists.

The evaluation of this condition includes a search for ocular and vertebral signs, major psychiatric disturbances, and other neurologic conditions with which it may be associated. Definable conditions account for only a small percentage of cases. In most, no known cause is uncovered.

There is no specific therapy for torticollis except when an underlying correctible disease process is found. Many measures have been recommended to ameliorate the symptoms. In mild cases or in the initial stages, a combination of drugs previously discussed under the treatment of parkinsonism has proved useful. Symptoms may be reduced to a tolerable degree, and it can be hoped that spontaneous remission will intervene. In those more severely affected a variety of surgical measures have been attempted with inconsistent results. Denervation of the affected muscles by section of the anterior cervical roots and/or the spinal accessory nerve has been utilized. Although the movements decrease on the operated side, they frequently recur in the contralateral group of muscles. Bilateral procedures may result in extensive disability. Recently thalamotomy has been performed with encouraging results. One is hesitant, however, to recommend a procedure of this magnitude except in extreme situations.

Herz, E., and Glaser, G. H.: Spasmodic torticollis. Clinical evaluation. Arch. Neurol. Psychiatry, 61:227, 1949.

376. HEMIBALLISM

Melvin D. Yahr

This rather violent involuntary movement occurs when lesions involve the contralateral subthalamic nucleus, the corpus Luysii. Although a variety of pathologic processes such as tumor and infectious diseases have been found as underlying causes, most are a result of vascular lesions, either hemorrhagic or occlusive. In consequence, they are encountered in older patients, sometimes after a transitory hemiparesis. The event leading to the onset of this movement disorder often is an acute cerebrovascular accident with weakness and/or sensory deficit. As the neurologic signs clear or at a variable interval afterward, the ballistic movements begin. The movements do not occur during sleep, are localized to one side of the body, and involve the limbs in a forceful throwing movement, a result of almost continuous activity of the proximal musculature. Initially, their violence may exhaust and incapacitate the patient to such an extent that death may ensue. However, in most instances, the initial intensity decreases gradually so that they become tolerable, and in approximately six to eight weeks the movements stop spontaneously. Surgical measures, such as thalamotomy, are rarely needed for control. In this regard, it is interesting to note that hemiballism has followed attempted thalamotomy for other extrapyramidal disorders when poor localization for lesion placement has occurred. In such instances, the surgeon has inadvertently placed a lesion in the region of the corpus Luysii.

Carpenter, M. B.: Ballism associated with partial destruction of the subthalamic nucleus of Luys. Neurology, 5:479, 1955.
Hyland, H. H., and Forman, D. M.: Progress in hemiballismus. Neurology. 7:381, 1957.
Martin, P. J., and McCaul, I. R.: Acute hemiballism treated by ventrolateral thalamolysis. Brain, 82:104, 1959.

377. IDIOPATHIC AUTONOMIC INSUFFICIENCY (Idiopathic Orthostatic Hypotension, Shy-Drager Syndrome)

Fred Plum

Definition. This is an uncommon disorder first clearly described by Bradbury and Eggleston in 1925 as idiopathic orthostatic hypotension; it has been more recently emphasized as including more generalized autonomic and nervous system defects. The cause is unknown and the course progressive; severe disability or death usually occurs within five to ten years after onset.

Pathology and Pathogenesis. Detailed examination of the central and peripheral nervous system at autopsy discloses degenerative changes in the intermediolateral column of the spinal cord, the dorsal motor nuclei, and the pigmented nuclei of the brainstem. In addition, some patients have abnormalities which resemble olivopontocerebellar degeneration, whereas others show striatal-nigral degeneration. Peripheral autonomic structures are morphologically normal in most patients. The cause is unknown.

Several observations indicate that the disease begins as a defect in preganglionic autonomic transmitter function. Most of the patients demonstrate a blood pressure hypersensitivity to injected levarterenol, implying the absence of the humoral agent in the sympathetic ganglia. Also, patients with neurogenic orthostatic hypotension have been found not to synthesize norepinephrine and its metabolic products in normal amounts and to have below normal urinary catecholamine levels. Since the drug tyramine, which acts to release norepinephrine from peripheral autonomic nerve terminals, is effective in elevating the blood pressure, at least some epinephrine synthesis must be going on in postganglionic peripheral nerve terminals, but whether this is of a normal or reduced amount is unknown.

Clinical Manifestations. Symptoms of autonomic insufficiency predominate initially. These include impotence in males, constipation, heat intolerance with anhidrosis, and, above all, weakness or faintness or rising to an erect position or during quiet standing. Urinary urgency or retention is common. As the disease progresses, symptoms of more generalized neurologic dysfunction appear. Some patients develop a Parkinson-like illness with hypokinesia, rhythmic postural tremor, and mild to moderate rigidity. Others develop a cerebellar type of incoordination plus a gross rhythmic tremor in the lower extremities. The mind remains clear.

Physical signs include prominent evidence of autonomic insufficiency. Pupillary abnormalities with Horner's syndrome can alternate from side to side. Even with a high environmental temperature there is diffuse anhidrosis of the trunk and extremities. The blood pressure is normal when the subject lies supine, but when he stands, systolic and diastolic pressures drop 20 to 40 mm Hg or more but the pulse fails to accelerate. In the early stage of illness the blood pressure can gradually climb during continued standing, but as the disease advances, autonomic compensation decreases and then fails altogether, and syncope with unobtainable blood pressure tends to interrupt any sustained effort to be erect. By this time, many patients have associated signs of generalized neurologic dysfunction, including the Parkinson-like signs mentioned above as well as a cerebellar type of incoordination, muscle wasting and fasciculations, coarse tremors, and extensor plantar responses. Signs of peripheral neuropathy are notably lacking in the idiopathic disease.

Laboratory tests of the usual type are valueless except to exclude other disorders, but confirmation of the autonomic insufficiency makes the diagnosis.

Briefly, the evaluation of autonomic insufficiency investigates the blood pressure response to tilting and quiet standing, the patient's ability to sweat when heated, a cold pressor test (the response is absent), the blood pressure response to injected levarterenol and sublingual nitroglycerin (the responses are hyperactive), and the response to the Valsalva maneuver (the normal blood pressure overshoot with its accompanying tachycardia fails to occur).

Differential Diagnosis. Orthostatic hypotension can accompany acute cardiac failure (as with myocardial infarction or severe aortic stenosis), blood volume depletion (as with gastrointestinal or other massive hemorrhage), or vasodepressor syncope, but in all these conditions other signs of autonomic activity such as tachycardia and sweating are present and signs of diffuse neurologic illness are absent. Autonomic insufficiency also accompanies some clearly identifiable neurologic diseases, including central thiamin deficiency (Wernicke's encephalopathy), tabes dorsalis, syringomyelia, surgical sympathectomy, the neuropathies of diabetes, amyloidosis, and the Guillain-Barré syndrome, and a small fraction of patients who have vascular occlusive disease producing infarction or ischemia of brainstem autonomic centers. The differentiation from most of these illnesses is readily made by the typical signs, symptoms, and laboratory findings of each, and particularly by the fact that most of them produce sensory impairments in the extremities and other peripheral nerve abnormalities which are altogether lacking in idiopathic autonomic insufficiency.

Course and Treatment. Although treatment is rarely completely satisfactory and does not affect the disease itself, much can be done to help these patients symptomatically during the early phase of the illness. Nine-α-fluorohydrocortisone given regularly by mouth is often effective in counteracting the orthostatic hypotension; it presumably operates partly by increasing the blood volume. Elastic bandages on the legs may help by reducing venous pooling. Placing the head of the bed on six-inch blocks for sleeping has been found to lessen the next day's degree of orthostatic hypotension. Pressor agents have generally been useless because of their short, intense action and undesirable side effects. However, a combination of monoamine oxidase inhibitors (which reduce the deamination of catecholamines in sympathetic nerve storage pools) and amphetamines (which stimulate norepinephrine release) has been found effective in maintaining the erect blood pressure of some patients previously bedridden from their illness.

Bannister, R., and Oppenheimer, D. R.: Degenerative diseases of the nervous system associated with autonomic failure. Brain, 95:457, 1972.
Bradbury, S., and Eggleston, C.: Postural hypotension: Report of 3 cases. Am. Heart J., 1:73, 1925.
Lewis, R. K., Hazelrig, C. G., Fricke, F. J., and Russell, R. O.: Therapy of idiopathic postural hypotension. Arch. Intern. Med., 129:943, 1972.
Shy, R. M., and Drager, G. A.: A neurological syndrome associated with orthostatic hypotension. Arch. Neurol., 2:511, 1960.
Stead, E. A., Jr., and Ebert, R. V.: Postural hypotension: Disease of sympathetic nervous system. Arch. Intern. Med., 67:546, 1941.

Section Eleven. CEREBROVASCULAR DISEASES

Fletcher H. McDowell

378. INTRODUCTION

It is estimated that there are 2 million persons alive today who have neurologic manifestations of cerebrovascular disease and that cerebrovascular disease of all varieties is annually responsible for approximately 200,000 deaths in the United States. Fully a half million Americans each year suffer a new, acute cerebrovascular attack. The over-all problem is even more imposing than the annual incidence and mortality figures. Recurrent vascular accidents are common in nearly all forms of cerebrovascular disease, each recurrence carrying a high risk of mortality. For the survivors, disability and dependency are the usual result. The need for medical care and hospital facilities for these patients is enormous and is an imposing challenge to medical and social service agencies alike.

In the following chapters, the cerebral vascular diseases are divided into two general groups, those producing ischemic *cerebral infarction* and those producing *intracranial hemorrhage.* Much of the material is derived from observations on 966 patients with clinically diagnosed cerebral vascular disease undergoing long-term study at the Cornell Division of Bellevue Hospital in New York City. As a rough index of the frequency of the different types of cerebral vascular accident or "stroke," 88 per cent of these patients had acute infarction or less severe cerebral ischemic attacks, and 12 per cent had intracranial hemorrhage. Of the infarctions, about one in eight was attributed to cerebral embolism.

379. CEREBRAL ISCHEMIA AND INFARCTION

DEFINITION AND ETIOLOGY

Cerebral thrombosis and cerebral emboli produce clinical symptoms by causing cerebral infarction, which means neural death from ischemia. Cerebral ischemia is the result of either a generalized or a localized prolonged reduction of blood flow to the brain. If ischemia is transient, less than 10 to 15 minutes, usually no discernible neurologic deficit remains. If it lasts longer than that, neural damage results, producing neurologic dysfunction, disability, and death.

The causes of cerebral infarction are numerous. The following are the most common ones:

1. Atherosclerotic disease of the intra- and extracranial arteries
2. Cerebral emboli with: (a) rheumatic heart disease, (b) myocardial infarction, (c) cardiac disease and atrial fibrillation, (d) subacute bacterial endocarditis, (e) nonbacterial thrombotic endocarditis
3. Reduced cerebral blood flow from severe hypotension or dysrhythmia of cardiac disease
4. Cerebral arterial spasm following subarachnoid hemorrhage
5. Generalized cerebral hypoxia from (a) cardiopulmonary insufficiency, (b) pulmonary emboli, (c) carbon monoxide poisoning
6. Cerebral thrombosis due to arteritis: (a) collagen vascular disease, (b) giant cell arteritis, (c) bacterial arteritis, including syphilis
7. Cerebral thrombosis due to polycythemia or ischemia caused by severe anemia
8. Cerebral thrombosis adjacent to intracerebral hemorrhage
9. Cerebral arterial vasoconstriction associated with migraine
10. Dissecting aneurysm of the aorta or great vessels in the neck

INCIDENCE AND EPIDEMIOLOGY

Cerebral infarction is most commonly the result of cerebral atherosclerosis and cerebral emboli. In the Cornell-Bellevue series of 873 cases with nonhemorrhagic stroke, 92 per cent were clinically related to cerebral atherosclerosis and 8 per cent to cerebral emboli. In the group with cerebral emboli 20 per cent occurred in association with myocardial infarction, 26 per cent with rheumatic heart disease, most commonly with mitral stenosis, and atrial fibrillation, and the remainder in patients with atrial fibrillation associated with other varieties of heart disease.

Cerebral infarction is almost twice as frequent in males as in females. The peak age period is 60 to 69 years, but the incidence of stroke rises linearly with increasing age. In the Cornell-Bellevue study, stroke occurred earlier than the age of 50 in only 8 per cent of the patients.

NEUROPATHOLOGY

The brain is exquisitely dependent on its oxygen supply. There is no reserve of oxygen in cerebral tissue to sustain cerebral metabolism during periods of reduced or absent cerebral blood flow. When the brain is acutely and completely deprived of oxygen generally or locally, the electroencephalogram changes within 10 to 20 seconds, and irreversible and extensive neural damage occurs in the cerebral hemispheres after three to ten minutes. The determinants of brain ischemia are hypoxia and reduced general or local cerebral perfusion. The more important of the two is a decrease in perfusion. When ischemia is prolonged, the ischemic tissue softens, and the usually distinct margins between gray and white matter become unclear and occasionally hemorrhagic. Under the microscope, neurons are seen to be necrotic and shrunken, i.e., infarcted.

Cerebral infarctions that follow ischemia may be "pale" (nonhemorrhagic) or hemorrhagic. The extravasation of blood into tissues more commonly follows an embolic arterial obstruction, and pale infarcts more frequently follow atherosclerotic or thrombotic arterial obstruction. Often the two varieties of infarction blend together, and there is little advantage in extensively weighing the difference of causation.

A variable amount of *cerebral edema* accompanies cerebral infarction. With large infarctions the edema may be so extensive that portions of the swollen hemisphere shift under the falx or down through the tentorium cerebelli. This change in intracranial space relationships further impairs the flow of blood and cerebrospinal fluid, thus increasing the ischemia and neurologic deficit. This is often followed by secondary congestion and ischemia of the upper brainstem, which is almost invariably fatal.

It is common to find numerous old, small cerebral infarctions in patients dying from other causes, indicating that cerebral infarctions need not always give rise to symptoms. Old infarctions that have been hemorrhagic are identified at postmortem examination by the presence of hemosiderin in the wall of the infarct. As the infarct ages, the necrotic area breaks down, is absorbed, and eventually may be replaced by a fluid-filled cavity lined with glial and fibrovascular tissue.

MECHANISMS

Cerebral infarction is usually accompanied by abnormalities in the state of the arterial conducting system from the heart to the brain or the venous system draining the brain; the efficiency of the heart as a pump in producing a constant blood flow at a sufficient arterial pressure; and the character of the circulating medium (blood), its viscosity, its oxygen-carrying capacity, and its capacity to change from a colloidal suspension to a gel. Most cerebral infarctions are due to simultaneous changes in several of these factors.

The arterial conducting system is most often altered by atherosclerotic disease. In the third decade of life atherosclerosis is usually evident in the arteries leading to the brain, particularly in the larger cerebral arteries. Sites of predilection for plaques (Fig. 1) are the origins of the common carotid artery; just above the common carotid bifurcation; the internal carotid in its siphonous portion; the origin of the middle cerebral artery; and the vertebral arteries just after they enter the skull and the basilar artery. The atheromatous process in cerebral arteries is the same as that found elsewhere in the body, with lipid deposition in the intima, fibrous tissue overgrowth, hemorrhage into the plaques, ulceration of the plaques, and vessel obstruction.

Although atheromatous vascular disease begins early, it is a silent process for most of the life of the patient, and rarely produces symptoms until the middle years, when myocardial infarction, cerebral infarction, and lower extremity infarction occur. Most postmortem studies show

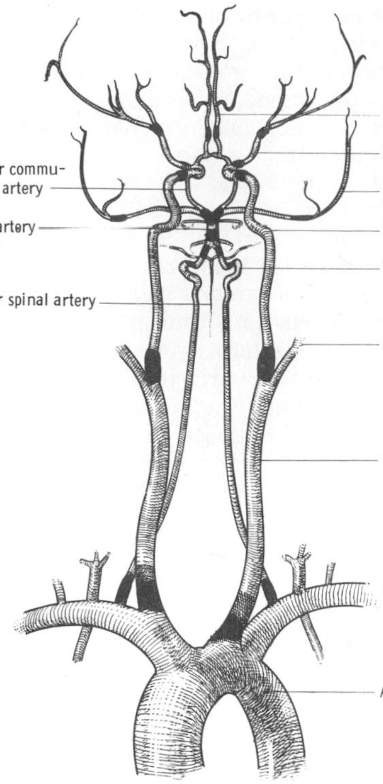

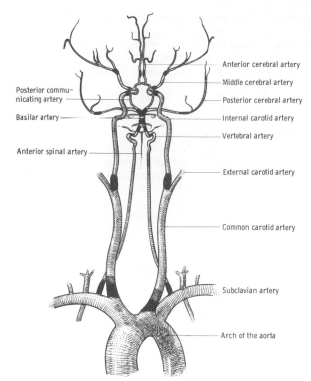

Figure 1. The darkened areas on the arterial diagram show the common sites of atherosclerosis and obstruction in the cerebral vessels.

that 80 to 90 per cent of all adult patients examined at autopsy have significant atheromatous disease. Since by no means all of these had experienced adverse clinical effects, the factors determining symptomatic complications assume major importance.

The first factor of importance is the degree and extent of atheromatous vascular disease, both in the arteries in the neck leading to the head and in the intracranial cerebral arteries. In general, persons who have cerebral infarctions have the most extensive cerebrovascular disease in the arteries in the neck and in the head. However, the pathogenesis of infarction depends on several mechanisms, and patients with only small or moderate amounts of vascular disease sometimes suffer serious cerebral infarcts. Conversely, extensive atheromatous disease can be found in large and small intracranial and extracranial cerebral arteries in patients without cerebral infarction.

Diabetes or *hypertension* can be detected in over two thirds of patients who have had cerebrovascular accidents. Patients with either diabetes or hypertension develop atherosclerosis at an earlier age, and the process develops more rapidly than in patients without these complicating illnesses. The atherosclerotic disease is extensive and is found in the smaller intracranial arteries.

The condition of the *cerebral collateral circulation* influences the development of cerebral infarction in persons with atherosclerosis. Most collateral circulation from one major intracerebral arterial system to another is through the circle of Willis via the posterior communicating arteries or the anterior communicating artery. Other sites of collateral circulation include the interconnections of the pial arteries on the cerebral surface between the anterior, middle, and posterior cerebral arteries. Sites of collateral circulation that become functional only when circulation through other routes is impaired are also found between the external and the internal carotid artery system, via the ophthalmic artery, and through muscular branches between the vertebral arteries and the external carotid artery in the neck.

Anomalies of the circle of Willis occur in nearly half the population. The most common is atresia of the posterior communicating artery, which tends to isolate the anterior (carotid system) circulation from the posterior (vertebral basilar) circulation. Anomalies in the circle of Willis are even more common in patients with cerebral infarction, and thus are believed to increase the chances of stroke in patients with cerebral atherosclerosis.

Inflammatory states involving the cerebral arteries are another cause of cerebral infarction. Inflammation produces edema and fibrosis of the vascular wall, which reduces the carrying capacity of the vessel and causes a decrease in cerebral blood flow distally. Collagen-vascular disease is the most common vascular inflammation causing cerebral infarction. Syphilis was formerly the most common inflammation of the cerebral arteries and a frequent cause of cerebral infarction, especially in young persons. Rarely, acute bacterial infections of the pharynx have been followed by vasculitis of the carotid arteries and cerebral infarction. Another uncommon illness is Takayasu's disease, which affects the origin of the cerebral arteries from the aortic arch and its branches, and often results in cerebral infarction, especially in young to middle-aged women.

CEREBRAL EMBOLI

Cerebral infarction can occur without intrinsic arterial disease when emboli block arteries and impair blood flow. The most common cause of cerebral emboli in patients under 50 is rheumatic heart disease with mitral stenosis and atrial fibrillation. Other conditions associated with embolus formation are myocardial infarction with mural thrombi, atrial fibrillation of unknown cause, subacute bacterial endocarditis, thyrotoxicosis with atrial fibrillation, and nonbacterial thrombotic endocarditis. Fat emboli are rare. Paradoxical emboli have been reported as a cause of cerebral infarction. These arise in distal veins, and are shunted through the heart to the brain through a patent foramen ovale.

The neuropathologic changes in the brain that follow embolic infarction are not different from those found with infarction from other causes except that hemorrhage into the infarct is found more often with emboli than with vascular occlusion from atherosclerotic disease. The actual embolic material is often not retrieved from the cerebral vessels at autopsy unless the embolus is large, presumably because most small emboli are lysed. This evanescence means that many instances of embolic cerebral infarction must be inferred by finding a source of emboli in other sites. Multiple small areas of cerebral infarction are commonly found at autopsy in patients with embolic disease.

Cerebral emboli that originate from infected material with bacterial endocarditis or pulmonary infections may cause local inflammation as well as infarction. Infected emboli may produce cerebral abscess, local encephalitis, or mycotic aneurysm.

Recurrent emboli have been postulated as a cause for the transient attacks of neurologic dysfunction often seen in patients with cerebrovascular disease (see below). The surface of atheromatous plaques in the internal carotid artery is frequently ulcerated. A granular lipid debris is present on the ulcer, and the surface of some plaques has been noted to be covered with collections of platelets or organizing blood clot. It is believed that some of the granular or thrombotic material on the surface breaks off, is carried into and obstructs small cerebral vessels, and produces small areas of ischemia. Because only minute vessels are occluded, infarction usually does not occur. In support of this concept is the observation in the optic fundi of some patients having transient ischemic attacks of small white or yellow refractile bodies moving through or blocking the retinal arteries. These emboli have been identified as platelet collections or cholesterol crystals; it is believed that they represent atherosclerotic debris from plaques in proximal vessels and that similar emboli go to brain vessels causing transient occlusion without necrosis. Embolic material from ulcerated atherosclerotic plaques can cause transient ischemic attacks in the absence of significant vascular obstruction.

Cerebral Venous Inflammation and Thrombosis

Cerebral infarction can result from thrombosis of one of the major venous sinuses, i.e., the superior sagittal sinus, the lateral sinus, or the cavernous sinus, or it can follow extensive thrombotic occlusion of cortical veins. The causes of cerebral venous thrombosis include dehydration, head injury, intracerebral hemorrhage, polycythemia vera, leukemia, infection, and the puerperal state. The most common cause is infection of the mastoid, the frontal sinus, or the subdural space. If the superior sagittal sinus is thrombosed anteriorly, both cerebral hemispheres become markedly congested, swollen, and hemorrhagic. The cerebral white matter may be involved, with small hemorrhages and edema. The surface veins become distended and filled with clot.

Thrombosis of surface veins is usually associated with cerebral or subdural abscess. The histologic picture is that of an acute inflammatory reaction with vascular congestion, edema, and neuronal loss.

Cavernous sinus thrombosis usually follows infection of the eye, face, or nose, and in many instances the thrombus extends through the perihypophyseal veins to involve the opposite cavernous sinus as well. Meningitis may follow spread of the infectious process through the sinus to the subarachnoid space.

Cardiac Disease

Hypotension and Hypertension

Cardiac disease contributes to infarction in patients with cerebral atherosclerosis as the result of periods of hypotension after myocardial infarction, congestive failure, and cardiac arrhythmia. In the Cornell-Bellevue series, clinical heart disease not only preceded cerebral infarction in half the patients, but was the actual cause of at least half the deaths after cerebral infarction.

Hypotension. Both hypotension and hypertension have been implicated in the production of cerebral ischemia and infarction. Although cerebral blood flow in the normal person is relatively independent of the systemic blood pressure down to levels of 50 to 60 mm of mercury, it has been suggested that a lesser drop in blood pressure may produce cerebral ischemia when a significant obstruction is present in a vessel leading to the brain. A localized obstruction must reduce the vessel lumen by nearly 80 per cent to produce a significant distal drop in pressure, but luminal encroachment that extends over long distances theoretically could significantly decrease the distal arterial pressure with less severe grades of obstruction. However, the contribution to cerebral infarction of obstruction and distal decreases in blood pressure and flow is still an unsettled matter. Thus Marshall has reported that when patients with transient ischemic attacks were made briefly hypotensive with hexamethonium and tilting, nearly one half showed evidence of generalized cerebral ischemia only, and another one fourth developed evidence of generalized cerebral ischemia before any focal ischemia.

Failure to maintain the blood pressure may occur with cardiac arrhythmias and after myocardial infarction. The asystole that occurs in Stokes-Adams attacks, if prolonged, can reduce the cerebral blood flow so markedly that cerebral ischemia or infarction results.

Hypertension. Longstanding hypertensive cardiovascular disease is probably the single biggest risk factor in stroke; the place of hypertension in the production of acute cerebral ischemia and infarction is less clear. Rapid elevations of blood pressure evoke an increase in cerebrovascular resistance, and model experiments have demonstrated that stenosis coupled with this increased resistance significantly reduces blood flow. In animal experiments, marked hypertension causes constriction in small cerebral vessels leading, in turn, to areas of cerebral infarction. Transient marked increases in blood pressure may contribute to cerebral infarction.

Other physiologic changes in cerebral hemodynamics may contribute to cerebral ischemia. Osteoarthritis in the cervical spine may compress the vertebral arteries so that extension, flexion, or rotation of the head can reduce vertebral artery blood flow to the point that ischemic symptoms occur. Cerebral ischemia will be augmented in these instances if anomalies or extensive atherosclerotic deposits compromise the circle of Willis.

Changes in Blood: Clotting, Viscosity, and Anemia

A variety of blood changes have been linked to cerebral infarction. The most frequent is *thrombus formation,* although in many instances it is unclear whether this is primary or secondary to the ischemic process. Thus infarction is not invariably associated with clot-filled vessels, and when thrombi do occur, they arise most commonly in association with ulcerated atherosclerotic lesions or atherosclerotic plaques, which by themselves produce a marked degree of vessel obstruction. In vessels with greatly reduced or absent flow, clots form readily, and long, wormlike clots have been removed from the distal segment of a partially or completely obstructed internal carotid artery shortly after the development of symptoms and signs of cerebral ischemia. A plausible reconstruction of this sequence suggests that marked stenosis was present first and was suddenly increased by hemorrhage into the atherosclerotic plaque, after which clotting occurred distally to the occlusion.

Alterations in blood clotting suggesting hypercoagulability have been described in patients with cerebral infarctions. However, a state of altered clotting has not been observed before an infarction, and some evidence suggests that hypercoagulability is an epiphenomenon that follows, rather than precedes, infarction.

Other potentially deleterious changes in blood include *increased viscosity* with polycythemia and *decreased oxygen-carrying capacity* with anemia. About 15 per cent of patients with polycythemia die from thromboembolism in the brain. Transient ischemic attacks that occur in patients with polycythemia are believed to result from the increase in blood viscosity that occurs when the hematocrit rises above 55.

Severe *anemia* sometimes precipitates cerebral ischemia, particularly if the hematocrit falls below 20, i.e., if the oxygen-carrying capacity drops more than half. Any degree of anemia may supplement severe atherosclerosis, cardiac disease, or hypotension in causing cerebral ischemia.

Cerebral Infarction and Medication

Stroke in young women of child-bearing age has been related to the use of oral contraceptive agents. The risk of developing stroke in women of this age group is small, but with oral contraceptive agents it is increased an estimated fivefold. Evidence has accumulated relating the increased risk to the estrogen content of the medication which is known to alter blood clotting. Particularly susceptible women are those with migraine and hypertension. In this group, when contraception is needed other means should be used.

THE PATHOGENESIS OF SYMPTOMS AND SIGNS IN CEREBROVASCULAR DISEASE

To make accurate clinical diagnoses in patients suspected of having cerebrovascular disease, the clinician requires an effective working knowledge of the structural and vascular anatomy of the brain. This is presented in the following paragraphs and diagrams, reference to which will explain why patterns of neurologic dysfunction after infarction or ischemia are related more to arterial territories than to specific neuroanatomic systems.

The brain is supplied by four large arteries, the two common carotids and the two vertebrals. One common carotid artery arises from the aortic arch and the other from the innominate artery in the upper thorax. The two vertebral arteries originate from the right and left subclavian artery. The common carotid artery bifurcates in the neck, forming the internal and external carotid arteries. Each internal carotid artery enters the skull through the homolateral foramen lacerum, passes through the cavernous sinus, and gives off branches in the following order: ophthalmic, anterior choroidal, and posterior communicating. It then bifurcates into the anterior and middle cerebral arteries.

The Anterior Cerebral Artery

As may be seen in Figures 2 and 3, the anterior cerebral artery supplies the medial and superior surfaces of the cerebral hemisphere and the whole of the most anterior portion of the frontal lobes. This area contains the motor and sensory cortex for the foot and leg and the supplementary motor cortex. The anterior cerebral artery also supplies several deep structures of importance, including the anterior nucleus of the thalamus and a portion of the anterior limb of the internal capsule.

The Middle Cerebral Artery

The middle cerebral artery (Figs. 3 and 4) supplies the lateral surface of the cerebral hemisphere with the exception of the occipital and frontal poles. The cortex supplied includes the primary motor and sensory area for the face, hand, and arm, the optic radiations, and, in the dominant hemisphere, the cortical areas for speech. The perforating branches of the middle cerebral artery reach the center of the cerebral hemisphere supplying the internal capsule and basal ganglia.

The Posterior Cerebral Artery

As shown in Figures 2 and 3, the posterior cerebral artery supplies the posterior pole of the lateral surface of the cerebral hemisphere and the posterior portion of the medial and inferior surfaces of the hemispheres. This area contains the calcarine cortex or the primary visual receptive area. The short perforating branches of the posterior cerebral artery supply the thalamus, part of

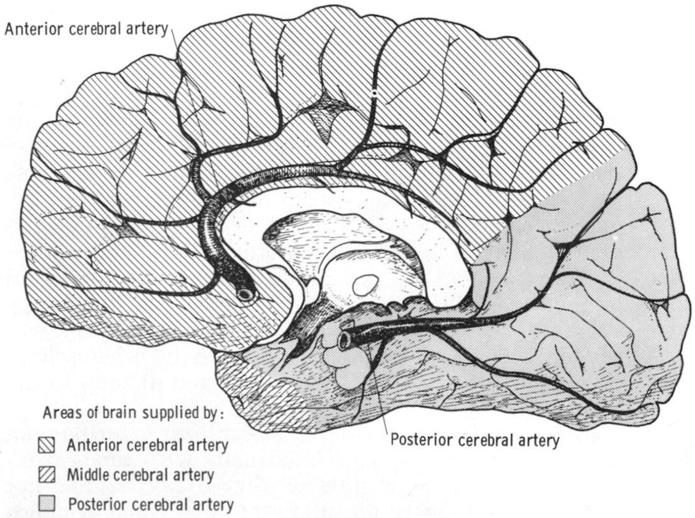

Figure 2. The medial surface of the cerebral hemisphere, showing the course of the anterior and posterior cerebral arteries and the area of brain supplied by each.

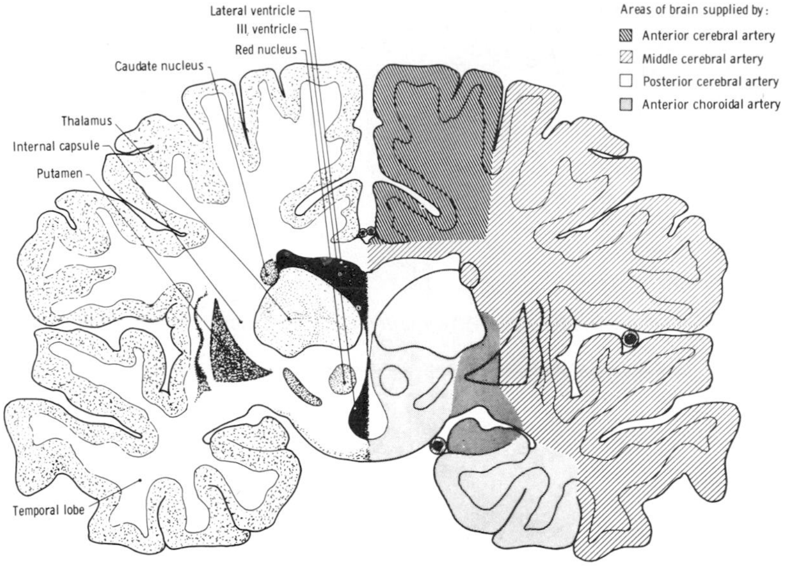

Figure 3. The cerebral hemispheres and the vascular supply, in coronal section.

the optic pathways, and other diencephalic structures including the midbrain.

The Vertebral and Basilar Arteries

The vertebral arteries reach the head via a bony canal in the transverse processes of the sixth through the second cervical vertebrae and enter the skull through the foramen magnum. Immediately after entering the skull each vertebral artery gives off a medial branch (these unite to form the anterior spinal artery) and, just distal to this, the posterior inferior cerebellar artery. At all levels along the brainstem, the ventral medial portion is supplied by short paramedian vessels. The ventrolateral portion of the brainstem is supplied by short circumferential branches from the vertebrals or basilar artery. The dorsal lateral portion and cerebellum are supplied by long circumferential branches: the posterior inferior, the anterior inferior, and the superior cerebellar arteries.

The vertebral artery lies on the ventral lateral surface of the medulla oblongata, and from it and the anterior spinal artery short paramedian branches supply the pyramids, the inferior olives and medial lemniscus, the medial longitudinal fasciculus, and the emerging fibers of the hypoglossal nerve as shown in Figure 5.

The more dorsal portion of the medulla includes the spinothalamic tract, the vestibular nuclei, the sensory nucleus of the fifth cranial nerve, the restiform body, and the emerging fibers of the vagus and glossopharyngeal nerves, and is supplied by longer branches from the vertebral artery and branches from the posterior inferior cerebellar artery. The most cephalad and dorsal segment of the medulla includes the vestibular and cochlear nuclei, and it and the posterior portion of the cerebellum are supplied by the posterior inferior cerebellar artery.

At the lower border of the pons, the two vertebral arteries unite to form the basilar artery. From this artery in the pons, short perpendicular branches enter the brainstem to supply paramedian structures including the corticospinal tracts, the pontine nuclei, the medial lemniscus, the medial longitudinal fasciculus, and the pontine reticular nuclei (Fig. 6). Circumferential branches supply the lateral portion of the pons, which includes the

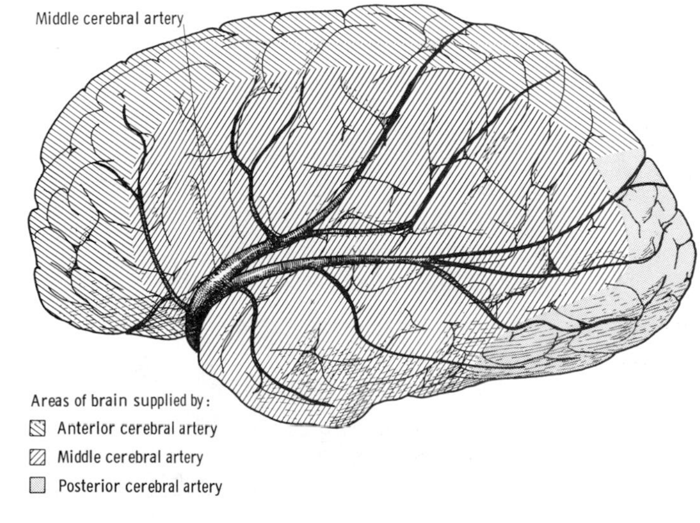

Figure 4. The lateral surface of the cerebral hemisphere and the course of the middle cerebral artery. The sylvian fissure has been opened to better illustrate the course of the vessel.

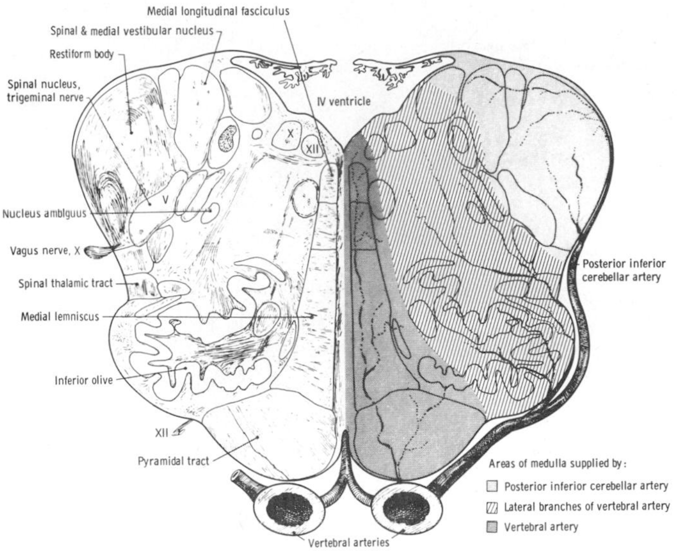

Figure 5. Cross section of the medulla oblongata seen from above at the level of the hypoglossal nuclei. The medial structures are supplied by short branches arising from the vertebral arteries and anterior spinal arteries. The lateral portions are supplied by longer branches and the dorsal and lateral areas by long circumferential branches, at this level called the posterior inferior cerebellar artery.

emerging seventh and eighth cranial nerves, the trigeminal nerve root, the vestibular and cochlear nuclei, and the spinothalamic tracts. The anterior inferior cerebellar artery, the long circumferential branch at this level, also gives branches to the most dorsal and lateral of these structures as it runs dorsally to the cerebellum.

At the level of the midbrain the basilar artery lies in the interpeduncular fossa (Fig. 7). Short branches pass laterally and dorsally to both sides to supply the cerebral peduncles, the emerging third nerve roots, the medial portions of the red nuclei, the medial longitudinal fasciculus, oculomotor nuclei, and the midbrain reticulum. Branches of the posterior cerebral artery supply the lateral portions of the peduncles, the red nuclei, and the medial lemnisci. The superior cerebellar arteries supply some of the dorsal portions of the midbrain, including the colliculi and the anterior portion of the cerebellum on each side.

It will be clear from this review of neurologic and vascular anatomy that infarction can produce a large variety of clinical pictures, depending on the vessels involved. The pattern of most syndromes is helpful in localizing the area of the nervous system damaged by infarction, but only a few reliably indicate exactly which portion of the vascular tree is involved. As an example, diagnoses are often made of middle cerebral artery occlusion, but a review of the vascular anatomy of the brain quickly reveals why, with both anterior cerebral arteries filling from either side, an identical clinical picture can be associated with occlusion of the internal carotid artery at any point along its course.

SIGNS AND SYMPTOMS IN CEREBROVASCULAR DISEASE: STROKE SYNDROMES

An adequate exposition of the symptoms and signs of cerebrovascular disease requires a classification of the various clinical entities that make up the stroke syndrome.

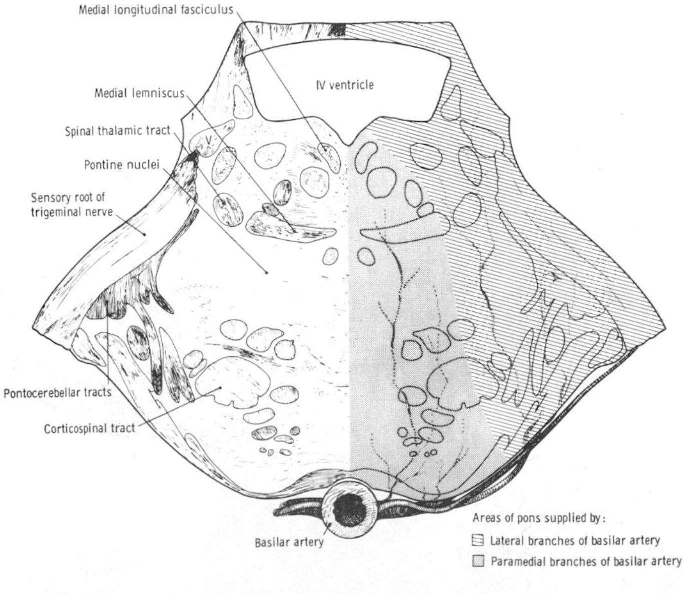

Figure 6. Cross section of the midpons. The most medial regions are supplied by short perforating branches from the basilar artery. The more lateral regions are supplied by lateral branches of the basilar artery. At this level, the more dorsal structures are supplied by the long circumferential branch, the anterior inferior cerebellar artery.

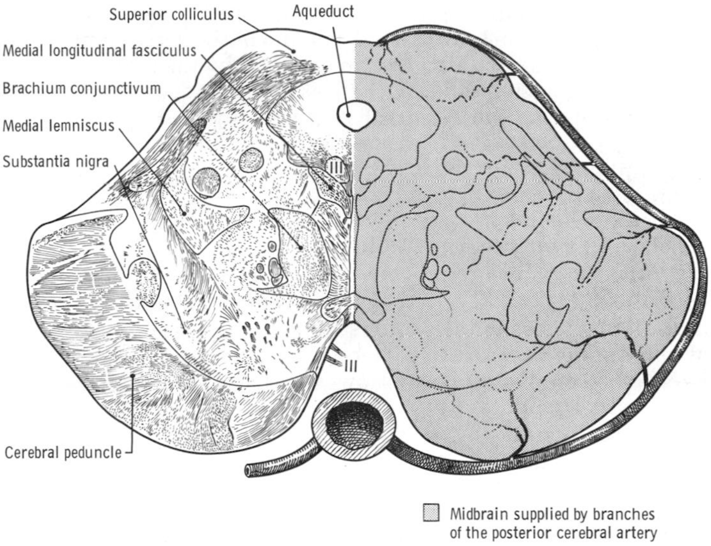

Figure 7. Cross section of the midbrain seen from below. The medial, lateral, and dorsal regions are supplied by short branches from the posterior cerebral artery as it passes around the midbrain.

Cerebrovascular accidents are classified on the basis of the anatomic site of ischemia or infarction, the cerebral vessels occluded or obstructed, and the temporal character of the entire clinical episode. The latter is clinically the most valuable in that the indicated therapy is often different for the three kinds of temporal profiles found. The three profiles have been defined as *transient ischemic attack, stroke-in-evolution* or *progressive stroke,* and *completed stroke.*

The term *transient ischemic attack* or incipient stroke refers to transient episodes of neurologic dysfunction caused by cerebrovascular disease. The attacks are believed to be caused by cerebral ischemia, and consist of fleeting, 5- to 30-minute disturbances in neurologic function that leave no permanent residue.

Stroke-in-evolution or progressive stroke refers to increasing neurologic dysfunction caused by cerebral ischemia over a period of minutes, hours, or, rarely, days.

Completed stroke refers to the clinical picture seen in patients who have ceased to show further progression in neurologic deficit or in those who have developed a neurologic deficit earlier that is now stable or improving. *Cerebral embolism* is one cause of completed stroke in which the onset is an abrupt monophasic event, and there is clinically a demonstrable source of emboli.

Cerebral Transient Ischemic Attacks

The symptoms vary, depending upon which area of the brain is ischemic, but there are two main types: those associated with ischemia of parts or the whole of a cerebral hemisphere and those associated with ischemia of the brainstem. The symptoms most often include transient contralateral weakness of the lower face, fingers, hand, arm, or leg, but such patients may also experience fleeting sensory symptoms such as tingling, "pins and needles," or numbness in parts of the body contralateral to the ischemia. Ischemia in the dominant hemisphere may cause dysphasia, with impairment in the context of speech and, at times, a transient lack of understanding.

Patients with ischemia in the portion of the brain supplied by the posterior cerebral artery may suffer blurred vision, or may notice transient hemianopic or altitudinal visual field defects or impairment of visual acuity.

Ischemia or insufficiency caused by internal carotid artery stenosis often produces transient retinal ischemia, resulting in monocular blindness or reduced acuity on the side of the stenosis, combined with contralateral weakness of the face, arm, or leg.

Ischemic attacks which result from involvement of the brain supplied by the vertebral and basilar arteries have an extremely wide range of symptoms. Common symptoms include vertigo, tinnitus, diplopia, dysarthria, dysphagia, and dysphonia. Patients may complain of unilateral or bilateral face, arm, and leg weakness and unilateral or bilateral sensations of numbness and tingling in the face, arms, or leg. There may be tinnitus, hearing loss, and ataxia. In addition, patients with brainstem ischemia may experience "drop attacks," in which they suddenly lose postural tone and fall to the ground without losing consciousness, then immediately regain postural control and rise quickly. The most common complaint with transient ischemic attacks from vertebrobasilar insufficiency is dizziness. However, dizziness is commonly associated with other physiologic disturbances and is rarely the only symptom of brainstem ischemia. When patients describe intermittent neurologic episodes with symptoms suggesting a generalized decrease in cerebral blood flow such as dizziness, lightheadedness, and generalized weakness, they should be carefully examined for cardiac dysrhythmia before being studied for the presence of extracranial arterial disease. Cardiac dysrhythmia, with a drop in cardiac output and subsequently in general cerebral blood flow, is a common cause of nonfocal transient ischemic attacks.

Symptoms of vertebral basilar artery ischemia, although variable, tend to occur in combinations that aid in their diagnosis. Vertigo, ataxia, dysarthria, paresthesia, diplopia, tinnitus, dysphagia, and focal weakness in the face, jaw, or pharynx tend to coexist, although not always in the same sequence or combination. Another grouping of symptoms is that of unilateral or bilateral weakness of the extremities with drop attacks and diplopia. The reason for these differences in symptom combinations can be found by referring to the diagrams of the blood supply to the brainstem. Ischemia of the dorsal and lateral portions of the brainstem supplied by the circumferential arteries produces the first group of symptoms. Ischemia of the more ventral portions supplied by the medial perforating arteries causes the second group.

Symptomatic vertebral basilar artery ischemia may occur with stenosis of the subclavian artery proximal to the origin of the vertebral artery. The arm on the side of the stenosis may be supplied by retrograde flow in the ipsilateral vertebral, and, during exercise, enough blood can be diverted from the vertebral system to the arm to cause symptoms of brainstem ischemia. This mechanism of producing brainstem ischemia has been called the *subclavian steal syndrome.* However, most instances of reversed vertebral artery flow with subclavian artery stenosis or occlusion are asymptomatic.

Ischemic attacks may occur many times a day or at weekly or monthly intervals. They may be intermittently present over several months or several years. Some patients with internal carotid artery occlusion have transient ischemic attacks for as long as two years before cerebral infarction occurs. Others have clusters of attacks lasting only a few hours or days before carotid occlusion becomes complete and causes infarction. *The major importance of transient ischemic attacks is that they signal the existence of significant cerebrovascular disease and clearly indicate the potential danger of cerebral infarction.* Studies of the natural history of transient ischemic attacks indicate that about one fourth to one third of patients afflicted will suffer a cerebral infarction within two to five years of onset of the attacks. It cannot always be predicted which patients with cerebral ischemia will develop cerebral infarction or even when it will occur. Transient ischemic attacks become more significant predictors of cerebral infarction if accompanied by extensive atherosclerosis as evidenced by abnormalities in the neurovascular examination, such as arterial bruit in the neck, absent temporal pulse, retinal embolization, and reduction of retinal artery pressure on the appropriate side. Some varieties of cerebral ischemic attacks carry a better prognosis than others. Thus symptoms suggesting involvement of the dorsal and lateral portion to the brainstem, the lateral medullary area, imply the best prognosis. Attacks suggesting ventral brainstem involvement, such as bilateral paresis or unilateral transient paresis or drop attacks, connote a considerably poorer prognosis. Carotid ischemic attacks that occur close together in clusters carry a poor prognosis, for in a large percentage of such patients cerebral infarction rapidly follows.

In the interval between transient ischemic attacks, the neurologic examination is usually entirely normal. During a transient ischemic attack, patients commonly have neurologic deficits corresponding to their symptoms. Thus with ischemia of a cerebral hemisphere, there may be a hemiparesis with reflex asymmetry and an extensor plantar response, or a mild hemisensory or visual field deficit. If the dominant hemisphere is affected, dysphasia may be noted: the patient has difficulty in naming and recognizing objects. Patients examined during a brainstem ischemic attack often exhibit nystagmus, complete facial weakness, palate and tongue weakness, and deviation, dysconjugate eye movements, sensory defects, and weakness on one side or on both sides of the body. The evaluation of patients with transient ischemic attacks must always include careful examination of the optic fundus through a dilated pupil, searching for cholesterol (bronze debris) or platelet emboli (white or invisible plugs) in the arterial tree. The presence of such emboli in one eye is important evidence of an embolic source in the carotid artery. Patients with such emboli should have cerebral angiography, and the presence of ulcerated atherosclerotic plaques should be determined.

Consciousness is usually unimpaired during transient ischemic attacks, although thinking is sometimes slowed. This lack of alteration of consciousness coupled with the absence of either aura or convulsive movements helps to distinguish these attacks from convulsive seizures. Other conditions that must be considered in the differential diagnosis are Meniere's syndrome (which is rare in the elderly), migraine headache, cerebral emboli, or the progressive neurologic deficits caused by cerebral neoplasm.

Stroke-in-Evolution
(Progressive Stroke)

The evolving stroke is characterized by the gradual development of paralysis and sensory impairment over a period of several hours and, at times, one to two days. The symptoms and signs may develop as a series of steplike changes or as an unbroken continuum of worsening. When first examined, a patient may have mild weakness which, as the hours pass, is found to be more and more marked and to involve more and more of the body. The symptoms and signs found are identical to those of completed stroke; only the time course of onset is different. This course also occurs with subdural hematoma and brain tumor, but, for these disorders, the duration usually extends over several days or weeks.

Cerebral Infarction
(Completed Stroke)

Cerebral infarctions resulting from cerebral emboli or from cerebral atherosclerosis and thrombosis, respectively, cannot be distinguished by the neurologic disorders they produce. Differences between these two causes of infarction do exist, however, in the mode of onset of symptoms and in the general physical evaluation.

The pattern of onset of neurologic symptoms and signs in cerebral infarction often suggests the cause. Cerebral embolism causes an abrupt onset of symptoms, and headache often precedes other neurologic symptoms by several hours. Cerebral infarction caused by atherosclerotic vascular obstruction or occlusion often has a less sudden onset. There may be a distinct series of steplike increases in neurologic symptoms and signs, or infarction may be preceded by a series of transient ischemic attacks. A gradual onset with increasing neurologic deficit over several (one to five) hours is characteristic of the progressing stroke. A gradual onset of symptoms and signs over two days or, occasionally, one week, does occur but is uncommon. The frequency of these different patterns can be inferred from the experience of one large series of patients with ischemic infarction; about one third had a sudden onset of symptoms, about one fifth had symptoms that progressively increased over one to 12 hours, and only about one in 20 had symptoms that progressed for as long as 12 to 24 hours. One fifth of the patients with occlusive vascular disease and cerebral embolism had the onset of neurologic signs during sleep.

Headache is present in many patients with embolic or atherosclerotic infarction. The headache is usually mild and localized to the side of the infarction. Headache is believed to be caused by vasodilation of unoccluded vessels near the infarcted area, and is most common when vessels near the base of the brain are occluded.

Consciousness is usually not lost at the onset of infarction of the cerebral hemispheres, but may be reduced, particularly when large infarcts strike the dominant hemisphere. When unconsciousness is present from the onset or is the initial symptom, brainstem infarction is the most likely cause. When large hemispheric infarctions are complicated by rapidly developing and severe brain edema, loss of consciousness caused by diencephalic and upper brainstem compression may occur shortly after the onset of symptoms. This may give the false impression of loss of consciousness from the onset unless a careful history documents a lucid period at the very beginning of symptoms. Convulsive seizures are rare at the onset of cerebral infarction, but they occur in about 8 per cent of patients sometime in the course of the acute or convalescent phase of the illness. They are usually focal, but may be generalized.

When infarction is limited to the cerebral hemisphere, there is weakness or paralysis in the extremities contralateral to the infarction. Patients may also be aware that sensory perception on the side of weakness is impaired and may complain of heaviness or numbness in the arm or leg. They rarely have other sensory symptoms such as pain or paresthesias. Defects in visual fields are common but often escape the patient's notice. The defect is suspected when patients pay little attention to visual stimuli on one side of the body. At times, the eyes may be constantly deviated to the side away from the neurologic deficits.

The most serious consequence of infarction in the dominant hemisphere is dysphasia, which can range from a mild deficit of expression to aphonic mutism. The dysphasia is almost invariably a mixture of difficulty with expression (expressive dysphasia) and difficulty in understanding what is said, written, or indicated by gesture (receptive dysphasia); one or the other may predominate. In patients who have infarction in the nondominant hemisphere, lack of awareness or concern about paralysis of the contralateral side is often evident. Such subjects may, at times, be so completely unaware of their neurologic disabilities that they are hospitalized only after family or friends notice their disabilities. This phenomenon, *anosognosia,* is most common when a patient is obtunded and when there is a significant sensory deficit on the paretic side as a result of infarction of the parietal lobe. It accompanies nearly one fourth of all large strokes, but usually persists only if the patient remains obtunded or confused or has little return of sensation.

Infarctions in the brainstem produce a wide variety of symptoms. Among the most conspicuous are vertigo, diplopia, dysarthria, dysphagia, and ataxia. In addition, the patient may note unilateral or bilateral sensory impairment or weakness. Often patients note clumsiness and difficulty in performing skilled acts without paresis.

Specific Vascular Syndromes

Internal Carotid Artery Occlusion

Occlusion of the internal carotid artery at its origin from the common carotid or intracranially is the site of the major vascular lesion in nearly 20 per cent of strokes. The usual lesion is atherosclerotic with, at first, partial obstruction and, finally, occlusion with a thrombus. Occasionally the internal carotid artery is obstructed by a large embolus.

Symptoms and signs specific for internal carotid artery occlusion in the neck are intermittent visual impairment or blindness in the eye on the side of the occlusion (retinal artery insufficiency) combined with a contralateral hemiparesis and sensory loss (middle cerebral artery insufficiency). This clinical picture often begins with a series of transient ischemic attacks and only later causes permanent weakness and sensory loss. Unless the history of intermittent blindness can be obtained, it is difficult, on clinical grounds alone, to distinguish occlusion of the internal carotid artery from middle cerebral artery occlusion.

On neurologic examination, patients with cerebral infarction caused by internal carotid artery occlusion have paresis of voluntary movement, with weakness most noticeable in the contralateral face and upper extremity. Infarcts produce motility defects as their main manifestations, but there is usually some impairment of sensory perception and, at times, visual field impairment as well.

In the paretic extremities, deep tendon reflexes are hyperactive, and pathologic reflexes such as the Babinski sign (extensor plantar response) are found. Muscle tone becomes increased on the weakened side, and spasticity may be so marked that early contracture is evident. Sensory impairment is most evident in modalities such as position sense, vibration sense, two-point discrimination, and tactile perception of shape and texture. Touch and pain perception may be moderately impaired, and extinction of stimuli on the involved side may be evident on double simultaneous stimulation. The size of the cerebral infarction produced by internal carotid occlusion is extremely variable. When there is no collateral circulation through the anterior communicating, posterior communicating, ophthalmic, or surface collateral arteries, the infarct can involve nearly the whole cerebral hemisphere, both lateral and medial surfaces. With a richer collateral circulation, smaller infarcts and proportionately fewer neurologic defects result. Occasionally occlusion of the internal carotid is asymptomatic, and is discovered only as an incidental finding at autopsy or when cerebral angiograms are done.

Internal carotid artery occlusion or stenosis sometimes causes a partial Horner's syndrome (slight ptosis and miosis) on the side opposite the paresis. The eye changes have been attributed to ischemia of the sympathetic fibers that lie in the adventitia of the arterial wall adjacent to the occlusion, but are more probably due to direct hypothalamic damage, for they can also be observed in patients with similar infarcts who do not have occlusion of the carotid arteries. An audible bruit in the neck at the angle of the mandible is a helpful indicator of stenosis of the internal carotid artery at that site. Occlusion of the internal carotid artery is also suggested when the retinal artery pressure on the affected side, as measured with an ophthalmodynamometer, decreases 25 per cent or more below the arterial pressure in the other eye. Some physicians find that palpation of the internal carotid artery in the pharynx behind the posterior tonsillar pillar is helpful in the diagnosis of carotid artery disease, as the pulse is absent when the artery is occluded. However, patients are often unable to cooperate for the examination, so that the usefulness of the test is limited.

Middle Cerebral Artery Occlusion

The cerebral tissue supplied by the middle cerebral artery is the most common area for infarction from emboli or vascular insufficiency, and the neurologic picture produced by either is the same.

When a middle cerebral artery is occluded, infarction occurs in the lateral portion of the hemisphere and produces varying degrees of contralateral paresis and sensory loss, mainly in the face, the upper extremities, and the hand, and often blindness in the contralateral, homonymous visual field. Occlusions at the origin of the middle cerebral artery produce extensive neurologic disturbance with profound contralateral hemiplegia and sensory loss. Occlusions in branches of the middle cerebral artery may produce a variable clinical picture. At times, only paresis is evident in the arm and face. In some patients, sensory impairment is the dominant and occasionally the only neurologic abnormality, and some patients have only dysphasia.

Anterior Cerebral Artery Occlusion

Anterior cerebral artery occlusion causes infarction in the cortical areas that control motor and sensory functions of the contralateral lower extremity, and impairs voluntary movement and sensory perception of that leg. The upper extremity and face are spared. Cerebral infarction caused by occlusion of the proximal portion of the anterior cerebral artery is uncommon because collateral circulation through the anterior communicating artery is usually adequate to supply both hemispheres.

Posterior Cerebral Artery Occlusion

Posterior cerebral artery occlusion causes infarction of the posterior lateral and posterior medial surfaces of the cerebral hemisphere, including the calcarine cortex. Proximal occlusions of the artery result in infarction of the thalamus and upper brainstem as well. Extensive infarctions in the occipital cortex cause homonymous hemianopic field defects, and those involving the dominant hemisphere may produce disturbances in reading, visual learning, visual recognition, and visual spatial orientation.

Infarction of both occipital poles can follow basilar artery stenosis or occlusion. The result is a double hemianopia and cortical blindness, a striking feature of which is that the patient is usually unaware that he is blind and may vigorously deny it (Anton's syndrome).

Brainstem Infarction

Brainstem infarction, although not as common as hemisphere infarction, produces several distinct clinical syndromes, best categorized by noting whether the clinical picture suggests involvement of ventral paramedian, ventrolateral, or dorsal brainstem structures. As noted in the discussion of neurovascular anatomy, these three areas receive blood supply through different groups of arteries.

Many of the particular groupings of symptoms and signs associated with various brainstem infarctions that have been given eponyms are believed to be common occurrences with brainstem infarction. However, in an analysis of 50 patients with brainstem infarction from the Cornell-Bellevue series, only two clearly fitted into these syndromes as originally described. The remaining 48 had an extensive mixture of symptoms and signs indicating an overlap in the areas believed to be infarcted with occlusions in specific arteries.

Midbrain Infarctions

Occlusion of the paramedian branches from the apex of the basilar artery or of the proximal posterior cerebral arteries causes infarction of portions of one or both cerebral peduncles, the oculomotor nerves, the oculomotor nuclei, the brachia conjunctivae, the red nuclei, and the midbrain reticular formation. The resulting symptoms and signs may be unilateral or bilateral, depending on the extent of the infarction. Unilateral signs include (1) ipsilateral oculomotor palsy and contralateral hemiparesis (Weber's syndrome), (2) ipsilateral oculomotor palsy, ipsilateral ataxia of gait, and poorly coordinated arm and hand movements (Nothnagel's syndrome). Bilateral signs include impaired consciousness, quadriparesis, divergent gaze, impaired vertical eye movements and midposition, or dilated pupils unresponsive to light. Purposeless, flail-like, involuntary movements (hemiballismus) may occur, and usually involve the upper extremity more than the lower. Patients in coma caused by infarction of the midbrain often have an unusual appearance, seeming to be almost awake although unable to communicate in any manner. This state has been called *coma vigil* or *akinetic mutism.* Such patients, although unresponsive, may exhibit a sleep-walking cycle.

When the dorsal area, supplied by the posterior cerebral artery, is ischemic or infarcted, the spinothalamic tract, the red nucleus, the descending sympathetic tracts, and the medial lemniscus are involved. The clinical picture consists of slight ptosis and miosis (Horner's syndrome), ipsilateral ataxia, and choreiform adventitious movements and contralateral impairment of all modalities of sensory perception of the entire body, including the face. This clinical picture is often called the superior cerebellar artery syndrome.

Pontine Infarction

Infarction in the pons is usually associated with basilar artery obstruction. Occlusion of the paramedian branches of the basilar artery causes necrosis of the corticospinal tracts, the pontine nuclei, the medial lemniscus, the medial longitudinal fasciculus, the abducens nucleus, the pontocerebellar tracts, and the pontine reticulum. Ipsilateral abducens palsy, facial weakness, and contralateral corticospinal tract dysfunction (Millard-Gubler syndrome) and the same findings with lateral conjugate gaze palsy (Foville's syndrome) are two unilateral syndromes that occur with occlusion in the paramedian arteries to the pons. Bilateral signs include quadriparesis, reduced reaction to noxious stimuli, and abducens paresis. Other signs include coma, hyperventilation, apneustic or ataxic breathing, small pupils, and internuclear ophthalmoplegia. If only the most ventral portion of the pons is damaged, awareness may be maintained even though the patient is quadriparetic.

With occlusion of arteries to the lateral pons, the signs and symptoms are unilateral and include tinnitus, deafness, nausea, vertigo, impairment of facial sensation, complete ipsilateral facial paralysis, nystagmus, miosis and ptosis (partial Horner's syndrome), and impaired conjugate gaze toward the side of the lesion. Impaired pain and temperature perception of one half the contralateral body below the face is usually found. This clinical picture is often referred to as the syndrome of anterior inferior cerebellar artery occlusion.

Medullary Infarction

Occlusion of the paramedian branches of the vertebral artery in the medulla causes contralateral paresis of the arm and leg, contralateral impaired sensory perception to touch, position sense and vibration sense in the arm, trunk, and leg, and ipsilateral tongue paralysis. With occlusion of arterial branches to the lateral medulla, the clinical picture includes vertigo, nausea, vomiting, dysarthria, dysphagia, nystagmus, ipsilateral Horner's syndrome, ipsilateral vocal cord paralysis, and impaired ipsilateral facial sensory perception to pain with impairment of pain sensation on the contralateral half of the body below the face. This clinical picture is referred to as the syndrome of posterior inferior cerebellar artery occlusion or Wallenberg's syndrome. It results from occlusion of the vertebral artery itself as frequently as or more frequently than it does from occlusion of its branches.

Basilar Artery Occlusion

When the basilar artery is completely occluded, infarction is found mainly in the ventral pons, midbrain, and occipital lobes. The clinical picture is like that seen with occlusion of the paramedian midbrain or pontine branches, but may include various defects in the visual fields and, at times, cortical blindness in addition. The brainstem tegmentum is almost invariably involved, causing major disturbances in consciousness.

Cerebral Embolism

The diagnosis of cerebral embolization is usually not difficult when it is remembered that the onset of neurologic symptoms and signs is abrupt, that they are often preceded by headache for a few hours before paresis is evident, and that a potential source for emboli is usually found on physical examination. Convulsive seizures occur at the onset, but they are uncommon. They are at first focal and later generalized in most patients. Loss of consciousness occurs in nearly one fourth of patients and is usually present for only a few minutes, but, after onset, patients may be confused. The neurologic signs depend upon which artery is occluded; the most common clinical picture is that of middle cerebral artery occlusion. Cerebral emboli can lodge in any major cerebral artery, and emboli commonly recur, often to the same artery. The cerebrospinal fluid is usually clear and without cells. When protein elevation and cells are found, subacute bacterial endocarditis should be suspected. Mitral stenosis with atrial fibrillation, myocardial infarction with mural thrombus, and subacute bacterial endocarditis are the cardiac disorders most commonly found. Normal sinus rhythm does not exclude the diagnosis of cerebral emboli, for it may be found in more than one third of such patients, particularly with a "tight" mitral stenosis or with past myocardial infarcts, respectively. Evidence of embolization to other sites strengthens the supposition that the cause of cerebral infarction is embolic.

Cerebral Venous Thrombosis

The symptoms of local cerebral venous thrombosis are headache, delirium, drowsiness, diplopia, and convulsions. The signs are usually those of increased intracranial pressure with papilledema and focal neurologic abnormalities. Focal fits are common, as are paresis and hemisensory loss. Such patients are restless, confused, and obtunded.

Superior sagittal sinus occlusion produces a somewhat similar clinical picture. At the New York Hospital, 21 patients with noninfective sagittal sinus thrombosis have been studied. Nine had terminal disease and marasmus, six had cyanotic congenital heart disease, and four had other, unexplained episodes of venous or arterial thromboses. Eleven of the 21 patients were children. Below the age of ten, cerebral infarction is more often due to venous than to arterial occlusion. Nearly all patients had fever, and their cerebrospinal fluids were under increased pressure, averaging 260 mm of fluid, and contained more than ten red blood cells. Neurologic symptoms appeared abruptly or progressed rapidly to a maximum, usually within 36 hours. Most patients were obtunded or confused and had headache. The white blood count was elevated in ten patients; in seven it was over 20,000. Nuchal rigidity was common, and papilledema, hemiparesis, and focal epileptic seizures occurred in about half the cases. Two patients presented later with signs of pseudotumor cerebri. The occurrence of hemiparesis or focal epilepsy was usually associated with cortical venous thromboses in addition to the sinus occlusion.

Cavernous sinus occlusion, usually a complication of sinus or paranasal skin infection, is characterized by proptosis, orbital chemosis, and edema, pain around the eye, papilledema, retinal hemorrhages, and fever. Extraocular palsy may be present. The disease carries a high risk of spread to the opposite cavernous sinus. Complications include meningitis and brain abscess.

Transverse or lateral sinus thrombosis, usually secondary to mastoiditis, is now uncommon with the decline in the incidence of that disease. When it does occur, it is usually manifested by headache, tenderness over the mastoid process, and, occasionally, paresis of the structures supplied by the glossopharyngeal and accessory nerve, with dysphagia, dysphonia, and weakness of the ipsilateral sternomastoid and trapezius muscle.

In all varieties of cerebral venous thrombosis, there is usually some evidence of sepsis with fever, malaise, headache, and leukocytosis.

Although the condition is uncommon, a diagnosis of cerebral venous thrombosis should be kept in mind for patients with evidence of cerebral infarction who have focal seizures, increased intracranial pressure, or evidence of infection. Cerebral venous thrombosis is particularly likely as a cause of postpartum cerebral infarction.

PHYSICAL AND LABORATORY FINDINGS

The general evaluation of the patient with cerebral infarction usually reveals evidence of vascular disease at other sites as well as a variety of associated diseases. About one fifth of patients with atherosclerotic cerebral infarction in the Cornell-Bellevue series had had previous strokes, half of which had occurred in the preceding year. Another fifth had had myocardial infarction, usually within the previous year. Over one half of the patients were hypertensive, but the diastolic pressure was above 100 mm of mercury in only one third of the patients. Nearly one fifth of the patients had diabetes mellitus, and one in ten gave a history of peripheral vascular occlusive disease.

Physical Examination. The physical examination of most patients with cerebral infarction discloses a normal or slightly elevated body temperature. Careful examination of the heart should never be overlooked because the presence of cardiac enlargement, atrial fibrillation, and cardiac murmurs, suggesting rheumatic heart disease with mitral stenosis, aids in detecting the presence of cerebral emboli. Patients with cerebral infarction often have atherosclerotic coronary heart disease, and perhaps one fifth have had recent or associated myocardial infarcts.

Palpation may reveal absence of pulsation in easily felt peripheral arteries. In the lower extremities, this is indicative of atherosclerotic vascular disease in the aorta, iliac, femoral or popliteal arteries. In the upper extremities, it may indicate occlusions in the major branches of the aorta, such as the innominate or subclavian arteries. Absence of pulses in one or both upper extremities should alert the physician to such diagnoses as "pulseless disease" (Takayasu's syndrome) or the "subclavian steal syndrome."

Auscultation for bruit over the neck is helpful in identifying sites of extracranial stenosis. A bruit heard in the neck under the angle of the mandible suggests atherosclerotic disease of the carotid artery, and bruit heard just above the clavicles is associated with vertebral or subclavian artery stenosis. Bruit, when loud and localized, is associated with atherosclerotic obstruction at that site in more than three fourths of patients.

Laboratory Examinations. Laboratory tests are aimed at both confirming the diagnosis and identifying complications. Every patient suspected of stroke should have a lumbar puncture and skull roentgenograms, and, if there are any unusual features at all about the illness, an electroencephalogram (EEG) should be obtained.

The cerebrospinal fluid should be examined promptly, for there is no other way to determine the presence of intracranial bleeding or an unsuspected infection. The lumbar puncture must be approached cautiously, however, when patients are in stupor or coma or when it is uncertain whether the illness is caused by stroke or by brain tumor, with increased intracranial pressure. In such instances, it is preferable to proceed with roentgenograms, electroencephalogram, radioactive brain scan, or an arteriogram, because lumbar puncture can inadvertently precipitate tentorial or foraminal herniation when there is an expanding intracranial mass.

The cerebrospinal fluid pressure is rarely over 200 mm of CSF in cerebral infarction. The fluid is usually clear and colorless, but bleeding and xanthochromia from hemorrhagic infarction may be found. The CSF protein level is usually normal, although slight elevations to 60 to 75 mg per 100 ml are found in perhaps one fifth of the patients. Elevations to 80 mg per 100 ml or above are found in less than 10 per cent, but particularly in those with basilar artery disease. With massive cerebral infarction, the protein may be raised to values of nearly 100 mg per 100 ml. Diabetes occasionally accounts for pronounced CSF protein elevations with stroke, probably by a leak of protein through damaged small vessels. Patients with high values should always be carefully reviewed for the possibility of brain tumor.

Skull roentgenograms should be examined for evidence of fracture, erosion of the posterior clinoids (suggesting chronically increased intracranial pressure), abnormal calcification, and pineal shift.

The *electroencephalogram* (EEG) offers potential help both in differential diagnosis and in distinguishing infarction of the brainstem from that of the hemispheres. The EEG is usually abnormal in patients with cerebral infarction, and the degree of abnormality generally parallels the size of the lesion and the severity of the neurologic deficit. With hemispheric lesions, the abnormality is focal and the normal frequency of brain waves is slowed, so that, acutely at least, the records may resemble those found with brain tumor. In infarction, however, a decrease in the EEG abnormality is expected in serial recordings as the patient improves. With brainstem infarction, the EEG may be entirely normal, paroxysmally abnormal, or generally and diffusely abnormal.

The general evaluation of patients with cerebral infarction should include an electrocardiogram (EKG) and a chest roentgenogram. The EKG may confirm the presence of an arrhythmia or may disclose a silent myocardial infarction. (A potentially confusing point is that the EKG may show minor T wave and S-T segment changes caused by cerebral infarction and not by primary cardiac disease.)

Special Investigations

Arteriography

The technical quality and safety of arteriography has improved to the point that complications develop only in about 1 to 2 per cent of patients with cerebrovascular disease, and permanent worsening and death follow arteriography in less than 1 per cent of patients.

Cerebral angiography is indicated only for certain patients with cerebrovascular disease and has two main values. The first is in differential diagnosis for the patient with an atypical history and findings, or who is unable to give an accurate history because of dysphasia or depressed consciousness.

The second and more important value of cerebral angiograms is the accurate demonstration of the site, extent, and incidence of arterial obstructions and ulcerated atherosclerotic plaques that might be susceptible to surgical correction. Patients with such lesions include predominantly those who suffer transient ischemic attacks or incomplete strokes from which recovery has been substantial. In such cases, it is necessary to outline both the neck vessels and the nature and extent of the intracranial collateral circulation and the collateral channels from extracranial to intracranial vessels.

Rapid roentgenographic exposures have clarified some aspects of the physiology of cerebral blood flow in patients with cerebrovascular disease. Cerebral angiography may identify unusual patterns of blood flow in cerebral vessels, such as retrograde flow down one vertebral artery with proximal subclavian artery stenosis (subclavian steal). Ulceration of plaques can be demonstrated in about 41 per cent of patients with transient ischemic attacks coming to operation. The accuracy of the angiographic diagnosis when compared to findings at surgery is 90 per cent.

Brain scanning, using radiomercury-chlormerodrin or

Tc^{99m} Pertechnetate, shows a high uptake of radioactive material in the area of a cerebral infarction. This technique may aid in accurate localization of the infarcted area, but an identical picture can result from brain tumor, thereby limiting its usefulness in differential diagnosis. A normal brain scan during the first few days after the onset of symptoms suggesting a stroke, followed by a positive brain scan, is highly suggestive of cerebral infarction.

Echoencephalography is often helpful in the diagnosis of cerebral infarction. Reflected ultrasound waves are recorded to demonstrate whether midline structures are shifted. Shift of midline structures is uncommon immediately after cerebral infarction, although cerebral edema occurring 24 to 48 hours later can be responsible for a considerable shift. Acutely, at least, a midline shift of more than 2 mm should make one suspect brain tumor or subdural hematoma.

DIFFERENTIAL DIAGNOSIS

The most common sources of error in the diagnosis of cerebral infarction are brain tumors, subdural hematomas, intracerebral hemorrhages, cerebral traumatic lesions, and cerebral infections.

When a clear history of the onset is available, cerebral infarction is seldom confused with other disorders. Stroke caused by cerebral emboli or cerebral thrombosis characteristically produces a maximal neurologic deficit initially, with gradual improvement in function over days, weeks, or months. The first symptoms of brain tumor and subdural hematoma occasionally are mistaken for stroke, but the general tendency is for these two disorders to cause gradually progressive worsening, even though the first symptoms may seem to begin suddenly. In addition, both brain tumor and hematoma tend to produce disturbances in consciousness that are as prominent as or more prominent than focal neurologic defects, which helps in their differentiation from cerebrovascular disease. Often the problem in differential diagnosis is reversed in that the onset of stroke may include a gradual steady progression of symptoms and signs of focal neurologic defects, making the physician think first of tumor and only later of cerebral infarction. When doubt occurs about the diagnoses of infarction, subdural hematoma, and neoplasm, cerebral angiograms and other tests should be done.

Clinically, it is easier to confuse cerebral infarction with intracranial hemorrhage, for the onset is often similar. The cerebrospinal fluid examination usually helps, but blood can be found in both states – although considerably less often in cerebral infarction. Large amounts of blood in a CSF under increased pressure is always caused by intracranial hemorrhage. Angiography helps to settle the problem by demonstrating aneurysm, A-V anomaly, or intracerebral hematoma.

When it is not known whether the patient could have suffered head trauma, it is often impossible to eliminate this as a cause of clinical states resembling cerebral infarction. Careful inspection for scalp lacerations and localized scalp edema and good quality skull roentgenograms identify most instances of trauma if it has been severe enough to cause neurologic injury. If trauma cannot be eliminated and the patient becomes progressively worse, angiography must be done to eliminate consideration of subdural or epidural hematomas. Angiography is preferable to exploratory burr holes, for it will not only indicate a hematoma but will also define other causes of illness such as tumor, intracerebral hemorrhage, or vascular occlusion.

Among the forms of intracranial sepsis only brain abscess is likely to be confused with cerebral infarction. The points that should alert the physician to the possibility of an abscess are a source of infection elsewhere in the body such as an ear, sinus, or chest infection; persistent headache; persistent low-grade fever; white cells, especially polymorphonuclear leukocytes, that persist more than 24 hours in the cerebrospinal fluid; a focal, highly abnormal EEG; and worsening of the clinical state. If abscess is suspected, angiograms performed on the side opposite to the paresis will demonstrate the presence or absence of an intracerebral mass, which, if present, then must be surgically explored and drained to prove the diagnosis.

COURSE

Some improvement in function after the initial neurologic deficit can be expected after almost every cerebral infarction. During the first 72 hours, however, gradual worsening of neurologic deficits and increasing or beginning impairment of consciousness are frequent. This change may indicate extension of the cerebral infarction, but usually is associated with cerebral edema in and around the necrotic area. *Some degree of cerebral edema complicates every infarct.* It appears almost immediately, and with large infarctions may be so extensive as to shift the brain laterally and downward to produce herniation through the tentorium cerebelli and subsequent brain stem compression. This course of events, with its associated impairment of consciousness and other vital functions, is a common cause of death in patients with extensive infarction. The diagnosis of cerebral edema is especially likely when a patient shows a decline in awareness without a significant increase in focal neurologic deficits. Other causes of lethargy and stupor in patients with cerebral infarction are fever, electrolyte imbalance, the injudicious use of sedatives, tranquilizers or narcotics, and malnutrition.

In patients whose course is not complicated by severe cerebral edema, there is usually an early improvement in neurologic function. If some voluntary movement is preserved, there is a good chance for return of more. When function improves rapidly after the onset, the outlook for a good recovery is excellent. A slow return of function over weeks or months is associated with a less complete recovery. If flaccid paralysis is present from the onset with no return of increased muscle tonus over 30 to 60 days, the outlook for recovery is poor, because a gradual change from flaccidity to spasticity always precedes the advent of voluntary movement. Significant sensory loss impairs the chances of recovery of motor function. With brainstem infarction, the course is usually one of gradual improvement if the infarct is localized in the lateral medullary area. Symptoms of nausea, diplopia, and ataxia lessen and eventually disappear. Although some residual impairment of eye and extremity movement may be detected on examination, such patients often have little physical limitation. It is important to realize that recovery from cerebral infarction with impaired neurologic function may continue for as long as one to two years.

PROGNOSIS

About one fourth to one fifth of patients with either thrombotic or embolic cerebral infarction die with their first attack. This figure varies somewhat with the cause of the infarction and especially with other factors such as age, cardiac status, and the degree of neurologic disability. The mortality rises sharply with increasing age; for patients over the age of 70 with cerebral infarction from atherosclerotic thrombosis or emboli the initial mortality is nearer 50 per cent. Patients with marked neurologic defects, coma, or extensive vascular disease elsewhere have an initial mortality of nearly 50 per cent. Infarction of the ventral portions of the brainstem after basilar artery occlusion, especially with quadriplegia, carries a poor outlook, although good medical and good nursing care may preserve a vegetative existence for long periods.

The prognosis with cerebral infarction is better in younger patients, in those with the least evidence of vascular disease at other sites, especially cardiovascular disease, and in those who do not have hypertension, diabetes, or severe neurologic defects.

About one fifth of patients who survive a cerebral infarction from atherosclerotic vascular disease suffer another cerebrovascular accident within the next 12 to 24 months. However, the most significant limiting factor on survival is not recurrent stroke but cardiovascular disease. Thus in the Cornell-Bellevue series, fully half of the patients who survived the initial cerebral infarction died at a later date from myocardial infarction or cardiac failure.

Recurrence of cerebral infarction is common with cerebral emboli. In the New York Hospital series about 22 per cent of patients with cerebral emboli suffered recurrences, and nearly all the patients had more than one embolus if extracerebral sites were included. There is a strong chance that each cerebral recurrence will cause death or further neurologic disability.

TREATMENT

General. Treatment of cerebral infarction has four goals: to preserve life, to limit the amount of brain damage, to lessen disability and deformity, and to prevent recurrences.

The treatment program designed to preserve life is similar to that outlined for all seriously ill patients with neurologic illness. Efforts are directed toward maintaining a clear airway, an adequate fluid, electrolyte, and caloric intake, and an adequate urine output. Constant care is required to protect the skin from ischemia and necrosis resulting from pressure. Such a program is necessary for the obtunded or comatose patient, and must often be continued for the remainder of his life.

In patients with hemispheric infarction *cerebral edema* can impair consciousness and vital function early in the course of the illness. When cerebral edema subsides, the patient may again be able to cough, swallow, and voluntarily move paretic parts. A variety of measures can often temporarily reduce the brain swelling and carry the patient through a period of severe difficulty. Hypertonic urea solution, 1 to 1.5 grams per kilogram of body weight given intravenously, rapidly reduces cerebral edema and causes a marked diuresis. The effect is transient, and a rebound effect attributed to recurrence of swelling has been reported. Hypertonic invert sugar, mannitol, has been used with similar results except that less rebound has been reported. One and one half to 2 grams per kilogram of body weight is given intravenously in a 20 per cent solution. In patients with cerebral infarction and brain edema this therapy is reserved until there is a serious threat to life with declining brainstem function, for the benefits are transient, and most patients can be carried through periods of depressed consciousness with careful nursing care alone. Although glucocorticoids such as methylprednisolone are often dramatically effective in improving patients with brain edema from primary and metastatic brain tumor, they have been found in carefully controlled studies to be ineffective in reducing cerebral edema after infarction.

Several agents have been utilized to increase cerebral blood flow in an effort to decrease the amount of ischemic tissue and limit the extent of cerebral infarction. Nearly all known agents that produce vasodilatation, including aminophylline, papaverine, tolazoline hydrochloride, nicotinic acid, and histamine, have been used without clear evidence of success in cerebrovascular disease. The only agent that produces effective vasodilatation in cerebral vessels is carbon dioxide. Although it has been used to treat acute stroke, there is no evidence that it reduces the neurologic defects.

Treatment for the late acute and convalescent phase of a stroke is directed toward lessening deformity and disability, a goal that requires daily passive exercise of paretic parts to prevent joint fixation and to maintain normal muscle and tendon length. Some increase in muscle tone with spasticity invariably accompanies hemiplegia and tends to be most marked in the flexor muscles in the upper extremities and in the extensor muscles in the lower extremities. If this increase in tone in one muscle group over another persists and cannot be overcome by voluntary movement, daily passive movement of weakened or paralyzed parts through the full range of motion must be carried out by a nurse, physician, physiotherapist, or member of the family to prevent muscle and tendon contracture that may be nearly impossible to correct later on.

Rehabilitation. After cerebral infarction, *programs of retraining and rehabilitation should begin as soon as there is no longer evidence of increasing infarction.* Stabilization of the neurologic findings for 12 to 24 hours with some evidence of improvement is usually sufficient evidence to permit a start. Rehabilitation programs have as their goal the retraining of the remaining functions for maximal effectiveness. Although a few patients do require and benefit from special hospital facilities for rehabilitation, most such programs can be carried out on medical services without the aid of extensive equipment. An internist or general physician who is interested in rehabilitation can direct programs of activity and exercise, and can achieve results in rehabilitating hemiplegic patients that are nearly as effective as those of specialized centers.

An active program of rehabilitation begins by increasing the patient's tolerance to sitting and standing, which is impaired both by weakness and by changes in the sense of balance. Patients are allowed to sit up and then stand for increasingly long periods, beginning with five to ten minutes. During this period daily active and passive exercises of weakened extremities are carried out. When patients begin standing they need firm support and often splinting or bracing of the knee on the weakened side; marked quadriceps weakness may even demand a long leg brace. Ambulation is one of the main goals of rehabilitation. Gait training should begin when the patient can comfortably stand for 15 to 20 minutes without fatigue, and the support of parallel bars or a walker should be depended upon at first. After ambulation has started, it may be necessary to brace the foot to avoid the foot drop and supination that commonly occur after hemiplegia. At the same time that the patient is relearning to walk he should be trained in developing new skills with his unaffected arm and improving the strength and function in the paretic arm. This is done by an active program of exercise and by observing and retraining the patient in the activities of daily living such as eating, dressing and undressing, and personal hygiene. More complete details of programs of rehabilitation are outlined in other sources such as Covalt (1965) and can be followed by patients and their families under the direction of the physician. Usually, the maximal effect is gained in six to eight months, but some patients continue to show improvement over periods lasting as long as two years. Passive exercise must be continued indefinitely for severely paralyzed patients if contractures are to be avoided.

For patients with cerebral infarction who have mild to moderate dysphasia, speech therapy may be helpful. With severe dysphasia, therapy is rarely able to restore usable speech.

PREVENTION

The probability of an asymptomatic individual developing an atherosclerotic cerebral infarction has been analyzed by the Framingham study. The risk of developing stroke is increased in either sex and at any age by hypertension, diabetes, electrocardiographic evidence of heart enlargement, hypercholesterolemia, and cigarette smoking. The risk is higher with more than one of these factors operant and increases with the age of the individual. At the moment, the only factor which, if altered, is clearly related to a reduced risk of cerebral infarction is hypertension. In view of this, careful control of blood pressure in hypertensive individuals emerges as an important factor in prevention of signs and symptoms of cerebral ischemia. For management of hypertension, see Ch. 564.

Prevention of recurrent attacks and of cerebral infarction in patients with transient ischemic attacks and prevention of recurrent infarction in patients with cerebral atherosclerosis and cerebral emboli are the goals of much of the currently recommended treatment for stroke. Two methods to achieve this have been extensively evaluated: anticoagulation and surgical correction of arterial obstruction.

Anticoagulant Drugs or Surgery in Transient Ischemic Attacks. *Anticoagulant therapy* was introduced to treat transient ischemic attacks after its use in myocardial infarction suggested a beneficial action. A controlled study of anticoagulants in transient ischemic attacks indicates that as long as patients receive anticoagulants and their prothrombin times are kept at two to two and a half times the normal value, they have fewer ischemic attacks and less chance of having a cerebral infarction. As a result, anticoagulants are now generally accepted as effective in treating patients with transient ischemic attacks. The question is, which patients should receive the anticoagulants and for how long? The natural history of attacks is variable; attacks often stop spontaneously; some varieties carry a better prognosis than others. Even admitting these differences, anticoagulants should be given to the patients with transient ischemic attacks who do not have contraindications to their use. They should be continued for six months to one year and then gradually discontinued. If transient ischemic attacks recur, they should be given again. The management of patients on anticoagulants is discussed in Ch. 543 to 545.

Drugs which inhibit platelet aggregation have been used to reduce platelet emboli as a cause of transient ischemic attacks. These agents include aspirin, dipyridamole, sulfinpyrazone, and cyproheptadine. Use of these agents has been shown to reduce the frequency of transient ischemic attacks, especially amaurosis fugax, and they are now being extensively evaluated to determine their effect on reducing strokes in patients with transient ischemic attacks.

Surgical correction of extracranial arterial obstruction has been extensively tried in the United States in treating patients with transient ischemic attacks. Most carefully evaluated series show that transient ischemic attacks are relieved after surgical removal of the obstruction and that chances of cerebral infarction are reduced. Patients with transient ischemic attacks who have evidence of an ulcerated atherosclerotic plaque should undergo surgical removal of this source of cerebral emboli. If skilled, experienced surgeons are unavailable or referral is impossible for other reasons, anticoagulants are the treatment of choice. Patients with transient ischemic attacks in whom arteriography demonstrates no surgically correctable lesion are best treated with anticoagulants.

Anticoagulant Drugs or Surgery in Progressing Stroke or Stroke-in-Evolution. Anticoagulants have been shown by Carter to significantly reduce mortality and morbidity among patients with stroke-in-evolution. Such situations are emergencies and, unless specifically contraindicated, anticoagulation must begin with heparin and must be continued with coumarin derivatives. Anticoagulants are usually given for four to six weeks. Surgical correction of an arterial obstruction for the patient with progressing stroke has sometimes been attempted as a means of reducing neurologic disability, but with poor results, except in those patients in whom it can be demonstrated that showers of emboli from an ulcerated atherosclerotic plaque in the carotid artery are the cause of the progression.

Anticoagulant Drugs or Surgery in Completed Stroke. For the patient with an already completed stroke, there is no clear treatment for preventing recurrences. Most series of patients with completed stroke studied by angiograms illustrate the widespread nature of atherosclerotic obstructive vascular disease. Intra- and extracranial vessels are commonly affected simultaneously and impose limiting factors on the successful outcome of surgical correction of extracranial arterial defects. A controlled evaluation of surgical therapy in this group of patients has been carried out and shows that surgical correction of an isolated carotid stenosis in patients with a mild neurologic defect is effective in reducing future mortality and morbidity. Surgical correction of arterial obstruction in patients with severe neurologic defects or with evidence of extensive atherosclerotic disease and occlusion does not reduce future mortality or morbidity.

Anticoagulants, given for one to four months, are

useful during the acute and early convalescent period after a cerebrovascular accident to prevent pulmonary emboli in paralyzed, bedridden patients. The use of anticoagulants has also been recommended on a long-term basis for prevention of recurrent stroke. However, most studies of this problem indicate that there is no benefit from this form of treatment and that the complication rate is too high to warrant its use. Anticoagulation, therefore, can be recommended only for highly selected patients after cerebral infarction.

Anticoagulant Drugs in Cerebral Embolization. Anticoagulants greatly reduce the mortality and morbidity associated with recurrent embolization, and patients with a well established diagnosis of cerebral embolus should be placed on these drugs if there are no contraindications. If the source of emboli is rheumatic heart disease, anticoagulants are given continuously. When emboli follow myocardial infarction, treatment is usually given for one year. Coumarin anticoagulants are used and should be started immediately after the diagnosis has been made and the lumbar puncture has revealed bloodless cerebrospinal fluid.

Patients with cerebral emboli who have atrial fibrillation are often considered for conversion to normal sinus rhythm. This may be valuable in increasing cardiac output, but does not clearly reduce the chance of recurrent cerebral emboli.

General management of anticoagulant therapy is outlined in Ch. 543 to 545.

Hemorrhagic complications from anticoagulants are serious in about 2 to 4 per cent of patients and fatal in 2 per cent. Minor bleeding does not require that the medication be discontinued, but with serious bleeding it should be. Minor surgical procedures can be undertaken safely in most patients on anticoagulants if the prothrombin time is slightly lowered.

Heparin is the anticoagulant of choice for the initial treatment of patients with progressing stroke.

Patients with transient ischemic attacks, progressing strokes, or established strokes who also have hypertension should be treated with antihypertensive medication. Studies of patients with atherosclerotic cerebrovascular disease and hypertension show that when the blood pressure is returned to normal or nearly normal levels the recurrence rate and mortality rate of stroke are reduced. Hypertension, depending on its severity, should be continuously treated with reserpine, chlorothiazide, or hexamethonium, and the blood pressure should be maintained as nearly normal as possible.

To sum up the prophylaxis of strokes: Patients with transient ischemic attacks should be treated with anticoagulants. If arteriography indicates significant extracranial vascular disease, especially ulceration of an atherosclerotic plaque, and experienced surgical care is available, the patient should be offered this form of treatment. Patients with completed strokes are not likely to benefit from any prophylactic treatment. If they are to remain bedridden for long periods, anticoagulants help to reduce the chances of pulmonary embolism.

HYPERTENSIVE ENCEPHALOPATHY

Hypertensive encephalopathy is an uncommon, acute neurologic syndrome characterized by headache, nausea and vomiting, convulsive seizures, transient focal neurologic defects, retinal artery spasm, papilledema, stupor, and coma. The cerebrospinal fluid pressure and protein content are commonly elevated. The syndrome is encountered in patients with longstanding hypertension. Its occurrence is associated with sudden marked increases in blood pressure from various causes, including malignant hypertension, eclampsia, and glomerulonephritis.

The mechanism by which hypertension causes neurologic dysfunction is believed to be acute cerebral vasospasm causing cerebral ischemia and edema. Similar changes have been observed in hypertensive rats.

Mild transient focal neurologic defects can be encountered in this syndrome. When neurologic defects are severe and sustained, the correct diagnosis is more likely to be cerebral ischemia or cerebral hemorrhage. When the blood urea nitrogen is above 100 mg per 100 ml, hypertensive encephalopathy can be difficult to distinguish from uremia, or can blend into that state.

The outlook for patients with hypertensive encephalopathy has been greatly improved with the use of antihypertensive medication, and temporary recovery is now frequent. The appearance of the syndrome, however, is usually associated with the end-state phases of advanced hypertensive vascular disease.

Hypertensive encephalopathy is a medical emergency, and treatment should be given to rapidly lower the blood pressure, for this is the only effective way to eliminate the symptoms. Initial treatment should be intramuscular reserpine, 2 to 5 mg per day. Blood pressure will begin to fall in two to three hours after administration of reserpine, and it can be maintained at desired levels with daily injections. Care must be exercised to avoid cerebral ischemia from hypotension. Permanent medical therapy must be instituted to maintain the blood pressure at more nearly normal levels, utilizing hydrochlorothiazide, reserpine, or alpha methyldopa (see Ch. 564).

PROGRESSIVE SUBCORTICAL ENCEPHALOPATHY

Progressive subcortical encephalopathy, described by Binswanger, is a rare disorder that occurs in patients with hypertension and atherosclerotic vascular disease. Progressive dementia, seizures, and focal neurologic signs characterize the clinical picture. The diagnosis is usually made at necropsy; the brain shows atrophy mainly in the temporal and occipital regions and patchy demyelination in the white matter of the hemispheres.

Carter, A. B.: Cerebral Infarction. New York, Pergamon Press and the Macmillan Company, 1964.
Kannel, W. B., et al.: Risk factors in stroke due to cerebral infarction. Stroke, 2:423, 1971.
McDowell, F. H. (ed.): Treatment of Strokes. *In* Modern Treatment. New York, Harper & Row, 1965, pp. 15–24, 84–92.
McDowell, F. H., and Brennan, R. W. (eds.): Cerebral Vascular Disease. Transactions of the Eighth Princeton Conference, 1972. New York, Grune & Stratton, 1973.
Millikan, C. H.: Reassessment of anticoagulant therapy in various types of occlusive cerebrovascular disease. Stroke, 2:201, 1971.
Toole, J. F., Moossy, J., and Janeway, R. (eds.): Cerebrovascular Disease. Transactions of the Seventh Princeton Conference, 1970. New York, Grune & Stratton, 1971.
Vinken, P. J., and Bruyn, G. W.: Handbook of Clinical Neurology. Vols. 11 and 12: Vascular Diseases of the Nervous System. New York, American Elsevier Publishing Company, 1972.

380. INTRACRANIAL HEMORRHAGE

DEFINITION

Intracranial hemorrhage, or apoplexy, comprises about one tenth of all acute cerebral vascular illness. Regardless of cause, intracranial hemorrhage is a serious illness with a high rate of mortality. At the bedside the physician can only suspect the diagnosis, which must be confirmed by finding blood in the cerebrospinal fluid or by the demonstration of a hematoma at surgery. The causes of intracranial hemorrhage are numerous, and the clinical pictures are similar regardless of the cause. It helps to understand the clinical problem better if one remembers that nontraumatic bleeding within the cranium takes one of four separate anatomic courses and that these produce three relatively distinct clinical pictures:

1. Bleeding emanating from vessels on the surface of the brain and limited to the cerebrospinal fluid–filled space between the pial and arachnoid membranes is called *subarachnoid hemorrhage.*
2. *Subarachnoid hemorrhage with intracerebral extension* occurs when the sudden force of bleeding from a surface vessel also penetrates into the brain itself; signs and symptoms of both the subarachnoid and the parenchymal lesions result.
3. Bleeding from ruptured vessels within the substance of the brain is called *intracerebral hemorrhage.* This may remain isolated therein as a *cerebral hematoma.*
4. Intracerebral hemorrhage may extend through brain tissue to the ventricles or subarachnoid space, causing signs and symptoms of both the parenchymal and the subarachnoid lesions.

ETIOLOGY

Bleeding from ruptured arteries is the usual source of intracranial hemorrhage, although veins also may bleed. The accompanying table lists the common causes.

Arterial Aneurysms

Berry Aneurysms. These are small, round, or saccular berry-shaped dilatations that form characteristically at arterial bifurcations at or near the circle of Willis. Their cause is uncertain, for aneurysms are not familial and they are rarely found in infants. They arise, however, from what are thought to be congenital defects in the media of cerebral vessels. The wall of an aneurysm is thin, composed usually only of intima and subintimal connective tissue. Muscle or elastic tissues may be evident at the origin of the aneurysmal sac from its parent vessel, but these tissues thin out and disappear as the sac enlarges. Most aneurysms are less than 1 cm in diameter; a few, however, dilate to as much as 2 to 5 cm. As the aneurysm enlarges, it may develop a narrow neck or may remain broadly attached to the vessel wall.

Most berry aneurysms, approximately 85 per cent, develop around the anterior portion of the circle of Willis, arising from the internal carotid, the posterior communicating, the middle cerebral, the anterior communicating, or the anterior cerebral artery, as shown in Figure 8. The most common site is the point of junction of the posterior communicating artery and the internal carotid. About 15 per cent of aneurysms arise from the vertebral-basilar artery system. Multiple aneurysms are found in about one of every six patients. Not all aneurysms bleed, and some are found incidentally at postmortem examination. Occasionally, they become so large that they compress adjacent cerebral tissue or cranial nerves, and, rarely, they enlarge sufficiently to cause a clinical state that simulates brain tumor.

What makes an aneurysm rupture at any given instant is not clear, although several factors seem important. These lesions gradually enlarge with time under the stress of the arterial blood pressure. They are more frequent in patients who are hypertensive, and their incidence is high in subjects with coarctation of the aorta and polycystic renal disease, both of which cause early hypertension. Atheromatous plaques form in their walls, and clots line the aneurysms, but whether either of these conditions increases the chance of rupture is problematic. Probably a change in the blood pressure is the single final event that precipitates perforation of the sac.

Fusiform Aneurysms. These spindle-shaped dilatations along the course of an artery, usually the basilar, sometimes the carotid artery in the cavernous sinus, are due to atherosclerosis. The resulting elongated and tortuous dilatation may be large enough to compress adjacent cranial nerves or the brain itself. Hemorrhage from such an aneurysm is unusual, but characteristically damages the brain fatally when it does occur.

Mycotic Aneurysms. Mycotic aneurysms are produced

Causes of Intracranial Hemorrhage

1. Arterial aneurysms
   a. *"Congenital" berry aneurysms*
   b. *Acquired arterial aneurysms*
      (1) Fusiform aneurysms
      (2) Mycotic aneurysms
2. Arteriovenous (A-V) anomalies
3. Hypertensive vascular disease
4. Vascular lesions associated with primary or metastatic brain tumors
5. Systemic bleeding diatheses
6. Undetermined and miscellaneous causes

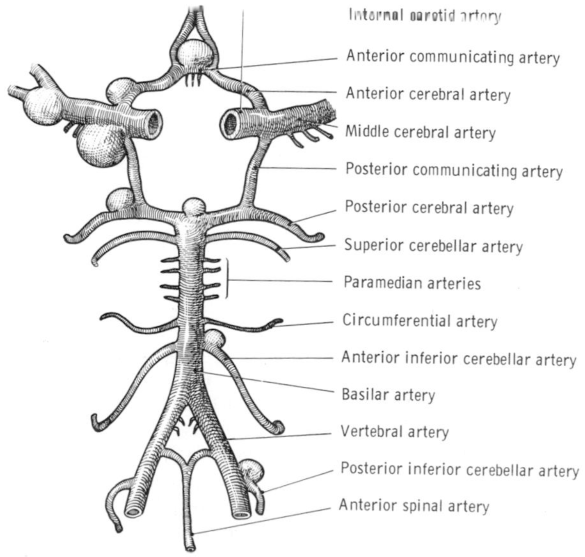

Figure 8. The more common sites of berry aneurysm. The size of the aneurysm at the various sites is directly proportional to the frequency at that site.

by septic emboli associated with bacterial endocarditis. A local necrotic vasculitis occurs at the site where the embolus lodges and results in thinning and dilatation of the vessel wall, which may eventually rupture. Such lesions tend to be multiple, and they are the only aneurysms found distally in the smaller branches of the middle cerebral artery.

Arteriovenous Anomalies or Cavernous Angiomas

Arteriovenous anomalies or cavernous angiomas are tangled, interconnected networks of vessels in which arterial blood passes directly to venous drainage without intervening capillaries. These lesions tend to be supplied by more than one parent cerebral artery, and they range in size from the microscopic to a huge cavernous network large enough to cover most of one cerebral hemisphere or to occupy an entire lobe of the cerebellum. The vessels in an A-V anomaly are themselves malformed so that some structurally resemble arteries, others veins. Since these vessels are usually thin-walled, circulating blood at arterial pressure distends and often eventually ruptures them, with a resultant subarachnoid hemorrhage, intracerebral hemorrhage, or both. Even without hemorrhage, large A-V malformations expand, and the neural tissue adjacent to the anomaly characteristically suffers an uneven pressure necrosis, causing progressively more abnormal neurologic signs of epilepsy. Hemorrhage can destroy all clinical evidence of a malformation of microscopic size and make antemortem diagnosis impossible.

Hypertensive Vascular Disease

Hypertension causes thickening and fibrinoid degeneration of the cerebral arterioles. Red cells can be found free in the perivascular spaces around many of the vessels, and microaneurysms have been described along the arteries since the time of Bouchard and Charcot in the nineteenth century. What part each of these abnormalities contributes to the eventual necrosis and rupture is still debated, although most contemporary pathologists view the fibrinoid degeneration as most important.

When hemorrhage occurs, it usually results from rupture of small arteries in the substance of the brain. This may occur anywhere; it is most common in the cerebrum and least common in the cerebellum and brainstem. In the cerebral hemispheres, small branches of the middle cerebral artery penetrating the region of the basal ganglia are most susceptible, and the lenticulostriate artery has even been termed "the artery of cerebral hemorrhage." In the brainstem, hemorrhages arise from paramedian perforating branches of the basilar more often than they do from the long circumferential branches of either the basilar or the vertebral arteries.

Hemorrhage in Brain Tumors

Hemorrhage may occur in either primary or metastatic lesions, usually in rapidly growing tumors with a large amount of vascular overgrowth. This complication is perhaps most common in glioblastoma multiforme and metastatic neoplasms from the lung. Among the more benign tumors pituitary adenomas have a tendency to cause apoplexy. Of the total number of cerebral hemorrhages, however, those from tumor contribute but a small fraction.

Bleeding Diatheses and Miscellaneous Causes

Leukemia, thrombocytopenia, and the ingestion of excessive amounts of anticoagulants all predispose to cerebral hemorrhage. In some patients it is difficult or impossible to establish what caused a cerebral hemorrhage. As mentioned, in some cases the hemorrhage may have erased the malformation. A hemorrhagic cerebral infarct can be so liquefied that it resembles a primary hemorrhage. However, with the increasing use of cerebral angiography, more and more intracranial aneurysms and malformations are being demonstrated in all age groups as the cause of intracranial hemorrhage.

PATHOLOGY AND PATHOGENESIS

Subarachnoid Hemorrhage. Subarachnoid hemorrhage most commonly comes from rupture of a berry aneurysm, less commonly from an A-V anomaly or a mycotic or fusiform aneurysm. Blood suddenly released in this manner has several deleterious effects, each contributing to the seriousness of the disease. The sudden high pressure jet raises the intracranial pressure and sometimes acts like an acute concussion, causing sudden unconsciousness or, occasionally, rapid brain displacement and death. Blood is also a noxious agent, particularly as it hemolyzes and breaks down into its pigments. It irritates blood vessels, meninges, and the brain itself. Meningeal irritation causes the characteristic headache of subarachnoid hemorrhage, and later, within hours or days, the blood produces a sterile meningitis. This hemogenic meningitis itself becomes a source of considerable disability, for it not only causes subjective discomfort and systemic toxicity but leads to meningeal exudation, thickening, and scarring that can impair cerebrospinal fluid absorption and cause subacute or chronic communicating hydrocephalus. Moreover, the blood may irritate the underlying brain so as to evoke adverse descending autonomic discharges, causing hypertension and cardiac arrhythmias.

In addition to the brain destruction caused by the physical action of the hemorrhage, ischemic changes and infarction of brain tissue are found in as many as two thirds of patients dying from subarachnoid hemorrhage. The ischemia and infarction have been attributed to vascular spasm or vessel wall edema, and they are encountered most commonly in the area of the brain supplied by the artery with the ruptured aneurysm. Evidence for arterial spasm in subarachnoid hemorrhage comes from angiographic studies showing segmental vessel narrowing that correlates with a high incidence of clinical and pathologic evidence of cerebral infarction. The causative mechanism is believed to be a combination of the irritating effect of free blood plus vessel injury. During surgery, mechanical stimulation of cerebral arteries causes significant and sustained vessel narrowing. Presumably, vascular spasm has a potentially protective action in reducing the amount of bleeding from a ruptured artery. Why in some instances it lasts long enough and is severe enough to reduce distal cerebral blood flow to the point of ischemia and neural death is unknown. The possibility that persistent vessel narrowing may be due to edema of the vessel wall and not spasm needs consideration.

Extension of bleeding into the brain occurs in about half of all surface aneurysms and in nearly all A-V anomalies. The complication is particularly likely when the bleeding site lies close to cerebral tissue, as is true with aneurysms of the anterior communicating or anterior cerebral arteries, which are interposed between the frontal lobes, or of branches of the middle cerebral artery, which are buried within the sylvian fissure. Rupture from the anterior communicating vessel tends to damage one or both frontal lobes, and rupture of middle cerebral artery aneurysms tends to lacerate the temporoparietal or posterior frontal lobes.

Intracerebral Hemorrhage. Intracerebral hemorrhage is most often caused by hypertensive vascular disease or ruptured aneurysm, less often by a bleeding arteriovenous malformation. The path that the blood takes with these lesions and the amount of bleeding are somewhat unpredictable. Some hemorrhages dissect the brain along fiber tracts, destroying relatively little brain tissue along the way. Others damage considerable amounts of neural tissue in the region of bleeding. All hemorrhages enlarge the brain and evoke cerebral edema. When the enlargement occurs rapidly, it displaces cerebral structures laterally across the midline under the falx and downward through the tentorium cerebelli, with resulting brainstem compression. Such a course of events is often fatal; at postmortem examination smaller areas of bleeding are found in the midbrain and pons in addition to the massive intracerebral hemorrhage. These secondary brainstem lesions have been attributed to venous obstruction and ischemia from transtentorial herniation.

Small intracerebral hemorrhages can remain entirely confined within the brain substance. Occasionally, the hematoma absorbs fluid, and this plus the surrounding edema can create the clinical picture of an expanding new growth. More often, however, the fluid is resorbed, and the remaining cavity shrinks almost to the point of disappearance.

Most large cerebral hemorrhages rupture into the subarachnoid space, the ventricular system, or both. Although serious consequences have been attributed to this course of events, it is likely that the large size of the hemorrhage causes the disastrous clinical effects rather than the fact that bleeding penetrated into the cerebrospinal fluid spaces.

CLINICAL MANIFESTATIONS OF INTRACRANIAL BLEEDING

Subarachnoid Hemorrhage. Subarachnoid hemorrhage has as its most common initial symptom a sudden violent headache. Initially the headache is usually described as an excruciating, intense, aching pain. Later it becomes dull and throbbing but remains severe, and most patients describe it as the most intense headache they have ever experienced. Even if it is at first localized, it soon becomes generalized, and frequently patients complain of severe neck and back pain. The initial localized headache is due to vascular distortion and injury. The later generalized headache is due to meningeal irritation from blood in the subarachnoid space.

Localization of headache at the onset is helpful in determining the site of the bleeding. Headache that begins in the back of the head suggests a posterior fossa origin of bleeding, and headache that begins in the anterior part of the head suggests a supratentorial bleeding source. If the initial headache is localized to one side, bleeding usually has occurred from a vessel on that side.

Other symptoms include dizziness, vertigo, vomiting, drowsiness, sweating and chills, stupor, and loss of consciousness.

Shortly after the onset of symptoms, the patient may lose consciousness for a few moments. With massive subarachnoid hemorrhage and intracerebral extension, the patient may lapse into and remain in coma until death. In some instances of subarachnoid hemorrhage death may be sudden and is related to intraventricular hemorrhage and sudden intense transtentorial herniation and brainstem compression. When hemorrhage is confined to the subarachnoid space or when intracerebral extension of bleeding is minor, consciousness is regained in a few minutes to a few hours. Delirium and lethargy often follow and may persist for as long as two weeks; severe mental clouding, delirium or coma usually indicates severe bleeding and brain damage.

Patients with subarachnoid hemorrhage usually complain of neck stiffness; this does not appear immediately in most patients but begins with the onset of the meningeal inflammatory reaction 6 to 12 hours later. When neck stiffness is evident shortly after the onset of symptoms, it is ominous and suggests that the meninges in the posterior fossa are stretched by beginning herniation of the cerebellar tonsils into the foramen magnum.

Although subarachnoid hemorrhage does occur during sleep, it most commonly occurs when patients are engaged in their usual activities. Many patients have reported that headache began during activity such as straining at stool, heavy lifting, or coitus.

Convulsions may occur, usually at onset, but sometimes during the acute phase of the illness. When present, they almost invariably indicate that the site of bleeding is in the anterior or middle fossa.

On examination the most conspicuous sign is marked neck rigidity and pain on attempting head movement. The most common localizing neurologic abnormality is pupillary inequality or paresis of vertical and medial movements of one eye that follows oculomotor nerve compression by aneurysms of the internal carotid artery.

Lateralizing neurologic signs, such as hemiparesis or hemiplegia, hemisensory defects or hemianopia, indicate either an intracerebral extension of bleeding or vascular spasm. The distribution of signs of neurologic dysfunction, particularly at onset, may be helpful in localizing the site of bleeding. Marked hemiparesis and severe hemisensory defects suggest bleeding from an aneurysm on the middle cerebral artery in the sylvian fissure. Unilateral oculomotor paresis with ptosis, diplopia, and mydriasis suggests that the bleeding source is from the region of the posterior communicating artery where it joins the internal carotid artery. This junction lies in close approximation to the oculomotor nerve as it passes from the posterior to the middle fossa. Bilateral paresis of the extremities suggests that the bleeding site is near the anterior cerebral-anterior communicating artery junction and suggests extension of bleeding into both frontal lobes. Paresis or sensory impairment present from onset is most likely to be caused by intracerebral extension of bleeding, whereas neurologic signs developing later are more often due to arterial spasm.

Examination of the optic fundi in patients with subarachnoid hemorrhage may reveal smooth rounded hemorrhages near the optic nerve head, "subhyaloid hemorrhages." They are often unilateral and, when present on one side, indicate the side of the bleeding. They are venous in origin and result from sudden increase in intracranial venous pressure at the time of the intracranial bleeding.

Fever caused by the hemogenic aseptic meningitis is common in patients with subarachnoid hemorrhage, appearing usually one to three days after onset and reaching 38 to 39° C (100.4 to 102.2° F). Greater elevations of body temperature usually suggest intraventricular or intracerebral extension of bleeding. Subsequent elevations of temperature during the course of the illness may suggest recurrent bleeding, but they are more often related to intercurrent infections.

Rupture of an Arteriovenous Anomaly. The symptoms and signs of a subarachnoid hemorrhage from a ruptured A-V anomaly are identical to those from a ruptured aneurysm, because both bleed into the subarachnoid space or into the brain tissues. Bleeding into surrounding brain is common for a ruptured A-V anomaly, and symptoms and signs are like those of intracerebral hemorrhage from other causes. Seizures may occur at the onset of bleeding and are nearly always focal in pattern. The diagnosis of arteriovenous anomaly is suggested by a history of pre-existing focal seizures or focal neurologic signs and of recurrent, always unilateral, vascular headache, each of which occurs in about a third of the patients. Rupture of arteriovenous anomalies is more frequent at a younger age than is rupture of aneurysms, so that a history of focal seizures in a young patient with subarachnoid hemorrhage makes the diagnosis of arteriovenous anomaly particularly likely.

When the patient with an arteriovenous malformation is examined, in addition to signs of meningeal irritation and focal neurologic defects, careful auscultation may disclose an audible bruit over the eyes or skull. Although bruits may be present with either arteriovenous anomalies or aneurysms, they are more common with the former.

Intracerebral Hemorrhage. When intracranial hemorrhage occurs directly into the substance of the brain, the onset of symptoms is usually abrupt. Severe headache, nausea, and vomiting occur and sometimes precede other signs of a neurologic deficit or loss of consciousness by several hours. These early symptoms are the result of an acute increase in intracranial pressure. Focal neurologic dysfunction follows, with hemiplegia or hemisensory defects; this results from disruption or distortion of the main motor and sensory pathways in the cerebrum. Loss of consciousness within minutes after the onset occurs in more than one third of patients and indicates a large hemorrhage, intraventricular bleeding, or both. Among patients who are not initially in coma, half deteriorate with decline of awareness and eventually lapse into coma. With the progressive decline in consciousness, patients may show neurologic signs at first, indicating functional decortication and later indicating decerebration. This sequence follows herniation of the brain through the tentorial space with secondary brainstem compression.

In patients who retain consciousness but have motor or sensory deficits, it can be difficult to differentiate intracerebral hemorrhage from cerebral infarction until the cerebrospinal fluid is examined and found to be bloody. In about 20 per cent of patients, the intracerebral hemorrhage is circumscribed, and the fluid never becomes bloody. In these instances, except for the higher incidence of headache with intracerebral hemorrhage, it may be impossible to differentiate intracerebral hemorrhage from cerebral infarction.

The clinical picture produced by intracerebral hemorrhages at various sites is often characteristic and may enable an accurate localization of bleeding.

Capsular or Putamen Hemorrhage. Intracerebral bleeding into the region of the internal capsule causes abrupt flaccid hemiplegia, loss of sensory perception, and homonymous hemianopia. Capsular hemorrhages in the dominant hemisphere produce aphasia. When the hemorrhage is large, loss of consciousness promptly follows. With small hemorrhages changes are less severe. Paralysis is usually more prominent than sensory impairment, and paralysis of gaze to the side opposite the hemorrhage may be found.

Thalamic Hemorrhages. Hemorrhage into the thalamus also produces abrupt motor deficits, but in addition an impairment of all modalities of sensory perception is common and more prominent than deficits in motility or the visual fields. Consciousness is less likely to be lost with a thalamic than with a capsular hemorrhage. Thalamic hemorrhages are associated with distinct disturbances in eye movements. Patients commonly show paralysis of upward gaze. At rest, their eyes deviate downward and laterally and they are unable to look up on command or reflex. The pupils may be unequal and react poorly to light. There may be partial oculomotor palsy with ptosis and loss of convergence. The mechanism that causes the gaze palsy is compression of the region of the posterior commissure and the adjacent upper brainstem nuclei. Because the disturbances in gaze gradually clear, actual tissue destruction from extension of the hemorrhage into this area is probably not the cause of the defect.

Cerebellar and Brainstem Hemorrhage. Parenchymal hemorrhage in the posterior fossa can occur either in the cerebellar hemispheres or in the brainstem (usually pons). With intracerebellar hemorrhage, the patient may experience sudden severe occipital headache, diplopia, nystagmus, and ataxia. Examination reveals miosis, conjugate gaze palsy, and irregular respiration. In some subjects, these symptoms and signs may be present for several hours before any loss of consciousness; in others, loss of consciousness is immediate. When warning symptoms occur, the diagnosis can often be made from the clinical examination alone, and prompt evacuation of the hematoma can be lifesaving. Hemorrhage into the brainstem causes immediate impairment of consciousness, irregular breathing, pinpoint pupils, and quadriplegia followed by a rapid decline to death.

LABORATORY FINDINGS IN INTRACRANIAL BLEEDING

Cerebrospinal Fluid Examination. Intracranial hemorrhage can be diagnosed ante mortem with certainty only when blood is found in the cerebrospinal fluid or in the brain substance at operation. Lumbar puncture can be safely carried out on most patients suspected of having intracranial hemorrhage, but should be done with caution when there is evidence of impaired consciousness or a progressive decline in awareness and focal neurologic defects. These signs indicate both extensive brain damage and the possibility of brainstem compression. With suspected intracerebral hemorrhages and hematoma, there is always the possibility of tentorial herniation, which may be precipitated or accentuated by changes in cerebrospinal fluid pressure after puncture. In such instances lumbar puncture is best postponed until after other studies have been carried out.

Examination of the cerebrospinal fluid shortly after

the onset of intracranial bleeding (1 to 24 hours) reveals red cells with a constant red cell count in sequential samples. The supernatant fluid of a centrifuged specimen will have a pink color owing to the presence of oxyhemoglobin. The fluid reacts positively with benzidine. Cerebrospinal fluid examined after 24 hours will begin to show, in addition, a yellowish coloration (xanthochromia) caused by the degradation of oxyhemoglobin to bilirubin. This intensifies over a period of several days and usually reaches peak intensity at 36 to 48 hours after the onset of bleeding.

Bloody fluid caused by a traumatic lumbar puncture is indicated by the absence of pink or yellow discoloration of the centrifuged supernatant cerebrospinal fluid, i.e., not xanthochromic, by failure to obtain a positive benzidine test for hemoglobin in the supernatant fluid, and by a decreasing red cell count in sequential samples of the fluid.

The white cell count in the CSF, when determined shortly after bleeding, will be commensurate with the amount of bleeding—usually one white cell for every 1000 red cells. When the white cell count is made on specimens collected 12 hours or more after the onset of bleeding, it may be elevated. This increase in white cells is caused by the inflammatory reaction in the meninges and may reach levels as high as 500 per cubic millimeter. Early in the course of the inflammatory reaction the cells may be polymorphonuclear leukocytes and lymphocytes; later, the cells are all lymphocytes.

An exudative reaction accompanies intracranial hemorrhage, and the cerebrospinal fluid protein is usually elevated to levels around 100 mg per 100 ml or more. During fresh bleeding, for each 10,000 red cells in the fluid, the protein is said to rise 15 mg per 100 ml. Protein elevations are maximal eight to ten days after bleeding and decline thereafter. The cerebrospinal fluid pressure is often elevated to levels of 200 to 300 mm (of CSF) with subarachnoid hemorrhage. Elevations may be much higher, 300 to 500 mm with large intracerebral hemorrhages. The white count in the peripheral blood can be elevated to levels up to 15,000, and some patients have a transient albuminuria and glycosuria.

Arteriography. It is often impossible on clinical grounds alone to distinguish between a bleeding aneurysm, a bleeding A-V anomaly, or intracerebral bleeding of unknown cause. Once the clinical diagnosis of intracranial hemorrhage has been made, cerebral arteriography is necessary to demonstrate the cause and site of bleeding. Thus if the patient is a satisfactory operative risk, arteriography should be performed as soon as possible with the hope that specific treatment can be instituted.

Arteriography is most useful in demonstrating aneurysms and A-V anomalies. In patients with suspected ruptured aneurysm, cerebral angiograms will demonstrate the aneurysm in over 80 per cent of instances. They may also indicate whether the aneurysm can be approached surgically. In addition to the aneurysm, the angiogram may reveal distortion of the usual vessel patterns near the aneurysm, indicating a hematoma, and frequently there will be arterial narrowing. The technical details of arteriography are discussed elsewhere; however, the physician should see to it that the intracranial branches of both the right and left carotid arteries are visualized to determine whether more than one aneurysm is present. When more than one aneurysm is present, it is often difficult to determine which one ruptured. Points that are helpful are that the bleeding aneurysm is often irregular in outline and, in the surrounding area, there may be distortion of other vessels, suggesting a local hematoma, or the nearby vessels may show narrowing. Local hematoma is the most reliable evidence of bleeding. If an aneurysm is not seen in the carotid arterial tree, the vertebral and basilar arteries and their branches should be visualized. The demonstration of an aneurysm on the distal branches of the middle or anterior cerebral arteries is almost diagnostic of mycotic aneurysm.

Arteriovenous anomalies are readily demonstrated in cerebral angiograms, as the usually large flow of blood through these structures produces a characteristic picture of early arterial filling and venous drainage of the anomalous vessels.

Intracerebral hemorrhage often can be visualized on cerebral angiograms. Shift of midline vessels, widening of the space between the anterior and middle cerebral arteries, and downward or upward displacement of the middle cerebral branches are helpful evidence. However, roughly a quarter of small hematomas (20 to 30 per cent) escape detection by angiograms.

When hemorrhage has occurred into a cerebral neoplasm, angiograms help in demonstrating vascular changes suggestive of tumor. In addition to vessel distortion and shift of midline vessels, abnormal vessels in the tumor may fill with contrast media and produce a so-called "tumor stain."

PROGNOSIS

Ruptured Aneurysm. Subarachnoid bleeding from a ruptured aneurysm is extremely serious; the mortality rate is 45 per cent for each major attack, and there is a high risk of recurrence. Among those who succumb to bleeding, about one third do so within the first 48 hours, another one third within the next month, and the remainder from later major recurrences. Recurrence strikes about one patient in three, with the maximal danger during the first two weeks after the initial bleeding, when about 60 per cent of all rebleeding occurs. However, some patients bleed during the third and fourth weeks and about 20 per cent have late recurrences, most of which are within the first six months after leaving the hospital. Fatal recurrences have been reported as long as 20 years after the initial bleeding, and there is no way to predict which patient will have a recurrence of bleeding or when he is likely to have it. The high mortality and the frequency of recurrence make accurate statements of prognosis impossible for individual patients. In general, the longer a patient survives after the initial bleeding, the less are his chances of recurrence. Data submitted to the National Co-operative Study of Subarachnoid Hemorrhage indicate that if a patient with subarachnoid hemorrhage is alive one week after onset, the chance of his surviving five more weeks is 65 per cent. If he lives two weeks without recurrence, he has a 76 per cent chance of living four more weeks. Patients 20 to 50 years of age have a better chance of survival than those over 60. As might be expected, patients with the least neural damage and the least impairment of consciousness have the best chance of survival.

Ruptured A-V Anomaly. The prognosis for bleeding from arteriovenous anomalies is better than for aneurysm. The initial mortality is about 25 per cent and the possibility of recurrence less than that. Because of their location and the tendency to bleed into brain tissue, the neurologic disability among survivors of bleeding A-V anomalies tends to be high. Seizures with A-V anomalies are common before bleeding, and patients who do not have seizures often develop them after bleeding.

Hypertensive Vascular Disease. The prognosis for intracerebral hemorrhage from hypertensive vascular disease is poor; the over-all mortality is more than 50 per cent. Mortality is highest with hemorrhage into the ventricle or when severe brain edema causes temporal lobe herniation with resultant compression of the midbrain. The initial mortality rises with the age of the patient. It is about 40 per cent for patients in the 40 to 60 age range, 50 per cent in patients over 60, and 80 per cent in patients over 70. Patients who are in coma when first seen have a mortality rate of 70 to 100 per cent. Recurrence of intracerebral hemorrhage is uncommon, but tissue destruction and displacement at the time of bleeding cause serious neural damage and residual neurologic dysfunction. Patients with small intracerebral hemorrhages usually are left with only slight disability.

TREATMENT

The treatment of intracranial hemorrhage has three goals: preserving life, reducing disability, and preventing recurrence. Treatment directed toward preservation of life is similar for all causes of intracranial hemorrhage and for most other life-threatening neurologic illnesses. During the acute phase of intracranial hemorrhage, the patient should be in bed for as long as the symptoms of headache, stiff neck, and prostration require. Rebleeding is unlikely with ruptured A-V anomaly and hypertensive vascular disease, and a patient with one of these disorders need not be kept in bed for a long period once he feels well enough to get up. Just when to mobilize the patient with subarachnoid hemorrhage from intracranial aneurysm is a question more difficult to answer. Four to six weeks of bed rest is usually recommended, because this is the period of maximal danger from rebleeding. Recurrent hemorrhage has been noted to occur with straining at stool and with other activity, and rest in bed is believed to lessen the chances for potentially dangerous activity.

When the patient is in coma or has impaired consciousness after intracranial hemorrhage, meticulous care must be taken to maintain an adequate airway, blood pressure, and fluid and electrolyte balance. The skin and eyes must be protected from pressure and irritation. The urinary bladder should not be allowed to become distended from urinary retention. These are common problems for all patients with neurologic illness and depressed consciousness; they are discussed more fully elsewhere.

Patients with intracranial hemorrhage who are conscious usually complain of severe headache and stiff neck. They also frequently are restless and delirious. Analgesics such as codeine sulfate by mouth or codeine phosphate intramuscularly in doses of 60 mg may be needed as often as every two hours to relieve headache; in most instances this also relieves restlessness. Other narcotics for analgesia should be avoided because they depress respiration. *Delirium may persist for as long as two weeks.* No specific treatment is indicated, but having a member of the family present at all times and reducing examinations and procedures to a minimum greatly reduce the patient's anxiety and restlessness.

Initially, patients with intracranial hemorrhage should not take fluid or food by mouth for 24 to 48 hours because of the danger of vomiting and aspiration. Subsequently, it is best to give clear fluids for another 24 to 48 hours and then a soft diet. During the period of restricted fluid and food intake, intravenous fluids should be given in the usual physiologic quantities.

Constipation must be avoided. When patients require codeine for relief of pain, mild laxatives or stool softeners should be given if the patient is able to take medication by mouth. Otherwise, small enemas should be given every other day.

When the blood pressure is elevated, it should be returned to nearly normal levels, particularly in patients with bleeding from intracranial aneurysms. This should not be done rapidly, however, because of the risk of precipitating a hypotension-induced cerebral ischemic infarct. Methyldopa or reserpine orally or parenterally is usually an effective antihypertensive.

Ruptured Aneurysm. Prevention of recurrent bleeding from aneurysms is the primary goal of treatment and, in view of the close approximation of recurrent bleeding to the initial hemorrhage, should be attempted as soon as possible. Thus angiograms to identify the source and site of bleeding should be made as soon as practicable, once the diagnosis of intracranial hemorrhage has been made. Similarly, if the aneurysm is believed to be amenable to surgical therapy, this is performed as soon as the patient's condition allows. Patients with no depression of consciousness, who are under 60 and normotensive, who have no evidence of arterial spasm on angiograms, and who have minimal neurologic deficits are considered good surgical risks and can be treated surgically immediately if this form of therapy is indicated for the particular aneurysm. Patients with depressed levels of consciousness or coma or with major neurologic deficits are very poor candidates for surgery; operative mortality in this group is extremely high; operation, if indicated, should be postponed until improvement occurs. Patients over the age of 60 who are hypertensive and who have arterial spasm on angiograms also are poor operative risks, and surgery should be delayed until their condition improves.

The possibility that rebleeding is related to lysis of a clot plugging the aneurysmal sac has been suggested. Agents which inhibit the enhanced intrathecal fibrinolytic state that often follows subarachnoid hemorrhage are being evaluated to see if they decrease the chances of rebleeding. These agents include epsilon-aminocaproic acid and p-aminomethylbenzoic acid. Epsilon-aminocaproic acid must be given in large quantities, 20 to 36 grams per day intravenously, to be effective. Studies indicate that it is useful in the prevention of rebleeding.

Surgical therapy is directed toward removal of the aneurysm or control of the bleeding by a direct surgical attack or toward decreasing the blood pressure in the feeding arterial tree by ligation of a proximal artery. Not all aneurysms can be treated surgically.

Some forms of surgical therapy are more suitable than others. In the past six years, several clinics and hospitals have worked together in a cooperative study to determine the type of surgery most suitable for a particular bleeding lesion. It has been concluded, through carefully controlled studies in the United States and England, that aneurysms arising from the internal carotid artery at the junction with the posterior communicating artery should be treated surgically, the procedure of choice being ligation of the common carotid artery in the neck or direct surgical attack on the aneurysm in good-risk patients.

The controlled studies indicate that patients with anterior cerebral artery aneurysms probably do not benefit from surgery and may actually do worse. However, some surgeons still believe that, in properly selected patients, surgical correction of an aneurysm of the anterior cerebral or anterior communicating artery is beneficial.

The outcome of surgical treatment of middle cerebral artery aneurysms is more uncertain. In the controlled treatment series, direct surgical attack provided better results in male patients, whereas women with middle cerebral aneurysms fared less well with surgery than when treated conservatively. The explanation of this difference appears to be that women are more prone to cerebral infarction after surgery than men. In addition, women have smaller, more fragile aneurysms that make surgery more difficult.

Aneurysms on the vertebral basilar vascular tree are difficult to reach surgically. The most successful surgery reported has been for aneurysms arising from the vertebral artery near the branching of the posterior inferior cerebellar artery.

Current surgical techniques include a large number of methods for dealing with ruptured aneurysms. Most of the carefully controlled treatment trials have utilized either common carotid ligation or clipping or tying of the neck of the aneurysm or its feeding vessels. To reinforce the aneurysm and prevent recurrent bleeding, plastic coating and gauze wrapping have been utilized, but their superiority over other methods of surgical treatment has yet to be proved.

If the patient is not suitable for surgical treatment or if surgery must be delayed, a program of medical treatment should be instituted as outlined above.

Arteriovenous Anomaly. Surgery for A-V anomalies require the tying of feeding vessels or the amputation of a portion of the brain containing the anomaly. The latter treatment is curative if the whole A-V malformation can be removed, but it is limited to those instances in which the anomaly lies entirely in or on the occipital pole or the frontal pole. The chance of neurologic disability associated with removal of A-V anomalies in other sites is usually too great to justify surgical therapy unless major disability had been present before bleeding.

Ligation of vessels feeding the anomaly has been recommended, but no carefully controlled evaluation of this form of surgical therapy has been done. Carotid ligation to reduce the blood pressure in the anomaly is also believed to reduce the chance of recurrent bleeding. Recently, artificial embolization with plastic spheres introduced into the feeding arteries has been reported to be successful in obliterating the anomaly.

Fortunately, the chance of recurrent bleeding with arteriovenous anomalies is less than with aneurysm. Also, bleeding carries a relatively low mortality, so that for most patients with arteriovenous anomaly and intracranial hemorrhage, medical management identical to that described for ruptured aneurysm is the treatment of choice. The frequency of disability and mortality associated with surgical treatment are too high to justify its use except in highly special instances. Convulsive seizures are common with arteriovenous anomalies and should be treated with anticonvulsants as outlined in Part X, Section Sixteen.

Intracerebral Hemorrhage. Cerebral hemorrhage is a severe disease and one for which there is no satisfactory form of treatment. The immediate medical treatment was outlined earlier. It must include meticulous attention to the problems imposed by impaired consciousness and abrupt neurologic disability.

Whether and when to operate on cerebral hemorrhage is a recurrent question, and efforts have been made in this direction for years, although generally with poor results. Recently, McKissock and his colleagues in England carried out a carefully controlled evaluation of surgical treatment of acute cerebral hemorrhage caused by hypertensive disease, in which they showed that patients treated surgically fared less well than those treated conservatively. No matter what the treatment, patients in deep stupor or coma from intracerebral hemorrhage rarely survive. For patients who survive the initial cerebral insult and become stable clinically, removal of a persistent encapsulated hematoma may lessen neurologic disability and hasten improvement.

Surgical removal of an intracerebral hematoma caused by bleeding from a ruptured aneurysm has been no more encouraging than when hypertensive vascular disease causes the hemorrhage. Patients with intracerebral hematoma from ruptured aneurysm are usually in coma and have severe neurologic dysfunction; survival in these circumstances is unlikely.

Removal of an intracerebral hematoma caused by bleeding from a ruptured A-V anomaly has been recommended for patients with neurologic disability. The results are difficult to appraise objectively, but surgical treatment has its best chance of offering relief if the patients have become stable clinically and have a well localized, encapsulated hematoma causing symptoms and signs of a mass lesion.

Patients who recover from intracerebral hemorrhage should begin programs of rehabilitation as soon as the effects of acute brain damage have subsided. Such a program begins with passive exercise of the paretic extremities to help avoid contractures and progresses to active exercises as voluntary movement returns. The program is as outlined under Treatment in Ch. 379.

Dinsdale, H. B.: Spontaneous hemorrhage in the posterior fossa. Arch. Neurol., 10:200, 1964.

McKissock, W., Richardson, A., and Taylor, J.: Primary intracerebral hemorrhage. A controlled trial of surgical and conservative treatment in 180 selected cases. Lancet, 2:221, 1961.

McKissock, W., Richardson, A., and Walsh, L.: Anterior communicating aneurysms. A trial of conservative and surgical treatment. Lancet, 1:873, 1965.

McKissock, W., Richardson, A., and Walsh, L.: Middle-cerebral aneurysms. Further results in the controlled trial of conservative and surgical treatment of ruptured intracranial aneurysms. Lancet, 2:417, 1962.

Pool, J. L., and Potts, D. G.: Aneurysms and Arteriovenous Anomalies of the Brain: Diagnosis and Treatment.. New York, Hoeber Medical Division, Harper & Row, 1965.

Sahs, A. L., Perret, G. E., Locksley, H. B., and Nishiotia, H.: Intracranial Aneurysms and Subarachnoid Hemorrhage. Philadelphia, J. B. Lippincott Company, 1969.

Toole, J. F., Moossy, J., and Janeway, R.: Cerebral Vascular Diseases. Transactions of the Seventh Princeton Conference, 1970. New York, Grune & Stratton, 1971.

Toole, J. F., Siebert, R. G., and Whisnant, J. P.: Cerebral Vascular Diseases. Transactions of the Sixth Princeton Conference, 1968. New York, Grune & Stratton, 1971.

Walton, J. N.: Subarachnoid Hemorrhage. London, E. & S. Livingstone, Ltd., 1956.

Section Twelve. INFECTIONS AND INFLAMMATORY DISEASES OF THE CENTRAL NERVOUS SYSTEM AND ITS COVERINGS

381. INTRODUCTION

Philip R. Dodge

The seriously ill patient with symptoms and signs of disease of the central nervous system and evidence of leptomeningeal inflammation presents a challenging diagnostic and therapeutic problem. Of crucial clinical significance is the determination of whether the involvement of meninges is primary, as in bacterial meningitis, or secondary, as in a variety of parenchymatous and parameningeal infections (e.g., encephalitis, brain abscess, subdural empyema). Central to this clinical problem is some degree of pleocytosis. Various bacteria, fungi, rickettsiae, viruses, and parasites may excite such a cerebrospinal fluid response. In addition, a similar reaction may be produced by a variety of noninfectious processes, including chemical irritation, hypersensitivity responses, and, occasionally, tumors. Elsewhere in this text many of the specific diseases that evoke an inflammatory response in the central nervous system and meninges are discussed. In this section emphasis will be placed on a systematic clinical approach to differential diagnosis and on the manner in which functions of the nervous system are deranged by such inflammatory processes.

382. AIDS TO DIAGNOSIS IN INTRACRANIAL AND INTRASPINAL INFLAMMATORY DISEASE

Philip R. Dodge

CEREBROSPINAL FLUID EXAMINATION

Because diagnosis rests in many instances on the cerebrospinal fluid findings, the importance of a carefully performed lumbar puncture and of meticulous study of the cerebrospinal fluid cannot be overstressed. The cerebrospinal fluid findings characteristic of various inflammatory diseases of the central nervous system and meninges are outlined in Tables 1 and 2. Measurement of the initial pressure should be part of every cerebrospinal fluid examination. In the presence of high pressure, just enough fluid should be removed slowly to allow for an adequate examination. Jugular compression (Queckenstedt's test) should be avoided except in cases of suspected spinal cord compression. Deeply yellow (xanthochromic) fluid derives its color primarily from

TABLE 1. Initial Cerebrospinal Fluid Findings in Suppurative Diseases of the Central Nervous System and Meninges

	Pressure (mm H_2O)	Leukocytes per cu mm	Protein (mg per 100 ml)	Sugar (mg per 100 ml)	Specific Findings
Acute bacterial meningitis	Usually elevated; average, 300	Several hundred to more than 60,000; usually few thousand; occasionally less than 100 (especially meningococcal or early in disease); polymorphonuclears predominate	Usually 100 to 500, occasionally more than 1000	Less than 40 in more than half the cases	Organism seen on smear usually; recovered on culture in more than 90% of cases
Subdural empyema	Usually elevated; average 300	Less than 100 to few thousand; polymorphonuclears predominate	Usually 100 to 500	Normal	No organisms on smear or by culture unless concurrent meningitis
Brain abscess	Usually elevated	Usually 10 to 200; rarely fluid is acellular; lymphocytes predominate	Usually 75 to 400	Normal	No organisms on smear or by culture
Ventricular empyema (rupture of brain abscess)	Considerably elevated	Several thousand to 100,000; usually more than 90% polymorphonuclears	Usually several hundred	Usually less than 40	Organism may be cultured or seen on smear
Cerebral epidural abscess	Slight to modest elevation	Few to several hundred or more cells; lymphocytes predominate	Usually 50 to 200	Normal	No organisms on smear or by culture
Spinal epidural abscess	Usually reduced with spinal block	Usually 10 to 100; lymphocytes predominate	Usually several hundred	Normal	No organisms on smear or by culture; may enter abscess on L.P. and get pus
Thrombophlebitis (often associated with subdural empyema)	Often elevated	Few to several hundred; polymorphonuclears and lymphocytes	Slightly to moderately elevated	Normal	No organisms on smear or by culture
Bacterial endocarditis (with embolism)	Normal or slightly elevated	Few to less than 100; lymphocytes and polymorphonuclears	Slightly elevated	Normal	No organisms on smear or by culture
Acute hemorrhagic encephalitis	Usually elevated	Few to more than 1000; polymorphonuclears predominate	Moderately elevated	Normal	No organisms on smear or by culture

TABLE 2. Comparative Cerebrospinal Fluid Findings in Nonsuppurative Meningitis

	Pressure (mm H_2O)	Leukocytes per cu mm	Protein (mg per 100 ml)	Sugar (mg per 100 ml)	Specific Findings
Tuberculous	Usually elevated; may be low with dynamic block in advanced stages	Usually 25 to 100, rarely more than 500; lymphoyctes predominate except in early stages when polymorphonuclears may account for 80% of cells	Nearly always elevated, usually 100 to 200; may be much higher if dynamic block	Usually reduced; less than 50 in 3/4 of the cases	Acid-fast organisms may be seen on smear of protein coagulum (pellicle) or recovered from inoculated guinea pig or by culture
Cryptococcal	Usually elevated; average, 225	0 to 800; average, 50; lymphocytes predominate	Usually 20 to 500; average, 100	Reduced in more than half of cases; average, 30; often higher in patients with concomitant diabetes mellitus	Organisms may be seen in India ink preparation and on culture (Sabouraud's medium); will usually grow on blood agar; may produce alcohol in CSF from fermentation of glucose
Syphilitic (acute)	Usually elevated	Average 500; usually lymphocytes; rarely polymorphonuclears	Average, 100; gamma globulin often high with abnormal colloidal gold curve	Normal (reduced rarely)	Positive reagin test for syphilis; spirochete not demonstrable by usual techniques of smear or by culture
Sarcoid	Normal to considerably elevated	0 to less than 100 mononuclear cells	Slight to moderate elevation	Normal	No specific findings
Tumor	Usually elevated; may be considerably so	0 to several hundred mononuclears	Elevated often to high levels	Normal or greatly reduced; (low in 3/4 of carcinomatous meningitis cases)	Neoplastic cells may be identified on smear, by Millepore filter technique or by tissue block
Viral	Normal to moderately elevated	5 to few hundred; but may be more than 1000, particularly with mumps or echovirus 9; lymphocytes predominate but may be more than 80% polymorphonuclears in first few days	Frequently normal or slightly elevated, less than 100; may show greater elevation in recovering stages (particularly poliomyelitis)	Normal (reduced rarely)	Viral agent may be recovered in tissue culture, embryonated egg or animal inoculation

bilirubin pigment. In the absence of prior hemorrhage, this is most frequently associated with high concentrations of protein, and is often seen with impaired cerebrospinal fluid circulation. Intense bilirubin staining of the cerebrospinal fluid may also occur in jaundiced patients with meningitis (as in Weil's disease).

As few as 200 to 300 leukocytes per cubic millimeter will impart an opalescence to the fluid, and fluid containing thousands of cells will be turbid. The fluid should be examined promptly for cells in a counting chamber, and an accurate differential count should be performed on a stained smear of the sediment after centrifugation. In the event of a traumatic lumbar puncture, care must be exercised to ensure that an underlying pleocytosis is not missed. A gram-stained smear for bacteria should be studied. Quellung and agglutination reactions with type-specific antisera may provide an almost certain, immediate etiologic diagnosis when *D. pneumoniae, N. meningitidis, or H. influenzae* organisms are responsible for meningitis. Whenever tuberculous meningitis is a consideration, a Ziehl-Neelsen or Kenyon stain should be performed on the sediment and on the protein coagulum or pellicle that frequently forms on standing. The India ink technique may outline *C. neoformans* in cases of cryptococcal meningitis (torulosis). The finding of budding forms of the yeast in cerebrospinal fluid will help distinguish cryptococci from lymphocytes, with which they may be confused even by experienced observers; however, confirmation by culture is always necessary.

The cerebrospinal fluid should be cultured whenever leukocytes are found or when an inflammatory process is suspected. A variety of media (blood agar, chocolate agar, thioglycollate broth) and various environmental conditions (reduced oxygen tension, increased CO_2 tension) are used routinely. Special media should be employed for the recovery of fungi or *M. tuberculosis.* The latter may also be injected into guinea pigs. Tissue culture techniques and inoculation of mice and embryonated eggs are used for virus isolation.

The concentration of protein in the cerebrospinal fluid increases whenever there is interference with the blood-CSF barrier, as occurs with inflammation. In bacterial, tuberculous, mycotic, and carcinomatous meningitis the glucose concentration in the cerebrospinal fluid is commonly reduced (hypoglycorrhachia). Although the mechanism of hypoglycorrhachia is incompletely understood, the high metabolic activity of rapidly growing cells, phagocytosis, and impaired glucose transport may all be involved. The gamma globulin concentration may be disproportionately increased in certain inflammatory disorders such as syphilis, subacute inclusion body encephalitis, and certain demyelinating disorders (postinfectious encephalomyelitis, multiple sclerosis). In addition to the time-honored tests for syphilis reagin, a new immunologic test applicable to the CSF is countercurrent immunoelectrophoresis. This is a reliable and simple test which permits identification of certain bacterial antigens within an hour or so of a diagnostic lumbar puncture.

RELATIONSHIP OF CEREBROSPINAL FLUID FINDINGS TO ANCILLARY CLINICAL AND LABORATORY DATA

An immediate etiologic diagnosis is possible only when the responsible agent is identified. However, the clinical and cerebrospinal fluid data can help to exclude certain clinical entities early in the diagnostic study. For example, when the symptoms and signs reflect involvement of the meninges and there is no evidence of cerebral or spinal cord disease, primary meningitis is probable. If, in addition, the cerebrospinal fluid contains about 100 or so lymphocytes, a normal quantity of sugar, and an only slightly elevated protein concentration, then bacterial, including tuberculous, and cryptococcal meningitis are less likely, and some form of aseptic meningitis should be suspected. (However, it should be emphasized that the cerebrospinal fluid sugar may be normal on initial examination of patients with tuberculous meningitis and may be reduced in samples obtained subsequently. It should also be appreciated that on occasion the cerebrospinal fluid glucose may be reduced in aseptic meningitis.) A history of exposure to mumps and manifest parotitis make a diagnosis of mumps meningitis probable. On the other hand, the same findings in the CSF in a patient recovering from varicella, especially if there are symptoms and signs of cerebellar ataxia, suggest a diagnosis of postinfectious (varicella) encephalitis. In addition to primary meningeal disease, parameningeal infections can produce cerebrospinal fluid abnormalities similar to those just described. The coexistence of a progressive dysphasia, superior quadrantanopsia, and hemiparesis on the right side and a history of a chronic draining left ear should immediately direct the physician's attention to the diagnosis of a left temporal lobe abscess. Unfortunately, however, a definite diagnosis cannot be made from either the initial clinical or cerebrospinal fluid findings in many cases. Every attempt should be made to amplify the immediate and remote history, including epidemiologic data. One should search for foci of infection adjacent to or remote from the meninges. The extent of the dysfunction of the nervous system should be defined by repeated neurologic examinations and by laboratory studies. In addition to culturing the cerebrospinal fluid, blood cultures should be obtained, because bacteremia is present in about half the cases of primary bacterial meningitis, and similar cerebrospinal fluid changes may occur in bacterial endocarditis. Secretions of the upper and lower respiratory tracts should also be cultured for bacteria and fungi. Enteroviruses cause aseptic meningitis and encephalitis, and recovery of these agents from the stools of patients may aid in establishing the diagnosis. The development of specific neutralizing and complement-fixing antibodies will help confirm the diagnosis. Acute phase sera should be obtained on admission, and a convalescent serum sample obtained two to three weeks later. A fourfold rise in complement-fixing or neutralizing antibody titer is usually evidence of a recent infection with that agent.

Roentgenograms of the skull, sinuses, chest, or spine may be helpful in establishing a diagnosis by disclosing a related focus of disease. An electroencephalogram or isotope scan may direct attention to a region of the brain that clinically is relatively silent. Roentgenographic contrast studies (myelography, pneumoencephalography, ventriculography, and angiography) have their place in diagnosis, but are reserved for the more precise localization of a focal mass lesion that has already been suspected on clinical grounds. Occasionally the clinician must resort to a tissue biopsy; for example, the granulomatous lesions of sarcoidosis may be demonstrated in a lymph node or liver biopsy, and trichina, toxoplasma, or an unusual arteritis may be identified in microscopic sections of muscle tissue. Biopsy of the meninges or brain should be resorted to only rarely, but will at times help to establish the diagnosis in an obscure case. The pathologic findings in herpes, subacute sclerosing panencephalitis, and acute necrotizing hemorrhagic encephalitis are histologically specific enough to permit an exact diagnosis. Whenever tissue is obtained for routine histologic study, appropriate methods for the recovery of an infective agent should also be employed.

383. PARAMENINGEAL INFECTIONS

Morton N. Swartz

The three major localized intracranial suppurative lesions are *cerebral abscess, subdural empyema,* and *cerebral extradural abscess.* Of paramount importance in their early recognition and subsequent management is an understanding of the nature of the predisposing suppurative conditions and of the portals by which infection has spread intracranially. Not only must these conditions be distinguished from one another but they must also, from a therapeutic viewpoint, be clearly distinguished from meningitis caused by bacteria or other infective agents.

CEREBRAL ABSCESS

Definition. Brain abscess represents a poorly or sharply delineated suppurative process of brain substance, resulting from extension from adjacent foci or from hematogenous spread.

Incidence. Despite the introduction of effective antimicrobial therapy, the over-all incidence of brain abscess has not changed significantly over the past two decades (about 7 per 1000 neurosurgical operations). It is seen approximately one fifth as frequently as bacterial meningitis in a large general hospital.

Predisposing Factors. More than one third of intracerebral infections are a consequence of an adjacent primary focus of infection: middle ear, mastoid, paranasal sinuses, face or scalp and skull (osteomyelitis, compound fracture with wound contamination, or craniotomy wound infection). Another one third or so are a consequence of bronchiectasis, lung abscess, empyema, skin infections, acute bacterial endocarditis, or congenital heart disease with right-to-left shunt. In the remainder of brain abscesses an underlying cause cannot be determined.

Subacute and Chronic Middle Ear Infection and Mastoiditis. Over one third of all brain abscesses stem from ear and sinus infection. Infection usually spreads from the ear by either of two routes: direct extension to the roof of the tympanic cavity or mastoid bone (osteomyelitis) and then through the meningeal covering of the brain, or by extension along veins of the inner ear through diploic vessels of the skull and through intracranial venous channels into the substance of the brain. Thrombophlebitis of the pial vessels and dural sinuses, by impairing cerebral circulation, may cause infarction of brain tissue and facilitate development of local infection. The temporal lobe and cerebellum adjacent to the ear and mastoid are the most common sites of otogenic abscess.

Infections of the Paranasal Sinuses. Frontal and sphenoid sinuses are most frequently implicated in "rhinogenic" brain abscess of the frontal and temporal lobes, respectively. Infection may erode the sinus wall and invade the brain directly or, as with otogenic infection, may spread by way of veins communicating with the cavernous sinus and brain.

Infections of the Face and Skull. Intracranial spread of infection from the face or nose to the frontal lobe occurs by way of a septic thrombophlebitis. Compound fractures of the skull may result in brain abscess, particularly when the dura and brain are lacerated, leaving a nidus of bone or foreign body in the devitalized tissue. Occasionally the original traumatic episode has seemed trivial and has been overlooked. Several cases of brain abscess caused by a pencil point introduced through the orbit have been reported. Brain abscess may complicate stereotactic surgery and ventriculovascular shunts.

Etiology. A wide variety of microorganisms cause brain abscesses, and a careful attempt to establish a bacteriologic diagnosis should be made in every case. A gram-stained smear of purulent material should be studied at the time of surgery, and aerobic and anaerobic cultures, as well as cultures for fungi, should be obtained. In about 20 per cent of brain abscesses cultures are sterile. In about 25 per cent, most often when there is a contiguous extracerebral focus, two or more microbial species are isolated.

Various streptococci (either anaerobic or non-group A strains) and *Staphylococcus aureus* are the most frequently isolated organisms. Pneumococcus, formerly a leading cause of brain abscess, is only rarely incriminated today. Species of the Enterobacteriaceae (*E. coli,* Proteus, Klebsiella) are sometimes isolated. Anaerobic bacteria (particularly streptococci and Bacteroides) are frequently found. Rarely Actinomyces, *Nocardia asteroides,* and other fungi may be recovered from an abscess cavity. Of interest is the frequent association of pulmonary alveolar proteinosis with pulmonary and occasionally cerebral nocardiosis. *Hemophilus aphrophilus* and the fungus *Cladosporium trichoides* rarely infect human beings, but when they do, they show a curious affinity for the central nervous system.

When *Entamoeba histolytica* causes brain abscess, there are associated lesions of the liver or lung in virtually every case. In Central and South America and parts of Europe and Asia cerebral cysticercosis (usually solitary cysts containing the larval form of the pork tapeworm *Taenia solium*) should be considered in patients presenting with symptoms of brain tumor. In the racemose form of disease, obstructive hydrocephalus results from the growth of cysts in the third or fourth ventricle. The clinical picture may suggest a diagnosis of pseudotumor cerebri. Very rarely the brain is the site of echinococcal cysts and the solitary or multiple granulomas of schistosomiasis.

Pathology. Abscesses resulting from direct spread of infection are found in the brain adjacent to the primary extracerebral site; those resulting from retrograde venous propagation are often located at some distance from the primary focus in the distribution of the nearest venous sinus. Thus, for example, cerebellar abscess from otitis media is the result of spread of infection from the middle ear to its deep venous drainage into the transverse sinus, and thence medially into the veins draining the anterior superior portion of the ipsilateral cerebellar hemisphere. Metastatic abscesses are usually found in the distribution of the middle cerebral artery.

Initially, the site is edematous and infiltrated with polymorphonuclear leukocytes. The lesion is poorly demarcated at this stage and represents a local suppurative encephalitis. Usually within two weeks of onset the center undergoes liquefaction necrosis. The surrounding zone of fibroblasts becomes progressively thicker and contains more collagen; this constitutes the wall of the abscess, and astrocytes proliferate in the adjacent cerebral tissue. Multiple satellite abscesses may develop and frequently communicate with the principal cavity. Since abscess cavities usually spread through the central white matter, they often extend to and through the ventricular wall, producing the dire complications of ventricular empyema and meningitis. Brain abscess seldom if ever results from primary bacterial meningitis. Coincidental occurrence of brain abscess and meningitis is usually related to intraventricular leakage of the abscess. In support of this view, the three most common organisms in primary pyogenic meningitis (pneumococcus, *H. influenzae,* and *N. meningitidis*) occur only rarely as the cause of brain abscess.

Clinical Manifestations. *Age Incidence.* Brain abscesses are most common in the second to fifth decades, but may occur at any age. They are rare in infancy, even in patients with congenital heart disease.

General Features. The natural history of brain abscess consists either of a subacute to acute febrile illness with headache accompanied or followed by localizing neurologic symptoms, or of a "stroke-like" or tumor-like development of focal signs and symptoms in which evidence of infection is lacking. A history of fever at the time of invasion of the brain by the infective agent may be elicited; but a third of patients will lack a history of fever and remain afebrile under observation. Blood cultures are usually sterile except in those with an underlying acute bacterial endocarditis.

Headache, the most frequent initial symptom of brain abscess, may develop suddenly or insidiously while the attention of the patient and physician is directed toward the primary infection of ear, sinus, or lung. The development of unexplained headaches in a child with congenital cyanotic heart disease should be regarded as due to abscess until proved otherwise. The headache may be localized to the side of the abscess, but it is often generalized and increases in severity as the infection progresses. Heightened intracranial pressure, manifested by nausea, vomiting, drowsiness, bradycardia, confusion, and stupor, is common. Papilledema is a relatively late finding that is recognized in a minority of cases. The increased intracranial pressure may result in signs of sixth- and, less often, in those of third-nerve palsy. They are often false localizing signs, because the abscess may be remote from the cranial nerves. Although, pathologically, brain abscess progresses through several phases, there is no clear correlation with the clinical course of most patients. In some patients, usually those with metastatic brain abscesses, the illness runs a fulminating course, ending fatally in 5 to 15 days. In most, however, the course is considerably prolonged, and a diagnosis of cerebral neoplasm is often suspected.

Specific Neurologic Syndromes. TEMPORAL LOBE ABSCESS. Most temporal lobe abscesses are secondary to ear infection. Involvement of the dominant temporal lobe may produce a nominal (inability to name objects) or Wernicke's (inability to read, write, or understand spoken words) aphasia. Homonymous upper quadrantic or hemianopic field defects may occur. The only motor deficit may be a slight contralateral faciobrachial monoparesis. Herniation of the temporal lobe through the tentorium may develop precipitously and cause a homolateral third-nerve paralysis, coma, and bilateral pyramidal tract signs.

CEREBELLAR ABSCESS. Cerebellar abscesses are almost exclusively otogenic. Increased intracranial pressure, suboccipital headache, and stiff neck may be the only manifestations. The patient may stagger and veer to the side of the lesion. Impaired coordination of extremities on the same side, with poor performance of rapid, alternating movements and with intention tremor, may be present. Nystagmus is frequent and usually coarser when the gaze is directed to the side of the abscess. Associated diseases of the inner ear may contribute to the unsteady gait and nystagmus, and may produce vertigo. Seizures do not occur with abscesses restricted to the cerebellum.

FRONTAL LOBE ABSCESS. Frontal lobe abscesses are most commonly associated with disease of the frontal or, less frequently, the ethmoid sinuses. Drowsiness, inattention, disturbed judgment, and impaired intellectual functions are common; the findings may suggest a psychiatric diagnosis. Mutism and increased grasp, suck, and snout reflexes are often present. In about a fourth of cases focal or generalized convulsions occur; deviation of the head and eyes to the side opposite the lesion is a common pattern of seizure. When the abscess is large or in the posterior frontal region, a contralateral hemiparesis usually develops. Rarely, dysphasia results from a lesion on the dominant side.

PARIETAL LOBE ABSCESS. Parietal lobe abscesses are usually hematogenous but large otogenic temporal lobe abscesses may extend to the parietal lobe. Impaired position sense, two-point discrimination, and stereognosis are characteristic signs of an anterior parietal lobe abscess. Focal sensory and motor seizures occur. Homonymous hemianopia, visual inattention (often demonstrated by bilateral simultaneous stimulation of visual fields), and impaired opticokinetic nystagmus are encountered with more posterior and deep lesions. Dysphasia is a feature of inferior parietal lobe abscess on the dominant side. When the posterior parieto-temporo-occipital region is affected, there may be impaired recognition of fingers, difficulty in differentiating left from right, acalculia, and agraphia (Gerstmann's syndrome).

BRAIN ABSCESS PRESENTING AS "ACUTE MENINGITIS." Occasionally patients with brain abscess present signs of meningitis, including fever, headache, stiff neck, and pleocytosis; focal neurologic signs are usually in evidence also. The syndrome is most often due to leaking of the abscess into the lateral ventricle. Massive rupture into the ventricle is a catastrophic event, with high fever, shock, and coma, and should be easily recognized. Pleocytosis with cell counts of more than 30,000 per cubic millimeter and reduced sugar concentrations are usual. Bacteria can often be seen on Gram stain and can be grown on culture.

In some patients with a similar clinical picture organisms are not found, and the syndrome may represent the phase of "bacterial encephalitis." The important point to be stressed is that one should be alert to the possibility of a brain abscess in any patients with chronic ear or sinus disease who develop meningitis. These patients often improve on treatment of the meningitis only to develop evidence of an intracranial mass lesion one or two weeks later as encapsulation of the abscess progresses.

Laboratory Diagnosis. Modern neuroradiologic techniques presently provide the preferred and safest first step in laboratory diagnosis. When the diagnosis is suspected on clinical grounds and preliminary x-rays of chest, skull, sinuses, and mastoids are completed, brain scanning should be the next step; it will be abnormal in 75 to 80 per cent of cases. Once the abscess has localized, cerebral angiography is generally diagnostic, but in some instances the avascular areas of the abscess can be mistaken for neoplasm.

The EEG in brain abscess is localizing in the great majority of cases, showing high voltage slow waves and, occasionally, sharp discharges over the margins of the abscess.

The cerebrospinal fluid may require examination when meningitis is suspected, but lumbar puncture should be approached cautiously when clinical signs point to a mass lesion already being present. Cerebrospinal fluid pressure is commonly 200 to 300 mm H_2O, but may be considerably higher, particularly in the presence of intraventricular rupture. The cell count varies from a few to several hundred, with lymphocytes predominating. In cases of intraventricular rupture of the abscess, cell counts may be in excess of 50,000 or 100,000 (mainly neutrophils). Also, cell counts of several thousand, with neutrophils predominating, may occur during the early phase of brain abscess ("bacterial encephalitis"). The sugar level is not reduced unless there is a simultaneous suppurative meningitis. The protein may be increased up to several hundred milligrams per 100 ml.

Treatment. Early diagnosis and prompt antimicrobial treatment are crucial. Some workers use mannitol to reduce brain edema. Surgery is usually required once acute cerebral inflammation and edema are brought under control, and consists of initial aspiration of the abscess cavity, followed in some cases by excision at a later time, or primary total excision of the abscess. The method employed depends, to some extent, on the site of the lesion and the state of the patient, but whenever feasible, primary excision is probably preferable.

Since in brain abscesses penicillin-susceptible organisms predominate, 10 million to 20 million units of penicillin per day intravenously should be started prior to operation. If there is reason to suspect an organism not susceptible to penicillin, e.g., gram-negative bacilli from a chronic ear infection, then chloramphenicol or similar drugs should be given concurrently. One of the semisynthetic penicillins, e.g., oxacillin, should be used if a penicillin-resistant Staphylococcus is suspected. The antimicrobial therapy should be modified as necessary at the time of operation, based on examination of a gram-stained smear and culture of the abscess.

Mortality from brain abscess remains high (40 per cent) despite antimicrobial and surgical treatment. Residual neurologic damage is frequent, and seizures are a significant sequela (up to 70 per cent) so that all patients should receive anticonvulsants for 24 months.

SUBDURAL EMPYEMA

Definition. The designation subdural empyema (less accurately termed a subdural abscess) refers to a collection of pus in the potential space between the dura and the arachnoid. It usually results from extension of infection from primary foci in the ears or sinuses. It is an infrequent complication of intracranial surgery, and may rarely represent a metastatic infection from a remote focus.

Incidence. Subdural empyema is about one fifth as common as brain abscess. Its prevalence has not changed in the past two decades.

Predisposing Factors and Pathologic Features. More than half the cases of subdural empyema develop in patients with chronic paranasal sinus infection, usually frontal. An acute exacerbation of the sinusitis just prior to the development of the subdural infection is common. Osteomyelitis of the frontal bone and an epidural abscess often accompany subdural empyema. Chronic otitis media and mastoiditis result in subdural empyema less often than formerly. Postoperative infection, penetrating wounds, infection in subdural hematomas, bacteremia, pulmonary infection, and (very rarely) bacterial meningitis are other sources of subdural empyema.

Infection spreads from the sinuses or mastoid by direct erosion of bone and dura or through infected veins. Thrombosis of cortical veins is observed in 90 per cent of fatal cases. Once pus forms in the subdural space it spreads widely over the convexity of the hemisphere and mesially along the falx. Rarely, the exudate extends beneath the falx to the opposite side. Purulent subarachnoid exudate is usually present immediately subjacent to the subdural exudate.

Etiology. Streptococci, often non-group A or anaerobic strains, are implicated most commonly, but a wide variety of gram-negative organisms are also found. Postoperative infections are usually due to *Staphylococcus aureus.*

Clinical Manifestations. The symptoms and signs of antecedent sinusitis, otitis, or osteomyelitis often blend into those of subdural empyema. Swelling and erythema of the tissues overlying the primary infection may be prominent, and percussion of the underlying bone may evoke considerable pain. In the early stages, pain or headache is mild and is limited to the area over the subdural infection. As the illness progresses, headache becomes generalized and severe; concomitantly high fever, chills, vomiting, and nuchal rigidity develop. Progressive obtundation, culminating in coma within 48 to 72 hours, occurs in untreated cases. Focal or generalized seizures and hemiparesis are common. Sensory deficits and visual field defects and dysphasia also occur. Although these signs are in part attributable to the compressive effects of a mass lesion, the associated thrombophlebitis of cortical veins and the consequent infarction of cerebral tissue are probably of equal importance. In the late stages, the intracranial pressure is severely increased, but papilledema is rare except in chronic cases in which the clinical course has been modified by antimicrobial therapy. Without treatment, death usually occurs within a few days of onset of focal neurologic signs.

Laboratory Diagnosis. The cerebrospinal fluid pressure is elevated, and the fluid characteristically contains a few hundred to a thousand or more neutrophils, a normal amount of sugar, and no organisms. Roentgenograms of the skull may show destructive changes in the frontal or mastoid bones. Carotid angiography and/or burr hole examination are diagnostic and distinguish subdural empyema from brain abscess.

Treatment. The patient with a subdural empyema requires prompt and adequate surgical drainage by multiple burr holes or craniotomy. Surgical treatment of the accompanying sinusitis, frontal osteomyelitis, or mastoiditis is a secondary consideration and is usually postponed until the acute intracranial infection has subsided. Vigorous systemic therapy with penicillin (10 million to 20 million units daily) and/or other antimicrobials, depending on the background of the case, is begun before surgery and continued until the infection has been completely controlled. The results of smear and culture of pus obtained at the time of operation may dictate changes in the antimicrobial regimen. Bacitracin or other antimicrobial drugs are commonly instilled into the subdural space at the time of operation and for a variable period thereafter.

CEREBRAL EPIDURAL ABSCESS

Epidural abscess is usually secondary to mastoiditis, sinus infection, osteomyelitis of the skull, skull fracture, or infection of an operative wound. Etiologic and pathogenetic considerations are identical to those described for subdural empyema. The close adherence of the dura to bone limits the size of the epidural abscess. It often represents granulations rather than a frankly purulent collection. Rarely, an extensive destructive osteomyelitis of the frontal bone ("Pott's puffy tumor") may be associated with an epidural abscess.

Diagnosis may be difficult. The patient is not as ill as with a subdural empyema, and the size of the collection is rarely sufficient to produce focal neurologic signs or increased intracranial pressure. Fever, pain, and tenderness over the affected area are the common manifestations. In most cases the cerebrospinal fluid is sterile, and contains few cells (lymphocytes predominating) and a normal concentration of sugar. Many times the diagnosis is made incidentally at the time of sinus or mastoid surgery or when intracranial surgery is performed for an associated subdural empyema or brain abscess. Some cases of epidural abscess are probably cured by antimicrobial therapy alone. Spread of infection from the mastoid along the ridge of the petrous bone may result in a small epidural granuloma or abscess that gives rise to a homolateral sixth-nerve palsy and temporoparietal pain from involvement of the sensory fibers of the fifth nerve (Gradenigo's syndrome).

THROMBOPHLEBITIS AND THROMBOSIS OF MAJOR VENOUS SINUSES

Cortical Thrombophlebitis. The syndrome of cortical thrombophlebitis characteristically appears some three to ten days after the onset of bacterial meningitis. The signs include a secondary rise in temperature, focal or generalized seizures, and focal neurologic deficits, such as a hemiparesis. In some instances at least, the underlying phlebitis has its inception earlier and is the basis for many of the seizures and signs of focal cortical disease encountered in the early stages of meningitis. Treatment includes continuation of the antimicrobial therapy and anticonvulsants. Anticoagulant drugs have no established place in therapy. In most cases the process is limited in extent and the patient recovers, but, when the process is widespread, substantial neurologic deficits and death may result.

MAJOR DURAL SINUS THROMBOSIS

Thrombosis of the large dural sinuses may occur in meningitis, may complicate epidural or subdural abscesses, or may develop during the intracranial spread of infection from extracerebral veins. (For spontaneous sinus thrombosis, see Ch. 379.) The thrombotic process may spread to connecting sinuses and cortical veins. Abscess formation within the thrombosed vessel may result in septicemia and infected emboli that travel to distant sites. The cavernous, lateral, and superior sagittal sinuses are most frequently involved.

Cavernous Sinus Thrombosis. Infection can spread to the cavernous sinus through venous channels by three routes: (1) from lesions of the upper half of the face through the facial veins communicating with the angular and superior ophthalmic veins, (2) from infections of the sphenoid and posterior ethmoid sinuses, inferiorly, and (3) from the ear, posteriorly. The initiating infection is usually an intranasal or facial furuncle, acute sinusitis, or an infection of the ear or mastoid. The widespread use of antimicrobial drugs in the treatment of superficial infections has markedly reduced the incidence of this disease. The majority of infections are due to *Staphylococcus aureus,* particularly in the presence of nasal furuncles.

Clinical Manifestations. The general clinical features are those of severe systemic infection: chills, fever, headache, nausea, lethargy, marked polymorphonuclear leukocytosis, and bacteremia. The specific findings are unilateral initially but become bilateral as the process extends to the opposite cavernous sinus via the connecting circular sinus. They include, in the case of infections about the face, unilateral edema of the forehead, eyelids, and base of the nose, as well as proptosis and chemosis—all caused by obstruction of the ophthalmic vein as it enters the cavernous sinus. The superficial veins over the forehead may be distended. The retinal veins become engorged or even thrombosed. Retinal hemorrhages and papilledema occur but may be late manifestations. Involvement of the ophthalmic branch of the fifth nerve produces pain in the eye, photophobia, and hyperesthesia of the forehead. Partial or even complete paralysis of the ocular muscles develops as a result of involvement of the third, fourth, and sixth cranial nerves as they pass through the sinus. The pupils are usually dilated but may be small; the pupillary reactions are often lost.

In infection spreading by the inferior route (e.g., sphenoid sinusitis) the process may be less acute initially. A meningeal reaction commonly occurs, usually without organisms in the cerebrospinal fluid, but pyogenic meningitis sometimes occurs. Rarely, infarction and abscess of the pituitary complicate septic cavernous sinus thrombosis.

Differential diagnosis includes other causes of proptosis, especially orbital cellulitis, abscess, or acute carotid-cavernous fistula. Retinal hemorrhages, papilledema, and palsies of cranial nerves innervating extraocular muscles rather than general restriction of ocular movement from the mechanical effects of orbital swelling are useful differential points.

Lateral Sinus Thrombosis. Thrombosis of the lateral sinus is almost always a complication of acute or chronic otitis media, of mastoiditis, or of cholesteatoma formation. Rarely, infection may spread in a retrograde fashion from a focus in the neck or from a tonsillar abscess. Streptococci, predominantly group A, and staphylococci have been implicated most frequently. The clinical manifestations include chills, fever, and signs of increased intracranial pressure. Pain, venous engorgement, and edema behind the ear may result from associated involvement of the mastoid emissary vein and may extend into the neck over the jugular vein. Papilledema is common; it may be unilateral as a consequence of extension to the cavernous sinus on that side. A generalized increase in intracranial pressure is more frequent with occlusions of the right lateral sinus, which is commonly larger and more important for venous drainage than the left. Convulsive seizures and obtundation occur, but focal neurologic findings are rare except when the thrombophlebitis extends into cortical veins over the convexity of the hemisphere. Rarely, ninth-, tenth- and eleventh-nerve palsies develop, presumably owing to involvement of the jugular bulb and related venous channels.

Cerebrospinal fluid pressure is elevated, and the fluid contains several to many hundred leukocytes (lymphocytes predominating) but no bacteria.

Superior Sagittal Sinus Thrombosis. The superior sagittal sinus is less commonly involved in septic thrombosis than are the lateral and cavernous sinuses. Infection may spread from the lateral or cavernous sinuses, from the pelvis by way of the vertebral veins, from a primary meningitis, or from a contiguous osteomyelitis and peridural infection. If thrombosis is restricted to that portion of the sinus anterior to the rolandic veins, and there is no associated involvement of cortical veins, then the process is usually asymptomatic. Thrombosis of the posterior portion of the sinus results in increased intracranial pressure; at times there are engorgement of scalp veins and edema of the forehead. Extension of the inflammatory process into the cortical veins results in infarction of the underlying cortex. Focal seizures, which alternately involve one and then the other side of the body, are characteristic. Because the superior and mesial surfaces of the cerebral hemispheres are particularly liable to infarction, weakness and sensory changes are frequently more prominent in the legs. However, hemiparesis, homonymous hemianopia, aphasia, and paresis, or conjugate deviation of the eyes may occur.

The cerebrospinal fluid findings are similar to those in lateral sinus thrombosis. A suspected diagnosis of major venous sinus thrombosis can often be confirmed by angiographic study.

Treatment of Dural Sinus Thrombophlebitis. Appropriate antimicrobial drugs in high dosage and surgical drainage, with removal of infected bone and extradural or intrasinus abscess, constitute proper treatment for major sinus thromboses. Ligation of the jugular vein in lateral sinus thrombosis to prevent spread of infected emboli is usually not necessary. Because of the frequent involvement of penicillinase-producing staphylococci, the use of semisynthetic penicillins (nafcillin, oxacillin) or the combination of penicillin and methicillin is warranted until cultures are reported. Since infarction of cerebral tissue from venous thromboses tends to be hemorrhagic, anticoagulants are not employed. The prognosis for recovery is reasonably good when optimal treatment is given, although there are frequently residual neurologic symptoms and signs.

CEREBRAL MANIFESTATIONS OF BACTERIAL ENDOCARDITIS

Neurologic symptoms or signs occur in about 30 per cent of patients with bacterial endocarditis, and a patient may present as a diagnostic neurologic problem. The neuropathologic findings of subacute bacterial endocarditis (usually due to *Streptococcus viridans)* are distinct from those of acute bacterial endocarditis (see Ch. 192). Diffuse embolic infarctions, with a variable and usually limited inflammatory response about involved blood vessels and adjacent meninges, constitute the major neurologic findings in subacute bacterial endocarditis. Pyogenic brain abscess and purulent meningitis do not occur. The clinical picture can resemble that of diffuse encephalitis, or there may be focal signs such as hemiplegia and hemianopia. The cerebrospinal fluid contains modest numbers of polymorphonuclear leukocytes (sometimes red cells as well) and a normal concentration of sugar; bacteria are absent. Subarachnoid hemorrhage may result from rupture of a mycotic aneurysm.

In acute bacterial endocarditis caused by invasive pyogenic organisms (usually *Staphylococcus aureus*), brain abscess (usually small and multiple), acute purulent meningitis, and embolic infarction of cerebral tissue may occur.

Cerebral Abscess

Ballantine, H. T., Jr., and Shealy, C. N.: The role of radical surgery in the treatment of abscess of the brain. Surg. Gynecol. Obstet., 109:370, 1959.

Garfield, J.: Management of supratentorial intracranial abscess: A review of 200 cases. Br. Med. J., 2:7, 1969.

Gates, E. M., Kernohan, J. W., and Craig, W. M.: Metastatic brain abscess. Medicine, 29:71, 1950.

Heineman, H. S., and Braude, A. I.: Anaerobic infection of the brain. Am. J. Med., 35:682, 1963.

Matson, D. D., and Salam, M.: Brain abscess in congential heart disease. Pediatrics, 27:772, 1961.

Samson, D. S., and Clark, K.: A current review of brain abscess. Am. J. Med., 54:201, 1973.

Swartz, M. N., and Karchmer, A. W.: Infections of the central nervous system. *In* Balows, A., et al. (eds.): Anaerobic Bacteria. Role in Disease. Springfield, Ill., Charles C Thomas, 1974.

Subdural Empyema

Conrood, D., and Dans, P. E.: Subdural empyema. Am. J. Med., 53:85, 1972.

Hitchcock, E., and Andreadis, A.: Subdural empyema: A review of 29 cases. J. Neurol. Neurosurg. Psychiatry, 27:422, 1964.

Cerebral Manifestations of Bacterial Endocarditis

Jones, H. R., Siekert, R. E., and Geraci, J. E.: Neurologic manifestations of bacterial endocarditis. Ann. Intern. Med., 71:21, 1969.

Kerr, A., Jr.: Subacute Bacterial Endocarditis. Springfield, Ill., Charles C Thomas, 1955, Chap. V, p. 92.

Ziment, I.: Nervous system complications in bacterial endocarditis. Am. J. Med., 47:593, 1969.

Thrombophlebitis and Thrombosis of Major Venous Sinuses

Brown, P.: Septic cavernous sinus thrombosis. Bull. Hopkins Hosp., 109:68, 1961.

Kalbag, R. K., and Woolf, A. L.: Cerebral Venous Thrombosis. London, Oxford University Press, 1967.

Krayenbuhl, H.: Cerebral venous and sinus thrombosis. Clin. Neurosurg., 14:1, 1967.

Ray, B. S., and Dunbar, H. S.: Thrombosis of the superior sagittal sinus as a cause of pseudotumor cerebri: Methods of diagnosis and treatment. Trans. Am. Neurol. Assoc., 75:12, 1950.

384. SPINAL EPIDURAL INFECTIONS

Philip R. Dodge

Definition. Spinal epidural infections consist of purulent or granulomatous collections contained within the spinal epidural space and overlying or encircling the spinal cord, roots, and nerves. Infection may be localized or may extend widely, at times involving the length of the spinal canal. In one large series an average extent of 4.3 bony segments was reported.

Incidence. This is a rare type of infection, less than one twentieth as common as bacterial meningitis. Although persons of any age are susceptible, it occurs most frequently in young adults.

Etiology and Pathogenesis. *Staphylococcus aureus* is involved in more than 90 per cent of cases, but group A streptococci, other streptococci, pneumococci, Brucella, Salmonella, and various other gram-negative organisms may be responsible. *M. tuberculosis* is an important cause of chronic epidural infections in areas where tuberculosis is prevalent; occasionally fungi and parasites may be recovered from epidural granulomas. There is a primary infective site remote from the spine in most cases. This usually involves the skin, and furuncles, boils, and cellulitis are the common underlying infections. Less often infections of the upper respiratory tract, genitourinary system, or bone may be responsible. Hematogenous or lymphatic spread of infection to the highly vascular epidural space is postulated. Occasionally the responsible organism may be cultured from the blood. Minor injury to the back frequently antedates the symptoms of epidural abscess, and trauma may in some way determine the site of infection. The lack of restraining fibrous tissue in the epidural fat allows the infection to spread caudally and rostrally, and epidural abscesses may extend into the extraspinal tissues; in contrast, the dura is rarely penetrated. In less than half the cases the spine and adjacent soft tissues are primarily affected, and the infection spreads secondarily to the epidural space. Only in tuberculous infections is primary osteomyelitis the rule. Epidural abscess may rarely complicate a lumbar puncture, myelogram, or spinal operation.

Pathology. The purulent material or granulomatous tissue is usually most abundant over the posterior aspect of the spinal cord. When the primary lesion is in a vertebral body, intervertebral disc, or some other anterior structure, the abscess may be predominantly ventral. Epidural abscess occurs most commonly in the thoracic region, but may develop at any level of the spinal axis. The lesion may be purulent or granulomatous.

The mechanism of neural dysfunction in spinal epidural abscess is uncertain. Since the lesion occupies space, direct compression of spinal cord, roots, and nerves is a prime consideration, but the small size of many epidural abscesses, in association with severe impairment of neural function, demands consideration of other possibilities. The most plausible of these and the one for which there are some supporting facts is a vasculitis with secondary venous and arterial occlusions resulting in infarction of neural tissues.

Clinical Manifestations. Heusner has divided the clinical picture into four phases: spinal ache, root pain, weaknesses (voluntary muscles, sphincters, sensibilities), and paralyses.

Spinal Ache. The spinal ache, characteristically maximal at the level of the major pathologic process, soon spreads axially and may also include the paravertebral regions. Restricted movement of the spine, especially in the anteroposterior plane, is common. A functional or even a structural scoliosis may develop. The spines overlying the disease process are tender to percussion; pain so induced may be exquisite, particularly when there is vertebral caries. Signs of sepsis (fever, leukocytosis) are prominent, except in the more chronic cases. The diagnosis is rarely made at this stage.

Root Pain. Within two or three days (acute cases) nerve roots inevitably become encased by the purulent material, and radicular pains develop. Meningeal signs are present in most cases, and headache is a common symptom. At times reflex activity at the level of the involved segment may be depressed. An erroneous diagnosis of "neuritis" or "shingles" is frequently made, but at this stage of illness the combination of clinical symptoms and signs should permit an accurate diagnosis.

Weaknesses. The characteristic feature of this phase of the illness is progressive impairment of neural functions below the level of the lesion, the exact syndrome depending upon the site of maximal damage. If the abscess overlies the spinal cord, spastic weakness, heightened reflexes, and a sensory level over the trunk are to be expected. There may be urinary urgency and incontinence. Abscesses in the lumbosacral region exert their effects on spinal roots and nerves, giving rise to dysesthesias in dermatomes supplied by the implicated nerves, along with appropriate pareses and depressed stretch reflexes. Pain is usually excruciating and nuchal rigidity extreme. The skin and soft tissues overlying the abscess may be swollen, warm, and red. High fever and signs of systemic toxicity are often present.

The diagnosis may be made as late as this with reasonable anticipation that prompt laminectomy and drainage of pus or removal of granulomatous tissue will effect considerable if not total recovery.

Paralyses. Within hours or at most a few days, severe or even total paralysis of nervous functions below the site of the lesion supervenes. Immediate surgical treatment is mandatory at this stage. Procrastination may vitiate the effect of any subsequent therapeutic measures, for enduring paralyses are usual if the patient remains paraplegic for more than a few hours. When an epidural abscess remains unrecognized and untreated, death occurs in 25 to 33 per cent of cases.

It is axiomatic that the foregoing analysis of the clinical features of subdural abscess is arbitrary and somewhat artificial, because the various stages may merge one into the other. Yet, considered in this way the early stages are stressed and the importance of prompt diagnosis and treatment is underscored.

Differential Diagnosis. Spinal epidural abscess demands consideration in the patient with sepsis, back pain, and even minimal neurologic symptoms and signs. Confirmatory evidence may be obtained by tapping the epidural space with an ordinary spinal needle. This is most safely done in the lumbar area. Gentle suction is applied with a small (2 ml) syringe while slowly advancing the needle. If no purulent material is obtained, the stylet should be replaced in the needle and the subarachnoid space entered. The cerebrospinal fluid is characteristically clear and xanthochromic. It may be acellular, but more often a few cells or a moderate pleocytosis (lymphocytes predominating) will be found. Normal sugar content and elevated cerebrospinal fluid protein are the rule (several hundred to more than 2000 mg per 100 ml). A partial or complete manometric block below the lesion is found in most cases.

An acute viral, postinfectious, syphilitic, or necrotizing myelitis may produce a neurologic syndrome similar to that seen in stage 4 of a spinal epidural abscess, and may be associated with symptoms and signs of infection and cerebrospinal fluid pleocytosis. There may be back pain in acute myelitis, but the duration of illness is compressed in time. Furthermore, xanthochromic cerebrospinal fluid and manometric block are unusual in myelitis. They are seen, however, in progressive adhesive arachnoiditis, which may be confused with subacute or chronic epidural infections. Spinal caries, demonstrable by roentgenography in less than 20 per cent of cases of spinal epidural abscess, suggests the correct diagnosis. In questionable cases a myelographic study will confirm the presence of a space-occupying intraspinal lesion. Rarely, malignant tumors, especially lymphomas that lodge in the epidural space, may present with fever, backache, neurologic signs, and spinal block. Chronic epidural abscess in which evidence of an inflammatory disease is meager or wanting will, on occasion, be confused with the more benign intraspinal tumors.

Treatment. Prompt laminectomy with drainage of purulent material or removal or granulomatous tissue and the administration of appropriate antimicrobial drugs constitute proper therapy. The antimicrobials must be continued in high doses for a minimum of six weeks when pyogenic osteomyelitis is present.

Heusner, A. P.: Nontuberculous spinal epidural infections. N. Engl. J. Med., 239:845, 1948.

Hulme, A., and Dott, N. M.: Spinal epidural abscess. Br. Med. J., 1:64, 1954.

385. TRANSVERSE MYELITIS OR MYELOPATHY

Philip R. Dodge

Transverse myelitis refers to a clinical syndrome in which there is evidence of complete or partial loss of neurologic funtions below a lesion which pathologically usually has a limited longitudinal dimension in the spinal cord. Thoracic and cervical segments are most frequently involved. Although inflammation is implied, it should be appreciated that evidence for this is frequently lacking, and thus the term transverse myelopathy is preferred by many neurologists.

Etiology. As a syndrome rather than a disease, the spectrum of specific causes is broad (see accompanying table). However, the cause remains unknown in the majority of patients presenting with the typical clinical findings.

Prevalence. No precise epidemiologic data are available. Although rare in general medical practice, the syndrome is not uncommonly encountered in a neurologic setting. Sixty-seven cases (44 adults and 23 children) were encountered over a 25-year period at the Columbia Presbyterian Medical Center in New York. Males and females are affected about equally. Altrocchi,

Diseases Which May Present as an Acute or Subacute Transverse Myelitis or Myelopathy

I. Myelitis due to viruses
  A. Poliomyelitis
  B. Coxsackievirus
  C. Herpes zoster
  D. Rabies
  E. B virus myelitis
  F. EB virus
II. Myelitis of unknown etiology
  A. Demyelination myelitis (acute multiple sclerosis)
  B. Postinfectious or postvaccinal myelitis
  C. Necrotizing myelitis (? myelopathy)
III. Myelitis secondary to inflammatory diseases of the meninges
  A. Syphilitic myelitis
    1. Acute meningitis
    2. Meningovascular spinal syphilis
    3. Tabes dorsalis
    4. Gummatous meningitis, including chronic spinal pachymeningitis
  B. Pyogenic or suppurative myelitis
    1. Subacute or chronic meningomyelitis
    2. Abscess of the spinal cord
    3. Subdural abscess
    4. Acute epidural spinal abscess or granuloma
  C. Tuberculous myelitis
    1. Pott's disease with spinal cord compression
    2. Tuberculous meningomyelitis
    3. Tuberculoma of the spinal cord
  D. Miscellaneous
    1. Parasitic and fungal infections producing an epidural granuloma, localized meningitis, or meningomyelitis
    2. Idiopathic meningomyelitis (chronic adhesive arachnoiditis)
IV. Myelopathies
  A. Vascular
    1. Anterior spinal artery occlusion
    2. Dissecting aneurysm with occlusion of major radicular arteries
    3. Arteritis, e.g., polyarteritis nodosa, lupus erythematosus
    4. Malformations
  B. Nutritional deficiencies

who reported on this experience, excluded compressive lesions, serious trauma, radiation myelopathy, those with evidence of concomitant cerebral involvement, and those thought to probably have multiple sclerosis.

Pathology. The pathology of myelitis or myelopathy includes varying degrees of destruction affecting either white or gray matter or often both, usually in an asymmetrical fashion with this irregular pattern of involvement persisting over the longitudinal extent of the lesion. Patchy destruction frequently involves several segments of the spinal cord but may be even more extensive. Demyelination, neuronal injury, and incomplete or complete necrosis of neural tissue have been described and may at times be associated with inflammatory cells, macrophages, or proliferation of astroglia. The form of the reaction is probably related to the duration of the disease and its cause. Thickening of small arteries and veins within or adjacent to the parenchyma of spinal cord has been prominent in only a few of the recorded cases. Because death rarely occurs in the acute stage of the illness today, recent reports characteristically lack postmortem studies employing modern histochemical and cytologic techniques.

Clinical Manifestations. The onset is usually abrupt, with the neurologic deficit evolving from the initial symptoms to maximal disability within hours to a few days or occasionally a few weeks. A premonitory history of an upper respiratory or other infection or minor trauma is reported in about 25 per cent of cases. The earliest symptoms are (1) muscle weakness, usually involving the lower limbs, (2) sensory aberrations, (3) back discomfort, or (4) root pain, all occurring with about equal frequency. Signs may be asymmetrical, but bilateral involvement of the spinal cord is invariable at some time in the course of disease. Bladder and bowel dysfunction are nearly universal as paresis of the limbs and sensory disturbances progress.

The degree of paraparesis is variable, but moderate to severe weakness of the legs obtains in about two thirds of patients. Weakness may affect the arms in as many as one quarter of patients. Sensory loss is also seen in approximately two thirds of reported cases, pain and temperature being more often affected than position and vibratory sensation. Segmental paresthesias and dysesthesias may occur. Stretch reflexes are often lost in the acute stage of the disease but become exaggerated later. Babinski signs are usual. Meningeal signs are encountered in up to one third of patients. There is fever in about one half of patients, although this may be referable to complicating infections of lung or urinary tract.

The cerebrospinal fluid findings are extremely variable even during the acute stage of the disease. In some patients the CSF may be acellular with only a slight rise in the protein concentration, but there may be several hundred or a thousand or more leukocytes, often with a predominant polymorphonuclear reaction in the acute state. The protein concentration may be elevated to several hundred milligrams per 100 ml, and the percentage of gamma globulin can be increased significantly. The sugar content is typically normal. Spine radiographs are unrevealing, as is myelography, except in rare instances when spinal cord swelling is extreme, impeding the flow of dye. In such instances there can also be a manometric block.

Diagnosis. Although the diagnosis of transverse myelitis or myelopathy can be suspected on clinical grounds, it is incumbent upon the physician to consider first those diseases which demand specific and prompt treatment. Spinal epidural abscess can mimic closely transverse myelitis, although the course of the latter condition is usually more rapid. Contrast myelography should be performed if there is any question about the diagnosis. The risk of this procedure is minimal, and the danger of missing a compressive suppurative lesion which should be treated by surgery is of overriding concern. Intraspinal neoplasms and other compressive tumors will also be excluded by myelography except in those rare instances in which an acutely inflamed, swollen cord may mimic an intra-axial mass. Syphilis, especially the meningovascular form, may mimic nonspecific myelitis and deserves immediate treatment. The treatable nutritional myelopathies evolve more slowly and have a pattern of spinal cord involvement which is more diffuse. Other evidence of vitamin B_{12} deficiency or of pellagra should make exclusion of these disorders relatively easy. A vascular nevus at the segmental level of the spinal cord lesion should signal the possibility of an intraspinal vascular malformation which can be defined by selective spinal cord angiography. Every effort should be made to establish the diagnosis of specific viral infections by appropriate cultural and serologic means. A diagnosis of multiple sclerosis may become obvious only when lesions of the central nervous system disseminated in time and space appear.

Treatment. There is no specific treatment for transverse myelitis or myelopathy of unknown cause. The efficacy of pharmacologic doses of the glucocorticoids is unproved but might be considered, particularly if there is evidence of swelling of the spinal cord. Prevention or appropriate treatment for the complications of paraplegia is criterial.

Prognosis. Proper supportive care, including therapy for complicating infection, prevention of pressure sores, and attention to urinary tract function, renders the prognosis for survival excellent. According to Altrocchi, one third of patients make a good or complete recovery, one third do moderately well, and a poor recovery characterizes the course in the other third. Lipton and Teasdall found similar results. Recurrent neurologic problems are rare among the survivors.

Altrocchi, P. H.: Acute transverse myelopathy. Arch. Neurol., 9:112, 1963.
Greenfield, J. G., and Turner, J. W. A.: Acute and subacute necrotic myelitis. Brain, 62:227, 1939.
Hoffman, H. L.: Acute necrotic myelopathy. Brain, 78:377, 1955.
Lipton, H. L., and Teasdall, R. D.: Acute transverse myelopathy in adults. Arch. Neurol., 28:252, 1973.

386. SYPHILITIC INFECTIONS OF THE CENTRAL NERVOUS SYSTEM

Philip R. Dodge

A general exposition of *T. pallidum* infection is presented in Ch. 246. The following presentation is restricted to a discussion of neurosyphilis.

Although the spirochete invades the nervous system and its coverings during the early weeks of infection in nearly every case, neurosyphilis develops in less than 10 per cent of untreated cases.

Pathology. Involvement of the leptomeninges is an essential feature of all forms of neurosyphilis. A meningitis of varying severity and extent is present in every case of active neurosyphilis regardless of the neurologic syndrome. The cerebrospinal fluid reflects this involvement. Even in cases of *asymptomatic neurosyphilis,* in which the presence of syphilis reagin constitutes the sole abnormality, rare postmortem examinations have disclosed definite meningeal inflammation and ependymal granulations. Similarly, in chronic tabes dorsalis with negative cerebrospinal fluid examination, evidence of prior active meningeal disease will be revealed by pathologic study.

Postmortem study of a few cases of acute *syphilitic meningitis* has shown a meningeal inflammatory reaction in which lymphocytes and plasma cells predominate. Cellular aggregates collect about blood vessels, and evidence of early arteritis may be found, although cerebrovascular accidents are rare in this stage of the disease. Reactive fibrosis of the leptomeninges, especially about the base of the brain, is also seen. This accounts for the cranial nerve palsies and for impaired cerebrospinal fluid circulation that can result in increased intracranial pressure. A granular ependymitis is commonly present, and, rarely, this may obstruct cerebrospinal fluid flow through the aqueduct.

In so-called *meningovascular syphilis,* which is typically a more chronic disorder occurring months or a few years after the primary lesion, the inflammatory response is usually less acute and meningeal fibrosis more prominent. As the name suggests, there is an associated arteritis (usually small vessels) that predisposes to arterial occlusion and consequent infarction of neural tissue. When larger arteries become occluded, infarction of brain or spinal cord may be extensive. In some cases damage to regions of neural tissue adjacent to meninges occurs without obvious vascular occlusions.

The neurologic syndromes of so-called parenchymatous syphilis (*tabes dorsalis, optic atrophy, general paresis*) also are due in part to this meningeal affection and in part to the direct invasion of neural tissue by the spirochete. In tabes dorsalis extension of the meningeal inflammatory reaction to the dorsal roots leads ultimately to their destruction and to secondary atrophy of sensory nerve fibers that ascend in the dorsal funiculi of the spinal cord. On gross inspection the dorsal roots appear gray and atrophic, and the dorsal aspect of the spinal cord appears wasted. Myelin sheaths are damaged as well, and demyelination of dorsal columns is easily demonstrated by appropriate stains. Involvement of anterior roots with resultant amyotrophy occurs also but is exceedingly rare. Why the syphilitic process shows a predilection for dorsal roots is unknown.

Treponema pallidum has been demonstrated only rarely in the spinal cords of patients with tabes dorsalis, and direct invasion by the spirochete is probably of little clinical and pathologic importance. In optic atrophy, also, it is probably the contiguous leptomeningitis that is primarily responsible for damage to visual fibers, and those in the periphery of the nerve are most often affected. Direct invasion of the optic nerve by the spirochete may produce additional damage, but the spirochete has been demonstrated in the optic nerve very infrequently.

In general paresis there are, on gross examination, meningeal thickening, atrophy of cerebral tissue (especially of frontal and temporal lobes), and enlargement of ventricles; a granularity of the ependymal surface is consistently present. Microscopically, diffuse destruction and loss of neurons, especially in the cortex, are found, and special stains may demonstrate a heavy infestation with *Treponema pallidum.* Reactive gliosis is often extreme, pleomorphic microglia being characteristically abundant. Inflammation of the meninges is prominent, and varying degrees of arteritis can be anticipated. Collections of subependymal astroglia account for the granularity noted grossly.

Focal *granulomatous accumulations* (gummas) are rare, but may occur in the meninges and extend into the parenchyma of the central nervous system. More diffuse granulomas of the dura (hypertrophic pachymeningitis) assume significance when they compress neural structures, especially the spinal cord.

CLINICAL SYNDROMES IN NEUROSYPHILIS

Asymptomatic Neurosyphilis

As the term suggests, the patient lacks symptoms or signs of neurologic disease, although pathologic involvement of the meninges and possibly of the nervous system parenchyma is implied. The diagnosis rests on the finding of cellular, chemical, or immunologic abnormalities of the cerebrospinal fluid. This is the most common form of neurosyphilis and constituted about 30 per cent of cases in one large neurosyphilis clinic. With adequate treatment (see Treatment) the development of neurologic symptoms can be prevented in most cases.

Symptomatic Neurosyphilis

Meningitis

Symptoms and signs of an acute meningitis are encountered only rarely by physicians, an incidence of less than 2 per cent among syphilitic patients being reported from one general hospital series. It seems likely that some patients with mild or even moderate symptoms go unnoticed. Symptomatic syphilitic meningitis usually occurs during the early weeks or months of infection, often during the period of the secondary rash or concurrently with a mucocutaneous relapse in a patient previously but inadequately treated. The illness is usually of less than a month's duration, but symptoms may persist for longer periods. Headache, vomiting, malaise, and irritability are prominent symptoms. Kernig and Brudzinski signs develop. Occasionally, confusion, delirium, seizures, and cranial nerve palsies (seventh and eighth nerves most common) occur. Argyll Robertson pupils are not part of the constellation of findings in acute syphilitic meningitis. Acute syphilitic hydrocephalus with evidence of increased intracranial pressure, including papilledema, may lead to confusion with other inflammatory and neoplastic conditions. But the diagnosis should not be difficult if the physician considers the possibility of syphilis. The cerebrospinal fluid will always contain an increased number of white blood cells (average about 500 per cubic millimeter – usually mononuclear, rarely polymorphonuclear), elevated total protein (average, about 100 mg per 100 ml), normal sugar concentrations (reduced rarely), and syphilitic reagins. An abnormal goldsol (Lange) curve will be found in 70 per cent of cases. The serologic tests for syphilis are usually but not always positive.

The response to therapy is generally prompt and gratifying, although an occasional patient will subsequently develop some other form of neurosyphilis.

Meningovascular Syphilis

Although the incidence of this form of neurosyphilis is difficult to ascertain, a figure of 3 per cent of syphilitic patients has been recorded. As with the other forms of neurosyphilis, men are more often affected than women (3:1). Patients with meningovascular syphilis present most commonly from two to ten years after the primary lesion. Symptoms and signs of meningitis are lacking, although headache is a frequent complaint. The major neurologic abnormalities result from the arteritis and consequent arterial thromboses. The neurologic deficits may develop slowly as the circulation through small vessels becomes compromised, or there may be an abrupt loss of function consequent upon occlusion of a major vessel. The specific syndromes depend upon the distribution of infarction within the brain or spinal cord. The patient may develop hemiplegia, hemisensory defect, dysphasia, or homonymous hemianopia. Involvement of the cortex accounts for seizures in a small percentage of cases. Various spinal cord syndromes have been described. A transverse myelopathy can be expected to produce varying degrees of paraparesis, sensory loss, and impaired function of bladder and bowel. Infarction of the anterior two thirds of the cord, with resultant paraplegia and loss of pain sensation below the lesion, follows occlusion of the anterior spinal artery. Sensory functions subserved by the posterior columns are usually preserved. Asymmetric infarction of one half of the spinal cord will result in weakness and impairment of light touch and position sense on that side and diminished pain and temperature sensation on the opposite side below the anatomic lesion (Brown-Séquard's syndrome).

Some abnormality of the cerebrospinal fluid is always found in meningovascular syphilis. A lymphocytic pleocytosis (few to 100 cells per cubic millimeter) and/or an elevated protein concentration is characteristic. The globulin content is often elevated; this is reflected in an abnormal Lange curve. Syphilitic reagins are nearly always present in the cerebrospinal fluid as well as in the blood.

The progress of meningovascular syphilis can usually be halted by specific treatment, but the degree of functional recovery depends upon the extent and location of the infarcts and upon the many complex physiologic factors that condition recovery in cerebrovascular disease of any type.

General Paresis

(Dementia Paralytica, General Paralysis of the Insane)

This dread complication of syphilis makes its appearance from 2 to 30 (usually 10 to 25) years after the primary lesion. It occurs more often in men than in women (3:1), and 89 per cent of cases occur between the ages of 30 and 60 years. In one large series about 60 per cent of patients presented with simple dementia, and less than 20 per cent displayed manic symptoms and megalomania. Often faulty judgment, impaired memory (recent memory affected first), disturbed affect (depression or euphoria), or paranoia suggests the presence of a serious mental disturbance. This behavioral change will be especially noticeable when the afflicted individual has been a competitive member of society. Delusions and hallucinations occur less often but, when present, prompt a quick referral to the physician. The patient himself may complain of "nervousness," but characteristically lacks insight into the nature of his difficulty. Fine or coarse tremors, often affecting facial muscles and tongue, are present in about two thirds of the patients with fully developed general paresis. Abnormal pupillary responses, including Argyll Robertson pupil (see Tabes Dorsalis, below), impassive facies, slurred or dysarthric speech, exaggerated stretch reflexes, and extensor plantar responses are additional neurologic signs. Convulsions occur in 10 per cent of patients, and strokes secondary to vasculitis are also seen. When symptoms and signs of tabes dorsalis accompany those of paresis, the designation taboparesis is used.

The cerebrospinal fluid is always abnormal, containing in excess of 5 white blood cells per cubic millimeter (mononuclear) in 85 per cent of untreated cases, and more than 30 cells per cubic millimeter in about a fourth of cases. An elevated total protein concentration (greater than 50 mg per 100 ml) of cerebrospinal fluid can be anticipated in 75 per cent, and a level of 100 mg per 100 ml or higher in about 20 per cent of cases. An elevated gamma globulin level accounts for the first zone colloidal gold (Lange) curve, e.g., 5554433211, which is frequently found in general paresis. Nearly every patient will have a positive reagin test for syphilis in the cerebrospinal fluid, and in more than 90 per cent of cases the blood serologic test will also be positive. Incomplete, prior treatment may modify but will not restore to normal the cerebrospinal fluid.

General paresis, once established, evolves rapidly, and

patients soon become disabled mentally, socially, and, in the late stage, physically. The term general paralysis of the insane derived from observations of patients helpless and bedridden in the terminal stages of the disease. Untreated general paresis is universally fatal, usually within three years.

If the disease is recognized early and treated vigorously, about 80 per cent of patients will return to some form of work, but only in about one half will complete recovery be achieved. There is little hope of a satisfactory result when treatment is delayed until the patient is demented, incontinent, and bedridden.

Tabes Dorsalis
(Locomotor Ataxia)

Tabes dorsalis develops in less than 5 per cent of patients with untreated syphilis, and symptoms usually become manifest 10 to 20 years after the primary infection. Rarely, there is a latent period of 30 or more years. Men are more often affected than women.

Dysfunction of affected posterior roots accrues slowly, and symptoms develop insidiously. Impaired joint position sense frequently results in stumbling and difficulty in walking, especially in the dark when visual compensation is imperfect. As the disease progresses, this sensory ataxia worsens, and a broad-based gait is assumed. Profound hypotonia, secondary to a lack of modulation of muscle tension by afferent fibers, is expressed frequently in a slapping gait. Paresthesias usually appear early in the disease but may be ignored by the patient until the appearance of lightning pains. These pains are characteristic of tabes dorsalis but are in no way specific, because they occur in other diseases affecting dorsal roots, e.g., diabetic neuropathy. Lightning pains develop in at least 75 per cent of patients and may appear in any area of the body, although they are most common in the lower extremities. Some patients insist that they are more troublesome when the barometric pressure is low. They may be described as sharp, burning, or aching. However, sharp jabs of pain are characteristic. These may be mild or excruciating, and frequently flit from one region to another. At times they are so transitory that by the time the patient has made the natural move to rub or massage the involved part, pain has disappeared. For a period of hours or days one spot will seem particularly vulnerable, but then the site of attack shifts to another place. Involvement of thoracoabdominal nerve roots gives rise to visceral pains *(gastric or visceral crises),* which may simulate intrinsic visceral disease and may lead to unnecessary surgery; in one series an estimated 25 per cent of tabetic patients had undergone operation for tabetic pain. The converse is also true: on rare occasions visceral pain has been ascribed to tabes dorsalis and suppurative appendicitis, or a ruptured peptic ulcer has gone undiagnosed. As the disease advances, pain sensation may be so dulled that recurrent trauma is unnoticed by the patient and indolent ulcers of the skin develop; the toes and balls of the feet are especially vulnerable. Weight-bearing joints and adjacent bone, deprived of pain sensation, are destroyed by the constant trauma of use in 5 to 10 per cent of tabetic patients (Charcot joints).

Unless general paresis coexists, as it does in a small percentage of cases (*taboparesis*), tabetic patients are mentally normal. Optic atrophy complicates tabes dorsalis in about 10 per cent of cases or occurs as an isolated disorder. Pupillary abnormalities, including meiosis, irregularity, poor responsiveness to light and mydriatics, but retained reaction in accommodation (Argyll Robertson pupils), are present in most cases of tabes dorsalis. Involvement of other oculomotor functions is occasionally seen. Hypotonia, ataxia, and broad-based gait can usually be demonstrated. Affection of the sensory arc of the myotatic reflexes accounts for the greatly diminished or absent stretch reflexes. The Achilles reflex is affected most constantly. The plantar responses are normal in most cases of uncomplicated tabes dorsalis. Loss or diminution of position and vibratory sensation is found in every case. Increased swaying when the eyes are closed and the patient is standing with feet together (Romberg's sign) results from the impaired position sense. Variable degrees of hypesthesia and hypalgesia in a root distribution can be anticipated but may be difficult to plot. Isolated areas of hypalgesia (Hitzig zones) are sometimes found. Delayed perception of a pain stimulus (from one to several seconds) often can be demonstrated. Impaired deep pain sensation may account for a dramatic lack of responsiveness to squeezing of the Achilles tendon or testicles. Because of involvement of sacral nerve roots, functions of the urinary bladder and bowel are impaired in up to one third of cases; overflow incontinence and constipation develop. Impotence is a major complaint in the male. Characteristically a cystometrogram shows an absence of, or reduction in, the normal muscular contractions of the bladder in response to filling; the patient may be unaware of a volume in excess of 500 ml. Hydronephrosis and pyogenic infection are common complications of a hypotonic bladder.

Early in the course of tabes dorsalis, the serologic tests for syphilis are, as a rule, strongly positive. The cerebrospinal fluid may reflect the meningeal inflammatory process with pleocytosis, an elevated total protein, and a positive reagin test. Late in the disease, especially after some antisyphilitic treatment, the serologic tests may be negative (in 25 to 50 per cent of cases), and even the cerebrospinal fluid is negative in up to 20 per cent of cases.

The course of tabes dorsalis is unpredictable, and the response to antisyphilitic therapy is variable. In general, patients who have had symptoms for a few months or at the most a few years, with significant cerebrospinal fluid abnormalities and no prior therapy, are most likely to improve with treatment. Patients with far-advanced disease and severe degeneration of dorsal roots and who suffer from the painful complications will not benefit significantly from antisyphilitic therapy. At least partial relief of pain may be achieved by analgesics, but when narcotics are used the risk of addiction is significant. Recently, some benefit has been reported with diphenylhydantoin (Dilantin) treatment (200 mg per square meter per day). Recourse to spinal cordotomy and other surgical measures to relieve pain should be deferred until all medical measures have failed. Urologic assistance may be required to deal effectively with the tabetic uropathies, and surgery may be required for management of penetrating ulcers of the skin and Charcot joints.

Optic Atrophy

Visual impairment in syphilis may result from iritis, choreoretinitis, increased intracranial pressure (consecutive optic atrophy), or primary optic atrophy. Optic atrophy occurs in 1 per cent of patients with untreated syphilis and is five times more common in males than in females. It is stated that blacks are more prone than whites to optic atrophy, whereas the reverse is reported in other forms of neurosyphilis.

Because the outer portions of the optic nerve are first affected, the visual impairment tends to be peripheral in the early stages. Ultimately, however, the papillomacular bundle lying in the center of the nerve becomes involved, and impaired visual acuity and central and paracentral scotomas develop. It has been estimated that, without treatment, 50 per cent of patients will be blind in two years and 90 per cent in ten years. One eye is typically affected before the other. Optic pallor is usually present by the time symptoms appear, but in the early stages it is recognizable only by the reduced vascularity. A chalk-white disc with sharp margins and prominent lamina cribrosa constitute the fully developed appearance of optic atrophy. The optic atrophy of syphilis is indistinguishable from that caused by other diseases of the optic nerve in which there has been no antecedent papillitis or papilledema. The cerebrospinal fluid is abnormal in most patients with active disease of the optic nerve. Intensive antisyphilitic therapy may arrest the disease process and preserve what vision remains, but return of vision already lost should not be anticipated.

Gumma

This rare complication of syphilis usually declares itself as an intracranial or intraspinal mass lesion and behaves in every way as a slowly growing neoplasm. The correct diagnosis may be suspected from a positive serologic test for syphilis or from cerebrospinal fluid abnormalities. Frequently, however, the diagnosis is not made until the patient is operated upon, and histopathologic studies are made. Removal of the tumor mass, supplemented by antimicrobial therapy (see Treatment), should alleviate symptoms and prevent spread of the disease.

Congenital Neurosyphilis

Syphilis acquired by the fetus from an infected mother after the first trimester of pregnancy tends to be a fulminant disease. Miscarriages and stillbirths are common, and a wide spectrum of clinical manifestations may be recognized in the infant or child who survives. *Neurosyphilis* develops in an estimated 10 to 20 per cent of infants and children with congenital syphilis. *Asymptomatic neurosyphilis* may be diagnosed in the early months or years of life by doing routine cerebrospinal fluid examinations on children of syphilitic mothers. But, as with acquired neurosyphilis, symptoms and signs develop only after a latent period that, in the case of *juvenile paresis,* may be as long as 20 years. More often symptoms first appear late in the first decade or during adolescence. Clinical syndromes and cerebrospinal fluid findings mirror those found with the acquired disease except that *tabes dorsalis* is exceedingly rare and *choreoretinitis* more common. Hydrocephalus, cranial nerve palsies (eighth cranial nerve especially), and seizures may complicate congenital syphilitic meningitis, and syphilis should be remembered as a cause of cerebrovascular accidents in children. Previous studies emphasize that more than a third of all children presenting with juvenile paresis have been retarded mentally since early life. Although mental retardation is very likely due to other factors in some cases, such statistics emphasize the vulnerability of the developing nervous system to syphilitic infection.

Other non-neurologic stigmata of congenital syphilis include dental deformities (Hutchinson's teeth), saddle nose, frontal bossing of the skull, saber shins, and interstitial keratitis (usually developing during the second decade). These signs are not seen in acquired syphilis. Fortunately, the current practice of doing routine serologic tests on all pregnant women and on infants of syphilitic mothers has all but eliminated congenital neurosyphilis in many areas of the world. In this regard it should be remembered that the mother can acquire syphilis at any time during pregnancy and that negative serologic studies obtained early do not exclude the possibility that they might become positive later in the course of pregnancy. In some institutions blood from the umbilical cord is routinely tested for the reagin of syphilis.

Early and intensive treatment of infants with congenital syphilis materially reduces the morbidity (see Treatment) from neurologic complications. Unhappily, results from even optimal treatment of patients with juvenile paresis remain poor.

TREATMENT

Penicillin is the preferred drug for treating neurosyphilis. Reasonable therapy for adults with all forms of neurosyphilis, except general paresis, is a total dose of procaine penicillin G of 9 to 12 million units given over two to three weeks. A total dose of 18 to 24 million units administered over the same period of time is used to treat patients with general paresis. For children, approximately one half of the adult dose is employed, and one quarter of the adult dose is given to infants. We prefer to treat patients with active neurosyphilis in hospital (mandatory in general paresis), but this is not always feasible. When outpatient treatment is necessary, an initial dose of 3 million units of long-acting penicillin (benzathine penicillin G, Bicillin) should be given. The sole use of benzathine penicillin G at weekly intervals in doses equivalent to those presented above has been advocated by some in the treatment of neurosyphilis. It must be stressed that these therapeutic regimens are empirical. Nevertheless, they are reasonable and have stood the test of time. The author suspects that early diagnosis of syphilitic infection is far more critical than the precise dosage and the time course of therapy.

Alternative drugs include the tetracyclines and chloramphenicol (3 to 4 grams per day for 15 days), but they should be reserved for cases in which there is a clearly proved allergy to penicillin. Sensitivity to penicillin should not be confused with the Jarisch-Herxheimer reaction, which occurs within a few hours of the first injection of the drug in 50 per cent or more of patients (see Ch. 246). During therapy, neurologic symptoms and signs may exacerbate temporarily—notably in paresis—presumably because of the Jarisch-Herxheimer reaction.

Clarke, E. G., and Danbolt, N.: The Oslo study of the natural history of untreated syphilis. J. Chronic Dis., 2:311, 1955.

Green, J. B.: Dilantin in the treatment of lightning pains. Neurology, 11:257, 1961.

Hahn, R. D., et al.: Penicillin treatment of general paresis (dementia paralytica)—Results of treatment in 1086 patients, the majority of whom were followed for more than 5 years. A.M.A. Arch. Neurol. Psychiat., 81:557, 1959.

Hooshmand, H., Escobar, M. R., and Kopf, S. W.: Neurosyphilis. A study of 241 patients. J.A.M.A., 219:726, 1972.

Idsøe, O., Guthe, T., and Willcox, R. R.: Penicillin in the treatment of syphilis. Geneva, Bull. WHO, Supplement to Vol. 47, 1972.

Merritt, H. H., Adams, R. D., and Solomon, H.: Neurosyphilis. New York, Oxford University Press, 1946.

Montgomery, C. H., and Knox, J. M.: Antibiotics other than penicillin in the treatment of syphilis. N. Engl. J. Med., 261:277, 1961.

Section Thirteen. VIRAL INFECTIONS OF THE NERVOUS SYSTEM

387. INTRODUCTION

Richard T. Johnson

Viral infections of the nervous system, in general, represent uncommon but important complications of systemic infections. With a few exceptions such as rabies or B virus (*herpes simiae*), nervous system infections are caused by agents which often infect man. Some of these viruses, such as polioviruses and arthropod-borne encephalitis viruses, cause clinically significant disease only on the rare occasion when the nervous system is involved. Others, such as herpes simplex and mumps virus, are frequent causes of mild disease that assumes a more serious form when the central nervous system is infected.

Experimentally, viruses have been shown to invade the nervous system by centripetal growth or movement in peripheral nerves, by penetration across the olfactory mucosa, or by a viremia. In man most viruses which infect the nervous system spread to the brain and meninges from blood, although neural spread appears to be important in rabies, B virus, and varicella-zoster virus infections. The infrequency of nervous system involvement can be attributed to a variety of host defense mechanisms, including cellular and humoral responses, interferon production, anatomic barriers of nonsusceptible cells, and the activity of the reticuloendothelial system which clears viruses from the blood. Youth, severe nutritional deficiency, and defects of cellular immunity have been shown to increase the risk of nervous system infection with some viruses, but in the majority of patients the factors which have permitted central nervous system invasion are not evident.

Viral infections of the nervous system can lead to diverse clinical signs and symptoms, varied clinical courses, and protean pathologic changes. This diversity can be explained by the following two principles: (1) the varied cell populations of the nervous system have different susceptibilities to different viruses; and (2) viral infections can have varied effects on susceptible cells. If infection is limited to the meninges covering the nervous system, then signs of headache, fever, stiff neck, and CSF pleocytosis (i.e., meningitis) may be the only clinical manifestations. If the infection spreads to the parenchymal cells of the brain, in addition to signs of meningeal irritation, there may develop a depression of the state of consciousness, seizures, focal neurologic deficits, or increased intracranial pressure (i.e., encephalitis). Some viruses cause even more selective involvement of specific cell populations in the brain and spinal cord and thus evoke characteristic clinical symptoms and signs. For example, in poliovirus infections the selective vulnerability of anterior horn cells leads to a characteristic clinical finding of acute meningitis with lower motor neuron paralysis. On the other hand, rabies virus infections in animals tend to spare the cortical neurons involved in most types of encephalitis and infect neurons of the limbic system. Therefore, instead of obtundation, seizures, and motor or sensory deficits, the infected animal shows alertness, loss of timidity, aberrant sexual behavior, and aggressive activity. This selective infection of cells of the limbic system appears to be a diabolic adaptation of the rabies virus to specific cell populations, so that the clinical disease in animals can drive the host to transmit the virus to another host by biting. Glial cell populations may also be selectively involved, such as in progressive multifocal leukoencephalopathy in which virus infection and cell lysis appear limited to the oligodendrocytes, causing a slowly progressive demyelinating disease.

The virus-cell interaction may be quite varied. There may be *acute lysis* of the infected cell, transformation of the cell with production of neoplasm, or *chronic infection* causing cellular dysfunction, cellular degeneration, or no abnormality. In acute viral infections the clinical and pathologic abnormalities may result either from an acute viral destruction of cells, as in acute viral meningitis or encephalitis, or from the host's immunologic response to the infection, as has been postulated in postinfectious encephalomyelitis. A *latent infection* is a virus-host relationship in which the virus remains present in some form in the host without giving rise to any signs of infection, but which can, when some trigger mechanism comes into play, emerge as an acute infectious process. This appears to occur in herpes zoster and possibly in some cases of herpes simplex encephalitis. *Chronic viral infections* are those in which there is an ongoing active infection, which may give rise to a somewhat irregular or unpredictable course extending over many months or years. Chronic inflammatory disease of the central nervous system is seen with fetal infections by rubella and cytomegaloviruses. In these indolent infections virus can be recovered for long periods of time postnatally and may or may not cause continuing or evolving clinical signs of disease. *Slow infections* have a more predictable course than chronic infections. They are defined as infections with an incubation period lasting for months to years, followed by a protracted but predictable clinical course ending in death. Slow viral infections of the nervous system in man include kuru, Creutzfeldt-Jakob disease, subacute sclerosing panencephalitis, and progressive multifocal leukoencephalopathy (see Ch. 398 to 403).

388. HERPES ZOSTER

Richard T. Johnson

Herpes zoster is an acute viral infection of sensory ganglia and the corresponding cutaneous areas of innervation. The disease is characterized by localized pain along the distribution of the nerve and a vesicular skin eruption over a single or adjacent dermatomes. The disease is due to the same virus that causes chickenpox (varicella) and is thought to represent an acute localized recrudescent infection by the varicella virus that has remained latent in the sensory ganglia since the primary attack of chickenpox. Herpes zoster is also called shingles or zona.

Etiology. The varicella or varicella-zoster virus is a herpesvirus. The virus core measures 45 to 50 mμ and contains deoxyribonucleic acid. This is surrounded by a capsid with a diameter of 50 to 100 mμ and an outer envelope, giving a total diameter of the virion of 150 to 250 mμ. The virus is naturally pathogenic only for man, although chickenpox has been seen in anthropoid apes in zoos. There is some evidence of experimental transmission of the virus to several species of monkeys. The virus can be grown in a variety of cell cultures of human and primate origin but not in nonprimate cells. The virus is avidly cell-associated and can usually be transmitted in the laboratory only by the inoculation of infected cells, although the virus is stable in a cell-free form in the vesicular fluid. Morphologically, varicella virus resembles herpes simplex virus, with which it shares some common antigens, but it is markedly different from herpes simplex virus in its inability to infect nonprimates and nonprimate cell cultures and in its loss of infectivity in most cell-free preparations.

Incidence. Herpes zoster occurs at a rate of three to five cases per thousand persons per year. The attack rate increases with age. The disease is rare in childhood and is most frequently seen in persons over the age of 50 years. It is estimated that half the people reaching 85 years of age have suffered from at least one attack of herpes zoster. Rates are higher in persons with malignancies, particularly those involving the reticuloendothelial system.

Epidemiology, Pathogenesis, and Pathology. It has long been recognized that chickenpox may develop after exposure to a patient with herpes zoster, although this is less likely than development of chickenpox after exposure to chickenpox. In contrast, zoster rarely develops after exposure to chickenpox or other cases of zoster. These observations are supported by the epidemiologic findings that chickenpox is a seasonal disease occurring mainly in the winter and spring and occurs in epidemic proportions every two to four years. In contrast, zoster is not a seasonal disease, and there is no increase in incidence during the years of chickenpox epidemics. There is, in fact, some evidence that the incidence of zoster decreases slightly during years when there are large numbers of cases of chickenpox.

The precise pathogenesis of herpes zoster is unknown, but the following hypothesis is widely accepted. Chickenpox is transmitted from man to man by respiratory spread, and in the susceptible person the virus is probably disseminated throughout the body by a viremia. Infection of the skin occurs through the blood, and vesicles develop most prominently over the face and trunk. It is postulated that virus then spreads centripetally via sensory nerve fibers to the sensory ganglia, where it becomes latent in some form within the neurons or stellate cells. This latency of varicella virus in ganglia has not been documented in man or laboratory animals, but the recent demonstration of latency of herpes simplex virus in sensory ganglia has added credence to this hypothesis for varicella virus. Virus replication is later activated. In some cases activation is associated with the development of malignancy, local x-irradiation, immunosuppressive therapy, trauma, treatment with arsenicals, neurosyphilis, or tumor entrapment of the dorsal root ganglia or nerve root. Nevertheless, in most patients, there is no obvious exciting cause, and it is thought that the decline of immunity with age and the lack of exposure to children with chickenpox may promote reactivation. When virus multiplies in the ganglia, an active ganglionitis develops, causing pain along its sensory distribution. Virus is then thought to pass down the nerve and multiply again in the skin, causing characteristic clusters of vesicles. The localized zoster lesions are most common over trigeminal or thoracic dermatomes corresponding to the areas of major eruption during the antecedent chickenpox infection. The more rapid secondary immune response may prevent hematogenous dissemination. Resolution and limitation of the rash of herpes zoster do not correlate well, however, with the development of antibody but appear to correlate with the collection of inflammatory cells and the presence of interferon in the vesicular fluid. This theory of pathogenesis is consistent with the occurrence of the disease with increasing age or development of malignancy, the lack of seasonal association with chickenpox, the observation that pain usually precedes the skin eruption, the dermatomal localization of the lesions of herpes zoster, and the pathology and patterns of distribution of herpes zoster.

Pathologic studies of herpes zoster have shown an acute ganglionitis with an intense inflammatory response, cell necrosis, and occasionally hemorrhages within the ganglia. In addition, there is inflammation in the adjacent segments of the cord or brainstem which is predominantly unilateral, more prominent in gray matter, and involves the posterior more than the anterior horns. A mild leptomeningitis is generally found which is most intense over the segments of involvement. Inflammation in the roots distal to the ganglia is also present, representing a true peripheral mononeuritis.

In the skin innervated by the nerve there is degeneration of the basal and deep prickle cell layers of the epidermis. Ballooning degeneration of these cells causes the formation of the intradermal vesicles. Giant cells and eosinophilic intranuclear inclusions are found in the base of the vesicles.

Clinical Manifestations. The eruption of herpes zoster is often preceded by malaise and fever for two to four days. Pain or dysesthesia along the segmental dermatome also precedes the rash usually for four to five days. The pain is often a superficial tingling or burning sensation, but may vary from severe deep pain, suggesting appendicitis, cholecystitis, or pleurisy, to very mild itching. The pain may be intermittent or constant. Tenderness or hypesthesia may be detected along the dermatome on examination during this pre-eruptive stage. The cutaneous lesions present first as small, red macules which rapidly vesiculate, becoming tense, clear vesicles on an erythematous base. On about the third day, the vesicular fluid becomes turbid as inflammatory cells collect within the vesicles. Within five to ten days, the vesicles dry and crusts develop. However, in severe cases the vesicles may become confluent with a gangrenous appearance, and healing may be delayed for many weeks. During the course of the rash, there is usually enlargement of the regional lymph nodes, and there is often spread of a few vesicles to adjacent dermatomes but seldom to the other side of the body. The pain or dysesthesia usually persists for one to four weeks, but approximately 30 per cent of the patients over the age of 40 have pain that persists for months to years. This postherpetic neuralgia is more common in the elderly when there has been a prolonged period of pain prior to cutaneous eruption and a more severe rash.

Although herpes zoster may occur over any sensory nerve distribution, the thoracic dermatomes are the sites in over two thirds of cases. Cranial nerve involvement is next in frequency, and this tends to be more severe, with greater pain, frequent signs of meningeal irritation, paralysis, and sometimes involvement of the mucous membranes. The ophthalmic division of the trigeminal nerve is the most common site of cranial involvement, accounting for 10 to 15 per cent of all cases of herpes zoster. Fortunately, the eye is usually spared, but occasionally a keratoconjunctivitis develops. With ophthalmic zoster it is not uncommon to have involvement of oculomotor function, with extraocular muscle weakness, ptosis, and paralytic mydriasis. The fourth and sixth cranial nerves may also be involved, indicating that the infection is not confined to the trigeminal ganglia and its ophthalmic fibers, but may involve the brainstem and other nerve roots. The association of vesicles in the external ear and ipsilateral facial palsy (Ramsay Hunt's syndrome) was originally ascribed to infection of the geniculate ganglia. This localization of zoster may be accompanied by hearing loss, vertigo, loss of taste, or vesicles on the tongue, and probably represents involvement of multiple cranial ganglia and the associated localized encephalitis and neuronitis.

Since the primary lesion of herpes zoster is in the nervous system, the cerebrospinal fluid commonly shows a pleocytosis and elevation of protein, even when clinical signs of meningeal irritation or encephalomyelitis are absent. Not infrequently, the peripheral mononeuritis or local encephalomyelitis may cause muscle paralysis and atrophy in the area of the segmental rash. Acute urinary retention and hemidiaphragmatic paralysis have also been seen. Signs of major central nervous system infections with herpes zoster are rare, but cases of acute transverse or ascending myelitis, disseminated encephalitis, and acute cerebellar ataxia have been described.

Zoster sine herpete is typical pain in an appropriate sensory area which is not followed by the development of the characteristic vesicles. Whether some of the common transient intercostal pains represent activation of varicella virus in ganglia without spread to the skin is a matter of speculation. An antibody response to varicella virus has been demonstrated in the absence of a rash in patients with transient facial pain resembling trigeminal neuralgia and in patients with facial palsy (Bell's palsy). However, these are rare occurrences, and the vast majority of cases of trigeminal neuralgia and Bell's palsy are not associated with serologic evidence of activation of the varicella or any other known viral infection.

Cutaneous dissemination is rare, occurring in less than 2 per cent of the cases. Dissemination is more common in patients with underlying malignancies, and about one quarter of the patients with Hodgkin's disease show a progressive spread of vesicles beyond the original one or two dermatomes of involvement. Such cutaneous dissemination, however, generally does not progress for more than six days, and spontaneous recovery occurs in most patients.

Diagnosis. Characteristic development of pain and vesicular eruptions over single or adjacent dermatomes served by a segmental or cranial nerve branch usually presents no problem in differential diagnosis. However, similar zosteriform lesions can be caused by herpes simplex virus in infants.

Diagnosis can be confirmed by the demonstration of multinucleated giant epithelial cells with intranuclear inclusions in Giemsa-stained scrapings from the base of an early vesicle. Virions can also readily be found in vesicular fluid by electron microscopic examination. However, neither of these tests differentiates zoster from herpes simplex virus infections, although they can be helpful in differentiating zoster or chickenpox from smallpox infections. Varicella and herpes simplex virus infections can be differentiated by fluorescent antibody staining of cells in scrapings from vesicles.

Virus can be isolated from vesicular fluid and, in some cases, from cerebrospinal fluid by inoculation of fluid onto cultures of human or primate cells. Serologic diagnosis can also be made, but in human sera some cross-reactions are found with herpes simplex virus, so that simultaneous serologic tests should be carried out against both viruses.

Treatment. Little can be done to treat the acute eruption of herpes zoster other than symptomatic application of powder or calamine lotion to the rash and the use of analgesics for the pain. A variety of previously advocated treatments such as protamide, vitamins, x-irradiation, vasodilators, antimicrobials, and gamma globulin have proved to be useless. In a controlled study corticosteroids have been shown not to affect the rate of healing of skin lesions but to shorten the period of the acute pain. This benefit must be weighed against the potential hazard that corticosteroids may promote dissemination. One study has indicated that 5-iodo-2′-deoxyuridine (IUDR) in dimethylsulfoxide applied topically to the lesions shortens the healing time and the duration of pain, but IUDR without the dimethylsulfoxide is of no value, and dimethylsulfoxide is not available for general use in the United States.

Recently, systemic cytosine arabinoside, a drug inhibitory against DNA virus replication in vitro, has been advocated for the control of severe and disseminated herpes zoster infections. However, in a placebo-controlled study, cytosine arabinoside was found to actually prolong the duration of dissemination in some patients compared to the placebo group. This adverse effect of cytosine arabinoside appeared to be related to its depression of antibody response, delay in vesicle interferon appearance, and possibly its effect on the cellular immune response.

Postherpetic Neuralgia. The development of prolonged postherpetic neuralgia after recovery from herpes zoster presents a difficult problem in management. Although this pain usually abates over a period of months to years, it is very refractory to the usual analgesics. Application of cold to the area by use of an ethyl chloride spray may give some transient relief. Tranquilizers or sedatives can sometimes be of help, and tricyclic antidepressants (amitriptyline) in combination with substituted phenothiazines have been effective in relieving pain in some cases. Local injection or section of the nerve root is of no value, and narcotics should be avoided because of the problem of addiction. In the most severe cases when pain persists over long periods, the use of transcutaneous peripheral nerve stimulation or even cordotomy may be considered (see Ch. 349).

Prognosis. There is a popular misconception that herpes zoster does not recur. However, zoster does not give immunity to further attacks, and the likelihood of a second attack is about the same as, if not slightly greater than, that of having suffered the first. Most patients recover uneventfully, although severe vesiculation may lead to permanent scarring. Scarring of the cornea after ophthalmic involvement may result in permanent visual impairment. Motor paralysis of the local nerves recovers to adequate function levels in over 75 per cent of cases.

Even in patients with severe encephalomyelitis, the mortality rate appears to be less than 10 per cent, and permanent sequelae are rare. The prognosis, however, must be more guarded in those patients who have underlying neoplastic disease, in which both the disease and the chemotherapeutic agents used in the treatment of neoplasms may increase the possibility of cutaneous and visceral dissemination.

Prevention. No vaccine is available for varicella virus. Chickenpox can be modified if gamma globulin is given after exposure, and sera obtained from patients recuperating from herpes zoster can totally prevent chickenpox in children if given within 72 hours of the time of exposure. This zoster immune globulin is recommended for children on immunosuppressive therapy or with leukemia who have been exposed to chickenpox or herpes zoster. Similar measures are not recommended for disabled adults exposed to chickenpox or to zoster, although contact should be avoided in the adult patient with a compromised immune system, because it is in this group that occasional cases of zoster have been thought to be related to exposure to chickenpox or zoster.

Hope-Simpson, R. E.: The nature of herpes zoster: A long-term study and a new hypothesis. Proc. R. Soc. Med., 58:9, 1965.
Juel-Jensen, B. E., MacCallum, F. O., Mackenzie, A. M. R., and Pike, M. C.: Treatment of zoster with idoxuridine in dimethyl sulphoxide. Results of two double-blind controlled trials. Br. Med. J., 4:776, 1970.
McCormick, W. F., Rodnitzsky, R. L., Schochet, S. S., and McKee, A. P.: Varicella-zoster encephalomyelitis. Arch. Neurol., 21:559, 1969.
Stevens, D. A., Jordan, G. W., Waddell, T. F., and Merigan, T. C.: Adverse effect of cytosine arabinoside on disseminated zoster in a controlled trial. N. Engl. J. Med., 289:873, 1973.
Taub, A.: Relief of postherpetic neuralgia with psychotropic drugs. J. Neurosurg., 39:235, 1973.
Taylor-Robinson, D., and Caunt, A. E.: Varicella virus. Virol. Monogr. 12. New York and Vienna, Springer-Verlag, 1972.

389. VIRAL MENINGITIS AND ENCEPHALITIS

Dorothy M. Horstmann

Definitions. The term *viral meningitis* is used to describe a syndrome characteristic of acute viral infections of the central nervous system manifested by signs of meningeal irritation, cerebrospinal fluid pleocytosis, and a short, uncomplicated course. In *viral encephalitis* the brain is involved in the inflammatory process; it is a more serious disease than viral meningitis, being commonly characterized by disorientation, alteration in consciousness, tremors, convulsions, coma, and, in a significant number of patients, death. Both syndromes can be induced by a variety of different viruses.

Etiology. *Aseptic Meningitis.* At present a specific cause can be established in up to two-thirds of the cases of presumed viral origin. The relative frequency and importance of the many agents which have been implicated vary in different parts of the world. In the United States and in temperate climates generally, the *enteroviruses* are the most common causes, accounting for approximately 75 per cent of cases in which a cause is established. The agents most frequently associated with meningitis are echovirus 4, 6, and 9; coxsackievirus A 7 and 9; and coxsackievirus B 1 to 5. In all, more than 60 enteroviruses have been identified. Not all have yet been associated with meningitis; but in view of the frequent additions from among previously known and newly recognized members of this family of agents, the list can be expected to grow. *Mumps virus* is the next most frequent cause of aseptic meningitis; *herpes simplex* and *adenoviruses* (mainly types 1, 2, 3, 5, and 7) and *lymphocytic choriomeningitis* viruses are infrequently responsible; rarely, the syndrome may be seen as a complication of *infectious mononucleosis* (Epstein-Barr virus), *herpes zoster,* and possibly *viral hepatitis.* Aseptic meningitis associated with the *arthropod-borne* group of viruses follows the geographic distribution of these agents, which is dependent upon specific arthropod vectors.

TABLE 1. Viruses Associated with Acute Infections of the Central Nervous System in the United States

Enteroviruses
Polioviruses
Coxsackievirus A
Coxsackievirus B
Arboviruses (arthropod-borne)
St. Louis
Eastern equine
Western equine
Venezuelan equine
California
Powassan
Mumps virus
Measles virus
Rubella virus
Herpesviruses
Herpesvirus hominis
Varicella-zoster virus
Epstein-Barr virus
Cytomegalovirus
Viruses associated with respiratory illness
Adenoviruses
Influenza
Lymphocytic choriomeningitis virus
Encephalomyocarditis virus
Rabies virus
Hepatitis viruses (?)

Encephalitis. In not more than a third of the cases can a specific viral agent be identified as the cause (Table 2). The geographic distribution of the viruses involved is similar in both aseptic meningitis and encephalitis, but their relative importance is different. Thus mumps virus accounts for more reported cases of encephalitis than any other agent; the arboviruses are also prominent, whereas enteroviruses are infrequently recovered from patients with this syndrome. Herpes simplex virus is a significant cause, both in primary infections and in reactivation of latent infections which involve the central nervous system (see Ch. 390). Encephalitis may also occur with influenza, adenovirus, and other respiratory infections, and rarely lymphocytic choriomeningitis (LCM), toxoplasmosis, infectious mononucleosis, and herpes zoster. When it occurs in association with measles, chickenpox, and rubella, it has been commonly believed to be of the postinfectious type rather than the result of a primary viral invasion, but recent evidence suggests that in mumps and measles encephalitis both mechanisms may be involved in some cases. Rubella meningoencephalitis occurs occasionally in infants with congenital rubella; it is caused by direct viral invasion and tends to be chronic.

Epidemiology. In the United States some 4000 to 6000 cases of aseptic meningitis and approximately 2000 cases of encephalitis are reported annually; however,

TABLE 2. Reported Cases of Encephalitis by Cause—United States, 1967–1971*

Year	Total Number	Arbo-viruses	Entero-viruses	Herpes Simplex	Associated with Childhood Diseases				Associated with Respiratory Infection†	Other Known Causes‡	Unknown Causes
					Mumps	*Measles*	*Varicella*	*Rubella*			
1971	1891	150	45	54	310	69	54	3	17	10	1179
1970	1950	110	52	37	288	27	46	7	9	14	1360
1969	1917	108	31	29	218	35	48	3	7	20	1418
1968	2283	130	66	35	408	19	69	6	17	23	1510
1967	2368	83	26	30	849	62	77	7	2	14	1218

*From Center for Disease Control, U.S. Public Health Service, Neurotropic Virus Disease Surveillance Reports, 1969–1973.
†Includes infections due to influenza, *M. pneumoniae*, and adenoviruses.
‡Includes infections due to lymphocytic choriomeningitis, varicella-zoster, Epstein-Barr virus, and cytomegalovirus.

these represent only a fraction of the total number, because marked under-reporting is the rule. Both syndromes, whether of known or unknown cause, have their peak incidence in the period from July through October, but sporadic cases may be seen at any time during the year. In temperate climates, aseptic meningitis caused by enteroviruses occurs most characteristically in small or large outbreaks during the summer and autumn, whereas in tropical and semitropical areas there is no striking seasonal incidence. Children are more frequently affected than adults; but in some epidemics caused by enteroviruses which have been absent from circulation for long periods, as many as 50 per cent of cases have been in individuals over 15 years of age. The agents are often widely disseminated in the population, giving rise chiefly to inapparent infections or minor febrile illnesses. Spread is primarily by contact with an infected person, and the healthy individual with an inapparent infection is as infectious as the frank case. Dissemination is greatest in areas of poor sanitation with a high density of preschoolchildren, who are the most frequent virus spreaders. Although one enterovirus type tends to be dominant and to account for the bulk of illness at any given time and place, it is not unusual during epidemic or endemic periods to find several agents circulating at the same time, causing similar illnesses, including meningitis. *Mumps meningitis* and *meningoencephalitis* follow the epidemiologic pattern of mumps infections generally, with the highest incidence in winter and spring. On rare occasions, they appear in epidemic form, without accompanying parotitis. *Lymphocytic choriomeningitis* is a relatively uncommon disease, occurring in the late autumn and winter. The infection is endemic in the common house mouse, *Mus musculus,* and is probably spread to man through dust or food contaminated by mouse excreta. *Adenovirus* and *herpes simplex meningitis* and *encephalitis* occur sporadically in children as primary infections spread by contact; encephalitis caused by herpes virus also occurs in older individuals as a reactivation of latent infection.

Infections caused by the arthropod-borne viruses (arboviruses) occur in epidemics during summer and fall, causing a range of illness which includes minor febrile episodes, aseptic meningitis, and, more characteristically, encephalitis. In the United States, California virus has recently been a prominent cause of this disease in children living in rural areas of the north-midwestern part of the United States, and Powassan virus has been recovered sporadically from cases in the northeast. Eastern equine encephalitis virus is found predominantly along the East and Gulf coasts, and western equine usually occurs west of the Mississippi River. St. Louis encephalitis is endemic in California and parts of the southwest; it has occurred in epidemic form in widely separated urban and suburban areas of New Jersey, Florida, and Texas. In 1971, Venezuelan encephalitis virus moved up from Mexico through Texas and the southern United States, causing epidemics in humans and in horses. Most cases of encephalitis reported in the United States each year (60 to 75 per cent) are of unknown cause. These occur the year round, but there is a concentration in summer and fall, paralleling the pattern of arbovirus and enterovirus infections.

Pathogenesis and Pathology. Like the epidemiology, the pathogenesis of the two syndromes varies with the nature of the infecting agent. The general pattern for enteroviruses is thought to be similar, the sequence being primary multiplication in the alimentary tract, spread to regional nodes, a viremic phase, and eventual invasion of the central nervous system. There is evidence that in enterovirus infections in humans as well as in experimentally infected primates, viremia precedes the onset of illness by several days and has usually disappeared by the time neurologic signs appear. In mumps, LCM, primary herpes simplex, and arbovirus encephalitis, the agents probably reach the central nervous system through the bloodstream, after initial multiplication in extraneural tissues. Spread by neural pathways occurs in rabies and herpes zoster, and possibly secondarily in certain other infections in which the blood-borne route is the major one.

Since *aseptic meningitis* is not a fatal disease, the extent of the pathologic lesions in the central nervous system is not accurately known, but is presumed to be limited mainly to the meninges. However, in the experimental disease induced in monkeys by poliovirus, neuronal lesions are commonly found in the precentral gyrus of the cerebral cortex (and the brainstem and spinal cord), indicating that the difference between aseptic meningitis and encephalitis is merely one of degree and concentration of nerve cell damage. In *encephalitis,* the meninges are also involved in an inflammatory reaction, but the most significant lesions are neuronal. The brain and cord are swollen and congested, and histologic examination of the brain parenchyma reveals changes in the neurons, ranging from slight alterations in the nuclei and cytoplasm to complete necrosis and neuronophagia. The involved areas contain polymorphonuclear leukocytes and microglia, and there is marked perivascular cuffing. The distribution of lesions tends to be characteristic for given agents or groups of agents, although, with the exception of poliomyelitis, it is usually not possible to distinguish between the various viruses on the basis of pathology alone. In arbovirus infections the lesions may be widely distributed, often involving the entire cerebral cortex, cerebellum, brainstem, and spinal cord. Fatal mumps encephalitis is rare, but in a recently reported case acute inflammatory lesions and necrosis attributed to direct viral action were revealed, along with demyelination characteristic of postinfectious encephalitis.

Clinical Manifestations. *Viral Meningitis.* Whatever the specific viral cause, the symptoms and signs are similar to, and not readily distinguished from, the pattern of aseptic meningitis of other causes. The onset is commonly abrupt. The most constant features are severe headache, fever, and stiff neck; other symptoms may occur, including sore throat, nausea and vomiting, listlessness, drowsiness, vertigo, pain in the back and neck, photophobia, paresthesias, myalgias, abdominal pain, and chills or chilly sensations. With certain echo- and coxsackievirus infections a striking skin eruption may appear. In general the severity of symptoms increases with the age of the patient. Although sudden onset is characteristic, in some patients there is a prodromal nonspecific "minor illness," followed by several days of well-being before the reappearance of fever and the development of signs of central nervous system involvement. This occurs most commonly with poliovirus infections in young children, but may be associated with other enteroviruses and with lymphocytic choriomeningitis.

On physical examination there are few findings. The temperature is elevated (38.5 to 40°C), but the patient does not appear as ill as one with bacterial meningitis. Neck and back stiffness are the only neurologic signs in the typical case; Kernig and Brudzinski signs are sometimes positive. Nuchal rigidity may be minimal and apparent only in the last degrees of neck flexion. The deep tendon reflexes are normal or hyperactive. Transient weakness (rarely frank paralysis) has been noted with the coxsackievirus B group, coxsackievirus A 7, and certain echoviruses, notably 7 and 9. *Rash* is encountered chiefly in young children. It has been a prominent feature of certain epidemics in which aseptic meningitis has also occurred, including outbreaks associated with echovirus 4, 6, 9, and 16 and coxsackievirus A 9 and 16, rash has also been observed occasionally with many other enterovirus types. The eruption usually appears with the fever and lasts four to five days (in severe cases, eight or nine days). Characteristically it is maculopapular, discrete, erythematous, and nonpruritic. The lesions may be confined to the face and neck or may spread over the chest and extremities and sometimes involve the palms and soles. At times the rash is petechial (echovirus 9) or vesicular (coxsackievirus A 9 and A 16), but the character is not constant, and a single virus type may induce any of the various forms of eruptions, even during the same epidemic. An *enanthem,* consisting of grayish white dots on the buccal mucosa, has been described in as many as one third of the patients in certain outbreaks caused by echovirus 9, but only occasionally with the other types (echovirus 6 and 16).

Viral Encephalitis. The characteristic signs of encephalitic involvement include mental confusion, delirium, stupor, convulsions, and coma. The onset of the disease may be sudden or gradual, with chills, fever, headache, lethargy, dizziness, vomiting, and stiffness of the neck. A prodrome consisting of headaches, fever, vague aches and pains, and sometimes sore throat may last for several days before the more typical neurologic signs appear. The severity of the clinical picture varies with the etiologic agent and the site and extent of the neuronal lesions. Mumps is commonly associated with a relatively benign meningoencephalitis in which the clinical picture is one of aseptic meningitis with the addition of mild encephalitic signs. Encephalitis caused by arboviruses (Ch. 144 to 152) may also be mild, particularly in infections with California virus, or the disease may be ushered in with severe headache, vomiting, hyperpyrexia, twitchings, tremors, convulsions, disorientation, and drowsiness followed by coma. There may also be ataxia caused by cerebellar involvement, as well as hyperactive reflexes, spasticity, and weakness of the extremities if the neurons of the spinal cord are attacked. In herpes simplex encephalitis, the illness is frequently catastrophic; convulsions are common, and signs suggesting a space-occupying lesion of the temporal lobe may be present. Variations in severity from mild to rapidly fatal may also occur when the disease is associated with other agents, as well as in the two thirds or more cases presumed to be of viral origin, although implication of a specific agent is not possible.

Laboratory Findings. *Viral Meningitis.* The blood count is commonly within normal range, but leukopenia or moderate leukocytosis without marked shift to the left may be present. The cerebrospinal fluid findings are diagnostic: the fluid is clear, with an elevated cell count ranging from 10 to 3000 or more cells per cubic milliliter, most frequently 30 to 300; no organisms are seen when the stained sediment is examined microscopically. Early in the disease the cells may be predominantly polymorphonuclear, but within a few hours there is a shift, with 80 to 90 per cent or more being lymphocytes. In contrast to bacterial meningitis, the glucose content is normal, although transient depression below 40 mg per 100 ml may be encountered early in the course, particularly in mumps meningitis. The protein level is normal or moderately elevated. The height of the cell count bears no fixed relation to the severity of the disease or to signs of meningeal irritation such as neck stiffness. The number of cells tends to return to normal within a few days, except in mumps and echo 9 meningitis, in which pleocytosis may persist for seven to ten days, often after nuchal rigidity has disappeared.

Viral Encephalitis. In encephalitis the peripheral white cell count is usually moderately elevated, but in eastern equine encephalitis marked leukocytosis as high as 60,000 cells with 90 per cent polymorphonuclears has been reported. Cerebrospinal fluid findings are commonly similar to those in viral meningitis, although in some cases the fluid may be entirely normal.

Diagnosis and Differential Diagnosis. *Viral Meningitis.* Recognition of the aseptic meningitis syndrome is not difficult except in young infants who frequently do not have the classic signs of meningeal irritation. There are a number of clinical and epidemiologic features which may suggest the viral agent involved, but a specific etiologic diagnosis can be established only in the laboratory. With enterovirus infections, virus isolation is the usual means of accomplishing this; serologic identification based on antibody rises is impracticable because of the multiplicity of virus types. Enteroviruses are readily isolated from fecal specimens and throat swabs, and coxsackie- and echoviruses (in contrast to polioviruses) may be found in the cerebrospinal fluid in

50 per cent or more of cases associated with these agents. Adenoviruses and herpes simplex virus can be recovered from the same sources as enteroviruses, except that herpes virus is very rarely found in the cerebrospinal fluid. Both blood and cerebrospinal fluid are sources of lymphocytic choriomeningitis virus. Infections caused by mumps, lymphocytic choriomeningitis, and the arthropod-borne viruses are usually diagnosed serologically (rising titers of complement-fixing, neutralizing, or hemagglutination-inhibiting antibodies), although virus isolation is also possible, if more difficult.

DIFFERENTIAL DIAGNOSIS OF CLINICAL EVIDENCE. A careful analysis of the history is most likely to suggest the correct etiologic diagnosis. The season of the year, the presence or absence of an epidemic, and the geographic location (particularly with respect to the arthropod-borne viruses) should be considered. In the United States, epidemics are most often associated with enteroviruses, whereas sporadic cases are likely to be induced by mumps, herpes simplex virus, adenoviruses, or other agents. In the summer and fall, leptospiral meningitis enters into the differential diagnosis, for it has the same seasonal incidence as enterovirus infections. In an epidemic in which there are many patients with paralysis, a relatively high percentage of aseptic meningitis cases will be due to polioviruses. In family epidemics caused by coxsackie- and polioviruses, most infections are inapparent, with only a single individual exhibiting overt illness such as meningitis. By contrast, with certain echoviruses (particularly echo 4, 6, and 9) it is common to find that all members of the family have recently experienced some febrile episode with or without meningeal signs.

The age and sex of the patient are also helpful. Mumps meningitis is much more common in males than in females (at least 3:1), and a similar but smaller difference has been noted in meningitis caused by enteroviruses in individuals under 20 years of age. Herpes simplex meningitis is seen primarily in young infants and in adults. Lymphocytic choriomeningitis occurs in the 20- to 40-year age group; mumps, adenovirus, and enterovirus meningitis affect chiefly children and young adults.

The appearance of parotitis, salivary gland enlargement, or orchitis in patients with aseptic meningitis strongly suggests mumps, but occasionally orchitis has been noted with coxsackievirus B infections and infectious mononucleosis; lymphocytic choriomeningitis virus has been isolated from a patient with meningitis, orchitis, and parotitis. The presence of pleurodynia (with or without orchitis) in a patient with aseptic meningitis is characteristic of coxsackievirus B infection, but occurs on rare occasions with echoviruses also.

CEREBROSPINAL FLUID FINDINGS. An immediate practical problem in dealing with a patient who is thought to have viral meningitis is to exclude the presence of leptospirosis or a bacterial infection which might be susceptible to antimicrobial therapy. A stained smear of the cerebrospinal fluid sediment should be examined carefully for microorganisms, which can usually be detected if the infection is a bacterial one. The question of a bacterial cause arises particularly in cases in which polymorphonuclear leukocytes are predominant in the cerebrospinal fluid and especially if the total count is high, i.e., more than 1000. If the cerebrospinal fluid is examined very early in the course of viral meningitis, the finding that 60 to 85 per cent of cells are polymorphonuclears is not unusual, but the pattern then shifts rapidly to approximately 90 per cent lymphocytes; a repeat lumbar puncture after 12 to 24 hours will thus help clarify the diagnosis. In meningitis caused by echo 9 virus, moderate predominance of polymorphonuclears may persist for a week or more. Echo 9 viral meningitis has been associated with unusually high cell counts (occasionally 6000 to 8000) in the cerebrospinal fluid. Relatively high counts, i.e., between 500 and 1000 cells, are also characteristic of mumps and lymphocytic choriomeningitis.

SIMULATION OF BRAIN ABSCESS OR BACTERIAL MENINGITIS. Confusion with meningococcal and other bacterial meningitis may also arise in echo 9 or other enterovirus infections, particularly if there is a petechial rash. The milder clinical course, the absence of significant papilledema, the lower cerebrospinal fluid cell count and normal glucose, and the peripheral blood picture usually indicate a viral infection. However, meningococcal meningitis presents occasionally with the clinical picture and laboratory findings of aseptic meningitis; the correct diagnosis is established only when meningococci are recovered from the cerebrospinal fluid. If reasonable doubt exists, the case should be treated as one of purulent meningitis until this has been excluded by appropriate cultures. *Inadequately treated bacterial meningitis* and mechanical irritation of the meninges caused by *brain abscess* (or other intracranial lesions) may also produce an aseptic meningitis syndrome. The possibility of a silent brain abscess is suggested by a history of recent pneumonia, chronic pulmonary infection, congenital heart disease, bacterial endocarditis, otitis media, or infection of the paranasal sinuses. *Tuberculous meningitis* in its early stages is another possibility. Aseptic meningitis caused by *neurosyphilis* may present as an acute illness, although the course is more typically subacute, with papilledema, cranial nerve palsies, and little or no fever.

OTHER FORMS OF ASEPTIC MENINGITIS. Among other causes of aseptic meningitis, the presence of severe sore throat, generalized lymph node enlargement, mild icterus, and a transient rash are compatible with *infectious mononucleosis. Leptospirosis* is to be considered in areas in which the infection is common and when there is a history of exposure to dogs, guinea pigs, and particularly rats, which excrete the agent in their urine. Wild rodents are also the probable source of infections with *encephalomyocarditis virus,* which may rarely be associated with typical aseptic meningitis. Involvement of the meninges may also occur in leukemia, Hodgkin's disease, metastatic carcinoma, and cat scratch disease.

Viral Encephalitis. As in viral meningitis, epidemiologic characteristics often point to one or another group of agents. Diseases of the central nervous system besides bacterial meningitis that may be confused with viral encephalitis include tuberculoma, toxoplasmosis, leukemia, primary or metastatic malignancies, and brain abscess. Skull films, electroencephalography, brain scan, and a pneumoencephalogram may be required to exclude these conditions. In the case of tuberculoma, a chest film and tuberculin skin test are helpful. In Reye's syndrome, i.e., encephalopathy and fatty degeneration of the liver occurring in children, the clinical picture is dominated by vomiting, convulsions, and coma. This diagnosis is suggested by the presence of hypoglycemia and deranged liver function tests; the disease usually follows a respiratory infection, notably influenza B, chickenpox, or other viral illness (See Ch. 397). Rabies is a rare disease in the

United States, but it may begin with the symptoms and signs of encephalitis (see Ch. 393).

Both *aseptic meningitis* and *encephalitis* occur in association with infections caused by *Mycoplasma pneumoniae.* They have been reported with increasing frequency, and, as with other syndromes caused by this agent, are seen most often in the fall of the year, primarily in individuals under 20 years of age. The neurologic signs are usually preceded by the characteristic respiratory illness, but nervous system involvement may be the only evidence of infection. The severity of the clinical picture varies widely; coma, seizures, and decorticate posturing may occur in the more severe cases. The cerebrospinal fluid findings are variable, but elevated protein and cell counts with a predominance of lymphocytes are usual at some time during the course; the glucose content is normal. A striking feature is that complete recovery is the rule, although this may require many months in those with extensive involvement. *M. pneumoniae* meningitis and encephalitis can be differentiated from viral central nervous system infections by demonstration of rises in antibody (by complement fixation or metabolic inhibition) and by the presence of high cold agglutinin titers. The agent can be cultured from the throat, and its recovery from the cerebrospinal fluid has recently been reported.

Treatment. There is no specific therapy for viral meningitis or encephalitis, nor is there evidence that steroids are beneficial. Bed rest, adequate fluid intake, and symptomatic treatment are indicated as in any acute febrile illness. In encephalitis, supportive therapy is of prime importance. Respiratory distress may require the use of a respirator. Tracheostomy is essential for comatose patients and for those who require mechanical aids for respiration and who also have problems with pooling of pharyngeal secretions. If secondary bacterial infection develops after tracheostomy, appropriate antimicrobial therapy should be instituted. Attention to fluid and electrolyte balance and to bladder function is essential. Urinary retention usually requires either intermittent or chronic catheterization, and infection is therefore common. The prophylactic use of antimicrobials for prevention of either respiratory or urinary tract infections is not effective and promotes the emergence of resistant organisms.

Prognosis. Aseptic meningitis caused by viruses is a self-limited disease, complete recovery occurring in 3 to 5 days in mild cases, and in 7 to 14 days in the more severe ones. Mortality rates and sequelae from encephalitis depend on the agent involved, the severity of the illness, and the age of the patient. Herpes simplex encephalitis results in death in up to 50 per cent of patients, and survivors are frequently severely damaged. Among the arboviruses, eastern equine and western equine infections are accompanied by significant mortality and neurologic sequelae in survivors, particularly children. Few deaths occur from California encephalitis, but minor sequelae follow in approximately 15 per cent of patients. In encephalitis caused by mumps or enteroviruses other than poliovirus, death is rare, as are residual neurologic deficits. In cases presumed to be viral but of unknown cause, the over-all mortality is approximately 15 per cent, but is higher in young children and in those over 40 years of age.

Balfour, H. H., Siem, R. A., Bauer, H., and Quie, P. G.: California arbovirus (La Crosse) infections. I. Clinical and laboratory findings in 66 children with meningo-encephalitis. Pediatrics, 52:680, 1973.

Casals, J., and Clarke, D. H.: Arboviruses: Group A. *In* Horsfall, F. L., and Tamm, I. (eds.): Viral and Rickettsial Infections of Man. 4th ed. Philadelphia, J. B. Lippincott Company, 1965, p. 583.

Clarke, D. H., and Casals, J.: Arboviruses: Group B. *In* Horsfall, F. L., and Tamm, I. (eds.): Viral and Rickettsial Infections of Man. 4th ed. Philadelphia, J. B. Lippincott Company, 1965, p. 606.

Feigin, R. D., and Shackelford, P. G.: Value of repeat lumbar puncture in the differential diagnosis of meningitis. N. Engl. J. Med., 289:571, 1973.

Gunderman, J. R., and Stamler, R.: Follow-up study of acute encephalitis residuals. Clin. Pediatr., 12:4, 1973.

Jamieson, W. M., Kerr, M., and Sommerville, R. G.: Echo type-9 meningitis in East Scotland. Lancet, 1:581, 1958.

Johnson, R. T., and Mims, C. A.: Pathogenesis of viral infection of the nervous system. N. Engl. J. Med., 278:23, 84, 1968.

Johnstone, J. A., Ross, C. A. C., and Dunn, M.: Meningitis and encephalitis associated with mumps infection. A 10-year survey. Arch. Dis. Child., 47:647, 1972.

Lepow, M. L., Coyne, N., Thompson, L. B., Carver, D. H., and Robbins, F. C.: A clinical epidemiologic and laboratory investigation of aseptic meningitis during the four-year period 1955–1958. I. Observations concerning etiology and epidemiology. N. Engl. J. Med., 266:1181, 1962. II. The clinical disease and its sequelae. Ibid., 266:1188, 1962.

390. HERPES SIMPLEX ENCEPHALITIS

J. Richard Baringer

Definition. Adult encephalitis caused by herpes simplex virus is usually encountered as a sporadic illness, the consequence of infection by the antigenically distinct type 1 herpes simplex virus. Recently it has become apparent that most if not all of the cases previously designated as acute necrotizing encephalitis are related to infection by this virus. Electron microscopic examination of tissues from a number of these cases has revealed characteristic herpes simplex virus particles.

In newborn infants, herpes simplex virus encephalitis is seen as a consequence of maternal genital herpes infection. Usually the infection is due to type 2 herpes simplex virus, but some cases are related to infection by type 1 virus. The type 1 adult infection remains confined to the central nervous system, whereas in newborns the process is commonly disseminated in a variety of other organs, and the virus may be recovered from blood and cerebrospinal fluid. Type 2 virus may also occasionally produce a meningitis or polyradiculitis in adults, frequently in association with genital infection by the same strain.

Rarely the related B virus of monkeys has been incriminated as a cause of encephalitis in humans, usually as a result of accidental transmission of the virus to laboratory workers or attendants. This condition in humans is notable for its high mortality.

Incidence. Because of the difficulty in establishing the diagnosis of herpes simplex encephalitis by currently available means, the precise incidence of the condition is unknown. It has been estimated that 4000 cases may occur in the United States each year. Herpes simplex virus probably causes fewer cases than either mumps or the arthropod-borne viruses. However, the considerable mortality and morbidity resulting from herpes simplex virus infection rank it as the most common cause of sporadic viral encephalitis with severe sequelae. In view of the tendency for some infections to undergo spontaneous resolution and the difficulty in establishing the virologic diagnosis, it is possible that herpes simplex virus may be a more frequent cause of mild encephalitic illness than is currently recognized.

Etiology. Herpes simplex virus is a large, 180 mμ, enveloped deoxyribonucleic-acid-containing virus which is antigenically related to B virus of monkeys but antigenically quite distinct from other herpesviruses. Herpes simplex virus has man as its natural host. It is known for its ability to cause recurrent cutaneous and oral or genital mucosal lesions. Recently it has been demonstrated that the virus commonly remains latent in trigeminal ganglion tissue of humans.

Early observations in man and animals suggested that various strains of herpes simplex virus behaved differently in regard to their ability to produce disease. Subsequent work has demonstrated that there are at least two distinct serotypes of herpes simplex virus (types 1 and 2) which differ not only antigenically but also in distribution. Type 1 is commonly isolated from oral and cutaneous lesions above the waist and from sporadic adult cases of herpes simplex encephalitis, whereas type 2 strains are commonly associated with genital infections and cutaneous lesions below the waist. Exceptions to these general rules are not uncommon. The two strains differ in several other respects. Type 1 has a slightly lower DNA density, produces smaller pocks on chick chorioallantoic membrane, produces a higher yield of virus in most tissue culture systems, possesses slightly less neurovirulence for mice and rabbits, and is slightly more sensitive to idoxuridine in tissue culture systems.

Pathogenesis. Many aspects of the pathogenesis of herpes simplex encephalitis in adults caused by type 1 virus are poorly or incompletely understood. Although most such infections appear to have resulted from a primary infection with the virus, in several cases a previous history of recurrent cutaneous or oral herpes simplex lesions has been obtained. Rare cases have been reported in patients whose immune systems were compromised by disease or immunosuppressive drugs, but most cases are encountered in previously normal adults.

In adults, there is usually no evidence of involvement of other viscera. Within the cerebrum the pathologic process has a characteristic bilateral distribution, necrotic and hemorrhagic lesions being most prominent in the hippocampus, amygdala and medial temporal lobe, orbital surface of the frontal lobe, insular cortex, and cingulum. The distribution is usually asymmetric. The posterior portions of the cerebrum, the cerebellum, the brainstem, and the spinal cord are characteristically spared. Histologically, the lesions are characterized by severe necrosis of all elements of the tissue. The presence of eosinophilic intranuclear inclusions in neurons, oligodendrocytes, and astrocytes is suggestive but not diagnostic of herpes simplex encephalitis. There is a brisk inflammatory reaction, consisting of mononuclear cells and lymphocytes and usually a mild to moderate meningeal exudate. Small hemorrhages within the lesions and on the pial surface are common.

The route by which the virus produces nervous system involvement has been the subject of much speculation. The consistent involvement of portions of the brain subserving olfactory functions has suggested that the virus may enter the nervous system by way of olfactory mucosa whence it may travel along the olfactory tract to reach the brain. The ability of herpes simplex virus to travel within nerves has long been recognized, but there is little evidence from human studies to indicate that the olfactory bulb or tract is uniformly or even commonly involved in cases of herpes simplex encephalitis. The possibility that the nervous system involvement might be the consequence of a viremia and a special affinity or susceptibility of neurons in the limbic system to hematogenous virus has also been considered, but there is little evidence from human or experimental data to support this hypothesis. Futher information concerning the pathogenesis of the disease awaits careful studies of the distribution of lesions and virus in human cases of herpes simplex encephalitis.

Clinical Manifestations. Encephalitis caused by type I herpes simplex virus is a sporadic disease of the nervous system which often has devastating effects and a fairly characteristic clinical course. It is uncertain whether or not the virus also causes a mild form of encephalitis, because the laboratory tests necessary to provide a definitive diagnosis are seldom feasible in patients with benign illness.

In contrast to other viral encephalitides in the United States, herpes simplex encephalitis is nonepidemic. In its severe form, the disease produces a combination of nonspecific signs and symptoms of an acute encephalitis plus focal manifestations of damage to the limbic system and frontal lobes. The onset in some patients is abrupt, with headache, fever, delirium, and, often, generalized or focal convulsions. Few illnesses can produce so much neurologic devastation in so short a time; within hours of the onset some patients may lose consciousness or undergo progressive unilateral or bilateral motor weaknesses.

Alternatively, the disease may have a subacute course. Behavioral changes have often been seen as early signs of disease and at times have prompted admission to psychiatric facilities. Some patients experience olfactory or gustatory hallucinations, presumably as a consequence of the focal involvement of temporal lobe structures. In others memory is impaired out of proportion to other cognitive functions, reflecting the bilateral involvement of the hippocampal system. Seizures are common and may take the form of generalized, focal motor, temporal lobe, or occasionally myoclonic phenomena. Involvement of larger or deeper portions of the cerebrum is signaled by the appearance of hemiparesis, conjugate deviation of the eyes, or aphasia. The illness characteristically undergoes fluctuation in its intensity, and such fluctuation may help in distinguishing herpes simplex encephalitis from involvement of the cerebrum by tumor or abscess.

The type 2 herpes virus, which is the major cause of fatal disseminated herpes infections in the newborn, causes more benign neurologic disease in adults. This virus in adults has been associated with aseptic meningitis and with radicular pain, often over lower lumbar and sacral dermatomes. The pain may mimic symptoms of a herniated intravertebral disc but is often temporally associated with the eruptions of genital herpes.

Diagnosis. The diagnosis of herpes simplex encephalitis rests upon clinical suspicion confirmed by laboratory data.

The cerebrospinal fluid (CSF) findings are of considerable importance. In most cases there are up to 500 cells per cubic millimeter, with lymphocytes or mononuclear cells predominating. Occasional cases, confirmed by isolation of the virus from the brain, have lacked cells in the CSF. Red cells in the CSF and/or xanthochromia may be frequently encountered; this reflects the hemorrhagic nature of the lesions. The CSF protein concentration is commonly elevated, but this does not serve to distinguish the process from a number of other affections.

Although the CSF sugar is usually within the normal range, several cases have been encountered in which the sugar is low.

Recent reports of the identification of herpesvirus antigen by fluorescent antibody study of cells in the CSF suggested a specific and convenient way of confirming that the illness is due to this virus. Further experience will be necessary before it is certain that such procedures correctly identify cases of herpes simplex involvement of the nervous system. Attempts to isolate virus from the cerebrospinal fluid have usually been unrewarding.

Serologic tests for confirmation of the diagnosis have frequently been employed, but have several inherent disadvantages. Comparison of acute and convalescent titers is of little practical value in the management of the acutely ill patient. Furthermore, fluctuations in the titer of antibody to herpes simplex virus are commonly encountered as a reaction to a variety of stimuli. Less than fourfold increases in titer do not necessarily signify recent herpes simplex virus infection; conversely in some confirmed cases of herpes simplex virus encephalitis, the titers have failed to rise. Recently, attempts have been made to confirm the presence of active herpes simplex infection by the use of a complement requiring neutralizing antibody in serum or by passive hemagglutinating antibodies in the CSF. The utility of these tests which require specialized and somewhat complicated techniques must await further experience with them from a variety of laboratories.

The electroencephalogram is virtually always abnormal, although the abnormality may not be specific. Diffuse slowing accentuated in one or both temporal lobes and the appearance of sharp waves or spikes in temporal areas are findings consistent with the diagnosis. Several cases have been associated with relatively specific, periodic sharp and slow wave complexes; such findings are highly suggestive of the disease, but their absence does not exclude it.

Brain scans frequently reveal unilateral or bilateral uptake of the tracer substance, a reflection of the increased permeability of vessels in the lesions. Cerebral arteriography usually demonstrates an avascular mass in the temporal lobe with or without shift of midline structures.

A certain diagnosis of herpes simplex encephalitis requires the use of cerebral biopsy. This is a technique which has several limitations and also some considerable hazard, and it should be performed only in major medical centers possessing the necessary facilities for proper processing of the tissue. The limitations arise from the fact that the encephalitic process is often confined to the medial and undersurfaces of the temporal and frontal lobes, so that biopsy of the lateral or superior portions of temporal or frontal lobes or other portions of the brain may fail to demonstrate the process or identify the agent. The time at which the biopsy is performed is of additional importance. Herpes simplex virus disappears from neural tissue within a short time and cannot be recovered thereafter by ordinary techniques. Thus the biopsy should be performed as early as possible in the course of the illness, and the tissue should be subjected to histologic study, fluorescent antibody study, electron microscopy and viral culture. If the tissue is fixed in Bouin's solution for histology, intranuclear inclusions are stained to better advantage and can be more easily recognized than with formalin-fixed tissue. Fluorescent antibody study has the advantages of relatively great sensitivity for detection of viral antigen, and specificity for the virus when appropriate controls are included. In addition, the test may be completed within a few hours after the tissue is removed. Electron microscopy is less sensitive because of the inherent sampling problems. Viral culture offers the most sensitive method for recovery of virus from nervous system tissue. The technique of inoculating trypsinized cells from the biopsy tissue onto indicator cultures may offer a better opportunity for recovery of virus than does inoculation of clarified suspension of homogenized brain.

Among conditions which must be distinguished from herpes simplex encephalitis, cerebral abscess presents the most difficult problem. Fever, headache, and seizures are all seen in cases of cerebral abscess, and these features do not serve to differentiate abscess from herpes encephalitis. The presence of another site of pyogenic infection, especially in sinus or mastoid, should alert the clinician to the possibility of abscess. However, unusual psychiatric changes or an isolated disorder of memory are less common in cerebral abscess than in herpes, and abscesses usually produce more focal and fewer diffuse signs than herpes. Cerebrospinal fluid changes may be quite similar; there is some tendency for the protein to be higher and the cell count lower in cases of abscess than in encephalitis. In doubtful cases, the arteriogram, electroencephalogram, and brain scan are more apt to reflect the bilateral pathology in encephalitis, and periodic high voltage sharp waves which appear and disappear over a few days are characteristic of encephalitis but are not a feature of abscess. Sometimes proper diagnosis is not reached until after craniotomy, but this is usually in patients in whom the diagnosis of encephalitis has not been given sufficient preoperative consideration.

The distinction between herpes encephalitis and a pyogenic or tuberculous meningitis is somewhat easier because of the prominence of meningeal signs, the more regular lowering of the CSF glucose, the presence of organisms, and the lesser frequency of focal signs in the latter conditions. Distinction between herpes simplex encephalitis and the postinfectious encephalitides may be difficult and rests with the history of one of the common viral exanthems or mumps in the weeks preceding the onset of the cerebral disorder. Cerebral neoplasm can usually be distinguished by its more slowly progressive course, by the absence of fever and of CSF findings suggestive of encephalitis, and by the appearance on scan and arteriographic studies.

Treatment. The difficulties in establishing the diagnosis of herpes simplex encephalitis, the infrequency with which cases are seen at any one medical center, and the great variation in course from one case to another have thwarted attempts to arrive at a reasonable evaluation of treatment. In any given case there is considerable uncertainty concerning the stage in the evolution of the disease at which treatment is instituted. In addition, recent improvements in supportive treatment may tend to invalidate comparisons between series of cases.

Since the original reports of the efficacy of idoxuridine (IUDR) in the treatment of herpetic keratitis in rabbits and humans, individual reports involving single or small numbers of patients have appeared in which IUDR has been used to treat human encephalitis caused by herpes simplex virus. IUDR, a thymidine analogue, presumably exerts its antiviral effect by becoming incorporated into the viral DNA, thus producing a fraudulent molecule which cannot be replicated. Although the experience of some has suggested that the drug is effective, others have found less convincing evidence of its efficacy; to this must be added the known tendency for the disease to subside spontaneously. Side effects of the drug include stomatitis, alopecia, and bone marrow depression with leukopenia and thrombocytopenia. The evaluation of the efficacy of IUDR on herpes simplex encephalitis in humans must await the results of carefully controlled large-scale studies now in progress.

Recently cytosine arabinoside (Ara-C), a pyrimidine nucleoside, has been shown to possess activity against herpes simplex virus both in tissue culture and in studies with herpes simplex keratitis in animals. Although the drug has the practical advantages of being readily available and easily solubilized and there is more experience with its use, it retains some of the toxic effects of IUDR, including granulocytopenia and thrombocytopenia. Experience with Ara-C in treatment of herpes simplex encephalitis is limited to a few largely favorable reports. Further carefully controlled experience with the use of both of these antiviral drugs will be necessary to determine their efficacy in man; at present their use must be regarded as experimental.

It has been suggested that corticosteroids may be helpful in the management of herpes simplex encephalitis in man on the basis of a close temporal association between administration of the steroids and improvement in neurologic function. Although the use of steroids for their antiedematous effect may be appropriate in the patient with brain swelling and impending tentorial herniation, this effect must be weighed against the potential for corticosteroids to enhance the spread and delay the clearing of herpes and virus from lesions. Further data bearing upon this topic are necessary; in the meantime it would seem reasonable to use steroids in situations in which brain swelling seems to be a critical factor threatening the patient's life; an attempt to discontinue their use should be made as soon as is feasible.

Prognosis. Because of the very great difficulty in establishing the diagnosis of herpes simplex encephalitis with certainty, as well as the tendencies for biopsy to be performed in more seriously ill patients and for cases to be reported only if they are confirmed by biopsy or autopsy, the outcome of herpes simplex encephalitis is quite difficult to predict. Published reports from many sources suggest that an over-all mortality of between 30 and 70 per cent is to be expected and that among survivors severe sequelae are common, including prominent impairment of memory. A few reports, however, emphasize that nearly complete recovery is possible even without any specific treatment.

Adams, H., and Miller, D.: Herpes simplex encephalitis: A clinical and pathological analysis of twenty-two cases. Postgrad. Med. J., 49:393, 1973.

Craig, C. P., and Nahmias, A. J.: Different patterns of neurologic involvement with herpes simplex virus types 1 and 2: Isolation of herpes simplex virus type 2 from the buffy coat of two adults with meningitis. J. Infect. Dis., 127:365, 1973.

Dayan, A. D., and Stokes, M. I.: Rapid diagnosis of encephalitis by immunofluorescent examination of cerebrospinal fluid cells. Lancet, 1:177, 1973.

Gilbert, D. N., Johnson, M. T., Luby, J. P., and Sanford, J. P.: Herpesvirus hominis type 1 encephalitis treated with cytarabine, an unresolved problem in encephalitis. Medicine (Baltimore), 52:331, 1973.

Johnson, K. P., Rosenthal, M. S., and Lerner, P. I.: Herpes simplex encephalitis: The course of five virologically proven cases. Arch. Neurol., 27:103, 1972.

Johnson, R. T., Olson, L. C., and Buescher, E. L.: Herpes simplex virus infections of the nervous system: Problems of laboratory diagnosis. Arch. Neurol., 18:260, 1968.

Nolan, D. C., Lauter, C. B., and Lerner, A. M.: Idoxuridine in herpes simplex virus (type 1) encephalitis: Experience with 29 cases in Michigan, 1966 to 1971. Ann. Intern. Med., 78:243, 1973.

Rappel, M.: The management of acute necrotizing encephalitis: A review of 369 cases. Postgrad. Med. J., 49:419, 1973.

Sarubbi, F. A., Sparling, P. F., and Glezen, W. P.: Herpesvirus hominis encephalitis: Virus isolation from brain biopsy in seven patients and results of therapy. Arch. Neurol., 29:268, 1973.

Shope, T. C., Klein-Robbenhaar, J., and Miller, G.: Fatal encephalitis due to herpesvirus hominis: Use of intact brain cells for isolation of virus. J. Infect. Dis., 125:542, 1972.

391. CYTOMEGALOVIRUS INFECTIONS

James B. Hanshaw

Definition. Cytomegalic inclusion disease (CID), generalized salivary gland virus disease, cytomegaly, and inclusion disease are synonyms for an illness caused by cytomegalovirus infection. Although frequently an inapparent infection, it is a cause of fetal encephalitis with irreversible damage to the central nervous system. Disease also occurs in patients on immunosuppressive therapy and others subject to opportunistic infections. The virus has been associated with a mononucleosis-like illness in previously well patients and in individuals receiving transfusions of blood.

Etiology. Cytomegalovirus (CMV) infection is caused by a species-specific agent with the physiochemical and electron microscopic characteristics of a herpesvirus. It was isolated in human fibroblastic tissue culture in the mid-1950's from infants with CID as well as from the adenoid tissue of schoolage children. A cytopathic effect was noted in tissue culture which was characterized by large intranuclear inclusions. The propagation of the virus provided the basis for the development of specific serologic tests.

Epidemiology. Cytomegalovirus infection is worldwide in distribution. The prevalence of complement-fixing antibodies is especially high in communities where crowding and poor living conditions are extant. Although approximately 50 per cent of women in the childbearing age group are seropositive, this may vary from 20 to 90 per cent. Approximately 4 per cent of pregnant women excrete the virus in the urine. In the several studies that have been done in this country and in the United Kingdom, 0.5 to 1.5 per cent of newborns are virus positive. Thus cytomegalovirus is the most common known fetal infection. In some countries infection occurs in the majority of infants at some time during the first year of life. In the United States complement-fixing antibody is present in approximately 5 to 15 per cent of infants from 6 to 24 months of age.

Pathogenesis and Pathology. Cytomegalovirus does not induce a highly communicable infection. Thus a substantial number of individuals remain susceptible to the infection in adult life. The virus has been isolated from saliva, the upper respiratory tract, urine, milk, cervical secretions, semen, feces, and circulating lymphocytes. Virus is probably transferred by intimate contact with an infected individual or by infusion of blood from an asymptomatic blood donor. Nursing personnel working on infant wards and newborn nurseries do not have a higher prevalence of complement-fixing antibody than women in the general population. There is evidence that the placenta itself is infected with the virus prior to transmission to the fetus.

The symptomatic newborn is rarely without neutralizing, complement-fixing, and immunofluorescent IgM antibodies in the cord serum. The presence of specific IgM antibody is of value in differentiating maternal from fetal antibody because of the failure of maternal macroglobulin to pass the placental barrier. Antibody in the serum of the congenitally infected infant does not prevent the persistence of virus excretion for years after birth. The precise mechanism of this remarkable persistence is not known.

Among adults undergoing immunosuppressive therapy after renal homotransplantation, over 90 per cent develop an active cytomegalovirus infection if they have cytomegalovirus antibody prior to surgery. Approximately half of the seronegative patients subsequently become infected on immunosuppressive therapy.

Cytomegalovirus infection tends to be focal in character with spread of the virus from cell to cell. Infected cells may be greatly enlarged and contain eosinophilic intranuclear and basophilic cytoplasmic inclusions.

Clinical Manifestations. *Congenital Infection.* The most frequently encountered signs of the infection in symptomatic newborns are hepatosplenomegaly, jaundice, purpura, microcephaly, cerebral calcifications, and chorioretinitis – in approximate order of decreasing frequency. Any one of these signs may occur alone. A petechial rash on the first day of life is suggestive of CID. Occasionally there are no physical findings other than increased irritability or a general failure to thrive. Some infants have repeated respiratory infections. The incidence of various congenital abnormalities in infants with CID is increased. These include clubfoot, inguinal hernia, strabismus, high-arched palate, microcephaly, and deafness. There have been reports of associated congenital heart disease, but this coexistence may be coincidental.

The major complications of congenital cytomegalovirus infection relate to central nervous system sequelae. There is little evidence that extraneural involvement of viscera such as the liver, spleen, kidney, or lungs results in any permanent damage to these organs. Blindness is associated with macular chorioretinitis or optic atrophy. Deafness may be complete or limited to the higher frequencies. Spastic quadriplegia or hypotonia are common manifestations in severely affected infants. Psychomotor function may range from the vegetative state with no meaningful communication to milder abnormalities with minimal effect on speech, behavior, and motor coordination.

Acquired Infection. Cytomegalovirus acquired after birth is often inapparent but may also produce respiratory symptoms with pneumonia, paroxysmal cough, petechial rash, hepatomegaly, and splenomegaly. Central nervous system disease caused by infection acquired after birth has not been frequently demonstrated, although there are reports of associated myoclonic seizures in infants and infectious polyneuritis. Chorioretinitis has been documented after acquired infection.

Hepatomegaly and mildly abnormal liver function tests are found in well individuals excreting CMV in the urine as well as in patients with cytomegalovirus mononucleosis. The latter patients may experience malaise, fever, chills, myalgia, sore throat, headache, anorexia, and abdominal pain. On physical examination, pharyngeal edema without exudate, lymphadenopathy, and splenomegaly may be present. Atypical lymphocytosis is common. Some patients have maculopapular rashes, especially if ampicillin is administered, and abnormal serologic reactions, including cold agglutinins, antinuclear antibody, and cryoimmunoglobulins, have been described. An illness similar to cytomegalovirus infection has been described in patients who have received blood transfusions. This condition, referred to as post-transfusion mononucleosis, occurs two to four weeks after the administration of blood.

Acquired cytomegalovirus infection has also been associated with autoimmune hemolytic disease, ulcerative lesions of the gastrointestinal tract, post-transplantation pneumonia, and thrombocytopenic purpura.

There is equivocal evidence that the mild liver dysfunction associated with acquired CMV infection is capable of progressing to chronic hepatitis, granulomatous hepatitis, or cirrhosis of the liver. Children with chronic hepatitis or chronic liver disease may have a higher prevalence of active infection, but the relationship of this infection to the pathogenesis of chronic liver disease is uncertain. For the majority of CMV infections acquired after birth, recovery is without significant complications. Patients with CMV mononucleosis may experience recurrent or protracted periods of malaise, pharyngitis, and cervical adenopathy.

Diagnosis. *Congenital Infection.* The diagnosis of congenital infection is usually not suspected at birth, because 90 per cent of infected infants are asymptomatic. The presence of infection (not necessarily disease) can be established by (1) virus isolation in human fibroblastic tissue culture from the urine, blood, upper respiratory tract, or biopsy material; (2) demonstration of cytomegalovirus 19S antibody in the cord or neonatal serum; (3) persistent cytomegalovirus complement-fixing or hemagglutination-inhibition antibody beyond the sixth month of life; or (4) demonstration of large nuclear inclusion-bearing cells in the urine sediment at birth.

Differential Diagnosis of Congenital Infection. TOXOPLASMOSIS. Cytomegalovirus infection resembles toxoplasmosis in striking detail. Toxoplasmosis, however, is more likely to be associated with microphthalmia, *scattered* cerebral calcifications, hydrocephalus, and chorioretinitis. The demonstration of specific toxoplasma antibody titers persisting beyond six months of age or the presence of toxoplasma IgM antibody is tantamount to isolation of the organism.

RUBELLA. Congenital CMV and congenital rubella may be difficult to distinguish in the neonatal period. Both can be associated with a purpuric rash, jaundice, microcephaly, and deafness. The presence of central cataracts, however, is strong presumptive evidence for rubella. If these are associated with a congenital heart lesion, the probability of rubella is high. Specific laboratory tests for rubella virus, rubella 19S antibody, or serial hemagglutination-inhibition antibody tests are required for a definitive diagnosis.

HERPESVIRUS HOMINIS (HERPES SIMPLEX). *Herpesvirus hominis* infection is usually transmitted to the infant during labor and has its onset in the second week of life. The disease is often fulminant in character and may present as a meningoencephalitis, pneumonitis, or undiagnosed vesicular rash. The virus is readily isolated from vesicular lesions (see Ch. 390).

BACTERIAL SEPSIS. Infants with bacterial sepsis usually are more lethargic than infants with CID and rarely have a petechial rash. Although the diagnosis rests on a positive blood culture, the decision to treat with antimicrobial drugs must be made on the basis of the early clinical findings.

Acquired Infection. The diagnosis of cytomegalovirus infection in a patient with mononucleosis-like symptoms can be established by virus isolation as described above. Serologic determinations, such as the presence of specific immunofluorescent IgM antibody or a fourfold rise or decline in complement-fixing antibody, must be interpreted with more caution than in the newborn period because of cross-reactions with other cell-associated herpesviruses, and a tendency for CF antibody to fluctuate widely in normal subjects. Patients with cytomegalovirus mononucleosis are always heterophil antibody negative.

INFECTIOUS MONONUCLEOSIS. Cytomegalovirus mononucleosis may be difficult to distinguish from heterophil antibody-negative infectious mononucleosis, because both conditions occur in young adults and both have atypical lymphocytosis, anginal symptoms, abnormal liver function tests, splenomegaly, and fever. In addition, the cytomegalovirus IgM (FA) test is positive in cytomegalovirus and infectious mononucleosis, presumably because Epstein-Barr virus (EB virus) and cytomegalovirus share common antigens. A patient with cytomegalovirus mononucleosis usually has virus in the urine, upper respiratory tract, and peripheral lymphocytes. EB virus antibody can be measured by an indirect immunofluorescence technique. The complement-fixation tests for EB virus and CMV are specific for each agent.

SERUM AND INFECTIOUS HEPATITIS. A jaundiced patient with CMV mononucleosis may clinically resemble one with infectious or serum hepatitis. A serum glutamic oxaloacetic transaminase level above 800 units is unusual for CMV infections at any age and common in icteric infectious hepatitis. Both conditions may be associated with mild atypical lymphocytosis. Jaundice in an adult is far more unusual in CMV infections than in infections with the hepatitis viruses. A history of recent contact with a jaundiced person is strong evidence in favor of infectious hepatitis. Serum hepatitis (SH) antigen may be detected in the serum of many patients with serum hepatitis.

Prognosis. *Congenital.* The prognosis is guarded for completely normal psychomotor development in an infant with symptoms of CID at birth. Approximately 75 per cent or more usually have some central nervous system sequelae. Although asymptomatic infants discovered on routine surveys have a more favorable outlook, there is evidence that approximately 50 per cent of infants with cytomegalovirus IgM in the cord serum have detectable CNS sequelae five years after birth. Unilateral or bilateral deafness may become apparent after the second year of life. The absence of cytomegalovirus IgM antibody in the cord serum and a birth weight above 3000 grams are favorable prognostic signs.

Acquired. Although acquired cytomegalovirus infections are usually benign, they may be life-threatening in a patient subject to opportunistic infection. This usually is manifest as a progressive pneumonitis but may take the form of a hemolytic anemia, purpura, gastrointestinal ulceration, hepatitis, pericarditis, and rarely encephalitis.

Treatment. There is no satisfactory treatment for cytomegalovirus infections. The use of corticosteroids, gamma globulin, and antiviral drugs such as deoxyuridine, floxuridine, cytosine arabinoside, and adenine arabinoside have been reported with equivocal, beneficial, or no effect on the clinical course. These reports are difficult to evaluate because of the small numbers of individuals treated, the multiple factors operating simultaneously, and the variability of virus excretion in individuals tested at different times.

Prevention. It is not possible to prevent cytomegalovirus infection at present. Handwashing and gown technique should be used in working with patients with cytomegalovirus infection in a hospital setting. Usually this is ineffectual because of the difficulty the physician has in making the diagnosis. Almost everyone in a given population will acquire CMV at some decade in life. The infection cannot be prevented by a live or killed vaccine, although this approach is under active investigation.

Benyesh-Melnick, M.: Cytomegaloviruses. *In* Lennette, E. H., and Schmidt, N. J. (eds.): Diagnostic Procedures for Viral and Rickettsial Infections. 4th ed. New York, American Public Health Association, Inc., 1969, pp. 701–732.

Hanshaw, J. B.: Congenital cytomegalovirus infection: A fifteen-year perspective. J. Infect. Dis., 123:555, 1971.

Jordan, M. C., Rousseau, W. E., Stewart, J. A., Nobel, G. R., and Chin, T. D. Y.: Spontaneous cytomegalovirus mononucleosis: Clinical and laboratory observations in nine cases. Ann. Intern. Med., 79:153, 1973.

Plummer, G.: Cytomegaloviruses in man and animals. *In* Melnick, J. L. (ed.): Progress in Medical Virology. Basel, S. Karger, 1973, pp. 92–125.

Weller, T. H.: The cytomegaloviruses: Ubiquitous agents with protean clinical manifestations. N. Engl. J. Med., 285:203, 267, 1971.

392. ACUTE ANTERIOR POLIOMYELITIS

Fred Plum

Definition. Acute poliomyelitis is a highly contagious viral disease which ranges in severity from inapparent infection to overwhelming paralytic illness and death. The illness may take a number of forms. An *inapparent infection* consists of an invasion by poliovirus that produces an antibody response but no systemic symptoms. An *abortive infection* produces transient nonspecific symptoms of a minor illness without central nervous system involvement with a rise in antibody. In *nonparalytic poliomyelitis,* the major illness develops with signs and symptoms of central nervous system invasion and meningitis but no paralysis. *Paralytic poliomyelitis* consists of the major illness, often with a biphasic pattern, associated with flaccid weakness in one or more muscle groups, the result of the attack by the virus on the somatic motor and autonomic neurons of the spinal cord and lower brainstem.

Initially endemic in character, poliomyelitis became epidemic during the first half of this century, especially in the highly developed countries of Western Europe and North America. Since the advent of effective vaccines in the 1950's, major epidemics have disappeared, but minor outbreaks have reappeared in groups of nonimmunized children and in specific areas such as the American-Mexican border.

Etiology. The polioviruses are small enteric viruses of the picornavirus group. The virus is naturally infectious only for selected primates, particularly man, and has no other known natural reservoir. Poliovirus can be classified immunologically into three distinct types. Infection with type I, type II, and type III confers immunity against subsequent infection with the same type, but cross-immunity from type to type is minimal, a fact reflected by well documented cases of second attacks of poliomyelitis. Occasionally cases of an acute paralytic illness clinically are caused by coxsackie- and echoviruses (see Ch. 126 to 136).

Epidemiology. The virus of poliomyelitis is worldwide, and the infection is spread largely if not entirely by human contact. Naturally occurring poliomyelitis epidemics tend to be both geographically localized and seasonal in nature. In nonepidemic areas with poor sanitation and largely unvaccinated populations, the illness is mainly confined to infants and children ("infantile paralysis"). In these areas, children come in contact with fecal-borne virus during the early months of life. Such children have a high infection rate with all three types of virus. Presumably they get some protection from maternal antibody, and there is very little serious illness. Under the circumstances, a large percentage of the population develop antibodies early in life and, despite repeated exposures, become immune from epidemic spread. However, once sanitation improves and infant mortality falls in a region, the average age incidence progressively rises, with a concomitant increase in the number of paralytic cases. Prior to the extensive use of preventive vaccines, as many as 35 per cent of affected patients in the northeastern United States were over 14 years old.

Individual epidemics are predominantly the result of a single virus type, although different types of virus may attack the same community in successive years. During epidemics, poliovirus can be recovered readily from the pharynx, nasopharyngeal secretions, and stools of both patients with clinical cases and those with inapparent infection. The ratio of inapparent infection to disease ranges from 50 to 1 to 500 to 1. Thus inapparent infections are by far the largest reservoir for transmission.

Pathogenesis and Pathology. Naturally occurring poliomyelitis infection is transmitted by human contact. Poliovirus enters the body through the alimentary tract and multiplies in the oropharynx and lower intestinal tract. No symptoms accompany this early proliferative stage. From the alimentary canal, the virus disseminates to regional lymph nodes with subsequent viremia which corresponds to the early, nonspecific phase of the abortive illness. With inapparent and abortive attacks, although viremia occurs, the virus apparently fails to penetrate the barriers of the central nervous system.

Both virus and host factors influence whether poliomyelitis virus invades the central nervous system and the severity of CNS involvement. Different strains of the virus vary widely in virulence. Host factors are perhaps even more important. Recent evidence indicates that susceptibility to paralytic poliomyelitis in man is genetically determined. The conclusion stems from studies in tissue culture in which poliovirus was found able to infect only hybridized human cells that contained on their surface a receptor that made it possible for the virus to attach. The sensitive cells contained chromosome 19, whereas resistant hybrids did not, implying that chromosome 19 contains the gene for the receptor. Age, excessive physical activity during the prodromal illness, and pregnancy all unfavorably influence the severity of paralysis. Local injections received during the preceding six weeks appear to increase the risk of paralysis in the injected extremity, and previous tonsillectomy enhances the risk of bulbar poliomyelitis. Inapparent and abortive poliomyelitis infections presumably never invade the nervous system at all, because these tissues undergo no pathologic changes when such mild illnesses are induced in experimental primates. In nonparalytic and paralytic cases, the distribution of lesions in the neural parenchyma is roughly similar, although the intensity of the changes increases proportionately to the degree of paralysis. No one knows just what factors govern the special susceptibility of the motor gray matter and the distribution of the virus along the neuraxis in any given patient. However, in paralytic cases, the spinal cord gray matter is diffusely affected, appearing reddened, swollen, and congested, particularly in the anterior horns; the involvement in some fatal cases commonly extends rostrally to the hypothalamus and thalamus. Lesions in the cerebral cortex are confined to mild alterations of the motor area. Microscopically in regions of maximal damage there are marked perivascular cuffing and diffuse infiltrates of mononuclear cells. The anterior horn cells of the spinal cord and the motor nuclei of the lower brainstem show abnormalities ranging in severity from mild chromatolysis and pericellular infiltration to total destruction. Small areas of necrosis commonly dot regions of intense inflammation. Ouside the anterior horns, the inflammatory reaction sometimes spreads into the intermediate horn of the spinal cord; posterior column demyelination and neuronolysis of dorsal root (sensory) ganglia are rare but well documented. In the brainstem, severe abnormalities can be found in the vestibular nuclei, the roof nuclei of the cerebellum, and especially that part of the reticular formation which regulates autonomic, respiratory, and circulatory functions.

Chronically active neural lesions do not follow poliomyelitis, although collections of lymphocytes may remain in devastated anterior horns for two years or more after the acute illness. In patients dying of motor neuron disease several years after poliomyelitis (see below), the pathologic changes have a degenerative rather than inflammatory character.

Outside the nervous system, pathologic changes of myocarditis may be found. Complications and secondary effects of the illness produce abnormalities in the lungs, gastrointestinal tract, urinary tract, bones, and muscles.

Cerebrospinal Fluid. The cerebrospinal fluid (CSF) in poliomyelitis is characterized by pleocytosis, a moderate increase in protein content, and normal values for sugar and electrolytes. The pressure is not significantly elevated. As many as 10 per cent of patients may have an initially normal fluid, but persistently negative findings are rare.

The white cell counts range from 5 to 10 to as many as 3000 per milliliter in acutely ill patients (more than 1 to 2 lymphocytes per milliliter of CSF is abnormal in a carefully examined fluid). Polymorphonuclear cells predominate at first but give way to a lymphocytosis within 72 hours. The concentration of sugar is not lowered. The initial protein content ranges between 30 and 100 mg per 100 ml, values over 150 mg per 100 ml being unusual. After the first week of the disease, however, the CSF protein often rises to 100 to 150 mg per 100 ml or even more, and by this time the cell count often has returned to normal.

Clinical Features. One would not suspect that a systemic infection was caused by poliovirus unless the virus invaded the nervous system. Furthermore, once central nervous system invasion has taken place, the severity of the naturally occurring disease still has wide limits. Poliovirus will cause a relatively mild attack of aseptic meningitis in one patient, whereas the most fulminating acute paralytic and encephalitic processes will be encountered in another infected with the same virus and during the same epidemic. The illness of poliomyelitis often pursues a bimodal course. The early stage is the time of viremia and dissemination of virus in the tissues. The later phase reflects the effects of later damage to the cells of the nervous system. Nothing specific characterizes the early illness of poliomyelitis; vague malaise, low-grade fever, muscular aching, and sometimes headache are accompanied by coryza or moderate gastrointestinal difficulties with anorexia, sometimes nausea, and, often diarrhea. This prodromal phase may subside in one to three days or can progress directly into the major illness. If it subsides, three to ten or more days may pass during which the individual feels healthy, only to fall ill again, this time usually with even more severe symptoms.

Nonparalytic Poliomyelitis. The major illness progresses with more severity and intensity. As a rule, moderate nonspecific malaise develops first, often with a sense of muscular aching or stiffness that may lead to unwise exercise to "work off" the discomfort. Generalized headache appears early and is usually nonthrobbing. Children may have coryzal upper respiratory symptoms. In contrast, anorexia, nausea, diarrhea, constipation, and sometimes vomiting are frequent in adolescents and adults. Chilliness is frequent, but shaking chills are rare. Other visceral symptoms are also prominent; many patients have insomnia as well as excessive and localized sweating. Some report urinary hesitancy or retention even before paralysis develops elsewhere.

As the illness progresses, *muscle pain* becomes prominent, usually antedating paralysis. (Meningeal irritation, involvement of the brainstem reticular formation, and direct inflammation of sensory structures are all present and are potential causes of muscle pain and shortening.) Patients also complain of a deep-seated low back discomfort that repeated changes in position fail to alleviate. Occasionally, frank *muscle twitching and cramping* develop in the early stages of the illness, and *diffuse fasciculations* can be seen.

Fever ranges between 38.5 and 40° C. The pulse is elevated commensurately, usually between 100 and 120 per minute. Most patients have mild hypertension. Patients with poliomyelitis usually look acutely ill. Their skin is flushed, and the lips of those with severe illness may show a dark cherry hue, associated with circumoral pallor. There is usually some facial sweating, and sweating in localized dermatomes or restricted bodily parts may be intense. Many patients are restless and express great anxiety, even at a stage when the diagnosis has not been made and paralysis has not set in. The pathogenesis of these feelings of agitation and fear is a matter of speculation. Along with the diffuse autonomic changes of the early stages of the illness, the psychologic symptoms may reflect the widespread involvement of the brainstem reticular formation or hypothalamus.

A stiff neck and back along with tight hamstring muscles are usually prominent in the early stages of nonparalytic or preparalytic disease. The muscles may be diffusely tender, and cutaneous hyperesthesia is often complained of. Early in the illness, muscle stretch reflexes are often hyperactive.

Paralytic Poliomyelitis. Paralysis in poliomyelitis may develop with overwhelming rapidity, proceeding from barely detectable weakness to tetraplegia in but a few hours, or it may pursue a more indolent course in which additional weaknesses appear over a four- or five-day period. Rarely this indolent progression may last for as long as 10 to 12 days. In general, the more rapid the early progression, the more severe the eventual involvement.

The virus has a predilection for large motor neurons, with weakness about large joints usually being noted first. Spread of the disease from this point shows no consistent pattern; although there is a tendency for adjacent spinal and brainstem segments to be involved together, paralysis is nearly always asymmetric and at times may be widely scattered in distribution. The lower extremities and lower trunk are involved most frequently, whereas upper extremities and cranial nerves are seriously paralyzed less often. These general incidences are of no help in predicting how the individual case will progress.

Poliomyelitis causes flaccid paralysis. After an initial brief period during which local stretch reflexes may be heightened, the involved part becomes toneless and inert. The stretch reflexes become reduced, and then disappear. Fasciculations are inconstant and transient, and the paralyzed part is initially painless. Indeed, in the first few days of the paralytic disease the absence of soreness or stretch pain usually stands in sharp contrast to the earlier discomfort and the marked degree of weakness that ensues. Sensory loss does occur in acute poliomyelitis, but it is extremely rare, and in most instances the finding of reduced sensation indicates some other illness.

Bulbar Poliomyelitis. Cranial nerve paralysis may develop at any time. When bulbar palsy initiates the paralytic disease, it is a dangerous sign, for the progress of paralysis seldom halts in less than four to five days. With bulbar poliomyelitis certain signs herald trouble. During the early hours, agitation and fear may become pronounced. Delirium is prone to occur at night. Fulminating bulbar polioencephalitis can produce stupor, acute excitement, or myoclonic twitches. Nystagmus on the extremes of gaze is frequent and carries no serious significance. More severe forms of ophthalmoplegia with opsoclonia or even total external ophthalmoplegia are usually limited to fulminating cases. The pupils, if they show any abnormality at all, tend to be constricted. Funduscopic abnormalities are absent during the acute stage of the disease.

Abnormalities in the rest of the motor cranial nerves are more common than those in the oculomotor nerves. Trismus may precede paralysis of the jaw. Facial paralysis is usually restricted to one or more muscles and rarely extends to produce a total facial diplegia. Paralysis of swallowing is the most frequent abnormality in cranial nerve function. Many such patients later show little or no residual pharyngeal weakness, implying that the acute dysfunction results from involvement of the integrating center for swallowing in the reticular formation of the medulla.

In addition to impaired swallowing, involvement of other somatic motor functions of the vagus is frequent. Muscle paralysis of the larynx creates the danger of respiratory obstruction. Total aphonia is rare, but laryngeal involvement may be so severe that the voice sounds are limited to hoarse cries. Vagal autonomic disturbances occur much more often than do actual cranial skeletal muscle paralyses, and include anorexia during the acute phase as well as vomiting in many subjects. Constipation is almost invariable both during the acute illness and for several weeks thereafter. Diarrhea is rarely persistent.

Autonomic Abnormalities. Many autonomic abnormalities complicate acute poliomyelitis. Hypertension and excessive sweating have already been mentioned. Over 50 per cent of adults suffer at least transiently from bladder paralysis with acute urinary retention. Sialorrhea and bronchorrhea are usually profuse in patients with severe bulbar disease. Indeed, the autonomic instability in such individuals is sometimes overwhelming and can progress into fulminating elevations of blood pressure, tachycardia, and fatal pulmonary edema. Cardiac arrhythmias are frequent with bulbar poliomyelitis and consist of partial heart blocks, wandering cardiac pacemakers, supraventricular tachycardias, or auricular flutter. Electrocardiographic tracings on such bulbar cases usually show abnormalities in the configuration of the T waves.

Differential Diagnosis. Poliomyelitis is singular in producing an acute febrile illness with headache, stiff neck, and asymmetric, flaccid, multifocal, and progressive muscle paralysis. However, unless poliomyelitis invades the nervous system, it cannot be differentiated clinically from many other viral diseases producing myalgia or influenza-like symptoms. Similarly, aseptic meningitis can be caused by mumps, coxsackieviruses and echoviruses that can be identified only by tissue culture or serologic studies (see Ch. 132). Bacterial or fungal meningitides can usually be separated from nonparalytic poliomyelitis by their characteristic cerebrospinal fluid alterations, including the reduction of sugar.

Many diseases may mimic some phase of poliomyelitis. However, those in which muscle pain is combined with weakness and fever provide the greatest difficulty in diagnosis. Of non-nervous system diseases, osteomyelitis or acute arthritis may sometimes produce focal pain and paresis. Here, the non-neurologic nature of the illness is usually evident within a few hours, and the CSF is normal. *Acute polyneuritis* can be differentiated by the presence of sensory changes in approximately 80 per cent of cases. Furthermore, patients with polyneuritis are seldom systemically ill or febrile, and the CSF rarely shows a persistent or significant pleocytosis. Protein elevations in the CSF above 100 mg per 100 ml are frequent in polyneuritis but unusual in polio. Paralysis in poliomyelitis usually lacks the symmetry which characterizes polyneuritis. *Epidemic neuromyasthenia* (benign myalgic encephalomyelitis, Iceland disease) has many clinical similarities to early poliomyelitis. It is characterized by insidious onset, headache, fever, diffusely aching and tender muscles, and the development of muscular weakness in approximately one quarter of the cases. The disease comes in epidemics, predominantly affects adolescents and young adults, and produces considerable emotional instability and lassitude. However, the cerebrospinal fluid is normal, and sensory paresthesias as well as mild sensory loss are often prominent. Paresis fails to progress to severe paralysis, and stretch reflexes are preserved. Viral, bacterial, and serologic studies have thus far failed to identify a cause for this obscure illness.

The course of *acute viral encephalitis* usually differs sharply from poliomyelitis. Although headache and some stiff neck are present in encephalitis, such patients usually have drowsiness, lethargy, convulsions, or mental changes. There may be pupillary changes, ophthalmoplegia, or spastic pareses, but lower motor neuron involvement is absent. The cerebrospinal fluid often is normal in acute encephalitis. Specific neutralizing antibodies can be detected in the blood within seven to nine days after attacks of equine, St. Louis, or herpes simplex encephalitis.

Acute porphyria is characterized by a symmetric motor polyneuropathy and sometimes has an abrupt onset with diffuse peripheral pain. However, fever is usually lacking and there is no CSF pleocytosis. Patients with porphyria often have a history of recurrent attacks, abdominal pain, and prominent psychiatric disturbances. Appropriate urine studies will usually demonstrate porphobilinogen.

Hysteria will occasionally present a difficult clinical picture. This may be particularly the case when the subject has had direct contact with paralytic poliomyelitis or during an epidemic. The hysteric has a normal cerebrospinal fluid and rarely looks severely ill. Hysterical paralyses commonly involve an entire body part rather than selective muscles, and reflex loss is rarely commensurate with weakness. Autonomic changes are seldom prominent in hysteria. Finally, in the face of paralysis persisting for more than three to four weeks, electromyographic studies in the hysteric will fail to detect the expected presence of motor unit degeneration.

Treatment. There is no specific treatment for the poliomyelitis viral infection. Patients with known or suspected acute anterior poliomyelitis are best kept at bed rest and should be hospitalized if signs of nervous system involvement are detected. Since there is no prognostic value in knowing the exact extent of the weakness until progression has ceased, serial studies of muscle function can be restricted to pertinent examinations of bulbar function, respiration, and circulation. Patients with paralytic and nonparalytic poliomyelitis are most comfortable if placed on a firm bed with the back and head supported. A low head pillow helps relieve neck pain, and a thin pad placed beneath the small of the back minimizes lumbar discomfort. Footboards to support the weight of bedclothes help to prevent foot drop.

During the acute illness, aspirin and other non-narcotic analgesics should be used for pain relief. Narcotics and sedatives, with the exception of small and occasional doses of codeine, are dangerous and should be avoided. Hot packs provide comfort to painful muscles and should be gently laid on with minimal manipulations. More vigorous physical therapy should be deferred to the convalescent phase, although the joints should be moved passively through their full range of motion in an effort to prevent contractures.

Patients should be on liquid or minimal diets until their appetite returns. If necessary, parenteral fluids totaling 2000 to 2500 ml should be given in order to maintain a high fluid intake and counteract the risks of immobilization. Either indwelling or intermittent catheterization can be employed to deal with urinary retention, parasympathomimetic drugs not being of much help at this stage.

Complications. The acute complications of poliomyelitis result mainly from the effects of damage to motor neurons and autonomic centers in the upper spinal cord and the brainstem. *Swallowing paralysis* is common in bulbar poliomyelitis and is treated by a combination of withholding oral intake and postural drainage. If respiratory failure coexists, tracheostomy should be performed. *Respiratory failure* can result either from paralysis of the muscles of breathing (peripheral failure) or from damage to the respiratory centers in the medulla oblongata (central failure). Peripheral respiratory failure is characterized by a falling vital capacity and a progressively increasing respiratory rate with shallow breathing. Central failure is characterized by a progressive slowing and irregularity of the respiratory rhythm, with intermittent periods of apnea, especially when drowsy or asleep. The treatment in either instance is the early and effective use of artificial respiration. *Cardiovascular complications* in poliomyelitis include hypertension, centrally induced arrhythmias, pulmonary edema, and shock, all of which are practically confined to patients with fulminating bulbar disease. Rarely, cardiac arrhythmias may persist for years after the severe attack. The management of circulatory problems in poliomyelitis is similar to their management in other diseases.

During convalescence from acute poliomyelitis *urinary tract complications* are common, almost all catheterized patients developing infections and many of the severely paralyzed ones subsequently developing urinary calcium phosphate stones caused by the combination of skeletal demineralization and the alkaline, infected urine. Treatment should include effective antimicrobial therapy, and stones should be prevented by maintaining a high fluid intake and turning severely paralyzed subjects so that gravel drains from the posterior renal calyces. Other complications are less frequent. Papilledema occurs in 5 to 10 per cent of patients during convalescence and has no serious significance. An equal number of patients develop an unexplained but usually reversible increase in various muscle weaknesses as late as three to four weeks after the acute disease. A more severe complication is *late motor neuron disease after poliomyelitis*. This is the uncommon but well documented occurrence of clinically typical progressive muscular atrophy or amyotrophic lateral sclerosis developing 30 to 40 years after acute paralytic poliomyelitis. The frequency of the occurrence is several times that of spontaneous motor neuron disease and strongly suggests an association between the two illnesses. The pathogenesis is unknown.

Prognosis. At the peak of the acute illness it is impossible to predict accurately how much recovery will take place. Less than 10 per cent of patients with paralytic poliomyelitis die when treated with modern methods. Only a few fail to recover significant strength during convalescence. It can generally be estimated that muscle groups which function partially at the end of the acute illness will recover considerably. Recovery or improvement in areas of total paralysis is less certain.

Muscle strength recovers through three mechanisms: recovery of partially damaged anterior horn cells; hypertrophy and increased strength in the muscle fibers of residual undamaged motor units; and peripheral branching from the axons of intact motor cells, the branches reinnervating muscle fibers in denervated motor units. Recovery of partially damaged anterior horn cells appears to provide the greatest return, the maximal rate of recovery usually occurring in the first three to four months after acute illness. Significant improvement in strength is unusual after the end of the first year, and improvement after this time is largely a matter of learning to use existing strength with greater skill. Muscles that show no voluntary motion at all by three months after the illness only rarely later develop functional usefulness.

Increased neuromuscular excitability is sometimes a more or less permanent residuum of poliomyelitis. Such patients experience diffuse muscle cramping on exercise or night cramps in the legs. They may be troubled by muscle tremulousness on exercise, and some have hyperactive stretch reflexes but not spasticity or pathologic reflexes. Many patients who have partially denervated muscles have fasciculations at least intermittently, and these are sometimes so prominent and enduring as to suggest active motor neuron disease. In most instances, such fascicular activity is benign and unaccompanied by any progression of weakness over the years.

Prevention. Natural infection from any of the three types of poliovirus induces lifelong immunity to the specific infecting strain. Proper vaccination with either the killed- or the live-virus vaccine appears to achieve a similar result and has largely eliminated epidemic poliomyelitis from the developed countries of the world.

Widespread use of poliovirus vaccines since 1955 has resulted in the virtual elimination of paralytic poliomyelitis from the United States. Paralytic poliomyelitis declined from 18,308 cases in 1954 to 17 cases in 1971 and 29 cases in 1972. A national survey in 1971 showed that 77 per cent of individuals 1 to 19 years old had received at least three doses of oral or inactivated poliovirus vaccine. Nevertheless, low immunization rates still prevail in certain disadvantaged population groups, and these represent the principal populations at future risk of paralytic disease.

Both live attenuated virus vaccines which are taken orally and inactivated virus vaccines which must be injected parenterally are effective in creating immunity against poliomyelitis. Because it is easier to administer and supervise, trivalent oral poliomyelitis vaccine has almost completely replaced both the inactivated and monovalent vaccines in this country. Oral poliomyelitis vaccine produces an immune response like that induced by natural poliovirus infection, and a primary series of three adequately spaced doses will produce immunity against the three poliovirus types in well over 90 per cent of recipients. Very rarely, paralysis has occurred in recipients of oral polio vaccine or in their close contacts within two months of administration. The estimated frequency of this complication is 1 case per 5 million doses distributed.

The desirable time to immunize against poliomyelitis is in infancy, when the three-dose series should start at 6 to 12 weeks of age, with the second dose 6 to 8 weeks later and the third 8 to 12 months after that. In older persons, a similar program may be given at any time, and when circumstances demand it, the third dose may be given as early as six weeks after the second. Routine immunization is not recommended for adults residing in the United States. In the event of an epidemic outbreak of poliomyelitis (two or more cases caused by the same virus type in a circumscribed population), immunization with either trivalent or homotypic monovalent oral poliovirus vaccine is recommended for all persons over six weeks of age who have not been completely immunized or whose immunization status is unknown.

In general, vaccination is contraindicated for patients with abnormal immune states caused by disease or drugs. Single booster doses of trivalent oral poliovirus vaccine are recommended for children just entering school and for persons traveling to a high risk area or having an occupational hazard such as employment in hospitals or medical laboratories.

Grist, N. R., and Bell, E. J.: Enteroviral etiology of the paralytic poliomyelitis syndrome. Arch. Environ. Health, 21:382, 1972.
Horstmann, D. M.: Lagging immunity of our children. N. Engl. J. Med., 285:1432, 1971.
Miller, D. A., et al.: Human chromosome 19 carries a poliovirus receptor gene. Cell, in press.
Mulder, D. W., Rosenbaum, R. A., and Layton, D. P.: Late progression of poliomyelitis or forme fruste amyotrophic lateral sclerosis? Mayo Clin. Proc., 47:756, 1972.
Paul, J. R.: A History of Poliomyelitis. New Haven, Yale University Press, 1971.
Plum, F., and Olson, M. E.: Myelitis and myelopathy. *In* Baker, A. B., and Baker, L. H. (eds.): Clinical Neurology, Vol. 3. New York, Harper & Row, 1973, Chap. 36, pp. 2–20.
Sencer, D. J., et al.: Supplement. Collected recommendations of the Public Health Service Advisory Committee on Immunization Practices. U.S. Department of Health, Education, and Welfare. Morbidity and Mortality Weekly Report, Vol. 21, No. 25, June 24, 1972.

393. RABIES (Hydrophobia, Lyssa)

Hilary Koprowski

Definition. Rabies is an acute infectious disease of the central nervous system to which all warm-blooded animals and man are susceptible. The virus, frequently present in the saliva of an infected host, is usually transmitted by bites, by licks, and occasionally by the respiratory route. The disease is characterized by a profound dysfunction of the central nervous system and ends almost invariably in death.

History. Rabies is one of the oldest diseases of man. First mention of it dates to the twenty-third century B.C., when it was referred to in the pre-Mosaic Eshunna Code. In the Americas, rabies as a bat-transmitted disease fatal to man was probably first described in the sixteenth century. Since 1753, when it was first recorded, its presence has been evidenced throughout the North and South American continents.

In 1971, 73 countries in the world reported rabies. In most countries, dogs were the main source of bite wounds or other human contact that required treatment. Cats were the second most frequent source of exposure to rabies, with rats, squirrels, foxes, jackals, cattle, and bats a main source in several countries. On the basis of species, the total number of rabid animals reported was as follows: dogs, 35,370; cats, 3737; foxes, wolves, and jackals, 6057; bats, 500; mongooses, 273; farm animals, 12,766; and others, 4767.

The total number of human deaths from rabies reported in 1971 was 769, as compared to 770 in 1970. However, 920,084 were reported to have received antirabies treatment in 1971 as compared to 448,512 in 1970. In 1971, antirabies treatment resulted in 42 paraplegic accidents, including four deaths; out of 16,779 who received the combined serum-vaccine protection against rabies, there were 1532 cases of serum sickness.

Etiology, Host Range, and Experimental Infection. Virus recovered in nature, the so-called *street virus,* is characterized by extremely variable, usually long incubation periods and by its ability to invade salivary glands as well as central nervous tissue. The term *fixed virus* is used for strains of rabies that have been adapted to laboratory animals by means of serial intracerebral passages. Fixed virus is characterized by a short incubation period (usually four to six days) and by its apparent inability to multiply in salivary glands. Prolonged cultivation of some strains of rabies virus in the developing chick embryo or in tissue culture has resulted in modification to the point of complete loss of pathogenicity for animals injected extraneurally.

The physicochemical properties of the virus are shown in Table 1. In addition, the virus is readily inactivated by sunlight, ultraviolet irradiation, formalin, 50 to 70 per cent alcohol, and 0.1 to 1.0 per cent quaternary ammonium compounds, bichloride of mercury, and strong acids. It is relatively resistant to phenol. In aqueous solutions, its thermal death point is reached at 56° C after an exposure of one hour. It survives desiccation from the frozen state, and rabies-infected tissue may be stored successfully at 4° C in 50 per cent glycerol saline or kept frozen at temperatures below −20° C.

TABLE 1. Specific Biologic Activities, Gross Chemical Composition, and Some Physical Properties of Purified Rabies Virus

Property	Observation
Specific infectivity	1×10^{10}–5×10^{10} PFU/mg protein
Specific hemagglutinating activity	10^4 HAU/mg protein
Specific complement-fixing activity	5×10^3 CFU/mg protein
Gross chemical composition	22% lipids 3% carbohydrates 1% RNA 74% protein
Protein composition	Four major proteins, one of which is glycoprotein and the other phosphoprotein
Sedimentation coefficient	600 S
Buoyant density in sucrose solution	1.17 grams per cm^3
Genome	Single-stranded RNA, 4.6×10^6 daltons molecular weight

PFU = Plaque-forming unit.
HAU = Hemagglutinating unit.
CFU = Complement-fixing unit.

All warm-blooded animals are susceptible to rabies. It is principally a disease of mammals, including bats. The virus is also pathogenic for birds, but to a lesser degree than for mammals. As far as we know, the disease is not transmissible by insects or arthropods. It has been found in all parts of the world, in all climates and seasons. The virus apparently cannot invade the body through intact skin, and is supposedly harmless when ingested; however, infection through unabraded mucosa seems possible. An airborne infection occurring in caves inhabited by rabid bats has been described.

Rabbits, guinea pigs, mice, and hamsters are most commonly employed for experimental infection. Hamsters are remarkably susceptible to intramuscular infection with street virus, but intracerebral injection of mice is usually employed for diagnostic purposes.

Epizootics of rabies occur in any climate during any season of the year. Wars and mass movements of men and animals favor the geographic spread of the disease. Man becomes an accidental host upon exposure to the infected saliva of the biting animal, and wild animals are often sources of human rabies. The attack rate in man, after exposure, depends to a certain extent on the location and on the severity of the inflicted wounds. Head and neck bites lead to a higher incidence of infection than bites on other parts of the body. The bites of rabid wolves are apparently very dangerous; an attack rate of

47 per cent was observed in 32 persons who were bitten by the same animal and did not receive antirabies treatment in time to be of any protective value.

Pathology. At autopsy, the brain is friable, edematous, and congested; the convolutions are broad and flattened. Severe vascular congestion of the white and gray matter may extend to the medulla and the spinal cord. Virus-infected salivary glands are usually soft and swollen. On microscopic examination of the central nervous system, the nonspecific findings consist of hyperemia, perivascular and perineuronal infiltration with mononuclear cells, and considerable neuronal degeneration. Mononuclear cell infiltration of periacinal interstitial tissue accompanied by degeneration of acinar cells may be observed in the parotid and sublingual and submaxillary salivary glands.

In the absence of Negri bodies (see below), the lesions are indistinguishable from those observed in some of the other viral encephalitides. The exact nature of the virus-host relationship is unknown.

Incubation. The incubation period in man varies from ten days to over twelve months. As minor and seemingly insignificant contacts with rabies virus in the saliva of an animal not obviously sick at the time of exposure are sometimes forgotten, claims of extended incubation periods (one to two years) have to be critically evaluated. In dogs, signs of rabies may appear after an incubation period of ten days to several months.

The length of the incubation period is related to the amount of virus introduced at the time of exposure and to the severity of the laceration. The site of the original exposure does not seem to affect the duration of the incubation period.

Clinical Manifestations. *Dogs.* In dogs the prodromal phase of the disease lasts two to three days and consists of fever, anorexia, and, very frequently, a change in the tone of the bark. However, these signs are often so slight that only a trained observer may note them. The animal's disposition is altered, and symptoms give way to the excitation phase, usually lasting three to seven days, during which time the animal grows unnaturally restless and agitated. General tremor owing to stimulation of the muscular system appears frequently. In the furious type of the disease, agitation intensifies as the illness progresses. The animal, erratic and aggressive, growls and barks constantly. It will grab viciously at any object or animal encountered. At this stage, an unrestrained animal sometimes leaves home and travels great distances, inflicting damage on other animals and humans along the way. Convulsive seizures are often observed, and the animal may become completely paralyzed. In many cases, however, the excitation phase predominates until the time of death.

In the paralytic type of rabies, the excitation phase may be slight or totally absent, and the disease is characterized only by the paralytic syndrome. Paralysis of the lower jaw, accompanied by excessive salivation, appears as an early symptom, and the animal acts as though it were choking on a foreign body. Paralysis of the muscles of phonation may lead to loss of the bark. As the disease progresses, paralysis of the posterior extremities sets in, followed by general paralysis and death. The time from the onset of the disease to the death of the animal ranges from one to eleven days. On the other hand, dogs may die suddenly without noticeable signs of illness.

Man. In man, the prodromal phase is marked by fever, anorexia, headache, malaise, nausea, and sore throat. *Abnormal sensations around the site of infection,* such as intermittent pain, tingling, or burning, are of diagnostic significance. Extreme stimulation of the general sensory system is manifested by hyperesthesia of the skin to temperature changes and to drafts, and by acute sensitiveness to sound and light. Other symptoms include increased muscular tonus, prompt gag and corneal reflexes, dilation of pupils, and increased salivation.

As the disease progresses, spasmodic contractions of the muscles of the mouth, pharynx, and larynx on drinking—and later at the mere sight of fluid—are observed in the majority of cases. This dysfunction of deglutition gave the disease its common name, *hydrophobia,* or fear of water. Spasms of respiratory muscles and convulsive seizures leading to opisthotonos also may occur. The pulse is very rapid. Periods of irrational and often maniacal behavior are interspersed with those of alertness and responsiveness. Paralysis of the muscles of phonation may lead to hoarseness or loss of voice.

The excitation phase may remain predominant until the time of death. However, in many cases it gives way shortly before death to cessation of muscle spasms, to hyporeflexia or areflexia, and to general paralysis of the flaccid type.

In rabies in man *resulting from vampire bat infection,* the excitation phase is almost totally absent, and the disease is characterized by ascending paralysis without hydrophobia. Without an adequate history of exposure, clinical diagnosis of this type of infection may be difficult.

Diagnosis. Profound dysfunction of the central nervous system, accompanied by impairment in deglutition, in persons who either were exposed to a bite or lick of any animal or may have recently visited caves harboring bats, facilitates the clinical diagnosis. Isolation of virus from saliva obtained in the course of the disease and from brain tissue obtained at autopsy, followed by proper identification of the agent by means of neutralization test, will confirm the diagnosis. Syrian hamsters, rabbits, guinea pigs, and, preferably, suckling mice are used for diagnostic purposes. Demonstration of rabies virus antigen in smears of brain tissue obtained from either patient or animal (preferably brainstem, cerebellum, or Ammon's horn) by means of specific staining with antibody coupled with fluorescein isothiocyanate is of diagnostic significance. The presence of intracytoplasmic inclusion bodies in the neuron (Negri bodies) is pathognomonic, but their absence does not exclude the diagnosis of rabies, as the presence of virus may be demonstrated by other means.

Prognosis. Although inapparent infection with street virus may be induced artificially in laboratory animals, and although animals have recovered completely after exhibiting signs of the disease, there is only one case reported of the recovery of a human from rabies after showing unmistakable signs of disease. In all other reported cases, the disease proved fatal to humans.

Treatment. *General Considerations.* Confinement and observation of the biting animal, preferably under the supervision of a veterinarian, for a period of not less than ten days for dogs and cats, is one of the most important steps in deciding whether an individual has been exposed to rabies. Biting wild animals should be sacrificed and their brain tissue examined properly by immunofluorescent staining. Treatment of severely exposed persons should be started without awaiting results of the laboratory diagnosis. If the absence of rabies infection in the biting animal is reported, treatment may be stopped.

Local Treatment of Wounds. Since the most effective available mechanism of protection against rabies is the elimination of the virus at the site of infection, all bite wounds, as well as scratches and other abrasions exposed to licks of animals, should be treated immediately by thorough cleansing and adequate mechanical flushing of the wound with soap solution followed by treatment with substances such as 40 to 70 per cent alcohol, tincture or aqueous solutions of iodine, or 0.1 per cent quaternary ammonium compounds, which are lethal to rabies virus. If debridement is necessary, infiltration with local anesthetics is not contraindicated. Bite wounds should *not* be sutured immediately. After determination of sensitivity to antirabies serum, the serum should be used in local application upon the wound.

Preliminary application of antimicrobial drugs is of no value as a prophylactic measure. However, antitetanus treatment and local application of antiseptics and antimicrobials should be instituted if indicated.

Indications for Specific Treatment. These are summarized in Table 2, prepared by the Expert Committee on Rabies of the World Health Organization. Emphasis is placed on the condition of the biting animal at the time of exposure and during the ensuing ten days. It is assumed that the saliva of an animal that is not obviously ill at the time of exposure may be infectious during a maximal period of five days preceding the appearance of clinical signs of the disease.

Passive-Active Immunization. Passive-active immunization by the administration of antirabies serum of animal or human origin and immunogenically potent vaccine in repeated doses is the most effective protective specific treatment of the exposed persons. Because of the existence of various vaccine preparations, no emphasis is placed on the use of any special type of vaccine, provided it meets the standard potency requirements and is known to induce antibodies in humans.

Administration of Preventive Treatment. The administration of preventive treatment may give rise to local allergic reactions, to serum sickness (if combined serum-vaccine therapy was used), and to nervous system reactions caused by the presence of nervous tissue in most of the vaccines. These occur most frequently during a repeated course of protective treatment. Treatment should be interrupted if signs of dysfunction of the central or peripheral nervous system are observed. *Avian embryo vaccines* and vaccines prepared from brains of suckling mice, rats, or rabbits are less apt to induce allergic reactions and have been used for preventive treatment in man. Many problems can be avoided if treatment is given only when specifically indicated (Table 2). All courses of vaccine should include booster doses at 10, 20, and 90 days after the regular course of vaccine.

Treatment Once Clinical Signs Are Apparent. Although no specific therapeutic measures are available to save the life of a person exhibiting symptoms of the disease, the survival of one patient with human rabies indicates that all the tools of modern medicine should be used in the attempt to save the patient's life. These therapeutic measures should consist of (1) starting treatment immediately after signs of rabies appear; (2) placing the patient in the intensive medical care unit in a quiet environment, with constant monitoring to prevent cardiac failure; (3) using sedatives for the relief of anxiety and pain; (4) performing a tracheostomy and applying artificial breathing to maintain respiratory function; (5) using curare-like drugs to alleviate spastic muscular contractions if they occur; and (6) instituting intravenous perfusions and administering diuretics to assure proper hydration and diuresis. *Note:* Since rabies virus may be present in the saliva of the patient exhibiting signs of the disease, all attending personnel should be protected against contamination through the use of goggles, masks, and rubber gloves.

Pre-exposure Immunization. Effective immunization with three injections of a potent antirabies vaccine given at five- to seven-day intervals, followed by a booster injection one month after the last dose, is important for persons engaged in veterinary practice, experimental surgery involving handling of dogs and cats, spelunking, dog catching, or any other activity involving unusually high risk of exposure. The vaccine used should be free from paralytic factors, and the vaccinated person should be bled one month after the last vaccination to check his sera for the presence of antirabies antibodies. Such persons upon exposure may be given one booster dose of a

TABLE 2. Specific Systemic Treatment

Nature of Exposure	Status of Biting Animal Irrespective of Previous Vaccination: At Time of Exposure	During 10 Days*	Recommended Treatment†
I. Contact, but no lesions; Indirect contact; no contact	Rabid	–	None
II. Licks of the skin; scratches or abrasions; minor bites (covered areas of arms, trunk, and legs)	(*a*) Suspected as rabid‡	Healthy	Start vaccine; stop treatment if animal remains healthy for five days*§
		Rabid	Start vaccine; administer serum upon positive diagnosis and complete the course of vaccine
	(*b*) Rabid; wild animal¶ or animal unavailable for observation		Serum + vaccine
III. Licks of mucosa; major bites (multiple or on face, head, finger, or neck)	Suspect‡ or rabid domestic or wild animal,¶ or animal unavailable for observation		Serum + vaccine; stop treatment if animal remains healthy for five days*§

*Observation period in this chart applies only to dogs and cats.
†See Explanatory Notes.
‡All unprovoked bites in endemic areas should be considered suspect unless proved negative by laboratory examination (brain FA).
§Or if its brain is found negative by FA examination.
¶In general, exposure to rodents and rabbits seldom if ever requires specific antirabies treatment.

potent vaccine. Persons without antibody should receive full treatment if re-exposed to rabies.

Control Measures. Although the presence of rabies-infected bats in the Northern Hemisphere presents a difficult problem for rabies control, most human exposure can be prevented by the use of control measures that will rid an area of enzootics or epizootics of rabies.

The following measures should be applied in an efficiently organized rabies control program conducted by public health authorities: control of the canine population (registration, restraint, elimination of stray dogs), reduction in number of susceptible dogs by mass vaccination, reduction in number of wildlife species that are a reservoir of the virus, and continuous educational campaigns for the general public.

Explanatory Notes to Table 2. Practice varies concerning the volume of vaccine per dose and the number of doses recommended in a given situation. In general, the equivalent of 2 ml of a 5 per cent brain tissue vaccine, or the dose recommended by the producer of a particular vaccine, should be given daily for 14 consecutive days. To ensure the production and maintenance of high levels of serum-neutralizing antibodies, booster doses should be given at 10, 20, and 90 days after the last daily dose of vaccine in *all* cases.

Combined serum-vaccine treatment is considered by the Committee as the *best* specific treatment available for the postexposure prophylaxis of rabies in man. Experience indicates that vaccine alone is sufficient for minor exposures. Serum should be given in a single dose—40 IU per kilogram of body weight for heterologous serum, and 20 IU for human antirabies gamma globulin; the first dose of vaccine is inoculated at the same time as the serum but at another site. Sensitivity to heterologous serum must be determined before its administration.

Treatment should be started as early as possible after exposure, but in no case should it be denied to exposed persons arriving late.

In areas in which antirabies serum is not available, full vaccine therapy, including three booster inoculations, should be administered.

Expert Committee on Rabies: Sixth Report. WHO Techn. Rep. Ser., No. 523, 1973.

Hattwick, M. A. W., Weis, T. T., Stechschulte, C. J., Baer, G. M., and Gregg, M. B.: Recovery from rabies. A case report, Ann. Intern. Med., 76:931, 1972.

Hummeler, K., and Koprowski, H.: Investigating the rabies virus. Nature, 221:418, 1969.

Johnson, H. N.: Rabies. *In* Horsfall, F. L., Jr., and Tamm, I. (eds.): Viral and Rickettsial Infections of Man. 4th ed. Philadelphia, J. B. Lippincott Company, 1965.

Kaplan, M., and Koprowski, H. (eds.): Laboratory Techniques in Rabies. 3rd ed. Geneva, World Health Organization, 1973.

ENCEPHALITIC COMPLICATIONS OF VIRAL INFECTIONS AND VACCINES

Donald Silberberg

394. INTRODUCTION

Acute disseminated encephalomyelitis may be associated with banal viral diseases or may follow immunization. Postrabies vaccinal encephalomyelitis resembles acute disseminated encephalomyelitis, but specifically follows immunization against rabies. Reye's syndrome seems to be related to banal viral infections, but has distinctive features. Despite some points in common, these entities are best considered separately.

395. ACUTE DISSEMINATED ENCEPHALOMYELITIS

Definition. Acute disseminated encephalomyelitis (postinfectious encephalomyelitis, postvaccinal encephalomyelitis, acute perivascular myelinoclasis, acute hemorrhagic leukoencephalitis) is an acute or subacute disease of the central nervous system which most commonly occurs after viral infections that do not normally affect the nervous system, or as a complication of immunization. Involvement of the brain and spinal cord may be widespread, or may be limited to discrete areas, such as optic nerves (optic neuritis, papillitis) or a single spinal cord level (transverse myelitis). Acute disseminated encephalomyelitis is characterized by varying degrees of perivenous mononuclear cellular infiltration and demyelination.

Etiology and Pathogenesis. Predisposing factors to acute disseminated encephalomyelitis include exposure to measles, mumps, varicella, rubella, influenza, infectious mononucleosis, smallpox, and poorly characterized upper respiratory infections. Similar disease has been associated with pertussis, tetanus, streptococcal infections, and mycoplasma pneumonia. Acute disseminated encephalomyelitis also follows immunization against smallpox, rabies, influenza, and tetanus. Disease occurring after immunization is often termed postvaccination encephalomyelitis, and the central nervous system disease which may follow immunization against smallpox with attenuated vaccinia virus is termed postvaccinal encephalomyelitis.

The neurologic complications of childhood viral diseases usually occur 4 to 18 days after the appearance of a skin rash or other systemic signs. However, it is important to recognize that encephalomyelitis can occur before, concomitant with, and even in the absence of systemic signs of viral infection.

The pathogenesis of acute disseminated encephalomyelitis may be viewed as the direct consequence of viral infection, as an immune disorder, or as the result of interaction of these two mechanisms. Historically an immune pathogenesis was considered first because of the histopathologic resemblance of acute disseminated encephalomyelitis to postrabies vaccine encephalomyelitis and to experimental allergic encephalomyelitis (see Ch. 396).

There have been few attempts to recover an infectious agent from the central nervous system of patients with acute disseminated encephalomyelitis using modern virologic techniques. Measles virus was isolated from the brain of a patient with postmeasles acute disseminated encephalomyelitis, using co-cultivation techniques. The patient's neuropathologic abnormalities included the typical histologic features of acute disseminated encephalomyelitis. Long after vaccination, vaccinia virus was isolated from the cerebrospinal fluid of a number of patients without neurologic symptoms, suggesting that persistent virus may play a role in postvaccinal encephalomyelitis. Mumps virus may be isolated from cerebrospinal fluid during the first few days of systemic illness in over half the patients.

At present no definite direct evidence exists for primarily immune pathogenesis of human acute disseminated encephalomyelitis, except for the form that follows rabies immunization (see Ch. 396).

Incidence. Approximately 30 per cent of the reported cases of encephalitis in the United States are associated with childhood diseases. Published reports from Great Britain indicate that deaths caused by acute disseminated encephalomyelitis exceed deaths from known encephalitis viruses. The incidence of neurologic complications may vary from epidemic to epidemic, but is approximately 1:1000 cases in measles, 1:5000 in rubella, 1:800 in scarlet fever, and probably exceeds these figures in pertussis. The fact that abnormalities in the electroencephalogram occur in approximately 50 per cent of neurologically uncomplicated cases of measles suggests that asymptomatic involvement of the nervous system is common. A variety of neurologic complications occur in approximately 1 per cent of patients with infectious mononucleosis, but acute disseminated encephalomyelitis is rare. In general, males are affected somewhat more frequently than females, approximating a ratio of 2:1 in some series. Infants younger than two years of age and the elderly are rarely affected; the age incidence reflects the age incidence of the precipitating disease.

Mumps resembles lymphocytic choriomeningitis in its central nervous system involvement. An increase of cells in cerebrospinal fluid is very common in neurologically asymptomatic children with mumps. As many as 18 per cent of patients with mumps have convulsions, and signs of meningeal irritations are frequent. Despite this, the incidence of acute disseminated encephalomyelitis associated with mumps remains very low.

Postvaccinal encephalomyelitis, which is practically unknown in infants under two years of age, occurred in 17 of 800,000 people who were vaccinated during the 1962 epidemic of smallpox in South Wales, suggesting an over-all incidence of approximately 1 in 50,000 vaccinations. Several other series report similar figures. There is a greater incidence of postvaccinal complications after primary vaccination than after revaccination, with the highest incidence among children of school age (3 per 100,000). A long interval between primary vaccination and revaccination increases the incidence.

Pathology. The basic lesion in acute disseminated encephalomyelitis is the presence of mononuclear cells around small veins, chiefly in white matter, but to a lesser extent in gray matter as well. This is accompanied by varying degrees of perivenous demyelination. Individual lesions are scattered and rarely coalesce to give large lesions. Severe cases may include destruction of axons and nerve cell bodies, serous exudate, fibrin impregnation of vessel walls, polymorphonuclear infiltration, and hemorrhages. The inclusion of hemorrhages as well describes acute hemorrhagic leukoencephalitis.

Clinical Manifestations and Course. Acute disseminated encephalomyelitis usually begins with fever, headache, vomiting, and drowsiness. This is quickly followed by depressed consciousness and often coma. Irritability, behavior disturbances, and convulsions are common. Ataxia, involuntary movements, paralyses of one or more extremities, visual impairment, or other focal neurologic signs occur, often accompanied by signs of meningeal irritation. Lesions restricted to the optic nerves producing optic papillitis or retrobulbar neuritis occur. The duration of symptoms varies from a few days to weeks and sometimes months.

Myelitis predominates in approximately 10 per cent of instances of acute disseminated encephalomyelitis. The lesion may affect only one cord level (transverse myelitis), or may progress to involve the entire spinal cord, producing successive backache, urinary retention, paraparesis, paraplegia, quadriplegia, and bulbar signs.

The cerebrospinal fluid may be normal or may show increased pressure and pleocytosis up to 1000 cells per cubic millimeter. The cell counts usually range from 15 to 250. Most cells are mononuclear, although polymorphonuclear cells may predominate during the first several days of illness. Approximately 60 to 70 per cent of patients with neurologic complications have pleocytosis, but over 10 per cent of patients with neurologically uncomplicated exanthemata also have pleocytosis. Cerebrospinal fluid protein may be normal. It is rarely elevated to more than 100 mg per 100 ml. The CSF changes have no prognostic significance and no relation to the type or severity of neurologic disorder.

The electroencephalogram is almost always diffusely abnormally slow. Interestingly, the EEG is reportedly abnormal in 50 per cent of neurologically asymptomatic patients with measles.

Neurologic manifestations may precede signs of systemic infection by up to ten days or follow signs of systemic infection by up to 24 days. The average latent period is about five days. The occurrence and severity of neurologic symptoms appear to bear no relation to the severity of the systemic disease.

The immediate and long-term prognosis varies somewhat with the individual virus. Encephalitis associated with rubella, measles, and mumps has a somewhat higher mortality (20 to 50 per cent) than in scarlet fever (13 per cent) or varicella (10 per cent). Sequelae are most common in scarlet fever (45 per cent) and measles (35 per cent), and less so in varicella (20 per cent) and rubella (2 to 5 per cent). The clinical sign which correlates best with prognosis is the level of consciousness.

Diagnosis. Identification of acute disseminated encephalomyelitis is not difficult when neurologic symptoms are preceded by a recognizable viral illness. Differential diagnosis includes acute infectious encephalitis and acute multiple sclerosis. Encephalitis caused by neurotropic viruses is almost always accompanied by increased cells and protein in the cerebrospinal fluid, which are often lacking in acute disseminated encephalomyelitis. Fever and meningeal signs are rare in multiple sclerosis. Correct diagnosis in the absence of precipitating illness may depend entirely on direct virus isolation from all possible sites and by serum antibody determinations during the course of the illness in an attempt to detect evidence of a virus infection. Fatal cases provide the opportunity for attempts at direct recovery of virus.

Treatment. Corticosteroid therapy appears to produce improvement in some patients with acute disseminated encephalomyelitis. However, no controlled studies have been feasible because of the low frequency of cases, and there is no convincing evidence to support the use of steroids in the absence of increased intracranial pressure. Appropriate measures to reduce increased intracranial pressure, including intravenous mannitol, high doses of corticosteroids, and hyperventilation, may be required to sustain life during severe acute illness. Appropriate symptomatic support includes reduction of fever with aspirin, the use of anticonvulsants and antimicrobial drugs when indicated (such as for pneumonia), and management of fluid and electrolyte balance.

Prevention. Initial smallpox vaccination during infancy reduces the danger of postvaccinal disease. The use of measles, mumps, and pertussis vaccines to induce active immunity to these diseases will reduce the frequency of acute disseminated encephalomyelitis.

396. POSTRABIES VACCINAL ENCEPHALOMYELITIS

The production of neurologic disease is a dreaded complication of immunization against rabies. Postrabies vaccinal encephalomyelitis resembles acute disseminated encephalomyelitis in its clinical manifestations and histology but is related to the presence of nervous system antigen in the vaccine rather than to the presence of virus.

It seems clear that the risk of developing postrabies vaccinal encephalomyelitis is proportional to the amount of brain tissue in the vaccine. The over-all incidence of postvaccinal encephalomyelitis varies from 1 in 2000 to 1 in 9000 of those receiving brain-containing vaccines. Practically no cases occur in young children, but as many as 1 per cent of young adults (20 to 40 years) developed encephalomyelitis after immunization with neural vaccines. The incidence after immunization against rabies with vaccines prepared in avian embryos is low, approximating 1 in 50,000.

With rare exceptions in which live rabies virus was accidently introduced with vaccines, the pathogenesis of postrabies vaccinal encephalomyelitis seems to be immunologic. The low incidence and the age-related incidence strongly suggest that immune responsiveness plays a role in disease production. In addition, an experimental disease which is very similar histologically, experimental allergic encephalomyelitis (EAE), can be induced in a variety of animals by injection of homologous or heterologous brain tissue or myelin basic protein.

Postrabies vaccinal encephalomyelitis may be divided into encephalitic and myelitic forms. Both are distinguished by widely spread foci of demyelination and cellular infiltration throughout white and gray matter, but more pronounced in white matter. Brain lesions (encephalitic form) tend to be larger, and many are periventricular as well as perivenous. These lesions resemble plaques of multiple sclerosis very closely. More acute lesions are distinguished by perivenous mononuclear cell invasion. Axis cylinders are spared in most instances. The myelitic form resembles acute disseminated encephalomyelitis more closely, with smaller scattered areas of perivenous demyelination and cellular infiltration.

The interval from the last injection to the onset of symptoms averages 15 days with the myelitic form, and about 35 days with the encephalitic form. Headache, fatigue, and changes in mental function commonly precede the appearance of such focal neurologic signs as visual disturbance, hemiplegia, or paraplegia. Progression of neurologic signs and symptoms may proceed for days or weeks. Mortality is approximately 20 per cent, but most cases were reported before the availability of corticosteroids which may increase survival. Permanent sequelae occur, including changes in mentation or behavior.

If any signs of the possible development of postrabies vaccinal encephalomyelitis develop during a course of immunization against rabies, immunization should be stopped. High doses of corticosteroids may be effective in reducing the morbidity of the acute process once postvaccinal encephalomyelitis has started. If a neural vaccine has been used, immunization can be continued with avian embryo vaccine.

Immunization against rabies should be undertaken only when it is reasonably certain that there has been a bite by a rabid animal. Vaccines prepared in avian embryos carry the least risk of producing postvaccinal encephalomyelitis.

397. REYE'S SYNDROME

Definition. Reye's syndrome describes an acute and often fatal encephalopathy of childhood that is characterized by acute brain swelling associated with hypoglycemia and fatty infiltration and dysfunction of the liver. Reye's syndrome may follow a variety of common viral infections.

Etiology and Pathogenesis. Reye's syndrome has been reported after infections with influenza B, varicella, adenovirus type 3, coxsackievirus A and B, reovirus, echovirus, herpes simplex, and parainfluenza. Viral infection is suggested as the initiating factor by recovery of virus from a few patients, by the frequency of varicella as the prodromal illness in sporadic cases, and by the reported increased incidence concurrently with outbreaks of influenza B infection in two epidemiologic studies. The pathogenic relationship between virus infection and the encephalopathy and hepatic injury is unknown.

It is possible that the encephalopathy is secondary to metabolic effects of the hepatic lesion. The combination of hypoglycemia and ammonia retention, together with other abnormalities of intermediary metabolism, may be sufficient to produce the coma and cerebral edema which occur. The early occurrence of mitochondrial abnormalities in liver suggests that induction of a partially reversible mitochondrial injury may be instrumental in the evolution of Reye's syndrome. It is not known whether similar changes in brain mitochondria occur concomitantly.

Incidence. Reye's syndrome occurs in children 6 months to 15 years of age. Approximately 500 cases have been reported. Large series have been described from Australia, Canada, Thailand, and the United States. It occurs both as a sporadic, rare disease, and in minor outbreaks in a particular area. It is a leading cause of death in children one to six years old in Thailand.

Pathology. Marked cerebral edema occurs, with or without anoxic neuronal changes and neuronal degeneration, but with no cellular infiltration or demyelination. The liver is swollen and orange to pale yellow. Fatty infiltration occurs initially as diffuse small vacuoles in the periportal areas, and spreads to cause massive involvement in fatal cases. Electron microscopic examination of liver biopsy specimens shows swollen pleomorphic mitochondria and small droplets of triglycerides in hepatocytes. Fat deposition also occurs in the renal tubules and in the myocardium.

Clinical Manifestations and Course. Typically, Reye's syndrome starts with an upper respiratory infection or mild gastrointestinal disturbance. A symptom-free interval of hours to several days is followed by persistent vomiting and then by delirium and coma. Convulsions are common. Hyperpnea or irregular deep respiration is common. There are no meningeal or focal neurologic signs. Decerebrate posturing may occur as increased intracranial pressure supervenes. Mild to moderate hepatomegaly is the only clinical suggestion of hepatic involvement, and even this is lacking in 50 per cent of cases.

Hypoglycemia, with decreased cerebrospinal fluid glucose, is common in children of less than five years, but is rarely found in older children. Cerebrospinal fluid protein is normal. Elevation of serum transaminases, hyperammonemia, and prolongation of the prothrombin time reflect hepatic damage. Bilirubin levels rise in a minority of patients. Hypocapnia, hyponatremia, hypokalemia, and ketosis are common. Elevation of plasma free fatty acid levels have been present whenever sought.

Deepening coma leading to death occurs in 25 to 80 per cent of patients. More recent reports indicate the lower mortality rates, perhaps because of improved management or because milder cases are being diagnosed. Severe neurologic sequelae, such as mental impairment, seizures, or hemiplegia, occur in some survivors.

Diagnosis. The diagnosis of Reye's syndrome is suggested by the clinical manifestations described above. Biopsy or autopsy demonstration of fatty infiltration of the liver can be considered as a confirmatory abnormality.

Treatment. Treatment is empirical. Hypoglycemia, acidosis, and electrolyte disturbances should be corrected. Enemas, neomycin and low protein intake as employed in hepatic encephalopathy are commonly used. Peritoneal dialysis and exchange transfusions have been used to correct refractory metabolic abnormalities and to correct clotting factor deficiencies. Corticosteroids, mannitol, and hyperventilation may be used to reduce intracranial pressure.

Alvord, E. C.: Acute disseminated encephalomyelitis and "allergic" neuroencephalopathies. *In* Vinken, P. J., and Bruyn, G. W. (eds.): Handbook of Clinical Neurology. New York, American Elsevier Publishing Company, 1970, Vol. 9, pp. 500–571.

Miller, H. G., Stanton, J. B., and Gibbons, J. L.: Para-infectious encephalomyelitis and related syndromes. Quart. J. Med. *25*:426, 1956.

Mowat, A. P.: Encephalopathy and fatty degeneration of viscera. Arch. Dis. Child., 48:411, 1973.

Reye, R. D. K., Morgan, G., and Baral, J.: Encephalopathy and fatty degeneration of the viscera: A disease entity in childhood. Lancet, 2:749, 1963.

Shiraki, H.: The comparative study of rabies post-vaccinal encephalomyelitis and demyelinating encephalomyelitides of unknown origin with special reference to the Japanese cases. *In* Bailey, O. T., and Smith, D. E. (eds.): The Central Nervous System: Some Experimental Models of Neurological Diseases. Baltimore, Williams & Wilkins Company, 1968, pp. 87–123.

ter Mullen, V., Käckell, Y., Müller, D., Katz, M., and Meyermann, R.: Isolation of infectious measles virus in measles encephalitis. Lancet, 2:1172, 1972.

SLOW INFECTIONS OF THE NERVOUS SYSTEM

Richard T. Johnson

398. INTRODUCTION

Recently, slow viral infections have been related to several chronic and subacute neurologic diseases in which clinical signs of infection are lacking and in which the pathologic changes are those of degenerative or demyelinative processes. The term slow infection was originally coined in the veterinary literature to describe several transmissible diseases of sheep. Two of these sheep diseases, *scrapie* and *visna*, are the prototypes of slow infections of the nervous system. Both these diseases are transmissible. After inoculation of sheep with tissue from an affected sheep, there is a latent period of one to four years during which the sheep appear well. This is followed by the insidious onset of neurologic signs which progress without fever from one to six months and lead inevitably to death. Scrapie is clinically characterized primarily by ataxia and visna by progressive paralysis. Pathologically the diseases are very different. The lesions of scrapie are confined to the nervous system, where there is marked proliferation of astrocytes and the degeneration of neurons with vacuolization of their cytoplasms. Inflammation and primary demyelination are not present. By contrast, central nervous system lesions of visna are characterized by marked inflammation and demyelination. The agents responsible for these two slow infections of sheep are also very different. The scrapie agent has been transmitted to a variety of other animals, but the agent does not cause cytopathic changes in cell culture, and no virus-like particles have been found in infectious tissue by electron microscopy. The infectivity of this tissue remains remarkably stable on exposure to physicochemical treatments which inactivate classic viruses. Furthermore, animals naturally or experimentally infected with scrapie fail to develop any evidence of an immune response against the agent. In contrast, the visna virus is an enveloped RNA virus. Although transmissible from sheep to sheep, it has not been transmitted to other animals but can be grown in a variety of tissue cultures. Of the four slow infections of the human central nervous system described below, kuru and Creutzfeldt-Jakob disease resemble scrapie pathologically, and the agents responsible for these diseases have properties similar to those described for the scrapie agent. Therefore scrapie, kuru, and Creutzfeldt-Jakob disease have been classified together as the subacute spongiform encephalopathies. Subacute sclerosing panencephalitis and progressive multifocal leukoencephalopathy, like visna, are due to classic viruses. These viruses have been visualized by electron microscopy, are antigenic in natural and experimental hosts, and can produce rapid cytolytic infection in some cell cultures even though they are capable of causing slow infections in man.

399. KURU

Kuru is an endemic disease of Melanesian tribal people inhabiting a remote area of the Eastern Highlands of central New Guinea. The disease has been seen only among the Fore linguistic group and several neighboring groups with whom the Fore have intermarried. However, within this limited area, kuru, until recently, was the most common cause of death. The disease predominantly affected adult women, but children over age five were also affected but without sexual predilection. Adult males were least involved. The disease begins insidiously with unsteadiness of stance and gait. A progressive symmetrical cerebellar ataxia develops over a period of months and follows a relentless, afebrile course until the patient is unable to make the slightest movement without violent ataxic tremors. Late in the course of the disease, abnormalities of extraocular movement and mental changes develop. The disease invariably leads to death in three to six months. Extensive laboratory examinations have failed to show any abnormalities, and the cerebrospinal fluid remains normal. Pathologic changes are confined to the brain where there is a marked increase of astrocytes and degeneration of neurons with vacuolization. The brain is diffusely affected, but the findings are most prominent in the cerebellum and pons and, to a lesser degree, in the hypothalamus and basal ganglia. Inflammation is not found.

Because of the similarities between kuru and scrapie in terms of epidemiology, clinical progression, and pathologic changes, brain tissue from patients dying of kuru was inoculated into a variety of primates for long-term observations. After incubation periods of 18 months to 4 years, a similar disease developed in chimpanzees, and this disease has subsequently been transmitted from chimpanzee to chimpanzee and to several other species of primates. The agent can be transmitted with serial dilutions, proving that it replicates within the primate host. However, like scrapie, the agent of kuru has not been seen by electron microscopy, does not induce cytopathic changes in cell culture, is resistant to physical and chemical treatments that usually inactivate viruses, and fails to evoke a demonstrable immune response in man or experimentally infected primates.

In recent years, there has been a striking decline in the incidence of kuru, particularly among children, in whom the disease has essentially disappeared. This decreasing incidence has been coincident with the suppression of cannibalism in this primitive culture, and there is considerable circumstantial evidence indicating that kuru was transmitted during the practice of ritual cannibalism.

400. CREUTZFELDT-JAKOB DISEASE

Creutzfeldt-Jakob disease is an uncommon form of rapidly progressive dementia accompanied by myoclonus and other neurologic signs. The disease usually develops between ages 40 and 65, is worldwide in distribution, and usually occurs sporadically, although a few familial cases have been reported. The dementia develops rapidly, so that deterioration from day to day or week to week is evident. Myoclonic jerks usually develop early in the disease, and often massive symmetrical myoclonic jerks of the limbs occur when the patient is startled by unexpected light or sounds. Pyramidal tract signs, cerebellar ataxia, visual disturbances, and muscle wasting with fasciculations are common but inconstant features. The disease is inexorably progressive, usually reducing the patient from good health to total helplessness or death in less than a year. The cerebrospinal fluid shows no abnormality; but the electroencephalogram becomes abnormal early in the disease, showing diffuse slowing with superimposed bursts of sharp waves.

Neuropathologic findings include diffuse loss of cortical neurons with a remarkable increase in fibrous astrocytes. Vacuoles are present in neurons and astrocytes, and this may give a spongiform appearance to the cerebral cortex. Inflammatory reactions and inclusion bodies are absent. Thus, despite clinical and epidemiologic differences, the pathologic findings in Creutzfeldt-Jakob disease are very similar to those of kuru and scrapie.

A similar disease develops in chimpanzees inoculated with brain tissue of most patients with Creutzfeldt-Jakob disease after an incubation period of about one year. The chimpanzees developed somnolence, ataxia, tremor, fasciculations, and intermittent jerking of the extremities. The pathologic changes in the brains resembled those of Creutzfeldt-Jakob disease. The disease has also been transmitted from chimpanzee to chimpanzee, to a variety of other primates, and to the domestic cat. Little information is available on the agent of Creutzfeldt-Jakob disease, but the absence of virus-like particles on electron microscopic examination of infectious tissues, the failure to demonstrate cytopathic changes in cell cultures, and the absence of a demonstrable immune response suggest that the agent is similar to those causing kuru and scrapie.

The natural mode of transmission is unknown, but the development of the disease in primates inoculated with brain tissue from several familial cases has raised the possibilities that the familial cases of disease may be dependent on genetically determined susceptibility to a common agent, vertical transmission, or common environmental or dietary factors in families.

401. SUBACUTE SCLEROSING PANENCEPHALITIS (Dawson's Encephalitis, Subacute Inclusion Body Encephalitis)

This is an uncommon, subacute encephalitis that usually occurs in children or young adults between the ages of 4 and 20 years. The onset is usually insidious and is characterized by deterioration in school work and behavioral disorders. This is followed in weeks or months by overt mental deterioration and neurologic signs, the most characteristic of which is myoclonus. The disease usually terminates after a third stage of stupor, blindness, dementia, and decorticate rigidity, which may last months to several years. Characteristically, the cerebrospinal fluid is under normal pressure and shows no pleocytosis, but an increased concentration in gamma globulin results in a first zone colloidal gold curve. During the stage of active myoclonus, the electroencephalogram usually shows a typical pattern of general suppression of activity, with periodic (8 to 15 seconds) synchronous bursts of high-voltage slow and sharp waves. The clinical course is usually characterized by progressive deterioration, but occasionally an apparent arrest of the disease process or even transient clinical improvement is seen.

Although the disease follows a protracted afebrile course, a viral cause has long been suspected because of the pathologic changes. Perivascular infiltrates of mononuclear cells are characteristic, and eosinophilic intranuclear inclusion bodies are found in neurons and glial cells. Because of these inclusions, a herpesvirus was long suspected of being the etiologic agent. However, electron microscope studies of cerebral biopsies show virus-like particles resembling the nucleocapsids of the measles-distemper group of paramyxoviruses. Astonishingly high levels of antibodies against measles virus can be demonstrated in the serums of most patients, and measles virus antigen is present in the brain. Nevertheless, the isolation of measles-like viruses from brains of patients with subacute sclerosing panencephalitis is difficult, requiring the establishment of cell cultures from brains of patients with the disease and subsequent cocultivation of these cultures with other cells. The measles virus associated with the disease is apparently defective.

The pathogenesis of subacute sclerosing panencephalitis is obscure. This disease bears little resemblance clinically or pathologically to the fulminating forms of measles virus infections, in which virus dissemination may lead to giant-cell pneumonia. Furthermore, it is quite distinct from parainfectious encephalomyelitis that occasionally complicates measles virus infections, in which acute neurologic disease occurs and perivascular demyelination is found in the brain and spinal cord. Epidemiologic studies have shown that subacute sclerosing panencephalitis is more common in males than females, in children of rural than of urban origin, and in patients with a history of measles during the first two years of life. These findings suggest that environmental factors and presence of residual transplacental passive immunity may play roles in inducing defective infection or precipitating disease.

Treatment of patients with antiviral agents and synthetic interferon inducers has been attempted, but without definite beneficial effects. It is not yet evident whether or not the measles vaccine has altered the incidence of the disease.

402. PROGRESSIVE MULTIFOCAL LEUKOENCEPHALOPATHY

This is a rare demyelinating disease of the central nervous system. It usually develops in patients having preexisting disorders of the reticuloendothelial system such as leukemia, lymphoma, or sarcoidosis, but has also developed in patients immunosuppressed therapeutically or after organ transplantation. Although the underlying systemic disorder may be of long standing, the neurologic abnormalities develop rather suddenly and follow a subacute progressive course until death. The findings usually suggest multifocal disease. Abnormalities of motor function, sensation, vision, or speech are common, and dementia frequently develops. The cerebrospinal fluid shows little if any abnormality, and the electroencephalogram shows only nonspecific slowing. Pathologic lesions in the brain consist of multiple foci of demyelination in various stages of evolution. Oligodendrocytes are depleted within the foci, but surrounding the foci they are enlarged and contain eosinophilic intranuclear inclusions. The astrocytes within the demyelinated areas are often bizarre and contain mitotic figures. Inflammatory cells are usually not prominent.

The presence of the inclusion bodies and the occurrence against a background of disorders associated with impaired immunologic responses led to speculation that the disease might be caused by a viral infection. Electron microscopic examination in almost all cases has shown particles in the oligodendrocyte inclusions resembling small papovaviruses. Two small deoxyribonucleic acid viruses related to simian-virus 40 have been isolated from brain tissue of patients dying from progressive multifocal leukoencephalopathy. The JC virus, a new human papovavirus to which the majority of people have antibody since childhood, appears to be the causative agent in most cases. Viruses antigenically indistinguishable from simian-virus 40 have been related to two cases. Neither of these viruses has been associated with any disease in man except progressive multifocal leukoencephalopathy. Therefore progressive multifocal leukoencephalopathy apparently results from opportunistic infection of the brain by normally nonpathogenic agents. The viruses appear to selectively infect and lyse oligodendrocytes, the glial cells which maintain the myelin sheaths, and cause demyelination. The disease occurs in patients with impaired cellular immune responses, but it is not known whether this disease represents a primary infection of an immunologically incompetent patient or whether it represents a reactivation of a latent or persistent papovavirus infection.

Evaluation of possible therapeutic agents has not been possible because of the rarity of cases and the infrequency of diagnosis during life.

403. OTHER NEUROLOGIC DISEASES

Since viruses can cause disease after a long incubation period, can produce disease with a subacute or relapsing course, and can give rise to noninflammatory pathologic changes, the possible role of slow or latent viral infection in a variety of neurologic diseases has been entertained.

In several chronic or relapsing inflammatory diseases of the nervous system, a viral cause has been suspected. *Chronic focal epilepsy* (epilepsia partialis continua, Kozhevnikov's epilepsy) is, in some cases, associated with a chronic focal inflammatory process in the brain. In the Soviet Union, this has been thought to represent a persistent focal infection with tick-borne viruses after acute encephalitis; and in several Soviet laboratories, tick-borne encephalitis virus has been isolated from surgically removed cerebral epileptogenic foci. No viruses have been isolated from similar cases in other countries. Chronic focal epilepsy can be a manifestation of focal disease processes such as neoplastic, vascular, or traumatic lesions, but chronic infection may play a role in some cases.

Recurrent acute meningitis or encephalitis occurs in three clinical syndromes of unknown cause in which latent viral infection has been suspected. *Mollaret's meningitis* is a rare, recurrent meningitis characterized by repeated attacks of headache, fever, and nuchal rigidity. Each attack is abrupt in onset and lasts for two to three days; the patient is entirely well between episodes. During attacks, the cerebrospinal fluid may contain large numbers of both polymorphonuclear and mononuclear cells and also large, poorly staining "epithelial cells," characteristic but not pathognomonic of this disease. More severe recurrent neurologic involvement can occur in *Behçet's syndrome* and in the *Vogt-Koyanagi-Harada syndrome.* Behçet's syndrome is a chronic disease characterized by recurrent oral and genital ulcers and inflammatory ocular lesions, usually taking the form of acute recurrent iritis. In about one quarter of the patients neurologic signs develop, consisting either of cranial nerve palsies, focal seizures, hemiparesis, or other focal signs or of severe depression of consciousness, coma, or meningeal signs, suggesting more diffuse neurologic involvement. Neurologic deficits usually remit and relapse but may be progressive. Neuropathologic findings include meningeal inflammatory reactions, perivascular inflammation, and focal areas of necrosis. The Vogt-Koyanagi-Harada or uveoencephalitic syndrome is characterized by depigmentation of skin and hair, inflammatory ocular lesions (usually consisting of iridocyclitis or exudative retinal detachment), and meningitis. Unlike Behçet's syndrome, neurologic involvement occurs in all cases, often precedes the ocular inflammation, and usually consists only of headache, nuchal rigidity, and a mononuclear cell pleocytosis. However, transient decrease in hearing and tinnitus may accompany the meningitis, or a severe encephalitis may develop, leaving permanent neurologic deficits. Neuropathologic findings have consisted only of a chronic arachnoiditis. Reports have been made of isolations of unidentified viruses from patients with Mollaret's, Behçet's, and Vogt-Koyanagi-Harada syndrome; but none of these claims have been entirely convincing. An allergic cause has also been postulated in each of these disorders, and consequently treatment with corticosteroids has been advocated.

Considerable interest in a possible viral cause of *multiple sclerosis* has been stimulated by epidemiologic data that indicate the role of a common exposure factor, serologic studies showing higher antibody levels against measles virus in patients with multiple sclerosis, observation of viral-like particles in brains, and unconfirmed claims of virus isolations. These data are still inconclusive. A notion that Parkinson's disease might have a viral cause has been entertained ever since the observation was made that a form of parkinsonism was a frequent sequela of encephalitis lethargica (von Economo's disease). Similarly, the possible role of a slow infection in amyotrophic lateral sclerosis and in a variety of other demyelinating and degenerative diseases has also been postulated. Although the spectrum of neurologic disease that can be potentially attributed to slow, latent, or chronic viral infections has greatly broadened in recent years, evidence is still scant for incriminating a transmissible agent in these chronic neurologic diseases.

Detels, R., Brody, J. A., McNew, J., and Edgar, A. H.: Further epidemiological studies of subacute sclerosing panencephalitis. Lancet, 2:11, 1973.

Freeman, J. M.: The clinical spectrum and early diagnosis of Dawson's encephalitis. Pediatrics, 75:590, 1969.

Johnson, R. T., and Herndon, R. M.: Virologic studies of multiple sclerosis and other chronic and relapsing neurological diseases. Prog. Med. Virol., in press.

Lampert, P. W., Gajdusek, D. C., and Gibbs, C. J., Jr.: Subacute spongiform virus encephalopathies. Scrapie, kuru, and Creutzfeldt-Jakob disease: A review. Am. J. Pathol., 68:626, 1972.

Narayan, O., Penney, J. B., Jr., Johnson, R. T., Herndon, R. M., and Weiner, L. P.: Etiology of progressive multifocal leukoencephalopathy: Identification of papovavirus. N. Engl. J. Med., 289:1278, 1973.

Roos, R., Gajdusek, D. C., and Gibbs, C. J., Jr.: The clinical characteristics of transmissible Creutzfeldt-Jakob disease. Brain, 96:1, 1973.

Section Fourteen. NUTRITIONAL DISORDERS OF THE NERVOUS SYSTEM

Pierre M. Dreyfus

404. INTRODUCTION

Malnutrition, undernutrition, and the deficiency of specific nutrients such as vitamins are known to affect normal function of some parts of the central and/or the peripheral nervous system. It is well established that an isolated or combined deficiency of vitamins B_1, B_6, B_{12}, niacin, pantothenic acid, and perhaps riboflavin can be associated with a variety of neurologic disorders. However, despite increasing knowledge regarding the role of these vitamins in general metabolism, the specific mechanisms by which a deficiency state affects the normal development and function of the nervous system remain essentially unknown.

Most of the neurologic disorders discussed in this section, although commonly associated with chronic alcoholism, have also been described in malnourished, chronically debilitated, nonalcoholic patients. The inveterate drinker is frequently the victim of a primary nutritional deficiency which alters the normal metabolic activity of the nervous system. During periods of heavy drinking, the chronic alcoholic patient may change the composition of his diet, sharply decreasing vitamin and other essential nutrient intake, because of decreased appetite. Vitamin absorption, intestinal transport, tissue storage, utilization, and conversion to metabolically active forms may be curtailed while the need for many vitamins and essential nutrients increases. In addition to causing abnormal vitamin metabolism, the prolonged and abusive intake of alcohol leads to a somewhat unusual and extreme state of nutritional imbalance characterized by an excess of carbohydrate, fatty acid, cholesterol, glycerol, glycogen, and calories combined with a severe deficiency of B vitamins and other essential nutrients. The chronic alcoholic patient may also suffer from a secondary nutritional deficiency which may be the result of a chronic illness, such as infection, anemia, or blood loss, which increases his over-all metabolic demands.

The various nutritional syndromes described in this section may present separately in relatively pure form, but more frequently they occur together in varying combinations, some more prevalent than others. It is not known why, under seemingly identical circumstances, one nutritionally depleted patient develops one or several neurologic syndromes whereas another emerges essentially unscathed. Basic constitutional and genetic differences combined with as yet unknown metabolic factors may underlie the individual response of patients to malnutrition and the chronic ingestion of alcohol.

Nutritional disorders of the nervous system are associated with one or more biochemical lesions which invariably antedate the appearance of symptoms and signs and histopathologic changes. These diseases all share the common neuropathologic attributes of other metabolic disorders of the nervous system by virtue of their predilection for specific areas or parts of the nervous system and because of the bilateral symmetry of the lesions.

405. NUTRITIONAL POLYNEUROPATHY (Dry Beriberi, Alcoholic Neuropathy)

Clinical Manifestations. Nutritional polyneuropathy, the most common of all the nutritional diseases of the nervous system, is characterized by progressive weakness and muscle wasting of varying degrees, involving, symmetrically, the legs more than the arms and the distal muscles more than the proximal ones. Weakness may be almost imperceptible or so severe that the legs are virtually paralyzed and the hands useless. Motor signs and sensory manifestations most frequently occur concomitantly. Abnormalities of sensation are usually striking. Patients complain of aching, coldness, hotness, deadness, numbness, prickliness, and tenderness, most commonly in the calves, on the plantar surfaces of the feet, and in the fingers. Deep pressure or light touch may be extremely unpleasant. In the most severe cases, the muscles become wasted, atrophic, flabby, and tender, and the skin may be dry, red, and shiny. Excessive perspiration of feet and hands is occasionally noted. The deep tendon reflexes, which may be exaggerated in some patients at the onset of the illness, are usually greatly diminished or totally abolished. The sensory loss is symmetrical, most severe distally, and diminishes gradually over more proximal parts; all modalities are involved, some more than others. On rare occasions, severe burning, shooting, lightning, or "electric" types of pain can occur in the absence of clear-cut signs of neuropathy. The term "burning feet syndrome" has been applied to this variety of neuropathic disorder. This syndrome has been encountered in inmates of prison camps, chronic alcoholics, and patients undergoing dialysis for chronic renal failure. In rare instances, nutritional polyneuropathy may be accompanied by vertigo, deafness, hoarseness, dysphagia, and amblyopia.

The mode of evolution and the severity of nutritional polyneuropathy can be quite variable. Usually the onset is insidious, and the progression is slow. Sometimes the course is rapid and abrupt, crippling the patient in a matter of weeks. Recovery requires months and is sometimes incomplete. A temporary worsening of paresthesias and of weakness may follow the start of therapy. In early or mild cases, a prolonged nerve conduction velocity may be the only objective manifestation of the disease. Examination of the cerebrospinal fluid reveals a normal level or a very slight elevation of the protein content.

Pathology. The salient pathologic changes suggest segmental demyelination of peripheral nerves involving distal parts to a greater degree than proximal ones. Occasionally dorsal root ganglia reveal a loss of nerve cells, and axonal reaction may be seen in some of the anterior horn cells of the spinal cord. In patients afflicted with hoarseness and dysphagia, degeneration of the vagus nerve and of the paravertebral sympathetic chain has been observed. It has been speculated that in nutritional polyneuropathy, primary axonal degeneration or a process of "dying back" results in destruction of both the axon and myelin sheaths in the periphery of the largest and longest nerve fibers.

Pathogenesis and Treatment. Nutritional depletion probably alters the normal metabolism of peripheral nerves in several different ways. Both experimental and clinical studies support the view that a deficiency of several of the B vitamins can result in neuropathy. Certain neuropathies respond to the administration of thiamin alone. Recent studies have shown decreased levels of thiamin in the blood, urine, and muscles of patients afflicted with alcoholic neuropathy. Prior to nutritional replenishment, the activity of blood transketolase is usually reduced, and blood pyruvate levels, measured before and after the administration of glucose, may be elevated. The fact that biochemical evidence of thiamin deficiency in nutritional polyneuropathy cannot always be obtained is explained by the slow evolution of this disorder. Whereas the biochemical lesion antedates all clinical manifestations of neuropathy, the latter linger on for many months after the metabolic insult has been removed. A deficiency of pyridoxine has also been blamed for nutritional polyneuropathy. A neuropathic disorder has been observed in patients who were given desoxypyridoxine, a metabolic antagonist of vitamin B_6. The neuropathy that develops in the course of isoniazid (isonicotinic acid hydrazide, INH) therapy can be reversed by pyridoxine alone. Isoniazid causes a deficiency of the essential cofactor pyridoxal phosphate by interfering with phosphorylation of the vitamin. Pyridoxal phosphate is an essential cofactor for a number of enzymatic reactions known to participate in protein metabolism. The specific role of these enzymatic reactions in the metabolism of peripheral nerves remains to be defined. A deficiency of pyridoxal phosphate results in the inadequate synthesis of nicotinic acid from tryptophan. Reduced blood levels of nicotinic acid and nicotinamide have been measured in some patients with nutritional polyneuropathy. Pantothenic acid deficiency may also be involved in the production of some forms of nutritional polyneuropathy. It has been claimed that the administration of pantothenic acid relieves the burning feet syndrome, regardless of its cause.

406. WERNICKE-KORSAKOFF SYNDROME

Of all the disorders of the central nervous system associated with the protracted and abusive intake of alcohol and nutritional depletion, Wernicke's disease and Korsakoff's psychosis are the most frequent. The term "cerebral beriberi" has sometimes been applied to these conditions.

Clinical Manifestation. *Wernicke's disease* is characterized by disturbed ocular motility, ataxia, impaired mentation, and, occasionally, polyneuropathy. The patient may complain of diplopia and unsteadiness of gait, but is usually unaware of his deficit. On examination, bilateral weakness or paralysis of the external recti muscles and paralysis of lateral conjugate gaze are common. Horizontal nystagmus is almost always present, although it sometimes cannot be elicited until abducens function has improved. Vertical nystagmus, particularly on upward gaze, is frequently present. Occasionally there are ptosis, complete paralysis of eye movements, miosis and, very rarely, unreactive pupils. The ataxia, which is almost always present, affects stance and gait primarily. It may be so slight that only special tests for cerebellar function betray its existence. When it is severe, the patient cannot stand or walk without help. Advanced polyneuropathy usually masks cerebellar ataxia. Intention tremor is less common and tends to affect the legs more than the arms. Scanning speech is a rarity. A mild to severe mixed sensory-motor polyneuropathy exists in at least 50 per cent of cases. When first seen, the patient with Wernicke's disease may display symptoms and signs attributable to alcohol withdrawal: i.e., delirium, tremulousness, confusion, agitation, hallucinosis, altered sense perception, and autonomic overactivity. More often, he lacks spontaneity, is apathetic, listless, indifferent, disoriented in time and place, and tends to misidentify objects and people around him. Dull mentation, impaired retentive memory, and general lack of grasp are more common than drowsiness or unconsciousness. With improved nutrition and supplemental thiamin the patient becomes more alert, more attentive, and more readily testable. He may then display a characteristic amnestic confabulatory syndrome known as *Korsakoff's psychosis.* In addition, the patient with Korsakoff's psychosis reveals a number of abnormalities of cognitive function. He may have a great deal of difficulty in forming visual and verbal abstractions. His capacity to shift from one mental set to another and his ability to learn are defective. Perceptual function and concept formation are affected. However, the most prominent and serious mental abnormality seen in Korsakoff's psychosis is the disordered memory function that renders some patients incapable of performing any but the simplest tasks. Recent retentive memory and the ability to learn newly presented material are strikingly impaired. An extensive retrograde amnesia covering a variable period of time is also common. Finally, the patient confabulates and fabricates fictitious stories. Confabulation is by no means unique to Korsakoff's psychosis and tends to disappear in the chronic stages of the illness.

Features of Wernicke's disease and Korsakoff's psychosis are frequently encountered in the same patient. In many instances of Korsakoff's psychosis, slight, residual nystagmus and ataxia may be detected years later. The Wernicke-Korsakoff syndrome may be complicated by other stigmata of chronic malnutrition, including cirrhosis of the liver, anemia, and mucocutaneous lesions of various types. Many patients suffer from postural hypotension, dyspnea, and tachycardia, but full-blown beriberi heart disease is rare. The Wernicke-Korsakoff syndrome usually begins abruptly. Some degree of recovery is the rule, except in the most advanced cases and in those complicated by other illnesses. During the acute stage of the disease the mortality may be as high as 17 per cent. The ocular manifestations, except for nystagmus, respond promptly and dramatically to vitamin therapy. Ataxia improves more slowly, and incomplete recovery occurs in over half the patients; complete recovery from Korsakoff's psychosis occurs in less than one third of patients. The recovered patient usually shows permanent amnesia for the acute phase of the illness.

Pathology. The pathologic alterations that affect the cerebrum and the brainstem are remarkably constant. They almost always involve structures in a bilaterally symmetrical manner. Lesions are invariably seen in the mamillary bodies and the terminal fornices. Lesions in the periaqueductal region of the midbrain, in the floor of the fourth ventricle, in the vicinity of the dorsal motor nucleus of the vagus, and in the anterior superior parts of the cerebellar vermis probably account for the paralysis of gaze, nystagmus, and ataxia. The lesions involving thalamic nuclei (anteromedial, lateral dorsal, and pulvinar) and the hypothalamus and those seen in the mamillary bodies and fornices may underlie some of the psychologic abnormalities, particularly the amnestic syndrome. Microscopically, the lesions consist of necrosis of both nerve cells and myelinated structures. A striking glial reaction involves the center of the lesion. Both endothelial proliferation and hemorrhages are found, but the latter are usually fresh and may represent a nonspecific, terminal change. In the vermis of the cerebellum the principal changes consist of a loss of Purkinje cells and gliosis of the molecular layer of the cortex.

Pathogenesis. There is now an overwhelming body of evidence that favors a specific lack of vitamin B_1 (cocarboxylase) as the main nutritional factor in the Wernicke-Korsakoff syndrome. Most patients give a history of inadequate nutrition and weight loss. Other stigmata of malnutrition, such as loss of subcutaneous fat and skin turgor, mucocutaneous manifestations, and an enlarged liver, are frequent. Clinical studies have shown that the continued intake of alcohol is not followed by aggravation of symptoms, provided adequate nutritional repletion is undertaken promptly. Thiamin alone, given orally or parenterally, can dramatically reverse some of the symptoms and signs. Victor and Adams maintained patients with Wernicke's disease on either glucose or a boiled rice diet containing no vitamins for brief periods, then gave them B vitamins selectively. Ophthalmoplegia, apathy, listlessness, and inattentiveness began to improve within a few hours and cleared completely within a few days after thiamin had been added to the regimen. Nystagmus and ataxia diminished, but Korsakoff's psychosis did not improve significantly. Other B vitamins were ineffective. The improvement of neurologic signs can be closely correlated with levels of blood transketolase activity, which are reduced prior to thiamin administration and increase toward normal with clinical improvement, sometimes within four to five hours after the injection of 25 to 50 mg of thiamin.

Although most commonly associated with chronic alcoholism, Wernicke-Korsakoff syndrome has been observed in clinical settings totally unrelated to abusive drinking. It has been described as a complication of chronic hemodialysis, pernicious vomiting of pregnancy, thyrotoxicosis, and gastric carcinoma.

407. NUTRITIONAL AMBLYOPIA (Tobacco-Alcohol Amblyopia, Nutritional Retrobulbar Neuropathy)

Clinical Manifestations. A remarkably uniform and stereotyped disorder of vision is encountered occasionally in persons who are chronically undernourished. Characteristically it evolves slowly and subacutely, the mode of onset of symptoms being much the same from patient to patient. Visual impairment usually starts insidiously and reaches a maximum in several weeks to months. Blurred or dim vision, difficulty in reading, photophobia, and retrobulbar discomfort on moving the eyes are the common presenting complaints. On examination, the patient has bilaterally symmetrical central, centrocecal, or paracentral scotomata. Ophthalmoscopic changes are restricted at first to slight redness of the temporal margins of the optic discs; minimal pallor is observed at a later stage. Often, no abnormality is visible. The peripheral visual fields are usually intact. The visual disorder is, to a large extent, reversible with improvement of nutrition.

Pathology. The pathologic change in nutritional amblyopia consists of bilaterally symmetrical loss of myelinated fibers in the central parts of the optic nerves, chiasm, and optic tracts, corresponding in location to the papillomacular bundle. In severe cases, the retina loses macular ganglion cells, probably secondary to the "zonal" destruction of medullated fibers in the retrobulbar parts of the optic nerve.

Pathogenesis. This type of visual disturbance has been encountered in undernourished populations all over the world. It is commonly seen during famine, and among civilian and military prisoners of war. It is endemic in certain parts of Africa, Asia, and South America. Among the more privileged populations in the western world, the syndrome is seen in persons chronically addicted to alcohol or, occasionally, to tobacco, who neglect their nutrition. A similar syndrome also occurs as a complication of vitamin B_{12} deficiency and diabetes mellitus, as well as in patients treated with isoniazid for tuberculosis. This visual disorder accompanies other neurologic syndromes believed to have a nutritional cause, such as *Strachan's syndrome,* in which amblyopia is combined with paresthesias of the feet, hands, trunk, and, occasionally, face, loss of reflexes, dizziness, deafness, hoarseness, spasticity, ataxia, and a variety of mucocutaneous lesions (genital dermatitis, corneal degeneration, glossitis, and stomatitis). In the chronic alcoholic patient, amblyopia may occur in conjunction with Wernicke's disease, cerebellar degeneration, Marchiafava-Bignami's disease, and peripheral neuropathy. In recent years, a nutritional deficiency rather than a toxicity has been held responsible for so-called tobacco-alcohol amblyopia. Detailed clinical and pathologic studies fail to distinguish this type of amblyopia from nutritional amblyopia. In clinical experiments, patients with amblyopia continued their usual consumption of alcohol and tobacco, but ate an adequate diet supplemented by B vitamins. All showed some recovery of visual acuity and a reduction in the size of the scotomata. As yet, the metabolic aberration or specific vitamin deficiency responsible for the development of amblyopia has not been defined. A lack of vitamin B_{12}, thiamin, riboflavin, and pyridoxine or a failure in the detoxification of cyanide present in tobacco smoke has been implicated in the genesis of the syndrome. Except for isolated findings of reduced serum vitamin B_{12} levels, the abnormal urinary excretion of methylmalonic acid and low levels of blood transketolase activity, no specific biochemical abnormalities have been reported in cases of amblyopia.

Treatment. Treatment with oral or parenteral B vitamins and improved nutrition are usually followed by improvement, depending upon the severity of the amblyopia and its duration before therapy is instituted.

408. CEREBELLAR CORTICAL DEGENERATION

Cerebellar cortical degeneration, or parenchymatous cerebellar degeneration, has often been referred to as alcoholic cerebellar degeneration, although well documented instances of cerebellar cortical degeneration have occurred as a result of chronic nutritional depletion not attributable to alcohol. This disorder can be set apart from all other known forms of acquired or familial cerebellar degeneration because of the uniformity of the clinical and pathologic manifestations. The clinical and pathologic findings are discussed in Ch. 431 to 440.

A substantial body of evidence favors the contention that cerebellar degeneration is due to nutritional factors. The history of chronic alcoholic patients is admittedly unreliable, yet most admit improper eating habits. Many patients with cortical cerebellar degeneration give a history of progressive weight loss before the onset of their symptoms. Signs of malnutrition are common, and the cerebellar syndrome frequently occurs in conjunction with cirrhosis and other nutritional complications of alcoholism. Furthermore, a number of nonalcoholic patients develop cortical cerebellar degeneration in the setting of other diseases associated with nutritional depletion, such as pellagra, amebiasis, and protracted vomiting. In general, improved nutrition and supplementary B vitamins result in some degree of improvement of ataxia.

409. CENTRAL PONTINE MYELINOLYSIS

Central pontine myelinolysis is a relatively rare disease characterized by demyelination of the central portion of the pons. It was described originally in patients afflicted with chronic alcoholism and malnutrition but has since been encountered in nonalcoholic patients who were nutritionally deprived. The illness affects adults mainly, but has been reported in children; males and females are equally afflicted. Although the precise clinical course has not yet been defined, the principal neurologic abnormalities are progressive weakness of facial muscles and tongue, causing severe impairment of speech and deglutition. In a number of cases, pseudobulbar phenomena such as emotional lability and pathologic crying have been noted. Quadriparesis at the onset of the illness usually leads to a flaccid and areflexic quadriplegia with Babinski signs. Lack of response to painful stimuli and absence of corneal reflexes are said to be common. Urinary incontinence, decerebrate posture, and respiratory paralysis have been reported in isolated cases. The illness evolves rapidly over a period of two to three weeks, usually ending in coma and eventual death; slow and partial recovery has been observed in rare instances. Examination of the cerebrospinal fluid is unremarkable.

Pathologic examination reveals a focus of demyelination, variable in size and extent, involving the center of the basal portion of the mid and upper pons. Axis cylinders, nerve cells, and blood vessels are relatively well preserved. An appropriate glial and phagocytic reaction is seen within the lesions. Vascular or inflammatory changes are absent. The clinical symptoms and signs depend upon the size of the lesion and, in general, correlate with its anatomic localization.

The pathogenesis of this curious disorder has been much debated, toxic and nutritional factors being the causes most frequently cited. The lesion has been found at postmortem examination in patients suffering from alcoholism, other forms of chronic malnutrition, neoplasia, renal disease, hepatic insufficiency, and a variety of infectious processes. To date, no biochemical data have been obtained.

410. MARCHIAFAVA-BIGNAMI DISEASE

Marchiafava-Bignami disease is among the rarest disorders complicating chronic alcoholism. Few cases have been examined in detail, and it is difficult to state the precise nature of the clinical manifestations. The disease affects males of middle age predominantly. The course is variable; it may evolve over a period of a few days or several months. Complete recovery, although rare, has been documented. The patients are agitated, confused, and have hallucinations (visual, auditory, and gustatory), disturbance of memory, negativism, impaired judgment, and progressive dementia. Neurologic symptoms and signs suggest bilateral involvement of frontal lobes and include disturbance of language, gait and motor skills, seizures, incontinence, rooting, grasping, sucking, and delayed initiation of action. Tremulousness of the hands and dysarthria have been reported.

Pathologically, Marchiafava-Bignami disease is characterized by symmetrical zones of demyelination affecting the central parts of the corpus callosum, beginning in the most anterior parts and extending caudally. Similar changes affect the central parts of the anterior commissure, the optic chiasm and tracts, and, in severe cases, the central white matter of the frontal lobes. In zones of demyelination, axis cylinders tend to be preserved. Occasionally, there are extensive tissue destruction and cavitation. The degree of glial reaction in these areas depends on the chronicity of the process.

Originally, it was assumed that the disease occurred exclusively in males of Italian descent who consumed excessive amounts of crude red wine. The illness has since been encountered in patients of varied ancestry, some of whom were addicted to other types of alcoholic beverages. The characteristic pathologic changes of Marchiafava-Bignami disease have been encountered in conjunction with Wernicke's disease and nutritional amblyopia as well as in malnourished, nonalcoholic patients. It is probable that Marchiafava-Bignami disease is yet another example of a nutritionally determined disease entity characterized by symmetrical and zonal demyelination.

411. VITAMIN B_{12} DEFICIENCY

Definition. Insufficient absorption of vitamin B_{12} from the gastrointestinal tract can result in a subacute degeneration of the spinal cord, optic nerves, cerebral white matter, and peripheral nerves. Although the neurologic manifestations of vitamin B_{12} deficiency are frequently associated with a macrocytic anemia (pernicious anemia), the latter is not always present. Neurologic symptoms develop in approximately 80 per cent of patients between the ages of 25 and 75 years afflicted with pernicious anemia. They rarely occur as a result of secondary vitamin B_{12} deficiency complicating fish tapeworm *(Diphyllobothrium latum)* infestation, sprue, vegetarianism, or gastrointestinal surgery. (This subject is also dealt with in Ch. 731.)

Clinical Manifestations. Symptoms and signs of spinal cord involvement *(combined system disease)* constitute the most common neurologic manifestations, and their mode of onset and progression is remarkably uniform. Symmetrical progressive paresthesias of the feet or hands in the form of numbness, tingling, burning, tightness and stiffness, and a feeling of generalized weakness constitute the most frequent initial symptoms. Vague asthenia and lameness progress to a measurable weakness and stiffness of the legs and an unsteadiness of gait that tends to be worse in the dark. The lower limbs may give way unexpectedly. The hands may be stiff and clumsy. When untreated, the illness progresses slowly and relentlessly. Spasticity, ataxia, and paraplegia ensue, often followed by bowel and bladder dysfunction. In the early stages of the disease, examination of the patient often reveals a few objective changes, but eventually signs of disturbed peripheral nerve and posterior and lateral column function become readily apparent. Diminution or loss of position and vibratory sense involves the legs, the hands, and, occasionally, the trunk, and tends to be pronounced. Pain, temperature, and tactile sensation are sometimes blunted over the distal parts of the legs in a pattern suggestive of peripheral nerve involvement. The motor examination reveals weak and, later, spastic legs and extensor plantar responses. The activity of the deep tendon reflexes is variable and appears to depend upon the severity of the illness. The knee jerks are often hyperactive and the ankle jerks absent. In advanced cases, all stretch reflexes may be diminished or absent, but may return when vitamin therapy has been promptly instituted. Psychologic symptoms range from apathy, irritability, and suspiciousness to confusion and dementia, and at times are the presenting neurologic abnormality. On rare occasions, failing vision caused by symmetrical centrocecal scotomata may be the presenting neurologic symptom of vitamin B_{12} deficiency.

Pathology. The lesions associated with subacute combined degeneration involve in sequence the posterior columns, the lateral columns, and the cerebral white matter. The earliest visible change consists of swelling of individual myelinated nerve fibers in small foci. These lesions subsequently coalesce into large, irregular, spongy, honeycomb-like zones of demyelination. Fibers with the largest diameter are predominantly affected. Axis cylinders tend to be spared. Myelin destruction frequently begins in the cervical and upper thoracic segments of the cord, spreading axially to involve other segments. The cerebral white matter is affected last. The large fibers of the peripheral nerves may show minimal loss of myelin.

Diagnosis. A number of diseases other than vitamin B_{12} deficiency affect the posterior and lateral columns of the spinal cord, the most important being multiple sclerosis, tumors, cervical spondylosis, syphilitic meningomyelitis, and familial spastic paraplegia. These entities can usually be differentiated from one another clinically, but ancillary examinations such as myelography and special tests involving the cerebrospinal fluid may be necessary to establish a correct diagnosis. In B_{12} deficiency of the nervous system, the cerebrospinal fluid is usually normal. The electroencephalogram is often abnormal. The serum vitamin B_{12} content correlates well with the severity of the neurologic impairment and is invariably low in untreated cases. The Schilling test, using radioactive cyanocobalamin, is always positive, and gastric achlorhydria can be demonstrated in almost every instance. Blood and bone marrow examinations are of limited value, particularly when the patient has been treated with folic acid, which corrects the anemia but not the neurologic manifestations. The urinary excretion of methylmalonic acid, an intermediary metabolite in the conversion of propionic acid to succinic acid, is a sensitive indicator of vitamin B_{12} deficiency, but its relation to the lesions in the nervous system is as yet unknown.

Pathogenesis. The pathogenesis of the neurologic manifestations of vitamin B_{12} deficiency is unknown, although it probably differs from the biochemical lesion affecting the hematopoietic system, because the neurologic manifestations are independent of the anemia and may appear when folic acid corrects the anemia. The specific biochemical role of vitamin B_{12} in the nervous system has not yet been elucidated. It is an essential cofactor for at least two enzyme systems which exist in mammalian tissue, including brain: (1) methylmalonyl-CoA isomerase, which converts methylmalonyl-CoA to succinyl-CoA, a step in the utilization of propionic acid, and (2) methylfolate-H_4 methyltransferase, which is responsible for the synthesis of methionine from homocysteine. In experimentally induced vitamin B_{12} deficiency, the activity of both of these enzyme systems is reduced in brain. These enzymes may be essential to the maintenance of the myelin sheath. Recently it has been shown that sural nerve specimens obtained from patients with pernicious anemia incorporate radioactively labeled propionate into abnormal fatty acids that have been identified as C_{15} branched-chain and C_{17} odd-chain acids. The presence of these abnormal fatty acids may explain, in part, the structural changes observed in central and peripheral myelin. An experimental approach to the pathogenesis of the neurologic manifestations of vitamin B_{12} deficiency in animals has been hampered by the absence of white-matter lesions in deficient animals.

Treatment. Prompt initiation of therapy is of the utmost importance, because the early neurologic manifestations can be rapidly and completely reversed. The greatest degree of improvement is achieved in patients treated within three months of onset of symptoms, although variable degrees of amelioration can be attained after longer untreated periods (six to twelve months). In the first two weeks, daily intramuscular injections of 50 μg of cyanocobalamin, or an equivalent amount of liver USP, should be administered. During the next two months, 100 μg of cyanocobalamin should be injected twice a week. For the remainder of his life, the patient should receive a minimum of 100 μg intramuscularly every month to prevent a relapse that might be caused by metabolic stress such as systemic illness or surgery. The administration of oral vitamin preparations containing folic acid must be avoided for patients with pernicious anemia, because folic acid may actually precipitate neurologic complications.

PELLAGRA AND PROTEIN-CALORIE DEFICIENCY

These entities are described in Ch. 715 and 719.

Denny-Brown, D.: Neurological conditions resulting from prolonged and severe dietary restriction. Medicine, 26:41, 1947.

Dreyfus, P. M., and Geel, S. E.: Vitamin and nutritional deficiencies. *In* Albers, R. W., Siege, G. J., Katzmann, R., and Agranoff, B. W. (eds.): Basic Neurochemistry. Boston, Little, Brown & Company, 1972, p. 517.

Gyorgy, P., and Pearson, W. N.: The Vitamins. New York, Academic Press, 1967.

Mayer, R. F., and Garcia-Mullin, R.: Peripheral nerve and muscle disorders associated with alcoholism. *In* Kissin, B., and Begleiter, H. (eds.): The Biology of Alcoholism. New York, Plenum Press, 1972, Chap. 2.

Pant, S. S., Asbury, A. K., and Richardson, E. P., Jr.: The myelopathy of pernicious anemia—a neuropathological reappraisal. Acta Neurol. Scand., 44 (Suppl. 35), 1968.

Victor, M.: The effects of nutritional deficiency on the nervous system. A comparison with effects of carcinoma. *In* Brain, R. L., and Norris, F. H., Jr. (eds.): The Remote Effects of Cancer on the Nervous System. New York, Grune & Stratton, 1965.

Victor, M., and Adams, R. D.: The effects of alcohol upon the nervous system. Am. Res. Ment. Dis. Proc., 32:526, 1953.

Victor, M., Adams, R. D., and Collins, G. H.: The Wernicke-Korsakoff Syndrome, Philadelphia, F. A. Davis Company, 1971.

Wolstenholme, J. E. W.: Thiamine Deficiency: Biochemical Lesions and Their Clinical Significance. Boston, Little, Brown & Company, 1967.

Section Fifteen. THE DEMYELINATING DISEASES

Labe C. Scheinberg

412. INTRODUCTION: THE BIOLOGY OF MYELIN

Demyelination or myelin breakdown may be a secondary feature of many disorders of the nervous system such as infections, intoxications, degenerations, vascular lesions, trauma, or deficiency states. However, what concerns us here are the demyelinating diseases, in which the myelin is primarily affected. These have as a common feature the selective involvement of the myelin sheaths with relative sparing of the axons. The distribution of the lesions is random and the cause is unknown. Electrophysiologic studies of the axon have not been made in these diseases; the criteria for the functional and structural integrity of the axon are usually those established by light microscopy. Recently biopsy material of chronic areas of demyelination in the cerebral cortex and subcortical white matter has been studied by means of electron microscopy. These areas reveal denuded axons, vacuolization of the endoplasmic reticulum of oligodendrocytes, fibrous astrocytosis, and evidence of remyelination.

The devastating consequences of myelin breakdown indicate the vital importance of this structure. Recent work has provided much new information about the formation, structure, chemistry, and metabolism of myelin. There is also much new information about its pathology, and many studies have been made of experimental demyelinating disorders.

The neuroglia, namely the oligodendrocyte and astrocyte, are now recognized as more than supporting elements in the brain. They appear to participate in myelin formation, transport of material to the neurons, and the maintenance of the neurons' ionic environment.

The formation of myelin in both the central and peripheral nervous system follows a similar pattern. Central myelin is formed by an extension of the external plasma membrane of the oligodendrocyte wrapping the axons, whereas peripheral myelin is formed by the extension of the Schwann cell membrane. This wrapping produces a structure comprised of layers of concentric, tightly packed membranes of uniform thickness. If one examines the C fibers of the peripheral nerve with the electron microscope, one sees the axon-myelin relationship in its simplest form. The individual membranes of the Schwann cell and the axon membrane of the C fiber each represent "unit membranes," which are equivalent to the plasma membranes of the cells. The unit membrane of the Schwann cell or oligodendrocyte closes upon itself to form the major and minor period lines of myelin. The internal surface becomes apposed to form the dark major line, and the external surfaces give rise to the intraperiod line. The results of studies employing x-ray diffraction, electron microscopy, and lipid analyses suggest that each unit membrane consists of a sandwich of a bimolecular lipid leaflet between parallel layers of hydrated protein, in close contact with the polar groups of the lipids. The lipids that make up this leaflet appear to be interdigitated molecules of cerebroside, phospholipid, and cholesterol. Detailed chemical analysis of myelin reveals protein (primarily proteolipid protein) 22 per cent of dry weight, and lipid 78 per cent of dry weight. The lipids are in approximately equal molar ratios of cholesterol and phospholipids with about one half as much galactolipid. The lipids in the myelin sheath, once deposited at the time of its formation, undergo little subsequent turnover. The biologic half-life of cholesterol in myelin is about one year, compared to about ten days in other biologic membranes.

The myelin sheath is a compact, highly organized membrane structure that must be regarded as one of the more permanent tissue elements of the body. However, myelin should not be considered as metabolically inactive, because white matter accounts for about 30 per cent of total cerebral oxygen consumption and the glial cells utilize about two thirds of this.

THE DEMYELINATING DISORDERS

413. INTRODUCTION

The foregoing considerations suggest that demyelination must be considered as a basic disorder of the oligodendrocyte or the Schwann cell. To consider demyelination solely as myelin breakdown, ignoring the fact that the myelin lamellae are an integral part of the parent glial cell, may be contradictory to the pathogenesis. The etiologic agent may attack either the perikaryon of the glial cell or its plasma membrane to produce demyelination.

Prior to a consideration of the pathogenesis of demyelinative disorders, one must make some attempt to classify the varied primary disorders of myelin. In 1957 Poser suggested classification into two basic types. One, a so-called "myelinoclastic" or demyelinating type, includes disorders in which myelin forms normally to a certain age and then for unknown reasons breaks down. This includes the most common demyelinating disease, multiple sclerosis, and also acute disseminated encephalomyelitis and certain other disorders. The other, the "dysmyelinative" type, includes disorders in which a presumed familial inborn error of metabolism results in defective myelin formation. The category includes the so-called leukodystrophies or some of the diffuse scleroses and lipidoses of the nervous system and the aminoacidurias resulting from genetic enzymatic disorders.

Pathogenesis. In most demyelinating disorders, the cause remains unknown. Demyelination is the typical response of white matter to noxious stimuli not severe enough to cause complete necrosis of the tissue, and almost any infectious, nutritional, vascular, or toxic disorder can result in demyelination. At present there is insufficient evidence to incriminate any one cause. Some workers interpret present evidence as supporting most strongly an allergic basis for most of the primary demyelinating disorders, with genetic and geographic factors influencing susceptibility, whereas others favor a viral cause based on epidemiologic, electron microscopic, and tissue culture studies. Autoradiographic studies in experimental allergic encephalomyelitis, using tritiated precursors of DNA, RNA, and protein, have shown a rise in circulating plasma-like cells prior to onset of neurologic signs. Supernatant from cultures of these cells produces demyelination in tissue culture of rat cerebellum similar to that produced by serum from multiple sclerosis patients.

The strongest stimulus for suspecting allergic factors in the pathogenesis of the demyelinating diseases lies in the similarity of their pathologic changes to those of rabies encephalomyelitis. Rivers and co-workers in 1933 showed that multiple injections of normal rabbit brain tissue in monkeys resulted in encephalomyelitis with lesions similar to those seen in rabies postvaccinal encephalomyelitis. This was followed by the extensive investigations of Kabat, Wolf, and co-workers in the 1940's, who demonstrated that experimental allergic encephalomyelitis (EAE) could be produced in monkeys by a few injections of adult homologous, heterologous, or autologous central nervous system tissue mixed with paraffin oil and killed mycobacteria (Freund's adjuvant). White matter appeared more encephalitogenic than gray, whereas peripheral nerve and fetal (unmyelinated) brain were ineffectual as encephalitogens. EAE is not transferable to other animals by serum, although the serum contains complement-fixing antibodies to brain. The pathologic change is primarily in the white matter of the central nervous system, with perivascular and meningeal inflammation and demyelination. These findings are in many instances indistinguishable from those in certain human demyelinating disorders.

TABLE 1. Primary Disorders of Myelin

A. Demyelinating (myelinoclastic or leukoencephalopathic): breakdown of normally constituted myelin
   1. Postimmunization encephalomyelitis (smallpox and rabies vaccination, other immunizations)
   2. Parainfectious encephalomyelitis (postinfectious, postexanthematous, etc.)
   3. Acute necrotizing hemorrhagic encephalomyelitis (rare)
   4. Multiple sclerosis (disseminated sclerosis) and possible variants, including:
      a. Acute disseminated encephalomyelitis
      b. Optic and retrobulbar neuritis
      c. Transverse myelitis, including necrotizing myelopathy
      d. Neuromyelitis optica (Devic's)
      e. Transitional sclerosis
   5. Diffuse sclerosis (Schilder's cerebral sclerosis)
   6. Concentric sclerosis (Balo's) (rare)
   7. Progressive multifocal leukoencephalopathy (viral)
   8. Subacute sclerosing panencephalitis (viral)
   9. Central pontine myelinolysis (nutritional deficiency?) (see Ch. 409)
   10. Progressive subcortical encephalopathy (Binswanger's disease, vascular)
B. Dysmyelinating (leukodystrophic): Failure to form normally constituted myelin, possibly secondary to genetically determined errors of myelin anabolism
   1. Simple storage type (metachromatic leukodystrophy, glial insufficiency type of sulfatidosis)
   2. Sudanophilic type (Pelizaeus-Merzbacher disease)
   3. Globoid cell type (Krabbe's disease)
   4. Spongy degeneration of white matter (spongy sclerosis or Canavan's disease)
   5. Other lipidoses (Tay-Sachs disease, Gaucher's disease, gargoylism, etc.)
   6. Aminoacidurias (phenylketonuria, maple syrup urine disease, etc.)

This pioneering work has been followed by genetic, immunologic, biochemical, and ultrastructural investigations. It has been shown that there are variations in susceptibility to EAE among various species and strains within species. Other workers have successfully transferred EAE by means of sensitized lymphoid cells in isologous (inbred) strains. Finally, workers have found that serum from EAE animals or from some patients with multiple sclerosis causes destruction of myelin in cultures of transplanted brain tissue.

The nature of the encephalitogen in EAE has been extensively studied, and most work indicates that it is a basic protein of myelin (Kies and Alvord, 1965). Specifically sensitized lymphocytes are found in immunofluorescence studies to take up this myelin protein. The demyelination in EAE has recently been shown in electron microscopic studies to be a result of the phagocytosis of oligodendroglial cells and dissolution of the myelin lamellae by mononuclear cells.

The relationship of EAE to the spontaneous demyelinating disorders is still conjectural. Since the brain lacks a lymphatic drainage, myelin antigens are inaccessible to the body's reticuloendothelial system. It is plausible to assume that in certain situations the body could produce myelin autoantibodies (cellular or humoral) that would react with central nervous system myelin and produce demyelinating lesions. How the normally inaccessible myelin autoantigens reach the antibody-forming site and under what circumstances this occurs are still unknown.

The other major theory on the etiology of multiple sclerosis based on epidemiologic studies is that it is of viral origin related to exposure in late childhood or early adolescence. Higher familial incidence is consistent with exposure in early life, whereas twin studies suggest little if any genetic influence. Family and migration studies of individuals who have moved from high risk areas to low risk areas suggest a latency period of 3 to 23 years between exposure and clinical onset.

The role of a myxovirus was first suggested by the finding of significantly higher concentrations of measles antibodies in patients with multiple sclerosis. Recently paramyxovirus-like particles have been found as intranuclear inclusions in the macrophages about acute lesions in multiple sclerosis autopsy and biopsy material. Using tissue culture techniques, paramyxovirus has been isolated from the brains of patients with multiple sclerosis.

POSTVACCINAL AND PARAINFECTIOUS ENCEPHALOMYELITIS

These disorders are considered in Ch. 394 to 397.

414. ACUTE NECROTIZING HEMORRHAGIC ENCEPHALOMYELITIS

This is a rare and fulminant variant of demyelinating disease that often progresses to death in days or weeks. The disease is characterized by a rapid course, fever, headache, convulsions, progressive change in state of consciousness from drowsiness to coma, nuchal rigidity, and hemiplegia or quadriplegia. The cerebrospinal fluid examination reveals a pleocytosis up to several thousand white blood cells that are predominantly polymorphonuclear leukocytes, and an elevated protein content. On pathologic examination, there are large foci of hemorrhagic necrosis of white matter. Although most patients succumb within a few weeks, there are rare alleged reports of recovery. There appears to be an experimental allergic model of this disorder with similarities on histologic examination. The only therapy that can be offered is supportive, though ACTH and corticosteroids should be tried.

415. ACUTE DISSEMINATED ENCEPHALOMYELITIS

Occasionally acute neurologic symptoms may occur without apparent preceding infection. The clinical picture is dependent on the location of the lesions and may include the symptoms and signs of meningitis, encephalitis, myelitis, or any combination of the preceding. Some cases blend indistinguishably into chronic, typical multiple sclerosis and so may represent the initial acute attack of that disease. Other cases may be uniphasic, and the patient may recover with or without neurologic residua and have no further attacks. Only prolonged follow-up with a recurrence or progression of neurologic symptoms can enable one to diagnose acute multiple sclerosis and exclude acute disseminated encephalomyelitis.

416. MULTIPLE SCLEROSIS

Definition. Multiple or disseminated sclerosis is the most common demyelinating disorder. It is usually pleomorphic and difficult to define completely in the absence of specific diagnostic tests. There are a number of well recognized and readily diagnosed syndromes, but borderline cases may be difficult to categorize clinically and pathologically. Generally it is chronic and relapsing, but fulminating attacks occur and as many as 30 per cent of patients tend to progress steadily from the onset. The symptoms and signs reflect involvement of central myelin, but occasionally symptoms are typical of neuronal or gray-matter involvement. Multiple sclerosis is a disease of the central white matter with "lesions separated in time and space."

Incidence. The prevalence of multiple sclerosis in the United States varies from about 10 per 100,000 in the South to 60 per 100,000 in the North, with similar prevalence and distribution in Europe. The disease affects males and females about equally. About 67 per cent of cases begin between the ages of 20 and 40 years and 95 per cent between 10 and 50 years.

Populations residing between latitudes 40° N and 40° S (tropical and subtropical zones) have a low risk of multiple sclerosis. With a few notable exceptions, all populations residing north of this latitude in North America and Europe are at higher risk. Other exceptions to these generalizations are found in other parts of the world; e.g., a low incidence is reported in the Union of South Africa and in Japan. Efforts have been made to correlate these geographic variations with dietary intake, temperature, solar radiation, and geomagnetic latitude, without success. Racial factors seem to play little part in the United States, because the incidence in blacks is almost the same as in whites.

Genetic studies have contributed indirectly to theories on the etiology of multiple sclerosis. There are occasional reports of a greater family incidence than could be expected by chance, but these fail to exclude the common effects of environmental factors. A purely hereditary basis seems to be excluded by concordance studies in identical twins.

Pathology. The external surface of the brain and cord generally shows no abnormality. Occasionally there is atrophy of the optic nerves, and rarely there is focal or generalized atrophy of the cerebral hemispheres. Acute large lesions may cause swelling of the cord. Rarely there may be sufficient focal swelling of the cerebrum to give the appearance of a neoplasm in roentgenologic contrast studies.

Cut sections of the brain or spinal cord reveal numerous scattered, grayish, well defined lesions that are

TABLE 2. Frequency of Occurrence of First Symptom of Multiple Sclerosis in Cases Proved by Clinical Study and Autopsy

Symptom	Autopsy (Carter et al.) (46 Cases)	Autopsy (Poser) (111 Cases)	Clinical Diagnosis (Carter et al.) (539 Cases)
	per cent	*per cent*	*per cent*
Weakness	42	39	54
Diplopia, impaired vision	35	32	21
Tremor, ataxia, incoordination	20	6	19
Paresthesias	13	16	32
Pain	11	1	–
Sphincter impairment	11	1	7
Dizziness or vertigo	7	1	8
Changes in muscle tone	7	–	–
Facial pain	2	–	–
Mental changes	2	2	–
Seizures	–	–	3

slightly depressed and vary in diameter from a few millimeters to a few centimeters. These are found throughout the white matter of the brain, optic nerves, and spinal cord and occasionally extend into gray matter. The number of lesions is usually greater than would be expected from the clinical picture.

Microscopic abnormalities depend on the age of the lesion. Acute lesions show an infiltration of microglial phagocytes and mononuclear cells about vessels, as well as scattered in the lesion itself. The myelin sheaths are affected to varying diagnostic procedures. The disease is chronic, often characterized by exacerbations and remissions, with evidence of multiple lesions in central white matter occurring in young adults without other systemic disorders. The symptoms of central white matter involvement are usually those of supranuclear weakness, incoordination, paresthesias, and visual complaints. Other symptoms and signs that are more characteristic of lesions in gray matter, e.g., aphasia, seizures, fasciculations, and neurogenic atrophy, are rare. Mental changes have an intermediate incidence and affect perhaps 30 per cent of patients.

The onset may be acute, with symptoms appearing within minutes to hours, or it may be insidious, with gradual, slow progression of symptoms over a period of months.

The frequency of occurrence of the first symptom of multiple sclerosis is given in Table 2.

The weakness usually begins or is most prominent in the lower extremities, but the upper extremities may be involved. When both lower extremities are involved, there are usually accompanying urinary complaints such as urgency or frequency. The weakness may be minimal, or there may be a total paralysis. There are usually upper motor neuron signs such as spasticity, hyperreflexia, and pathologic reflexes.

Visual complaints include blurring of vision with a central scotoma and decreased visual acuity or diplopia with extraocular paresis and nystagmus.

The incoordination is seen as ataxia or clumsiness and intention tremor of the upper extremities. Often a combination of spastic-ataxic gait is seen.

The paresthesias may involve any or all of the extremities. Usually there is impairment of vibratory sense and position sense in the lower extremities, whereas cutaneous sensation is relatively spared.

The typical clinical course of multiple sclerosis is one of exacerbations and remissions over a period of years, with increasing neurologic deficits caused by an increasing number of disseminated lesions. Less frequent are (1) an acute, severe course progressing to death in a few days or weeks; (2) a chronic, progressive course over a period of years; and (3) a benign form with relatively few presenting symptoms and signs and long-lasting remissions. In middle age the insidious onset of a progressive spastic paraparesis is often seen as the major clinical manifestation, particularly in women.

Multiple sclerosis is sometimes divided into clinical types, depending upon which portion of the neuraxis is most involved, e.g., spinal, cerebral, brainstem-cerebellar, or mixed. The most common form is spinal with prominent features of spastic paraparesis, lower extremity paresthesias, and urinary complaints. The brainstem-cerebellar variety with prominent visual complaints, cranial nerve signs, nystagmus, vertigo, and incoordination is also common, but the cerebral form with mental changes and hemiparesis and hemisensory changes is uncommon.

Although most cases may be classified as one of these forms early in the course, almost all patients appear to have a mixed type of involvement after about 15 years.

In Table 3 may be noted the frequency of various symptoms and signs of multiple sclerosis in clinical and autopsy series reported by Carter et al. and by Poser.

Certain uncommon symptoms and signs such as nausea, vomiting, facial pain, seizures, dysphagia, atrophy, hearing loss, tinnitus, and changes in states of consciousness occur in 2 to 10 per cent of cases. Signs such as internuclear ophthalmoplegia are highly characteristic of multiple sclerosis; headache and aphasia are rare.

Laboratory Data. Abnormal findings in multiple sclerosis are usually confined to the cerebrospinal fluid. In the acute disease, there may be a mild mononuclear pleocytosis of as much as 200 to 300 cells per cubic millimeter, but usually less than 40. The protein content is usually normal or slightly elevated (50 to 100 mg per 100 ml); values higher than this are rare. The gamma globulin content is elevated in about two thirds of the cases and, correspondingly, there is often an abnormal colloidal gold curve (first or second zone), accompanied by a negative serologic test for syphilis.

The electroencephalogram may be mildly abnormal in about two thirds of cases, revealing either focal or generalized abnormalities.

Diagnosis. Because of the pleomorphic nature of the disease, it is often necessary to exclude many other

TABLE 3. Frequency of Occurrence of Symptoms and Signs in Course of Multiple Sclerosis

	Carter et al. (46 Cases)	Poser (111 Cases)
	per cent	*per cent*
Weakness (symptom or sign)	89	96
Abnormal movements	67	
Abnormal reflexes (absent superficials, Babinski signs, or hyperreflexia)	99	95
Sphincter and genital difficulties	78	82
Visual disturbance (symptom or sign)	100	85
Nystagmus (any type)	85	70
Disc pallor, atrophy, decreased acuity	75	85
Third nerve impairment (and internuclear ophthalmoplegia)	67	
Tremor, ataxia	93	79
Impaired vibration and position sense	81	58
Impaired touch, pain, temperature sense	35	35
Mental changes (symptom or sign)	61	45
Paresthesias	44	65
Pain	42	19
Vertigo or dizziness	18	15

neurologic disorders. Most often one must consider spinal cord, brainstem or cerebellar tumors, degenerative diseases such as the spinocerebellar degenerations, and combined system disease.

The fact that multiple sclerosis has a remitting nature in many instances and the dissemination of symptoms and signs should indicate that one is not dealing with an expanding lesion involving the nervous system. If all the symptoms and signs can be explained by a single lesion, then one should assume that the condition is not multiple sclerosis. If the patient complains of headache, seizures, or progressive focal neurologic signs, which are uncommon in multiple sclerosis, and if these are accompanied by abnormalities such as increased cerebrospinal fluid pressure, roentgenographic changes in the skull or spine, and marked elevation of cerebrospinal fluid protein, then one must proceed further to exclude a neoplasm. This can be done in most cases by a neuroroentgenologic procedure such as myelography, pneumoencephalography, cerebral angiography, or computerized transaxial tomographic scan. Vascular disease, particularly that involving the brainstem, can be confused with multiple sclerosis in middle-aged patients. In some of these cases only prolonged follow-up reveals the true diagnosis.

Certain degenerative disorders of the nervous system can be confused with multiple sclerosis. However, the former tend to have a family history, to be slowly progressive without remission, and to confine themselves to systems, e.g., cerebellar, extrapyramidal, or motor system. In the differential diagnosis of spastic paraparesis of middle age, one should consider, respectively, motor neuron disease (amyotrophic lateral sclerosis), cervical spondylosis, or spinal cord tumor. The first has no sensory abnormalities, and the latter two both have characteristic roentgenologic abnormalities. Combined systemic disease can be excluded in most cases by hematologic studies and gastric analysis.

Treatment. There are several aspects to the management of multiple sclerosis. The first is the possible benefit to be gained from ACTH or corticosteroids during acute exacerbations. Many authorities advise a course of three to four weeks of therapy with suitable precautions against complications, and some recent controlled studies have shown that this treatment has some benefit in the acute symptom complex. There are no indications for long-term maintenance therapy on ACTH or corticosteroids, and the risks outweigh any possible benefit. Preliminary studies with other immunosuppressive agents indicate that the course of the disease may be stabilized with fewer exacerbations. From a consideration of the pathology it is unreasonable to expect alleviation of symptoms that have been static for many months.

The second aspect is the general management of the patient. During acute exacerbations, especially severe ones, there may be some benefit from bed rest, although the demoralizing effects of prolonged immobilization must be avoided. The prevention of complications, especially genitourinary infections, bedsores, contractures, and flexor spasms, requires adequate nursing care, physiotherapy, and occasionally more specific measures such as rhizotomy, tenotomy, antimicrobials, and other indicated measures. Exhausting physiotherapy with active exercises offers no benefit and may even be harmful. Certain other measures such as unnecessary catheterization have serious consequences and should be avoided.

The third aspect of patient care is the management of long-term disabling illness with an unpredictable course. Initially there arises the question of informing the patient, and this must be dealt with on an individual basis after considering the emotional makeup of the patient and his family, the patient's responsibilities, and other factors. This is particularly important in relation to pregnancy. The route of delivery is an obstetrical decision.

One must encourage and support the patient to remain active and yet protect him from constantly seeking untried and potentially harmful therapies or unnecessary diagnostic tests and operations.

Prognosis. In the early stages of the disease it is not possible accurately to predict the course, although certain symptoms seem to indicate a better prognosis. Monosymptomatic and acute symptoms lasting hours to weeks tend to give a better prognosis than polysymptomatic or slowly progressive manifestations. Cranial nerve, visual, and sensory symptoms carry a better prognosis for remission or a benign course than do motor or cerebellar symptoms. More than half the cases remit after an initial attack, but one cannot predict the next attack. The remission of certain symptoms, e.g., retrobulbar neuritis, may be so complete as to make the clinician doubt the history.

Within the first five years after onset, about 70 per cent of patients are able to be employed, although with occasional interruptions in some cases. By the end of ten years this drops off to 50 per cent. At the end of 20 years 35 per cent are still employed, with minor interruptions, and about 20 per cent of patients succumb to complications of the disease by this time. The major disabilities are spasticity, disturbances of coordination, and disturbance in bladder and bowel function.

Life expectancy varies considerably, ranging from a few weeks to over 50 years regardless of whether one considers hospitalized, severe cases or the more benign forms. The average life expectancy is from 13 to more than 25 years after onset. The cause of death is often an intercurrent infection, usually respiratory or genitourinary.

417. POSSIBLE MULTIPLE SCLEROSIS VARIANTS

OPTIC AND RETROBULBAR NEURITIS

Optic neuritis is a term used to describe involvement of the optic nerve as a result of inflammation, demyelination, or degeneration. When the site of the lesion is intraocular, ophthalmoscopy reveals papilledema and the terms *papillitis* or intraocular neuritis are employed. *Retrobulbar neuritis* indicates involvement of the orbital or intracranial optic nerve behind the eye. There is often a predilection for the papillomacular bundle, producing a characteristic central scotoma but usually with minimal or absent ophthalmoscopic abnormalities in the acute stage.

Optic neuritis has many known causes, such as nutritional deficiency, intoxications (tobacco, alcohol), local inflammatory conditions (sinusitis, meningitis, orbital infections), and metabolic diseases (diabetes mellitus, pernicious anemia, other vitamin deficiencies). Once these have been excluded, demyelinating disease must be considered as a likely cause. In several large series of patients who presented with retrobulbar neuritis and were followed for many years, 15 to 30 per cent later developed other manifestations of multiple sclerosis. Conversely, about 50 per cent of patients with multiple sclerosis exhibit symptoms of optic neuritis at some time during the course of the disease.

Both optic and retrobulbar neuritis are characterized by an abrupt or progressive loss of vision that is rarely total and is usually unilateral. Associated with the visual loss may be pain in and around the eye that is accentuated by ocular movement. There may be tenderness on palpation of the eyeball. Visual testing reveals decreased acuity and central or paracentral scotomas. In *intraocular neuritis* or *papillitis,* the optic disc appears inflamed, and there may be hyperemia, blurred margins, and even elevation. A few hemorrhages may be seen in the retina adjacent to the disc. In *retrobulbar neuritis* the ophthalmoscopic picture is normal, but the features are otherwise similar to those of optic neuritis.

It is essential to differentiate optic neuritis from papilledema associated with increased intracranial pressure or other conditions. Papilledema is almost always bilateral, and vision is usually well preserved until late in the course. The disc elevation is usually greater in papilledema, and the only visual field defect is an enlarged blind spot. In optic neuritis the cerebrospinal fluid pressure is almost always normal, and there may be other findings indicative of multiple sclerosis.

Optic and retrobulbar neuritis may be treated with ACTH or corticosteroids. However, almost complete spontaneous recovery often occurs, and the benefits of therapy are difficult to assess.

The prognosis in a single attack of optic or retrobulbar neuritis is usually good. There may be complete recovery, or there may be residual visual field defects, temporal pallor of the discs, or optic atrophy. The visual acuity may be further impaired with subsequent attacks, but complete visual loss is rare.

ACUTE TRANSVERSE MYELITIS

Acute transverse myelitis may appear as the initial event in a subsequently typical form of multiple sclerosis, or it may develop during the course of the disease. The findings include complete or partial paralysis of both legs or of all four limbs, variable sensory loss, and bladder and bowel involvement. The condition is described in detail in Ch. 385.

Subacute necrotizing myelopathy is often associated with vascular malformations of the spinal cord or thrombophlebitis (Foix-Alajouanine syndrome). In acute necrotizing myelopathy there is hemorrhagic necrosis of the spinal cord without any associated vascular malformation. Such cases, which are rare, show a rapidly ascending motor and sensory paralysis with polymorphonuclear cells in the cerebrospinal fluid, and death may occur in weeks or months.

NEUROMYELITIS OPTICA (DEVIC'S DISEASE)

This clinical syndrome is characterized by acute transverse myelitis and optic neuritis. It may be considered to be a variant of multiple sclerosis and may occur as the initial illness or later during the course of the disease. There may be sudden loss of vision in both eyes, with central scotoma or sudden onset of paraplegia with sensory loss. The ocular involvement may be due to optic or retrobulbar neuritis, and the transverse myelitis may be partial or complete. Days or weeks may elapse between the onsets of the two symptom complexes. In severe cases the motor symptoms tend to be permanent, but otherwise the course, laboratory data, and treatment are similar to those of multiple sclerosis.

TRANSITIONAL SCLEROSIS

Transitional sclerosis is probably a pathologic variant of multiple sclerosis in which the disseminated plaques tend to become confluent, creating large areas of myelin loss. Clinically these cases are indistinguishable from cases of typical multiple sclerosis. Transitional sclerosis probably represents an intermediate pathologic form between multiple sclerosis and Schilder's cerebral sclerosis.

418. DIFFUSE SCLEROSIS

There is a group of progressive neurologic disorders of young patients who manifest severe neurologic deficits of various types and progressive visual and mental deterioration. In three publications from 1912 to 1924, Schilder described three cases of diffuse disease of white matter that he proposed grouping under the name *encephalitis periaxialis diffusa* (now called Schilder's disease). Actually, Schilder had described three distinct entities, and these, plus cases subsequently described, are of three types: (1) the myelinoclastic group, closely related to multiple sclerosis, referred to hereafter as Schilder's cerebral sclerosis; (2) the leukoencephalitides, which are probably of viral origin; and (3) the dysmyelinating group or leukodystrophies, which are probably due to genetically determined enzymatic defects.

SCHILDER'S CEREBRAL SCLEROSIS

The demyelinative disorders in this group are related pathologically to multiple sclerosis. The characteristic lesions are large, bilateral areas of demyelination in the cerebral hemispheres with preservation of the subcortical "U" fibers, a relative sparing of the axons, and a replacement gliosis. Recent lesions show a perivascular inflammatory reaction. Swelling of the cerebral hemispheres in acute, fulminant cases may rarely cause increased intracranial pressure and may mimic brain tumor. In more chronic lesions there is a suggestion of confluence of smaller plaques to make the large areas of demyelination. In some cases there are, in addition, randomly scattered small lesions in other areas of the central nervous system, and these have been called "diffuse-disseminated sclerosis" or transitional sclerosis. These cases may represent an intermediate form of the same process, diffuse sclerosis representing one extreme whereas multiple sclerosis represents the other.

The disease may occur at any age, but unlike multiple sclerosis the majority of cases begin in childhood. About half the cases begin prior to the age of 10 years, and three fourths begin before the age of 20. The disease is relatively rare; fewer than 50 autopsied cases have been reported. Both sexes are equally involved.

The onset is usually insidious but may be acute. It is usually slowly progressive, but there may be successive bursts to simulate the course of multiple sclerosis. A typical presenting picture is of insidious mental deterioration with loss of recently acquired intellectual achievements, and this progresses slowly to dementia. Many patients develop aphasia, apraxia, and dysarthria. Various psychiatric syndromes may be manifested. Visual loss with cortical blindness is characteristic, and auditory complaints with cortical deafness may follow involvement of the cortical radiations. Motor symptoms such as hemiparesis may be prominent, and seizures of various types tend to appear during the course. Other neurologic symptoms and signs such as vertigo, ataxia, nystagmus, paraplegia, or extraocular palsies are less frequent.

The course varies from days to many years, with an average duration of about three years. Terminally patients are severely demented and often in a decerebrate state.

Laboratory findings are usually abnormal only in the cerebrospinal fluid and electroencephalogram. The CSF pressure may be elevated, and there may be mild pleocytosis and elevation of protein content. The gamma globulin content is usually abnormal. The EEG findings vary from paroxysmal discharges to focal slowing. Patients with increased intracranial pressure may have misleading indications of a mass lesion in encephalographic or angiographic studies. There is no specific therapy.

BALO'S CONCENTRIC SCLEROSIS

Some cases of demyelinating disease have an unusual concentric arrangement of the demyelinating lesions of the cerebrum. Balo gave these the name *encephalitis periaxialis concentrica.* This rare entity probably represents a variant of Schilder's cerebral sclerosis.

419. LEUKODYSTROPHIES

This group includes heredofamilial diseases in which normal myelin is probably not formed because of some genetically determined enzymatic defect. The classification is not completely satisfactory; the group tends to merge with the lipidoses of the nervous system, so that authorities differ in their classifications. Only further elucidation of the enzymatic defects of myelin metabolism in these disorders will lead to a satisfactory classification.

METACHROMATIC LEUKOENCEPHALOPATHY

These are otherwise known as the glial insufficiency forms or the sulfatide lipidoses. This group includes those cases in which large amounts of metachromatic material accumulate in the central nervous system. The disease is inherited as an autosomal recessive and begins in the first ten years of life, usually with gait disturbances, convulsions of various types, hypotonia, ocular palsies, and dysarthria. There are coarse tremors of the extremities and, terminally, severe mental deterioration and spasticity or rigidity.

The cerebrospinal fluid protein is usually elevated (100 to 200 mg per 100 ml), and metachromatic material (staining red with toluidine blue) can be found in the urinary sediment. The metachromatic material also collects in the kidney, liver, gallbladder, spleen, or peripheral nerves, and biopsy confirms the diagnosis. Gallbladder function studies may be abnormal. The course is one of progressive neurologic deterioration leading to death in one to four years, although some patients have survived 10 to 20 years. Some cases may begin later in childhood and run a more protracted course. The disorder is one of the more common leukodystrophies and can often be diagnosed in life. There is no therapy.

SUDANOPHILIC LEUKODYSTROPHY
(Pelizaeus-Merzbacher Disease)

This is a very rare, familial leukodystrophy, predominantly of males. The pathologic changes consist of extensive diffuse demyelination in the cerebral hemispheres and cerebellum. The disease appears to be transmitted as a sex-linked recessive and begins in early life with a slowly progressive course. Disturbances of coordination such as intention tremor, gait disturbances, dysarthria, spasticity, abnormal movements, and mental deterioration occur. The illness lacks pathognomonic features, but the predominant progressive cerebellar symptoms in a male with a positive family history should make one suspect the entity. It runs a course of several years or more before fatal termination. There is no therapy.

GLOBOID CELL LEUKODYSTROPHY
(Krabbe's Disease)

This rare familial type of leukodystrophy begins in infancy and rapidly progresses to death. The typical pathologic feature is the deposition of cerebrosides in globoid cells of the brain. These may be glial or another type of macrophage. The cases described by Krabbe began at about four months of age with seizures, spastic quadriplegia, abnormal startle responses, cortical blindness, and optic atrophy, and progressed rapidly to death in one or two years. The protein in the cerebrospinal fluid is usually elevated. There is no therapy.

SPONGY DEGENERATION OF WHITE MATTER
(Canavan's Disease)

In this rare familial leukodystrophy there is widespread demyelination accompanied by microscopic vacuolation that gives rise to a spongy appearance. It appears to be transmitted as an autosomal recessive and seems to be most common among Jews. Usually it begins early in infancy with atonia of the neck muscles, spastic paraplegia, severe mental retardation, optic atrophy, abnormal reflexes, and enlargement of the head. Laboratory studies, except for skull roentgenograms showing enlargement, are usually normal. Death usually occurs at about 18 months of age. There is no therapy.

LIPIDOSES OF THE CENTRAL NERVOUS SYSTEM

These comprise disturbances of metabolism that result in an increase of lipids in the brain. Included are amaurotic idiocy, or Tay-Sachs disease (gangliosidoses) (see below); Niemann-Pick disease (sphingomyelin) (see Ch. 777); Gaucher's disease (cerebrosides) (see Ch. 776); and Hurler's disease (mucopolysaccharides) (see Ch. 934).

The dividing line is by no means sharp between the dysmyelinating diseases, characterized by faulty myelin formation, and the lipid storage diseases, characterized by the accumulation of lipid-staining materials within nerve cell bodies. The distinction is further blurred by the fact that demyelination also occurs in many of the lipidoses, particularly amaurotic idiocy.

Amaurotic idiocy, or cerebromacular degeneration, can have an infantile (Tay-Sachs), late infantile (Bielschowsky), or juvenile (Batten-Spielmeyer-Vogt) onset. The Tay-Sachs variety is found chiefly among children of Jewish descent and has a recessive genetic pattern. The incidence of the other forms is genetic recessive and nonracial. All three are characterized by a progressive decrease in vision leading to complete blindness within one to two years. Concomitantly, there is a progressive and usually severe dementia combined with convulsions and advancing weakness, leading eventually to the patient's being bedridden with paralysis. Diagnosis in all three forms depends upon the characteristic clinical combination of dementia and blindness plus, in the Tay-Sachs and Batten-Spielmeyer-Vogt varieties, either a cherry-red or red-purple discoloration, respectively, marking the area of macular degeneration in the retina. An adult form (Kufs') has also been recognized. This group of late onset neuronal storage disorders without organomegaly is characterized by seizures, pigmentary degeneration or cherry-red spot changes in the retina, pyramidal signs, basal ganglia signs, cerebellar signs, and dementia. The problem remains whether these disorders are examples of identical or different genetically determined enzymatic defects of the nervous system. Clinicopathologic changes are not diagnostic. Rectal biopsy disclosing fat-packed ganglion cells in Meissner's plexus provides morphologic confirmation of the diagnosis.

Adams, J. M., and Imagawa, D. T.: Measles antibodies in multiple sclerosis. Proc. Soc. Exp. Biol. Med., 111:562, 1962.
Carter, S., Sciarra, D., and Merrit, H. H.: The course of multiple sclerosis as determined by autopsy proven cases. Am. Res. Nerv. Ment. Dis. Proc., 28:471, 1950.
McAlpine, D., Lumsden, C. E., and Acheson, E. D.: Multiple Sclerosis. A Reappraisal. London, E. & S. Livingstone Ltd., 1965.
Miller, H. G., Stanton, J. B., and Gibbons, J. L.: Parainfectious encephalomyelitis and related syndromes. Quart. J. Med., 25:427, 1956.
Poser, C. M.: Recent advances in multiple sclerosis. Med. Clin. North Am., 56:1343, 1972.
Prineas, J. W.: Paramyxovirus-like particles associated with acute demyelination in chronic relapsing multiple sclerosis. Science, 178:760, 1972.
Raine, C. S., Powers, J. M., and Suzuki, K.: Acute multiple sclerosis. Confirmation of "paramyxovirus-like" intranuclear inclusions. Arch. Neurol., 30:39, 1974.
Vinken, P. J., and Bruyn, G. W. (eds.): Multiple Sclerosis and Other Demyelinating Diseases. Handbook of Clinical Neurology, Vol. 9. Amsterdam, North-Holland Publishing Company, 1970.
Wolfgram, F., et al. (eds.): Multiple Sclerosis: Immunology, Virology and Ultrastructure. New York, Academic Press, 1972.

Section Sixteen. THE EPILEPSIES

Gilbert H. Glaser

Definition and Prevalence. Epilepsy is derived from the Greek *epilepsia* meaning a "taking hold of" or "a seizing." It refers to the many types of recurrent seizures produced by paroxysmal excessive neuronal discharges in different parts of the brain that can be due to a variety of cerebral and general bodily disorders. Designation of "the epilepsies" as symptom complexes, therefore, is more appropriate, and the term encompasses convulsions or convulsive disorders with loss of consciousness as well as nonconvulsive seizures with only slight changes in conscious awareness.

An accurate epidemiology of the epilepsies is difficult, but various studies indicate an over-all incidence of between 0.5 and 1.0 per cent in general populations involving all age groups. The experience of a single seizure is more common, especially in early childhood, but recurrence is necessary for the diagnosis of an epilepsy.

Pathogenesis. *Basic Mechanisms of Epileptic Discharge.* Given the sufficient and proper electrical and chemical stimuli, abnormal discharges and seizures can arise in even the normal brain. Certain regions of the brain are particularly sensitive to seizures, having a low threshold and a high susceptibility. These include particularly the motor cortex and the structures within the limbic system. The temporal lobe and its deeper nuclear aggregates, the amygdala and hippocampus, are especially susceptible; their vascularity is vulnerable to compression, and the tissues themselves are especially sensitive to biochemical disturbances. It sometimes is difficult to separate cause from effect in temporal lobe lesions, because morphologic abnormalities in these regions may result when a severe seizure produces secondary vascular insufficiency and hypoxia.

Factors related to age and development are important in the genesis of the epilepsies, and brain lesions acquired during the perinatal period often mature and produce clinical epileptic phenomena only years later. Certain seizure types such as massive spasms are more common in infants; petit mal seizures appear in childhood rather than later in life. This is reflected by different electroencephalographic patterns associated with seizures in infancy and childhood, compared with those in older age groups. The immature brain also is more susceptible than that of the adult to biochemical disturbances such as hypoxia, hypocalcemia, hypoglycemia, and hyponatremia. The occurrence of seizures with high fever is almost confined to early childhood. The periodicity of epilepsy correlates with sleep or menstrual cycles in some patients.

Seizures may be *focal,* arising from an abnormal focus or a number of foci, or *generalized from the onset,* seemingly without focal origin. However, generalization throughout the brain of an initially focal paroxysmal discharge may occur so rapidly that the focal origin can be obscured, and the attacks of many patients with fixed cerebral lesions and *secondary or symptomatic seizures* are in this category. It is still uncertain whether generalized seizures, such as some idiopathic grand mal convulsions and the brief seizures of petit mal absence (see below), develop immediately as generalized cerebral discharges involving specific pathways, or whether initially a localized discharge occurs. Convulsions caused by metabolic disturbances such as water intoxication, hypocalcemia, or hypoglycemia may be considered examples of those generalized from the onset. In these instances, the initial detonation starting the seizure is believed to be in the subcortical mesodiencephalic nonspecific reticular systems, with diffuse propagation bilaterally into the cerebral cortex. The rapid loss of consciousness that first occurs and the marked memory disturbance after the seizure can be related to this spread.

Hughlings Jackson concluded many years ago from clinical observations that most seizures develop from a focus or aggregate of abnormally excitable neurons, and many studies since his time have supported this hypothesis. It is postulated that the nerve cells of patients with epilepsy contain intrinsic intra- and extracellular metabolic disturbances which produce excessive and prolonged depolarization of the membrane, producing a defect in the recovery process after excitation. The cortical regions containing such cells generate shifts in slow or standing wave potentials as a result of abnormal electrical activity arising in the region of neuronal dendrites. The neurons in the abnormal, epileptic focus are a hyperexcitable aggregate, and they tend to discharge paroxysmally. Clinical seizures develop if the discharge propagates along neural pathways or if sufficient local recruitment occurs. The abnormal discharges, once initiated, spread through essentially normal brain; the manifestations of the particular seizure then depend upon both the focus of origin and the region of the brain subsequently involved in the propagated discharge. In certain cases, seizures may be provoked by various sensory stimuli ("reflex" or sensory-induced epilepsy), especially flickering light or visual patterns and sound. At other times, peripheral sensory stimulation has been found to arrest the development of a seizure.

The metabolic environment of epileptogenic neurons is most important in the genesis of attacks, and many metabolic disturbances may be associated with seizures. For example, a balance of electrolytes is required to maintain the resting potential of the neuronal membrane. An alteration in membrane permeability with an increased, intraneuronal sodium content could be a significant change preceding seizure discharge. Initiation and maintenance of neuronal hyperexcitability have been related to increases in extraneuronal potassium. Depletion of available calcium ions upsets membrane stability and causes oscillations; conversely, an increase in calcium has a depressant, anticonvulsive effect. Both hypoxia and hypoglycemia deprive neurons of basic substrates, allowing insufficient energy for the maintenance of appropriate ionic gradients. However, if effects of excessive muscle metabolism and apnea during generalized convulsive seizure activity are eliminated, such seizures do not induce cerebral hypoxia; actually, cerebral blood flow increases to meet cerebral oxygen demands in this state.

An excess of excitatory transmitter, such as acetylcholine, produces repetitive discharges and seizure activity. This may be induced experimentally by anticholinesterase drugs, but it is not found significantly in naturally occurring epilepsy.

The coenzyme function of pyridoxal phosphate is directly involved in the metabolic pathway of gamma-aminobutyric acid, which has neuronal inhibitory activity. Experimental alterations of this system can be produced by such substances as the antimetabolite methoxypyridoxine and the hydrazides, but pyridoxine deficiency seizures occur only rarely and in infants. Isoniazid toxicity occurs with an overdosage by this mechanism.

Etiology. It is customary to divide epilepsy into two categories, *idiopathic* and *symptomatic or acquired.* A diagnosis of idiopathic epilepsy is made when no specific cause is found; in acquired epilepsy the cause can be determined by available diagnostic procedures. Present techniques fail to uncover a specific structural or biochemical cause of epilepsy in up to 75 per cent of patients.

Idiopathic Epilepsy. Idiopathic epilepsy has been designated as *genetic,* with the implication that a transmitted predisposition for seizures is present. A family history of seizures exists in high incidence for some groups of seizures, particularly those with an onset in early life. The relatives of patients with idiopathic epilepsy have a 3 to 5 per cent incidence of epilepsy, six to ten times that in the ordinary population. There is also an increased incidence of electroencephalographic abnormality in the relatives of seizure patients, particularly in monozygotic twins, in whom the incidence of concordant abnormalities may exceed 20 per cent. Since epilepsy may be but a symptom associated with other neurologic abnormalities, an inheritance pattern for a specific cerebral disease must be considered in some cases. There are also a number of indirect factors, such as cerebral birth trauma resulting from a narrow maternal pelvis, that tend to produce seizures in families.

Acquired Epilepsy. Most diseases or structural abnormalities of the brain may be associated with seizures. *Congenital malformations* induced chromosomally or otherwise, such as microgyria, porencephaly, and hemangiomas, have a varying incidence of associated epilepsy, depending upon the intensity of the abnormality and possibly on more general genetic factors. Maternal infection, as by rubella, can produce multiple cerebral abnormalities, and severe toxemia of pregnancy also can affect the fetus. Perinatal difficulties causing *birth trauma* and *asphyxia* are relatively common causes of cerebral damage and later epilepsy.

Acute, subacute, and chronic infections of the brain and its coverings, such as meningitis, encephalitis, and abscess, cause seizures, both during the active process and later as healing leaves cerebral scars. Acute viral encephalitis often causes seizures, and convulsions, caused by cerebral tuberculomas (more often by tuberculous meningitis) remain common in certain countries such as India. Cysticercosis and schistosomiasis have specific geographic distributions and are frequent causes of seizures in highly endemic areas.

Febrile convulsions commonly accompany nonspecific infections in infants and young children and are to be distinguished from direct infection of the nervous system. The seizure usually accompanies a high rise in fever in an otherwise neurologically normal child. However, at least 30 per cent of these children may develop epilepsy later without fever. Sometimes febrile convulsions precipitate status epilepticus, which, in turn, contributes to permanent cerebral damage. The deep temporal lobe structures are particularly sensitive to these effects; the lesions occurring therein may later produce a temporal lobe–psychomotor seizure state.

Head injury is a major cause of acquired epilepsy, the seizures occurring both in the acute phase and as a chronic residual. The incidence of epilepsy after head injury is difficult to determine, because of the great variability of injury. General surveys report an incidence of up to 10 per cent after closed-head injury and between 30 and 40 per cent after open-head injuries, seizures developing in most cases within three years. The seizure incidence is highest when the wound is severe, when the dura is penetrated, and when the injury involves the rolandic or parietal regions.

Brain tumors are an important cause of seizures, particularly in adults, but it has been difficult to ascertain the relative incidence of brain tumor within the large population of epileptics. Between 30 and 40 per cent of all patients with cerebral tumors have seizures, especially if the tumor is supratentorial. The seizure is apt to be focal and, in 15 to 20 per cent of cases, is the first symptom. The brain tumors most likely to cause seizure are astrocytomas, meningiomas, and metastatic neoplasms, especially those from the lung.

Cerebral vascular disease is a relatively common cause of seizures, particularly in the older age groups. The attacks may result either from localized vascular insufficiency and secondary ischemic hypoxia or from a chronic residual scar, left after thrombosis, embolism, or hemorrhage. Episodes of loss of consciousness owing to diminished cerebral blood flow may progress into seizures, as in severe states of carotid sinus sensitivity and Adams-Stokes syndrome caused by heart block. Seizures appear in up to 20 per cent of patients with the various collagen disorders, i.e., systemic lupus erythematosus and periarteritis nodosa, and are the result of small vascular lesions involving the brain.

Various *allergic reactions* may be related to single seizures, but usually not recurrent epilepsy. Convulsions have been reported after immunizations, in drug sensitivity reactions, and after insect bites.

Certain generalized *cerebral degenerative and demyelinating diseases* carry a significant incidence of seizures; in multiple sclerosis this is 5 per cent, and patients with Alzheimer-Pick dementia may experience generalized and myoclonic seizures. The complex cerebral lesions of tuberous sclerosis often produce seizures, including infantile massive spasms. The cerebral lipidoses, such as Tay-Sachs disease, may cause generalized and myoclonic seizures.

Toxic and metabolic disorders are an important cause of seizures since treatment may be directed quite specifically. Seizures are prominent during withdrawal from chronic drug intoxications, particularly from barbiturates (and other sedatives and tranquilizers), and from alcohol. Seizures developing in association with alcoholism usually appear within 48 hours after cessation of drinking and may precede delirium tremens. Carbon monoxide intoxication and other forms of hypoxia may cause seizures. Lead poisoning has been a common cause of convulsions in young children. Water intoxication or excessive hydration, with hemodilution, can produce seizures, again especially in the young. Other pertinent metabolic causes are pyridoxine deficiency, phenylketonuria, hypocalcemia (with or without hypoparathyroidism), porphyria, and hypoglycemia. Hypoglycemia may be a complication of the treatment of diabetes or may accompany islet cell tumors of the pancreas and other endocrine disturbances such as hypopituitarism. Seizures, especially myoclonic, are common in acute and chronic renal insufficiency but are relatively unusual in hepatic failure. Secondarily induced magnesium deficiency, such as that after severe gastrointestinal fluid loss, has been implicated in the production of seizures.

It is likely that, in many patients, several factors combine to produce attacks: a genetically determined predisposition, an increased cerebral excitability related to a general metabolic disturbance, the presence of a focal brain lesion or a tendency to vascular insufficiency, and a triggering disturbance such as an emotional crisis or an excessively flickering light. Each patient, therefore, must be evaluated from many different aspects in order to establish causation on different levels and to develop appropriate total therapy.

Clinical Manifestations. The classification of seizures employed here is based, whenever possible, on a combination of clinical manifestations and electroencephalographic correlates.

Generalized Seizures (Grand Mal or Major Convulsions). The major tonic-clonic seizures have many causes and arise in all age groups. These seizures usually start with a *prodromal phase* that lasts minutes or even hours, with a change in emotional reactivity or affective responses, such as increasing anxiety or depression, often difficult to recognize. More commonly, the specific onset of the seizure is the *aura*, a brief experience directly related to the locus of origin of the seizure. Frequently experienced auras are a sense of fear, a peculiar epigastric sensation welling up into the throat, an unpleasant odor, various visual and auditory hallucinations, and strange sensations in an arm or leg. At times, localized movements of an extremity or portions of the face precede the onset of the general convulsion. The *convulsion* itself occurs with sudden vocalization (the "epileptic cry"), loss of consciousness, tonic extensor rigidity of the trunk and extremities, then clonic movements, a brief cessation of respiration, cyanosis, and then heavy, stertorous breathing. Incontinence of urine and feces occurs; there is often biting of the tongue and cheeks in the clonic phase. After some minutes, the excessive motor activity ceases, breathing becomes more normal, and consciousness gradually returns. Frequently a *postictal state* appears, characterized by confusion, general fatigue, headache, and, at times, certain specific, residual neurologic signs such as hemiparesis or monoparesis, sensory disturbances, and dysphasia. Automatic behavior may be present. As with the aura, these postictal phenomena have significance with regard to possible focal origins of the generalized seizure. The postictal paralysis, sometimes called "Todd's paralysis," ordinarily lasts for several minutes to hours after the seizure. In general, there is amnesia for a generalized seizure with the exception of possible recollections of the prodromal phase or the aura.

The designation *fragmentary seizure* is given to the occurrence of brief components of the generalized complex. For example, only auras may appear and may or may not be followed by abortive tonic movements or loss of consciousness. Such fragments occur particularly during therapy with anticonvulsant drugs and reflect incomplete control.

Grand mal seizures vary in their frequency from once

or twice yearly to many times daily; 20 per cent of patients may have only nocturnal seizures. In women the seizures may appear cyclically with or immediately before the menstrual periods, and the incidence may increase or decrease with pregnancy, being increased by toxemia and water retention.

The *electroencephalographic (EEG) patterns associated with generalized seizures* during the attack are difficult to distinguish from movement artifact. Between attacks, the EEG often contains paroxysms of bilateral, essentially synchronous, 4- to 7-cycle-per-second discharges from all areas, interspersed with nonspecific patterns of high amplitude spikes and slow waves. A paroxysmal or slow wave discharge localized to one region of the scalp suggests that a focal cerebral lesion may be present. Between seizures up to 25 per cent of patients have an electroencephalogram within the normal range.

Petit Mal (Absence Attack). The petit mal seizure is a specific form of minor epilepsy, consisting of a sudden brief lapse of consciousness, usually lasting no longer than 30 seconds, more commonly 5 to 10 seconds. Petit mal almost always appears in childhood, with onset usually between the ages of three and ten. Its incidence diminishes during postpuberty, and persistence into adult life after the age of 30 is rare. Usually, no specific cause is found. In rare instances a specific brain lesion such as a vascular calcified tumor of the frontal lobe or diffuse cerebral lipidosis has been reported with petit mal seizures, but the EEG was seldom entirely characteristic.

Clinically, the patient with petit mal has a sudden cessation of activity and stares blankly, making no movements, except at times a 3 per second blinking of the eyelids, a slight deviation of the eyes and head, or brief minor movements of the lips and hands. The end of the spell is equally abrupt. More complex behavioral disturbances or postictal confusion or drowsiness suggest another type of minor seizure such as psychomotor automatism rather than petit mal. The attacks of petit mal can be as few as a flurry every several days to as many as 100 or more per day. As the frequency increases, the repeated absences sometimes produce difficulties in continuing motor tasks and in learning. The designation *petit mal status* or absence state refers to many attacks occurring close together for minutes to hours and producing confusion and disorientation.

The electroencephalographic correlate of the petit mal or absence seizure is a rhythmic 3-cycle-per-second spike and wave discharge appearing synchronously from all scalp regions both during and between seizures. Usually, a discharge of more than a few seconds' duration is associated with a clinical absence. The characteristics of the seizure and the typical electroencephalographic discharge have led to these seizures being designated as "centrencephalic," implying an origin in the centrally placed, "integrating," mesodiencephalic regions of the brain. Experimentally, there is evidence to support this hypothesis, although direct confirmation in the human is inconclusive.

Akinetic Seizure. The term akinetic attack is applied to a generalized seizure associated with loss of consciousness and simple falling. It may be accompanied by an absence and minor movements, but generally there is a marked diminution of postural tone with falling and, often, self-injury. Afterward, the reappearance of normal posture and mental clarity is common, although there may be a brief period of confusion. Electroencephalographically, there is a diffuse abnormality with slow wave discharges or atypical spike waves, often slower than 3 per second.

Myoclonic Seizures. These are characterized by sudden involuntary contractions involving an integrated response of a single muscle or several muscle groups, producing relatively simple arrhythmic jerking movements about a single joint or several joints, or of a segment of the body. The jerks may exist as an independent entity, as a phenomenon preceding and building up to a generalized grand mal convulsion or as an accompaniment to petit mal absences in children. Myoclonic attacks are often sensitive to sensory stimulation and may be precipitated or accentuated by sound or light, by change in posture, by movement of an extremity, by drowsiness, or by an emotional upset. Myoclonic jerks occur as a normal phenomenon in normal subjects during drowsiness.

Myoclonus Epilepsy. The myoclonus epilepsy of Unverricht refers to generalized myoclonus and mental deterioration secondary to a diffuse degenerative metabolic disorder of undetermined origin. Other forms of myoclonus appear in diseases of cerebral lipid metabolism, in subacute encephalitis, and with rare forms of cerebellar disease. A severe myoclonus appearing in the first 18 months of life and associated with general cerebral deterioration is called *infantile massive spasms* or jackknife seizures. In this condition, the infant develops severe flexion spasms of the head, neck, and trunk and extension of the legs and arms. Some known causes of this disorder are phenylketonuria, tuberous sclerosis, and Down's syndrome, but in most instances neither a biochemical nor an anatomic abnormality can be found.

The *electroencephalographic correlates of the myoclonic seizure* are variable, depending on the severity of the seizure state; in mild instances, generalized, synchronous slow spike and wave complexes or sharp and slow wave elements occur intermittently, with relatively clear electroencephalographic patterns interspersed. Infantile massive spasms are commonly associated with *hypsarhythmia,* which consists of more or less continuous, nonsynchronous, asymmetric discharges of spike and sharp wave elements along with slow waves from all regions.

Focal or Partial Seizures. Involvement of a specific region of the brain may be manifested by characteristic signs and symptoms. They are typical of acquired epilepsy, although occasionally no definite morphologic lesion is found. As indicated above, a focal onset seizure can occasionally spread extremely rapidly to become generalized, but in seizure states specifically classified as focal or partial, the attack usually remains limited. There often is a disturbance of consciousness or awareness with varying degrees of amnesia, but total loss of consciousness occurs only with general spread.

Lesions involving any of the motor regions of the brain, but particularly the so-called motor cortex, produce focal motor seizures. The classic *jacksonian motor seizure,* caused by a lesion sharply localized in a specific region of the motor cortex, begins as a repetitive movement of a distal portion of an extremity, such as the fingers or toes, and then spreads by a march of the clonic contractions up the extremity toward the trunk. Such a seizure usually remains limited to the extremity, but it may spread to the rest of the ipsilateral side, the face, and the contralateral side. Occasionally, these seizures begin at the corner of the mouth and are associated with masticatory movements and speech disturbances. Other focal motor seizures involve gross movements of the arms or legs without the classic jacksonian march. *Adversive seizures* produce turning movements of the head, eyes, and trunk toward the side opposite the cerebral lesion, which is usually in the prefrontal cortex.

Focal seizures originating from the *supplementary motor area* of the mesial frontal supracingulate cortex are not common; they are characterized by gross body movements, especially raising of the contralateral arm with the head turning toward that arm, rhythmic bilateral arm and leg movements, and repetitive speech, usually of syllables, not words. Occasionally, speech is slowed or totally inhibited during such a seizure. Other experiences are peculiar sensations in the abdomen, generalized flushing, and palpitations.

Focal sensory seizures caused by a lesion involving the sensory cortex may be jacksonian with a march of abnormal sensations such as numbness and tingling spreading up an extremity. Other sensory areas of the cerebral cortex produce more complex seizures with paroxysmal visual, auditory, olfactory, gustatory, and vertiginous components in varying degrees of organization. As with other types of focal attacks, the pattern of onset is often the most accurate guide to the locus of an abnormal cerebral lesion.

Autonomic seizures are produced by focal lesions in the regions of the brain associated with autonomic representation, namely the deep temporal, limbic, and diencephalic (hypothalamic) areas. Many autonomic symptoms are associated with other focal or generalized seizures, but they also appear in attacks more or less by themselves, as paroxysms of abdominal pain, sweating, piloerection, incontinence, salivation, and, rarely, fever.

Psychomotor (temporal lobe, limbic system) epilepsy is due to seizure activity involving the temporal lobe, its deeper nuclear masses (the amygdala and hippocampus), and their associated limbic system structures. Psychomotor epilepsy is common in both children and adults and occasionally coexists with grand mal seizures. Evidence of an acquired lesion is found in more than half the patients, with a frequent history of trauma at birth or, later, encephalitis or neoplasm. Some patients with psychomotor seizures are found to have focal frontal or occipital lobe lesions, but even with these there is evidence that the discharges produce their eventual manifestations by propagation through temporal-limbic lobe structures.

Psychomotor-temporal-limbic seizures are manifested by an initial aura of anxiety and visceral symptoms, especially by a peculiar epigastric sensation welling up into the throat. An alteration in consciousness follows, associated with many varied, complex feeling and thinking states, as well as automatic somatic and autonomic motor behavior. Activity is first arrested or suspended, then simple movements ensue, such as chewing, swallowing, sucking, lip smacking, and aimless twistings of the arms and legs. Automatisms then appear which are of varying complexity and involve either partially purposeful or inappropriate and bizarre behavior. Usually, the automatism is stereotyped, but, despite this, the movements usually interplay with the environment, and occasionally they appear to be determined in part by psychologic factors. The activities in this phase of the seizure may merge into normal behavior. The complex attack beginning with unpleasant olfactory hallucinations caused by lesions of the mesial portions of the temporal lobe, the uncus, was specifically called an uncinate seizure by Jackson, who also described the "dreamy" and confused state of the patient. Visceral manifestations are common in young patients, who experience hunger, nausea, vomiting, and abdominal pain as well as urinary incontinence. Destructive aggressive behavior occasionally occurs but usually is not goal-directed. Affective disturbances may be present, particularly expressions of fear, anger, and depression. Occasionally, prolonged fuguelike states with running or wandering may last many minutes. During some psychomotor-temporal lobe seizures, patients experience hallucinations, visual or auditory as well as interpretive illusions involving their own bodies or the immediate environment. These symptoms frequently are associated with ideational blocking and forced thinking as well as peculiar feelings of familiarity called "déjà vu" and "déjà pensée." Amnesia is usually present.

ELECTROENCEPHALOGRAPHIC CONCOMITANTS OF FOCAL SEIZURES. These are represented by discharges of slow waves, spikes, and sharp and slow complexes localized over the particular cerebral region involved. Frequently, the abnormalities are bilateral but asynchronous, representing transmission and diffusion of the abnormal discharge from one hemisphere to its mirror point on the other. At times, deeply situated lesions produce only minimal or no significant alteration in the ordinary electroencephalogram recorded from the scalp.

Status Epilepticus. The rapid repetitive recurrence of any type of seizure without recovery between attacks is called status epilepticus. The term is usually applied to attacks of generalized epilepsy in which the patient remains unconscious and in continuous seizures, with tonic and clonic fluctuations, incontinence, severely disturbed breathing, high fever, excessive sweating, and elevation of blood pressure. Such status may last for hours, even days, and requires emergency medical treatment because of the possible dangers of cerebral damage, thought to be due to ischemic anoxia (or "consumptive" hypoxia) and cardiac and renal failure. The onset of status epilepticus can be spontaneous, but frequently withdrawal from anticonvulsant medication or a too rapid shift of medication is the precipitating cause.

Focal motor seizures may appear in continuous fashion, lasting many hours; this state has been called *epilepsia partialis continua.*

Petit mal status is associated with sustained 3-cycle-per-second spike-wave discharges in the electroencephalogram. The patient is in a state of confusion, has a continuously dazed expression, and has minor movements around the lips or in the arms and legs. *Psychomotor* or *temporal lobe status* also occurs, but less frequently. Such patients are found in a confused state with persistent, inappropriate, bizarre complex behavior patterns lasting over many hours, occasionally associated with fluctuating visceral symptoms.

The Interseizure State. A patient with a progressive cerebral degenerative disease, an extensive cerebral malformation, a severe encephalitis, or an expanding brain tumor may develop changes in behavior and intellectual functioning, primarily because of the underlying structural lesions and not directly because of any seizures that might be present. However, in the past much attention has been paid to the possibility of a specific personality distortion in epileptic patients. Most patients subject to seizures have normal behavior and intellectual functions between attacks and adjust appropriately to society, often excelling. In some instances, however, severe emotional problems do develop, usually in response to environmental restrictions. *Neurotic, maladjusted behavior* occurs, along with obsessional, particularly religious, preoccupations. Often, under these circumstances, the seizures increase and become more difficult to control.

An undetermined number of patients with frequent recurrent generalized seizures, especially status epilepticus, or with recurrent psychomotor temporal-limbic seizures, develop continuing *defects in intellectual function.* Psychologic tests reveal persistent impairments of concentration and attention, memory lapses, word-finding distortions, subtle losses in the ability to associate, and perceptual difficulties. It is possible that prolonged subclinical seizure activity contributes to these disturbances.

More severe personality disturbances, ranging all the way to *psychosis with schizophrenic manifestations,* complicate the interseizure course of a few patients with either psychomotor or severe grand mal epilepsy. The psychotic reactions often have psychologic precipitating factors; occasionally, they follow control of the actual seizures by medication, and these instances may be related, in part, to a reaction to the drug. The symptoms include paranoid, depressive, and hallucinatory reactions, catatonic disorders, flattening of the affect, and severe obsessional states. The patients suffer marked difficulty in concentration and disorientation of time sequences. Defects in memory are present and are accompanied by abnormalities in perception as well as difficulties in word finding, in calculating, and in analyzing the thought content of written material. However, the patients usually attempt to maintain contacts with reality, and major withdrawal is not present, in contrast to most examples of spontaneous schizophrenic illness. Diffuse electroencephalographic abnormality, with either bilateral temporal lobe involvement or diffuse spike wave paroxysms, accompany some of these clinical phases, but with others, the electroencephalogram remains normal.

Diagnosis in Epilepsy. The patient with epilepsy should receive a thorough diagnostic evaluation to determine causative factors and precipitating circumstances. This requires a thorough history, a detailed medical and neurologic physical examination, and selected laboratory investigations, with particular reference to blood chemistry tests, cerebrospinal fluid analysis, electroencephalography, and special roentgenologic studies. Every effort should be made to identify a specific medical illness or a focal cerebral lesion.

History. The history must contain a detailed description of the attacks to help establish the fact of recurrent seizures. As much recollection as possible should be obtained from the patient, particularly of experiences of the aura and the onset of the seizure. The patterning or course of events during and after the seizure should be documented, especially by eyewitness accounts, with special attention to any phenomena that might possess localizing significance. Information should be sought as to the various circumstances under which seizures occur, such as the time of day or night, the frequency of attacks and how medication influences them, their relationship to the menstrual cycle, pregnancy, food intake, sound or light stimulation, intake of alcoholic drinks, or psychologic stresses. All symptoms of neurologic disturbances should be described, such as headache, hemiparesis, hemisensory disturbances, dysphasia, visual difficulties, or vertigo.

The *past medical and developmental history* is of great aid in establishing the cause. Information should be obtained concerning pregnancy, delivery, the neonatal period, the developmental neurologic milestones, head injuries, and reactions to immunizations and the various childhood illnesses such as measles, mumps, and chickenpox. The occurrence of any severe illness with delirium or coma that might be considered an encephalitis should be inquired about, as well as any exposure to toxic substances. Drug intake needs particular investigation, particularly with adults suspected of taking barbiturates or tranquilizer drugs. One must inquire into the patient's social development and behavior in and out of the family setting, his intellectual performance at school, and his vocational adjustments and performance. Any alteration in these phases of existence should be related to seizure occurrence, to the interseizure state, and to the possible effects of medication.

A *family history* of susceptibility to seizures may delineate a significant number with a history of febrile seizures in early childhood as well as of generalized and focal seizures extending into later life. The family history may reveal not only genetically determined cerebral disorders associated with seizures but also other neurologic abnormalities as well.

The *general medical history* can reveal evidence of pertinent cardiovascular disease, blood dyscrasias, and metabolic and endocrine disorders; a seizure may be the first manifestation of a cerebral metastasis or of a generalized vascular disease.

Clinical Examination. In most patients with seizures, physical examination fails to disclose significant physical or neurologic abnormalities. Nevertheless, a thorough general examination is warranted; careful examination of the skin, for example, may produce the diagnosis in cases of tuberous sclerosis, neurofibromatosis, or cerebral hemangioma. Examination of the lungs provides evidence for consideration of metastatic tumor or abscess; evaluation of the peripheral circulation and blood pressure gives an indication of the possibility of the various types of cerebral vascular lesions or aids in differentiating between syncope and seizure.

The *neurologic examination* serves two purposes: to elicit signs of any general neurologic disorder and to determine whether or not focal signs of a localized cerebral lesion are present. A neurologic examination is particularly valuable at the time of, or shortly after, a seizure if it reveals a transitory hemiparesis or related signs.

A battery of *psychologic tests* can aid the evaluation of both intellectual capabilities and psychologic adjustments. Simple tests of memory and perception are part of the regular neurologic examination. For more complete studies, the most useful tests include the Wechsler Intelligence Scale (especially the Kohs block test), the memory scales, the Bender-Gestalt, the Rorschach, and the Thematic Apperception tests. Attention should be paid to the patient's performance during these tests as well as to the actual scores.

Laboratory Investigations. Each patient with recurrent seizures, no matter the age, should be examined with certain laboratory investigations at least once and more often if changes develop in seizure patterns or neurologic signs. At different ages certain tests are more apt to produce results leading to specific etiologic diagnosis. Additional studies are necessary to evaluate the general health of the patient and follow the potentially toxic effects of medication.

There are no abnormal laboratory findings associated directly with seizure activity except electroencephalographic discharges. Urine analysis is necessary to determine the state of kidney function; if abnormal, a specific renal disorder may be present, and certain drugs cannot be administered. Similarly, a complete blood count is necessary. Severe seizure states such as status epilepticus may be associated with proteinuria, leukocytosis, and fever as secondary manifestations. In certain instances, special blood chemistry studies are warranted, such as the blood sugar for the diagnosis of suspected hypoglycemia and in the evaluation of a diabetic with epilepsy, and the serum calcium determination for infants and young children with seizure states. Evaluation of fluctuations in serum electrolytes and acid-base balance is necessary to study both children and adults with disorders of the kidney, liver, heart, and lungs. Serologic tests help to diagnose past infections.

The *cerebrospinal fluid* is apt to be normal in all constituents and pressures, except in the minority of patients who have specific neurologic disease. After severe seizures, there may be a slight increase in the cerebrospinal fluid protein and white cell count. In structural neurologic disorders with seizures, the protein and/or pressure may be elevated persistently, and the specific diagnosis then depends on other tests, such as contrast roentgenologic studies. Chronic nervous system infection can be associated with an increase in the white cell count of the cerebrospinal fluid; occasionally, a cerebral tumor may be revealed by neoplastic cells in the fluid.

Roentgenograms of the skull and chest must be taken of all patients. The film of the skull may reveal asymmetry caused by early injury or maldevelopment, abnormal calcifications, shift of the calcified pineal, or signs of increased intracranial pressure. The chest film potentially detects pulmonary infection or tumor and aids in evaluating the cardiac status. Roentgenologic studies of the intracranial contents employing contrast media are extremely useful diagnostic procedures if employed at the proper time, but must be selected with care because of their morbid potential. Such procedures are considered when a focal intracranial lesion is suspected. *Ventriculography* is the procedure of choice when there is increased intracranial pressure, particularly when a lesion is suspected in the posterior fossa. Ordinarily, when the pressure is normal, a fractional *pneumoencephalogram* gives more information about a lesion occupying space within the skull or distorting the ventricular or subarachnoid systems. Pneumoencephalography also discloses focal brain atrophy as reflected by selective enlargements of important specific space such as the temporal horns. *Cerebral arteriography* is useful for patients with or without evidence of increased pressure and can demonstrate localized abnormal vascular patterns in neoplasms as well as intracranial hematomas, vascular malformations, and the location of vascular occlusions.

Radioactive isotopic brain scanning may be of use. A negative brain scan often eliminates the immediate necessity for performing a contrast roentgenologic procedure, whereas an abnormal study requires further investigation.

Electroencephalography. The various electroencephalographic correlates of the different types of seizures have been described. The electroencephalogram is an indicator of a certain kind of cerebral activity determined by recording electrodes upon the scalp. This is important to realize, because electroencephalograms from up to 25 per cent of patients with seizures are normal; yet, abnormal discharges are disclosed in many of these same patients by depth electrodes recording from deeper cerebral structures such as the amygdala and hippocampus. The electroencephalogram, therefore, has limited diagnostic applications and must be correlated with other information from the various physical and neurologic examinations. It can be utilized to confirm the presence of a seizure disturbance, particularly if paroxysmal discharges are recorded during and correlated with a seizure. An example of this specificity is that up to 85 per cent of children with petit mal will have the typical 3-cycle-per-second spike and wave discharges both during and between seizures and, in many instances, these discharges can be precipitated during the recording by overventilation and light stimulation.

In other instances of epilepsy, the electroencephalogram contains generalized, nonspecific slow wave discharges that merely indicate the presence of cerebral dysfunction, but not a definite seizure disorder. Focal slow wave abnormalities in the electroencephalogram suggest a localized structural lesion and ordinarily lead to further investigations. Finally, in certain forms of focal epilepsy, the electroencephalogram may show focal discharges of spikes, sharp waves, and complex components indicative of the epileptogenic nature of the focus. Yet, in some of these instances, such an abnormality might be transmitted, the basic discharging focus being elsewhere.

In most laboratories of electroencephalography the test procedure involves recording in the waking state and during voluntary overventilation. Additional attempts are usually made to provoke generalized and focal paroxysmal discharges by means of sleep, sensory stimulation with light and occasionally sound, and sometimes by utilizing certain metabolic and pharmacologic adjuvants.

The recording of the electroencephalogram during sleep is useful in the attempt to demonstrate focal temporal lobe discharges in patients with psychomotor–temporal lobe epilepsy. In adults, such discharges are increased during sleep in up to 75 per cent of patients, but the results in children are less definitive, the increase occurring in only 30 per cent. In many patients, sleep produces increased bilateral appearance of abnormal temporal discharges. The use of sphenoidal electrodes is occasionally of some help in lateralizing temporal lobe discharge, particularly when patients are being evaluated for surgical therapy. At times, barbiturate-induced fast wave activity is found to be diminished on the side of the involved temporal lobe. Photic stimulation identifies patients with light-sensitive epilepsy and, occasionally, produces lateralized discharges in patients with a sensitive focus. There have been many attempts to alter the electrical activity of the brain in susceptible patients by inducing metabolic changes, such as hydration after an injection of Pitressin. Various stimulant drugs have been used, such as Metrazol and Megimide. All these methods, particularly the use of the drugs, may produce paroxysmal discharges as well as clinical seizures, usually generalized. However, attempts to measure seizure discharge threshold have been unsuccessful because of great variability, and many normal subjects respond with seizures to these procedures. Accordingly, these methods are not recommended for general use in the diagnosis of epilepsy. Occasionally, it may be important in the evaluation of a specific patient to study in detail the phenomena of the seizure and to determine focal components either in the electroencephalogram or clinically. In selected cases, this can be accomplished by the administration of a controlled dose of a seizure-producing drug.

The use of the electroencephalogram in following patients with epilepsy is limited, because in many instances some degree of electroencephalographic abnormality persists even though seizures are controlled. This is most often the case in patients with psychomotor–temporal lobe epilepsy and least often in children with petit mal and myoclonic seizures.

Differential Diagnosis. The diagnosis of epilepsy has profound implications, medically and psychologically, as it affects the total life situation of the patient and his family. Consequently, careful attention must be given to make this diagnosis positively and specifically, and to differentiate it from other disturbances that producc somewhat similar abnormalities of neurologic function that are not seizures.

Consciousness may be disturbed episodically by inadequate cerebral blood flow in attacks of *cerebrovascular insufficiency* or of *syncope* of various types, particularly the vasodepressor form. Disturbances of cerebral circulation affect older persons especially, and such patients generally suffer other evidence of hypertension and cerebral arteriosclerosis. Periodic blackouts and recurrent confusional states are manifestations of basilar artery insufficiency, as are other episodic signs of brainstem and cerebellar dysfunction. Patients with carotid arterial insufficiency characteristically experience transitory hemiparesis and hemisensory disturbances along with dysphasia, but the clonic movements of a paroxysmal disorder usually are absent. The electroencephalographic findings of paroxysmal discharge do not occur with cerebrovascular disease although, at times, bilateral rhythmic discharges are observed related to vascular lesions of the upper brainstem. The differential diagnosis is sometimes difficult and may require arteriographic confirmation of a vascular lesion as well as the usual evaluation of the history and general medical state of the patient.

Syncopal episodes may resemble akinetic or brief motor seizures; prolonged syncope can progress into a convulsion resulting from the persistence of cerebral ischemia and hypoxia. The patient with syncope usually has indications of disturbed vasomotor reactivity with excessive sweating, pallor, and tachycardia. Specific precipitating factors often are present such as fear or other psychologic upset. The confusion, headache, and drowsiness that occur after a generalized seizure usually do not appear in syncope. The electroencephalogram during simple syncope consists of diffuse asynchronous slow waves without paroxysmal or focal discharges.

Certain *psychogenic disorders* resemble epileptic states and can be difficult to differentiate. Hysterical "seizures" not only occur as independent problems, but also complicate the course of a limited number of patients with known seizures, the combination being called "hysteroepilepsy." The clinical problem is difficult to unravel because of the interrelationships between the actual seizure and the reactive psychologic disturbance. The hysterical seizure is not associated with neurologic signs of reflex abnormality and, during it, the electroencephalogram contains no paroxysmal discharges. The pattern of hysterical seizures is often bizarre and not a stereotyped tonic-clonic movement sequence. Self-injury is an unusual result of the seizure, and the postictal states of confusion, headache, and drowsiness are absent. Hysterical or psychotic fugue disturbances and dissociative reactions must be distinguished from psychomotor–temporal lobe seizures. The diagnosis of an hysterical seizure state requires careful psychiatric evaluation because of the severe neurotic process involved.

Treatment. Treatment of the epilepsies must take into account not only the patient and his disorder, but his family and general life situation. Much depends on the diagnostic evaluation and the finding of specific causes whenever possible that can be treated directly. This is clearly defined in instances in which metabolic disturbance is obvious, such as hypoglycemia and hypocalcemia, or when an operable cerebral tumor is found. However, in many cases of acquired epilepsy, the basic cause of the seizure cannot be treated directly. Seizures may continue in patients even after removal of a brain tumor because of scarring, or when the tumor is found to be inoperable or incompletely removable. The diagnosis of an acquired epilepsy after head injury or encephalitis usually does not lead to specific therapy. Only a limited number of patients with post-traumatic epilepsy are satisfactory candidates for surgical removal of a localized meningocerebral scar. The administration of anticonvulsant drugs is necessary, therefore, for the majority of patients.

Medical Therapy. There are many available anticonvulsant drugs, as shown in the accompanying table. None is capable of achieving total seizure control in all patients, but careful selection and utilization in each case often leads to optimal results. Each physician should learn to use a number of these drugs well and to recognize disturbing side effects as early as possible. Periodic blood counts, urinalyses, and liver function tests are necessary with certain drugs.

The basic mechanisms of anticonvulsant drugs are not definitely known. Most of the drugs are neuronal depressants with certain variations in action. The hydantoin drugs reduce the synaptic activity of post-tetanic potentiation; the oxazolidine (methadione) drugs decrease nerve transmission during repetitive stimulation. The drugs are believed to increase the stability of excitable neuronal membranes by acting upon electrochemical characteristics involved in ion permeability and membrane polarization. Such stabilizing effects would decrease the activity of the hyperexcitable neuronal aggregates in an epileptogenic focus and prevent the spread of discharge through normal neuronal circuits.

The anticonvulsant drugs are administered to achieve the desired effect of seizure control and must be built up in dosage while not producing untoward toxic reactions. It is best to start with one drug of choice, but usually a single drug is not totally effective, and a second is necessary. Two drugs might be needed initially for patients with two different types of seizure such as grand mal and petit mal. This occurs fairly frequently (from 25 to 50 per cent in some series, especially in adolescents [see Lennox, 1960]). The process may require weeks of adjustment and, during this time, the patient's or parent's cooperation in reporting effects on seizure frequency or side-reactions is most important. Determination of anticonvulsant blood levels, i.e., diphenylhydantoin, phenobarbital, primidone, may be very helpful in identifying patients who are obtaining unsatisfactory control be-

Anticonvulsant Drugs: Dosage, Indications, and Toxic Effects

Bromides
- Daily dosage: 1.0 to 3.0 grams for adults; not recommended for children
- Indications: All types of seizures, especially grand mal and psychomotor; may be combined with hydantoins
- Toxic effects: Drowsiness, dulling, rash, psychosis; rarely used now

Celontin
- Dose: 0.3 gram capsules
- Daily dosage: Children: 0.6 gram; adults: 1 to 1.5 grams
- Indications: Petit mal, psychomotor seizures, myoclonic seizures, massive spasms
- Toxic effects: Ataxia, drowsiness; rarely, blood dyscrasias

Dexedrine (dextroamphetamine)
- Dose: 5 mg tablets; 5 mg, 10 mg, and 15 mg long-acting Spansules
- Daily dosage: Children: 5 to 15 mg; adults: 15 to 30 mg
- Indications: To counteract sedative effects, hyperkinetic behavioral disturbances in children, narcolepsy
- Toxic effects: Anorexia, irritability, sleeplessness

Diamox (acetazolamide)
- Dose: 250 mg tablets
- Daily dosage: Children: 0.75 to 1.0 gram; adults: 1.0 to 1.5 grams. Use intermittently; tolerance occurs
- Indications: As an adjuvant in all types of seizures, especially those in females related to menstrual cycles
- Toxic effects: Anorexia, acidosis, drowsiness, numbness of extremities; rarely, blood dyscrasias

Dilantin (diphenylhydantoin)
- Dose: 0.03 gram and 0.1 gram capsules; 0.05 gram tablets; 0.1 gram delayed action capsules; 0.025 gram per ml suspension; 0.1 gram in oil, capsules; 0.25 gram ampules for parenteral use
- Daily dosage: Children: 0.15 to 0.3 gram; adults: 0.3 to 0.6 gram. Effective blood level 10 to 20 μg/ml
- Indications: Grand mal, psychomotor and focal seizures; most useful in combination with phenobarbital or primidone
- Toxic effects: Rash, fever, gum hypertrophy, gastric distress, diplopia, ataxia, hirsutism (young females); drowsiness, uncommon; megaloblastic anemia (due to secondary folic acid deficiency); lymphadenopathy

Mebaral (mephobarbital)
- Dose: 0.03 gram, 0.1 gram tablets
- Daily dosage: Children: 0.06 to 0.3 gram; adults: 0.3 to 0.6 gram
- Indications: Grand mal, petit mal, psychomotor, focal seizures; similar to phenobarbital; most useful in combination with hydantoins
- Toxic effects: Drowsiness, irritability, rash

Mesantoin (methylphenylethylhydantoin)
- Dose: 0.1 gram tablets
- Daily dosage: Children: 0.1 to 0.4 gram; adults: 0.4 to 0.8 gram
- Indications: Grand mal, psychomotor, and focal seizures
- Toxic effects: Rash, fever, drowsiness, ataxia, gum hypertrophy (less than Dilantin), neutropenia, agranulocytosis

Milontin (methylphenylsuccinimide)
- Dose: 0.5 gram capsules; 250 mg per 4 ml suspension
- Daily dosage: Children: 0.25 gram to 1.5 grams; adults: 2.0 to 4.0 grams
- Indications: Petit mal, myoclonic and akinetic seizures; occasionally psychomotor seizures
- Toxic effects: Nausea, dizziness, rash, hematuria (may be nephrotoxic)

Mysoline (primidone)
- Dose: 0.05 gram, 0.25 gram tablets; 250 mg per 5 ml suspension
- Daily dosage: Children: 0.25 gram; adults: 0.75 to 2.0 grams. The daily dosage should be built up very slowly. Effective blood level range 5 to 15 μg/ml
- Indications: Grand mal, psychomotor and focal seizures; occasionally, petit mal; useful in combination with Dilantin
- Toxic effects: Drowsiness, ataxia, dizziness, rash, nausea, leukopenia (rare)

Paradione (paramethadione)
- Dose: 0.15 gram, 0.3 gram capsules; 0.3 gram per ml solution
- Daily dosage: Children: 0.3 gram to 1.8 grams; adults: 1.2 grams to 2.4 grams
- Indications: Petit mal, myoclonic and akinetic seizures, massive spasms, occasionally psychomotor seizures (in children); often useful in combination with Dilantin and phenobarbital; somewhat less effective and less toxic than Tridione
- Toxic effects: Rash, gastric distress, visual symptoms (glare, photophobia), neutropenia, agranulocytosis

Peganone (ethylphenylhydantoin)
- Dose: 0.25 gram, 0.5 gram tablets
- Daily dosage: Children: 0.5 gram to 1.5 grams; adults: 2.0 to 3.0 grams
- Indications: Grand mal, psychomotor and focal seizures
- Toxic effects: Similar to those of Dilantin but less frequent; may be substituted for Dilantin, but is generally less effective

Phenobarbital
- Dose: 0.015 gram, 0.030 gram, 0.060 gram, 0.1 gram tablets; 4 mg per ml elixir
- Daily dosage: Children: 0.045 gram to 0.1 gram; adults: 0.1 gram to 0.3 gram. Effective blood level range 15 to 30 μg/ml
- Indications: All seizure states: grand mal, petit mal, psychomotor and other focal; most useful in limited dosage in combination with other drugs such as Dilantin
- Toxic effects: Drowsiness, dulling, rash, fever; irritability, and hyperactivity in some children

Phenurone (phenacemide)
- Dose: 0.5 gram tablets; 0.3 gram enteric-coated tablets
- Daily dosage: Children: 0.5 gram to 2.0 grams; adults: 1.5 grams to 3.0 grams
- Indications: May be effective in all types of seizures, especially psychomotor–temporal lobe seizures, should be used only in very resistant cases
- Toxic effects: A highly toxic drug, producing liver damage, agranulocytosis, psychotic reactions, and rashes

Tridione (trimethadione)
- Dose: 0.15 gram tablets; 0.3 gram capsules; 0.15 gram per 4 ml solution
- Daily dosage: Children: 0.3 gram to 1.8 grams; adults: 1.2 grams to 2.4 grams. Effective blood level range 10 to 30 μg/ml
- Indications: Petit mal, myoclonic and akinetic seizures, massive spasms; often useful in combination with Dilantin and phenobarbital
- Toxic effects: Rash, gastric distress, visual symptoms (glare, photophobia) neutropenia, agranulocytosis, nephrosis

Zarontin (ethosuximide)
- Dose: 0.25 gram capsules
- Daily dosage: Children: to 0.75 to 1.0 gram; adults: 1.5 grams. Effective blood level range 40 to 80 μg/ml
- Indications: Petit mal seizures (now the drug of choice); used with Dilantin in mixed seizure states
- Toxic effects: Blood dyscrasias (pancytopenia, leukopenia) unusual; dermatitis, anorexia, nausea, drowsiness, dizziness

The following drugs may be used in the emergency treatment of status epilepticus:

- Diazepam (Valium): 2.5 to 10 mg intravenously
- Sodium phenobarbital: 0.25 to 0.50 gram intravenously
- Sodium amytal: 0.25 to 0.50 gram intravenously
- Paraldehyde: 3.0 to 5.0 ml intravenously (diluted in 10 to 20 ml saline)
- Dilantin sodium (parenteral): 0.25 gram intravenously or intramuscularly (to 0.5 gram per 24 hours in patients previously receiving this drug or as much as 1.0 to 1.5 in previously untreated patients). *Caution*: Dilantin intravenously must be given slowly in 0.05 gram increments to avoid vasodepression

General anesthetics such as ether, Avertin, and xylocaine have a limited usefulness in the treatment of status epilepticus. Careful nursing and attention to fluid and electrolyte balance, airway, cardiac and renal functions, and temperature control are essential in the over-all management of status epilepticus.

cause they either fail to take the drug or metabolize it abnormally. Frequent and rapid shifting or replacement of drugs is to be avoided. Following blood levels in each individual patient and adjusting medication dosage into the therapeutic range have significantly improved seizure control as well as increased our understanding of overdosage and toxic effects.

Diphenylhydantoin metabolism is impaired in patients with acute and chronic liver disease, resulting in elevations of blood levels when standard doses of the drug are taken. By contrast, in the presence of uremia, the blood level of diphenylhydantoin is reduced; however, apparently adequate amounts of the drug unbound to plasma protein may be achieved with administered low dosage.

There also is increasing evidence that other drugs can alter the rate of diphenylhydantoin metabolism induced in liver microsomal enzymes so as to lead to an increase in diphenylhydantoin blood levels even to toxicity (see Ch. 20). These drugs include isoniazid, bishydroxycoumarin, phenyramidol, disulfiram, methylphenidate, diazepam, chlordiazepoxide, phenylbutazone, chlorpromazine, prochlorperazine, and some estrogens. Carbamazepine and ethanol have been reported to lower diphenylhydantoin blood levels. On the other hand, diphenylhydantoin has been reported to lower blood levels of digitoxin, bishydroxycoumarin, metyrapone, and DDT. Diphenylhydantoin also has been found to stimulate enzymes which rapidly turn over endogenous or exogenously administered adrenocorticosteroids; this has resulted, in some instances, in increased adrenocorticotrophic and cortisol production by negative feedback effects.

A specific anticonvulsant drug for each type of seizure is not available. However, there is one major therapeutic division; petit mal absences respond best to either succinimide or oxazolidines (methadiones). These drugs are not effective in the treatment of major generalized (grand mal) or focal cerebral seizures, nor are the hydantoins (used in grand mal and other seizures) effective in petit mal. It is stated that the drugs used in the therapy of petit mal may worsen a generalized seizure state, but this has not been proved.

Generalized grand mal and focal motor seizures are best treated by diphenylhydantoin sodium and phenobarbital. Initially, either drug may be administered to patients who have infrequent attacks, but generally the combination of diphenylhydantoin and phenobarbital produces the most effective seizure control. The average dose of diphenylhydantoin is 0.3 to 0.4 gram per day, usually administered as 0.2 gram in the morning after breakfast and 0.2 gram after dinner. The dosage of phenobarbital is initially 60 mg at bedtime, with 30 mg increments over the day, up to three times daily, if necessary, limited by the unwanted sedative effect.

Patients with psychomotor–temporal lobe epilepsy are often more difficult to control. Many trials of different agents and different doses may be necessary in these cases; the best results are to be expected with diphenylhydantoin and either phenobarbital or primidone. Although in some clinics the two latter drugs are used together, primidone is partially converted to phenobarbital, and their sedative effects combine to make such administration difficult. It is most important with primidone to start therapy with small doses, such as 125 mg, increased at weekly intervals to reach a maximal dosage of 0.75 gram for children or 1.0 to 2.0 grams per day for adults. If untoward side effects to diphenylhydantoin occur, substitution with the less reactive Peganone is sometimes successful, although this drug has less anticonvulsant effect. Mesantoin and phenacemide are used only for the most difficult cases and even then with extreme care because of their high degree of toxicity.

Acetazolamide is an adjuvant to the treatment of any type of seizure. It seems to have a general effect upon hyperexcitable cerebral neurons because of its properties of inhibition of carbonic anhydrase and production of acidosis. Because tolerance develops, the drug should be administered intermittently. It is occasionally useful, for example, in helping to control seizures appearing periodically in females at the time of menstruation. Under these circumstances, acetazolamide is administered for a week prior to and during menses.

The *results of drug therapy* are difficult to predict. With careful attention to individual details and general management, most patients with occasional generalized and psychomotor seizures achieve either complete or nearly complete reduction of seizures. Satisfactory or complete control can be achieved in most children with petit mal absences. However, each group of patients, especially those with grand mal and psychomotor epilepsy, contains a refractory number who suffer from troublesome side effects of drugs and from increasing psychologic and sociologic difficulties as the years go by.

In a relatively small but significant number of patients under treatment with diphenylhydantoin and occasionally phenobarbital-related drugs, a paradoxical increase in seizures occurs, along with depressed mentation and increased electroencephalographic abnormalities. The blood levels of the drugs are usually in a "toxic" range, but not always, and other signs of "toxicity," such as nystagmus and ataxia, may not be present. Reduction of anticonvulsant drug dosage, in these instances, leads to a diminution of seizure activity and clearing of mental functions.

When to stop drugs for a patient whose seizures are completely controlled is a recurrent question. Some authorities recommend cautiously withdrawing anticonvulsants if patients have been free of attacks for two years, but in relatively few cases can drugs be withdrawn without seizures recurring even after symptom-free periods of three to five years. Thus continued treatment is indicated for most adults with grand mal and psychomotor epilepsy. The electroencephalogram may remain abnormal in clinically seizure-free patients, indicating persistent seizure potentiality, but even in patients with normal electroencephalograms drug withdrawal may be unsuccessful. Yet, in the management of some patients, it is understandable that a calculated risk of drug withdrawal be considered if this represents a psychologic achievement of great magnitude. Under these circumstances, the drug should be withdrawn carefully with small decrements over many weeks. Drug elimination may be carried out more successfully in children with controlled petit mal, particularly because there is a natural tendency for the absences to diminish with age and maturity.

A presentation of drugs used in the medical treatment of epilepsy is given in the accompanying table in alphabetical order, with statements concerning dose administration, indications for different seizure types, and toxic effects.

Adrenocorticotrophic hormone (ACTH) and adrenocortical steroids are now used in the treatment of massive spasms in infancy associated with the "hypsarhythmic" electroencephalogram. Such therapy is administered after primary causes of massive spasms, such as phenylketonuria, have been excluded. Although initial improvements in the spasms and the electroencephalogram may occur, the prognosis is poor, particularly with regard to the mental deterioration accompanying this condition. Nothing is known about the mechanism of action of the hormones in this disorder; this is somewhat paradoxical because these hormones are known to raise cerebral excitability and precipitate seizures in older persons and in experimental situations.

Dietary Treatment. In general, there are no dietary restrictions for the patient with epilepsy, nor is there a specific diet capable of aiding most patients. However, a diet high in fat content producing significant ketosis, the *ketogenic diet,* occasionally is helpful in treating young children, particularly those with intractable petit mal and generalized motor seizures. Anticonvulsant drugs usually have to be continued, and the diet is difficult to maintain because it is unpleasant.

Psychologic Therapy and Sociologic Management. Many basic problems in the over-all life adjustments of the patient need additional management even though drugs can achieve significant control of seizures. In many cases, the coexistence of seizures and personality problems requires a combination of medical anticonvulsant therapy and psychologically oriented management.

The sedative properties of anticonvulsant drugs usually are not used directly. The so-called tranquilizing drugs have limited usefulness in the management of seizure patients; chlordiazepoxide (Librium) and diazepam (Valium) may reduce disturbed behavior, particularly in children. The phenothiazine drugs have variable effects; an alerting phenothiazine, fluphenazine, is of some use in controlling abnormal behavior in certain patients with psychomotor seizures. However, other drugs in the chlorpromazine group are known to provoke seizures and paroxysmal discharges in the electroencephalogram.

There is often a direct interplay between emotional disturbances and clinical seizure activity. Some patients in a state of psychologic turmoil experience increased seizures and require greater amounts of anticonvulsant drugs. The subsequent achievement of psychologic adjustment decreases the frequency of seizures and lessens the drug requirement. This needs to be developed in various ways, depending on the patient's age and his family and social circumstances. Family understanding is of primary importance, because the child with seizures has to live, insofar as possible, as a normal person within home and school settings. A great problem, still to be overcome, is the stigma attached by society to the diagnosis of epilepsy, and the lack of understanding that not only exists among people in general but is reflected by various restrictive legal practices. Most children with seizures are able to attend schools and vocational programs successfully; most adults with controlled seizures are capable of developing productive careers and engaging in the activities that are so much a part of our culture, such as marriage, childbearing, obtaining an education, driving an automobile, traveling from country to country, and working with appropriate safeguards, protected by insurance and worker's compensation programs. Only a relatively small number of patients require a protected environment, such as that in schools or colonies specifically developed for epileptic patients. Even these no longer should be institutions where many hundreds or thousands of epileptic patients are kept in essentially custodial care. "Colonies" with schools, homelike units, and small villages exist in Great Britain, Holland, and Denmark and take care of relatively small numbers of patients (up to a few hundred at most in each), involved in intensive programs of medical therapy, psychologic management, education, and vocational training. From these places increasing numbers of adequately controlled patients are sent out into the general community, where they live well adjusted and productive lives.

Only a few occupations are contraindicated for patients with seizures. These include activities of potential danger to either the patient or others, such as work requiring unprotected climbing to great heights and utilizing heavy power equipment or dangerous chemical substances.

Informal and formal psychotherapeutic measures can be undertaken in order to reduce emotional disturbances. The role of the family physician is all-important in these considerations. Often he alone can judge the problems that exist in a family, school, or social setting. His understanding and guidance help both the patient and his family to overcome the feelings of despair, anxiety, fear, and self-consciousness that otherwise interfere with the normal adjustments of everyone involved. It is only when anxieties and depressive tendencies develop into more severe reactions, associated with paranoid states, increased withdrawal, and excessive obsessional tendencies, that more intensive psychiatric treatment becomes necessary. Occasionally, brief periods of hospitalization help in the evaluation of the intensity of the psychologic disturbance and any associated intellectual difficulties that may interfere with the patient's performance. Drug schedules may be revised at the same time, under controlled conditions.

Even the child with epilepsy and behavioral disorder can be cared for best if he attends a regular school in an understanding environment and is associated with a clinical outpatient service in which the physician and social service department work together with both the child and the family. It is becoming less necessary to arrange for either home tutoring or the placement of such children into schools or other facilities for the maladjusted.

Surgical Therapy. The patient with a potentially remediable lesion, such as a brain tumor, usually is considered for operation, whatever the state of the seizures. Surgical intervention for the removal of a focus of abnormal discharge is appropriate only for selected patients who have focal epilepsy that remains intractable after intensive medical therapy. A constant focally discharging area should be confirmed by serial electroencephalographic studies, and the region of brain considered for excision must be such that the patient will not be left afterward with a severe speech, memory, or other disabling neurologic deficit.

Patients so evaluated usually do not have gross space-occupying lesions, but the epileptogenic region eventually excised may contain a small tumor, a vascular lesion, or a scar secondary to trauma or previous encephalitis. The surgical approach has been utilized particularly for patients with focal motor and psychomotor–temporal lobe seizures. Even though many patients are considered for surgical therapy, relatively few are chosen, and the numbers of patients so treated are still only in the hundreds the world over. In carefully selected series, about half the patients enjoy significantly improved control of seizures postoperatively, although this sometimes merely represents less anticonvulsant drug requirement. In some patients, generalized seizures appear instead of previous psychomotor–temporal lobe attacks. A small number experience relief from severe personality disturbances, particularly aggressive psychotic behavior, but this is an uncertain effect, and surgical intervention usually is not primarily directed toward this. Bilateral operations on the temporal lobe have been of limited success and have produced severe memory disturbances.

Cerebral hemispherectomy has been accomplished in a small number of carefully selected children with severe infantile hemiplegia, intractable convulsions, and behavior disturbances. Improvement in the seizures and behavior has occurred despite the persistence of motor and sensory neurologic disability.

Much more must be learned about the natural history of the epilepsies in order to evaluate thoroughly the different therapies. Adequate seizure control can be achieved now for most patients. The drugs involved are increasingly less toxic, but anticonvulsant medication remains essentially nonspecific and is directed against mechanisms of neuronal hyperexcitability that are little understood. A relatively small number of cases not responding to other management can be selected for surgical intervention. It is hoped that combined physiologic and biochemical studies of disturbed cerebral and bodily functions in the epilepsies will lead eventually to more rational and effective therapy.

Epilepsia (Journal of the International League Against Epilepsy), H. Gastaut. G. H. Glaser. M. Lennox-Buchthal (eds.). Raven Press. New York.

Gowers, W. R.: Epilepsy and Other Chronic Convulsive Disorders: Their Causes, Symptoms and Treatment. London, J. & A. Churchill, 1881. Reprinted by Dover Publications, New York, 1964.

Jasper, H. H., Ward, A. A., and Pope, A.: Basic Mechanisms of the Epilepsies. Boston, Little, Brown & Company, 1969.

Lennox, W. G.: Epilepsy and Related Disorders. Boston, Little, Brown & Company, 1960.

Lennox-Buchthal, M. A.: Febrile convulsions. A reappraisal. Amsterdam, Elsevier Scientific Publishing Company, 1973.

Penfield, W. G., and Jasper, H. H.: Epilepsy and the Functional Anatomy of the Human Brain. Boston, Little, Brown & Company, 1954.

Schmidt, R. P., and Wilder, B. J.: Epilepsy Contemporary Neurology Series Monograph No. 2. Philadelphia, F. A. Davis Company, 1968.

Woodbury, D. M., Penry, J. K., and Schmidt, R. P. (eds.): Antiepileptic Drugs. New York, Raven Press, 1972.

Section Seventeen. INTRACRANIAL TUMORS AND STATES CAUSING INCREASED INTRACRANIAL PRESSURE

Robert A. Fishman

420. INTRACRANIAL TUMORS

Intracranial tumors include neoplasms, both benign and malignant, and other space-taking lesions of chronic inflammatory origin that develop in brain, meninges, or skull. Their clinical manifestations are diverse and vary greatly according to tumor type and location. Errors in diagnosis are relatively common because the clinical manifestations of tumor may simulate a variety of neurologic disorders. Brain tumors occur at any age; they are common in children under ten, but have their peak incidence in the fifth and sixth decades of life. Race, occupation, and history of trauma have not been established as predisposing factors in the occurrence of intracranial tumors. Genetic factors are relevant, however, to the occurrence of a few tumor types, e.g., hemangioblastoma and neurofibromatosis.

Classification and Pathology. A great number of tumor types have been variously classified. Most classifications include (1) primary tumors originating in brain, (2) meningeal tumors, (3) vascular tumors, (4) pituitary tumors, (5) congenital tumors, (6) adnexal tumors, (7) metastatic tumors, and (8) granulomas and parasitic cysts.

Primary Brain Tumors. The largest group of primary brain tumors are the gliomas, composed of malignant glial cells. These include the following:

GLIOBLASTOMA MULTIFORME. These most malignant gliomas are composed of very undifferentiated cells. Complete surgical removal is impossible. The average life expectancy is 12 months. They have a very rapid growth rate and are characterized by much tissue necrosis and brain edema.

ASTROCYTOMA. Astrocytomas are composed of astrocytes that infiltrate the brain and are often associated with cysts of varying size. They are generally slow growing and may occasionally run a course of many years or even decades. They may infiltrate normal brain widely but with relatively little effect on brain function early in the illness. Complete surgical excision of cystic astrocytomas of the cerebellum may be possible, particularly in children, but in most other instances their marked invasiveness of brain prevents complete removal. Astrocytomas may undergo malignant change, and a highly malignant glioblastoma may develop within a relatively benign astrocytoma.

OLIGODENDROGLIOMA. Oligodendrogliomas, composed of oligodendroglial cells, are similar in behavior to astrocytomas and are distinguishable only on histologic study.

EPENDYMOMA. Ependymomas are derived from ependymal cells. They arise from the walls of the ventricular system, filling or obstructing the ventricles and invading adjacent tissues. They are malignant and cause death in about three years.

MEDULLOBLASTOMA. Medulloblastomas develop from a primitive cell within the cerebellum. They are chiefly tumors of childhood but can occur in older patients. They are highly malignant and frequently metastasize throughout the subarachnoid space to involve the cerebrum or spinal cord.

Meningeal Tumors. The most important tumor arising in the meninges is the *meningioma,* which may invade the adjacent bone as well as compressing and distorting the brain. It is slow growing, well circumscribed, often highly vascular, and may be calcified. It is benign, and complete removal is often possible unless the tumor involves critical structures.

Vascular Tumors. Tumors composed of vascular elements include the arteriovenous malformations (angiomas) and hemangioblastomas. The angiomas are congenital malformations composed of an abnormal collection of blood vessels of adult structure. They are present from birth but slowly enlarge and may not cause symptoms for many years. They may compress normal brain, may bleed intracerebrally or into the subarachnoid space, may be manifest only as a source of seizures, or may be an incidental finding at autopsy. Hemangioblastomas are true neoplasms composed of primitive vascular elements that may be quiescent for many years or may enlarge very slowly. They are most commonly found in the cerebellum but occur also in the cerebrum. Cerebellar hemangioblastoma may be associated with angiomatosis of the retina and cysts of the kidney and pancreas (the von Hippel–Lindau syndrome).

Pituitary Tumors. Pituitary tumors may arise from chromophobe, eosinophil, or basophil cells of the anterior pituitary. Of these, chromophobe adenomas are the most common. Chromophobe adenomas are nonfunctioning tumors that give symptoms by compression of the normal pituitary gland as well as the optic chiasm, the hypothalamus, and the adjacent brain with their suprasellar growth. Eosinophilic adenomas give rise to hyperpituitarism, acromegaly in adults, and gigantism in children, but do not generally compress suprasellar structures unless the tumor is mixed with chromophobe elements. Basophil adenomas are small and, although associated with Cushing's syndrome, are not responsible for symptoms by compression of adjacent tissues. *Craniopharyngiomas* derived from Rathke's pouch may be intrasellar or suprasellar in location, may compress the pituitary and optic chiasm, and are similar in effect to the chromophobe adenoma. They are frequently calcified and often contain cysts filled with thick, lipid-laden fluid.

Congenital Tumors. These tumors develop from congenital rests and include craniopharyngiomas of the pituitary, chordomas, dermoids, and teratomas. Chordomas are composed of cells derived from the embryonic notochord. They are midline and usually arise on the clivus, posterior to the sella. They grow slowly, but are highly invasive, and their total extirpation can seldom be accomplished. Dermoids and teratomas may occur anywhere in the central nervous system, particularly near the midline, adjacent to the ventricular system, or at the distal end of the cord. They tend to become symptomatic during the first decade of life, but may be silent for many years.

Adnexal Tumors. These tumors include those originating within the pineal body and those derived from the choroid plexus, the choroid papilloma. Pinealomas are rare tumors that cause symptoms by compressing the aqueduct, resulting in obstructive hydrocephalus and giving paralysis of vertical gaze by involvement of the pretectum of the midbrain. They may compress the hypothalamus and give rise to precocious puberty or diabetes insipidus. Choroid plexus papillomas are benign lesions that may cause intraventricular bleeding. They may cause increased intracranial pressure by obstructing the ventricular system or, it has been suggested, by excessive formation of cerebrospinal fluid.

Metastatic Tumors. Metastatic tumors constitute 10 to 25 per cent of brain tumors. They may originate from almost any primary tumor, most commonly those of breast and lung, but also from neoplasms of the gastrointestinal and genitourinary tracts, bone, thyroid, or nasal sinuses. They may be single or multiple, well encapsulated or diffuse, spread by extension from adjacent tissues or hematogenously. They may occur as a late manifestation in widespread carcinomatosis or as the first manifestation of an unrecognized primary visceral malignancy.

Granulomas and Parasitic Cysts. Granulomas affecting the nervous system include those associated with tuberculosis, mycotic infection, sarcoidosis, parasitic infestation, and syphilis. *Tuberculoma* may present as a solitary mass lesion within the brain; although rare in the United States, it is common in some areas, including Central and South America. Tuberculoma usually develops without evidence of tuberculous meningitis, although evidence of pulmonary tuberculosis is common. Favorable results with surgical excision and antituberculosis therapy have been reported. *Toruloma* is the most common mycotic granuloma affecting brain. This is usually associated with some evidence of meningeal involvement as well. The *granulomas of sarcoidosis* have been reported to occur in the brain; there is usually evidence of meningeal or posterior pituitary involvement, although the evidence for systemic sarcoid may be minimal. *Cysticercosis,* caused by the larvae of *Taenia solium* or *Taenia saginata,* may be responsible for single or multiple cerebral masses. This is seen chiefly in South America and in the Middle East and India. *Syphilitic gummas* are extremely rare, but have been reported, presenting like slow-growing cerebral gliomas.

Pathophysiology. Intracranial tumors give rise to focal disturbances in brain function and to increased intracranial pressure. Focal manifestations occur because brain is compressed or infiltrated by tumor, because the blood supply of the region is compromised, resulting in tissue necrosis, and because of cerebral edema. Tumors may be located either within or outside brain parenchyma, i.e., intra-axial or extra-axial in location. Brain dysfunction is generally greatest with rapidly growing, infiltrative intra-axial tumors, e.g., glioblastoma, because of marked infiltration, compression, and necrosis of brain. Cyst formation within tumors also compresses adjacent normal brain. Cerebral edema about tumors increases the neurologic deficit. In edema, the water and sodium content of the brain are increased owing to their accumulation in the extracellular space and in glial cells. Extra-axial tumors, e.g., meningioma, which slowly compress brain, may reach great size with few, if any, clinical signs.

Tumors cause a generalized increase in intracranial pressure when they reach sufficient mass, because of the fixed volume of the intracranial cavity. Obstruction of the ventricular system also increases intracranial pressure and causes hydrocephalic dilatation of the proximal ventricles and thinning of the cerebral hemispheres. Tumors that obstruct the intracranial venous sinuses also cause increased intracranial pressure. Complete compensation with very little or even no rise in pressure can occur with slowly growing neoplasms, but with rapidly growing malignant tumors, increased intracranial pressure is an early sign. Increased intracranial pressure becomes life threatening when there is sufficient displacement of brain to cause herniation of the uncus or cerebellum. In *uncal herniation,* the most medial gyrus of the temporal lobe, the uncus, is displaced inferiorly by a hemispheric mass through the tentorial notch, thus causing compression of the midbrain, which results in depression of consciousness and ipsilateral or bilateral dilated and fixed pupils owing to compression of the third nerve. In *cerebellar herniation,* the tonsils are displaced downward through the foramen magnum by a posterior fossa mass, causing compression of the medulla and respiratory arrest. Characteristic vasomotor changes ensue with increased intracranial pressure, only if rapid or severe. These include *progressive bradycardia* caused by vagal slowing of the heart; *systemic hypertension,* which occurs as the intracranial pressure begins to approach arterial diastolic pressure, inducing medullary ischemia and compensatory systemic vasoconstriction; and, finally, *central respiratory failure.* Any degree of CO_2 retention will further increase intracranial pressure because of its cerebrovasodilator effects, and therefore adequate ventilation with maintenance of a clear airway is essential for the patient with increased intracranial pressure. (Drugs such as morphine, which depress respiration sufficiently to raise arterial CO_2 levels, are therefore contraindicated.)

Clinical Manifestations. The natural history of intracranial tumor is characterized by insidious onset and progression of focal or general neurologic deficits, or both. Many tumors have rather characteristic manifestations that point to the diagnosis (see below). There is great variation, depending upon location and rate of growth. Occasionally symptoms may be explosive in onset, suggesting a vascular lesion, and there may also be variations in course, suggestive of a remission. The symptoms and signs of intracranial tumor are discussed below.

Headache. Headache is a major but not invariable symptom of intracranial tumor. Patients with extensive tumors may not complain of headache, particularly if they have slowly growing infiltrative tumors (astrocytoma) or slowly growing extra-axial tumors (such as meningiomas, acoustic neuromas, or pituitary tumors). Similarly, when tumors interfere with the higher intellectual functions, headache may not be reported. Tumors give rise to headache by displacement of the pain-sensitive structures within the cranial cavity. Rarely, tumors give rise to a chronic meningeal inflammatory response that also may be responsible for pain. The problem of headache with brain tumor is discussed more extensively in Ch. 350.

Mental Changes. Mental changes may occur either early or late in the history of brain tumor, depending upon tumor location. Subtle evidence of personality change may be the first manifestation of a mass in the cerebral hemispheres, particularly involving the frontal lobes. This may take several forms. The symptoms may be chiefly affective, simulating an involutional depression. Some patients develop confusional states, at times associated with episodes of bizarre behavior. The most common mental changes are progressive impairment of abstraction, recent memory and judgment, and a shortened attention span (see Ch. 326 to 331). However, some patients, particularly those with slowly growing neoplasms in the right (nondominant) hemisphere, may harbor huge tumors with only minimal impairment of intellect. Drowsiness progressing to stupor and coma accompanies severely increased intracranial pressure.

Disturbances of Speech. Various forms of aphasia occur with neoplastic involvement of the dominant hemisphere. The aphasic disorders are insidious in their development, and minor disturbances may be overlooked or erroneously attributed to psychologic factors. The various discrete forms of apraxia and agnosia may occur in evolution of the tumor syndrome, and may be the initial symptom in otherwise well persons.

Papilledema and Vision. The presence of the characteristic ophthalmoscopic appearance of papilledema suggests increased intracranial pressure; however, the funduscopic findings may be indistinguishable from those of optic neuritis or pseudopapilledema. Pseudopapilledema is a congenital change in the funduscopic appearance of the disc that simulates the swelling associated with increased intracranial pressure. Differential points include the late loss of visual acuity in increased intracranial pressure as opposed to early and more severe visual loss in optic neuritis. Visual acuity is generally unaffected in pseudopapilledema. Episodes of *amaurosis fugax,* fleeting moments of dimming vision, may be associated with a marked degree of papilledema and are a dangerous warning sign of potential loss of vision. The visual fields in true papilledema or pseudopapilledema may show enlargement of the blind spots. Disturbance of vision in patients with intracranial tumor also can be caused by extraocular muscle palsies, disturbances of the central visual pathways (see below), and disorders of visual interpretation, as in the alexias and visual agnosias. Uniocular papilledema with contralateral optic atrophy occurs characteristically, with subfrontal tumors that cause optic atrophy by direct involvement of the nerve and papilledema in the opposite eye owing to increased intracranial pressure. The fundi may not reveal papilledema despite very elevated intracranial pressure; this may be attributable to glaucoma when present, but may also occur for unexplained reasons.

Diplopia and Hemianopia. Diplopia with brain tumors is due to involvement of one or both sixth cranial nerves, either directly by the tumor or, more commonly, indirectly because of generalized increase in intracranial pressure (see False Localizing Signs, below). Third-nerve palsy may be due to involvement of the superior orbital fissure by meningioma, although the nerve may be involved by a variety of other lesions anywhere along its course. Hemianopias result from involvement of the visual pathways. Lesions affecting the optic chiasm, most notably originating in or near the pituitary, give rise to bitemporal hemianopia. Lesions of the optic tract, optic radiation, or occipital cortex give rise to contralateral homonymous hemianopias. Lesions of the anterior temporal pole characteristically cause a contralateral homonymous, superior quadrantopsia.

Ataxia and Hemiplegia. Unsteadiness in walking may occur with tumor in various intracranial sites.

Lesions affecting the midline cerebellum cause a characteristic truncal ataxia with lateralized ataxia of the extremities if the cerebellar hemispheres are also involved. Disease in the frontal lobes may give rise to unsteadiness in walking, an apraxia of gait, which may simulate cerebellar truncal ataxia. Drug intoxication caused by diphenylhydantoin or barbiturates may potentiate ataxia. Tumors of the hemisphere characteristically cause contralateral spastic hemiparesis; initially the signs may be so minimal as to be easily overlooked.

Sensory Disturbances. Hemisensory defects occur with intracranial tumors affecting the contralateral sensory pathways. The primary sensory modalities of touch, pain, temperature, and proprioception are impaired when the thalamus or the ascending spinothalamic pathways are involved. Tumors of the parietal sensory cortex cause loss of cortical sensory functions that results in impairment of sensory localization, two-point discrimination, graphesthesia, stereognosia, and position sense. Tumors of the thalamus may be manifested by episodes of pain affecting the contralateral side of the face or body. Tumors of the cortex may cause focal sensory seizures with a jacksonian march; these may be reported as an aura before a grand mal seizure. Pain in the face occurs with tumors affecting the base of the skull, particularly those arising in the nasopharynx and paranasal sinuses. Tumors affecting the trigeminal nerve may give rise to paroxysms of pain in the face simulating trigeminal neuralgia (tic douloureux), but unlike the latter there is also some loss of facial sensation.

Seizures. Seizures may serve as the first clinical manifestation of brain tumor, or may occur at any time in the course of the illness. The types include classic grand mal seizures and various forms of focal seizures. Typical petit mal is probably never due to neoplasm; minor seizures with brain tumor that at first may resemble petit mal generally are, in fact, either fragmentary grand mal seizures or a variety of psychomotor attack. With any cerebral seizure, it is extremely important to note its aura or the pattern of its onset, for this often provides a reliable indicator of the location of the neoplasm. Focal motor and sensory seizures may be limited to one region of the body or may progress (jacksonian seizures) to involve the entire body. Lesions in the temporal lobe characteristically give rise to psychomotor seizures. These may be associated with olfactory hallucinations (uncinate fits), disorders of visual or auditory perception, experiential attacks such as déjà vu and various types of automatic behavior, for which the patient is generally amnesic (see Part X, Section Sixteen). The onset of convulsions in an otherwise healthy subject over the age of 20 without history of convulsions raises the possibility of an expanding lesion. This possibility is greater if focal signs can be detected in the neurologic examination; if so, additional specialized neurologic diagnostic studies are warranted.

Nausea and Vomiting. Nausea and vomiting occur as a result of direct or reflex stimulation of the emetic center of the medulla. This is most likely to occur in association with increased intracranial pressure, particularly with displacement of the brainstem owing to herniation or the presence of bleeding into the cerebrospinal fluid. The vomiting may occur without preceding nausea and may be projectile. Brain tumor is not suggested by the occurrence of nausea and vomiting alone, i.e., there are invariably other clinical manifestations of the tumor. Antiemetic drugs, e.g., the phenothiazines, inhibit this type of centrally induced vomiting.

Stiff Neck. Signs of meningeal irritation may occur in brain tumor, as a manifestation of cerebellar herniation through the foramen magnum, because of the effects of bleeding into the subarachnoid space, or with meningeal involvement. Cervical rigidity may be striking but Kernig's sign is generally absent (see Tumors of the Cerebellum, below).

Vasomotor and Autonomic Changes. These occur as ominous late signs. They include bradycardia and hypertension, as described above. Apnea generally precedes cardiac arrest in fatal cases. Autonomic manifestations of brain tumor include gastric ulceration (Cushing's ulcer), which may present as a massive gastrointestinal hemorrhage. This may occur with mass lesions anywhere in the intracranial cavity. (The use of adrenocortical steroids in the management of patients with brain tumor may further increase this hazard.) Fever may also occur in patients with mass lesions in the absence of pulmonary, urinary, or other infection, because of a central disturbance, presumably of hypothalamic origin. Hyperthermia is not uncommon just prior to death, but hypothermia may also occur. Fever commonly accompanies the presence of blood in the subarachnoid space. This may occur with rapidly growing neoplasms or as a result of surgery. Disturbances of sweating may occur, lesions of hypothalamus and brainstem giving rise to contralateral signs of sympathectomy.

Metabolic Manifestations. The complex interrelationships between the hypothalamus and the anterior and posterior pituitary may be deranged with intracranial tumors, giving rise to various systemic metabolic disorders. These include diabetes insipidus, inappropriate secretion of antidiuretic hormone, hypopituitarism, and precocious puberty (see Ch. 834, 805, 831, and 858, respectively).

False Localizing Signs. These may occur with increased intracranial pressure or with shift of intracranial structures. The most common such sign is unilateral or bilateral lateral rectus palsy due to sixth-nerve compression. This need not imply neoplastic involvement of the nerve, for it frequently occurs as a pressure palsy of the nerve resulting from increased intracranial pressure itself. Signs of hemiplegia can occur ipsilateral to the tumor owing to compression of the opposite cerebral peduncle on the tentorium; i.e., hemiplegia need not be contralateral to the mass. There are relatively silent areas in brain, wherein tumors reach large size with relatively little clinical deficit; these are the right frontal and temporal lobes. This must be considered in evaluating patients with the syndrome of increased intracranial pressure without localizing signs (see below).

Diagnosis. Patients suspected of having an intracranial tumor require complete medical evaluation to establish the relationship of the neurologic findings to possible coexisting systemic disease. Appropriate laboratory studies should be obtained to search for a primary systemic neoplasm, e.g., lung, breast, gastrointestinal, genitourinary, or thyroid malignancies. The major neurologic diagnostic techniques are described below.

Skull Roentgenograms. The films should be examined for the following: (1) changes suggestive of increased intracranial pressure, (2) bone destruction, (3) bony thickening or hyperostosis, (4) abnormal vascular channels, (5) abnormal calcifications, (6) the shape of the sella turcica, (7) the position of the pineal if calcified, and (8) the relationship of the skull to the cervical spine in suspected platybasia, basilar impression, and related disorders (see Ch. 424).

Characteristic roentgenographic changes may occur with chronically increased intracranial pressure as a result of pressure atrophy of bone, which produces a beaten-silver appearance in the cranial vault, decalcification of the clinoid processes, and separation of the sutures in children. Bone destruction is characteristic of metastatic neoplasms arising from distant organs and of directly invasive tumors that arise in the paranasal sinuses and nasopharynx. Focal hyperostosis of the skull, i.e., thickening of the inner or outer tables of the skull, or both, with increased calcification, is characteristic of meningioma. Generalized thickening of the skull occurs with Paget's disease. Hyperostosis frontalis interna, localized bilateral thickenings of the inner table of the skull, is generally considered an incidental finding without clinical significance. The vascular markings of the skull, which accompany arterial and venous channels, vary greatly in the normal subject. Focal enlargements of the markings occur characteristically with meningioma involving adjacent meninges and skull. Abnormal calcifications characteristically occur in very slowly growing primary neoplasms (astrocytoma, oligodendroglioma, craniopharyngioma, meningioma), in arteriovenous malformations, in aneurysmal walls, and in the glial nodules associated with tuberous sclerosis. Calcifications may also occur in the gliotic walls of old abscesses, in hemorrhagic cavities, and in granulomas of cerebral toxoplasmosis. Displacement of the pineal laterally more than 2 mm is pathologic, and this or a shift superiorly or inferiorly suggests the presence of a space-taking lesion.

Electroencephalography. The electroencephalogram is useful in screening for possible brain tumor. Focal changes, particularly slowing in frequency of the record, are common with tumors in the cerebral hemispheres. Rapidly growing tumors with adjacent cerebral edema are more likely to evoke focal changes than are slowly progressive tumors with only minimal clinical manifestations, and with the latter the record may be entirely normal. The electroencephalogram is often normal with posterior fossa neoplasms.

Cerebrospinal Fluid. Examination of the cerebrospinal fluid (CSF) for pressure, protein, sugar, cell count, cultures, serologic tests, and cytologic analysis is often helpful in the diagnosis of intracranial tumor. The incidence of abnormalities varies with the stage of the illness and the site and nature of the neoplasm. The fluid is crystal clear unless the protein exceeds about 150 mg per 100 ml or unless bleeding has occurred. With slowly growing neoplasms the intracranial pressure will remain normal, less than 200 mm, until late in the illness, whereas in rapidly growing tumors increased pressure may be an early manifestation. Jugular compression for the Queckenstedt test is contraindicated in patients who are suspected of having brain tumor. A protein content greater than 100 mg per 100 ml is frequently associated with rapidly growing tumors near the ventricles or subarachnoid space. With slowly growing tumors, the protein may be normal despite the presence of a huge mass. Of the posterior fossa neoplasms, acoustic neuroma commonly results in marked elevation of the protein, 100 to 500 mg per 100 ml. The fluid is normal in most patients with brainstem gliomas. The cell count is elevated from 5 to 100 white cells per cubic millimeter in about one third of the cases, and may exceed 1000 white cells, particularly when the tumor involves the ventricular wall and has undergone necrosis. Malignant cells may be detected with suitable techniques. The glucose content is normal with brain tumor, apart from patients with diffuse neoplastic involvement of the meninges, when it is characteristically reduced to levels below 40 mg per 100 ml; in some cases this may be the sole abnormality, although commonly 10 to 100 mononuclear cells are seen, and with special cytologic techniques malignant cells may be detected.

Lumbar puncture may be hazardous; it is *contraindicated* in critically ill patients with clinical signs of incipient herniation because the removal of fluid from the lumbar sac may increase the degree of *pre-existing* herniation of the temporal lobe or of the cerebellar tonsils.

Roentgenographic Contrast Studies. *Pneumoencephalography* by the lumbar route, *ventriculography,* and *arteriography* are of major importance in the diagnosis and localization of brain tumor. Lumbar pneumography delineates the ventricular system and the subarachnoid space and thus may reveal the presence of a mass lesion. In ventriculography, air is injected via burr holes in the skull directly into the lateral cerebral ventricles; this may prove necessary for patients with increased intracranial pressure, in whom the lumbar route is deemed hazardous, and for patients in whom there is nonfilling of the ventricular system by the lumbar route. Cerebral angiography may yield much information concerning the location and size of a tumor. Major advances in neuroradiology have established angiography as the most useful of the contrast studies. The vascular patterns of the tumor, arterial, capillary, and venous, may give indications of its histology. The decision as to which contrast technique is most likely to give maximal information in any patient depends upon the specific circumstances of the diagnostic problem in question and must be resolved individually. Some patients need more than one such study.

Noninvasive Radiographic Procedures. Various scanning techniques have become available that permit the recording of the radioactivity present over regions of the skull after intravenous administration of radioiodinated human serum albumin, technetium, and other gamma emitters. The isotope may enter more rapidly and in greater concentration into the tumor and its adjacent area of edema because of the greater permeability of the capillaries and adjacent cellular membranes. The isotope scan does not readily differentiate between focal changes caused by neoplasm, sepsis, or infarction, and is often negative with slowly growing tumors. A recent development in this field is *computerized axial tomography,* which accurately outlines both normal and abnormal intracranial structures without the necessity to employ contrast materials. Although presently available only in a few major centers, the technique promises to add greatly to accurate and safe diagnosis of brain tumor and other lesions.

Echoencephalography. This technique is useful in determining the position of midline structures, i.e., whether there is a shift of the intracranial contents. This is particularly valuable in patients without a calcified pineal. Although the technique gives no information regarding the cause of a shift, it is a useful screening device for patients with suspected mass lesions.

Ancillary Laboratory Tests. Audiometry and vestibular tests are necessary in evaluating patients with suspected tumor of the eighth nerve, and visual fields are valuable in assessing lesions of the visual system.

Tumor Syndromes. *Tumors of the Skull.* Benign osteomas rarely reach a size sufficient to compress underlying brain; generally these can be extirpated. Malignant tumors arising in the paranasal sinuses or nasopharynx directly invade the base of the skull and cause chronic facial pain and multiple cranial nerve involvement. Tumors of the glomus jugulare (nonchromaffin paraganglioma) arise near the jugular bulb and often lead to progressive deafness and a bloody discharge in the external auditory canal. Other lesions that give roentgenographic evidence of bone destruction and that must be differentiated include Paget's disease, Hand-Schüller-Christian disease, eosinophilic granuloma, and cholesteatoma (epidermoids).

Diffuse Meningeal Neoplasia (Neoplastic Meningitis). Carcinomas, gliomas, sarcomas, melanomas, and lymphomas may diffusely infiltrate the leptomeninges and subarachnoid space to produce a syndrome of chronic meningitis, which may simulate chronic meningitis caused by fungi, tuberculosis, sarcoidosis, and meningovascular syphilis. Common manifestations include headache, mental changes, cranial nerve palsies, areflexia, and minimal if any signs of meningeal irritation. The cerebrospinal fluid findings generally will establish the diagnosis. The pressure is usually normal; sugar content may be below 45 mg per 100 ml and as low as 10 mg per 100 ml; protein content is normal or elevated; cell count reveals from 5 to several hundred mononuclear cells; cultures are negative; cytologic studies may reveal malignant cells. The diagnosis may not be apparent at autopsy because gross lesions are generally absent, and microscopic sections are needed to verify the diagnosis.

Tumors of the Cerebral Hemispheres. Tumors affecting the cerebral hemispheres are characterized by progressive focal neurologic deficits and, commonly, by generalized or focal convulsive seizures. Hemispheric tumors involving any lobe may be associated with contralateral hemiplegia; when located in the parasagittal region the paralysis is greater in the leg than in the arm. Tumors of the frontal lobes are also characterized by early impairment of intellectual function. Tumors in the parietal region cause contralateral cortical (interpretive) sensory deficits, impairment of primary sensation, and homonymous hemianopia. Tumors in the occipital region also cause contralateral homonymous hemianopia plus disorders of visual interpretation. Tumors in the temporal lobe, in the nondominant hemisphere, are relatively silent apart from contralateral superior quadrantopsia. Tumors of regions adjacent to the sylvian fissure of the dominant hemisphere give rise to aphasic disorders; anterior lesions in the frontal lobe cause expressive aphasia, posterior lesions in the parietal region cause the receptive aphasias, and lesions in the superior temporal gyrus cause anomic aphasia.

Tumors of the Cerebellum. The common tumors of the cerebellum include medulloblastomas, which affect the midline vermis most commonly in childhood, and tumors of the cerebellar hemisphere, chiefly gliomas and metastatic tumors. Early manifestations of tumor of the midline vermis include truncal ataxia on tandem walking and symptoms of increased intracranial pressure. Tumors of the cerebellar hemisphere cause ipsilateral limb ataxia as an early manifestation. Tilting of the head to one side may be an early sign as well. Stiffness of the neck is often seen in posterior fossa neoplasms as an early sign of herniation.

Brainstem Tumors. These intrinsic tumors of midbrain, pons, and medulla are most commonly gliomas. The initial symptoms are those of cranial nerve dysfunction, most commonly affecting the extraocular muscles (nuclear or internuclear ophthalmoplegia), chewing and swallowing, as well as the long tracts, ascending and descending. Headache and other manifestations of increased intracranial pressure occur late in the course. The cerebrospinal fluid is often normal.

Pituitary Tumors. The earliest symptoms may be those of endocrine disturbances (see above) or may be due to effects on the visual system. Frontal headache may be an early symptom, as well as progressive bitemporal hemianopia caused by chiasmatic involvement. Pituitary tumors may invade the sphenoid sinus and thus permit the development of bacterial meningitis. The cysts associated with craniopharyngioma may release lipid-laden fluid into the subarachnoid space, thus causing bouts of sterile meningitis.

Optic Nerve Glioma. Gliomas may develop in the intraorbital, retro-orbital, or chiasmatic region of the optic nerve, the first of these being the most common location. These tumors usually occur in early childhood with uniocular loss of vision as the most common presenting symptom. Proptosis is seen in about one third of cases. Uniocular optic atrophy or papilledema may be noted. Roentgenographic evidence of enlargement of the optic foramen is common. The tumor is most often a slowly growing astrocytoma and may be associated with neurofibromatosis.

Acoustic Neuroma (Cerebellopontine Angle Tumor). These neurofibromas (schwannomas) of the eighth nerve begin within the auditory canal or in the subarachnoid space. They are slowly growing and characteristically cause progressive tinnitus and nerve deafness. The vestibular portion is more seriously involved than the acoustic portion, and in patients who do not have a dead labyrinth on caloric testing, the diagnosis is suspect. There are few symptoms referable to loss of vestibular function. A mild sensation of giddiness or unsteadiness is common, but recurrent episodes of vertigo are very rare in acoustic tumors. Adjacent cranial nerves are also commonly involved, particularly the fifth, sixth, and seventh nerves. Large tumors cause ipsilateral cerebellar signs and manifestations of increased intracranial pressure. Meningiomas of the cerebellopontine angle may give a similar clinical picture without, however, enlargement of the auditory canal on roentgenograms of the skull.

Metastatic Tumors. The clinical pictures that result from metastatic neoplasms are very variable, depending on the site and number of metastases and their rate of growth. The diagnosis is readily made in patients with evidence of widespread metastatic disease who then develop focal neurologic signs. However, frequently the metastatic tumor may become symptomatic in brain with few if any manifestations of systemic malignant disease. Therefore patients with an apparently single intracranial mass lesion should be studied for a hidden neoplasm.

Differential Diagnosis. A wide variety of neurologic diseases may simulate brain tumor because they are also characterized by progressive focal neurologic signs or signs of increased intracranial pressure. Some of the more common problems in differential diagnosis are considered in the following paragraphs.

Syndrome of Increased Intracranial Pressure Without Localizing Signs. A major diagnostic problem is seen in the patient who presents with increased intracranial pressure manifested by headache and papilledema and who is otherwise apparently normal. The many diagnostic possibilities (see Ch. 422) include extra-axial neoplasms that obstruct the ventricular system, such as tentorial meningioma and pinealoma, and intraventricular tumors like ependymoma and glioma. Some patients have the syndrome of aqueduct stenosis, generally a manifestation of congenital forking (see Ch. 423). Tumors of relatively silent areas like the right frontal and temporal lobes must be excluded. Arteriography and ventriculography and/or lumbar pneumography are generally required to establish the diagnosis.

Tumor vs. Vascular Disease. The differential diagnosis between tumor and vascular disease is generally made on the basis of history: most tumors have an insidious onset and progress slowly, but most vascular lesions characteristically have an abrupt onset. However, some neoplasms such as glioblastoma or metastatic tumors may have a very abrupt onset, most often caused by bleeding into the tumor. Also, the stepwise progression ("stuttering onset") of hemiplegia in some patients with vascular disease of the extracranial portions of the internal carotid and vertebral arteries and, at times, of the intracranial arteries, may pose diagnostic uncertainty. Careful analysis of the history, the laboratory studies, and observation of the patient's course will clarify the diagnosis.

Tumor vs. Chronic Subdural Hematoma. The clinical picture in these patients simulates an expanding hemispheric mass: e.g., headache, drowsiness, papilledema, hemiparesis. About one third of patients with chronic subdural hematoma provide no significant history of head injury. The differential diagnosis can be made almost always with arteriography.

Tumor vs. Demyelinating Diseases, Multifocal Leukoencephalopathy. The more common forms of multiple sclerosis do not usually simulate expanding intracranial lesions. There are occasional cases of acute multiple sclerosis or Schilder's disease that may simulate a progressive hemispheric deficit. Diagnostic difficulty also may be encountered in patients with another disorder of white matter, multifocal leukoencephalopathy, which has been reported in association with the lymphomas and malignant disease arising in lung and other organs. In this disorder, multiple foci of demyelination are associated with electron microscopic evidence of viral infection. Clinically, there are signs of multiple lesions in the brain that can simulate metastatic disease. However, despite clinical evidence of multiple lesions and rapid progression, signs of increased intracranial pressure are absent. Although the diagnosis may be suspected, pathologic confirmation is necessary and usually comes only after death.

Tumor vs. Presenile Dementia. Progressive development of an organic dementia in middle age may be caused by many diseases, including frontal or bifrontal neoplasms. Tumors most likely to present with dementia include frontal and subfrontal tumors (olfactory groove meningioma and tumors of the corpus callosum, "butterfly glioma"). Roentgenographic contrast studies may be necessary to establish the diagnosis. A CSF protein greater than 100 mg per 100 ml favors tumor over the degenerative dementias.

Tumor vs. Abscess, Granuloma. Encapsulated brain abscess and the granulomas associated with cysticercosis may simulate brain tumor. Cysticercosis must be considered in any patient in an endemic area having signs of a cerebral mass lesion. An eosinophilic pleocytosis in the cerebrospinal fluid favors cysticercosis. Differentiation between tumor and abscess may be particularly difficult because patients with encapsulated brain abscess generally do not have systemic manifestations of infection (fever, leukocytosis), and the primary source of infection may be obscure. The cerebrospinal fluid may show little, if any, inflammatory change. The correct diagnosis of abscess or granuloma may not be made until surgery is performed.

Tumor vs. Epilepsy. The common occurrence of convulsive seizures with intracranial tumors requires consideration of this diagnosis when patients develop seizures (apart from true petit mal, which is never due to brain tumor). This is particularly true of patients in whom seizures first develop after the age of 20. The occurrence of transient focal neurologic signs in the postictal state (Todd's paralysis) favors the presence of a structural lesion as basis for the attacks. It is estimated that about 20 per cent of patients who develop seizures after the age of 20, who do not have post-traumatic seizures, will in time be shown to have intracranial tumors. The likelihood of a brain tumor diminishes with the passage of years if focal signs do not appear. There are differences of opinion as to how far one should proceed with diagnostic tests in a patient otherwise normal, with onset of seizures after the age of 20, particularly with regard to the indications for contrast studies. The occurrence of focal seizures, a focal neurologic deficit on clinical examination, or focal EEG slowing all increase the likelihood of the presence of tumor; in the absence of any of these, air study or arteriography is generally unrewarding.

Treatment. *Surgical Therapy.* Total surgical removal without sacrifice of normal cerebral tissue is possible only with tumors that are extra-axial in location, such as some meningiomas, osteomas, neurofibromas, and pituitary tumors. Total surgical extirpation of the primary tumors of brain, glioblastomas, and the less malignant gliomas, is not possible, although there are rare exceptions, e.g., cystic astrocytomas of the cerebellar hemisphere. Complete surgical removal of angiomas may be possible. Therefore it is essential to establish the precise location and tumor type to allow optimal therapy. Surgical attack on primary brain tumors may be helpful as palliative therapy, e.g., internal decompression or partial removal of tumor and edematous brain may relieve headaches and prolong useful life, particularly if the tumor is cystic and in the nondominant frontal or temporal lobes. There is no absolute rule for the surgical treatment of metastatic tumors. In some patients with major symptoms caused by an apparent single brain tumor without widespread systemic disease, surgical excision may offer useful palliation.

Radiotherapy. The gliomas may have a high degree of sensitivity, and x-ray therapy is generally indicated for palliation. Although biopsy and tissue diagnosis are highly desirable prior to instituting radiotherapy, a specimen is not always obtainable, particularly when the tumor is located in an inaccessible area like the brainstem. In such cases, diagnosis must be made on clinical and roentgenographic grounds. Unfortunately, the response of the gliomas to radiation is often brief, and recurrent growth supervenes. Chromophobe adenomas of the pituitary are generally radiosensitive, and radiotherapy is often the treatment of choice unless there is a rapidly progressive threat to vision, in which case surgical therapy is indicated.

Supportive Measures. Anticonvulsant drugs are indicated for patients with a history of convulsive seizures and for patients who have had intracranial surgery. Diphenylhydantoin, 300 to 500 mg per day, and phenobarbital, 30 to 60 mg three times a day, are common dosages. Higher dosages of these and other anticonvulsant drugs may be necessary for seizure control. The use of hypertonic intravenous solutions such as 30 per cent urea or 25 per cent mannitol to lower intracranial pressure has a limited place in management of patients with increased intracranial pressure. This is chiefly for very acute situations while the patient awaits neurosurgical intervention. Adrenal corticosteroids, such as dexamethasone, in high dosages help to reduce cerebral edema associated with brain tumors, particularly in the postoperative period and during radiotherapy; gastrointestinal bleeding, however, is a potential complication. Dosages of dexamethasone of 22 mg in the first 24 hours are recommended. The administration of parenteral fluids must be planned carefully when hydrating patients with increased intracranial pressure, because intravenous infusion of 5 per cent glucose in water can result in a significant increase in intracranial pressure. This danger can be avoided by use of normal saline, 5 per cent glucose in saline, or 5 per cent glucose in 0.42 per cent saline. The phenothiazines may be used as antiemetic agents for patients with severe vomiting. These drugs are depressants and must be used cautiously. Parenteral administration of caffeine transiently reduces intracranial pressure (it causes cerebral vasoconstriction and reduces cerebral blood flow) and may be useful in controlling brain tumor headaches. A variety of chemotherapeutic agents for the treatment of brain tumor are under active study, but their value has not yet been established.

Dastur, H. M., and Desai, A. D.: A comparative study of brain tuberculomas and gliomas based upon 107 case records of each. Brain, 88:375, 1965.

Dixon, H. B. F., and Lipscomb, F. M.: Cysticercosis: An Analysis and Follow-up of 450 Cases. Medical Research Council Special Report, Series No. 299. London, Her Majesty's Stationery Office, 1961.

Jelsma, R., and Bucy, P. C.: Glioblastoma multiforme: Its treatment and some factors affecting survival. Arch. Neurol., 20:171, 1969.

Richardson, E. P.: Neurologic effects of cancer. *In* Holland, J. F., and Frei, E. (eds.): Cancer Medicine. Philadelphia, Lea & Febiger, 1973.

Rubinstein, L. J.: Tumors of the Central Nervous System. Atlas of Tumor Pathology. Second series. Fascicle 6. Washington, D.C., Armed Forces Institute of Pathology, 1972.

Samson, D. S., and Clark, K.: A current review of brain abscess. Am. J. Med., 54:201, 1973.

Zulch, K. J.: Brain Tumors. Their Biology and Pathology. 2nd ed. New York, Springer Publishing Company, 1965.

421. RADIATION INJURY OF THE NERVOUS SYSTEM

Radiation injury of the nervous system occurs as a complication of x-ray therapy wherein tissue dosage has been excessive. Signs of injury may appear within hours or days of high-dosage irradiation in laboratory animals; in man, with the doses used therapeutically, the onset is delayed. Characteristically, a progressive neurologic deficit develops after a latent period of many months or years after the termination of radiotherapy. This complication occurs when irradiation has been directed at neoplasms of the brain or at other tumors in the head and neck. The spinal cord is also subject to injury from excessive radiation, whether directed at a primary cord tumor or at tumors overlying the spine and paraspinal regions, e.g., tumors of the thyroid or mediastinum. Peripheral nerves are relatively radioresistant but are injured also by high doses.

Pathology. The response of the central nervous system to ionizing radiation can be recognized in three phases: an acute phase of meningoencephalitis, a period of apparent normalcy, and a period of late nerve cell damage, demyelination, and vascular change. The lesions in the nervous system attributed to irradiation are extensive in both white and gray matter. There are hyaline thickenings in the walls of blood vessels that may partially or completely occlude the lumen. There is a variable degree of cellular necrosis and degeneration of myelin. Astrocytosis and thickening of the leptomeninges are common. The long latent period between the time of irradiation and the onset of progressive signs is poorly understood; it has been attributed to progressive ischemia caused by gradual narrowing of the vascular lumen. Latent radiation effects in skin are readily attributable to vascular and connective tissue damage; this lends weight to the primary importance of the vascular injury in the brain, although it is likely that neuronal degeneration is not due to progressive ischemia alone. It has been suggested that autoimmune mechanisms play a role in the tissue damage that develops after a latent period.

Dosages. The precise tissue dosage that will induce radiation injury is uncertain. The minimal dose in Lindgren's series of 71 cases that produced pathologic evidence of brain necrosis was 4500 to 5000 roentgens, with delivery through medium-sized fields over a period of 30 days. The spinal cord is vulnerable to somewhat lower doses; radiation myelopathy has been reported after 4000 r in 28 days directed toward the mediastinum. Boden has defined the tolerance of the brainstem and spinal cord from a review of his own material. With small treatment fields of 10 by 7 cm or less, tissue doses up to 4500 r in 17 days or their biologic equivalent seem to be tolerated by the cord and brainstem. With large fields, a tissue dose of 3500 r is considered as the maximal tolerance dose to the brainstem and cord. There is considerable biologic variation in susceptibility of normal tissue to radiation damage, and precise definition of the effects of various dosages on normal tissue is difficult.

Clinical Manifestations. When radiotherapy has been administered to tumors close to, but sparing, the brain and spinal cord, the development of a focal neurologic deficit after a latent period raises the possibility of radiation injury. After radiotherapy to brain or spinal cord tumors, clinical improvement that persists for one to five years with subsequent regression suggests the possibility of late radiation damage to normal nervous tissue. A transient form of radiation myelopathy is not uncommon; its major manifestation is the occurrence of Lhermitte's sign 2 to 37 weeks after radiation. Symptoms most often appear about a year after irradiation. The onset is insidious, and the rate of subsequent progress is unpredictable. The process may become arrested or may progress to cause a major cerebral hemispheric deficit or complete functional spinal cord transection. The clinical differentiation between radiation injury and recurrent tumor growth may be very difficult and uncertain pending pathologic confirmation at autopsy, and both may be coexistent. A repeated roentgenographic contrast study may help in differentiation. There is no specific therapy for radiation injury of the nervous system.

Boden, G.: Radiation myelitis of the brain-stem. J. Fac. Radiol., 2:79, 1950.
Coy, P., Baker, S., and Dolman, C. L.: Progressive myelopathy due to radiation. Can. Med. Assoc. J., 100:1129, 1969.
Lindgren, M.: On tolerance of brain tissue and sensitivity of brain tumours to irradiation. Acta Radiol. (Stockholm), (Suppl. 170):1, 1958.
Locksmith, J. P., and Powers, W. E.: Permanent radiation myelopathy. Am. J. Roentgenol., 102:916, 1968.
Reagan, T. J., et al.: Chronic progressive radiation myelopathy. J.A.M.A., 203:106, 1968.

422. BENIGN INTRACRANIAL HYPERTENSION (Pseudotumor Cerebri)

Definition. Benign intracranial hypertension (BIH) describes the syndrome of increased intracranial pressure in which intracranial mass lesions, obstruction of the cerebral ventricles, intracranial infection, and hypertensive encephalopathy have been excluded. It has also been termed pseudotumor cerebri, serous meningitis, and otitic hydrocephalus. BIH includes a heterogenous group of disorders in which a number of different etiologic factors have been identified, although in most cases the cause and pathogenesis of these syndromes are poorly understood. They are termed "benign" because spontaneous recovery generally occurs; however, serious threats to vision may occur.

Clinical Manifestations. The presenting symptoms are headache and disturbance of vision. The headache is often worse on awakening and is aggravated by coughing and straining. It is often relatively mild and may be entirely absent. The most common ocular complaint is visual blurring, a manifestation of papilledema. Some patients complain of brief, fleeting movements of dimming or complete loss of vision, occurring many times during the day (amaurosis fugax), at times accentuated or precipitated by coughing and straining. The ominous symptom indicates that the patient's vision is in serious jeopardy. Visual loss may be minimal despite severe chronic papilledema, including retinal hemorrhages; however, blindness rarely may develop very rapidly—in less than 24 hours. Visual fields characteristically show enlargement of the blind spots, and may show constriction of the peripheral fields and central or paracentral scotoma. Diplopia caused by unilateral or bilateral sixth nerve palsy may develop as a result of increased intracranial pressure. The neurologic examination is otherwise normal. A major clinical point is that patients with BIH commonly look well; that is, their appearance and apparent well-being belie the ominous appearance of the papilledema.

Pathophysiology. The signs and symptoms of BIH are due to the effects of increased intracranial pressure; pressures between 300 and 600 mm are frequent. The intracranial pressure is normally between 50 and 180 to 200 mm of water as measured in the lumbar sac or ventricles with the patient in the lateral recumbent position. This pressure is dependent upon the pressure-volume relationships within the intracranial and spinal cavities. The intracranial cavity contains about 1400 ml of brain, 75 ml of blood, and 75 ml of CSF, and an additional 75 ml in the spinal subarachnoid space. The CSF pressure is directly dependent upon the intracranial venous pressure; changes in the latter pressure are readily transmitted to the CSF, and thus a sustained increase in intracranial venous pressure may result in the syndrome of chronically increased intracranial pressure. The intracranial pressure is largely independent of the systemic arterial pressure, and it is normal in essential hypertension; however, it falls with acute systemic hypotension and rises acutely with very acute increases in systemic blood pressure, e.g., with the administration of vasopressor drugs or in the syndrome of acute hypertensive encephalopathy. Increased intracranial pressure also accompanies increased cerebral blood flow resulting from CO_2 retention, as in acute asphyxia or with chronic pulmonary insufficiency. In patients with BIH apart from those with obstruction of the intracranial venous system and chronic pulmonary insufficiency, the mechanism of the increase in intracranial pressure is unknown. Two different kinds of changes have been noted on pneumoencephalography. The first has been normal air studies except for narrowed, slitlike ventricles and little air in the cortical subarachnoid space, which has been interpreted to mean that the brain volume is increased owing to "edema." The second has been normal air studies apart from normal or enlarged ventricles with an excessive amount of air in the cortical subarachnoid spaces, implying an increased volume of CSF. It is not clear whether these differences represent separate entities or whether the differences can be attributed to variation in time, i.e., the first type may develop into the second type after sufficient time has elapsed. Although cerebral edema has been suspected, there are few clinical manifestations of cerebral dysfunction in these patients to denote any functional changes as a result of the edema.

There are new methods available that permit measurement of the rates of formation and of removal of CSF in man, but to date these have not been applied to patients with this syndrome. (The only disease in which there is any evidence in favor of a pathologic increase in CSF formation i papilloma of the choroid plexus.) The calculation of the Ayala index at lumbar puncture, an old clinical guide to the volume of CSF, favors an increased CSF volume in many patients with BIH. (Ayala index $= \dfrac{\text{Final pressure}}{\text{Initial pressure}} \times 10$ ml removed. 5.0 to 7.0 is normal. Values greater than 7.0 denote increased CSF volume; values less than 5.0 denote decreased CSF volume.) The index is almost always increased in patients with benign intracranial hypertension. Although there are clinical correlations between various endocrinopathies (see below), the mechanism wherein the adrenal, parathyroids, ovaries, or anterior pituitary might affect brain or CSF volumes is obscure.

Etiologic Factors and Associated Disorders (Table). *Intracranial Venous Sinus Thrombosis.* Increased intra-

Benign Intracranial Hypertension: Etiologic Factors and Associated Disorders

1 Intracranial venous sinus thrombosis
   a. Mastoiditis and lateral sinus thrombosis
   b. After head trauma
   c. Pregnancy and postpartum
   d. Oral progestational drugs
   e. "Marantic" sinus thrombosis
   f. Cryofibrinogenemia
2. Endocrine dysfunction
   a. Obesity and menstrual irregularities
   b. Pregnancy and postpartum (without sinus thrombosis)
   c. Menarche
   d. Addison's disease
   e. Hypoparathyroidism
3. Drugs and toxins
   a. Adrenal steroids and steroid withdrawal
   b. Female sex hormone
   c. Vitamin A
   d. Tetracycline and nalidixic acid
4. Hematologic disorders
   a. Iron deficiency anemia
   b. Infectious mononucleosis
   c. Wiskott-Aldrich syndrome
5. Pulmonary encephalopathy
   a. Paralytic hypoventilation
   b. Pulmonary emphysema
   c. Pickwickian syndrome
6. High cerebrospinal fluid protein
   a. Spinal cord tumors
   b. Polyneuritis
7. Miscellaneous
   a. Roseola infantum
   b. Sydenham's chorea
   c. Familial
8. Idiopathic

cranial pressure as a result of occlusion of the intracranial venous sinuses occurs as a consequence of otitis media with extension of the infection into the petrous bone and to the wall of the lateral sinus. This syndrome has been termed otitic hydrocephalus. It occurs as a complication of both acute and chronic infection; at times the evidence for otitis media is minimal and readily overlooked. The sixth cranial nerve may also be involved, giving rise to diplopia on lateral gaze. Thrombosis of the superior longitudinal sinus may occur as a consequence of relatively mild closed head injury and may give rise to a pseudotumor syndrome. (Occlusion of this sinus that drains both cerebral hemispheres is more likely to result in hemorrhagic infarction in the cerebrum as the thrombosis extends into the cerebral veins, giving rise to bilateral signs. In such cases, the course is frequently fulminant and the prognosis guarded, although occasionally complete recovery may occur.) Aseptic or primary thrombosis of the superior longitudinal sinus may also be responsible for a pseudotumor syndrome.This develops as a complication of pregnancy and has been reported to occur during the first two to three weeks post partum, at the end of the first trimester of pregnancy, and with the use of oral progestational drugs. A disorder of the blood clotting mechanism has been suggested as basis for these events during the postpartum period, although this has not been substantiated. Sinus thrombosis occurs as a complication of cachexia ("marantic" thrombosis), and in association with cryofibrinogenemia.

Endocrine Dysfunction. The most common association is the occurrence of BIH in women with a history of menstrual dysfunction. The women are frequently moderately to markedly overweight (without evidence of alveolar hypoventilation). Menstrual irregularity is common, often with amenorrhea. Galactorrhea is a rare associated symptom. The histories usually emphasize excessive premenstrual weight gain. Endocrine studies thus far have not revealed any abnormalities of urinary gonadotrophins or estrogens, and the pathogenesis is unknown. BIH has been reported as a complication of Addison's disease, improvement occurring with replacement therapy. The mechanism is obscure. Hypoparathyroidism may present with evidence of increased intracranial pressure. The presence of hypocalcemic seizures or cerebral calcifications roentgenographically may further complicate the clinical picture. Increased intracranial pressure disappears with replacement therapy.

Drugs and Toxins. BIH has been reported in patients treated with adrenal corticosteroids for prolonged periods. Many of the patients have been children with allergic skin disorders or asthma. The syndrome is more likely to occur when the steroid dosage is reduced, suggesting that relative adrenal insufficiency might have been present, but this has not been substantiated. BIH has been reported in women taking oral progestational drugs when angiography has excluded sinus thrombosis. BIH has been reported in otherwise healthy adolescents taking huge doses of vitamin A for the treatment of acne. Doses as low as 25,000 units per day orally have been noted to cause headache and papilledema; there is rapid improvement after cessation of the therapy. The syndrome is said to have occurred in Arctic explorers who consumed polar bear liver, a great source of the vitamin. A few cases of BIH, manifested by bulging fontanelle and papilledema, have been reported in children after the administration of tetracycline or nalidixic acid. The mechanisms involved are obscure. Spontaneous rapid recovery occurs when the drugs are stopped.

Hematologic Disorders. Papilledema and increased intracranial pressure have been attributed to severe iron deficiency anemia, with striking improvement after treatment of the anemia. The mechanism presumably is dependent upon the marked increase in cerebral blood flow that accompanies profound anemia. BIH occurs with infectious mononucleosis and the Wiskott-Aldrich syndrome, but its mechanism is not known.

Pulmonary Encephalopathy. BIH can be a major complication of chronic hypoxic hypercapnia caused by paralytic states such as muscular dystrophy and cervical myelopathy, as well as of obstructive pulmonary disease and the pickwickian syndrome. The mechanism is dependent upon the chronic increase in cerebral blood flow resulting from the anoxemia and carbon dioxide retention.

High Spinal Fluid Protein. BIH occurs rarely with spinal cord tumors and polyneuritis without any evidence of pulmonary insufficiency. Papilledema and headache have disappeared with treatment of the spinal lesion. The mechanism may involve the effects of a very high CSF protein upon CSF absorption at the arachnoid villi, both in the cranial and spinal subarachnoid spaces.

Idiopathic. One of the more common forms of BIH is its occurrence in otherwise healthy subjects in the absence of any of the etiologic factors described above. Both sexes are involved and the occurrence is most often between the ages of 10 and 50 years. These cases represent the idiopathic form of BIH; its pathogenesis is a mystery. There are rare case reports of BIH with roseola infantum and Sydenham's chorea in which the mechanism is unknown.

Diagnosis. The patient with headache and papilledema without other neurologic signs must be considered to have an intracranial mass, ventricular obstruction, or intracranial infection until proved otherwise. Although the diagnosis of BIH may be suspected by the appearance of apparent well-being and by the history of some of the associated features listed above, the diagnosis is essentially one of exclusion dependent upon ruling out the more common causes of increased intracranial pressure. Brain tumor, particularly when located in relatively silent areas such as the frontal lobes or right temporal lobe or when obstructing the ventricular system, may be manifest only by headache and papilledema. Patients with chronic subdural hematoma, without history of significant trauma, may present in the same way. Diagnostic evaluation requires skull films, electroencephalography, and arteriography and/or air studies (see Ch. 420). Lumbar puncture is necessary in these patients, but is generally deferred until arteriography has revealed that the ventricular system is normal in size and location. Laboratory studies regarding possible hypoadrenalism or hypoparathyroidism may be rewarding in rare cases of these disorders that present with the pseudotumor syndrome. The cerebrospinal fluid pressure is elevated, between 250 and 600 mm, but the fluid is otherwise normal. The protein content is generally low normal, and lumbar CSF protein levels below 15 mg per 100 ml are common, suggesting that such patients have increased rates of CSF absorption. The electroencephalogram is normal in BIH. Pseudopapilledema may be a source of diagnostic confusion. It is a developmental anomaly of the fundus wherein the ophthalmologic appearance may be indistinguishable from that of the true papilledema; there is elevation of the optic disc, but exudates or hemorrhages are absent. The visual acuity is normal, although visual fields may show some enlargement of the blind spots. The unchanging appearance of the fundus in subsequent examinations favors the diagnosis of pseudopapilledema, as does the finding of normal CSF pressure on lumbar puncture.

Treatment. In patients with lateral sinus thrombosis caused by chronic infection in the petrous bone, surgical decompression is often indicated. When the pseudotumor syndrome is a manifestation of hypoadrenalism or hypoparathyroidism, replacement therapy is indicated. Vitamin A intoxication disappears when administration of the vitamin is stopped. Anticoagulation therapy has been recommended for patients with dural sinus thrombosis; however, for patients with extension of the clot into cerebral veins with infarction of tissue, anticoagulation is hazardous because it increases the likelihood of hemorrhagic infarction.

The idiopathic form of BIH and its occurrence in patients with menstrual disorders and obesity require individualized management. This syndrome is self-limited in most cases, and after some weeks or months spontaneous remissions occur, making evaluation of therapy difficult. In rare instances, the illness may last as long as two years. In the very obese, weight reduction is recommended. The use of daily lumbar punctures has been advocated to lower pressure to normal levels by removing sufficient fluid; 15 to 50 ml of fluid may be required, but its value is dubious. Subtemporal decompression has been widely used in the past. This procedure may be necessary for patients with serious threat to vision caused by pressure, although its efficacy has been questioned in a number of reports. The use of dexamethasone has been advocated because it minimizes cerebral edema of diverse causes. However, many patients with BIH appear to have a large volume of CSF and adrenal steroids have uncertain effects on CSF volume or the rate of CSF formation. Acetazolamide has been used because this carbonic anhydrase inhibitor has been shown to reduce CSF formation. Digoxin has been suggested for the same reason. Hypertonic intravenous solutions (20 per cent urea or 25 per cent mannitol) to lower intracranial pressure can be used in acute situations when there is rapidly failing vision, while one awaits neurosurgical intervention; however, prolonged dehydration therapy is impossible because of its deleterious systemic effects. The use of oral glycerol has the disadvantage of high caloric intake for obese patients. Management of these patients is difficult and requires the attention of neurologists and neurosurgeons experienced in these problems.

Feldman, M. H., and Schlezinger, N. S.: Benign intracranial hypertension associated with hypervitaminosis A. Arch. Neurol., 22:1, 1970.

Greer, M.: Benign intracranial hypertension. I. Mastoiditis and lateral sinus obstruction. II. Following corticosteroid therapy. III. Pregnancy. IV. Menarche. V. Menstrual dysfunction. Neurology, 12:472, 1962; 13:439, 670, 1963; 14:569, 668, 1964.

Lysak, W. R., and Svien, H. J.: Long-term follow-up on patients with diagnosis of pseudotumor cerebri. J. Neurosurg., 25:284, 1966.

Miller, A., Bader, R. A., and Bader, M. E.: The neurologic syndrome due to marked hypercapnia with papilledema. Am. J. Med., 33:309, 1963.

Neville, B. G. R., and Wilson, J.: Benign intracranial hypertension following corticosteroid withdrawal in childhood. Br. Med. J., 3:554, 1970.

423. HYDROCEPHALUS

Definitions. Hydrocephalus is a pathologic state characterized by dilatation of the cerebral ventricles with an increase in volume of cerebrospinal fluid (CSF), almost always caused by an obstruction in the circulation of this fluid. In children, prior to fusion of the cranial sutures, there is enlargement of the skull. Hydrocephalus must be distinguished from other causes of macrocephaly in infancy, including subdural hematoma. In older subjects, cranial enlargement cannot occur. Hydrocephalus is termed "active," i.e., progressive and associated with increased intraventricular pressure, or "arrested" when the intraventricular pressure has returned to normal and is no longer a stimulus for ventricular enlargement. These forms of hydrocephalus are distinguished from hydrocephalus ex vacuo, which is characterized by an increase in the volume of CSF under normal pressure that is compensatory to a primary atrophy of the brain. "Normal" pressure occult hydrocephalus refers to the syndrome of ventricular dilatation associated with inadequacy of the subarachnoid spaces without evidence of increased intracranial pressure (see below).

Etiology and Pathophysiology. There are three possible mechanisms for the development of hydrocephalus: overproduction of CSF, defective absorption of CSF, and obstruction of the CSF pathways. *Overproduction* of the fluid has not been documented, although it may occur with the rare papilloma of the choroid plexus. *Defective absorption* of the CSF at the arachnoid villi, where the fluid passes through valvelike structures to enter the venous sinuses, may occur with subarachnoid hemorrhage, meningitis, and with a very high CSF protein. *Obstruction* of the CSF pathways, which results in dilatation of the channels proximal to the site of obstruction, is the most common underlying mechanism in both the hydrocephalus of infancy and in adults. When the block is within the ventricular system, the process is termed *noncommunicating hydrocephalus,* whereas *communicating hydrocephalus* describes ventricular dilatation in which there is free flow of fluid and air between the ventricular system and the spinal subarachnoid space. Communicating hydrocephalus is characterized by extraventricular obstruction of the CSF pathways, most commonly in the subarachnoid spaces about the brainstem at the incisura of the tentorium or in the subarachnoid spaces about the cerebral hemispheres, or both. Ventricular dilatation develops in hydrocephalus because the intraventricular pressures (both the mean pressure and the pulsatile pressures, synchronous with cardiac systole) are pathologically increased; these give rise to a transmural pressure gradient across the cerebral mantle sufficient to cause characteristic compression of the adjacent white matter that has a loss of protein and lipid but an increase in water and sodium content. The magnitude and duration of the transmural pressure gradient necessary to induce ventricular dilatation have not been well defined. These changes may be reversible if surgical therapy can successfully relieve the increased intraventricular pressure (see below).

The major causes of obstruction in the CSF pathways that produce hydrocephalus are neoplasms, congenital malformations, and post-traumatic and postinflammatory lesions.

Neoplasms most likely to give rise to hydrocephalus are those that arise within or adjacent to the ventricular system and obstruct the flow of CSF. These include gliomas and ependymomas of the third and fourth ventricles and of the aqueduct (see Ch. 420). Congenital malformations give rise to hydrocephalus by causing a variety of obstruction, the most common being "forking" or stenosis of the aqueduct. This may give rise to symptoms early in life, or manifestations may be absent until adulthood. Congenital malformations of the craniovertebral junction also may be associated with hydrocephalus (see Arnold-Chiari Malformation in Ch. 424). Most frequently, hydrocephalus is related to postinflammatory or post-traumatic obstruction of the basilar cisterns, particularly in the region of the tentorium. In infancy, this follows intracranial bleeding at the time of birth, at times unrecognized, or episodes of bacterial meningitis or toxoplasmosis. These processes lead to progressive fibrosis of the subarachnoid pathways at the base of the brain, with subsequent obstruction. In adults, postinflammatory hydrocephalus may develop with or after purulent, tuberculous and mycotic meningitis or with cysticercosis, and also may follow subarachnoid hemorrhage caused by trauma or ruptured congenital aneurysm.

Clinical Manifestations. The major signs and symptoms of hydrocephalus are those of increased intracranial pressure (see Ch. 420). In infancy, this is manifest by a greater than normal growth rate and size of the head and by distended scalp veins; in severe cases there is downward displacement of the eyes and mental retardation. Although the head size (occipitobregmatic circumference) in comparison with the chest circumference is of importance, repeated observations of the *rate* of head growth are more significant. Additional information can be obtained from measurements of the anterior fontanelle, as active hydrocephalus does not occur in conjunction with a closing fontanelle. On the other hand, a fontanelle enlarging from month to month is evidence for increased intracranial pressure, and further investigations are warranted.

In older children and adults, the major manifestations include headache, diplopia caused by sixth nerve palsy, papilledema, visual blurring, nausea, and vomiting. Thus occult hydrocephalus that is due to a benign process must be differentiated from intracranial mass lesions, including tumor without localizing signs and chronic subdural hematoma, as well as from the various forms of benign intracranial hypertension and the chronic meningitides, including fungal meningitis, sarcoidosis, and diffuse meningeal neoplasia (carcinomatous meningitis).

Occult "Normal Pressure" Hydrocephalus. In recent years, a new syndrome has been delineated as occult "normal pressure" hydrocephalus. Typically, there is a gradual development over weeks or months of a mild impairment of memory with mental and physical slowness which progresses insidiously to a severe dementia with unsteady gait and urinary incontinence. The patients are usually headache-free and have no signs of increased intracranial pressure, e.g., they have normal fundi and normal CSF pressure at lumbar puncture. Pneumoencephalography reveals enlarged ventricles and a lack of filling of the subarachnoid space over the hemispheres. Isotope cisternography (intraspinal injection of RISA with serial scanning of the skull) has revealed a pathologic reflux of the isotope into the ventricular system with delayed and inadequate visualization of the cortical subarachnoid space. Some patients have a previous history of head injury or subarachnoid bleeding; in others, the cause is obscure. Striking improvement in the mental state and gait has been noted to follow ventriculoatrial or other shunting procedures. This treatable syndrome is uncommon but must be differentiated from the more frequent forms of organic dementia as discussed in Ch. 326 to 331.

Diagnosis. Detailed neurologic study is necessary to determine the cause of increased intracranial pressure and ventricular dilatation. Skull films show characteristic signs of increased intracranial pressure in young children; the signs in adults are generally less striking and may be absent. Electroencephalograms may be normal or may demonstrate bilateral slowing of nonspecific nature. Carotid angiography will show displacement of the arteries and veins characteristic of ventricular enlargement. Air contrast studies are essential to establish the diagnosis of hydrocephalus in most cases. Ventriculography via a parietal burr-hole or lumbar pneumoencephalography, or both, will reveal the degree of ventricular enlargement, the presence of obstructive lesions in the cerebrospinal fluid pathways, and the adequacy of the subarachnoid spaces about the brainstem, base, and cerebrum. Precise neuroradiologic analysis is essential to establish the diagnosis. The cerebrospinal fluid pressure is characteristically, but not invariably, increased in the cerebral ventricles and lumbar sac. The protein content is generally normal; elevated protein levels favor an underlying neoplastic process in the absence of bleeding or chronic meningitis.

Treatment. The treatment of hydrocephalus is surgical; it is directed toward reducing the volume and pressure of cerebrospinal fluid by bypassing obstruction. A wide variety of shunting procedures have been used. The choice of procedure will depend upon technical factors and the skill and experience of the operating surgeon. If the block exists in the third ventricle, aqueduct, or fourth ventricle (as with intraventricular tumors or with "aqueduct stenosis"), the Torkildsen procedure is often employed (ventriculocisternal shunt), wherein a catheter is placed from one or both lateral ventricles over the occiput into the cisterna magna to enable normal CSF reabsorption into the intracranial venous sinuses. In patients with communicating hydrocephalus, direct shunting of the ventricular fluid into the venous system is generally used, particularly the ventriculoatrial shunt wherein the fluid exists from the ventricle through a valved tube, which extends into the superior vena cava and right atrium of the heart. There are many variations of these procedures in use, including shunting to other body cavities, e.g., ventriculopleural, ventriculoureteral, and ventriculoabdominal shunts. Infections and recurrent obstruction of the shunt are common complications of the various shunting procedures, and the results of treatment particularly in young children are frequently discouraging. Acetazolamide, a carbonic anhydrase inhibitor, reduces the rate of formation of CSF; but there is no convincing evidence that it is useful in the management of the various forms of hydrocephalus. Some hydrocephalic children will have spontaneous arrest and may function within the normal range with only a prominent forehead and large hat size as residual defects. Shunting procedures have established occult "normal pressure" hydrocephalus as a treatable dementia.

Benson, D. F., Le May, M., Patten, D. H., and Rubens, A. B.: Diagnosis of normal pressure hydrocephalus. N. Engl. J. Med., 283:609, 1970.
Milhorat, T. H.: Hydrocephalus and Cerebrospinal Fluid. Baltimore, Williams & Wilkins Company, 1972.
Ojemann, R. G., Fisher, C. M., Adams, R. D., Sweet, W. H., and New, F. P. J.: Further experience with the syndrome of "normal" pressure hydrocephalus. J. Neurosurg., 31:279, 1969.
Wolinsky, J., Barnes, B. D., and Margolis, M. T.: Diagnostic tests in normal pressure hydrocephalus. Neurology, 23:706, 1973.

424. ANOMALIES OF THE CRANIOVERTEBRAL JUNCTION, SPINE, AND MENINGES

A wide variety of neurologic syndromes are associated with morphologic anomalies in the region of the foramen magnum of the skull that are due to distortion of the brainstem, cervical cord, and cerebellum. The most common of these are: (1) Arnold-Chiari malformation, (2) fusion of the cervical vertebrae (Klippel-Feil syndrome), (3) basilar impression and platybasia, and (4) spina bifida and meningocele. These defects may occur singly or together, with or without clinical symptoms. Symptoms result from compression, distortion, or malformation of adjacent neural structures. These are most often congenital lesions, but acquired defects caused by bone disease or neoplasms of this region may give rise to similar syndromes.

ARNOLD-CHIARI MALFORMATION

This congenital anomaly is characterized by downward displacement of the cerebellum through the foramen magnum of the skull and by similar caudal elongation of the medulla. These cases can be divided into two major types, the infantile and the adult.

Infantile Form. The infantile form is commonly associated with other midline defects such as spina bifida and meningocele, hydrocephalus caused by aqueductal or fourth ventricular obstruction, and other congenital malformations of the brain and cord. The infantile form of the Arnold-Chiari malformation usually presents itself because of hydrocephalus in the early months of life, with evidence of spina bifida or frank paraparesis resulting from myelomeningocele. Therapy is directed toward surgical relief of the hydrocephalus with a ventricular shunting procedure and repair of the meningomyelocele. Prognosis is poor for patients with extensive defects.

Adult Form. The malformation may be asymptomatic until adult life, when there is the onset of symptoms and signs of damage to the cerebellum, lower cranial nerves, pyramidal tracts, and posterior columns. The presenting signs may be due to hydrocephalus secondary to obstruction of the cerebrospinal fluid pathways or to coexisting syringomyelia of the cervical spinal cord and medulla (see Ch. 423 and 452). Commonly, there is evidence, clinical or roentgenographic, of fusion of the cervical vertebrae, platybasia, or basilar impression. The Arnold-Chiari malformation in adults may simulate syndromes produced by tumors near the foramen magnum and by multiple sclerosis. Surgical enlargement of the foramen magnum and decompression of the cervicomedullary junction are beneficial in selected cases.

CONGENITAL FUSION OF CERVICAL VERTEBRAE
(Klippel-Feil Syndrome)

Fusion of one or more of the cervical vertebrae is a congenital malformation that may be an asymptomatic finding, detected only with roentgenograms of the cervical spine; malformation of the atlas and axis may coexist. Multiple fusions and condensation of vertebrae result in shortening of the cervical spine, which produces a characteristic appearance of a short, thick neck, head set low on the shoulders, and limitation of neck movements.

Coexisting abnormalities are common, including undescended scapula (Sprengel's deformity), platybasia, basilar impression, Arnold-Chiari malformation, and other "dysrhaphic" disorders such as syringomyelia and meningomyelocele. Clinical evidence of spinal cord involvement is most likely to be due to coexisting syringomyelia. "Mirror movements" may occur with the Klippel-Feil syndrome, and other anomalies of the craniovertebral junction and high cervical cord, in which voluntary movements of one upper extremity are involuntarily imitated by the other upper extremity. Surgical decompression may be indicated if there is evidence of spinal cord compression.

BASILAR IMPRESSION AND PLATYBASIA

Basilar impression refers to abnormal invagination of the cervical spine into the base of the posterior fossa of the skull. The diagnosis is made from lateral roentgenograms of the skull when there is excessive protrusion of the tip of the odontoid process of the axis above Chamberlain's line, that is, a line drawn from the back of the hard palate to the posterior margin of the foramen magnum. Other radiologic criteria are also useful. *Platybasia* refers to flattening of the base of the skull, wherein lateral roentgenograms of the skull reveal flattening of the angle between the orbital plates of the anterior fossa and the clivus, the sloping anterior floor of the posterior fossa. The angle is normally 135 degrees, and becomes 145 degrees or more in platybasia. Platybasia alone is asymptomatic.

These malformations, which commonly coexist or may exist alone, are usually developmental in origin, and there may be hereditary transmission. Occasionally, these deformations of the base of the skull may result from metabolic bone diseases such as rickets, osteitis deformans, osteomalacia, or osteogenesis imperfecta. The congenital form may be associated with the Klippel-Feil syndrome, Arnold-Chiari malformation, and other congenital malformations of the atlas and axis, such as fusion of the atlas to the base of the skull, malpositioning of the odontoid process, or atlantoaxial subluxation. Minor degrees of deformity of the base of the skull give rise to no symptoms. The neck appears shortened, and its movements may be limited. With more severe invagination, there may be signs of impaired function of the cerebellum, lower cranial nerves, pyramidal tracts, and posterior columns. Syringomyelia and syringobulbia may also be present. Increased intracranial pressure may develop owing to obstruction of the foramina of the fourth ventricle and the basal cisterns. The clinical manifestations must be differentiated from those caused by neoplasms in the region of the foramen magnum and multiple sclerosis. When neurologic signs are progressive, surgical decompression of the posterior fossa and upper cervical cord may be indicated.

SPINA BIFIDA AND MENINGOCELE

Various malformations of the meninges and spinal cord result from developmental defects in the closure of the bony canal. Although many of these are obvious at birth, some may not be symptomatic until adult life. The classification of these defects would include the following: (1) *Complete rachischisis,* in which the bony vertebral arches are missing in the lumbar region, the cord is undeveloped or aplastic, and the nerve elements have no covering. (2) *Meningomyelocele,* an obvious soft tissue saccular mass which extends over the lumbosacral spine. The cerebrospinal fluid may leak from a defect which may be responsible for bacterial meningitis. (3) *Meningocele,* a bony defect in the spine associated with a meningeal diverticulum covered by atrophic skin. The spinal cord and roots are generally not involved and there may be no associated neurologic defect. (4) *Spina bifida occulta,* a defect in the bony arches in the lumbar region often discovered incidentally on roentgenographic examination. In most cases, neither cord nor roots are involved. The overlying skin may be the site of a tuft of hair, a pilonidal dimple, or a dermal sinus, which is continuous with the subarachnoid space. The latter may serve as a portal of entry for recurrent bouts of meningitis. It should be sought in all patients presenting with bacterial meningitis. These malformations may be associated with Arnold-Chiari malformation and with hydrocephalus. There may also be evidence of syringomyelia. The neurologic deficit varies with the degree of involvement of the spinal cord, conus medullaris, and cauda equina. In adults the chief manifestation may be a neurogenic bladder and defective anal sphincter. Asymptomatic spina bifida requires no therapy. Dermal sinuses, when responsible for bacterial meningitis, require surgical excision. In patients with neurologic deficits, attempts at surgical correction may be indicated.

Appleby, A., Foster, J. B., Hankinson, J., and Hudgson, P.: The diagnosis and management of the Chiari malformations in adult life. Brain, 91:131, 1968.
Bharucha, E. P., and Dastur, H. M.: Craniovertebral anomalies (a report on 40 cases). Brain, 87:469, 1964.
Greenberg, A. D.: Atlanto-axial dislocations. Brain, 91:655, 1968.
Gunderson, C. H., Greenspan, R. H., Glaser, G. H., and Lubs, H. A.: The Klippel-Feil syndrome: Genetic and clinical re-evaluation of cervical fusion. Medicine, 46:491, 1967.
McRae, D. L.: Bony abnormalities at the cranio-spinal junction. Clin. Neurosurg., 16:356, 1969.

Section Eighteen. NONMETASTATIC EFFECTS OF CANCER ON THE NERVOUS SYSTEM

Jerome B. Posner

When patients with systemic cancer develop nervous system dysfunction, metastasis is usually the cause. However, cancer also exerts deleterious effects on the nervous system in the absence of direct metastatic involvement. Recognition of these nonmetastatic neurologic complications can prevent inappropriate and perhaps harmful therapy directed at a nonexistent metastasis. Since at times the nervous system symptoms precede the discovery of the cancer, they can also lead the physician to the diagnosis of an otherwise occult neoplasm.

An almost bewildering variety of neurologic disorders have been ascribed to effects of systemic cancer, as shown in the accompanying table. Many of these bear only an indirect nutritional or metabolic (e.g., hepatic coma) relationship to cancer and are discussed elsewhere in this book. The term "remote effects of cancer on the nervous system" as used in this section applies to nervous system dysfunction of unknown cause occurring in association with cancer (see accompanying table). The classification is similar to that of Brain and Adams (see Brain and Norris), but progressive multifocal leukoencephalopathy is not included because its cause (a viral infection by a papovavirus) is known.

Remote effects of cancer on the nervous system are uncommon. Croft and Wilkinson found remote effects in 96

Nonmetastatic Effects of Systemic Cancer on the Nervous System

I. "Remote effects," cause unknown
  A. Brain and cranial nerves
    1. Dementia
    2. Bulbar encephalitis
    3. Subacute cerebellar degeneration–opsoclonus
    4. Optic neuritis
  B. Spinal cord
    1. Gray matter myelopathy
      a. "Amyotrophic lateral sclerosis"
      b. Poliomyelitis-like syndrome
    2. Subacute necrotic myelopathy
  C. Peripheral nerves and roots
    1. Dorsal root ganglionitis
    2. Sensorimotor peripheral neuropathy
    3. Acute polyneuropathy, "Guillain-Barré" type
  D. Neuromuscular junction and muscle
    1. Polymyositis and dermatomyositis
    2. "Myasthenic" syndrome
II. Metabolic encephalopathy
  A. Destruction of vital organs
    1. Liver (hepatic coma)
    2. Lung (pulmonary encephalopathy)
    3. Kidney (uremia)
    4. Bone (hypercalcemia)
  B. Elaboration of hormonal substances by tumor
    1. "Parathormone" (hypercalcemia)
    2. "Corticotrophin" (Cushing's syndrome)
    3. Antidiuretic hormone (water intoxication)
  C. Competition between tumor and brain for essential substrates
    1. Hypoglycemia (large retroperitoneal tumors)
    2. Tryptophan (carcinoid)
III. Infections (usually associated with lymphomas)
  A. Parasites
    1. Toxoplasma cerebral abscess
  B. Fungi
    1. Meningitis (cryptococcosis)
    2. Encephalitis (aspergillus, mucormycosis)
  C. Bacteria
    1. Meningitis (*Listeria monocytogenes*)
  D. Viruses
    1. Herpes zoster (radiculitis, myelitis, encephalitis)
    2. Progressive multifocal leukoencephalopathy
IV. Vascular disease
  A. Intracranial hemorrhage (secondary to bleeding disorders)
    1. Subdural hematoma
    2. Subarachnoid hemorrhage
    3. Intracerebral hemorrhage
  B. Cerebral infarction
    1. Thrombotic (due to "disseminated intravascular coagulation")
    2. Embolic (tumor emboli, marantic endocarditis)
V. Effects of therapy
  A. Steroids
    1. Myopathy
    2. Psychosis
  B. Chemotherapy
    1. Central effects (asparaginase encephalopathy)
    2. Peripheral effects (vinca alkaloid neuropathy)
  C. Radiation
    1. Encephalopathy
    2. Myelopathy
    3. Neuropathy

of 1465 patients, an incidence of 6.6 per cent, but a rather ill-defined weakness and wasting of proximal muscles associated with diminished deep tendon reflexes accounted for two thirds of their patients. The incidence varied according to the type of cancer, with ovary (16.4 per cent) and lung (14.2 per cent) leading the list. Rectal (0.5 per cent) and uterine (1.3 per cent) cancer rarely caused remote effects. Since carcinoma of the lung is much more common than ovarian carcinoma, about half of all their patients with remote effects had lung cancer, usually of the oat cell type. Shy and Silverstein found a 3.5 per cent incidence of "neuromyopathy" in 1500 patients with cancer. In patients with hematologic malignancies, the incidence of "remote effects" was 2.2 per cent; polyneuropathy was the most common syndrome, and polymyositis next. My experience is that "remote effects" are less common than the aforementioned series suggest, and the diagnosis should never be accepted until a thorough evaluation has excluded metastatic or other nonmetastatic (e.g., infection, vascular disease) causes of neurologic dysfunction.

The etiology and pathogenesis of these disorders are unknown; suggestions for their cause have included autoimmune reactions, viral infections, toxins secreted by the tumor, and nutritional deprivation. It is possible that different mechanisms are responsible for the several types of remote effects. Although the neurologic disorders described below are separated into anatomic categories, there is often an overlap. This is particularly true of the dementias, which are often lumped together with brainstem, cerebellar, and spinal cord lesions as "carcinomatous encephalomyelitis," and of myopathy and peripheral neuropathy associated with cancer, often called "carcinomatous neuromyopathy." The latter term was also applied by Brain to all the remote effects of cancer on the nervous system.

BRAIN AND CRANIAL NERVES

Cerebrum. Dementia, with or without other neurologic signs, characterizes about 40 per cent of patients with remote effects of carcinoma. The dementia is insidious in onset and progressive. There is usually a striking loss of recent memory and an alteration of the affect, either anxiety or depression. Generalized seizures are prominent in some patients, and others have a fluctuating confusional state mimicking metabolic encephalopathy. When other abnormal neurologic signs are present, they usually point to brainstem, cerebellar, or peripheral nerve involvement (see below). The electroencephalogram in the demented patients is diffusely slow, and there are sometimes 10 to 40 lymphocytes per milliliter in the cerebrospinal fluid and a slight elevation of the protein.

Pathologically, there are two main groups: In some patients, particularly those who also have subacute cerebellar degeneration, bulbar encephalitis, or carcinomatous neuropathy (q.v.), no significant pathologic changes can be found in the cerebrum despite clinical dementia. Other patients demonstrate widespread cerebral neuronal loss with perivascular collections of lymphocytes, particularly in the temporal lobes (limbic encephalitis) or the thalamus.

The etiology of the dementing illness is unknown, but the inflammatory changes have led some to propose that a virus is responsible. The differential diagnosis includes metastatic disease of the brain or meninges, fungal or parasitic infections of the brain, a metabolic encephalopathy, and multifocal leukoencephalopathy. In the first three, focal cerebral signs other than dementia are present, and appropriate contrast and cerebrospinal fluid studies support the diagnosis of infectious or metastatic disease of the brain. Metabolic encephalopathy can usually be diagnosed by appropriate laboratory tests, as indicated in Ch. 320. The presence of a progressive dementia in middle age accompanied by cerebellar, brainstem, or peripheral nerve dysfunction but no other focal cerebral signs suggests carcinomatous dementia. There is no treatment for the dementias associated with carcinoma.

Bulbar Encephalitis. Henson et al. have reported a few patients with brainstem dysfunction and usually dementia, which develops insidiously or subacutely and is progressive. The brainstem signs include vertigo, nystagmus, dysphagia, ophthalmoplegia, and at times ataxia and extensor plantar reflexes. The pathologic changes, predominantly in the lower pons and medulla, are those of neuronal loss and perivascular lymphocytic cuffing. The lymphocytic infiltration is responsible for the term encephalitis. The cause is unknown, and there is no effective treatment.

Cerebellum. Subacute cerebellar degeneration represents about 3 per cent of the remote effects of cancer but has a clinical picture sufficiently characteristic to suggest strongly that cancer is present even if the neurologic symptoms predate the appearance of the tumor. There is a subacute onset of bilateral and symmetrical cerebellar dysfunction, the patient being equally ataxic in arms and legs. Severe dysarthria is usually present, but nystagmus is generally absent or mild. Many patients have neurologic signs pointing to disease outside the cerebellum: extensor plantar responses are common; tendon reflexes may be either diminished or exaggerated; and dementia occurs in about half. The cerebrospinal fluid is usually normal, but there may be as many as 40 lymphocytes and an elevated protein content. The disease, which is usually associated with either carcinoma of the lung or of the ovary, precedes the discovery of the neoplasm by periods of from weeks to three years in more than half the patients, and it tends to run a progressive course over six to eight weeks, rendering the patient severely disabled. Characteristic pathologic changes consist of diffuse loss of Purkinje cells in all areas of the cerebellum with lymphocytic cuffs around blood vessels. There is often additional neuronal degeneration of brainstem nuclei and subthalamic structures as well. This illness can be distinguished from cerebellar metastases by the symmetry of its signs and the absence of increased intracranial pressure, and from alcoholic-nutritional cerebellar degeneration because dysarthria and ataxia in the upper extremities are prominent in the carcinomatous cerebellar degenerations, and are usually mild or absent in the alcoholic variety. The hereditary cerebellar degenerations rarely run so rapid a course. There is no treatment for this disorder, and its cause is unknown. There is no evidence that treatment of the tumor reverses the neurologic disability.

Another, less common, cerebellar syndrome is that of opsoclonus (spontaneous, conjugate, chaotic eye movements most severe when voluntary eye movements are attempted). Opsoclonus is frequently associated with cerebellar ataxia and myoclonus of the trunk and extremities. It has been reported in adults as a remote effect of cancer, but is more common in children as a remote effect of neuroblastoma. In children, the neurologic symptoms respond to adrenocorticosteroid therapy and to removal of the tumor.

Optic Nerves. Acute optic neuritis is a rare remote effect of cancer which may precede the discovery of the cancer by months or years. The disease is bilateral, acute or subacute in its onset, and associated with decreased vision, central scotomas, and papilledema. The cerebrospinal fluid is normal, and vision usually does not improve. Pathologically, there is widespread demyelination of the optic nerves with relative preservation of the axis cylinders and occasional perivascular cuffings with lymphocytes. The illness cannot be distinguished from the optic involvement which is a common accompaniment of meningeal carcinomatosis except by examination of the cerebrospinal fluid, which in meningeal tumor usually reveals increased protein and decreased glucose concentrations and the presence of malignant cells. Treatment of the acute optic neuritis with corticosteroids is not helpful.

SPINAL CORD

Two rare but distinct myelopathies complicate cancer. The first, which involves spinal gray matter (particularly anterior horn cells), has clinical and pathologic findings at times indistinguishable from amyotrophic lateral sclerosis, except that the patients with cancer are usually older and suffer a more indolent course. Alternatively, the course may be subacute, more like poliomyelitis, but with sensory changes. In these patients, there are inflammatory changes in the spinal gray matter as well as neuronal loss. Rarely, gray matter myelopathies with clinical courses resembling syringomyelia or autonomic insufficiency (q.v.) complicate systemic cancer. The second myelopathy is that of a subacute necrotic destruction of the spinal cord in which both gray and white matter are affected to an equal degree. Clinically, there is a rapidly ascending sensory and motor loss, usually to midthoracic levels, the patient becoming paraplegic and incontinent within hours or days of the onset of symptoms. The neurologic symptoms often precede the discovery of the neoplasm, and the illness is clinically and pathologically indistinguishable from idiopathic subacute necrotic myelopathy. Since epidural spinal cord compression from metastatic tumor or arteriovenous spinal cord anomalies may present similar clinical signs, a myelogram is essential to the diagnosis. In addition to the two aforementioned entities, many patients with carcinomatous cerebellar degeneration develop extensor plantar responses, mild sensory changes, and reflex asymmetries and weakness associated with degenerations of long tracts and anterior horn cells of the spinal cord. However, spinal cord symptoms do not predominate in these patients.

PERIPHERAL NERVES

Three types of peripheral nerve disorders occur in association with cancer. Characteristic of carcinoma is a subacute sensory neuropathy (dorsal root ganglionitis) marked by loss of proprioception and cutaneous sensory modalities with relative preservation of motor power. The illness sometims precedes the appearance of the carcinoma and progresses over a few months, leaving the patient with a moderate or severe disability. The cerebrospinal fluid protein is usually elevated. Pathologically, there is destruction of posterior root ganglia with perivascular lymphocytic cuffing. There is wallerian degeneration of sensory nerves. Many of the patients have inflammatory and degenerative changes in brain and spinal cord as well. The entity is rare; in one series no examples were found on examination of 1476 patients with cancer. The illness is of interest, however, both because it is almost pathognomonic of cancer and because four such patients have been reported to have complement-fixing antibodies to brain tissue in their plasma. These findings suggest an autoimmune disorder, but the exact pathogenesis is unknown. There is no treatment.

More common than sensory neuropathy is a distal sensorimotor polyneuropathy characterized by motor weakness, sensory loss, and reflex absence distally in the extremities. Croft et al. subdivided their 33 patients with cancer and sensorimotor polyneuropathy into three groups: (1) a mild neuropathy often occurring in terminal patients (10 patients), (2) a more severe subacute or acute neuropathy at times preceding discovery of the cancer (15 patients), and (3) a remitting or relapsing neuropathy (8 patients). The illness is pathologically characterized by both segmental demyelination and wallerian degeneration of sensory and motor peripheral nerves. Dorsal root ganglia are never involved to the same degree that they are in the purely sensory neuropathy. Pathologically and clinically, the sensorimotor neuropathy is indistinguishable from nutritional polyneuropathies as well as those associated with uremia and other metabolic defects. Indeed, some have suggested that the late or terminal polyneuropathy may be due to nutritional deprivation associated with cancer. Its etiology, however, is not clear, and it does not respond to treatment with vitamins and other nutritional supplements.

A polyneuritis clinically and pathologically indistinguishable from acute postinfectious polyneuropathy (Guillain-Barré syndrome) also complicates cancer, but the association may be coincidental because both acute polyneuropathy and carcinoma are common illnesses.

NEUROMUSCULAR JUNCTION AND MUSCLES

Neuromuscular Junction. *Myasthenia gravis* is associated with thymomas but not other systemic tumors. However, Lambert and Eaton described a "*myasthenic syndrome*" occurring predominantly in men over 40 and associated with intrathoracic tumors in 70 per cent of the patients (see Brain and Norris). The patients complain of weakness and fatigability of proximal muscles, particularly of the pelvic girdle and thighs. The cranial nerves and respiratory muscles are involved less. In addition, patients complain of dryness of the mouth, impotence, pain in the thighs, and peripheral paresthesias. On examination there is weakness of the proximal muscles, but strength increases over several seconds of a sustained contraction. The deep tendon reflexes are diminished or absent. The diagnosis is made by electromyographic studies in which repeated nerve stimulations at rates above ten per second cause a progressive increase in the size of the muscle action potential (exactly the opposite of the effect of myasthenia gravis). The neuromuscular defect in this illness is believed to be deficient release of acetylcholine. The illness responds poorly to anticholinesterase drugs, but does respond to guanidine hydrochloride given in doses of 35 to 50 mg per kilogram per day. There is no direct relationship between treatment of the tumor and change in the myasthenic syndrome.

Muscle. Typical *polymyositis* and/or *dermatomyositis* may appear as a remote effect of cancer. About 20 per cent of patients with this disorder have cancer, and although polymyositis is considerably more common in women, the illness is more commonly associated with cancer in men over the age of 50. In at least 60 per cent of males over 50 with polymyositis, a cancer either can be found when the disease develops or will appear within a few months or years. The clinical picture is indistinguishable from that of dermatomyositis or polymyositis. Pathologically there may be two groups: one with the typical inflammatory lesions of polymyositis, and one with little inflammation but severe muscle necrosis. The latter group may suffer an explosive clinical course. The patients respond somewhat less well to corticosteroid therapy than do those with dermatomyositis unaccompanied by cancer, although improvement with steroid treatment does occur in some.

MUSCLE WEAKNESS

A small number of patients with cancer complain of weakness and fatigability which seems worse than can be accounted for by their cancer alone. The weakness is usually proximal and produces particular difficulty in climbing stairs and getting out of low chairs. Ankle reflexes may be diminished or absent. Further neurologic evaluation does not yield findings diagnostic of one of the remote effects of cancer described above. Brain and his colleagues have labeled this entity a "neuromyopathy" because its exact anatomic locus is unclear, but Hildebrand and Coers have suggested that it is a nonspecific accompanniment of cachexia and systemic illness. The cause and treatment of the weakness are unknown, but a recent report by Sloane and Truong suggests that some of the patients have mild neuromuscular transmission disorders of the "myasthenic syndrome" type and respond to guanidine HCl.

Brain, R., and Norris, F. H., Jr.: The Remote Effects of Cancer on the Nervous System. New York, Grune & Stratton, 1965.

Croft, P. B., and Wilkinson, M.: The course and prognosis in some types of carcinomatous neuromyopathy. Brain, 92:1, 1969.

Curries, S., Henson, R. A., Morgan, H. G., and Poole, A. J.: The incidence of the nonmetastatic neurological syndromes of obscure origin in the reticuloses. Brain, 93:629, 1970.

Henson, R. A., Hoffman, H. L., and Urich, H.: Encephalomyelitis with carcinoma. Brain, 88:449, 1965.

Hildebrand, J., and Coers, C.: The neuromuscular junction in patients with malignant tumors. Brain, 90:67, 1967.

Section Nineteen. INJURIES OF THE HEAD AND SPINE

Russel H. Patterson, Jr.

425. INJURIES OF THE HEAD

Trauma claims over 110,000 lives each year in the United States and ranks in frequency as a cause of death after heart disease, cancer, and stroke. Head injury accounts for death in 70 per cent of cases and surpasses all other causes in persons between the ages of 1 and 35. Good management can benefit many of these patients, but often responsibility for their care falls first on someone who lacks formal training in the field of cerebral trauma. This need not be a disadvantage if the physician follows a few simple principles of management based on an understanding of the pathophysiology of the injury. Properly prepared, he can recognize the indications for specialized diagnostic procedures and possible surgery.

Pathophysiology. The scalp, hair, skull, and bones of the face protect the brain from trauma by absorbing energy from blows to the head. When struck by a blow of moderate velocity, the calvaria bends inward, but a few centimeters away the skull bends outward, and linear fractures radiate toward and away from the point of impact. A blow of higher kinetic energy may comminute or penetrate the skull to cause a depressed fracture.

Beneath the point of impact intracranial pressure may increase for a few milliseconds to as much as 5000 mm Hg, and low or even negative pressure can be recorded simultaneously in the brain at the opposite side of the skull. Cavitation occurs in the brain in regions of low pressure, which accounts for many contrecoup injuries. The pressure gradients distort the brain, which attempts to flow toward the foramen magnum, inducing shear stresses in the brainstem and upper cervical spinal cord. Other shearing forces, induced by rapid acceleration and deceleration of the head, tear axonal processes; this is manifest pathologically by chromatolysis in the cell body of the neuron and microglial proliferation in the white matter associated with abnormalities of the myelin sheath. These changes may not be visible macroscopically at autopsy but account for widespread dysfunction in the cerebral hemispheres, basal ganglia, and brainstem.

The brain and skull respond at different rates to forces of acceleration and deceleration produced by a blow which results in mass movements of the brain. Sharp and irregular surfaces inside the cranial cavity such as the orbital surface of the frontal fossa, the sphenoid ridge, the falx, and the tentorium lacerate and contuse the moving brain. Rotational forces shear nervous tissue around arterioles and result in parenchymal hemorrhages; fragile cerebral veins draining into the dural venous sinuses may tear and fill the subdural space with blood. Fractures that divide meningeal arteries or major venous sinuses commonly cause bleeding in the epidural space.

After brain injury cerebral blood flow may decrease in some areas owing to vasospasm, whereas in other areas the arterioles dilate and lose their capacity to regulate flow in response to change in arterial blood pressure. Loss of the normal autoregulatory mechanism accompanies many, but by no means all, severe head injuries. The resulting dilation of the vascular bed combines with cerebral edema and any hematoma that might be present to increase the intracranial pressure. The elevated intracranial pressure fluctuates rhythmically and, in cases of severe injury, periodically may rise further to levels of 50 to 100 mm Hg for 15 to 20 minutes. These additional pressure elevations, known as *plateau waves,* are often associated with a transient deterioration in neurologic status.

Cerebral contusions and lacerations accompany 90 per cent of severe nonpenetrating injuries. Blood stains the cortical surface and subarachnoid space over both cerebral hemispheres, areas of hemorrhage are found in the brain parenchyma, and clots form in the subdural and epidural spaces. Edema further crowds the contents of an unyielding cranium. The swollen cerebrum displaces the uncus of the temporal lobe through the tentorial notch to compress the oculomotor nerve and the midbrain. Continued pressure obstructs the posterior cerebral artery and basilar vein, inducing ischemia and augmenting edema.

The supratentorial structures generally are most susceptible to damage from head trauma because a heavy layer of muscle protects the contents of the posterior fossa. But should the effects of an injury swell the cerebellum, the tonsils herniate downward through the foramen magnum to compress the medulla while the vermis pushes upward through the apex of the tentorial notch to squeeze the vein of Galen against the corpus callosum, which is backed by the rigid falx.

Increased intracranial pressure causes constriction of the peripheral vascular bed, bradycardia, and increased return of venous blood to the heart. The left ventricle of the heart may be unable to increase cardiac output sufficiently to prevent the development of high pressure in the left atrium and pulmonary edema. Even in the absence of pulmonary edema, pulmonary arteriovenous shunts may open in response to both the increased blood flow in the pulmonary artery and increased sympathetic tone in the pulmonary vascular bed. The consequence is frequently arterial hypoxemia even if the patient's ventilation is adequate to maintain normocapnia or hypocapnia. If the tongue or secretions obstruct the airway, hypoxia develops in association with hypercapnia. Hypercapnia augments cerebrovasodilatation and causes a further increase in intracranial pressure with the grave consequences outlined above. In addition, blood flow may be shunted to one area of the brain through a portion of the vascular bed that is dilated and of low resistance, thereby reducing circulation to other areas that become relatively ischemic.

Hemorrhages are found about the pituitary gland and hypophyseal stalk in about two thirds of patients dying of craniocerebral trauma. Necrosis of the anterior lobe is present in more than a fifth of cases and has been attributed to shock, swelling of the gland, and obstruction of the portal vessels. The consequence may be some combination of diabetes insipidus, absence of thirst, and hypoadrenalism producing a varied picture of abnormal fluid and electrolyte metabolism which can range from hypernatremia to water intoxication.

CONCUSSION

Concussion is a clinical term that may be defined as loss of consciousness after an injury to the head without macroscopic damage to nervous tissue. Recovery is usually prompt after less severe injuries, but long periods of unconsciousness or death may occur, and amnesia for events before and after the accident is common. Concussion implies that contusions and lacerations of the brain have not accounted for the symptoms, but the diagnosis must be presumptive except in occasional fatal cases studied at autopsy. Information about the pathophysiology of concussion therefore is derived largely from experiments with animals.

How an injury to the head causes unconsciousness is not entirely clear. Transmitted pressure gradients and rotational forces distort the brainstem, but bilateral injury to the cerebral hemispheres may be equally important. Changes in the brainstem probably account for the apnea and bradycardia that immediately follow the blow as well as for the unsteadiness and giddiness with change in position of which patients often complain for a time. Amnesia, forgetfulness, irritability, fatigue, and impaired memory are attributed to neuronal damage in the cerebrum, although long persistence of these vague symptoms after cerebral trauma may be hard to evaluate, particularly if a lawsuit is unsettled.

Microscopic changes in the brain after a concussive blow are observed in the neurons and glia within a few hours. Some cells may recover, but others do not, and thus permanent damage to the nervous system occurs. Psychologic tests and neurologic examination may not reveal evidence for the loss of a relatively few neurons, but the effects of repeated small injuries are cumulative as the dull, querulous behavior of the punchdrunk fighter testifies.

EVALUATION OF THE ACUTE HEAD INJURY

The diagnosis of an intracranial clot may be difficult and often depends on the demonstration of an increasing neurologic deficit. Consequently, the initial examination of the patient assumes importance as a baseline for subsequent observations.

Details of the accident suggest what parts of the brain may be injured. The duration of unconsciousness is a rough index to the severity of the injury; even brief unconsciousness is evidence of enough damage to merit hospitalization and careful observation. The neurologic examination is repeated at intervals to detect any change in consciousness, breathing, pupillary diameter, motor strength, speech, or vision, which may signal the presence of an expanding intracranial mass.

The blood pressure, pulse, respirations, and temperature should be recorded frequently after an injury to the head. However, the classic response to increasing intracranial pressure of bradycardia and arterial hypertension may not occur, and any instability of vital signs implies a change in intracranial homeostasis.

Continuous monitoring of intracranial pressure by a ventricular catheter can be of substantial value in following patients with acute head injury. The appearance of plateau waves (described earlier) may signal the need for the lowering of intracranial pressure either by the drainage of ventricular fluid or by the administration of an osmotic diuretic.

As death after trauma is usually due to failure of the respiratory and circulatory centers, the physician must be particularly alert to the early signs of damage to the brainstem. Coma may result from extensive injury to both cerebral hemispheres, but stupor that progressively deepens usually results from distortion of the brainstem caused by an enlarging clot or progressively edematous brain. The evolution of these signs of dangerous rostral-caudal deterioration is emphasized later in this discussion. Grave signs, however, are fixed pupils, impaired oculovestibular responses, and decerebrate posturing.

If edema or a clot herniates the temporal lobe through the tentorial notch, the uncus compresses the ipsilateral third cranial nerve, and the pupil first dilates, then fixes to light. Occasionally the contralateral third nerve is first affected, but eventually both nerves are paralyzed, and both pupils dilate. Later, when sympathetic centers in the midbrain are damaged, the pupils may contract to become fixed in midposition. Treatment, to be fully effective, must reverse the process before this advanced stage.

Sometimes retinal hemorrhages follow intracranial bleeding, or an occluded venous sinus causes papilledema, but mydriatics alter pupillary responses and for this reason should not be used to obtain a better view of the ocular fundus.

Diagnostic Procedures. *Roentgenograms.* Roentgenographic examination of the skull should be performed without undue delay in all cases of injury to the head. Fractures of the calvaria are generally visible, but most basilar fractures are obscured in the bony detail. The presence of skull fracture is reason enough to admit a patient to the hospital after an injury even if he appears to have sustained no brain damage. Roentgenograms perhaps will reveal an indriven fragment of bone, a displaced pineal gland, or intracranial air if a fracture through a paranasal sinus tears the dura and arachnoid. The patient is a likely candidate for an intracranial blood clot if fracture is found which crosses a venous sinus or meningeal artery.

Lumbar Puncture. Lumbar puncture is helpful in the differential diagnosis of coma because the cerebrospinal fluid is commonly xanthochromic after being centrifuged in cases of trauma. However, if a good history is available, lumbar puncture is better avoided because in a patient with an edematous brain or an intracranial clot the withdrawal of fluid can precipitate transtentorial or foramen magnum herniation.

Echoencephalography. A shift of the midline structures of the brain caused by edema or hematoma can be identified by a displaced pineal gland on roentgenograms of the skull or by echoencephalography if the gland is uncalcified. After evacuation of a clot, the displaced midline structures return to their normal position unless the clot reaccumulates. The absence of a shift does not necessarily mean that an intracranial clot is not present; bilateral subdural hematomas are common and may cause transtentorial herniation of the temporal lobes without shift of the midline structures.

Electroencephalography. The electroencephalogram

is rarely helpful in the management of acute injury to the head. An abnormal tracing is common immediately after the trauma and tends to improve as recovery takes place. In cases of chronic subdural hematoma the electroencephalogram may be of value if low voltages and abnormal wave forms are recorded from the scalp overlying the hematoma.

Radioactive Scan. Chronic subdural hematomas are often well demonstrated by the radioactive scan technique. In acute injuries a scan is less helpful because the study does not differentiate space-occupying lesions from contused areas of brain.

Cerebral Angiography. Angiography is widely used in evaluating trauma to the head, and in some cases, such as subdural hematoma, the films are almost diagnostic. The procedure is not without danger, particularly when the circulation to a region of the brain is already impaired by an injury. Consequently, angiography is best reserved for patients in whom progressive deterioration or focal signs such as hemiparesis raise suspicion that a blood clot may be present.

Burr Holes. Burr holes placed in the skull can be used to diagnose and treat subdural and epidural hematoma. The advantages of the procedure lie in low risk and speedy evacuation of the clot if the patient's condition is rapidly worsening. Unfortunately, a subdural hematoma in an unusual location may escape detection unless the burr holes are judiciously placed, and a parenchymal hematoma will not be revealed by inspection of the surface of the brain. Angiography remains the most useful diagnostic tool in head trauma. Diagnostic burr holes are reserved for emergencies or occasions when angiography is not available.

Air Encephalography. Air encephalography provides less information than angiography in patients with trauma and carries more risk because of the possibility that a change in pressure relationships in the head may precipitate an unfavorable shift in the brain with serious consequences. As a result, air studies are employed infrequently in the management of head injury.

MANAGEMENT OF ACUTE HEAD INJURY

Although it sometimes accompanies a severe head injury, hypovolemic shock is rarely the consequence of moderate head trauma or a scalp laceration. Consequently, a patient with a head injury who is in shock deserves investigation for a source of an occult hemorrhage, such as a pelvic fracture with retroperitoneal bleeding. Scalp lacerations are best repaired in the emergency room before roentgenograms are obtained in order to control bleeding and to prevent infection. This is the time to initiate baseline observations of vital signs and neurologic status and to examine the patient for associated injuries of the skeleton, viscera, and soft tissues. Prophylaxis against tetanus is administered, as are antimicrobial agents if open fractures are present.

Respiration. A number of steps may be taken to reduce edema in the brain after an injury. The most important is the establishment of an adequate airway. Hypoxia and hypocarbia have grave consequences on cerebral homeostasis as outlined earlier. If a stuporous patient is unable to clear his own airway, the trachea should be intubated.

Blood gases should be monitored even in patients who appear to be respiring adequately, because pulmonary edema and shunting in the lung, described above, may result in low values of arterial P_{O_2} that the administration of oxygen can correct. When spontaneous respirations cease, even if cardiac action continues, death is inevitable, and mechanical ventilation is unavailing.

Opiates and sedatives are avoided for patients with injuries to the head. These drugs further depress an already damaged nervous system, impair respirations, and increase stupor. Urinary retention often accounts for restlessness in drowsy patients and is readily treated by catheterization.

Blood and Fluid Replacement. Motor vehicle accidents commonly result in multiple injuries. Hypovolemic shock occurs and is best treated by the ordinary measures except that the head-low position is avoided if the brain is damaged. Elevation of the extremities increases the return of blood to the heart without contributing to cerebral edema.

Cerebral swelling is increased when hypotonic fluids are administered. Five per cent dextrose in water becomes hypotonic as the sugar is metabolized, and therefore should not be given in large quantities. Isotonic saline is less hazardous because sodium chloride passes the blood-brain barrier poorly. Consequently, fluids are mildly restricted for patients with brain injury, and more saline is employed than in ordinary practice.

Patients with head injury sometimes develop inappropriate secretions of antidiuretic hormone with consequent water intoxication, even if fluids are replaced with care. The resulting symptoms of stupor and seizures are often mistakenly attributed to extensive parenchymal damage. Water intoxication is confirmed by demonstrating a serum sodium of 120 mEq per liter or less. The primary treatment consists of restricting water and perhaps giving small amounts of intravenous 5 per cent saline.

Occasionally trauma damages homeostatic centers in the hypothalamus so that diabetes insipidus results. A patient who is alert ordinarily will drink enough to prevent dehydration. However, if osmoreceptor mechanisms are also disturbed or the subject is in stupor with a lack of thirst, serum hyperosmolarity with high electrolyte levels occurs if adequate fluids are not administered. Replacement of water, restriction of salt, and administration of Pitressin are indicated until the condition corrects itself, as it usually does.

Severe injuries to the brain are sometimes associated with impaired renal function despite the absence of shock, or a reaction to blood transfusion, or other common causes of damage to the renal tubules. Characteristically the output of urine remains good, but the specific gravity is fixed at 1.010, albuminuria is present, and the sediment contains red cells, white cells, and casts. Death from renal failure may occur in spite of treatment. The mechanism of the renal damage is not entirely clear, but stimulation of certain cortical areas and destructive lesions in the hypothalamus cause similar renal lesions in laboratory animals.

Osmotic Diuretics. By administering a hypertonic solution it is possible to establish an osmotic gradient across the blood-brain barrier that removes water from the brain and reduces cerebral edema. Drugs that penetrate the brain slowly are employed, such as a 30 per cent solution of urea in 10 per cent invert sugar or 20 per cent mannitol given intravenously or glycerin given by mouth.

The administration of an osmotic diuretic often stabilizes or improves the neurologic status of a patient who is deteriorating rapidly after a head injury. The beneficial effects, if observed, are only temporary, but respite even for an hour or two may be enough to perform angiography or emergency burr holes. If the patient is sufficiently ill to warrant the use of osmotic diuretics, his state is serious enough to deserve prompt and vigorous management. Any temporary improvement that might follow their use should not lull the physician, because the patient's neurologic status once again may worsen rapidly when the drug effect wears off.

During the first several days after injury, osmotic diuretics may also be of value to treat episodes of neurologic deterioration of the sort associated with the plateau waves of increased intracranial pressure. They also are helpful in controlling the cerebral edema that sometimes follows removal of a compressive hematoma.

Steroids. Steroids effectively reduce cerebral edema and are used when intracranial pressure persists for several days, a circumstance that limits the utility of the osmotic diuretics. Doses equivalent to more than 1000 mg of cortisone daily are employed; dexamethasone, which has less salt-retaining property, is frequently prescribed in doses of 16 to 40 mg daily. The incidence of pituitary necrosis after severe head injury ranges around 25 per cent, which is an additional reason to administer steroids. However, the hoped-for benefits are often unrealized because extensive structural brain damage is present.

COMPLICATIONS OF HEAD INJURY

Cranial Nerve Injury. Damage may occur to the cranial nerves as they exit from the skull. Among the more common complications, anosmia and blindness are often permanent in contrast to extraocular palsies and facial paralysis, which usually improve.

Depressed Fractures. The incidence of epilepsy is 30 per cent or more after depressed fractures and penetrating wounds, but the risk is reduced if the fracture is elevated, and fragments of bone and other foreign bodies are promptly removed. As seizures may occur even if the site of fracture is remote from the motor areas of the cerebral cortex, all depressed fractures should be elevated except possibly a small depression over a major venous sinus. If a laceration of the scalp overlies a depressed fracture, antimicrobial agents are administered to prevent the occurrence of osteomyelitis and intracranial infection.

Debridement of a depressed fracture or penetrating missile wound often leaves an unsightly cranial defect that a properly executed cranioplasty will correct. The current use of synthetic material such as tantalum, acrylic plastic, and stainless steel has simplified this operation and improved its cosmetic results. Some have thought that cranioplasty both ameliorates such subjective symptoms as headache and giddiness and reduces the frequency of convulsive seizures, but properly controlled studies do not bear this out.

Basilar Skull Fracture and Cerebrospinal Fluid Fistula. Because they are often not visible on skull roentgenograms, basilar fractures are usually diagnosed by clinical signs such as anosmia, Battle's sign, bilateral periorbital ecchymoses, and the drainage of blood or cerebrospinal fluid from the nose or ears. Cerebrospinal fluid can be distinguished from a mucoid nasal discharge by testing for sugar, which can be done conveniently with the paper test strips used in urinalysis. Patients with cerebrospinal fluid fistulas should be treated prophylactically with antimicrobial agents to prevent meningitis until the leak stops, as it does in 75 per cent of cases of rhinorrhea and almost all cases of otorrhea. The ear or nose should not be probed or packed, and sealing of the leak may be hastened by repeated lumbar punctures in which 30 ml or more of cerebrospinal fluid is withdrawn. A fistula which persists more than 10 to 14 days demands surgical repair.

Epilepsy. The incidence of epilepsy after head injury varies with the severity of the injury to the brain. Seizures occur in 40 per cent of patients who sustain penetrating missile wounds, but follow only 10 per cent of the blunt injuries characteristic of civilian life. Depressed skull fracture is associated with an increased incidence of epilepsy, which reaches 40 per cent if accompanied by evidence of severe brain damage such as traumatic amnesia lasting more than 24 hours. Elevation of the depressed fracture, debridement of the wound, and prevention of the infection can reduce this toll.

The first convulsive seizure occurs within the first week after injury in 95 per cent of cases. These early seizures are typically focal motor in type and many do not recur. Late epilepsy, meaning seizures which occur after the first week, has a more ominous prognosis. It is treated by anticonvulsants. Fortunately in many patients the attacks decrease in frequency as the years pass and ultimately stop in half the cases. A persistent, debilitating convulsive disorder can sometimes be improved by surgical excision of the epileptogenic focus.

Intracranial Hematomas. Both increasing edema and an enlarging hematoma cause neurologic signs that progress. As the two are difficult to distinguish, progressive signs are a justifiable reason in any patient to search for a clot by angiography or trephination of the skull.

Epidural Hematoma. Although small amounts of blood are often found in extradural space after fracture of the skull, large hematomas are uncommon, occurring in only 1 or 2 per cent of injuries to the head. Despite their rarity, epidural hematomas are important because they are potentially fatal, yet proper treatment is followed by recovery with little or no neurologic deficit if the brain has not sustained other injuries.

Epidural hematomas most frequently occur in the temporal region from a tear in the middle meningeal artery but are sometimes found in the frontal parietal, occipital, and suboccipital areas. Typically, a patient receives a blow on the temple that results in transitory unconsciousness. After a lucid interval of a few minutes or hours the expanding clot causes headache, drowsiness, contralateral hemiparesis, and paralysis of the ipsilateral third cranial nerve. Signs of decompensation of the brainstem soon follow, and death results.

The classic case is easily recognized but not often encountered. The patient may relate that the blow was light and unconsciousness brief. His prompt recovery and normal roentgenograms apparently substantiate the unimportance of the injury. Yet an epidural hematoma may be present and may reach a critical size some hours later, and death may ensue if the patient has been sent home with inadequate observation.

Variations from the typical pattern are common. An associated serious brain injury may cause the patient to remain stuporous without the lucid interval, or symptoms may be delayed several days if the bleeding is slow or intermittent. Progressive coma without localizing signs is the rule with clots over the cerebellum, and occasionally occurs with supratentorial clots. At times a hematoma is missed at operation, especially in children in whom the dura adheres to the suture lines of the skull and restricts the spread of blood over the convexity.

About 40 per cent of patients with epidural hematoma die or are permanently incapacitated. Because the hematoma often occurs in patients with other severe injuries to the brain, some morbidity doubtless is inevitable. But the gratifying recovery that may follow surgery justifies a meticulous evaluation of every patient with severe head injury in a search for this infrequently occurring intracranial clot.

Subdural Hematoma. Subdural hematomas are conveniently divided into categories of acute, subacute, and chronic, which differ in both symptomatology and prognosis. A subdural hematoma is called acute when a rapid progression of symptoms leads to its discovery within hours or a day or two after the injury. Prospects for recovery depend on the severity of the associated brain damage. The fatality rate is 90 per cent in patients whose symptoms warrant operation within 12 hours of injury, but the outlook is much improved if the need for surgery is evident only after several days have passed.

Chronic Subdural Hematoma. Chronic subdural hematoma in adults usually occurs after the age of 50 and often in alcoholics because of their unsteadiness and frequent falls. With age the brain shrinks away from the dural lining of the skull and leaves a space that can fill with blood if a fragile vein should tear. The trauma that initiates the bleeding is often trivial and even forgotten when symptoms commence several weeks later. Headache occurs in 90 per cent of cases. Even if a confused patient denies it, the family may testify to his earlier complaints of pain or to his increased consumption of aspirin. Fatigue and irritability are followed insidiously by drowsiness, urinary incontinence, and stupor, which may be attributed erroneously to a natural deterioration in senescence. Hemianopsia, hemiparesis, or pupillary abnormality are observed in less than half the cases. Lumbar puncture usually reveals normal pressure, but in 50 per cent of cases the fluid is xanthochromic. Bruises about the head are frequently present, but a fracture of the skull is identified in only one third of cases, and a calcified pineal is displaced in only one fifth.

The patient usually deteriorates at an irregular rate. Intervals of substantial improvement interrupt the gradual decline and give hope of recovery, but sudden decompensation and unexpected death may occur.

Small clots may be tolerated or occasionally resorbed, but a persistent mass causes edema and irreversible anoxic-ischemic demyelination of the underlying brain. Subdural hematomas are therefore best treated by surgical drainage. The diagnosis, when suspected, is readily confirmed by arteriography or trephination. The results of treatment are good except that irreversible effects of pressure on the brain may leave a noticeable defect in mentation after recovery, particularly in elderly patients. If treatment is delayed until stupor signals dysfunction of the brainstem, evacuation of the clot and the administration of steroids and osmotic diuretics may be unable to reverse progressive transtentorial herniation that results in death.

Intracerebral Hematoma. Scattered petechial hemorrhages are commonly observed in fatal injuries to the brain, but large parenchymal hematomas occur in only 1 to 2 per cent of cases and are usually located in the frontal or temporal lobes or, less frequently, in the occipitoparietal region or cerebellum. The diagnosis is difficult because stupor from associated concussion or contusions may mask the focal neurologic signs produced by the hematoma. The mass is best demonstrated by arteriography, after which it can be removed through a small craniotomy. The results of surgery are often disappointing because the hemorrhage has destroyed sufficient cerebral tissue to leave a substantial neurologic deficit.

Vascular Complications. A blow to the head may rupture the carotid artery within the cavernous sinus and establish a *carotid–cavernous sinus fistula.* The arterial pressure dilates the tributaries of the sinus such as the orbital veins, with the result that the eye protrudes and pulsates, a bruit is usually heard, and chemosis and extraocular palsies occur. Altered arterial circulation to the eye causes loss of vision and, eventually, blindness. If the fistula is small, the symptoms may progress slowly, but spontaneous cure is uncommon. Repair by a direct approach through the cavernous sinus is not often attempted because of the threat of serious bleeding and injury to the nerves supplying the extraocular muscles. Ligation of the carotid artery in the neck or trapping of the fistula by proximal and distal ligation of the carotid artery is sometimes successful. Good results have been obtained by embolizing the fistula with bits of muscle floated up from the carotid bifurcation in the neck, possibly after first ligating the internal carotid artery intracranially just beyond the cavernous sinus in order to prevent the muscle embolus from migrating into the anterior or middle cerebral artery.

Trauma about the head occasionally leads to *thrombosis of the internal carotid artery* in the neck, resulting in hemiplegia. Less frequently, *thrombosis of the middle cerebral artery* by a dissecting aneurysm accounts for an unexpected paralysis several days after the injury.

Depressed fractures may cause *occlusion of the superior longitudinal sinus,* blocking venous drainage from the cerebral hemispheres and thereby raising intracranial pressure and causing the rapid appearance of papilledema and hemorrhages in the ocular fundus. Patients display paralysis of both lower limbs and often of one or both upper limbs.

Infection. Osteomyelitis of the skull, meningitis, and abscesses of the brain occasionally complicate open injuries of the head, and may recur for years after the injury. Antimicrobial therapy and proper debridement of the wound greatly reduce the incidence of these infectious complications.

Cerebral Swelling. Enthusiasm for aggressive surgery to cope with cerebral edema in patients with serious head injury waxes and wanes. Current interest lies in the removal of large areas of the skull and opening the dura to allow room for brain swelling, particularly in young patients with advanced signs of transtentorial herniation. Good results are sufficiently infrequent to leave the merit of such surgery in doubt.

Cerebral Fat Embolism. Fat embolism is an infrequent complication observed after severe trauma in which a long bone is fractured, or occurs occasionally with just extensive soft tissue injury. Symptoms start between 12 and 48 hours after the accident; a frequent history is that a patient has remained comatose after general anesthesia to reduce a fractured extremity. Cerebral symptoms and signs consist of rapidly progressive stupor often associated with extensor plantar responses and decerebrate posturing but with preservation of pupillary responses. Petechiae may appear on the chest and in the conjunctivae; dyspnea, tachypnea, and cyanosis are evidence that the lungs are affected. The diagnosis is best made by bedside examination, but the finding of fat globules in urine and sputum can lend laboratory support to the clinical impression.

Although cerebral fat embolism has an ominous prognosis, some patients recover even after long periods of coma. Treatment consists of taking measures to prevent shock and hypovolemia, providing ventilatory support, and perhaps administering steroids to reduce cerebral edema. The value of intravenous ethanol or of anticoagulation with heparin, which have been suggested, remains to be seen.

Prognosis in Severe Head Injuries. The young are more likely to recover from the effects of severe head injury than are adults. Patients between 20 and 50 years old who remain in coma for as long as two weeks rarely make a good recovery, whereas patients less than age 20 sometimes recover from coma lasting several weeks. The presence of nonpurposeful motor responses to noxious stimuli in young patients in coma is an unfavorable sign, and in patients over age 30, the combination of abnormal motor responses and coma makes recovery unlikely.

After head injury some patients remain in a *persistent vegetative state* that also has been called the *apallic syndrome*, or *coma vigil* or *akinetic mutism* if the patient appears alert but is unresponsive to his environment. At autopsy, multiple lesions are likely to be present throughout the brain, with the most consistent pathologic changes to be found in the periaqueductal gray matter of the rostral brainstem. Unfortunately, it is not possible to predict with certainty soon after injury which survivors will persist in a vegetative state. This often obligates the physician and the family to embark on supportive treatment which results in the great cost and heartache that accompany prolonged coma.

Less severely damaged patients profit from intensive care in a rehabilitation center where their physical, emotional, and social disabilities receive appropriate attention. Recovery from the injury continues for a long time, even several years. Ultimately 80 per cent can be returned to work, but others remain handicapped by permanent neurologic defects. Even some who appear to make a good recovery have subtle defects in memory, concentration, and comprehension which prevent their achieving their expected potential at work. Others manifest distressing psychopathology ranging from mildly asocial behavior through psychosis or dementia.

426. INJURIES OF THE SPINE

General Considerations. The first morphologic changes in the spinal cord after injury are observed in the microvasculature of the gray matter and in the myelin sheaths of the white matter. Small hemorrhages occur in the gray matter within an hour, spinal cord blood flow falls, and hypoxia develops. Catecholamines are released at the site of injury and appear to contribute hemorrhage and necrosis. Based on these observations, a variety of experimental treatments are now under study. These include longitudinal myelotomy to permit the injured spinal cord to swell, the administration of drugs such as corticosteroids and osmotic diuretics to prevent edema, epsilon-aminocaproic acid to inactivate proteolytic enzymes, and compounds such as reserpine to inactivate catecholamines.

The Cervical Spine. Forced flexion of the cervical spine often compresses the vertebral bodies, dislocates a vertebra forward on the one below, and interlocks the articular facets. Either the squeeze between the upper lamina and the lower body or displaced fragments of bone or intervertebral disc then compress the spinal cord. A prolapsed intervertebral disc does not usually damage the cord in a flexion injury unless the force is sufficient to cause a fracture-dislocation as well.

Flexion injuries tend to block circulation in the branches of the anterior spinal artery as the result of either direct pressure or injury to the radicular or vertebral arteries in the intervertebral foramen. The resulting ischemic injury is most severe in the central portion of the spinal cord. Actual thrombosis of the anterior spinal artery is rarely observed.

Hyperextension of the neck, on the other hand, buckles the ligamentum flavum forward, pinching the cord, especially if an arthritic spur bridges the interspace anteriorly. Several centimeters of the central portion of the cord can be damaged by such an injury even though roentgenograms of the spine remain normal. The upper limbs are left weaker than the lower, and a variable loss of sensation occurs with relative sparing of touch, position, and vibration sense. Bleeding into the central cord (hematomyelia) may complicate the injury and has similar clinical effects.

Patients with injury to the cervical spine must be handled carefully to prevent an unfavorable shift of the fracture-dislocation from further damaging the spinal cord. A conscious patient usually gives warning of his plight, but the possibility of an unstable spine is easily overlooked if the patient is unconscious. A gentle pull on the head in line with the spine is advisable to keep traction on the neck whenever the patient is moved. Spine boards to which the head and trunk can be strapped commonly are used to protect the spinal cord when removing a patient from a wrecked automobile. If one is not available, a bulky wrapping about the neck which supports the chin and occiput will help reduce motion that might be dangerous. A firm board or a door makes a better litter than a sagging canvas stretcher that flexes the neck. Roentgenograms are best obtained on the litter to avoid the manipulation of a transfer to the x-ray table.

The primary treatment of fracture-dislocation of the cervical spine is traction with tongs or wires inserted in the skull to achieve and maintain the reduction. The pull should be in the line of the spine, and weights exceeding 30 pounds should be used with care to prevent a sudden shift from causing further damage.

After reduction is obtained, traction can be continued for six weeks, after which the patient is ambulated in a collar that is worn for three months. An acceptable alternative that shortens the period of immobilization is to perform an operation at which loose fragments of bone and disc are removed and the vertebral bodies fused anteriorly. Atlantoaxial dislocations are characteristically unstable and are appropriately treated by early fusion of the first three cervical vertebrae.

The Thoracolumbar Spine. Hyperflexion in a fall characteristically causes compression of one or more vertebral bodies between T12 and L3. Unless neoplasm or osteoporosis has softened the bone, a heavy direct blow is needed to fracture the midthoracic vertebrae.

Hyperextension, plaster jackets, and operation were formerly used in an often futile effort to restore a normal roentgenographic appearance to the fractured spine. At present the deformity of a stable fracture is accepted and treated by bed rest until the pain subsides; this is followed by progressive ambulation. The occasional unstable fracture-dislocation requires open reduction and fusion.

Surgical Decompression. Whether surgical decompression restores function to a traumatized spinal cord is a matter of controversy. Here the initial neurologic examination assumes importance because almost no patient with complete loss of motor power and sensation that persists more than 24 hours ever regains much useful function regardless of treatment. Examination should include the testing of perianal sensation, and current clinical research includes efforts of record electrical activity in the cerebral cortex when sensory nerves below the level of the lesion are stimulated. If either a trace of motor activity or persistent sensation confirms that the cord has been only partially interrupted, surprising improvement may take place and may continue as long as two years, even without surgery.

All agree that the rare patient who shows progression of the neurologic defect after an injury should have a decompressive operation. Surgical debridement and closure prevent a spinal fluid fistula in open fractures, and possibly damaged nerve roots of the cauda equina benefit from decompression. At present many patients with fracture-dislocation of the cervical spine are operated upon by the anterior approach to achieve decompression of the cord and fusion of the vertebral bodies. The results are difficult to assess because of the relatively good prognosis without surgery when the damage to the cord is incomplete, and a conservative approach is usually justified.

Dresser, A. C., Meirowsky, A. M., Weiss, G. H., et al.: Gainful employment following head injury. Arch. Neurol., 29:111, 1973.
Jennett, B., Teather, D., and Bennie, S.: Epilepsy after head injury. Residual risk after varying fit-free intervals since injury. Lancet, 2:652, 1973.
Kornblum, R. N., and Fisher, R. S.: Pituitary lesions in cranio-cerebral injuries. Arch. Path., 88:242, 1969.
Leech, P. J., and Paterson, A.: Conservative and operative management for cerebrospinal fluid leakage after closed head injury. Lancet, 1:1013, 1973.
Lewin, W.: Vascular lesions in head injuries. Br. J. Surg., 55:321, 1968.
Maloney, A. F. J., and Whatmore, W. J.: Clinical and pathological observations in fatal head injuries. Br. J. Surg., 56:23, 1969.
Ommaya, A. K., Grubb, R. L., Jr., and Naumann, R. A.: Coup and contrecoup injury: Observations on the mechanics of visible brain injuries in the rhesus monkey. J. Neurosurg., 35:503, 1971.
Osterholm, J. L.: The pathophysiological response to spinal cord injury. The current status of related research. J. Neurosurg., 40:5, 1974.
Overgaard, J., Christensen, S., Hvid-Hansen, O., et al.: Prognosis after head injury based on early clinical examination. Lancet, 2:631, 1973.
Raynor, R.: Severe injuries of the cervical spine. Treatment by early anterior interbody fusion and ambulation. J. Neurosurg., 28:311, 1968.
Symposium on head injuries. Clin. Neurosurg., 19:1, 1972.
Weiss, G. H., and Caveness, W. F.: Prognostic factors in the persistence of posttraumatic epilepsy. J. Neurosurg., 37:164, 1972.
Weisz, G. M., and Barzilai, A.: Nonfulminant fat embolism: Review of concepts on its genesis and physiopathology. Anesth. Analg. (Cleve.), 52:303, 1973.

427. SEVERE SPINAL CORD DYSFUNCTION AND PARAPLEGIA

Many disorders, including spinal trauma, neoplasms, acute myelitis, poliomyelitis, and multiple sclerosis, can result in extensive spinal paralysis and cause similar problems in care and in the management of complications.

Antimicrobial agents and improved medical care have greatly reduced the mortality among patients with paraplegia or other forms of extensive spinal paralysis. Life expectancy is related to the severity of the neurologic deficit. Patients who are partially paraplegic have a mortality which approaches the normal population; partial quadriplegia carries a mortality twice normal, complete paraplegia four times the normal, and complete quadriplegia twelve times the normal.

Prognosis. The degree of independence that a paraplegic achieves largely depends on how many muscle groups escape paralysis. The lower the spinal level of the injury or disease, the more skills a well motivated patient can develop if good care prevents the complications of muscle spasm, decubitus ulcers, and infection of the urinary tract.

An understanding of how much recovery is possible sets goals and supplies a yardstick with which to measure progress during rehabilitation. The patient with a complete or extensive lesion of the spinal cord just below C5 retains innervation of the neck musculature and some of the shoulder girdle. He is unable to move in bed, and becomes easily fatigued because of poor respiratory reserve, but he may be able to feed himself with special equipment. With lesions of the lower cervical cord, function of more muscles of the upper limb is preserved; thus the patient is able to roll over, sit up, propel a wheelchair and possibly learn a job at home that does not require strength and dexterity of the hands. He depends upon an attendant for most of his needs.

High levels of thoracic spinal cord injury leave a functional upper limb, but the trunk is unstable, and intercostal breathing is not possible. The patient can transfer to and from a wheelchair, but even with bracing cannot develop a useful gait. Lower thoracic injuries, which leave a strong pectoral girdle and good respiratory reserve, permit the patient to be independent in all his daily activities. Bracing is still cumbersome, and ambulation is generally not practical.

Patients with lesions at T12 to L3 can usually walk in long leg braces and even negotiate stairs, but depend heavily on wheelchairs. Even with an injury below L3 a patient may sometimes use a wheelchair because such acts as arising from the sitting position, climbing steps, and standing for prolonged periods are difficult.

Emotional Aspects. Severe depression may accompany the realization that paralysis and partial dependency are permanent. Progress in rehabilitation is slowed, and recently learned skills may be temporarily lost, but emotional support from the hospital staff does much to reduce the depth and length of the depression. The environment of a center where others face and overcome similar hurdles also bolsters the morale of the paraplegic.

Cardiorespiratory System. Injuries in the cervical

region paralyze the intercostal muscles and leave only diaphragmatic respiration. Exercise quickly results in dyspnea, so that the usefulness of a hand-driven wheelchair or braces for walking is limited.

Interruption of motor pathways in the cervical spinal cord isolates the thoracic sympathetic centers from higher control. Consequently, the patient cannot constrict peripheral arteries when he sits or stands. Blood pools in the limbs and viscera, thus reducing venous return to the heart, and even elastic supports cannot adequately compensate. Venostasis in the lower limbs also accounts for a higher incidence of pulmonary embolus in paraplegics who are confined to bed.

Gastrointestinal System and Nutrition. Paralytic ileus commonly follows spinal injury or acute poliomyelitis for a few days. In treatment oral feedings should be omitted until bowel activity returns. If abdominal distention occurs, a nasogastric tube is advisable to decompress the intestinal tract.

Most paraplegics eventually begin to defecate without an enema. However, fecal impactions are frequent in patients with acute spinal paralysis, so that stool softeners, gentle laxatives, or low enemas may be needed at first. As recovery progresses, a regular dietary schedule and adequate fluids are important to achieve spontaneous evacuation. Some patients initiate reflex evacuation by abdominal massage or digital stimulation of the rectum.

Adequate nutrition is imperative for recovery but is difficult to attain, particularly for patients confined to bed. A diet high in protein and calories helps repair injured tissue and prevent bedsores. A reasonable goal at first is 2000 to 2500 calories daily, although this may have to be lowered later to avoid obesity. During the early months the daily calcium intake should be kept below 0.5 gram to minimize the likelihood of urinary calculus. Transfusions to correct anemia and low blood volume in poorly nourished patients are often beneficial.

Skin. Decubitus ulcers are a serious problem for paraplegics and can occur in any paralyzed, immobilized patient who is neglected. The danger of an anesthetic region is that it tolerates continuous pressure without the pain that ordinarily prompts a shift in position. After about two hours of immobility, ischemic changes begin in the subcutaneous tissue and are manifested by erythema of the overlying skin. Repeated ischemic insults are followed by ulceration.

Bedsores can be prevented by turning the patient at least every two hours, protecting reddened skin from further pressure, and maintaining adequate nutrition. Alternating air mattresses and rotating frame beds help to vary pressure points but are not by themselves guarantees against ulcers forming over the occiput, heels, trochanters, and sacrum. The weight of bedding is sometimes sufficient to erode the tips of the toes. Plaster casts over anesthetic areas may ulcerate the skin, and even supporting braces are dangerous.

Bedsores that heal with scar tissue remain particularly vulnerable to pressure. Therefore the most satisfactory coverage of a sizable decubitis ulcer is obtained by rotating pedicle tissue into the defect after trimming off any underlying bony prominence.

Musculoskeletal System. Many operations and mechanical devices have been used to compensate for paralyzed muscles. Crutches, braces, or wheelchairs restore mobility. An automatic lift enables anyone to transfer a patient from bed to chair. Bracing or surgery can reconstruct the loss of pinch between the thumb and index finger and thus allow the patient to feed and shave himself.

Kyphosis or lordosis is a grave consequence of the unequal pull of partially paralyzed muscles that distorts the growing spine of a child. Spinal fusion halts progression of such deformity, and often can correct a moderate curvature. Good results have been reported with internal fixation of the spine to avoid the complications of plaster immobilization.

Although a certain amount of muscle spasm may help a paraplegic to support the trunk or to position an extremity, painful or recurrent spasms that forcibly flex or adduct the lower limbs interfere with sitting and ambulation and thus prevent rehabilitation. As flexor spasms are reflex responses, the first step is to remove sources of noxious, afferent stimuli such as infection of the bladder and bedsores. If these measures plus physical therapy fail, more drastic procedures may be required, such as myelotomy, excision of the distal end of the spinal cord, anterior rhizotomy, subthecal injections, peripheral neurotomy, or division of muscles and tendons. Any procedure that increases the neurologic deficit of an already paralyzed subject is undesirable. Accordingly, division of spastic muscles and tendons or a myelotomy that disconnects the afferent sensory input from the efferent limb of the spinal reflex is appropriate if motor or sensory function is present. Subthecal alcohol, anterior rhizotomy, or excision of the cord is suitable only for those who have no useful spinal cord function.

Urinary Tract. Renal calculi, pyelonephritis, and hydronephrosis are the major causes of death in paraplegics and are sources of considerable disability in patients with lesser paralysis. These renal complications follow incomplete emptying of the bladder, which initially necessitates catheterization. Secondary infection and vesicoureteral reflux follow. These complications can be minimized by providing a low calcium diet, intermittently turning patients soon after the onset of paralysis, forcing fluids to achieve 1500 to 2000 ml of daily urine output, and treating culturally proved urinary tract infections promptly—but not prophylactically—with antimicrobial drugs. During recovery, nearly all patients with poliomyelitis and about 80 per cent of paraplegics become able to void without catheterization. Patients with poliomyelitis regain essentially normal bladder function. In paraplegics with high lesions of the spinal cord, reflex micturition occurs, mediated through the distal spinal segments. If an injury has destroyed sacral roots, suprapubic pressure may be necessary to empty the bladder.

Regaining spontaneous voiding after spinal injury is always difficult. In many patients a fluid intake of 3000 to 4000 ml daily and either intermittent catheterization or intermittent clamping of an indwelling catheter may establish spontaneous, automatic voiding. Intermittent catheterization using aseptic technique has given the best results as the urine remains sterile in three quarters of patients; if a catheter is left indwelling, one of the Gibbon type is preferred to the more irritating Foley. Some may need a transurethral resection of obstructing tissue at the bladder neck. If there is spastic hypertrophy of the bladder, especially with vesicoureteral reflux, satisfactory voiding usually cannot be obtained without partially interrupting the reflex arc. If there are no undesirable muscle spasms of the lower limbs, graded sacral rhizotomy is the most satisfactory procedure for enabling some patients to master bladder training. Myelotomy, as described earlier, is useful in managing patients with disabling spasticity of both the bladder and lower limbs. The more extensive procedures will also relieve autonomic hyperreflexia manifested by unpleasant episodes of sweating, hypertension, and headache triggered by contraction of bladder, bowel, or skeletal muscle. Recently, electrical stimulation of the conus medullaris to induce micturition has shown some promise, although the stimulus may also induce unwanted motion of lower limbs and penile erection.

Even patients who have apparently established satisfactory micturition may have slowly progressive hydronephrosis that, if unrecognized, will eventually cause death. Consequently, all patients should be evaluated periodically by intravenous pyelography. Progressive renal damage is an indication for urinary diversion, usually by implantation of the ureters into an ilial conduit.

Bosch, A., Stauffer, S., and Nickel, V. L.: Incomplete traumatic quadriplegia. A ten year review. J.A.M.A., 216:473, 1971.
Grimes, J. H., Nashold, B. S., and Currie, D. P.: Chronic electrical stimulation of the paraplegic bladder. J. Urol., 109:242, 1973.
Guttman, L.: Spinal cord injuries, comprehensive management and research. Oxford, Blackwell Scientific Publications, 1973, p. 696.
Kottke, F. J., Kubicek, W. G., Olson, M. E., and Hastings, R. H.: Studies on the parameters of cardiovascular performance of quadriplegic patients. Arch. Phys. Med. Rehabil., 44:635, 1963.
Laitinen, L., and Singounas, E.: Longitudinal myelotomy in the treatment of spasticity of the legs. J. Neurosurg., 35:536, 1971.
Long, C., II, and Lawton, E. B.: Functional significance of spinal cord lesion level. Arch. Phys. Med. Rehabil., 6:249, 1965.
Wilcox, N. E., and Stauffer, E. S.: Follow-up of 423 consecutive patients admitted to the spinal cord centre, Rancho Los Amigos Hospital, 1st January to 31st December, 1967. Paraplegia, 10:115, 1972.

Section Twenty. DEGENERATIVE AND HEREDOFAMILIAL DISEASES OF THE CENTRAL NERVOUS SYSTEM

Donald J. Reis

MOTOR NEURON DISEASE

428. INTRODUCTION

The motor neuron diseases are a group of disorders of the motor system of unknown cause whose principal pathology is a degeneration of lower motor neurons in spinal cord and brainstem. Clinically, several distinctive syndromes can be recognized on the basis of heredity, age of onset, and course and associated signs, particularly of upper motor neuron dysfunction. These syndromes are amyotrophic lateral sclerosis, progressive muscular atrophy, including the infantile, juvenile, and adult forms, and the Mariana type of amyotrophic lateral sclerosis. In the absence of any knowledge of the cause of the disorders, a clinical classification is useful, particularly because each nosologic entity tends to be true to type. However, cases intermediate to the major groups are occasionally found so that in "atypical" cases classification may be difficult.

429. AMYOTROPHIC LATERAL SCLEROSIS

Definition. Amyotrophic lateral sclerosis is a chronic progressive disease of the nervous system of unknown cause. It is usually sporadic but rarely familial, and is characterized pathologically by degeneration of motor neurons in the spinal cord and the lower brainstem, and often of Betz cells in the motor cortex. Clinically, it appears in its usual form as a disturbance in motility, reflecting dysfunction of both lower and upper motor neurons.

Pathology. On gross inspection, the most obvious abnormality of the spinal cord is thinning of the ventral roots and reduction of the size of the cervical enlargement. In the brain, atrophy of the hypoglossal nerve and occasionally of the precentral gyrus is evident. Microscopically, there is a diffuse pallor of myelin staining, most noticeable in the lateral columns of the spinal cord, the bulbar pyramids, and the anterior limb of the internal capsule. Loss or degeneration of neurons occurs in the ventral horns and in the nuclei of some cranial nerves. The motor nucleus of the trigeminal nerve and nuclei of the facial and hypoglossal nerves are particularly involved. Affected muscles show the typical features of neurogenic atrophy with intermingling of small, atrophic muscle fibers and fibers of normal size. The structure and staining of the affected fibers are preserved until late in the disease when they finally disappear, leaving residual clumps of hyperchromatic sarcolemmal nuclei. Myopathic changes may sometimes be observed as well.

Clinical Manifestations. Amyotrophic lateral sclerosis is a disorder of later life with a peak incidence in the fifth and sixth decades. It is slightly more common in men than in women and is found in all races and on all continents. For reasons unknown it has a higher incidence in patients afflicted many years earlier with poliomyelitis. It has been estimated that in the United States there are about 3000 new cases occurring annually and a total of about 8000 to 10,000 persons afflicted with the disease at any given time. The clinical picture of the disorder reflects the underlying pathologic changes of the lower and upper motor neurons. Lower motor neuron dysfunction causes weakness and wasting of the afflicted muscles. An additional consequence of the disease process may be a spontaneous irregular discharge of motor neurons, reflected peripherally by irregular twitchings in the distribution of one or several motor units. This is termed fasciculation. Fasciculations may be observed as continuous movements of portions of muscles anywhere in the body and may be perceived by the patient. Characteristically, fasciculations are widely distributed, extending beyond the territory of a single nerve root or peripheral nerve, and are ominous when associated with weakness. Involvement of the upper motor neuron leads to spastic rigidity, augmented deep tendon reflexes, and extensor plantar responses. When the corticobulbar tracts are involved bilaterally, the syndrome of *pseudobulbar palsy* may ensue. In this state, voluntary swallowing, tongue movements, or facial mimicry may be impaired. In addition, the patient may have episodes of inappropriate crying or laughing which are often provoked by an innocuous stimulus and are dissociated from feelings of excessive sadness or mirth.

There are several clinical variations of the disease that depend upon the regional distribution and the relative involvement of lower and upper motor neurons. Most commonly the disease presents in the distal muscles of the upper limb. The anterior horn cells in the cervical region are the first affected, and this leads to the appearance of wasting and fasciculation in the upper limbs which is particularly obvious in the small muscles of the hand. Involvement of both lateral and medial thenar groups leads to the thumb falling into the plane of the palm of the hand—the "simian hand." Although bilaterally symmetrical in later stages, the disease may be unilateral or even hemiparetic early in its course. As the disease progresses, proximal muscles and then muscles of the trunk and bulb become weak. In some cases involvement of motor units in the leg may be the earliest sign of the disease. The disease may present as footdrop, which is confused in its earliest stage with palsy of the lateral peroneal nerve. As the signs of lower motor neuron dysfunction are progressing, some associated signs of upper motor neuron disease become evident, particularly in the lower extremities.

Less commonly, bulbar signs may predominate in the early stages of the disease, producing the syndrome of *progressive bulbar palsy.* The muscles of the palate, pharynx, and tongue are most commonly affected. Jaw movement and facial expression are impaired somewhat later. Extraocular movements are rarely involved in the disease. Involvement of the hypoglossal nucleus is an early sign, resulting in a slurring dysarthria and weakness of tongue movements. As the disease progresses, the tongue, small and shriveled, lies immobile but fasciculating in the floor of the mouth. The palatal and pharyngeal musculature becomes weak, and aphagia, nasal speech, and regurgitation of liquids result. Later there is often wasting of the facial muscles, especially the orbicularis oris, which may be coupled with the signs of pseudobulbar palsy. Usually some signs of involvement of upper or lower motor neuron innervation of the trunk and limbs are evident in later stages of the disease.

Rarely, the disease may present as a progressive spastic paraparesis in which the evident signs of the disorder can be attributed to dysfunction of the upper motor neuron. This form of the disease has sometimes been called *primary lateral sclerosis.* At this stage it is not possible to make the diagnosis of amyotrophic lateral sclerosis, and full investigation, particularly to exclude spinal cord compression, is mandatory. If there is no evidence of denervation, it is probably not amyotrophic lateral sclerosis. Only the subsequent development—perhaps a number of years later—of fasciculations, of electromyographic evidence of denervation, or of the characteristic pattern on muscle biopsy permits the proper diagnosis to be made with certainty. By then, the disease is no longer confined to the upper motor neuron.

Despite the massive involvement of upper and lower neurons of the cortical spinal system, there are no adventitious movements, signs of cerebellar dysfunction, sensory disturbances, or involvement of sphincteric function. In a few patients dementia may occur.

Diagnosis. In making the diagnosis of amyotrophic lateral sclerosis the only laboratory test of value is electromyography. A sampling of affected muscles will reveal a reduction in the number of motor units active on contraction, as well as fasciculations and fibrillation potentials which represent the electrophysiologic consequence of denervation. Nerve conduction velocities are normal until advanced stages of the disease. There are no characteristic chemical changes in the blood or the cerebrospinal fluid. Serum creatine phosphokinase activity may be elevated. A muscle biopsy is useful in distinguishing between a neurogenic and amyopathic process. However, the histologic findings in muscle are nonspecific for any neurogenic atrophy.

Differential Diagnosis. Because of the bleak prognosis of amyotrophic lateral sclerosis, it is imperative that all efforts be made to establish with certainty the diagnosis of the disease. The disease can be diagnosed without difficulty when presenting in its most typical form as progressive, painless, diffuse muscle weakness with atrophy, fasciculations, and an associated spasticity, enhanced stretch reflexes, and extensor plantar responses. In the earliest stages, when presenting as a more localized disease, it is necessary to distinguish amyotrophic lateral sclerosis from other conditions which may produce lower motor neuron dysfunction, particularly when signs of corticospinal tract involvement are evident. When presenting as localized wasting of muscles, particularly in the hand, the disease must be distinguished from *lesions of peripheral nerves.* Mononeuritis or multiple mononeuritis will have a distribution characteristic of the involved nerve or nerves, reduced or absent deep tendon reflexes, and sensory abnormalities in the territory of the sensory innervation of the nerve. The metabolic polyneuritides, such as diabetic polyneuritis, tend to involve the feet before the hands, and sensory abnormalities are common. Conduction velocity in those peripheral nerves that can be tested is commonly abnormal in these conditions. Polyneuritis of the Guillain-Barré variety will have a more rapid onset; it is unassociated with fasciculations and is usually accompanied by elevation of the cerebrospinal fluid protein. *Compression of the brachial plexus by cervical rib* may present itself with weakness and wasting of intrinsic muscles of the hand. The relatively static and localized nature of the disease, the presence of pain, and confirmatory roentgenographic evidence of bony abnormalities will establish the diagnosis. Compression of cervical or lumbar *nerve roots* by osteoarthritic spurs or a herniated intravertebral disc may result in painless wasting, and in limb muscles is often associated with fasciculations. A differential diagnosis from amyotrophic lateral sclerosis in this condition may be further complicated by evidence of spasticity in the extremities, occurring as a result of extradural compression of the spinal cord by bony ridges of the vertebra. Pain, sensory abnormalities, a fixed location of the defect, and localized EMG abnormalities, as well as the characteristic roentgenographic changes of the vertebral column, may help to establish this diagnosis. However, in some cases the differential diagnosis may be extremely difficult and may only be resolved by following the evolution of the disease. *Epidural compression* of the spinal cord by tumor, by arachnoidal thickening secondary to syphilis or other infectious processes of the meninges, or in cervical spondylosis may lead to segmental weakness, atrophy, and long tract signs in the legs. Most such lesions cause pain, and the fixed nature of the lower motor neuron disorder and the evidence on myelography of a compressive lesion of the cord can usually establish the diagnosis. *Intramedullary* lesions of the spinal cord, including tumors or syringomyelia, usually interrupt segmental reflex arcs and also produce sensory signs. The sensory loss may occasionally be of the dissociated type with selective loss of pain sensation and preservation of touch and deep sensibilities over several segments. When presenting as *bulbar palsy,* myasthenia gravis can be diagnosed by appropriate pharmacologic tests. The syndrome of *primary lateral sclerosis* is most commonly due not to amyotrophic lateral sclerosis, but to multiple sclerosis or spinal cord compression. Investigation of such a case must include careful cerebrospinal fluid examination and myelography. The diagnosis of motor neuron disease becomes established only when signs of lower motor neuron involvement are unequivocally demonstrated. *Benign fasciculations* or myokymia is a troublesome but innocuous syndrome of migrating or static fasciculations of skeletal muscles. It may be localized, often to one eyelid, or it can be more generalized. It is common in younger patients. The distinguishing feature in the differential diagnosis in that weakness or wasting of muscles does not occur with benign fasciculations. However, the overt fasciculations may alarm both the patient and unwary physicians, and may sometimes lead to a misguided clinical diagnosis of amyotrophic lateral sclerosis. However, such patients lack EMG evidence of muscle denervation. Degeneration of the lower motor neuron may occasionally occur as a remote effect of cancer on the nervous system, and is discussed in Part X, Section Eighteen.

Course and Prognosis. Amyotrophic lateral sclerosis almost always has a dismal prognosis. In most cases death occurs within three to four years after the onset of symptoms. There are atypical cases in which the condition may appear to become arrested with little or no progression of symptoms over many years. In general the prognosis is worse when the initial symptoms are bulbar; survival in these cases seldom exceeds two years. Inability to handle secretions and weakness of the respiratory muscles are the predisposing causes of the usual terminal event, bronchopneumonia.

Treatment. The absence of any treatment that could influence the course of motor neuron disease only increases the physician's responsibility for the symptomatic care of these patients. In advanced cases, tracheostomy may be indicated to prevent the patient from drowning in his own secretions. Tube feeding or gastrostomy may prolong survival.

THE MARIANA FORM OF AMYOTROPHIC LATERAL SCLEROSIS

In the early 1950's it was discovered that the Chamorro Indians in the Mariana Islands had an unusually high incidence of a disease very similar in both its clinical and pathologic features to amyotrophic lateral sclerosis. Subsequent studies have demonstrated that this disease deviates from the classic form of amyotrophic lateral sclerosis (1) clinically, by its appearance at a generally younger age and its more prolonged course, and (2) pathologically, by the presence, in most cases, of neurofibrillary changes and granulovacuolar bodies, an uncommon finding in sporadic cases. Of particular interest is the fact that 10 per cent of patients with the Mariana form of amyotrophic lateral sclerosis show evidence, in the course of the disease, of either dementia or extrapyramidal types of motor dysfunction, particularly parkinsonism. At present it has not been conclusively determined whether the disease is truly genetic or is caused by environmental factors.

430. THE PROGRESSIVE MUSCULAR ATROPHIES

PROGRESSIVE MUSCULAR ATROPHY OF INFANCY
(Werdnig-Hoffmann Disease)

Definition. Infantile progressive muscular atrophy is a heredofamilial disorder of early onset and progressive course, characterized pathologically by degeneration of anterior horn cells and bulbar motor nuclei, and clinically by signs of disease of the lower motor neuron.

Etiology. The cause is unknown. However, the disorder is genetically determined and transmitted as an autosomal recessive trait.

Clinical Manifestations. The disease may begin in utero or in early or even late infancy. The features that draw attention to the disease are profound hypotonia and absence of volitional movements in an infant. An observant mother may note a lack of intrauterine movements, and soon after birth the infant, though bright and alert, is seen to lie immobile. The legs lie abducted and externally rotated at the hips and flexed at the knees. The arms hang limply at the sides. A few feeble movements may occur in the distal parts of the extremities. With handling the hypotonia is revealed. It may be so marked that when supported under the arms, the infant tends to slip through the examiner's hands. Painful stimuli are clearly appreciated, but there is little, if any, movement of withdrawal. The deep tendon and superficial reflexes are uniformly absent as a consequence of denervation. The limbs do not appear unduly thin, because the wasting of the muscles may be obscured by normal infant fat. Within a few months, weakness of the respiratory muscles leads to a characteristic retraction of the ribs on inspiration, and such accessory muscles as remain are brought into play. The disease spreads to involve the hypoglossal nuclei, and typical fasciculations of the tongue are observed. If life is prolonged beyond a year, contractures may occur, but death often supervenes before their advent. Less commonly, the paucity of movement is noted toward the end of the first year of life or even later when the child fails to stand or to talk at a normal age. In these cases the disease may be limited to the lower limbs, and the course may be slow. In general, the older the child at the onset of the disease, the more gradual its evolution. The natural rate of maturation of movement patterns may exceed the rate of destruction of anterior horn cells, so that apparent improvement occurs. Rarely, after development of paralysis, contractures, and wasting, the progress of the disease is apparently arrested for years. The occurrence of anterior horn cell disease during intrauterine life may result in *arthrogryposis multiplex congenita,* a clinical syndrome of multiple congenital contractures of the extremities that may also be caused by congenital muscular dystrophy, developmental defects of the spinal cord, intrauterine polyneuritis, or any disease which produces joint immobilization prenatally.

Differential Diagnosis. The diagnosis of the infantile form of progressive muscular atrophy is made on the basis of muscle biopsy and electromyographic findings, in addition to the clinical features of the disease. Generalized hypotonia may occur in a number of other disorders of infancy and lead to the syndrome of the "floppy infant." Malnutrition, chronic diseases, and lipidosis may all manifest hypotonia, which is also occasionally seen in retarded children. A small number of cases may be due to congenital myopathy, central core disease of muscle, or polyneuritis. In *benign congenital hypotonia,* unlike progressive muscular atrophy, there are spontaneous movements of the limb and reflexes that may be preserved. Recovery or improvement is the rule, and muscle biopsy shows no abnormality.

JUVENILE FORM OF PROGRESSIVE MUSCULAR ATROPHY
(Kugelberg-Welander Disease)

The juvenile form of progressive muscular atrophy may be inherited as an autosomal recessive or an autosomal dominant trait, and it has pathologic features similar to infantile spinal muscular atrophy. Indeed the presence of both diseases in members of a single family suggests that they may be variants on a continuum of motor neuron diseases.

Clinical Manifestations. The onset of the disease usually occurs in two peaks, in the preschool years or in adolescence. With an early onset there is no clear distinction from cases of infantile spinal muscular atrophy of late onset. When appearing in adolescence the clinical manifestations of the disease can be strikingly similar to those of the limb girdle form of muscular dystrophy. The initial complaint is usually clumsiness in walking. The gait is waddling and lordotic, and the child has difficulty rising from the lying position. There are weakness and wasting of the proximal muscles of the legs and pelvic girdle, with relative preservation of the distal musculature. Weakness of the arms usually does not appear until several years later and is also proximal. Muscles innervated by the cranial nerves are often spared, with the exception of the sternomastoid. Fasciculations, when evident, help to establish the diagnosis as neurogenic. Deep tendon reflexes are impaired or lost in proportion to the muscular atrophy. Mental and sensory functions are unimpaired. Skeletal abnormalities, such as scoliosis, a high arched palate, or pes cavus, are sometimes seen. The course is long, and a number of patients are still able to walk more than 20 years after the onset of the disease. Many patients enjoy a normal life span despite this ailment.

Diagnosis. The diagnosis of neurogenic atrophy rather than muscular dystrophy can be made on the basis of the clinical history and of electromyographic and muscle biopsy findings characteristic of disease of the lower motor neuron.

ADULT FORMS OF PROGRESSIVE MUSCULAR ATROPHY

A number of patients have been described with progressive muscular atrophy with onset in adult life. The disorder may occur spontaneously or can be inherited as an autosomal dominant, recessive, or sex-linked trait.

Clinical Manifestations. In the familial form there is some interfamilial variation in the disease. In general, the disorder presents as progressive weakness, which may begin either proximally or distally, or rarely with preponderant involvement of the scapuloperoneal muscle groups. Bulbar involvement is variable. Weakness, atrophy, fasciculations, reduction or disappearance of deep tendon reflexes in the affected muscles, and the preservation of sensation are characteristic in this disorder as in other progressive muscular atrophies. Unlike amyotrophic lateral sclerosis, the course is prolonged and the prognosis generally favorable.

Diagnosis. The diagnosis of progressive muscular atrophy in the adult is clearly established when it presents as a familial disorder with clinical, electromyographic, and biopsy evidence of lower motor neuron disease. It is distinguished from rare familial forms of amyotrophic lateral sclerosis by the absence of any evidence of corticospinal tract disease, specifically spasticity, enhanced deep tendon reflexes, and extensor plantar responses. Sporadic cases of progressive muscular atrophy occur, although uncommonly, and present difficult diagnostic distinctions from amyotrophic lateral sclerosis early in the disease. The absence of both upper motor neuron dysfunction and a prolonged course marks these cases as different from that of the typical patient with amyotrophic lateral sclerosis. However, until a cause is found, it will not be possible to know whether such cases represent a separate disease or cases of amyotrophic lateral sclerosis with an uncommonly prolonged course.

Bobowick, A. R., and Brody, J. A.: Epidemiology of motor-neurone diseases. N. Engl. J. Med., 288:1047, 1973.

Dubowitz, V.: Infantile muscular atrophy, a prospective study with particular reference to a slowly progressive variety. Brain, 87:707, 1964.

Fenichel, G. M.: The spinal muscular atrophies. *In* Norris, F. H., Jr., and Kurland, L. T. (eds.): Motor Neuron Diseases. New York, Grune & Stratton, 1969, p. 122.

Kugelberg, E., and Welander, L.: Heredofamilial juvenile muscular atrophy. Arch. Neurol. Psychiatry, 75:509, 1956.

Kurland, L. T., Choi, N. W., and Sayre, G. P.: Implications of incidence and geographic patterns on the classification of amyotrophic lateral sclerosis. *In* Norris, F. H., Jr., and Kurland, L. T. (eds.): Motor Neuron Diseases. New York, Grune & Stratton, 1969, p. 28.

THE SPINOCEREBELLAR DEGENERATIONS

431. INTRODUCTION

The spinocerebellar degenerations are a group of closely related neurologic disorders, usually heredofamilial, but not infrequently sporadic, which manifest themselves clinically as progressive disorders of gait, posture, equilibrium, and movement. Pathologically they are

The Spinocerebellar Degenerations*

A. Spinal forms
1. Friedreich's ataxia
2. Roussy-Levy syndrome
3. Hereditary spastic paraplegia
4. Bassen-Kornzweig syndrome

B. Spinocerebellar forms
1. Hereditary spastic ataxia
2. Subacute spinocerebellar degeneration (carcinogenic)

C. Cerebellar forms
1. Olivopontocerebellar atrophy
2. Cerebello-olivary degeneration
3. Parenchymatous cerebellar degeneration (nutritional-toxic)
4. Bassen-Kornzweig syndrome
5. Dyssynergia cerebellaris myoclonica

*Modified from Greenfield.

characterized by a simple neuronal atrophy, affecting primarily the cerebellar cortex and peduncles, the inferior olivary nuclei, and the long motor and proprioceptive tracts of the spinal cord. Degeneration of the cerebral cortex, basal ganglia, anterior horn cells, and optic and peripheral nerves is sometimes associated, producing appropriate symptoms. The rich variety of signs and symptoms in this heterogeneous collection of disorders – over 50 "syndromes" may be found in the literature – reflect differences in the regional patterns of distribution of lesions as well as in age of onset and course. Certain neuropathologic and clinical forms of spinocerebellar degeneration are found more commonly than others. These have been recognized as single disease entities. However, even in families with the purest of clinical syndromes, some members may have a clinical disorder typical of another symptom complex. Because of intrafamilial variations in the clinical and pathologic manifestations, the spinocerebellar degenerations have been viewed as a continuum of inherited diseases linking the degenerative disorders of peripheral nerve at one extreme to those of the cerebral cortex at the other. The cause of this group of diseases is unknown. In the absence of any identifiable biochemical defects it is not possible to state whether the varying clinical pictures are due to different biochemical abnormalities or just represent a different expression of a common metabolic defect. A useful clinicopathologic classification of the spinocerebellar degeneration, modified from Greenfield, is presented in the accompanying table.

432. FRIEDREICH'S ATAXIA

Definition. Friedreich's ataxia is a heredofamilial disease of early onset. It is characterized pathologically by degeneration of the lateral corticospinal tract and the posterior columns and the spinocerebellar pathways in the spinal cord, and clinically by progressive ataxia, nystagmus, absent or diminished deep tendon reflexes, and extensor plantar responses.

Etiology. The disease is transmitted as an autosomal recessive, and rarely as a dominant trait, with equal incidence in both sexes.

Pathology. The disease predominantly affects the posterior columns and peripheral nerves, where there is a selective degeneration of the large primary sensory neurons, the spinocerebellar tracts, and the lateral corticospinal tracts. Degeneration of the axis cylinders and their myelin sheaths with gliosis occurs. In the posterior columns, the degeneration is most obvious in the middle root zone. There may be associated loss of nerve cells in the dorsal root ganglia, and less commonly in the retinal ganglion cell layer. There are often diffuse fibrosis and focal degeneration of the myocardium.

Clinical Manifestations. Friedreich's ataxia usually presents in the first decade of life as an abnormality of gait. At first, stumbling and awkwardness are seen, but as the disease progresses, the gait becomes markedly ataxic, with superimposed truncal titubation. Unsteadiness remains the most prominent and disabling symptom throughout the course of the disease. Later, ataxia in the arms and a progressive ataxic disorder of speech become evident. Words are unevenly scanned and syllables explosively uttered. As the disease progresses, the patient becomes confined to a chair and is unable to feed himself, and speech becomes unintelligible. Examination discloses signs referable to the three primary neuronal systems involved. Degeneration of the spinocerebellar pathways results in a profound ataxia of all extremities. Until its final stages, the disease is most pronounced in the lower limbs. Impairment of function of the posterior columns leads to a loss of position sense, particularly in the lower extremities, which may further aggravate the ataxia. Corticospinal tract dysfunction is indicated by extensor plantar responses. Spasticity is not a feature of the disease. Weakness, as a consequence of combined cerebellar and pyramidal tract dysfunction, is evident. Deep tendon reflexes at the ankle are usually lost; those in the arms are diminished, but those of the knees may be retained for considerable periods. Choreic and pseudoathetoid movements are sometimes observed. Nystagmus is almost invariably present and is usually horizontal, but vertical nystagmus is occasionally seen. Involvement of other neuronal symptoms occurs rather commonly. Primary optic atrophy and, rarely, retinitis pigmentosa are sometimes seen in afflicted members of some families. Intellectual impairment is not uncommon and can be progressive. Loss of anterior horn cells in cervical and lumbar enlargements of the spinal cord may, in rare cases, lead to distal wasting of the extremities, suggesting a link to familial amyotrophic lateral sclerosis. Skeletal defects are commonly associated. Pes cavus with clawing of the toes may be evident before ataxia develops, and is thought by some to be caused by muscle imbalance. Kyphoscoliosis is usual as the disease develops. Cardiac abnormalities, including cardiac enlargement, murmurs, and congestive failure, are well recognized and may cause the patient's death. Bundle branch block, complete heart block, and inversion of the T wave are the common electrocardiographic abnormalities. Patients with this disease have an unusually high incidence of diabetes mellitus.

Course and Prognosis. The usual course of Friedreich's ataxia is steadily progressive. Although some patients with mild forms of the disease may live a normal life span, it is more common for the disease to run a progressive, downhill course. Total disability occurs within five to ten years in most cases, and death from intercurrent infection, cardiac failure, or, rarely, from complications of associated diabetes usually occur sometime in the third or early part of the fourth decade. There is no specific treatment, and therapy is primarily effected through symptomatic treatment of the cardiac or metabolic abnormalities. However, in patients with very slowly evolving disease, physical therapy may offer useful training to help the patient compensate for his progressive motor impairment.

Laboratory tests are of little specific value in establishing the diagnosis. The cerebrospinal fluid, on examination, is usually normal. Electromyography may demonstrate signs of denervation in patients in whom anterior horn cell disease is evident. Nerve conduction velocity may be impaired. The differential diagnosis between Friedreich's ataxia and multiple sclerosis must be made in patients with a sporadic form of the disease characterized by late onset and minimal skeletal abnormalities. The principal features by which the two diseases may be distinguished are the progressive course and the absence of deep tendon reflexes in Friedreich's ataxia.

433. THE ROUSSY-LEVY SYNDROME (Hereditary Areflexic Dystaxia, Hereditary Ataxia with Muscular Atrophy)

This disease is transmitted as an autosomal dominant trait. It is characterized by the development in childhood of an unsteadiness of station and gait, associated with a general loss of deep tendon reflexes, club foot, and kyphoscoliosis. A static tremor of the hands may be a prominent sign. There is occasionally some evidence of wasting of muscles of the legs and small muscles of the hand. Nerve conduction velocities may be reduced. It differs from Friedreich's ataxia in that nystagmus and dysarthria are absent, sensation is usually preserved, and there is a tendency for this syndrome to remain static or evolve slowly throughout life. However, since this particular combination of symptoms has been reported in relatives of patients with pure forms of both Friedreich's ataxia and peroneal muscular atrophy, some have considered the disease an intermediate between these two disorders.

434. HEREDITARY SPASTIC PARAPLEGIA

Definition. This is a rare, genetically determined disease transmitted as an autosomal dominant, and, less commonly, as an autosomal recessive or sex-linked recessive trait. It is characterized pathologically by degeneration in the spinal cord of the corticospinal tracts and dorsal columns, and occasionally of other spinal tracts as well, and clinically by the onset in early life of progressive spasticity.

Clinical Manifestations. The disease is more common in males than in females. Its onset is gradual and usually occurs in the first decade of life, but may occur later. The disease is characterized by a progressive bilateral and symmetrical spastic impairment of gait. Weakness of dorsiflexion of the feet results in the toes being dragged along the ground in a scissor gait. The patient has difficulty in climbing stairs because of weakness and rigidity of hip flexors. There is evident spasticity in extensor muscles with increased deep tendon reflexes and extensor plantar responses. Sensory disturbances are absent. Involvement of the bladder, upper limb, and bulbar musculature, when present, occurs late. The course may extend over many decades. Rarely, families have been described in which affected members, although presenting in early life with spastic paraplegia, have later developed wasting of the small muscles of the hand with lesser involvement of the peripheral musculature of the legs. Additionally such subjects usually have mild sensory loss of the modalities of touch-pressure, vibration, and joint position. The characteristics of the EMG in such patients suggest an axonal degenerative process. The distribution of this wasting, so suggestive of that of peroneal muscular atrophy, and the occasional association of pes cavus, scoliosis, and nystagmus indicate the close tie of this syndrome to the other spinal cerebellar degenerations. In the sporadic case the disease must be distinguished from multiple sclerosis and progressive muscular atrophy.

435. HEREDITARY SPASTIC ATAXIA (Sanger-Brown's and Marie's Ataxia)

Definition. Hereditary spastic ataxia, a usually heredofamilial disease, is characterized pathologically by atrophy of the cerebellum, cell loss in the dentate and olivary nuclei, and degeneration of the spinocerebellar tracts, and clinically by progressive ataxia associated with spasticity.

Clinical Features. This is an uncommon form of spinocerebellar degeneration. It is usually hereditary with several clinical and pathologic variants. Clinically and pathologically, these variants represent an intermediate between Friedreich's ataxia, which is principally spinal, and olivopontocerebellar degeneration, primarily a cerebellar disease. The age of onset varies according to the pedigree, and often may not occur until the fifth and sixth decades of life. The disease consists of a mixture of ataxia and spasticity. The onset is most usually characterized by ataxia of gait, which may progress to incoordination of the upper extremities. There may be associated optic atrophy, ptosis, diplopia, and extraocular muscle palsies. Deep tendon reflexes are preserved and are often hyperactive, and ankle clonus and extensor plantar responses are frequently seen. In some patients spasticity may be the prominent finding. Unlike Friedreich's ataxia, nystagmus and abnormalities of the skeleton are usually absent. Dementia may sometimes be prominent. Phenotypic variation of the disease within a family may be striking.

Course and Prognosis. The course, although progressive, is often slow so that impairment may be delayed over many years. There is no specific therapy.

436. OLIVOPONTOCEREBRAL ATROPHY

This disorder, first described by Déjérine and Thomas in 1900, is characterized by the onset in late life of a progressive disorder of cerebellar function. The disease, when hereditary, is inherited as either an autosomal dominant or recessive trait. It is often sporadic.

Pathology. There is loss of the Purkinje cell layer, which may be limited to the lateral lobes of the cerebellum or may involve the vermis only slightly. In addition, there is atrophy of the middle cerebellar peduncle and pontine nuclei. In a number of cases loss of pigmented cells in the substantia nigra has been seen. In rare cases, there is degeneration of the corticospinal and spinocerebellar pathways in the spinal cord and of ganglion cells in the retina.

Clinical Manifestations. The clinical syndrome is characterized by the development in late middle life of slowly progressive cerebellar deficiency. This includes a cerebellar ataxia of trunk and limbs, dysmetria, action tremor, impairment of rapid rhythmic alternating movements, dysarthria, and sometimes a static tremor of the head and trunk. Nystagmus is usually absent. Volitional movements are usually unimpaired, and the deep tendon reflexes are usually normal, although loss of ankle jerks and an occasional extensor plantar response are sometimes seen. A number of patients may display signs of an extrapyramidal nature, including rigidity, bradykinesia, and a parkinsonian tremor. A progressive dementia may also be associated. Infrequently, retinal degeneration leads to blindness. The diagnosis is made clinically, laboratory findings usually being normal. The course of the disease is progressive, incapacitation usually occurring within five to ten years after the onset of clinical signs. There is no specific therapy.

437. CEREBELLO-OLIVARY DEGENERATION
(Holmes Type of Hereditary Ataxia, Late Corticocerebellar Atrophy)

Cerebello-olivary degeneration is a rare form of spinocerebellar degeneration, characterized pathologically by atrophy of the cerebellum and shrinkage of the medulla and pons, and histologically by the almost complete disappearance of Purkinje cells diffusely throughout the cerebellum, with atrophy of the inferior and accessory olivary nuclei. The disorder is usually familial and inherited as an autosomal dominant trait. It is characterized by the onset, in early middle life or even later, of a progressive cerebellar syndrome, with gait ataxia, action tremor, dysmetria, dysarthria, and static tremor of the trunk and head. Deep tendon reflexes are normal, and the plantar responses are flexor. Nystagmus may occur late in the course of the disease. There are no visual, sensory, or skeletal disturbances. The diagnosis is made clinically. There is no specific therapy.

438. BASSEN-KORNZWEIG SYNDROME
(Acanthocytosis, Abetalipoproteinemia)

In 1950, Bassen and Kornzweig described a heredofamilial disease inherited as a recessive trait, in which a progressive ataxic disturbance of gait in childhood (similar in its clinical symptoms to Friedreich's ataxia) was associated with thorny erythrocytes (acanthocytes) and a marked diminution in the serum β-lipoproteins. These children usually first develop celiac disease with fatty stools as the presenting symptom. Somewhat later the patient becomes progressively more unsteady. The neurologic abnormalities include kyphoscoliosis, cerebellar ataxia, and distal sensory loss, involving especially dorsal column functions. Bilateral ptosis, paresis of extraocular muscles, and retinitis pigmentosa have been reported. The relationship among the abnormal erythrocytes, the absence of β-lipoprotein, and the neurologic syndrome remains to be determined. This disorder is also discussed in Ch. 817 and in Part XIV, Section Three.

439. PARENCHYMATOUS CEREBELLAR DEGENERATION

Degeneration of cerebellar neurons, particularly of the Purkinje cells, may result in an acute, subacute, or chronic cerebellar syndrome. The disease usually occurs in late middle life, and is sporadic. Pathologically, there is atrophy of the cerebellum which can be demonstrated microscopically to be due to disappearance of Purkinje cells in atrophic areas, to the reduction of the granular and molecular cells, and to some reduction of the white matter. No changes in the brainstem nuclei are seen. The etiology of the syndrome is multiple, the most common cause being prolonged and excessive intake of alcohol. This form of cerebellar degeneration occurs in chronic alcoholics, and its onset is usually subacute. Maximal disability is reached over weeks or months, and if the patient is abstinent the disorder may stabilize. The usual symptom is unsteadiness, which on examination may be demonstrated to be due to severe cerebellar impairment of the lower extremities. The gait is slow and lurching, and on heel-knee-shin tests there is an evident ataxia of the legs. The arms are usually mildly affected, if at all, and nystagmus and dysarthria are usually mild or absent. Pure cerebellar degeneration may sometimes occur in association with carcinoma of ovary or lung. Heat strokes and intoxication with some heavy metals, particularly with organic mercuric compounds and lead, may also result in isolated degeneration of the cerebellum.

440. DYSSYNERGIA CEREBELLARIS MYOCLONICA
(Familial Myoclonus and Ataxia)

This rare disease of children and young adults is both sporadic and familial and is characterized by myoclonic jerks, epilepsy, and progressive cerebellar ataxia. Postmortem examination has shown degeneration of the dorsal columns and atrophy of the dentate nucleus and the superior cerebellar peduncle. When familial, the inheritance appears to be by an autosomal dominant with incomplete penetrance.

Bell, J.: Hereditary ataxia and spastic paraplegia. Treasury of Human Inheritance. Vol. IV, Part 3. London, Cambridge University Press, 1939.
Boyer, S. H., Chisholm, A. W., and McKusick, V. A.: Cardiac aspects of Friedreich's ataxia. Circulation, 25:493, 1962.

Gach, J. V., Adriange, M., and Franck, G.: Hypertrophic obstructive cardiomyopathy and Friedreich's ataxia. Am. J. Cardiol., 27:436, 1971.
Gilbert, G. J., McEntee, W. J., and Glaser, G. H.: Familial myoclonus and ataxia. Neurology, 13:365, 1963.
Greenfield, J. G.: The Spino-cerebellar Degenerations. Springfield, Ill., Charles C Thomas, 1954.
Konigsmark, B. W., and Weiner, L. P.: The olivopontocerebellar atrophies: A review. Medicine, 49:227, 1970.
Oelschlager, R., White, H. N., and Schimke, R. N.: Roussy-Levy syndrome. Acta Neurol. Scand., 47:80, 1971.
Podolsky, S., and Sheremata, W. A.: Insulin-dependent diabetes mellitus and Friedreich's ataxia in siblings. Metabolism, 19:555, 1970.
Schwartz, J. F., Rowland, L. P., Eder, H., Marks, P. A., Osserman, E. F., Hirschberg, E., and Anderson, H.: Bassen-Kornzweig syndrome: deficiency of serum β-lipoprotein. Arch. Neurol., 8:438, 1963.
Sperling, M. A., Hengslenberg, F., Kunis, E., Kenny, F. M., and Drash, A. L.: A-betalipoproteinemia: Metabolic, endocrine and electron-microscopic investigations. Pediatrics, 48:91, 1971.
Victor, M., Adams, R. D., and Mancall, E. L.: A restricted form of cerebellar cortical degeneration occurring in alcoholic patients. Arch. Neurol., 1:579, 1959.

441. SYRINGOMYELIA

Definition. Syringomyelia is a chronic disease of the spinal cord, characterized pathologically by cavitation of the spinal cord with gliosis and clinically by a mixture of segmental and suprasegmental motor and sensory abnormalities and trophic disturbances. When a syrinx occurs in the brainstem, the disease is called *syringobulbia.*

Etiology. The cause of syringomyelia is unknown. Several theories have been proposed to explain its pathogenesis, but none are entirely satisfactory. Because of the common association of syringomyelia with other congenital abnormalities of the neuraxis and skeleton, the most popular hypotheses have attributed the disease to developmental anomalies. One hypothesis has suggested that the disease is due to abnormal closure of the neural tube; another, that it results from the persistence of ependymal cell rests which later proliferate and cavitate. A third, based on the frequent association of intramedullary vascular malformations, vascular neoplasms, and gliomas with syrinxes, is that focal ischemia within the spinal cord resulting from abnormalities of the microcirculation is pathogenic. Finally, a theory first elaborated by Gardner and since modified by others has proposed that the cavitation is hydrodynamic in origin and is caused by distention of the central canal by ventricular fluid displaced caudally from the fourth ventricle as a consequence of atresia of the foramina of Luschka and Magendie.

Pathology. On gross inspection the spinal cord may appear normal, enlarged, or flattened in its anteroposterior axis, depending upon the size and state of the syrinx. The syrinx itself, when intact, is filled with clear, slightly yellow serous fluid. The walls of the cavity are irregular, and consist of degenerated neural and neuroglial elements. The cavity is usually surrounded by gliosis, composed for the most part of glial fibers. Abnormal blood vessels with hyalinized walls may sometimes be seen. There is usually secondary degeneration and demyelination of long ascending and descending tracts of the spinal cord and brainstem as a result of extension of the syrinx. The syrinx most commonly runs over several segments in the cervical cord. It may extend into thoracic segments for a varying distance and may even terminate at lumbar levels. The cavity often begins in the gray matter adjacent to the central canal, and tends, as it enlarges, to interrupt the decussating fibers and destroy neurons in the dorsal and ventral horns. Within the thoracic cord, the cavity is commonly seen in the dorsal horns, and may affect the intermediolateral cell column, producing autonomic deficiencies. Syrinxes of the lumbar cord are uncommon. *Syringobulbia* is associated with cavitation that is usually slitlike and often in communication with the fourth ventricle. Bulbar syrinxes commonly involve several cranial nerve nuclei, notably the descending root of the trigeminal nerve, and the solitary, ambiguous, and hypoglossal nuclei. They also may involve the medial longitudinal fasciculus, the pyramidal tract, and the medial lemniscus. Extensions into the pons are rare. A *secondary syrinx* consisting of central cavitation of the spinal cord and sometimes associated with gliosis may occur as a result of chronic arachnoiditis, spinal tuberculosis, or meningeal or vascular syphilis. It may also be found after trauma of the spinal cord, the cavitation gradually extending many cord segments above or below the lesion and leading, clinically, to a post-traumatic myelopathy.

Clinical Manifestations. The clinical manifestations of syringomyelia depend upon the localization and size of the lesion. The disease most commonly presents in the second decade, but sometimes the onset may be delayed until the patient is in his sixties or seventies. In its most usual form the signs and symptoms of the disease are referable to a *syrinx in the cervical cord.* The presenting symptoms are often wasting and weakness in the muscles of the upper extremity, associated with mild burning dysesthesias and loss of pain sensation distally in the arms. There are sometimes complaints of weakness of the legs, and bowel and bladder symptoms. On examination the patient may have Horner's syndrome as a consequence of interruption of the sympathetic pathways in the spinal cord. Nystagmus resulting from damage to the spinal projections of the medial longitudinal fasciculus may also be seen. Muscle weakness in the upper extremity is usually associated with obvious atrophy, and frequently involves the small muscles of the hand. If the syrinx has extended into the corticospinal tract, weakness and spasticity in the lower extremities are evident. At the level of the lesion, the deep tendon reflexes may be absent or reduced. Because of the interruption of the second order afferent fibers arising from cells in the dorsal horn and crossing to the contralateral ventrolateral spinothalamic tracts, there may be a dissociated segmental type of sensory loss, often in a shawl- or capelike distribution over the shoulders, upper trunk, and arms. In this zone, light touch, vibration, and deep sensibility are preserved with a striking absence of pain and temperature sensation. When the lesion has extended to include the dorsal columns or the spinothalamic pathways, there are appropriate sensory abnormalities in the trunk and lower extremities. Trophic changes, particularly involving the hands, are common. Their pathogenesis is not known, but may in part be related to the absence of pain sensation and to the interruption of vasomotor outflow to the limb. Unfelt burns from cigarettes or light bulbs may lead to tissue destruction and severe scarring. Cyanosis, hyperkeratosis, and thickening of subcutaneous tissues may result in puffy, swollen fingers. True hypertrophy of body parts may occur. Traumatic osteoarthropathy (Charcot's joint) is common. Sometimes the distal phalanges may atrophy and be lost painlessly, a condition known as Morvan's disease. The common clinical features of *lumbosacral syrinxes* are atrophic weakness of the lower limbs, loss of deep tendon reflexes, dissociated anesthesia, and fecal and urinary incontinence. If the lesion lies high in the lumbar cord, it may be associated with an extensor plantar response. Trophic changes of the lower extremity, particularly club foot deformities, are common. In *syringobulbia* the syrinx formation in the medulla may be unassociated with the syrinx in the cervical cord. Common findings in this disorder are atrophy of the tongue, nystagmus, impairment of pain and temperature sensation on one side of the face, dysphonia, and respiratory stridor. In addition, sensory and spastic motor abnormalities of the extremities may be seen.

There are many associated findings in syringomyelia. Papilledema may result from an associated hydrocephalus. Skeletal abnormalities are common and include cervical rib, spina bifida, premature closures of the skull, Klippel-Feil syndrome, basilar impression, and kyphoscoliosis. The association of syringomyelia with intramedullary gliomas or vascular tumors has long been recognized.

Diagnosis. The diagnosis may often be made clinically by the observation of muscular atrophy and weakness, dissociated sensory loss, trophic changes, and long tract signs attributable to a lesion in the cervical cord. The laboratory findings in this disorder are nonspecific. The cerebrospinal fluid may be under increased pressure as a result of an associated hydrocephalus. A mild pleocytosis or increased protein in the cerebrospinal fluid may sometimes be seen. Elevated cerebrospinal fluid protein is more commonly associated with intramedullary gliomas or cysts. Electromyography may reveal evidence of denervation in affected muscles. Roentgenographic evidence of bony deformities may be helpful. Pantopaque x-ray myelography may sometimes give evidence of a swollen syrinx. Gas myelography has proved useful in distinguishing a syrinx from an intramedullary cyst.

Differential Diagnosis. Syringomyelia must be differentiated from tumors of the spinal cord or cervical ribs, other bony anomalies, amyotrophic lateral sclerosis, multiple sclerosis, and tabes dorsalis. Intramedullary tumors of the cord, which produce comparable symptomatology because of a similar location, and extramedullary tumors, which can sometimes simulate an intramedullary lesion by compressing the anterior spinal artery, can often be differentiated from syringomyelia by myelography. Cervical rib may be identified roentgenographically, although the fact that this abnormality may be associated with a syrinx sometimes complicates the differential diagnosis. Amyotrophic lateral sclerosis is never associated with sensory abnormalities. Multiple sclerosis can be differentiated by its remitting course and by the fact that muscular wasting, trophic changes, and dissociated sensory abnormalities are uncommon. Tabes dorsalis can be differentiated by the serology and by a different pattern of sensory loss.

Course and Prognosis. The course of syringomyelia is variable, but is usually protracted over many years. In some patients there may be gradual deterioration; in others, changes may occur in a stepwise fashion. In some patients, after an initial attack, the disease may appear to have become arrested. In syringobulbia, death from respiratory paralysis may sometimes occur.

Treatment. At present there is no satisfactory treatment for syringomyelia. Some surgeons recommend decompression of the syrinx, but the therapeutic results have been at best doubtful.

Barnett, H. J. M., Botterell, E. H., Jousse, A. T., and Wynn-Jones, M.: Progressive myelopathy as a sequel to traumatic paraplegia. Brain, 89:159, 1966.

Ellertson, A. B.: Semiologic diagnosis of syringomyelia related to roentgenologic findings. Acta Neurol. Scand., 45:385, 1969.

Gardner, W. J.: Hydrodynamic mechanism of syringomyelia: its relationship to myelocele. J. Neurol. Neurosurg. Psychiatry, 28:247, 1965.

McIlroy, W. J., and Richardson, J. C.: Syringomyelia. A clinical review of 75 cases. Can. Med. Assoc. J., 93:731, 1965.

Netsky, M. G.: Syringomyelia. A clinicopathological study. Arch. Neurol., 70:741, 1953.

Williams, B., and Weller, R. O.: Syringomyelin produced by intramedullary fluid injection in dogs. J. Neurol. Neurosurg. Psychiatry, 36:467, 1973.

NEUROCUTANEOUS SYNDROMES

442. MULTIPLE NEUROFIBROMATOSIS (Von Recklinghausen's Disease)

Multiple neurofibromatosis is a congenital defect of the ectoderm, usually heredofamilial, characterized by cutaneous pigmentation and multiple tumors of the spinal and cranial nerves and skin. The cutaneous and osseous manifestations of the disease are described in Ch. 921. Tumors of the peripheral nerve are most characteristic, and occur as nodules along the course of the nerve or nerve roots, usually without interfering with nerve conduction. Occasionally diffuse involvement of the nerve trunk in its distal branches produces a plexiform neuroma which, when it occurs, is particularly common in the cervical and occipital regions. Other tumors of the nervous system, particularly meningiomas and gliomas, are often associated. Neurofibromas may undergo sarcomatous degeneration. The signs and symptoms of neurofibromatosis depend upon the localization and rate of growth of the tumors. When lying within the spinal canal, they may produce a syndrome of spinal cord compression. Cranial nerve tumors are often found. When tumors of the eighth nerve are bilateral, they are almost invariably a manifestation of neurofibromatosis, and optic nerve gliomas are frequently associated with that disease. Tumors of other cranial nerves may occur, particularly the trigeminal vagus, and hypoglossal.

443. TUBEROUS SCLEROSIS (Epiloia, Bourneville's Disease)

Definition. Tuberous sclerosis is a congenital disease characterized by the presence of congenital tumors and malformations of the brain, skin, and viscera, and clinically by epilepsy and mental retardation.

Etiology. The disease is both sporadic and heredofamilial and is probably inherited through a single dominant trait.

Pathology. The brain, although usually normal in size, is studded by many small nodules or tubers. These are firm, and occasionally calcified. Sometimes they distort the normal configuration of gyri and may project into the cerebral ventricles, where they present as characteristic "candle gutterings." Microscopically, the tubers are composed of nests of glial fibers and abnormal ganglion cells. They may undergo gliomatous degeneration or develop into meningiomas. Glial tumors of the retina (phakomas) and gliomatous tumors of the nerve head and optic tract are also found in some cases. Adenoma sebaceum, the characteristic skin lesion, is a small firm tubercle often found over the nose and cheeks. They are rarely present at birth, but usually develop during the first decade toward puberty. Although tending to cluster over the bridge of the nose and the cheeks, they may be found elsewhere over the head. In addition, a variety of other polyps, subcutaneous nodules, pigmented warts, and café-au-lait spots similar to those of von Recklinghausen's disease are found. Hypopigmented macules may be the earliest cutaneous manifestations. Mesodermal tumors of the kidney, liver, pancreas, lung, and thyroid gland are seen, along with rhabdomyoma of the heart.

Clinical Manifestations. The presenting symptom of this disease is usually epilepsy, which appears in the first few years of life. The attacks may present as minor or focal seizures, but in time generally progress to major motor convulsions. Mental retardation is usually noticed during the early years of life and may vary in degree, differing in no way from mental retardation from any other cause. Some patients, however, may have normal I.Q.'s. The adenoma sebaceum usually appears toward the end of the second or the beginning of the third year of life as small, lightly pigmented, shiny papules that appear vascular. They may first appear on the malar areas, but as they proliferate they become confluent and more deeply pigmented, and extend in a butterfly distribution over the nose and cheeks. The retinal lesions are flat, white or gray, round or oval areas, and are present in almost half the patients. Subungual fibromas on the toes or fingers may be seen but most commonly not until after puberty. Patients with mild or partial forms of the disease are not uncommon.

Diagnosis. The clinical triad of seizures, mental retardation, and adenoma sebaceum will establish the diagnosis. Roentgenographic examination of the skull may often reveal scattered calcifications in areas of increased or decreased density in the skull vault. Pneumoencephalography may sometimes demonstrate the tubers projecting into the ventricles.

Course and Prognosis. The disease is usually progressive. The outlook in individual cases, however, depends on the severity of the mental impairment and the frequency and intensity of seizures. It must be emphasized that the three cardinal features of the disease may occur singly or in any combination with varying degrees of severity in members of the same family. Often the defects are progressive, and death occurs in the second decade of life. The development of gliomatous changes in the brain may also shorten the course of the disease, as may progressive pulmonary insufficiency from pulmonary tumors. Sudden death from rhabdomyoma of the heart may occur.

Treatment. The treatment is the same as that for epilepsy with appropriate measures for the mental retardation. Institutionalization is sometimes indicated.

444. STURGE-WEBER-DIMITRI DISEASE (Encephalotrigeminal Angiomatosis)

The Sturge-Weber-Dimitri disease is characterized by a unilateral, port-wine, facial nevus usually confined to the distribution of the first and occasionally the other divisions of the trigeminal nerve, together with a capillary hemangioma of the ipsilateral cerebral cortex. The full clinical picture consists of the nevus, a contralateral hemiparesis, smallness of the affected limbs, epilepsy—often consisting of jacksonian seizures beginning in the paralyzed limbs—ipsilateral exophthalmos, angiomas of the retina, and some degree of mental retardation. Incomplete manifestations of the disease may be observed, and there is great variability in the severity of the retardation, the frequency of the seizures, the profoundness of the hemiplegia, and the extent of the cutaneous abnormalities. Extensive linear calcification of the cortex often occurs in parallel lines, and, when visible roentgenographically, may help to establish the diagnosis. The films may also show hemiatrophy of the skull reflecting the maldevelopment of the underlying cerebral hemisphere. The cause of the disease is unknown, and there is no evidence of hereditary transmission. The diagnosis can be made clinically without difficulty.

445. VON HIPPEL–LINDAU DISEASE

This is a rare, usually heredofamilial disease, consisting of a hemangioblastoma of the brain (usually in cerebellum, but occasionally elsewhere) in association with an angioma of the retina and, less commonly, cysts of the pancreas, kidneys, and other viscera and a pheochromocytoma. The disease is inherited as an autosomal dominant trait. Its onset usually occurs in the third decade of life with symptoms referable to the retinal or cerebral tumors. The angioma of the retina (von Hippel) is usually peripheral, and is supplied by a large, entering artery and drained by a single vein. Hemorrhages, exudates, and papilledema may occur in association with the lesion. The hemangioblastoma is usually a solitary cystic vascular tumor. It is most commonly localized to the cerebellum, but may occur in the medulla, brainstem, or spinal cord. The hemangioblastoma of the cerebellum presents with the usual signs of cerebellar deficiency. The protein content of the cerebrospinal fluid tends to be unusually high, and a polycythemia of unknown cause is commonly associated. However, it should be emphasized that the majority of cases of proved cerebellar hemangioblastoma present no evidence of von Hippel–Lindau disease. The diagnosis is established in patients with a positive family history by the onset of retinal or brainstem symptoms. Diagnosis of a tumor in the brainstem is made by the usual roentgenographic methods of pneumoencephalography or angiography. Early recognition of cerebellar tumors in afflicted members of the family is important, for early surgical resection may effect a cure.

446. ATAXIA TELANGIECTASIA (Louis-Bar Syndrome)

Ataxia telangiectasia is a heredofamilial disease manifested by ocular and cutaneous telangiectasia, a progressive cerebellar ataxia, and various immunodeficiencies which are discussed in Ch. 69. This rare disease is linked clinically and pathologically with both the neurocutaneous syndromes and the hereditary ataxias.

The neuropathologic changes of the disease consist of widespread atrophy of the cerebellar cortex, with loss of Purkinje cells and thinning of the internal granular layer. There is chronic neuronal degeneration of the dentate and inferior olivary nuclei, as well as demyelination affecting particularly the posterior columns of the spinal cord.

The onset of the disease is usually marked by the appearance in infancy of the cerebellar ataxia first noted as the child begins to walk. The gait is reeling and wide based. The loss of equilibrium persists, and is later aggravated by the onset of limb ataxia. At about the age of four, telangiectasia appears, first being noted in the bulbar conjunctiva and then spreading over the malar surfaces in a butterfly distribution, on the ears, the palate, along the neck, and in the antecubital and popliteal fossae. Occasionally, café-au-lait spots are seen. Patients also suffer from sinusitis and frequent pulmonary infections. As the disease progresses, other neurologic signs, including opsoclonus, choreoathetoid movements, and, rarely, myoclonic jerks, may be observed. The disease is slowly progressive, and patients rarely live beyond the age of 25.

Aguliar, M. J., Kamoshita, S., Landing, B. H., Boder, E., and Sedgwick, R. P.: Pathological changes in ataxia-telangiectasia. J. Neuropathol. Exp. Neurol., 27:659, 1968.

Alexander, G. L.: Sturge-Weber syndrome. *In* Vinken, P. J., and Bruyn, G. W. (eds.): The Phakomatoses. New York, American Elsevier Publishing Company, 1972, pp. 223–240.

Bundey, S., and Evans, K.: Tuberous sclerosis: A genetic study. J. Neurol. Neurosurg. Psychiatry, 32:591, 1969.

Canale, D. J., and Bebin, J.: Von Recklinghausen's disease of the nervous system. *In* Vinken, P. J., and Bruyn, G. W. (eds.): The Phakomatoses. New York, American Elsevier Publishing Company, 1972, pp. 132–162.

Donegani, G., Grattarola, F. R., and Wildi, E.: Tuberous sclerosis. *In* Vinken, P. J., and Bruyn, G. W. (eds.): The Phakomatoses. New York, American Elsevier Publishing Company, 1972, pp. 340–389.

Dwyer, J. M., Hickie, J. B., and Garvan, J.: Pulmonary tuberous sclerosis. Quart. J. Med. (N.S.), 40:115, 1971.

Grossman, M., and Melmon, K. L.: Von Hippel–Lindau disease. Von Recklinghausen's disease of the nervous system. *In* Vinken, P. J., and Bruyn, G. W. (eds.): The Phakomatoses. New York, American Elsevier Publishing Company, 1972, pp. 241–259.

McFarlin, D. E., Strober, W., and Waldmann, T. A.: Ataxia-telangiectasia. Medicine, 51:581, 1972.

Section Twenty-One. MECHANICAL LESIONS OF THE NERVE ROOTS AND SPINAL CORD

Albert J. Aguayo

447. SYMPTOMS OF NERVE ROOT AND SPINAL CORD COMPRESSION

Certain diseases result in compression of the nerve roots or spinal cord within the spinal canal. In general the symptoms and signs that accompany such intraspinal lesions may be classified into two groups: radicular syndromes caused by spinal root injury, and myelopathy caused by compression of the spinal cord; but a combination of both syndromes is also common.

RADICULAR SYNDROMES

Compression of nerve roots causes pain, paresthesia, sensory loss, weakness, atrophy, and reflex changes which are confined to a radicular anatomic distribution. A single nerve root can be compressed, as in most cases of intervertebral disc protrusion, but several roots are often involved in arachnoiditis or when there is neoplastic invasion of the spinal canal.

The pain caused by root compression is experienced in the overlying spine, deep in certain muscles, or along the cutaneous distribution of the injured root *(dermatome)*. This pain is often influenced by movement and increases with strain. Radicular pain is usually unilateral, but some intraspinal lesions, by compressing roots bilaterally, can give rise to pain in both limbs or on both sides of the thorax or abdomen. The most common sensory symptoms are hypesthesia and paresthesia, both of which may be described by patients as numbness. These sensory symptoms are usually accompanied by sensory impairment in the distribution of the compressed root or roots. Because of the more extensive overlapping of adjacent innervation for touch, this sensory loss is better outlined by testing responses to pinprick than to light touch.

Muscles supplied by roots that originate from the same spinal cord segment constitute a *myotome.* Because most muscles are supplied from more than one segmental level, compression of a single root causes different degrees of weakness and atrophy in different muscles. The effects of a root lesion on a muscle ultimately depend on the importance of the innervation provided by the injured root; weakness of certain muscles within a particular myotome may be difficult to elicit, whereas other muscles may be severely affected. For example, although fibers from the L5 root innervate approximately 30 different muscles in the lower limb, severe changes after

TABLE 1. Clinical Findings in the Four Most Common Radicular Syndromes

Root	Usual Distribution of Pain	Principally Affected Muscles	Sensory Loss	Muscle Stretch Reflexes Affected
C6	Neck, parascapular, lateral aspect of arm and forearm	Biceps, brachioradialis, wrist extensors and flexors	Radial border of forearm, thumb	Biceps and/or brachioradialis may be diminished
C7	Neck, parascapular, posterolateral arm, dorsum of forearm	Triceps, wrist, finger flexors and extensors	Dorsum of forearm; index and middle fingers	Triceps
L5	Low back, buttock, lateral thigh, dorsum of foot	Dorsiflexors of foot and toes	Anterolateral aspect of lower leg, dorsum of foot	Usually none, but ankle jerk may be diminished
S1	Low back, buttock, posterior thigh	Calf muscles, plantar flexors	Outer edge of foot and sole	Ankle jerk

compression of this root may be clearly apparent in only two: the extensor hallucis longus and extensor digitorum brevis muscles.

Muscle stretch reflexes are diminished or absent when reflex arcs are interrupted by root compression. At the levels at which they can be clinically tested, reflex changes have an important localizing value (Table 1).

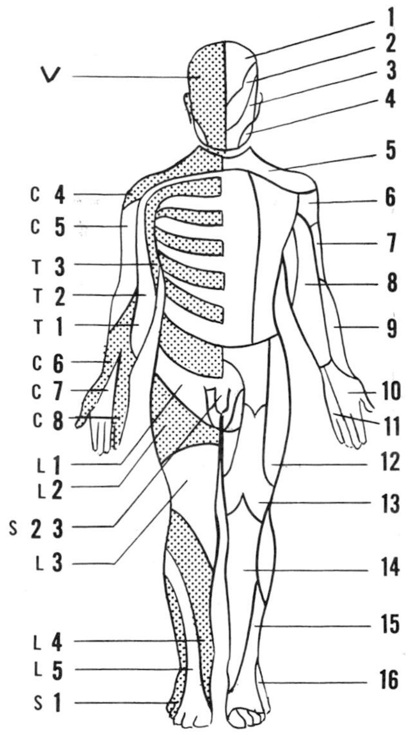

Schematic representation of dermatomes and peripheral nerve sensory areas:

1. Trigeminal 1st division
2. Trigeminal 2nd division
3. Trigeminal 3rd division
4. Greater auricular nerve
5. Branches from cervical plexus
6. Axillary nerve
7. Radial nerve
8. Medial brachial cutaneous nerve
9. Musculocutaneous nerve
10. Median nerve
11. Ulnar nerve
12. Lateral femoral cutaneous nerve
13. Femoral nerve
14. Saphenous nerve
15. Peroneal nerve
16. Sural nerve

Differentiation between symptoms caused by nerve root and peripheral nerve lesions must follow anatomic guides (see figure and Table 2). In radiculopathy, as mentioned above, weakness and atrophy of muscles occur within a myotome. In a neuropathy, weakness and reflex changes are confined to the anatomic distribution of the nerve, and sensory deficits do not fully correspond to individual dermatomes. Differentiation is made easier when the affected muscles are supplied by different nerves (e.g., the deltoid and biceps may be weak in lesions of the C5 root; these muscles are supplied by different nerves: axillary and musculocutaneous nerves, respectively). Because of the proximity of roots and spinal cord within the spinal canal, both structures may be compressed together. Associated signs of spinal cord compression are not a feature in peripheral neuropathies except in rare disorders such as familial hypertrophic neuropathy, in which pathologically enlarged roots may encroach upon the spinal cord (Symonds and Blackwood).

SPINAL CORD COMPRESSION

The clinical symptomatology depends on the speed of compression, the transverse and longitudinal extent of the lesion, the functional role of the compressed level of the spinal cord, and the cause of compression.

The spinal cord accommodates to slow forms of compression such as occur with meningiomas and neurofibromas. As a result these tumors in their early stages may cause few symptoms and signs. However, an acute intervertebral disc protrusion or an epidural hematoma will result in rapid impairment of function with severe paralysis, sensory loss, and loss of bladder and bowel control.

The effects of compression may be limited to only a portion of the transverse area of the cord. When one half of the spinal cord is injured at levels higher than the tenth thoracic level, the symptoms and signs that follow are designated the *Brown-Séquard syndrome.* Such patients have spastic weakness, exaggerated muscle stretch reflexes, and an extensor plantar response (Babinski sign) all on the same side as the lesion. Joint position and vibration sense are decreased ipsilaterally, but pain and temperature are impaired on the opposite half of the body. The contralateral loss of pain and tempera-

TABLE 2. Peripheral Nerve and Radicular Innervation of Muscles

Upper Limb:

Nerves	Radicular Innervation					
	C-4	*C-5*	*C-6*	*C-7*	*C-8*	*T-1*
Suprascapular	– –Supraspinatus– –					
Axillary	– –Deltoid– – – – –					
Musculocutaneous		– –Biceps– – – – – – – –				
Median			– –Flexor carpi radialis– –			
			– – – –Flexor pollicis longus– –			
				– –Flexor digitorum– –		
				– –Abductor pollicis longus– –		
				– –Opponens pollicis– – – –		
Ulnar				– –Flexor carpi ulnaris– – – –		
				– –Opponens digiti quinti– –		
				– –Abductor digiti quinti– – – –		
					– –Interossei– – – – – –	
Radial			– –Triceps brachialis– – – – – – – – – – – –			
		– –Brachioradialis– –				
			– –Extensor carpi radialis– –			
			– –Extensor carpi ulnaris– –			
			– –Extensor digitorum longus– –			

Lower Limb:

Nerves	Radicular Innervation						
	L-1	*L-2*	*L-3*	*L-4*	*L-5*	*S-1*	*S-2*
	– –Iliopsoas– – – – –						
Gluteal				– –Gluteus maximus– – – – –			
Femoral		– – – – – – – – – –Quadriceps femoris– –					
Obturator		– –Adductors– – – – –					
Sciatic				– – – –Hamstrings– – – – –			
C. Peroneal			– –Tibialis anterior– –				
			– –Extensor digitorum brevis– –				
Tibial					– – – – –Gastrocnemius– –		
				– –Abductor hallucis			
					– –Abductor digiti quinti– –		

ture sensation is due to crossing of spinothalamic fibers subserving these modalities. Spinothalamic fibers are somatotopically arranged within the ventrolateral columns of the spinal cord, with fibers originating at lower levels lying most laterally. Because of this anatomic organization, extrinsic compression tends to first produce symptoms well below the site of the lesion, the level of sensory impairment gradually ascending as the compression affects deeper parts of the spinal cord. Conversely, because deep-seated lesions may spare superficially arranged fibers, sensation may be normal in the lower dermatomes in patients with intramedullary lesions (sacral sparing).

In addition, intramedullary lesions may give rise to sensory dissociation with loss of pain and temperature sensation and relative preservation of touch. This occurs when mainly crossed fibers are interrupted by a central cord lesion *(commissural or syringomyelia-like syndrome).* In addition, by predominantly disturbing postural sensibility, cord compression may cause ataxia.

LEVELS OF INTRASPINAL COMPRESSION

Foramen Magnum and Upper Cervical Spine. Compression at this level may cause symptoms resulting from spinal cord, nerve root, or intracranial involvement. Pain in the neck and back of the head is the most common and earliest sign. The pain is made worse by head movement, particularly nodding. There may be weakness and atrophy of muscles of the neck and shoulder girdle with spasticity in the lower limbs. Paresthesia and sensory deficits may also occur in the occipital head region (C2 dermatome) and the neck (C3 dermatome). Radicular-like motor and sensory signs may even extend to involve the hands (C6 to C8 segmental level); this extension to the mid- and lower cervical cord has been thought to be due to impaired circulation from compression of spinal vessels. Tumors of the foramen magnum may also extend intracranially and cause increased intracranial pressure, cerebellar dysfunction, nystagmus, trigeminal sensory loss, and atrophy of the tongue.

The most common causes of compression at the craniocervical junction are bony abnormalities which result in basilar invagination, dislocation of the atlantoaxial and atlanto-occipital joints, and neoplasms, meningiomas in particular.

Cervical Region. Compression at this level characteristically produces segmental and radicular signs in the upper limbs combined with long tract signs in the lower extremities.

There is loss of power and bulk in muscles of the shoulder girdle and arms. The biceps, brachioradialis, or triceps jerks mainly depend on the integrity of the C5, C6, or C7 reflex arcs, respectively, and may be diminished or absent. In addition, there can be "inversion" of the brachioradialis reflex; tapping the tendon of this muscle elicits a brisk reflex contraction of the hand and finger flexor muscles and not a normal flexion and supination of the forearm. This unusual response is due to efferent interruption of the segmental reflex arc; the spread of the response and hyperreflexia at lower spinal levels results from pyramidal tract involvement.

When sensory symptoms extend along the radial border of the forearm and thumb ("numb thumb"), they suggest involvement of the C6 cord segment or nerve root. Symptoms in the index and middle fingers point to C7, and sensory impairment in the ring and little fingers suggest C8. Lesions at the cervicothoracic junction can cause unilateral Horner's syndrome which can be associated with wasting of the small muscles of the hand and a sensory deficit on the ulnar border of the hand and forearm (C8, T1).

The most common causes of compression at this level are cervical spondylosis and protrusion of an intervertebral disc, but intramedullary and extramedullary tumors also occur.

Thoracic Region. Compression is suggested by the finding of normal upper limbs and spasticity in the legs. When thoracic radicular symptoms are present, a more precise localization is possible. It is useful to remember that the projection of the thoracic segments coincides with that of the intercostal spaces. Important landmarks are the level of the nipples for the fourth thoracic, the xiphoid process for T7, and the umbilicus and groin for T10 and T12, respectively. Patients will often complain of a tight, bound feeling which usually coincides with the compressed root or segment. In addition, intercostal muscles may be wasted. In low thoracic lesions the umbilicus may elevate when the patient, in the supine position, raises his head against resistance (Beevor's sign).

Common causes of compression at the thoracic spine level are metastatic tumors, meningiomas, and neurofibromas. Intervertebral disc protusions are comparatively rare at this level.

Lumbosacral Region. *Lower Spinal Cord.* There is a close relation between the segments in the lower cord and the roots that form the cauda equina. As a result, pain, sensorimotor signs in the lower limbs, and loss of sphincter control can result from the involvement of either cord or roots. It is seldom that a discrete spinal cord segmental lesion can be clinically identified at this level. When they occur, lesions at the first lumbar segment usually cause referred pain to the groin, and there may be loss of the cremasteric cutaneous reflex, weakness of hip flexion, and spasticity in the lower legs. A compression localized at L2 and L3 may give rise to weakness of the quadriceps and adductors of the thigh, loss of knee jerks, brisk ankle reflexes, and bilateral Babinski signs. Involvement of L5 and S1 results in weakness and atrophy of the peroneal, calf, and intrinsic foot muscles. Knee jerks may be present, but, because the lower segmental reflex arcs are interrupted, ankle jerks and Babinski signs cannot be elicited.

Normal power in the legs, preservation of knee and even ankle jerks, but loss of sensation in the perianal and genital (saddle) area, together with impaired bladder and bowel control, are characteristic of lesions that involve the lower sacral segments. When this localization is suspected, sensory function over the buttocks must be carefully examined, and rectal sphincter tone should be tested.

Cauda Equina. Compression of nerve roots forming the cauda equina is difficult to differentiate from signs caused by involvement of the lower segment of the spinal cord. In cauda equina compression, dull, aching pain may be experienced in the sacrum or perineum or can radiate to the legs in a sciatic distribution. Symptoms depend on the level of compression and number of motor and sensory roots affected. Often there is atrophic, areflexic paralysis combined with asymmetrical bilateral radicular sensory impairment. Sensory dissociation does not occur. Progression of signs is usually slow, and loss of bladder and bowel control may occur late.

Presumably because of interference with blood supply to the roots of the cauda equina by compression, some patients with a narrowed lumbar spinal canal experience transient radicular signs or pain in the calf muscles when walking or after prolonged standing. This syndrome has been named intermittent claudication of the cauda equina.

The most important cause of single or multiple root compression at the low lumbar and sacral level is an intervertebral disc protrusion. Cauda equina compression occurs in congenital spinal stenosis and lumbar spondylosis, Paget's disease, and achondroplasia. Ependymomas, teratomas, and lipomas may constrict the lower segments of the cord and cauda equina. Tabes dorsalis, diabetic neuropathy, and other lesions affecting peripheral nerves to the lower limbs must be differentiated from lesions compressing the lumbosacral roots.

Aids to the Investigation of Peripheral Nerve Injuries. London, Her Majesty's Stationery Office, 1960.

Haymaker, W.: Bing's Local Diagnosis in Neurologic Diseases. 15th ed. St. Louis, C. V. Mosby Company, 1969.

Keegan, J. J., and Garett, F. D.: The segmental distribution of the cutaneous nerves in the limbs of man. Anat. Rec., 102:409, 1948.

Klenerman, L.: Cauda equina and spinal cord compression in Paget's disease. J. Bone Joint Surg., 48B:365, 1966.

Rewcastle, N. B., and Berry, K.: Neoplasms of the lower spinal canal. Neurology (Minneap.), 14:608, 1964.

Symonds, C. P., and Blackwood, W.: Spinal cord compression in hypertrophic neuritis. Brain, 85:251, 1962.

448. LABORATORY AIDS TO INVESTIGATION

To localize and establish the nature of lesions causing intraspinal compression, several diagnostic tests may be used. Roentgenographic investigations are the most important, but electrophysiologic techniques, radioisotope scanning, and cerebrospinal fluid examination are also helpful.

ROENTGENOGRAPHIC METHODS

Roentgenographic investigation should begin with plain films of the suspected site of spinal cord or root compression. Frontal, lateral, and oblique views are required for examination of the cervical spine; frontal and lateral views are generally satisfactory for visualization of the thoracic and lumbosacral spine. Lateral films of the cervical spine in flexion and extension are needed if recurrent subluxation is suspected. In certain situations, tomography may be necessary to define a bone lesion more precisely.

Plain films of the spine should be systematically examined, noting the number, shape, density, and alignment of the vertebrae and the contour of the pedicles, the size of the intervertebral foramen, the size and shape of the spinal canal, the width of the disc spaces, and the presence of abnormal soft tissue shadows or calcifications. The anteroposterior depth of the spinal canal is a particularly important measurement. Sagittal diameters of less than 10 mm at any level of the cervical spine usually indicate spinal cord compression; bony compression of the cord is also possible with canals measuring 10 to 13 mm but improbable if measurements are greater than 13 mm. Increases in the transverse diameter of the spinal canal may be associated with thinning of the pedicles and are seen with syringomyelia or intramedullary tumors. Narrowing of the spinal canal with compression of the spinal cord or roots may occur in spondylosis, achondroplasia, and Paget's disease.

Plain x-rays of the vertebral column may suggest certain specific conditions. Dumbbell-shaped neurofibromas which enlarge the intervertebral foramen will become readily apparent in such x-rays. Congenital anomalies of the vertebral bodies are at times associated with intraspinal teratomas or lipomas. Bone caries suggests an infectious process such as tuberculosis, typhoidal infection, or brucellosis. Vertebral bone destruction by infection often involves the intervertebral discs; conversely, tumor metastases to the vertebral column spare the discs.

When surgical treatment is contemplated, radiopaque *oil myelography* by lumbar or cisternal injection is required for precise localization. In expert hands, *air myelography* is also a useful tool for the assessment of spinal cord size and for a diagnosis of small tumors. *Spinal angiography* is a specialized technique necessary for the detailed investigation of tumors and vascular malformations.

SCANNING AND ELECTROMYOGRAPHY

Bone scanning after radioisotope injection may be helpful if metastases are suspected as a cause of bone destruction. However, fractures, infection, and ankylosing spondylitis may also cause increased radioisotope uptake.

Electromyography is useful for the localization of intraspinal lesions affecting the motor unit at the anterior horn cell or the nerve root levels, as noted in Ch. 358.

CEREBROSPINAL FLUID EXAMINATION

Cerebrospinal fluid examination rarely provides specific diagnostic information about compressive spinal cord or root lesions. Therefore because satisfactory myelograms are difficult to obtain in patients who have had lumbar puncture in the preceding week, cerebrospinal fluid examinations are usually best performed at the time of myelography. In general, the examination of cerebrospinal fluid may suggest certain diagnostic possibilities. Xanthochromic fluid is seen with intraspinal hemorrhage or block of cerebrospinal fluid circulation. Intraspinal bleeding may originate from vascular malformations, ependymomas, or melanomas. Inflammatory cells indicate an infectious process or chemical meningitis caused by a ruptured teratoma or dermoid cyst. Tumor cells may be identified in the cerebrospinal fluid of patients with carcinomatous infiltration of the meninges.

In the absence of a block in the circulation of cerebrospinal fluid, elevations of CSF protein over 60 mg per 100 ml suggest other intraspinal lesions than an intervertebral disc protrusion or spondylosis. Spinal fluid blocks are best established by myelography; because irreparable damage to the spinal cord may result from displacement of an intraspinal mass after pressure changes resulting from jugular compression (Queckenstedt test), this procedure should not be done if spinal cord compression is suspected.

Aguilar, J. A., and Elvidge, A. R.: Intervertebral disc disease caused by the Brucella organism. J. Neurosurg., 18:27, 1961.
Ambrose, G. B., Alpert, M., and Neer, C. S.: Vertebral osteomyelitis. A diagnostic problem. J.A.M.A., 97:101, 1966.
Charkes, N. D., Sklaroff, D. M., and Young, I.: A critical analysis of strontium bone scanning for detection of metastatic cancer. Am. J. Roentgenol. Radium Ther. Nucl. Med., 96:647, 1966.
DiChiro, G., and Doppman, J. L.: Differential angiographic features of hemangioblastomas and arteriovenous malformations of the spinal cord. Radiology, 93:25, 1969.
Elsberg, C. A., and Dyke, C. G.: Diagnosis and localization of tumors of the spinal cord by means of measurements made on x-ray films of vertebrae and the correlation of clinical and x-ray findings. Bull. Neurol. Inst., 3:359, 1934.

449. MANAGEMENT OF PATIENTS WITH SUSPECTED NERVE ROOT OR SPINAL CORD COMPRESSION

The specific management of intraspinal compression of nerve roots or cord depends on the suspected diagnosis, the severity of the symptoms, and the extent of the neurologic signs.

Conservative Management Aimed at Reducing Pain and Preventing Future Recurrences. Patients in this category have acute localized pain in the spinal or paraspinal region with or without peripheral radicular radiation; they do not have neurologic deficits indicative of spinal cord or severe root compression. The most likely diagnosis is an acute intervertebral disc protrusion, and with time complete recovery can usually be anticipated. This approach is particularly justified when there is no history of similar previous episodes and when the pain follows minor trauma, effort, or strain.

Patients may stay at home and should rest on a firm bed and make no physical effort. Analgesics and muscle relaxants are given for symptomatic relief. When pain subsides, exercises aimed at strengthening the muscular support of the spinal column may help prevent recurrences.

Plain x-rays of the involved segment of the spine help ascertain changes in the vertebral bodies or discs. Initially, however, these investigations can be deferred if the patient is in considerable pain.

Conservative Management Aimed at Deciding If the Course of Intraspinal Root Compression Is Progressive. Acute pain may be accompanied by signs of moderate sensory or motor deficit in a root distribution. Such signs are represented by some loss of strength, paresthesia, and mild sensory impairment or a loss of muscle stretch reflexes. If these signs worsen or do not subside after a trial of conservative treatment, admission to hospital should be arranged to assure immobilization and rest and to arrange further investigations.

Management Aimed at Possible Surgical Decompression. This approach is indicated for patients showing signs of spinal cord compression. It is also advisable for patients with nerve root compression if there is intractable or severe recurrent pain or if there are signs of severe neurologic deficit, particularly marked weakness and muscle atrophy. These patients should be admitted to hospital for investigation. If there are no contraindications to surgery, myelography should be performed to establish a diagnosis and determine the site and extent of compression. If indicated, operative treatment should soon follow.

Prompt Investigation and Surgical Decompression. This approach is required for patients who rapidly develop spinal cord or cauda equina compression. A particular emergency is represented by impaired bladder or rectal control. Patients should be immediately admitted to hospital to undergo only those investigations which enable a localization of the lesion. Such investigations usually include plain films of the spine and an emergency myelogram. In the course of these investigations, patients should be kept fasting to allow for immediate anesthesia if surgical intervention is decided upon.

SPECIFIC DISORDERS THAT CAUSE NERVE ROOT OR SPINAL CORD COMPRESSION

450. INTERVERTEBRAL DISC PROTRUSION

Each intervertebral disc consists of fibrocartilage and has a soft center, the nucleus pulposus, surrounded by thicker fibrous tissue, the anulus fibrosus. The nucleus pulposus constitutes most of the disc substance in the young, but with age it loses volume and resilience. When, during effort or trauma, the disc is suddenly compressed and the nucleus pulposus is caused to protrude through the anulus, fragments of disc may be extruded into the spinal canal. The herniated disc is usually directed toward the spinal canal because the anulus and longitudinal ligament are thinner posteriorly. Disc disease is more common in the cervical and lumbar spine where there is greater mobility; in the thoracic spine, where movement is limited, disc herniations are rare.

The signs and symptoms of disc herniation result from compression of pain-sensitive structures within the spinal canal, including nerve roots or the spinal cord itself. Posterolateral disc herniations tend to involve individual nerve roots at the intervertebral foramina, whereas central protrusions may compress the spinal cord or cauda equina. Commonly the compressed root approximately corresponds to the level of the protruded disc, but this may not be the case in the lumbosacral region where several roots can be compressed by a single disc. Furthermore, extruded disc material may move several centimeters along the dural sac and compress roots situated below the site of disc rupture.

Clinical Manifestations. Pain is the main symptom of an intervertebral disc protrusion. It is usually severe and accompanied by local reflex contraction of paraspinal muscles. Other symptoms and signs depend upon the localization of the protruded disc.

Herniated Cervical Discs. Cervical disc herniations occur most frequently at the fifth and sixth interspaces with fewer protrusions at C4 and C7 interspaces. Symptoms are often precipitated by sudden twisting, hyperextension, or hyperflexion of the neck. The pain may radiate to the shoulder and parascapular region and usually has a boring, aching quality. If nerve roots are compressed below the midcervical level, pain may extend into the upper extremity. Movements of the neck, but particularly hyperextension and tilting toward the affected side, are limited by pain. Symptoms caused by compression of the C6 and C7 roots are summarized in Table 1, Ch. 447. More rarely cervical disc protrusion results in cord compression. In such patients, long tract signs which develop below the level of the lesion are mainly due to involvement of the corticospinal tract.

Herniated Lumbar Discs. The most common disc protrusions are in the low lumbar region and affect the L5 and S1 roots (Table 1). There is often a poorly localized low backache (lumbago), and pain may radiate into the buttocks, thigh, and lower leg (sciatica). The pain is generally severe and follows effort, such as lifting. In some patients, however, the pain may be spontaneous; occasionally sensory and motor deficits caused by disc herniation occur in the absence of pain. In most patients, the radiation of pain is unilateral; when there is a central disc protrusion, however, pain may occur in both lower extremities.

On examination patients show straightening of the normal lumbar curvature, and the pelvis may be tilted away from the side of the protrusion. Paraspinal muscles and vertebral spinous processes are tender to palpation. Straight leg raising (Lasègue's maneuver) on the side of compression is limited by back pain. In addition, the pain can occur with raising of the opposite leg ("crossover pain"). There may be tenderness on palpation of the sciatic notch.

Cord compression occurs when disc herniation occurs higher than the first lumbar intervertebral space. Compression of several of the roots of the cauda equina is more common, however, and gives rise to pain, asymmetric bilateral sensory and motor changes, and even to loss of sphincter control. Occasionally, bladder control may be lost in the absence of other symptoms.

Diagnosis. The symptoms of an intervertebral disc protrusion must be differentiated from those caused by arthritis of the spine and other bone and joint diseases. Neuropathies caused by entrapment, neuralgic amyotrophy, and diabetic neuropathy may enter the differential diagnosis because they may present with localized pain, sensory, and motor deficits.

Plain x-rays of the spine reveal narrowing of disc spaces in less than half the patients. In the cervical spine, oblique views are necessary to establish whether there is a reduction in the size of intervertebral foramina. Myelography should be performed only when the cause of compression is doubtful or when surgical treatment is contemplated. Disc protrusions are evidenced by myelography as a filling defect at the level of the interspace. Obliteration of the root sleeve by a protruded disc may also be demonstrated by this procedure. The cerebrospinal fluid protein may be normal or increased; in the absence of complete block of cerebrospinal fluid circulation, protein values are usually below 60 mg per 100 ml.

Treatment. Patients presenting with acute pain should be treated with analgesics, muscle relaxants, rest, and immobility. A cervical collar or a lumbar brace may reduce mobility, and rest in bed on a hard mattress is often helpful. If improvement follows such measures, usually no investigations other than plain x-rays of the spine are necessary. If pain and other symptoms persist after a period of rest, hospitalization must be considered to ensure immobilization. Intractable pain, persistent disability, or development of progressive sensory or motor signs of radicular compression requires consideration of surgical treatment. Prompt operative treatment is mandatory when signs of progressive cord involvement or impairment of bladder or rectal sphincter control develop.

Recurrent symptoms after discoidectomy may be due to arachnoiditis or to a recurrent intervertebral disc prolapse. In addition the possibility that a herniated disc may have been associated with another type of intraspinal disease must be considered.

Fisher, R. G.: Protrusions of thoracic disc. The factor of herniation through the dura mater. J. Neurosurg., 22:591, 1965.
Kessler, L. A., and Stein, W. Z.: Posterior migration of a herniated disc. Radiology, 76:104, 1961.
Love, J. G., and Emmett, J. L.: "Asymptomatic" protruded lumbar disc as a cause of urinary retention. Mayo Clin. Proc., 42:249, 1967.
Love, J. G., and Schorn, V. G.: Thoracic disc protrusions. J.A.M.A., 191:627, 1965.
Scott, P. J.: Bladder paralysis in cauda equina lesions from disc prolapse. J. Bone Joint Surg., 47B:224, 1965.
Spanos, N. C., and Andrew, J.: Intermittent claudication and lateral lumbar disc protrusions. J. Neurol. Neurosurg. Psychiatry, 29:273, 1966.
Spurling, R. G.: Lesions of the Lumbar Intervertebral Disc. Springfield, Ill., Charles C Thomas, 1953.
Spurling, R. G.: Lesions of the Cervical Intervertebral Disc. Springfield, Ill., Charles C Thomas, 1956.

451. MYELOPATHY AND NERVE ROOT COMPRESSION DUE TO SPONDYLOSIS

Spondylosis refers to degenerative changes in the spine which may be neurologically asymptomatic or may cause symptoms by compression of nerve roots or spinal cord.

Spondylotic changes consist of intervertebral disc narrowing, osteophyte formation, and thickening of spinal ligaments. These changes most frequently involve the cervical or lumbar spine and are rare in the thoracic region. The term spondylosis is not generally used to describe acute protrusion of intervertebral discs, although the two conditions may be associated.

Pathogenesis. Spondylosis presumably results from the "wear and tear" of repeated spinal movement. Although more than one half of people older than 50 years of age have cervical spine osteophytes, associated neurologic symptoms and signs are much less frequent. The single most important factor in the development of clinical manifestations caused by spondylosis is the size of the spinal canal. If the canal is congenitally narrow, the spinal cord or roots may be compressed by relatively small osteophytes or ligamentous hypertrophy; on the other hand, a wide spinal canal may accommodate extensive spondylotic changes without causing appreciable neurologic signs of compression.

When the cervical spinal cord is compressed by osteophytes from the vertebral bodies or by thickening of the posterior longitudinal ligament and ligamentum flavum, symptoms and signs may follow trauma caused by neck movement or from impairment of spinal cord circulation. The cauda equina may also be injured in lumbar spondylosis. At both the cervical and lumbar levels, nerve roots are compressed by degenerative changes in bone and soft tissues adjacent to the intervertebral foramina.

Clinical Manifestations. *Cervical Spondylosis.* The most important symptoms and signs of cervical spondylosis are due to spinal cord (cervical myelopathy) and root (cervical radiculopathy) compression.

Cervical Myelopathy. Cervical myelopathy commonly develops insidiously, but symptoms may be precipitated by minor trauma. Sensory abnormalities are usually less striking than signs of disturbed motor function. Spastic paresis, clonus, and hyperreflexia in the legs as well as extensor plantar responses are the most common neurologic signs of this myelopathy.

In the upper limbs, there may be segmental muscle weakness and atrophy, as well as loss of muscle stretch reflexes, particularly if there is an associated radiculopathy. Vibration sense may be diminished in the lower limbs, but loss of joint position sense or pain and temperature sensation is uncommon. As a rule, bladder and bowel control are normal in patients with cervical myelopathy.

Cervical Radiculopathy. Cervical radiculopathy may occur in the absence of cervical myelopathy. Various radicular syndromes may develop, depending on the particular root affected. In the cervical spine the most common radiculopathies are those of the C6 and C7 root (Table 1, Ch. 447).

Pain and limitation of neck movement are common in cervical spondylosis, and some patients may present with occipital headaches.

Diagnosis. X-rays of the cervical spine confirm the presence of cervical spondylosis. However, there is a high incidence of asymptomatic spondylotic changes, and careful clinical correlation is required for interpretation of such radiologic findings. To prove the diagnosis of cervical spondylotic myelopathy, the anteroposterior diameter of the cervical canal must be measured. If this measurement is less than 10 mm, there is almost certain cord compression. The extent of compression can best be determined by myelography which also shows soft tissue changes in spondylosis. Oblique x-ray views demonstrate narrowing of the intervertebral foramina.

Prognosis and Treatment. Because of wide variations in the natural course of cervical spondylotic myelopathy, it is difficult to assess the relative merits of conservative and surgical management. Recent advances in surgical techniques have been accompanied by more effective relief of spinal cord compression in patients with advancing or rapidly progressing disability. Other patients can usually be managed effectively with analgesics, muscle relaxants, and cervical immobilization.

LUMBAR SPINAL STENOSIS DUE TO SPONDYLOSIS

In addition to compression of individual nerve roots by osteophytes encroaching upon intervertebral foramina, spondylosis of the lumbosacral spine may significantly reduce the size of the spinal canal. In such circumstances, spinal canal stenosis may cause injury to the cauda equina.

The pathogenesis of neurologic symptoms in patients with lumbar stenosis is similar to that in other bone diseases resulting in shallow lumbar canals, namely, congenital spinal stenosis, achondroplasia, and Paget's disease. In all these disorders, further narrowing by osteophytes, disc herniation, or ligamentous hypertrophy may give rise to compression of the cauda equina.

Clinical Manifestations. The only symptom in patients with lumbar spinal stenosis may be backache after prolonged standing or effort. Signs of single or multiple root compression may develop gradually or have a sudden onset. These radicular symptoms are similar to those of intervertebral disc herniation and other causes of lumbosacral nerve root compression. Patients with lumbar spinal stenosis may suffer acute compression of the cauda equina after minor trauma or when subjected to prolonged hyperextension as during anesthesia for certain surgical procedures.

Intermittent Claudication of the Cauda Equina. Intermittent claudication of the cauda equina is a rare syndrome which may present in association with narrowing of the spinal canal. Typically, symptoms and signs are evoked or accentuated by walking and disappear soon after stopping. In other patients symptoms follow prolonged standing. In both varieties of intermittent claudication of the cauda equina, roots are compressed within a narrow spinal canal. The onset of symptoms has been explained by postulating that transient additional spinal narrowing is caused by the lordotic posture adopted during walking and standing. Patients usually present with pain in the low back and legs and may show weakness and sensory symptoms. During examination signs of motor and sensory deficit, as well as diminished reflexes, may be temporarily elicited by asking the patient to walk until symptoms reappear.

The absence of signs of vascular insufficiency in the iliofemoral and other arteries to the lower extremities helps differentiate claudication caused by compression from that which results from primary vascular disease.

Diagnosis. The diagnosis of lumbar spinal stenosis requires radiologic demonstration of a narrow lumbar canal and myelographic confirmation of cauda equina compression.

Treatment. In advanced lumbar spinal stenosis, progressive signs of individual root or cauda equina compression can be relieved by surgical decompression.

Crandall, P. H., and Batzdorf, U.: Cervical spondylotic myelopathy. J. Neurosurg., 25:57, 1966.
Ehni, G., et al.: Significance of the small lumbar spinal canal: Cauda equina compression syndromes due to spondylosis: (Parts I to V). J. Neurosurg., 31:490, 1969.
Stoltmann, H. F., and Blackwood, W.: The role of the ligamenta flava in the pathogenesis of myelopathy in cervical spondylosis. Brain, 87:45, 1964.
Turnbull, I. M.: Microvasculature of the human spinal cord. J. Neurosurg., 35:141, 1971.
Waltz, T. A.: Physical factors in the myelopathy of cervical spondylosis. Brain, 90:395, 1967.
Wilkinson, M. (ed.): Cervical Spondylosis. Its Early Diagnosis and Treatment. Philadelphia, W. B. Saunders Company, 1971.

452. SPINAL CORD TUMORS

Depending upon their anatomic relation to the dura mater, tumors affecting the spinal cord may be classified as *extradural tumors,* which usually arise in the bone of the spinal column or within the extradural space; *intradural extramedullary tumors,* which lie between the dura mater and the spinal cord; and *intramedullary tumors,* which arise within the substance of the cord itself. The relative incidence in a general hospital population is approximately 50, 40, and 10 per cent, respectively.

EXTRADURAL TUMORS

Such tumors are usually manifested by symptoms and signs of spinal cord compression and are most often caused by extradural bone metastases. Common primary sources are carcinomas of the lung, breast, kidney, and prostate; less frequent sources are the gastrointestinal tract and thyroid gland. Spinal extradural compression may also occur in multiple myeloma, sarcomas, or lymphomas. Most metastases give rise to localized compression, but a few, particularly lymphomas and sarcomas, may extensively infiltrate the epidural space.

Pain resulting from bone destruction or root compression is the first symptom in over 90 per cent of patients with extradural tumors. It is usually dull, constant, and localized, is made worse by movements of the spine or pressure over the vertebral spinal processes, and is often exacerbated by bed rest. Radicular symptoms usually follow the local pain and are often bilateral. Pain alone is usually present for weeks or months before signs of spinal cord dysfunction develop; but once spinal cord signs appear, they usually progress rapidly over a few days or weeks to produce, if untreated, complete paralysis. More rarely, compression develops acutely, because of pathologic collapse of an infiltrated vertebral body or from hemorrhage within the metastasis. In either event, spastic weakness and loss of vibration and joint position sense below the level of the lesion are the first spinal cord signs to develop, whereas disturbances of bladder and/or bowel control generally occur late.

Radiologic changes are present on the plain x-ray films of most patients with malignant extradural metastases. Signs vary from osteoporosis to frank destruction of bone. When ordinary x-ray films of the spine are normal, evidence of bone involvement may be provided by radioisotope scanning. A definitive diagnosis of malignant extradural metastasis, however, can be made only by myelography, which must be carried out promptly if there is clinical suspicion of spinal cord compression, no matter what the plain radiograms reveal.

As a rule the cerebrospinal fluid protein is elevated, but there are no malignant cells. The CSF glucose is normal, in contrast to the decreased levels often seen in patients with carcinomatous invasion of the subarachnoid space.

Because metastatic tumors are a frequent cause of spinal cord compression in adults, this possibility should always be considered in patients with signs or symptoms of compression. In particular, the lungs and breasts should be carefully examined as sources of a possible primary malignancy. Anemia, bone pain, mediastinal enlargement, hepatomegaly, or splenomegaly all suggest metastatic disease or lymphomas. Bone x-rays, serum electrophoresis, testing for Bence Jones protein in the urine, and bone marrow examinations are all of help in diagnosing multiple myeloma.

Hormones, radiotherapy, and/or chemotherapy are used in the treatment of most metastatic tumors involving the spine. Surgical decompression is indicated when such therapy is ineffective or when there are signs of rapidly progressing compression of the cord. Whatever form of treatment is chosen, it must be begun promptly and be vigorous, because if neurologic signs are mild, the chances of maintaining or improving neurologic function are better.

INTRADURAL EXTRAMEDULLARY TUMORS

The two most important tumors in this category are meningiomas and neurofibromas, which together account for almost two thirds of all primary intraspinal neoplasms. Less common tumors are teratomas, arachnoid cysts, some lipomas, and meningeal invasion by carcinoma.

Meningiomas show a high incidence among middle-aged women. They are usually single, relatively small, and located posterior or lateral to the spinal cord. Excluding those that occur in the region of the foramen magnum, approximately 90 per cent are found in the thoracic region. Signs of spinal cord compression develop insidiously so that an ataxic, spastic syndrome, which superficially resembles subacute combined degeneration of the spinal cord, may result. Moderate localized or segmental pain is presented in only 50 per cent of patients and is the central symptom in only 20 per cent. Tenderness on percussion of the vertebral spinous processes may be present. Tumors of the foramen magnum are particularly difficult to diagnose. Spastic ataxia and nystagmus are often early symptoms and may suggest multiple sclerosis rather than tumor. With tumor there may be pain or sensory loss in the C2 distribution, and the CSF protein is elevated.

X-rays may show bone erosion or calcification within a meningioma (4 per cent). Myelography is required for a precise localization of intraspinal meningiomas. In tumors of the foramen magnum a routine myelogram may be negative; therefore if such a tumor is suspected, myelography must be done in the supine as well as in the prone position to localize high, posteriorly placed tumors.

Neurofibromas arise from dorsal nerve roots, affect both sexes equally, occur at all ages, and may be present at any level of the spinal canal. Neurofibromas may extend extradurally but may also arise from within the substance of the spinal cord. In some cases the tumors are part of a generalized neurofibromatosis. A small percentage of neurofibromas undergo sarcomatous changes and become invasive or metastasize.

Patients with intraspinal neurofibromas often give a history of longstanding radicular pain, and this symptom usually long precedes any sign of cord compression. When neurofibromas extend on either side of an intervertebral foramen, they may adopt a dumbbell or hourglass shape. X-rays, including oblique views of the spine, may often show enlargement of a foramen and thinning of the adjacent pedicle. The degree of radiographic change may be out of proportion to the presenting symptoms. When the intraspinal portion of the tumor is small in comparison to the extraspinal, the latter may grow to such a large size that it is palpable externally even when there are few signs of cord compression.

As with meningiomas, the cerebrospinal fluid protein is almost always elevated. Myelography is essential for precise localization. A complete recovery usually follows the early surgical removal of both meningiomas and neurofibromas.

INTRAMEDULLARY TUMORS

Most of these tumors arise from constituent cells of the spinal cord. Ependymomas are the most common, followed by astrocytomas, glioblastomas, and oligodendrogliomas. In addition, vascular tumors (hemangioblastomas), lipomas, and even metastases may occur as intramedullary tumors.

Ependymomas arise at all levels of the spinal cord but have a preference for the caudal region. They represent more than two thirds of the tumors of the conus medullaris and are even more common as causes of tumors of the filum terminale. Ependymomas may extend through several segments of the spinal cord; in rare instances the entire length of the cord is involved. Syringomyelia may develop in association with these and other intramedullary tumors. Spontaneous hemorrhages into ependymomas and hemangioblastomas occur and may give rise to sudden pain and neurologic deficit. Excluding glioblastomas and metastases, most intramedullary tumors have a slow progression. Radicular signs are not an early manifestation. Dull, localized aching pain, muscle weakness or atrophy, impotence in males, and sphincter disturbances in both sexes are common early symptoms. Intramedullary tumors affecting the cervical or thoracic cord may cause sensory dissociation with predominant pain and temperature impairment. In such cases the sacral dermatomes are usually spared. Rarely, increased intracranial pressure with headache and papilledema is the first sign of spinal tumor. The symptoms result from hydrocephalus, believed to result from blocking of CSF absorptive pathways by elevated CSF protein.

Longstanding intramedullary tumors may cause radiologically visible widening of the spinal canal and erosion of the pedicles. Contrast myelography usually demonstrates an enlarged spinal cord. In the lumbosacral region tumors may present as a pedunculated mass involving the cauda equina. Tumors of the filum terminale may be mobile and be a source of confusion for myelographic localization.

Successful surgical removal of intramedullary tumors is sometimes possible. Operative success is particularly high with ependymomas and hemangioblastomas, but recurrences may occur; gliomas respond poorly to any form of treatment, and lipomas are technically difficult to remove.

Davis, R. A., and Washburn, P. L.: Spinal cord meningiomas. Surg. Gynecol. Obstet., 131:15, 1970.
Harries, B.: Spinal cord compression. Br. Med. J., 1:611, 673, 1970.
Posner, J. B.: Neurological complications of systemic cancer. Med. Clin. North Am., 55:625, 1971.
Thomas, J. E., and Miller, R. E.: Lipomatous tumors of the spinal canal. Mayo Clin. Proc., 48:393, 1973.
White, W. A., Patterson, R. H., Jr., and Bergland, R. M.: Role of surgery in the treatment of spinal cord compression by metastatic neoplasm. Cancer, 27:558, 1971.

453. SPINAL ARACHNOIDITIS

Spinal arachnoiditis results from a low grade inflammation of the spinal meninges with formation of fibrous adhesions and loculation of cerebrospinal fluid. The changes extend throughout the length of the subarachnoid space or may be confined to a few segments. The adhesions may compress roots or the spinal cord itself.

Arachnoiditis may result from spinal surgery or spinal anesthesia and, more rarely, from myelography. It can be a late complication of subarachnoid hemorrhage, syphilis, tuberculosis, or other bacterial or parasitic spinal meningitides. In some cases no cause is found.

The development of symptoms and signs is insidious, the earliest symptoms usually reflecting multiple root involvement. This is particularly true if the adhesions extend into the lumbosacral spinal region, thereby involving the cauda equina. Pain is common and may be unrelated to movement; sensory symptoms usually exceed motor deficit. Signs of cord compression gradually develop and may progress to paraplegia; in other cases the disease process spontaneously arrests.

The diagnosis of spinal arachnoiditis depends upon the clinical course, as well as on examination of the cerebrospinal fluid and myelography. The CSF protein is elevated, and there may be pleocytosis. On myelography there are spotty, irregular collections of oil and an impairment of the flow of contrast material in the subarachnoid space.

When a specific infectious agent is identified, appropriate chemotherapy is indicated. Surgical exploration may provide histologic evidence as to the diagnosis, but laminectomy and removal of adhesions are not always beneficial for the relief of spinal and root compression.

Davidson, S.: Cryptococcal spinal arachnoiditis. J. Neurol. Neurosurg. Psychiatry, 31:76, 1968.
Guidetti, B., and LaTorre, E.: Hypertrophic spinal pachymeningitis. J. Neurosurg., 26:496, 1967.
Seaman, W. B., Marder, S. N., and Rosenbaum, H. E.: The myelographic appearance of adhesive spinal arachnoiditis. J. Neurosurg., 10:145, 1953.
Weiss, R. M., Sweeney, L., and Dreyfuss, M.: Circumscribed adhesive spinal arachnoiditis. J. Neurosurg., 19:435, 1962.
Wise, B. L., and Smith, M.: Spinal arachnoiditis ossificans. Arch. Neurol., 13:391, 1965.

454. ARTERIOVENOUS MALFORMATIONS AND OTHER VASCULAR LESIONS OF THE SPINAL CORD

Vascular malformations may be present on the surface of the spinal cord or within its substance. They may thus give rise to subarachnoid hemorrhage, intramedullary hemorrhage (hematomyelia), or both. Rarely, a spinal epidural hematoma results from such bleeding. The sudden development of partial or complete transverse myelopathy is the most common form of onset. This is manifested by paralysis, sensory impairment, and loss of sphincter control. If there is bleeding into the subarachnoid space, pain in the neck and back and other signs of meningeal irritation occur. Sudden headache, neck stiffness, and blood in the cerebrospinal fluid may be mistakenly attributed to hemorrhage of intracranial rather than intraspinal origin.

Arteriovenous malformations may also compress the spinal cord or give rise to hemodynamic changes that result in spinal ischemia. Distortion and compression of the cord by enlarged, abnormal vessels occur only gradually, and patients present with slowly progressive symptoms of spinal cord dysfunction. In some patients transient exacerbation of symptoms may occur in association with menstrual periods or pregnancy, but in others exacerbations occur spontaneously.

Complete or partial recovery of function can follow episodes of spinal cord ischemia or even small hemorrhages. The unchanging localization of the attacks and the prominence of pain help to differentiate those symptoms caused by arteriovenous malformations from other recurrent neurologic disorders such as multiple sclerosis. In some patients a spinal bruit may be heard by auscultation over the site of the malformation.

Cavernous angiomas of the spinal cord are vascular hamartomas which may be associated with cysts and tumors in other organs or with hemangioblastomas of the cerebellum. Retinal vascular changes (von Hippel–Lindau syndrome) and cutaneous vascular nevi may be associated with spinal vascular malformations. The presence of these associated signs lends support to the assumption that, in a patient who presents them, spinal symptoms may be due to a vascular malformation.

Intraspinal bleeding caused by vascular malformation must be differentiated from bleeding that occurs as a complication of hemorrhagic diathesis, anticoagulant therapy, or collagen diseases such as polyarteritis nodosa. In these conditions, however, there are usually signs of a more general disorder, cutaneous hematomas or other skin lesions, hematuria, or abnormal laboratory investigations.

In most patients with vascular malformations presenting with acute symptoms, examination of the cerebrospinal fluid reveals body or xanthochromic fluid, but, when there has been no recent bleeding, the only finding may be an elevated protein. Plain x-rays of the spine may show erosion, coexistent vertebral hemangiomas, or calcification within the spinal canal. On myelography, serpentine streaks within the column of oil may reveal the site of the vascular malformation. Angiography with regional catheterization of radicular vessels is a necessary preliminary to surgical treatment. Advances in microsurgery have increased considerably the chances for a satisfactory removal of spinal vascular malformations.

Antoni, N.: Spinal vascular malformations (angiomas) and myelomalacia. Neurology, 12:795, 1962.
Fine, R. D.: Angioma racemosum venosum of spinal cord with segmentally related angiomatous lesions of skin and forearm. J. Neurosurg., 18:546, 1961.
Henson, R. A., and Parsons, M.: Ischaemic lesions of the spinal cord: An illustrated review. Quart. J. Med., 36:205, 1967.
Matthews, W. B.: The spinal bruit. Lancet, 2:1117, 1959.
Taylor, J. R., and Van Allen, M. W.: Vascular malformation of the cord with transient ischaemic attacks. J. Neurosurg., 31:576, 1969.

455. SPINAL EPIDURAL HEMATOMA

Bleeding into the spinal epidural space may occur spontaneously but is more commonly associated with trauma, bleeding diathesis, or vascular malformations. It is a particular risk in patients receiving anticoagulants. The hemorrhage usually originates in the epidural venous plexus, and the hematomas tend to collect over the dorsum of the thoracic dura mater. Epidural hematomas vary in size, but the larger ones cause spinal cord compression. The clinical picture is characterized by the sudden onset of severe, localized back pain. Cord compression, when it occurs, results in the rapid development of flaccid paralysis, sensory loss, and impaired bladder and bowel control. The sudden onset of signs of cord compression in a patient on anticoagulants should allow few doubts as to the likelihood of a spinal epidural hematoma.

In epidural hematomas the cerebrospinal fluid may be clear or very slightly hemorrhagic.

Emergency surgical evacuation of the hematoma is essential. Although myelography is of great help in the diagnosis and localization of epidural hematomas, this and other investigations should not take the place of prompt surgical intervention in order to avoid irreversible spinal cord damage.

Bidzinski, J.: Spontaneous spinal epidural hematoma during pregnancy. Case report. J. Neurosurg., 24:1017, 1966.

Jacobson, I., McCabe, J. J., Harris, P., and Dott, N. M.: Spontaneous spinal epidural hemorrhage during anticoagulant therapy. Br. Med. J., 1:522, 1966.

Markham, J. W., Lynge, H. N., and Stahlman, G. E. B.: The syndrome of spontaneous spinal epidural hematoma. Report of three cases. J. Neurosurg., 26:334, 1967.

Section Twenty-Two. DISEASES OF THE PERIPHERAL NERVOUS SYSTEM

Peter James Dyck

456. BIOLOGY OF THE PERIPHERAL NERVOUS SYSTEM

Peripheral nerves are made up of bundles of nerve fibers whose cell bodies lie within the ventral gray horn of the spinal cord (motor fibers), within the dorsal root ganglion (sensory fibers), and within autonomic ganglia. Myelinated and unmyelinated fibers are surrounded by longitudinally directed collagen fibrils (endoneurium). A bundle of fibers (a fascicle) is surrounded by a tough sheath (the perineurium) made up of neuroepithelial cells and collagen. Between the fascicles and surrounding them is the epineurium.

Peripheral nerves receive their blood supply along their length from various regional blood vessels. Anastomatic arteries, which lie in the epineurium, are formed by the branches from regional arteries. Only the arterioles penetrating the perineurium are thought to be end-arteries. Because of the nature of the blood supply, large-artery disease, unless extensive, does not usually cause infarction within the nerve, but small-artery and arteriolar disease may do so. The collateral blood supply also explains why a peripheral nerve may be undercut for long distances and placed into a new bed without becoming infarcted.

The peripheral nervous system includes all the cranial nerves (except the olfactory and the ocular) from their point of exit from the brainstem to their termination. It further includes all segmental nerve roots from their point of exit from the spinal cord; dorsal root ganglia; autonomic ganglia; mixed spinal nerves; brachial, lumbar, and sacral plexuses; and peripheral nerves. A knowledge of the anatomic arrangement of these structures is essential for adequately assessing the signs of motor, sensory, and autonomic dysfunction in disease of the peripheral nervous system. Since portions of both motor and sensory neurons lie within the spinal cord, it is apparent that diseases of these neurons may affect both the central and the peripheral nervous systems.

The electron microscope has clarified the nature of the structure of myelinated and unmyelinated fibers. Both myelinated and unmyelinated fibers are clothed along their length by a series of Schwann cells of neuroectodermal origin. Unmyelinated fibers, first described by Remak, usually occur in clusters. In transverse sections, individual fibers may be seen occupying invaginations of the Schwann cell cytoplasm; but they remain extracellular. Myelinated fibers in their development also extend into invaginations of Schwann cell cytoplasm, but in addition—either by rotation of Schwann cells or by differential growth—wrap Schwann cell membrane around themselves to form myelin. Especially from the x-ray diffraction and electron microscopic studies of nerve, it is now known that myelin is layered Schwann cell membrane and that nodes of Ranvier are constituted by abutment of two Schwann cells along a fiber.

There is evidence that certain macromolecules, such as enzymes and various proteins, are synthesized in the cell body and flow down the axis cylinder. In addition, Schwann cells have a trophic influence on the axis cylinder.

A lower motor unit is the anterior horn cell (including its axon and terminal branches) and the muscle fibers it innervates. Primary sensory units might be thought of as the nerve cell within the dorsal root ganglion which innervates a small region of skin by its peripheral axon and terminal branches. Its central axon makes connections within the spinal cord.

From the work of Gasser and Erlanger, it is known that if a peripheral nerve is laid on a series of electrodes in the appropriate environment, a rapidly conducted wave (usually called the A-α potential) evoked by low-voltage stimulation of large myelinated fibers can be detected. As the voltage is increased, other deflections appear that correspond to groups of small myelinated fibers (A-δ) and finally of unmyelinated fibers (C fibers). The modality of sensation lost in diseases of primary sensory neurons usually falls into one of three types: (1) selective decrease or loss of touch-pressure, two-point discrimination, and perception of joint position and motion, with preservation of pain and temperature sensation, from selective loss of large myelinated fibers; (2) sensory loss inverse to that just mentioned, from loss of unmyelinated and small myelinated fibers; and (3) loss of all sensory modalities, from loss of all groups of fibers.

457. PATHOLOGY OF THE PERIPHERAL NERVOUS SYSTEM

Pathologic changes in peripheral nerve tissue can be divided broadly into interstitial and parenchymatous. Interstitial pathologic changes arise outside the nerve and Schwann cells and may damage these cells secondarily. Usually in interstitial neuropathies the initial change is in the supporting tissue of the nerve or in its blood vessels. Examples of such neuropathies are amyloidosis, necrotizing angiopathy, and acute, chronic, and relapsing inflammatory polyradiculoneuropathy. In parenchymatous neuropathies the nerve and Schwann cells are primarily affected from various causes such as inherited metabolic diseases, toxic substances, deficiency states, and other metabolic diseases. Examples of parenchymatous neuropathies are those caused by alcohol, lead, arsenic, diphtheria, and metachromatic leukodystrophy.

Two histologic features of especial importance in peripheral nerve disease are, respectively, the formation of linear rows of myelin ovoids and myelin balls (wallerian degeneration or axonal degeneration) and the focal absence of myelin with preservation of the axis cylinder along the length of myelinated fibers (segmental demyelination). Linear rows of myelin ovoids and balls are formed in distal nerve fibers after crush or transection of nerve fibers. In parenchymatous neuropathy similar linear rows of myelin ovoids and balls are seen, but no mechanism of acute transection has been demonstrated, and the electron microscopic abnormalities of axis cylinders are not identical to wallerian degeneration. For these reasons a distinction should be made between the terms wallerian degeneration consequent to transection and the histologic changes of acute axonal degeneration. Segmental demyelination is usually interpreted as evidence of Schwann cell disease. Actually, however, segmental demyelination may also occur secondary to axis cylinder atrophy and degeneration. In many neuronal disorders such segmental demyelination and remyelination are clustered on degenerating fibers, especially at the distal aspect of the neuron. When demyelination and remyelination occur repetitively on fibers, "onion bulb" formations and increased collagen are formed. These characteristics of hypertrophic neuropathy therefore are found to varying degrees in a variety of neuropathies.

Although in many parenchymatous neuropathies the main symptoms, signs, and morphologic changes suggest involvement of the distal processes of the peripheral nervous system neurons only, this reflects more generalized disease of these neurons. Recently, peripheral nerve biopsy has been used to evaluate selected patients with peripheral neuropathy. Nerve biopsy, especially in patients with mild neuropathy, is often followed by a disagreeable or painful numbness and with a small region of sensory loss. The procedure should be done sparingly and only at centers which can adequately evaluate the tissue.

Fascicular or whole biopsy of such nerves as the sural may provide diagnostic information in leprosy, amyloidosis, angiopathic vasculopathy, inflammatory polyradiculoneuropathy, and various lipidoses. It may provide unequivocal evidence of the presence and of the type and severity of fiber degeneration. A subclinical or mild neuropathy may be recognized by good histologic evaluation of nerve biopsy tissue even when clinical examination and nerve conduction and electromyography are normal. Furthermore, an examination of teased-out fibers helps to identify the exact type of neuropathy. Nerve biopsy tissue may be studied electrophysiologically by recording the compound action potential, thus giving information not only about A-α fibers (which are also studied in vivo) but also about A-δ and C fibers. Nerve biopsy tissue may also be utilized for biochemical studies of lipids and of transport of such substances as dopamine beta hydroxylase.

458. MANIFESTATIONS OF PERIPHERAL NEUROPATHY

The hallmarks of peripheral neuropathy are muscle weakness with or without atrophy, sensory changes, autonomic manifestations, or mixtures of these, all in the appropriate anatomic distribution. Conventionally, peripheral neuropathy is considered to be a disorder of the peripheral nerves that affects predominantly the distal muscles of the extremity, and is associated with sensory loss of all modalities, which also is greatest distally and shades off to normal in more proximal regions of extremities. Although this is a common clinical pattern, not all neuropathies conform to it. Some polyradiculoneuropathies (for example, the Guillain-Barré syndrome) affect the ventral roots and varying amounts of the posterior roots and peripheral nerves, producing weakness in axial and proximal limb muscles as well as in the distal limb muscles. In other diseases such as Friedreich's ataxia or in subacute combined degeneration, the dorsal root ganglia neurons (in addition to other CNS structures) are particularly affected. In some maladies such as metachromatic leukodystrophy or Krabbe's disease, the central nervous system manifestations so dominate the clinical pattern that the disorder in nerve may be overlooked unless one subjects the nerve to histologic examination or measures its conduction velocity.

Patients with neuropathy may not have symptoms or may attribute them to other disease. Commonly the patient with an inherited neuropathy or a chronic neuropathy has no symptoms, or attributes them to a past accident or poliomyelitis. The insidious development of many neuropathies allows for accommodation to the disease. Motor symptoms in such patients are usually described as clumsiness of gait, difficulty in picking up the toes in walking, frequent tripping or stumbling, or inability to perform some ordinary act such as combing the hair, turning a key in a lock, or fastening a safety pin. Some patients notice muscle atrophy, but in chronic neuropathy many of them do not—presumably because the development is so gradual.

Patients with sensory nerve involvement may have symptoms of tightness, burning, jabbing, searing, pricking, tingling, and numbness. These are particularly common in the neuropathies associated with diabetes mellitus, vitamin deficiency, vasculitis, arsenic intoxication, and sprue. In other neuropathies, the predominant symptoms are not of pain or discomfort but rather of a decrease or loss of function, evident as inability to locate a pill in the mouth or to recognize a comb in the pocket, or as unsteadiness in walking owing to kinesthetic loss. Patients with a very slow course tend to have fewer symptoms. Patients with acute axonal degeneration of small and large fibers tend to have discomfort, whereas those with segmental demyelination predominantly usually have little if any. Loss of sympathetic nerve function, such as occurs in such diseases as diabetes mellitus and amyloidosis, results in postural hypotension, loss of sweating, and bladder and bowel incontinence.

459. DEFINITION, DIFFERENTIAL DIAGNOSIS, AND CLASSIFICATION OF PERIPHERAL NEUROPATHY

The cells of the peripheral motor nerves lie in the anterior horn of the spinal cord or in autonomic ganglia, and the cells of sensory fibers lie in the dorsal root ganglia. Many diseases that start in the peripheral nerve sooner or later affect the perikaryon (cell body) and vice versa, so that peripheral neuropathies, anterior horn cell diseases, radicular sensory disorders, and even diseases of the dorsal columns have a certain biologic overlap. This chapter arbitrarily gives attention to conditions in which the peripheral nerve is heavily affected. The relations among these several disorders can be seen by examining the accompanying table.

In evaluating a patient with possible peripheral nerve disease, it is first necessary to establish that there is disease of the peripheral nerves. In some cases the clinical symptoms, the diffuse muscle weakness and atrophy, and the sensory loss may unequivocally suggest a disorder of peripheral nerves. In patients with only muscle weakness and atrophy with either no or equivocal sensory loss, it may be difficult to decide whether the disease is neurogenic or myogenic, but there are three types of study that may help. (1) Concentrations of such serum enzymes as phosphocreatine kinase and the transaminases are often elevated in muscle disease but are usually normal or only slightly elevated in neurogenic muscular atrophy. (2) A particularly helpful study is determination of the conduction velocity of nerves and electromyography. In disease of muscle, conduction velocity of nerves should be normal, unless spuriously decreased by low temperature or by pressure palsies from the patient's remaining in bed for a long time. Conduction velocities may be normal in neurogenic muscle atrophy as well, but in this situation the characteristics of the

Classification of Peripheral Neuropathy

I. Mononeuropathy and plexus neuropathies
   - A. Cranial nerves
   - B. Peripheral nerves
     - 1. Physical injury
     - 2. Entrapment neuropathies
       - a. Carpal tunnel syndrome
       - b. Tardy ulnar nerve palsy
       - c. Acute radial nerve palsy
       - d. Acute and tardy peroneal nerve palsy
       - e. Tarsal tunnel syndrome
       - f. Meralgia paresthetica
       - g. Thoracic outlet syndrome
     - 3. Mononeuropathy multiplex
     - 4. Plexus neuropathy
       - a. Brachial plexus neuropathy
       - b. Lumbar and sacral plexus neuropathy

II. Multiple neuropathy
   - A. Associated with malnutrition and vitamin deficiency
     - 1. In alcoholism
     - 2. In malnutrition
     - 3. In pellagra
     - 4. In celiac disease
     - 5. In pernicious anemia
     - 6. In postgastrectomy condition
   - B. Associated with carcinoma and other malignancy
     - 1. Primary sensory neuropathy with carcinoma
     - 2. Mixed neuropathy with carcinoma
     - 3. Peripheral neuropathy with lymphoma
   - C. Associated with mesenchymal disease and with necrotizing arteritis
   - D. Associated with diabetes mellitus
   - E. Associated with drugs and toxins
     - 1. Heavy metals
       - a. Lead
       - b. Arsenic
       - c. Thallium
       - d. Mercury
       - e. Copper, antimony, and zinc
     - 2. Organophosphate compounds (TOCP)
     - 3. Industrial poisons
     - 4. Drugs
   - F. Neuropathy associated with hormonal disturbances
   - G. Neuropathy associated with possible immunologic disorders
     - 1. Acute inflammatory polyradiculoneuropathy of the Guillain-Barré-Strohl type
     - 2. Chronic and relapsing inflammatory polyradiculoneuropathy
     - 3. Serum neuropathy
   - H. Neuropathy associated with infection
     - 1. Diphtheria
     - 2. Leprosy
   - I. Neuropathy associated with inborn errors of metabolism (hereditary disorders)
     - 1. Predominant involvement of lower motor neurons
       - a. Hereditary proximal motor neuropathy
         - Infantile
         - Juvenile
         - Adult
       - b. Hereditary distal motor neuropathy
       - c. Hereditary scapuloperoneal motor neuropathy
       - d. Hereditary facioscapulohumeral motor neuropathy
       - e. Motor neuron disease
       - f. Progressive bulbar paresis of childhood
     - 2. Predominant involvement of primary sensory neurons
       - a. Inherited sensory neuropathy, Type I (dominantly inherited sensory radicular neuropathy)
       - b. Inherited sensory neuropathy, Type II (recessively inherited congenital sensory neuropathy)
       - c. Inherited sensory neuropathy, Type III (Riley-Day syndrome)
       - d. Inherited sensory neuropathy, Type IV
       - e. Angiokeratoma corporis diffusum (Fabry's)
     - 3. Involvement of lower motor or primary sensory neurons and other systems
       - a. Spinocerebellar degeneration
       - b. Friedreich's ataxia
       - c. Spastic paraplegia with peroneal muscular atrophy
       - d. Hypo-β-lipoproteinemia (Bassen and Kornzweig)
       - e. Hypo-α-lipoproteinemia (Tangier disease)
       - f. Hereditary motor and sensory neuropathy, Types I–VII
       - g. Acute intermittent porphyria
       - h. Dominantly inherited amyloidosis (Portuguese)
       - i. Dominantly inherited amyloidosis (Indiana)
   - J. Associated with peripheral vascular disease
   - K. Associated with uremia
   - L. Of unknown cause

electromyographic examination may be distinguishing (see Ch. 358). (3) Biopsy of muscle or nerve. The diagnostic usefulness of these methods of examination varies considerably in different clinics, primarily because of differences in the experience of the persons doing the studies. Neither enzyme tests nor electrophysiologic studies ever provide a specific diagnosis, and the muscle and nerve biopsies do so only infrequently.

A second differential to be made is between disorders of peripheral nerve and disorders of central nervous system disease. In peripheral disorders, muscle weakness is usually associated with atrophy, denervation in electromyographic studies, decrease or absence of the tendon reflexes, and a pattern of sensory loss compatible with disease of multiple nerves. In central lesions muscle weakness is usually unaccompanied by atrophy, tendon reflexes are hyperactive with corticospinal and corticobulbar tract signs, and sensory loss is of the type seen in spinal cord or cerebral hemisphere disease.

Probably the most satisfactory method of classifying the peripheral neuropathies would be based on etiology. Unfortunately, however, the precise etiologic factors for most neuropathies are unknown. Additionally, the diagnosis of many other neuropathies depends entirely on an association with a disease, such as diabetes mellitus, carcinoma, or uremia.

Neuropathies may also be classified by the anatomic site of involvement: cranial neuropathy and peripheral neuropathy, mononeuropathy (single nerves) and multiple neuropathy (multiple nerves), radiculopathy (roots), and plexus neuropathy (brachial, lumbar, or sacral plexus). They may be classified as motor, sensory, and autonomic neuropathy, depending on the predominant type of fiber involvement. On the basis of their rate of progression, neuropathies may be divided into acute, subacute, and chronic categories. In general, they may further be divided into those associated with diffuse low conduction velocity of peripheral nerves (a velocity less than 60 per cent of the mean for normal nerves probably signifies a demyelinating type of fiber degeneration), and those in which the conduction velocities are borderline or only slightly reduced but in which there is other electrophysiologic evidence of fiber degeneration (probably an axonal type of fiber degeneration). Another classification is based on the nature of the sensory loss: in one type there is a selective loss of touch-pressure, two-point discrimination, and joint position, indicating involvement of large myelinated fibers; in another type there is a selective loss of pain and temperature sensation and of autonomic function, indicating loss of unmyelinated fibers; and in a third type there is loss of all sensory modalities, indicating loss of all groups of fibers. Pathologic classifications are based on the nature of the fiber degeneration (wallerian, axonal degeneration, segmental demyelination) or site of pathologic changes, as well as on the specific histologic pattern (vasculitis, granulomatous reaction, hypertrophic neuropathy, amyloidosis, and specific infective organism).

MONONEUROPATHY AND PLEXUS NEUROPATHIES

460. CRANIAL NERVES

Olfactory. Anosmia is most often the result of local disease in the nasal passageways, skull fracture, or brain tumor and is usually reported by the patient as a defect in taste.

Optic. Any visual field defect is a serious matter and demands thorough investigation. Permanent visual impairment or blindness can occur because of unnecessary delay in the diagnosis and treatment of benign and removable compressive lesions such as meningiomas, craniopharyngiomas, cholesteatomas, and chromophobe adenomas. Intrinsic lesions of the optic nerves, such as occur in multiple sclerosis, tend to produce scotomas, whereas compressive lesions like tumors and carotid aneurysms predispose to monocular and binasal or bitemporal visual field defects. Homonymous field defects are usually the result of lesions of the optic pathways posterior to the chiasm, generally as the result of lesions involving the brain itself.

Oculomotor, Trochlear, and Abducens. The motor nerves to the eye may be damaged by a variety of diseases anywhere in their long course from brainstem to orbit. Tumor, aneurysm, and temporal lobe herniation often cause oculomotor palsy, usually with pupillary involvement. A slightly dilated pupil and sluggish response to light may be early, subtle signs of third-nerve compression. Either purulent or granulomatous meningitis may impair third- or, more commonly, sixth-nerve function. Increased intracranial pressure may cause unilateral or, especially, bilateral abducens palsy.

Loss of normal eye movement can be a difficult diagnostic problem. The rapid onset of oculomotor palsy associated with pain around or behind the eye immediately suggests diabetic mononeuropathy, migraine, or intracranial aneurysm. However, in as many as one third of such cases no satisfactory cause is found. The pupil is usually dilated with aneurysm and migraine, but not in diabetes or in the idiopathic types. Aneurysm is frequently, but not always, accompanied by hypertension and subarachnoid hemorrhage. A history of typical headache, previous ocular palsy, and occurrence in childhood favors migraine. Diabetic ophthalmoplegia occasionally also includes the sixth nerve and may occur with only mild glucose intolerance; improvement usually begins within three to five weeks, though diplopia persists until motor balance is nearly perfect. Occurrence of other neurologic deficits, along with impaired ocular motility, is common with aneurysm or tumor, and is expected with a midbrain infarct. *Myasthenia gravis* can affect extraocular muscles as an isolated symptom and should be considered, especially when the weakness differs from typical cranial nerve patterns, is inconstant, includes eye opening and closing, does not involve the pupil, and is bilateral.

Abnormalities of pupillary size, shape, and reaction are not confined to third-nerve injuries. The *Argyll Robertson pupil* is small, irregular, usually bilateral, responds to convergence accommodation but not to light, and responds poorly to mydriatics; it is common with neurosyphilis and rare with diabetes. The pupils of diabetics are often unequal and may be completely nonreactive. *Adie's myotonic pupil* may cause confusion. It reacts only slowly to light or accommodation convergence, but constricts to fresh 2.5 per cent mecholyl instilled in the conjunctival sac, whereas a normal pupil does not.

Bilateral external ophthalmoplegia of rapid or sudden onset occurs with four diseases, all of which are potentially serious and demand prompt treatment: *acute myasthenia gravis, acute thiamin deficiency with Wer-*

nicke's syndrome, botulism, and *acute idiopathic cranial polyneuropathy.*

Trigeminal. Impairment of function peripherally in the sensory components of the trigeminal nerve may result from a variety of neoplastic and inflammatory processes. Divergence of the third division from the first and second, which pass forward through the cavernous sinus, frequently allows precise localization.

Trigeminal neuralgia is described in Ch. 349.

Facial. Brain injury above the facial nucleus usually spares the brow and forehead muscles because they are bilaterally represented at higher nervous levels; injury to the facial nerve at, or peripheral to, its nucleus paralyzes all the ipsilateral facial muscles. An intrapontine lesion causing facial weakness usually also affects abducens nerve function. As the facial nerve leaves the pons and enters the internal auditory meatus along with the acoustic nerve, it also carries fibers for lacrimation, salivation, and taste. As the nerve descends through the petrous bone, fibers to the lacrimal glands branch off first, then salivary and taste fibers depart in the chorda tympani and cross the middle ear. Only motor fibers to the face emerge from the stylomastoid foramen. Thus the syndrome of seventh nerve damage varies according to the site of injury. Acoustic neurinomas and other tumors of the cerebellopontine angle often involve the facial nerves, as do infections and neoplasms of the meninges.

Bell's palsy is a peripheral facial weakness of unknown cause and rapid onset, occasionally attended by aching pain about the angle of the jaw or behind the ear. Recent work has shown that the point of nerve conduction block is usually in the vicinity of the internal auditory meatus. Retraction of the angle of the mouth and eye closure are impaired, and the forehead is smooth on the affected side. Taste perception on the anterior part of the involved half of the tongue may be distorted. Rarely, hyperacusis results from paralysis of the stapedius muscle. Recovery usually begins within a week, and three of four patients fully recover over a period of several weeks. Occasionally, some permanent deficit remains after a protracted course. In these cases, distressing facial spasms may accompany voluntary facial movement. Adrenal corticosteroids begun near the onset of the illness and continued for seven to ten days may favor a more rapid and complete recovery.

Herpes zoster affecting the geniculate ganglion produces a severe facial paralysis that is associated with a painful eruption within the external ear canal. This, often referred to as the *Ramsay Hunt syndrome,* may also involve the auditory nerve.

Chronic facial hemispasm affects middle-aged or older women somewhat more commonly than men, with spontaneous, unilateral, frequent, sudden, strong, brief contractions of part or all of the facial musculature. The condition usually begins with the orbicularis oculi muscle and, over many years, spreads to involve more of the face. The cause is not known, but a slowly progressive, degenerative condition of the facial nucleus in the pons has been postulated. Relief can be obtained by alcohol injection or section of the facial nerve, but it must be weighed against the facial paralysis necessarily produced.

Auditory. Disturbances of eighth nerve function are discussed in Ch. 351 and 352.

Glossopharyngeal, Vagus, and Spinal Accessory. The glossopharyngeal and vagus nerves supply sensory and motor innervation to the pharynx. They may be involved by tumor or aneurysm along with the spinal accessory nerves in their common exit through the jugular foramen. Hoarseness and asymmetric elevation of the soft palate result from lesions of the vagus nerve, and weakness and atrophy of sternocleidomastoid and superior trapezoid muscles result from disruption of the spinal accessory.

Glossopharyngeal neuralgia is described in Ch. 349.

Hypoglossal. This motor nerve to the tongue is rarely involved in its peripheral course. Atrophy and fasciculation of the ipsilateral half of the tongue are seen, and the tongue deviates toward the affected side upon protrusion.

461. PERIPHERAL NERVES

Physical Injury. Spinal nerves, plexuses, and peripheral nerve trunks may be injured by traction, compression, contusion, and laceration. Nerves may be damaged by electricity and radiation. Fractured bones may lacerate or compress nerves. Excessively tight casts or tourniquets may damage nerves by direct compression or by ischemia. Injection of penicillin or other medications into the sciatic nerve can cause serious injury. In Sunderland's textbook (1968) details on these and other nerve injuries are presented.

Entrapment Neuropathies. Peripheral nerves may be injured by compression or ischemia at points where they pass through rigid anatomic canals or beneath tight fascial bands. Such injury occurs more readily when inflammation or degeneration develops in adjacent joints and tendons (as may happen in rheumatoid arthritis, myxedema, and acromegaly), and when the nerves lie in shallow grooves allowing them to be compressed or repeatedly traumatized.

Carpal Tunnel Syndrome. In the carpal tunnel syndrome the median nerve is compressed as it passes through the canal made by the carpal bones and ligament. Some cases are idiopathic, and, in these, surgeons report a flattening of the median nerve just distal to the crease of the wrist and either thickening of the ligament or, more commonly, noninflammatory thickening of the synovia of the flexor tendons. The median nerve may be compressed within the carpal tunnel by a ganglion or by degenerative joint and synovial changes from rheumatoid arthritis, myxedema, and acromegaly.

This common disorder especially affects women. Pricking numbness and pain in the fingers and hands, coming on especially during the night and relieved by changing the position of the hands (shaking them), are characteristic. It is uncommon for patients to localize the numbness to the exact cutaneous distribution of the median nerve. Furthermore, the aching discomfort that may accompany the numbness may extend up the arm. Atrophy of the muscles innervated by the median nerve (for example, the thenar muscles) is not an early sign. In many cases it is possible to reproduce the painful numbness by holding the wrist in extreme flexion for a short period *(Phalen's sign).* Also a burst of tingling may occur when the skin over the nerve at the wrist is percussed *(Tinel's sign).* There may be sensory loss in the distribution of the median nerve, though more frequently none is detected.

An important confirmatory test can now be done in most electromyographic laboratories. It consists in determining the time from stimulation of the median nerve at a point above the carpal ligament to the appearance of the thenar muscle action potential. Similarly, one can determine the time from stimulation of digital fibers to the obtaining of an action potential in electrodes overlying the median nerve above the carpal ligament. In the carpal tunnel syndrome, the latency of both responses is usually prolonged.

Since the carpal tunnel syndrome may be brought on by an excess of gardening, ironing, sewing, crocheting, or similar activity, relief may follow their discontinuance. Immobilization of the wrist during the hours of sleep with a posterior splint of forearm and hand may give relief. Injections of corticosteroid preparations beneath the carpal ligament sometimes help. Treatment for an associated disease (myxedema, rheumatoid arthritis, acromegaly) may effect an improvement. However, in most instances the treatment of choice is surgical section of the carpal ligament, which usually provides almost immediate relief.

Tardy Ulnar Nerve Palsy. The ulnar nerve may be injured at the elbow, especially in persons with a shallow ulnar groove, those who rest their weight on their elbows excessively, and those who are cachectic and lie in bed.

Contrary to the finding in the carpal tunnel syndrome, muscle weakness and atrophy characteristically predominate over sensory symptoms and signs, possibly because the ulnar nerve at the elbow has relatively fewer sensory fibers than the median nerve at the wrist. Characteristically, the patient notices atrophy of the first dorsal interosseous muscle or difficulty in performing fine manipulations. There may be numbness of the small finger and contiguous half of the proximal and middle phalanges of the ring finger and ulnar border of the hand. Treatment consists in prevention of further injury. A doughnut cushion for the elbow may be helpful. Mobilizing and transplanting the nerve to a position in front of the median epicondyle may prevent further progression of the disorder.

Acute Radial Nerve Palsy. The radial nerve may be compressed against a hard edge or surface after digesting an excess of alcohol or sedatives (Saturday night palsy) or may be compressed for excessive periods by the weight of the head of another (bridegroom's palsy). With time, complete recovery may be expected.

Acute and Tardy Peroneal Nerve Palsy. The common peroneal nerve is vulnerable where it crosses the head of the fibula, and can be injured when a person falls asleep in the sitting position with the knees crossed. A more chronic form occurs in cachectic patients who lie for prolonged periods with the legs externally rotated. In this disorder, dorsiflexion of the foot at the ankle and extension of the toes are weak, but usually little or no sensory loss is found over the lateral surface of the leg and on the dorsum of the foot.

Tarsal Tunnel Syndrome. In fractures of the ankle, compression of the posterior tibial nerve may occur, resulting in pain and numbness of the sole of the foot.

Meralgia Paresthetica. Fat people wearing tight corsets, people wearing gun belts, and people with pendulous abdomens may develop superficial paresthesia and burning discomfort in the distribution of the lateral cutaneous nerve of the thigh. Presumably the trouble results from compression of this nerve as it passes beneath the inguinal ligament.

Thoracic Outlet Syndrome. Formerly, paresthesias of the fingers were frequently attributed to compression of the brachial plexus by a cervical rib or a tight scalene anterior muscle. However, most such patients prove to have either a cervical disc or carpal tunnel syndrome.

Mononeuropathy Multiplex. The term "mononeuropathy multiplex" implies that a process involves several individual peripheral nerves in different regions of the body. Characteristically, the disorder begins with pain, paresthesias, or weakness in the distribution of a peripheral nerve which progresses to a maximal deficit within a few hours to several days. Other nerves become affected within days. The nerves of the lower extremities are affected more often than those of the upper, and signs are usually asymmetric. After the initial involvement the disorder may improve, relapse, or deteriorate. This type of neuropathy is a common manifestation of polyarteritis nodosa, but is also encountered in diabetes mellitus, rheumatoid arthritis, disseminated lupus erythematosus, and scleroderma.

The pathologic changes in most instances affect the interfascicular arteries of nerves, which may show degeneration of the media, fragmentation of the internal elastic lamina, thickening of the intima, and infiltration of the media and adventitia by mononuclear cells and polymorphonuclear cells (especially eosinophils). At necropsy arterioles with an occluded lumen may be widespread along the length of the nerve. Regions of fiber degeneration do not coincide with these occluded vessels, but begin in isolated central regions of fascicles at watershed zones of poor blood supply. For the ulnar and median nerves these zones are at mid-upper arm; for the peroneal and tibial nerves they are at midthigh. Because of separation and recombination of fascicles at more distal levels of the nerve, degenerating fibers in a section from the nerve taken distal to these regions of fiber degeneration may contain in many of its fascicles degenerating fibers that come from the same circumsected origin.

Plexus Neuropathy. *Brachial Plexus.* The brachial plexus can be injured by traction, penetrating wounds, or compression. *Acute nontraumatic brachial plexus neuropathy* is a disorder of unknown cause. Antecedent needle injections into shoulder muscles, intercurrent infections, and an allergic basis have been suggested as possible etiologic factors. Typically this disorder begins with aching pain in the lateral aspect of the shoulder or, less often, in the region of the elbow or arm. Muscle weakness develops within a few hours or days, and atrophy follows; sensory loss is usually minimal and is restricted to a small patch in the cutaneous distribution of the axillary nerve. The upper brachial plexus is much more commonly affected than the lower, and therefore the weakness and atrophy are more often located in the region of the shoulder. In mild cases, improvement begins in a few weeks, and clinical recovery is complete within months. More characteristically, improvement does not begin for several months and may not be complete for years. Recently it has been shown that the likelihood of eventual complete or almost complete recovery is good. Sometimes, as improvement on one side occurs, the other brachial plexus becomes affected. Careful examination by electromyography may reveal much more extensive involvement of nerves as expected from the clinical examination. The cerebrospinal fluid is usually normal. There is no known treatment.

Lumbar and Sacral Plexus and Roots. Under the term *femoral neuropathy,* a disorder has been described which in many cases arises from the lumbar plexus.

Many such cases occur in association with diabetes, but sometimes no associated illness is found. Pain centered in the thigh and extending to the medial side of the leg may herald the onset of muscle weakness and atrophy, which usually develops rather rapidly over the next week. If the onset is abrupt and the neurologic signs are restricted to the distribution of the femoral nerve, an infarction of that nerve is a possibility. Careful examination and electromyography, however, often indicate that the condition is more widespread. Such studies often indicate that multiple lumbar and sacral roots are affected with or without involvement of lumbar and sacral plexuses (in reality a lumbosacral radiculoplexus neuropathy). The cerebrospinal fluid protein may be elevated. Although recovery may not occur before months or years have passed, the prognosis is good.

Occasionally, patients with lumbosacral plexus neuropathy present with the symptoms of sciatica, which differs from that caused by disk disease in the lack of a history of injury, the lack (usually) of marked back symptoms, and the clinical and electromyographic evidence of involvement of multiple roots and the negative myelogram. Although marked muscle weakness and wasting may occur, the outlook is usually favorable. The cause, pathology, and treatment are unknown.

MULTIPLE NEUROPATHY

462. NEUROPATHY ASSOCIATED WITH MALNUTRITION AND VITAMIN DEFICIENCY

The common feature of these disorders is deficiency of one or more essentials in the diet owing either to inadequate intake (as in alcoholism, hyperemesis of pregnancy, food fads, and starvation) or failure of absorption (as in pernicious anemia, sprue, or gastrointestinal cancer). The pathologic changes in the peripheral nerves are similar in that distal axons of large fibers are affected first and more severely than proximal parts. Rows of myelin breakdown products are seen along peripheral nerves. At the dorsal root ganglion level there may be some slight decrease in the number of neurons. The posterior columns may show some demyelination. Ordinarily the conduction velocities of the nerves are not markedly abnormal. These disorders are also discussed in Ch. 404 to 411.

463. NEUROPATHY ASSOCIATED WITH CARCINOMA AND OTHER MALIGNANCY

In malignancy, peripheral nerves may be affected by direct implantation, by compression against bony structures, and by remote unknown mechanisms (see Part X, Section Eighteen). Sites at which peripheral nerves may be compressed are the foramina of exit of the segmental nerves, the retroperitoneal space, and the nasopharynx. Neuropathy in a patient with malignancy may also develop from drugs used in treatment, as from vinca alkaloids in treatment of lymphoma.

Mixed Neuropathy with Carcinoma. Mixed sensory motor neuropathies have been found in association with carcinoma of the bronchus, gastrointestinal tract, thyroid, ovary, and other organs. Whether this is a specific association or is due to nutritional effects is still unknown.

Peripheral Neuropathy with Lymphoma. Peripheral neuropathies have been found in association with multiple myeloma and various leukemias and lymphomas. The lack of pain and the symmetry of the disorder are usually interpreted as indicating that the peripheral nerve involvement is a remote effect and not due to direct invasion. However, such invasion has been demonstrated in a few cases, particularly when meticulously searched for. The treatment for the neuropathy is the treatment for the primary tumor.

464. NEUROPATHY ASSOCIATED WITH MESENCHYMAL DISEASE AND NECROTIZING ANGIITIS

The neuropathy associated with these disorders is usually a mononeuropathy multiplex as described above. However, in a small percentage of cases the onset is that of a symmetrical multiple neuropathy. With the latter presentation, the correct category of disease is suggested by the painful nature of sensory symptoms and the associated signs of multiple tissue involvement.

465. NEUROPATHY ASSOCIATED WITH DIABETES MELLITUS

It is now known that most patients with diabetes mellitus have some dysfunction of the peripheral nerves, and that even those who are asymptomatic may have an abnormality of conduction velocity. The neuropathies fall into two types: mononeuropathy, involving single cranial nerves such as the oculomotor or large single peripheral nerves and plexuses, as described in Ch. 460 and 461, and polyneuropathy, as described here.

Pathology. Neither the pathogenesis nor the pathology of diabetic neuropathy is fully understood. The greater amount of atherosclerosis of limb vessels of diabetic patients probably does not account for the neuropathy. If the polyneuropathy is due to ischemia, it is more likely to be due to a specific angiopathy involving small arteries or arterioles. Thickening of the basement membranes of such vessels has been described. It is not clear whether the observed segmental demyelination is due to ischemia or to deranged metabolism selectively affecting Schwann cells, or whether it is secondary to nerve fiber change.

Clinical Manifestations. Many diabetics have asymptomatic polyneuropathy. Symptomatic polyneuropathy is typically a symmetric, distal sensorimotor neuropathy occurring in elderly patients with mild diabetes. Sensory symptoms in the toes and feet predominate and include numbness, burning paresthesia, and stabbing pains. The soles of the feet are often excessively sensitive to tactile or painful stimuli, rendering walking unpleasant. In the majority of patients with diabetic neuropathy, touch-pressure, vibration, and joint position sensations are predominantly affected, presumably because of a greater involvement of large myelinated fibers. If the loss of position sensation is severe, locomotor ataxia develops (pseudotabes diabetica). The ataxia is worse in the dark. Those patients with much discomfort are usually found to have loss of pain sensation, temperature sensation, and autonomic function, presumably owing to loss of small myelinated and of unmyelinated fibers. The disorder usually develops insidiously and may remain static or progress over the course of many years. It is unlikely to remit, as are the femoral, lumbar, and lumbosacral radiculoplexus, and oculomotor neuropathies. It has not been established that good control of the blood sugar with insulin or with oral hypoglycemic agents prevents the development or results in improvement of symptomatic neuropathy. Charcot joints, although rare, do occur. Disturbances of intestinal motility, loss of hair, and shiny tight dry skin are attributable to autonomic nerve damage.

One clinical variant of the neurologic complications of diabetes has been called diabetic amyotrophy. Older males with recent substantial weight loss are said to be predominantly affected. Bilateral asymmetric proximal weakness of the lower limbs, with anterior thigh pain, myalgia, and muscle wasting, is seen. Some have extensor plantar responses. Based on the characteristics of the electromyographic examination, patients with the aforementioned symptoms usually can be shown to have involvement of multiple lumbar nerve roots or of the lumbar or sacral plexus. The relatively abrupt onset and good prognosis exclude spondylosis as a cause. Most of the cases described under this term would probably fall under the previously described category of femoral neuropathy, which in reality is a lumbosacral radiculoplexus neuropathy.

The protein concentration of the cerebrospinal fluid in diabetic neuropathy is often elevated from 50 to 400 mg per 100 ml.

Treatment. It is the current practice to maintain good control of the blood sugar in order to prevent or improve neuropathy in spite of the lack of evidence of such prevention or improvement. There is a suggestion from some reports that repeated hypoglycemic attacks may hasten the onset or worsen the existing neuropathic state. To prevent trophic ulcers of the feet in patients with loss of pain and temperature sensation, good foot care and special shoes are needed.

466. NEUROPATHY ASSOCIATED WITH DRUGS AND TOXINS

Many drugs and toxins can damage peripheral nerves, and new agents constantly join the list. Publicity, legislation, and education have reduced the frequency of poisoning by some of the older chemicals.

Heavy Metals. Peripheral neuropathy has been reported in association with lead, arsenic, thallium, mercury, copper, antimony, and zinc. However, only the first two occur with any frequency.

Lead poisoning was formerly a common occurrence, but is becoming rare. Lead ingestion or inhalation may occur among farm workers using insecticides (for example, arsenate of lead), among painters using lead paint, among children who chew lead-containing paint from cribs and walls, among factory workers burning batteries or working with white lead, and among persons who drink beer or water stored in lead-lined containers or sent through lead pipes. Upper abdominal colic, joint pain, peripheral neuropathy, and encephalopathy develop. The encephalopathy is particularly characteristic of toxicity in children. The neuropathy is mainly motor and asymmetric, beginning in the upper extremity with wrist drop and weakness of the extensor muscles of fingers.

The peripheral nerves in lead neuropathy undergo axonal degeneration and segmental demyelination. The normal amount of lead in the urine ranges from 0.00 to 0.06 mg per liter. For a diagnosis of lead poisoning the value should be at least twice this. (See Ch. 29.)

Arsenic has been a favorite choice for homicide. Arsenic poisoning has also resulted from drinking illegal alcohol ("moonshine") and from eating food sprayed with insecticides. It is manifested by vomiting and other gastrointestinal symptoms, a scaly exfoliating rash, and evidences of neuropathy. White lines in the fingernails (Aldrich-Mees lines) may provide a diagnostic clue.

Arsenic poisoning produces a mixed motor and sensory neuropathy which is symmetric and distal and affects the lower extremities preferentially. The nerve fibers undergo an axonal type of degeneration. Diagnosis is made by identifying increased levels of arsenic in the nails, hair, or urine. (See Ch. 28.)

Thallium neuropathy has the clinical features of arsenic neuropathy but is associated with loss of hair.

Organophosphate (Triorthocresylphosphate) Compounds. Widespread ingestion of fluid extract of ginger in the United States in 1930 was followed by thousands of cases of severe polyneuropathy, mostly motor and distal in distribution. It was established that adulteration with triorthocresylphosphate was responsible and, since that time, periodic outbreaks have occurred traceable to adulterated cooking oil. Usually, stolen motor oil has been sold for cooking purposes. The neuropathy is delayed 10 to 14 days after poisoning. Imperfect recovery is the rule. Years after the acute poisoning, spastic paraparesis emerges, indicating that damage to the spinal cord occurs but is not immediately apparent because of the severe neuropathy. There is no effective treatment.

Industrial Poisons. Trichlorethylene, an anesthetic agent, is also a powerful solvent used in industry. In toxic amounts, it produces multiple cranial nerve palsies and trigeminal nerve analgesia. Particularly in Japan, n-hexane, an organic solvent used in printing, extraction of vegetable oil, and cleaning, has been associated with peripheral neuropathy. Acrylamide is a chemical that is pumped into soil to render it waterproof. In both man and animals, it produces peripheral neuropathy by an axonal type of degeneration of myelinated fibers. A recent outbreak of peripheral neuropathy in Japan was traced to the eating of fish which contained an excessive content of organic mercury.

Drugs. Many medicaments can produce numbness in

distal extremities and neurogenic weakness, including isoniazid, diphenylhydantoin sodium, nitrofurantoin, and the vinca alkaloids. Arsenic in Fowler's solution, mercury in various antisyphilitic preparations, and gold in treatment for rheumatoid arthritis also can produce peripheral neuropathy. The medication clioquinol, used frequently in Japan for nonspecific gastrointestinal disturbances, has now been implicated in subacute myelo-opticoneuropathy (SMON). Dosages of 1 gram or more per day for a period of one week or longer may lead to abdominal colic and numbness of the feet. Prolonged use may lead to severe neuropathy, spasticity, and optic atrophy.

467. NEUROPATHY ASSOCIATED WITH HORMONAL DISTURBANCES

Myxedema and acromegaly both predispose to the syndrome of the carpal tunnel. In myxedema a more diffuse peripheral neuropathy may occur.

468. NEUROPATHY ASSOCIATED WITH POSSIBLE IMMUNOLOGIC DISORDERS

ACUTE INFLAMMATORY POLYRADICULONEUROPATHY
(Postinfectious Polyneuritis, Guillain-Barré-Strohl Syndrome)

Etiology. The cause is unknown, although a similar illness has been produced in animals by inoculating extracts of peripheral nerve plus adjuvants. This, plus the characteristic postinfectious timing, has led many workers to postulate an autoimmune mechanism.

Pathology. The pathologic changes bear some resemblance to those of experimental allergic neuritis. There are foci of mononuclear cells in the roots and in the peripheral nerves, and these are associated with segmental demyelination. Proximal slowing of conduction velocity may be seen in about a third of the cases. In others the low conduction velocities are more generalized.

Clinical Manifestations. Many, but not all, patients give a history of a banal, nonspecific, febrile illness, usually respiratory, preceding the neurologic disorder by 10 to 21 days. The polyneuropathy usually begins insidiously and without fever, malaise, nausea, or prostration. In most instances, motor weakness is predominant. A few patients suffer muscle pain or, occasionally, stiff neck. Weakness may start in the face or hands but is most common in the lower extremities, and always is bilateral, though sometimes asymmetrical. The motor paralysis is flaccid and has a considerable tendency to ascend the body *(Landry's ascending paralysis)* and to involve both the trunk and upper limbs. Less frequently, paralysis affects the face, the muscles of swallowing, or the oculomotor muscles. About 5 per cent of patients develop urinary retention. Sensory symptoms and signs affect 90 per cent of patients. Paresthesias usually begin in the toes and fingers, and may spread proximally, but *demonstrable sensory* deficits are usually modest. Variant onsets are common, and weakness may begin in the upper limbs or even in the oculomotor muscles. Progression may cease at any point in the course. Once weakness reaches its maximum, a plateau occurs that lasts for several days to several weeks, depending on the individual. After this, improvement begins and continues for weeks or, rarely, many months. About one patient in 20 develops papilledema.

An acute inflammatory polyradiculoneuropathy of dorsal roots may produce the sensory counterpart of the same illness that affects ventral roots (usually called the Guillain-Barré-Strohl syndrome). Like the predominantly motor form, the development of the sensory disorder can be acute or subacute, the maximal deficit developing over days to a few weeks. The disorder may first be heralded by lancinating pain. Subsequently pain may continue, but its quality may turn into a more constant hyperpathia. Additional symptoms may come from sensory ataxia. The sensory loss sometimes persists—possibly because the perikarya of cells have been irreversibly damaged. Areflexia, cutaneous sensory loss, and absence of compound nerve action potentials from afferent fibers of median, ulnar, and sural nerves are characteristic.

The classic cerebrospinal fluid findings are of a normal pressure with an elevated protein concentration but without increased numbers of leukocytes. However, many exceptions exist, and the protein concentration may be normal at any time in the course of the illness, particularly at the onset. Rarely, a mild lymphocytosis is discovered in the cerebrospinal fluid at the outset of the disease.

The prognosis for full recovery from paralysis is good but not invariable, and perhaps one of ten patients is left with muscle weakness of some degree. Without mechanical ventilation, there is 10 to 20 per cent mortality, the result of respiratory and vasomotor failure. Thus, upon first encounter with the patient, even one in whom weakness may be slight and distal, the physician must anticipate a possible need for a respirator and vasopressor agents within a day or so.

Treatment. Adrenal steroids have been widely used to treat severe cases, but there are no controlled studies by which to judge their effectiveness, and it is difficult to know whether they are beneficial. Skilled nursing care is imperative, as is the availability of an intensive care unit to manage potential respiratory insufficiency. Full convalescence may require months, and a few patients suffer recurrent bouts of weakness and a relapsing course that may go on for years.

CHRONIC AND RELAPSING INFLAMMATORY POLYRADICULONEUROPATHY

This disorder may be the same as the preceding one, except that possibly the pathogenic mechanisms persist, and so the disorder continues. Typically, the onset is much more protracted, and the disease is more prolonged; but the symptoms are symmetric and predominantly motor. In some patients spontaneous remissions and relapses occur. When sensory loss is present, it affects the modalities of touch-pressure, joint position, and vibration in particular. Occasionally papilledema develops, but usually without headaches or focal cerebral disorders. In addition, a tremor with the features of essential tremor may develop. The cerebrospinal fluid protein is elevated and without cells. Conduction velocities are usually diffusely low. In nerve biopsies, segmental demyelination and remyelination are evident. In some cases, corticosteroids bring a remission; in others they worsen the disorder. Controlled studies to determine the long-term beneficial and adverse effects of corticosteroids in this condition have not been done.

SERUM NEUROPATHY

The use of antitetanus serum is sometimes associated with a diffuse and severe peripheral neuropathy, but more often it has the characteristic features of a brachial plexus neuropathy.

469. NEUROPATHY ASSOCIATED WITH INFECTION

Diphtheria is commonly complicated by paralysis of the nasopharynx and oculomotor and ciliary muscles. More widespread cranial polyneuropathy is uncommon. Paralysis of the extremities and trunk can also occur, usually appearing later and sometimes with cutaneous rather than the pharyngeal infection. The disease is discussed fully in Ch. 205.

Leprosy causes a characteristic peripheral neuropathy resulting from invasion of nerves by *M. leprae.* The neuropathy, in which selective pain and temperature loss are often striking, is discussed along with other manifestations of the disease in Ch. 245.

470. DISORDERS OF PERIPHERAL SENSORY NEURONS

Patients with disorders of peripheral sensory neurons characteristically suffer from pain, cutaneous injury from lack of sensation, unsteady movement from kinesthetic sensory loss, or combinations of these. Frequently they also have autonomic dysfunction. The nature of these symptoms and the kind of sensory loss correspond reasonably well with the populations of fibers affected. Thus it is generally true that patients with loss of pain and temperature sensation and with autonomic impairment have degeneration, particularly of unmyelinated and of small myelinated fibers, whereas patients with loss of touch-pressure sensation have degeneration of large myelinated fibers of cutaneous nerves. The nature of the sensory loss, particularly early in the course of the disorder, may be of help in differential diagnosis. In advanced disease this selectivity of involvement by fiber size tends to be lost.

Mild degrees of these disorders can be difficult to recognize, because clinical methods of determination of sensation are imprecise and nerve conduction studies have only recently been applied to their analysis.

Acquired disorders of sensory neurons include those of herpes zoster (see Ch. 388), acute inflammatory polyradiculoneuropathy (Guillain-Barré-Strohl syndrome) (see Ch. 468), and carcinomatous neuropathy (see Ch. 463).

Hereditary Sensory Neuropathy, Type I. Hereditary sensory neuropathy, Type I, is a dominantly inherited sensory radicular neuropathy. It has been variously described as perforating ulcers of the feet, mutilating acropathy, lumbosacral syringomyelia, acrodystrophic neuropathy, and hereditary sensory radicular neuropathy. Great variability in severity of involvement is commonplace. Sensory loss is usually much more severe over the feet and legs than in the hands and forearms, and some patients have lancinating pains. Pain and temperature sensation are affected more than touch-pressure sensation, and sensory ataxia is not a feature. Loss or decrease of sweating usually corresponds to the region of sensory loss. Nerve conduction of motor fibers is usually normal, but it is usually not possible to record compound action potentials of afferent fibers. Denervation may be seen in foot and leg muscles. The ankle tendon reflex may be absent. Life expectancy is probably normal in most cases. The treatment is described below. Late in the disorder, perforating ulcers of the foot may develop, especially when there has been poor foot care. In kinships, signs such as pes cavus, hammer toes, plantar calluses, inability to walk on heels, and sensation loss of acral parts of lower limbs point to the affliction.

Hereditary Sensory Neuropathy, Type II. This is a recessively inherited disorder, also called congenital sensory neuropathy, which usually manifests itself in infancy or childhood with a mutilating acropathy characterized by paronychia, whitlows, ulcers of the fingers and plantars of the feet, and frequently unrecognized fractures of the extremities. Sensory loss affects all types of cutaneous and sometimes kinesthetic sensation and is most marked distally in all four limbs. Tendon reflexes are usually absent. Sweating loss usually occurs over the distal limbs. Nerve action potentials of afferent fibers of cutaneous and limb nerves cannot be detected. Pathologically, there is an almost complete absence of myelinated fibers from the cutaneous nerves of the distal lower limb with preservation of decreased numbers of unmyelinated fibers. Treatment is discussed below.

Hereditary Sensory Neuropathy, Type III (Dysautonomia of Riley-Day). Familial dysautonomia is a recessively inherited disorder of Jewish infants and children. It affects peripheral autonomic neurons, peripheral sensory neurons, peripheral motor neurons, and probably other central nervous system neurons. Characteristics are an onset in infancy, premature death, a history of poor feeding, repeated episodes of vomiting and pulmonary infections, and autonomic disturbances. The last-named include defective lacrimation, defective temperature control, skin blotching, excessive perspiration, hypertension, and postural hypotension. There are also insensitivity to pain, areflexia, corneal insensitivity, and an absence of the fungiform papillae of tongue. In infants the symptoms reported by mothers are poor sucking, poor swallowing, failure to thrive, lack of tears, and unexplained fevers. At an older age one notes delay in development, stunted growth, corneal abrasions, kyphoscoliosis, clumsiness, excessive sweating, and blotching of skin, with emotion and lack of pain from stimuli usually considered painful. Evidence for involvement of peripheral neurons comes from the observed hyporeflexia and the finding of a decrease of unmyelinated fibers of cutaneous nerves. An abnormality of catecholamine metabolism has been demonstrated.

Hereditary Sensory Neuropathy, Type IV. In this recessively inherited sensory neuropathy insensitivity to pain, anhydrosis, and mental retardation are found. This disorder has been attributed to an abnormality of differentiation of the neural crest.

Angiokeratoma Corporis Diffusum (Fabry's). This rare disorder, described in Ch. 918, is characterized by angiokeratomas, impaired renal function, and small purple to black spots distributed especially over the lower trunk and buttocks along segmental lines. Typically, patients have pain and numbness in the limbs but no motor symptoms. A deposition of glycolipids in the cell bodies of peripheral sensory neurons and a decrease in the number of small neurons of spinal ganglia and of unmyelinated and small myelinated fibers have been observed and may be important in explaining the painfulness of the disorder.

Treatment of Insensitive Hands and Feet. Persons with pain and temperature insensitivity of hands and feet are vulnerable to many injuries which potentially can result in a chain of events, including ulceration, cellulitis, lymphangitis, osteomyelitis, and osteolysis. These events are seen particularly in the disorders of leprosy, inherited amyloidosis, and other inherited and acquired neuropathies with this type of sensory loss. Congenital neuropathies with such sensory loss are particularly difficult to manage, because they occur at an age when it is difficult to obtain the cooperation of the patient. The goal in treatment is to prevent the onset of tissue damage or, when it has occurred, to promote healing and prevent further damage. Persons with such sensory loss should not engage in most forms of manual labor or perform repetitive tasks with hands and feet which can cause bruising. Repeated inspection of feet and hands is necessary. Any bruise or ulcer should be taken seriously and, if on the foot, one should stop weight bearing until healing has occurred. Shoes should be wide and well constructed. The inside of the shoes must be inspected before the foot is placed inside in order to remove retained objects or nails. The feet of such patients should be soaked in lukewarm water for 15 minutes twice a day and lightly covered with petrolatum lotion so that the moisture in the softened skin is retained.

471. INHERITED DISORDERS OF PERIPHERAL MOTOR, SENSORY, AND AUTONOMIC NEURONS

In this group of disorders, the predominant involvement is of peripheral motor neurons. The disorders are usually inherited, are usually progressive, and usually have signs which are symmetrical. Neurons of similar structure and function are affected. The pathologic features are nonfocal, and the nature of the fiber degeneration is that of an axonal atrophy and degeneration. Although an inborn error of metabolism probably underlies these disorders, for the most part this has not been elucidated.

Hereditary Motor and Sensory Neuropathy, Type I (Hypertrophic Neuropathy Type of Peroneal Muscular Atrophy). This is a fairly common, mild, dominantly inherited variant of peroneal muscular atrophy. Affected persons may have no symptoms or signs, but yet be known to have the disorder by their position in the kinship and by characteristic low conduction velocities of all nerves.

Pathologically the disorder affects myelinated fibers predominantly, producing segmental demyelination and remyelination and varying degrees of onion-bulb formation (the hallmark of hypertrophic neuropathy). An actual loss of myelinated fibers probably occurs.

In kinships with the disease an affected person may be recognized by high arches of the feet, hammer toes, curled-up toes (with convexity upward), frequent corns or calluses, and a high-stepping, awkward gait caused by paresis of the dorsiflexor muscles of the ankle and instability of the ankle joint. Persons with greater weakness may have weakness and wasting of the intrinsic hand muscles and weakness of the plantar flexor muscles of the ankles. Ankle joint instability makes it difficult for such persons to stand still. The amount of muscle atrophy is usually not great. Typically, the tendon reflexes are reduced or absent, disappearing successively from the Achilles tendon, the quadriceps, and the upper extremity. Sensory loss is mild, affecting the modalities of touch-pressure, two-point discrimination, and joint position and motion in the distal parts of the extremities. Clinical enlargement of peripheral nerves may be detected in about one fourth of the cases. Some members of kinships have, in addition to the clinical features mentioned, a tremor of the head and outstretched hands which is indistinguishable from essential tremor (Roussy-Levy syndrome). Foot ulcers occur in occasional persons with this disorder. Osteomyelitis and mutilation of the feet develop only if the ulcers are neglected. There is no specific treatment. Corrective surgery should be reserved for those affected persons who develop ulcers at pressure points owing to excessively high arches and for those with excessive inversion of the foot. Foot-drop springs or braces may be used to elevate the toes in walking and to stabilize the ankle. When foot ulcers develop, a program of ulcer debridement and rest in bed should be begun immediately. Weight-bearing should not be resumed until the ulcer is completely healed. Then shoes should be fitted which have sufficient width, an adequate arch support, and a fit that distributes the weight to all parts of the foot.

Hereditary Motor and Sensory Neuropathy, Type II (Neuronal Type of Peroneal Muscular Atrophy, Charcot-Marie-Tooth Disease). This dominantly inherited disorder begins in the second decade of life or later. Not uncommonly it begins in the fifth or sixth decade. Symmetric muscle weakness with atrophy begins in small foot muscles, peroneal, long toe extensor, and ankle dorsiflexor muscles. Pes cavus and hammer toes may or may not be associated with the weakness. Initial symptoms include inability to pick up the toes in walking, instability of the ankle, difficulty in standing still in one position, and visible atrophy of muscles. Some patients tend to stand with their feet spread apart, and shift the position constantly to maintain balance. Others tend to stand with their knees bent to lock the ankles. Later weakness of small hand muscles may make such acts as unlocking a door with a key, unscrewing the top of a glass jar, or buttoning difficult. The muscle atrophy of the lower limbs may be typical of peroneal muscular atrophy, with a greater degree of atrophy in the distal aspect of thigh muscles and with much atrophy of leg muscles. Most frequently tendon reflexes are diminished or absent in the lower limbs. Touch-pressure, joint position, and vibration sensation are mildly decreased distally in lower limbs. Conduction velocities of motor fibers are within the limits of normal in upper limbs and only slightly reduced in lower limbs.

Sporadic cases similar in every way to the above are seen. These cases may be a different disorder or the same disorder in which the inherited nature has not been detected. However, Charcot-Marie-Tooth disease is genetically and morphologically entirely distinct from either Friedreich's ataxia or spastic paraplegia with peroneal muscular atrophy, disorders discussed in Ch. 432 and 434.

These patients can often be helped significantly by leg braces that stabilize the ankle joint. Their use permits these patients to stand still without losing their balance for such acts as shaving.

Hereditary Motor and Sensory Neuropathy, Type III (Recessively Inherited Hypertrophic Neuropathy). This is a rare disorder transmitted as an autosomal recessive trait and beginning in infancy. The children learn to walk late, have great difficulty in walking even at their best point of neuromuscular development (ages 8 to 12), and are usually in wheelchairs by the age of 20 years. The patients are usually short, and most have a severe, symmetrical, sensory motor neuropathy affecting predominantly the distal extremities with enlarged peripheral nerves. Some weakness of proximal muscles of the extremities usually is present also. Sometimes there are associated miosis and nystagmus. The conduction velocity of motor and sensory fibers of peripheral nerves is among the lowest determined in electromyographic laboratories. Pathologically, marked segmental demyelination and remyelination are found in myelinated fibers; unmyelinated fibers are not decreased in number but are probably affected also. A systemic biochemical abnormality involving ceramide hexoses and their sulfates has been found. No specific treatment is available.

Hereditary Motor and Sensory Neuropathy, Type IV (Recessively Inherited Hypertrophic Neuropathy with Excess of Phytonic Acid; Refsum's Disease). This rare progressive or relapsing disorder is inherited as an autosomal recessive trait and is due to the inability of affected subjects to alpha-oxidize ingested phytanic acid. Clinical manifestations usually begin in the second decade with night blindness and constriction of the visual fields owing to an atypical retinitis pigmentosa. Additionally, symptoms caused by a distal sensorimotor neuropathy develop, as well as an ataxia which is thought to be greater than that accounted for by kinesthetic loss. Ichthyosis, skeletal abnormalities, and sudden death in the third or fourth decade from involvement of the heart all provide evidence of systemic extraneural involvement. The cerebrospinal fluid protein is usually markedly elevated. Pathologically, the peripheral nerves contain evidence of segmental demyelination and remyelination and onion-bulb formation. Pathognomonic is the occurrence of 3,7,11,15-tetramethylhexadecenoic acid (phytanic acid) in the serum, red blood cells, liver, heart, kidneys, and skeletal muscles. Treatment consists of withholding dietary phytols (chlorophyll-free diet); if begun early it can result in dramatic improvement.

Hereditary Spastic Paraplegia with Motor and Sensory Neuropathy, Type V. Symptomatic onset and severity of this dominantly inherited disorder are extremely variable. Difficulty in walking and running because of stiffness is the usual manifestation. The progression is slow, and life expectancy is probably normal. The most prominent changes consist of a spastic, scissoring gait, hyperreflexia, and Babinski signs. However, careful examination usually gives evidence of involvement of lower motor and peripheral sensory neurons.

Hereditary Motor and Sensory Neuropathy with Optic Atrophy, Type VI. In this very rare dominantly inherited disorder, there is optic atrophy in addition to peroneal muscular atrophy.

Hereditary Motor and Sensory Neuropathy with Retinitis Pigmentosa, Type VII. This disorder has many of the features of the syndrome described by Refsum, but elevated plasma phytanic acids are not found.

472. AMYLOIDOSIS

Dominantly Inherited Amyloidosis (Portuguese). Amyloid neuropathy has been noted most often in countries surrounding the Mediterranean Sea, although kinships are sometimes encountered in the United States, Japan, and other countries. The disorder usually begins in the late second or third decade with loss of the sensations of pain, cold, and heat in the lower extremities accompanied by anhydrosis and, sooner or later, loss of sphincter control. Males become impotent. Nerve biopsy studies disclose selective loss of small myelinated and unmyelinated fibers, accounting for the selective sensory loss. Subsequently other fibers are also affected so that sensory loss becomes more generalized, and motor weakness and atrophy develop. The disorder progresses relentlessly to death, usually in the fourth or fifth decade. Amyloid deposits may be found in many tissues, including peripheral nerve, muscle, vitreous of the eye, and many other organs.

Dominantly Inherited Amyloidosis (Indiana). In contradistinction to the Portuguese type of dominantly inherited amyloidosis, the symptoms of the Indiana type usually begin in the upper extremities, and may suggest the diagnosis of carpal tunnel syndrome. Eventually, a more generalized neuropathy develops.

473. NEUROPATHY ASSOCIATED WITH PERIPHERAL VASCULAR DISEASE

Besides the vasculitis previously described in polyarteritis nodosa and other collagen diseases, there are alterations produced in the peripheral nerves by atherosclerosis of larger vessels. Patients who experience claudication when walking or who have evidence of peripheral gangrene may also have a distal sensory and motor neuropathy that appears to be due to inadequate blood supply and infarction of nerves. All sensory modalities are affected, and there may be burning, pricking, and jabbing pains in the feet. Depending on the site and distribution of vascular involvement, the neuropathy may be symmetric or asymmetric.

474. NEUROPATHY ASSOCIATED WITH UREMIA

Particularly since the development of dialysis programs for the treatment of chronic renal disease, severe peripheral neuropathy has appeared in many patients with uremia, affecting approximately one half of the patients receiving dialysis. This neuropathy is mixed motor and sensory, symmetric, and more severe in the distal parts. Bladder and bowel disturbances are unusual. The pathogenesis is unknown. Frequent and apparently adequate dialysis does not always produce a remission, but with successful kidney transplantation the peripheral nerve function returns toward normal.

Asbury, A., Victor, M., and Adams, R.: Uremic polyneuropathy. Arch. Neurol. 8:413, 1963.
Austin, J.: Recurrent polyneuropathies and their corticosteroid treatment. Brain, 81:157, 1958.
Cooke, W., and Smith, W.: Neurological disorders associated with coeliac disease. Brain, 89:683, 1966.
Croft, P., Urich, H., and Wilkinson, M.: Peripheral neuropathy of sensorimotor type associated with malignant disease. Brain, 90:31, 1967.
Denny-Brown, D.: Primary sensory neuropathy with muscular changes associated with carcinoma. J. Neurol. Neurosurg. Psychiatry, 11:73, 1948.
Dyck, P., and Lambert, E.: Lower motor and primary sensory neuron diseases with peroneal muscular atrophy. I. Neurologic, genetic, and electrophysiologic findings in hereditary polyneuropathies. Arch. Neurol., 18:603, 1968.
Dyck, P., and Lambert, E.: Lower motor and primary sensory neuron diseases with peroneal muscular atrophy. II. Neurologic, genetic, and electrophysiologic findings in various neuronal degenerations. Arch. Neurol., 18:619, 1968.
Dyck, P., and Lambert, E.: Dissociated sensation in amyloidosis. Compound action potential, quantitative histologic and teased-fiber, and electron microscopic studies of sural nerve biopsies. Arch. Neurol., 20:490, 1969.
Engel, W., Dorman, J., Levy, R., and Fredrickson, D.: Neuropathy in Tangier disease. Arch. Neurol., 17:1, 1967.
Lovelace, R., and Horwitz, S.: Peripheral neuropathy in long-term diphenylhydantoin therapy. Arch. Neurol., 18:69, 1968.
Moress, G., D'Agostino, A., and Jarcho, L.: Neuropathy in lymphoblastic leukemia treated with vincristine. Arch. Neurol., 16:377, 1967.
Nickel, S., et al.: Myxedema neuropathy and myopathy. A clinical and pathological study. Neurology (Minneap.), 11:125, 1961.
Raff, M., Sangalang, V., and Asbury, A.: Ischemic mononeuropathy multiplex associated with diabetes mellitus. Arch. Neurol., 18:497, 1968.
Steinberg, D., Mize, C. E., Herndon, J. H., Fales, H. M., Engel, W. K., and Vroom, F. O.: Phytanic acid in patients with Refsum's syndrome and response to dietary treatment. Arch. Intern. Med., 125:75, 1970.
Sunderland, S.: Nerves and Nerve Injuries. Edinburgh and London, E. and S. Livingstone Ltd., 1968.
Swanson, A. G., Buchan, G. C., and Alvord, E. C., Jr.: Anatomic changes in congenital insensitivity to pain. Arch. Neurol., 12:12, 1965.
Thomas, P., and Lascelles, R.: The pathology of diabetic neuropathy. Quart. J. Med., 35:489, 1966.
Tyler, H.: Neurological complications of dialysis, transplantation and other forms of treatment in chronic uremia. Neurology (Minneap.), 15:1081, 1965.
Wiederholdt, W., Mulder, D., and Lambert, E.: The Landry-Guillain-Barré-Strohl syndrome or polyradiculoneuropathy. Historical review, report on 97 patients, and present concepts. Mayo Clin. Proc., 39:427, 1964.

Section Twenty-Three. DISEASES OF MUSCLE AND NEUROMUSCULAR JUNCTION

Lewis P. Rowland

475. INTRODUCTION

Definitions. Muscles can be weakened by many different disorders. When muscles become weak, they may waste away. Until recently it has been conventional to ascribe the varied causes of weakness and wasting to neurogenic and myopathic disorders, a fundamental distinction originally made a century ago when diseases were defined by pathologists. In the neurogenic disorders, the brunt of pathologic change was seen in the motor neuron or peripheral nerve; changes in muscle were less pronounced or could be attributed to secondary effects of denervation. In the myopathic disorders, on the other hand, the histopathologic changes in muscle were of different type and there was little abnormality in nerve cell or peripheral nerve.

Pathologic criteria, however, have limitations when one is dealing with living people. Muscle biopsy is possible, but there is no way of obtaining a sample of the spinal cord. Other criteria were therefore introduced to separate neurogenic and myopathic disorders: clinical and genetic characteristics, electromyography, nerve conduction velocity, and assay of serum activity of sarcoplasmic enzymes. Together, these criteria have provided a reasonably consistent basis for continued separation of those syndromes characterized by weakness into neurogenic and myopathic groups.

The concept, however, has been shaken in recent years. Denervation and cross-innervation studies of fast and slow muscles have shown that physiologic and biochemical characteristics of muscle are under neural control. A new kind of electrophysiologic evidence has been adduced to indicate a neurogenic cause for the muscular dystrophies, long held to be the prototype of myopathy. Unsurprisingly, there is confusion. Nevertheless, the traditional separation of neurogenic and myopathic disease may be more than an editorial convenience and will be perpetuated in this section.

Because of these conceptual problems, an air of vagueness pervades the language used to describe neuromuscular diseases, and the same words have different meanings to different authorities. It is not mere nit-picking to attempt definitions; the ideas are important. It is therefore appropriate to define some of the more prevalent words before going on with this discussion.

The word *atrophy* means, literally, "lack of nourishment." It has come to mean wasting of muscle, or loss of muscle bulk from any cause, and it is also used to denote single muscle fibers that are smaller than normal when viewed microscopically. But when used in the name of a disease, it always implies that the muscle wasting is secondary to a neural disorder, e.g., infantile spinal muscular atrophy, progressive spinal muscular atrophy, or peroneal muscular atrophy. To avoid ambiguity, it is therefore appropriate in examining patients to use "wasting" rather than "atrophy" to describe diminution in muscle bulk unless the cause is known to be neurogenic. *Myopathies* include disorders characterized by weakness that is not due to emotional or neurogenic cause. Some authors speak of "primary" or "secondary" myopathies but there is little evidence that any muscle disease is really "primary," in the sense that there is an abnormality in muscle and nowhere else. In some myopathies, as in thyrotoxic myopathy, the fundamental disorder is elsewhere, and this could be true even in genetically determined diseases. The *dystrophies* are a subgroup of myopathy with two special characteristics: they are genetically determined, and the weakness is progressive. There are other genetic disorders of muscle in which the weakness seems to be stationary, and some in which progressive weakness is not the dominant symptom (transient attacks of weakness in periodic paralysis, cramps, and myoglobinuria in some glycogen diseases, or myotonia); other names are given to these conditions individually.

DIFFERENTIATION OF NEUROPATHIC AND MYOPATHIC DISEASE

When muscles are sick, they are usually weak. Few other symptoms result; sometimes muscles ache (myalgia); sometimes they relax with difficulty (myotonia); sometimes they shorten abruptly and painfully (cramp or contracture). Weakness is the most common symptom of muscle disease, but it is also the symptom that results from neurogenic diseases affecting corticospinal pathways, motor neurons, or peripheral nerves. The differential diagnosis of muscle disease is therefore a problem in distinguishing myogenic from neurogenic causes. Corticospinal disorders have characteristic signs that immediately identify them, and therefore they do not often enter into this differential diagnosis. Disorders of the lower motor neuron or peripheral nerve may be difficult and sometimes impossible to separate from muscle disease. In this kind of neurogenic disorder and in myopathies, weakness, wasting, and depression of myotatic reflexes are common to both groups. Neurogenic disorders are apt to affect distal muscles primarily, whereas myopathic disorders are more likely to affect proximal muscle, but there are so many exceptions that this is an unreliable guide. (Distal myopathy is rare but does occur; proximal weakness is not so rare in motor neuron disease or peripheral neuropathy.) Twitching of muscle is probably a reliable guide to motor neuron disease, but it is not yet definitely excluded as a myopathic sign. The combination of active reflexes in a limb with weak, wasted, and twitching muscles is almost pathognomonic of amytrophic lateral sclerosis, especially if there are also Babinski signs. Sensory loss and an increased protein content of the cerebrospinal fluid are reliable guides to peripheral neuropathy, but once it is established that there is a peripheral neuropathy, it may be difficult or impossible to state whether there is also a concomitant myopathy. Because of these ambiguities in clinical diagnosis, increasing attention has been directed to three laboratory aids: serum enzymes, electromyography and nerve conduction velocities, and muscle biopsy. Some syndromes are virtually defined by electromyography: distal myopathy and "juvenile muscular atrophy simulating muscular dystrophy."

Serum Enzymes. Several different enzyme activities are increased in the serum of patients with X-linked dystrophies and polymyositis, whereas they are not increased in neurogenic diseases. It is often stated that determination of creatine phosphokinase (CPK) activity is the "best" because it is the most sensitive. This enzyme is significantly increased in almost all muscle diseases, but it is, if anything, too sensitive; it picks up all the myopathic cases, but it is sometimes also increased in neurogenic disease. Other serum enzyme levels, e.g., SGOT or lactate dehydrogenase, LDH, and others, do not rise so much in myopathies, but neither do they give falsely positive reactions in neurogenic disorders. For this reason, it is useful to couple determinations of CPK with SGOT or LDH in evaluating individual cases. CPK has one other considerable advantage: it is not present in erythrocytes or liver and is therefore normal in serum contaminated by hemolysis or in patients with liver disease.

Electromyography. Needle electromyography, the amplification of action potentials from muscle, has been refined to a very useful technique. Normal muscle is electrically silent at rest, and patterns of potentials evoked by voluntary contraction have been analyzed in terms of frequency, duration, and amplitude of individual motor unit potentials. In denervated muscle, there is spontaneous activity (fibrillations from single muscle fibers or fasciculations from motor units), the number of potentials during a voluntary contraction is reduced, and the duration of potentials is increased. In myopathic disorders, there is usually no spontaneous activity, there is no reduction in the number of potentials under voluntary control, and the potentials are reduced in duration. These signs are usually reliable, but in some cases the results are equivocal, and there may be features of both a neurogenic and myopathic disorder.

Nerve Conduction Velocities. The speed of conduction along motor nerves can be recorded accurately, and slowing of conduction is a reliable guide to neuropathy. A normal conduction velocity, however, does not exclude a nerve lesion.

Muscle Biopsy. The features of neurogenic and myopathic diseases can usually be differentiated in a muscle biopsy, especially when one utilizes the new techniques of the rapid examination of frozen tissue and the application of histochemical methods. The electron microscope has opened new approaches that are still in the process of refinement. Only a few diseases can be definitively identified by muscle biopsy: periarteritis nodosa, trichinosis, sarcoidosis, and most (but not all) cases of glycogen storage disease. The congenital myopathies are best identified by histochemical and other special procedures.

In most cases, the results of all these special studies are consistent, one with the other. In some cases, however, the results are conflicting, and problems of classification remain.

Dubowitz, V., and Brooke, M. H.: Muscle Biopsy: A Modern Approach. Philadelphia, W. B. Saunders Company, 1973.

Hausmanowa-Petrusewicz, I., and Jedrzejowska, H.: Correlation between electromyographic findings and muscle biopsy in cases of neuromuscular disease. J. Neurol. Sci., 13:85, 1971.

Lenman, J. A. P., and Ritchie, A. E.: Clinical Electromyography. Philadelphia, J. B. Lippincott Company, 1970.

McComas, A. J., Sica, A. E. P., and Campbell, M. J.: "Sick" motoneurones. A unifying concept of muscle disease. Lancet, 1:321, 1971.

Rowland, L. P.: Are the muscular dystrophies neurogenic? Ann. N.Y. Acad. Sci., 228:244, 1974.

INHERITED DISEASES

476. MUSCULAR DYSTROPHIES

Definition. Muscular dystrophies are inherited myopathies, characterized primarily by progressively severe weakness.

Etiology. Although it is generally believed that inherited diseases must be due to a missing or structurally abnormal protein (either an enzyme or a structural protein), this abnormality has not been identified in any form of dystrophy. Indirect evidence implicates the muscle membranes in several forms, but this hypothesis cannot now be put to direct test. Pathologic and biochemical abnormalities can be detected in muscle, and there is no clear evidence of neural abnormality in traditional terms. It is conceivable, however, that the funadmental abnormality is in another organ (such as the liver or bowel) and that the muscular abnormalities are secondary. Some authors have postulated a debatable vascular cause, one of chronic and relative ischemia.

Classification. No classification of the muscular dystrophies is entirely satisfactory, but the application of clinical and genetic analysis provides the best approach at present. The classification in the accompanying table is based upon the clearly identifiable features of Duchenne dystrophy, facioscapulohumeral dystrophy, and myotonic muscular dystrophy. Limb-girdle dystrophy is probably not a single disease, but merely encompasses cases that do not fall into the other categories.

Incidence. None of the muscular dystrophies are common. Incidence rates vary from 5 per million births for facioscapulohumeral dystrophy to about 250 per million births for Duchenne dystrophy. Many cases seem to be sporadic; the mutation rate of Duchenne dystrophy is high, 7×10^{-5}, and about two thirds of the cases appear sporadically, with no other affected individual in the family.

Pathology. Pathologic abnormalities are restricted to skeletal muscle, sometimes involving cardiac muscle. The brain, spinal cord, and peripheral nerves are devoid of histologic change, although some authors have implicated the brain because of a seemingly high incidence of mental retardation in children with Duchenne dystrophy. Terminal pneumonia may cause changes in the lungs, and there may be a variety of associated diseases not directly linked to the dystrophy. In myotonic muscular dystrophy, however, baldness and testicular atrophy are integral parts of the disease in men, and corneal opacities affect both sexes.

The abnormalities in muscle seem to involve all fibers in random fashion. Early, there is scattered evidence of necrosis and regeneration, with prominent variation in fiber size, including many fibers much larger than normal. Later, fibers disappear, to be replaced by fibrous connective tissue and fat. "Pseudohypertrophy" is probably due to both "true" hypertrophy (large fibers) and

Classification of Human Muscular Dystrophies

	Duchenne Dystrophy	Facioscapulohumeral Dystrophy	Limb-Girdle Dystrophy	Myotonic Dystrophy
Genetic pattern	X-linked, recessive	Autosomal, dominant	Autosomal, recessive	Autosomal, dominant
Age at onset	Before age 5	Adolescence	Adolescence	Early or late
First symptoms	Pelvic	Shoulders	Pelvic	Distal; hands or feet
Pseudohypertrophy	+	0	0	0
Predominant weakness, early	Proximal	Proximal	Proximal	Distal
Progression	Relatively rapid; incapacitated in adolescence	Slow	Variable	Slow
Facial weakness	0	+	0	Occasional
Ocular, oropharyngeal weakness	0	0	0	Occasional
Myotonia	0	0	0	+
Cardiomyopathy	0 or late	0	0	Arrhythmia, conduction block
Associated disorders	None (?mental retardation)	None	None	Cataracts; testicular atrophy and baldness in men
Serum enzymes	Very high	Slight or no increase	Slight or no increase	Slight or no increase
Prevalence (per million population)	38	5	20	25
Incidence (per million births)	251	5	47	–
Mutation rate	9×10^{-5}	5×10^{-7}	3×10^{-5}	10×10^{-6}

increased accumulations of fat and connective tissue. In myotonic dystrophy, unusual figures form "ring fibers" (with one fiber running at right angles, encircling the other fibers in the same bundle) and "sarcoplasmic masses," or accumulations of sarcoplasm that are free of myofilaments. However, these abnormalities occur occasionally in other diseases and are not pathognomonic of myotonic dystrophy. In Duchenne dystrophy, the myocardium may be affected by similar changes at autopsy, but cardiac symptoms are rarely evident in life, a discrepancy that has been attributed to the sedentary life imposed upon the patients by advanced muscular weakness. Myopathic changes in the heart are common in myotonic dystrophy. There is no good evidence that smooth muscle is affected in any form of dystrophy. Ultrastructural investigations have not provided any clues to the initial lesion. Disruption of myofibrillar structure, alterations of mitochondria, and degeneration of tubules and sarcoplasmic reticulum all seem to proceed together.

Clinical Manifestations. The symptoms and signs of all forms of the muscular dystrophies are related to weakness alone, except that additional systems are involved in myotonic dystrophy. In other forms, the symptoms depend upon the distribution of weakness and the age at onset. In *Duchenne dystrophy* weakness is primarily proximal at onset, and symptoms begin early. By definition, girls are not affected. There are no symptoms in the first year of life, but walking may be somewhat delayed beyond 18 months. Once the child walks, some abnormality is usually evident to an experienced observer (either a parent with a previously affected child or a skilled physician). The boys tend to waddle when they walk, or walk on their toes, or fall frequently and have difficulty rising. They are probably never able to run, because they have difficulty raising their knees. These symptoms become more evident as the children grow older, and even the most unsuspecting parent becomes aware of some abnormality by age five, or teachers sometimes may be the first to recognize the difficulty when the child starts school. Some cases are averred to start between ages five and ten, but these must be exceptional. It is difficult to examine individual muscles of a young child, but the waddling gait, the typical method of rising from the ground by "climbing up" himself (Gowers' sign), enlargement of calf or other muscles, and inability to run are characteristic. Myotatic reflexes may be normal at first, but by three years the knee jerks are usually lost, and later the ankle jerks disappear. As the child grows there are two countervailing influences; increased growth and coordination may compensate temporarily for the concurrent progressive weakness and wasting, but the disease always wins. There is increased difficulty walking. Going up grades or stairs first requires aid, then becomes impossible. Weakness of the trunk muscles leads to increased lordosis and a protuberant abdomen. Then the arms become weak. Finally, in early adolescence, the child becomes unable to walk. This is inevitable, but may be accelerated by a period of inactivity after an injury or an orthopedic operation. Contractures appear, at first in the feet, as the gastrocnemius muscles tighten. When the child stops walking, flexion contractures limit motion of the knees, and scoliosis becomes more a problem with prolonged sitting. Ultimately respiration becomes shallow and the child is increasingly subject to pulmonary infection. Sooner or later, one of these infections is fatal, usually in the third decade. Although muscles are ravaged from the neck down, the cranial muscles are entirely spared, an apparently important clue to the nature of the disease, but presently uninterpretable. Congestive heart failure and abnormalities of cardiac rhythm are rare.

Becker dystrophy has manifestations similar to those of Duchenne dystrophy, but the onset is later in childhood or in adolescence, and the tempo is slower and more variable. This form may also be devastating, but some patients are able to function, albeit with limitations, well into adult life. The clinical similarities include pseudohypertrophy of calf muscles. However, it is clear that although the two forms are similar, they are genetically separate; there are no mildly affected individuals in typical Duchenne families, nor are children affected severely in Becker families.

The manifestations of *limb-girdle dystrophy* are also similar because weakness of muscles of the pelvic girdle usually initiates the syndrome, but symptoms start in late childhood or adolescence. Girls are affected as often as boys, and pseudohypertrophy is rare. Waddling gait, difficulty in walking and climbing, and frequent falls are common. Occasionally, symptoms may begin in the shoulder girdle. In either case, there is usually weakness in all four limbs by the time the patient seeks medical attention. The severity, age at onset, and rate of progression vary considerably, suggesting that this category contains more than one disease.

Facioscapulohumeral dystrophy is distinct. Symptoms vary in severity so that some affected individuals never have any disability (but can be recognized by the signs), whereas others become incapacitated early; there are all grades in between. The first symptoms are apt to be related to difficulty in raising the arms or to prominence of the scapulae. Weakness of the legs may affect pelvic girdle muscles, or equally prominent weakness of the anterior tibial muscles may lead to a steppage gait. Truncal weakness may lead to prominent scoliosis. The face is always involved on examination; the perioral muscles may be more affected than those of the upper face, but ultimately patients develop difficulty in closing the eyes. The sternal head of the pectoral muscle is affected earlier than the clavicular head, a selectivity that can be detected on testing the individual muscles, and leads to a peculiar appearance of the axillary folds when the arms are dependent, because the anterior axillary fold of normal people is formed by the sternal portion of the pectoral muscle. Winging of the scapulae can be seen when the patient leans against a wall with the arms extended, and the weakness of shoulder girdle muscles leads to an unusual appearance because, viewed from the front, the superior margin of the scapula is higher than the clavicle.

Myotonic muscular dystrophy diverges from the preceding types in several respects. (1) The distribution of weakness differs in that cranial muscles are often affected and limb weakness is initially more marked in distal muscles. Thus weakness of the hands (as in twisting bottle caps or using tools) precedes shoulder weakness, and footdrop or steppage gait precedes symptoms of pelvic muscle weakness. *Ptosis, facial weakness,* and *dysarthria* are signs not seen in the other forms of dystrophy. Moreover, there is almost always selective weakness of the sternomastoids. The masticatory muscles either are poorly developed or waste early (even when not symptomatically weak), causing a characteristic facial appearance. The long, lean look has led physicians to use several callous descriptive phrases that are best not perpetuated. (Among the more foolish designations is "myopathic facies," but the facial appearance of a patient with myotonic dystrophy differs from facioscapulohumeral dystrophy or from myasthenia gravis.) (2) Myotonia, or difficulty in relaxation, may be symptomatic, and after a firm grip the patient may have difficulty letting go. Myotonia may cause other symptoms in patients with mytonia congenita (see below), but in the dystrophy only the hands are affected by this kind of stiffness. Myotonia of grip may be evident on examination, and can also be elicited by percussing the thenar eminence. In normal persons this evokes a rapid twitch, whereas in patients with myotonia, a sustained contraction of the adductor pollicis muscle persists for several seconds, only gradually relaxing. Similar responses to percussion may be elicited uncommonly in other limb muscles, but can often be seen in the tongue. Although myotonia is a dramatic sign and a symptom that can be relieved by drugs, it is not the symptom that causes the major disability in myotonic dystrophy; weakness is the problem. (3) Other systems are involved in this pleomorphic disorder; cataracts appear sooner or later in all patients, and are sometimes the only sign of the disease; most of the men (but not the women) have frontal baldness; testicular atrophy affects most of the men, but often after they have sired children to perpetuate the disease (there is no definite evidence of gonadal insufficiency in affected women); the basal metabolic rate is often low, but other tests of thyroid function are normal (extrathyroidal hypometabolism). The incidence of diabetes mellitus may be increased. (4) Conduction defects are common in the electrocardiogram, and may lead to clinically significant arrhythmia or congestive heart failure.

Certain rare forms of muscular dystrophy are named after the prominent manifestations. *Ocular dystrophy* is a slowly progressive disorder in which ptosis of the eyelids and progressive immobility of the eyes are the cardinal features. The pupils are spared, and both eyes are usually affected symmetrically so that diplopia is uncommon (but may occur). Other muscles of the head, neck, and limbs may also be affected, varying from family to family. This syndrome raises problems of definition; some cases probably are myopathic in origin, but this kind of ophthalmoplegia is often associated with other manifestations that are clearly neurogenic (such as spinocerebellar degeneration or peripheral neuropathy). The final distinction as to the origin of the ophthalmoplegia is often difficult or impossible to make because the ocular muscles normally differ so much from limb muscles that signs of myopathy in muscle biopsy or electromyography are not valid in studying them. In some, but not all, patients with myopathic ophthalmoplegia, structural and biochemical abnormalities may be found in limb muscles. Abnormally large mitochondria are present in increased numbers; this can be seen dramatically in electron microscopy, and the numbers are sufficient to stain fibers red in the trichrome stain for light microscopy, leading to the appellation "ragged red fibers." In these cases there is apt to be an accumulation of glycogen, but the biochemical cause of this has not been ascertained.

Distal myopathy, as the name implies, affects distal leg and hand muscles first. It is probably the rarest form of dystrophy, and can be identified only by characteristic signs of myopathy in electromyography and muscle biopsy.

In the *scapuloperoneal syndrome* distal weakness in the legs resembles that of neurogenic peroneal muscular atrophy, but sensory loss is lacking, and there is proximal weakness in the shoulder girdle very similar to that of facioscapulohumeral dystrophy. Some of these cases are myopathic and some seem to be neurogenic as distinguished by electromyography, muscle biopsy, and serum enzymes. In either case, autosomal dominant inheritance and a relatively slow progression seem characteristic.

Diagnosis. The clinical picture of Duchenne dystrophy is so characteristic that it entails little diagnostic confusion. In its first stages, some children are merely regarded as clumsy, and some receive orthopedic care because of toe-walking; otherwise the diagnosis becomes obvious. As noted, the trait is transmitted as a sex-linked recessive, and once a case is recognized, members of the family rapidly detect the signs in subsequently affected youngsters. Once a family is known, affected individuals can be identified in the neonatal period because the serum enzymes are already markedly abnormal. Limb-girdle and facioscapulohumeral dystrophy must be differentiated from neurogenic diseases, from congenital myopathies, and from polymyositis, as will be discussed below. Myotonic dystrophy may be confused with endocrine disorders or, because of the distal weakness, with neuropathy or amyotrophy, or with hypothyroidism or gonadal disorders. Ocular myopathy must be differentiated from myasthenia gravis; this is usually not a problem because there is no fluctuation of symptoms in the myopathy, and the weakness does not respond to cholinergic drugs. The differential diagnosis of the dystrophies depends also upon the age of the patient. In childhood and adolescence, the major problems involve peroneal muscular atrophy (Charcot-Marie-Tooth) and "muscular atrophy simulating muscular dystrophy" (Wohlfart-Kugelberg-Welander). In adults, amyotrophic lateral sclerosis is the major problem. At all ages, polyneuritis must be considered.

Treatment. There is no specific treatment for the weakness of any form of dystrophy. Physical medicine, exercises, splints, braces, and corrective orthopedic surgery are applied in different centers with varying degrees of enthusiasm. Some therapeutic activists claim that walking can be prolonged into late adolescence in Duchenne dystrophy. They may be correct, but it is difficult to prove. The most poignant decisions concern the use of antimicrobial drugs or supported respiration for young men paralyzed from the neck down and with no hope of ultimate recovery. The myotonia of myotonic dystrophy can be relieved by diphenylhydantoin (0.3 to 0.6 gram daily), quinine (0.3 to 1.5 grams daily), or procainamide (4 to 6 grams daily), but this is rarely the problem, and nothing can be done for the weakness. Cataracts are treated surgically upon appropriate indication, and cardiac arrhythmias or congestive heart failure are managed accordingly.

Prophylaxis. Genetic counseling offers the only possibility to control muscular dystrophy at present. Carriers of Duchenne dystrophy may often but not always be identified by abnormally increased serum enzyme activity (higher than normal, but not as high as in affected boys). In some centers, antenatal detection of sex allows selective prophylactic abortion. There is presently no way to determine whether a male fetus is affected, however. Birth control ought to be effective in dominantly inherited diseases such as facioscapulohumeral and myotonic dystrophy, but since many cases are mild, the families go on interminably. The high rates of mutation do not encourage optimism that genetic restriction can be the ultimate goal.

Caughey, J. E., and Myrianthopoulous, N. C.: Dystrophia Myotonica and Related Disorders. Springfield, Ill., Charles C Thomas, 1963.

Dyken, P. R., and Harper, P. S.: Congenital dystrophia myotonica. Neurology, 23:465, 1973.

Emery, A. E. H., Watt, M. S., and Clacl, E. R.: The effects of genetic counseling in Duchenne muscular dystrophy. Clin. Genet., 3:147, 1972.

Gardner-Medwin, D., Pennington, R. J., and Walton, J. N.: The detection of carriers of X-linked muscular dystrophy genes. J. Neurol. Sci., 13:459, 1971.

Research Committee, Muscular Dystrophy Group (eds.): Research in Muscular Dystrophy. London, Sir Isaac Pitman & Sons, Ltd., 1969.

Rowland, L. P.: Muscular dystrophies. DM, November 1972, p. 1.

Walton, J. N.: Disorders of Voluntary Muscle. 2nd ed. Boston, Little, Brown & Company, 1969.

477. CONGENITAL MYOPATHIES

Definition. These are rare diseases characterized by weakness that is usually relatively mild but persists throughout life, either progressing slowly or remaining stationary.

Etiology. The cause is not known. A few of these disorders are familial and are suspected of having a genetic basis, but so many cases are sporadic that other causes are not excluded, and there are no clear clues.

Pathology. These diseases are defined in terms of pathology, and most of them have been delineated within the past 15 years since the introduction of histochemical techniques to study muscle biopsy. The names of the diseases reflect the predominant anatomic disorder.

In *central core disease,* the central portion of the muscle fiber appears rather amorphous, in contrast to the fibrillar appearance of the surrounding normal portion. In cross-section, the central portion appears blue when stained with Gomori's trichrome, in striking contrast to the red periphery. The central areas lack all oxidative enzyme activity, and there are no mitochondria in this region. In *nemaline myopathy or rod myopathy,* small threadlike or rod bodies are scattered throughout the fiber. The rods are barely visible in conventional hematoxylin and eosin stains, but can be seen readily in phase contrast or with the trichrome stain. In electron microscopy the structures seem to originate in the Z-band, and circumstantial evidence suggests that they are composed of tropomyosin. *Myotubular myopathy* designates the appearance of myofibers that resemble a stage in the early development of fetal muscle, with nuclei located centrally rather than at the periphery and surrounded by a halo of apparently empty space. Because the pathogenesis of this appearance is uncertain, some investigators prefer the name *centronuclear myopathy.* In other disorders mitochondria have appeared abnormal, either in number (too many) or size (too large), often associated with accumulations of lipid droplets.

Clinical Manifestations. Although designated "congenital," these disorders are only exceptionally symptomatic in the first year of life, except that the onset of walking may be delayed. Later, the symptoms of proximal limb weakness become evident: waddling gait, difficulty in climbing stairs, frequent falls, and scoliosis. Later, there may be weakness of the arms. There are few clinical clues to each specific histologic abnormality. Among the nemaline cases there have been skeletal abnormalities (kyphoscoliosis, pigeon breast, pes cavus, high palate, and an unusually elongated face). In two families with myotubular disease, ophthalmoplegia was present as well as limb weakness. Central core and mitochondrial disorders have not been assciated with distinctive clinical signs other than proximal limb weakness. In two unrelated patients, similar morphologic alterations of mitochondria were found in muscles of patients with nonthyroidal hypermetabolism; these disorders were neither familial nor congenital, however, and hypermetabolism has not been a manifestation of the congenital disorders. In none of the structurally defined congenital myopathies, therefore, is it possible to link the morphologic abnormality to a biochemical or physiologic cause of the weakness.

Diagnosis. Proximal limb weakness in a young child is usually myopathic in origin, but must be distinguished from the neurogenic Wohlfart-Kugelberg-Welander syndrome and from polyneuritis. Myopathic abnormalities in the EMG, an abnormal family history, an incidence in girls, and especially the histologic abnormalities define the individual entities. The serum enzymes may be normal or slightly increased. In some clinics most cases of apparently congenital myopathy fail to meet the specific histologic criteria, showing only nonspecific myopathic changes in biopsy. There is no better designation for these cases than "congenital myopathy," but it is likely that there is more than one cause.

In infancy, the major cause of weakness is a form of motor neuron disease (Werdnig-Hoffmann disease). Among infants with multiple congenitally fixed joints (arthrogryposis multiplex), some prove to have myopathic disease as defined by muscle biopsy and electromyography. In some cases, neonatal difficulty in swallowing is followed by delayed onset of walking, possibly persistent weakness, obesity, childhood diabetes, mental retardation, and a characteristic facial appearance (Prader-Willi syndrome), but there is no abnormality on muscle biopsy or electromyogram.

Treatment and Prognosis. There is no specific treatment for any of these disorders. Physical therapy and orthopedic corrective measures are of value. There are too few cases to generalize about the course of these illnesses; most seem to be mild and nonprogressive, but occasional cases are more severe.

Afifi, A. K., Ibrahim, M. Z. M., Bergman, R. A., Haydar, N. A., Mire, J., Bahuth, N., and Kaylani, F.: Morphologic features of hypermetabolic mitochondrial disease. J. Neurol. Sci., 15:271, 1972.

Bharucha, E. P., Pandya, S. S., and Dastur, D. K.: Arthrogryposis multiplex congenita. J. Neurol Neurosurg. Psychiatry, 35:425, 1972.

Dubowitz, V.: The Floppy Infant. London, Spastics International Medical Publications, 1969.

Hall, B. D., and Smith, D. W.: Prader-Willi syndrome: A résumé of 32 cases. J. Pediatr., 81:286, 1972.

Hefferman, L. P., Rewcastle, N. B., and Humphrey, J. G.: The spectrum of rod myopathies. Arch. Neurol., 18:529, 1968.

Kinoshita, M., and Cadman, T. E.: Myotubular myopathy. Arch. Neurol., 18:265, 1968.

478. MYOTONIA CONGENITA (Thomsen's Disease)

Definition. Myotonia congenita is a disorder characterized by difficulty in relaxation of skeletal muscle after forceful contraction, present from early childhood.

Incidence. This is one of the rarest of all muscular disorders.

Etiology. There are occasional sporadic cases, but most are inherited in a pattern corresponding to an autosomal dominant trait. In a few families, the disease seems to be autosomal recessive. The biochemical fault is not known, but the muscle membrane is electrically unstable and tends to fire repetitively. The abnormality must be inherent within the muscle, because myotonic phenomena may be elicited after all neural influences are abolished by spinal anesthesia, block of motor nerves by local anesthesia, or blockade of the neuromuscular junction by intra-arterial injection of d-tubocurarine. Myotonia is abolished, however, by the intramuscular administration of procaine. That the membrane is abnormal is suggested by the myotonia that occurs in otherwise normal individuals taking diazacholesterol, a substance that interferes with the biosynthesis of cholesterol. How this affects the membrane, however, is not known, and membranes of other organs are not functionally altered.

Clinical Manifestations. The difficulty in relaxation in this disorder, in contrast to that in myotonic dystrophy, is widespread. Difficulty in relaxing the grip may lead to prominent and sometimes embarrassing symptoms. Ocular muscles may also be affected, so that the eyes seem momentarily "stuck" in one position, or the eyelids may remain closed after forceful closure. Sometimes oropharyngeal muscles are affected, with difficulty in speaking or swallowing. Startle reactions may induce stiffness of the legs, thwarting sudden attempts to catch a bus or run from home plate. There is no weakness, and one unexplained characteristic is the unusual muscular development of many patients, causing a Herculean appearance, and perhaps related to involuntary and repeated isometric exercise. The myotonia can be elicited by tapping any muscle in severely affected cases. Reflexes are unaltered.

Diagnosis. The major problem is in distinguishing these patients from those with myotonic muscular dystrophy. Here the only symptoms and signs are related to myotonia. There is no weakness, no cataract, no baldness, no gonadal atrophy. Some authors have described "transitional cases," but these are probably patients in families with myotonic muscular dystrophy who are only mildly affected and show only myotonia before the other manifestations. There may be some weakness in families with the rare autosomal recessive form of myotonia congenita. In general, families with myotonia congenita breed true.

Treatment. Drug therapy is effective. For many years, quinine was the staple treatment in doses of 0.3 to 1.5 grams daily. Recently, diphenylhydantoin has proved equally effective and less apt to cause disagreeable side effects in therapeutic doses of 0.3 to 0.6 gram daily. Should this fail, procainamide may also be used, in doses of 4 to 6 grams daily, but this drug is prone to cause drug-induced lupus erythematosus.

Landau, W. M.: The essential mechanism in myotonia. Neurology, 2:369, 1952.
Lipicky, R. J., Bryant, S. H., and Salmon, J. H.: Cable parameters, sodium, potassium, chloride and water content, and potassium efflux in isolated external intercostal muscle of normal volunteers and patients with myotonia congenita. J. Clin. Invest., 50:2091, 1971.

479. FAMILIAL MYOGLOBINURIA

Most cases of myoglobinuria are sporadic, and they will be described in Ch. 484. Some persons, however, have repeated attacks from early childhood, suggesting some genetic fault, and sometimes more than one individual in a family is affected. Some of these familial cases are due to lack of muscle phosphorylase or phosphofructokinase. They can be recognized by the ischemic work test in which contracture is induced and venous lactate fails to rise. (See Ch. 809). In one family, an abnormality of fatty acid oxidation associated with attacks of myoglobinuria was shown to be due to lack of carnitine palmityl transferase deficiency. Several families have been studied, however, in which glycogen metabolism was normal, and contracture could not be induced. The genetic abnormality in these patients has not been identified.

DiMauro, S., and DiMauro, P. M.: Muscle carnitine palmityltransferase deficiency and myoglobinuria. Science, 182:929, 1973.
Rowland, L. P., DiMauro, S., and Bank, W. J.: Glycogen storage diseases of muscles. Problems in biochemical genetics. Birth Defects, 7:43, 1971.

480. FAMILIAL PERIODIC PARALYSIS

Definition. Periodic paralysis is characterized by recurrent attacks of flaccid weakness usually associated with abnormally high or low serum potassium concentrations. Many cases are familial. In sporadic cases the abnormality may be secondary to identifiable aberrations of potassium metabolism.

Etiology and Pathogenesis. Familial cases are distributed in a pattern consistent with autosomal dominant inheritance. Hypokalemia during attacks was the first metabolic abnormality to be recognized, with no loss of potassium in urine. It was therefore presumed that potassium shifted from extracellular to intracellular compartments, especially muscle. This has been difficult to prove, and the anticipated hyperpolarization of the muscle membrane potential has not been substantiated by direct measurement with intracellular electrodes. Abnormalities of glucose metabolism have been suspected, because attacks can be precipitated by infusions of glucose and insulin, by eating a large meal, or by administration of epinephrine. However, biochemical studies have failed to pinpoint the abnormality.

During the past two decades it has been recognized that the serum potassium tends to rise in some patients, and attacks in these individuals are induced by the ingestion of potassium. This variety is therefore called "hyperkalemic periodic paralysis," and is generally considered to be the mirror image of the hypokalemic type, with potassium presumably shifting out of muscle and into blood during attacks. Why this should happen is not clear, but at least in the hyperkalemic type there are alterations of the intracellular potential in the direction required by theory. There are clinical differences between the two forms of periodic paralysis, but there are so many areas of overlap and so many common features that it is difficult to decide just how many genetically distinct forms there really are.

Pathology. In both forms of periodic paralysis there may be vacuoles within muscle fibers. These may be numerous or scanty, and it is not clear that they are more frequent in paralyzed muscle. Most electron microscopists believe that the vacuoles are derived from the sarcoplasmic reticulum, but others think they originate in the T-system in areas of necrotic muscle. Glycogen seems to be increased in amount in ultrastructural studies, but the results of biochemical analysis have been inconsistent. There is no evidence that other organs are affected in either form of the disease. The heart is usually spared pathologically.

Clinical Manifestations. There are clinical differences between the two forms. In the hypokalemic variety, attacks tend to start in late childhood or adolescence, frequently occur at night, are apt to be severe, and last for a day or more. In the hyperkalemic variety, attacks start at an early age, occur much more frequently, tend to be milder, and may last minutes or hours. Moreover, patients with hyperkalemic periodic paralysis usually have some evidence of myotonia, which is rarely symptomatic and often limited to percussion myotonia of the tongue. Lid-lag and Chvostek's sign are identified with the hyperkalemic type. These clinical distinctions may break down in application to individual cases and are therefore only crude guides. Moreover, many features are common to both types: a dominant pattern of inheritance, a susceptibility to attacks during periods of rest after vigorous exercise, the ability to ward off attacks by mild exercise after a mild attack has begun, persistent weakness between attacks, vacuoles in muscle, a lack of clear relation between the serum potassium concentration and the severity of paresis, the induction of local weakness by cooling, and protection against attacks by acetazolamide. Some patients are affected by attacks in which the serum potassium may be either high or low.

Typical attacks start with weakness of the legs that ascends to the arms. Cranial muscles are affected in severe attacks only, and respiratory insufficiency is exceptional. The attacks may be mild and brief, or severe and prolonged, with all gradations in between. During severe attacks, the myotatic reflexes are lost, and the muscles are electrically inexcitable. Attacks are rarely apoplectic in onset and usually take an hour or more to develop, except that attacks beginning in sleep may be fully developed when the patient awakes. Paresthesias and myalgia may be prominent at the onset, or may be completely lacking. Some patients are aware of oliguria during the attack and of diuresis afterward.

The serum potassium is in the range of 2.5 to 3.5 mEq per liter in hypokalemic attacks, and 5.0 to 7.0 mEq per liter in the hyperkalemic type. Between attacks serum potassium values may be normal. The electrocardiogram is altered as would be predicted from the serum values, with low T waves in hypokalemia and peaked T waves in hyperkalemia.

Patients with hyperkalemic periodic paralysis may have mild symptoms attributable to myotonia, especially of the hands. When individuals in a family are studied, some may be found to have myotonia without any history of periodic paralysis.

In both types of the disease, there may be persistent weakness between attacks, most often proximal, sometimes distal. In the past this has been attributed to a permanent "myopathy," but experience with acetazolamide therapy indicates that even longlasting weakness may be reversible, regardless of pathologic changes in muscle. A few patients with intermittent normokalemic or hyperkalemic paralysis have had persistent cardiac arrhythmia, especially bigeminy, and bouts of ventricular tachycardia. The cardiac disorder is neither temporally related to attacks of limb weakness nor related to serum potassium content.

Diagnosis. Periodic paralysis can be recognized by the history of typical attacks; no other disease causes this pattern of recurrent weakness. In myasthenia gravis, weakness may come and go, but less abruptly and with a duration of weeks rather than hours or days; remissions are less frequent so that it is less "periodic." Polymyositis may be transient, but episodes are rarely shorter than several weeks or months. Attacks of myoglobinuric weakness could conceivably be confusing if the pigmenturia were not recognized, but myalgia and malaise are so prominent that is rarely mistaken for periodic paralysis. Hysterical attacks might be confusing.

If the patient is seen during the attack and the serum potassium is abnormal, other causes of hypo- or hyperkalemia must be considered. Low serum potassium concentrations with paralysis are also encountered in hyperaldosteronism, potassium-losing nephritis, potassium depletion caused by laxative abuse, diuretics, or diarrhea, and thyrotoxicosis. *Thiazide* and *thalidone diuretics* are in such widespread use nowadays that these drugs are likely to be an increasingly frequent cause of hypokalemic weakness; in one series, about 25 per cent of randomly chosen patients receiving these drugs had serum potassium contents below normal. Hyperkalemia is most often due to renal insufficiency, but may also occur in adrenal insufficiency, after administration of spironolactone, or as a manifestation of aldosterone deficiency.

The signs of these other disorders usually provide appropriate diagnostic clues. A family history of periodic paralysis is useful in diagnosis, but apparently sporadic cases may be indistinguishable from the familial disorder. If the patient is not having a spontaneous attack when studied, the only way to distinguish the two forms is to provoke an attack. The techniques to be described have been used in numerous centers with many patients, without serious complications. But induced attacks may be frightening to patient and physician, and should be left to experienced investigators. Facilities for supported respiration should be immediately available. Appropriately informed consent is mandatory. Because of the uncertainty of clinical distinction, it is advisable to start with glucose (100 grams) given intravenously in one hour, with 20 units of regular insulin either in the infusion or given subcutaneously. Hypoglycemic symptoms should be anticipated, and the electrocardiogram should be monitored. Hypokalemia is induced as the blood sugar falls, usually within one hour after the infusion is completed. If an attack is induced, it can be terminated with administration of 7 to 10 grams of potassium chloride (KCl) by mouth. Whether or not an attack is induced by glucose and insulin, but especially if it is not, the patient should then be challenged with potassium. This poses delicate problems because it is not clear how much potassium constitutes an adequate challenge. We start with 3 grams of KCl by mouth. If this fails we gradually increase the dose on successive days to a maximum of 8 or 10 grams. Patients with hyperkalemic paralysis have attacks with serum potassium levels between 5 and 8 mEq per liter.

Other members of the family should be investigated clinically and electromyographically for evidence of myotonia.

Treatment. Acute attacks of hypokalemic paralysis are best treated with oral KCl, 5 to 10 grams. Relief of weakness usually commences within 30 minutes but may take several hours, and some attacks are peculiarly refractory. Hyperkalemia may be relieved by infusions of glucose and insulin. Chlorothiazide and calcium gluconate have also been reported to be effective. In severe attacks, weakness may persist even after the serum potassium has returned to normal concentrations.

The traditional method used to protect patients

against hypokalemic paralysis was, until recently, a low-sodium diet supplemented by oral KCl, or perhaps by spironolactone or dexamethasone. Then, acetazolamide in small doses, sometimes only 250 per mg daily, sometimes more, was found to be effective prophylaxis in the hyperkalemic type. Subsequently, it was found that similar doses of acetazolamide were equally effective in the hypokalemic variety, so a single drug is beneficial in both forms. How it exerts this effect is not known. The best-known effects of this compound relate to its ability to inhibit carbonic anhydrase, but muscle lacks this enzyme, and no definite systemic effects of the drug have been recognized in the doses used, but metabolic acidosis may be responsible.

Gordon, R. M., Green, J. R., and Lagunoff, D.: Studies on a patient with hypokalemic familial periodic paralysis. Am. J. Med., 48:185, 1970.

Griggs, R. C., Engel, W. K., and Resnick, J. S.: Acetazolamide treatment of hypokalemic periodic paralysis: Prevention of attacks and improvement of persistent weakness. Ann. Intern. Med., 73:39, 1970.

Pearson, C. M., and Kalyanaraman, R.: Periodic paralyses. *In* Stanbury, J. B., Wyngaarden, J. B., and Fredericksou, D. S. (eds.): The Metabolic Basis of Inherited Disease. 3rd ed. New York, McGraw-Hill Book Company, 1972, pp. 1180–1203.

Satoyashi, E., Murakami, K., Kowa, H., Kinoshita, M., and Hishiyama, Y.: Periodic paralysis in hyperthyroidism. Neurology, 13:746, 1963.

Zierler, K. L.: Speculations on hypokalemic periodic paralysis. Am. J. Med. Sci., 266:131, 1973.

481. MYOSITIS OSSIFICANS

This rare disorder is most dramatic in its consequences, producing the "stone man" of circus sideshows. Symptoms usually begin in early childhood, with transient and localized swellings of the neck and back. Ultimately there is progressive rigidity of the neck, trunk, and limbs. Palpable plates are discernible beneath the rigid parts. Severely affected patients may be able to stand and walk, and yet be totally unable to bend so that they must be raised from bed with assistance. The bars beneath the skin are visible roentgenographically. Microscopically, muscle is replaced by bone and connective tissue. Whether the primary disorder is in the fibroblasts (leading to abnormal ossification) or in the muscle itself is not resolved. Muscle biopsy early in the disease may show widespread necrosis and inflammation, but serum enzymes are not always elevated, nor is the electromyogram always myopathic. Few cases are familial, but the disorder is believed to be inherited because digital abnormalities are almost always present in both the patients and other members of the family in a pattern suggesting an autosomal dominant inheritance. Microdactyly commonly affects the great toe, and clinodactyly (curved digits) may affect the hands. There is no detectable systemic abnormality of calcium and phosphate metabolism, and there has been no effective therapy, but recent reports suggest that administration of disphosphonates may prevent the deposition of bone. Once bone is formed, however, these drugs are ineffective.

Bassett, C. A. L., Donath, A., Macagno, F., Preisig, R., Fleisch, H., and Francis, M. D.: Diphosphonates in the treatment of myositis ossificans. Lancet, 2:845, 1969.

Lutwak, L.: Myositis ossificans progressiva. Am. J. Med., 37:269, 1964.

SPORADIC DISORDERS

482. DERMATOMYOSITIS AND POLYMYOSITIS

The main discussion of these conditions is found in Ch. 80. However, the concept of polymyositis is central to the analysis and concepts of acquired myopathies of adult life, and thus it is appropriate to review some of the problems here.

Definition. These conditions are usually considered together, but this practice may prove imprudent. *Dermatomyositis* is a recognizable syndrome of unknown cause, characterized by a rash and myopathy, both with distinctive clinical features. The name is derived from the inflammatory cellular response that is usually found in skeletal muscle, but lymphocytic infiltration is not present in all cases. This lack causes problems in defining *polymyositis,* a disorder presumably identical with dermatomyositis but without the rash. There probably is such a disease, because the rash of dermatomyositis may be so mild that it could be overlooked by parents or inexperienced clinicians, and there are patients with no history of rash who develop subcutaneous calcinosis, implying that the skin had been involved even without visible dermatitis. But once the rash is taken away, an essential sign of dermatomyositis is withdrawn, and it becomes impossible to define polymyositis as the same condition. Polymyositis, therefore, is a syndrome, probably of diverse causes, and is identifiable by the following set of diagnostic criteria.

Diagnosis. At the outset it should be noted that the diagnosis of dermatomyositis is a clinical diagnosis, depending upon the characteristic rash and muscular weakness. In some patients the features of scleroderma may also be prominent, warranting the name "sclerodermatomyositis." But there is no overlap with lupus erythematosus or periarteritis nodosa, and the visceral lesions of these conditions do not occur in dermatomyositis.

Problems arise when there is no rash. The syndrome must be differentiated from the dystrophies by lack of family history, onset after age 35 (because no familial limb-girdle dystrophy starts so late), rapidity of onset in weeks or months rather than years, spontaneous improvement (which does not occur in dystrophy, by definition), distribution of weakness affecting cervical and cranial muscles, or systemic symptoms such as arthralgia or Raynaud's syndrome. The muscle biopsy ought to be crucial, but inflammatory lesions may be lacking in dermatomyositis, and may occasionally be seen in dystrophies; severe inflammation, when present, supports the diagnosis of polymyositis, but lack of leukocytic infiltration does not exclude the diagnosis. The electromyogram is helpful, but, again, not distinctive; there are the usual features of myopathy with the additional evidence of irritable muscle (increased insertional activity and some spontaneous activity). Serum enzymes tend to be high. There may also be an increased erythrocyte sedimentation rate, increased serum gamma globulin concentration, or a positive latex fixation test for rheumatoid factor. But there are no antibodies to muscle. Evidence of lymphocytes sensitized to muscle may be demonstrable, but this has not yet attained diagnostic reliability.

The problem of diagnosis is best exemplified by a patient with limb weakness commencing at age 40 and evidence of myopathic disease in muscle biopsy and EMG. Search must be made for the known causes of muscle disease, to be discussed below. If none is found, the diagnosis of exclusion is polymyositis, no matter what the laboratory data show or do not show. That this residual group is all due to one disease seems unlikely, not only because there is clinical heterogeneity, but also because if there are so many known causes of the syndrome, there are some others still to be recognized. Because inflammatory cells are not always seen in the muscle biopsy, some authorities eschew the word "polymyositis" and prefer "myopathy of unknown cause." This, at least, identifies the problem, but for the present "polymyositis" seems to be entrenched. Clinicians should recognize, however, that "polymyositis" is no more a specific diagnosis than "headache," "polyneuritis," or "convulsive disorder," terms that also imply inadequately defined syndromes of diverse etiology.

483. OTHER ACQUIRED MYOPATHIES

Proximal limb weakness in patients with no rash, with or without inflammatory lesions in muscle, and with or without increased serum enzyme activity, occurs in several disorders. These may be considered diseases associated with polymyositis or causes of polymyositis. To identify these disorders, appropriate diagnostic tools must be utilized.

Carcinomatous Myopathy. Muscle weakness without rash may occur in patients with carcinoma of the lung or of any other primary site. Myeloma, macroglobulinemia, and other gammopathies may also be associated with myopathy. The tumor itself may or may not be symptomatic, and treatment of the tumor may or may not affect the muscular symptoms.

Collagen Diseases. Proximal limb weakness may occur in the course of systemic lupus erythematosus, progressive systemic sclerosis, rheumatoid arthritis, and, rarely, periarteritis nodosa or giant cell arteritis. In these circumstances, the myopathy is treated as part of the general disorder.

Endocrine Disease. Thyrotoxic myopathy is a well-recognized syndrome. Usually there is clinical evidence of hyperthyroidism, but not always ("apathetic hyperthyroidism"). Signs of hypermetabolism are especially apt to be lacking in elderly patients. This myopathy inevitably disappears when the patient is rendered euthyroid by treatment. Similarly, weakness may complicate hypothyroidism. Another muscle syndrome of hypothyroidism is Hoffmann's syndrome, a peculiar difficulty in relaxing muscles that lack the characteristic electromyographic abnormalities of myotonia and is therefore called "pseudomyotonia," but may appear similar clinically. This, too, disappears with appropriate replacement therapy. Infants with cretinism may have unusually well developed muscles but not the disorder of relaxation.

Hyperparathyroidism and hyperadrenacorticism may also be responsible for weakness that looks like any other proximal myopathy. Surprisingly, because asthenia has so long been regarded as prominent, Addison's disease seems not to be a cause of this syndrome. Weakness may be part of hyperpituitarism, but acromegalic features always overshadow the myopathy. Myalgia, with or without weakness, may be a prominent symptom in patients with osteomalacia, and the muscular disorder may respond dramatically to administration of vitamin D.

Infections. Structures resembling viral particles have been seen with the electron microscope with polymyositis, and sometimes there are acute myopathic disorders in individuals with influenza or encephalomyelitis, but no specific virus has been isolated from these cases. Muscle may be affected by a variety of organisms, but the only one of practical importance in the differential diagnosis of acute or subacute myopathy is trichinosis. Toxoplasmosis may affect muscle in the course of a syndrome that looks like severe infectious mononucleosis with adenopathy, rash, mucosal lesions, and hepatomegaly. In tropical countries, trypanosomiasis and schistosomiasis are important causes of muscle involvement.

Sarcoidosis. In muscle clinics, sarcoidosis is recognized as a significant cause of polymyositis. Usually there is other evidence of the disease, but sometimes the first symptoms are due to weakness, and in a few cases only muscle seems to be involved. Myalgia may be severe in these patients.

Drugs. A variety of drugs used to treat more common disorders may themselves cause muscular weakness, especially triamcinolone and other fluorinated adrenal steroids (but probably all steroids), vincristine, chloroquine, bretylium, and guanethidine. Repeated injections of narcotics and other drugs may lead to fibrosis of muscle that simulates a diffuse myopathy.

Alcoholic Myopathy. The clearest myopathic disorder in alcoholic persons is acute myoglobinuria. Some of these individuals, and some who never have an attack of pigmenturia, also suffer from proximal limb weakness, especially affecting the legs. The serum creatine phosphokinase is often elevated. The problem in some of these patients, however, is that they also suffer from the typical polyneuritis of alcoholism, and it then becomes difficult to prove that the muscular weakness is not also secondary to a neurogenic disorder. Too few patients have been evaluated to know whether abstinence and a good diet will reverse the persistent weakness. Chronic hypokalemia from any cause may be associated with the syndrome of polymyositis: weakness of relatively abrupt onset, muscle necrosis in biopsy, and high serum enzymes. This is most commonly seen in patients taking thiazide diuretics, but may also occur in hypokalemic states caused by chronic diarrhea. Hypokalemia may also contribute to some cases of alcoholic myopathy. (Other acquired disorders of potassium metabolism are discussed under Diagnosis in Ch. 480).

Byers, R. K., Bergman, A. B., and Joseph, M. C.: Steroid myopathy. Report of five cases occurring during treatment of rheumatic fever. Pediatrics, 29:26, 1962.

Dawkins, R. L., and Mastaglia, F. L.: Cell-mediated cytotoxicity to muscle in polymyositis. Effect of immunosuppression. N. Engl. J. Med., 288:434, 1973.

Frame, B., Heize, E. G., Block, M. A., and Manson, G. A.: Myopathy in primary hyperparathyroidism. Ann. Intern. Med., 68:1022, 1968.

Hall, W. H.: Proximal muscle atrophy in adult celiac disease. Am. J. Dig. Dis., 13:697, 1968.

Mastaglia, F. L., Gardner-Medwin, D., and Hudgson, P.: Muscle fibrosis and contractures in a pethidine addict. Br. Med. J., 4:532, 1971.

Perkoff, G. T.: Alcoholic myopathy. Ann. Rev. Med., 22:125, 1971.

Scarpalezos, S., et al.: Neural and muscular manifestations of hypothyroidism. Arch. Neurol., 29:140, 1973.

Silverstein, A., and Siltzbach, L. E.: Muscle involvement in sarcoidosis. Arch. Neurol., 21:235, 1969.

Trojaborg, W., Frantzen, E., and Andersen, I.: Peripheral neuropathy and myopathy associated with carcinoma of the lung. Brain, 92:71, 1969.

484. SPORADIC MYOGLOBINURIA

Definition. Sporadic myoglobinuria comprises a group of disorders characterized by injury of muscle and excretion of myoglobin in the urine. *Rhabdomyolysis* has been proposed as a more precise term, but it is used to mean "myoglobinuria," and therefore is of dubious value.

Pathogenesis. Myoglobin may be released from muscle whenever there is extensive and rapid destruction. Sometimes the cause is evident, as in the *crush injuries* of World War II when individuals were pinned beneath the timbers of buildings destroyed in bombing raids. Similar pressure injuries may occur in comatose persons who lie on one side without moving for prolonged periods. This kind of injury is perhaps more apt to occur when there are other causes of *metabolic depression;* for instance, in coma after suicidal ingestion of barbiturates or carbon monoxide intoxication, or prolonged unconsciousness in the snow. A similar effect may be induced by *arterial occlusion* by tourniquet or embolism, or even by prolonged knee-chest posture under anesthesia.

In other patients, the cause is less discernible. In every series of patients with myoglobinuria, a disproportionate number are *alcoholics,* but why this should occur is not known. Sometimes there has been exposure to a known *membrane toxin,* such as the bite of the Malayan sea snake. In some addicts, heroin itself seems to cause myoglobinuria. Or there may be *metabolic alterations* that do not ordinarily cause this kind of trouble, such as diarrhea with hypokalemia; potassium depletion caused by diuretics, amphotericin, or licorice; diabetic acidosis; or systemic infection with fever. In many attacks, however, not even these clues prevail.

The most common cause of myoglobinuria is probably unusually *vigorous exercise* by an otherwise normal person. Most cases have been reported by military physicians, and local designations include such titles as the "squat-jump syndrome." Some cases are attributed to "march hemoglobinuria." When large numbers of recruits endure these tortures, a certain number will have attacks of myalgia followed by pigmenturia. Why these individuals have attacks and others are spared is not clear, but this seems to be a "normal" variation. In civilians, cases have been caused by the excess muscular activity of an initiation rite into a club or fraternity, and isolated attacks have occurred after the vigorous muscular activity induced by succinylcholine before it achieves relaxation. In *malignant hyperthermia,* there is a rapid rise in temperature, widespread muscular rigidity, hyperkalemia, and metabolic acidosis, with a fatal outcome in about 75 per cent. The offending agents are usually halothane and succinylcholine. Increased serum activities of sarcoplasmic enzyme are the rule, and often there is myoglobinuria. The intense muscular contraction may be the proximate cause of myoglobinuria in this syndrome, but the widespread metabolic disorder probably contributes. Spontaneous convulsions and electroconvulsive therapy have also been followed by myoglobinuria. If an individual is subject to repeated attacks, it may be suspected that there is some kind of undiscovered genetic defect, although the only ones recognized now are deficiencies of phosphorylase, phosphofructokinase, or carnitine palmityl transferase.

Clinical Manifestations. In attacks other than those caused by local crushing or arterial occlusion, the clinical picture is similar. Affected muscles are apt to be the ones subject to greatest physical strain (the legs in squat-thrusts, the arms after chinning or push-ups, the arms and legs after wrestling matches). The muscles ache, may be swollen, and are weak. Sometimes there is so much edema that local vascular abnormalities are suspected. There may be fever and considerable malaise. Symptoms persist for several days even though pigmenturia rarely lasts more than 48 hours. Recovery may be gradual. Cranial muscles are rarely involved, and although respiratory failure is uncommon it is a hazard. The most important threat to life is renal injury secondary to excretion of heme. There may be red cells or myoglobin in the urine as well as casts. Oliguria is followed by azotemia and hyperkalemia. This may be treated by appropriate measures.

Diagnosis. The diagnosis of myoglobinuria can be made on clinical grounds and with relatively simple tests, but precise identification of the pigment depends upon biochemical analysis. The urine may appear red-brown because of hemoglobin, myoglobin, or porphyrins. The latter would not give a positive test with benzidine (or other heme-reacting reagents), and would not give a positive Watson-Schwartz test for porphobilinogen. Besides, the neurologic disorder of porphyria is neuropathy, not an acute myopathy. If the urine gives a positive test for heme and contains no or few erythrocytes, the pigment is either myoglobin or hemoglobin. If it is hemoglobin, the serum would be pink (after a hemolytic reaction), whereas the color of the serum in myoglobinuria is normal. (This distinction depends upon the affinity of serum haptoglobin for hemoglobin and not for myoglobin. Hemoglobin is not excreted until haptoglobin is saturated by visible amounts of the pigment, whereas myoglobin is excreted at much lower concentrations.) Furthermore, in attacks of myoglobinuria, the muscular weakness and myalgia are distinctive, and serum enzymes are greatly increased, whereas they are not in hemolysis. Positive identification of myoglobin can be achieved by several tests: absorption spectrophotometry is direct and simple, but in many laboratories the most convenient method is electrophoresis on starch gel or cellulose acetate. In the future, immunochemical methods are apt to gain favor. In all patients presenting in coma, especially after drug ingestion or carbon monoxide intoxication, it is important to check the urine for heme pigment and to assay serum for sarcoplasmic enzyme activity because of the possibility of a crush syndrome; if recognized, mannitol diuresis may prevent renal injury.

Treatment. If there is no renal injury, myoglobinuria is not threatening. The hazards of renal injury are not directly correlated to the amount of pigment excreted, and other factors are probably involved. Once an attack starts, it is useful to encourage excretion of dilute urine, and some authorities still favor alkalinizing agents although it has not been clearly demonstrated that these treatments protect the kidneys. Few patients are left with residual weakness, but in some the syndrome is characterized by prolonged weakness punctuated by attacks of myoglobinuria.

Gordon, R. A., Britt, B. A., and Kalow, W. (eds.): International Symposium on Malignant Hyperthermia. Springfield, Ill., Charles C Thomas, 1973.

Greenberg, J., and Arneson, L.: Exertional rhabdomyolysis with myoglobinuria in a large group of military trainees. Neurology, 17:216, 1967.

Kagen, L. J.: Immunologic detection of myoglobinuria after cardiac surgery. Ann. Intern. Med., 67:1183, 1967.

Rowland, L. P., and Penn, A. S.: Myoglobinuria. Med. Clin. North Am., 56:1233, 1972.

Vertel, R. M., and Knochel, J. P.: Acute renal failure due to heat injury: An analysis of ten cases with a high incidence of myoglobinuria. Am. J. Med., 43:435, 1967.

485. MYASTHENIA GRAVIS

Definition. Myasthenia gravis is usually defined as a state of abnormal fatigability. This definition has the merit of being consistent with the characteristic electrophysiologic disorder found in patients with this condition, but there are serious disadvantages. "Normal" fatigue is not defined, muscles weakened from any cause are apt to fatigue more readily than normal, and myasthenic muscle may be completely paralyzed (especially ocular muscles), with no signs of fatigue. Moreover, emphasis on fatigue has led to the treatment of many psychoneurotic patients with cholinergic drugs. An alternative definition has therefore been proposed:

"*Myasthenia gravis* is a disease characterized by weakness that has special characteristics: predilection for ocular and other cranial muscles; tendency to fluctuate during brief periods of observation (in the course of a single day) or for longer periods (remissions and exacerbations); with no signs of neural lesion, and partial reversibility by the administration of cholinergic drugs."

Etiology. The cause of myasthenia gravis is not known. Several disorders tend to occur more frequently in patients with myasthenia gravis, such as hyperthyroidism or other thyroidal disorders, and a significant number of patients with myasthenia gravis have thymomas. But neither in these situations nor in others has a causal relationship been proved. Whether or not there is a significant association with "autoimmune" diseases remains to be proved; rheumatoid arthritis and systemic lupus erythematosus have been reported in patients with myasthenia gravis, but the statistical significance of these associations is uncertain.

Several lines of evidence suggest an immunologic disorder in myasthenia gravis. Thymomas occur in about 15 per cent of all patients, more often in patients older than 40 years. Germinal centers are seen frequently in the thymus glands of patients who have no tumor. Infiltration of muscle by monocytes is characteristic, especially in perivascular collections called lymphorrhages. Antibodies to muscle can be demonstrated by immunofluorescent techniques in approximately a third of all patients with myasthenia, and in almost all patients with concomitant myasthenia and thymoma. However, the nature of the antigen that elicits these antibodies is uncertain, and it seems quite clear that the antibodies are not responsible for the symptoms of myasthenia. Thus antibodies may be present in patients with thymoma who have no evidence of myasthenia. There is no correlation between the presence of antibodies in serum and the appearance of transient neonatal myasthenia, and the concentration of serum antibodies does not correlate with the severity of symptoms. Finally, physiologic evidence indicates a disorder of neuromuscular transmission in myasthenia, and the antibodies react with proteins in the myofiber, but not at the neuromuscular junction. The significance of these human antibodies is therefore uncertain. The possibility that lymphocytes are sensitized to some component of muscle is currently being evaluated. No one has yet succeeded in designing a fully reproducible experimental model of the disease by immunologic techniques; however, injections of muscle and thymus may produce an experimental disorder, and injections of acetylcholine receptor from electric eel have induced a myasthenic state in rabbits.

Neuromuscular Disorder. The symptoms of myasthenia gravis resemble those of curare intoxication. This observation led to the use of curare antagonists in the treatment of myasthenia gravis. All effective therapies have been derived from this initial observation, and all drugs currently in use are inhibitors of the enzyme cholinesterase. These drugs also partially repair a physiologic defect that can be detected in patients by relatively simple techniques. When the ulnar nerve of normal individuals is stimulated at rates of 25 per second or less, the action potential of the hypothenar muscles is sustained at a constant amplitude. In patients with myasthenia, however, there is a rapid decline in the height of the evoked potentials. If the patient is then given neostigmine, the amplitude of the evoked potentials is restored to normal. This pattern could be consistent with either excessive cholinesterase activity, inadequate release of acetylcholine, or blockade of the junction by some curare-like compound. Microelectrode studies have been performed upon intercostal muscle fibers of patients with myasthenia (after excision of these muscles, they can be studied in vitro with the most advanced techniques). Investigations of this nature suggest that the basic defect is a reduced amount of acetylcholine released in each quantum from the motor nerve terminal. This could be caused by either some defect in the binding of acetylcholine or the presence of a "false transmitter," but how the defect comes about is not known.

Incidence and Prevalence. The prevalence of myasthenia gravis is about 33 per million population and the annual incidence about 2 to 5 per million. Translated into the experience of a busy 1000-bed general hospital, about 20 new cases are encountered each year, or about the same incidence as for lupus erythematosus. Cases occur in all decades of life, most frequently at about age 40. Among young adults, the disease affects women about three times more frequently than men. Among children and older persons, however, there is no sexual predilection.

Pathology. Pathologic changes in myasthenia gravis are limited to muscle and thymus. Skeletal muscles may appear completely normal, but there are often collections of lymphocytes around blood vessels. In some cases there is evidence of degeneration of muscle fibers, and the inflammatory cellular response may be more extensive. Rarely, similar lesions are encountered in the myocardium. The thymus gland is often abnormal. Encapsulated tumors (thymoma) occur in about 15 per cent of the cases, almost all after age 30. In about 25 per cent of these tumors there is evidence of local invasion, but distant metastases are virtually unknown in patients with myasthenia, and the local invasiveness is not a cause of symptoms. Lymphocytic proliferation, in the form of germinal centers, is seen in the thymus glands of almost all other patients, but sometimes the gland appears normal, and in some older individuals the gland is so involuted that it cannot be found. Patients dying of this disease usually have some pulmonary disorder (edema, atelectasis, infection) but this is secondary to the terminal events. Patients with myasthenia may live long enough to develop a carcinoma of any organ, but it has not been shown that myasthenia occurs more frequently in patients with cancer than might be expected on the basis of chance.

Clinical Manifestations. The symptoms of myasthenia gravis are all due to weakness. The most common presenting symptoms relate to weakness of eye muscles, ptosis, or diplopia. At the onset these symptoms may last only a few days, then disappear, only to return weeks or months later. Ptosis frequently varies even in the course of a single day. Diplopia may be noted in particular directions of gaze. Difficulty in chewing, dysarthria, and dysphagia are other common initial symptoms. Limb weakness is perhaps more often proximal in accentuation, so that patients have difficulty climbing stairs or rising from chairs, or have difficulty lifting heavy objects or raising the arms overhead. However, distal weakness is not uncommon, and the initial symptoms may be related to the strength of the hands or fingers. Selective respiratory weakness is most unusual. There is no alteration of consciousness, no pain, and, in untreated patients, no cramps or muscular twitching. Difficulty in eating and swallowing may lead to considerable loss of weight, but there is no specific wasting of muscle except in patients with severe chronic weakness.

On examination, evidence of weakness of the appropriate muscle groups is found. If any sensory abnormality is found, there must be some other disorder, alone or in combination with myasthenia. Similarly, hyperactive reflexes and Babinski signs imply some other disorder, as does the complete loss of reflexes. Weakness is responsible for all the signs of myasthenia. Ptosis may be unilateral or bilateral. The patient may experience diplopia even when there is no obvious weakness of the ocular muscles; more often, there is weakness of several muscles in a pattern that cannot be explained by disorder of a particular ocular motor nerve and is not usually symmetrical in the two eyes. In addition, there is frequently weakness of eye closure because of paresis of the orbicularis oculi. Muscles of the lower face are involved later. Lingual and palatal weakness are evident in patients with dysarthria. A nasal twang and indistinct speech imply that dysarthria has facial, lingual, palatal, and, sometimes, respiratory components. In advanced cases, patients support the chin with one hand to help them talk, a maneuver that seems almost pathognomonic of myasthenia. Neck weakness may be mild or severe enough to cause difficulty in holding the head erect. Limb weakness may be mild or so severe that the patient cannot walk or even turn in bed. Respiratory weakness does not occur alone; ventilatory insufficiency occurs only in severely affected patients and usually in generalized disease, but some patients with oropharyngeal weakness may be unable to breathe unassisted even though limb muscles are strong. Even though weakness fluctuates, a normal neurologic examination is inconsistent with the diagnosis of myasthenia gravis if the patient is symptomatic at the time.

SPECIAL FORMS OF MYASTHENIA

Neonatal Myasthenia. Infants born to myasthenic women may have a transient syndrome of weakness. The most prominent symptom is difficulty in sucking and swallowing. This may be the sole manifestation, or there may also be noticeable reduction in spontaneous movement and in the vigor of the baby's cry. Only rarely is there respiratory difficulty, but unrecognized neonatal myasthenia has been fatal in exceptional cases. The condition can be identified by the intramuscular injection of neostigmine (0.1 to 0.25 mg), followed by improved sucking, a louder cry, better response to the Moro reflex, and stronger spontaneous movements. Small doses of cholinergic drugs may be administered therapeutically, but more often all that is needed is a nasogastric tube to ensure adequate nutrition. Symptoms subside within a week, or at most, a month.

Congenital Myasthenia. Myasthenia gravis may commence at any age. But there are some children who seem to have had ophthalmoplegia from birth, with or without other signs of myasthenia. Although presumably congenital, this disorder rarely causes concern in the first year of life. It is only later, when the ophthalmoplegia is recognized, that the parents state the child's eyes have always been that way. There may be a disproportionate number of familial cases among children with congenital myasthenia; ophthalmoplegia occurs in almost all of them, and there may be somewhat less tendency for crisis and remission. Otherwise, there are no characteristics that distinguish this syndrome from myasthenia at any other age.

Thyrotoxicosis. About 5 per cent of patients with myasthenia have thyrotoxicosis at some time. Usually the two disorders occur simultaneously, but sometimes hyperthyroidism is evident for weeks or months before there are myasthenic symptoms. Only rarely does myasthenia come first, long before the thyrotoxicosis, and patients who appear euthyroid do not ordinarily have laboratory evidence of thyroid overactivity. Treatment of the two disorders is directed according to the usual indications for each. (There is still talk of a "seesaw" relationship, the myasthenia worsening if the patient is rendered euthyroid; this may have been a consideration years ago when surgery was the only treatment for hyperthyroidism, but it is not important now.)

Diagnosis. In almost all cases the diagnosis of myasthenia is obvious from the history and examination. The diagnosis is immediately confirmed by the response to cholinergic drugs. For adults, 1 ml of edrophonium (10 mg) is given by vein intermittently; after injection of 2 to 3 mg, specific muscle groups are evaluated. If there is no response within 30 seconds, the injection is continued to a total of 6 mg and the patient is evaluated once again. If there is still no response, the remainder is given, a total of 10 mg. This drug is preferred when cranial muscles are being tested because the response is prompt and dramatic. Cranial weakness cannot be simulated voluntarily, and placebo injections are therefore not necessary. If it is desired to evaluate limb strength, the injection of neostigmine has advantages because the effect lasts longer, permitting more leisurely testing. The adult dose is 1.5 mg intramuscularly, and it is usually combined with atropine, 0.5 mg, to avoid the muscarinic symptoms of abdominal cramps and sweating. When limb strength is evaluated, it is sometimes advisable to evaluate placebo responses by giving the atropine 30 minutes before the neostigmine. In all cases of myasthenia gravis there is some response to these drugs, but the response is sometimes slight, and the test may have to be repeated on several occasions to provide convincing evidence.

To provide confirmatory evidence in some cases, the electromyographic response to ulnar nerve stimulation may be studied. The characteristic decline in amplitude of the evoked potential is usually seen in affected muscles, but the response may be normal when the disease is restricted to the eyes. Rarely, it is desirable to administer d-tubocurarine, a drug to which myasthenics are unusually sensitive. There are hazards in the administration of this drug, however, and it should probably be left to research centers; d-tubocurarine should never be given without appropriate precautions to support respiration.

No other laboratory tests provide diagnostic information, but it is useful to perform a standard series of studies. Thymomas can almost always be identified in standard roentgenograms of the chest, supplemented by oblique views. Laminagrams rarely provide more information, and there is little need for thymic venography or mediastinal pneumography as practiced in some centers. Thyroid function should be tested in all myasthenics, and it is useful to evaluate immunologic disorders by serum protein electrophoresis, LE cell preparation, latex fixation test for rheumatoid factor, and antinuclear antibodies. Tests for muscle antibodies or lymphocyte sensitivity are performed in special centers.

The differential diagnosis of myasthenia includes most of neurology, but a few conditions require special consideration. Probably the most frequent error in diagnosis concerns patients with emotional fatigue states and hysterical weakness. There are no cranial muscle symptoms in these patients (except globus hystericus), whereas cranial muscles are involved in virtually all myasthenics. Their symptoms are not those of weakness but of exhaustion, and in tests of strength against resistance there is apt to be marked variation in effort, or dramatic giving way. The diagnosis of myasthenia may be mistakenly made in a patient with botulism. As the discovery of botulism calls for urgent action, for both patient and eating companions, the physician should be aware of this diagnostic pitfall whenever he first sees a patient with apparent myasthenia gravis (see Ch. 23). Amyotrophic lateral sclerosis and peripheral neuropathy may be confused with myasthenia when these disorders affect cranial muscles, but signs indicative of a neurogenic disorder distinguish them from myasthenia. Polymyositis may be confusing, but ocular muscle paresis is not found. There is some debate about the specificity of the therapeutic effect of cholinergic drugs, but for practical purposes it may be taken that an authentic (not placebo), convincing (not equivocal), and reproducible (not seen by one examiner only) effect is found only in myasthenia gravis.

Treatment. *Cholinergic Drug Therapy.* The major drugs used to treat myasthenia gravis are inhibitors of cholinesterase, neostigmine, and pyridostigmine. Another drug, ambenonium, is also used in some clinics, but has no special advantages. It is best to use only one drug; there is no benefit from combinations of two or more. Neostigmine is provided in 15 mg tablets, and pyridostigmine in 60 mg tablets; these are essentially interchangeable. The choice of drug is arbitrary because there is no evidence that the maximal benefit achieved by one is more than that of the other. Most patients, but not all, prefer pyridostigmine because it is less apt to cause abdominal cramps and diarrhea, and it is less apt to cause noticeable peaks and valleys of strength. But these advantages have never been proved objectively, and some patients do very well with neostigmine. Pyridostigmine is also provided in a slow-release capsule (Timespan) of 180 mg, said to provide 60 mg immediately and the remainder in 8 to 12 hours. Some clinicians use the prolonged-action preparation throughout the day, but because of uncertainties of release, it seems advisable to use this only at bedtime for patients who would otherwise have to awaken at night or who are very weak on waking in the morning. (For patients who cannot swallow pills, both drugs may be administered parenterally, and pyridostigmine may be given as a syrup. The intramuscular dose is about one tenth of the oral dose, and the intravenous dose is one thirtieth of the oral dose.) Decisions about optimal dosage are sometimes difficult. Some authorities advocate the use of edrophonium to evaluate oral drug therapy; a test dose of 2 mg is given intravenously. If the patient improves, oral therapy has been too little. If there is aggravation of weakness, oral therapy has been too much. If there is no change, oral therapy has been just right. But other authorities find this test an unreliable guide. If edrophonium is not used, there is nothing but clinical observation to guide the therapist. For mild cases, two tablets of either neostigmine or pyridostigmine three times daily, with meals, is useful. If there is inadequate response, the dose may be increased, first by shortening the interval between doses, then by increasing the quantity of drug with each dose. Problems arise because these drugs never completely reverse symptoms. Therefore the dose should be increased only so long as there is clear-cut response, and it should not be increased beyond the amount giving some percerptible benefit.

The question of proper dosage is important because overtreatment itself can cause weakness; cholinesterase inhibitors may cause a depolarizing block at the neuromuscular junction. How often this happens is a matter of debate among experts, but that it can happen is unquestionable.

Because drugs currently available have limited effect, the search for better agents continues. Drugs advocated as "adjuvants" include potassium chloride, ephedrine, and guanidine; they may have some effect in individual patients, but their true value is unproved.

Steroids and Immunosuppressive Drugs. The use of adrenocorticosteroid drugs in myasthenia has had a curious history. For almost 15 years after the introduction of these agents, they were viewed with skepticism. Then, after a favorable report at an international symposium in 1965, there was an avalanche of confirmations, none the result of controlled trial. These papers appeared in such rapid succession and included such a variety of doses and combinations that it is difficult to make precise recommendations. Corticotrophin (ACTH) is given in short courses (100 units daily or more for 10 to 14 days), sometimes followed by maintenance therapy, 100 units weekly. Because significant worsening may precede the anticipated improvement, this treatment is best reserved for patients with severe myasthenia who already have a tracheostomy in place. Prednisone has been given in doses of 80 to 100 mg daily for variable periods, then gradually tapered. Most recently alternate-day treatment, 100 mg every other day, has been favored, but some investigators omit cholinergic drugs and some continue them. Whether this form of treatment will avoid the steroid-induced weakness or the long-term ill effects of steroids remains to be seen. Other investigators start with small amounts of prednisone and gradually increase. Whether steroid treatment should be used before or after thymectomy is another undecided variable.

A reasonable program starts with thymectomy for patients who are significantly disabled despite cholinergic drug treatment. If there is no further improvement promptly after thymectomy, prednisone is used, 100 mg every other day, for an indefinite period. Because of the possible worsening, the introduction of prednisone should be done with the patient in the controlled setting of a hospital equipped with respiratory care facilities.

The mechanism of action of steroids in myasthenia is not known, but current theories favor an immunosuppressive role. More specific immunosuppressive drugs such as azathioprine, methotrexate, or cyclophosphamide have also been used. There is no indication that these drugs are any better than prednisone, and evaluation of them is probably best performed in research centers.

Surgical Treatment. Thymectomy is followed by significant improvement in about two thirds of patients with myasthenia and no tumor. Patients with thymoma fare worse whether the tumor is excised or not. Chest surgeons, anesthesiologists, and respirator units for postoperative care are now so skillful that the risks of operation are almost negligible, and recent attempts to remove the gland through an incision in the neck rather than by splitting the sternum should reduce the morbidity considerably. Because not all patients improve, and because it is difficult to predict which patients will benefit, there is still some uncertainty in the selection of patients. Some recommend the operation for all patients who are incapacitated in daily living for more than six months despite adequate drug therapy. In preparing patients for operation, their usual oral dosage is continued until the day of operation, then stopped. Endotracheal intubation is used for all patients with oropharyngeal weakness, and intermittent positive pressure breathing is used in the postoperative period. The endotracheal tube may have to be replaced by tracheostomy after a few days, but often tracheostomy can be avoided. Specific drug therapy is withheld for several days, until fever subsides, and then started again at a level of one half or less of the preoperative dose.

Crisis. Patients with myasthenia gravis may suddenly develop difficulty breathing, severe enough to require artificial ventilation. This may be induced by systemic infection or major surgical procedures, but often there is no apparent cause. Patients with oropharyngeal weakness are especially liable to this threat, perhaps because of aspiration. Whenever there is doubt about the need for a tracheostomy, it is best to err on the side of caution and perform it. Increasingly, however, endotracheal intubation is being used for short periods of respiratory support, obviating the need for tracheostomy. The insertion of a cuffed tube makes intermittent positive pressure breathing feasible, and also reduces the hazard of aspiration. Patients are best transferred to a respiratory intensive care unit. Cholinergic drugs are stopped. After several days, usually after fever (an almost inevitable concomitant of crisis and tracheostomy) has started to subside, drugs may be started once again, at half the precrisis dosage. The cause of crisis is not clear, but it is usually transient, and will subside if the patient can be kept alive. The mortality rate of crisis was formerly about 50 per cent, but since the advent of intensive care units, only about 10 per cent die, and these are mostly elderly patients with complicating cardiac and renal disease.

Some patients require assisted ventilation for prolonged periods, some longer than one year. For these patients, trial programs of ACTH or prednisone seem advisable.

Prognosis. The course of myasthenia is variable. The disease may be restricted to ocular muscles for many years, with no threat to life. Other patients are disabled to a variable degree by oropharyngeal or limb weakness, and a few are crippled. Crisis occurs in about 25 per cent of the cases. The over-all mortality is probably about 15 per cent, and although myasthenia itself was formerly the main hazard, intercurrent and unrelated disease is now more often the cause of death.

Elmqvist, D., Hofmann, W. W., Kugelberg, J., and Quastel, D. M. J.: An electrophysiological investigation of neuromuscular transmission in myasthenia gravis. J. Physiol., 174:417, 1964.

Fields, W. S. (ed.): Myasthenia gravis. Ann. N. Y. Acad. Sci., 183:3, 1971.

Flacke, W.: Treatment of myasthenia gravis. N. Engl. J. Med., 288:27, 1973.

Harvey, A. M.: Myasthenia gravis: The first 100 years in perspective. Trans. Am. Clin. Climatol. Assoc., 82:149, 1970.

Namba, T., et al.: Corticotropin therapy in myasthenia gravis: Effects, indications, and limitations. Neurology, 21:1008, 1971.

Osserman, K. A., and Genkins, G.: Studies in myasthenia gravis: Review of a twenty-year experience in over 1200 patients. Mt. Sinai J. Med. N.Y., 38:497, 1971.

Papatestas, A. E., et al.: Studies in myasthenia gravis. Effects of thymectomy. Am. J. Med., 50:465, 1971.

486. EATON-LAMBERT SYNDROME (Myasthenic Syndrome)

Definition. Eponyms are in disfavor these days, but they are still useful when there is no other satisfactory name for a syndrome and when the eponym pays homage appropriately, without arguments of priority. This syndrome qualifies on both counts. The originators regarded it as "myasthenic" because of a disorder of neuromuscular function, but there are so many important differences from myasthenia gravis that this term may be confusing. The syndrome is defined essentially in terms of electromyography. In the Eaton-Lambert syndrome, the amplitude of the muscle action potential evoked by stimulation of its nerve is markedly reduced, and with repetitive stimulation the action potential is augmented.

Pathogenesis. The first cases were all associated with oat-cell carcinoma of the lung, but cases have been found with other tumors, other diseases, and sometimes with no complicating disorder. Microelectrode studies indicate that the defect is due to impaired release of acetylcholine at the nerve terminals. How the tumor effects this syndrome is not known.

Clinical Manifestations. The first evidence of the Eaton-Lambert syndrome may be prolonged apnea after curarization for surgery. Formal testing with d-tubocurarine also indicates that patients are unduly sensitive. Other patients may have symptoms of limb weakness, but cranial muscle weakness is never prominent. The response to cholinergic drugs is usually equivocal at best. Pain in the limbs may be prominent. Movements may be peculiarly slow. In tests of strength it may seem as though the patient gets stronger with continued effort. Myotatic reflexes are frequently depressed.

Diagnosis. The signs listed above diverge sufficiently from myasthenia to avoid confusion; only limb weakness and curare sensitivity are similar. The remainder of the syndrome resembles polymyositis, and polyneuritis would also have to be considered. The diagnosis is made by electromyography.

Treatment. Under a variety of experimental conditions, guanidine promotes the release of acetylcholine. It was therefore a logical choice to treat this rare syndrome, and the drug is effective in daily doses of 35 mg per kilogram of body weight, given orally. This drug may suppress bone marrow, and appropriate precautions should be taken.

Eaton, L. M., and Lambert, E. H.: Electromyography and electric stimulation of nerves in diseases of motor unit: Observations in myasthenic syndrome associated with malignant tumors, J.A.M.A., 163:1117, 1957.

Elmqvist, D., and Lambert, E. H.: Detailed analysis of neuromuscular transmission in a patient with myasthenic syndrome sometimes associated with brochogenic carcinoma. Mayo Clin. Proc., 43:689, 1968.

487. UNUSUAL CAUSES OF NEUROMUSCULAR BLOCK

Botulism and *tick paralysis* are described in Ch. 23 and 51. Both cause a syndrome of flaccid quadriplegia with paresis of cranial muscles, and must be differentiated from polyneuritis, myasthenia gravis, and periodic paralysis. In neither is there a sensory disorder, but autonomic fibers may be affected in botulism, especially pupilloconstrictor fibers (resulting in a dilated, fixed pupil). The physiologic disorder in both syndromes is impaired release of acetylcholine from motor nerve terminals. The electromyogram in botulism may resemble that in the Eaton-Lambert syndrome, an observation that may be diagnostically important. Guanidine has been used with benefit to treat botulism and might also be effective in tick paralysis. Supportive therapy (tracheostomy and assisted respiration) is mandatory in severe cases. Tick paralysis is reversed by removal of the organism.

Several *aminoglycoside antimicrobial drugs* interfere with the release of acetylcholine, and may cause clinical syndromes in man. The offending drugs include neomycin, streptomycin, colistin, polymyxin, and kanamycin. The most common manifestation is postoperative apnea without other evidence of paralysis. This is most apt to occur in patients with renal failure, presumably with unusually high blood levels of the antimicrobial drug. In occasional cases, however, there may be flaccid quadriplegia. Administration of calcium and guanidine may be helpful, but the essence of management is supportive treatment and use of a safer antimicrobial.

Cherington, M., and Ryan, D. W.: Botulism and guanidine. N. Engl. J. Med., 278:931, 1968.

de Jesus, P. V., Slater, R., Spitz, L. K., and Penn, A. S.: Neuromuscular physiology of wound botulism. Arch. Neurol., 29:425, 1973.

McQuillen, M. P., Cantor, H. E., and O'Rourke, J. R.: Myasthenic syndrome associated with antibiotics. Arch. Neurol., 18:402, 1968.

488. SYNDROMES OF MUSCULAR OVERACTIVITY: CRAMPS AND RELATED DISORDERS

Cramps, caused by painful, abrupt shortening of muscle, affect almost everyone at some time or other. Electromyographic investigation indicates that motor units fire at a rate of about 300 per second, much higher than the most vigorous voluntary contraction. It is presumably the high rate of discharge that causes the palpable muscle tautness and the pain. Anyone who has had more than one cramp knows that the pain can be relieved by stretching the affected muscle, or by massage. The stimulus responsible for cramps is not known; relief by stretching suggests that some central mechanism is involved, since this is the stimulus for receptors in muscle that inhibit discharge of the motor neuron to the same muscle. Certain conditions are known to be associated with a propensity to cramps: denervation (especially amyotrophic lateral sclerosis), pregnancy, and electrolyte disorders (especially water intoxication and hyponatremia). Some people are more susceptible than others for reasons which are not known. Sometimes cramps occur only at night, and can be prevented by quinine sulfate, 0.3 gram orally at bedtime. Sometimes cramps occur frequently during the day, occasionally so often that the individual is effectively crippled. Diphenylhydantoin, 0.3 to 0.6 gram daily, may be helpful to these patients, but some are resistant to this and to other drugs that may be tried, including diazepam and procainamide.

Tetany is a special form of cramp, identified by its predilection for flexor muscles of the hand and fingers, its association with laryngospasm, and its relationship to hypocalcemia. Tetany can be painful. It differs from other cramps electromyographically because of the characteristic rhythmic grouping of discharging potentials.

Contracture is the term reserved for the painful shortening of muscles in glycogen storage diseases, in which the muscles are electrically silent although maximally shortened.

Myokymia has been used to describe a variety of apparently different disorders characterized by cramps in association with spontaneous twitching of muscle. In some cases there are prolonged trains of spontaneous potentials, whereas in others there is grouping of potentials. Some of these patients have difficulty in relaxing grip, but, unlike myotonia, the muscular activity is abolished by neuromuscular blocking agents, indicating a neural rather than a muscular origin. Hyperhidrosis is prominent in some patients and is secondary to the increased muscular activity.

Continuous shortening of the muscle would lead to abnormal postures and abnormally increased resistance to passive movement. These abnormalities, of course, are often due to central neurologic disorders. In recent years, however, an increasing number of patients have been described because of fluctuating rigidity of axial and limb muscles. For want of a better name, and lacking understanding of the pathogenesis, this has been called the *stiff man syndrome.* The diagnosis requires that there be no signs of cerebral or spinal cord disease, and there must be continuous electromyographic activity despite authentic attempts to relax. Ordinary cramps may be superimposed upon the persistent stiffness. Diazepam, 30 to 60 mg daily, may bring dramatic relief.

A variety of other names have been applied to these syndromes, including *quantal squander, armadillo disease, neuromyotonia,* and *continuous muscle fiber activity.* Some cases of brief duration may be related to mild cases of tetanus. It will take some time to sort out the variety of causes. If these unusual forms can be analyzed, we may yet understand why an otherwise normal individual occasionally has a cramp.

Editorial: Writer's cramp. Br. Med. J., 1:67, 1972.

Garner-Medwin, D., and Walton, J. N.: Myokymia with impaired muscular relaxation. Lancet, 1:127, 1969.

Geschwind, N.: Skeletal muscle cramps. J. Clin. Pharm. Therap., 5:859, 1964.

Gordon, E. E., Januszko, D. M., and Kaufman, L.: A critical survey of stiff man syndrome. Am. J. Med. 42:582, 1967.

Layzer, R. B., and Rowland, L. P.: Cramps. N. Engl. J. Med., 285:31, 1971.

Wallis, W. E., Van Poznak, A., and Plum, F.: Generalized muscular stiffness, fasciculations and myokymia of peripheral nerve origin. Arch. Neurol., 22:430, 1970.

Part XI
RESPIRATORY DISEASE

489. INTRODUCTION

M. Henry Williams, Jr.

In recent years, there have been dramatic changes in the field of chest medicine. New techniques, advances in therapy, and awareness of new diseases have changed and greatly increased the demands upon the knowledge and skill of both internist and pulmonary specialist.

Major advances have been made in the treatment of tuberculosis. Modern chemotherapy has led to substantial decrease of morbidity and mortality and has made it possible to treat the disease successfully on an ambulatory basis. Nevertheless, tuberculosis remains prevalent in the large cities, and it is apparent that many social and personal factors are important in its pathogenesis and in response to therapy. In treating tuberculosis the physician must concern himself with the frequently coexistent problems of alcoholism, drug addiction, and, particularly, failure of the patient to take prescribed medication regularly and for a sufficient period. Because the treatment of tuberculosis belongs rightfully within the province of the internist, because it should be treated as an infection in general hospitals instead of in sanatoriums, and because it still ranks as a major cause of undiagnosed febrile, pulmonary, or hematologic disease, the practicing physician must be thoroughly familiar with its manifestations and with the principles of therapy. This disease is discussed in detail in Ch. 227.

Pneumonia also remains a common problem in medical practice, and the mortality among patients sick enough to be hospitalized is still distressingly high, despite antimicrobial therapy. Pneumococcal infection is the most common cause of pneumonia, but infections with Staphylococcus, Klebsiella, and other organisms are sufficiently frequent and the proper choice and use of antimicrobial drugs is so important that the physician must be familiar with the clinical features of the different infections (see Ch. 175, Ch. 179 to 183 inclusive, Ch. 188, and Ch. 195).

In particular, he must be skilled in obtaining and interpreting sputum smears so as to institute appropriate therapy at the earliest possible moment and to avoid the use of unnecessary drugs.

Lung cancer and chronic obstructive pulmonary disease (COPD), discussed in detail in Ch. 540 and Ch. 502 to 507, respectively, have both emerged as major health problems during the past two decades. Treatment is far from satisfactory for either. The physician can provide some measure of comfort to the patient with COPD, can successfully treat life-threatening episodes of ventilatory failure, and by discriminating radiographic study can select an occasional patient whose cancer can be resected. Nevertheless, hope for cure of these diseases is bleak, and efforts must be directed at prevention, especially by combating cigarette smoking.

The interstitial pneumonias and alveolar proteinosis are some of the newly described diseases with which the physician must now be familiar, and they are discussed in Ch. 520. Sarcoidosis, particularly as manifested by asymptomatic hilar adenopathy, has emerged as an extremely common disease, rivaling tuberculosis in prevalence in many places. Although sarcoidosis commonly involves the lung and hilar lymph nodes, it can involve any organ of the body; it is discussed in Ch. 102.

The organization of Part XI has been based partly on common anatomic features (bellows, airways, air spaces, lung parenchyma, pleura, and pulmonary circulation) and partly on common clinical features (irritants and neoplasm). Major emphasis is placed on principles of pathophysiology; diseases which have been well studied and which illustrate important principles have received special emphasis.

Evaluation and treatment of respiratory disease requires an understanding of pulmonary physiology and of the meaning and value of tests of pulmonary function. Section One (Ch. 490 to 497), which concerns pulmonary structure and function, is not a complete exposition of anatomy and physiology, but it is designed to build on a framework of basic knowledge and to relate the basic material to clinical phenomena. The purpose of Section One is to emphasize pulmonary physiology as it relates to clinical medicine, to refresh the reader about important physiologic principles, and to bridge the gap between the basic text and the clinical problem. In addition to understanding how the lung works, the physician should know when and why to perform various tests. Serial studies of arterial blood gas composition are essential to the appropriate management of ventilatory failure; measurement of peak expiratory flow provides useful, moment-to-moment evaluation of the patient with asthma; spirographic measurement is as much a part of the evaluation of the chest patient as an electrocardiogram is part of the evaluation of the cardiac patient; and a measurement of diffusing capacity may be the only clue to the presence or extent of diffuse interstitial pulmonary disease. Abnormalities of pulmonary function have differing degrees of therapeutic urgency. Arterial oxygen unsaturation is a potentially lethal condition which requires treatment, whereas impaired diffusion is seldom of consequence to the patient, but knowledge of its presence is vital for accurate diagnosis and prognosis.

A number of clinical problems and diagnostic techniques cut across the material presented here and elsewhere. The emergence of respiratory failure as a common problem requiring skilled, intensive therapy warrants a separate chapter on the subject (Ch. 507), but it is also a serious complication of many types of neuromuscular disease, and is discussed in Part X as well as here under COPD. Hemoptysis is a significant clinical entity requiring appropriate diagnostic study and management (see Ch. 227, 516, and 540). The physician must be familiar with the specific physical findings in each illness, but today it is even more important to have a working familiarity with the x-ray film of the chest. Every patient with pulmonary disease should have an anteroposterior, lateral, and apical lordotic film, and the physician should know when to request oblique views, tomograms, bronchograms, and angiograms and how to evaluate localized and diffuse densities when they are present. Specialized procedures, such as needle biopsy of lung and pleura and, now, bronchoscopy, are important tools for the chest physician, who should also be aware of the value, limitations, and risks of bronchography, mediastinoscopy, and thoracic surgery. As in all medicine, the risk and discomfort of a thoracic diagnostic procedure must be balanced carefully against the likelihood of obtaining useful and important information.

Section One. STRUCTURE AND FUNCTION

490. INTRODUCTION

M. Henry Williams, Jr.

The primary function of the lung is the exchange of respiratory gases—the elimination of carbon dioxide and the uptake of oxygen. The actual gas exchange occurs in the alveoli and is governed by the physical laws which govern the diffusion of gases. In order for gas exchange to occur and for arterial blood gas composition to be maintained at normal, the alveolar gas composition must be kept constant and normal despite the continuing extraction of oxygen and addition of carbon dioxide. This is achieved by periodic ventilation of the alveolar gas with fresh air containing 21 per cent oxygen and essentially no carbon dioxide. Closely related to this primary function is the maintenance of a normal partial pressure of oxygen and of carbon dioxide in the arterial blood. For this system to operate successfully, all the blood perfusing the tissues must come from the lung, and all the blood leaving the tissues must be pumped to the lung for repletion of oxygen and removal of carbon dioxide.

Since all the blood leaving the cells is pumped through the lungs, the pulmonary cells and capillaries are subject to assault by a variety of potentially noxious materials: blood clots, foreign proteins, and other toxins. Mechanisms must be present to deal with these insults. Likewise, the air which ventilates the alveoli may contain organic and inorganic materials which are capable of producing disease, and the lung must maintain an effective defense against these invaders. In addition, the lung itself is an organ that must remain viable and maintain itself by cellular replication and other metabolic functions. Although the following chapters are organized around consideration of the primary, gas-exchanging function of the lung, mention will be made of important metabolic functions as well as of the structural characteristics of the system which are essential to its proper functioning.

In studying pulmonary function, physiologists have developed a battery of tests which have proved useful to the physician. Sometimes these tests provide direct and critical insight into pathophysiologic processes; they often shed light on the ways in which the primary function of the lung is faulty, but even more often provide quantitative information of clinical significance even when the over-all function of the system remains adequate to maintain normal arterial blood gas composition.

491. VENTILATORY FUNCTION

M. Henry Williams, Jr.

LUNG VOLUMES, PLEURAL PRESSURE, AND THE RESPIRATORY CYCLE

The most obvious and easily measured aspect of pulmonary function is ventilatory function. Inspiration consists in the enlargement of the thorax by contraction of the diaphragm and intercostal muscles. By forceful contraction of inspiratory muscles, it is possible to inspire considerably more air than the tidal volume. Chest expansion is limited largely by the structural, fibrous restraints within the lung parenchyma. Measurement of the *total lung capacity* (TLC), the volume of air in the lung at the end of a maximal inspiration, provides useful clinical information. In some patients with emphysema, destruction of lung tissue and reduced resistance to lung expansion is associated with an increased TLC. Reduction of the TLC results from imperfect function of the thoracic bellows (chest deformity, pleural disease, muscle paralysis), from increased resistance of the lung to stretch (pulmonary fibrosis), or from diseases in which air-containing tissue is replaced by abnormal tissue (inflammation, neoplasia, or granulomatous disease).

Expiration is largely the result of the passive recoil of the lung which becomes greater as the lung is stretched by an inspiration. The tendency of the lung to collapse is counterbalanced by the tendency of the thoracic cage to enlarge. As the lung empties and gets smaller, its elastic recoil becomes less, whereas the outward recoil of the thorax increases. When these opposing forces become equal, expiration ends. The lung volume at which this occurs, the *functional residual capacity* (FRC), is determined by the mechanical properties of the lung and the thorax. Increased retractive force of the lung or decreased retractive force of the thorax causes reduction of the FRC, whereas reduced retractive force of the lung or increased retractive force of the thorax leads to an increase of the FRC. The inherent tendency of the lung to collapse at all volumes above residual is responsible for the negative intrapleural pressure, the magnitude of

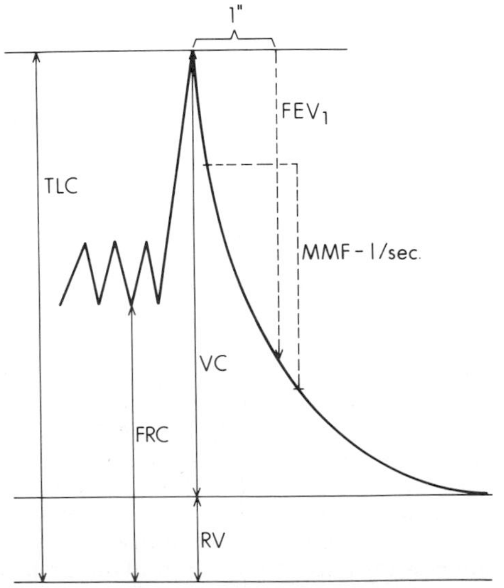

Schematic representation of lung volumes and a maximal forced expiration with depiction of one-second forced expiratory volume (FEV_1) and maximal midexpiratory flow rate (MMF).

which is directly proportional to the lung volume. Normally the pleural pressure is minus 2 cm H_2O at FRC, decreasing to minus 6 cm H_2O at the end of an inspiration and to less than minus 20 cm H_2O at TLC. Although the pleural pressure is always negative, the alveolar pressure is atmospheric at the end of inspiration and of expiration. During inspiration, enlargement of the thorax generates additional negative intrapleural pressure which, transmitted to the alveoli, causes air to enter the lung. The opposite occurs during expiration when the tendency of the chest to collapse makes the intrapleural pressure less negative and the alveolar pressure positive so that air leaves the lung.

By forceful contraction of expiratory muscles, additional air can be expelled from the lung. Forced expiration is limited by airway closure, by loss of lung recoil, or by weakness of the muscles of expiration. Generally, however, an increase of residual volume (RV), the volume of air left in the lung after maximal expiration, signifies airway obstruction. The *vital capacity* is the maximal volume of air expired from full inspiration and is one of the oldest and most useful indices of pulmonary function. It is determined by the total lung capacity and by the degree to which the lung can be emptied. The vital capacity is reduced in patients whose respiratory muscle strength is abnormal, in patients in whom the lung is rendered indistensible by fibrous tissue or by chest wall deformity, in patients whose air-containing tissue is replaced by tumor or inflammatory disease, and in patients with obstructive disease leading to complete occlusion of airways at an increased residual volume.

EXPIRATORY FLOW RATES AND LUNG MECHANICS

The dimensions of the conducting system through which air must move in and out of the lung are so large that inspiration and expiration can be accomplished easily and quickly. In various types of obstructive pulmonary disease, the airways become so narrow as to limit the rate of air flow into and out of the lung. This impairment is easily assessed by spirometry, which involves recording inspiration and expiration as the patient breathes in and out of a cannister or bellows (see accompanying figure). Obstruction to air flow is particularly obvious during expiration, both because the diameters of the airways narrow as lung volume becomes smaller and because the positive intrapleural pressure which tends to drive air from the lungs during a forced expiration also tends to collapse the conducting airways. As a result, attention is generally focused on air flow during a forced expiration. Useful indices of airway obstruction include the *timed vital capacity,* the percentage of the total which can be expired in one, two, and three seconds (normally at least 70, 85, and 95 per cent), and the volume of air expired in the first second, the *forced expiratory volume* (FEV_1), or during the middle half of expiration, the *maximal midexpiratory flow rate* (MMF: normal 2 to 4 liters per second). Patients with chronic obstructive pulmonary disease always have an MMF below 1 liter per second, and generally below 0.5 liter per second. In these patients the MMF is relatively constant and little improved by administration of a bronchodilator. In patients with bronchial asthma, the MMF may or may not be very low, and when low generally increases with therapy.

The *peak expiratory flow rate* (PEFR) is a very simple and convenient method of evaluating ventilatory function, particularly when one wishes to obtain frequent serial measurements, as in asthma. The PEFR is measured by having the patient inspire maximally and then expire as forcefully as possible into a portable meter which registers the maximal velocity of air flow. Since this is achieved early during the forced expiration, the patient need not empty his lungs completely, but he must fill his lungs at the start and employ maximal expiratory effort. Normally, the PEFR exceeds 400 liters per minute, and in asthma associated with such severe airway obstruction as to cause death from asphyxia the PEFR is less than 80 liters per minute. In general, asthmatic patients with a PEFR less than 120 liters per minute should be considered seriously ill and in need of constant medical attention.

The presence of audible rhonchi and wheezes signifies turbulent air flow, suggesting the presence of obstructive disease, and the physician can obtain a semiquantitative index of the problem by timing the duration of a forced vital capacity by listening over the larynx. By measuring intrapleural (esophageal) pressure, and simultaneously recording the air flow at the mouth, the physiologist can obtain more precise measurements of respiratory mechanics. *Lung compliance,* defined as change of volume per change of pressure, is an index of the mechanical properties of the lung, and *airway resistance,* defined as the pressure required to generate flow through the airways, is an index of the dimensions of the tracheobronchial tree. Both these measurements vary with lung volume, the lung becoming stiff (less compliant) as it is inflated and the airways becoming wider and less resistant to flow as the lung volume increases. Although these measurements provide interesting information, a study of expiratory flow rates and vital capacity generally provides adequate clinical assessment of restrictive and obstructive disease so that the more precise measurements are seldom necessary.

INSPIRATORY FLOW RATE

Fixed narrowing of airways, particularly of the extrathoracic trachea and larynx, produces just as much impedance to inspiration as to expiration. Lesions such as vocal cord paralysis and tracheal stenosis characteristically cause similar reductions of inspiratory and expiratory flow rates and are easily detected on spirometry. Patients with this type of obstruction may be surprisingly asymptomatic, since dyspnea in obstructive pulmonary disease appears to result from the extreme narrowing and closure of airways that occur during expiration, and a fixed degree of obstruction may cause significant increase of the work of inspiration without extreme expiratory limitation. This may result in hypercapnia, predominantly related to the inspiratory work cost of breathing, and measurement of inspiratory flow rates is strongly indicated in the patient with unexplained elevation of the arterial P_{CO_2}.

MINUTE VENTILATION

Measurements of the lung volumes, expiratory flow rates, and lung mechanics provide useful information about the respiratory system. They do not, however, indicate whether or not the minute ventilation is normal. Patients with severe abnormality of lung volumes or mechanics may or may not have reduced ventilation. The effectiveness of ventilatory function must be considered in terms of the purpose of the minute ventilation, which is to add oxygen to the alveolar air and to remove carbon dioxide in accordance with the metabolic needs of the body. The ventilation is regulated to meet these metabolic needs by maintaining a normal alveolar gas composition: a Pco_2 of 40 mm Hg and a Po_2 of 100 mm Hg. Increased metabolic rate, as in fever or muscular exercise, is matched by an appropriate increase of ventilation so that alveolar gas composition remains constant. Under a variety of conditions, to be discussed subsequently, ventilation may not be maintained at the appropriate level, resulting in increase of alveolar Pco_2 and a decrease of alveolar Po_2. It should be emphasized that the alveolar Pco_2 and the arterial Pco_2, which are essentially identical, actually measure the effectiveness of ventilation. Hypercapnia indicates that ventilation is reduced, and hypocapnia means that ventilation is increased in relationship to metabolic needs.

The alveolar Po_2 also reflects the level of ventilation, a high Po_2 indicating hyperventilation and a low Po_2 hypoventilation. Hyperventilation will cause the alveolar Po_2 to be elevated about as much above 100 mm Hg as the Pco_2 is reduced below 40 mm Hg, and in hypoventilation the Po_2 will be as much below 100 mm Hg as the Pco_2 is above 40 mm Hg. However, alveolar gas is often neither uniform nor measurable, and assessment of hypoventilation is best based on arterial blood measurements. Since many abnormalities can cause reduction of arterial Po_2 but not hypercapnia, adequacy of ventilation is best assessed by the arterial Pco_2.

Although the clinician may form some conclusions about ventilatory function by listening to the breath sounds generated by movement of air in and out of the lungs and by observation of the movement of the chest cage, these observations are grossly inexact, and accurate assessment of total ventilation requires a measurement of tidal volume and respiratory rate. Evaluation of the adequacy of the ventilation, which depends upon the size of the physiologic dead space (see Ch. 493) as well as the minute ventilation, requires a measurement of arterial Pco_2.

ALVEOLAR VOLUME

Although gas exchange actually occurs across the walls of individual alveoli, the basic unit of the lung is now considered to be the acinus, the alveolar ducts and alveoli supplied by a terminal bronchiole. This unit of respiratory function is ventilated with each inspiration, and the air spaces are so small as to allow practically instantaneous diffusion of gases within the unit so that alveolar gas composition is essentially uniform throughout. Indeed, alveolar "ventilation" is largely the result of diffusion of gas molecules within the small airways and alveoli, and is not due to mass movement of air much beyond the large bronchi. Only a small portion of the lung volume within the acinus is actually turned over with each breath. The existence of a large alveolar volume, even at the end of a maximal expiration, may be considered to be a homeostatic adjustment to the fact that gas exchange across the alveolar capillaries is continuous, whereas ventilation is discontinuous – fresh air enters the alveoli only during inspiration. If the volume of the unit were not large compared to the amount of gas exchanged, the alveolar Po_2 would fall and the alveolar Pco_2 would rise from the end of one inspiration until the beginning of the next, and there would be large fluctuations of arterial blood gas composition. Thus one may consider that the function of the lung volume is to maintain constancy of the alveolar and arterial blood gas composition throughout the respiratory cycle.

RESPIRATORY CONTROL

Respiration serves several purposes, including metabolic gas exchange, communication, and heat regulation. In addition, the respiratory system is endowed with a number of protective reflexes, some of which influence the respiratory rate and depth; others induce coughing, sneezing, and yawning. The principal integration and regulation of these several functions are achieved by respiratory neurons located in the medulla oblongata and lower pons. This "respiratory center" is, in turn, influenced by structures at higher levels of the nervous system as well as by changes in its local chemical environment. In the metabolic regulation of ventilation, priority is awarded to the maintenance of a normal Pco_2. Increased arterial Pco_2 leads to increase of the Pco_2 within tissue fluids and, hence, to a decreased pH within the chemosensitive neurons of the respiratory center. This is followed by increased respiratory activity. The resultant increase of ventilation causes decreased Pco_2 and, hence, decreased respiratory drive. This feedback control system maintains the arterial Pco_2 within narrow limits unless there is gross disturbance of the effector system (the lungs and the chest cage) or of the respiratory center itself. In addition, chemosensitive arterial receptors respond to hypercapnia, to an increased hydrogen ion concentration, and to hypoxia, the last accounting for the mild hyperventilation which exists at altitude or in subjects with hypoxemia. This is generally considered to be an emergency mechanism, and it plays little part in normal regulation of ventilation. A variety of reflex pathways also exist in lungs and other tissues which directly or indirectly affect respiration. Of these the most important clinically are afferent stimuli from pulmonary vessels stretched by pulmonary hypertension or from lungs stiffened by edema, fibrosis, or granulomatous disease.

Increased respiratory drive in excess of CO_2-determined stimulation leads to increased ventilation and hypocapnia. Decreased respiratory drive causes hypoventilation and hypercapnia and is usually the result of depressant drugs or impaired mechanical performance of the lung and chest bellows so that extra muscular effort is needed to achieve a given minute ventilation.

A clear distinction should be made between hyperventilation and dyspnea. The latter is the patient's *subjective awareness* of respiratory discomfort. This symptom, which is present in many diseases, may have as its physiologic basis an inappropriate shortening of respiratory muscle fibers in response to respiratory need. Respiratory need is determined by all the chemical and nervous stimuli to respiration and cannot be measured. However, one can measure the mechanical properties of the lung and ascertain that excessive muscular effort is being spent on the act of ventilation or that excessive ventilation is indeed taking place, in which case the patient might be "entitled" to dyspnea. But beyond that, the subjective nature of the symptom, attenuated and amplified by emotional factors, precludes quantitative assessment.

492. ABNORMALITIES IN RESPIRATORY CONTROL

Fred Plum

Neurologic or neuromuscular disorders frequently produce breathing abnormalities. Diseases of the cerebrum or upper brainstem commonly induce disturbances in the respiratory rate and rhythm which do not interfere with gas exchange. Diseases of the lower brainstem, spinal cord, nerve, or muscles can produce respiratory failure, and this is often the most serious aspect of such illnesses.

Abnormal Respiratory Rhythms in Neurologic Disease. The abnormal, irregular breathing rhythm of medullary disease is discussed below.

Patients with disease at upper pontine or low midbrain levels sometimes show *central neurogenic hyperventilation.* Such patients are usually in stupor or coma, and their metronomically regular hyperpnea must be distinguished from the other causes of hyperpnea listed in Table 1.

Cheyne-Stokes respiration is a regularly oscillating pattern of respiratory rhythm in which hyperpneic and apneic periods alternate, one full cycle requiring twice the circulation time. Usually such periodic breathing reflects bilateral neurologic damage at subcortical or diencephalic brain levels. Occasionally, particularly when the hyperpneic phase is brief and the apneic phase relatively long, periodic breathing can be a manifestation of severe lower brainstem injury at pontine levels.

Respiratory Failure in Neurologic Disease. Neurologic or muscular disease may cause either peripheral or central respiratory failure.

Peripheral respiratory failure results when the skeletal musculature of the diaphragm, chest wall, abdomen, and neck becomes so weakened that the chest bellows cannot move sufficient air to ventilate the lungs. Potential causes of peripheral respiratory failure are listed in Table 2; those that are most frequent or tend to create medical emergencies are marked with an asterisk.

The symptoms of peripheral respiratory failure depend partly upon which muscles are affected first. Patients suffering progressive paralysis of chest wall or abdomen may have few symptoms until their diaphragms are involved, at which time no respiratory reserves are left. On the other hand, patients whose diaphragms are paralyzed first may feel breathless almost immediately. Those who need to cough may become incapacitated rapidly if they lose their abdominal muscles. These considerations imply that whenever faced with the diseases listed in Table 2, the alert physician must evaluate respiratory function, using serial vital capacity measurements to estimate the quantitative functional impact of paralysis. Gross indices of respiratory function such as attention to respiratory rate, inspecting the apparent magnitude of chest expansion, and checking for dyspnea usually are unreliable. Patients with acute peripheral respiratory failure almost never become anoxemic or hypocarbic until ready to collapse, so that therapy, to be effective, must be started before cyanosis appears or abnormalities appear in blood gases.

Central respiratory failure results when the respiratory integrating neurons in the medulla oblongata become damaged or diseased. Common causes are listed in Table 2. Central respiratory failure produces defects in the respiratory rate and rhythm, and symptoms usually evolve through progressive stages. At first, a subtle respiratory irregularity appears, which is most pronounced during drowsiness or rest. Patients may report that it is impossible to sleep or that they must concentrate on the breathing act. By this time, the pattern of breathing may be frankly irregular. In those with drug-induced depression, the respiratory rate is slow and the volume shallow; intermittent, irregular apneic periods may occur. Respiratory sensitivity to carbon dioxide is reduced, and an-

TABLE 1. Conditions Causing Hyperpnea with Stupor or Coma

Respiratory Alkalosis	Metabolic Acidosis
Central neurogenic hyperventilation:	Diabetic coma
Brainstem infarcts	Uremia
Secondary brainstem compression	Ingested organic acids
Severe hypoglycemia	Methyl alcohol
Acute anoxia	Ethylene glycol
Hepatic coma	
Salicylate poisoning (adult)	
Sepsis	

TABLE 2. The Neurologic Causes of Respiratory Failure

A. Peripheral

I. Diseases of the respiratory muscles
- Progressive muscular dystrophy
- Myotonic muscular dystrophy
- Polymyositis

II. Diseases and disorders of the myoneural junction
- Myasthenia gravis*
- Botulism*
- Anticholinesterase poisons* (parathione, DFP etc.)
- Hypersensitivity to curare in patients with pseudomyasthenia (malignancy)

III. Peripheral neuropathies
- Guillain-Barré syndrome*
- Diphtheria
- Acute intermittent porphyria

IV. Anterior horn cell diseases
- Poliomyelitis*
- Amyotrophic lateral sclerosis

V. Lesions of the spinal conducting pathways
- High cervical trauma*
- Acute myelitis
- High spinal compression or malignancy

B. Central

I. Infections
- Encephalitic poliomyelitis
- Postexanthematous or disseminated encephalomyelitis

II. Trauma, brainstem hemorrhage, or neoplasm (rare)
- Craniovertebral abnormalities

III. Drug depression
- Barbiturates
- Opiates
- Other depressants

oxia or CO_2 retention may develop unless treatment is instituted. By this point, progressive failure and decompensation are usually rapid.

The treatment of respiratory failure is artificial respiration. There are many satisfactory respirators. Both the "iron lung" and positive-pressure types create intrapulmonary pressures that cyclically exceed external pressures on the chest. However, individual models vary widely, and the physician would do well to familiarize himself with available devices before trying to use them in emergencies. When treating respiratory failure, careful and constant attention is required to see that the airway is unobstructed. If there is any doubt, tracheostomy should be performed.

Bendixin, H. H., Egbert, L. D., Hedley-Whyte, J., Laver, M. B., and Pontoppidan, H.: Respiratory Care. St. Louis, C. V. Mosby Company, 1965.

Campbell, E. J. M., Agostini, E., and Newsom Davis, J.: The Respiratory Muscles. London, Lloyd-Luke, 1970.

Plum, F.: The neurologic integration of behavioral and metabolic control of breathing. *In* Porter, R. (ed.): Ciba Foundation Symposium: Breathing. Hering Breuer Centenary Symposium. Boston, Little, Brown & Company, 1970.

493. CONDUCTING AIRWAYS

M. Henry Williams, Jr.

The airways leading to the acini are tubes which branch by irregular dichotomy and provide increasing surface area at each branching. As a result, the highest resistance to flow through the conduction system occurs in the major bronchi and trachea, the smaller airways actually contributing relatively little resistance to airflow. Narrowing of the large bronchi has more effect on expiratory air flow than a similar narrowing of peripheral bronchioles, and a patient must develop widespread occlusive disease of peripheral airways before symptoms of chronic obstructive disease develop.

The airways are designed to conduct tidal volume in and out of the alveoli, and their size must represent a compromise between a large surface for conducting air with little resistance and a minimal dead space, the latter being that portion of the inspired air which remains in the airways and is not available for gas exchange. Normally about a third of each breath is so wasted. The *physiologic dead space* is measured by relating the expired to the arterial carbon dioxide tension, the difference between the two being essentially a measure of the amount of dead space air which dilutes the alveolar gas to form the expired air. Measurement of physiologic dead space is useful in determining total ventilatory requirements of a patient. The measurement also has clinical value, since an increase of physiologic dead space rarely stems from increased volume of the conducting airways but, rather, reflects ventilation of alveoli which are not perfused with blood. Air going to such units remains unaltered in composition and is wasted ventilation. The physiologic dead space is extremely variable, even in a single subject, but is closely related to the tidal volume, and the ratio of dead space to tidal volume (V_D/V_T) is essentially constant. This ratio is normally less than 0.30, and increase or decrease signifies worsening or improvement of matching of ventilation to perfusion.

Because, as mentioned above, inspired air contains a variety of inorganic and organic pollutants which may settle anywhere along the tracheobronchial tree, mechanisms must be present to remove these potential pathogens from the lungs. The bronchial mucus, secreted by goblet cells and mucous glands, serves this function. The mucus is propelled up the tracheobronchial tree by the constant beating of cilia. Any material which settles on the airways, or is brought there by alveolar macrophages, is carried up this mucous escalator to the mouth and is expectorated or swallowed. Normally, about 100 ml of mucus is produced per day, and this amount is greatly increased in those exposed to air pollution, particularly cigarette smoke. Excessive secretion of mucus, which is accompanied by morphologic evidence of hypertrophied mucous glands, is the cardinal symptom of chronic bronchitis.

494. ALVEOLAR STRUCTURE AND FUNCTION

M. Henry Williams, Jr.

DIFFUSION

The actual process of gas exchange takes place in the 300 million alveoli. The alveolar wall consists of a thin epithelial lining separating the air space from the pulmonary capillary. The design of the structure provides maximal exposure of circulating blood to alveolar gas over some 80 square meters of surface area and through a minimal layer of separating tissue. This permits such rapid diffusion of gases that, in normal subjects, there is no discernible difference between the partial pressure of oxygen in the alveolar air and in the blood leaving the alveolar capillary. In patients with extensive loss or thickening of this diffusion surface, by emphysema or inflammatory disease respectively, diffusion may be imperfect, leading to measurable reduction of the end-capillary P_{O_2}. It is rare for this impairment to be so severe as to cause detectable unsaturation of arterial blood. As carbon dioxide is 20 to 30 times as "diffusible" as oxygen, hypercapnia is never a result of diffusion impairment. Although diffusion is rarely a cause of blood gas abnormality, measurement of the *diffusing capacity* of the lung is a very useful index of pulmonary structure and function. In many patients with diffuse lung disease, reduction of the diffusing capacity may be the only indication that parenchymal disease is present, and the measurement provides useful information about prognosis and the effects of therapy.

METABOLIC FUNCTION

The alveolar walls are not dry, but are lined by a complex substance, *surfactant,* which has the property of reducing surface tension, particularly at small lung volumes when the high surface tension would tend to collapse the small alveoli into larger units with correspondingly lower internal pressure. This surfactant is undoubtedly important in maintaining stability of alveolar structure and in preventing atelectasis, but the role of surfactant deficiency in human disease is uncertain. The surface-active material is apparently synthesized by alveolar lining cells, one of the many metabolic functions of the lung that are essential to maintenance of its functional integrity.

VENTILATION-PERFUSION RELATIONSHIPS

One of the extraordinary features of pulmonary function is the correspondence between ventilation and circulation in individual lung units. Although there is considerable variation of ventilation to various parts of the lung, the upper lobes receiving less than the lower, normally there is, in general, a matching of perfusion so that the well-ventilated units receive more circulation than those that are poorly ventilated. This is very important, since ventilation of nonperfused lung would be wasted dead-space ventilation, and perfusion of nonventilated lung would, in effect, constitute a right-to-left shunt of venous blood through the lung. Imbalance of ventilation and perfusion is common in chronic pulmonary disease and, indeed, represents the major cause of arterial unsaturation (see Ch. 497). A number of mechanisms provide for the matching of ventilation and diffusion. It is likely that an alveolus of normal size represents the least resistance to blood flow so that alveoli which are collapsed and nonventilated because of complete obstruction, or which are overexpanded because of partial obstruction, hinder blood flow and so are correspondingly poorly perfused. In addition reduction of the oxygen tension in the alveolar air is capable of causing vasoconstriction which prevents perfusion of poorly ventilated alveoli. Likewise, reduction of the P_{CO_2} in the alveoli elicits bronchial constriction, tending to reduce the alveolar ventilation to a unit of lung which has been deprived of circulation. These mechanisms are imperfect in extreme disease but are valuable contributors to normal pulmonary function.

OXYGEN AND CARBON DIOXIDE TRANSPORT

The function of the lung is to maintain an appropriate alveolar environment with respect to oxygen and carbon dioxide and to permit the rapid diffusion of oxygen into the blood and of carbon dioxide from the venous blood into the alveoli. Maintenance of cellular function by provision of adequate oxygen supplies and carbon dioxide removal also depends upon the transport function of the blood.

Most of the carbon dioxide is carried in the form of bicarbonate (HCO_3), which is in equilibrium with carbonic acid (H_2CO_3). The concentration of the latter is determined by the concentration of CO_2 in the blood, which is, in turn, dependent upon the P_{CO_2}. These relationships are discussed in more detail in Ch. 805.

Although a little oxygen is dissolved in blood (approximately 0.03 ml per 100 ml), most of the oxygen is bound to hemoglobin, which has the unique property of combining with large amounts of oxygen when the P_{O_2} is high and of releasing oxygen as the P_{O_2} falls. At a normal arterial P_{O_2} of 100 mm Hg and in the absence of anemia, approximately 20 ml of oxygen is carried in 100 ml of blood. In the tissues, where the oxygen tension is lower, substantial quantities of oxygen are given up to the cell. Furthermore, the oxyhemoglobin dissociation curve has the additional feature of a flat, upper portion so that there can be considerable reduction of arterial oxygen tension before appreciable hypoxemia develops.

495. PULMONARY CIRCULATION

M. Henry Williams, Jr.

PRESSURE FLOW AND RESISTANCE

The pulmonary circulation is unique in two important respects: the entire cardiac output passes through the lung, and the function of this circulation is to replenish the blood with oxygen rather than to deliver oxygen to metabolically active tissue. The pulmonary artery and its branches are so capacious as to offer minimal resistance to blood flow and to permit passage of blood through the large alveolar capillary network with a pressure head only one fifth of that required to pump blood to the rest of the body. Since there is no need to vary blood flow in the lung with the metabolic needs of competing tissues, the muscular arterioles which are present in the other organs of the body are not needed here. Another characteristic of the pulmonary circulation is its enormous capacity for expansion. Doubling of cardiac output by muscular exercise or of the blood flow through one lung by occlusion of the contralateral pulmonary artery is associated with relatively little increase of pulmonary artery pressure because the total cross section area of the pulmonary vascular bed expands in response to a small rise of intraluminal pressure. In acute experiments, 75 per cent of the pulmonary vascular bed must be obstructed before pulmonary hypertension develops, and the presence of severe pulmonary hypertension implies the existence of widespread vascular disease.

REGIONAL CIRCULATION

Because of the low pressure in the pulmonary artery, variation of hydrostatic pressure caused by gravity has a relatively large effect on the perfusion pressure at the apex and the base of the lung. At the top of the lung, the pressure inside the small arteries may actually be less than the atmospheric pressure within the alveoli, so that the vessels are totally occluded and there is no blood flow. At the bottom of the lung, the hydrostatic pressure is large, and blood flow is correspondingly great. The gravitational effects on the lung volume also tend to divert more ventilation to the lower lung zones than to the upper. This is due to the fact that the pleural pressure is less negative at the bottom of the lung than at the top. As a result, at FRC the upper lobes are under greater stretch, are larger and less compliant, so that they fill less with a given inspiratory change of pleural pressure than do the less expanded and more compliant lower lobes.

A number of isotope techniques have been developed

for studying regional circulation through the lung, of which the most widely used is lung scanning with I^{131}-labeled microaggregates of albumin. Aggregates of albumin are injected into the pulmonary circulation where they embolize functioning capillaries and are detected by appropriate scintillation counting. Albumin aggregates do not embolize areas of lung not perfused with blood; hence these appear as nonradioactive areas on the lung scan. Such filling defects are encountered in patients who have suffered pulmonary embolization or in patients in whom areas of the pulmonary circulation have been obstructed because of inflammation, collapse, or even overinflation, as in bronchial asthma.

BRONCHIAL CIRCULATION

The main nutritive circulation to the lung is provided by the systemic blood brought by the bronchial arteries. As a result, total occlusion of a pulmonary artery does not necessarily lead to necrosis of pulmonary tissue, or even to x-ray changes so long as the bronchial circulation remains intact. The bronchial circulation assumes clinical importance when it becomes excessive, as in chronic suppurative lung disease (bronchiectasis) or after interruption of the pulmonary artery circulation. An expanded bronchial circulation represents a flow load on the left ventricle which pumps blood round and round through the affected pulmonary tissue, and an expanded bronchial circulation is a rare cause of left ventricular failure. Of greater importance is the fact that these systemic vessels are a potential source of serious hemoptysis. Modern techniques of angiography have made it possible to visualize the main bronchial arteries radiographically after injection of contrast material.

PULMONARY HYPERTENSION

As mentioned, significant elevation of the pulmonary artery pressure implies the presence of severe obstruction to the pulmonary circulation. This subject is considered in detail in Ch. 546 to 550.

496. DISABILITY EVALUATION

M. Henry Williams, Jr.

PULMONARY FUNCTION TESTING

As is the case with dyspnea, disability evaluation can only be partially aided by pulmonary function testing because of the importance of subjective factors. The physician can learn whether or not an abnormality which might limit performance is present, but he cannot say that it does or will. For example, patients with apparently similar degrees of severe obstruction to airflow show marked variation in their exercise capacity.

In normal subjects, physical activity is limited largely by cardiac rather than by pulmonary performance. Even at maximal exercise, the limits of ventilation are not reached, and there is no decrease of arterial oxygen tension, implying that total pulmonary performance is perfectly adequate. Theoretically, severe obstruction of airways or severe stiffening of the lungs might make it impossible to achieve levels of adequate ventilation commensurate with the high metabolic rate induced by heavy exercise, but one rarely encounters patients in whom exercise is actually associated with worsening hypercapnia and hypoxemia. In practical terms, there is a rough correlation between the severity of obstructive airway disease and extent of disability so that a patient with a maximal midexpiratory flow rate (MMF) of 1 liter per second may be expected to be unable to do heavy work and a patient with an MMF of 0.2 liter per second can probably do no more than walk slowly on the level. Likewise, when the vital capacity is reduced to 1 liter by severe restrictive lung disease, the effort to achieve more than a slight increase of minute ventilation, such as that induced by slow walking, may become intolerable.

Disability is not synonymous with disease. Extensive involvement of the lung by metastatic disease or with granulomatous disease, as in sarcoidosis, may be associated with little impairment of pulmonary function because of preservation of large areas of normal lung. On the other hand, diffuse microscopic alteration of the alveolar capillary membrane may lead to sufficient impairment of oxygen diffusion as to result in arterial unsaturation, particularly with exercise, and to sufficient stiffening of the lung as to make breathing difficult on mild effort. It may be important for the physician to know that an inhaled pollutant, such as beryllium, has led to extensive lung disease which may be evident only by measurement of the diffusing capacity; but this need not imply that the patient has limited ability to work. A careful assessment of the type and extent of lung disease and evaluation of whether or not the disease has led to mechanical impairment of the respiratory system and/or to blood gas abnormalities at rest or on exercise are the essential ingredients of disability evaluation.

PREOPERATIVE EVALUATION

A special type of disability evaluation is represented by the patient who is being considered for pulmonary resectional surgery. In performing this evaluation, the physician must first determine whether or not the resected tissue is functioning, since nonfunctioning tissue can be removed with relative impunity. Isotope studies of regional ventilation and perfusion now make this estimation possible. Indeed, if it is determined that an area of lung is ventilated but not perfused, resection may be of benefit in that this tissue is of no value to the patient, and its ventilation actually represents wasted effort. Likewise, a perfused but nonventilated lung contributes to hypoxemia and is of little value to the patient.

Since, as in the case of the pulmonary circulation, there is a tremendous reserve of pulmonary function available for ventilation and for gas diffusion, large amounts of pulmonary tissue may be resected from a normal individual without causing hypoxemia or even respiratory discomfort. Often, however, one must decide whether a patient with restrictive or obstructive lung disease is capable of withstanding removal of some functioning lung tissue, generally in connection with cancer surgery. One useful guide is a study of exercise tolerance. If a patient can sustain exercise requiring twice the normal resting oxygen consumption, one can anticipate that he could tolerate removal of half his functioning lung. Calculation of the extent to which the lung to be resected is contributing to gas exchange, most easily based on studies of regional perfusion with lung scan coupled with measurements of ability to increase oxygen uptake with exercise, permits a reasonable assessment of whether or not surgery can be carried out. Other evidence of severe functional impairment may represent compelling contraindications to surgery. Most physicians feel that a patient with resting hypercapnia represents enough of a risk to preclude a thoracotomy. Likewise, pulmonary hypertension, at rest or after balloon occlusion of the segment of lung to be resected, is considered a contraindication to surgery. Beyond that, although severe obstructive or restrictive diseases represent relative contraindications to surgery, assessment must be made on the basis of the patient's general health, age, and vigor and of the indications for operation.

497. HYPOXEMIA

M. Henry Williams, Jr.

HYPOXIA

Tissue hypoxia occurs when the supply of oxygen to the cells is inadequate to meet metabolic needs. The two general causes of hypoxia are reduction of blood flow and reduction of oxygen concentration within the blood. Reduction of blood flow may be localized, as in occlusive arterial disease, or general when the cardiac output is reduced. Arterial oxygen concentration may be diminished if there is impairment of the transport function of the blood. Impaired transport is most commonly the result of anemia, and the oxygen-carrying capacity is reduced in direct proportion to the reduction of hemoglobin concentration. Reduced transport also results from replacement of normal hemoglobin by abnormal hemoglobin such as methemoglobin or carbon monoxide hemoglobin. Heavy smokers may have as much as 10 per cent of their hemoglobin combined with carbon monoxide instead of with oxygen, and they are at a further disadvantage in that the carbon monoxide hemoglobin affects the oxygen dissociation curve of the remaining hemoglobin so that there is interference with release of oxygen to the tissues. Impaired transport also occurs when the amount of oxygen in the arterial blood is reduced because the oxygen tension is reduced. Reduced arterial oxygen tension and saturation is always, with the exception of right-to-left intracardiac shunts, the result of impaired pulmonary function.

ARTERIAL UNSATURATION

Reduced arterial oxygen saturation may, if severe, be evident clinically as cyanosis of the skin or mucous membranes. Since mild degrees of arterial unsaturation are not detectable as cyanosis and since cyanosis can result from any condition which will lead to increased amounts of reduced hemoglobin in the capillaries, such as polycythemia and reduced blood flow, accurate assessment of the arterial oxygen saturation requires its measurement. Since arterial oxygen unsaturation may be an important cause of tissue dysfunction and since it also has clinical implications concerning the type and extent of pulmonary disease present, the measurement should be carried out routinely in patients in whom hypoxemia is suspected to be present.

Hypoxemia may result from four types of impairment of pulmonary function: reduced alveolar ventilation, impaired diffusion of oxygen, right-to-left shunts, and abnormal ventilation-perfusion relationships. Two or more of these abnormalities often coexist in a given patient.

Alveolar hypoventilation is characterized by hypercapnia out of proportion to hypoxemia. Reduction of alveolar ventilation causes proportional increase of arterial P_{CO_2} and reduction of arterial P_{O_2}, but the flat portion of the oxygen dissociation curve of hemoglobin permits substantial reduction of arterial P_{O_2} before the arterial oxygen saturation falls appreciably. Thus a patient with an arterial P_{CO_2} elevated from 40 up to 80 mm Hg would have significant respiratory acidosis, but the concurrent reduction of the arterial P_{O_2} from 100 to about 50 mm Hg would be associated with only mild arterial unsaturation of little clinical significance. Alveolar hypoventilation may occur after overdosages of drugs, in acute paralytic disease of muscles, or, rarely, in individuals with isolated abnormality of the respiratory center (alveolar hypoventilation syndrome), but it is associated most commonly with severe obstructive pulmonary disease, which leads to hypoxemia for other reasons.

The diffusing capacity of the lungs for oxygen is so large that even during heavy exercise the arterial oxygen tension is only slightly lower than the alveolar oxygen tension, and the diffusing capacity must be severely reduced by disease before arterial oxygen unsaturation develops. When hypoxemia is present because of impaired diffusion, as in advanced pulmonary fibrosis, it is characteristically exaggerated by exercise and is not accompanied by hypercapnia.

Right-to-left shunts produce hypoxemia in direct proportion to the magnitude of the shunt, and they are found most commonly in patients with intracardiac defects. Since the venous carbon dioxide tension is only 6 mm higher than the arterial, even a large shunt leads to little elevation of the arterial P_{CO_2}. A 50 per cent shunt would cause the arterial P_{CO_2} to be increased by only 3 mm Hg, whereas the oxygen saturation would be substantially reduced because of the much lower venous oxygen saturation.

Mismatching of ventilation and perfusion is the most important cause of hypoxemia. Arterial unsaturation results from the fact that well-perfused but poorly ventilated alveoli have a very low oxygen tension and the blood leaving these alveoli contains low concentrations of oxygen. Since these alveoli are relatively well perfused, they contribute large amounts of blood to the total cardiac output and, hence, cause substantial reduction of arterial oxygen saturation. Hypercapnia is also a feature of this condition, but is mitigated by the fact that alveoli which are excessively ventilated but underperfused contain correspondingly low concentrations of carbon dioxide, and the blood coming from these alveoli tends to counterbalance the CO_2-rich blood from underventilated alveoli. There is no similar compensation for oxygen because the extra ventilation does not serve to increasse the oxygen saturation above the normal 98 per cent.

OXYGEN THERAPY

Most types of hypoxemia are corrected completely and easily by oxygen breathing. Inspiration of air containing a higher than normal concentration of oxygen will lead to an increase of the oxygen concentration in all the ventilated alveoli. Thus if a patient breathes 31 per cent oxygen instead of 21 per cent oxygen, the inspired air will contain an oxygen tension which is 70 mm Hg higher than normal, and all except the very poorly ventilated alveoli will have an oxygen tension which is elevated by approximately 70 mm Hg. This will more than suffice to raise the oxygen tension to a level capable of saturating the hemoglobin passing through these alveoli whether the hypoxemia is due to total alveolar hypoventilation, regional hypoventilation, or impaired diffusion. Hypoxemia caused by a right-to-left shunt will not be corrected fully by this treatment since the inspired oxygen fails to affect the blood passing through the shunts. Inspiration of 100 per cent oxygen will have some effect on arterial oxygen saturation because it will dissolve an extra 2 volumes per cent of oxygen in the blood which does circulate through ventilated lung. This will increase the arterial oxygen saturation 10 per cent in a patient with a normal hematocrit.

Knowledge of arterial blood gas composition during air and oxygen breathing makes possible an accurate assessment of the type of pulmonary malfunction which is causing hypoxemia, and it also provides an indication of the severity of the disease. Since high concentrations of oxygen increase the tendency for atelectasis to develop and adversely affect the metabolic functions of the lung, the physician should use as little additional inspired oxygen as necessary to correct hypoxemia. Measurement of the arterial oxygen saturation is the proper guide to rational oxygen therapy.

ACCLIMATIZATION

One of the extraordinary adaptations of which man is capable is the acclimatization to chronic hypoxia. Whereas acute reduction of arterial oxygen saturation to 70 per cent in a normal subject is associated with gross evidence of cerebral dysfunction and slightly lower levels of saturation will cause death, patients with chronic hypoxia, due either to chronic pulmonary disease or to prolonged residence at high altitude, are capable of normal function with an arterial oxygen saturation as low as 25 per cent. Some of this acclimatization results from polycythemia, which increases the oxygen-carrying power of the blood and from a change in the oxygen-combining character of hemoglobin, which releases oxygen more readily to the tissues. Arteriolar dilation and increased cardiac output permit a more rapid flow of blood and oxygen to the tissues. A fundamental and major adaptation undoubtedly resides in the expansion of the capillary network throughout the body. This brings the oxygen in the capillaries nearer to the cells and makes possible the diffusion of oxygen into the cells even though the partial pressure of oxygen in the capillaries is very low.

Bates, D. V., Macklem, P. T., and Christie, R. V.: Respiratory Function in Disease. 2nd ed. Philadelphia, W. B. Saunders Company, 1971.

Briscoe, W. A.: The current status of pulmonary function tests. Arch. Environ. Health, 16:531, 1968.

Comroe, J. H. Jr., Forster, R. C., DuBois, A. B., Briscoe, W. A., and Carlsen, E.: The Lung. Clinical Physiology and Pulmonary Function Tests. 2nd ed. Chicago, Year Book Publishers, 1962.

Howell, J. B. L., and Campbell, E. J. M. (eds.): Breathlessness. Philadelphia, F. A. Davis Company, 1966.

Hugh-Jones, P., and Campbell, E. T. M. (eds.): Respiratory physiology. Br. Med. Bull., 19:1, 1963.

Liebow, A. A., and Smith, D. C. (eds.): The Lung. Baltimore, Williams & Wilkins Company, 1968.

Section Two. THE DIAPHRAGM

J. B. L. Howell

The diaphragm is the most powerful muscle of inspiration and is responsible for the major part of the tidal volume in quiet breathing. Developmentally, the mesodermal partition which separates the thoracic and abdominal cavities, the septum transversum, is invaded by premuscular tissue derived principally from the fourth cervical myotome, and forms the muscular diaphragm. The motor nerve supply is bilateral and is derived from the third, fourth, and fifth cervical segments via the phrenic nerves. Sensory fibers are also derived from the lower six or seven intercostal nerves.

Congenital Defects. The posterolateral foramen of Bochdalek and less commonly the anterior foramen of Morgagni, owing to persistence of the pleuroperitoneal canal, may be the sites of herniation of abdominal viscera into the thoracic cavity. Herniation may also occur through normal foramina, especially the esophageal opening (see Ch. 635).

Paralysis of the Diaphragm. Paralysis of the diaphragm may occur from interruption of its nerve supply, from muscular atrophy, or temporarily from diaphragmatic pleurisy. Unilateral diaphragmatic paralysis is usually the result of phrenic nerve interruption in the mediastinum by bronchial carcinoma or other tumors. Unilateral or bilateral diaphragmatic paralysis occurs in high cervical cord injuries, motor neuron disease, paralytic poliomyelitis, infectious polyneuritis (Landry-Guillain-Barré syndrome), or peripheral neuritis associated with diphtheria, tetanus, measles, typhoid, and rheumatic fever; or it may occur after antitetanus serum injection into the deltoid region as part of a cervical radiculitis. Phrenic crush or section was once used therapeutically in the treatment of pulmonary tuberculosis; it may still occur inadvertently during cervical sympathectomy.

Congenital atrophy, called *eventration,* of one half of the diaphragm is a rare and usually symptomless finding on routine roentgenography; its prevalence is about 1 in 12,000. It is more common on the left side. Its main significance is that it may be confused with the potentially more sinister phrenic paralysis. Occasionally, left-sided eventration is associated with mild dyspepsia.

Phrenic paralysis causes elevation of the affected hemidiaphragm, which shows paradoxic movement on sniffing, the basis of its fluoroscopic diagnosis.

The main disturbance of pulmonary function tests in

diaphragmatic paralysis is reduction in the vital capacity, especially when the patient is supine. Symptoms are orthopnea and difficulty in inspiration. Arterial oxygen saturation may be reduced, but hypoventilation does not occur.

Inflammation of the Diaphragm. Inflammation of the diaphragm and its serous surfaces may occur in viral infections, e.g., epidemic pleurodynia, or as extensions of pneumonia, pleurisy, or peritonitis. The clinical significance is that of the underlying condition, except that diaphragmatic, like thoracic wall, pleurisy may cause pain referred to the abdomen or to the shoulder, leading to diagnostic confusion.

Rupture of the Diaphragm. Rupture of the diaphragm is due to trauma, especially when associated with abdominal compression injuries. Direct trauma to the chest may also be responsible. On the right side, the liver may herniate into the thorax. The diagnosis should be suspected when roentgenographic features of paralysis of a hemidiaphragm follow thoraco-abdominal injury, especially if breathlessness is disproportionately severe.

Myotonia Dystrophica and Hemiplegia. The diaphragm may also be involved as part of generalized muscular disease in myotonia dystrophica. Unless extremely severe, spirometry, resting ventilation, and the ventilatory response to CO_2 are normal; however, sedatives readily induce respiratory depression. In hemiplegia, diaphragmatic movement is in a normal direction. Chest movements are reduced on voluntary breathing maneuvers, but not when breathing is stimulated by CO_2. This indicates that although supramedullary innervation of the respiratory muscles is bilateral, it is not symmetrically represented.

HICCUP

Hiccup is an involuntary spasm of the inspiratory muscles followed by abrupt closure of the glottis which is responsible for the characteristic sound. Normal subjects may experience hiccup, especially after eating or drinking, but it may also be a symptom of disease. It may occur in conditions which irritate vagal nerve endings in the abdomen or thorax. These include gastritis, peritonitis, pleurisy, pericarditis, and mediastinitis. It may occur in lateral brainstem ischemia (Wallenberg's syndrome), and as a very troublesome symptom in uremia when it is also thought to have a central origin. When no cause is found, the psyche may be blamed, but there is no evidence to support this. In most instances, hiccup is a short-lived symptom and can sometimes be induced to stop by a variety of maneuvers such as taking a deep breath, breath holding, or drinking cold water. Rebreathing from a paper bag may sometimes help. If symptoms still persist, chlorpromazine, 25 to 50 mg intravenously, may be successful. In the small number of cases in which hiccup has proved resistant to these simple measures, local anesthesia of one of the phrenic nerves has been successful, block of the left nerve usually being tried first.

Section Three. THE CHEST WALL

J. B. L. Howell

498. SCOLIOSIS

Definition. Scoliosis means lateral curvature of the spine which may occur in the lumbar, thoracolumbar, or thoracic regions. The higher the location of the scoliosis in the vertebral column, the greater the likelihood of severe deformity and of disturbance of cardiopulmonary function (heart failure of the hunchback). Lumbar scoliosis is relatively benign. Thoracic scoliosis is associated with rotation of the spine and prominence of the posterior angles of ribs which form the hump or gibbus, and gives rise to the hunchback appearance. Although commonly called kyphoscoliosis, forward angulation of the spine or kyphosis is usually not the major component of kyphoscoliosis; indeed marked lumbar or cervical lordosis is characteristic.

Etiology and Mechanism. Four types of scoliosis are recognized. The largest group is *idiopathic,* developing in childhood and forms 80 per cent of all scoliosis. When idiopathic scoliosis occurs in infancy, boys predominate in the ratio of 6 to 4, and the curvature is usually to the left; when it occurs in adolescence, girls predominate in the ratio of 9 to 1 and the curvature is usually to the right.

Congenital scoliosis results from a variety of developmental abnormalities, including hemivertebrae, fused vertebrae, spina bifida, and absent ribs. Other congenital abnormalities are commonly associated. *Paralytic* scoliosis resulting from poliomyelitis is especially likely to cause deformity and disability owing to the associated muscular paralyses.

Genetic abnormalities may be due to autosomal dominant conditions such as neurofibromatosis, osteogenesis imperfecta, Marfan's and Ehlers-Danlos syndromes, or autosomal recessive conditions, including Morquio's disease, Hurler's syndrome, and diatrophic dwarfism. The mechanism of the deformity is probably a combination of abnormal bone growth, usually in the vertebrae, and altered distribution of muscular forces. The importance of each factor will vary according to the type of scoliosis. The degree of deformity varies between individuals and at different ages. In one series, two thirds of the patients with thoracic idiopathic scoliosis had curvature of the spine greater than 70 degrees, and in over a fourth it was greater than 100 degrees. Scoliosis may also follow fibrotic disease of the lungs and pleura, e.g., tuberculous empyema. This is not as severe as the scoliosis that may develop in the aforementioned varieties, and cardiopulmonary disturbances are due largely to the thoracic disease.

Clinical Manifestations. Deformities with less than 70 degrees of angulation rarely cause symptoms other than those due to their psychologic effects. When more severe deformities interfere with pulmonary function the first symptom is breathlessness on exertion. With progression of the deformity or with superadded bronchitis, disturbance of pulmonary function increases, and arterial hypoxia develops; breathlessness now becomes more severe. If ventilatory failure supervenes, more severe cyanosis and signs of congestive cardiac failure develop. These findings are similar to those of chronic cor pulmonale developing in association with chronic obstructive bronchitis; however, symptoms of morning chest tightness and bronchial irritability are not present in scoliosis unless bronchial disease coexists. Abnormal physical signs are those associated with congestive cardiac failure, but allowance must be made in their elicitation and interpretation for the deformity and displacement of the viscera.

Laboratory Tests. In all patients with significant deformity, total lung capacity, vital capacity, and residual volume are reduced in relation to the degree of deformity. The FEV_1/VC is essentially normal. Airway resistance in relation to lung volume is normal or slightly raised. Maximal breathing capacity is particularly reduced in paralytic scoliosis. In patients with mild deformity, Sa_{O_2} is normal. With increasing severity, Sa_{O_2} becomes reduced while Pa_{CO_2} first remains normal; but when congestive cardiac failure develops Sa_{O_2} is reduced further, Pa_{CO_2} is elevated, CO_2 sensitivity is reduced, and polycythemia may develop. Intrapulmonary gas mixing and diffusing capacity are usually not markedly abnormal. The electrocardiogram may show evidence of right ventricular hypertrophy. Interpretation of the chest film may be very difficult owing to the distortion of the bony cage and displacement of the thoracic contents.

Mechanism of Cardiorespiratory Failure. The deformity of the bony thoracic cage reduces its capacity; it also impairs the action of the inspiratory muscles, resulting in reduced total lung capacity and its component volumes. The work of breathing is increased largely because of increased elastic resistances in the chest wall and altered mechanical advantage of the muscles. This results in more rapid shallow breathing which increases dead space ventilation and causes arterial unsaturation. Initially, over-all alveolar ventilation is maintained, but with progression of the deformity the work of breathing and arterial desaturation are further increased, and alveolar hypoventilation develops in association with impaired ventilatory response to CO_2. Hypoxemia becomes more severe, resulting in polycythemia and increased pulmonary vascular resistance. This, together with the reduction in the pulmonary vascular bed resulting from the low lung volumes, causes pulmonary hypertension and congestive cardiac failure. The end result is similar to the cardiorespiratory failure of primary alveolar hypoventilation, and of chronic obstructive bronchitis ("blue bloater" form).

Pathologic Conditions of Lungs and Heart in Scoliosis. Characteristically, the lungs are small and may appear atrophic; areas of atelectasis are common. Emphysema is not a feature. When the deformity has arisen in infancy, hypoplasia of the air spaces and vascular bed may be found. In patients dying with cardiorespiratory failure, there is usually right ventricular hypertrophy as well as other evidence of pulmonary hypertension.

Prognosis. The factors which influence the progression of minor degrees of scoliosis in childhood are poorly understood. In some it may disappear, but in others, apparently similar, rapid deformity may develop. Cardiopulmonary abnormalities are most likely with thoracic deformities, especially when due to muscular paralysis and when the deformity has occurred in infancy and early childhood rather than later in life.

Treatment. *Prophylaxis.* Progress of the deformity is usually preventable by a Milwaukee brace (frame) in growing patients with idiopathic curves of less than 50 degrees. With more severe curves operation may be required to reduce the curvature. At best about 50 per cent reduction in the curvature may be obtained, but there is no general agreement on the best surgical procedure. Prevention and treatment of recurrent bronchitis (see Ch. 503) is important as the pulmonary damage is additive to the effects of the deformity.

Cardiopulmonary Failure. The treatment of acute cardiopulmonary failure is similar to that provided in chronic obstructive bronchitis (see Ch. 503). It includes the treatment of bronchial infection and retained secretions with antimicrobial drugs and physiotherapy, controlled administration of oxygen, venesection for polycythemia, and diuretics. Chronic cardiopulmonary failure requires attention to bronchial toilet, diuretics, and digitalis, and repeated venesection to maintain the hematocrit below 55 per cent. Surgical correction of the deformity at this late stage is not feasible; surgery is usually restricted to the prevention of paraplegia if early signs of spinal cord damage appear. A period of assisted ventilation may be necessary for acute cardiorespiratory failure, but intubation may be difficult owing to the marked cervical lordosis. Intermittent positive pressure inspirations have caused increased lung compliance, but the effect lasted only up to three hours, and the clinical significance, if any, has not been assessed.

499. ANKYLOSING SPONDYLITIS

Ankylosing spondylitis results in bony ankylosis of posterior intervertebral, costovertebral, and sacroiliac joints; there is also ossification of the spinal ligaments and the margins of the intervertebral discs. As a result, the bony thoracic cage becomes rigid and immobile, and respiratory movement becomes increasingly dependent upon diaphragmatic movement. It was once thought that respiratory illnesses were unduly common in this condition, but this has been shown not to be the case. Respiratory symptoms are not common, and pulmonary function shows few abnormalities. In the most severely affected patients, the vital capacity and maximal breathing capacity may be reduced to approximately two thirds of normal. Total lung capacity remains normal, but the residual volume and functional residual capacity are increased, suggesting that the chest is fixed in an inspiratory position. Diffusing capacity for carbon monoxide is reduced only in the most severely affected group. At autopsy, the lungs are normal.

DEFORMITIES OF THE ANTERIOR CHEST WALL

Three types of deformity are recognized: depression of the sternum (pectus excavatum or funnel chest), prominence of the sternum (pigeon chest), and depression of the rib cage anterolaterally in the region of the sixth rib (Harrison's sulcus). Of these deformities, only the first-named may cause any disturbance of cardiopulmonary function.

Pectus excavatum is a congenital abnormality of the anterior chest wall in which the sternum is depressed, being most marked just above the xiphisternal junction, with symmetrical or asymmetrical prominence of the ribs on either side. Occasionally, the xiphoid may project backward as a xiphoid horn. The cause of this deformity is uncertain; some believe that it is due to excessive diaphragmatic traction on the lower sternum, but others believe it is secondary to displacement of the heart into the left hemithorax. Symptoms are not common and appear to be of cardiac origin. They include breathlessness on exertion, precordial pain, palpitation, and dizziness; rarely congestive cardiac failure has been reported. The electrocardiogram may show arrhythmias and changes suggestive of ischemia, but there is no supporting evidence of myocardial disease. Hemodynamic studies have rarely demonstrated restriction of ventricular filling similar to that which occurs with constrictive pericarditis. It is unlikely that disturbed pulmonary function ever plays any part in the disability. Tests are usually normal, but with very severe deformity the vital capacity and maximal breathing capacity may be reduced. Surgical correction has been reported to afford immediate symptomatic benefit, although there is a high incidence of recurrence of the deformity. Surgery is contraindicated if there are serious psychiatric manifestations.

500. PRIMARY OR IDIOPATHIC ALVEOLAR HYPOVENTILATION

Definition. The term primary or idiopathic alveolar hypoventilation denotes a rare clinical syndrome occurring in patients with normal pulmonary and thoracic cage mechanics in whom the primary abnormality is alveolar hypoventilation. It is sometimes referred to as Ondine's curse. The syndrome is characterized by symptoms of headache, drowsiness, or somnolence, exertional dyspnea, and signs of cyanosis and congestive heart failure.

Etiology. The causes of this syndrome are not known. Resistances to breathing and respiratory muscular power are essentially normal, which distinguishes it from hypoventilation occurring in chronic bronchitis, in neuromuscular disorders, in skeletal abnormalities of the thorax, e.g., kyphoscoliosis, or in extreme obesity. Associated central nervous system disorders, such as the sequelae of encephalitis, neurosyphilis, and mental retardation with or without epilepsy, have been reported in over half the patients, but no specific lesions have been found in the region of the respiratory center at autopsy. Alveolar hypoventilation has also been reported in a small proportion of patients after bulbar poliomyelitis, sometimes many years after apparent recovery, and it seems likely that in these patients central nervous system disease is responsible.

Incidence and Prevalence. Primary or idiopathic hypoventilation is a rare disease; it was first described in 1955, and since then fewer than 50 cases have been reported. The majority of patients have been between 30 and 50 years, with a preponderance of males.

Clinical Manifestations. Symptoms have usually been present for many years, but occasionally the presentation has been more acute, usually in response to a respiratory infection or after surgical anesthesia. The dominant symptoms include breathlessness on exertion, drowsiness, or even somnolence suggesting narcolepsy. When the symptoms are severe, the patient is cyanosed, the face being dark and suffused, sometimes with chemosis; tachycardia, raised jugular venous pressure, hepatomegaly, and peripheral edema are present. Crepitations at the bases are common. Clinical evidence of cardiac enlargement, pulmonary hypertension, and right ventricular hypertrophy is commonly present. Periodic breathing and snoring may be prominent during sleep. Laboratory findings include raised Pa_{CO_2} (55 to 75 mm Hg), usually with good compensation of the respiratory acidosis; there is arterial desaturation (70 to 80 per cent), mainly resulting from ventilation-perfusion abnormality, and the hematocrit is usually greater than 60 per cent. The ventilatory response to inhaled CO_2 is markedly depressed and, in one recent report, to hypoxia as well. The vital capacity may be slightly reduced, but the FEV_1/VC ratio is normal. Physiologic dead space ventilation is increased.

Diagnosis. The aforementioned findings in the absence of other disorders of the lungs and thorax are highly suggestive of idiopathic alveolar hypoventilation. This diagnosis is supported if the patient can temporarily restore the blood gas tensions to normal by a period of voluntary hyperventilation. Differential diagnosis includes other causes of congestive cardiac failure, cyanosis, polycythemia, and somnolence, the most common being chronic obstructive bronchitis ("blue bloater" form) and cyanotic congenital heart disease; the syndrome may also be confused with primary polycythemia or narcolepsy. Severe metabolic alkalosis caused by prolonged vomiting, as in anorexia nervosa or chronic pyloric stenosis, may be accompanied by severe hypoventilation. It is not certain whether the cardiorespiratory failure of extreme obesity is an essentially different disorder or not.

Pathology. No specific disease has been found in the central nervous system. In two patients substantial increase in the number and size of capillaries was found at autopsy in the floor of the fourth ventricle, reticular substance, periaqueductal region, mamillary body, and hypothalamus. There was no evidence of neuronal loss. There are usually right ventricular hypertrophy and evidence of chronic pulmonary hypertension. Thromboses of large branches of the pulmonary artery with pulmonary infarcts are common.

Pathogenesis. The primary abnormality in primary alveolar hypoventilation is impaired responsiveness of the respiratory center to carbon dioxide, leading to ventilatory failure. As a result of this reduced CO_2 sensitivity, the center is unable to increase its motor output to the inspiratory muscles by the normal amount when alveolar ventilation is reduced by increased resistances to breathing. Although the normal subject will double or treble the resting power (rate of work) of the inspiratory muscles in response to a rise in the P_{CO_2} of only 1 mm Hg, these patients are unable to do so even with a rise in

Pco_2 of 20 to 30 mm Hg. Consequently, normally trivial events like acute bronchitis or increase in body weight may cause profound underbreathing, with further elevation of alveolar Pco_2 and fall in alveolar Po_2. Because of altered ventilation-perfusion relationships which accompany underbreathing, Pa_{O_2} is reduced even further until it becomes the dominant ventilatory stimulus and stabilizes ventilation at a new reduced level. Administration of oxygen is likely to be harmful by reducing or removing ventilatory drive, increasing hypercapnia, and leading to increased drowsiness or even unconsciousness. A similar response may follow small doses of sedatives or narcotics, and a number of cases have been recognized for the first time by this striking response. The hypoxemia causes polycythemia, increased pulmonary vascular resistance, and increased cardiac output, resulting in pulmonary hypertension, right ventricular hypertrophy, and systemic venous congestion. Although most patients have various degrees of ventilatory failure, some patients with this syndrome maintain alveolar ventilation at virtually normal levels, alveolar Pco_2 and Po_2 being only slightly abnormal, providing that they do not have respiratory obstruction. It is the failure to maintain adequate alveolar ventilation in the face of increased mechanical hindrance that characterizes the syndrome.

Mechanism of Impaired Sensitivity of the Respiratory Center to Carbon Dioxide. Reduced CO_2 sensitivity is not peculiar to this syndrome. It has been reported in association with a wide range of disorders, including chronic bronchitis and airway obstruction, scoliosis and kyphoscoliosis, obesity, and brainstem disorders; it also occurs as a normal event during sleep. Experimentally, reduced CO_2 sensitivity has been observed in man after vagal blockade and narcotic drugs, and has been thought to occur during partial curarization. The control of breathing is a complex process involving the integration of a variety of sensory inputs from mechanical and chemical receptors, and of motor outputs to the ventilatory apparatus. Theoretically, control may be impaired at any of a number of points, and it is possible that in different diseases interruption of normal control mechanism occurs at different sites. It is generally believed that the abnormality in primary alveolar ventilation is in the central nervous system, but its nature is unknown.

Treatment. Treatment of congestive cardiac failure usually improves the ventilatory failure as well. Oral diuretic therapy with, for example, chlorothiazide, 1 gram, or furosemide, 40 to 80 mg daily; venesections to reduce the hematocrit to between 50 and 55 per cent; and digoxin, ~~0.25 mg once~~ or digitoxin ~~1 mg daily~~ will reduce pulmonary congestion and peripheral edema, with improvement in arterial Pco_2 and Po_2. Sometimes, when these measures are not successful, a short period of artificial or assisted ventilation to reduce the arterial Pco_2 and raise Po_2 may be followed by prompt diuresis. Cuirass ventilators permit ventilation to be assisted without endotracheal intubation, and in some patients regular artificial ventilation at night in a cuirass ventilator may maintain them in an improved state. Attempts to increase ventilation with acetazolamide, progesterone, aminophylline, and analeptics have not been successful. Instruction in voluntary increased breathing and electrophrenic stimulation with surface electrodes have been successful in the short term only. All other abnormalities likely to hinder breathing, e.g., bronchitis, asthma, and obesity, should be treated as effectively as possible. If upper airway obstruction occurs during sleep (see Ch. 501) despite weight reduction and withdrawal of all central nervous system depressant drugs, tracheostomy should be considered.

Prognosis. There is insufficient information at present to estimate the prognosis with accuracy. Without effective treatment of congestive cardiac failure, the prognosis is very poor. With treatment, patients may continue in reasonable health for several years, requiring only intermittent therapy for acute pulmonary infections and venesections if polycythemia becomes severe. One patient has been reported to have maintained normal arterial Pco_2 for nine months after three years of continuous hypercapnia and repeated episodes of ventilatory and cardiac failure; this was attributed to voluntary increase in ventilation.

501. CARDIORESPIRATORY FAILURE OF EXTREME OBESITY

Cardiorespiratory failure similar to that of primary alveolar hypoventilation has been described in association with extreme obesity, the average weight being approximately 325 pounds. The similarity in appearance and behavior of these patients to the description of the fat boy, Joe, in *Pickwick Papers,* has led to this association being termed the pickwickian syndrome. The main symptoms are breathlessness on exertion and somnolence. Apart from obesity, the physical signs and physiologic abnormalities are similar to those in idiopathic alveolar hypoventilation. Periodic breathing is common during sleep. Prominent cyanosis, tachycardia, raised central venous pressure with cardiac dilatation, functional tricuspid incompetence, hepatomegaly, and peripheral edema may be observed. Investigations reveal diminished total lung capacity and its component volumes, decreased lung compliance, and increased airway resistance at functional residual capacity owing to the low lung volume. Physiologic dead space is increased. Arterial saturation is reduced to about 80 per cent; this is due partly to underbreathing but mainly to increased venous admixture. The Pco_2 is usually 60 to 70 mm Hg. Ventilatory response to CO_2 is markedly reduced. Cardiac output is normal or increased; there is pulmonary hypertension usually of the order of 75 systolic and 30 diastolic in mm Hg. There may also be systemic hypertension, which is common in obesity. With voluntary overbreathing patients can restore the blood gases to normal.

Pathogenesis. The mechanism of the cardiorespiratory failure associated with obesity is obscure. First, it has been attributed to the increased work of breathing which occurs in obesity. Two observations make this unlikely; only a minority of patients with this degree of obesity develop the syndrome, and small amounts of weight reduction of the order of 25 pounds may be associated with marked improvement. Second, this syndrome may be essentially similar to the idiopathic alveolar hypoventilation syndrome, obesity being either a fortuitous association or the result of an underlying central nervous system lesion, e.g., in the hypothalamus, which is responsible for both features. Against this are reports of the restoration of normal ventilatory control in those patients in whom weight has been restored to normal. Third, a combination of increased respiratory work resulting from obesity and low sensitivity to carbon dioxide, which occurs in a proportion of normal people, may initiate a vicious circle of events. Thus gross obesity may cause a small reduction in ventilation with increase in P_{CO_2} and arterial unsaturation; this leads in turn to further reduction in CO_2 sensitivity, further underbreathing, and more severe arterial unsaturation and the development of congestive cardiac failure. This increases respiratory work and causes further ventilatory failure. A sequence of events such as this would explain the reversibility of the condition, but at present insufficient knowledge is available concerning the range of CO_2 sensitivity in these patients when nonobese. Recently a small number of cases have been reported in which intermittent asphyxia caused by collapse of hypotonic pharyngeal muscles occurred during sleep; the resulting hypoxia caused arousal and prevented the patient from reaching deep sleep. Permanent tracheostomy resulted in marked clinical improvement, including disappearance of somnolence.

Treatment. Weight reduction and the measures described under idiopathic alveolar hypoventilation, i.e., diuretics, venesection, digitalis, and antimicrobial drugs, as well as attention to bronchial toilet result in marked reduction in ventilatory failure and circulatory abnormalities, and improvement in the ventilatory responsiveness to CO_2. Uncontrolled administration of oxygen is likely to cause severe underbreathing and CO_2 narcosis. If pharyngeal obstruction is present and persists despite weight reduction and withdrawal of CNS depressant drugs, tracheostomy may be necessary.

Diaphragm, Scoliosis, and Ankylosing Spondylitis

Bergofsky, E. H., Turino, M., and Fishman, A. P.: Cardiorespiratory failure in kyphoscoliosis. Medicine, 38:263, 1959.

Borgeskov, S., and Raahave, D.: Long-term result after operative correction of funnel chest. Thorax, 26:74, 1971.

Fluck, D. C.: Chest movements in hemiplegia. Clin. Sci., 31:383, 1966.

Gacad, G., and Hamosh, P.: The lung in ankylosing spondylitis. Am. Rev. Respir. Dis., 107:286, 1973.

Gillam, P. M. S., Heaf, P. J. D., Kaufman, L., and Lucas, B. G. B.: Respiration in dystrophia myotonica. Thorax, 19:112, 1964.

McCredie, M., Lovejoy, F. W. J. R., and Kaltreider, N. L.: Pulmonary function in diaphragmatic paralysis. Thorax, 17:213, 1962.

Nordwall, A.: Studies in idiopathic scoliosis. Acta. Orthop. Scand. (Suppl. 150), Copenhagen, 1973.

Wachtel, F. W., Ravitch, M. M., and Grishman, A.: The relation of pectus excavatum to heart disease. Am. Heart J., 52:121, 1956.

Idiopathic Hypoventilation Syndrome and Obesity

Burwell, C. S., Robin, E. D., Whaley, R. B., and Bickelman, A. G.: Extreme obesity associated with alveolar hypoventilation—A pickwickian syndrome. Am. J. Med., 21:811, 1956.

Proceedings of a Symposium: Hypersomnia with Periodic Breathing, Rimini, May, 1972. *In* Bull. Physiopathol. Respir. (Nancy), 1972. This reference contains many papers on primary alveolar hypoventilation and the cardiopulmonary syndrome of obesity.

Severinghaus, J. W., and Mitchell, R. A.: Ondine's curse. Failure of respiratory center automaticity while awake. Clin. Res., 10:122, 1962.

Section Four. AIRWAY OBSTRUCTION

GENERALIZED AIRWAY OBSTRUCTION: CHRONIC OBSTRUCTIVE LUNG DISEASE

502. INTRODUCTION

J. B. L. Howell

The term chronic obstructive lung disease embraces a number of clinical syndromes of varying etiology and pathology, with the common feature of increased hindrance to the flow of air out of the lungs resulting from an intrapulmonary pathologic condition. In some, airflow obstruction is intermittent, and the clinical presentation is one of asthma; in others, airflow obstruction is continuous, often associated with chronic bronchitis or emphysema or both, and the clinical presentation varies depending upon the degree to which the pulmonary condition results in disturbance of pulmonary and circulatory function. In recent years, considerable advances have been made toward understanding the basic pathophysiology of airflow obstruction and of gas exchange in these various conditions; many studies have correlated the clinical features, pulmonary pathology, and disturbances of pulmonary function. It is now possible to recognize a number of different patterns of disorder within the ill-defined group called chronic nonspecific lung disease, which includes simple chronic bronchitis and chronic obstructive disorders associated with chronic bronchitis, emphysema, and allergic disorders of the bronchi.

Ultimately, an etiologic classification of generalized obstructive disorders of the lungs may be possible, but at present, knowledge is incomplete and classification depends largely on differences in clinical presentation supplemented by what is known about their mechanism and pathology.

503. CHRONIC BRONCHITIS

J. B. L. Howell

Definition. Chronic bronchitis is characterized by increased mucous secretion by the tracheobronchial tree, resulting in cough productive of mucus present at some time of the day for at least three months of two consecutive years. It may be diagnosed on this history providing that a localized pulmonary cause such as bronchiectasis, tuberculosis, or tumor has been excluded. The definition is often interpreted less rigidly to include those with chronic or recurrent cough productive of sputum of unspecified duration. It is therefore a clinical diagnosis made solely upon the history. It has a close pathologic counterpart in an increase in the mucus-secreting glands and goblet cells of the bronchial mucosa.

Etiology and Epidemiology. The United Kingdom has the highest recorded mortality attributed to chronic bronchitis in the world. It is 4 to 5 times that of Western Europe and more than 15 times that of Scandinavia and the United States.

Factors predisposing to chronic bronchitis have been identified from epidemiologic studies carried out mainly in Europe and North America. Cigarette smoking has been shown to be the most important single factor; because of its almost overwhelming effect, the contributions of other factors have been partly obscured. Studies comparing the prevalence of chronic bronchitis in urban and rural communities, in workers in different occupations and of different social classes, have shown that, in addition to cigarette smoking, air pollution, dusty occupations, poorer social and economic circumstances, and, especially, increasing age all lead to a higher prevalence of chronic bronchitis. An indication of the magnitude of these factors can be seen from recent statistics of death rates attributable to chronic bronchitis in England and Wales. The standard mortality rate (SMR) was six times greater in males living in a heavily air-polluted area of the industrial Northwest of England compared with a South coast holiday resort. It was five times greater in the lowest social class (Class V) compared with social class I. Recent reduction in air pollution in certain areas in North America and Europe has already been associated with a reduction in the prevalence of chronic lung disease. The effect of occupation is shown by an approximately tenfold increase in SMR in coal miners and laborers compared with clergymen, teachers, and doctors.

There is mounting evidence that during childhood environment is important in influencing both the frequency of lower respiratory tract infections and the ventilatory capacity. In recent epidemiologic studies in the United Kingdom, peak flow rates were found to be significantly lower in children living in areas of high air pollution and were further reduced in those with a past history of bronchitis or pneumonia. The prevalence of acute bronchitis in children is similarly increased by air pollution and also by cigarette smoking; it has been reported also to be more common among children of smokers than of nonsmokers. These influences in childhood probably play an important part in the development of chronic bronchitis and obstructive lung disease in adult life, a view which is supported by the observation that deaths attributed to this cause are higher in male immigrants from Europe to the United States of America than in native-born males. In addition, a history of lower respiratory tract illness occurring under the age of two years has recently been shown to be more important than social class or air pollution in influencing the tendency to winter bronchitis in young adults; but current smoking habits had an even greater effect. As only a proportion of individuals exposed to adverse provoking factors develop chronic bronchitis, other factors which make the individual more susceptible to their effects and which might be termed endogenous must exist, although we have little information about them in most instances.

There are two special circumstances about which more is known. First, the genetically determined abnormality of mucus production, mucoviscidosis, impairs bronchial clearance and protective mechanisms leading to recurrent or, more commonly, chronic bronchial infection. Second, and more common, bronchial allergies may themselves increase secretion of mucus by direct stimulation of the glands, or alternatively, cause increased liability to bronchial infections.

Pathology and Pathogenesis. In the majority of patients with chronic productive cough, mucous gland hyperplasia and increased numbers of goblet cells, especially in the smaller bronchioles, are present. The degree of mucous gland hyperplasia and hypertrophy may be expressed as the ratio of the thickness of the mucous glands to thickness of the bronchial wall between cartilage and epithelium (Reid index) and is normally between 0.14 and 0.36. In chronic bronchitis the ratio is increased; for example, in patients with symptoms of five years' duration or longer, the ratio was found to be from 0.41 to 0.79. In the epithelium increased numbers of goblet cells and areas of squamous metaplasia reduce the numbers of ciliated cells. Scanning electron microscope studies have revealed unsuspected marked irregularities of the bronchial surface even in the absence of gross infection. If infection is present, the bronchial wall is infiltrated with inflammatory cells and congested by dilated capillaries and lymphatics, and, if severe, small abscesses may form. Healing of these more severe infections may lead to fibrosis and deformity of the bronchial wall: bronchitis deformans, stenosans, or obliterans; or bronchiectasis. The combination of increased bronchial mucus, fewer cilia, and irregularities of the bronchial wall impairs the rate of mouthward movement of mucus, and the bronchial protective mechanisms are therefore less effective.

Normally the trachea and bronchi yield no bacteria on culture, but in chronic bronchitis a variety of organisms may be isolated, and pus cells may be seen on microscopy. The organisms include those which are normally commensals in the oropharynx and recognized pathogens such as *D. pneumoniae* and *H. influenzae.* Any factors which further impair the clearance mechanisms or other defenses against infection may lead to the development of acute purulent bronchitis. This is presumably a common mechanism of the recurrent "winter" bronchitis to which these patients are prone, although in a number of cases various respiratory viruses, especially respiratory syncytial virus and *Mycoplasma pneumoniae,* have been isolated. Many exacerbations are not associated with recognizable infecting agents. When resulting from an allergic cause, a purulent appearance of the sputum may be due not to bacterial infection with pus cells but to heavy infiltration with eosinophils.

Diagnosis. The diagnosis of chronic bronchitis is made on the history. Confirmation of the associated pathologic changes of mucous gland hyperplasia may be made by bronchial biopsy, but this is a research, not a routine, procedure. Bronchography may reveal dilated enlarged ducts of hypertrophied glands, and the bronchi themselves may be irregular, giving a "concertina" appearance.

Clinical Manifestations. The productive cough of chronic bronchitis is often not regarded as abnormal and is dismissed as a "smoker's cough." The patient expectorates mucus each morning shortly after rising and may produce only a few pieces of mucoid sputum at times during the remainder of the day. This stage is called *simple chronic bronchitis.* However, two other manifestations may occur, and standard terminology has been recommended by the Chronic Bronchitis Committee of the Medical Research Council of Great Britain. First, the sputum may become purulent, either continuously or for at least a part of the day, usually in the morning; this is termed *chronic or recurrent mucopurulent bronchitis.* Second, airflow obstruction may develop, the condition becoming *chronic obstructive bronchitis,* which will be discussed in more detail later. All forms of chronic bronchitis may be subject to acute exacerbations with increased volumes of sputum with or without purulence. These acute exacerbations frequently follow a head cold, exposure to smog, or other irritants.

Treatment. *Simple Chronic Bronchitis.* A careful history to establish the likely role of smoking, occupational hazard, or presence of allergies must be taken. The patient must be urged to stop smoking, and realization that only a minority will succeed should not deter the attempt. Most patients are unlikely to change occupations, and the physician must not lightly advise it without also considering the social and economic circumstances of the patient. Chronic bronchitis occurring in a nonsmoker is unusual; it should raise the suspicion of bronchiectasis, or of an allergic cause. Mucoviscidosis is a much less common cause of chronic bronchitis. In the relatively small number of patients in whom there is suspicion of allergy, the diagnosis is strengthened by the finding of eosinophils in the sputum or blood or both; attempts to identify the allergen by history and skin testing then may be worthwhile. (For treatment of bronchial allergies, see Ch. 505.)

Mucopurulent Bronchitis. In addition to the aforementioned measures, administration of the appropriate antimicrobial drug may be successful in removing evidence of infection. Occasionally, despite administration of the whole range of antimicrobials, the infection persists. This usually implies structural damage to the bronchi, possibly with bronchiectatic areas and grossly impaired bronchial clearance. In some such patients, infection is due to organisms such as *P. aeruginosa,* Proteus, and *E. coli.* (For management of the last-named group of infections, see Ch. 181 to 183).

In nonhospital practice, it is not necessary or feasible to obtain sputum culture during each acute exacerbation. Treatment should be started with a minimum of delay and is best achieved by self-administration at the earliest sign of infection of either tetracycline, 500 mg four times a day, or ampicillin, 500 mg four times a day, for seven to ten days. The patient must be instructed that, should his condition not improve within 48 hours, or deteriorate within this time, he should seek medical advice without further delay.

A variety of other antimicrobials may be used. These are usually variants of tetracycline or penicillin. If the patient is intolerant of these drugs or the organisms are resistant, cephalothin, clindamycin, erythromycin, or trimethaprim with sulfamethoxazole may be substituted. Tetracycline is particularly effective in mycoplasma infections. In infections with *H. influenzae,* ampicillin, 1 gram every six hours for seven to ten days, is particularly effective when started in the acute phase, and may reduce the frequency of subsequent exacerbations. Chloramphenicol, 250 to 500 mg four times a day, is very effective, but fear of blood dyscrasia has limited its use to situations in which delay in using an effective drug would be very dangerous, e.g., in association with ventilatory failure.

Long-Term Antimicrobial Therapy for Mucopurulent Chronic Bronchitis. In controlled studies, long-term treatment with oxytetracycline, 2 grams daily, did not affect the frequency of acute exacerbations but reduced the duration of illness. Pneumonias were less frequent but did occur; there was no change in the frequency of isolation of *H. influenzae.* Superinfection with drug-resistant bacteria was not found to be a problem. Equally good results have been obtained from prompt intermittent therapy, and most physicians consider that unless the frequency of recurrences is so great that virtually continuous therapy is being given, individual therapy of exacerbations is the method of choice.

Chronic Obstructive Bronchitis. The special additional features of management in patients with chronic obstructive bronchitis are considered later.

Prognosis. Reduction in cough and sputum may be expected if the provoking irritant can be removed, and some regression of the histologic changes has been recorded. Mortality depends largely on whether generalized obstructive changes develop in the bronchi.

Prevention. Chronic bronchitis is usually a preventable disease. Education in the dangers of cigarette smoking, control or elimination of dusty atmospheres in occupations with known hazards, and prompt effective treatment of bronchial infections in childhood are measures that would reduce chronic bronchitis to a minor disorder. Although the medical profession has a leading role to play in alerting the public to the dangers, in the last analysis it is the community as a whole which must provide the solutions. There is one exception: recognition of allergic factors and their elimination or effective treatment comprise one area in which the physician alone is responsible.

Air Pollution and Health. Summary and Report on Air Pollution and Its Effects on Health by the Committee of the Royal College of Physicians of London on Smoking and Atmospheric Pollution. London, Pitman Medical and Scientific Publishing Company, Ltd., 1970.
American Thoracic Society: Chemoprophylaxis of chronic bronchitis. A Statement by the Committee on Therapy. Am. Rev. Respir. Dis., 104:776, 1971.
Bates, D. V.: Air pollution, chronic bronchitis and emphysema. Am. Rev. Respir. Dis., 105:1, 1972.
Colley, J. R. T.: Respiratory disease in childhood. Br. Med. Bull., 27:9, 1971.
Ferris, B.: Chronic bronchitis and emphysema. Classification and epidemiology. Med. Clin. North Am., 57:637, 1973.
Holland, W. W., Bennett, A. E., and Elliot, A.: Factors influencing the onset of chronic respiratory disease. Br. Med. J., 2:205, 1969.
Medical Research Council Report of the Committee on Etiology of Chronic Bronchitis: The definition and classification of chronic bronchitis for clinical and epidemiological purposes. Lancet, 1:775, 1965.
Reid, L.: Emphysema with chronic bronchitis. *In* Pathology of Emphysema. London, Lloyd-Luke, 1967, Chap. 12, p. 158.
Report to Medical Research Council – The value of chemoprophylaxis and chemotherapy in early chronic bronchitis. Br. Med. J., 1:1317, 1966.

504. BRONCHIECTASIS

J. B. L. Howell

Definition. The Greek word "ectasia" means widening; hence bronchiectasis means widening of the bronchi. There are no symptoms or signs directly related to widening of the bronchi. However, to the clinician, bronchiectasis usually means more than the anatomic lesion; it includes in addition the chronic or recurrent bronchial infection and hypersecretion of mucus which usually accompanies it.

Etiology. The causes of bronchiectasis are varied and their relative frequency has changed since the introduc tion of antimicrobial drugs and the control of pulmonary tuberculosis. In the prechemotherapy era, the most common causes of bronchiectasis were postbronchopneumonic atelectasis and pulmonary tuberculosis. Aspiration of a foreign body, pulmonary complications of surgery, pertussis, and measles were also responsible, but in approximately 25 per cent of cases no cause could be identified. Since the advent of antimicrobial drugs the incidence and the problems in management of bronchiectasis have become much less. It now occurs mainly after the pneumonias that may complicate pertussis or measles, although all the previous causes may still occasionally be responsible. Bronchiectasis secondary to infected obstructive atelectasis resulting from bronchial neoplasm is being seen more frequently. So-called congenital bronchiectasis is probably the result of infections and collapse in infancy, but bronchiectasis associated with chronic sinusitis and situs inversus (Kartagener's syndrome) is probably truly congenital. Mucoviscidosis may also result in widespread bronchiectasis, the ectatic regions sometimes tending to extend more centrally. Bronchiectasis localized to a proximal region of a segmental bronchus, with normal bronchial distribution distal to it, is sometimes seen with pulmonary aspergillosis when the bronchial wall is infiltrated and weakened by the fungus.

Pathogenesis. The caliber of intrapulmonary bronchi depends upon a balance between the inward acting forces of the connective tissues of the bronchial wall and the outward traction of surrounding lung tissue. An increase in outward traction is insufficient to cause dilatation; weakening of the wall resulting from chronic inflammation must also occur. Both these factors may occur after obstructive atelectasis with chronic infection; the atelectasis tends to increase traction and the chronic infection causes damage to the connective tissue and bronchial smooth muscle. Irregular dilatation of the bronchus and damage to the epithelial lining interfere with bronchial drainage; secretions are retained and chronic bronchial suppuration becomes established.

Pathology. Bronchiectasis usually affects segmental bronchi and may involve one or more segments, a lobe, or rarely a whole lung. It is often distributed in patches over a number of segments, and is frequently bilateral. The regions most frequently involved are the basal segments, right middle lobe, and lingula. Upper lobe bronchiectasis is usually secondary to tuberculosis.

The affected bronchus may become dilated into thick-walled sacs, *saccular bronchiectasis,* cyst-like spaces, *cystic bronchiectasis,* or may cause irregular widening over the affected length to form *fusiform* or *cylindrical bronchiectasis.* In saccular bronchiectasis approximately only four generations of bronchi, widely dilated and distorted, can be identified; the distal generations of bronchi and alveoli are usually obliterated by inflammatory tissue and fibrosis. In fusiform bronchiectasis, the distal bronchi are occluded with mucus and pus but are usually not obliterated. Extension of infection to the pleural surface causes pleurisy and adhesions to the chest wall. Histologically, some bronchi are infiltrated with lymphocytes and have lymphoid nodules in their walls; mucus-secreting glands and cells are prominent. This is likely in children with fusiform bronchiectasis of lower lobe bronchi. In saccular bronchiectasis particularly, the walls of the sacs are fibrous and contain granulation tissue in places lined with metaplastic squamous epithelium. The normal structures of the bronchial walls are destroyed. The bacterial flora is similar to that of chronic mucopurulent bronchitis. The usual commensals of the nasopharynx are present, and *H. influenzae,* pneumococci, and staphylococci may also be found. Sometimes various species of spirochete, the fusiform bacilli, and other anaerobic bacteria are present and are largely responsible for the offensive fetor (see Ch. 211).

Clinical Manifestations. The clinical manifestations of bronchiectasis are dominated by the chronic infection and hypersecretion of mucus in the ectatic bronchi. *Cough* productive of copious purulent sputum, occurring especially with changes of posture, is the classic symptom. In a minority of cases, infection is minimal (dry bronchiectasis), and recurrent hemoptysis associated with episodes of infection is the major symptom.

In the heavily infected extensive case, the sputum may have a fetid odor and volumes of 400 to 500 ml daily may be seen. After adequate drainage and control of infection this may be reduced to a few milliliters a day. Hemoptysis is common and occasionally may be profuse. Coexisting chronic sinusitis, especially of the maxillary antrum, is common, but its relationship to the bronchiectasis is uncertain. *Chest pain* usually occurs as a result of pleurisy during an infective episode, but occasionally there may be a continuous ache in the region of the bronchiectasis. Shortness of breath on exertion and edema of the ankles may occur when the bronchiectasis is complicated by chronic cor pulmonale. General symptoms caused by chronic infection include tiredness, fatigue, and, in children, stunted growth. Sometimes, bronchiectasis is entirely without symptoms and is a fortuitous finding on routine chest roentgenography or on physical examination.

The physical signs depend on the extent and degree of purulence of the bronchiectasis and on whether generalized obstructive bronchial changes have developed.

If the bronchial changes are extensive and associated with airway obstruction, the patient may be dyspneic and cyanosed. With extensive purulent bronchiectasis the fingers are clubbed. There may be flattening of the thorax and the mediastinum may be deviated to the side of the lesion. Movement is diminished, tactile fremitus is reduced, and there may be dullness to percussion. Breath sounds may be bronchial in quality over consolidated segments. Crepitations occur over affected regions and have a characteristic coarse character, well expressed by the term "leathery" crepitations; they do not clear but may be altered by coughing.

Complications. These include recurrent pneumonia, hemoptysis, lung abscess, brain abscess, empyema, pyopneumothorax and, if longstanding, amyloid disease. The frequency of these has been greatly reduced with the improved management of bronchiectasis.

Disturbance of pulmonary function is more frequent in bronchiectasis than is generally realized but is due mainly to the associated generalized bronchitis. In a recent study, increased airway resistance and residual volume – total lung capacity ratio and reduced maximal breathing capacity were present in over half the patients. Physiologic dead space – tidal volume ratio and nitrogen washout, indicating alteration in the distribution of inspired gas, was abnormal in the majority. However, arterial oxygen saturation below 90 per cent and slightly raised arterial P_{CO_2} was seen in only 10 to 15 per cent. These disturbances of pulmonary function were rarely severe but increased in proportion to the number of segments involved. The effects of cylindrical and saccular bronchiectasis on pulmonary function tests were similar. The persistence of *H. influenzae* was correlated with a lower maximal breathing capacity, but no deterioration was observed over a period of three years in any of these patients irrespective of whether *H. influenzae* was eliminated from the sputum by antimicrobial drugs. The rate of deterioration is related to the frequency of lower respiratory infections.

Diagnosis. The clinical diagnosis may be confirmed by roentgenography, and the chest roentgenogram is nearly always abnormal in some respect. Increased, coarse-meshed lung markings are seen in over half the patients. Evidence of lobar atelectasis occurs particularly in young patients; a honeycomb appearance is less common. Sometimes with saccular and cystic bronchiectasis, ring shadows with fluid levels are present. The diagnosis, extent, and location of the bronchiectasis is established by *bronchography* in which a radiopaque oil is introduced into the trachea and allowed to spread evenly through the tracheobronchial tree, followed by chest roentgenograms in the anteroposterior, lateral, and right anterior oblique positions. It is inadvisable to fill both sides at one examination if there is evidence of impaired pulmonary function. If a primarily endobronchial cause of the bronchiectasis is suspected, bronchoscopy must be performed. A microcytic anemia, neutrophil leukocytosis, and an elevated erythrocyte sedimentation rate, all due to chronic infection, may be present.

There is a spectrum of chronic purulent disease of the bronchi, ranging from mucopurulent bronchitis with little ectasia at one end to gross bronchiectasis at the other. In certain intermediate cases therefore the categorization is arbitrary.

Treatment. *Medical.* After identification of the affected segment or segments, a rational program of postural drainage can be introduced, usually twice or thrice daily. In selected cases of basal bronchiectasis, drainage throughout the night by elevation of the foot of the bed may be beneficial. After improvement has occurred, postural drainage should be continued routinely even if it is unproductive of sputum during drainage; the secretions are often moved and coughed up later. Antimicrobial drugs appropriate to the sputum culture should be administered for a limited course, but should not be administered continuously because of possible superinfection, although admittedly this rarely seems to occur. With adequate postural drainage, sputum should be reduced to small quantities daily even though it remains purulent. The drugs should be reserved for acute exacerbations when they should be administered with minimal delay. The choice of drug regimen is the same as in the treatment of chronic bronchitis and is discussed in Ch. 181 to 183 and Ch. 503.

Surgical. If bronchography shows localized unilateral bronchiectasis which is causing sufficient symptoms to be troublesome, usually as a socially disturbing productive cough, surgical removal of the affected segment or lobe should be considered, providing that over-all lung function is adequate. Rarely, bilateral disease may be treated in this way. Sequential resections for recurring disease will result in a greater loss of lung function than if the diseased segments had been removed at one point in time. Prognosis is poorer with left lobe bronchiectasis owing to frequent recurrence in the lingula. The best results are obtained with unilateral bronchiectasis affecting patients less than 30 years old.

Incidence and Prevalence. There is little recent information about the prevalence of bronchiectasis. It has been estimated to affect 1.3 per 1000 persons, but certainly significant clinical problems arising from this cause are becoming rare. Cylindrical bronchiectasis is reported to complicate bronchopneumonia in approximately 4 per cent of cases.

Prognosis. The prognosis has altered substantially since the introduction of antimicrobial drugs. With good control of infection, either by medical or surgical treatment, life expectancy is normal. If extensive suppuration cannot be controlled, the outlook is poor, and it has been estimated that approximately one third will die within ten years. The development of chronic airway obstruction is a serious complication and affects prognosis accordingly.

Cherniak, N. S., and Carton, R. W.: Factors associated with respiratory insufficiency in bronchiectasis. Am. J. Med., 41:562, 1966.
Gudbjerg, C. E.: Bronchiectasis—Radiological diagnosis and prognosis after operative treatment. Acta Radiol. (Suppl. 143), 1957.
James, U., Brimblecombe, F. S. W., and Wells, J. W.: The natural history of pulmonary collapse in childhood. Quart. J. Med., 25:121, 1956.
Perry, K. M. A., and Holmes Sellers, T. (eds.): Chest Diseases. London, Butterworth, Ltd., 1968.
Prolonged antibiotic treatment of severe bronchiectasis. Clinical Trials Committee of the British Medical Research Council. Br. Med. J., 2:255, 1957.

505. ASTHMA: ACUTE REVERSIBLE AIRWAY OBSTRUCTION

J. B. L. Howell

Definition. Asthma has proved difficult to define. It is not a disease entity, but one form of clinical presentation of bronchial disorder associated with airway obstruction. It is characterized by marked changes in bronchial caliber occurring over short periods of time, either spontaneously or in response to treatment.

Because the degree of reversibility of bronchial narrowing may vary widely from complete to barely measurable, it is not possible, nor even desirable, to define asthma in more quantitative terms. The term merely describes that end of the spectrum of reversibility of bronchial narrowing at which the changes both in the bronchi and in the clinical state of the patient are unequivocal. Many cases are encountered in which the variability in the caliber of the bronchi and in the state of the patient is such as to make categorization as asthma uncertain. However, the management of the individual patient does not require that this uncertainty be resolved; it is the cause and mechanism by which the disorder is produced that must be recognized if effective therapy is not to be withheld. Most patients with this clinical entity have an allergic basis for their bronchial disorder. Nevertheless, other nonallergic mechanisms are sometimes responsible so that the presence of asthma is not in itself unequivocal evidence of the presence of an allergic disorder.

Mechanism and Etiology. In asthma, there is a continuous state of hyper-reactivity of the bronchi, during which exposure to a wide variety of bronchial irritants will precipitate an asthmatic attack.

Bronchial Hyper-reactivity. In normal subjects, inhalation of histamine or carbachol may cause small increases in airway resistance. By contrast, the bronchi of patients with asthma are highly reactive and show marked bronchoconstriction in response to these substances. This phenomenon is termed *bronchial hyper-reactivity.* Bronchial hyper-reactivity has also been shown to occur with a variety of nonspecific irritants such as dusts and cold air. This reaction is not restricted to asthmatic patients; it may also occur in many patients with chronic bronchitis and chronic airflow obstruction. It may sometimes be seen in normal subjects, especially for short periods after an acute tracheobronchial infection. This state of hyper-reactivity may be reversible; in subjects with seasonal grass-pollen asthma, hyper-reactivity increases during the pollen season whether attacks are occurring or not. In children with perennial asthma, removal from an urban environment to the Swiss Alps has been followed by progressive reduction in the degree of hyper-reactivity; appropriate therapy with sodium cromoglycate may also have the same effect. In subjects with hyper-reactivity associated with nonallergic states, e.g., chronic bronchitis, clinical observation of the effects of removal of inhaled irritants such as smoking or moving to a less polluted environment suggests that some degree of reversibility is possible.

At least two types of mechanism are involved in hyper-reactivity. The bronchoconstriction induced by cold air, for example, is blocked by atropine, indicating that a nervous reflex is involved. By contrast, the actions of histamine and So_2 are less affected by atropine, and the mechanism resides partly in the tissues. The nature of the changes in allergic or nonallergic states is not known.

Bronchial Irritants. A number of "trigger factors" may cause hyper-reactive bronchi to constrict. Although the end-result of their action is similar, it is important clinically to decide whether they act by inducing an allergic reaction or by some other mechanism, because specific therapy is available only for the allergic type.

Allergic or Presumed Allergic Factors. Allergic or presumed allergic factors are involved in most cases of asthma. They may induce either bronchial hyper-reactivity or trigger attacks, or both. The most common and best recognized reaction is the immediate (Type I) reaction in which antigen combines with reaginic antibody (IgE) present on the surface of bronchial mast cells, causing their degranulation and release or formation of a number of "spasmogens." In some patients, possibly as many as 20 per cent, the reaginic antibody appears to be an IgG. The spasmogens include histamine, slow-reacting substance of anaphylaxis (SRS,A), bradykinin, rabbit aorta contracting substance, and possibly 5-hydroxytryptamine which cause increased mucus secretion, edema, and bronchial muscle contraction. Common antigens include grass and tree pollens, mold spores, fungi including Aspergillus, animal dander, and house dust mite (*Dermatophagoides pteronyssinus*). Food allergies, e.g., to eggs, shellfish, and chocolate, may cause asthma but are more likely to cause urticaria.

After exposure, airway obstruction develops over minutes, and the immediacy of the response may enable the patient to recognize the relationship between exposure and attack. This contrasts with a different type of late allergic reaction (Type III) in which there is a delay, usually of 6 to 12 hours, between exposure and the development of airway obstruction. The late reaction involves circulating precipitating antibodies, and has been found to occur with a variety of antigens, e.g., Aspergillus, house dust mite, *B. subtilis* in the manufacture of biologic detergents. With some antigens, e.g., Aspergillus and house dust mite, both immediate and late reactions may occur in the same individual.

Contrasting Features of Extrinsic and Intrinsic Asthma

	Extrinsic	Intrinsic
Age of onset	Childhood or young adulthood	Middle age
Family history of allergies	Positive	Negative
Nasal symptoms	Hay fever	Nasal polyps
Aspirin sensitivity	Not a feature	Significant association
Skin tests	Positive	Negative
IgE levels	Raised	Normal

In some individuals, often in those in whom asthma has occurred for the first time in middle age, there may be no evidence of an IgE-mediated mechanism. IgE levels are normal, and skin tests to a wide range of antigens are negative. Because of this, their asthma is often called "intrinsic." However, in many cases sputum eosinophilia and response to sodium cromoglycate and/or steroid therapy suggest underlying allergic reactions. Some workers have denied any fundamental difference between intrinsic and extrinsic asthma, believing that if only the appropriate antigen were used for testing, all asthmas would be found to be extrinsic in origin. However, there are other features which indicate differences between the two types, as listed in the accompanying table. A clear-cut separation as suggested by this table is not always evident, but there can be little doubt that the distinction between the two types is a valid one. It does not necessarily follow that these are two diseases. It is also well recognized that some patients with extrinsic asthma in childhood may develop intrinsic asthma in middle age.

Physical or Chemical Irritants. Irritants such as inert dusts, sulfur dioxide, and other atmospheric pollutants are often responsible for asthma; for example, so-called Tokyo-Yokohama asthma is believed to be due to the high levels of atmospheric irritants in these cities, acting on individuals with pre-existing bronchitis or asthma. A number of industrial chemicals, for example, aluminum solder flux and toluene diisocyanate (TDI), a chemical widely used in the plastics industry, may induce asthma, almost certainly on an allergic basis.

Psychologic and Nervous Factors. Psychologic stress and conditioned reflexes have been shown to be important in precipitating attacks in subjects with bronchial hyper-reactivity, presumably through an exaggerated response to efferent autonomic nervous activity. Effective drug therapy may remove or override these influences, but if this fails, "verbal deconditioning" as reported by Moore (1966) should be considered for intractable cases. Hypnosis probably has little place.

Physical Exertion. Although the immediate effect of brief exercise may be to induce bronchodilatation in an asthmatic subject, many patients experience chest tightness and breathlessness if exercise is prolonged for several minutes; this may be especially noticeable after stopping the exercise. It is due to bronchoconstriction and is particularly common in children and young adults with mild asthma. The mechanism is uncertain and may be caused by different factors in different people. Hyperventilation with a lowering of Pco_2 or release of a circulating bronchoconstrictor substance during exercise has been suggested, but neither mechanism will explain all cases. The response is usually not blocked by the administration of atropine, but isoproterenol and cromolyn sodium are effective in the majority, the latter suggesting that mast cell degranulation may be the final common pathway. Occasionally exercise-induced attacks are the only clinical manifestation of asthma for years before spontaneous attacks begin to occur.

Infections. Respiratory infections, especially viral, are commonly associated with attacks of asthma. Whether this represents an allergic reaction to the infecting agent or is merely a nonspecific response of hyper-reactive bronchi to the infection is uncertain. There is still no firm evidence that chronic infections such as chronic sinusitis, tonsillitis, or dental sepsis are a cause of asthma in those patients in whom clear evidence of allergy is lacking (intrinsic or "infective" asthma). Lack of correlation between exacerbations of asthma and degree of activity of infection, together with failure of removal of infected foci or of long-term antimicrobial therapy to influence the course of the disease, casts doubt on the relevance of this mechanism. Skin tests to bacterial antigens are usually negative, but this may merely mean that an immediate Type I allergic reaction is not involved; delayed skin reactions to killed bacterial antigens have been reported in many patients with intrinsic asthma.

Pathology. Pathologic studies of asthma are largely related to the lungs of patients who die in status asthmaticus. The lungs are voluminous, and the smaller bronchi are largely occluded by mucous plugs. Histologically, large numbers of eosinophils are present in the bronchial walls together with varying numbers of lymphocytes and neutrophils and plasma cells. Hypertrophy of bronchial mucous glands and bronchial smooth muscle is usual; shedding of the epithelium is common.

Clinical Manifestations. Asthma occurs characteristically as episodes which may last from a few minutes to several days with a wide range of severity; between attacks the patient is well. Frequently asthma begins in childhood, and in about 30 per cent of the cases it is associated with eczema. Asthma may be particularly troublesome once the child begins school, possibly because of additional emotional stress and respiratory tract infections. Exercise-induced asthma may prevent the child from participating in games. It is at this stage that the etiologic role of psychologic factors is likely to be overrated; instead they should be recognized as only one of several possible provoking factors. Parental anxiety is especially likely to be blamed but only leads to even greater stress if not dealt with sympathetically. Alternatively, asthma may appear for the first time in middle age or later, sometimes after a lower respiratory tract infection. In some patients, especially with intrinsic asthma, there is a gradual change in the character of the disorder. Attacks become less frequent and less severe, but the degree of recovery between them is less complete. The patient develops chronic narrowing of the bronchi with airflow obstruction, and his capacity for physical exertion is progressively reduced. This chronic airway obstruction is usually associated with chronic cough and sputum (chronic bronchitis) and liability to episodes of purulent bronchitis.

The Attack of Asthma. The attack may begin within minutes of exposure to antigen and may or may not be associated with symptoms of hay fever. Alternatively, it may be precipitated by exertion, irritants, emotional stress, excitement, or infection; often there is no known precipitating factor. The patient experiences a sensation of chest tightness, with coughing and wheezing, which increases in severity. Dyspnea may become severe, and expiration is usually felt to be more difficult than inspiration. If untreated, the attack may last a variable time from a few minutes to several hours, but the prompt inhalation of an aerosol of isoproterenol or similar substance may abort the attack.

In some patients, attacks occur only at night, usually between 2 and 4 A.M., and in older subjects may then be mistaken for left ventricular failure. Nocturnal attacks may occur sporadically for months or years before also occurring during the day.

In a severe attack, the patient is extremely dyspneic, orthopneic, and often cyanosed. He is agitated and may be confused. He is often most comfortable sitting forward with his arms leaning on some support, a point to remember when asking the patient to lean back on the pillows to be examined. There is indrawing of the soft tissues of the neck, and the accessory muscles are active. Retraction of the sternomastoid muscle has been reported to be the only consistent accompaniment of severe asthma. The chest is overinflated with diminished hepatic and cardiac dullness to percussion, and respiratory movement is reduced. The larynx is pulled downward and the lower lateral rib cage inward with inspiration. High pitched, sibilant rhonchi, often associated with coarse crepitations in some areas, occur during inspiration as well as expiration. It is important to remember that when airflow obstruction becomes extreme, rhonchi may disappear. The pulse is rapid and blood pressure is normal. Pulsus paradoxus may be present, and indicates at least a 60 per cent reduction in the FEV_1; unlike the situation in pericardial tamponade, there is no associated engorgement of the cervical veins on inspiration. The sputum is usually viscid and difficult to expectorate; it may contain branched white bronchial casts and spirals of condensed mucus up to a few millimeters long, so-called Curschmann's spirals. A purulent appearance is commonly due to infection but may be due solely to the presence of large numbers of eosinophils. If the attack has been present for many hours or days without remission despite treatment, the patient has "status asthmaticus." This is often associated with signs of exhaustion and dehydration. Tachycardia is the rule, and, if greater than 130 per minute, indicates severe hypoxemia. Rarely, in patients with very prolonged severe airflow obstruction, edema of the feet and ankles may occur without other clinical evidence of heart failure.

The severity of an attack of asthma is often misjudged. Disturbance of consciousness, general exhaustion, marked pulsus paradoxus, any elevation of the Pco_2*, very low* FEV_1*, pneumothorax, and pneumomediastinum are signs of great severity and indicate need of urgent effective therapy.*

Laboratory Tests. Vital capacity, FEV_1, and FEV_1/VC ratio are diminished. Residual volume is increased, and, if airflow obstruction is severe and prolonged, total lung capacity may also be increased. Airway resistance is markedly increased. Arterial Po_2 is reduced owing to disturbed ventilation-perfusion relationships. An FEV_1 of less than 1 liter is almost always associated with reduction in arterial Po_2, and in status asthmaticus the arterial Po_2 may reach alarmingly low levels but is usually above 50 mm Hg. In moderate asthma, the Pco_2 is often low, indicating hyperventilation. Any elevation of the Pco_2 is of grave significance, for it indicates that the resting ventilation is virtually the maximum of which the patient is capable and that further increase in airway resistance, or reduction in drive to breathe, either through exhaustion or because of the use of sedatives or opiates, may be rapidly lethal. During recovery, symptoms disappear when the FEV_1 is still less than 50 per cent of predicted normal; signs disappear between 60 and 70 per cent. The Pa_{O_2} may not return to normal between attacks owing to persisting ventilation-perfusion disturbances.

The peripheral blood often shows eosinophilia. A slight polymorphonuclear leukocytosis is not uncommon. Microscopy of the sputum reveals eosinophilia and also long narrow crystals, Charcot-Leyden crystals, which are believed to be derived from eosinophils and with which they are always associated. The chest roentgenogram usually shows signs of overinflation, but occasionally patchy radiopacities may be present. These are particularly common in association with aspergillosis. Heart size is normal.

Prognosis and Prevalence. It is usual for attacks to become less frequent and severe during middle and late adolescence, and they may disappear completely. Approximately 50 per cent of children with asthma will become symptom free before adult life, and only 5 to 10 per cent continue to have severe disability, this unfortunate outcome being more likely when asthma has begun in infancy in association with eczema. This presumably reflects their greater tendency to develop hypersensitivity reactions. Often those not wholly symptom free in adulthood will experience only occasional mild attacks at infrequent intervals, but sometimes severe attacks may recur years or decades later. In adult asthmatics of the intrinsic type, followed for at least 15 years. Rackemann found that 22 per cent were symptom free, 44 per cent were improved, 33 per cent were unimproved, and 3 per cent had probably died of their asthma. Sinusitis and nasal polyps were more common in the unimproved group. There is general agreement that deaths are most common in patients with severe disabling chronic symptoms.

Asthma occurs in approximately 1 to 2 per cent of the population. There is a higher prevalence in childhood which varies between countries, as follows: Sweden, 0.73 per cent; United Kingdom, 3.8 per cent; United States, 6.9 per cent; and Australia, 11 per cent. Asthma occurs more frequently in boys up to ten years of age, and the ratio becomes even wider during adolescence. Severe childhood asthma is much more common among boys.

Between 1959 and 1966, the death rate from asthma in the United Kingdom in the age group 5 to 34 years increased threefold from 0.7 to 2.2 per 100,000, and this rise corresponded with increased sales of pressurized bronchodilator aerosols. Asthma then accounted for 7 per cent of all deaths in persons 10 to 14 years old. A study of the possible causes was initiated, but the "epidemic" rapidly declined, and by 1969 the death rate was only slightly higher than it had been ten years earlier. Fifty-two deaths in the age group 5 to 34 years were analyzed. Below 15 years there were four males to each female death, but over 30 years females predominated. Death was unexpected in 79 per cent, about one third being judged by their doctors not to have been severely ill. Eighty-one per cent died at home or on the way to hospital. There was no evidence to incriminate excessive use of pressurized aerosols. Indeed, the duration of the final attack was considerably longer in those who had used their aerosols excessively compared with those who had not. It was noted that the "epidemic" of asthma deaths had not occurred in countries like the United States, where a concentrated form of pressurized aerosol was not available; but epidemiologic studies, particularly in Australia, do not support the hypothesis that the concentrated aerosol was responsible for the "epidemic." Severe reactions have been recorded resulting from hypersensitivity to penicillin, aspirin, indomethacin, and radiopaque contrast media.

Differential Diagnosis. States of increased ventilation may be confused with asthma. These include severe metabolic acidosis, e.g., "renal" asthma, hyperventilation syndrome, and pulmonary embolism in which bronchospasm may also occur. Airflow obstruction with wheezing also occurs in certain patients with left ventricular failure, and inhalation of isoproterenol may give temporary relief. Paroxysmal nocturnal dyspnea caused by left ventricular failure may be confused with asthma. Large airway obstruction, e.g., laryngeal carcinoma and tracheal growths or compression from lymph nodes, may sometimes cause confusion, but inspiratory stridor should indicate the mechanism. Asthma may sometimes occur in association with other disorders of immunologic mechanisms; in association with polyarteritis nodosa, marked eosinophilia is characteristic. Carcinoid tumors are a rare cause of asthmatic attacks associated with flushing.

Management of Asthma. Obviously the most direct form of management of the patient with asthma is to terminate the exposure to responsible allergens or irritants. This may give complete relief and is most likely to be effective with occupational exposures or specific sensitivities, e.g., to animal dander. If avoidance of the allergen is not feasible, attempts may be made to *hyposensitize* the patient by injections of graded doses of the antigen at regular intervals. This is believed to induce IgG antibody, which competes for the antigen and prevents it from reaching IgE-sensitized mast cells. This procedure, which is particularly successful for hay fever, is less successful for the relief of asthma, although sometimes dramatic success occurs with complete relief of symptoms for varying periods up to several years. Further courses of antigen injection may not be so successful. It is not possible to predict which patients will benefit, and therefore it is always worth trying in patients with continuing disability whenever other methods of treatment have failed.

Reversal of the Asthmatic Reaction. Acute exacerbations of asthma may be promptly relieved by inhalation of 0.1 mg of isoproterenol, or 0.1 ml of 1:1000 epinephrine subcutaneously or 1:100 by nebulizer. Longer-acting beta-adrenergic drugs, such as orciprenaline, salbutamol, and terbutaline, are available in some countries as pressurized aerosols. The latter two are largely beta-2 (bronchial) stimulators and have relatively little effect upon the heart. All tend to cause a further small reduction in the Pa_{O_2}, but there is no unequivocal evidence that this is dangerous; if necessary, it can be corrected by oxygen administration. Unfortunately, the more severe the asthmatic reaction, the less is the response to these drugs, and the shorter their duration of action. It is in these circumstances that repeated doses are taken at short intervals and the danger of overdosage is present. In some individuals, a rebound bronchoconstriction occurs as the bronchodilator effect wears off.

For continuous symptoms, the most successful drugs are those which stimulate β-adrenergic receptors. Ephedrine, 15 to 30 mg, may be given twice or three times daily. This should be first given in low dosage as it may cause palpitation and tremor and, in the elderly male, urinary retention. Other effective drugs are isoproterenol, 5 to 20 mg sublingually as required, aminophylline, 100 to 300 mg three times a day, and salbutamol, 2 to 4 mg, terbutaline, 5 mg, aminophylline, 100 to 300 mg three times a day, or orciprenaline 20 mg four times a day. Aminophylline is liable to cause gastric irritation, but there are several proprietary chemical analogues which are better tolerated. Nocturnal symptoms may be relieved by suppositories of aminophylline, 360 mg rectally on retiring at night. In persistent asthma, potassium iodide, 0.6 gram three times a day after meals, is often valuable in thinning tenacious sputum.

Although the aforementioned drugs are often given in combination, they should be first administered singly and with caution to patients with heart disease, hypertension, and hyperthyroidism. Antihistamines are rarely of much value in asthma and may cause drowsiness, but because of occasional successes should be considered in special situations.

Suppression of Allergic Reactions. If the asthmatic response is not controlled by simple measures, suppression of the allergic reaction should be attempted. Three types of drugs may be employed: corticosteroids, corticotrophin (ACTH), and cromolyn sodium. The mode of action of *corticosteroids* in asthma is uncertain. They will not suppress the acute asthmatic response to inhaled antigen but are effective in suppressing clinical extrinsic and intrinsic asthma in most cases. It has been suggested that they reduce the inflammatory reaction and may therefore act mainly by reducing edema and mucous secretion as well as bronchial hyper-reactivity. A large number of different corticosteroid preparations are available, each with different dosage schedules. For simplicity, dosages will be described for prednisone or prednisolone; dosages of other preparations should be adjusted accordingly.

ACUTE ATTACK. *For the treatment of an acute attack* comparatively large doses, 30 to 60 mg daily, may be given for a few days with safety, and after relief has been obtained reduction in dosage at a rate of 5 mg daily is usually possible without early recurrence. The occasional use of large doses of prednisone in this way is without significant risk of side effects except in patients with peptic ulceration in whom gastrointestinal bleeding may be induced. In children, as many as 15 courses of steroids have been given in a year without any detectable side effects developing.

CONTINUOUS SYMPTOMS. For continuous symptoms which recur during or shortly after the course of corticosteroids administered as described above, there are two alternative forms of dosage, continuous or intermittent.

CONTINUOUS THERAPY. An initial dose of prednisolone is given sufficient to produce effective, rapid suppression of symptoms, for example, 10 mg three times a day (range usually 20 to 60 mg daily). When definite improvement has occurred (usually within four days) the daily dosage may be reduced by 2.5 mg (half tablet) daily (or at longer intervals if experience indicates). When the daily dosage is down to 15 mg daily (that is, one to two weeks after start), reduction by 1 mg once or twice weekly may be continued until either symptoms begin to recur or it has been found possible to discontinue treatment. If troublesome symptoms recur while reducing dosage, the daily dose may be increased by 3 to 5 mg, and the procedure restarted.

INTERMITTENT THERAPY. Treatment is given for one to three days with the lowest dose of corticosteroids which will permit them to be omitted for a similar period without return of symptoms. The patient will usually find a dosage below which reduction is always followed by recurrence of symptoms.

Whether the intermittent or the continuous regimen is being used, superimposed acute exacerbations should be treated promptly with a large increase in dosage for a few days; then a progressive reduction may be followed as before.

Corticotrophin, natural or synthetic, may be used in place of corticosteroids for continuous symptoms. By using depot preparations, a satisfactory regimen of intermittent injections can usually be achieved. Initially, 1 mg of depot ACTH may be given daily and reduced to once weekly. The need for reducing the dose to the minimum which will maintain adequate control is the same as for oral corticosteroids. Corticotrophin has been reported to cause less retardation of growth in children than oral corticosteroids. Suppression of pituitary secretion of ACTH may occur and abrupt cessation of therapy may lead to acute adrenocorticoid insufficiency. Allergic reactions have occurred to the natural hormone, and a case of sensitivity to the synthetic preparation has recently been reported.

Recently, beclomethasone dipropionate and betamethasone 17-valerate, widely used for topical therapy in dermatology, have been prepared in pressurized aerosol form and shown to be effective substitutes in many patients for oral corticosteroid therapy without causing suppression of the hypophysial-pituitary-adrenal (HPA) axis. The usual initial dose is 100 μg every six hours, slowly reducing to minimal requirements. In patients already receiving long-term oral therapy in moderate dosage (e.g., less than 15 mg per day), it may be possible to substitute completely with an aerosol preparation, but care must be taken that hypocorticism caused by existing HPA suppression is not induced by too rapid withdrawal of oral steroid. Sometimes troublesome allergic rhinitis and eczema may recur as systemic steroid effects are reduced, and may require reinstitution of some oral therapy. The only side effect reported to date is an increased incidence of oral and laryngeal candidiasis which may occur in up to 10 per cent of patients.

CROMOLYN SODIUM (SODIUM CROMOGLYCATE). Cromolyn sodium, a bis-cromone derived from khellin, is a new type of compound used for prophylaxis of allergic asthma. When inhaled prior to antigen provocation challenge in sensitized subjects, it has the unique property of inhibiting the development of the immediate (Type I) asthmatic reaction. It is effective only when inhaled. Cromolyn sodium acts by stabilizing mast cells; it does not prevent antigen and reaginic antibody from combining but prevents the combination from triggering the degranulation of mast cells and thereby releasing spasmogens. Cromolyn sodium also inhibits the late (Type III) precipitin-mediated asthmatic and febrile reactions to inhaled house dust, Aspergillus, avian, and other proteins. In a recent study of subjects in whom both Types I and III reactions occurred after exposure to Aspergillus or house dust, prior inhalation of cromolyn sodium inhibited both reactions, whereas corticosteroids inhibited only the late (Type III) reaction. Cromolyn sodium does not possess anti-inflammatory or bronchodilator properties and does not antagonize histamine, SRS(A), bradykinin, serotonin, or prostaglandins F_{2alpha} and E_1. It may possess alpha-adrenergic blocking properties, but these also may be mediated through its effects upon the mast cell membrane.

Because of its mode of action, cromolyn sodium is used to prevent rather than treat attacks. Despite extensive trials there are still no firm criteria for the selection of patients who will benefit. Young patients with strong evidence of allergy are most likely to respond, about 80 per cent showing worthwhile improvement. Recent work has shown that patients who do not respond to cromolyn sodium may possess IgG rather than IgE mediated allergic reactions. Up to two thirds of older patients with "intrinsic" asthma are likely to benefit to some extent. In general, clear evidence of allergic factors, e.g., seasonal history, positive skin tests, sputum and/or blood eosinophilia, or the presence of exercise-induced asthma, especially if inhibited by cromolyn sodium, make benefit from cromolyn sodium likely; associated chronic bronchitis and irreversible airway obstruction make improvement less likely.

Improvement may be reflected in a number of ways such as reduction in the number of attacks, reduced cough and sputum, and reduced bronchodilator and corticosteroid requirements. These changes may sometimes occur without corresponding improvement in the results of spirometry.

In a group of patients already receiving continuous corticosteroid therapy, cromolyn sodium permitted an average reduction of steroid dosage of 40 per cent in approximately two thirds of cases; it was rarely possible to discontinue corticosteroids. The only known side effect is irritation of the throat by the dry powder.

Cromolyn sodium is prepared as a powder in capsules containing 20 mg of drug dispersed with lactose, and is inhaled through a specially designed turbo-inhaler (Spinhaler). For patients in whom the dry powder induces irritation of hyper-reactive bronchi, a preparation containing 0.1 mg of isoproterenol is available in the United Kingdom only. The usual dose schedule is inhalation of the contents of one capsule (20 mg) four times a day, but this may be adjusted to the minimal dose that maintains suppression of symptoms.

IMMUNOSUPPRESSIVE THERAPY. Immunosuppressive therapy similar to that used in tissue or organ transplantation has been used in attempts to suppress the allergic reaction in asthma. In a small number of trials using azathioprine, chlorambucil, and methotrexate in chronic severe asthma, conflicting results have been reported, and their value has yet to be determined.

Status Asthmaticus. The majority of patients with asthma improve rapidly after admission to hospital, administration of corticosteroids, and bronchodilator therapy. Subcutaneous epinephrine should not be administered because the patient may already have taken large doses of isoproterenol before admission. Sedatives are potentially dangerous and are absolutely contraindicated if the P_{CO_2} is raised; with lesser degrees of severity, their cautious use may be helpful. When improvement is delayed, particular attention must be paid to humidification of the inspired air, preferably by an ultrasonic nebulizer, although occasionally this aerosol is itself a bronchial irritant. Oxygen may be administered freely since CO_2 sensitivity is not impaired. Hydration of the patient must be maintained, with intravenous fluids if necessary. Occasionally hypovolemia is present and requires more rapid rehydration.

Intravenous hydrocortisone, 100 to 200 mg, may be repeated hourly if necessary, and some workers advocate even higher dosage up to 1 gram repeated as necessary. However, gastrointestinal hemorrhage has been reported on such a regimen. If severe respiratory acidemia is present, intravenous sodium bicarbonate, 50 to 100 mEq, may be beneficial. Serial measurement of Pa_{CO_2} and Pa_{O_2} is helpful in monitoring ventilatory status and oxygen therapy.

A decision which is often difficult is that of when to use *assisted ventilation*. This is made on the basis of the overall state of the patient, with particular attention to whether he is becoming exhausted, is unable to cooperate in bronchial toilet, or if the Pa_{CO_2} is rising progressively. It should not be made on any arbitrary level of Pa_{CO_2} or Pa_{O_2}. Endotracheal intubation has replaced tracheostomy in this situation; in addition to assisting ventilation, it enables bronchial toilet to be improved if necessary by direct instillation of 5 to 10 ml of warmed saline a few minutes prior to tracheal suction. (For discussion of the general question of acute respiratory failure, see Ch. 507.)

Altounyan, R. E. C.: Changes in responsiveness to histamine and atropine as a guide to diagnosis and evaluation of therapy in obstructive airway disease. *In* Proceedings of a Symposium on Disodium Cromoglycate in Allergic Airways Disease. London, Butterworth & Co., Ltd., 1970.

Bernstein, L., Siegel, S. C., Brandon, M. L., Brown, E. B., Evans, R. R., Feinberg, A. R., Friedlander, S., Krumhelz, R. A., Hadley, R. A., Handelman, N. I., Thurston, D., and Yamate, M.: A controlled study of cromolyn sodium sponsored by the drug committee of the American Academy of Allergy. J. Allerg. Clin. Immunol., 50:235, 1972.

Brompton Hospital/Medical Research Council Collaborative Trial: Long-term study of disodium cromoglycate in treatment of severe extrinsic or intrinsic asthma in adults. Br. Med. J., 4:383, 1972.

DeVries, K., Booij-Noord, H., Goei, J. T., Grobler, N. J., and Orie, N. G. M.: Inhalation tests. The influence of nonspecific irritants on the airways. Acta Allergol. (Kbh), (Suppl. 8):131, 1967.

D'Souza, M. F., Pepys, J., Wells, I. D., Tai, E., Palmer, F., Overell, B. G., McGrath, I. T., and Megson, M.: Hyposensitization with *Dermatophagoides pteronyssinus* in house dust allergy: A controlled study of clinical and immunological effects. Clin. Allergy, 3:177, 1973.

Jones, R. S.: Assessment of respiratory function in the asthmatic child. Br. Med. J., 2:972, 1966.

McFadden, E. R., Kiser, R., and deGroot, W. J.: Acute bronchial asthma. Relations between clinical and physiologic manifestations. N. Engl. J. Med., 288:221, 1973.

McNeill, R. S., Nairn, J. R., Millar, J. S., and Ingram, C. G.: Exercise-induced asthma. Quart. J. Med. (N.S.), 35:55, 1966.

Moore, N.: Behaviour therapy in bronchial asthma: A controlled study. J. Psychosom. Res., 9:257, 1965.

Pepys, J.: Asthma. Br. J. Hosp. Med., 7:709, 1972.

Porter, R., and Birch, J. (eds.): Identification of Asthma. Ciba Foundation Study Group No. 38. Edinburgh and London, Churchill-Livingstone, 1971.

Rackemann, F. M., and Edward, M. C.: Asthma in children. N. Engl. J. Med., 246:815, 1952.

Rebuck, A. S., and Read, J.: Assessment and management of severe asthma. Am. J. Med., 51:788, 1971.

Sodium cromoglycate (cromolyn): A review of its mode of action, pharmacology, therapeutic efficiency and use. Drugs, 1974.

Szentivanyi, A.: The beta adrenergic theory of the atopic abnormality in bronchial asthma. J. Allerg. Clin. Immunol., 42:203, 1968.

506. CHRONIC AIRWAY OBSTRUCTION

J. B. L. Howell

Chronic airway obstruction denotes an alteration in the mechanical properties of the lungs characterized by poorly reversible increased hindrance to expiratory airflow; it is usually but not necessarily accompanied by increased resistance to inspiration. It occurs mainly in association with primary disorders of the lungs such as chronic bronchitis, emphysema, and asthma, but rarely may complicate systemic disorders such as polyarteritis nodosa. The two main abnormalities responsible for this obstruction are, first, generalized narrowing of the bronchi and, second, destruction of the pulmonary parenchyma. An understanding of the interaction of these two factors is important in order to appreciate the significance of the abnormalities involved and the nature of the disability experienced by the patient.

MECHANISMS OF AIRWAY OBSTRUCTION

During inspiration, the inspiratory muscles lower alveolar pressure, and air flows into the alveoli at a rate which depends upon the caliber of the bronchi. During expiration, recoil of stretched elastic tissues expels air from the lungs by raising intra-alveolar pressure above mouth pressure. The rate of flow depends upon the pressure difference and the resistance of the airways. In normal subjects, this mechanism is sufficient to meet ventilatory needs even under conditions of severe exercise. In subjects with increased resistance to airflow, elastic recoil alone may not be sufficient to achieve the ventilation required, and active expiratory muscular efforts may be made. However, the increased intrathoracic pressure which results from this expiration muscle effort introduces a new factor in expiratory airflow, a tendency to compression of the large airways. *The key to understanding this new factor is that elastic recoil of the lung alone is responsible for raising intrabronchial pressure above intrathoracic pressure.* Providing that the pressure within the bronchi is higher than intrathoracic pressure, there is no airway compression. However, when expiratory airflow is increased in subjects with raised airway resistance or diminished elastic recoil of the lungs, the greater pressure drop along the bronchial tree may cause the pressure inside the trachea and large bronchi to fall below the surrounding intrathoracic pressure, and these structures will be compressed unless there is sufficient rigidity in their walls to resist it. Once compression occurs, no amount of further effort will increase airflow because the pressure within the bronchi cannot be increased without simultaneously increasing the surrounding pressure. In this way, compression which usually occurs in the larger segmental or main-stem bronchi forms a flow-limiting mechanism (often called a Starling resistor), and determines maximal rate of expiratory airflow. This mechanism cannot operate during inspiration; the rate of inspiratory airflow is always effort-dependent.

The maximal rate of expiratory airflow will therefore be reduced by (1) increased resistance to airflow due to structural narrowing or increased tone; (2) decreased elastic recoil of the lung parenchyma; and (3) decreased rigidity of larger airways.

Increased Airway Resistance. Increased airway resistance may be due to increased secretions; thickening of the wall of the airways caused by infiltration, edema, or glandular hypertrophy; or constriction resulting from smooth muscle contraction or fibrosis; deformity of the bronchi may also contribute. The dominant mechanism varies in different circumstances. When associated with chronic bronchitis, there are both narrowing of the smaller bronchi and increased mucus, sometimes causing plugging. When emphysema is also present, there are both narrowing and a slight loss in the number of airways, with an increased tendency to mucus plugging. The role of infection is doubtful; it has not been possible to establish a correlation between the rate of progression of airway obstruction and the frequency of infective bronchial episodes, although during acute infections airway obstruction is temporarily increased. In some areas, complete occlusion of bronchi requires that ventilation of distal areas be by collateral channels, thereby increasing airway resistance. It is possible that narrowing of chronic airways may involve increased smooth muscular tone at least in the initial stages before irreversible structural changes develop. Two observations suggest that some process additional to the results of chronic inflammation and fibrosis may be involved. First, hyper-reactivity of the bronchi is a feature of most patients with narrowing of the small airways; second, airway resistance is reduced, albeit to a small degree, after administration of isoproterenol and atropine aerosols.

Decreased Rigidity of the Walls of Larger Airways. A diminished rigidity of the trachea and bronchi is a common feature of chronic mucopurulent bronchitis. In itself, it is not responsible for reducing maximal expiratory airflow but predisposes toward airway compression when the other factors are present.

Diminished Elastic Recoil: Emphysema

The most important cause of diminished elastic recoil is emphysema. This word is derived from the Greek word meaning "an inflation" and was introduced by Laennec to describe the overinflated and partially destroyed state of the lung "vesicles." Unfortunately, many workers later adopted this term for the clinical syndrome of breathlessness, cough, and sputum with which emphysema is often associated. This resulted in confusion because a similar clinical picture may occur without emphysema. *There is now general agreement to restrict the use of the word emphysema to its original meaning as a pathologic term.* The most generally accepted definition at present is that agreed on by the World Health Organization (1961): "Emphysema is a condition of the lung characterised by increase beyond the normal in the size of air spaces distal to the terminal bronchiole, with destructive changes in their walls." There is still difference of opinion whether dilatation caused by distention without destruction should be included in the definition.

Destructive changes and dilatation may be restricted to the respiratory bronchioles (centriacinar or centrilobular emphysema), or may be more extensive with destruction of the whole of the acinus (panacinar emphysema), involving both air spaces and vascular bed. These may coalesce or distend to form bullae and cysts. Changes restricted to the periphery of the acinus (paraseptal emphysema) are never extensive and are without functional significance.

Gradual stretching but not rupture of lung tissue occurs with age (senile emphysema) and with longstanding overdistention as in severe chronic airway obstruction or status asthmaticus. Rupture of connective tissue requires weakening or destruction of the connective tissue; but until Eriksson reported in 1965 that the electrophoretic alpha$_1$ globulin peak, of which alpha$_1$ antitrypsin (AAT) is the major component, was absent in some patients with emphysema, little was known about the factors responsible. The substance AAT is a nonspecific inhibitor of proteolytic enzymes such as trypsin, elastase, skin collagenase, thrombin, and bacterial and leukocyte proteases, and is normally responsible for 90 per cent of the total serum trypsin inhibitory capacity. The degree of plasma protease inhibitory activity depends upon the inheritance of certain genes. The normal gene is termed Pi^M, the gene associated with the lowest level of inhibitory activity is Pi^Z, and other genes, e.g., Pi^S, have lesser degrees of deficiency. The homozygous ZZ phenotype has marked deficiency, whereas the heterozygous ZM phenotype and the homozygous SS have intermediate levels. Eriksson originally thought that only the homozygous (ZZ) state developed emphysema and that this was rare. It is now known that the heterozygous state with intermediate levels of inhibitory activity may also show an increased incidence of emphysema, and in one recent series 26 per cent of patients with emphysema showed some degree of inhibitor deficiency. The characteristics of emphysema associated with AAT deficiency are its development at an earlier age (mean age for homozygotes and heterozygotes 45 and 57 years, respectively) and its tendency to be more severe in the basal regions. Diminished basal perfusion on lung scan is strongly supportive of the likelihood of its presence.

These findings have suggested a possible etiology for emphysema. Proteolytic enzymes are released in the lungs at sites of inflammation and leukocyte breakdown but are normally limited in their action by the serum inhibitors. Deficiency of inhibitors may permit a greater degree of proteolysis of lung parenchyma causing emphysema. Although bronchial infection and inhaled irritants may cause widespread low-grade acinar inflammation, the localization of centriacinar emphysema to the upper parts of the lobes is explained by increased alveolar wall tension at these sites owing to gravitational effects. Basal panacinar emphysema in AAT deficiency may be related to the reported sequestration of leukocytes in the lungs, especially at the bases, with failure to inhibit leukocyte proteases. In support of this concept, emphysema has been produced experimentally by inhalation of extracts of leukocytes in animals. The importance of this hypothesis is that all types of emphysema are seen as an imbalance between proteolysis and protease inhibition. This may occur either because of increased protease production in otherwise normal individuals or because of deficient protease inhibition.

Extensive emphysema may be a major factor in limiting the maximal rate of expiratory airflow by reducing elastic recoil. The reduction in recoil is not due to alteration in the properties of the elastic fibers themselves; it is due largely to the increased size of the affected air spaces, occupying a larger proportion of the thorax and allowing less room for distention of the normal parts of the lung. This is reflected in a reduction of the maximal intrathoracic pressure which may be developed at full inspiration from the normal of 20 to 30 cm of water to as low as 3 to 5 cm of water.

Diagnosis of Emphysema During Life. There are no clinical stigmas of emphysema, and the diagnosis cannot easily be made during life because it requires evidence of the pathologic lesion. Extensive emphysema, especially centrilobular, may be present without roentgenographic abnormality. The presence of emphysema may be inferred from the chest roentgenogram if it shows reduction in the caliber and number of the peripheral branches of the pulmonary artery, usually associated with increased transradiancy of the lung field. This is the most reliable radiologic sign. Other abnormalities such as low, flat diaphragm and increased retrosternal space, although commonly present, are actually evidence only of overinflation of the lungs.

CLINICAL FEATURES OF CHRONIC AIRWAY OBSTRUCTION

Typically, the patient with chronic airway obstruction is a male cigarette smoker, between 50 and 60 years old, who may or may not have a long history of chronic bronchitis with recurrent winter bronchitis. His cardinal symptom is breathlessness on exertion, often with wheezing; it is worse in the morning, associated with a sensation of tightness until he has expectorated the night's accumulation of sputum. Intolerance of sudden exposure to cold air or smoky atmospheres which induce coughing, tightness, and breathlessness (bronchial irritability) is usually present when dyspnea is of sufficient severity to interfere with everyday activity. Similar symptoms may be precipitated by involvement in argument or other emotional situations. There is often orthopnea, along with shortness of breath on stooping. These features are attributable to disturbance of the bronchi and are common to nearly all patients with chronic airway obstruction. However, in some patients varying degrees of disturbance of pulmonary gas exchange may occur, leading to a wider range of clinical presentation; some patients have little evidence of disturbances of cardiopulmonary function, but others become cyanosed and edematous.

Professor Dornhorst of London caught the clinical imagination when he described the extremes of this range as "pink and puffing" and "blue and bloated." A number of studies have correlated these presentations with pulmonary pathology and pulmonary function disturbances, leading to the introduction of other descriptive terms, for example, emphysematous or bronchitic, "fighters or nonfighters," Type A or Type B. It must be emphasized that these are not two distinct diseases but the extremes of a range of presentation; some patients intermediate in type might well be called "blue puffers."

Type A, Emphysematous Type, "Pink Puffers"

This patient is severely breathless on exertion. He is underweight, his appearance often suggesting hyperthyroidism. The mucous membranes are pink; there is no finger clubbing. The chest is overinflated, and the accessory muscles are prominent. Cardiac and hepatic dullness are diminished or absent, and resonance extends down to the region of the eleventh to twelfth rib posteriorly. The larynx and trachea are pulled down with each inspiration. On auscultation, breath sounds are quiet, expiration is prolonged, and forced expiration induces fine sibilant rhonchi. The forced expiratory time (the time taken to deliver the forced vital capacity) is prolonged beyond four seconds.

The apex beat is usually impalpable, but pulsation is often seen and felt in the epigastrium where the heart sounds are also heard best. The chest roentgenogram confirms the overinflated state of the chest and usually shows roentgenographic evidence of emphysema. The cardiac shadow is long and narrow.

Laboratory Findings. Total lung capacity, residual volume, and residual volume–total lung capacity ratio are increased. The vital capacity, FEV_1, and the FEV_1/VC ratio are reduced. Other indices of airflow obstruction such as peak flow rate and maximal midexpiratory flow rate are also reduced. Pa_{CO_2} is normal and Pa_{O_2} may be slightly reduced. The transfer factor (diffusing capacity) for carbon monoxide is reduced.

Many of these patients have little increase in inspiratory airway resistance, expiratory airflow obstruction being dominated by *reduced pulmonary elastic recoil.* Flow limitation may be present even during quiet breathing in severe cases, and is best seen when flow-volume curves of the lung are displayed. CO_2 sensitivity is characteristically normal or near normal, and this together with the reduction in ventilatory capacity accounts for the severe exertional dyspnea.

Pathology. Panlobular emphysema is the dominant pathologic lesion in most cases. Mucous gland hyperplasia and hypertrophy may or may not be present. The heart is usually normal.

Type B, Bronchitic Type, "Blue Bloaters"

Typically, the history can be considered in three stages. First, there is a long history of chronic bronchitis with recurrent mucopurulent exacerbations. At this stage there may be no reduction of exercise capacity, although spirometry may reveal reduction in maximal ventilatory capacity. The second stage usually merges gradually with the first as the reduction in ventilatory capacity progresses to the stage at which shortness of breath on exercise becomes noticeable. Sometimes, as in Type A, this may develop relatively suddenly after an acute infective exacerbation. Usually, before shortness of breath becomes very severe, the third stage begins when the patient notices ankle edema, at first in the evenings but gradually becoming more marked and persistent.

Characteristically, the patient is well covered with a plethoric appearance. He is cyanosed at rest with warm extremities. The chest is overinflated but usually less so than in Type A. The signs of increased airway obstruction may be similar to those of Type A, but breath sounds are usually well heard and rhonchi and basal crepitations may be prominent; expiration is prolonged. The forced expiratory time is prolonged. There may be cardiac enlargement, right ventricular hypertrophy, raised jugular venous pressure, and hepatic enlargement together with edema. These signs often become more prominent during an acute exacerbation.

Laboratory Findings. Although the type B patient may have severe airway obstruction, it is not uncommon for the airway obstruction to be relatively mild (FEV_1, 1 to 1.5 liters) even though the Pco_2 is raised. Total lung capacity is usually normal, but residual volume is raised. There is arterial desaturation of varying degree, but not often lower than 80 per cent. Secondary polycythemia occurs with the more severe degrees of desaturation. The Pa_{CO_2} is raised, usually less than 55 mm Hg in the early phases of the illness, but may progress to severe ventilatory failure with Pa_{CO_2} 65 to 75 mm Hg. This is usually well compensated but with higher levels of Pco_2 may fall below pH 7.35. During acute exacerbations more severe changes may develop.

Airway resistance is increased during both inspiration and expiration. Diffusing capacity may be normal if emphysema is slight; CO_2 sensitivity is depressed. The latter is not usually measured as a routine procedure, but can readily be observed if a rebreathing method for measuring Pco_2 is used.

The chest roentgenogram shows good bronchovascular markings with thickening of bronchial walls, but characteristically there is no roentgenographic evidence of emphysema. The heart is usually enlarged. The electrocardiogram may show evidence of right ventricular hypertrophy. In acute exacerbations, Kerley B lines, indicating edema of interlobular septa, may be seen; in addition to pulmonary hypertension, cardiac catheterization may reveal raised left ventricular end-diastolic pressure, indicating left ventricular failure. A raised blood urea is common during an acute exacerbation; this is temporary and is corrected when the patient improves.

Pathology. The lungs usually show a combination of centrilobular and panacinar emphysema, but centrilobular emphysema is the more prominent. Occasionally emphysema is absent, but mucous gland hyperplasia is said to be present always. The right ventricle is usually hypertrophied, and there may be evidence of hypertensive changes in the pulmonary artery. Thrombosis of branches of the pulmonary artery is common.

Mechanism and Significance of Differences Between the Type Extremes of Clinical Prototypes

The "pink puffer" may be regarded as an otherwise normal subject with severe reduction of ventilatory capacity resulting from the development of a flow-limiting mechanism. The pulmonary pathology does not lead to gross disturbance of ventilation-perfusion relationships, and arterial blood gas composition is virtually normal, at least at rest. Ventilatory control mechanisms are intact. By contrast, the "blue bloater" has, in addition to airflow obstruction, gross disturbance of ventilation-perfusion relationships and impairment of CO_2 sensitivity of the respiratory center. The ventilation-perfusion abnormality leads to a chain of abnormalities, beginning with arterial hypoxemia and followed by polycythemia, pulmonary hypertension, right ventricular hypertrophy, and systemic venous congestion with edema. The mechanism of impaired CO_2 sensitivity of the respiratory center is unknown; it leads to chronic ventilatory failure with hypercapnia and impairs the ability to maintain ventilation in the face of increased airway resistance.

DIAGNOSIS OF CHRONIC AIRWAY OBSTRUCTION

Clinical Diagnosis. When dyspnea is associated with symptoms of bronchial irritability and morning tightness, it strongly suggests that airway obstruction is responsible. Although rhonchi are highly suggestive, they may be absent even with severe airway obstruction. *Prolonged expiration and forced expiratory time are the only reliable signs of airway obstruction.*

Etiologic Diagnosis. A history of heavy smoking or occupational exposure to dust often suggests the causative mechanism. Radiographic evidence of emphysema in a younger person, especially basal, raises the possibility of $alpha_1$ antitrypsin deficiency. Occasionally, a striking improvement follows administration of corticosteroids or cromolyn sodium (see Ch. 505), suggesting that allergic factors are causing or contributing to the disability. *It is important never to overlook this treatable possibility; its presence is suggested if chest tightness tends to recur during the day, if there is nocturnal dyspnea, and especially if there is sputum and/or blood eosinophilia.* If there is any doubt, a therapeutic trial of these drugs should be given, but it is sometimes difficult to separate specific from general effects of corticosteroids.

Assessment of Severity of Airway Obstruction. Simple clinical assessment of the severity of airflow obstruction and reduction in ventilatory capacity may be obtained from the vital capacity and FEV_1, or from peak flows. More detailed measurements are seldom needed for initial clinical assessment. The following are rough correlations between FEV_1 and physical activity. If the FEV_1 is greater than 1.5 liters, the subject can usually undertake moderate exercise. With an FEV_1 between 1.0 and 1.5 liters, the subject can usually undertake light activity but is somewhat short of breath on hurrying or climbing stairs. With an FEV_1 below 1.0 liter, he is usually breathless on slight exertion, although there are wide differences according to clinical type and personality. If the degree of disability grossly exceeds the severity of the airway obstruction, other causes of shortness of breath should be sought. These include heart disease, pulmonary hypertension, anemia, thyrotoxicosis, and metabolic acidosis. An important but often overlooked cause is a psychologic disturbance. This diagnosis should be suspected if attacks of breathlessness also occur at rest and are associated with symptoms of hyperventilation, i.e., dizziness and paresthesia. This reaction tends to occur in patients with strong obsessional traits associated with an anxiety reaction or depression; the three most common precipitating factors are bereavement, illness or fear of illness, and resentment; less commonly it is an hysterical reaction.

Detection of Early Changes. Macklem has pointed out that because of the very low resistance of small bronchioles, considerable pathologic changes may be present without causing a significant increased airway resistance. Thus, doubling the resistance or halving the number of the peripheral airways will result in only a 10 per cent increase in over-all airway resistance, because this region normally contributes only 10 per cent of the total. This raises problems in the early detection of airway disease. Measurements reflecting airway resistance are relatively insensitive, and it is now considered that abnormalities in the distribution of inspired gas (single breath N_2 test), increased closing volume, or the demonstration of frequency dependent compliance are more likely to reveal early peripheral bronchial disease.

TREATMENT OF AIRWAY OBSTRUCTION

Despite ignorance of basic causes of chronic airway obstruction, it is nevertheless possible to reduce the effects of these disturbances by attention to detail in management.

Removal of Irritants and Treatment of Infection. Removing atmospheric irritants and stopping cigarette smoking may cause a gradual reduction in the volume of mucus and the degree of hyper-reactivity of the bronchi and a moderate decrease in airway obstruction. One of the most potent irritants is bronchial infection, and this should be eradicated or minimized by appropriate antimicrobial therapy.

Bronchodilatation. Oral and aerosol bronchodilator drugs as discussed in Ch. 505 may be helpful. However, more prolonged bronchodilatation in subjects without an allergic cause for their bronchial narrowing can sometimes be achieved with an aerosol of atropine methonitrate (0.04 mg). Its action is slower in onset, and for this reason commercial preparations combine isoproterenol or its variants and atropine.

Bronchial Toilet and Mucolytics. Attention to humidification of inspired air and active bronchial toilet with physiotherapy may induce considerable improvement in airway obstruction. Inhalation of mucolytic drugs such as acetylcysteine may occasionally be helpful, but in allergic subjects hypersensitivity reactions have been recorded. Bromhexine (8 mg three times a day) by disrupting the mucopolysaccharide fibers of noninfected sputum aids expectoration and in controlled studies has been shown to improve airway obstruction.

Respiratory Stimulants. Oral analeptics, e.g., amiphenazole, 100 to 200 mg thrice daily, and prethcamide, 400 mg three or four times daily, have been advocated for the treatment of chronic ventilatory failure. They may result in transient slight reduction in Pco_2, but there is no evidence that they afford clinical benefit. Acetazolamide, 250 to 500 mg, or dichlorphenamide, 50 to 100 mg twice a day, has been reported to improve the breathlessness of some patients with airway obstruction. These carbonic anhydrase inhibitors may cause reduction in Pco_2 up to 8 to 10 mm Hg, but this fall does not correlate with subjective improvement. Paresthesia, headache, and general malaise may occur as side effects which disappear rapidly on stopping the drug.

Circulatory Management. The use of diuretics, e.g., chlorothiazide, 0.5 to 1.0 gram, furosemide, 40 to 80 mg orally from twice weekly to daily, has greatly improved management of edematous patients. Adequate diuresis may cause considerable improvement in pulmonary gas exchange and mechanisms. Daily administration requires supplements of potassium (600 to 1200 mg four times a day). Alternatively, amiloride, triamterene, or spironolactone may be effective without the need of potassium supplements. Digoxin, ~~0.25 mg~~, or digitoxin, ~~1.0 mg daily~~, should be given only if clearly indicated because of the risk of inducing ventricular arrhythmias. These drugs should not be used during acute respiratory failure; routine monitoring of patients admitted to hospital with chronic obstructive lung disease recently showed an incidence of arrhythmia of 89 per cent, with 57 per cent requiring specific therapy; there was no correlation between the occurrence of arrhythmia and the Pa_{CO_2}, Pa_{O_2}, or pH. If the hematocrit is raised above 55 to 60 per cent, repeated venesection should be used to reduce the hematocrit to about 55 per cent.

see Ch 541

Oxygen Therapy. This has been used in two ways: first, intermittently during exercise and in the recovery phase. Portable oxygen cylinders which provide small supplements of O_2 in the inspired air are available, but self-consciousness in wearing the equipment often deters patients from using them. Second, long-term oxygen therapy has been studied in patients with the Type B, "blue bloater" form of the disease and has been shown to reduce the severity of the circulatory abnormalities, at least in residents of Denver at 5000 feet. Its value at lower altitudes is unproved, and clinical trials are presently in progress.

Surgery of Emphysema. Removal of large localized emphysematous bullae or regions may reduce airway obstruction by permitting increased inflation of the remaining lung tissue and therefore increased elastic recoil. Selection of suitable patients is difficult; the best results have been obtained after removal of a single large cyst or when emphysematous changes have been in lower rather than in upper lobes. When tests of over-all function suggest widespread emphysema, improvement after bullectomy is less likely.

PROGNOSIS IN CHRONIC AIRWAY OBSTRUCTION

The prognosis in chronic airway obstruction is related to the severity of the lung disease; it is worse when airway obstruction is severe, when the diffusing capacity is markedly reduced, and when cor pulmonale is, or has been, present. It is worse at altitude than at sea level, presumably because of the greater hypoxemia. The length of history and the age of onset of symptoms are not related to mortality.

In a group of patients with chronic bronchitis with or without airway obstruction in London, 54 per cent died within ten years; 57 per cent of these died of respiratory causes, and 8 per cent died of bronchial carcinoma. The prognosis of 200 patients with airway obstruction has been studied in more detail in a group of patients in Chicago. The severity of ventilatory impairment, resting pulse rate, and mixed venous P_{CO_2}, were the most predictive of poor survival. The conclusions were that if there is no resting tachycardia, chronic hypercapnia, or severe impairment of diffusing capacity, a five-year survival may be expected in 80 per cent of cases when the FEV_1 exceeds 1.2 liters; in 60 per cent when FEV_1 is close to 1 liter; and in 40 per cent when the FEV_1 is below 0.75 liter. If the factors listed initially are present, the survival figure is reduced by 25 per cent.

The development of weight loss is of bad prognostic significance. Intensive treatment with bronchodilator aerosols or with antimicrobial drugs is without influence on the rate of deterioration of airflow obstruction. Advances in therapy in the past 15 years have not improved survival rates after the onset of cor pulmonale, approximately two thirds of the patients being dead at five years in one series.

ACUTE RESPIRATORY FAILURE

The greatest risk to the life of a patient with chronic airway obstruction is the development of an acute increase in bronchial secretions and airway obstruction which occurs in response to an acute bronchial infection or on exposure to irritant atmospheres such as smog. In patients of the "blue bloater" type, a rise in P_{CO_2} will almost certainly occur; it is unusual in the "pink puffer" patient, in whom an elevation of P_{CO_2} implies very severe airway obstruction unless unwise sedation has been given. If P_{CO_2} rises above 50 mm Hg or Pa_{O_2} falls below 60 mm Hg, respiratory failure is said to be present. It is very unusual for the P_{CO_2} to exceed 80 mm Hg because of the concomitant development of hypoxemia. Higher values generally imply the prior administration of oxygen.

Management of this life-threatening situation requires appreciation of three things. First, the acute situation has been caused largely by increased secretions and increased airway obstruction. Second, the immediate danger is hypoxemia. Third, hypercarbia and acidemia, if present, may cause clouding or even loss of consciousness and an inability by the patient to cooperate in his therapy.

The assessment of the patient therefore requires the following two immediate decisions: Can the patient raise the secretions by coughing? And does the patient need oxygen?

Ability to Raise Secretions by Coughing. Ability of the patient to raise the secretions by coughing can only be ascertained by instructing the patient to cough; the response to this is the most useful single physical sign in this situation. If he is unable to do so unaided, skilled physiotherapy may yet be successful, especially if effective humidification can be achieved. Administration of aminophylline, 250 mg intravenously over three to five minutes, may enable an effective cough to be produced. If the patient is too drowsy to cooperate, he may be roused sufficiently by this treatment or by the administration of nikethamide, 500 to 1000 mg intravenously, or some equivalent analeptic. There is no place in this situation for continuous intravenous analeptics unless combined with intensive chest physiotherapy.

The expectoration of even a few pieces of sputum may result in dramatic improvement. If the patient cannot raise secretions despite all efforts, there is no alternative but bronchoscopy and tracheal suction or, preferably, endotracheal intubation with regular tracheal suction and a period of assisted ventilation. Tracheostomy should be avoided unless prolonged assisted ventilation becomes necessary.

Oxygen Need. The presence of severe hypoxemia does not *necessarily* mean that tissue damage is occurring because increased perfusion may transport sufficient oxygen to the tissues to permit aerobic metabolism to continue. It has been shown that an arterial P_{O_2} even below 30 mm Hg can be adequate for tissue oxygenation *providing that a good circulation is maintained;* but usually Pa_{O_2} values below this level are associated with evidence of tissue hypoxia in the form of lactic acidosis and raised serum transaminase levels. Because of the steep slope of the hemoglobin dissociation curve for oxygen at these levels, relatively small increases in inspired oxygen will move the patient away from the brink of tissue hypoxia.

The *danger* of administration of high concentrations of oxygen is that by correcting hypoxemia, the main source of ventilatory stimulation will be removed, thus converting a conscious, cyanosed patient capable of cooperation into a pink unconscious patient in whom secretions accumulate and in whom intubation and assisted ventilation become mandatory. With care, the cautious administration of oxygen in inspired concentrations of 24 to 28 per cent, e.g., using a Venturi device, will increase arterial oxygen tension sufficiently without seriously reducing ventilatory drives in the majority of patients. With improvement in ventilatory capacity, progressive increases in oxygen concentrations will be tolerated.

The absolute indications for oxygen may be taken as, first, evidence of poor peripheral circulation, i.e., poor volume pulse, low blood pressure, poor capillary filling; and second, an arterial Po_2 below 30 mm Hg. In practice, when arterial Po_2 levels may not be available, it is advisable to administer 24 to 28 per cent O_2, e.g., using a Venturi device, to all patients and to measure Pco_2 serially. If the Pco_2 does not rise more than a few millimeters over the next one to two hours, it may be possible to increase the concentration of oxygen further. If adequate improvement in Pa_{O_2} cannot be achieved by these means without causing a progressive rise in Pa_{CO_2}, then assisted ventilation must be considered.

Other Therapeutic Measures. While these more urgent measures are being instituted the sputum should be obtained for culture. A broad-spectrum antimicrobial drug should be started, e.g., tetracycline, 500 mg four times a day, or ampicillin, 500 mg four times a day orally or parenterally, unless there are clinical indications for a different drug. A diuretic, e.g., furosemide, 40 to 80 mg intravenously, should be given if there is any evidence of pulmonary congestion or peripheral edema. Digitalis should be given with caution in the acute severely hypoxemic state because of the danger of inducing a ventricular dysrhythmia.

Prophylaxis. In view of the seriousness of acute exacerbations, advice about minimizing their occurrence should be given. The patient and his relatives should be warned of the signs of acute exacerbation and the need for attention to bronchial toilet and prompt antimicrobial therapy. A patient with previous history of respiratory failure should be admitted to hospital without delay if no rapid improvement occurs. Influenza vaccination should be administered annually.

Bates, D. V., Macklem, P. T., and Christie, R. V.: Respiratory Function in Disease. 2nd ed. Philadelphia, W. B. Saunders Company, 1971.

Burns, B. H., and Howell, J. B. L.: Disproportionately severe breathlessness in chronic bronchitis. Q. J. Med., 38:277, 1969.

Burrows, B., and Earle, R. H.: Prediction of survival in patients with chronic airway obstruction. Am. Rev. Respir. Dis., 99:865, 1969.

Burrows, B., Fletcher, C. M., Heard, B. E., Jones, N. L., and Wootliff, J. S.: The emphysematous and bronchial types of chronic airways obstruction. Lancet, 1:830, 1966.

Cotes, J. E.: Lung Function: Assessment and Application in Medicine. 2nd ed. Oxford and Edinburgh, Blackwell Scientific Publications, 1968.

Filley, G. F., Beckwitt, H. J., Reeves, J. T., and Mitchell, R. S.: Chronic obstructive bronchopulmonary disease. II. Oxygen transport in two clinical types. Am. J. Med., 44:26, 1968.

Hogg, J. C., Macklem, P. T., and Thurlbeck, W. M.: Site and nature of airway obstruction in chronic obstructive lung disease. N. Engl. J. Med., 278:1355, 1968.

Lane, D. J., Howell, J. B. L., and Giblin, B.: Relation between airways obstruction and CO_2 tension in chronic obstructive airways disease. Br. Med. J., 3:707, 1968.

Lieberman, J.: Alpha$_1$-antitrypsin deficiency. *In* Symposium on Chronic Respiratory Disease. Med. Clin. North Am., 57:691, 1973.

Matsuba, K., and Thurlbeck, W. M.: Disease of the small airways in chronic bronchitis. Am. Rev. Respir. Dis., 107:552, 1973.

Nash, E. S., Briscoe, W. A., and Cournand, A.: The relationship between clinical and physiological findings in chronic obstructive disease of the lungs. Med. Thorac., 22:305, 1965.

Oswald, N. C., Medvie, V. C., and Waller, R. E.: Chronic bronchitis: A ten year follow up. Thorax, 22:279, 1967.

Pride, N. B., Barter, C. E., and Hugh-Jones, P.: The ventilation of bullae and the effect of their removal on thoracic gas volumes and tests of over-all pulmonary function. Am. Rev. Respir. Dis., 107:83, 1973.

Tarkoff, M. P., Kueppers, F., and Miller, W. F.: Pulmonary emphysema and alpha$_1$-antitrypsin deficiency. Am. J. Med., 45:220, 1968.

Uses and Dangers of Oxygen Therapy. Report of a Sub-Committee of the Standing Medical Advisory Committee. Edinburgh, Her Majesty's Stationery Office, 1969.

507. RESPIRATORY FAILURE AND ITS MANAGEMENT

James P. Smith

Definitions. *Respiratory insufficiency* indicates impaired ability of the lungs to eliminate carbon dioxide or to take up oxygen. The condition may be obvious at rest or may be manifested only by inability of the patient to meet increased demands of exercise. Respiratory insufficiency has progressed to *respiratory failure* when serious abnormalities of the arterial blood gases are present at rest.

Respiratory failure is characterized by an arterial carbon dioxide tension (Pa_{CO_2}) in excess of 50 mm Hg or an arterial oxygen tension (Pa_{O_2}) of 60 mm Hg or less. Normal or only slight abnormalities of the blood gases may be present until the immediate preterminal stages of widely different disorders, including neuromuscular respiratory paralysis and pure emphysema. In these and other disorders the clinical signs of respiratory insufficiency indicate treatment before the appearance of serious blood gas changes.

Etiology and Classification. The causes of respiratory failure are multiple and often coexist in the individual patient. The classification in the accompanying table identifies five groups of disorders according to the anatomic component of the breathing apparatus which has been primarily damaged. The table also separates the causes of failure based on the characteristic alteration in Pa_{CO_2} and Pa_{O_2} which they produce. *Ventilatory failure* is distinguished by carbon dioxide retention, and is always accompanied by hypoxemia, as long as air without supplemental oxygen is breathed (hypercapnic-hypoxemic respiratory failure). *Oxygenation failure* consists purely in hypoxemia with initially low Pa_{CO_2} (hypocapnic-hypoxemic respiratory failure).

Ventilatory failure is characteristic in neurologic disorders, in respiratory muscle disease, in other chest bellows conditions, and in chronic obstructive pulmonary disease.

Oxygenation failure is usual in infiltrative diseases of the lung, both diffuse and localized, in pulmonary vascular disorders, and in the extrapulmonary conditions which cause secondary respiratory failure. When extremely severe, oxygenation failure has been variously termed "shock lung," "wet lung," or "adult respiratory distress syndrome."

Pathophysiology. The essential difference between *ventilatory failure* and *oxygenation failure* is the occurrence in the former of CO_2 retention.

Hypercapnia in disorders of the central and peripheral nervous systems and the respiratory muscles is caused by simple alveolar hypoventilation and is accompanied by a necessary reduction in Pa_{O_2}, which is proportional to the increase in Pa_{CO_2} (see Ch. 491). Most commonly, *ventilatory failure* is due to chronic obstructive pulmonary disease (COPD), and the development of hypercapnia is more complex than over-all alveolar hypoventilation (West, 1971). Moreover, hypoxemia observed during ventilatory failure in COPD is much more severe than predicted from the Pa_{CO_2}. This "extra" reduction in Pa_{O_2} is caused by gross disturbances in ventilation–blood flow relationships ($\dot{V}_A/\dot{Q}$), which occur early

Causes of Respiratory Failure

I. Disorders of the central nervous system:
- A. Drug intoxication
  - Sedatives (barbiturates, glutethimide)
  - Tranquilizers (phenothiazines, meprobamate)
  - Analgesics (opiates, e.g., morphine, heroin, methadone)
  - Anesthetic gases
- B. Vascular disorders and hypoperfusion states
  - Brainstem infarction
  - Brainstem hemorrhage
  - Postcardiac arrest
  - Shock
- C. Trauma to the brainstem
  - Head injury
  - Increased intracranial pressure
- D. Infection
  - Encephalitis (viral)
  - Bulbar poliomyelitis
- E. Miscellaneous
  - Primary alveolar hypoventilation (with or without obesity)
  - Myxedema
  - Status epilepticus

II. Disorders of the peripheral nervous system and respiratory muscles:
- A. Anterior horn cell and peripheral nerve disorders
  - Guillain-Barré syndrome
  - Poliomyelitis
  - Amyotrophic lateral sclerosis
  - Other polyneuritides
- B. Myoneural junction disorders
  - Myasthenia gravis
  - Tetanus
  - Curariform drugs (succinylcholine, curare, polymyxin, Coly-Mycin, streptomycin, kanamycin)
  - Anticholinesterase drugs (insecticides, neostigmine)
- C. Muscular disorders
  - Polymyositis
  - Muscular dystrophies
  - Myotonia

III. Disorders of the chest wall and pleura:
- A. Scoliosis
  - Congenital
  - Idiopathic
  - Paralytic (postpolio)
  - Miscellaneous (post-thoracic surgery, post-tubercular, Marfan's syndrome, von Recklinghausen's disease)

These disorders produce *ventilatory failure*; hypoxemia precedes carbon dioxide retention

- B. Chest trauma
  - Flail chest
  - Multiple rib fractures
  - Post-thoracotomy
- C. Pleural disorders
  - Massive effusions
  - Tension pneumothorax
  - Massive fibrosis

IV. Intrinsic pulmonary disorders:
- A. Airway obstruction
  - Chronic obstructive pulmonary disease (chronic bronchitis, emphysema, asthma)
  - Acute obstruction (foreign body, acute epiglottitis and laryngitis, inhalation burns, noxious gases)

These disorders produce *either ventilatory or oxygenation failure;* ventilatory failure is more common

- B. Alveolar and interstitial disorders
  - Pneumonia (lobar, aspiration, interstitial)
  - The granulomatoses and fibroses
  - Pulmonary edema (left ventricular failure)
  - Lymphangitic metastases
- C. Vascular disorders
  - Embolic disease (thrombo-, fat, tumor)
  - Obliterative vasculitis (primary pulmonary hypertension, scleroderma)

V. Extrapulmonary disorders leading to pulmonary disease:
- Hepatic failure, shock, renal failure, acute pancreatitis, peritonitis, sepsis, postcardiopulmonary bypass, and post-traumatic states (extrathoracic injuries and surgery)

These disorders produce *oxygenation failure*; hypercapnia is usually a preterminal event

in chronic bronchitis and emphysema and during attacks of asthma.

The lungs in oxygenation failure are also characterized by $\dot{V}_A/\dot{Q}$ disturbances with regions of poorly or nonventilated alveoli. When perfusion continues through such areas, the issuing capillary blood has relatively high P_{CO_2} and low P_{O_2}. But by way of contrast to COPD, hyperventilation of the relatively large volume of alveoli remaining normal in the disorders causing *oxygenation failure* is sufficient to offset the increment of P_{CO_2}. However, the amount of oxygen which is added by hyperventilation to hemoglobin already normally saturated is limited by the shape of the oxyhemoglobin dissociation curve (see accompanying figure). This is never sufficient to counter the contribution of deoxygenated blood to the arterialized stream; thus low Pa_{O_2} results. Equally or perhaps more important in the genesis of hypoxemia in cases of very *severe oxygenation failure* (shock lung, wet lung, adult respiratory distress syndrome) is the impediment to oxygen diffusion which results from invasion of the interstitium by edema, inflammatory cells, fibrosis, granuloma, or tumor cells. Yet even in these cases with extreme hypoxemia, hyperventilation, sustained by hypoxic stimulation of the peripheral chemoreceptors and by stimulation of the respiratory centers via stretch receptors in the alveoli and chest wall, maintains normal or low Pa_{CO_2}.

Respiratory acidosis, acute or chronic, is typical of *ventilatory failure.* Not infrequently, however, the administration of diuretic agents to patients with *chronic ventilatory failure* without adequate chloride replacement may impose a *metabolic alkalosis.* Caution is necessary to avoid too rapid reduction of chronic hypercapnia by mechanical ventilation, especially in these circumstances, because myoclonus, seizures, coma, and dangerous cardiac arrhythmias may result. *Oxygenation failure* is characterized initially by *respiratory alkalosis.* In addition, a metabolic contribution to alkalosis may obtain from diuretic therapy, vomiting, gastric tube drainage, or multiple blood transfusions. The appearance of *metabolic acidosis* resulting from hypoxia, shock, sepsis, or renal failure is a dire and often preterminal complication of both *ventilatory* and *oxygenation* failure. The pathophysiologic bases and the clinical signs and symptoms associated with these important disturbances of acid-base equilibrium are discussed in Ch. 805. The important cardiovascular disorders, including pulmonary hypertension, cor pulmonale, and left ventricular failure, which commonly exist during respiratory failure are discussed in Ch. 546 to 550.

Clinical and Laboratory Evaluation. *Clinical Phenomena.* In respiratory failure the clinical indicators of disturbances in blood gases and pH are unreliable. Even a low order of suspicion of hypoxemia or hypercapnia

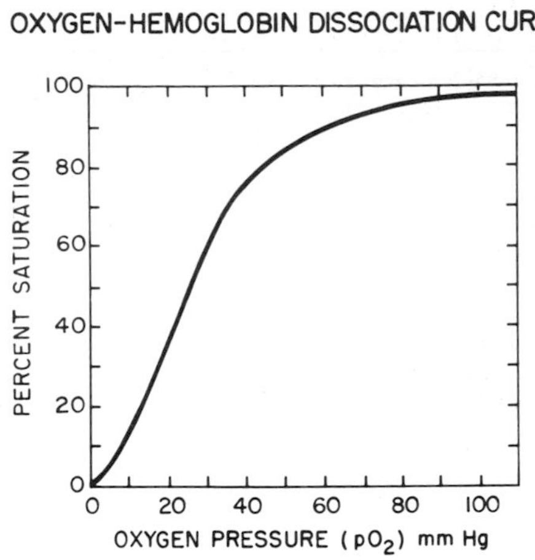

The clinical importance of a low Pa_{O_2} is determined by the reduction in arterial oxygen content it produces. Oxygen content in turn is dependent on hemoglobin concentration and the arterial oxygen saturation ($Sa_{O_2}\%$); i.e., oxygen content = grams of hemoglobin × 1.34 ml oxygen × $Sa_{O_2}\%$. Note that a decrease in Pa_{O_2} from 95 to 50 mm Hg causes only a 10 per cent decrease in Sa_{O_2} and O_2 content. However, at 50 mm Hg, a small reduction in Pa_{O_2}, as may occur with a minor decrease of alveolar ventilation, produces a sharp fall of Sa_{O_2} and content. *Arterial hypoxemia* then causes *tissue hypoxia* at some indefinite point over the steep portion of the curve and before the lethal limit of 30 per cent Sa_{O_2}. Moderate arterial oxygen unsaturation (75 to 85 per cent) is acceptable during treatment of respiratory failure, provided that tissue oxygen is adequate. The latter is generally assessed as follows: tissue oxygen = $\frac{\text{cardiac output} \times \text{arterial } O_2 \text{ content}}{\text{tissue } O_2 \text{ consumption}}$. Successful therapy of respiratory failure requires attention to all elements of this expression.

should prompt laboratory confirmation. Maximal information about the initial severity of respiratory failure is obtained if Pa_{CO_2}, Pa_{O_2} or Sa_{O_2}, and pH are measured before treatment is initiated. The inspired oxygen concentration ($F_{I_{O_2}}$), respiratory frequency (f), tidal volume (V_T) and whether breathing is spontaneous or supported by mechanical ventilation should be recorded. Often it is necessary to sample the arterial blood and to begin treatment before the history, physical examination, and other laboratory investigations are completed.

History taking should be directed at determining rapidly the nature of the disorder underlying the respiratory failure and the acute precipitating event. The precipitating event may be obvious in patients with an asthmatic attack, trauma, airway burn, or confessed drug overdose; however, concealed drug overdose, minor infection in chronic lung disease, or excessive transfusion during surgery may be detected only after meticulous questioning or search of the medical record. A history of taking narcotics, tranquilizers, or other respiratory depressants should be sought in all patients.

The level of consciousness manifested by the patient indicates the severity of failure. Mental cloudiness, apathy, headache, and depressed tendon reflexes comprise the classic "CO_2 narcosis syndrome," but diffuse myoclonus, asterixis, and papilledema may also be observed with hypercapnia. When the brain is hypoxic, irritability, insomnia, and impaired judgment usually precede delirium, convulsions, or coma. Bradypnea ($f<10$) is characteristic of central nervous system damage or depression by drugs, whereas tachypnea ($f>20$) occurs in failure from most other causes. The excursion of the chest bellows and diaphragm as evaluated by percussion and palpation gives some index of ventilatory ability. Auscultation of the neck and chest can detect obstruction of the upper airway, pneumothorax, pleural rub or effusion, or rales and wheezes in the lower airways. In chronic obstructive pulmonary disease wheezes may not be heard because of diminished airflow until the patient is directed to increase his depth and rate of breathing. This maneuver is also useful in other causes of *ventilatory failure,* because an increase in breath sounds suggests that alveolar ventilation might be improved by continued verbal or tactile stimulation without resorting to immediate mechanical ventilation. Rales and rhonchi are produced by bronchopulmonary infection in patients with *ventilatory failure* and by pulmonary edema causing *oxygenation failure.* These conditions must be differentiated, because treatment with high concentrations of oxygen and morphine is appropriate in some cases of pulmonary edema, but it may be lethal in hypercapnic subjects.

Examinations of the cardiovascular system may demonstrate systolic hypertension, flushed skin, and warm extremities which suggest the presence of hypercapnia, whereas hypotension implies severe acidemia, marked hypoxia, or a nonpulmonary disorder such as sepsis, hemorrhage, or low cardiac output. Cyanosis appears with reduction of peripheral blood flow and as a late sign of arterial hypoxemia, not appreciated by most observers until Sa_{O_2} is less than 75 per cent.

Laboratory Evaluation. Minimal laboratory survey of patients with acute respiratory failure includes complete blood count, urinalysis, measurement of blood urea nitrogen or serum creatinine and serum electrolytes, electrocardiogram, chest x-ray, vital capacity (VC), some measure of air flow, i.e., one-second forced expiratory volume (FEV_1), or peak expiratory flow rate (PEFR), and determinations of arterial blood gases. The hemoglobin determination may identify anemia and the potential for increase of blood oxygen content by transfusion, or it may reveal erythrocytosis secondary to chronic hypoxemia. If polycythemia is severe (HCT $>$ 60 per cent), therapeutic phlebotomy is warranted once oxygenation is adequate. The leukocyte count varies among the disorders causing failure, but it is usually normal during bronchial infection in patients with chronic obstructive pulmonary disease. A normal urinalysis and a normal serum creatinine exclude a renal contribution to acidosis. The importance of chloride and potassium levels has been discussed previously. The *electrocardiogram* during respiratory failure may be normal, or it may identify cardiac arrhythmia, right or left ventricular hypertrophy, or myocardial infarction. The chest roentgenogram can identify the presence of pneumonia, pleural effusion, pneumothorax, atelectasis, fibrosis, and pulmonary edema. The chest film is usually normal in neuromuscular disorders and is frequently normal or unchanged during acute ventilatory failure in patients with asthma or chronic bronchitis. Bedside measurements of vital capacity and FEV_1 or PEFR are useful in quantitating the extent of ventilatory impairment and changes with treatment. Decrease of FEV_1/VC per cent or PEFR suggests obstruction caused by chronic bronchitis, emphysema, or asthma. A reduced vital capacity without airway obstruction indicates a restrictive ventilatory defect caused by neuromuscular disease, diffuse pulmonary infiltration, massive pleural effusion, or other causes. Additional laboratory studies are selected according to the underlying cause and precipitating event of failure. Gram stain and culture of the sputum are indicated in all patients suspected of having a pulmonary infection. Monitoring of central venous pressure is a useful guide when correcting disturbances of fluid balance. A flow-directed pulmonary cardiac catheter can be used to monitor pulmonary artery pressure and pulmonary "wedge" pressure when it is considered necessary to assess pulmonary vascular dynamics and left ventricular performance.

TREATMENT OF ACUTE RESPIRATORY FAILURE

General Approach

Acute respiratory failure is prevented by identifying patients at risk, promptly starting ambulatory treatment, and immediately hospitalizing patients with respiratory insufficiency. This medical emergency is best managed in a respiratory intensive care facility. Such units, when staffed by specially trained physicians and nurses, permit close patient monitoring and the appropriate use of the many therapeutic modalities now available.

Immediate life-saving measures, such as establishing a patent airway and ensuring adequate ventilation and oxygenation, often must be implemented before the cause or the severity of the physiologic derangements is known in detail.

The upper airway is cleared by suctioning or manual removal of debris and secretions from the nose and mouth. Tactile and verbal stimulation of somnolent patients is employed to achieve a more wakeful state and to induce cough for clearing the lower airway. In patients with impairment of swallowing or severe obtundation, an oropharyngeal airway should be installed to facilitate suctioning and to prevent obstruction by the tongue. *Immediate endotracheal intubation* is indicated when the oropharyngeal airway appears inadequate or when the patient is comatose. An oral or nasal endotracheal tube with an inflatable cuff provides ready access for suctioning, prevents aspiration, and secures a reliable airway for mechanical ventilation if required. The cuff is pretested for leak and maintained in the inflated state to prevent aspiration of upper airway secretions. Periodic deflations for five minutes every two hours and use of minimal inflation pressure reduce injury to the tracheal mucosa. Meticulous attention to sterile techniques minimizes the risk of introducing bronchopulmonary infection when the airway is suctioned. With proper care, an endotracheal tube can be kept in place without being changed for several days.

Emergency tracheostomy is performed for obstruction of the airway at or above the level of the larynx (e.g. maxillofacial injury, laryngeal edema, foreign body), whereas in all other conditions it is deferred until the later care of respiratory failure. *Elective tracheostomy,* performed over the cuffed endotracheal tube in the operating room or intensive care unit with oxygenation and ventilation assured, is indicated when secretions are unmanageable or when mechanical ventilation is required for longer than one week.

Artificial ventilation is necessary in patients with apnea or obviously inadequate minute ventilation. This is accomplished by mouth-to-mouth breathing or a self-inflating bag-mask combination while the need for a mechanical respirator is assessed. A respirator is required for patients who remain apneic or fail to increase minute ventilation after several minutes of emergency ventilation. Other indications for mechanical ventilation vary greatly according to the disorder causing failure; these are considered below. Once the decision to employ a respirator is made, endotracheal intubation is required. *Attempts to provide prolonged mechanical ventilation by a face mask are ineffective and hazardous.* Essential features of any mechanical respirator include (1) reliable delivery of a preselected tidal volume despite changes in the patient's airway resistance and pulmonary compliance; (2) accurate control of the inspired oxygen concentration over the full range of 21 to 100 per cent; (3) efficient humidification; and (4) effective safeguards to prevent bacterial contamination. Other desirable features include the ability of the machine to provide periodic large tidal volumes ("sighs"), positive end-expiratory pressure, in-line nebulization of medication, and the "assist" and "controlled" modes of breathing. In the "assist" mode, inspiration is initiated by the patient and tidal volume is supplemented by the respirator. With "controlled" ventilation, both rate and depth are imposed by the apparatus; this mode of ventilation is preferred because it eliminates the patient's respiratory work and establishes adequate inspiratory time for delivery of the tidal volume. A machine setting of 12 to 20 cycles per minute and an inspiratory-to-expiratory-time ratio of 1:2 or 1:3 are acceptable for most adults. A longer time for expiration minimizes the increase in intrathoracic pressure and consequent decrease of venous return and cardiac output. Tidal volume settings and the inflation pressures required for their delivery should be varied according to the size of the patient and the specific disorder causing respiratory failure.

Oxygen is indicated whenever hypoxia is suspected, and this therapy should be started before arterial blood gas results are available. The initial oxygen concentration should be selected according to the cause of the failure.

When chronic obstructive pulmonary disease is likely and the patient is not in coma, 24 to 28 per cent oxygen is used to achieve adequate arterial saturation without inducing underventilation from complete loss of hypoxic ventilatory drive. Controlled low-dose oxygen is also suitable for immediate treatment of conscious patients with other causes of *ventilatory failure* and chronic hypercapnia, e.g., scoliosis and the primary hypoventilation syndromes. Although not all patients with chronic hypercapnia demonstrate reduction of ventilation with oxygen administration, those at risk cannot be readily identified. It is therefore safest to initiate treatment with an FI_{O_2} of 24 per cent, increasing to 28 to 35 per cent if there is failure to promptly achieve an Sa_{O_2} of 75 to 85 per cent. When *ventilatory failure* is associated with coma or one of the other indications for mechanical ventilation listed above, oxygen is delivered by the respirator and poses no threat of underventilation at any FI_{O_2}.

In conscious patients suspected of having *oxygenation failure,* an initial oxygen dosage of 30 to 40 per cent is appropriate. These concentrations are approximated by nasal cannulas with oxygen flow rates of 4 to 6 liters per minute, but more closely by Venturi-type masks. A much higher FI_{O_2} may be necessary in the treatment of severe *oxygenation failure;* concentrations between 40 and 100 per cent can be provided by several available bag-mask appliances with a nonrebreathing reservoir. Oxygen toxicity of the lung which is both dose- and time-related is a complication of prolonged therapy with FI_{O_2} above 40 per cent.

Neurologic Disorders

Drug overdose is the most important central nervous system cause of *ventilatory failure.* When respiratory depression by opiates (heroin, methadone, morphine) is suspected, a specific pharmacologic antagonist (naloxone HCl, 0.4 mg intravenously) is administered immediately and repeated at two- to three-minute intervals two or three times if necessary. With other drug intoxications (e.g., barbiturates), the nonspecific analeptic respiratory stimulants (e.g., nikethamide) have limited value, and serious side effects, especially seizure, may accompany their use.

Techniques for the care of the airway and the indications for endotracheal intubation in drug-induced and other neuromuscular causes of *ventilatory failure* are discussed above. In addition, the subject of abnormalities in the neurologic control of respiration is considered in Ch. 492.

In both neurologic and respiratory muscle disease, changes in the arterial blood gases are late and insensitive indications of impending ventilatory disaster. The time to institute mechanical ventilation, except in the obvious instance of apnea or grossly inadequate minute ventilation, is identified by changes in physical signs and vital capacity. Commonly the earliest signs of ventilatory insufficiency appear during sleep when Pa_{CO_2} rises and when the conscious effort to breathe, which may be a critically important ventilatory drive in neuromuscular disease, is eliminated. Rapid shallow breathing, the depth of which cannot be augmented on command, characterizes peripheral nervous system and respiratory muscle impairment. Dyspnea is usually prominent, and the patient frequently complains of air hunger before significant changes in minute ventilation occur. Total ventilation is maintained by the rapid rate, but dead space ventilation is favored. When the patient is exhausted, rapidly progressive hypoventilation supervenes. This sequence is prevented by serial measurements of vital capacity as a progressive decrease of VC long precedes the development of hypercapnia. Preparations for mechanical ventilation should be made when VC is less than one half of predicted, and use of a respirator should be considered when VC is one third of the predicted value. If alveolar hypoventilation and hypoxemia of a degree requiring therapy ($Sa_{O_2} < 75$ to 85 per cent) are demonstrated in acutely progressive neuromuscular disease, the patient has already been too long without mechanical support of ventilation.

Since the distribution of ventilation, airway resistance, and lung compliance are generally normal in patients with neurologic or respiratory muscle disease, the minute ventilation required from a mechanical respirator is predictable from conventional nomograms. Similarly, because ventilation/perfusion relationships and diffusion capacity are also typically normal, unless pneumonia or aspiration has occurred, an FI_{O_2} of 25 to 30 per cent is usually sufficient to maintain Pa_{O_2} and Sa_{O_2} at normal values. An important and common exception to these modest ventilatory and oxygenation requirements, however, is *heroin or methadone pulmonary edema.* Typically, the patient is in coma with pinpoint pupils, deep cyanosis, apnea or bradypnea, and hypotension. Pink, foamy edema fluid is present in the mouth, airway, and lungs, causing reduced lung volume, severe ventilation/perfusion disturbances, and abnormalities of diffusion. Acute hypercapnia, profound hypoxemia, and combined respiratory and metabolic acidosis result. Successful therapy requires endotracheal intubation, immediate mechanical ventilation with large tidal volumes, and minute ventilation of three or more times that predicted. Initially, an inspired oxygen concentration of 60 to 100 per cent is necessary to achieve adequate Sa_{O_2}; the oxygen concentration is lowered as rapidly as possible to avoid oxygen toxicity. Sodium bicarbonate may be required to correct the metabolic component of the acidosis, and rapidly acting diuretics may facilitate clearance of the edema. Temporary support of blood pressure with vasopressor agents may occasionally be necessary, but hypotension, shock, and the other clinical features of this dramatic syndrome are most effectively reversed by correction of the hypoxia and acidemia.

Chronic Obstructive Pulmonary Disease

Acute ventilatory failure in chronic obstructive pulmonary disease often develops insidiously, and consciousness remains relatively well preserved. Common precipitating events include bronchopulmonary infection, congestive heart failure, and injudicious administration of high-dose oxygen, sedatives, or tranquilizers to hypercapnic subjects.

Treatment of acute failure is guided by the patient's level of consciousness rather than the arterial blood gas values. Conscious patients should receive (1) controlled low dose oxygen, (2) intensive nursing care, and (3) general supportive measures without mechanical ventilation.

The objective of controlled low dose oxygen is prompt restoration of Sa_{O_2} to 75 to 85 per cent. This is achieved in the majority of patients with 24 per cent FI_{O_2}; increasing to 28 or 35 per cent only as necessary minimizes the risk of oxygen-induced depression of ventilation. The appropriate Venturi-type mask is the most reliable device for delivering oxygen in this low range; nasal cannulas at low flow rates with close monitoring of the blood gases are preferred by some physicians. When adequate Sa_{O_2} is established, time becomes available for intensive nursing care and general supportive measures to reverse the disturbances that led to acute failure.

Intensive nursing care is both one of the most important facets of treatment and the most difficult to ensure. During early treatment, techniques to reduce airway obstruction and improve the patient's level of consciousness are performed by a specially trained nurse assigned to the bedside. Secretions are often cleared by demanding the patient to cough and to breathe deeply and by striking the chest with a flat hand. The nurse also assists the patient with nebulizers that deliver bronchodilator aerosols, and she suctions the lower airway in precomatose patients. Verbal and tactile stimulation may be constantly required to increase alertness and ventilatory effort in the initial hours of care. Later, the patient is permitted to sleep for periods to avoid exhaustion and further hypercapnia.

Antimicrobials, bronchodilator drugs, diuretics, digitalis, and electrolyte preparations are administered to combat infection, reverse airway obstruction, improve heart failure, and correct metabolic disturbances. Bronchopulmonary infection is assumed to be present during *acute ventilatory failure* secondary to chronic obstructive pulmonary disease. In the absence of specific pneumonia and if the usual mixed bacterial floras are present in the sputum, treatment is begun with ampicillin or tetracycline. Bronchodilator drugs should also be tried in most patients. Aerosols of these drugs should be delivered by nebulizers that require minimal patient effort. For this purpose, conventional intermittent positive pressure breathing (IPPB) machines designed as respirators are best avoided, because they often produce fatigue and have not been demonstrated to be more effective than simple devices which employ a fluidic principle or other means to generate an aerosol. Solutions of 0.3 to 0.5 ml of 1:200 isoproterenol, or 0.5 ml of a mixture of isoetharine and phenylephrine diluted with 2 to 3 ml of saline may be given every two to six hours. Careful monitoring and caution in the use of these drugs are required to avoid cardiac arrhythmias. Orally or parenterally administered bronchodilators may be used in addition to aerosols. Of the xanthine derivatives, aminophylline by intravenous infusion or rectal suppository (250 to 500 mg every four to six hours), is most effective during severe failure. During convalescence, oral preparations of aminophylline alone or in combination with ephedrine sulfate may be useful.

Corticosteroids, unless specifically contraindicated, are used in all cases of asthma producing *ventilatory failure*. The equivalent of 60 to 80 mg of prednisone daily in divided doses is usually adequate in nonsteroid-dependent asthmatics, but much higher doses (to 1000 mg per day) have been recommended for patients already receiving these drugs. In chronic bronchitis and emphysema, corticosteroids are reserved for patients with intractable wheezing or those in whom the sympathomimetic effects of the other bronchodilator agents are not acceptable. An effective diuretic (furosemide, 40 to 120 mg intravenously) is indicated whenever edema is present. The value of a diuretic in patients without overt edema or signs of cor pulmonale is controversial, but its use has been recommended to eliminate occult increases in extravascular lung water and thereby to improve gas transfer.

Administration of adequate amounts of fluids facilitates clearance of tenacious secretions, but excessive parenteral fluids may precipitate or worsen cor pulmonale. It should be emphasized that patients with chronic hypercapnia and cor pulmonale who have received diuretics before the development of acute ventilatory failure are frequently depleted of potassium and chloride. Replacement of these ions, especially chloride, is recommended from the outset of therapy.

Digitalis is useful in cor pulmonale, but initiation of the drug early in *acute ventilatory failure* is hazardous and usually unnecessary. In patients who have already been given digitalis, maintenance on the drug is continued after severe hypoxemia has been relieved.

Conservative therapy with controlled low dose oxygen, intensive nursing care, and general measures is successful in most patients with *acute ventilatory failure* secondary to chronic obstructive pulmonary disease. Endotracheal intubation and mechanical ventilation are reserved for the small number of patients (10 per cent) with untreated ventilatory failure who present in coma and for those in whom conservative therapy either fails to provide adequate Sa_{O_2} or is associated with marked respiratory acidosis, shock, or coma. Endotracheal tubes are well tolerated for several days; performance of a tracheostomy is not likely to improve the outcome in patients with ventilatory failure secondary to COPD that is not corrected during respirator care for seven or more days. Mechanical ventilation is best achieved with a volume-cycled respirator operating in the "controlled" mode. Requirements for minute ventilation in this group cannot be predicted without reference to the Pa_{CO_2}, but tidal volume and rate should initially be set to deliver twice the minute ventilation needed as predicted from the patient's size. The immediate objectives of mechanical ventilation are to produce normal pH rather than normal Pa_{CO_2} and normal Sa_{O_2}. Normal Sa_{O_2} can usually be achieved with an FI_{O_2} of 35 to 40 per cent delivered by the respirator. Continuous mechanical ventilation is provided until the patient is fully conscious, the cardiovascular system is stable, and acid-base and electrolyte abnormalities are corrected. Complications of mechanical ventilation in addition to overcorrection alkalosis include gastrointestinal hemorrhage, local tracheobronchial injury from the tube or suctioning, and bronchopulmonary infection. Sedation and antacids may reduce the risks of gastrointestinal hemorrhage, and meticulous suctioning technique and cleaning of the respiratory equipment reduces the risk of injuring and contaminating the airway. Procedures for weaning patients from the respirator are not within the scope of this discussion; the general management of patients with chronic obstructive pulmonary disease and chronic hypercapnia may be found in Ch. 506.

Oxygenation Failure

The provision of adequate oxygen to the tissues without producing oxygen toxicity of the lungs is the main therapeutic goal in *oxygenation failure* (hypocapnic-hypoxemic respiratory failure). Concomitantly, other measures should be applied to reverse the underlying disorder. When hypoxemia is moderate (Pa_{O_2}: 45 to 60 mm Hg) and specific therapy is initiated early, as in bacterial pneumonia, 35 to 40 per cent FI_{O_2} (oxygen delivered by nasal cannulas, 6 liters per minute or Venturi mask) usually suffices. However, severe and progressive hypoxemia (Pa_{O_2}: 20 to 45 mm Hg), sometimes resistant to all forms of oxygen therapy, may be encountered with fulminant pneumonia and a wide variety of other clinical disorders (table). Typically with *severe oxygenation failure* ("shock lung," "wet lung," "adult respiratory distress syndrome") there are tachypnea and hyperventilation yet progressive hypoxemia despite administration of oxygen in increasing concentrations, decreased pulmonary compliance, and advancing opacification of the lungs in the chest films. Pathologically, interstitial pulmonary edema, fibrin accumulation, alveolar hemorrhage, and hyaline membrane formation are prominent. In some disorders (bacterial and viral pneumonia, hypersensitivity alveolitis, acute pancreatitis, uremia, pulmonary edema), the syndrome evolves steadily, whereas in other conditions (trauma, shock, respiratory burns, postcirculatory perfusion states) there is characteristically a latent period from the initial insult to the onset of *severe oxygenation failure.*

Preventive and early treatment measures in *severe oxygenation failure* include (1) prompt treatment of pneumonia, (2) avoidance of excessive parenteral fluid or blood transfusion, (3) early use of diuretics when an increase in extravascular lung water is suspected, (4) rapid correction of hypotension and shock, (5) use of ultrafilters during transfusion to prevent particulate matter from lodging in the pulmonary microcirculation, and (6) restriction of FI_{O_2} to 40 per cent to avoid oxygen toxicity.

The risk of lung damage notwithstanding, an FI_{O_2} as high as 100 per cent may be necessary to sustain life once *severe oxygenation failure* has developed. Many causes of this syndrome are accompanied by circulatory insufficiency, which further compromises tissue oxygenation; thus the acceptable levels of Pa_{O_2}, and Sa_{O_2} are higher than in hypoxemic states with normal circulation. The decision to increase $F_{I_{O_2}}$ above 40 per cent is made on the basis of clinical deterioration, including signs of cerebral hypoxia, with apprehension, disorientation, and poor cooperation with therapy, and blood gas measurements indicating severe and progressive hypoxemia. High-dose oxygen (50 to 100 per cent) delivered by a bag-mask with a nonrebreathing reservoir can be given to increase Pa_{O_2} and gain time for either the natural evolution of the underlying disorder or additional treatment to improve blood and tissue oxygenation. The time required for irreversible pulmonary damage to result from oxygen toxicity is unknown but is probably less than 72 hours with 100 per cent O_2. During this limited "safe" time, tissue oxygenation may be improved using one or a combination of the following measures: (1) increase of Pa_{O_2} by mobilization of pulmonary edema with a potent diuretic; (2) increase of arterial oxygen content by restoration of hemoglobin to normal levels with transfusion of red cells or whole blood; (3) increase of oxygen delivery by improving cardiac output and blood pressure (depending on the primary disorder and its complications, this may require either an increase or decrease in plasma volume or the use of vasoactive or cardioactive drugs); and (4) decrease of oxygen utilization by elimination of fever with antipyretics and hypothermia. Corticosteroids in large doses (methylprednisolone, 1.0 gram or more daily) have been recommended for this stage of *severe oxygenation failure,* but their use is controversial and may be hazardous in primarily infectious disorders.

Mechanical ventilation is indicated in *severe oxygenation failure* when the underlying cause is potentially reversible, $F_{I_{O_2}}$ has been in the toxic range but for less time than causes irreversible lung damage, and Pa_{O_2} and Sa_{O_2} remain inadequate. Commonly at this stage, consciousness is depressed and the rapid, shallow breathing no longer sustains hyperventilation as indicated by change in Pa_{CO_2} from low to a normal value. Extensive, bilateral opacification of the lungs with a mixed interstitial and alveolar pattern ("white lung") is typically seen radiographically. The appropriate time for endotracheal intubation and takeover ventilation is difficult to determine, but it should occur before the appearance of metabolic acidosis, shock, bradycardia, severe hypercapnia, or cardiac arrest. Ventilation is "controlled" (see General Approach, above) to eliminate respiratory muscle work and to improve the distribution of the inspired gas. A central respiratory depressant (morphine sulfate, 4 to 8 mg intravenously initially) or a neuromuscular blocking agent (pancuronium bromide, 0.04 to 0.1 mg per kilogram initially) may be required for intubation and subsequently to relax the patient and eliminate competition with the respirator. These agents may induce hypotension, and their use in shock is hazardous. During the initiation of mechanical ventilation and for a short period of stabilization thereafter, 100 per cent oxygen is delivered by the respirator to minimize the risk of hypoxia. Thereafter, $F_{I_{O_2}}$ is reduced as rapidly as is compatible with maintenance of satisfactory Sa_{O_2}. The application of positive end-expiratory pressure (PEEP) using 5 to 15 cm H_2O has been shown to increase Pa_{O_2} and allow reduction of $F_{I_{O_2}}$ to safe levels in patients in whom this was previously not possible. PEEP should be used cautiously, since cardiac output may fall, especially in hypovolemic patients, because of the increased mean intrathoracic pressure; despite an increase of Pa_{O_2}, oxygen delivery to the tissues is thereby worsened. Once $F_{I_{O_2}}$ is reduced to 40 per cent, the lung is no longer at risk of oxygen toxicity, and the outcome is largely determined by the response of the primary disorder.

In a small but important number of patients, despite mechanical ventilation with PEEP, no reduction below 100 per cent $F_{I_{O_2}}$ is possible. In these patients, the use of extracorporeal supplementation of oxygenation with a membrane oxygenator and pump has achieved limited success.

Filley, G. F.: Pulmonary Insufficiency and Respiratory Failure. Philadelphia, Lea & Febiger, 1967.

Moore, F. D., Lyons, J. H., Jr., Pierce, E. C., Jr., Morgan, A. P., Jr., Drinker, P. A., MacArthur, J. D., and Dammin, G. J.: Post-Traumatic Pulmonary Insufficiency. Philadelphia, W. B. Saunders Company, 1969.

Petty, T. L., and Ashbaugh, D. G.: The adult respiratory distress syndrome. Clinical features, factors influencing prognosis and principles of management. Chest, 60:233, 1971.

Smith, J. P.: Respiratory failure and its management. *In* Holman, C. W., and Muschenheim, C. (eds.): Bronchopulmonary Diseases and Related Disorders. Hagerstown, Md., Harper & Row, 1972, pp. 694-727.

Smith, J. P., Stone, R. W., and Muschenheim, C.: Acute respiratory failure in chronic lung disease: Observations on controlled oxygen therapy. Am. Rev. Respir. Dis., 97:791, 1968.

Sykes, M. K., McNicol, M. W., and Campbell, E. J. M.: Respiratory Failure. Oxford and Edinburgh, Blackwell Scientific Publications, 1969.

West, J. B.: Causes of carbon dioxide retention in lung disease. N. Engl. J. Med., 284:1232, 1971.

Williams, M. H., Jr., and Shim, C. S.: Ventilatory failure: Etiology and clinical forms. Am. J. Med., 48:477, 1970.

LOCALIZED AIRWAY OBSTRUCTION

J. B. L. Howell

508. INTRODUCTION

The causes of localized airway obstruction may be grouped as endomural, intramural, and extramural. Endomural causes include bronchial secretions and aspirated foreign bodies; intramural causes include benign and malignant neoplasms, edema, and fibrous strictures; extramural causes are mainly due to enlargement of lymph nodes and other structures which cause airway compression. The effects of obstruction vary according to its location and whether it is complete or partial.

Laryngeal Obstruction. Laryngeal obstruction may be caused by laryngeal spasm, carcinoma, partial paralyses of the vocal cords, or collapse of the cartilaginous elements of the larynx as in rheumatoid arthritis or polychondritis.

Tracheal Obstruction. Tracheal obstruction is uncommon. Foreign bodies either impact in the larynx or descend beyond the bifurcation. Tracheal carcinoma, benign cylindroma, and amyloid tumors are rare. An increasingly common cause is tracheal stricture after tracheostomy or endotracheal intubation. It occurs at the site of the cuff or lower end of the tube and, if severe, may cause marked airway obstruction both during inspiration when it is associated with stridor and during expiration when a Starling resistor mechanism may operate (see Mechanisms of Airway Obstruction in Ch. 506). Surgical excision may be required.

External compression of the trachea may occur from goiter, thymic tumors, or neoplastic lymph nodes. Such pressures initially cause an irritating nonproductive cough but may progress to severe obstruction with stridor.

Localized Bronchial Obstruction. Localized bronchial obstruction does not cause interference with resting airflow unless it is severe; it is more likely to cause infection distally by interfering with mucous flow. When obstruction is nearly complete, overdistention of the distal lung tissue (obstructive emphysema) may occur; complete obstruction results in atelectasis.

509. ATELECTASIS

Definition. Strictly, the word atelectasis means imperfect expansion, and pathologists often use the term in this sense to describe the failure of expansion of the lungs at birth. In clinical practice, it usually implies airlessness in lung which had once been normally aerated.

Etiology and Pathogenesis. Airlessness of lung tissue may arise in two ways. First, alteration in the alveolar surfactant material by increasing alveolar surface tension may permit alveoli to deflate completely, thus expelling the air through the bronchial tree. This occurs in the lungs of premature infants and contributes to the *respiratory distress syndrome of the newborn.* Damage to alveolar surfactant is believed to occur in oxygen toxicity when multiple atelectases and sometimes massive collapse may develop. Surfactant may also be reduced after severe pulmonary edema. Second, when a bronchus is occluded, e.g., by secretions, foreign body, or neoplasm, continued perfusion of the distal alveoli results in absorption of the air (absorption atelectasis). Alternatively, when the lung is permitted to relax to its minimal volume by large quantities of air or liquid in the pleural cavity, as in pneumothorax or pleural effusion, collapse of the small bronchi or bronchioles occurs. The final removal of air is again by absorption into the perfusing blood, but the atelectasis is termed "relaxation atelectasis."

Absorption of alveolar gas occurs because the total pressure of the gases in mixed venous blood is less than that in the alveoli since, in its passage through the tissues, oxygen tension falls by approximately 60 mm Hg and is replaced by a rise in carbon dioxide tension of only 4 to 6 mm Hg. The absorption of air takes a few hours because of its poorly soluble nitrogen content; if the subject has been breathing pure oxygen, absorption may be complete within a few minutes. After relaxation atelectasis, the lung tissue remains undamaged, and reinflation with normal function is said to be possible after prolonged airlessness. With obstructive atelectasis, obstruction may interfere with bronchial toilet and lead to infections, abscesses, and fibrosis.

Clinical Manifestations. Atelectasis of one or more pulmonary segments is a common complication of acute tracheobronchial infections and is diagnosed usually as a result of chest roentgenograms. The atelectatic areas usually disappear with recovery from the generalized bronchitis without any specific therapy. The sudden development of atelectasis in larger segments of lung, e.g., a lobe or even a whole lung, may cause severe symptoms of dyspnea and chest pain associated with cyanosis, and, if very large, with sweating and peripheral circulatory failure. This is common in the postoperative period, especially with upper abdominal operations. A similar picture may be seen with foreign body inhalation. Over a period of a few hours, the symptoms often subside as the circulation through the atelectatic area is reduced. Lobar or segmental atelectasis resulting from bronchial neoplasm is often symptomless presumably because of its slow evolution. Segmental or lobar atelectasis may occur in patients with mild asthma, and is attributed to obstruction by secretions; however, atelectasis is an uncommon finding at autopsy in status asthmaticus. Atelectasis may also be a component of pulmonary infarction resulting from embolism. Plate atelectases have been described in drug addicts who administer their drugs intravenously.

Physical signs depend upon the size of the atelectatic area. If large enough, chest movement and tactile fremitus are diminished, the mediastinum is deviated toward the affected side, the percussion note is impaired, and breath sounds are characteristically absent. Atelectasis is confirmed by roentgenography, but unless the cause is obvious, bronchoscopy is indicated. Aspiration of occluding material may occasionally be possible through the bronchoscope.

Treatment. Treatment of atelectasis is directed at the underlying cause. For conditions requiring medical treatment, antimicrobial drugs and chest physiotherapy are given. Specific therapy of the atelectasis is seldom indicated, most conditions resolving spontaneously. When associated with bronchiectasis, the treatment is the same as for bronchiectasis. In relaxation atelectasis, removal of fluid from the pleural cavity usually causes re-expansion, often associated with transient precordial pain and violent coughing.

Lemoine, J. M.: L'atelectasie pulmonaire. Étude critique. Bronches, 17:109, 1967.

510. RIGHT MIDDLE LOBE SYNDROME

The right middle lobe bronchus is especially prone to involvement during primary tuberculosis because its origin is surrounded by a ring of lymph nodes draining both the middle and lower lobes of the right lung. Enlargement of these nodes readily compresses the narrow bronchus, causing atelectasis; extension of the infection into the bronchial wall leads to subsequent stricture with the eventual development of bronchiectatic changes distally. In later life, these changes may lead to recurrent infection, and the combination of recurrent pneumonic illness, hemoptysis, and right middle lobe atelectasis has been given the name of right middle lobe syndrome.

However, post-tuberculous bronchostenosis is only one of the causes of this syndrome. Other causes include chronic suppuration, foreign body, and bronchial neoplasm. Full investigation including bronchoscopy is essential; if the cause remains uncertain, thoracotomy should be considered.

Albo, R. J., and Grimes, O. F.: The middle lobe syndrome: A clinical study. Dis. Chest, 50:509, 1966.
Brock, R. C., Cann, R. J., and Dickinson, J. R.: Tuberculous mediastinal lymphadenitis in childhood. Guy's Hosp. Rep., 87:295, 1937.
Clements, J. A., and Tierney, D. F.: Alveolar instability associated with altered surface tension. *In* Handbook of Physiology, Section 3: Respiration. Baltimore, Williams & Wilkins Company, 1965, p. 1565.
Graham, E. A., Burford, T. H., and Mayer, J. H.: Middle lobe syndrome. Postgrad. Med., 4:29, 1948.
Hinshaw, H. C.: Diseases of the Chest. 3rd ed. Philadelphia, W. B. Saunders Company, 1969, pp. 241 et seq.
Hutcheson, S., and Guerrant, J. L.: Atelectasis in asthma. A report of five cases and a review of the literature. Va. Med. Mon., 94:629, 1967.
Lindskog, G. E., and Spear, H. C.: Middle lobe syndrome. N. Engl. J. Med., 253:489, 1955.
Rahn, H.: The role of N_2 gas in various biological processes with particular reference to the lung. Harvey Lectures Series, 55:173, 1959–1960.

Section Five. ABNORMAL AIR SPACES

Richard V. Ebert

511. GIANT BULLOUS EMPHYSEMA (Vanishing Lung)

Lungs examined at autopsy frequently contain small blebs or bullae. These are most commonly found in older men. Bullae are air-containing structures resembling cysts but with a wall which is trabeculated and not lined with epithelium. The lesion is derived from the terminal air spaces of the lung, and the trabeculae represent remnants of the blood vessels and fibrous tissue of the lung. Similar lesions occurring just beneath the visceral pleura are called blebs. Occasionally these lesions may be of great size and give rise to a characteristic appearance on the chest roentgenogram. These giant bullae may or may not be associated with generalized emphysema of the lung.

Large solitary bullae are occasionally observed. The lesion is usually not associated with symptoms and pulmonary function studies may reveal no abnormality. If the bulla becomes huge, it may produce dyspnea and impair pulmonary function. The term "anepithelial air cyst" has been used to describe these lesions.

More commonly, multiple large bullae are found. These may be confined to one lobe or to one lung, or they may involve both lungs. They usually occur in the upper lobes. The lesions are commonly seen in relatively young persons, being found in approximately 1 in 1000 routine roentgenograms of the chest. The patient may be asymptomatic. If the lesions are large or if there is associated generalized emphysema, the patients may complain of exertional dyspnea. Physical examination may reveal increased resonance to percussion and diminished breath sounds over the involved area. Pneumothorax is a common complication. The bullae rarely become infected or filled with fluid. On the chest roentgenogram the area involved is devoid of lung markings. The wall of the lesion is extremely thin and may not be visible. This has given rise to the term *vanishing lung*. The roentgenographic appearance can be easily confused with a pneumothorax. Pulmonary function studies are variable because the lesions may be either well ventilated or poorly ventilated and because there may be generalized emphysema that is not visible on the roentgenogram. There may or may not be adequate expansion of the remaining normal lung. If the lesions are not accompanied by diffuse pulmonary emphysema, the usual findings are a relatively normal vital capacity, a considerable increase in functional residual capacity, a normal or only slightly impaired maximal breathing capacity and rate of expiratory air flow, and normal blood gases. With very large bullous lesions there may be more severe impairment of pulmonary function. Finally, some patients present the typical clinical picture of chronic obstructive lung disease, and in addition demonstrate giant bullous lesions on roentgenography.

The therapy of giant bullae is surgical excision, but there is little reason to remove these lesions if the patient is asymptomatic. Occasionally, repeated pneumothorax may be an indication for surgery. A difficult problem is presented by those patients who are symptomatic. The dyspnea may be related to diffuse pulmonary emphysema rather than to the bullae. In this case removal of the bullae will be of little or no benefit. In certain patients, however, the bullae may be important in the production of symptoms. This occurs if the bullae interfere with the function of the remaining normal lung. If the bullae reach sufficient size to occupy much of the thorax, the intrathoracic pressure may not be sufficiently negative to expand the remaining lung. The normal portion of the lung may be partially atelectatic and poorly ventilated. Removal of the bullae may lead to significant improvement. Careful evaluation of the chest x-ray and of pulmonary function is necessary for a proper decision as to the need for surgery.

Boushy, S. F., Kohen, R., Billig, D. M., and Heiman, M. J.: Bullous emphysema. Clinical, roentgenologic and physiologic study of 49 patients. Dis. Chest, 54:327, 1968.
Pride, N. B., Barter, C. E., and Hugh-Jones, P.: The ventilation of bullae and the effect of their removal on thoracic gas volumes and tests of over-all pulmonary function. Am. Rev. Respir. Dis., 107:83, 1973.

512. LUNG CYSTS

The classification of lung cysts is somewhat confusing, since any air-containing structure in the lung can enlarge and form a cyst or cavity. There is tension on the wall of all air-containing structures in the lung because the pressure within fluctuates about atmospheric pressure, whereas the intrathoracic pressure is negative. If there is obstruction to the egress of air from a cyst or cavity, the pressure within may be considerably in excess of atmospheric pressure. The tension on the wall of a sphere such as a lung cyst is proportional to both the pressure difference across the wall and to the radius of curvature. For this reason a thin-walled cyst or cavity in the lung tends to continue to enlarge.

Thin-walled cavities may form in the lung as a result of destruction of lung substance and formation of a communication with a bronchus. Such cavities may be seen in pulmonary tuberculosis, the pulmonary mycoses, and lung abscess. These are called cavities and not cysts, but their appearance on the roentgenogram may be similar to that of lung cysts. Cystlike lesions can also form in bronchiectasis.

Belcher, J. R., and Siddons, A. H. M.: Air-containing cysts of the lung. Thorax, 9:38, 1954.

513. BRONCHOGENIC CYSTS

These cysts arise from the bronchi, as indicated by the name. It is thought that in most instances they are caused by a congenital defect. The cyst is lined with epithelial cells. The wall of the cyst may contain glands, smooth muscle, and cartilage. The cysts may be located in the lungs or mediastinum.

The patient with a bronchogenic cyst may be asymptomatic. Symptoms are usually the result of secondary infection and consist of a productive cough, hemoptysis, and fever. The roentgenographic appearance is variable. The cyst may contain only air or may be filled with fluid. In the latter case the cyst may be confused with a solid tumor of the lung. The cyst may have an air-fluid level, in which case it is often mistaken for a lung abscess. The treatment of symptomatic lung cysts is surgical removal.

Congenital cysts in the lower lobe of the lung may be associated with an anomalous artery arising from the aorta near the diaphragm. This complex developmental abnormality is called *intralobar bronchopulmonary sequestration.* A knowledge of this abnormality is of some importance because the artery may be inadvertently cut during surgery, with serious hemorrhage.

514. HONEYCOMB LUNG

Honeycomb lung describes a pathologic state in which the lung contains many small cystic structures that are several millimeters in diameter. These cysts are derived from the bronchioles and are lined by epithelium. Fibrous tissue and smooth muscle are found about the cysts. Honeycomb lung has been described in association with eosinophilic granuloma, rheumatoid lung disease, and idiopathic interstitial pulmonary fibrosis. It occurs in association with advanced fibrosis and represents the end stage of the disease. A similar pathologic lesion may be found in association with tuberous sclerosis.

The major symptom is dyspnea. Spontaneous pneumothorax is a common complication. The chest roentgenogram reveals a fine or coarse reticular appearance. Small rounded translucencies may be seen.

Heppleston, A. G.: The pathology of honeycomb lung. Thorax, 11:77, 1956.

515. ACQUIRED CYSTS

As mentioned above, any air-containing structure in the lung can enlarge and form a cyst or cavity. Lung abscess as a cause of such cavities is discussed immediately below. The other necrotizing lung diseases are considered in Ch. 178 to 183, Ch. 211, and Ch. 227.

516. LUNG ABSCESS

Definition. Lung abscess is a suppurative infection of the lung resulting in destruction of lung parenchyma with the formation of a cavity containing fluid and air.

Etiology. *Aspiration of infectious material* into the lung is the most common cause of lung abscess (primary lung abscess). A history of an episode of stupor or unconsciousness is often obtained. This is most commonly the result of excessive drinking. Careful inquiry will reveal that a high proportion of persons with lung abscess are chronic alcoholics. Other causes of unconsciousness predisposing to aspiration lung abscess are convulsive seizures, anesthesia, diabetic coma, ingestion of large amounts of sedatives, and various neurologic lesions. The infected material aspirated is usually from the mouth. Most people with lung abscess will be found to have periodontal disease with accumulation of infected materials about the teeth and gums. Lung abscess is rare in an edentulous person. Aspiration of infected materials during surgery on the oral cavity or tonsils was common at one time, but is rare now because of improvements in anesthetic techniques. Aspiration is common in cancer involving the upper respiratory passages or esophagus.

As might be anticipated, the pus from a primary lung abscess contains a mixture of bacteria. Cultures performed on material aspirated from an abscess cavity prior to the use of antimicrobial drugs may demonstrate gamma streptococci, diphtheroids, and a variety of anaerobic organisms.

Pneumonia caused by *Staphylococcus aureus* or Klebsiella may be complicated by abscess formation. Primary pneumococcal pneumonia is rarely associated with abscess formation. Treatment of patients with therapeutic agents which interfere with the normal body defenses, such as high doses of corticosteroids or the chemotherapy for cancer, predisposes to necrotizing pneumonia with abscess formation. In many hospitals lung abscesses occur almost exclusively in patients with terminal cancer.

Bronchial obstruction may lead to a lung abscess. The obstructing lesion is most commonly a bronchogenic carcinoma but may be a foreign body or an enlarged lymph node causing compression of a bronchus.

Metastatic lung abscess may result from septic emboli

secondary to right-sided bacterial endocarditis or pelvic thrombophlebitis. Lung abscess may occur in association with septicemia.

Rare causes of lung abscess include amebic abscess of the lung, melioidosis, glanders, actinomycosis, and nocardiosis.

Incidence and Prevalence. The exact incidence of lung abscess has not been determined. Recent reports indicate that five to ten instances of primary lung abscess are seen each year in a large general hospital. The disease was more common prior to the introduction of antimicrobial drugs. Lung abscess occurs as a terminal event in a variety of illnesses.

Pathogenesis. The sequence of events to be described is thought to be the mechanism of formation of lung abscess in those cases in which aspiration of infected material is the initiating agent. Although this mechanism of abscess function cannot be proved in every case, there is a large body of circumstantial evidence in its support.

When infected material is aspirated into the tracheobronchial tree, it lodges in a small bronchus in the dependent portion of the lung. As aspiration usually occurs in the supine position, the posterior segment of the upper lobe and the superior segment of the lower lobe are most commonly involved. Pneumonia develops in the surrounding tissue. The critical event is the formation of a cavity. This occurs as a result of necrosis and liquefaction of the pneumonic lung. The cavity is created when this liquid is discharged into the bronchus. For the lung parenchyma to be disrupted the collagen and elastic framework of the lung must be destroyed. The frequent finding of fragments of elastic tissue in the sputum is evidence of this destruction. The exact means by which liquefaction necrosis occurs is not known. It has been suggested that thrombosis of small vessels leads to ischemia of the pneumonic area. The liquefaction and destruction of the connective tissue framework of the lung must result from the liberation of proteolytic enzymes.

Clinical Manifestations. Patients with primary lung abscess often give a characteristic history. The illness begins with fever, sweats, malaise, loss of appetite, and loss of weight. After a few days or weeks a productive cough develops. The amount of sputum increases until several hundred milliliters is produced daily. The patient and his associates may note a foul odor to the sputum. Some patients give a history of suddenly coughing up large amounts of foul sputum. Hemoptysis occurs in about 40 per cent of the cases. Pleuritic chest pain may occur. In some cases the characteristic abundant foul sputum may be absent. This is most commonly seen in patients receiving antimicrobial drugs. Careful questioning of both the patient and his relatives may elicit a history of a period of unconsciousness or of excessive use of alcohol. When lung abscess complicates pneumonia caused by Staphylococcus or Klebsiella, the symptoms are those of a severe pneumonia. Abscess formation is detected on the chest roentgenogram.

The patient with lung abscess usually appears acutely ill and is febrile. Periodontal disease is often present, and infected material may be seen about the teeth and gums. Examination of the lung most commonly shows fine or medium moist rales over the involved area. Dullness and change in breath sounds may or may not be detected. Clubbing of the fingers is seen in about one fourth of the patients.

In primary lung abscess the sputum is usually copious, forms several layers on standing, and has a putrid odor. Occasionally the sputum is scanty or absent. Culture of the sputum will reveal the specific organism if the abscess is caused by Staphylococcus or Klebsiella. In lung abscess resulting from aspiration, a mixed flora is found. In patients receiving penicillin a variety of gram-negative organisms may be cultured. The important anaerobic organisms described earlier are not cultured by the routine methods used in most clinical laboratories.

The diagnosis of lung abscess is usually made on roentgenography. A cavity containing fluid surrounded by alveolar infiltrate is found. A fluid level in the cavity can usually be demonstrated and can be confirmed by roentgenograms taken in different body positions. Approximately one third of the abscesses related to aspiration are found in the posterior segment of the right upper lobe. Other common locations are the superior segments of the right and left lower lobes and the posterior segment of the left upper lobe. With treatment the surrounding pneumonic infiltrate may rapidly disappear and fluid may no longer be seen if good drainage is obtained. Ultimately a thin-walled cavity is left. In most cases this will eventually disappear.

Complications. Empyema with or without bronchopleural fistula may complicate lung abscess. This usually occurs in the neglected cases, and rarely is seen once antimicrobial therapy has been started. If therapy of lung abscess is begun weeks or months after the onset of the disease, complete healing may not occur, and a residual thick-wall cavity remains. Scarring may be associated with local bronchiectasis. Recurrent infection may occur and lead to prolonged disability. Other complications are rare. Brain abscess and amyloidosis are almost never seen with present methods of therapy.

Diagnosis. The tentative diagnosis is made from the appearance of the chest roentgenogram, and particularly from the presence of a cavity with an air-fluid level. Differentiation from other diseases simulating lung abscess is made by analysis of the history, examination of the sputum, and careful study of serial roentgenograms after initiation of therapy.

The most common mistake in diagnosis is the confusion of bronchogenic carcinoma and primary lung abscess. Bronchogenic carcinoma can simulate lung abscess in two ways. A true lung abscess can develop peripheral to the obstructed bronchus, or a large tumor can undergo necrosis and cavitate. The latter event usually occurs with a squamous cell bronchogenic carcinoma but may occur with metastatic carcinoma. The diagnosis of an obstructing carcinoma can usually be made by bronchoscopy. Diagnosis of a peripheral cavitating carcinoma is difficult, and bronchoscopy is usually of no aid. The diagnosis may be suspected if the predisposing factors to an aspiration abscess are absent, if the sputum is not foul, if the location of the abscess is in the anterior portion of the lung, if the wall of the abscess is irregular, and if there is failure to respond to therapy. Examination of the sputum for neoplastic cells may be helpful. The diagnosis can be established in selected cases by the introduction under fluoroscopic control of a specially designed bronchial brush into the cavity. Tissue for histologic examination and culture can be obtained.

The differentiation of lung abscess from pulmonary tuberculosis is less difficult. Tuberculosis has a more insidious onset and less systemic symptoms. The sputum is not foul. The cavity usually does not contain a fluid level. Examination of the sputum for tubercle bacilli by microscopy and culture should always be done and will establish the diagnosis. Cavitating fungal infection of the lungs, such as histoplasmosis or coccidioidomycosis, can usually be distinguished from lung abscess without difficulty.

An infected lung cyst may simulate a primary lung abscess. Differentiation may be made by a careful history and by the lack of severe systemic symptoms or foul sputum. The wall of the cavity as seen by x-ray is thin and not surrounded by an area of pneumonitis. Previous films may show an air-containing cyst. Occasionally a bulbous lesion containing fluid may be seen in an area of resolving pneumonia and may be mistaken for a lung abscess.

Other lesions occasionally simulate lung abscess. At times an uninfected infarct of the lung will cavitate. Cystic bronchiectasis may be confused with lung abscess. There is a history of long-standing chronic cough, and the cavities are usually multiple and basal in location. Echinococcus cyst of the lung is extremely rare in the United States. Rheumatoid nodules and the lesions of Wegener's granulomatosis may cavitate, but are readily differentiated from lung abscess.

Treatment. The cornerstone of therapy in lung abscess is the administration of the appropriate antimicrobial drug in adequate dosage for a sufficiently long period. In abscesses complicating pneumonia caused by Staphylococcus or Klebsiella, the drug should be chosen on the basis of the susceptibility of the organism isolated from the sputum. In aspiration lung abscess, however, a variety of organisms are isolated. Moreover, the important anaerobic bacteria may not be cultured. Nevertheless, on an empirical basis penicillin in large doses has been found to be highly effective and is the antimicrobial drug of choice.

As a definable syndrome, primary lung abscess is usually quite readily distinguishable from the cavitation so prominent in the pneumonias produced by klebsiellae, staphylococci, or tubercle bacilli (for treatment of these three diseases see Ch. 182, 195, and 227). Moreover, selection of the proper drug therapy for primary lung abscess is quite a different type of medical judgment from that involved in selecting drugs for microbial diseases produced by a single clearly identifiable agent. In lung abscess the choice must be based on knowledge of the pathogenesis of the condition rather than on the identity of the microbial species isolated from the sputum. The latter, more often than not, have no etiologic significance or, at the very least, their relationship to the disease is by no means assured. Whether this syndrome of lung abscess is wholly microbial in origin and, if so, whether only a single microbial species is involved has not been established. Several lines of evidence, including the rarity of lung abscess in the edentulous person and the similarity of the flora in peridental and pulmonary abscesses, indicate that anaerobic microbes are significantly involved. Recent studies of secretions obtained by transtracheal aspiration, using special methods of culture, have revealed the constant presence of anaerobic bacteria in untreated primary lung abscess. *As a practical matter, lung abscess can be regarded as a cavitating pneumonia caused by anaerobic microbes.*

Since penicillin is known to maintain its effectiveness in anaerobic environments and is demonstrably of high effectiveness in lung abscess, it represents the major drug for the treatment of this condition. Five to ten million units of crystalline penicillin daily by continuous intravenous drip may be used initially. After improvement has occurred, 600,000 units intravenously every four to six hours can be substituted. Therapy should be continued until the lesion heals or until continued improvement fails to occur. This usually requires four to six weeks. An alteration in the bacterial flora of the sputum with penicillin therapy is to be expected, but change to another antimicrobial drug should not be made unless there is clear evidence that penicillin is ineffective. Clindamycin may be used in those individuals with primary lung abscess allergic to penicillin and those failing to respond to an adequate course of penicillin therapy. Postural drainage facilitates emptying of the cavity and may be useful early in the course of therapy.

Surgery is no longer performed early in the disease. The usual indication for surgical intervention is a residual thick-walled cavity persisting after antimicrobial therapy. Thin-walled cavities or cystic lesions need not be removed and will often heal spontaneously. Residual lesions requiring surgery usually occur in patients in whom antimicrobial therapy has been delayed or was inadequate.

Barnett, T. B., and Herring, C. L.: Lung abscess. Initial and late results of medical therapy. Arch. Intern. Med., 127:217, 1971.

Bartlett, J. G., Gorbach, S. L., Tally, F. P., and Finegold, S. M.: Bacteriology and treatment of primary lung abscess. Am. Rev. Respir. Dis., 109:510, 1974.

Bernhard, W. F., Malcolm, J. A., and Wylie, R. H.: The carcinomatous abscess. A clinical paradox. N. Engl. J. Med., 266:914, 1962.

Flavell, G.: Respiratory tract disease. Lung abscess. Br. Med. J., 1:1032, 1966.

Perlman, L. V., Lerner, E., and D'Esopo, N.: Clinical classification and analysis of 97 cases of lung abscess. Am. Rev. Respir. Dis., 99:390, 1969.

517. UNILATERAL HYPERLUCENT LUNG

Unilateral hyperlucent lung is discovered by roentgenography of the chest. One lung is translucent as compared with the other. The vascular markings of the hyperlucent lung are diminished, and the pulmonary artery may be inconspicuous. Fluoroscopy demonstrates a shift of the mediastinum away from the involved lung on expiration. Dilatation and irregularity of the small bronchi are visible on bronchograms. Histopathologic examination of the diseased lung demonstrates an extensive bronchitis and bronchiolitis. The alveoli may be enlarged, but typical destructive emphysema is not usually found. The pulmonary artery is present. One theory of pathogenesis is that a severe pulmonary infection occurred in childhood, with consequent altered development of the lung.

The patient usually gives a history of productive cough. Dyspnea and hemoptysis may be present. Breath sounds are often diminished over the affected lung, and rales may be heard. The perfusion and ventilation of the involved lung are impaired. This can be demonstrated by obtaining an image of the lungs with a scintillation camera following the administration of radioactive xenon.

Treatment consists of management of infection. Surgery is not usually performed.

Hamilton, C. R., Jr., Ballinger, W. F., II, and Cader, G.: The unilateral hyperlucent lung syndrome. Bull. Hopkins Hosp., 123:222, 1968.

Section Six. DIFFUSE LUNG DISEASE

Richard V. Ebert

518. INTERSTITIAL LUNG DISEASE

The normal alveolar wall is made up of capillaries, connective tissue, and thin alveolar epithelium. A network of delicate collagen, reticulin, and elastic fibers gives strength and support to the tissue. Coarser and more abundant connective fibers surround the alveolar ducts, bronchioles, and small bronchi. Except for the lobular septa there is surprisingly little fibrous tissue in the peripheral portions of the lung. A group of diseases is associated with cellular infiltration and increase in fibrous tissue in the walls of the alveoli. The cause of many of these diseases is unknown. All are associated with similar roentgenographic findings and have similar symptoms and physiologic findings.

ROENTGENOGRAPHIC, CLINICAL, AND PHYSIOLOGIC FEATURES

Roentgenographic Findings. The changes in the lungs are diffuse and consist of fine mottling and reticulation. Early in the disease the change may be subtle and can be readily overlooked. Later the shadows may be dense. Annular shadows may appear, giving a honeycomb appearance. In contrast to alveolar disease the vascular shadows persist and may be accentuated.

Clinical Manifestations. The major symptom is exertional dyspnea. This begins insidiously and in the early stages may be disregarded by the patient. The symptoms are usually progressive, and ultimately ordinary activities become limited by shortness of breath. In the advanced form of the disease dyspnea may be present at rest. Wheezing is not present, but a dry cough is common. Purulent sputum is not seen unless there is secondary bronchitis. Examination of the lungs may reveal no abnormal findings, or crackling fine rales may be observed over the lower portions of the lung. Clubbed fingers are common in diffuse interstitial pulmonary fibrosis. Cyanosis and evidence of right heart failure occur in the terminal phase of the illness.

Physiologic Features. The pulmonary function is usually altered. The changes in function differ from those in obstructive lung disease, there being no evidence of impairment of expiratory air flow. The breathing is rapid and shallow. The total pulmonary ventilation is increased both at rest and on exercise. The vital capacity and total lung capacity may be normal but are usually reduced to a variable degree. The maximal breathing capacity is normal or only slightly reduced, and the ratio of the volume of air forcibly expelled in one second to the vital capacity is normal. The diffusing capacity for carbon monoxide is reduced, and the reduction parallels the severity of the disease. In the milder forms of the disease the oxygen saturation of the hemoglobin of the arterial blood may be normal at rest and on exercise. In more severe disease the oxygen saturation is markedly decreased on exercise and may be abnormal at rest. The carbon dioxide tension of the arterial blood is normal or decreased. The basis for these changes in pulmonary function is complex. Capillaries are obliterated and alveoli destroyed by fibrosis. Some alveoli have thickened walls, and others are normal. Contrary to common opinion the alveolar capillary membrane is usually not thickened. These changes in the structure of the lung result in alterations in the mechanical properties of the lung and in gas exchange. The compliance of the lungs is reduced, resulting in an increased work of breathing. The irregular distribution of pathologic changes in the lung produces regional differences in ventilation-perfusion ratios, resulting in inadequate oxygenation of blood leaving certain regions of the lung (venous admixture).

CAUSES OF INTERSTITIAL LUNG DISEASE

Diffuse Interstitial Fibrosis. In 1944 Hamman and Rich described a group of patients with intense dyspnea, cyanosis, and right heart failure. The disease was rapid in its course, only a few months elapsing between the onset of symptoms and death. The lungs at autopsy showed thickening of the alveolar walls with edema, fibrin deposition, and cellular infiltration, together with extensive interstitial proliferation of fibrous tissue. The term Hamman-Rich syndrome was used to describe this clinical and pathologic entity. Subsequently it was found that there was a larger group of patients with diffuse thickening and fibrosis of the alveolar walls who exhibited a more prolonged clinical course. The term idiopathic diffuse interstitial fibrosis or fibrosing alveolitis has been used to describe these patients. Although no specific cause has been found, the presence of rheumatoid factor or antinuclear factor in the serum of a number of these patients has raised the question of whether this is an autoimmune disease.

Approximately 1 to 2 per cent of patients with *rheumatoid* arthritis will have diffuse interstitial fibrosis. Most of these have a high titer of rheumatoid factor in the blood. Approximately 20 per cent of patients with diffuse interstitial fibrosis in whom there are no joint changes have an elevated titer of rheumatoid factor in their blood. Diffuse interstitial fibrosis associated with rheumatoid arthritis or with rheumatoid factor in the blood does not differ from the idiopathic type of fibrosis. A peculiar type of fibrosis involving the upper portion of the lung and associated with cyst formation has been described in ankylosing spondylitis. This differs from diffuse pulmonary fibrosis complicating rheumatoid arthritis, and is not usually associated with a positive test for rheumatoid factor.

Diffuse interstitial fibrosis is also found to occur in association with *scleroderma* and less frequently with dermatomyositis. The fibrosis in scleroderma is not accompanied by a cellular reaction. The changes are usually more marked at the bases of the lungs.

Lymphoid Interstitial Pneumonia. The pathologic findings consist of extensive infiltration of the interstitial tissue of the lungs with mononuclear cells. The pathologic changes may be confused with those of lymphoma of the lung. Lymphoid interstitial pneumonia is often associated with alterations in the plasma gamma globulins and may be associated with Sjögren's syndrome or Waldenström's macroglobulinemia.

Eosinophilic Granuloma. Eosinophilic granuloma of the lung may produce clinical and roentgenologic findings which are indistinguishable from those in diffuse interstitial fibrosis. Bone lesions may or may not be demonstrable. (For further description see Ch. 108).

Idiopathic Pulmonary Hemosiderosis. Idiopathic pulmonary hemosiderosis is described in Ch. 520. In severe cases interstitial fibrosis of the lungs develops, and may resemble roentgenographically the other types of diffuse fibrosis.

Chemical and Physical Irritants. Chemical and physical irritants may lead to interstitial fibrosis (see Ch. 521 to 538).

Extrinsic Allergic Alveolitis. Diseases such as farmer's lung, bagassosis, and pigeon breeders' disease produce an interstitial inflammatory reaction and may lead to interstitial fibrosis (see Ch. 533).

Drug Reaction. Certain drugs such as nitrofurantoin, busulfan, methotrexate, bleomycin, and hexamethonium may produce interstitial edema which may be followed by diffuse interstitial fibrosis.

Sarcoidosis. Sarcoidosis involving the lung may lead to a diffuse interstitial involvement of the pulmonary parenchyma. Initially the lesions are granulomas, but later fibrosis may be present. The roentgenologic appearance of the lung may simulate diffuse interstitial fibrosis. The hilar lymph nodes are usually but not always enlarged (see Ch. 102).

Tuberculosis and Fungal Diseases of the Lungs. Tuberculosis and fungal diseases of the lungs may lead to a diffuse interstitial lesion with granuloma formation. Miliary tuberculosis results from hematogenous spread of the tubercle bacilli. Early in the illness the lesions may not be visible on chest roentgenography. Later diffuse fine miliary densities are seen. Healing occurs with chemotherapy, and the patient is usually left with no functional disability. Histoplasmosis may also give a diffuse granulomatous lesion of the lung. Healing is often associated with multiple small areas of calcification of the lung.

Neoplasm. Lymphangitic spread of primary or metastatic carcinoma of the lung may produce the clinical picture of interstitial lung disease. Occasionally, lymphoma involving the lung may present similarly.

DIAGNOSIS

The appearance of the chest roentgenogram usually establishes the pulmonary lesion as interstitial in character. The differentiation of the various interstitial lesion may be difficult. Inquiry should always be made regarding exposure to various dusts. This should include a review of the various jobs held during a lifetime of work. Special emphasis should be placed on possible exposure to silica or asbestos. Physical examination may give evidence of rheumatoid arthritis or scleroderma. Enlarged lymph nodes may be discovered and on biopsy show the lesions of sarcoid. Bone x-rays may demonstrate the lesions of eosinophilic granuloma or sarcoid. Serologic studies, including tests for rheumatoid factor and complement fixation tests for histoplasmosis and blastomycosis, should be done.

In spite of careful study, a group of patients remain in whom diagnosis is obscure. Most of these will fall into the category of diffuse interstitial fibrosis of unknown cause. A much smaller group will have eosinophilic granuloma or one of the other granulomatous diseases. A firm diagnosis in these doubtful areas can be established only by lung biopsy. This need not be done in every case but should be strongly considered if there is any question of the clinical diagnosis being correct.

TREATMENT

Treatment will depend on the cause of the interstitial lesion. Idiopathic diffuse interstitial fibrosis is often treated with corticosteroids. Immunosuppressant drugs have also been used. The best results have been reported in patients treated in the early stages of the disease. Results are difficult to evaluate, as no controlled clinical trials have been carried out.

The course of idiopathic pulmonary fibrosis is variable. The disease is fatal in a few months in some patients, and may continue with only slow progress for many years in others. Development of hypoxemia at rest usually means that the end of life is approaching. Cor pulmonale with right heart failure often follows and leads to death. A few patients die with alveolar cell carcinoma.

Fraire, A. E., Greenberg, S. D., O'Neal, R. M., Weg, J. G., and Jenkins, D. E.: Diffuse interstitial fibrosis of the lung. Am. J. Clin. Path., 59:636, 1973.

Liebow, A. A., and Carrington, C. B.: Diffuse pulmonary lymphoreticular infiltrations associated with dysproteinemia. Med. Clin. North Am., 57:809, 1973.

Livingstone, J. L., Lewis, J. G., Reid, L., and Jefferson, K. E.: Diffuse interstitial pulmonary fibrosis. A clinical, radiological, and pathological study based on 45 patients. Quart. J. Med., 33:71, 1964.

Nagaya, H., and Siecker, H. O.: Pathogenetic mechanisms of interstitial fibrosis in patients with serum antinuclear factor. Am. J. Med., 52:51, 1972.

Sharp, J. T., Sweaney, S. K., and Van Lith, P.: Physiologic observations in diffuse pulmonary fibrosis and granulomatosis. Am. Rev. Respir. Dis., 94:316, 1966.

Walker, W. C., and Wright, V.: Pulmonary lesions and rheumatoid arthritis. Medicine, 47:501, 1968.

519. DIFFUSE ALVEOLAR DISEASES OF THE LUNG

ROENTGENOGRAPHIC, CLINICAL, AND PHYSIOLOGIC FEATURES

A variety of diseases may lead to replacement of air in the alveoli and alveolar ducts by fluid. The alveoli may be filled by edema fluid (pulmonary edema), by inflammatory exudate (pneumonia), by blood (pulmonary infarct, bleeding from bronchi and aspiration, Goodpasture's syndrome), by exudate containing a high lipid content (alveolar proteinosis, lipoid pneumonia), or by cancer tissue (alveolar cell carcinoma). The roentgenographic appearance of the lungs is similar in all of these and can usually be differentiated from the changes produced by interstitial lung disease. The shadows form a homogeneous density with fluffy ill-defined edges. The infiltrates tend to obliterate the vascular markings, and at times an air bronchogram may be seen. In chronic lesions a pattern related to filling of acini is seen at the edge of the lesion. This is a rosette-like density measuring several millimeters in diameter.

The clinical manifestations of alveolar disease will depend on the nature of the underlying lesion, the duration of the disease, and the extent of involvement. Cough and dyspnea are the two major symptoms. Fever may or may not be present. If the cough is productive, examination of the sputum grossly and with the microscope may cast light on the nature of the alveolar lesion. The sputum in pulmonary edema is thin, and white or pink in color. The sputum in pneumonia is tenacious and purulent, and may contain blood. The sputum in pulmonary hemorrhage consists of pure blood. The degree of dyspnea is related to the acuteness of the lesion and the amount of lung involved. Diffuse pulmonary edema or pneumonia will be associated with rapid, shallow, labored breathing at rest. A chronic alveolar lesion such as alveolar proteinosis may result only in exertional dyspnea.

The physiologic changes will also be dependent on the extent of the lesions and whether they are acute or chronic. The vital capacity will be reduced. The change in blood gases will depend on whether blood flows through the capillaries of the involved alveoli or not. Blood often continues to flow through areas of lung involved by acute lesions, with resultant shunting of unoxygenated blood into the pulmonary venous system. In more chronic lesions the blood flow from the pulmonary artery into the involved area is diminished or absent. The decrease in oxygen saturation of the arterial blood will be dependent on the magnitude of the shunt. If the shunt is large, hypoxia will persist while the patient is breathing high concentrations of oxygen. With massive filling of alveoli with fluid, death occurs from hypoxia in spite of oxygen administration. Hypoxia may also result from alteration in the ventilation-perfusion ratio in alveoli adjacent to the lesion. These alveoli may be poorly ventilated and well perfused, resulting in inadequate oxygenation of blood in the pulmonary capillaries. Administration of oxygen will correct this type of hypoxia. In alveolar disease the carbon dioxide tension of the arterial blood remains low or normal until massive involvement of the lung occurs.

Felsen, B.: The roentgen diagnosis of disseminated alveolar diseases. Seminars Radiol., 2:3, 1967.
Goodman, N.: Differential diagnosis of pulmonary alveolar infiltrates. Am. Rev. Respir. Dis., 95:681, 1967.

520. CAUSES OF DIFFUSE ALVEOLAR DISEASE

PULMONARY EDEMA

Mechanism of Formation of Edema of the Lungs. The formation of edema in the lungs bears a certain similarity to the formation of edema in the subcutaneous tissues. In both instances the forces involved are the same, namely, the hydrostatic pressure in the capillaries, the colloid osmotic pressure of the plasma and interstitial fluid, and the interstitial fluid pressure. There are, however, major differences in the anatomy of the tissues and the hemodynamics in the two locations which lead to differences in the mechanism of formation of edema.

The anatomy of the lung is designed to permit efficient exchange of gas between the alveoli and the pulmonary capillaries. The alveolar septa are made up largely of capillaries. Between the capillaries is a very small amount of connective tissue, including ground substance, collagen, and elastin fibers. The plasma in the capillaries is separated from the air in the alveolus by a thin membrane consisting of capillary endothelium, basement membrane, and alveolar epithelial cells. There is more abundant connective tissue about the bronchi and blood vessels and in the interlobular septa. The pulmonary capillary pressure is below 10 mm Hg in normal human beings. As a result, the difference between pulmonary capillary pressure and colloid osmotic pressure of the plasma is large and creates a force tending to move fluid into the capillary. Another important force is created by the surface tension at the fluid-air interface in the alveoli. This force is related to the radius of curvature of the alveoli and the surface tension. The latter is influenced by a lipid on the surface of the alveolar wall (surfactant). The effect of this force is to make the interstitial fluid pressure negative.

Recent experimental work has elucidated the mechanism of formation of pulmonary edema. As a result of alteration in the hydrostatic forces or increase in capillary permeability to protein, fluid moves from the capillary into the interstitial space in the alveolar septum. As the interstitial fluid increases, it moves into the connective tissue about the blood vessels and bronchi and into the interlobular septa. Lymphatic flow is increased and removes some of this fluid. If the interstitial fluid continues to accumulate, fluid dissects between the capillary endothelial cells and the adjacent basement membrane, resulting in damage to the capillary wall. Finally, fluid moves through the alveolar epithelium into the alveolus. This fluid contains plasma protein and often fibrinogen and red cells.

Roentgenogram. The chest roentgenogram mirrors the pathologic changes. During the phase of interstitial edema linear shadows may be seen (Kerley's A and B lines) which represent edema of the septa of the lungs. There may be thickening and loss of definition of the shadows of the vessels. A perihilar haze may be seen. In some circumstances the edema may remain interstitial and not progress to intra-alveolar edema. Intra-alveolar edema results in confluent shadows of uniform density. These may be diffuse, confined to the lower portion of the lung, or seen at the hila of the lungs (butterfly pattern). Occasionally the shadows are unilateral.

Symptoms and Signs. During the period of development of interstitial edema there is intense suffocating dyspnea, and the breathing is rapid and shallow. A severe attack of paroxysmal nocturnal dyspnea resulting from left ventricular failure exemplifies the symptoms of interstitial edema. During the attack the patient is in the sitting position and breathing rapidly and in a labored manner. His face gives evidence of apprehension and is sweating. He may have difficulty in talking because of the urge to continue breathing. In spite of the intense dyspnea, examination of the lungs may fail to demonstrate rales, and the roentgenogram may not show intra-alveolar edema. If interstitial edema has been present for some time as in mitral stenosis, the patient may be free of dyspnea at rest, although exertional dyspnea is present.

With the development of intra-alveolar edema the patient continues to be severely dyspneic at rest and may cough up white or pink frothy sputum. Examination of the lungs reveals numerous moist rales. Cyanosis may be present if the edema is severe. If formation of edema fluid continues, the patient drowns in the edema fluid.

Alterations in Pulmonary Function. The rapid shallow breathing characteristic of developing pulmonary edema is believed to be related to neurogenic stimuli arising from receptors in the alveolar septa. As a result of the abnormal stimulus to ventilation, the carbon dioxide tension of the arterial blood is decreased. With interstitial edema the oxygen saturation of the arterial blood may show little change, but with the development of alveolar edema hypoxia occurs. The oxygen tension of the arterial blood may fall to extremely low levels in severe diffuse intra-alveolar edema in spite of the administration of high concentrations of oxygen. Increase in the carbon dioxide tension of the arterial blood may be present at this stage. A decrease in the pH of the arterial blood is common in severe pulmonary edema. This may be caused by metabolic acidosis related to increased lactic acid production as well as by carbon dioxide retention. Death results from hypoxia.

Edema of the lung leads to changes in the mechanics of ventilation. The vital capacity is decreased, and the course of pulmonary edema can be followed by repeated use of this simple bedside measurement. The total lung capacity is also reduced. This reduction is associated with a change in the elastic properties of the lung. A greater change in intrapleural pressure is required to produce a given volume change in the lung (decrease in compliance of the lung). This in turn leads to an increase in the work of breathing. With early edema there is usually no change in the resistance to air flow in the lung. Later, obstruction to flow of air may result from fluid in the bronchi. Occasionally this obstruction is severe and associated with wheezing, giving rise to the term cardiac asthma.

Causes of Pulmonary Edema. *Increase in Pulmonary Capillary Pressure.* This is the most common cause of pulmonary edema. The usual mechanism is failure of the left ventricle with rise in left ventricular end diastolic pressure. Hypertension, aortic valve disease, and acute myocardial infarction are common causes of acute failure of the left ventricle. Mitral stenosis leads to elevation in pulmonary capillary pressure by obstructing blood flow to the left ventricle. As a consequence the edema of the lungs is often chronic and interstitial in character. Mitral stenosis may also be associated with acute intra-alveolar edema usually precipitated by severe exertion or a sudden increase in heart rate.

The pulmonary capillary pressure may be elevated by an increase in blood volume. A general increase in blood volume is accompanied by an increase in pulmonary blood volume, which in turn leads to an elevation in pulmonary vascular pressures. Administration of large amounts of blood may precipitate pulmonary edema in a normal person. More commonly, the administration of blood or salt solution leads to pulmonary edema in an individual with previous disease of the heart or kidney. Great care must be taken in administering blood or saline to a person with a history of left ventricular failure, as small amounts of fluid may precipitate pulmonary edema. A combination of left ventricular failure and increase in blood volume may produce pulmonary edema in patients with severe chronic anemia who are receiving blood transfusions.

Pulmonary edema complicating renal disease involves fluid overload and left ventricular failure. If the patient is oliguric, as in acute tubular necrosis or acute glomerulonephritis, and receives excessive fluid orally or intravenously, the blood volume increases, and pulmonary edema may occur. Often hypertension is present and predisposes to left ventricular failure. In chronic renal disease left ventricular failure plays an important role in the formation of pulmonary edema. Uremic pneumonia is thought to be a form of pulmonary edema occurring in patients with severe renal insufficiency.

Pulmonary edema may complicate intracranial lesions. The most common cause is marked increase in intracranial pressure secondary to head injury or spontaneous intracranial hemorrhage. It has also been described in association with brain tumors and following generalized convulsive seizures. The mechanism of production of the edema is not completely understood, but is thought to be related to reflex effects on peripheral circulation and heart with massive peripheral vasoconstriction.

High altitude pulmonary edema is a poorly understood disorder. It occurs in those recently arrived at high altitude who have engaged in vigorous exercise. The clinical picture is similar to other types of pulmonary edema. Recovery is the rule with suitable treatment and evacuation to lower altitudes. The pathogenesis is believed to be related to the effect of hypoxia on the pulmonary vascular bed. Pulmonary edema may complicate self-administration of large doses of heroin or methadone. The mechanism of production of this type of edema may relate to hypoxia secondary to respiratory depression.

Lowered Colloid Osmotic Pressure of Plasma. Pulmonary edema is rarely caused by diminution in the concentration of plasma proteins unless other predisposing factors are present. In the nephrotic syndrome there may be massive peripheral edema, yet the lungs remain free of fluid. In edema of the lungs produced by massive infusion of saline, the lowered plasma proteins contribute to edema formation. This is particularly true if the plasma proteins have been depleted by hemorrhage. In renal disease decrease in the concentration of plasma proteins may be one of several factors contributing to pulmonary edema.

Negative Intrapleural Pressure. Sudden re-expansion of the lung by the rapid removal of large amounts of pleural fluid may result in unilateral pulmonary edema. Edema may also result from the rapid expansion of a lung collapsed by a pneumothorax. The edema is thought to result from the application of a large negative intrapleural pressure to the lung.

Increased Capillary Permeability. Certain gases when inhaled into the lungs damage the pulmonary capillaries and increase the permeability of the capillary wall to protein. Among these gases are phosgene, chlorine, and nitrogen dioxide. The latter may result from fermentation of corn in a closed space (silo-filler's disease). Certain herbicides such as paraquat may cause pulmonary edema.

Pulmonary edema may occur as an idiosyncratic reaction to certain drugs. Drugs reported to cause increased capillary permeability with edema include hexamethonium, nitrofurantoin, busulfan, and methotrexate. Pulmonary edema has been reported after a single blood transfusion as a result of hypersensitivity.

Pulmonary edema may complicate septic shock. It may also occur in patients being resuscitated from severe shock associated with nonthoracic trauma. The pathologic findings in the *shock lung* consist of focal areas of atelectasis as well as interstitial and alveolar edema. The mechanism of production of these pathologic changes in the lung is not well understood. Among the factors involved may be damage to the pulmonary capillaries and overzealous administration of intravenous fluids in the treatment of shock.

Certain pneumonias resemble pulmonary edema. Fulminating pneumonia may occur with influenza virus infection, and death may occur in 24 hours. The alveoli are filled with edema fluid, fibrin, red blood cells, and mononuclear cells. The pneumonia associated with *Pneumocystis carinii* infection is more chronic. The alveoli contain a foamy amorphous exudate.

There is considerable evidence that the administration of a high concentration of oxygen for long periods of time will cause damage to the pulmonary capillaries. It has been known for many years that damage to the lungs of animals could be produced by the prolonged administration of pure oxygen at atmospheric pressure. More recently interstitial edema and hyaline alveolar membranes have been described in patients receiving high concentration of oxygen in association with mechanical ventilation. During life there is a progressive fall in the oxygen tension of the arterial blood in spite of continuing high concentration of oxygen in the inspired air.

Treatment. The treatment of pulmonary edema consists of general measures and therapy specific for the underlying cause. Examples of specific therapy are digitalis for left ventricular failure, appropriate treatment of arrhythmias, and the use of antihypertensive drugs in heart failure precipitated by severe hypertension.

Morphine will produce dramatic relief of symptoms if administered during the interstitial phase of edema or in the early stages of alveolar edema. The pattern of breathing may return to normal, and apprehension is relieved. Morphine is of special value in attacks of pulmonary edema resulting from acute left ventricular failure. The drug is given subcutaneously in a dose of 15 mg. If rapid action is desired or shock is present, it may be given intravenously. The administration of morphine to patients with chronic obstructive lung disease under the mistaken impression that pulmonary edema is present should be avoided at all costs. Morphine should also be avoided in the late stages of pulmonary edema when respiration is depressed because of severe hypoxia.

Oxygen should be administered, as hypoxia may be present. In mild pulmonary edema an adequate concentration of oxygen in inspired air can be obtained with a nasal catheter. A high concentration of oxygen may be required in severe pulmonary edema. If pulmonary edema fails to respond to usual treatment and if hypoxia persists in spite of the use of oxygen, consideration should be given to intubation with an intratracheal tube and the application of intermittent positive pressure using positive end expiratory pressure (PEEP). Positive pressure breathing decreases cardiac output, inhibits the movement of fluid into the alveoli, and prevents the terminal airways from closing. The latter effect is believed to be the most important. The use of high concentrations of oxygen for prolonged periods of time in the treatment of pulmonary edema should be avoided, as further damage to pulmonary capillaries may ensue.

Reduction in pulmonary blood volume is imperative in pulmonary edema associated with high pulmonary capillary pressure. This can be accomplished by pooling blood in the extremities or by venesection. Placing the patient in the sitting position with legs dependent will pool blood in the legs. Additional blood can be pooled by the application of venous tourniquets to the upper thighs. Venesection of 500 to 700 ml of blood is particularly useful in those cases in which the attack of pulmonary edema has been precipitated by administration of blood or the excessive use of intravenous fluids. Diuretics have also been found valuable. Ethacrynic acid given intravenously in a dose of 50 mg will produce a prompt massive diuresis with consequent reduction of blood volume.

Aberman, A., and Fulop, M.: The metabolic and respiratory acidosis of acute pulmonary edema. Ann. Intern. Med., 76:173, 1972.

Fishman, A. P.: Pulmonary edema. The water-exchanging function of the lung. Circulation, 46:390, 1972.

Fishman, A. P.: Shock lung—a distinctive nonentity. Circulation, 47:921, 1973.

Heitzman, E. R., and Ziter, F. M.: Acute interstitial pulmonary edema. Radiology, 98:291, 1966.

McMahon, S. M., Halprin, G. M., and Sieker, H. O.: Positive end-expiratory airway pressure in severe arterial hypoxemia. Am. Rev. Respir. Dis., 108:526, 1973.

Robin, E. D., Cross, C. E., and Zelis, R.: Pulmonary edema. N. Engl. J. Med., 288:239, 292, 1973.

PULMONARY ALVEOLAR PROTEINOSIS

In pulmonary alveolar proteinosis the microscopic appearance of the lungs is typical. Large groups of alveoli are filled with a proteinaceous material containing a high concentration of phospholipid. The material gives a positive reaction with periodic acid–Schiff stain. A few large cells containing stainable lipid are present in the alveoli and along the alveolar septa. The septa themselves are remarkably normal. It is thought that the lipid material in the alveoli is derived from granular pneumocytes and may be related to surfactant.

Symptoms consist of gradually progressive dyspnea and a productive cough. Physical examination of the lungs may be normal. The roentgenogram reveals bilateral diffuse soft densities seen most commonly at the hila or bases of the lungs. The vital capacity is reduced to a variable degree. The maximal breathing capacity is normal or slightly reduced. The oxygen saturation of the hemoglobin of the arterial blood may be normal or reduced. Complicating infection occurs. Fungal infection is common, Nocardia being the most frequent offending organism. The disease may remain stable for considerable periods of time and spontaneous improvement may occur, but it is eventually fatal in about one third of the patients.

Pulmonary alveolar proteinosis must be differentiated from diseases of the heart with pulmonary edema and from the pulmonary fibroses, pneumoconioses, sarcoidosis, and fungal infections of the lung. *Pneumocystis carinii* infection can present with a similar clinical picture and similar pathologic findings. Lung biopsy is usually necessary to clarify the diagnosis.

Various methods of treatment have been attempted. These include the use of proteolytic enzymes and pulmonary lavage; of these, lavage appears to be the most promising. One lung is irrigated at a time using several liters of saline. The washings contain material with a high lipid content similar to that seen in the alveoli.

Davidson, J. M., and Macleod, W. M.: Pulmonary alveolar proteinosis. Br. J. Dis. Chest, 63:13, 1969.
Pulmonary alveolar proteinosis—editorial. Br. Med. J., 1:395, 1972.
Ramirez-R., J., and Harlan, W. R.: Pulmonary alveolar proteinosis. Nature and origin of alveolar lipid. Am. J. Med., 45:502, 1968.
Rosen, S. H., Castleman, B., and Liebow, A. A.: Pulmonary alveolar proteinosis. N. Engl. J. Med., 258:1123, 1958.

DESQUAMATIVE INTERSTITIAL PNEUMONIA

The tissue response in desquamative interstitial pneumonia consists of proliferation and desquamation of large alveolar cells with slight thickening of the walls of the distal air spaces.

Patients with this disease complain of cough and shortness of breath, which is gradually progressive. Rales may or may not be heard on physical examination of the chest. The roentgenogram demonstrates a ground-glass appearance in the basilar portion of the lungs. Diagnosis must be made by lung biopsy. The course is chronic, the lesions persisting for months or years. Steroids are said to have a beneficial effect.

There is some question whether this entity is distinct and separate from diffuse interstitial fibrosis (fibrosing alveolitis). Cases are seen which are intermediate between the two entities with varying degrees of alveolar wall thickening and varying numbers of cells in the alveoli. There is evidence that patients with typical desquamative interstitial pneumonia may develop interstitial fibrosis after several years.

Gaensler, E. A., Goff, A. M., and Prowse, C. M.: Desquamative interstitial pneumonia. N. Engl. J. Med., 274:113, 1966.
Liebow, A. A., Steer, A., and Billingsley, J. G.: Desquamative interstitial pneumonia. Am. J. Med., 39:369, 1965.
Scadding, J. G., and Hinson, K. F.: Diffuse fibrosing alveolitis (diffuse interstitial fibrosis of the lungs). Correlation of histology at biopsy with prognosis. Thorax, 22:291, 1967.

LIPOID PNEUMONIA

Lipoid pneumonia can be exogenous or endogenous in type. In the exogenous variety mineral oil or animal fats are introduced into the lung by aspiration. A common cause is the use of nose drops with a mineral oil as a base. The oil has ready access to the larynx and trachea when applied through the nose. Another cause is the habitual use of mineral oil to regulate bowel movements. In certain persons the mineral oil is aspirated into the trachea and lungs. This is most commonly seen in the elderly in whom the protective reflexes may be dulled. Animal fats may be introduced into the lungs in chronic disease of the esophagus where regurgitation of food occurs. Achalasia of the esophagus is often associated with a chronic pneumonitis as a result of aspiration (see Ch. 635).

In pneumonia caused by mineral oil the earliest reaction is phagocytosis of the oil by alveolar macrophages. The alveolar walls become thickened, and there is an increase in fibrous tissue. Lymphocytes and globules of oil are seen in the interstitial tissue. Ultimately extreme fibrosis of the involved area of the lung occurs.

The endogenous form of lipoid pneumonia consists of a chronic inflammatory process involving a segment or lobe of the lung. The alveoli contain large mononuclear cells with a vacuolated cytoplasm. These cells are also found in the walls of the alveoli. Lymphocytic infiltration and fibrosis of the alveolar walls are present. The lipid present in the lesion is cholesterol. This type of pneumonitis not infrequently occurs secondary to an obstructed bronchus. Occasionally it is present without evident cause.

The symptoms of lipoid pneumonia are extremely variable. The patient may be virtually asymptomatic and the lesion be detected on a routine chest film, or productive cough and dyspnea may be present. The earliest roentgenographic change is the presence of an alveolar type of infiltrate. An acinar pattern may be visible at the periphery of the lesion. Later evidence of fibrosis is present, and there may be contraction of the involved area of the lung. In the exogenous form of the disease the lesions are usually seen in the basilar or posterior segments of the lung.

An important method of diagnosis is the demonstration of oil-containing macrophages in the sputum. The sputum should be collected before breakfast and after cleansing the mouth. Appropriate fat stains should be used. In some cases bronchial brushing or biopsy may be necessary to establish the diagnosis.

There may be difficulty in differentiating lipoid pneumonia from bronchogenic carcinoma. The failure to demonstrate an obstructed bronchus is of great importance in diagnosis. The history of aspiration and the lack of tumor cells in the sputum or in specimens obtained by bronchial brushing of the involved area confirm the diagnosis of lipoid pneumonia.

There is no specific treatment except prevention of aspiration of oil or fat. If symptoms are troublesome and persistent or if the diagnosis is in doubt, resection of the segment or lobe involved should be considered.

Miller, A., Bader, R. A., Bader, M. E., Teirstein, A. S., and Selikoff, J.: Mineral oil pneumonia. Ann. Intern. Med., 57:627, 1962.
Padula, R. T., and Stayman, J. W., Jr.: Chronic interstitial pneumonia: Cholesterol type. Review of the literature and report of two cases. J. Thorac. Cardiovasc. Surg., 54:272, 1967.
Wagner, J. C., Adler, D. I., and Fuller, D. N.: Foreign body granulomata of the lungs due to liquid paraffin. Thorax, 10:157, 1955.
Weill, H., Ferrans, V. J., Gay, R. M., and Ziskind, M. M.: Early lipoid pneumonia. Roentgenologic, anatomic and physiologic characteristics. Am. J. Med., 36:370, 1964.

GOODPASTURE'S SYNDROME AND IDIOPATHIC PULMONARY HEMOSIDEROSIS

Goodpasture's syndrome is a rare disease characterized by repeated episodes of hemorrhage into the pulmonary alveoli associated with glomerulonephritis. The presenting symptoms are hemoptysis and dyspnea. Roentgenographic examination of the lungs demonstrates fluffy infiltrates in both lungs. An iron deficiency anemia is present, and the urine contains albumin, red blood cells, and casts. The course of the disease consists of remissions and exacerbations. Repeated episodes of hemoptysis and pulmonary infiltration occur. Progressive impairment of renal function is common, and uremia often results. The disease has a poor prognosis, and recovery is rare. There is no specific therapy. The pathology of the disease is of great interest. Red blood cells and hemosiderosin-containing macrophages are in the alveoli. The alveolar septa may be thickened with an increase in collagen. A proliferative type of glomerulonephritis is found in the kidneys. An important finding is the presence of gamma globulin and complement in the basement membrane of the renal glomeruli and of the pulmonary alveoli demonstrated by immunofluorescence. Globulins eluted from lung tissue react with glomerular basement membrane. These findings suggest that antibodies against kidney and lung basement membrane are important in the pathogenesis of the disease.

The pulmonary lesions of *idiopathic pulmonary hemosiderosis* bear considerable similarities to those of Goodpasture's syndrome, but no renal lesion is present. The disease occurs most commonly in children, but may occur in young adults. The earliest symptom is hemoptysis. This is associated with transient confluent infiltrates seen on chest roentgenography. The hemoptysis and pulmonary infiltrates come and go. Pallor develops which can be ascribed to an iron deficiency anemia. The patient ultimately develops chronic dyspnea. The chest roentgenogram now may show a reticular appearance with fine stippling. Biopsy of the lung will demonstrate hemosiderin-laden macrophages in the alveoli and an increase in interstitial fibrous tissue. Hemosiderin-containing macrophages can also be found in the sputum. Massive hemoptysis is not uncommon and may lead to death.

The mortality with both syndromes is high. Death in Goodpasture's syndrome may occur after a relatively brief period of time and results from uremia or from pulmonary hemorrhage. Corticosteroids and immunosuppressive agents have been used in therapy, but the results have not been dramatic. Bilateral nephrectomy followed by renal transplantation has been performed in Goodpasture's syndrome with some success.

Koffler, D., Sandson, J., Carr, R., and Kunkel, H.: Immunologic studies concerning the pulmonary lesions in Goodpasture's syndrome. Am. J. Path., 54:293, 1969.
McCombs, R. P.: Diseases due to immunologic reactions in the lungs (second of two parts). N. Engl. J. Med., 286:1245, 1972.
Proskey, A. J., Weatherbee, L., Easterling, R. E., et al.: Goodpasture's syndrome. A report of five cases and review of the literature. Am. J. Med., 48:162, 1970.
Repetto, G., Lisboa, C., Emparanza, E., et al.: Idiopathic pulmonary hemosiderosis. Pediatrics, 40:24, 1967.
Weiss, E. B., Earnest, D. L., and Greally, J. F.: Goodpasture's syndrome. Case report with emphasis on pulmonary physiology. Am. Rev. Respir. Dis., 97:444, 1968.

ALVEOLAR MICROLITHIASIS

Alveolar microlithiasis is a rare disease characterized by the presence of round calcified bodies in the alveoli. The origin and exact nature of these bodies are not known. The disease develops in young adults, and multiple cases may be seen in a family. It is most commonly discovered by examination of a routine roentgenogram of the chest. The appearance of the lungs is characteristic. Fine miliary calcific densities are distributed throughout the lung. The lesions are most prominent at the bases of the lung. The shadows may coalesce, giving a uniform density in portions of the lung. Early in the disease the patient is asymptomatic. Later dyspnea and cough are present. The course is prolonged over many years, and death occurs from pulmonary insufficiency.

Fulechon, F. J. D., Abboud, A. T., Balikian, J. P., and Nucho, C. K. N.: Pulmonary alveolar microlithiasis. Lung function in five cases. Thorax, 24:84, 1969.
Sears, M. R., Chang, A. R., and Taylor, A. J.: Pulmonary alveolar microlithiasis. Thorax, 26:704, 1971.

Section Seven. PHYSICAL AND CHEMICAL IRRITANTS

Margaret R. Becklake

521. INTRODUCTION

Man, in taming his environment, in developing his complex industrial society, and, more recently, in pursuit of his hobbies, has become increasingly exposed to a wide variety of materials which may act as chemical and physical irritants to his lungs. The industrial physician is sensitized to the need for a detailed occupational history. However, in many communities working men and women first seek medical advice from their personal physician who may easily fail to recognize an occupational exposure because it occurs in a small plant, using experimental materials, or in the processing as a secondary user of dangerous products whose hazards are not appreciated. Thus *a work history should always be exhaustive* and should cover every job ever held, even part-time or vacation jobs, together with the materials handled directly or indirectly, as well as safety measures recommended on the job and information about the health of co-workers. Place of residence is also important, as well as the occupation of other family members, because exposure may be only indirect.

Thus today *occupational lung disease* covers the reaction of the lung to *a variety of physical and chemical irritants,* extending beyond those conditions originally described by the term *pneumoconioses,* which refers to lung diseases consequent to the inhalation of dust, in keeping with its Greek derivation. Originally applied only to inorganic (mineral) dusts, it has subsequently been extended to cover organic (biologic) "dusts" as well, because exposure to the latter is also frequently occupational. However, these biologic "dusts" act as neither physical nor chemical irritants, but as stimulants to the subject's immune mechanisms. A large number of variants of the term have been coined to describe specific occupations at risk or specific dust diseases, and probably serve more to confuse than to clarify.

The classification of lung irritants outlined in the accompanying table, although it implies more precise understanding of mechanisms of lung response than is justified by current knowledge, does provide a working and essentially practical approach for diagnosis.

Physical and Chemical Irritants: Working Classification of Their Pulmonary Effects

Agent	Effect on the Lung	Produced by	Circumstances of Exposure, Including Occupation at Risk
Inorganic dusts	1. Noncollagenous pneumoconioses	Carbon, tin, iron, coal, graphite	Mining, welding
	2. Collagenous pneumoconioses		
	a. Nodular	Silica	Hardrock mining, sandblasting
	b. Diffuse	Asbestos, fume and fine silica	Mining, all secondary users of asbestos in industry
		Beryllium	Fluorescent light industry, space industry
	c. Complicated	An altered tissue response to a usually nonfibrogenic dust	Progressive massive fibrosis in coal miners
	3. Neoplasia	Asbestos, radioactive dusts	Asbestos mining, milling, and manufacturing; uranium mining
Organic "dusts"	1. Asthma-like reactions	Enzymes of *B. subtilis,* western red cedar	Manufacturers of detergents; wood workers and processors
	2. Delayed, eventually irreversible, airway obstruction	Cotton, hemp, flax, jute	Processors of vegetable fiber, particularly the carding of cotton
	3. Extrinsic allergic alveolitis	Spores of fungi, e.g., *Thermopolyspora polyspora*	Haymaking, sugar cane picking or processing the residue; mushroom and malt growing; maple bark stripping, etc.
	4. Chronic (lipoid) interstitial pneumonia	Blackfat tobacco (Guyana)	Smoking
Chemicals	1. Asthma-like reactions	Complex salts of platinum, aluminum soldering flux	Platinum refining
		Toluene diisocyanate (TDI)	Manufacturing and home use of polyurethane plastics
	2. Chemical bronchitis	TDI in heavier doses	Ditto
		SO_2	Pulp and paper mills
		NH_3	Refrigeration
	3. Chemical pulmonary edema	NO_2, phosgene	Silo filling, fire fighting
		Paraquat	Accidental ingestion of weed killer
Radiation	Pneumonitis	X-radiation	Medical treatment

INORGANIC DUSTS

522. DOSAGE, CLEARANCE, AND CELLULAR REACTION

Although a heavy inorganic dust load may produce some acute reversible obstruction in airways, the main biologic effects of inorganic dusts depend on their retention in the lungs of man for long periods of time, measured usually in years, not months. It has been suggested that any mineral dust, if relatively insoluble and not immediately toxic, can produce a pneumoconiosis when inhaled in sufficient quantities. The physician is probably better advised to adopt this oversuspicious attitude to mineral dusts than to fail in recognizing old as well as new pneumoconioses.

Human lungs have been aptly called *"size-selective dust samplers."* Airborne dust, when inspired into the lung, undergoes a process of separation based on size and falling rate. Likewise, breathing patterns and minute ventilation affect penetration and deposition. Over 80 per cent of larger particles (6 μ and over) impact on the mucous lining of the larger airways to be removed, usually quite rapidly (i.e., within hours), by ciliary escalation; however, some particles of considerable length, e.g., asbestos fibers up to as much as 100 μ in length, may penetrate as far as terminal respiratory units. Small dust particles penetrate more deeply, but only the fine particles (below 2 μ) penetrate the alveolar spaces. The retention rate is about 40 per cent in the 2 to 1 μ size, and higher for those below 0.2 μ (see Fig. 1).

Since the respiratory bronchioles and alveoli are lined with surfactant, not mucus, dust particles settling here are removed by alveolar phagocytosis; dust-laden phagocytes migrate toward the alveolar ducts and terminal bronchioles; if not extruded into the airways they may penetrate into lung interstitium and lymphatics. Furthermore, clearance mechanisms may be provoked, i.e., mucus and surfactant production, ciliary activity, and

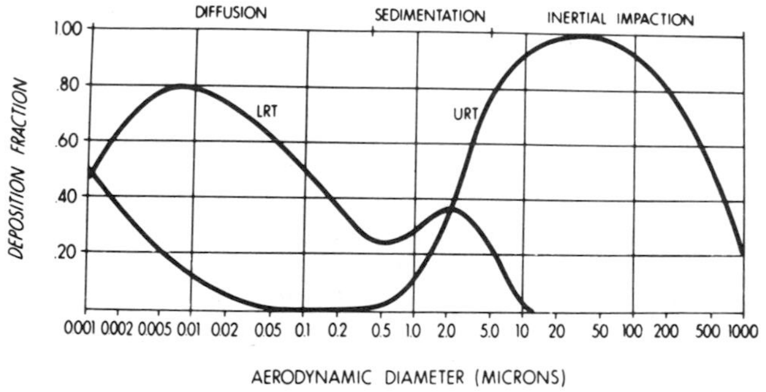

Figure 1. Deposition rate of particles in the human lung in the nose and supraglottic structures (URT) and in the tracheobronchial tree and lung parenchyma (LRT) in relation to aerodynamic diameter, a measurement which refers to the actual diameter in the presence of water vapor which may exceed the particle size in dry air. (Courtesy of Professor Paul Morrow, University of Rochester, N.Y.; reproduced from Lee, D. H. K. [ed.]: Environmental Factors in Respiratory Disease. New York, Academic Press, 1972.)

endocytosis all increase, in response to the inhalation of irritants, particularly if exposure is intermittent. Heavy doses, on the other hand, may overwhelm the removal mechanisms, and their efficiency may also be reduced by associated pollutants, either industrial or personal (tobacco smoke).

The *lung tissue response to inorganic dust* has been likened to the color spectrum to emphasize the variety in the type of response and its intensity, ranging from noncollagenous dust deposits to intense collagen fibrosis. The nature of the tissue response is thought to depend on the physicochemical properties of the dust as well as on its antigenic properties. It is almost certainly dose related, the consequence of the integrated personal exposure less the integrated clearance over the years, and probably relates to how long the dust has been resident in the lung. Other factors which may influence the response are the presence or absence of infection, and possible synergistic or antagonistic effects of other respirable materials in the environment. Finally, although dust dose is probably the most important factor determining the lung response, individual susceptibility undoubtedly plays a role.

The nodular pneumoconioses, either noncollagenous or collagenous, are caused by the relatively insoluble dusts, and the diffuse pneumoconioses by relatively soluble dusts.

523. DIAGNOSIS, LUNG FUNCTION, AND DISABILITY IN THE INORGANIC DUST PNEUMOCONIOSES

The *diagnosis* of the inorganic dust pneumoconioses depends on the characteristic changes in the chest roentgenogram, *provided that the subject in question has had a suitable history of dust exposure.* In other words, there may be no physical signs and no impairment of physical performance, even in the presence of marked radiographic changes. In no other field therefore is the quality of the chest radiograph more important, and the technique used should be appropriate; e.g., low kv to define pleural calcification, high kv to define the pulmonary parenchyma and noncalcified pleural changes. In addition, use of standard films in conjunction with the UICC/Cincinnati Classification of Radiographic Appearances of the Pneumoconioses (1970) will improve the accuracy of film interpretation. In the absence of an exposure history, it may be necessary to resort to *mediastinal node biopsy* or to *open* or *needle lung biopsy* to establish a diagnosis. However, the pathologic findings may also be inconclusive, because lung tissue has only a limited number of response patterns and a given response may be evoked by several stimuli, e.g., irritants and infections. Thus adequate tissue samples should be sent for chemical assay and mineralogic study with x-ray diffraction as well as histopathology. The electron microprobe may ultimately allow precise characterization of mineral in very small tissue samples, or even in the single ferruginous (asbestos) body. Since most pneumoconioses develop as a consequence of occupational exposure, *precise evaluation of disability* is frequently called for, with a view to establishing compensation; hence, the many studies of pulmonary function in pneumoconiosis. However, the interrelationship between the dyspnea and measurable disturbance of static or dynamic pulmonary function has not yet been satisfactorily defined in pneumoconiosis, or, indeed, in lung disease in general. To date, the most acceptable theory is that *dyspnea* is felt when the respiratory effort (either minute volume or muscular effort) for a given task is greater than the subject habitually experiences. In health there exists a tremendous reserve of cardiopulmonary function, indicated by the capacity to increase O_2 consumption (going from rest to maximal exercise) by a factor varying from 20 in the young athlete to perhaps 10 in the middle-aged man. In its early stages pneumoconiosis may produce only very minor measurable changes in function, affecting performance at high levels of exercise only, and this may well be interpreted by the subject as the natural consequence of aging. As the condition progresses, dyspnea may be more easily related to demonstrable changes in lung function. In the following chapters, an attempt is made to describe the usual clinical picture and lung function findings in the different pneumoconioses in their different stages of development. *In evaluating the individual case,* however, *there is no substitute for the detailed study of pulmonary function at rest and on effort,* with a view to determining performance at an average aerobic workload (such as many jobs demand) and possibly to determine maximal aerobic work capacity. This information can then be interpreted in the light of industrial history, dust exposure (quality and quantity), medical history (in particular, previous and present heart and lung disease), and appropriate laboratory investigations.

In a case of industrial lung disease, the physician's responsibility to his patient does not cease until he has assured himself that the case has been referred to the correct local authority in charge of industrial safety. This is important, not only from the point of view of the individual patient who may merit compensation because of already evident disease, but also from the point of view of others working in the same environment whose future health might be ensured by early and adequate preventive action.

524. NONCOLLAGENOUS INORGANIC DUST PNEUMOCONIOSES

Examples. Examples include *coal workers' pneumoconiosis; siderosis* in welders; *pneumoconiosis* in hematite and magnetite miners; *stannosis* in tin miners; *baritosis* in barium miners; *pneumoconiosis* in *chromite* and *china clay miners,* and in workers with *Fuller's earth.*

Pathogenesis and Mechanisms. The dusts mentioned above are those which elicit a virtually noncollagenous response in the lung; hence the diseases associated with such exposure have been called the "*benign*" *pneumoconioses.* The dusts concerned can accumulate in large amounts, usually in phagocytes which accumulate in the alveolar spaces or penetrate the interstitial pulmonary tissue to collect as discrete macules, or as thick sheaths of cells around the respiratory bronchioles. Although considerable amounts of dust (up to 20 grams) may be recoverable from the lungs at autopsy, only small amounts of fibrous tissue develop in these macules, usually in a radial rather than a concentric fashion. The intensity of the fibrosis, never marked, is thought to be related to quartz contamination in the dust, and variations in quartz content probably explain such regional differences as exist, for example, among the dust macule of the Welsh soft coal miner, the more fibrous macule of his counterpart in Belgium, and the *stellate "mixed dust" nodule* of the foundry worker. In addition, the radiodensity of the nodules appears to be related to their iron content, endogenous iron accumulating around dust as it does around other foreign bodies. In time the respiratory bronchioles around the dust foci dilate, perhaps because of the local traction of the dust-encased bronchioles on the surrounding lung parenchyma, and a characteristic form of *focal proximal acinar emphysema* develops, involving primarily the respiratory bronchioles.

The pathologic changes of generalized emphysema may also be seen in lungs which are affected by these nodular pneumoconioses, particularly when the nodulation is of the smaller variety (pinhead rather than micronodular). Such changes occur more frequently and to a more disabling degree (leading to pulmonary hypertension and right heart failure) in certain geographic areas, e.g., the iron mines of Lorraine and the coal mines of Belgium. Finally, pulmonary emphysema has been shown to occur more frequently in the lungs of miners than in the lungs of the nonmining population, even in the absence of pneumoconiosis, thus strengthening the evidence that dust exposure, particularly in the cigarette smoker, is an important factor contributing to the development of chronic obstructive lung disease.

Clinical Manifestations. The term "tattooing" of the chest roentgenogram has been applied to this group of *"benign" noncollagenous nodular pneumoconioses,* because even in the presence of diffuse radiologic nodular densities symptoms and signs of chest disease are rarely present. Likewise, most tests routinely used to evaluate pulmonary function such as measurements of lung volume, flow rates, diffusing capacity at rest, and even the pulmonary mechanics, have been found to be within the normal limits in keeping with the histology of the dust macules. However, abnormalities of gas exchange (reflected in increased A-a O_2 differences) have been shown to exist. These changes, demonstrable at rest and exaggerated during effort, presumably reflect regional inequalities in ventilation vis-à-vis perfusion. Such changes probably do not impair function enough to cause symptoms, and disability affecting performance, if present, is usually attributable to chronic obstructive airway disease.

Epidemiology and Prognosis. The prevalence rate of simple pneumoconiosis varies very much from operation to operation, even within the same industry; for example, rates range from 58 to 253 per 1000 underground workers in the coal mining industry of Great Britain, and from 100 to 400 per 1000 working coal miners in various American pits. In small uncontrolled operations prevalence may well be higher. These differences are thought to be related to the dust exposure levels, and prevalence usually falls dramatically as dust control becomes effective, e.g., in the Dutch coal miners rates fell from 270 to 160 per 1000 working miners over a seven-year period.

In addition to the pathologic evidence quoted above, there is also epidemiologic evidence that the prevalence of chronic obstructive lung disease (as measured by questionnaire or simple ventilatory tests, or both) is increased in coal miners and that this is related to their occupation since dose relationships have been shown. However, other factors which influence its prevalence include environment (e.g., in some areas bronchitis appears to be as common among miners' wives as among the miners themselves) and cigarette smoking, since miners are frequently heavy smokers. Thus attributability is a taxing and difficult problem for compensation commissions, especially as the noncollagenous nodular pneumoconioses in this group do not usually per se produce significant disability.

It is *unusual* for these pneumoconioses *to develop for the first time or to progress after exposure has ceased,* but this does occur. Likewise, the disappearance of radiologic changes after removal from exposure, though unusual, has been described, and is in keeping with animal experiments showing that dust nodules are not static structures but are the site of continuing phagocytic activity. Life expectancy does not appear to be affected by the presence of these "benign" pneumoconioses, especially if exposure stops and they are not complicated by obstructive lung disease.

525. COLLAGENOUS INORGANIC DUST PNEUMOCONIOSES OF THE NODULAR TYPE

Examples. Examples of these disorders include *classic silicosis of hardrock miners* and of *granite workers* and *cutters;* and silicosis in *iron and steel workers* and *sandblasters,* in the *pottery industry,* in industries using *silica flour,* and in those processing *bentonite.*

Pathogenesis and Mechanisms. If the dusts of carbon and coal represent those at the low end of the response spectrum, free crystalline silica dust represents the opposite end, with its almost unique biologic capacity to evoke a powerful fibrogenic tissue response. Reaction to silica appears to start with an alteration of the lung macrophages, though by what mechanism is not fully understood; neither a mechanical nor a simple solubility theory fully explains the biologic findings. There is support for the view that damaged macrophages release altered cell material which is antigenic and which activates the reticuloendothelial system. A fibroblastic reaction follows (peribronchiolar, perivascular, or both) which leads to the accumulation of hyaline material at the site of the macrophage collections, and ultimately to the development of the *characteristic fibrous silicotic nodule* made up of layers of whorled connective tissue, like an onion. Extensive and marked fibrosis may be present in the lungs at autopsy with only relatively small amounts of dust (up to 10 grams, of which perhaps half is silica). Involvement of the hilar and mediastinal lymph nodes is common, occasionally with *egg-shell calcification,* whereas abdominal nodes are occasionally affected. In nature, free crystalline silica occurs almost exclusively as quartz; however, other free crystalline silicas, e.g., crystobalite, tridymite, though rare in natural geologic formation, may be formed from quartz in steelmaking and in other high-heat smelting processes, and probably have a more powerful silicosis-producing action than quartz.

Conglomerate silicosis is the result of the matting together by fibrosis of silicotic nodules, frequently associated with caseous areas, which often but by no means always show conclusive histologic evidence of tuberculosis. These changes account for the right heart strain, hypertrophy, and failure which may develop subsequently, perhaps as a consequence of the pulmonary vascular bed's being reduced by the fibrosis and tissue loss and associated emphysematous changes in the adjacent lung. A reversible element in the pulmonary hypertension may also be present, related perhaps to hypoxia or hypercapnia or both.

Clinical Manifestations. Even in nodular silicosis (in which the radiologic lesions are fibrous nodules, not collagenous dust macules, as in the "benign" pneumoconioses) there may be no clinical manifestations, and no apparent impairment in pulmonary function. The proportion of cases without signs and symptoms is probably only about 20 per cent, in contrast to about 90 per cent in the "benign" pneumoconioses of equivalent radiologic category.

The first complaint in nodular silicosis is commonly *shortness of breath,* brought on by moderate, and then progressively less, exercise until it is present at rest. This symptom is probably due to the increased muscular work required to ventilate incompliant lungs and is aggravated by increased minute ventilation to offset impaired gas exchange. Lung volumes are reduced as the nodular disease becomes more widespread. However, miners who smoke may present with the symptoms, signs, and classic lung function pattern of chronic obstructive lung disease, even though the radiologic pattern is primarily that of diffuse nodular pneumoconiosis.

When *complicated pneumoconiosis* develops *on a background of classic silicosis,* the symptoms, signs, and clinical presentation usually represent a progression from an already symptomatic state, and the diagnosis is made from the chest radiograph which shows a conglomeration of existing lesions, usually in the upper midzones, often bilateral, with eventual progression to the characteristic bilateral "angels' wings" shadows. The lung function pattern may suggest restrictive disease but frequently shows a pattern characteristic of obstructive disease, or there may be a mixed picture. Infection with *M. tuberculosis* is more likely to be demonstrable in conglomerate silicosis than in the progressive massive fibrosis of coal workers, and is more likely to behave and progress as in the nonsilicotic lung with constitutional symptoms (see below). Right heart strain and failure may complicate the picture, particularly if chronic bronchitis and emphysema are present.

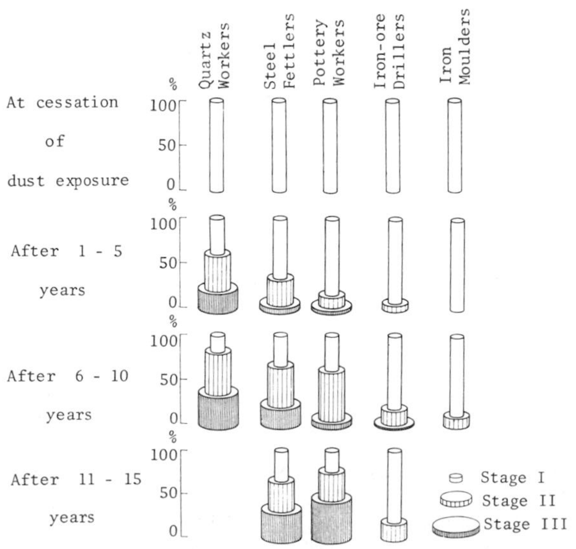

Figure 2. Rate of progression of different pneumoconioses after removal from dust exposure. The figures are based on five occupational groups of Swedish workers (each containing a minimum of ten cases) followed for 15 years after dust exposure ceased. (From Bruce, T., Nystrom, A., and Ahlmark, A. L.: Scand. J. Resp. Diseases, Supp. 63, 1968.)

Epidemiology and Prognosis. Prevalence rates vary from operation to operation, depending chiefly on the efficiency of dust control. Thus in the Witwatersrand gold mining industry, rates fell from 40 per 1000 underground miners in the 1920's to less than 10 per 1000 in the 1950's, and the average period of mining service prior to diagnosis rose from 10 to 23 years over this period. However, the simple silicosis of gold miners is undoubtedly a less benign disease than the simple pneumoconiosis of coal miners, despite the fact that it does not appear to affect life expectancy. Thus figures for Sweden indicate that, after withdrawal from exposure, x-ray changes never regress but progress in the majority of cases (Fig. 2). The prevalence of chronic obstructive lung disease does not appear to be occupationally related to classic silicosis, other than can be accounted for by a man's smoking habits.

526. COLLAGENOUS INORGANIC DUST PNEUMOCONIOSES OF THE DIFFUSE TYPE

Examples. These pneumoconioses include *asbestosis* in mining, milling, manufacturing, and all the secondary industrial uses of asbestos; *aluminosis,* as in shaver's disease; *talcosis* in miners and millers of talc; and *chronic beryllium disease of the lung.*

Pathogenesis and Mechanisms. Asbestos, the most important mineral in this group, occurs in several forms: *chrysotile* (a magnesium silicate, occurring as long, white, flexible fibers), the chief asbestos of commerce, mined primarily in Canada and the U.S.S.R. as well as in Italy and in Southern Africa; and the *amphiboles,* iron silicates (occurring as brittle fibers such as amosite, anthophyllite, and blue crocidolite) mined in South Africa, Australia, and Finland. Exposure occurs in mining and milling, and in the manufacture of a wide variety of the commodities used by modern man. *Asbestos cement products,* such as tiles and pipes, account for 70 per cent of production; and *insulation materials,* including floor tiles, for another 10 per cent; the rest is used in *paper, friction materials* (car brake and clutch linings), and *textiles* for use as protection against heat in industry and in homes.

The extent to which asbestos fibers penetrate the lung in all likelihood depends on their physical properties, the curly fibers of chrysotile being more likely to impinge on the mucus blanket than the short straight amphibole fibers. Some fibers appear to penetrate the interstitium directly and remain there, perhaps undergoing chemical and physical degeneration but nevertheless visible in much greater profusion than was ever suspected before the use of electron microscopy in their detection. Other fibers become engulfed by macrophages, and still others, but probably only a very small proportion, become enveloped in a smooth protein film which becomes iron-impregnated, giving rise to the typical drumhead, golden-brown *asbestos bodies,* a process also attributed at least in part to macrophage action. The pleura also appears to be a target organ, and *pleural reactions* to exposure include *effusion* (often bloody); dense, fibrous, *adhesive pleurisy; plaques* and *calcification* involving parietal rather than visceral pleura; and malignancy in the form of *mesothelioma* (see below).

It is not known which fibers are, or become, fibrogenic; nor is their precise mode of action known. Fibers deposited in alveolar structures elicit a cellular reaction similar to *desquamative alveolitis;* others at the level of the respiratory bronchiole produce an appearance of *bronchiolitis obliterans;* a third reaction is characterized by *interstitial edema* going on to *collagenization.* Nonspecific antinuclear antibodies may accelerate the fibrosis once it has started, and it eventually becomes confluent, obliterating air spaces and replacing them with cystic spaces lined by flattened epithelium *("honeycomb" lung).* Other mineral dusts which produce this pattern of diffuse fibrosis are talc, diatomaceous earth, and some of the very fine silicas currently used in industry, particularly if the exposure is heavy. *Caplan's syndrome* (see below), though more frequently recognized in coal workers, may be seen in relation to exposure to asbestos, silica, and probably most dusts.

Generalized pulmonary fibrosis may also be found in *chronic beryllium disease* of the lung, a manifestation of systemic poisoning with this mineral rather than a pneumoconiosis. The early signs are characterized by chronic interstitial pneumonitis, which is frequently granulomatous. The granulomas may vary from loose collections of histiocytes to large circumscribed granulomas, often containing giant cells with various inclusion bodies, indistinguishable histologically from sarcoidosis. The end result is frequently fibrosis of varying severity. Diagnosis can be made with certainty only by isolation of the element beryllium in tissues or body fluids. There is often a very long period of latency, up to 30 years, and initial exposure may only have been indirect, so that cases related to the manufacture of fluorescent light in the United States during World War II continue to be reported today, even though the use of beryllium in the fluorescent lamp industry ceased in 1949. Although its modern uses, particularly those concerned with space exploration, appear to be better controlled, physicians should remain vigilant because new cases continue to be added to the U.S. Beryllium Registry at the Massachusetts General Hospital.

Clinical Manifestations. These are no different from those of diffuse pulmonary fibrosis, whatever the underlying cause. In some subjects *dyspnea* is the first symptom, brought on at first by considerable exertion and then by progressively less effort, until it is eventually present at rest. In other subjects, an *irritating dry cough* precedes the awareness of shortness of breath, often by many years. With the progress of the disease, the cough may become productive, and *spells of chest pain* may be associated with the coughing. When the condition is advanced, there are usually diffuse basal rales, but these may also occur early before radiologic evidence of lung changes. The lung signs may be modified by the presence of pleural thickening or calcification. Respiratory failure may only appear late in the course of the disease, with pulmonary hypertension, right heart strain, and right heart failure. Nor is the victim of these diffuse pneumoconioses immune from the attack by general atmospheric pollutants—in particular, cigarette smoking—which may encourage the development of chronic bronchitis and bronchiectasis and increase the risk of bronchial neoplasm.

The *established case of asbestosis* is associated with changes in pulmonary function characteristic of restrictive lung disease, i.e., small volumes, impaired gas exchange with reduced diffusing capacity, and hyperventilation on effort and eventually at rest. The earliest function changes in response to asbestos dust exposure appear to be reduced vital capacity and increased exercise ventilation, tests which may eventually prove useful in the longitudinal surveillance of exposed workers. In addition, the function changes of chronic obstructive lung disease are not infrequently seen, particularly in workers who smoke.

In certain parts of the world, e.g., Finland, *pleural calcification* may appear as the only manifestation of exposure to asbestos, and less commonly to talc and mica. It is rarely seen under 20 years of industrial exposure, and neighborhood cases are seen with diminishing frequency as the circumferential distance of the place of residence from the industry increases.

Epidemiology and Prognosis. The *attack rate of asbestosis* varies in different industries (probably in relation to the heaviness of exposure) from under 10 per cent of working miners in open mining, as in Quebec, up to over 70 per cent in men with over 20 years' exposure in the insulation and construction industries.

The epidemiology of *population exposure to asbestos* has been established from the search for asbestos bodies in lung scrapings or extruded lung fluid in routine autopsies. Positive results are reported in many parts of the world, ranging from 1 per cent in rural Scotland to over 50 per cent in Finland, the site of the world's oldest known asbestos deposits. Insofar as the lung is an accumulator over time, and the world's use of asbestos is increasing dramatically, it is not surprising that this percentage is increasing in adults in London; New York studies by contrast report between 50 and 60 per cent both in recent and in 1934 autopsy material. It must be emphasized that the presence of *ferruginous bodies* (as experts now urge that they be called) indicates exposure, not disease. Nor are they specific for asbestos, because other types of fibers, e.g., glass, wool, cotton, talc, may constitute their core, and the lung probably uses this method to "inactivate" a large variety of inhaled particles. However, their presence in the sputum should alert the physician to the possibility of asbestos-related disease.

527. NEOPLASIA ASSOCIATED WITH EXPOSURE TO INORGANIC DUSTS

Asbestos. Exposure to asbestos increases the attack rate (probably in a dose-related fashion) of *bronchial carcinoma,* particularly and perhaps only in smokers, suggesting a synergism between carcinogens. The presence of asbestosis increases the risk, and some reports indicate that neoplasia will develop in 50 per cent of patients with already established asbestosis. Exposure to asbestos dust is also associated with increased risk of *gastric neoplasia,* presumably because of dust swallowing. Finally a rare tumor, *mesothelioma of the pleura and/or peritoneum,* occurs with greater frequency not only in industrially exposed populations, but also in association with indirect exposure, often after a long latent period, e.g., neighborhood exposure as a child 40 years before.

Although all types of asbestos fiber are implicated in the increased incidence of neoplasia, the order of increase varies, being on the whole higher for those engaged in processing and using than for those engaged in mining or milling. To what extent these differences are attributable to dust dose, fiber type, changes in physical and chemical properties with processing, and/or contamination by cocarcinogens remains to be determined.

Airborne Radioactive Particles. An increased number of deaths from lung cancer have been observed in American uranium miners, the risk being related to the radiation dose with a preponderance of small cell cancers. Increased deaths from lung cancer have also been observed in miners handling other materials, thought to be noncarcinogenic, in whom exposure has occurred to mine air contaminated by radon decay products from the ore-bearing rock or mine water, e.g., fluorspar miners of St. Lawrence, Newfoundland, and hematite miners in Cumberland, England.

Whether or not a neoplasm is occupation associated makes no difference to the outcome as far as the individual patient is concerned; *recognition of this association* on the part of the attending physician may, however, be important both from the patient's point of view (if there is a question of compensation) and from the point of view of the patient's working colleagues, since index cases serve to direct attention to occupational hazards.

528. COMPLICATED PNEUMOCONIOSIS

Examples. Examples of the complicated pneumoconioses include *progressive massive fibrosis of coal workers* and *Caplan's syndrome.*

Pathogenesis and Mechanisms. Most inorganic dust pneumoconioses can advance to progressive massive fibrosis whether or not exposure continues. Thus, although initially the response to dust exposure may be a macrophage reaction producing a noncollagenous response with little effect on the lung architecture, years later the same lung tissue may react to the same dust with severe fibrosis which obliterates and destroys all anatomic structure. The lesions of *progressive massive fibrosis in coal workers* (PMF) consist of dust irregularly mixed with bundles of coarse, hyaline collagen fibers. Few blood vessels and air passages are seen, but the persistence of internal elastic lamellae suggests that they have been obliterated by invading fibrous tissue. Sclerosis of the vessel walls and intimal thickening at the periphery of the lesions are common. At autopsy histologic and/or bacteriologic evidence of tuberculosis is found in about half the cases, even though in only a small proportion is it possible to recover tubercle bacilli in the sputum during life.

Several mechanisms may be operative in the development of complicated pneumoconiosis, of which infection by *M. tuberculosis* and/or atypical mycobacteria is probably the most frequent (the recovery rate of organisms both in life and at autopsy increases with increasing effort and has exceeded 50 per cent in some autopsy series). Other factors are the overwhelming of clearance mechanisms by lung dust; aseptic necrosis owing to interference with blood supply; significant silica contamination of the coal dust; and, finally, reaction on an immunologic basis, perhaps caused by liberation of antigenic material from macrophages damaged by dust. A comparable mechanism in the susceptible individual is thought to occur in *Caplan's syndrome.* Caplan observed an association between rheumatoid arthritis and a particular radiologic picture, characterized by well-defined opacities 0.5 to 5 cm in diameter, widely distributed and developing rather more suddenly than progressive massive fibrosis, often on a background of slight or no pneumoconiosis. Some lesions eventually cavitate, then shrink, perhaps with calcifications, and may later become incorporated into a mass radiologically indistinguishable from progressive massive fibrosis. Histologically, the rheumatoid nodule is distinguished by wide concentric bands of necrotic collagen separated by bands of dust, with a peripheral zone of active inflammation and a well-marked arteritis in the adjacent vessels. Caplan's syndrome, though first recognized and most frequently seen in coal miners, has been described in workers in foundries, asbestos, potteries, sandblasting, and boiler scaling.

Clinical Manifestations. In coal workers, the appearance of progressive massive fibrosis usually marks the onset of symptoms and signs of lung disease. The first symptom is commonly *dyspnea* on heavy effort, and subsequently at lesser work loads until it becomes evident at rest. The changes in function initially suggest loss of functioning volume, followed by a generalized restrictive lung disease. The symptom of cough does not appear to be more common in the earlier stages of complicated pneumoconiosis than in simple pneumoconiosis. *Melanoptysis* (sudden coughing up of a moderate amount of jet black fluid) is not uncommon, and frequently relates to cavitation. *Chest pain,* dull and aching, and diffusely located, is common, and there is an increasing tendency to *acute purulent bronchitis.* Pulmonary hypertension and right heart hypertrophy, leading ultimately to *right heart failure,* is present in many instances, with the usual symptoms and signs. When infection with *M. tuberculosis* appears to be the factor precipitating the development of the complicated pneumoconiosis, it is seldom accompanied by the usual systemic symptoms, i.e., fever, weight loss, and hemoptysis.

When the chest roentgenogram suggests Caplan's syndrome (see above), serum tests for rheumatoid factor are positive in 80 per cent of cases, whereas arthritis, already present in about 50 per cent of cases, may develop in others only after a delay of several years.

Epidemiology and Prognosis. Attack rates of progressive massive fibrosis in Welsh coal miners increase from 1 per cent in the lowest category of simple pneumoconiosis to 30 per cent in advanced simple pneumoconiosis, and appear to be highest in the younger men working on heavier jobs. Rheumatoid pneumoconiosis occurs in 2 to 6 per cent of United Kingdom coal miners affected by pneumoconiosis, and should be suspected when PMF develops suddenly in an individual with minimal or no pneumoconiosis. Prevalence rates of PMF relate to the prevalence of pneumoconiosis in that industry concerned (which, in turn, relates to dustiness), as well as to the prevalence of tuberculosis. It is therefore somewhat disappointing to find that vigorous antituberculosis measures in coal-mining communities have not reduced attack rates of progressive massive fibrosis as dramatically as hoped.

529. TREATMENT AND PREVENTION OF THE INORGANIC DUST PNEUMOCONIOSES

Treatment. There is *no specific treatment for the simple nodular or diffuse inorganic dust pneumoconioses.* The medical management of associated chronic obstructive lung disease and right heart failure and pulmonary heart disease is the same whether or not it coexists with pneumoconiosis (see Ch. 507). Progression of the condition, particularly to complicated pneumoconiosis, appears to depend as much on past as on subsequent exposure. Thus the physician faces the difficult question of *whether he should advise the individual patient to find other employment.* A reasonable decision must be based on an accurate knowledge of what determines progression of simple pneumoconiosis and the attack rates of complicated pneumoconiosis in the particular operation concerned. Such knowledge is accumulating in the larger industries which can mount well-planned research operations, e.g., the coal mining industries in Great Britain, Germany, and the United States, but cannot necessarily be applied to other situations, e.g., a welder in a small local plant. In general, most physicians, when faced with such a problem, permit continued employment, with the proviso that regular medical surveillance be available.

Likewise, in *complicated pneumoconiosis,* medical management is concerned with treatment of the complications. When active tuberculous infection or even a positive skin test to PPD can be demonstrated, appropriate chemotherapy should be instituted (see Ch. 228). However, controlled clinical trials do not support the routine use of tuberculosis chemoprophylaxis in all cases. Since complicated pneumoconiosis is invariably accompanied by disability, often associated with right heart failure, most patients with complicated pneumoconiosis will have already left the industry concerned. Opinion is divided on the advisability of withdrawal from exposure if the patient is still so occupied.

Dust Control. Inorganic dust pneumoconioses cannot be treated effectively, but they can be prevented, and *prevention* means, essentially, *dust control.* Attack rate increases with exposure, and there is a dust dose–disease relationship. Thus *control should be at an epidemiologic level,* aiming at controlling the exposure of the community at risk, not at a personal level with the use of masks or respirators which should be regarded only as temporary until the environment has been controlled. Dust can seldom be completely eliminated from industrial operations. However, disease could be controlled if the minimal exposure which produces health effects in a given industry were known. It is possible to envisage a future in which, using cumulative ongoing records of each worker's exposure, operations could be planned so that no worker would be likely to exceed the exposure known to produce disease within his working life. Such an ambitious scheme, already under way in the West German coal mining industry, is likely to be set up only in large industries able to mount extensive research programs. However, for smaller industries, it is quite valid to assert that *less dust means less disease;* definitions of low-risk levels of exposure for different dusts (threshold limit values) are annually revised by bodies such as the American Conference of Governmental Industrial Hygienists and provide general reference standards. There is, however, room for much more definitive action than has occurred in the past on the part of the treating physicians, communities, and governments concerned.

Tuberculosis Control. Medical attention should be directed toward reducing the attack rates of complicated pneumoconiosis and silicotuberculosis. All subjects with pneumoconiosis are at a higher risk in terms of tuberculosis than the general population; in addition the circumstances of employment may favor infection, e.g., recruitment of workers from populations in which infection with tubercle bacilli occurs relatively late in life. Case finding and control of tuberculosis should thus be of a particularly high standard in populations exposed to an inorganic dust hazard; at the very least this should include the annual chest roentgenogram. Finally, gastrectomy for peptic ulcer should be avoided in subjects with pneumoconiosis, because this increases the chance of developing PMF much in the same way that it constitutes a risk factor in developing active tuberculosis.

Prophylactic Substances. Studies in laboratory animals have indicated that certain substances (ferric oxide, iron, coal, aluminum, and more recently poly-2-vinylpyridine-N-oxide or PVNO) inhibit the biologic effects of silica dust. Of these materials only aluminum has received a trial in man when it was introduced into the gold mines of Ontario in 1943; however, no conclusive evidence on its effectiveness has come out of this experience, and this type of prophylaxis is a sorry substitute for proper environmental dust control. A therapeutic trial of PVNO has been started in West German coal miners, and a prophylactic trial may be undertaken in the future.

ORGANIC "DUSTS"

530. FACTORS INFLUENCING REACTIONS TO INHALED ORGANIC "DUSTS"

The inorganic "dusts" referred to here include fungal spores, components of plants, and a wide variety of other biologic material. Unlike the inorganic dusts, the effects of which are related primarily to exposure dose, the effects of exposure to inorganic "dusts" appear to depend to a major extent on the reactivity of the subject, atopic individuals usually showing both immediate and delayed responses (attributed to Type I and Type III allergy, respectively) and nonatopic individuals usually showing delayed responses only (attributed to Type III allergy). The list of organic "dusts" generated in industrial and commercial operations and capable of producing *asthma in the atopic individuals* is virtually limitless, and such subjects frequently withdraw voluntarily from an occupation involving exposure. Treatment of such patients is on an individual basis (see Ch. 505). However, with the relatively heavy exposures which occur in certain industrial and other commercial processes often involving large numbers of workers, *many nonatopic individuals* may also be affected, and the term *organic dust pneumoconioses* has come into use to underline their occupational association. Evaluation of the individual patient should therefore be made in terms of the following three factors considered by Pepys to be of prime importance in determining an individual's response: (1) his immunologic reactivity (whether or not atopic, since this may determine the approach to treatment); (2) the nature of the inhaled antigen, including particle size, which will influence its penetration in the respiratory tract; and (3) the nature and circumstances of exposure (obtained by careful history taking).

531. ASTHMA-LIKE REACTIONS TO ORGANIC "DUSTS"

Examples. Examples include asthma in workers exposed to the enzymes of *B. subtilis* in the manufacture of detergents and asthma in workers with Western red cedar *(Thuja plicata)*.

Pathogenesis and Mechanisms. Reactions to these occupational exposures occur usually within months of first exposure in the case of the enzymes, but often only after years in the case of *Thuja plicata*. The nonatopic individual is as much at risk as the atopic individual. In the case of *detergent workers who are atopic,* bronchial provocation tests invariably elicit a dual response, i.e., immediate and late (within hours), attributed to Type I (IgE-mediated) and Type III (precipitin-mediated) hypersensitivity, respectively. In *nonatopic workers* (usually the majority of the factory personnel), the immediate effects may be irritant rather than allergic, but there is growing evidence that the late effects are precipitin mediated (see Ch. 505). Skin reactions are positive in about half the workers, but do not distinguish the symptomatic from the nonsymptomatic.

Clinical Manifestations. In sensitized workers, symptoms follow exposure within minutes and include chest tightness, cough, and wheezing, with audible rhonchi. Without bronchodilators, the symptoms subside slowly over about four hours, to be followed by the development of *dyspnea, wheezing,* and *rhonchi,* and the general symptoms of headache, malaise, and muscle pains at about six hours. *Nocturnal exacerbations of wheezing* are also characteristic and have been attributed to inhibition of endogenous regulatory mechanisms, and their association with a daytime occupational exposure can easily be missed. There is no present evidence of chronic effects, but the manufacture of these detergents is too recent to be certain that such effects may not occur, particularly because animal exposures, admittedly to much higher doses, have produced diffuse emphysema. A case of chronic granulomatous lung disease attributed to the inhalation of cedar sawdust has been reported.

Treatment and Prevention. Sensitized individuals should be removed from exposure. However, since some 50 per cent of exposed workers appear to become sensitized, control must be environmental. In some instances this has been achieved by coating the enzyme particles to increase their size (from 0.5 to 1.0 mm), thus reducing the chance that they will be inhaled into smaller airways.

532. AIRWAY OBSTRUCTION (DELAYED, EVENTUALLY IRREVERSIBLE) DUE TO ORGANIC "DUSTS"

Examples. Examples include *byssinosis* in association with the processing of *cotton* (particularly spinning), *flax,* and *soft hemp dusts*; *jute* may be implicated; sisal probably is not.

Clinical Manifestations. An acute response to cotton dust may occur at first exposure or only after many years of exposure; the term *byssinosis* usually refers to the latter, and, again, the nonatopic individual appears to be as much at risk as the atopic one. The diagnosis is made on the basis of a characteristic symptom pattern in a subject with suitable exposure. Symptoms are *cough, tightness in the chest,* and *breathlessness,* occurring at first only occasionally on the first day of the working week (Grade $^1/_2$), then regularly on Monday morning (Grade 1), then persisting beyond Monday (Grade 2), and finally, after several years, persisting throughout the week (Grade 3), when it is indistinguishable from nonindustrial chronic obstructive lung disease. There are no specific radiologic changes. Attack rates may reach over 90 per cent of exposed populations; a family history of atopy, with hypersensitivity to inhaled histamine, is unusual; immediate skin reactions to cotton dust are infrequent. Cigarette smoking increases the risk and severity of the disease. In the nonsymptomatic worker, dust exposure may result in small decreases in airway conductance, suggesting a nonspecific effect on major airways. By contrast in the worker with the *Monday morning dyspnea* of byssinosis, exposure causes a reduction in forced expiratory flow rates and vital capacity with effects on flow volume curves which can be improved by isoproterenol inhalation. Antihistaminic drugs may also improve the flow rates in byssinosis without necessarily affording subjective relief, a finding pointing to the probable importance of small airway involvement. Pretreatment with orciprenaline, antihistamines, and ascorbic acid appears to diminish the biologic response to cotton dust.

Pathogenesis and Mechanisms. It is thought that some fraction of the offending dusts (probably the protein fraction) causes the nonantigenic release of histamine and perhaps of other pharmacologically active substances; these reduce the caliber of large and/or small airways, the site of action perhaps being related to dust size and site of maximal deposition. Whether the histamine release is entirely nonantigenic, as originally proposed, or whether there is an antigenic component to the reaction, as recently proposed, has not been determined. Information on the long-term effects comes from the few published autopsy reports in which chronic bronchitis and emphysema were noted, together with occasional "ferruginous" bodies containing what was assumed to be cotton fibers; in addition, the lungs contain somewhat increased amounts of nonspecific dusts, probably carbonaceous. A single report of extensive fibrosis with plasma cell infiltration suggests an immunologic background for the disease, indicating the need for further study.

Epidemiology. Attack rates of byssinosis vary widely, usually, though not invariably, in relation to exposure levels; in some instances plant modernization has even led to increased environmental dust. Reported rates for Egyptian workers vary from 0 to 90 per cent; for Swedish, Dutch, and British workers, about 50 per cent; and for American workers, up to 30 per cent; whereas a study of retired rural Spanish workers shows a high prevalence of chronic disease. There are no data on the rate and inevitability of progression from Grade I (essentially reversible) to Grade III (essentially irreversible) disease. However, it is not insignificant; indeed the recognition of byssinosis resulted from the observation of increased mortality and morbidity rates for cardiovascular and respiratory disease in certain Lancashire cotton workers.

Prevention. Present efforts to control byssinosis are directed toward dust control by means of environmental engineering, and its success depends on defining as accurately as possible the dust levels which constitute risk in respect of particle size and number in relation to toxic properties of the dust concerned. However, a recent study of cotton workers under controlled dust exposures has shown that *preprocessing the cotton* by autoclaving diminished by tenfold the incidence of the biologic response. Thus dust control of the future may well be a source intervention as envisaged many years ago by Schilling. Medical aspects of prevention include a *preemployment examination* (to eliminate those with pre-existing lung disease and those who show a marked response to dust) and *regular medical surveillance,* because this may be one of the few industrial exposures in which progression to chronic disease may be halted by removal from exposure at any early clinical stage of the disease.

533. EXTRINSIC ALLERGIC ALVEOLITIS

Examples. Examples of this disorder include *farmer's lung, bagassosis* in sugar cane workers, *mushroom-worker's lung, maplebark-stripper's lung, suberosis* of cork workers, *sequoiosis,* and *malt-worker's lung.*

Pathogenesis and Mechanisms. The term *extrinsic allergic alveolitis* is used to describe reactions produced in the gas-exchanging tissues of the lung, usually of nonatopic individuals, after inhalation of spores of a number of different fungi. It is thought to occur when the spores penetrate the alveoli in sufficient numbers initially to sensitize (with the production of serum precipitins) and subsequently to elicit an alveolitis. The reaction is thought to be a Type III or Arthus one on the basis of its time relationship to exposure, its correlation with the presence of serum precipitins and delayed skin reactions, and its inhibition by corticosteroid drugs. The presence of precipitins, however, is not decisive, and it is presumed that a critical balance between antigen exposure and antibody production is necessary for the formation of the damaging antibody-antigen complexes to occur which mediate the inflammatory and probably also the granulomatous response. Identification of the major source of allergen in *farmer's lung* (the spores of the thermophilic actinomyces, *Micropolyspora faeni* and *Thermoactinomyces vulgaris,* found in moldy hay) has led to the recognition of an increasing number of diseases of similar origin and of certain unusual exposure risks, e.g., contamination of air conditioner systems with spores; undoubtedly more will be documented in the future. The main examples currently recognized are *bagassosis,* from the spores of *T. sacchari* in moldy bagasse (sugar-cane residue used in the production of hard board, acoustic, and other thermal boards); *mushroom-worker's lung,* usually from the spores of both *T. vulgaris* and *M. faeni,* two of some 20 fungi found in mushroom compost; *malt-worker's lung* from the spores of *Aspergillus clavatus* and *A. fumigatus* in moldy barley and malt dust; *maplebark-stripper's lung,* from the spores of *Cryptostroma corticale; sequoiosis* from the spores of *Pullularia pullulans; cheese-washer's lung* from the spores of *Penicillium casei;* and *suberosis* from moldy cork dust. All these spores are of the order of 6 μ or less in size, but there is evidence that spores up to 10 μ may penetrate the lung in adequate numbers to elicit alveolitis. In addition, a number of heterologous serum proteins are implicated, e.g., those of avian origin occurring in bird droppings, causing *bird-breeder's lung,* and disease caused by antigens of insect origin, e.g., wheat weevil.

Lung biopsy in the early stages shows changes attributable to a foreign body reaction resulting from the cellular removal and sequestration of large antigen-antibody complexes, rather than implicating an additional Type IV allergy. The changes may resolve completely or may, particularly if associated with recurrent exposures, go on to fibrosis, which may also involve the organization of endobronchial exudates with bronchiolitis obliterans.

Clinical Manifestations. After a variable period of exposure, symptoms usually develop within six to eight hours of re-exposure, commonly appearing in the evening after a day's work with the particular spore source. *Fever, chills, malaise,* and generalized nonpleuritic *chest pain* are characteristic, together with a dry irritant *cough* productive of scanty sputum, and respiratory distress. *Weight loss* is common. On clinical examination in the acute stage, rales are heard, often less widespread than anticipated, and rhonchi are not usually prominent. The chest roentgenogram, though sometimes normal, usually shows a widespread interstitial pattern of a reticular nature, occasionally with fine, nodular shadows, which may become confluent. Pulmonary function measurements are in keeping with the location of the disease in alveoli and small airways, i.e., volumes are reduced, gas exchange is impaired, but expiratory flow rates are usually normal. Only occasionally does an obstructive function pattern predominate.

In the absence of further exposure, clinical, radiologic, and function changes usually resolve fully, or there may be minor residual changes; these, however, recur with re-exposure. A *chronic form* appears to follow the superimposition of repeated acute episodes, particularly if the initial acute episode is not severe (usually because spore dose is lower) and the victim is not aware of its association with his occupation. In these individuals the chest film is more suggestive of a diffuse pulmonary fibrosis, sometimes complicated by cystic changes and associated with appropriate effects on lung function. The long-term complications include pulmonary hypertension, right heart strain, and failure.

Diagnosis and Treatment. Diagnosis during the acute attack is made on the basis of a characteristic clinical pattern, providing that there is a suitable exposure history. The chest film and lung function tests may add confirmatory evidence. A high percentage of patients have positive serologic tests (such as the demonstration of precipitins, double diffusion tests, and immunoelectrophoresis) in the acute episode, but the number diminishes with time thereafter. Taken on their own, however, positive reactions are evidence of exposure rather than evidence of disease. In subjects seen in remission, in whom serologic tests are negative, the *cautious use of provocation tests* involving inhaled aqueous extracts of the appropriate allergen is suggested; these result in symptoms and in reduction of forced expiratory volumes and VC several hours after the challenge. The diagnosis of the chronic case may be more difficult because of its nonspecific character, particularly if there have been no acute episodes which are clearly exposure related.

In the treatment of the acute episodes, the usual general measures are advised, together with adrenal corticosteroids which, in some cases, produce very satisfactory remissions, though it is uncertain whether they can always prevent progression to fibrosis. Avoidance of reexposure is of prime importance to prevent repetitive episodes with progression to chronic form.

Epidemiology and Prevention. It is difficult to estimate attack rates in undefined exposed populations (as, for instance, in self-employed farmers). Furthermore, attack rates vary with spore dose, and this again will vary with the seasonal conditions predisposing to moldy hay, bagasse, or sequoia dust as the case may be. Bagassosis, once considered a rare entity, has been reported in half the workers in a Puerto Rican factory, and on another occasion in 10 per cent of employees of a West Indian plant.

Prevention at an epidemiologic level, i.e., by removal of exposure hazards, is not easy, because the conditions favoring spore formation occur only intermittently. Spraying with 2 per cent propionic acid, an inexpensive fungicide, has been suggested. Nor is the prevention at the individual case level practicable, since masks appear to be capable only of reducing, not of wholly excluding, particles of small size such as the 1 μ spores of *M. faeni.* Furthermore, the increased resistance to breathing on exercise imposed by even the best mask limits their regular use. The only safe course is to ensure that the subject who has suffered one acute episode avoid altogether any further exposure, a drastic recommendation which may involve a farmer, for instance, in giving up his means of livelihood.

534. CHRONIC INTERSTITIAL (LIPOID) PNEUMONIA

Example. Blackfat tobacco smokers' lung.

Pathogenesis and Mechanism. In Guyana, a high prevalence of diffuse interstitial pulmonary fibrosis in older individuals, recognized for at least 25 to 30 years, has recently been shown to be due to a chronic interstitial lipoid pneumonia, the consequence of many years of smoking blackfat tobacco. Blackfat tobacco is unusual in that certain oils are added to the leaf during processing, and smoking causes these to distil over into the lungs. Lung biopsy has shown the lipid to be present in alveolar phagocytes, lying free in alveoli or in collections in the interstitium in a peribronchiolar or subpleural location where they evoke first a cellular and eventually (if the dose is large) a collagenous response, with lesions resembling those of liquid paraffin granulomas. The end result is a diffuse interstitial fibrosis and vasculitis, with deposits of lipid and black material in the walls of blood vessels and in the interstitium. Immunologic studies have for practical purposes excluded hypersensitivity to the suspected agent, teichoic acid, and extrinsic allergic alveolitis as the background of the chronic interstitial fibrosis.

Clinical Manifestations. The symptoms are cough, dyspnea, and rather striking weight loss, with eventually pulmonary heart disease, in subjects with a long history (usually 20 to 30 years) of blackfat tobacco smoking. Basal crepitations are characteristic, and wheezing is unusual except during superimposed infection. Radiologic changes are those of diffuse interstitial fibrosis, whereas the pulmonary function changes are unusual in that an obstructive profile predominates in a diffuse pulmonary fibrosis.

Treatment, Epidemiology, and Prevention. Treatment, essentially palliative, is not different from that of other chronic interstitial lung diseases. Giving up smoking blackfat tobacco is apparently no guarantee that symptoms will not develop in the future. The steady decline in blackfat tobacco smoking in Guyana suggests that this local health problem is also on the decline. However, *recognition that inhaled additives to tobacco* can produce *long-term effects* of a *low-grade inflammatory type* on the lungs is of great importance to physicians the world over who are concerned with the health effects of tobacco smoking.

CHEMICAL IRRITANTS

535. CHEMICALS CAUSING ASTHMA-LIKE REACTIONS

Examples. Those affected include workers with *toluene di-isocyanate* (TDI) and other isocyanates used in the application of certain lacquers and resins and in the manufacture of polyurethane foams for cushioning, insulation, and soft toys; and *cable jointers* using certain aluminum soldering flux. *Platinosis* (describing rhinorrhea, asthma, and urticaria) results from exposure to complex platinum salts in refineries.

Pathogenesis and Mechanisms. From carefully controlled occupational-type provocation tests monitored by measurements of forced expiratory volumes, it has been shown that immediate, late, and dual asthmatic reactions occur in workers sensitized to the chemical vapors, fumes, and dusts listed above. The presence of reaginic and precipitating antibodies against platinum salts and against TDI in symptomatic subjects suggests an immunologic basis (Types I and III allergy) for these reactions, and others may well come to light in the future. Furthermore, it seems likely that Type I reactions occur in the atopic worker who is exposed, and Type III reactions in the nonatopic worker. These reactions, which may follow exposure to very low doses, should be distinguished from the well recognized irritant effects of the same chemicals in higher doses and other chemicals discussed subsequently. Thus sensitization to isocyanate vapors may occur at very low exposure levels (0.003 parts per million) which is well below the threshold limit value of 0.02 ppm, which is again below the level at which the irritant effects of isocyanates are seen.

Clinical Manifestations. Symptoms of asthma, immediate and/or late and often nocturnal, develop after periods varying from one week to several months after first exposure and if possible should be distinguished from those of high dose irritation, of which eye, nose, and throat irritation are the most common. Symptoms subside after removal from exposure, and function may return to normal within days or weeks. However, re-exposure regularly results in recurrence, often more violent. The number of people who become sensitized varies and may be related to exposure level (estimated at 4 per cent in a well-controlled plant and 100 per cent in a poor one). Most exposed persons show some reduction in expiratory flow rates during working hours, a change eliminated by the oral administration of an aminophylline compound.

Diagnosis and Treatment. Diagnosis depends on a high degree of suspicion particularly when symptoms occur predominantly at night, and can be confirmed using carefully controlled occupational-type provocation tests as suggested by Pepys. These can be carried out only under hospital supervision with monitoring of forced expiratory flow tests, together with observation of the effects of isoproterenol and dichromoglycolate on the reactions. Objective demonstration of sensitization is important, because it calls for removal from exposure with potential financial and other hardships for the worker. The suggestion that long-term exposure leads to chronic obstructive lung disease should be followed up, because it has been estimated, for example, that workers exposed to TDI number between 50,000 and 100,000 in the United States alone.

536. CHEMICAL BRONCHITIS

Examples. Those affected include workers exposed to sulfur dioxide (SO_2) in the *pulp and paper industry*; *refrigeration workers* exposed to ammonia (NH_3); and *chemical workers* exposed to sulfurous acid (H_2SO_3) and chlorine (Cl_2).

Pathogenesis and Mechanisms. The acutely irritant effects of these gases and mists can probably be attributed to their high solubility; of the physiologic gases, CO_2 is the most soluble (56.7 vols per cent in water at 37° C at 1 atmosphere); however, equivalent values for SO_2 (280 vols per cent), Cl_2 (257 vols per cent), and NH_3 (139 vols per cent) indicate their very much greater solubility. Accidental inhalation of high concentrations results in rapid solution in the mucous membranes of the upper airways with the formation of irritant compounds, e.g., H_2SO_3 from SO_2, NH_4OH from NH_3, HCl from Cl_2. The initial irritation causing *bronchorrhea* is rapidly followed by sloughing and a *frank necrotizing bronchitis.* If exposure is prolonged or unduly heavy, the lower respiratory tract becomes exposed, with the development of an *acute chemical pulmonary edema.* Recovery may be complete. However, residual mucosal scars and submucosal thickening are not uncommon, particularly if the mucosal sloughs were deep and secondary infection prominent. Acute chemical irritation may also result from the *aspiration of vomited or regurgitated material high in HCl content,* an event more common in the frail and elderly than is generally supposed, or in relation to blunting of the gag reflex as in anesthesia, head injuries, and alcoholic or other intoxications. If the aspirate is chiefly water or saline in small amounts, absorption is quick and the consequences usually slight. Large food particles on the other hand may obstruct large or small airways.

Clinical Manifestations. When exposure to a chemical irritant is heavy, clinical manifestations are invariably immediate, the patient is alerted to his exposure, and he makes every effort to remove himself therefrom. *Conjunctivitis, irritation* and *burning* in the *mucosa* of the mouth and throat, *cough, laryngitis, laryngospasm,* and *difficulty in breathing* are in keeping with the usual site of damage, i.e., upper respiratory tract, and coarse *rhonchi* are a characteristic physical finding, often with profound *mucorrhea,* which may be bloodstained. More profound *dyspnea* usually implies alveolar involvement resulting from either chemical edema or aspiration of bronchial sloughs. These complications can frequently be suspected from chest roentgenograms and may result in profound impairment of pulmonary blood gas exchange with *severe arterial hypoxemia* and a low arterial CO_2 tension. Nausea, vomiting, and stupor may complicate the picture.

If the patient survives the acute event, complete recovery is usual. However, some patients may be left with chronic bronchitis or saccular bronchiectasis or both, sometimes of considerable severity, with residual effects on pulmonary function.

Chronic irritation from long-term exposure to low doses, e.g., SO_2, as in city air pollution, Cl_2, as in chlorine plants, may perhaps be more important in terms of community health, particularly in relation to the etiology of chronic obstructive lung disease.

Treatment. *Acute chemical bronchitis* and *acute chemical pulmonary edema* are *medical emergencies.* In the acute phase, survival depends on maintaining airway patency and adequate oxygenation. To aspirate sloughs, it may be necessary to employ intubation, lavage with saline, using modest amounts only (10 ml at a single flush), and even bronchoscopy. Controlled oxygen administration is usually necessary, and frequently must be supplemented with positive pressure respiration, assisted in mild cases, controlled in the severe ones. Corticosteroids, thought to modify the acute inflammatory reaction at the gas-exchanging surface, should always be given in the presence of pulmonary edema and indeed are recommended by some in all cases of exposure on a prophylactic basis. Heavy initial doses should be reduced as the clinical picture improves. Infection should be controlled by the use of antimicrobial drugs.

537. CHEMICAL PULMONARY EDEMA

Examples. Chemical pulmonary edema can result from exposure to *oxides of nitrogen* such as may occur in freshly filled silos (*silo-filler's disease*); welding in poorly ventilated spaces; misfires in blasting operations carried out in closed spaces (e.g., mines); burning of N_2-containing materials in closed spaces; *exposure to phosgene* after its liberation from many chlorinated substances, e.g., carbon tetrachloride in fire extinguishers; or *accidental ingestion of the herbicide paraquat.*

Pathogenesis and Mechanisms. The immediate clinical effects of exposure of the oxides of nitrogen and phosgene may be mild, but a severe, chemical pulmonary edema, often fatal, may develop after a *delay of several hours to several days.* The physicochemical processes underlying this delay are not fully understood. If the acute event is not immediately fatal, healing by fibrosis may lead to the development of *bronchiolitis fibrosa obliterans,* usually four to eight weeks after initial exposure, often with a fatal result. Autopsy studies show widespread organization of exudates, primarily located in the terminal bronchioles; atelectasis is not seen, however, presumably because of the collateral ventilation now recognized to be extensive in man.

Acute chemical pulmonary edema of delayed onset (one to three days) may also follow the *accidental ingestion of the herbicide paraquat* (1,1′-dimethyl-4,4′-dipyridilium), a common constituent of commercial weed-killers. Thus the acute effects of this poison, which also include acute oral, esophageal, hepatic, and renal damage, become evident only after a delay of several days, i.e., after the peak blood levels and at a time when most of the material has been excreted. These characteristics have earned it the name of the "hit and run" poison, and once the pulmonary damage starts, it invariably runs a relentless course to death within weeks from respiratory failure caused by a *diffuse progressive pulmonary fibrosis* and replacement of gas-exchanging tissue by cystic changes. Its mechanism of action is unknown, but it has been suggested that the primary action is to inactivate or depress formation of surfactant.

Clinical Manifestations. Immediate effects of exposure to the oxides of nitrogen and phosgene, which may include cough, chest irritation, and sputum, are often so mild that the victim may even fail to report to the first-aid post, only to return from hours to several days later with the symptoms, signs, and chest roentgenogram of *acute, severe, pulmonary edema.* Hence it is reasonable to suggest observation in hospital for 48 hours after possible exposures (e.g., for firefighters who have been inside burning buildings), perhaps even giving steroid therapy if suspicion of exposure is strong. In the mild case of edema, symptoms may escape attention, changes on the chest film at the most may be equivocal, and the diagnosis depends on the finding of coarse rales, sometimes lasting over a short period only, with a transient hypoxemia. Clinical management has been discussed above; in cases of frank, severe edema, steroid therapy should probably be prolonged for six to eight weeks to cover the period when the subacute complication of bronchiolitis obliterans is likely to develop. This complication, probably avoidable if steroid therapy is given early, should be suspected when symptoms recur or appear at three to six weeks, and generally responds to steroid therapy.

Management of a patient known to have ingested paraquat should include heroic measures to prevent absorption. In laboratory animals bentylol and/or Fuller's earth by mouth has been shown to inactivate the material more effectively than charcoal. Forced diuresis and hemodialysis are recommended once blood levels have risen. There is some evidence that corticosteroids may be effective in the treatment of the pulmonary edema, and that O_2 therapy should be used with the utmost caution, experimental work indicating that it potentiates the action of the poison.

Epidemiology. Large-scale heavy exposure to, for instance, oxides of nitrogen occurs only in relation to mass disasters, e.g., in the Cleveland clinic fire in 1929 owing to the burning of stored x-ray film, and in the Cocoanut Grove fire in Boston in 1943 owing to the burning of nitrogen-containing plastics. Many modern plastics no longer contain nitrogen. However, in most fires involving domestic buildings in which wood is used, circumstances exist in which these fumes could be evolved, and three or four cases are seen annually in most city hospitals.

538. RADIATION

Increased use of x-irradiation in the treatment of cancer of the breast and of various intrathoracic organs led to the recognition that the lungs themselves may be affected by this procedure. It is thought that the *acute changes,* which may come on within weeks of the onset of treatment up to six months after its cessation, include an alveolar cellular reaction followed by desquamation and in some instances by hyaline membrane formation. Focal necrosis of the bronchial mucosa may develop as a result of damage to capillary endothelium with subsequent necrosis and vascular occlusion. These changes may resolve or go on to loss of lung volume, sometimes of marked degree, occurring rather suddenly, and usually ascribed to fibrosis, shrinkage, and hyalinization, particularly if there has been infection. Studies in animals suggest, however, that the loss of volume may, on occasion, be due to atrophy and that the hyalinization may be in part due to autohypersensitivity, the consequence of new cell antigens formed as a result of the ionizing radiation.

There may be no clinical manifestations of *radiation pneumonitis* even in the face of definite radiologic changes. The most common symptom is a persistent, hacking dry cough. Fever, some dyspnea, and weakness may be seen, and the symptoms of radiation esophagitis are common. On physical examination the effects of radiation on the skin of the thorax are usually evident; rales and a friction rub may be found. The chest film characteristically reveals regional or diffuse haziness, and pulmonary function tests indicate a restrictive pattern. Spontaneous remission over weeks is frequent. Recommended therapy includes steroids (to lessen the chances of healing by fibrosis) and anticoagulants (to lessen the ischemic effects of small-vessel thrombosis commonly seen at autopsy), though the value of these measures has not been conclusively demonstrated (see Ch. 543 to 545). When *radiation fibrosis* supervenes, clinical presentation will depend on how much functioning lung tissue is lost and on the function in the remaining lung. Respiratory failure, pulmonary hypertension, and right heart failure may all follow.

Some authors suggest that there is a parenchymal reaction to ionizing radiation of the thorax in 100 per cent of cases so exposed, that some degree of pneumonitis is common if not invariable, though symptoms occur in a small percentage of these cases only, and that progression to radiation fibrosis is rare. Factors thought to affect the attack rate include total dose as well as the time over which it is given, and the technique of application. Clinically important reactions are unusual at total doses below 2000 rads and invariable above 6000 rads. The age of the patient, the chest wall thickness, and the presence of complicating disease may also be important. Individual factors remain to be identified, however, since identical doses can be harmless to one person and cause a severe reaction in another.

Inorganic Dusts

Becklake, M. R.: Pneumoconioses. *In* Handbook of Physiology, Respiration II. Baltimore, Williams & Wilkins Company, 1965, Chapter 71, p. 1601.
Biological effects of asbestos. Ann. N.Y. Acad. Sci., 132:338, 1965.
Bruce, T.: Occupational diseases of respiratory system. Scand. J. Resp. Dis., 63(supp.):73, 1968.
Coalworkers' pneumoconiosis. Ann. N.Y. Acad. Sci., Vol. 200, 1972.
Fitzgerald, M., Carrington, C. B., and Gaensler, E. A.: Environmental lung disease. Med. Clin. North Am., 57:593, 1973.
Hatch, T. F., and Gross, P.: Pulmonary Deposition and Retention of Inhaled Aerosols. New York, Academic Press, 1964.
Leading article: Asbestos → lung cancer → mesothelioma. Lancet, 1:815, 1973.
Selikoff, I. J., Bader, R. A., Bader, M. E., Churg, J., and Hammond, E. C.: Asbestosis and neoplasia. Am. J. Med., 42:487, 1967.
Stoeckle, J. D., Hardy, H. L., and Weber, A. L.: Chronic beryllium disease: Long-term follow-up of sixty cases and selective review of the literature. Am. J. Med., 46:545, 1969.
Walton, W. (ed.): Inhaled Particles and Vapours. III. Surrey, England, Unwin Bros. Ltd., Gresham Press, 1971.

Organic Dusts

Bouhuys, A., Gilson, J. C., and Schilling, R. S. F.: Byssinosis in the textile industry. Arch. Environ. Health, 21:475, 1970.
Hearn, C. E. D.: Bagassosis: An epidemiological, environmental and clinical survey. Brit. J. Industr. Med., 25:267, 1968.
Hogg, J. C., Macklem, P. T., and Thurlbeck, W. M.: Site and nature of airway obstruction in chronic obstructive lung disease. N. Engl. J. Med., 278:1355, 1968.
Merchant, J. A., Kilburn, K. H., and O'Fallon, W. M.: Byssinosis and chronic bronchitis among cotton textile workers. Ann. Intern. Med., 76:423, 1972.
Miller, G. I., Ashcraft, M. T., Beadnell, H. M. S. G., Wagner, J. C., and Pepys, J.: The lipoid pneumonia of blackfat tobacco smokers in Guyana. Quart. J. Med., 160:457, 1971.
Nicholson, D. P.: Extrinsic allergic pneumonias. Am. J. Med., 53:131, 1972.
Schilling, R. S. F.: Byssinosis in cotton and other textile workers. Lancet, 2:261, 319, 1956.

Chemical Irritants

Bates, D. V., Macklem, P. T., and Christie, R. V.: Respiratory Function in Disease. 2nd ed. Philadelphia, W. B. Saunders Company, 1971, pp. 389–398.
Connor, E. H., DuBois, A. B., and Comroe, J. H.: Acute chemical injury of the airways and lungs. Anesthesiology, 23:538, 1962.
Leading article: Poisoning from paraquat. Br. Med. J., 3:690, 1967.
Morrow, P.: Adaptations of the respiratory tract to air pollutants. Arch. Environ. Health, 14:127, 1967.
Moskowitz, R. L., Lyons, H. A., and Cottle, H. R.: Silo-filler's disease: Clinical, physiological and pathological study of a patient. Am. J. Med., 36:457, 1964.
Peters, J. M., and Murphy, R. L. H.: Pulmonary toxicity of isocyanates. Ann. Intern. Med., 73:654, 1970.
Royal Society of Medicine: Symposium on isocyanates. Proc. R. Soc. Med., 63:365, 1970.
Walton, M.: Industrial ammonia gassing. Br. J. Ind. Med., 30:78, 1973.

Radiation

Fraser, R. F., and Paré, J. A. P.: Diagnosis of Diseases of the Chest. Vol. II. Philadelphia. W. B. Saunders Company, 1970, pp. 1076–1085.
Smith, J. C.: Radiation pneumonitis: A review. Am. Rev. Respir. Dis., 87:647, 1963.

Section Eight. NEOPLASMS OF THE LUNG

Alvan R. Feinstein

539. INTRODUCTION

The benign or malignant clinical consequences of pulmonary neoplasms do not depend on histologic type alone. Their biologic behavior is demonstrated by their site, dissemination, and functional effects. All are important. For example, a histologically "benign" tumor can become lethal by leading to such complications as exsanguinating hemoptysis, pneumonia, or lung abscess. Conversely, a histologically "malignant" tumor may not be fatal if it grows slowly enough to be found and removed before it disseminates. Uncommonly, a slow-growing carcinoma may be undetected during life and first found at necropsy after the patient has died of some other disease.

Tumors of the lung can arise from any part of the trachea, bronchi, bronchial tree, pulmonary parenchyma, or pleura. Although larger bronchi are the most common sites of primary lung tumors, only about 25 per cent of the tumors are central enough to be seen at bronchoscopy.

The lung is a frequent site of metastasis from carcinomas originating elsewhere, particularly in the kidney, thyroid, breast, testis, or intestine. The cellular types and biologic behavior of the metastases in the lung usually depend on the characteristics of the primary tumor. When multiple lesions are found on a chest roentgenogram, an extrapulmonary tumor can be suspected; when the lesion is solitary in an asymptomatic patient, its differentiation from a primary lung tumor may be difficult and is sometimes resolved only after surgical exploration.

Carcinomas are the most common type of primary lung neoplasm. Among 757 primary lung tumors diagnosed consecutively in adults at a single medical center in the United States, 708 were carcinomas, 18 were bronchial adenomas, 10 were hamartomas, 8 were pleural mesotheliomas, and 3 were primary tracheal tumors. The remainder consisted of 2 teratomas, 2 fibromas, 2 lymphosarcomas, 1 fibrosarcoma, 1 sarcoma, 1 neurofibroma, and 1 Hodgkin's disease. These patterns and ratios of occurrence are similar to those reported in England and in Israel. The proportion of different cellular types in primary carcinomas will vary at any medical center, in part reflecting differences in the histologic criteria used by the pathologist. In general, squamous cell tumors are the most common, followed in frequency by anaplastic tumors and adenocarcinomas. No current scheme of histologic classification is used universally, however, and diverse discrepancies have been reported in reclassifications of the same tumor.

Bronchial adenomas, which are particularly common in women, usually have a central location. With slow growth of the tumor, bouts of pulmonary infection or small hemoptyses may occur repeatedly for a long time before the patient seeks medical attention. Peripheral tumors are often detected before they become symptomatic, particularly in countries where diagnostic roentgenograms are readily available. A routine roentgenogram may show an unexpected circumscribed shadow that is often called a "coin lesion" if it happens to present in coinlike size and shape. *Hamartomas* of the lung are usually peripheral and are often found by surgical exploration of such a symptomatically silent coin lesion. *Adenocarcinomas* tend to be peripherally located, whereas most other types of primary carcinoma are central. *Mesotheliomas* arise in the pleura and produce clinical manifestations related to pleural effusion or invasion of the chest wall.

Aside from these morphologic distinctions, neoplasms of the lung show no constant correlations between histologic type and clinical manifestations. Primary carcinoma, as the predominant neoplasm in this group of tumors, will be the topic of the remainder of this discussion.

540. PRIMARY CARCINOMA OF THE LUNG

Occurrence. The occurrence rate of cancer of the lung is difficult to estimate because the annual statistics for a particular population depend on the likelihood of a correct diagnosis being established in members of the population who have the disease. The opportunity to establish a correct diagnosis has sharply increased in recent years, with the frequent use of chest roentgenograms and with the availability of such diagnostic techniques as bronchoscopy, biopsy of affected structures, and cytologic examination of sputum and other fluids. These better methods of diagnosis lead to the detection of many cases of lung cancer today that might have been unrecognized years ago. During the past few decades, the occurrence rates of lung cancer have risen markedly, particularly in countries where the cited diagnostic aids are available and in general use.

In addition to these distinctions, several other features of diagnostic selectivity tend to cloud the epidemiologic picture. Patients referred to medical centers for specialized modes of therapy, such as thoracic surgery, high voltage radiotherapy, and new chemotherapeutic agents, may not reflect the true distribution of lung cancer in that community or in other regions. Certain cancers formerly regarded as metastatic have been called primary in the past few decades, after pathologists recognized that nonbronchogenic lung cancers can arise peripherally and disseminate widely to other parts of the body. The opportunity for cancer to develop is enhanced by the increased life span of people who formerly might have died at a young age because of microbial diseases that today are prevented or cured by sanitation, vaccination, and the various agents of modern therapy.

For all these reasons, cancer of the lung is now diagnosed more frequently than ever before. The epidemiologic significance of the increase is difficult to evaluate, but the clinical significance of this increased occurrence rate is that lung cancer is now perhaps the most commonly recognized form of carcinoma in man.

Etiology and Prevention. No single cause for lung tumors has been identified. Although cigarette smoking has been generally accepted as a major factor, particularly for squamous cell tumors, tobacco has had a less striking role in undifferentiated tumors, and has not been proposed as a cause of human adenocarcinomas and other forms of lung neoplasia.

Among the other agents variously invoked as contributory factors in causing lung cancer are atmospheric fumes and pollution (among urban dwellers), airborne radiation (among uranium miners), and proliferating scar tissue (in patients with previous pulmonary infections). Inhalation of asbestos fibers appears to have a dose-related role in the lung cancers found in asbestos workers, and has been suspected as a cause of mesotheliomas. Genetic factors may be implicated by reports that relatives of lung cancer patients have a higher death rate from lung cancer than matched controls.

The Spectrum of Clinical Patterns. It is not possible to describe a set of clinical signs and symptoms that could be considered as typical of the disease and illness produced by lung cancer. This problem occurs because a lung cancer, by metastasis or by other mechanisms, can affect the structure or function of almost any system in the body. Consequently, the following discussion is intended to identify and indicate the relative frequency of the major phenomena that occur with lung cancer and to describe how this knowledge can be used in the diagnosis of that disease.

The functional disorders can be "direct" effects, caused by the physical presence of the tumor at the involved site, or "indirect" effects, occurring without anatomic dissemination of tumor to the affected site or system.

Some of the effects are *pulmonic,* arising from the affected lung, pleura, or chest wall. Others are *extrapulmonic,* arising more remotely from involvement of the mediastinum or of regions beyond the thorax. The extrapulmonic effects can be *systemic* or *metastatic,* or both. It is the fact that these different manifestations of cancer of the lung can occur alone or in various combinations that gives the disease its wide, protean spectrum with many different patterns of appearance.

The clinical spectrum of lung cancer according to the presence or absence of any of the described pulmonic, systemic, and metastatic features is best seen in the form of a Venn diagram (see accompanying figure). The numbers in each subset of this diagram indicate the proportionate distribution of these clinical features at the time of diagnostic detection of lung cancer in 1032 consecutive patients. The most common pattern of appearance was the combination of pulmonic and systemic symptoms, which were present in 340 patients. Of the other patients in this series, 271 had pulmonic symptoms only, 196 had a combination of pulmonic, systemic, and metastatic features, 70 were asymptomatic, 34 first pre-

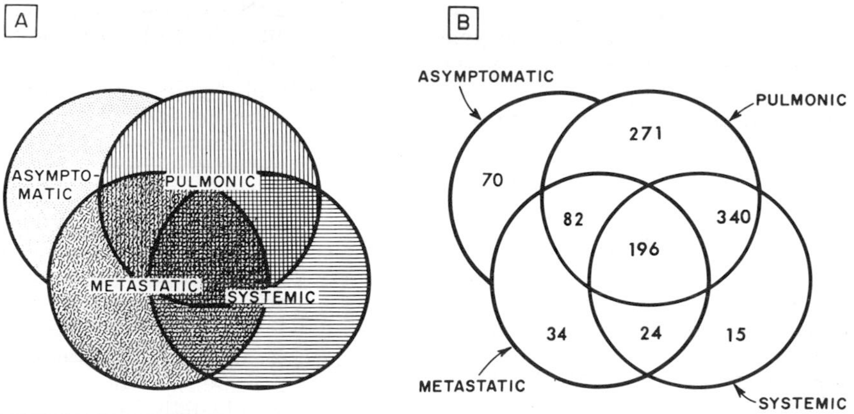

The clinical spectrum of lung cancer. The three main circles of the Venn diagram in part *A* are shaded to demonstrate sets of patients with pulmonic, systemic, or metastatic manifestations, as described in the text. The overlap of the circles produces seven subsets, in which these manifestations are present alone or in various combinations. An eighth subset, containing asymptomatic patients, is appended at the upper left of the diagram. Part *B*, for which the shading is removed, demonstrates the number of patients in each of these subsets at the time of clinical detection of lung cancer in 1032 cases.

sented only with metastatic features, and the remaining cases were distributed as shown.

Diagnosis. As shown in the figure, patients with lung cancer frequently seek medical attention after development of a cough, often with hemoptysis and with an associated infection or chest pain. Anorexia and weight loss may also be present, and the chest roentgenogram almost always shows an abnormal shadow or shadows.

Although no single pattern of clinical and roentgenographic features is either characteristic or pathognomonic for diagnosis, certain manifestations are particularly suspicious. Lung cancer is suggested clinically by the combination of hemoptysis, weight loss, and clubbing of the fingers in a patient who has no evidence of infection, congenital heart disease, or previous lung disease. The roentgenographic findings that most suggest lung cancer are (1) a mass arising in the hilar area; (2) an apparently pneumonic infiltrate that persists long after improvement of concomitant clinical symptoms; (3) a mass that obstructs a bronchus, usually demonstrated by tomography; and (4) a localized peripheral or coin lesion that shows no calcium in tomographic views. All of these and other clinical and roentgenographic manifestations associated with lung cancer can also be produced by such diseases as tuberculosis, various chronic pneumonias, granulomas, and other entities.

In diagnosis, therefore, the patient's signs and symptoms serve mainly to suggest the presence of a pulmonary lesion. The existence and extent of the lesion can be shown by roentgenography, which can also be used to detect lesions in asymptomatic patients. To specify the identity of any pulmonary lesion, however, requires additional tests. It is necessary to exclude causes other than cancer, and to provide cytologic or histologic evidence of the neoplasm. Many microbial or circulatory causes of lung lesions can be identified by appropriate examination of sputum or blood, although their demonstration does not exclude the possible coexistence of an underlying lung cancer.

Papanicolaou smears of the sputum are often positive in patients with primary carcinoma, particularly if special techniques are used to induce sputum when it is absent, and particularly when the tumor is centrally located. Peripheral cancers may not communicate well with the bronchial tree or may not exfoliate enough cells to yield positive results on cytologic examination. In these circumstances, the tests of sputum may produce "false negative" results; a rare "false positive" may occur in patients who have chronic bronchial inflammation rather than cancer.

Bronchoscopy is useful both for grossly visualizing the tumor (when possible) and for obtaining bronchial specimens for histologic or cytologic examination. Most other pathologic specimens used for the diagnosis of lung cancer are obtained by biopsy of metastatic sites or from the fluid of a neoplastic pleural or pericardial effusion. A favorite location of metastasis for lung cancer is the mediastinal and supraclavicular lymph nodes. Mediastinoscopy and biopsy of the scalene nodes are often done to obtain histologic evidence when none is otherwise available, and also to exclude metastasis, although a scalene node biopsy is seldom positive for tumor unless the node is palpably enlarged.

In some instances, when no other cytologic evidence is obtainable, needle biopsy of a peripheral lung lesion may disclose the tumor. More often, however, when diagnostic tests have failed to reveal the identity of the lesion disclosed by x-ray, exploratory thoracotomy is performed. Because the risk is low, surgical thoracic exploration is now a common diagnostic procedure in these circumstances. A benign tumor, granuloma, or a metastasis from a "silent" primary site may sometimes be found, but just as often a lung cancer is discovered in a still curable state. Among patients with "operable" lung cancer, about 70 per cent do not have a specific histologic diagnosis established until thoracotomy.

Correlation of Anatomic, Functional, and Clinical Manifestations. The direct and indirect effects of lung cancer can produce a variety of anatomic, clinical, and other manifestations.

Pulmonic Manifestations. Irritation of bronchial mucosa by tumor or by inflammation adjacent to the tumor may cause a change in the pattern of a chronic cough or may produce a wholly new cough. Hemoptysis of bright red blood, flecks of blood, or "rusty" sputum may be due to vascular invasion or to pneumonia developing behind the tumor. Occasionally, the tumor may occlude enough of a large bronchus to make the patient notice a respiratory wheeze.

An obstructed bronchial lumen may cause retention of secretions, predisposing to parenchymal infection. If the lumen is completely obstructed, the distal parenchyma may become atelectatic. Although roentgenographically apparent atelectasis may be asymptomatic, parenchyma that is infected or inflamed may produce all the classic clinical, bacteriologic, and roentgenographic manifestations of a pneumonia. With conventional treatment of the pneumonia, the patient may have a conventional symptomatic and bacteriologic response, but the roentgenogram may fail to clear because of the underlying neoplasm. In this circumstance, the "unresolved pneumonia" becomes the clue that leads to further tests and discovery of the tumor. A lung abscess can sometimes be produced at the site of such a pneumonia, although an alternative cause of lung abscess is necrosis of the interior of a large tumor.

As a parenchymal manifestation, dyspnea is the direct result of metastasis when the tumor either replaces large amounts of parenchymal tissue or, more commonly, invades the pleural surface, causing an effusion that reduces the space available for ventilation. In many other circumstances, however, dyspnea may be indirect, occurring because (1) parenchymal inflammation extending to the pleura initiates a pleural effusion, (2) the primary tumor may locally obstruct the trachea or carina, or (3) the amount of secondary parenchymal inflammation or atelectasis may be great enough to impair ventilation in a patient whose respiratory reserve had been reduced – by chronic lung disease or by poor cardiac compensation – before the tumor developed.

Involvement of *the pleural surface* can produce inspiratory chest pain, the physical findings of an effusion, or dyspnea if the effusion is massive. When pleural involvement is due to the inflammatory extension of pneumonia developing behind the primary tumor, the pleural fluid is often pink or bloody. Another form of indirect pleural involvement, usually associated with serous effusion, occurs when the primary tumor obstructs appropriate vascular and lymphatic channels draining the pleura. In both these indirect circumstances, the pleural fluid contains no tumor cells. In other circumstances, however, the pleura can be directly invaded via contiguous spread from a peripherally located tumor or by lymphatic metastases from a tumor in the bronchus. A neoplastic pleural effusion is seldom clinically different from one that is inflammatory or hydrostatic, but the fluid is more likely to be bloody and will usually contain cancer cells.

Although pleural involvement is the most common single cause of chest pain in lung cancer, inspiratory chest pain may also occur when a peripheral tumor extends through the pleura to the chest wall, involving muscle, bone, or both. Rib invasion may alternatively occur as a distant metastasis from a central tumor. Chest pain that lacks inspiratory accentuation can develop with invasion of an upper rib, sternum, or thoracic vertebra. The tumor may sometimes extend beyond the vertebra or rib to involve a thoracic nerve, with pain in the anatomic distribution of the nerve.

Extrapulmonic Manifestations. The many possible extrapulmonic manifestations of lung cancer include *systemic features,* which are often indirect, and *metastatic features,* which are due to direct spread of tumor to the affected site.

SYSTEMIC MANIFESTATIONS. Anorexia may occur indirectly because of persistent infection, pain, or other discomforts of the pulmonic features just cited. With decreased food intake, the patient may then lose weight and become easily fatigued. Alternatively, however, anorexia and other digestive disturbances can be the direct result of hepatic, peritoneal, or other intra-abdominal metastases.

Hypertrophic pulmonary osteoarthropathy, i.e., clubbing of the fingers and/or pain in the articular extremities of long bones, can occur with either central or peripheral tumors of the lung. They may sometimes be the earliest or the only clinical clues that suggest the presence of a lung cancer. The clubbing has no physical differences from the clubbing sometimes found in congenital heart disease, chronic lung disease, and other non-neoplastic entities. Careful criteria are often needed to distinguish "curving" of the nail bed from true clubbing.

The osteoarthropathy is actually a "periostopathy" and, when present, involves the distal third of a long bone, commonly in the leg. The bone becomes exquisitely tender to pressure, and an associated synovitis may make the subcutaneous tissues swollen and the joint painful on movement. Although the articular surface of the neighboring joint is not affected, the clinical manifestations may be attributed to arthritis until the periosteal changes are noted roentgenographically. By palpating tenderness in the bone well beyond the region of the joint, the clinician can suspect osteoarthropathy before the radiologist finds it. The mechanisms of clubbing and of hypertrophic osteoarthropathy are unknown. The manifestations may be improved by vagotomy or by direct treatment that removes or shrinks the primary tumor.

With the availability of modern laboratory techniques, many "hormonal" effects, although not common, have been reported with almost any type of lung tumor, most often with "oat cell" cancers. So many different systems have been involved that lung cancer seems to have the occasional capacity either for acting like an auxiliary pituitary gland or for producing other nonpituitary hormonal effects.

When a patient with lung cancer has an endocrine problem resulting from a *decrease* in hormone, the cause is usually destruction of the glandular site by metastasis. An *increase* in hormone may represent one of the functional "endocrinopathies" that can produce adrenal hyperfunction, inappropriate antidiuresis, hypercalcemia, or the carcinoid syndrome (see Ch. 869 and 870). The hypersecretive endocrine problems can often occur without metastasis and can sometimes be the first evidence of the tumor.

The weakness often associated with lung cancer was long regarded only as a nonspecific systemic effect until the discovery in recent years that many instances of weakness were due to *neurologic lesions,* occurring without metastasis and presumably caused by a secretory product of the tumor. The lesions can include cortical cerebellar degeneration, peripheral neuropathies, encephalomyelitis, and various myopathic syndromes.

METASTATIC MANIFESTATIONS. *Hoarseness* occurs when tumor impinges on the mediastinal portion of the recurrent left laryngeal nerve. The subsequent paralysis of the left vocal cord is demonstrated at laryngoscopy (or bronchoscopy).

The superior vena cava syndrome can be produced by metastases in mediastinal nodes. Lung cancer today is the most common cause of the suffusion and brawny edema that occur in the face, neck, or upper arms as a consequence of compression or invasion of the superior vena cava.

Involvement of the esophagus by lung cancer in the mediastinum can produce the same clinical pattern of *dysphagia* noted in esophageal carcinoma.

Although *myocardial involvement* is rare in lung cancer, direct invasion of the pericardium is more common. Neoplastic cells found in a bloody pericardial effusion may sometimes be the first evidence of the cancer.

Carcinomas arising in the apex of the lung—*superior sulcus tumors* (sometimes called Pancoast tumors)—can invade adjacent bone or the nerve bundles that pass through the thoracic inlet. Involvement of the first or second rib can produce local pain; involvement of the brachial plexus can produce sensory or motor disturbances in the arm; and involvement of the sympathetic nerve chain can produce Horner's syndrome on the affected side.

EXTRATHORACIC MANIFESTATIONS. Cancer of the lung can metastasize to any structure of the body. The brain has been a distant metastatic site so commonly that pulmonary examination is often performed to exclude metastasis from a lung cancer in any adult suspected of having a primary brain tumor.

Among the other diverse extrathoracic metastatic manifestations of lung cancer are pathologic fractures of bone, the development of multiple cutaneous nodules, enlargement of the liver, hypoadrenalism caused by metastatic replacement of the adrenal glands, diabetes mellitus resulting from destruction of the pancreas, gastrointestinal bleeding from metastasis to small bowel, jaundice from metastasis to periportal nodes, ascites from peritoneal invasion, and various peripheral neurologic manifestations from metastasis to vertebrae or to spinal cord.

Prognosis and Treatment. Therapeutic procedures in lung cancer begin with the diagnostic and epidemiologic effort to detect the tumor in a premetastatic state, suitable for surgical resection. The effort depends on the hope that symptomatic patients will seek medical aid promptly and that asymptomatic patients, not under medical surveillance, will be found by widespread use of routine roentgenography of the chest.

This hope of "early discovery" followed by surgical cure, which currently seems to be the most effective form of therapy, is often thwarted by diverse biologic behavior in the rate and direction of growth of the cancer. Symptomatic patients with a rapidly growing tumor may seek medical aid promptly but may already have metastases. Conversely, the initial symptoms of a slowly growing tumor may be so mild and unprovocative that a long time elapses before the patient decides to see a physician; yet the lesion may still be curable by surgical resection despite the apparently "late" treatment. Among asymptomatic patients with no previous roentgenograms, a shadow found unexpectedly in a routine film often represents a slowly growing curable tumor. If the shadow is found on the *subsequent* film of an asymptomatic patient, the increment of size in the interval between "negative" and "positive" film helps denote the rate of growth of the tumor; and for a rapid-growing tumor, even an "early" asymptomatic discovery may sometimes come too "late."

Because the clinical course and outcome of lung cancer depend on its diverse patterns of behavior, the disease does not have a single, clearly demarcated natural history. The differences in survival of different subgroups are shown in Table 1, in which 1032 consecutive patients with lung cancer are classified according to the evidence present at the time of diagnostic detection, before a therapeutic decision was carried out. The symptomatic manifestations are cited in four stages of ascending severity. The anatomic stage before treatment is classified as *localized* if none of the available roentgenographic or microscopic evidence showed spread of tumor; *regional,* if the spread was confined to the mediastinum or same hemithorax as the primary lesion; and *distant,* for contrathoracic or ultrathoracic dissemination. The six-month survival rates are shown, regardless of therapy, for the 12 symptomatic-anatomic subgroups and for the totals in each category of staging.

TABLE 1. Six-Month Survival Rates in 1032 Patients with Lung Cancer

Symptomatic Stage	Anatomic Stage			Totals
	Localized	*Regional*	*Distant*	
Asymptomatic	36/43 (84%)	19/25 (76%)	1/2 (50%)	56/70 (80%)
Pulmonic	90/114 (79%)	59/139 (42%)	7/18 (39%)	156/271 (58%)
Systemic	66/110 (60%)	76/194 (39%)	13/51 (25%)	155/355 (44%)
Metastatic	9/28 (32%)	55/144 (38%)	23/164 (14%)	87/336 (26%)
Totals	201/295 (68%)	209/502 (42%)	44/235 (19%)	454/1032 (44%)

The varying rates of survival in Table 1 indicate the diverse behavior of the disease. Less than half (44 per cent) of the 1032 patients in the entire series survived for six months or more. Among subgroups, the six-month survival rate was 26 per cent (87 of 336) in patients found with symptomatic evidence of metastasis, and 41 per cent (175 of 429) in the six subgroups of patients whose regional or distant spread was not accompanied by metastatic symptoms. On the other hand, of the 267 patients who had neither symptomatic nor anatomic evidence of metastasis, 72 per cent (192) survived six months. Within the anatomically localized group, the survival rates showed a distinctive prognostic gradient according to the associated symptoms. The rates were highest (84 per cent) in the asymptomatic patients; 79 per cent in those with pulmonic symptoms only; and 60 per cent in the systemic group. The symptomatic stages were associated with analogous survival gradients within the other two anatomic stages.

These biologic distinctions must be borne in mind for selecting and evaluating different modes of therapy. Unless patients are analyzed according to both morphologic and clinical features, the compared populations will not be similar, and many triumphs attributed to therapy may actually be due to unrecognized aspects of the neoplasm's biologic behavior. Table 2 contains quantitative evidence of the selective prognostic "bias" with which therapy is chosen. The patients in Table 2 are classified according to the same arrangement used in Table 1, but the rates show the relative frequency with which patients were regarded as "operable," with performance of exploratory thoracotomy and possible surgical resection. The highest rates of choice for thoracotomy in Table 2 occurred in those patients who, as noted earlier in Table 1, had the best prognostic expectations.

TABLE 2. Rate of Selection for Thoracotomy in 1032 Patients with Lung Cancer

Symptomatic Stage	Anatomic Stage			Totals
	Localized	Regional	Distant	
Asymptomatic	37/43 (86%)	13/25 (52%)	0/2 (0%)	50/70 (71%)
Pulmonic	92/114 (81%)	55/139 (40%)	0/18 (0%)	147/271 (54%)
Systemic	75/110 (68%)	70/194 (36%)	7/51 (14%)	152/355 (43%)
Metastatic	7/28 (25%)	16/144 (11%)	2/164 (1%)	25/336 (7%)
Totals	211/295 (72%)	154/502 (31%)	9/235 (4%)	374/1032 (36%)

Conversely, the lowest rates of thoracotomy occurred in patients with the worst prognoses.

These differences in case selection may demonstrate the skill with which surgeons choose relatively "healthy" patients for thoracotomy, but they also reveal that the surgically treated group had a major prognostic advantage over patients assigned to other modes of treatment. These natural prognostic distinctions must also be contemplated when the results of different forms of surgery are evaluated in the operable group or when different forms of radiotherapy and/or chemotherapy are appraised in patients whose tumor was not resected. For example, among all patients with surgical resection of the cancer, the five-year survival rate was 25 per cent (69 of 279); but the rate ranged from 34 per cent (12 of 35) in the asymptomatic, localized group, to 22 per cent (23 of 104) in patients with systemic symptoms, to 0 per cent (0 of 14) in those with metastatic symptoms. The results of different forms of surgical resection will obviously depend on the kinds of patients chosen for operation.

Similarly, among all patients with nonresected tumors (i.e., inoperable and/or surgically explored but not excised), the six-month survival rate was 31 per cent (237 of 753). This rate ranged, however, from 66 per cent (27 of 41) among patients with localized tumors and with no metastatic or systemic symptoms to 13 per cent (22 of 163) when symptomatic and anatomic evidence of distant metastasis was present. The neglect of these and other clinical distinctions can be an important source of ambiguous, misleading, or controversial results whenever one mode of therapy is compared against another without regard to the major pretherapeutic prognostic differences that can occur in subsets of patients with "unresected" or "inoperable" lung cancer.

As for specific considerations in choice of treatment, a morphologic prerequisite to surgical resection is location of the tumor at a resectable site, i.e., not in the trachea or carina. A functional prerequisite is the ability of the patient to tolerate both the operation itself and the subsequent reduction in functioning lung tissue. For the resection, some surgeons routinely perform pneumonectomy and radical dissection of mediastinal nodes regardless of the apparent gross extent of the tumor. Other surgeons—hoping to preserve as much normal lung tissue as possible—confine resection to the smallest amount of lung in which the tumor appears grossly contained. At operation, some surgeons may decide against resection of primary tumor if metastatic deposits are adjacent to the aorta, pericardium, or other critical mediastinal structures; other surgeons remove both the primary tumor and any deposits that do not actually invade the adjacent structures. A "palliative" resection of the primary tumor is sometimes performed despite apparent "incurability" in order to relieve hypertrophic pulmonary osteoarthropathy or lung abscess.

Irradiation may be used before or after surgery or when surgery is unfeasible. By "shrinking" a juxtacarinal lesion or mediastinal nodes, irradiation may sometimes permit subsequent surgery in a previously "inoperable" case. Radiotherapy is particularly valuable for pain caused by bony metastasis and for alleviating such symptoms as osteoarthropathy, superior vena cava syndrome, and vocal cord paralysis. Malignant pleural effusions are sometimes treated by instillation of nitrogen mustard radiotherapeutic or other chemotherapeutic substances.

Antineoplastic chemotherapy is usually reserved for widely disseminated tumors beyond help by either surgery or irradiation. In the panorama of available agents, adrenocortical steroids or nitrogen mustard have often had transiently good results with the superior vena cava syndrome and in cutaneous metastases. No antineoplastic agent has been consistently successful in metastatic cancer, but new agents are constantly becoming available. Cyclophosphamide has sometimes been beneficial, and adriamycin may prove useful.

Supportive care is needed to help the patient maintain good nutritional intake. Rhizotomy or cordotomy can be attempted for pain relief when other measures have failed, and narcotics or sedatives should be used liberally in appropriate circumstances. Such complications as infections and hormonal imbalances require appropriate treatment.

Many rapidly growing tumors produce death within six months. A patient who survives more than six months, however, is likely to have a slowly growing tumor. For such patients the best therapeutic attitude, even when metastases are present, is to regard the cancer as a chronic incurable disease for which a great deal can still be done. By maintaining an attitude of hope, by suitable attention to remediable or improvable situations, and by attention to the personal aspects of clinical care, the physician can often prolong useful life, prevent needless suffering, or permit death to come, when it must, in circumstances of tranquility and dignity.

Boucot, K. R., Cooper, D. A., Weiss, W., and Carnahan, W. J.: The natural history of lung cancer. Am. Rev. Respir. Dis., 89:519, 1964.

Carbone, P. P. (moderator): Lung cancer: Perspectives and prospects. Ann. Intern. Med., 73:1003, 1970.

Feinstein, A. R.: A new staging system for cancer and a reappraisal of "early" treatment and "cure" by radical surgery. N. Engl. J. Med., 279:747, 1968. See also Ann. Intern. Med., 61:127, 1964; Nature, 209:241, 1966; and Amer. Rev. Respir. Dis., 101:671, 1970, and 107:790, 1973.

Garland, L. R., Coulson, W., and Wollin, E.: The rate of growth and apparent duration of untreated primary bronchial carcinoma. Cancer, 16:694, 1963.

Kreyberg, L.: Histological lung cancer types. Acta Pathol. Microbiol. Scand., Suppl. 157, 1962.

LeRoux, B. T.: Bronchial Carcinoma. Edinburgh, E. & S. Livingstone, Ltd., 1968.

Selawry, O. S., and Primack, A. (eds.): First International Workshop for Therapy of Lung Cancer. Cancer Chemotherapy Reports, Part 3, Vol. 4, No. 2, 1973.

Watson, W. L. (ed.): Lung Cancer. A Study of Five Thousand Memorial Hospital Cases. St. Louis, C. V. Mosby Company, 1968.

Section Nine. DISEASES OF THE PLEURA

John H. McClement

INTRODUCTION

The pleura, a serous membrane of mesodermal origin, covers the lung, the chest wall, the diaphragm, and the mediastinum. It is a closed sac which encloses the pleural space and separates the lung from adjacent structures. The visceral pleura designates that portion of it which covers the lung; the remainder is the parietal pleura. The parietal pleura receives its blood supply from the systemic circulation, whereas the visceral is supplied by the pulmonary circulation. The normal pleural space contains no gas and only a small amount of serous fluid. During quiet breathing, the elastic recoil of the lung produces a subatmospheric pressure (−4 to −10 cm H_2O) in the pleural space.

Pleural pain and signs and symptoms secondary to collections of fluid and gas in the pleural space are principal indicators of pleural disease.

Pleural pain originates in the parietal pleura; stimulation of the visceral pleura does not cause pain. Typically, pleural pain is sharp, aggravated by respiration and thoracic motion, and relieved by splinting of the involved area. When it arises from the pleura of the chest wall, the pain is referred to the chest wall overlying the involved area; pain arising from the pleura of the central portion of the diaphragm is referred to the posterior part of the shoulder area; pain from the costal portions of the diaphragm is referred to adjacent parts of the chest wall and abdomen.

The formation and removal of pleural fluid are dependent on those forces which regulate the exchange of fluid into and out of capillary beds, and on lymphatic drainage. The hydrostatic pressure in the pleural capillaries (Pc), the hydrostatic pressure in the pleural space (Ppl), the oncotic pressures of the plasma (OPp) and the pleural fluid (OPpf), and the permeability of the pleural capillaries (K) are the factors which regulate the transport of fluid (F) into and out of the pleural capillaries. According to Starling's law of transcapillary exchange, this can be expressed as follows:

$$F = K(Pc - OPp) - (Ppl - OPpf)$$

The visceral pleura is supplied by arterioles from the low pressure pulmonary arterial system, whereas the parietal pleura is supplied by the higher pressure systemic arteries. There is evidence that the permeability (K) of the visceral capillaries is less than that of the parietal pleura. Normally a balance of these forces favors absorption of fluid by the visceral pleura at about the same rate it is formed. However, all these forces may be altered by disease, and the removal of fluid may be slowed or its formation increased. An increase in capillary permeability (K) from inflammation, a decrease in the oncotic pressure of the plasma proteins (OPp) from hypoalbuminemia, and an increase in the hydrostatic pressure in the pulmonary capillaries (Pc) are the common alterations that lead to pleural fluid collections. Uncommonly a decrease in the hydrostatic pressure in the pleura (Ppl) from a collapsed and nonexpandable lung will cause effusion. Protein, red blood cells, and particulate matter are removed from the pleural space by the pleural lymphatics. The absorption and transport of pleural fluid by way of the lymphatics is increased by diaphragmatic and intercostal activity. Decrease in this activity or obstruction of local or distant lymphatic channels may prolong or prevent reabsorption of pleural fluid.

METHODS OF EXAMINATION IN PLEURAL DISEASE

History and Physical Examination. Pleural pain and shortness of breath are the symptoms which most often call attention to pleural disease. A dry, irritating, nonproductive cough may sometimes accompany the pleural pain. Shortness of breath may sometimes be caused by severe pleural pain, but usually indicates the presence of fairly large amounts of intrapleural fluid or gas. Early in the course of pleural inflammation a friction rub may be heard over the involved area. As fluid forms, the friction rub and the pain disappear, and dullness to percussion and diminished breath sounds on auscultation appear. At the upper limits of pleural fluid, egophony is sometimes elicited. Pleural disorders for the most part arise from derangements in cardiac, hepatic, or renal function which lead to increased collections of fluid, or by extension of disease from adjacent structures such as the lung, mediastinum, chest wall, esophagus, or the upper abdomen. Evidence of disease in these structures must be searched for in the history and physical examination.

Radiologic Examination. Up to 300 ml of fluid may be present in a pleural space and not be apparent on the usual upright chest x-ray film. Small amounts of fluid may sometimes be suspected, especially on the left side, from the presence of a density or apparent widening of the diaphragmatic shadow as it is seen between the gas-containing stomach and the lower limits of the lung. Decubitus films taken with the involved side dependent may also sometimes make small amounts of fluid apparent on the x-ray film. With larger amounts of fluid the characteristic density of pleural fluid with its curvilinear upper border appears. However, if pleural fluid occurs in a pleural space in which previous inflammatory disease has produced adhesions, the distribution of the fluid may produce varied shadows. The x-ray shadows of pleural fluid are characteristically adjacent to the chest wall; rarely fluid will collect in or become encapsulated in one of the interlobar fissures and produce a pattern similar to a parenchymal pulmonary tumor.

Examination of Pleural Fluid. A detailed chemical, bacteriologic, and cytologic analysis of all pleural fluids aspirated is essential in patients in whom the diagnosis is not completely clear. Analysis for total protein and lactic acid dehydrogenase (LDH), a complete blood count with a differential count, cultures for bacteria including mycobacteria, a Gram-stained smear, and a search for malignant cells should be carried out initially on virtually all pleural fluids. Glucose, amylase, fat, and cholesterol measurements may also sometimes be indicated. The specific gravity of pleural fluid was once recommended as a measurement that would help differentiate between exudates and transudates. Because the specific gravity depends almost entirely on the protein content of the pleural fluid, and because it is a measurement that is frequently inaccurate, it can usually be omitted if an accurate measure of protein content is available.

The differentiation of pleural transudates and exudates is most helpful diagnostically and can usually be accomplished from examination of pleural fluid. Transudates are those fluids which occur in response to a decrease in the oncotic pressure of plasma, an increase in hydrostatic pressures in the pleural capillaries, or a decrease in intrapleural pressure. Exudates result from infections or from inflammatory or neoplastic processes which alter the permeability of pleural capillaries. Characteristically, transudates have a low protein content, a low specific gravity, and few white blood cells, whereas exudates have a high protein, high specific gravity, and increased numbers of white blood cells. Arbitrary limits have been chosen to separate transudates and exudates (e.g., total protein more than 3.0 ml per 100 ml and specific gravity greater than 1.015). Unfortunately, when these arbitrary limits are tested in patients who have pleural fluid in which the cause is certain, both transudates and exudates are sometimes misclassified. Light and his associates have examined the cellular and chemical characteristics of pleural fluid from patients in whom a definite diagnosis could be established. On this basis they were classified as transudates or exudates. The three measurements which they found most reliable in differentiating transudates and exudates were the pleural fluid to serum protein ratio (greater than 0.5 in exudates), the level of LDH (greater than 200 IU in exudates) and the ratio of pleural fluid to serum LDH (greater than 0.6 in exudates). Although white blood counts greater than 10,000 per cubic millimeter are usually found only in exudates and counts of greater than 2500 per cubic millimeter suggest that the fluid is an exudate, counts below 2500 per cubic millimeter do not distinguish transudates from exudates.

Chylothorax refers to the presence of chyle in the pleural space and results from trauma to or obstruction (most often by a neoplastic process) of the thoracic duct or some other major intrathoracic lymphatic. Chylous pleural effusions are characteristically milky in appearance and have a high fat content which can be identified both microscopically and chemically. The protein content is usually about half that of plasma.

Milky-appearing pleural collections may also occur late in the course of tuberculous pleural effusion, in the pleural effusions of rheumatoid lung disease, and in other chronic effusions from the accumulation of cholesterol and cholesterol crystals in these fluids. Chemical analysis of such fluids will show a high cholesterol content and a low fat content and distinguish them from chylous effusions.

Pleural Biopsy. Biopsy of the pleura with a Cope or Abrams needle is indicated in nearly every patient in whom the diagnosis is not clear, and who has sufficient pleural fluid to make this a safe procedure. Material from the biopsy should be submitted not only for histologic examination, but also for culture for tubercle bacilli. Pleural biopsy has been particularly useful in establishing the diagnosis of tuberculous pleurisy and malignant neoplastic implants in the pleura.

SIMPLE HYDROTHORAX

Pleural fluid collections occur more often as a result of cardiac, hepatic, or renal disease than from inflammatory or malignant disease of the pleura. These fluid collections most often result either from increases in hydrostatic pressures in the pleural capillaries, from a decrease in the oncotic pressure of the plasma, or from a combination of these factors. There is some exchange of fluid between the peritoneum and the pleura through the diaphragmatic lymphatics, and in patients with ascites this mechanism may result in pleural collections. Clinically these fluid collections are usually identified by physical examination, from x-rays of the chest, or, if they are large, from the appearance of dyspnea. They occur much more frequently on the right side than on the left. Pleural fluid in patients with simple hydrothorax will have those characteristics of a transudate which have been described. Because the parietal pleura is thin and uninvolved, pleural biopsy often fails to yield any identifiable pleural tissue. The treatment of these pleural collections is the treatment of the underlying disease, and pleural aspiration should be used therapeutically only if these measures fail and dyspnea requires relief.

PULMONARY EMBOLISM AND PULMONARY INFARCTION

Pulmonary embolism frequently produces pleural manifestations. In patients with pulmonary embolism, confirmed by pulmonary angiography, more than half will have a clinically detectable pleural effusion. The pleural effusion does not appear immediately and is usually identified more than 24 hours after the embolic event. The pleural effusion is an exudate and sometimes has moderate numbers of red blood cells; however, it is usually a clear amber fluid. Unless repeated embolization occurs, the pleural fluid disappears as the pulmonary infarction resolves.

PLEURAL EFFUSIONS WITH PNEUMONIA: EMPYEMA

Inflammation of the adjacent pleura occurs in most patients with pneumonia whatever the cause. Bacterial pneumonia frequently has clinically significant pleural involvement; in most pneumonias caused by viruses and mycoplasma, pleural disease is not clinically prominent.

The extent of pleural inflammation in bacterial pneumonia varies widely from case to case. There may be minor inflammation which produces pleural pain with clinically undetectable amounts of fluid, and which leaves no clinical residue; or large collections of grossly purulent fluid containing large numbers of bacteria (empyema) resulting in marked pleural fibrosis and fibrothorax. In practice one encounters patients who produce a continuum between these two extremes. Treatment of these effusions depends largely on the severity and intensity of the pleural inflammation, but is primarily the treatment of the associated pneumonia with appropriate antimicrobial drugs. The less intense small serous effusions with relatively small numbers of white blood cells and few organisms will usually respond to drug treatment alone. With larger collections of fluid and more white blood cells, aspiration by means of closed drainage through an intercostal tube may speed resolution and lead to smaller pleural residues. With grossly purulent fluid and larger numbers of bacteria, surgical rib resection and open dependent drainage may be necessary. Infrequently pleural inflammatory disease leads to persistent massive fibrous entrapment of the underlying lung even after the infection has been controlled. A so-called fibrothorax results; the affected lung has its volume greatly decreased; ventilation and perfusion are reduced; there is a shift in the mediastinum toward the entrapped lung, and overdistention of the contralateral lung occurs. In such cases surgical decortication may free the entrapped lung and restore pulmonary function.

TUBERCULOSIS OF THE PLEURA

Definition. Localized tuberculosis of the pleura probably occurs in most patients with pulmonary tuberculosis. It is usually clinically inapparent, but does result in pleural adhesions over the involved area.

Tuberculosis of the pleura with pleural effusion and without apparent pulmonary tuberculosis is the principal or first clinical manifestation of tuberculous disease in a few patients. Characteristically it is a febrile illness, accompanied by a serous pleural effusion. Although the acute illness, even if untreated, usually subsides in a few weeks with resorption of the fluid, it is very frequently followed by pulmonary tuberculosis or some other form of tuberculosis. Roper and Waring found that 65 per cent of patients with serofibrinous pleurisy who did not receive antituberculous chemotherapy developed tuberculosis during the next five years. Thus recognition of the tuberculous cause is of great importance. Infrequently pleural effusions that are grossly purulent and contain large numbers of tubercle bacilli are encountered; such cases are designated as tuberculous empyema.

Epidemiology. Tuberculous pleurisy with effusion can occur at any age but occurs most often in older children and young adults. It usually occurs soon after tuberculous infection, and is uncommon in patients who are known to have had tuberculous infection for a long time.

Pathology and Pathogenesis. Tuberculosis of the pleura in nearly all cases results from extension of disease from the lung. Extension from tuberculosis of adjacent bones or lymph nodes is rare. Usually this extension from the lungs results only in localized pleural disease, and pleural effusion is not significant. In an occasional patient there is a massive outpouring of pleural fluid, and tuberculous infection is generalized over the visceral and parietal pleura. Myriads of typical tubercles stud the pleural surfaces. The immunologic reasons why some patients have this acute, widespread disease whereas others have only insignificant localized disease are not known. In a few weeks the acute reaction subsides, the pleural fluid decreases and then disappears, and fibrous adhesions between the visceral and parietal pleura form. Infrequently the fluid persists, becomes more purulent, and has increased numbers of tubercle bacilli; a chronic tuberculous empyema is established, which may persist for many years. Perhaps because the adjacent subpleural area is richly supplied with lymphatics, there is easy access for the dissemination of tubercle bacilli. In any case the subsequent development of tuberculosis in the lung and in other organs is a common event after untreated tuberculous pleurisy with effusion.

Clinical Manifestations. The onset of tuberculous pleurisy with effusion is usually fairly sudden and acute. Sharp, fairly severe pleural pain is the most common first symptom. It is usually unilateral, made worse by breathing, and relieved by splinting the affected area. It is sharpest and most painful for the first few days, and then with the outpouring of pleural fluid it becomes duller and gradually subsides. Shortness of breath which is sometimes severe results from large collections of pleural fluid. Fever, which is sometimes as high as 39 to 40° C, is usually present in the first two or three weeks, and gradually subsides. Physical examination and x-ray examinations will identify the presence of variable amounts of fluid. In the typical case the parenchymal focus in the lung from which the disease originated is not apparent radiologically.

Diagnosis. The diagnosis of tuberculous pleurisy should be considered in every patient with a pleural effusion; should be strongly suspected if this is accompanied by skin reactivity to 0.0001 mg of PPD; and should be presumptively diagnosed if, in addition, the fluid has the characteristics of an exudate and another diagnosis cannot be firmly made. Fortunately, methods for making the diagnosis of pleural tuberculosis have improved to such an extent that, if they are all used in a concerted fashion before treatment is started, the number of cases in which only a presumptive diagnosis must be made is small. Tubercle bacilli can be cultured from pleural fluid in up to 20 per cent of cases, from the sputum in a similar number, and from pleural biopsy material in over 60 per cent of cases. Typical tuberculous granulation tissue is seen in over 60 per cent of pleural biopsies from cases of tuberculous pleurisy. Although none of these methods are diagnostic in all cases, if they are used together, bacteriologic or histologic evidence of tuberculosis will be found in most cases.

Congestive heart failure, metastatic carcinoma involving the pleura, pulmonary infarction, and the effusions of bacterial pneumonia are the most commonly encountered conditions from which tuberculous pleurisy with effusions must be differentiated. Pleural mesothelioma, subdiaphragmatic abscess with an associated pleural effusion, rheumatoid pleural disease, and disseminated lupus erythematosus are less common conditions that may resemble tuberculous pleurisy.

Treatment. The treatment of tuberculous pleurisy is the prolonged administration of isoniazid and at least one other antituberculous drug and is the same as that for pulmonary tuberculosis (see Ch. 228). Surgical decortication to free a lung trapped by pleural adhesions (fibrothorax) after chemotherapy has controlled the infection is rarely necessary. With prompt and adequate chemotherapy, pleural residues are usually minor and do not benefit from surgical correction.

NEOPLASMS OF THE PLEURA

Metastatic Carcinoma. Implants of metastatic carcinoma of the pleura are, especially in older age groups, a common cause of pleural effusions. Carcinomas of the lung and breast are the tumors that most commonly extend to the pleura, but almost any carcinoma can have this complication. If the primary tumor has already been identified, the diagnosis is usually quickly made. If the pleural effusion is the first indication of the tumor, the diagnosis may not be so apparent. Characteristically the pleural effusions of malignant implants in the pleura are not accompanied by fever, the fluid is an exudate and often contains a large number of red blood cells, and the course is marked by the continued outpouring of fluid. The diagnosis can be established by finding malignant cells in the pleural fluid, by the presence of tumor in the parietal pleura on pleural biopsy, or by open surgical biopsy of the pleura.

Treatment is aimed at preventing the accumulation of fluid in the pleural space and eliminating the need for repeated thoracenteses for the relief of dyspnea. Obliteration of the pleural space may be produced by the instillation of various irritating substances (e.g., atabrine, nitrogen mustard, cyclophosphamide, radioactive gold), followed by aspiration of the fluid to assure that the visceral and parietal layers are opposed. The insertion of an intercostal tube attached to suction is sometimes used for continuous aspiration after the irritating material has stimulated an inflammatory response.

Mesothelioma. Pleural mesotheliomas may be either localized or diffuse. The localized tumor, the so-called fibrous mesothelioma, is relatively benign, may grow to a very large size, is sometimes cured by surgical resection, but does have a tendency to recur. The diffuse mesothelioma is a highly malignant tumor which involves the pleura widely and produces massive encroachment on the pleural space with fluid and tumor. Formerly this was believed to be a very rare tumor. It is now being seen with increased frequency, and its association with exposure to asbestos has been established (see Ch. 527).

Other Pleural Tumors. Benign tumors of the pleura include lipomas, fibromas, vascular tumors, and pleural cysts. Primary malignant tumors of the pleura other than mesotheliomas include various sarcomas. They are all very uncommon.

Pleural effusions from intrathoracic lymphoma are not uncommon and apparently can result either from direct involvement of the pleura or from intrathoracic lymphatic obstruction. Chylothorax is sometimes seen when there is lymphatic obstruction.

SPONTANEOUS PNEUMOTHORAX

The pleural space normally does not contain gas, and if gas is instilled into the pleural space, it is absorbed. The total pressure of dissolved gases in venous blood is 54 mm Hg less than the atmospheric pressure which is transmitted to the pleura. This negative gradient keeps the intact pleural space gas free. Air may enter the pleural space through either the chest wall or the lung. Trauma to the chest wall or lung, medical procedures that permit the entry of air through the chest wall or that puncture the lung, and the spontaneous entry of gas from a ruptured emphysematous bleb are the most common causes of pneumothorax. The rupture of lung abscesses and tuberculous cavities into the pleura are less common causes. Spontaneous pneumothorax occurs in at least two distinct populations: the young, tall, otherwise healthy male, and the older person with underlying and usually clinically apparent chronic obstructive pulmonary disease or some other disease that has produced pulmonary fibrosis and localized emphysema.

Clinical Manifestations. Pleural pain and shortness of breath are the principal symptoms of spontaneous pneumothorax. The severity of the shortness of breath may vary from insignificant to very severe and depends on the amount of gas in the pleural space and the amount of underlying pulmonary disease which is present. Physical examination of the chest will sometimes show increased resonance to percussion over the affected side, but a decrease in the intensity of the breath sounds is a more definite and discernible sign. If the pneumothorax is large and there is a marked increase in intrapleural pressure, a shift in mediastinal structures away from the affected side may be detected. The chest x-ray will show air in the pleural space and the amount of collapse of the lung which has occurred.

Diagnosis. The possibility of spontaneous pneumothorax should be considered whenever there is the sudden onset of shortness of breath and particularly when it is accompanied by chest pain. It is a diagnosis which is usually made easily when it occurs in an otherwise healthy person and when the clinical findings which have been enumerated are present. The diagnosis is occasionally missed when it occurs in an asthmatic, a patient with obstructive pulmonary disease, or in other patients who have some other disease that seems to explain their shortness of breath. Because it can be lethal in such patients if untreated, the possibility of its occurrence should be kept prominent.

If a vessel in the lung or chest wall is torn when a pneumothorax occurs, a hemopneumothorax may result. When the chest x-ray shows the presence of fluid as well as air, this possibility should be considered, and a thoracentesis should be performed. Massive intrapleural bleeding is uncommon, but if present it requires surgical correction.

Treatment. The treatment of pneumothorax is concerned with its immediate and acute management, and with the prevention of recurrences.

The methods used in the early management of spontaneous pneumothorax will depend on the size and cause of the pneumothorax, the presence or absence of complicating pulmonary disease, and whether the leak between the lung and the pleura is closed or continuing. If the pneumothorax has occurred in a young healthy person, is small (e.g., 10 to 15 per cent), is causing few or minimal symptoms, and does not increase during the first 12 hours of observation, it requires no treatment. However, the fact that it has indeed resorbed should be confirmed by chest x-ray about two weeks later. In a similar patient with a larger pneumothorax, and especially if there is significant shortness of breath, the gas may be removed by inserting a small venous catheter through a thoracentesis needle and aspirating the intrapleural gas. This simple method will usually succeed in patients who do not have underlying pulmonary disease and who do not have a continuing leak. If there is significant pulmonary disease, pleural adhesions, or evidence of a continuing bronchopleural fistula, a larger intercostal tube should be inserted and attached to an underwater seal. The relief of an increasing and positive pressure – a *tension pneumothorax* – by prompt decompression is occasionally lifesaving. If there is a significant continuing leakage of air or evidence of respiratory insufficiency, continuous suction is required. If the lung cannot be reexpanded or there is continued leakage for more than a few days, an open thoracotomy with resection and closure of the bronchopleural fistula may be required.

Recurrence. Spontaneous pneumothorax may recur once or many times over several years after the first episode. Recurrences may be on the same side or the opposite side. The possibility of recurrence can be greatly reduced or eliminated by surgical treatment. Surgical treatment includes the resection of blebs and bullae if they are sufficiently localized to permit this and the obliteration of the pleural space. The removal of the parietal pleura, the application of irritating substances to the pleura, and the scarification of the pleura followed by intrapleural suction are methods which are used to obliterate the pleural space.

MISCELLANEOUS PLEURAL DISEASES

The pleura is involved in a great variety of systemic diseases and in diseases of the lung and adjacent structures.

Collagen Vascular Diseases. Systemic lupus erythematosus and rheumatoid arthritis are the collagen vascular diseases in which pleural effusions are most often encountered. In rheumatoid arthritis pleural effusions are usually seen in older men in whom the arthritis is of long duration. The fluid is an exudate and characteristically has a very low glucose content.

Pancreatitis. Pleural effusions secondary to acute and chronic pancreatitis are occasionally encountered. They may occur in either pleural space, but are more common on the left. There is often an associated pancreatic pseudocyst. The fluid is an exudate, may have extremely high amylase content (500 to 50,000 units per milliliter), and characteristically has a higher level of amylase than the serum.

Asbestosis. Inhalation of asbestos dust commonly leads to pleural disease. Serous pleural effusion, pleural fibrosis, pleural calcification, and pleural mesothelioma are all complications of asbestos dust exposure.

The pleural effusion of asbestos exposure is commonly bilateral and frequently recurrent; the fluid is usually an exudate and is often serosanguineous. Pleural effusion is often accompanied by clinically apparent parenchymal fibrosis, but can occur in the absence of obvious asbestosis. Duration and intensity of exposure to asbestos can vary widely.

Pleural fibrosis is a common accompaniment of pulmonary asbestosis and has been identified in up to 14 per cent of cases of asbestosis. Like pleural effusion it may be seen in patients who do not have evident parenchymal fibrosis.

Pleural calcification is common among asbestos workers and has been found in more than 10 per cent of workers with prolonged exposure. It is often bilateral, predominantly involves the basilar portions, is primarily in the parietal pleura, and usually occurs only after lengthy exposures to asbestos.

Although pleural mesothelioma has been reported to follow these more benign forms of pleural disease from asbestos, it is an uncommon complication.

Meigs' Syndrome. Ascites, pleural effusion, a benign fibroma, or fibroma-like ovarian tumor, with cure of the ascites and pleural effusion by removal of the tumor, is a syndrome that Meigs called attention to in 1934. It is an uncommon cause of pleural effusion, but many cases of the syndrome have been reported. Most often the fluid is found in the right pleural space, but it can be present in either or both pleural spaces. The fluid is usually a clear transudate, but exudative fluids and serosanguineous collections have been reported. The amount of fluid in both the pleural and peritoneal spaces is variable, and in some cases the amount of ascites has been quite small. The mechanism for the formation of the pleural and peritoneal fluid has not been completely explained, but it is suggested that somehow the fibroma causes the ascites which is then transported to the pleural space by diaphragmatic lymphatics. Because this uncommon condition can be cured by pelvic surgery, it should be considered in women with pleural effusion of obscure origin, especially if there is evidence of concurrent ascites and pelvic disease.

Subdiaphragmatic Abscess. Pleural effusion and pleurodiaphragmatic pain, particularly on the right side, are common manifestations of a subdiaphragmatic abscess, and are frequently the first indicators of the location of the infection. The pleural effusion is most often a serous exudate, and the organism in the subdiaphragmatic abscess is often not found in the pleural fluid. Amebic infection from the liver may also extend through the diaphragm and cause a pleural exudate, which is characteristically purulent and chocolate-colored and may contain amebae.

Besson, L. N., Ferguson, T. B., and Burford, T. H.: Chylothorax. Ann. Thorac. Surg., 12:527, 1971.

Black, L. F.: The pleural space and pleural fluid. Mayo Clin. Proc., 47:493, 1972.

Bruneau, R., and Rubin, P.: The management of pleural effusions and chylothorax in lymphoma. Radiology, 85:1085, 1965.

Gaensler, E. A., and Kaplan, A. I.: Asbestos pleural effusions. Ann. Intern. Med., 74:178, 1971.

Killen, D. A., and Gobbel, W. G., Jr.: Spontaneous Pneumothorax. Boston, Little, Brown & Company, 1968.

Light, R. W., MacGregor, M. I., Luchsinger, P. C., and Ball, W. C., Jr.: Pleural effusions: The diagnostic separation of transudates and exudates. Ann. Intern. Med., 77:507, 1972.

Meigs, J. V.: Fibroma of the ovary with ascites and hydrothorax—Meigs' syndrome. Am. J. Obstet. Gynecol., 67:962, 1954.

Mellins, R. B., Levine, O. R., and Fishman, A. P.: Effects of systemic and pulmonary venous hypertension on pleural and pericardial fluid accumulation. J. Appl. Physiol., 29:564, 1970.

Scharer, L., and McClement, J. H.: The isolation of tubercle bacilli from needle biopsy specimens of parietal pleura. Am. Rev. Respir. Dis., 97:466, 1968.

Selikoff, I. J.: The occurrence of pleural calcification among asbestos insulation workers. Ann. N.Y. Acad. Sci., 132:351, 1965.

Szucs, M. M., Brooks, H. L., Grossman, W., Banas, J. S., Meister, S. G., Dexter, L., and Dalen, J. E.: Diagnostic sensitivity of laboratory findings in acute pulmonary embolism. Ann. Intern. Med., 74:161, 1971.

Yeoh, C. B., Hubaytar, R. T., Conklin, E. F., Simpson, D. G., and Ford, J. M.: Spontaneous pneumothorax: Treatment with small lumen polyethylene tube. New York State J. Med., 70:779, 1970.

Index

Note: In this index the expression "vs." has been used to denote "differential diagnosis." Thus "Addison's disease, vs. acanthosis nigricans" is the equivalent of "Addison's disease, differential diagnosis from acanthosis nigricans." **Boldface entries and folios** in the index indicate main discussions in the text. *Italic folios* indicate illustrations and tables.